AF716691

PRAISE FOR THE SECOND EDITION OF THE ESSENTIAL GUIDE TO WESTERN BOTANICAL MEDICINE

"A master makes learning easy for others. After years of dedicated practice, Christa paints a glorious portrait of plant medicine using compelling photos and poetic language. *The Essential Guide to Western Botanical Medicine* invites the reader into an empowered landscape for sustained and vibrant health. For professionals, there is essential science, theory, and objective data. For everyone, there are simple answers to complex medical questions."

—AMANDA MCQUADE CRAWFORD, MA, Medical Herbalist, RH (AHG)
Licensed Marriage and Family Therapist, MCPP, MNZAMH

"*The Essential Guide to Western Botanical Medicine* is not only beautifully designed, it is also exceptionally well written and researched, and full of vibrant color photos. This book is an essential text for the herbal enthusiast or clinical herbalist—in fact, I would consider it required reading!"

—DAVID WINSTON, RH (AHG)
Author of *Adaptogens: Herbs for Strength, Stamina and Stress Relief*

"*The Essential Guide to Western Botanical Medicine* demonstrates a high level of excellence in the depth of material, practical clinical applications, usability of format, and sheer beauty of presentation. Many of the chapters are so extensive it is like having five books in one—history and lore, medical uses, combinations and formulation, safety, and pharmacy. I have been practicing for more than 50 years, and I have this book within reach for when my insatiable curiosity wants to know something more about an herb or something about an herb new to me. It is a core text in our school. It is an investment for a career, you may still be using it in 50 years."

—PAUL BERGNER
Director, North American Institute of Medical Herbalism, naimh.com
and the Medical Herbalism Journal, medherb.com

"*The Essential Guide to Western Botanical Medicine* is a welcome and extremely thorough compilation and vital resource on many of the major herbs recommended by herbalists today. Christa Sinadinos has made an important contribution in this essential guide that will save countless hours of research for clinicians and herb lovers as a gateway to expanding their herbal knowledge and repertoire. I will have it on hand with the resource books I consult daily. It is a milestone in the literature of herbal medicine along the same lines as the great herbals of Gerard and Parkinson, and in Traditional Chinese Medicine, the *Bencao Gangmu*."

—CHRISTOPHER HOBBS, PhD, LAc
Integrative Biology (University of California, Berkeley), Phylogenetics,
Natural Products Chemistry, Herbal Medicine, Ethnomedicine

"The lovingly detailed herbal monographs provide more than 1,000, often stunning photos. This substantial tome will be front and center for herbalists. Herbal medicine is a discipline requiring love, devotion, and surrender. Christa is a passionately committed agent to the relationship between humanity and the plant kingdom. Since 1994, Christa has been bringing her students and clients into a deep, joyful connection with plants. This book will serve that mission, reaching many more people who will benefit from her work. Christa's background in herbal medicine is among the greats of contemporary practice. This book offers pearls of clinical experience that will make it a regular companion on my journey."

—WILLIAM MORRIS, PhD, RH (AHG)
Author of *TCM Case Studies: Dermatology*

"I've been impatiently awaiting this book for years—it is truly an iconic work for our times! The resurgence of interest in botanical medicine ushered in a wave of introductory books geared toward the home herbalist, leaving serious herbal students and practitioners high and dry. *The Essential Guide to Western Botanical Medicine* remedies this with extensive herbal profiles and recipes, and thorough medicine-making tutorials. Lest you are daunted by the heft of Christa's opus, rest assured that the informative pages are artfully adorned with gorgeous botanical photography."

—JULIET BLANKESPOOR
Director of Chestnut School of Herbal Medicine

"*The Essential Guide to Western Botanical Medicine* is a comprehensive materia medica incorporating more than two decades of clinical practice in a lavish presentation with beautiful photography. The 129 monographs provide a deep dive into the pertinent professional and advocacy literature, infused with the wisdom of experience. Certainly, a book you will enjoy owning!"

—STEVEN FOSTER
Herbalist, photographer, author of *Herbal Renaissance,* and coauthor of *Peterson's Field Guide to Western Medicinal Plants Herbs, Desk Reference to Nature's Medicine,* and *Herbal Emissaries*

"*The Essential Guide to Western Botanical Medicine* is an immensely useful text and a must have for herbalists and students of herbal medicine. The combination of the extensive and in-depth materia medica, along with medicine making guidelines and useful therapeutic formulas makes for a valuable resource that compiles a large amount of easily accessible information. Christa has put together an impressive amount of herbal wisdom that will be on the book shelves of herbal enthusiasts for years to come."

—KAMI MCBRIDE
Author of *The Herbal Kitchen* and KamiMcBride.com

"This stunningly visual and information-packed herbal is destined never to gather dust on a shelf. Along with over 100 well-researched monographs, Christa has included not only recipes, but something that is not common: herb formulas! You'll be reaching for this colorful, 700+ page tome on a regular basis. Kudos for raising the bar on herbal publishing."

—ROBYN KLEIN, MS
Medical Botany

"The beautiful photographs are works of art that entice you to look deeper into the pages of this well-crafted masterpiece. This exquisite experience is enhanced by the detailed herbal wisdom shared in this comprehensive collection of herbal knowledge. *The Essential Guide to Western Botanical Medicine* offers more than an educational experience. It is a book that will lure you away from your daily schedule to sit down with a cup of tea, and peruse through the stunning beauty and volumes of knowledge."

—SHAROL TILGNER, ND
Author of *Herbal Medicine* and *Herbal ABC's—The Foundations of Herbal Medicine*

"What a gem! *The Essential Guide to Western Botanical Medicine* is essential for anyone wanting detailed herbal monographs with luscious photos, clear guidelines on medicine making, and over 35 pages of therapeutic formulas from an experienced practitioner and teacher—all in one book. A must-have for your herbal library."

—KARIN C. UPHOFF, Medical Herbalist, RH (AHG)
Author of *Botanical Body Care*

"From the pen of an expert herbalist, many years in preparation, *The Essential Guide to Western Botanical Medicine* is a comprehensive, well-documented and illustrated, easily read textbook covering the entire field of herbal medicine. Perfect for students and schools needing a comprehensive textbook in one volume; equally a reference book for the experienced herbalist."

—MATTHEW WOOD, MS (Herbal Medicine), RH (AHG)

Author of *The Book of Herbal Wisdom: Using Plants as Medicines* and *The Earthwise Herbal*

"*The Essential Guide to Western Botanical Medicine* offers us a reference guide that exceeds all expectations. The monographs cover some of our most clinically valuable herbs, bolstered by an extensive formulary, but what makes this book really shine, is that it's written by an extremely skilled practitioner."

—JIM MCDONALD

Herbalist and founder of herbcraft.org

"The long-awaited *Essential Guide to Western Botanical Medicine* is finally here, and it does not disappoint. The sheer beauty of this text is only outmatched by the content, which Christa Sinadinos has crafted based on her 25 years of clinical experience and nearly as many years teaching. The massive materia medica of more than 550 pages includes historical context, as well as modern and practical applications of 129 medicinal plants. I am very happy to see the inclusion of citations showing the rigor necessary for this text to be more than just another herb book, but one that lay herbalists and professionals will want on their shelves. Following an excellent section on how to prepare the plants she elucidates so beautifully, the author expertly guides the reader through formulation for the body systems, and covers a wide range of common conditions with presentations of formulas and preparation techniques that can be immediately applied. This is a welcome addition to the literature—a text I am sure I will reference often."

—THOMAS AVERY GARRAN

Director of East West School of Herbology, Author of *Western Herbs in Chinese Medicine: Methodology and Materia Medica,* translator of *Growing Chinese Herbs: Daodi Practices for Growing and Processing Chinese Herbs*

"A truly essential addition to any herbal library, from the budding to the lifelong herbalist. Christa beautifully blends the rich history of western herbalism with in-depth and applicable modern herbal research, easy-to-follow formulas and recipes, and tops it off with stunning images of each plant. It has an honored place with my most beloved and dog-eared herbal references."

—AUTUMN SUMMERS

Herbalist

"With detailed plant monographs, gorgeous photography, easy medicine-making instructions, and tried and true formulas for hundreds of common health concerns, this truly is the most useful western plant medicine reference I've seen (as a decades long shopkeeper of a retail herbal apothecary, I've seen many!). It's hands down my go-to choice for my customers."

—JULIE CALDWELL, MA

Founder and owner of Humboldt Herbals

"Aspiring and practicing herbalists need a detailed materia medica that can serve as an immediate reference, a text that can be pulled off the shelf and the required information found easily and efficiently. Christa's new book fulfills this job perfectly, with a gorgeous layout and amazing detail capturing everything needed in a reference manual of medicinal herbs, including a detailed formulary. This attractive book is a must for every serious herb student and a valuable addition to any researcher's library."

—TODD CALDECOTT, Dip. Cl.H., RH (AHG), CAP (NAMA)

Ayurveda practitioner and medical herbalist, author of *Food as Medicine*

"*The Essential Guide to Western Botanical Medicine* is a beautiful book—deeply satisfying intellectually and aesthetically. The monographs are useful for all levels of herbal inquiry. The extensive listing of historical uses of each herb around the globe with terrific lists of common names gives the herbs context, even as the language we use to talk about them changes from one culture to the next, evolving over time. The current western medicinal use with dosing, cautions, and preparation recipes are fully explored. Best of all are the superb photos of each plant."

—GAIL JULIAN
Medical herbalist and instructor

"Christa has created a defining text for western herbalism. Herbalists will be reaching for this impressive reference time and time again."

—ROSALEE DE LA FORÊT
Author of *Alchemy of Herbs: Transform Everyday Ingredients into Foods and Remedies That Heal*

"Christa's book delves into western medicinal herbs to a depth you won't find anywhere else. It's beautifully laid out with full-color photographs, medicinal uses and actions, botanical descriptions, constituents, history, energetics, annotated sources, safety, preparations, and doses—providing an intimate understanding of each plant and its nuances. It's packed with information, yet easy to read and understand. *The Essential Guide to Western Botanical Medicine* is destined to become a classic herbal medicine text for all levels of experience, and one of my top-recommended herbals."

—MARIA NOËL GROVES, Clinical Herbalist, RH (AHG)
Author of *Body into Balance, Grow Your Own Herbal Remedies,* and *Herbal Remedies for Sleep*

"As I read through each herb's extremely thorough presentation, I felt excited to enjoy the plant as though meeting it for the first time. Suggestions for formulation with each plant and medicine making instructions are concise. Cautions are stated simply and clearly. As a practitioner, the temperature and flavor notes are invaluable. It is so nice to see the common names and uses from other countries!"

—MARGI FLINT, RH (AHG), HM
Author of *The Practicing Herbalist* and founder of Earthsongherbals.com

"Christa is fully dedicated to the art and science of using herbs for medicine. Since she announced that she was taking on the immense work of this incredibly well-researched book, I have eagerly awaited its final completion as a valuable addition to my herbal resource library. You will find this book to be an essential addition to your herbal reference library, and it is beautiful enough to be displayed on the coffee table! I know this book will be well used in my own library as an important resource."

—GRETA DE LA MONTAGNE
Clinical herbalist, founder of MASHH Clinic Collective, and proprietor of Gentle Strength Botanicals

"With bated breath, we at Moonrise Herbs have awaited the publication of this book. Having practiced as a clinical herbalist for a quarter of a century, Christa holds a wealth of practical knowledge. Her writing is engaging and informative to read as she includes the historical uses, as well as the sources of plant names. Christa's monographs are written in great depth and thoroughly researched. Preparation and dosage are conveniently listed as a sidebar for ease of reference, and there are great recipes. Beautiful detailed pictures of each herb adorn the pages. This book was truly worth the wait!"

—IRENE LEWIS
Proprietor of Moonrise Herbs, herbalist, and aromatherapist

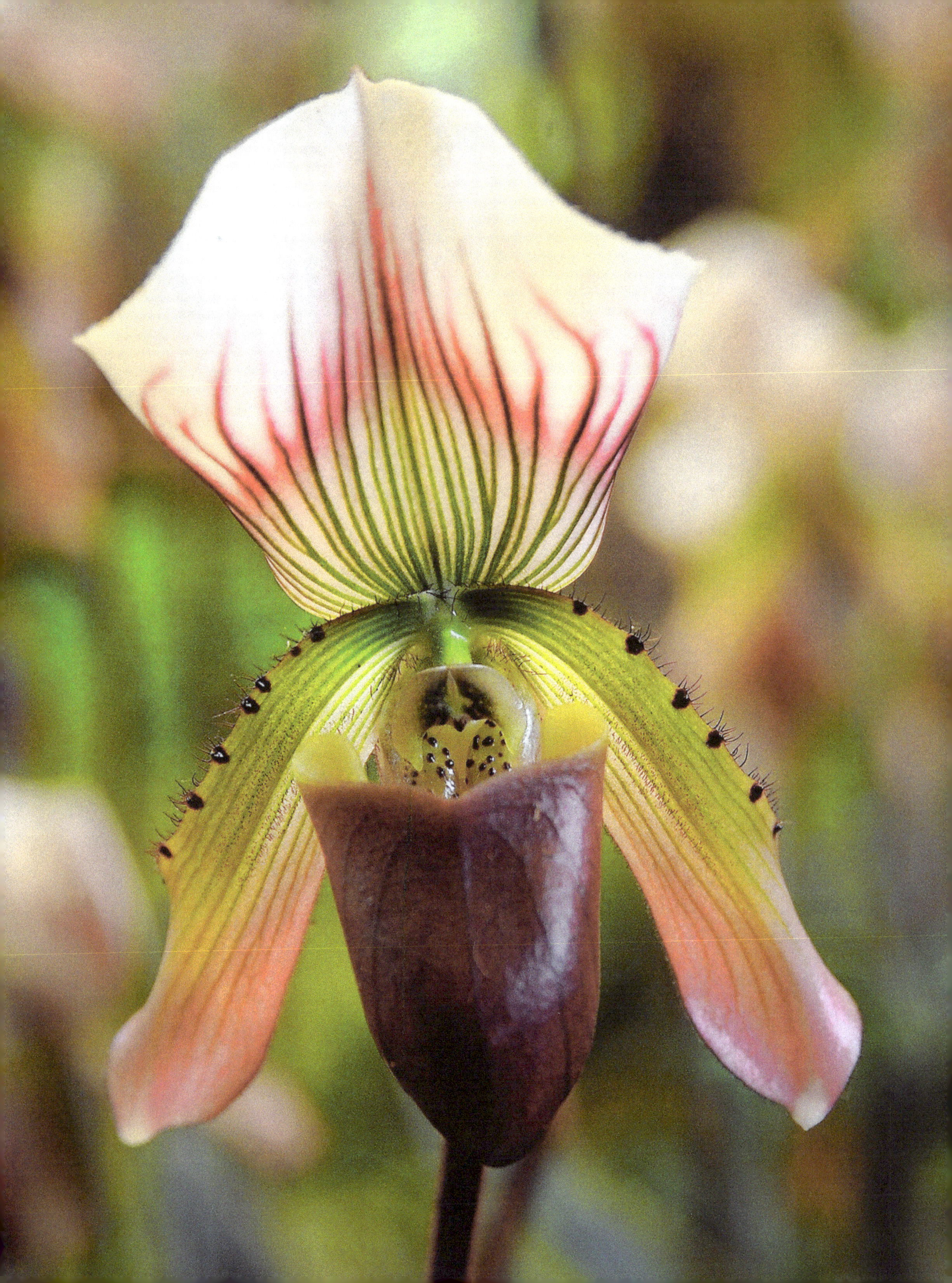

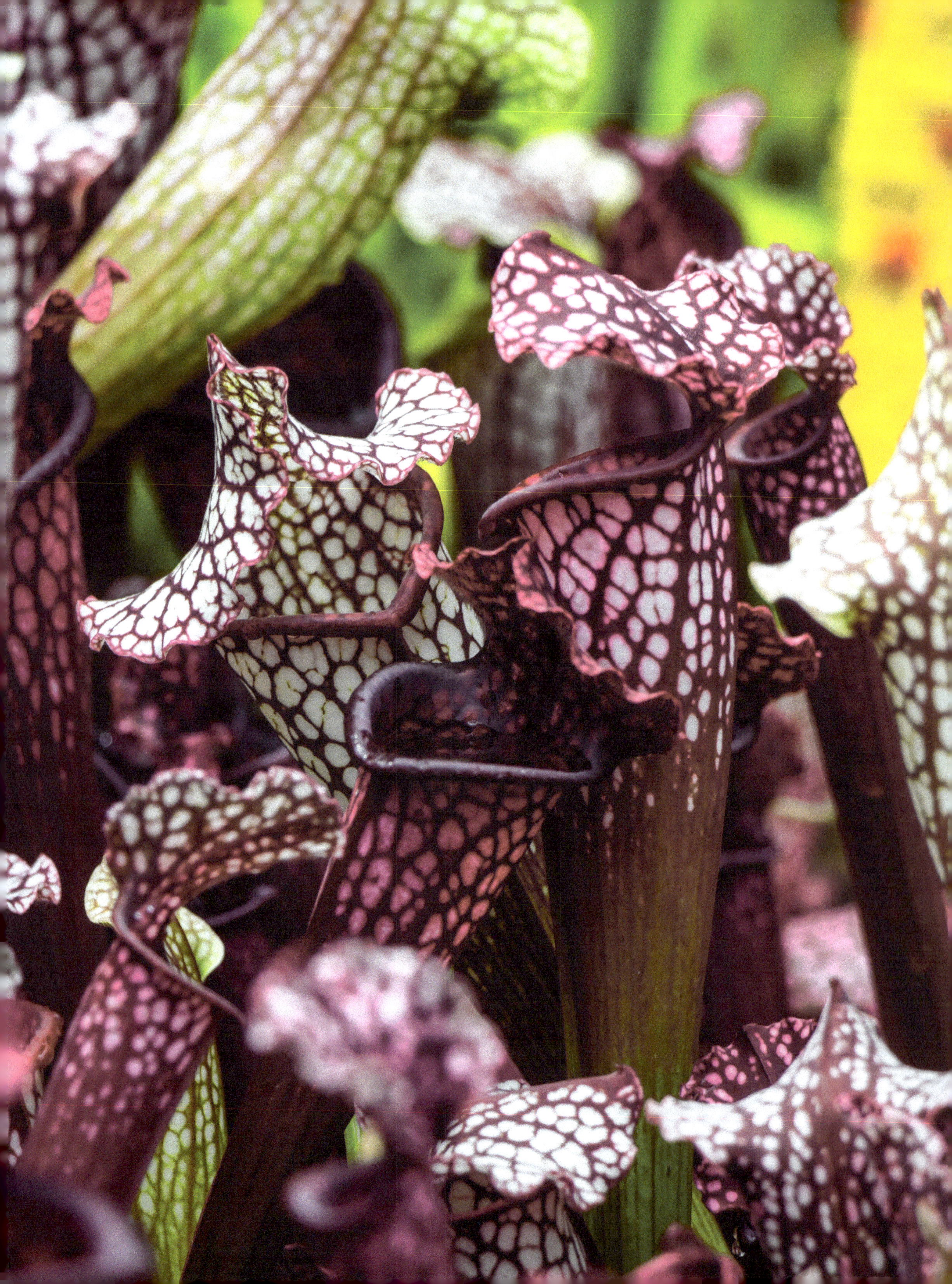

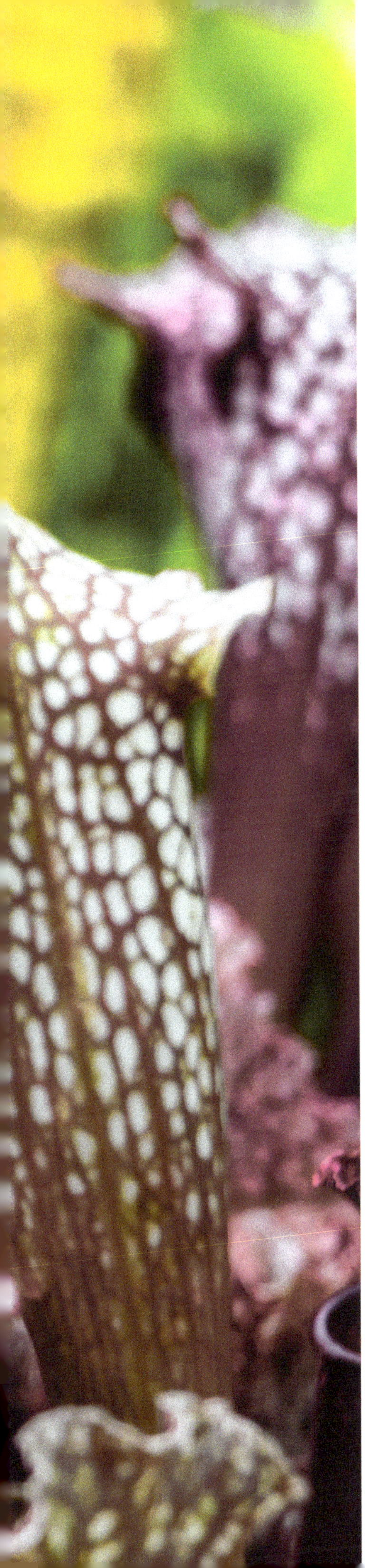

Second Edition

THE ESSENTIAL GUIDE TO WESTERN BOTANICAL MEDICINE

Second Edition

THE ESSENTIAL GUIDE TO WESTERN BOTANICAL MEDICINE

CHRISTA SINADINOS

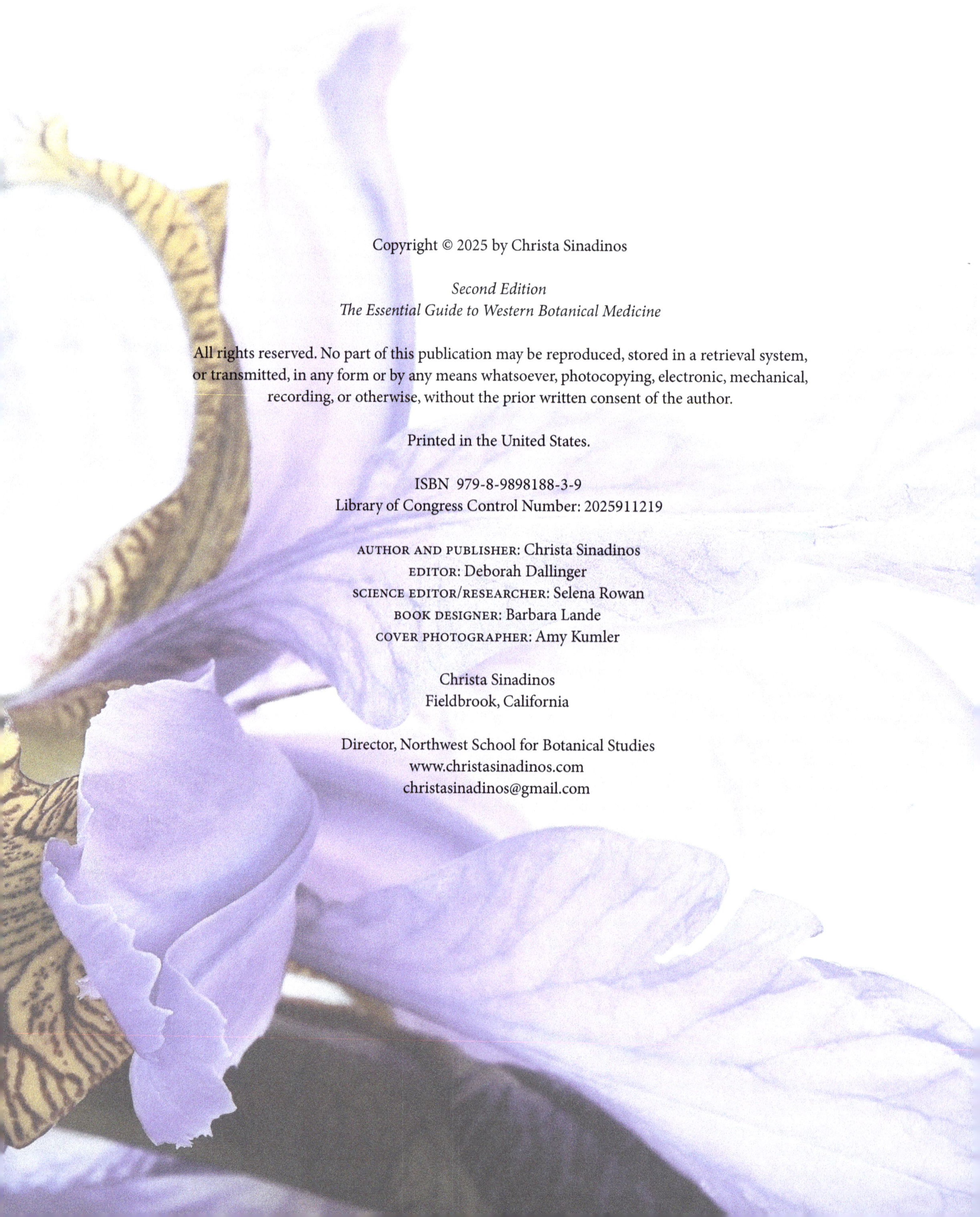

Copyright © 2025 by Christa Sinadinos

Second Edition
The Essential Guide to Western Botanical Medicine

All rights reserved. No part of this publication may be reproduced, stored in a retrieval system, or transmitted, in any form or by any means whatsoever, photocopying, electronic, mechanical, recording, or otherwise, without the prior written consent of the author.

Printed in the United States.

ISBN 979-8-9898188-3-9
Library of Congress Control Number: 2025911219

AUTHOR AND PUBLISHER: Christa Sinadinos
EDITOR: Deborah Dallinger
SCIENCE EDITOR/RESEARCHER: Selena Rowan
BOOK DESIGNER: Barbara Lande
COVER PHOTOGRAPHER: Amy Kumler

Christa Sinadinos
Fieldbrook, California

Director, Northwest School for Botanical Studies
www.christasinadinos.com
christasinadinos@gmail.com

CONTENTS

Foreword v
Preface vii
Acknowledgements xi

MATERIA MEDICA

Alfalfa 1
Aloe 4
Ambrosia 9
Anemone 12
Angelica 16
Anise 22
Aralia 26
Arnica 31
Artichoke leaf 34
Ashwagandha 38
Asparagus 41
Astragalus 45
Bayberry 49
Berberis 53
Black cohosh 59
Black haw 64
Blackberry 68
Blue cohosh 73
Bogbean 77
Boneset 80
Bugleweed 83
Burdock 87
Calamus 91
Calendula 97
California poppy 101
Cannabis 104
Cardamom 113
Carob 116
Cayenne 119
Chamomile 124
Chickweed 130
Cinnamon 133
Cleavers 137
Clove 140
Codonopsis 144
Comfrey 147
Coptis 152
Cordyceps 156
Corn silk 160
Couch grass 163
Cow parsnip 165
Cramp bark 168
Damiana 171
Dandelion 175
Dong quai 180
Echinacea 185
Elder 190
Elecampane 195
Eleuthero 199
Ephedra 205
Fennel 210
Fenugreek 215
Feverfew 218
Garlic 221
Gentian 226
Ginger 231
Ginkgo 236
Ginseng, Asian 241
Goldenrod 246
Gotu kola 249
Gravel root 253
Grindelia 255
Gymnema 258
Hawthorn 261
Hops 266
Horsetail 271
Hydrangea 275
Jamaican dogwood 278
Kava 281
Kelp and Bladderwrack 286
Lady's mantle 291
Lavender 295
Lemon balm 301
Licorice 305
Lobelia 312
Lomatium 316
Marjoram 320
Marshmallow 323
Meadowsweet 328
Milk thistle 331
Mint 335
Motherwort 341
Mullein 345
Myrrh 350

Nettle 354
Oats 361
Orange 365
Oregano 373
Oshá 377
Parsley 381
Partridge berry 386
Passion flower 389
Pedicularis 393
Pennyroyal 398
Peony 403
Plantain 408
Prickly ash 411
Propolis 415
Raspberry leaf 418
Red clover 421
Red root 424
Reishi mushroom 429
Rose 435
Rosemary 441
Sage 447
Saw palmetto 452
Schisandra 456
Shepherd's purse 461
Shiitake 464
Silk tassel 468
Skullcap 471
Spilanthes 475
St. John's wort 478
Stone root 482
Thyme 484
Tulsi basil 490
Turmeric 495
Usnea 501
Uva ursi and Manzanita 504
Valerian 508
Vitex 514
Wild cherry bark 518
Wild yam 522
Willow bark 527
Yarrow 532
Yellow dock 537
Yellow pond lily 542
Yerba mansa 545
Yerba santa 548

MEDICINE MAKING

WATER-BASED PREPARATIONS 555
Herbal Tea 555
Hot Infusions 556
Cold Infusions 557
Solar and Lunar Infusions 557
Decoctions 557
Topical Preparations 560
Fomentation and Poultice 560
Vaginal Irrigation and Enema 560

ALCOHOL-BASED EXTRACTS 561
Fresh Plant Extracts 561
Dry Plant Extracts 562
Menstruum Calculation Worksheet 563
Tincture Worksheet 564

GLYCERIN EXTRACTS 565
Fresh Plant Extracts 566
Dry Plant Extracts 566

ACETUM EXTRACTS 568
Internal Use 568
Fire Cider 568
Mediterranean Vinegar 570
Digestive Bitters 570
Pickled Herbs and Seaweed 570
Topical Preparations 571
Vinegar Liniments 571
Hair Rinses 571

HERBAL HONEY AND SYRUP 572
Honey 572
Fresh Herbal Honey 572
Dry Herbal Honey 575
Herbal Syrup 575

MEDICINAL OILS AND SALVES 577
Base Oils 577
Preparing Medicinal Oils 577
Simpler's Method 577
Alcohol Intermediary Oil Method 579
Salves 580
Salve Recipes 581

HERBAL THERAPEUTIC FORMULAS

ADRENAL AND IMMUNE SUPPORT 585
Adaptogenic Compounds and Teas 585
Adaptogen and Adrenal Tonic Compound 585
Adaptogen and Adrenal Tonic Tea I 585
Adaptogen and Adrenal Tonic Tea II 586
Adaptogen Delight 586
Calming Adaptogen Compound 586
Tonifying Teas 587
Delicious Immune Tonic Tea 587
Kidney and Liver Yin Tonic Tea 587
Lung Qi Tonic Tea 588
Spleen and Lung Qi Tonic Tea 588
Spleen Qi Tonic Tea 588

CARDIOVASCULAR SUPPORT 589
Circulatory Compounds 589
Atherosclerosis Compound 589
Circulatory Stimulant Compound 589
Circulatory Stimulant Tea 589
Diuretic Hypertension Compound 590
Nervine Hypertension Compound 590
Hypotension Relief Compound 590
Varicose Vein Tonic (Alkaloid-based) 591
Varicose Vein Tonic (Tannin-based) 591

DIGESTIVE SUPPORT 591
Carminative Formulas 591
Calm Belly Compound 591
Carminative Tea 592
Digestive Delight Tea 592
Digestive Soothing and Calming Tea 592
Digestive Formulas 593
Antidiarrhea Compound 593
Astringent Tea 593
Coating and Soothing Tea 593
Coating and Soothing Tea (Pyrrolizidine Alkaloid Free) 593
Delicious Digestive Tea 594
Digestive Healing Teas I and II 594
Liver and Gallbladder Support 595
Blood Sugar Balancing Formula 595
Christa's Favorite Liver Support Tea 595
Cooling Bitters Compound 596
Digestive Bitter Acetum Compound 596
Digestive Bitter Compound 596
Gallbladder and Liver-cooling Compound 597
Hemorrhoid Comfort Compound 597
Hepatodetoxifying Compound 598
Liver Decongestant Compound 598
Liver-heat Clearing Compound 598

NERVOUS SYSTEM SUPPORT 599
Analgesic, Antispasmodic, and Anti-inflammatory Compounds 599
Analgesic, Antispasmodic, and Sedative Compounds I and II (Alkaloid-based) 599
Anti-inflammatory Compound (Short-term) 599
Anti-inflammatory Compound (Long-term) 599
Cramp bark Compound 600
Headache Relief Compound 600
Samuel Thomson's Compound Tincture of Lobelia and Capsicum 600
Antidepressant, Anxiolytic, and Nootropic Compounds 601
Antidepressant Compound 601
Anxiolytic Compound (Alkaloid-based) 601
Anxiolytic Compound (Tannin-based) 601
Gentle Nervine Tea 602
Mental Clarit-Tea 602
Mental Clarity Compound 602
Mood Elevating, Trophorestorative, and Gentle Nervine Compound 603

REPRODUCTIVE SYSTEM SUPPORT, FEMALE 603
Perimenopause Support 603
Perimenopause Compound (with Adrenal Depletion) 603
Perimenopause Compound (Calming and Liver-decongesting) 604
Pregnancy Support 604
Pregnancy-safe Hemostatic Tea 604
Uterine Calming Compound I (for Threatened Miscarriage) 604
Uterine Calming Compound II (for Threatened Miscarriage) 605
Uterine Tonic Partus Preparator Compound 605
Premenstrual Syndrome and Menstrual Support 606
Reproductive and Hormone Deficiency Phase I and II Compounds 606
Reproductive and Blood Tonifying Tea 606
Estrogen Dominance Relief Compound 607
Hormone Excess Compound 607
Premenstrual Syndrome Relief Compound 607

REPRODUCTIVE SYSTEM SUPPORT, MALE 608
Male Reproductive Tonifying Tea 608
Benign Prostatic Hypertrophy Compound 608

RESPIRATORY, IMMUNE, AND LYMPHATIC SUPPORT 609
Acute Immune and Lymphatic Treatments 609
Immune Stimulant Compounds I and II 609
Lymphatic Compound 610
Lymphatic Alterative Compound I 610
Lymphatic Alterative Compound II—Hoxey Formula 610
Lymphatic Alterative Teas I and II 611
Sudorific Cold and Flu Tea 612
Respiratory, Lower 612
Hack-away Compound 612
Quitter's Crutch—Smoker's Mix 612
Respiratory Antispasmodic Compound 613
Respiratory Relief Tea 613
Respiratory Roots Blend 614
Respiratory, Upper 614
Allergy-ease Compound 614
Respiratory Decongestant Tea 614
Sinus Decongestant Compound 615
Sinus Decongestant Tea 615
Sinus Decongestant Steam 615
Throat Coat and Soothe Teas I and II 616
Throat Ease Compound 617
Throat Pastilles 617
Throat Spray 617

THYROID SUPPORT 618
Hyperthyroid Support Compound 618
Hypothyroid Support Compound 618
Hashimoto's Thyroiditis and Immune Modulating Compound 619

URINARY SYSTEM SUPPORT 619
Children's Bladder Strengthening Compound 619
Diuretic Tea 619
Diuretic Soothing Tea 620
Interstitial Cystitis Support Compound 620
Kidney and Bladder Soothing Tea 620

TOPICAL FORMULAS 621
Burn Relief Oil 621
Burn Relief Spray 621
Echinacea Clay Poultice 621
Earache Ease Glycerin- or Oil-based Compound 622
Earache Ease Oil 622
Plantain Clay Poultice 622
Topical Teething Compound 622

SALVES 623
Black Drawing Salve 623
Cayenne and Cinnamon Salve 623

APPENDICES AND INDEXES
Compendium of Herbal Therapeutic Uses and Conditions 627
Herbal Therapeutic Glossary 655
Botany Glossary 661
Plants by Family or Group 669
Index of Alternative Names (Common to Latin) 681
Reference of Alkaloid- and Tannin-containing Herbs 690
Endnotes 693
Index 731
Photography Credits 750

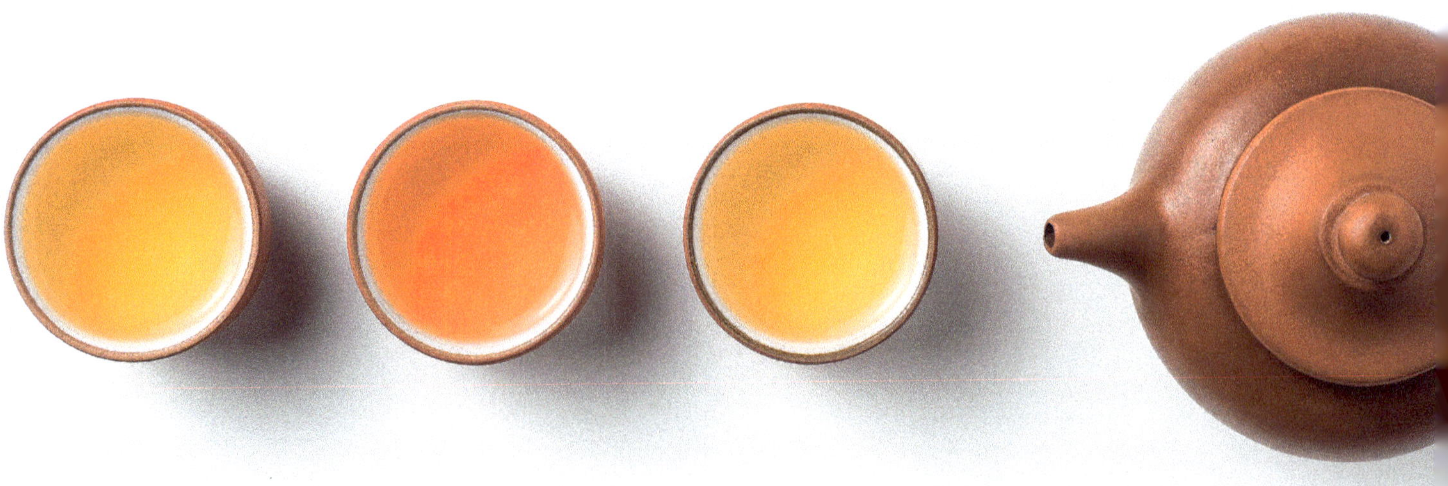

FOREWORD

Christa Sinadinos and I met several years ago through the American Herbalists Guild. We are both Greek-Americans from the Midwest, and founders of our own successful schools of herbal medicine (Christa in California and me in Georgia).

Early in our friendship, Christa shared with me her dream of writing a reference book for clinical herbalists that would encompass much of what she knows about medicinal herbs, clinical herbalism, medicine making, and formulation. As Christa's plans for the book grew, and her manuscript expanded into a 780-page book, she realized how much she had to share after 30 years as a practitioner and teacher. Christa is a devoted independent scholar, and her strong background in science, biochemistry, botany, medicine, and history enrich each herb profiled in this extraordinary book.

The result of Christa's dream is a sweeping resource that honors the complexity of medicinal herbs, describes their long history of use as medicines, and increases the field's ever-evolving understanding of how herbal medicine heals the body.

Christa knows what herbalists need in order to create safe, effective herbal protocols, and has written a comprehensive, invaluable reference for clinical herbalists. The format makes it easy to access information in minutes, and at the same time, the scope of the material invites one to read it cover to cover. Students just setting out on the herbal path need look no further for guidance to become competent clinical herbalists.

Always keeping in mind the inherent diversity of experience at the heart of herbalism, Christa's text gives equal attention to history, folklore, physiology, chemical constituents, and current research.

Detailed monographs, a series of appendices listing herbs according to their actions and the conditions they treat, body systems overviews with a collection of relevant formulas and recipes, and extensive glossaries for medical and botanical terms provide the foundation for the book. All of the data is meticulously footnoted. In addition, the book contains many pearls of wisdom Christa has gleaned in her 20 years of running an herbal extracts business and pharmacy, along with practical instructions for making herbal medicines, and guidelines for designing specific formulas.

Christa's passion for herbs as a gardener and herbalist is evident in the stunningly intimate photographs throughout the book. They capture the essence of the plants and awaken the reader's sense of wonder at their beauty. Thumbing through the pages, I found myself wanting to lean closer to the photographs so I could smell and touch the herbs. Her detailed botanical descriptions rival the best field guides, and I can imagine that many of us will be tempted to make room for this hefty volume in our packs when heading out for a day of botanizing.

The Essential Guide to Western Botanical Medicine provides a concise, in-depth record of current herbal practice, grounded in proven practical experience. Christa's contribution to the field deserves a place in the lineage of timeless herbal reference books such as *Grieve's A Modern Herbal, Hoffmann's Medical Herbalism*, and *Skenderi's Herbal Vade Mecum.*

– Patricia Kyritsi Howell, RH (AHG)
Mountain City, Georgia

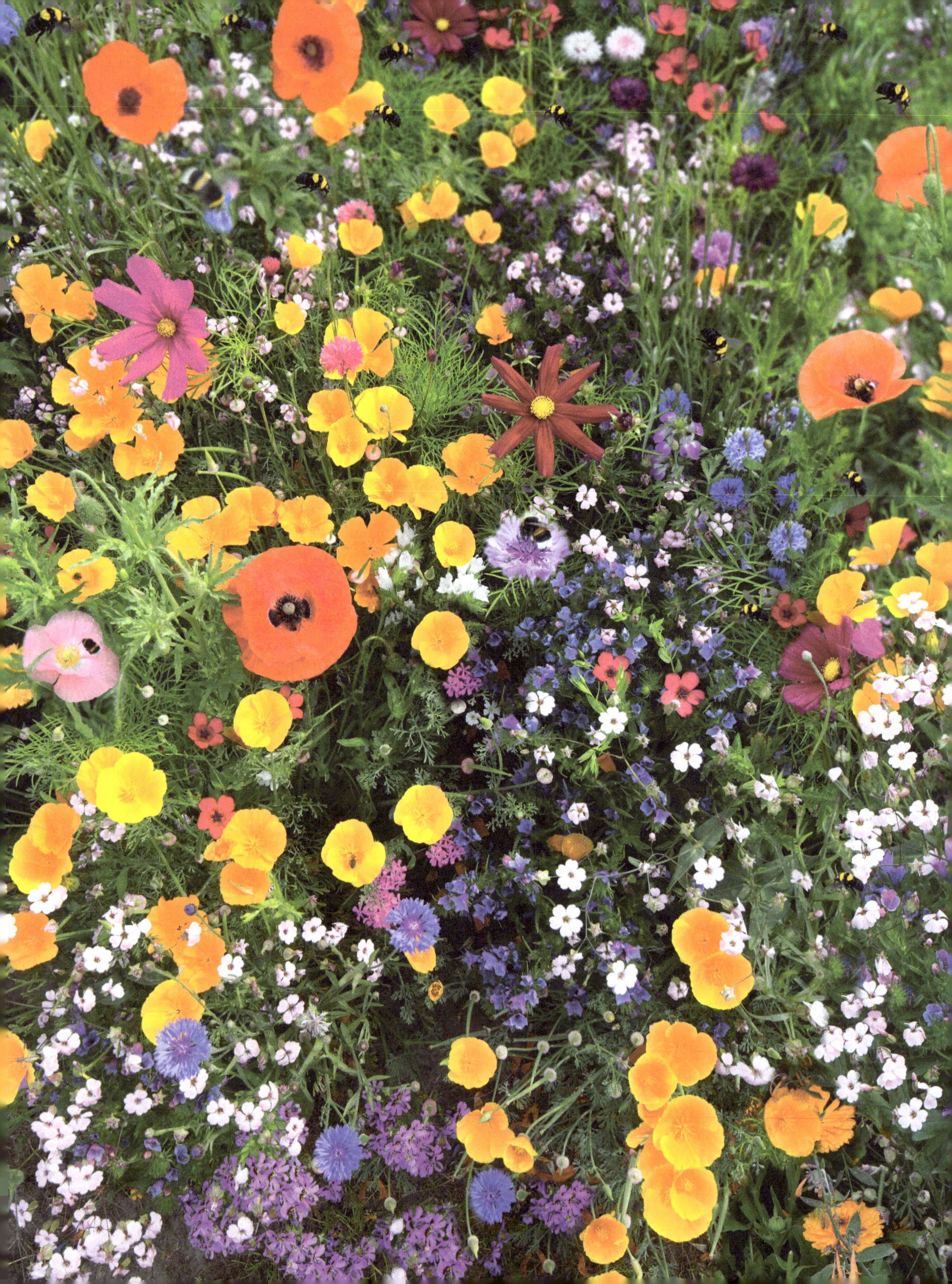

PREFACE

My inspiration to study herbal medicine was sparked by my elders, especially my beloved paternal Greek grandmother, Lefkothea Sinadinos. She was a kind, resilient, spirited woman deeply devoted to her family and faith. Living close to the earth, she was scarcely five feet tall and radiant, with a sparkle in her beautiful blue-green eyes. She'd walk into the house carrying an apron full of fresh vegetables and pockets full of herbs she gathered from her garden that she maintained until she was 99 years old.

Incredible aromas of Greek food filled her home. I can still smell her lemon-roasted chicken and potatoes seasoned with oregano and thyme, the cinnamon bark, clove, and onions simmering in beef stew *(kapama),* and her roasted garlic-rosemary-rubbed lamb. She kindled my love of gardening and cooking, and instilled the importance of maintaining vibrant health by incorporating herbs and nutritious foods into every meal. To this day, the herbs and spices she used remain among my favorites.

My maternal grandparents, Georgia and Clark Brown, were salt-of-the-earth, and cultivated my deep love of nature. Raised on farms in rural Illinois, they walked five miles to and from school in harsh midwestern winters, hand-pumped their water from wells, cultivated and harvested food by hand, and put food by in their cellars. My beloved grandmother had a heart of gold; she was loving and humble. My grandfather was a quiet, artistic tool-and-die maker, a woodworker, fisherman, and hunter. He taught me how to forage mushrooms, chop wood, build a fire, and catch, clean, and cook fish. During the summers, I spent considerable time with them in their hand-built, birch-framed cottage in northern Michigan, where I roamed the woods barefoot, climbed trees, swung from willow branches, caught turtles and frogs, fished, and swam in the lake. I gathered bushels of berries for my grandmother, who prepared delicious pies and preserves. All of these basic, but necessary life skills laid the foundation for becoming an herbalist.

Following the sudden death of my father just two weeks before I started high school, I was depressed and disheartened. Lacking the tools and time to properly grieve, I became very ill. My doctors offered no cure or reasonable solutions. Like many wounded healers, I took matters into my own hands, and began pursuing dietary, lifestyle, and herbal curatives that restored my health and led me to my life path, empowering me to take responsibility for my health.

As I began my healing journey, I sought every resource I could find on medicinal herbs and foods, but few herbal reference books were available. They included classics such as *The Herb Book* by John Lust, *School of Natural Healing* by Dr. John R. Christopher, and *A Modern Herbal* by Margaret Grieve. I was captivated by *A Modern Herbal* because it contained detailed accounts of the historical uses of plants, in-depth botanical descriptions, it was extremely well organized, and Grieve was among the few females who authored a brilliant herbal text. Several years later, I became acquainted with materia medica and dispensatory references by Eclectics and Physiomedics, thanks to my teacher Michael Moore who scanned thousands of pages of non-copyrighted texts, making them available to his students, and eventually, the public. These encyclopedic references profoundly influenced my clinical practice and teaching. They also inspired me to expand my contributions to the field more broadly by writing this book, in the hope that my expertise would be shared globally.

As a bibliophile and avid herbal enthusiast, my reference library grew considerably with the publication of numerous works during the herbal renaissance in the 1980s and '90s. Many of those books now have well-worn pages, with broken binders detached from frequent referencing. Among my favorite books were those written by practicing herbalists who administered and observed the effects of herbs in numerous patients, made self-care accessible, and cultivated, gathered, and prepared their own medicine. I thoroughly enjoyed reading well-researched, information-rich texts; however, I grew weary of reading books with generic materia medica descriptions that rattled off 50+ properties and multisystemic uses for an herb in one or two paragraphs without presenting an intimate relationship with the plants.

As I researched each herb to enrich my materia medica, I referenced an average of 20 – 50 books to acquire the information I sought, yet the information was often incomplete. I longed for a contemporary, comprehensive reference book written by a practicing herbalist with detailed monographs that emphasized medicinal and clinical uses of plants, and also contained accurate botanical descriptions, etymology, chemical constituents, nutritional properties, temperature and flavor, contraindications, preparations and dosages, as well as therapeutic compounds. In order to fill this gap, I became compelled to write the reference book I always wanted.

The Essential Guide to Western Botanical Medicine was designed to provide a clinically-based, efficiently organized, meticulously referenced book containing detailed, science-based plant monographs. I felt it was imperative to include beautiful color photos that captured plants in many stages from the lens of a plant-loving herbalist. I wanted to provide a comprehensive text of the western herbs I knew intimately, having grown, harvested, prepared as medicines, administered and observed them at least 20 years in clinical practice. I included herbs that were easily cultivated, accessible in commerce from reputable sources, and/or abundant. My goal was to provide a comprehensive, go-to reference to serve herbalists, students, and educational institutions, as well as a complete range of healthcare practitioners, botanists, gardeners, and naturalists, among others.

I've spent more than half my life as an herbalist, and what I love most about the eternally humbling process of studying plant medicine, is the realization that the more I learn, the more there is to know. I have worked for more than 30 years as an herbal practitioner, teacher, medicine-maker, and formulator. I've run a private practice for more than two decades, treating patients through the use of herbs, nutrition, and diet, and I've witnessed the profound healing capacity of plants, nutrition, and nature. I operated a wholesale herbal extract business and a compounding pharmacy that served thousands of clients throughout the West Coast. I continue to direct and instruct herbalist training programs at The Northwest School for Botanical Studies in California.

As a passionate plant lover, gardener, and outdoor enthusiast, I'm most fulfilled gardening, strolling in wild places, gazing at insects and birds pollinating plants, and teaching. Plants soothe, ground, and delight me, healing my family, friends, and community, and gracing my dreams. Whether they're emerging from sidewalk cracks, covering buildings, lining pathways and forest floors, or decorating gardens, plants are an indispensable part of my life.

The eight-year process of writing my book entailed thousands of hours of researching, writing, editing, and revising each monograph countless times. I met weekly with my dear editor for six years, and many times weekly with my designer for nearly two years. I gathered thousands of photos, many of which were often rejected by my meticulous designer. All the while, I ran my Northwest School for Botanical Studies, raised my beloved son who transformed from ages 5 to 13, and maintained my clinical practice, pharmacy, and demonstration garden containing hundreds of species of medicinal herbs. In spite of spending far too much time in front of a computer, I can honestly say that I was thrilled to write this book.

I'm grateful for the humble, wise practitioners who quietly passed their knowledge to their community, clients, students, apprentices, and others. I deeply respect those who've maintained practices, run clinics, herb shops, and apothecaries, made house calls, addressed acute and chronic health conditions, birthed babies, eased infants and children, gathered herbs from their gardens and the wild, unearthed roots, shaved barks, macerated plants, dried plants in their rafters and hand-woven racks, and cultivated and prepared herbal medicines. They are part of the evolving, living tradition of herbalism.

I'm delighted to share through this book, much of what I have been so fortunate to learn in my lifetime, about the practice and therapeutic uses of botanical medicine. I hope it deepens your understanding of herbs, inspires you to integrate them into your daily life, and empowers you to heal yourself, your family, friends, patients, and community.

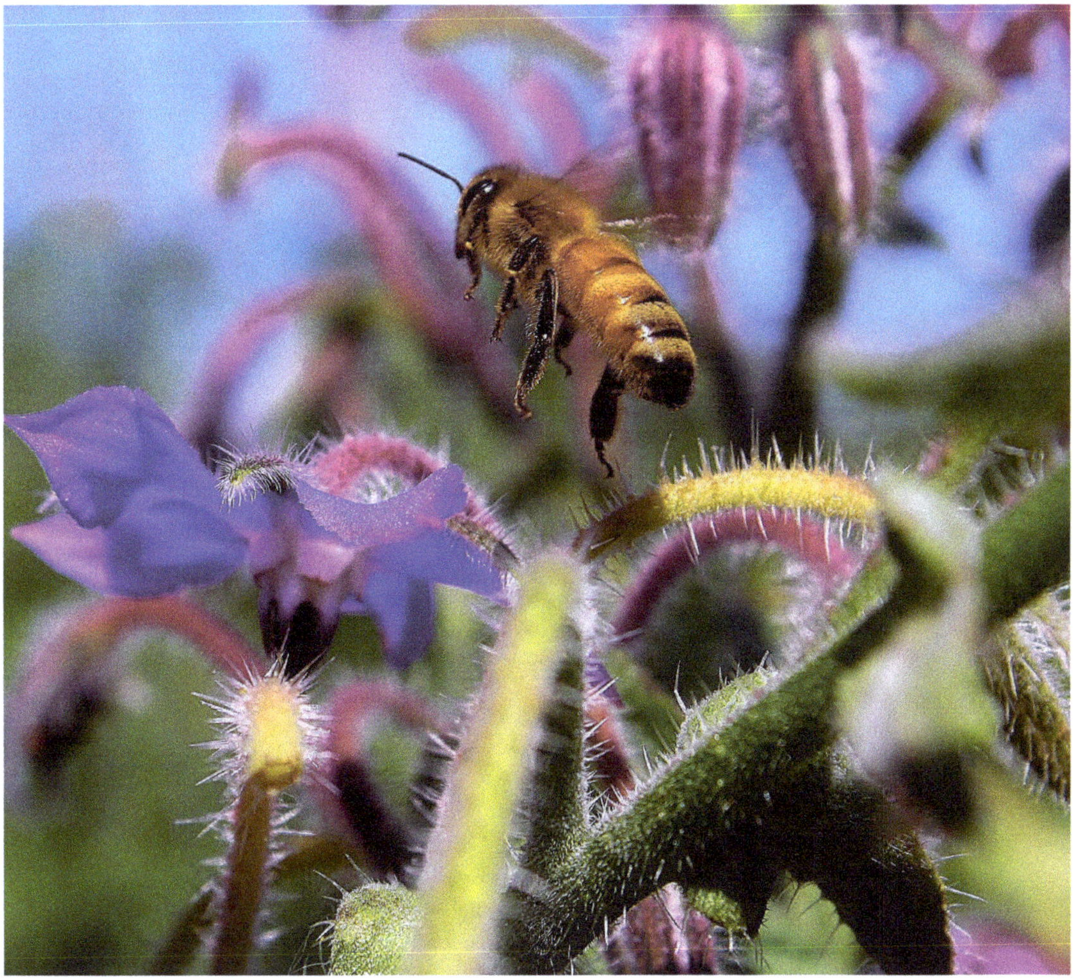

This book is dedicated to my son, Jayden George Kaufman. I love, adore, and admire you.

ACKNOWLEDGEMENTS

I am deeply indebted to three phenomenal women who contributed profoundly to *The Essential Guide to Western Botanical Medicine:* Deborah Dallinger, editor; Barbara Lande, designer; and Selena Rowan, scientific editor and researcher. This book would not be possible without your unwavering support and expertise.

An ever encouraging and grounding presence, Deborah Dallinger has gracefully guided all of the processes, from the book's conception, through countless revisions, eloquently condensing and polishing the content to create a beautiful final publication. After eight years of working extensively together, I'm extremely grateful for her tremendous dedication, impeccable editorial expertise, professionalism, wise counsel, and devoted friendship.

I'm especially grateful to Barbara Lande, a brilliant designer and type aficionado who devoted an incredible amount of time and intensely focused energy to create one of the most visually stunning herbal books. She meticulously edited more than 1,000 photos, and diligently tended to every detail.

A dear friend and respected colleague, herbalist and botanist Selena Rowan was instrumental in the content editing and peer review of this book. She generously contributed her expertise and countless hours of researching, organizing, formatting, and revising. Thank you immensely for your luminous intellect, dedication, integrity, support, and enduring friendship.

Patricia Kyritsi Howell, thank you for your wise counsel, moral support, friendship, and gentle nudges. You were instrumental in shaping my book. You are a colleague, practitioner, and teacher I respect and admire, and I am deeply honored to include your foreword.

Special thanks to my dear husband, Howie Kaufman, for your patience and support, as well as your efforts in maintaining our household and lovingly tending to our family. To my beloved son Jayden, thank you for your unwavering support, love, encouragement, and patience. Your hugs and check-ins were the best distractions from my work. I would like to thank my mom Charlotte, my sister Rachel, and my brother Stephen, for cheering me on every step of the way.

I'm grateful to my former students, especially Michelle Large, who devoted countless hours of editing. I'm deeply appreciative to these friends, colleagues, and fellow plant lovers who generously shared their photos: 7Song, David Bunting, Rosalee de la Forêt, Amy Kumler, Richard Mandelbaum, Darlyne Murawski, Selena Rowan, CoreyPine Shane, Richard Spjut, and Marie van der Schijff.

To my most influential herbal teachers, the late Michael Moore, Donna Chesner, and Adam Seller, thank you for humbly inspiring and training generations of herbalists. I am deeply appreciative for the lifetime contributions of all the many wise herbalists, colleagues, and friends who've enriched the world through their healing presence and teachings. Your compassion, dedication, knowledge, vision, and drive have made this world a better place. You and your many contributions hold a dear place in my heart; thank you immensely: Cascade Andersen-Geller, Paul Bergner, William Morris, Rebecca Ellis, Gaye Ayton, Faye Honoroff, Amy Bohner, Suzy Haggerty, and Kathryn Day.

To the patients and customers I've had the honor of serving for more than two decades, thank you for entrusting me with your health care. Because of you, I've witnessed the profoundly transformative, healing power of plants.

Lastly, I'm beholden to the plants for their eternal inspiration. They've captured my heart, mind, body, and soul, and have healed and nourished me and so many others in countless ways.

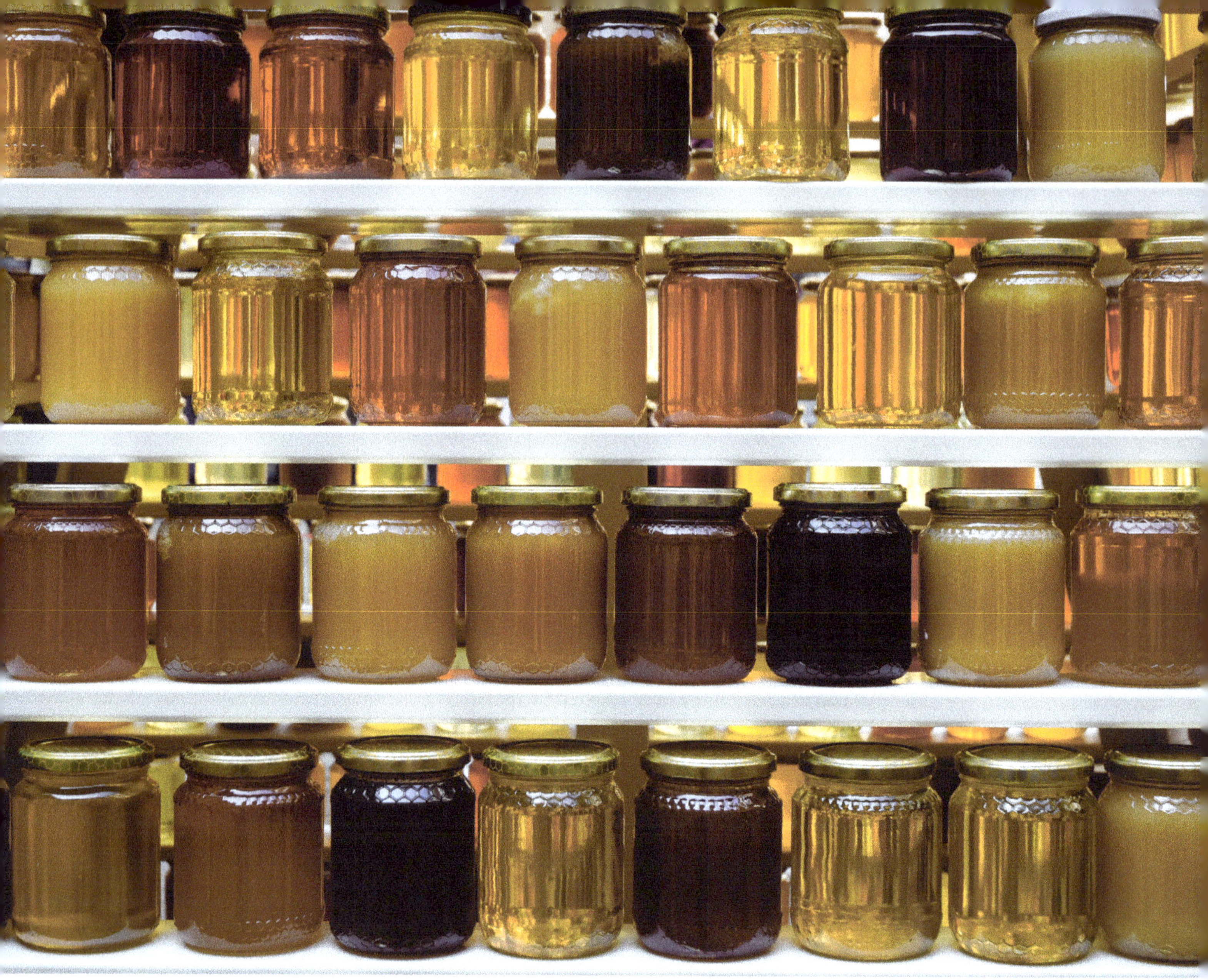

The information contained in this book is intended as a health-promoting, educational reference, and self-help guide. The author is not responsible for any adverse effects or consequences resulting from the use of the herbs, preparations, approaches, or procedures covered in this book. The information contained herein is not a substitute for professional medical care or treatment; nor can it replace the foundational aspects of health including adequate sleep, a nutritious diet, supplements, and exercise. The author recommends consulting a healthcare professional or physician for diagnosis and treatment of serious health concerns. The content of this book has not been evaluated by the FDA.

Prior to consuming a single herb or compound formula, the author encourages the reader to review the herb/s to make sure they suit you and have no ill side effects. This is especially important for individuals with pre-existing health conditions and/or those consuming medications. Consult a medical professional before combining herbs and medications.

The author recommends trying each herb individually to familiarize yourself with its effects before consuming compounded herbal formulas. The formulas and proportions listed in the "Herbal Therapeutic Formulas" are not fixed; they can easily be modified to suit the individual. When a patient has an aversion to a particular herb in a formula, or when an herb is contraindicated, replace or omit it. When an ingredient is unavailable, substitute it with a bioregional herb that has a similar effect, or omit it. If any of the herbs, compounds, or tea blends produce unpleasant side effects, discontinue them immediately.

Research on the use of botanical medicine by Indigenous peoples is ongoing, and our understanding continues to evolve as new studies and perspectives emerge. In this book, the *Historical Uses* sections are presented in the past tense, following the original sources, to reflect documented practices while acknowledging that Indigenous knowledge systems are living, dynamic, and culturally significant. This approach seeks to honor the peoples whose knowledge is represented, ensuring that their traditions are recognized, respected, and not inadvertently erased.

Throughout the text, the terms "female" and "male" are used in reference to biological sex as described in the sources. These terms are intended for clarity in describing physiological characteristics and historical documentation; they are not intended to be exclusionary. The author recognizes and affirms the diversity of gender identities and expressions, including gender fluidity and non-binary experiences, and affirms that these identities are valid and integral to contemporary understandings of human biology, culture, and social experience.

MATERIA MEDICA

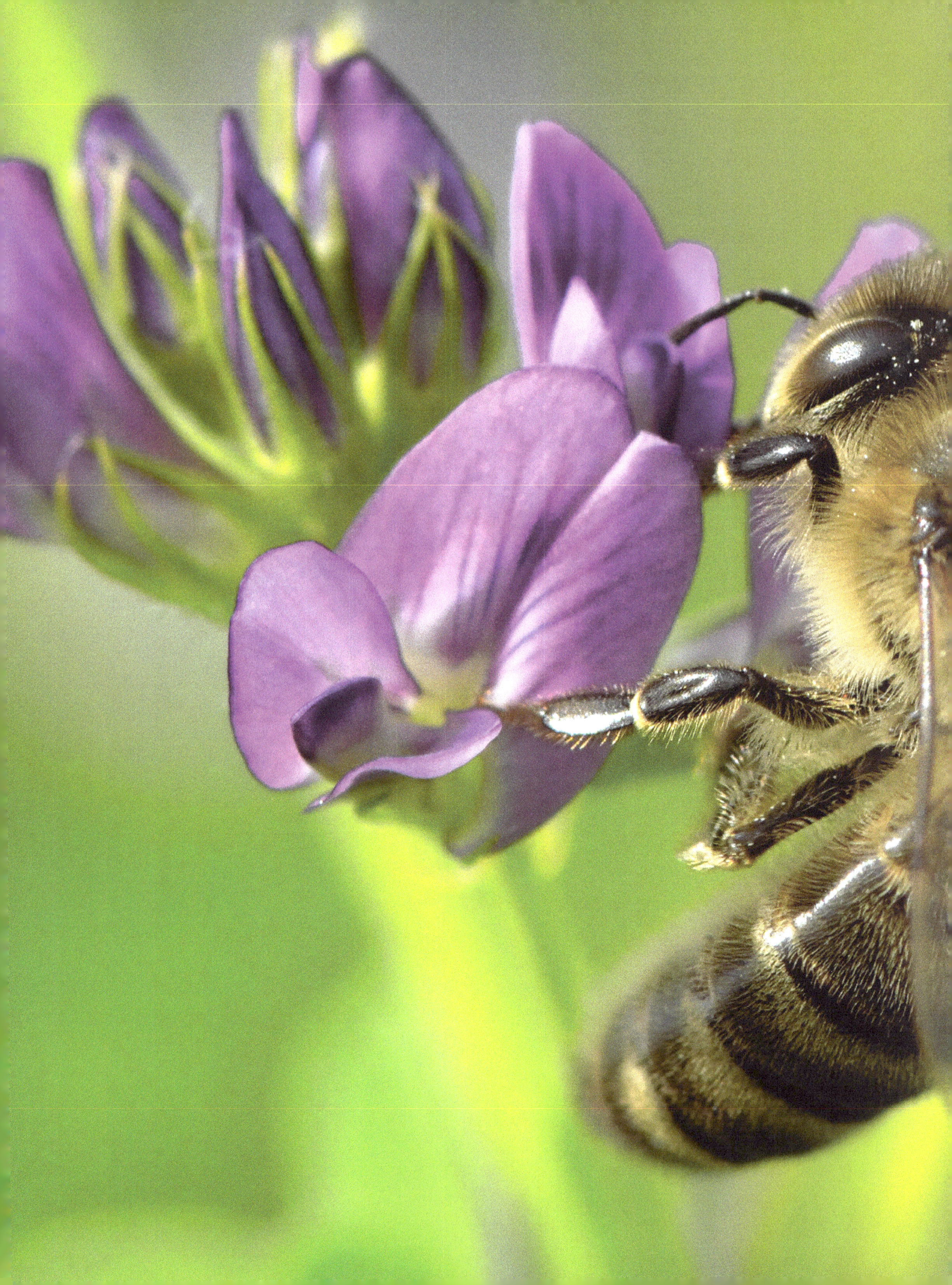

ALFALFA

DESCRIPTION

BOTANICAL NAME:
Medicago sativa

COMMON NAMES:
Alfalfa, lucerne, lusern, purple medic, buffalo grass, Chilean clover, Spanish clover, Spanish hay
gum fa choi (Cantonese)
lucerna (Croatian)
foder-lucerne (Danish)
kylvomailanen (Finnish)
lucerne (French)
luzerne (German)
midiki (Greek)
aspeset (Hebrew)
luzerna medica (Italian)
blalucern (Norwegian)
lucerna (Polish)
feno-de-borgonha (Portugese)
lasunghas (Sanskrit)
alfal (Spanish, Slovenian)
adi yonca, kaba yonca (Turkish)

FAMILY NAME:
Fabaceae (Leguminosae)

PARTS USED: Harvest the leaves and stems, or flowering tops in full bloom.

BOTANICAL DESCRIPTION AND HABITAT: Alfalfa is native to Asia, but now grows worldwide in cultivated and wild settings. Spanish conquistadors introduced it to Chile and Mexico, where it was cultivated as animal fodder. It is planted as a cover crop throughout the United States (U.S.). It is a perennial legume with deep roots containing symbiotic bacteria that fix nitrogen in the soil.

Alfalfa is an herbaceous perennial (20 – 100 cm tall) with slightly square stems.[1,2] The trifoliate leaves have prominent lanceolate stipules and obovate leaflets (10 – 30 mm long by 3 – 10 mm wide) with appressed hairs on the upper sides and glabrous undersides.[1,2] The racemes (1 – 2.5 cm long) bear many small, white to purple pea-like flowers on short petioles. Each flower has five fused sepals, five specialized petals, ten stamens with nine filaments fused to each other, and one carpel.[1,2] The fruit is a leathery, yellow-brown glabrous legume (5 – 9 mm diameter) that is sickle-shaped or coiled.[1,2]

THE NAME: The genus name *Medicago* derives from the Greek name for alfalfa *(medick)*, as it was brought to Greece from Media, Iran.[3] The epithet *sativa* ("sown") derives from the Latin, *sativus*. The common name alfalfa derives from the Arabic name for the plant, *al-facfacah*, meaning "father," or "father of all foods."[4] The Spanish modified the name to alfalfa.[4] Lucern ("lamp") refers to the bright, shiny seeds.

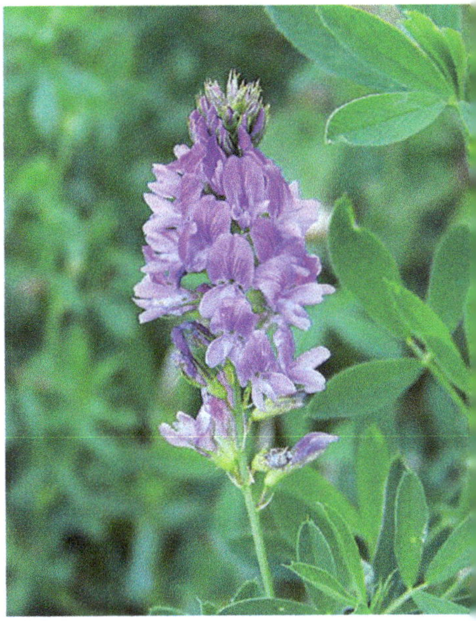

HISTORICAL USES: Alfalfa was cultivated in Armenia as early as 2,000 BCE. It was introduced to Greece around 500 BCE, and spread throughout Europe and northern Africa.[4] Europeans began cultivating alfalfa in the 17th century.[4] It was used by Chinese physicians to treat digestive and kidney disorders.[4] Ayurvedic practitioners administered alfalfa to enhance digestion, and the seed poultice was applied to boils.[4] Native Americans applied a hot alfalfa poultice to treat earaches.[4] Eclectic physicians administered alfalfa to malnourished mothers, and as a galactagogue.[9] The tea was prescribed as a diuretic, appetite stimulant, and laxative.[9] Eclectic physician Ben Bradley recommended alfalfa as an alternative to black tea and coffee, especially for individuals with digestive disorders.[9] Alfalfa was used as nutritious fodder for grazing animals, and was esteemed for increasing cow milk production.[3]

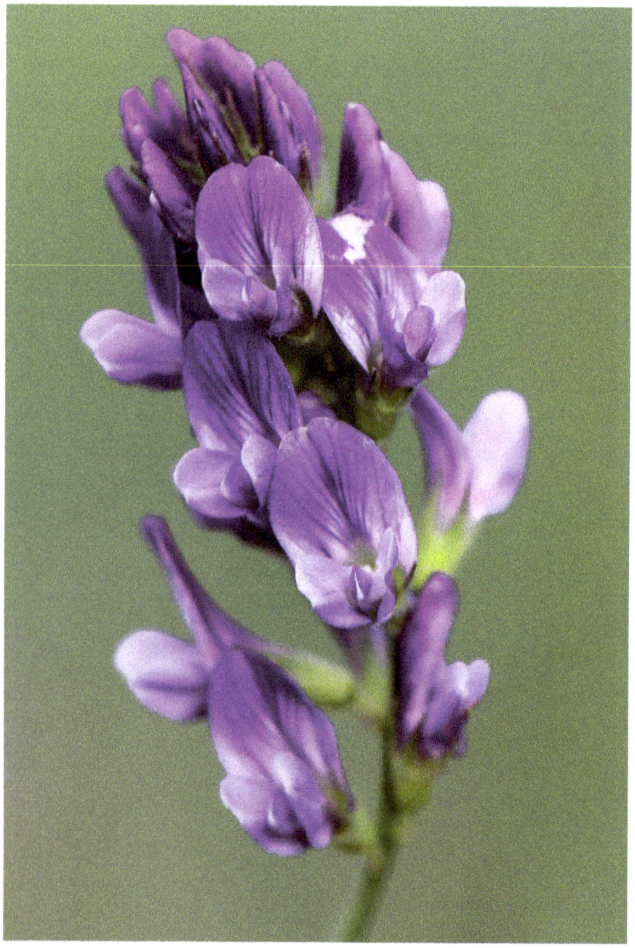

CONSTITUENTS: Alfalfa contains saponins that upon hydrolysis, yield aglycones (soyasapogenols A – E, medicagenic acid, and hederagenin) and glycones (glucose, arabinose, xylose, rhamnose, galactose, and glucuronic acid). It contains phytosterols (β-sitosterol, α-spinasterol, stigmasterol, cycloartenol, and campestrol), high molecular weight alcohols (octacosanol and triacontanol), a volatile oil (hexanal), paraffins (nonacosane, triacontane, and hentriacontane), fatty acids (lauric, myristic, and palmitic), flavones and isoflavones (genistein, tricin, daidzein, biochanin A, formononetin, and (-)-5'-methoxysativan), coumarin derivatives (coumestrol, medicagol, sativol, lucernol, trifoliol, and daphnoretin), alkaloids (homostachydrine, stachydrine, tricine, and trigonelline — in seeds only), and plant acids (malic, oxalic, malonic, maleic, and quinic).[5-7]

NUTRITIONAL PROPERTIES: Alfalfa contains high amounts of chlorophyll, protein, fiber, β-carotene, B vitamins (B_1, B_2, B_6, B_{12}, biotin, folic acid, niacin, and pantothenic acid), and vitamin C. It contains average amounts of vitamins D, E, and K, as well as amino acids (valine, lysine, arginine, leucine, isoleucine, tryptophan, phenylalanine, methionine, and threonine). Additionally, alfalfa contains trace minerals including calcium, chromium, cobalt, copper, iron, magnesium, manganese, phosphorus, potassium, silicon, sodium, and zinc.[6,7]

MEDICINAL PROPERTIES: Antiatherosclerotic, antiscorbutic, depurative, diuretic (mild), galactagogue, hemostatic, hypocholesterolemic, hypoglycemic, nutritive, restorative, stomachic, and yin tonic.

TEMPERATURE AND FLAVOR: Neutral, sweet, bitter, and mildly salty.

MEDICINAL USES

Alfalfa is a gentle, effective nutritive and restorative tonic, especially when tea or tablets are consumed daily. It contains high amounts of chlorophyll and easily assimilated nutrients.[6, 10] Alfalfa nourishes the blood and aids in treating anemia.[4,6,10] Combine it with nettle leaf *(Urtica dioica)*, oat straw *(Avena)*, red clover *(Trifolium)*, mint *(Mentha)*, and a small quantity of yellow dock *(Rumex)* as a daily tonic tea.

A subtle alterative, alfalfa is rich in alkalinizing minerals. The tea can be consumed long-term to reduce chronic conditions aggravated by an acid environment in the tissues. The high mineral content and chlorophyll in alfalfa help to relieve acid-aggravated conditions, such as rheumatoid arthritis, gout, joint pain, and uric acid kidney stones.[4] Skin conditions such as eczema, psoriasis, and acne are often alleviated by consuming a gentle cleansing tonic of alfalfa and red clover *(Trifolium pratense)*.

Alfalfa supports women in all phases of life, including teenage, childbearing, perimenopausal, and menopausal years.[10] Alfalfa tea is a nourishing tonic to consume during pregnancy and a postpartum restorative agent.[6,10] Combine it with raspberry leaf *(Rubus)*, oat straw *(Avena)*, nettle *(Urtica)*, and peppermint *(Mentha)* or lemon grass

(Cymbopogon) for flavor as a nutritive and uterine tonifying tea.[10] Consuming alfalfa tablets or tea aids in preventing hemorrhaging after birth.[4,10] Prepare a pregnancy-safe hemostatic tea by combining it with equal parts nettle *(Urtica)*, raspberry leaf *(Rubus)*, lady's mantle *(Alchemilla)*, and mint *(Mentha)* for flavor. Alfalfa is a galactagogue, increasing breast milk flow, and nourishing breast milk.[9]

Alfalfa has a balancing effect on digestion, enhancing salivary and digestive secretions, and improving digestion and assimilation.[10] An infusion regulates stomach acid levels when consumed 20 minutes prior to eating.[10] Alfalfa eases acid indigestion, heartburn, and gastric reflux.[10] Epithelial cells lining the mucous membranes in the digestive tract are strengthened due to the β-carotene content. Alfalfa is a gentle recuperative agent for individuals who are weak, fatigued, or convalescing from a febrile or chronic illness.[6] It tonifies yin, replenishing tissues and bodily fluids.

Alfalfa reduces cholesterol levels and decreases low density lipids (LDLs), but has little to no effect on high density lipids (HDLs).[4] This action may be attributed to the saponins that inhibit the intestinal absorption of cholesterol, lowering circulating cholesterol, and preventing atherosclerosis.[4] Animal studies show that alfalfa has hypoglycemic effects potentially beneficial for individuals with syndrome X and type 2 diabetes.[4]

CONTRAINDICATIONS

There are no known contraindications for alfalfa leaves, stems, or flowers. However, long-term, excessive consumption of alfalfa sprouts can cause erythrocytosis (breakdown of red blood cells) likely due to the high saponin content. Consuming large amounts of alfalfa seeds can induce reversible pancytopenia, lowering red and white blood cell counts.[4,5] Ingesting large quantities of alfalfa seeds or sprouts can initiate systemic lupus erythematosus (SLE).[4,5] Predisposed individuals or those with SLE should avoid or limit intake.[5] This action may be due to the amino acid canavanine content of the seeds and sprouts, not the leaves.[4]

PREPARATION AND DOSAGE

TINCTURE: Fresh leaves [1:3+, 60-95% alcohol]; dry leaves [1:5, 50% alcohol]; consume 15-60 drops, up to three times daily.

GLYCERITE: Fresh leaves [1:5, 40% glycerin, 40% water, 20% alcohol]; consume 15-60 drops, up to three times daily.

SYRUP: Consume 1 teaspoon to 1 tablespoon, up to three times daily.

TABLETS: Consume 2-4 tablets, one to three times daily, or use as directed. Consume 1-2 capsules, one to three times daily.

TEA: Prepare a hot or cold infusion; consume 8-12 ounces, three to four times daily. Tea is the ideal form for obtaining nutrients from alfalfa. Fresh leaves may also be added in small amounts as a salad green.

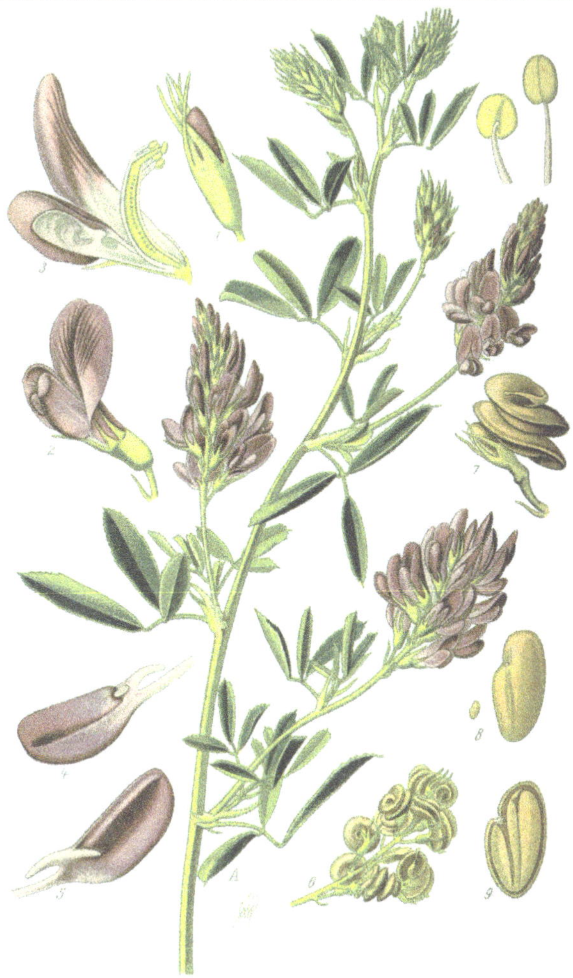

ALOE

DESCRIPTION

BOTANICAL NAMES:
Aloe vera (syn. *A. barbadensis*), *A. arborescens, A. ferox, A. africana, A. perryi, A.* spp.

COMMON NAMES:
Aloe, Barbados aloe, Curacao aloe, cape aloe, Bombay aloe, Turkey aloe, Zanzibar aloe, Socatrine aloe
moka, aalwee, aalwelyn (Afrikaans)
aloés, laegealoe, port (Danish)
laakeaaloe (Finnish)
aloes (French)
aloi, panini'awa'awa (Hawaiian)
ghikanvar, guar patha (Hindi)
rokai (Japanese)
nohwa (Korean)
lú hui (Mandarin)
ghiu kumari (Nepali)
aloes zwycajny (Polish)
aloes (Portuguese)
kumāri (Sanskrit)
acíbar (Spanish)
hang ta keh (Thai)
umhlaba (Zulu)

FAMILY NAME:
Xanthorrhoeaceae (formerly Liliaceae)

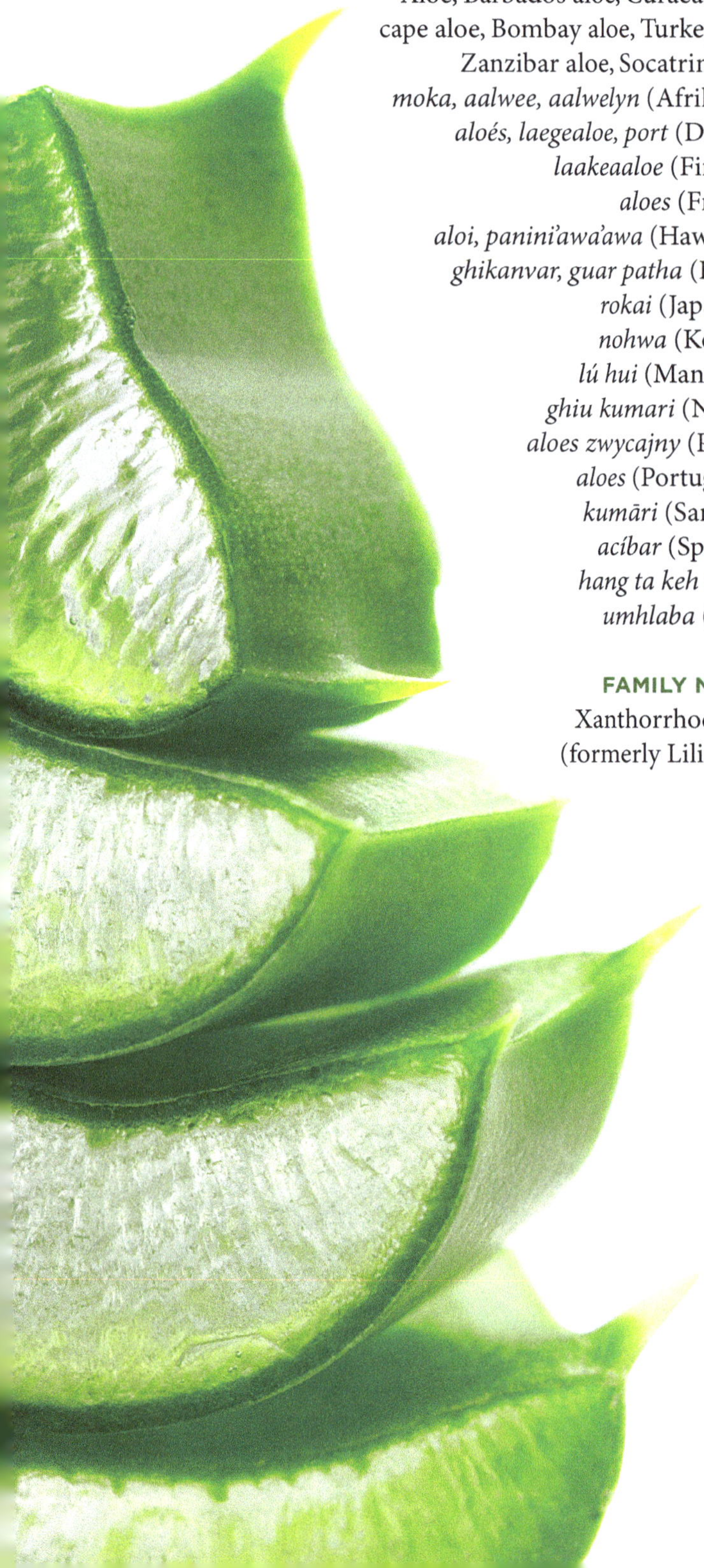

PARTS USED: The gel or juice.

BOTANICAL DESCRIPTION AND HABITAT: *Aloe*, a genus of perennial herbs and shrubs native to southern and tropical Africa and the Arabian Peninsula, is also naturalized in the Mediterranean region, India, China, and California.[1-3] There are more than 360 *Aloe* species.[4] Aloe often grows in basal rosettes; however, many are thicket-forming shrubs or arborescent, like *Aloe ferox*.[1] The thick, succulent leaves have hard spines along their margins, a pointed apex, and bases that clasp the stems.[1,2] When the leaf is cut, a bitter yellow-green sap (latex) oozes from the glabrous skin.[1] The inflorescence is an erect raceme or panicle with a sturdy peduncle. Growing on a short pedicel, the nodding, cylindric flower has six fused red, orange, or yellow tepals that separate at the tips.[1,2] Inside the flowers are six exserted,

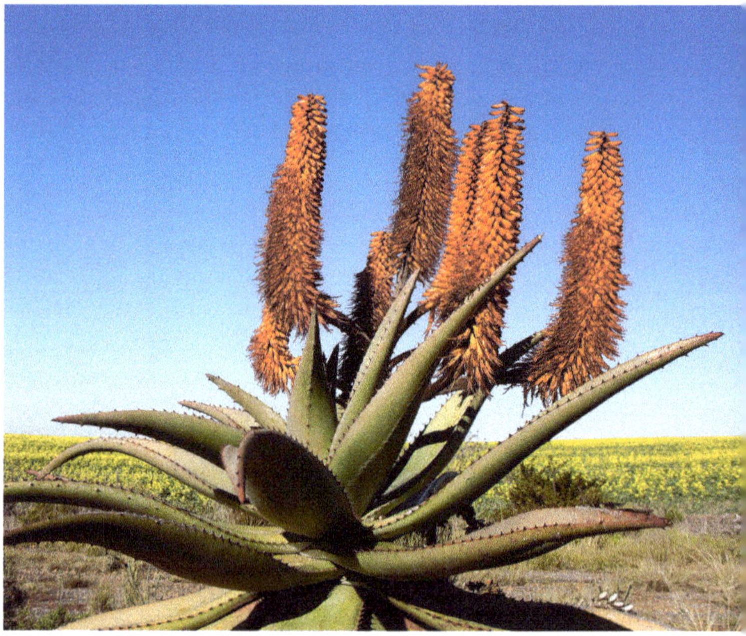

unequal stamens, and a superior ovary comprised of three fused carpels.[1] The fruit is a papery or woody capsule holding many seeds.[1-3]

THE NAME: Aloe derives from the Greek or Latin *alloeh*, originating from the Hebrew *ahalim* ("the fragrant resin from an East Indian tree"). The word *ahalim* may be borrowed from the Sanskrit *agaru*, the name for aloe wood, also known as aloeswood, agarwood, or lignaloes. *Ahalim* may have been applied to *Aloe vera* due to the resinous latex

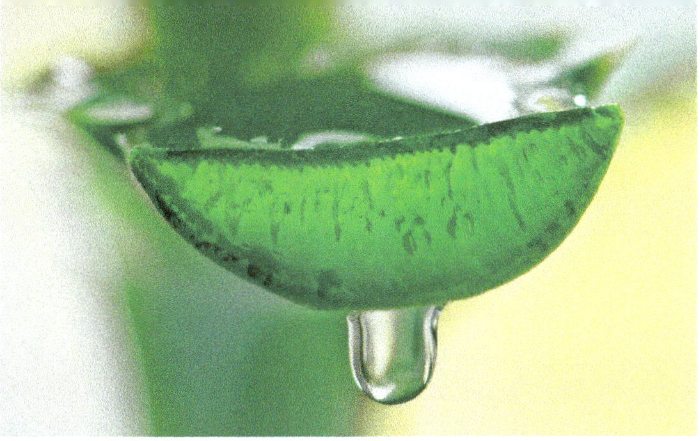

in the leaves; however, aloeswood is an entirely different plant that has been burned as incense since biblical times.[5-7] The epithet *vera* originates from the Latin *verus* ("true"), referring to *Aloe vera* as the true aloe, as opposed to agave, which was mistakenly given the name aloe in the 1680s.[8] The epithet *ferox* ("fierce") derives from Latin, likely referring to the spine-rimmed leaves.[9] Kumāri ("young maiden"), the Sanskrit name for aloe, alludes to its replenishing qualities in the female reproductive system.[10]

Aloe vera is commonly referred to as aloe, Barbados aloe, or Curacao aloe. Native to South Africa, *A. ferox* is known as Cape aloe. Socotrine aloe is the common name of *A. perryi.*

HISTORICAL USES: One of the earliest records of aloe dating back to 2200 BCE was carved into Sumerian clay tablets.[11] In 1550 BCE, the medicinal uses of aloe were recorded on ancient Egyptian papyri.[11] Egyptians incorporated aloe in embalming fluid.[11] Cleopatra prized aloe as a beautifying agent. The ancient Greek physicians Dioscorides and Pliny valued aloe's wound-healing qualities.[11,12] Dioscorides wrote about the laxative and stomach-cleansing actions of aloe juice. He also mentioned that aloe reduced inflammation in the mouth, throat, and eyes.[11] In the 4th century BCE, Aristotle attempted to convince his pupil Alexander the Great to conquer the island of Socotra in order to supply his army enough aloe to treat their wounds.[11] In the 10th century, aloe was imported in Europe.[11] Eventually, it was adopted as a medicine in many cultures worldwide.

In 1820, aloe preparations were included in the *U.S. Pharmacopoeia.*[12] Eclectic physicians administered aloe juice to stimulate peristalsis and increase secretions in the liver, pancreas, and intestinal glands.[13,14] For example, John King and John Scudder recommended aloe for torpid conditions, including chlorosis, hypochondria, indigestion, jaundice, scrofula, and habitual constipation.[14,15] Aloe and aloin were also prescribed to treat hemorrhoids and rectal prolapse caused by insufficient venous return and poor health, although it was contraindicated for active hemorrhoid inflammation.[14,16] Aloe juice was recommended to stimulate pelvic circulation, and as an emmenagogue to treat suppressed menstruation; however, it was contraindicated during pregnancy.[13,14,16] Aloin, a constituent of aloe, was recommended for excessive beer drinkers, as well as individuals who overate starchy foods or sugar.[13] The bitter latex of aloe juice was painted on children's fingertips to deter them from biting their nails.[11]

CONSTITUENTS

ALOE GEL: Aloe gel contains mucilaginous polysaccharides (acetylated galactomannan, acemannan = aloeverose, mannan, glucomannan, arabinan, arabinose, xylose, galactose, glucose, L-rhamnose, aldopentose, and cellulose), saponins, β-sitosterol, lectins, enzymes (oxidase, amylase, catalase, lipase, and alkaline phosphatase), amino acids (lysine, threonine, valine, methionine, leucine, isoleucine, and phenylalanine), vitamins (B_1, B_2, B_6, C, and E, folic acid, choline, and β-carotene), minerals (calcium, sodium, manganese, magnesium, zinc, copper, and chromium), lipids, fatty acids (gamma-linolenic acid), "biogenic stimulators," "wound-healing hormones," tannins, and small amounts of anthranoids. The polysaccharides can degrade within 48 hours at room temperature; therefore, fresh gel is superior.[4,10,12,17]

ALOE JUICE: Aloe juice contains cathartic anthraquinone glycosides (C-glucosides consisting primarily of barbaloin = aloin, a glucoside of aloe-emodin; emodin, isobarbaloin, anthranol, aloetic acid, anthracene, ester of cinnamic acid, chrysophanic acid, ethereal oil, and resistannol), chromone-C-glycosides *(A. vera*: aloeresin B = aloesin; *A. ferox*: aloeresin A and B, and its aglycone aloesone*),* resins, and bitter principles. The young leaf exudate contains higher concentrations of barbaloin; they decrease in older leaves towards the base of the plant.[4,10,12,17]

NUTRITIONAL PROPERTIES: Aloe contains high amounts of carbohydrates, crude fiber, dietary fiber, selenium, and vitamin C. It contains low to average amounts of aluminum, ash, calcium, carbohydrates, chromium, cobalt, fat, iron, magnesium, manganese, niacin, phosphorus, potassium, protein, riboflavin, silicon, sodium, thiamine, tin, vitamin A, and zinc.[18]

MEDICINAL PROPERTIES: Aloe gel is an anti-inflammatory, demulcent, emollient, moisturizer, laxative, immune modulator, antibacterial, antifungal, and vulnerary. Aloe juice is a bitter tonic, choleretic, cathartic laxative, and emmenagogue.

TEMPERATURE AND FLAVOR: Aloe gel is cool, bland, salty, and sweet. Aloe juice is cool and bitter.

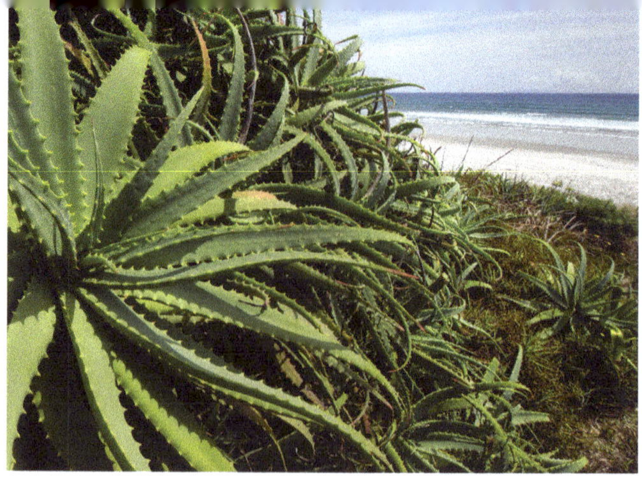

MEDICINAL USES

ALOE GEL

Aloe gel *(aloe vera* gel*)* is obtained from the parenchymatous tissue in the inner portion of the leaf. Also referred to as the inner fillet, aloe gel is often erroneously called "aloe juice." The gel is a clear, mucilaginous or jelly-like substance; aloe juice has a yellow to brown hue.

Aloe gel contains mucilaginous polysaccharides that have soothing demulcent actions, reducing inflammation in the mucous membranes and skin.[19] It coats the digestive tract and has antiulcer activity.[4,12] Aloe gel aids in treating upper digestive inflammatory conditions such as hyperacidity, peptic ulcers, ulcerative colitis, intestinal bleeding, and gastric lesions.[12] It also helps to reduce digestive tract inflammation caused by radiation or chemotherapy.[20] Aloe is best consumed 30 – 60 minutes before meals, or two hours after meals to protect mucous membranes. Aloe gel lubricates the digestive tract and has mild laxative actions.[12] It also soothes the respiratory tract and aids in treating a sore throat, dry cough, or laryngitis.[10]

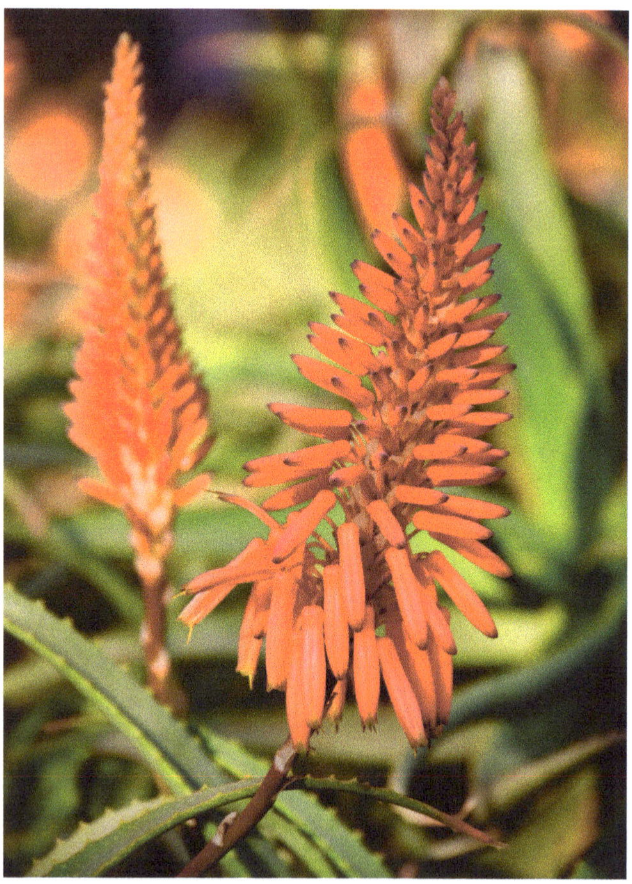

Aloe gel has yin tonifying actions, and is hydrating and moistening. Consume the gel to treat yin deficiency or yin deficiency with heat signs (hot flashes or night sweats). The gel is a recuperative agent following a debilitating illness, high fever, heat stroke, dehydration, or sunburn. In Ayurvedic medicine, it is administered as a female reproductive tonic to increase fertility, aid in recovery from childbirth, and treat menopausal symptoms such as vaginal dryness, hot flashes, and night sweats.[10] Aloe gel can be consumed to address *pitta* excess.[10,11]

The gel contains polysaccharides that have immune modulating actions.[4] Studies demonstrate that acemannan (acetylated mannose), a polysaccharide in aloe, has antiviral and immune potentiating actions.[12] Acemannan has antiviral actions against human immunodeficiency virus type 1 (HIV-1), influenza, and measles.[12] It enhances macrophage activity and T cell function, and increases the production of interferon and immune potentiating substances.[12] It also synergizes the effects of certain antiviral drugs.[12] For instance, acemannan improved the effectiveness of azidothymidine (AZT), an antiviral drug used to treat AIDS, as well as acyclovir (Zovirax) used to treat herpes simplex type 1 (HSV-1).[12] *In vitro* studies demonstrate that acemannan combined with AZT or acyclovir inhibits the replication of HIV and HSV-1.[12] It was also found to exert a direct antiviral action against HIV-1 by inhibiting glycosylation of viral glycoproteins.[12] Aloctin A (a constituent in *A. arborescens*) increases the production of lymphokines, including interleukin-2 (IL-2) and interferon-y (INF-y) produced by human T cells and accessory cells *in vitro*.[4] Aloctin A also increases natural killer (NK) cell activity, and stimulates cells cytotoxic to tumor cells *in vitro*.[4]

Fresh aloe gel also has antibacterial and antifungal actions.[5,12] It demonstrates antibacterial actions against *Pseudomonas aeruginosa, Klebsiella pneumoniae, Serratia marcescens, Citrobacter* spp., *Enterobacter cloacae, Streptococcus pyogenes, Streptococcus agalactiae, Staphylococcus aureus*, *Escherichia coli*, and *Streptococcus faecalis*.[12] It is a fungistatic, inhibiting *Candida albicans* growth.[12]

Aloe gel is an anti-inflammatory, vulnerary agent that aids in healing thermal burns, sunburns, and burns resulting from electrical injury or X-ray radiation exposure.[4,12,17,20] It works most effectively when applied immediately, or soon after a burn occurs. Aloe gel reduces the pain, redness, and inflammation of sunburn.[4,20] The fresh gel has hydroscopic properties that draw water from the subcutaneous membranes, preventing blistering.[21]

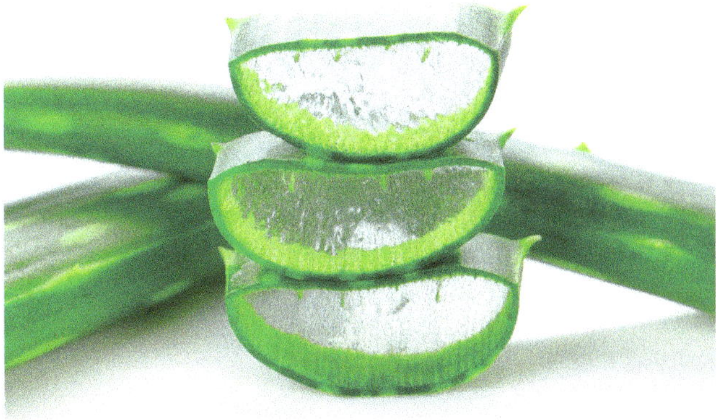

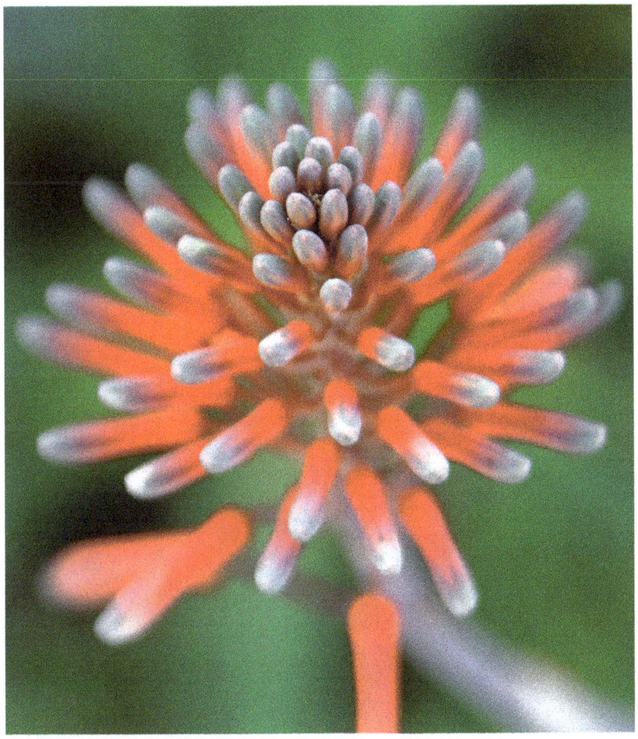

Aloe gel penetrates injured tissue, reducing inflammation and encouraging wound healing.[4] Topical applications of fresh gel alleviate pain and swelling by inhibiting the formation of inflammatory mediators, thromboxane and bradykinin.[5,12,22] Thromboxane is produced by red blood cells in response to injured tissue, and slows wound healing from burns.[5] Bradykinin is a polypeptide formed from plasma proteins that is also released following tissue injury. It increases capillary permeability, has vasodilating actions, increases smooth muscle spasms, and stimulates pain receptors. Aloe gel contains glycoproteins that inhibit bradykinin formation and enhance its catabolization.[12] It also stimulates epidermal growth and repair by increasing fibroblasts and connective tissue formation.[12] Aloe gel aids in maintaining healthy prostaglandin ratios, while preventing the collapse of injured blood vessels.[4] It contains unsaturated fatty acids, notably gamma-linolenic acid ($C_{18:3}$) that can be converted to a 1-series prostaglandin, producing more beneficial effects for inflammation, platelet aggregation, and wound healing.[12]

Topical applications of fresh aloe gel aid in treating psoriasis, dandruff, dry eczema, stretch marks, skin ulcers, and dry, inflamed eyes.[10] Aloe gel has an antiaging effect, and is often included in ointments, creams, and lotions as a cosmetic aid.[11] Fresh aloe gel applications aid in treating cuts, wounds, ulcers, stretch marks, and abrasions. It catalyzes the healing of skin conditions such as eczema, psoriasis, seborrheic dermatitis, urticaria, acne, and mouth ulcers. Aloe gel reduces itching and hastens healing in the final stages of poison oak or poison ivy. Applying the fresh gel to closed eyelids reduces swelling and inflammation. *Note:* When treating cuts or broken skin, use only fresh aloe vera gel, because commercial aloe preparations can encourage *Staphylococcus* bacteria.

ALOE JUICE

Aloe juice is obtained from the yellow bitter juice or latex in specialized cells beneath the thick epidermis. The leaves are cut at the base, then drained and dehydrated. The concentrate is light to dark brown. The dry juice is powdered and encapsulated or extracted. The juice of cape aloe is commonly referred to as aloe juice.

Aloe juice is a bitter choleretic and cathartic laxative.[4,11-13,16] Compared to other potent anthraquinone-containing laxative herbs such as rhubarb root *(Rheum palmatum)*, cascara sagrada *(Rhamnus purshiana)*, and senna *(Senna angustifolia)*, this form of aloe is considered one of the most irritating purgatives, due to its propensity to cause cramping, griping, and colon irritation.[11] It contains aloin (barbaloin), which stimulates the excretion of electrolytes and water from the intestinal lumen, increasing intestinal volume and stimulating peristalsis.[4,12] It also prevents the reabsorption of electrolytes and water from the large intestine.[4] Consume tea or extracts of carminative herbs such as fennel *(Foeniculum)*, cardamom *(Elettaria)*, or coriander

(*Coriandrum*) with aloe juice preparations to prevent intestinal cramping and griping pain.[16] *Note:* Results can take 12 – 18 hours following consumption; therefore, aloe juice should be consumed early in the evening to obtain results the following morning. Aloe juice should only be used short-term for treating constipation, because it has habituating potential.[16]

CONTRAINDICATIONS

Aloe juice should not be consumed during pregnancy or lactation, or by children.[10,13,16,23] Avoid consuming aloe juice with active intestinal inflammation.[13,21] Overdosing on aloe juice can cause abdominal pain, bloody diarrhea, hemorrhagic gastritis, or nephritis.[4]

Topical aloe gel preparations should be avoided in deep, vertical wounds such as those caused by laparotomy or cesarean delivery because it can delay healing.[12] Commercial preparations of aloe gel should not be applied to severe burns or wounds; use only fresh gel.[17] Expressed gel is the preferable method of extraction in store-bought aloe gel; otherwise, commercial products may contain solvents.

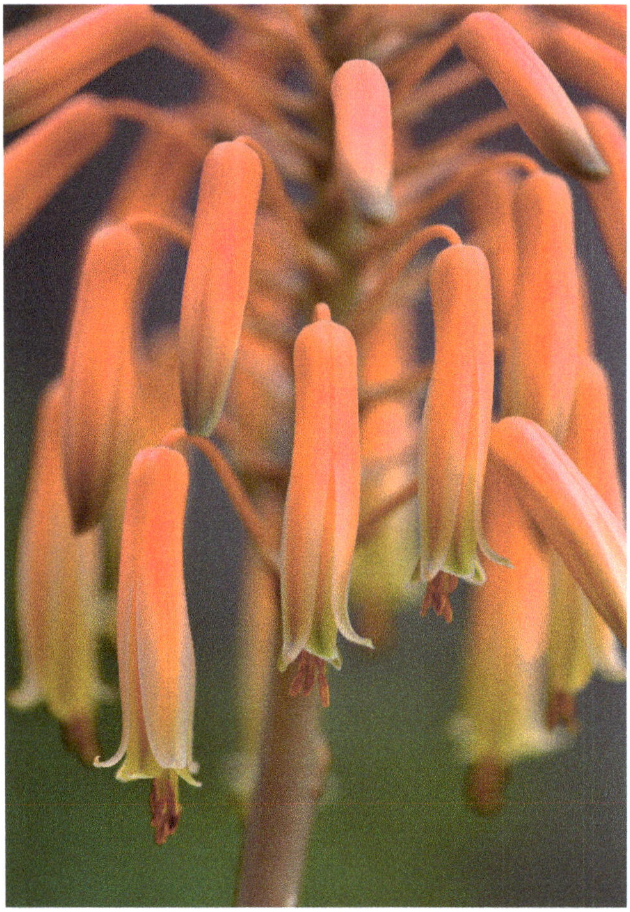

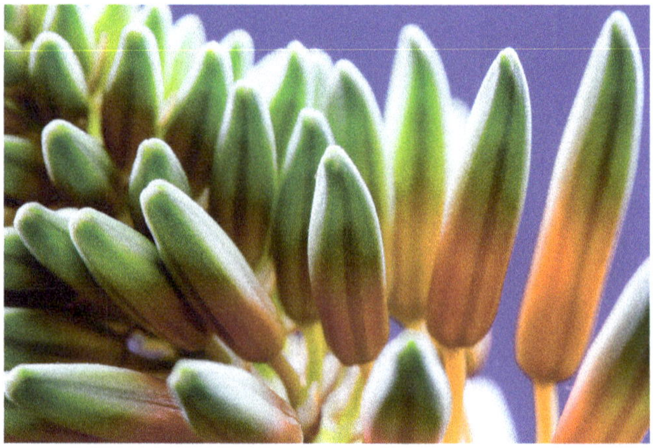

PREPARATION AND DOSAGE

TINCTURE: Dried juice extract [1:10, 50% alcohol]; consume 15 - 60 drops, once daily.

SUCCUS: Consume 1 - 4 ounces of gel from the inner fillet of *Aloe vera.*

CAPSULES: Consume 1 - 3 capsules of aloe juice powder, once daily.

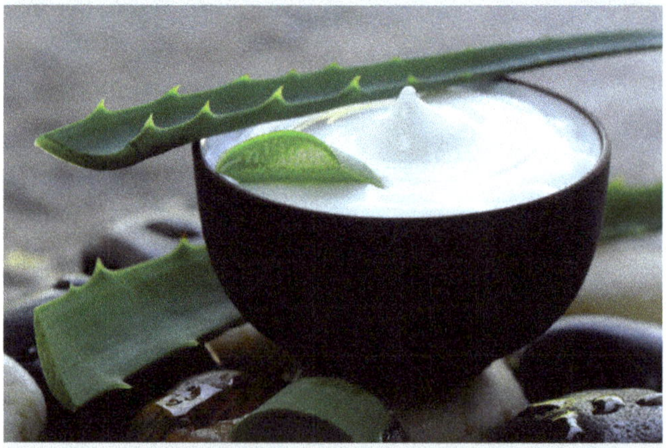

TOPICAL USE: Apply fresh aloe gel topically. Use a sharp knife or scissors to remove a thin strip of the spines along the sides of the leaves. Remove one side of the outer leaf and apply topically, or manually express the gel from between the outer portions of the leaves. Commercial gel preparations can be added to lotions, creams, water-based sprays, and other skin care products; however, they often contain citric acid or preservatives.

CULINARY USE: The inner fillet of *Aloe vera* can be cubed and prepared in stir fries and curries.

AMBROSIA

DESCRIPTION

BOTANICAL NAMES:
Ambrosia ambrosioides, A. acanthicarpa, A. artemisiifolia A. chamissonis, A. confertiflora, A. psilostachya, A. trifida A. spp.

COMMON NAMES:
Ambrosia, tall ambrosia, ragweed, canyon ragweed, coastal ragweed, great ragweed, western ragweed, bur ragweed, silver burweed, bitterweed, bloodweed, chicua, weakleaf, burrobrush, horseweed, horse cane, richweed, wild hemp, bursage *yerba del sapo* (Spanish)

FAMILY NAME:
Asteraceae (Compositae)

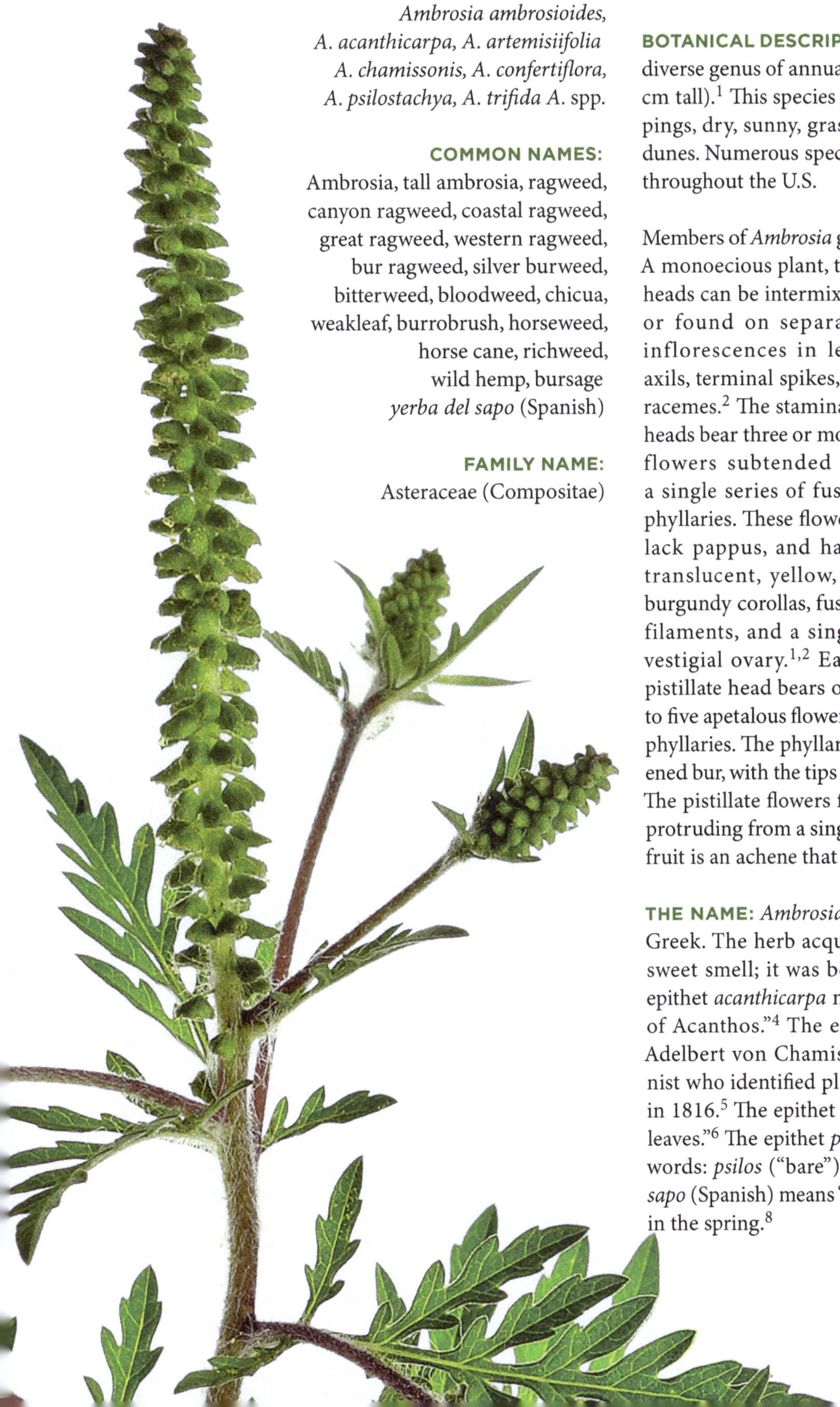

PART USED: Foliage harvested before flowering.

BOTANICAL DESCRIPTION AND HABITAT: *Ambrosia* is a diverse genus of annuals, perennials, and shrubs (10 – 400 cm tall).[1] This species grows on roadsides, rocky outcroppings, dry, sunny, grassy plains, riverbanks, and coastal dunes. Numerous species are considered common weeds throughout the U.S.

Members of *Ambrosia* genus feature highly variable leaves.[2] A monoecious plant, the staminate and pistillate discoid heads can be intermixed or found on separate inflorescences in leaf axils, terminal spikes, or racemes.[2] The staminate heads bear three or more flowers subtended by a single series of fused phyllaries. These flowers lack pappus, and have translucent, yellow, or burgundy corollas, fused filaments, and a single vestigial ovary.[1,2] Each pistillate head bears one to five apetalous flowers subtended by up to eight series of phyllaries. The phyllaries can fuse at the base into a hardened bur, with the tips hardening into nodules or spines.[1,3] The pistillate flowers feature a branched, elongated style protruding from a single ovary.[2] Found inside the bur, the fruit is an achene that lacks a pappus.[2]

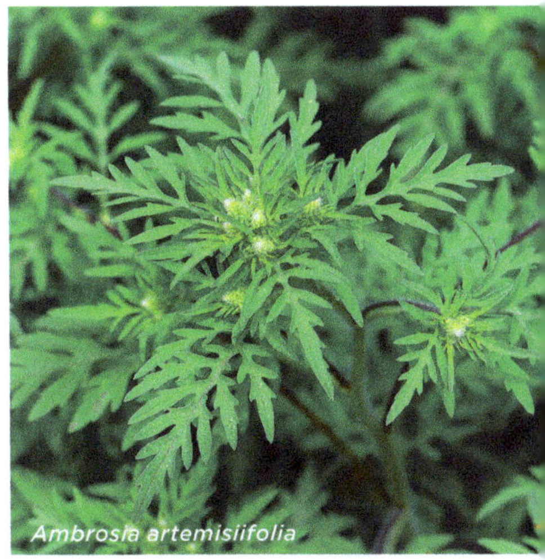
Ambrosia artemisiifolia

THE NAME: *Ambrosia* ("food of the gods") derives from Greek. The herb acquired the genus name based on its sweet smell; it was believed to increase longevity. The epithet *acanthicarpa* means "with thorny fruits like those of Acanthos."[4] The epithet *chamissonis* is named after Adelbert von Chamisso (1781 – 1838), a German botanist who identified plants in the San Francisco Bay Area in 1816.[5] The epithet *confertiflora* means "with crowded leaves."[6] The epithet *psilostachya* derives from two Greek words: *psilos* ("bare") and *stachys* ("a spike").[7] *Yerba del sapo* (Spanish) means "herb of the toad" because it appears in the spring.[8]

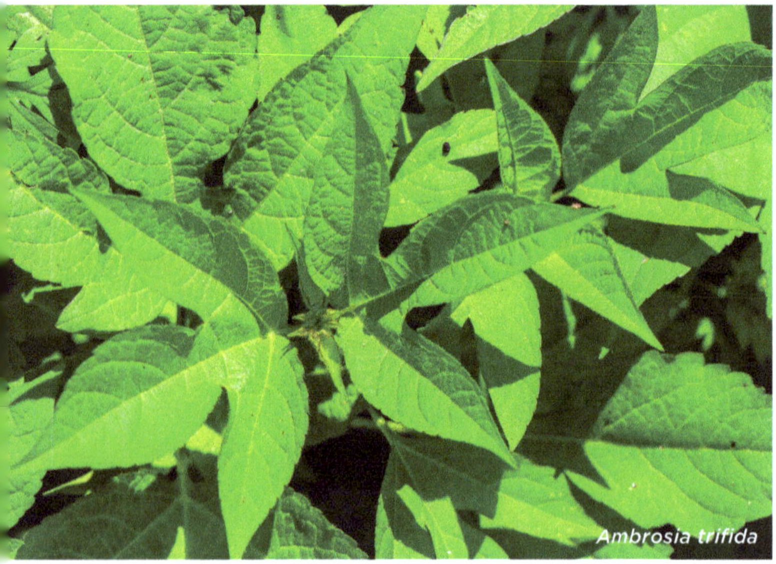

Ambrosia trifida

HISTORICAL USES: Numerous Native American tribes used the powdered leaves or leaf tea as a wash for sores and dandruff. A hot leaf poultice was applied to achy joints.[9] A warm poultice was applied to tired, sore eyes.[9] An infusion of leaf tea was consumed to treat constipation, bowel cramping, and bloody stools.[9] Zunis prepared a decoction of *Ambrosia acanthicarpa* roots to treat delayed menstruation.[8] The decoction was consumed internally and massaged on the abdomen.[8] The ground root poultice was placed in a hollow tooth to relieve a toothache.[8]

Eclectic physician Dr. John King administered ambrosia tea as an astringent, hemostatic, and diaphoretic.[10] The tea was prescribed to alleviate afterbirth pain, nervous disorders, and "hysteria."[10] Vaginal irrigation was used to treat leukorrhea, gonorrhea, gleet, and a prolapsed uterus.[10] A gargle alleviated a sore or ulcerated mouth and mercurial ulcers.[10]

CONSTITUENTS: Ambrosia contains sesquiterpene lactones (damsin, damsinic acid, franserin, parthinolide, and psilogstachyin C), and a flavonoid (hispidulin).[11]

MEDICINAL PROPERTIES: Antiallergenic, antihistaminic, anti-inflammatory, astringent, bitter tonic, counterirritant, and mild hemostatic.

TEMPERATURE AND FLAVOR: Cool, bitter, astringent, and pungent.

MEDICINAL USES

Ambrosia has antihistaminic, anti-inflammatory, and decongestant qualities that aid in treating seasonal allergies, especially those caused by pollen.[12,13,15] It stabilizes the mast cells and prevents the local histamine response.[13,15] Ambrosia reduces excessive mucus discharge from the nose, eyes, and throat.[12,15] The astringent properties decrease upper respiratory mucous membrane congestion and inflammation. The decongestant qualities also alleviate sinus infections or nasal congestion accompanying a cold or flu.[12,13,15] It is most effectively employed for acute or subacute conditions. Ambrosia is a substitute for eyebright *(Euphrasia)*, an herb often used to treat allergies that is difficult to cultivate and not readily available.[12]

An astringent, ambrosia tea reduces inflammation and edema in mucous membranes throughout the body, including respiratory, intestinal, urinary, and vaginal tissues.[12] It aids in treating short-term digestive flareups resulting from food sensitivities or digestive microbes.[12] However, it is not an anti-infective; additional antimicrobial herbs are necessary when an infection is present.

Apply a hot poultice, fomentation, or wash of ambrosia leaves as an anti-inflammatory and mild counterirritant for achy muscles or joints, bruises, sprains, or strains. Treat wounds and ulcers with a fomentation, and hemorrhoids with salve.[10]

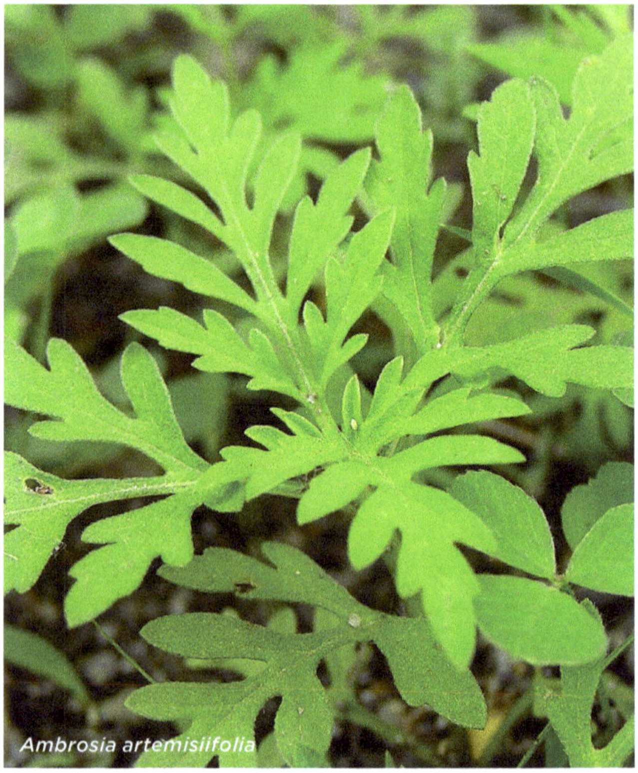

Ambrosia artemisiifolia

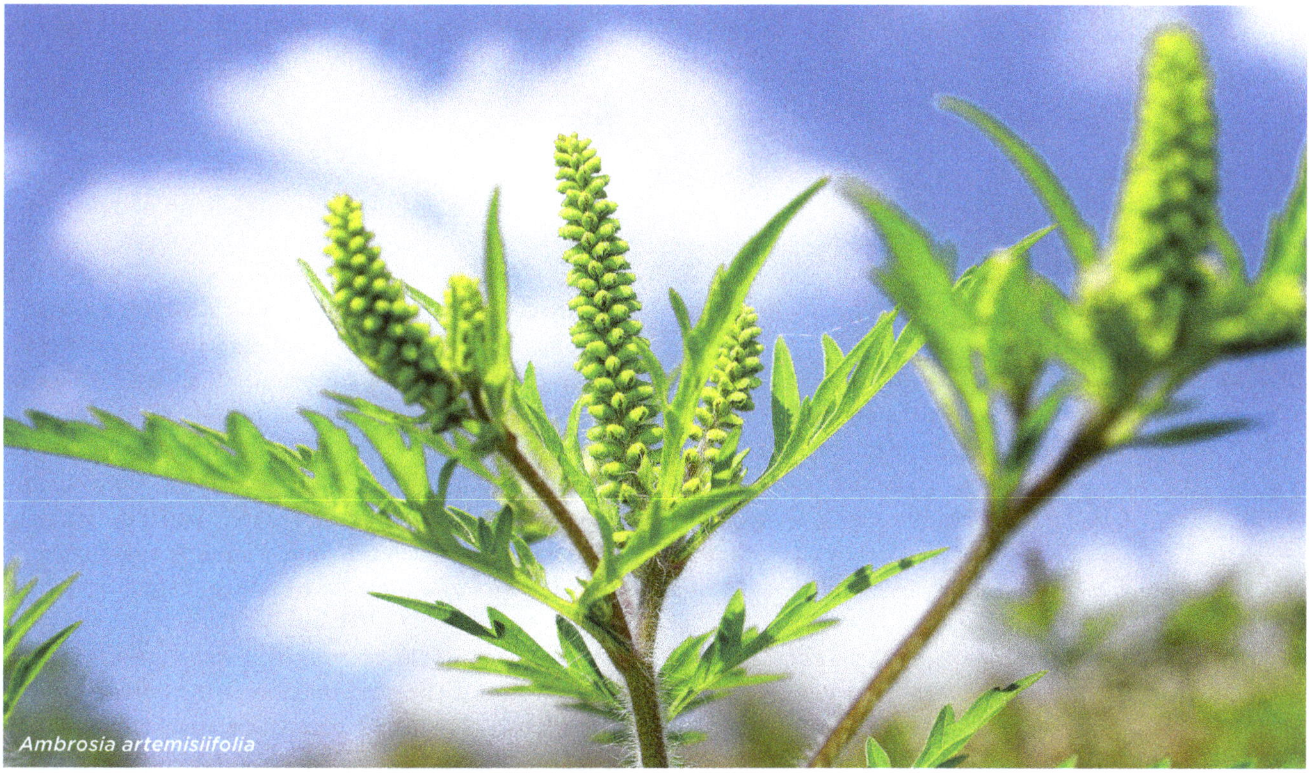

Ambrosia artemisiifolia

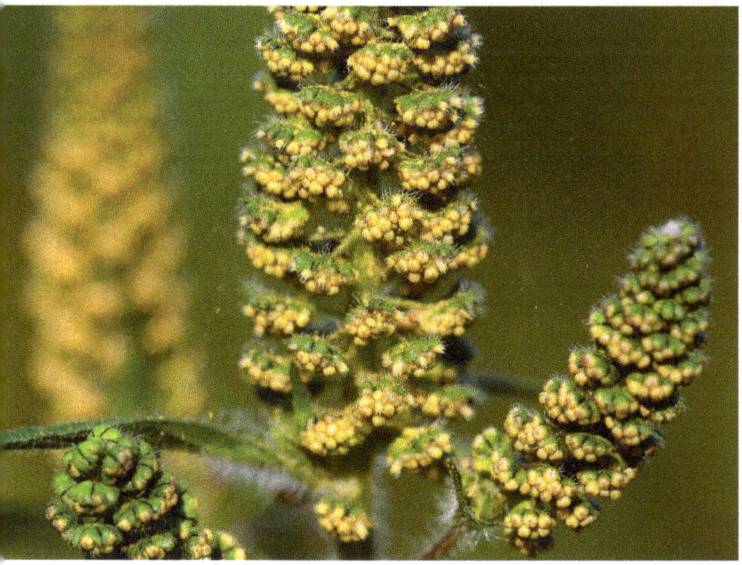

CONTRAINDICATIONS

During pregnancy, avoid using roots of the southwestern species of ambrosia *(A. acanthicarpa, A. ambrosioides,* and *A. confertiflora).* Ambrosia is well tolerated by people of all ages. Some individuals can experience an allergic response to the sesquiterpene lactones of numerous Asteraceae (Compositae) family plants. Some individuals have severe allergies to ambrosia pollen; inhaling, ingesting, or touching the pollen while the plant is flowering may cause an allergic reaction. For individuals with ambrosia allergies, it is best to harvest the plant before it flowers, and prepare it as a fresh tincture. Alcohol denatures the proteins in the pollen, and the tincture will not cause an allergic reaction. Avoid topical applications for individuals with ambrosia or sesquiterpene lactone allergies.

There are no known contraindications using ambrosia extract with allergy medication. Discontinue using ambrosia if it is too drying to the mucous membranes. In rare cases, ambrosia can be mildly stimulating to the nervous system.

PREPARATION AND DOSAGE

TINCTURE: Fresh leaves [1:2, 80-95% alcohol]; recently dried leaves [1:4, 60% alcohol]; consume 20-90 drops, up to four times daily.

FLUID EXTRACT: Dry leaves [1:1, 50% alcohol]; consume 10-30 drops, up to four times daily.

TEA: Prepare a hot infusion; consume 4-8 ounces, three to four times daily.

TOPICAL USE: Apply a fomentation, poultice, or wash to the affected area. Prepare ambrosia oil using the alcohol intermediary or double-boiler method.

ANEMONE

DESCRIPTION

BOTANICAL NAMES:
Anemone pulsatilla, A. tuberosa, A. occidentalis, A. patens

COMMON NAMES:
Pulsatilla, pasque flower, European pasque flower, western pasque flower, mountain pasque flower, pulsatille, Easter flower, shamefaced maiden, meadow anemone, wind flower, crow flower, crow foot, flower of death, desert anemone, tuber anemone, old man in the mountain, prairie crocus, crocus anemone, prairie anemone, ears of the earth, wind flower, blue tulip, gosling flower, prairie smoke, April fool, eastern pasqueflower, sandflower, tuber anemone
coquelourde (French)
gemeine küchenschelle, kuhschellenkraut (German)
flor de Paschoa (Portuguese)
pulsatila (Spanish)
backsippa (Swedish)[1]

FAMILY NAME:
Ranunculaceae

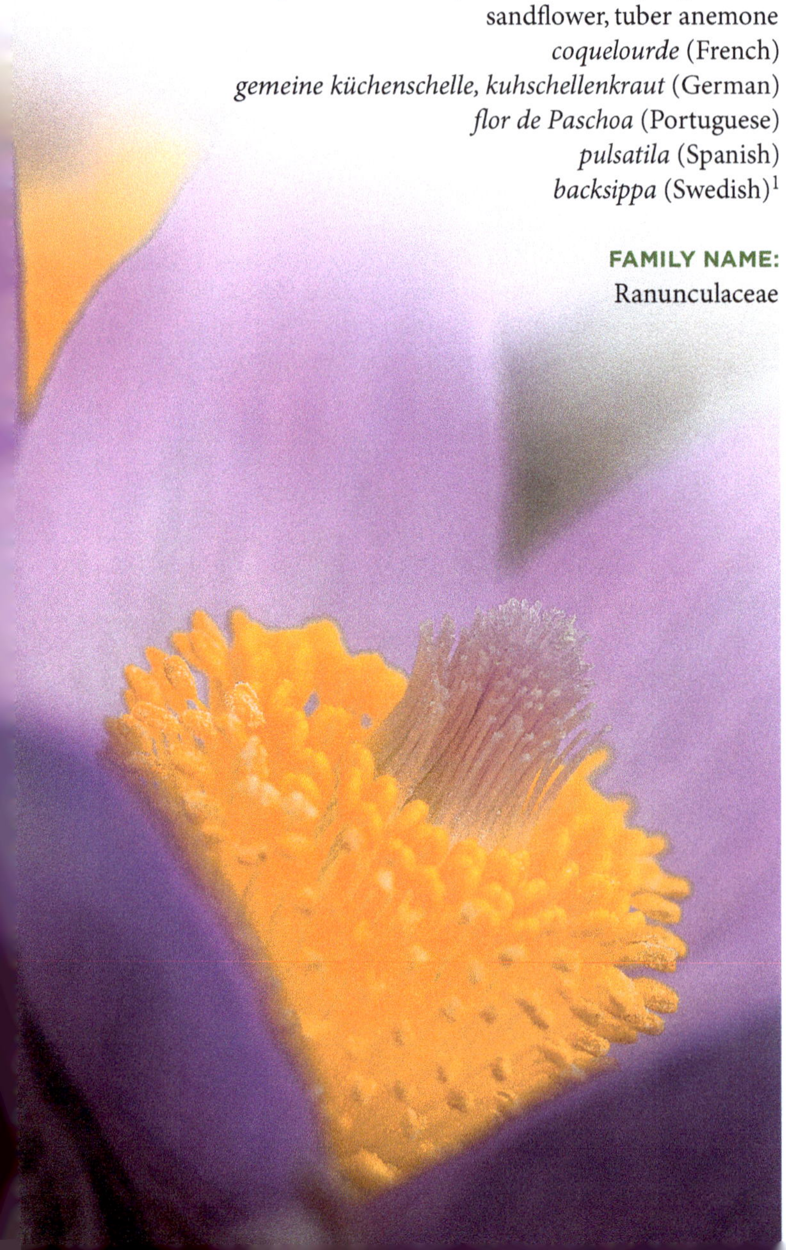

PARTS USED: The foliage or aerial portions.

BOTANICAL DESCRIPTION AND HABITAT: *Anemone* is a genus of herbaceous perennials found in the Arctic and cooler temperate areas around the world.[2,3] Some species have been domesticated as non-medicinal ornamentals. Depending on the species, they may have caudices, rhizomes, or tubers, and a clumping habit.[2] Leaves, found in basal rosettes, range from ternately lobed to ternately dissected (as are the commonly utilized *A. pulsatilla* and *A. occidentalis),* and some have toothed margins.[2]

Terminal cymes bear up to nine flowers, subtended by whorls of leaf-like bracts.[2] The radially symmetric flowers usually have 5 – 10 petal-like sepals in almost any color of the rainbow, and lack petals.[3] Flowers have many stamens and separate pistils.[2] The styles persist in fruit as beak-like or feather-like extensions of the achene (up to 4 cm long).[2,3] When fruiting, the plant can have the overall appearance of a mophead or of Dr. Seuss's truffula trees.

Note: Anemone is a very delicate plant that is extremely difficult to cultivate. Harvest only very small amounts of this herb (1 – 2 ounces), and leave the flowers to reseed. It is a rare, threatened plant.

THE NAME: The genus name derives from the Greek *anemos* ("the wind").[4] The epithet, former genus name, and common name *pulsatilla* derive from *pulsc* ("I beat"), referring to the seeds being pummeled about by the wind.[5] The epithet *tuberosa* refers to the plant's underground tuber. The epithet *occidentalis* ("western") indicates the species' distribution in the western U.S. The epithet *patens* ("spreading, lying open") derives from Latin. The common name pasque flower derives from the French word for Easter — *pasque,* as the flowers emerge during Easter in early spring.[6] Tow-headed babies and moptop refer to the white, hairy appearance of the fruits.[4]

The following common names correspond with the Latin names: pasque flower, wind flower, anemone, and pulsatilla (*Anemone* sp.*);* western pasque flower, mountain pasque flower, pasque flower, white pasque flower, old man in the mountain, moptop, and tow-headed baby *(A. occidentalis);* prairie crocus, crocus anemone, prairie anemone, ears of the earth, blue tulip, gosling flower, prairie smoke,

April fool, eastern pasqueflower, and sandflower *(A. patens);* European pasque flower, coquelourde (French), gemeine küchenschelle, kuhschellenkraut (German), flor de Paschoa (Portuguese), pulsatila (Spanish), and backsippa (Swedish) *(A. pulsatilla);* and tuber anemone, desert anemone *(A. tuberosa).*

HISTORICAL USES: The Romans picked anemone as a charm against fever. It was used to treat rheumatism, gout, and headaches. Homeopaths and Eclectics (influenced by homeopathy) prescribed anemone, otherwise known as pulsatilla, to treat chronic catarrh in the stomach with distention, pain, fullness, and discomfort or sensation of fullness following a meal.[7] It was used to treat indigestion and bilious attacks.[5] In these cases, the tongue was heavily coated with a dark brown center, red tip, and red edges.[7] Anemone was used to treat measles, earaches, nettle rashes, neuralgic toothaches, indigestion, and bilious attacks.[5]

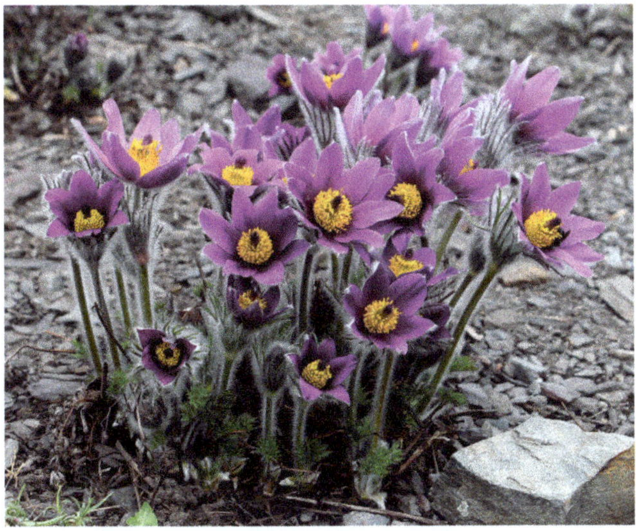

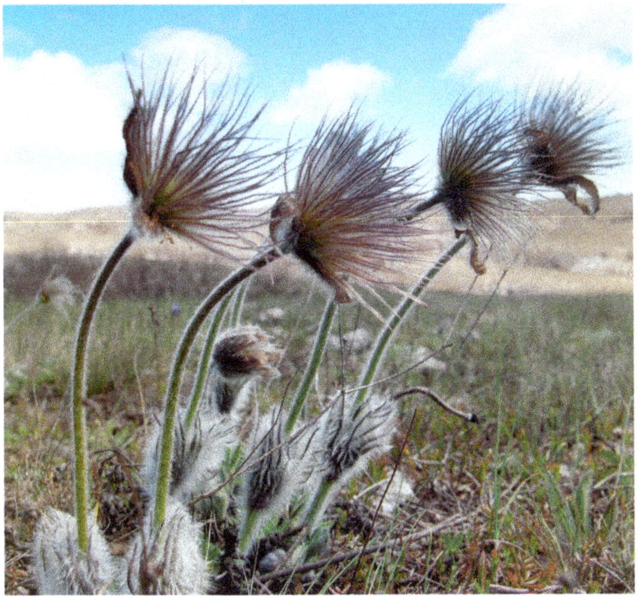

In 1710, English herbalist William Salmon described using the plant's juice as an anticatarrhal, and to "purge the Head and Brain of cold, thick, and tough flegmatick Humours."[8] He lauded its use for strokes, epilepsy, lethargy, vertigo, migraines, and other "cold head-aches."[8] He recommended other preparations for hastening birth and expelling afterbirth, clearing obstructions in the womb, as a diuretic for "expelling sand," and topically for aches and weakness of the nerves, tendons, ligaments, and joints.[8]

Eclectic physicians administered anemone for reproductive disorders aggravated by anxiety.[7] Anemone was used to

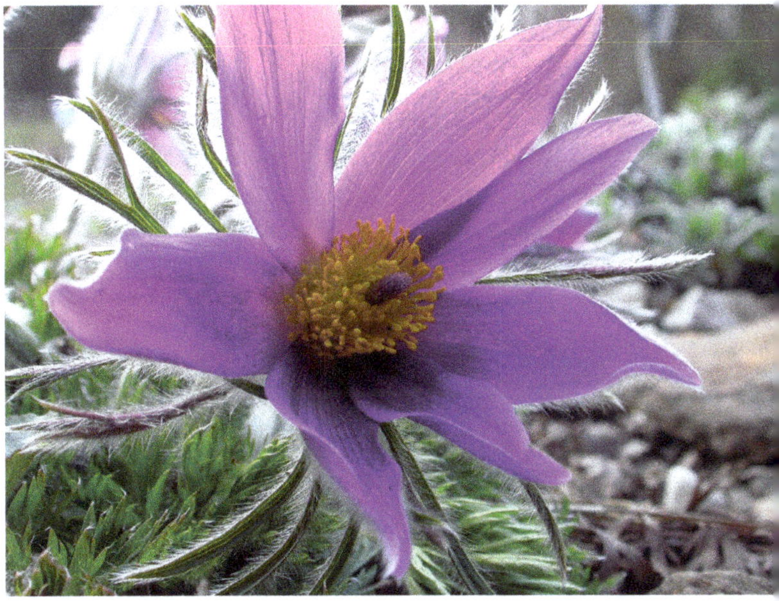

improve the tone and function of the female reproductive organs, and to overcome amenorrhea and irregular menstruation. It was also used to treat deficient, suppressed, or irregular menstruation. Anemone was often prescribed for women with "hysteria" or "melancholia," now recognized as premenstrual syndrome.[7] In males, it was used to treat sexual excess with spermatorrhea, impotency, and prostatorrhea.[7] It was also prescribed in low doses to alleviate gonorrheal epididymitis and orchitis.[7]

Anemone was administered to alleviate fevers accompanied by a rapid pulse and nervousness, and due to measles.[7] It was used to alleviate an earache, eye inflammation, neuralgic toothache, and acute or subacute respiratory congestion with thick yellow or yellow-green mucus.[7] Anemone was used to allay a severe cough, bronchial irritation, and asthma.[5,7]

Dr. Finley Ellingwood prescribed pulsatilla to enhance cerebral function and impart tone to the sympathetic nervous system.[7] It was often recommended to ease nervous exhaustion.[5-7] Ellingwood also used it to slow a rapid heartbeat due to nervousness, and increase the strength and pulse.[7]

Native Americans applied the tea as a wash to kill lice and fleas.[9] Anemone was applied as a poultice for boils, remaining in contact with the skin for a brief period, and removed prior to causing blisters. Native Americans chewed *A. cylindrica* leaves and applied it to rattlesnake bites to neutralize the venom.[10] *A. multifida* leaves were crushed, and the fumes were inhaled to allay colds and lung problems.[9] Smoke from the ripe seed head pappi was inhaled for headaches. The leaves were ingested prior to sweat lodges to ease rheumatic pain, and the tea was used to wash rheumatic joints.[9] The Upper Cowlitz consumed small quantities of anemone tea to treat tuberculosis.[4]

CONSTITUENTS: Anemone contains anemonin (protoanemonin dimer), protoanemonin (an unstable compound), anemonic acid, anemoninic acid, anemone camphor, glucose, resins, tannins, flavonoids, saponins, calcium and magnesium compounds, and organic acids.[10-12] It contains amenonin, a volatile oil that dissipates upon drying. Fresh anemone contains ranunculin, a poisonous compound. When the plant is crushed or chopped, it releases an enzyme that converts ranunculin to protoanemonin, a highly irritating volatile oil. Protoanemonin is unstable, and breaks down into a nontoxic substance called anemomin. Applied to the skin, protoanemomin is an irritant and vesicant.[5,10] If ingested in high dosages, it can damage the kidneys and urinary tract, or lead to central nervous system paralysis.[6]

NUTRITIONAL PROPERTIES: Not appropriate because moderate to high doses can be toxic.

MEDICINAL PROPERTIES: Alterative, anxiolytic, antispasmodic, counterirritant, diaphoretic, nervine, parasympathamimetic, sedative, vasodilator, and vesicant (topically).

TEMPERATURE AND FLAVOR: Hot, pungent, bitter, and sweet.

MEDICINAL USES

A very potent herb, anemone should be used with caution. An extract of the fresh plant should be administered in low doses, starting with 3 – 5 drops in two to four ounces of water, in order to avoid irritating the mucous membranes and digestive tract. The average dosage of the fresh herb extract ranges from 3 – 15 drops, up to three times daily, but can vary according to the species. Exceeding that dosage can be toxic. Constituents are altered upon drying the herb, and become inert.[12]

Anemone is a deeply calming nervine and sedative for extremely nervous individuals prone to anxiety, panic attacks, and insomnia.[12,13] It aids in treating post-traumatic stress disorder, hypervigilance, and obsessive compulsive disorder.[12,14] Anemone helps to induce peaceful sleep in individuals with insomnia, fear of sleeping due to nightmares, or night terrors.[12,14] It eases anxiety and panic attacks resulting from adrenalin surges, hyperthyroidism, or recreational drug use. Anemone aids in treating nervous exhaustion with symptoms including poor circulation, a feeble, thready pulse, cold, clammy, shaky hands, and paleness.[12]

Anemone alleviates more extreme forms of premenstrual syndrome and premenstrual anxiety, irritability, nervous exhaustion, and depression (conditions formerly known as "uterine disorders that cause hysteria and melancholia").[6,7,12,13] Eclectic physician Dr. Finley Ellingwood

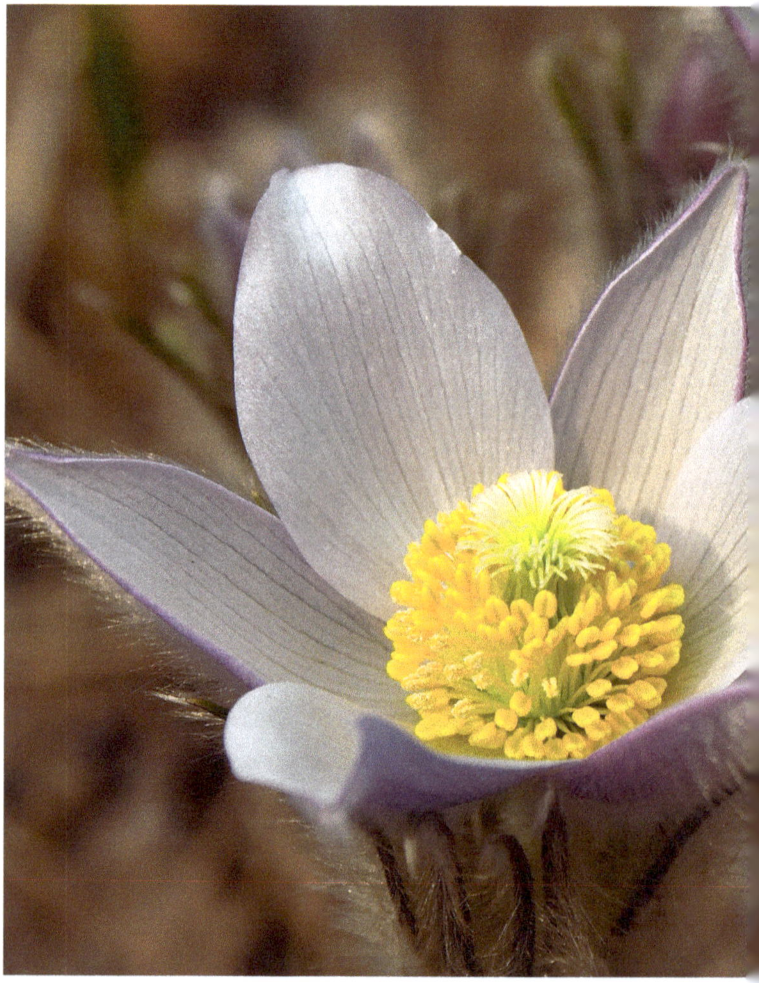

prescribed anemone to treat "menstrual disorders accompanied by a headache, chilliness, loss of strength, and nausea."[7,13] An antispasmodic, it alleviates menstrual cramping and ovarian pain.[6] Anemone serves as an emmenagogue that aids in treating stress-related amenorrhea and irregular menstruation.[5] It was also used to treat males with impotence, performance anxiety, spermatorrhea, and prostatorrhea.[7] Eclectic physician John Scudder utilized this remedy for involuntary ejaculation caused by nervous system excess.[13]

A cardiotonic, anemone calms a rapid heartbeat, reduces palpitations, and slows and strengthens the heart and pulse rate.[7,12] It increases cardiac proficiency and dilates peripheral blood vessels, increasing blood supply to tissues.[12] Anemone aids in treating stress-related vascular constriction.[7]

Anemone is a vasodilator that is often effective in treating one-sided, throbbing migraine headaches with visual disturbances, accompanied by anxiety. It works most effectively when consumed at the onset of a migraine.[7] Anemone also aids in treating tension headaches, and mild occipital headaches with a light, dull character, and a restless, rambling mind.[6,7] *Note:* Administer the herb in low doses (3 – 5 drops, depending on the species). If three to five drops aren't effective in 10 to 15 minutes, increase the dosage in 2 – 3 drop increments every 15 minutes for one hour, until the desired effect is achieved. Do not exceed a 15-drop dosage in one hour; wait another hour before consuming another dose.

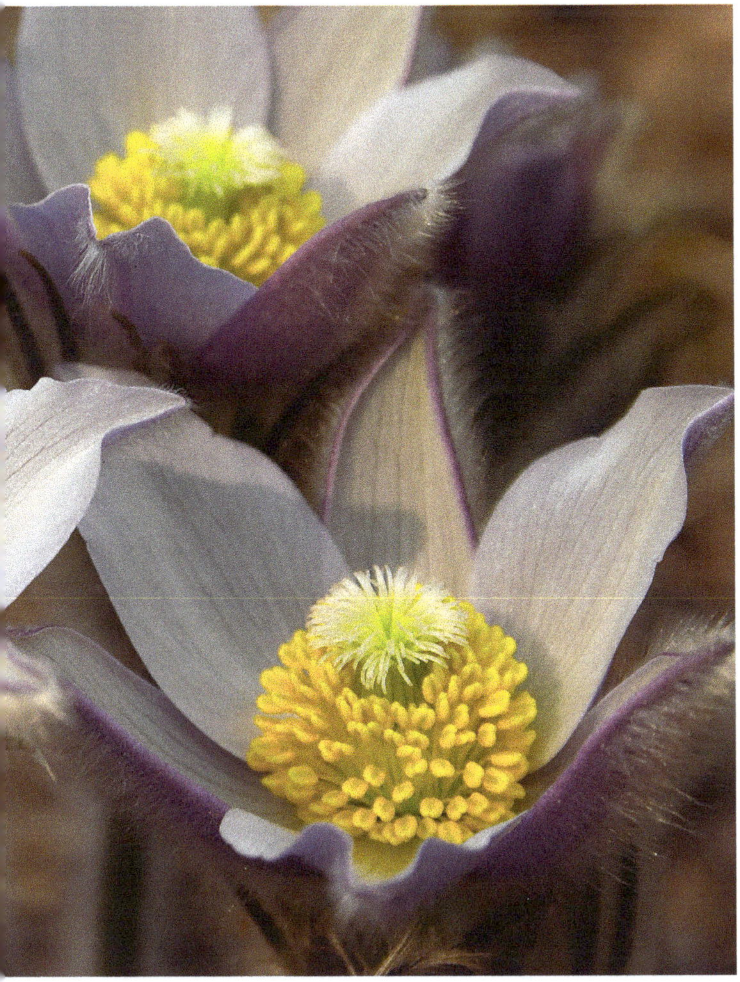

A moderate smooth muscle antispasmodic, anemone eases a spasmodic cough, treating asthma, dry bronchitis, and whooping cough.[5,6] However, there are numerous highly effective herbs that alleviate coughing, with far less potential for toxicity.

CONTRAINDICATIONS

Avoid use during pregnancy or lactation, and in young children (except homeopathic preparations).[12] A hypotensive agent, anemone should be avoided with bradycardia.[12] Exercise caution in individuals with low blood pressure. Avoid use in combination with parasympathamimetic pharmaceuticals.

Warning: Do not consume in quantities greater than 15 drops. High doses can act as a parasympathamimetic; it can lower blood pressure, and cause salivation, nausea, and dizziness.[12] Toxic doses of anemone can cause pupil dilation, depressed heart function, reduced body temperature, and in extreme cases, coma and convulsions.[7]

Due to the protoanemonin in the fresh herb, topical applications and consumption of moderate to high doses can irritate the skin and mucous membranes.[11] It can cause tingling, burning, and numbing sensations, and irritate the digestive tract, or cause violent gastroenteritis.[5,7] The plant is a vesicant and powerful counterirritant; external applications or topical contact is an irritant and can cause tissue blistering. Carefully wash hands and tools when harvesting and processing this plant. Avoid touching the eyes or tissues after handling anemone.

PREPARATION AND DOSAGE

TINCTURE: Fresh leaves or aerial portions [1:2 - 1:3, 70 - 90% alcohol]; consume 3 - 15 drops, up to four times daily.

ANGELICA

BOTANICAL NAMES:
Angelica archangelica (syn. *Angelica officinalis* and *Archangelica officinalis*), *A. arguta, A. atropurpurea, A. breweri, A. genuflexa, A. lucida, A. pinnata, A. sylvestris, A. tomentosa*

COMMON NAMES:
Angelica, garden angelica, wild angelica, European wild angelica, American angelica, brewer's angelica, hairy angelica, purple angelica, California angelica, archangel, wild archangel, root of the holy ghost, goutweed, bellyache root, sea watch, masterwort, wild celery
engelwortel (Dutch)
angeline angélique (French)
brustwurz, engelwurz (German)
arcangelica (Italian)
choraka (Sanskrit)
angelica, yerba del espiritu santo (Spanish)
kvanne (Swedish)

FAMILY NAME:
Apiaceae (Umbelliferae)

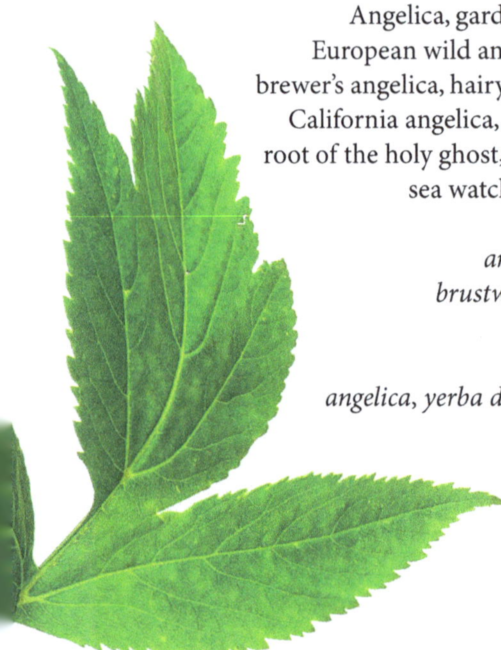

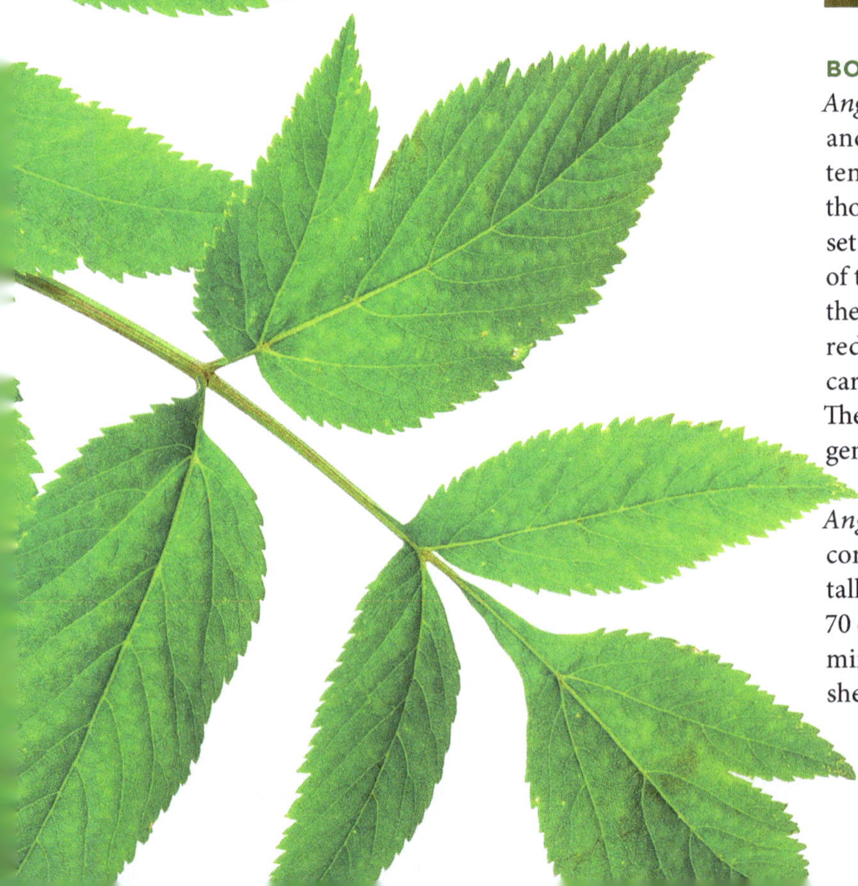

DESCRIPTION

PARTS USED: The roots, rhizomes, and seeds. The roots can be gathered in the fall or spring of the first year, before the plant flowers. They also can be gathered in the fall of the second year, or less ideally, before or immediately after it seeds, because the roots deteriorate and can become moldy or insect-ridden. The seeds are harvested in the fall of the second year. Cutting down the aerial portions before the seeds emerge can prolong the plant's life.

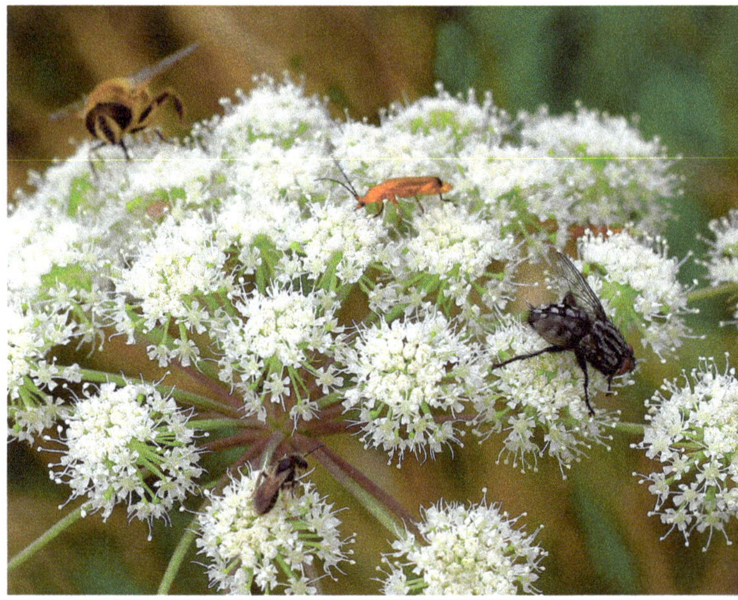

BOTANICAL DESCRIPTION AND HABITAT: The genus *Angelica* contains 50–60 species of herbaceous perennial and biennial plants with robust taproots. They grow in temperate regions of North America, Europe, and Asia, though this monograph only covers the uses of a restricted set of species.[1] Like other members of Apiaceae, the bases of the pinnately compound leaves strongly sheathe around the main stems. The asepalous flowers have five white, pink, red, or purple petals, five stamens, two styles, and two carpels. The flowers are produced in compound umbels.[1] The fruit, a two-part schizocarp, varies between species, but generally has a flattened oblong shape with winged ribs.[1]

Angelica archangelica, the species used most often in commerce, is a glorious, statuesque herb up to two meters tall.[2] It has large green pinnate or bipinnate leaves (up to 70 cm long) divided into oblong or lance-shaped, entire to minutely-toothed leaflets.[2] These leaves grow from dilated sheaths that surround the hollow, round, grooved stems.

The leaf veins extend from the midrib to the outer tips of the serrations. In the second year of growth, angelica bears large, greenish-white to white compound umbels (10 – 14 cm across) containing many tiny flowers (4 mm across) with a sweet, musky aroma.[2] The flattened, oblong fruit (up to 9 mm long) is green to tan and ribbed; the dual side ribs are more broadly winged than the midribs.[2] When crushed, the fruit releases volatile oil that exudes a bitter-sweet fragrance. The reddish-brown to brown taproots have hairy root crowns and a pungent, sweet, celery-like aroma.

This can serve as a basic description of angelica; however, before harvesting, accurately key the plant in a field guide. *Caution:* Misidentification can be fatal! Make sure to read the warning in the *Contraindication* section before harvesting.

Various angelica species grow wild along coastal regions, on riverbanks and rocky slopes, and in moist mountain ravines and meadows. *Angelica archangelica* makes a lovely addition to the garden. A biennial plant native to Europe, it can grow as a perennial when the stems are cut before the plant flowers in the second year.

European angelica and garden angelica are the common names for *Angelica archangelica.* The following common names correspond with the Latin names: wild angelica *(Angelica arguta);* American angelica, purple angelica, bellyache root, and masterwort *(A. atropurpurea);* brewer's angelica *(A. breweri);* sea-watch *(A. lucida);* wild angelica *(A. pinnata);* European wild angelica and goutweed *(A. sylvestris);* and hairy angelica or California angelica *(A. tomentosa).*

THE NAME: *Angelica* ("angel") derives from Latin. Following the onset of Christianity, angelica was associated with archangelic patronage.[3,5] Several beliefs are related to the origin of the epithet and the common name *archangelica.* Some individuals associated the name with Archangel Gabriel, believed to have appeared to the Virgin Mary during the Annunciation at the end of March.[3] Others associated the plant with Archangel Michael, who appeared in a visionary dream revealing angelica's curative powers against the plague.[3] In another association, the name *archangelica* emerged because it blooms around the feast of the Apparition of St. Michael (May 8), also known as Archangel Michael. It was believed to offer protection against bad spirits, witches, spells, and enchantment, as well as the cattle disease, elfshot.[3,5]

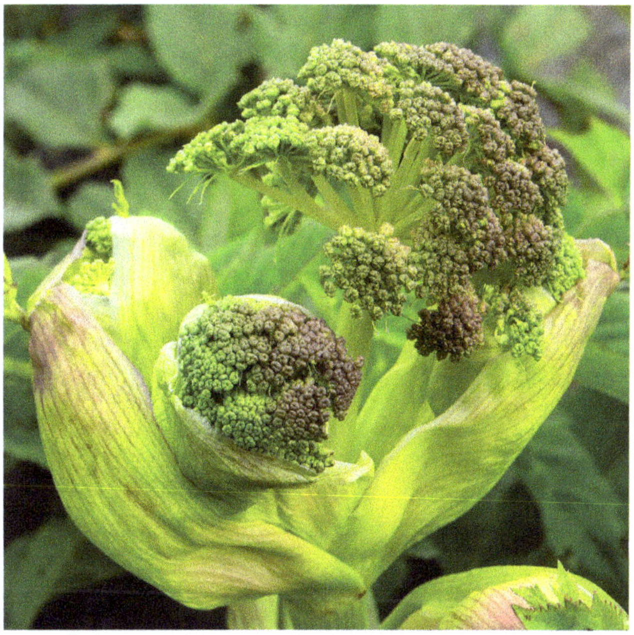

The epithet *arguta* derives from the Latin *argūtus* meaning "pungent, sharp, or producing a clear, constant sound." The epithet *atropurpurea* refers to the purple stems; *breweri* originates from the Middle English *brewen* ("to make beer or ale"), likely referring to the combination of angelica and hops in beer.[3] The epithet *genuflexa* ("to genuflect") refers to the bending knees at the leaf stalks; *lucida* means "glittering or shining."[5] *Pinnata* refers to the pinnate leaves. *Sylvestris* derives from the Latin *silvester* or *silva* ("woody, forest, or rural"). *Tomentosa* originates from the Latin *tomentum* ("cushion stuffing"), referring to the woolly coating formed by the densely-matted, flattened hairs.

HISTORICAL USES: More than 12 Native American tribes used angelica extensively for medicines and ceremonies. It was most commonly administered as a diaphoretic.[6] Tribes living in mountainous regions from central to northern California consumed the root decoction of *Angelica breweri* for colds, flu, coughs, bronchitis, tuberculosis, kidney ailments, and venereal disease.[6] The tea was occasionally mixed with whiskey for whooping cough and severe chest colds.[6] Dried root shavings were added to smoking mixtures to treat head colds.[6] A wash of the tea was applied for venereal diseases.[6] Crushed root poultices were applied to rheumatic joints, cuts, sores, and swelling, and to the chest for pneumonia.[6]

Aerial portions of *Angelica tomentosa* were burned and whipped onto aching joints.[6] A wash of the pounded, boiled roots and heated juice from the leaves were applied to sores.[6] In order to treat headaches, the root poultice was applied to the forehead, or smoke from the burning roots was inhaled.[6] Roots were chewed and held in the mouth to treat sore throats, hoarseness, halitosis, and stomachaches.[6] A decoction of the roots was consumed for menstrual cramps, stomachaches, diarrhea, and colds.[3,6]

Coastal tribes consumed a tea of *Angelica hendersonii* to ease the symptoms of food poisoning from mussels.[6] *A. atropurpurea* was administered for heartburn and flatulent colic.[7] A tea of *A. genuflexa* root was consumed for colds and respiratory ailments, and as a purgative.[6] The Bella Coola tribe used *A. genuflexa* stems as breathing tubes when hiding underwater.[5] They also consumed the stems and leaf stalks of *A. lucida.*[5]

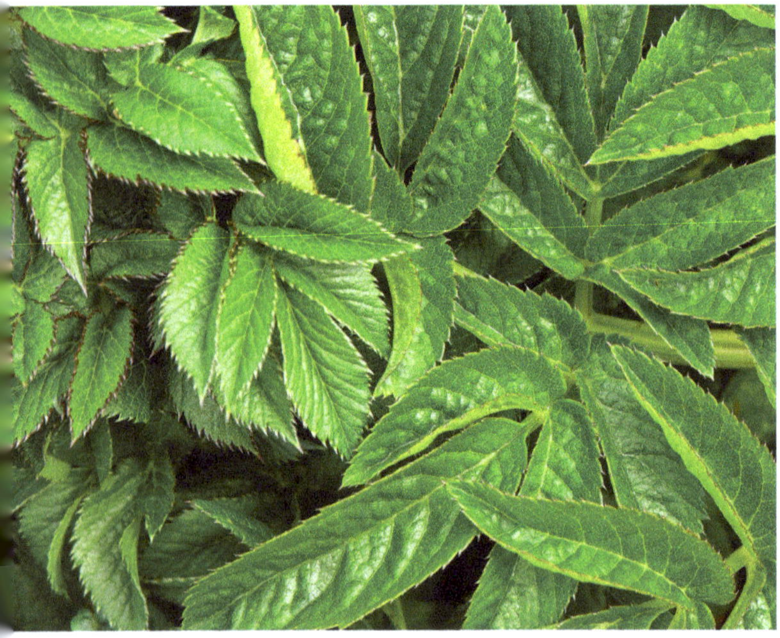

For centuries, angelica was an esteemed medicine in northern Europe. It cured nearly every conceivable health problem and contagious infection.[4] Angelica root and seed preparations were consumed to treat colds, coughs, pleurisy, bronchitis, respiratory catarrh, bronchial ailments, stomachaches, hyperacidity, indigestion, flatulent dyspepsia, intestinal disturbances, urinary disorders, nervous conditions, and insomnia.[7,8] They were also administered as an anti-inflammatory, diaphoretic, and diuretic. Angelica root and leaf were used as folk remedies for stomach cancer and indolent tumors.[9] The root was considered an antidote for poisons.[9]

Icelanders consumed raw roots and stems with butter. Laplanders regarded angelica stalks as a delicacy, gathering them before the plant flowered, removing the leaves, and serving them with relish. Finns ate young stems baked in hot ashes and consumed infusions of the herb. Norwegians incorporated the powdered root into flour for baking bread.[3]

During the 14th century, Carmelite nuns concocted a sweet drink with angelica called Carmelite water to treat headaches and neuralgia, and improve the complexion.[4] In the 16th century, London's Royal College of Physicians created another form of angelica water, "the King's Majesty's Excellent Recipe for the Plague," believed to be a cure for that highly contagious disease.[4] This remedy contained angelica root, nutmeg, and a treacle (sweet syrup) simmered over a fire and consumed twice daily.[4] The following recipe was consumed throughout northern Europe to treat typhus fever: six ounces of angelica root steeped in one quart of water and strained; then add the juice of two lemons, four ounces of honey, and ½ gill of brandy.[3]

Angelica was used in pagan rituals and worn as an amulet for protection against evil spirits and witches' spells.[3,4] Later, Christians adopted beliefs about the protective properties of angelica, and associated them with archangels and spring festivals. The root was regarded so highly, it was called "the root of the Holy Ghost."[3,4]

Angelica was applied topically to calm skin nerves and treat arthritis.[8] Bathing in angelica tea was believed to soothe the nerves.[10] Angelica salve was applied for rheumatic pains, and root compresses were used to treat gout.[10] Root decoctions were applied to the skin to treat gout, scabies, itching, and wounds.[10] The juice was applied to the gums for dental problems.[9]

Angelica continues to be incorporated as a flavoring for various alcoholic beverages, including digestive bitters, Benedictine, Chartreuse, gin, and vermouth.[3,4,8] It is also used to flavor nonalcoholic beverages, desserts, baked goods, gelatins, and puddings.[3,8] The tender leaves and

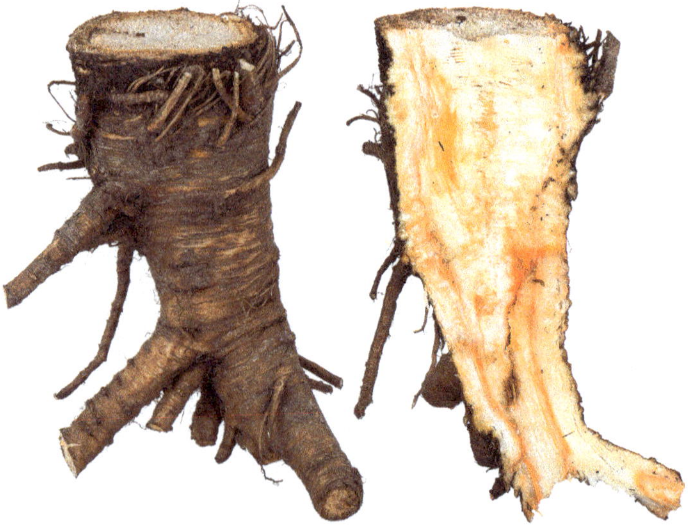

shoots were stewed with tart fruits and berries to reduce their acidity.[4] The seeds were added to cookies, and the candied stems were prized by confectioners.

CONSTITUENTS

ANGELICA ROOT: Angelica root contains volatile oils (d-α-phellandrene, β-phellandrene, α-pinene, β-pinene, *trans*-4-ethoxy-2-pinene, limonene, β-caryophyllene, linalool, borneol, acetaldehyde, D-3-carene, *p*-cymene, myrcene, *trans*-ocimene, α-copaene, camphene, ciso-cimene, and four macrocyclic lactones: tridecanolide, 12-methyl-ω-tridecanolide, ω-pentadecanolide, and ω-heptade-caonlide). The whole plant contains high amounts of coumarins; the root is the richest in coumarins (osthol, angelicin, osthenol, umbelliferone, archangelicin, bergapten, ostruthol, imperatorin, umbelliperinine, xanthotoxol, xanthotoxin, oxypeucedanin, oreoselone, phellopterin, marmesin, byakangelicol, and 2'-angeloyl-3'-isovaleryl vaginate, with osthol in major concentration). It contains plant acids (angelic, aconitic, citric, malic, oxalic, malonic, fumaric, succinic, caffeic, chlorogenic, quinic, lauric, tridecanoic, myristic, pentadecanoic, palmitic, palmitoleic, stearic, oleic, linoleic, linolenic, petroselinic, and behenic acids). Additional constituents include resin, starch, sugars (sucrose, fructose, glucose, and umbelliferose), a flavonone (archangelenone), β-sitosterol, palminate, and arachinate.[7-9,11] Herbalist Steven Foster notes that angelica's volatile oil content can increase up to 80% when it is planted as a companion with nettle.[12]

ANGELICA SEED: Angelica seed contains volatile oil (mainly β-phellandrene, α-pinene, and other terpenes similar to the roots), and coumarins (imperitorin, bergapten, iso-imperitorin, isopimpinellin, 8-hydroxy-5-methoxypsoralen, 4-methoxy-7-hydro-xypsoralen, phellopterin, xanthotoxol, and xanthotoxin, with the highest concentration of bergapten and imperitorin).[8,11]

NUTRITIONAL PROPERTIES: Unknown.

MEDICINAL PROPERTIES: Angelica roots are an antibacterial, antispasmodic, aromatic, bitter tonic, carminative, cholagogue, choleretic, circulatory stimulant, diaphoretic, emmenagogue, expectorant, mild diuretic, and stomachic. Angelica seeds are a carminative, diaphoretic, and diuretic.

TEMPERATURE AND FLAVOR: Warm, pungent, bitter, and sweet.

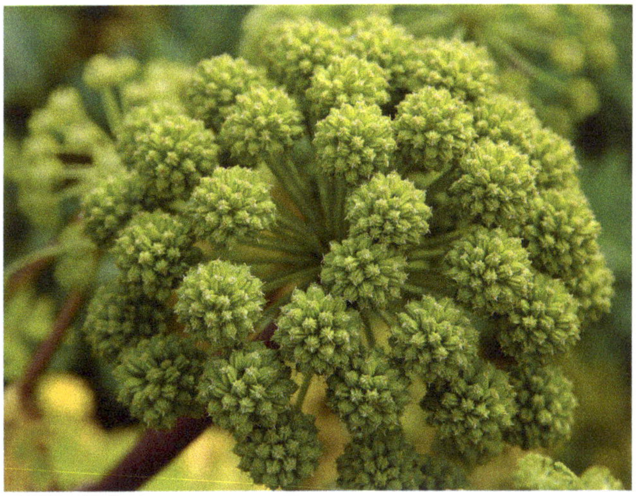

MEDICINAL USES

ANGELICA ROOT: Angelica is an aromatic digestive bitter tonic, choleretic, cholagogue, and carminative.[3,15,16] It stimulates secretions in the stomach and gallbladder, enhancing digestion and assimilation.[15] The root increases circulation in the digestive tract. It aids in treating gas, bloating, nonulcer dyspepsia, and indigestion.[3,4,15] Add a small quantity of angelica tincture (5 – 15 drops per dose) to digestive bitter tonic formulas, and consume 15 – 30 minutes before meals as an aromatic digestive aid. In *The Modern Herbal,* author Maude Grieve states that regular consumption of angelica is believed to create a distaste for alcoholic beverages.[3]

Angelica root exerts smooth muscle antispasmodic effects, reducing stomach, intestinal, and menstrual cramping.[7,8,11,13] The constituent angelicin relaxes smooth muscles, while the coumarin-based compounds are calcium channel blockers.[7,8] Angelica is effective for treating digestive cramps resulting from gastrointestinal microbes, poor food combining, or ingestion of inadequately cooked beans or grains.[13] It is a highly effective antispasmodic for slow-starting, crampy menses.[11] Angelica is especially efficacious when the skin above the reproductive region feels cold to the touch, when a woman feels chilled, has cold extremities, and/or when she experiences intestinal cramping with menstrual cramps. It aids in treating menstrual cramps that improve following topical heat applications. Angelica warms the womb and reduces blood stagnation in the reproductive organs. It acts as an emmenagogue and encourages shedding of the uterine lining.[3,11,13] Consume 8 ounces of hot decocted tea, or 30 – 60 drops of tincture in hot water, every two hours (up to four times daily) to obtain optimal antispasmodic and emmenagogue properties.

Midwives administer the herb to hasten detachment of the placenta following labor when the usual methods of standing, massaging downward over the uterus, or gently tugging on the umbilical cord are not effective. It often works in five to ten minutes. Angelica is highly effective in this circumstance, especially considering that a woman can go into shock if the placenta is not expelled within 30 minutes following delivery.

Angelica root is an aromatic expectorant and antitussive.[3,4] It is most effective for treating respiratory conditions with clear, white, or cloudy mucus that indicate an infection with a cold nature. It aids in treating hoarseness, tracheitis, laryngitis, colds, a dry, hacking cough, whooping cough (pertussis), bronchitis, asthma, and wheezing.[3,4,13] Combine with *Aralia californica*, gumweed *(Grindelia)*, anise *(Pimpinella)*, elecampane *(Inula)*, Senega snakeroot *(Polygala)*, and licorice *(Glycyrrhiza)* to alleviate respiratory spasms and breathing difficulties.

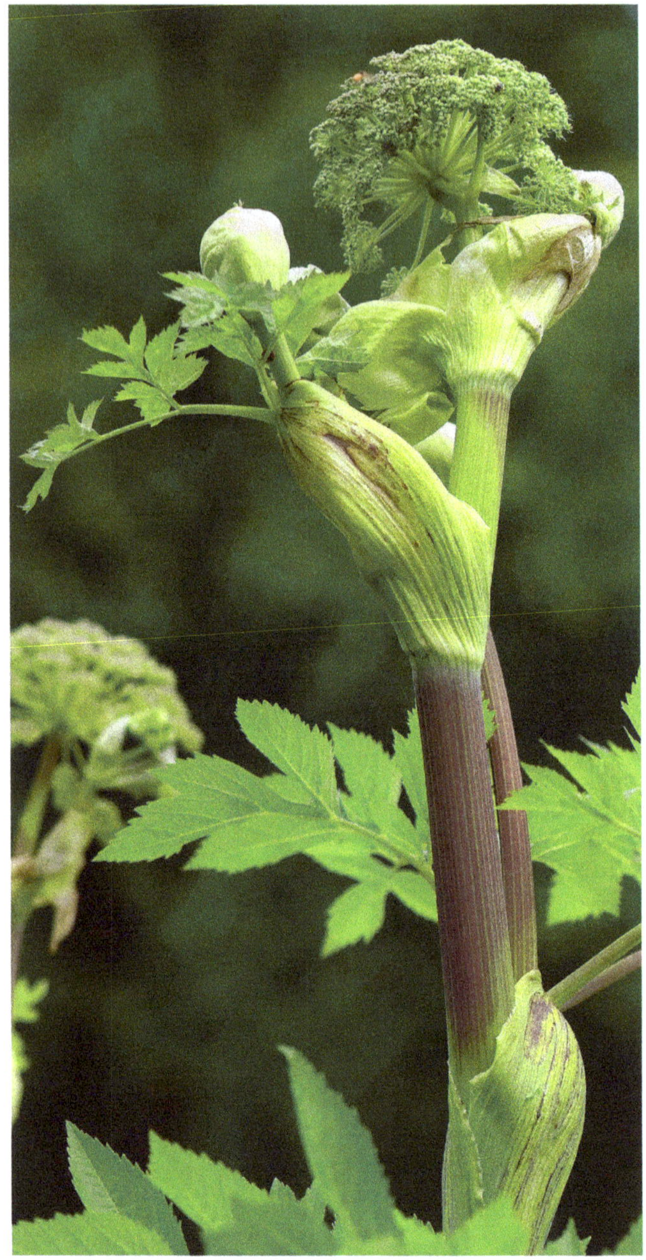

Angelica is useful as an immune stimulant and diaphoretic in the first phase of a cold or flu.[3,8,9] All parts of the plant contain coumarins that stimulate white blood cells and enhance their phagocytic capacity, aiding in the destruction of foreign particles and cancer cells.[7] Coumarins activate macrophages — cells that recognize and destroy tumor cells and offer protection against their growth.[7] Coumarins also have immune modulating activity. They have been found to increase white blood cell activity, stimulate interferon production, and increase non-specific host defense mechanisms.[7] The volatile oil in *Angelica archangelica* exhibits significant antifungal activity, but has limited antibacterial capacity.[7,8] Angelica is a warming diaphoretic that stimulates the resolution of a fever.[3,4] Consume 4–8 ounces of hot tea or 30–60 drops of tincture in hot water every hour until the fever breaks.

Angelica is a circulatory stimulant and peripheral vasodilator.[4,7] It increases circulation, warming cold hands and feet, as well as enhancing circulation to the internal organs.[4] For individuals with poor circulation, Raynaud's phenomenon, or Burger's disease, angelica is a well suited, warming winter tonic.[4] *Angelica archangelica* contains several constituents (dihydropyranocoumarins and dihydrofuranocoumarins) that act as calcium channel blockers in the heart, aiding in the treatment of high blood pressure, angina, and cardiac arrhythmias.[4,7,8]

Apply hot angelica compresses or fomentations to increase circulation in the tissues and reduce muscle or joint pain. This aids in treating bruises, sprains, strains, rheumatism, and arthritis.[15] Bathing the hands or feet in hot angelica tea effectively warms the extremities.

ANGELICA SEED: Angelica seeds have antispasmodic and antinauseant properties.[11] They anesthetize pain associated with acid indigestion, hiatal hernia, nausea, vomiting, food poisoning, and bloating.[11] Similar to the roots, the seeds have aromatic bitter tonic, carminative, digestive antispasmodic, and cholagogue properties.[11] Combine angelica seeds with cathartic herbs to prevent intestinal cramping. The seeds also stimulate circulation and act as a diaphoretic.[13] They are a more potent diuretic than the roots.

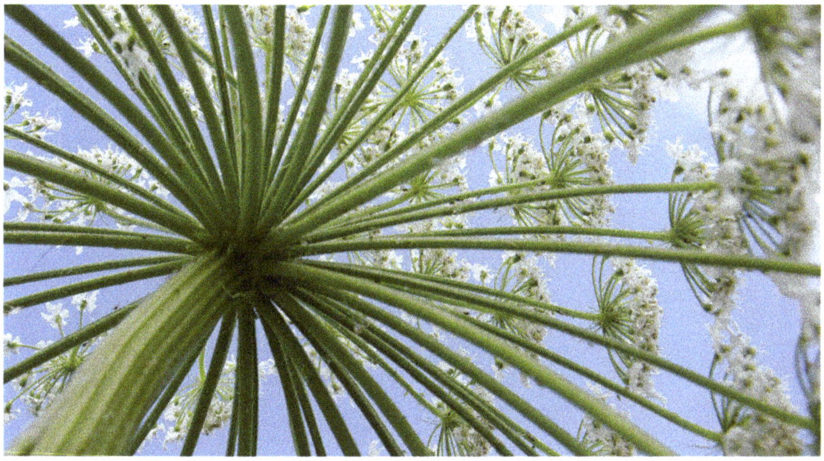

pretty hip." Water hemlock has chambered roots. Poison hemlock has glabrous stems and leaves that are covered in a bluish glaucous coating (though this may be rubbed off or not thickly developed). It often has purple splotches or lines on the stems, but this isn't a definitive indicator, because some non-poisonous members of the Apiaceae family also have purple splotches, and, importantly, other members of *Cicuta* genus may not always have splotches or lines.

CONTRAINDICATIONS

Angelica is contraindicated during pregnancy and should be used with caution during lactation.[11,13,15] Due to the coumarins, angelica can cause photosensitivity (sensitivity to sunlight, causing a rash upon sun exposure). Protect the skin and avoid subsequent exposure to ultraviolet rays or prolonged exposure to the sun.[7,8,15] Coumarins pass through breast milk and can cause infant photosensitivity. Exercise caution and avoid exposing infant's tender skin to the sun if you consume angelica while lactating. When administering this herb to children, protect their skin from sun exposure.

Because angelica root stimulates menstrual bleeding, women with excessive uterine bleeding from conditions such as fibroids, cysts, endometriosis, or menorrhagia (heavy menstrual flow), and during perimenopause should avoid or limit use. Angelica is a heating herb; long-term use is best avoided by individuals with heat-aggravated conditions, night sweats, or hot flashes. An overdose of angelica can cause nausea.[11]

Warning: Be sure to properly identify angelica and other members of the umbel family before harvesting; *misidentification can be fatal.* Angelica can be mistaken for poisonous members of the same family, such as poison hemlock *(Conium maculatum)* and water hemlock *(Cicuta maculata, C.* spp.*). Water hemlock is the most poisonous plant in North America; consuming ¼ teaspoon of the root can be fatal within 15 minutes. Accurate identification of the seeds, flowers, and leaves is critical!* Some distinguishing features are that water hemlock's leaf veins extend from the midribs and terminate in the notches of the serrations, while angelica's veins terminate in the outer tips of the serrations. This demonstrates the importance of the adage, "Vein to the cut, pain in the butt; vein to the tip,

PREPARATION AND DOSAGE

TINCTURE: Fresh roots [1:2, 70-95% alcohol]; dry roots [1:5, 60-70% alcohol]; consume 15-60 drops, up to four times daily. Fresh seeds [1:3, 70-95% alcohol]; consume 10-30 drops, up to four times daily.

GLYCERITE: Dry roots [1:5, 40% glycerin, 40% alcohol, 30% spring water]; consume 30-60 drops, up to four times daily.

CAPSULES: Consume 2-3 "00" capsules of ground root or seed, up to three times daily.

TEA: Prepare a seed infusion or root decoction; consume up to 8-12 ounces, three to four times daily.

HONEY AND SYRUP: Prepare honey with fresh roots [1:4, volume to volume]; dissolve 1 tablespoon of fresh root honey in hot water or tea, consume up to four times daily.

TOPICAL USE: Apply a poultice or fomentation of the root topically. Prepare root oil using the alcohol intermediary or double boiler method.

CULINARY USE: The leaves and stems have a pungent, celery-like flavor and can be added to tea, soup, fish, or vegetable dishes instead of celery. The stems or seeds can be candied by simmering on low in simple syrup. Place on parchment paper to dry, and store in a sealed glass container in a dark place. In *The Modern Herbal,* author Maude Grieve lists several more detailed recipes for preparing candied angelica.

ANISE

DESCRIPTION

BOTANICAL NAMES:
Pimpinella anisum
(syn. *Anisum vulgare; A. officinarum*)

COMMON NAMES:
Anise, anis, sweet cumin
kamun halu (Arabic)
anýz (Czech)
aniis (Estonian)
saunf (Hindi)
ánizs (Hungarian)
anís (Icelandic)
jinten manis (Indonesian)
anice (Italian)
anīss (Latvian)
anyż (Polish)
erva doce (Portugese)
anason (Romanian)
shatapushpa (Sanskrit)

FAMILY NAME:
Apiaceae (Umbelliferae)

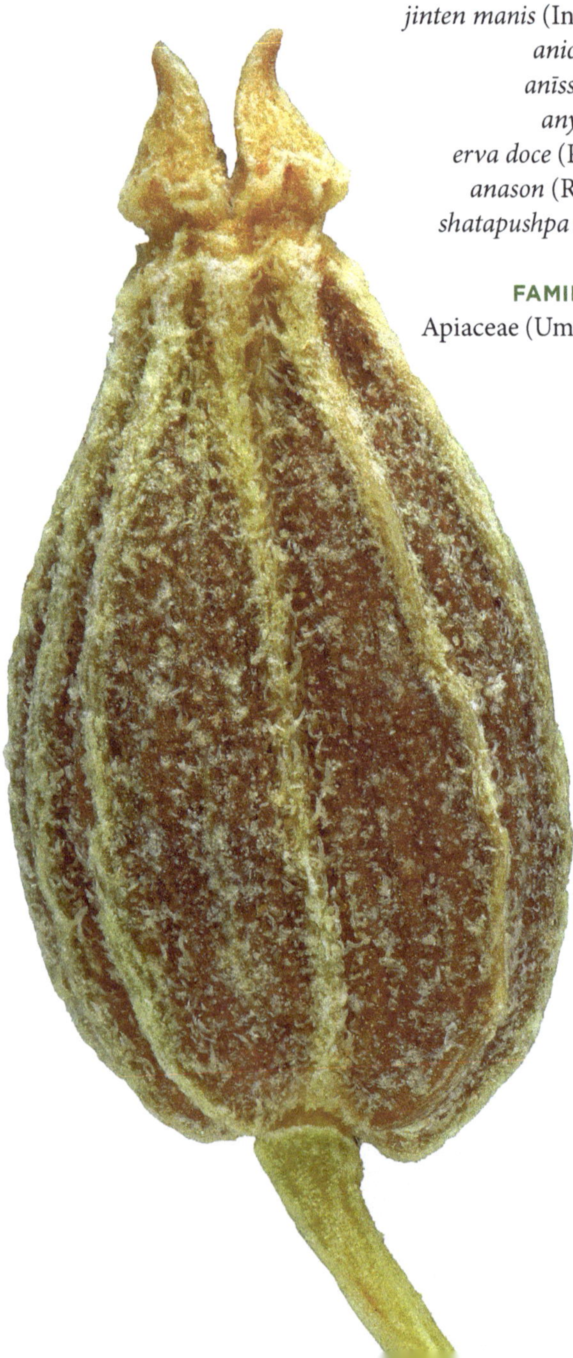

PART USED: The seeds.

BOTANICAL DESCRIPTION AND HABITAT: Anise is an annual herb native to the Mediterranean, including Egypt, Greece, and Asia Minor. It has been cultivated for more than 2,000 years.[1] Anise is delicate, and requires a warm climate and consistent watering or rainfall; excessive heat wilts it.

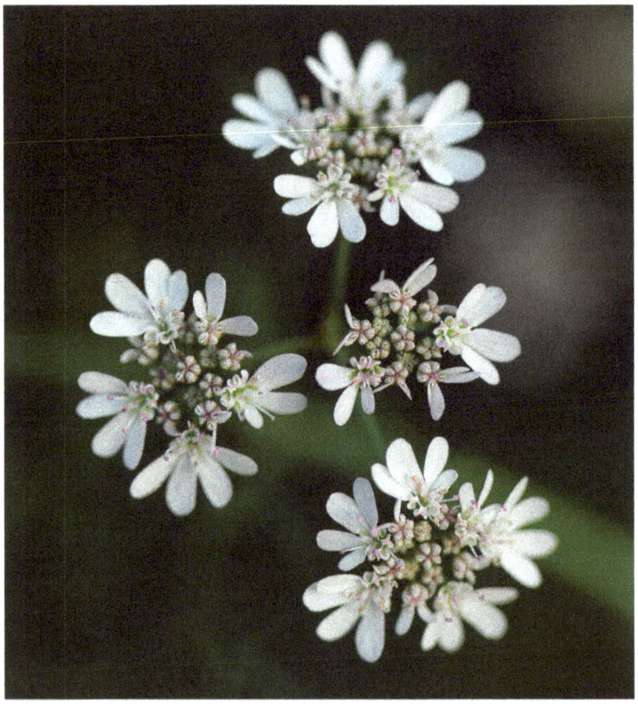

Pimpinella anisum is a strongly aromatic herb that grows 10 – 50 cm tall and has a slender taproot. The entire plant is sparsely covered in short hairs.[2] Leaves take different forms. Those at the base of the plant are simple and bear longer petioles (2 – 5 cm long); they are kidney-shaped to ovate (1 – 3 cm by 1.2 – 2.8 cm) with serrate margins.[2] The leaves on the stems are once- to twice-pinnate, with leaflets varied in shape.[2] Leaflets at the tip of the leaves are ovate (6 – 17 mm long by 2 – 7 mm wide) with three-lobed, serrate margins.[2] As leaves climb the stem, they reduce in size and their shape simplifies to three narrow lobes.[2]

The inflorescence is a compound umbel (1.6 – 6 cm diameter) with either one narrowly lanceolate bract (1 – 2 mm long), or none at all.[2] Seven to 15 unequal rays bear smaller umbels (5 – 10 mm across) consisting of ten flowers each.[2]

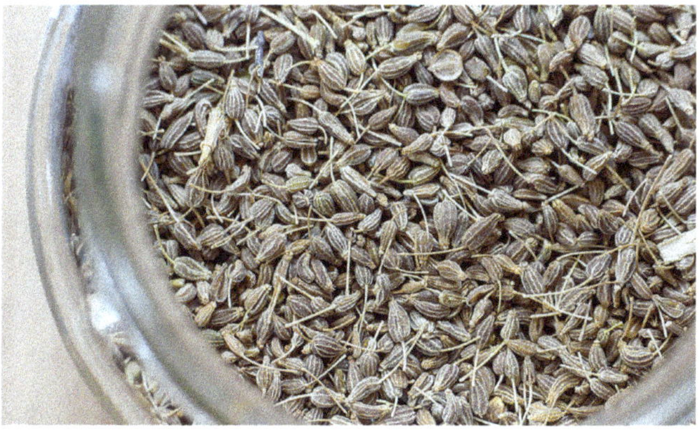

The flowers lack calyces and have white, heart-shaped petals. Within is an ovary topped by a stylopodium and two styles.[3] The seed-like, ribbed, oblong-ovoid fruit (3 – 5 mm by 2 – 2.5 mm) often retains the pedicel after it falls off the plant, appearing as a little tail at the end of the fruit.[2]

THE NAME: *Pimpinella* originates from the medieval *dipinella* ("twice pinnate"). The epithet *anisum* derives from the ancient Greek *anison* and *annēson,* as well as the Latin *anisum*. The Portuguese name erva doce means "sweet herb." The Sanskrit name shatapushpa means "a hundred flowers," referring to the many flowers of the umbel clusters. The Hindi name saunf is used interchangeably with fennel and anise, but properly denotes fennel. The Indonesian name jinten manis and the Arabic name kamun halu mean "sweet cumin."[4,5]

HISTORICAL USES: Romans served a spiced cake containing anise seed and other aromatic herbs for dessert following rich meals to prevent indigestion. This tradition is thought to be the origin of the spiced wedding cake, served at the end of wedding feasts.[4] Europeans use anise seed as a flavoring in cakes and soups.[4]

In Mediterranean and South American countries, anise-based cordials, liqueurs, brandies, and bitters are served as aperitifs and digestifs. Anise is the primary ingredient in numerous alcoholic beverages, including anisette (French), ouzo (Greek), aguar diente (Latin America), kummel (Latvian), and raki (Turkish). On hot days, Greeks pour ouzo liqueur over ice and the French add anisette to chilled water.[4] Mixing these clear liqueurs with ice or water transforms them into a cloudy, white liquid.

Pliny the Elder administered anise to cure sleeplessness. Gerard used anise tea as a remedy for hiccups, colic, and griping, as well as children's convulsions and epileptic seizures.[4] Anise was a traditional remedy for respiratory concerns such as asthma, bronchitis, and a cough with difficult expectoration. It was also given for digestive disorders including colic, indigestion, nausea, griping, and gallbladder disorders.[6] The seeds were chewed following a meal to freshen the breath. A preparation of anise seed tea called *yansoon* is given to nursing mothers in Egypt.

In some cultures, anise was thought to avert the evil eye. Among other spices, anise was used as a form of tax payment. Anise salve applications were used as a traditional treatment for scabies and lice.[7] The essential oil was applied to mouse traps as bait. Anise scent is applied to fishing lures and nets to attract fish.[4]

CONSTITUENTS

ANISE SEED: Anise seed contains volatile oil (transanethole, estragole, β-caryophyllene, and anise ketone), coumarins (bergapten, umbelliprenine, umbelliferone, and scopoletin), lipids including fatty acids (C_{16}, C_{18}, C_{20}, C_{22}, C_{24}, C_{26}, C_{30}), β-amyrin, stigmasterol and its salts (palmitate and stearate), flavonoid glycosides (quercetin-3-glucuronide, rutin, luteolin-7-glucoside, isoorientin, isovitexin, and apigenin-7-glucoside), myristicin, phenolic acids (caffeic and chlorogenic acids), protein, and carbohydrate.[6,8-11]

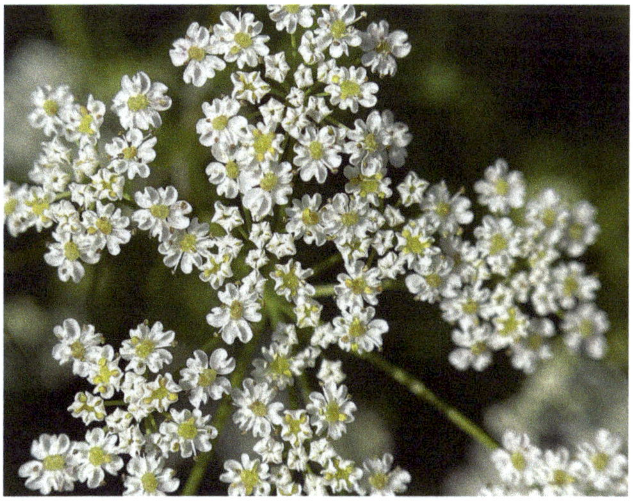

ANISE ESSENTIAL OIL: Anise seed essential oil contains phenylpropane = anethole, transanethole, estragole = methylchavicol, anise ketone = *p*-methoxyphenylacetone, β-caryophyllene, anisaldehyde, anisic acid, linalool, limonene, α-pinene, acetaldehyde, *p*-cresol, hydroquinine, β-farnesene, γ-himachalene, and *ar*-curmumene.[8,9] Anethole is attributed to the "licorice-like" flavor.

NUTRITIONAL PROPERTIES: Anise seed contains flavonoids (see above listing) and minerals including calcium, phosphorus, iron, sodium, potassium, and zinc.[6]

MEDICINAL PROPERTIES: Aromatic, antispasmodic, antitussive, carminative, expectorant, galactagogue, harmonizer, sialagogue, stomachic, diuretic, and mild antibacterial.

TEMPERATURE AND FLAVOR: Warm, sweet, salty, and pungent.

MEDICINAL USES

ANISE SEED: Anise has expectorant and antitussive properties that are useful for a variety of lung ailments.[9,10] It reduces respiratory spasms, treating tracheitis, laryngitis, asthma, whooping cough, bronchitis, smoker's cough, and a dry, irritating cough.[6,10] Anise can be consumed for acute or chronic lung conditions. It is a useful adjunct for individuals with chronic obstructive pulmonary disease (COPD) or asthma. Anise seed also reduces the wheal response and helps to lower immunoglobulin E (IgE) levels, reducing allergy-induced inflammation in mucous membranes.[12] It can be included in formulas for individuals with asthma or chronic bronchitis, with no noted interference with asthma medications.

Anise has carminative, stomachic, and smooth muscle antispasmodic actions.[6-10] It reduces gas, bloating, and digestive cramping, and enhances digestion.[6-8,10] Anise decreases colic, griping, nausea, and belching.[6-8] It also inhibits nausea accompanying the stomach flu, gastrointestinal microbes, or hangovers.[13] Combined with other bitter cholagogues and cathartic laxatives, anise prevents intestinal griping associated with their use.[10] The aromatics anesthetize the nerves in the digestive tract and reduce pain; however, anise's cousin, fennel, has more potent actions on the digestive tract. Chewing the seeds following a meal freshens the breath, treating halitosis.

Anise has galactagogue properties, increasing the supply of breast milk.[7,8,10] The aromatic carminative properties pass through breast milk, reducing infant colic.[7] Prepare a galactagogue compound by combining anise with fennel *(Foeniculum)*, fenugreek *(Trigonella)*, and blessed thistle *(Cnicus)*.

Anise is an aphrodisiac. The ground seeds are a delicious addition to cordials, elixirs, and herbal truffles. It can be combined with aromatic aphrodisiac herbs including: damiana *(Turnera)*, orange peel *(Citrus sinensis)*, cardamom *(Elettaria)*, cinnamon (*Cinnamomum*) and vanilla *(Vanilla)*. Anise seeds act as a harmonizing agent, enhancing the flavor of herbal blends.

Similar to the effects of licorice, but far milder, anise increases the reabsorption of sodium in the kidney nephrons. Because water follows sodium, the body will retain more water. This can be useful for individuals with frequent thirst, dry skin, and dry mucous membranes throughout the respiratory, digestive, or genitourinary tract. Prepare a moistening, hydrating decoction by combining marshmallow root *(Althaea)* and anise, with lesser amounts of licorice *(Glycyrrhiza)*.

ANISE ESSENTIAL OIL: Anise essential oil has similar actions to the seeds; it is a carminative, expectorant, and antispasmodic.[9,13] A sympatholytic, anise essential oil is high in anethole (up to 97%).[13] The aroma has a calming effect on the nervous system, encouraging relaxation.[13,14] Inhale the essential oil to ease nervous tension and anxiety.[13,14] Several constituents (anethole, anisaldehyde, and myristicin) have insecticidal properties.[9] *Note:* Review the *Contraindications* section before using the essential oil.

CONTRAINDICATIONS

Anise seeds are gentle, but limit their use during pregnancy. The seeds and seed preparations are safe for children and lactating women. In rare cases, anise causes allergic reactions in the skin and respiratory tract. Anethole, a component of the volatile oil, can cause allergic dermatitis in some individuals.[9] The seeds are not considered dangerous; however, the essential oil can be toxic in high doses.

Avoid internal use of anise, or exercise caution in individuals with edema, sodium-related hypertension. It should be avoided by those taking diuretic medications or blood pressure-lowering agents.

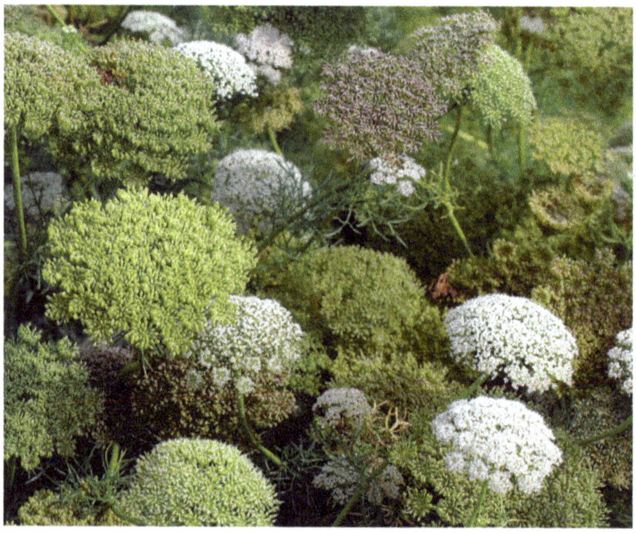

Due to the ketone content, internal use of anise seed essential oil should be avoided during pregnancy, by lactating women, and in children under the age of ten.[13] The essential oil is reported to have estrogen-like activities; therefore, some aromatherapists caution against internal consumption of it in individuals with estrogen-sensitive conditions (reproductive cancers, tumors, or cysts), and those who consume medications containing synthetic estrogen (birth control or hormone replacement therapy), or estrogen-blocking medications (Tomaxafen).[13] The potential estrogenic actions were initially thought to be caused by anethole. However, further study indicates that polymers of enthole, such as dianethole and photoanethole, are the estrogenic compounds.[9] Topical use of the essential oil may cause contact dermatitis in some individuals.

Star anise (*Illicium verum*) should not be confused with true anise *(Pimpinella anisum),* though they share some similar medicinal actions. Star anise has an oily, salty, sour, and astringent quality; while the actions may be similar, the flavor of star anise pales by comparison. *Note:* Japanese star anise *(Illicium lanceolatum)* is poisonous and cannot be used as a substitute.

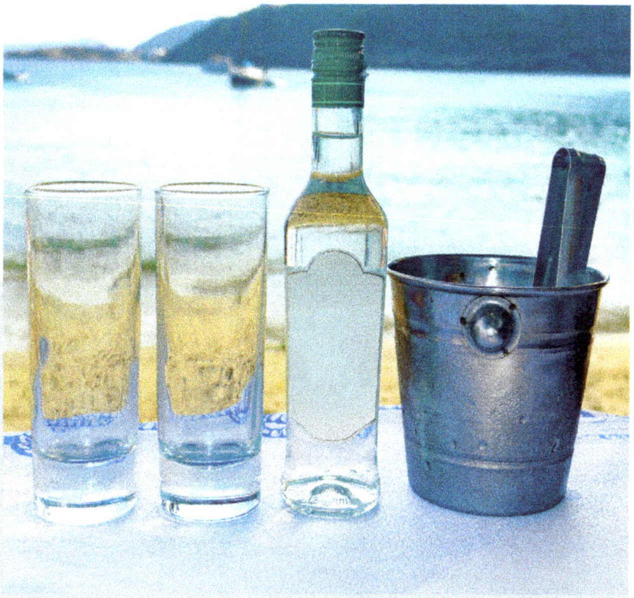

PREPARATION AND DOSAGE

TINCTURE: Fresh seeds [1:2, 70-95% alcohol]; dry seeds [1:5, 60% alcohol]; consume 15-60 drops, up to four times daily.

GLYCERITE: Dry seeds [1:5, 40% glycerin, 30% alcohol, and 30% distilled water]; consume 15-60 drops, up to three times daily.

CAPSULES: Consume 2-4 "00" capsules of recently ground seeds, up to three times daily.

TEA: Prepare a hot or cold infusion, or decoction; consume 8-12 ounces, up to four times daily. Anise milk decoction can be prepared by simmering the crushed seeds for 15-20 minutes at a low temperature.

HONEY AND SYRUP: To make infused syrup, decoct anise seeds in distilled water and cook to one-half the original volume; strain the seeds, and sweeten to taste with honey, maple syrup, or simple syrup. Consume 1 teaspoon, up to four times daily. Refrigerate the syrup up to one month. Another option is to add 1-2 drops of organic essential oil to 1 teaspoon of honey or simple syrup, and mix thoroughly. Consume or add to a cup of hot water or herbal tea.

CULINARY USES: The seeds and essential oil have long been used as flavoring agents in beverages, condiments, and foods. Anise seeds are a delicious addition to curries, breads, cookies, cakes, and other baked goods. Prepare a delicious digestive chew by combining anise seed, fennel seed, cardamom seed, orange peel, and chopped, crystalized ginger. Or consume the seeds following a meal to enhance digestion and freshen the breath. Dry roasting and crushing the seeds enhances the aromatics.

Many cultures consume anise-containing beverages and bitter formulas to enhance digestion. Anise seed oil is used to flavor black licorice candy and natural toothpaste.

ESSENTIAL OIL: Anise spirits can be made by adding one part by volume of anise essential oil to 10 parts by volume of organic alcohol. Consume 1-2 drops of spirits, one to three times daily. Place 1-2 drops of anise seed essential oil on a sugar cube or in one teaspoon of honey; dissolve into one cup of warm water and drink. Add 1-2 drops of essential oil per capsule, and consume one to two times daily. *Note:* Consuming capsules containing essential oil is for short-term use only (3-10 days). Place 1-4 drops of essential oil into 1 teaspoon of base oil, and massage into the belly (for adults); for children, only use one drop diluted in base oil, and massage into the belly.

ARALIA

DESCRIPTION

BOTANICAL NAMES:
Aralia californica, A. racemosa, A. nudicaulis

COMMON NAMES:
California spikenard, California ginseng, American spikenard, Indian spikenard, spikenard, small spikenard, false sarsaparilla, bristle-stem sarsaparilla, wild sarsaparilla, American sarsaparilla, dwarf elder, wild elder, elk clover, old man's root, spignet, petty morel, spiceberry, wild licorice, shot bush
terttuaralia (Finnish)
aralie (French)
espicanardo (Spanish)
lundaralia (Swedish)

FAMILY NAME:
Araliaceae

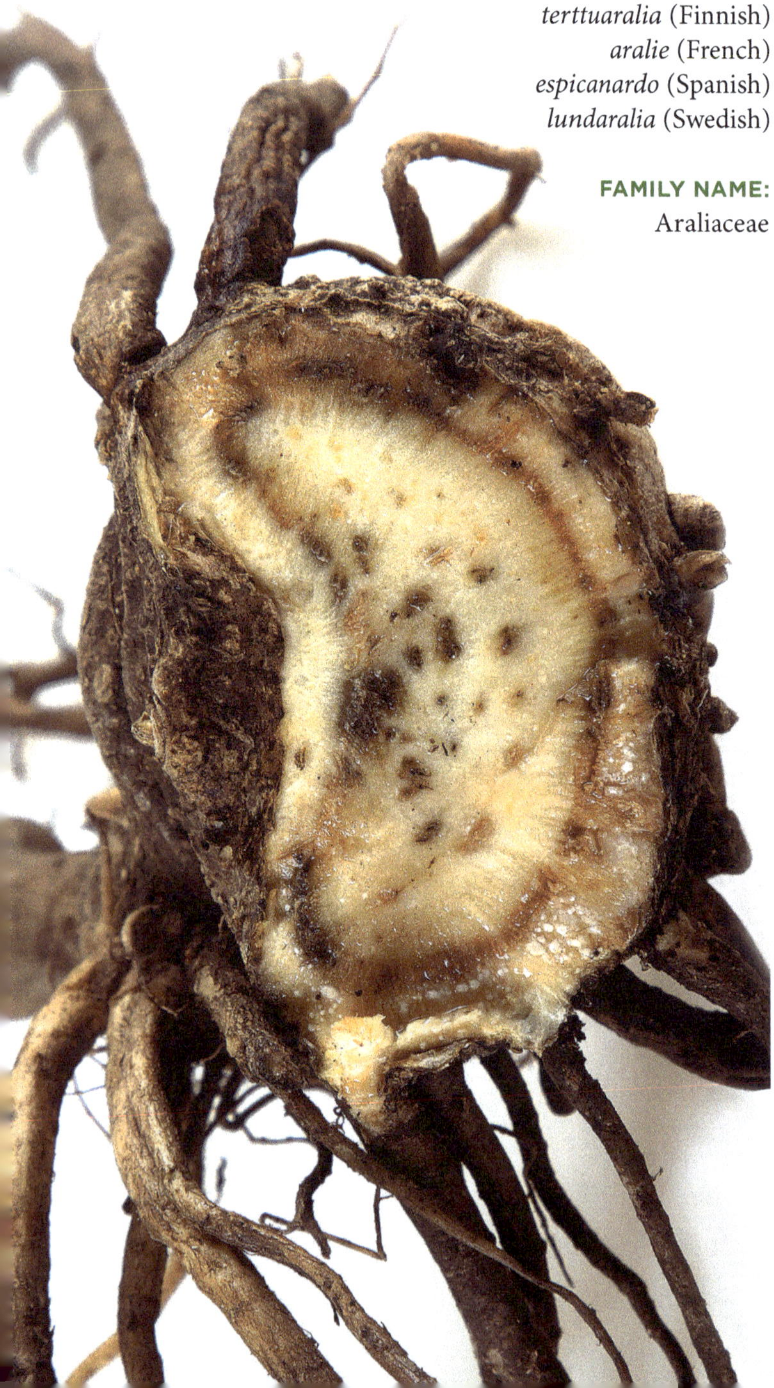

PARTS USED: The roots, berries, and leaves (prepare separately).

BOTANICAL DESCRIPTION AND HABITAT: The *Aralia* genus contains 36 species, six of which are indigenous to North America.[1] Species of *Aralia* vary in habit, from perennial shrubs to small trees, though the three medicinal species mentioned in this monograph are all herbaceous perennials.

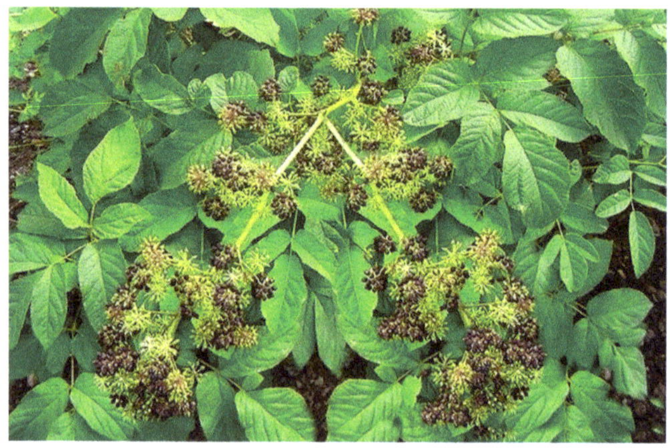

Aralia californica has large, twice pinnately compound, deciduous leaves. The ovate to oblong, serrated leaflets are 15 – 30 cm long. The cream-colored, bisexual flowers (<5 mm) have five sepals fused at the base, five greenish-white petals, five stamens, and an inferior ovary. The inflorescence grows in spreading, umbel-like panicles. The immature seeds are white, and mature into deeply purple-black berries. The coarse cortex of the roots is gray-brown; the inside is creamy white to light beige. The roots emit a sweet, pungent aroma and when cut, ooze a thick, viscous, whitish-yellow resin. Like all members of the ginseng family, each year of growth is represented by a leaf scar on the rhizome.[2]

Aralia californica is one of the largest herbaceous plants in North America. Its native habitat is northern California and southern Oregon. It can be found growing in the shade on the banks of creeks and streams.

THE NAME: The genus name is Latinized from the French Canadian *aralie*. The epithet *californica* indicates the origin. This monograph covers the medicinal uses of *A. californica;* however, *A. racemosa* and *A. nudicaulis* have many similar, interchangeable properties. *A. spinosa* and *A. hispida* contain more acrid irritants that lack the tonifying actions of the previously listed species. Their current medicinal uses are not described in this monograph; their historical applications are listed.

The following common names correspond with the Latin names: elk clover, California spikenard, California ginseng, and false sarsaparilla *(A. californica)*; spikenard, American spikenard, spignet, and petty morel *(A. racemosa)*; American, wild, or false sarsaparilla, small spikenard, wild licorice, and shot bush *(A. nudicaulis)*; and dwarf elder, wild elder, and bristle-stem sarsaparilla *(A. hispida)*.

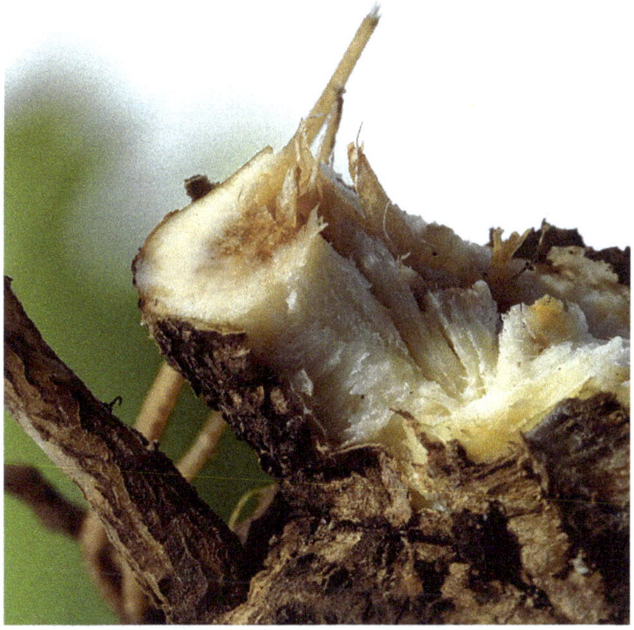

HISTORICAL USES: Native Americans used *Aralia* root for respiratory disorders including colds, fevers, asthma, and consumption.[1,3,4] Kwakiutl steeped the root in oil and consumed it as a cough medicine. Penobscot combined the crushed, dried roots with calamus *(Acorus calamus)*, and drank the tea for coughs.[3] The tea was widely utilized as a diaphoretic. Iroquois consumed *Aralia* tea to purify blood and alleviate rheumatic pain.[1] Warriors subsisted on root bundles during hunting quests and wars.[3] Cherokee, Miskwaki, and other tribes applied a root poultice as a vulnerary to treat wounds, cuts, sores, burns, swellings, and boils.[1,3] Tea prepared from the decocted roots was administered as a poultice to treat open sores and itching, and bathe arthritic joints.[4] Potawatomi, among other tribes, added the young shoots to soup.[1,3] Menominee prepared a dish containing wild onions, wild gooseberries, and spikenard root.[1] Montagnais fermented berries in water and consumed the preparation as a tonic.[3] The fruits were consumed raw or cooked.

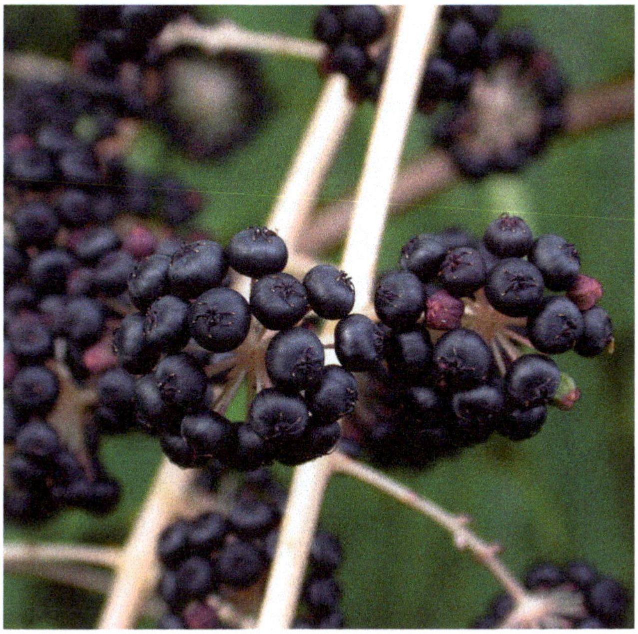

Several species of *Aralia* were included in American Pharmacopeias. Eclectic physicians administered *A. racemosa* as a stimulating, aromatic expectorant and diaphoretic in the early stages of a cough or cold.[5,6] Similar to *A. nudicaulis*, it was administered to treat a wide range of upper and lower respiratory conditions.[5,7] *A. racemosa* was given to treat suppressed menses and lochia.[5] It was also administered for more serious conditions, including scrofulous enlargement of the glands, rheumatism, gouty diathesis, and syphilis.[5] Tea prepared from the fresh root was applied topically as a stimulant and antimicrobial to treat skin ulcers and chronic skin diseases.[5] Vaginal irrigation was recommended as a antimicrobial to treat foul-smelling and acrid leucorrhoea.[5] *A. racemosa* and *A. nudicaulis* roots were ingredients in root beer.

Aralia nudicaulis was given as an alterative, and was frequently substituted for sarsaparilla root *(Smilax)*. It was also administered to relieve coughs and respiratory irritability, and to reduce catarrh in pulmonary complaints.[7] A wash made from the decoction was applied to indolent ulcers and shingles.[7]

Aralia hispida root was administered by Eclectic physicians as a renal stimulant and diuretic for treating dropsy, gravel, and suppressed urine.[5-7] It was also considered an alterative.[7] A hot infusion of the leaves was given as a sudorific.[7] When the root bark was consumed in large doses, it acted as a cathartic and emetic.[8]

The young shoots of two closely related species *(Aralia cordata* and *A. elata)* are cultivated and consumed in Japan and China.[1] The shoots of *A. cordata* are known as

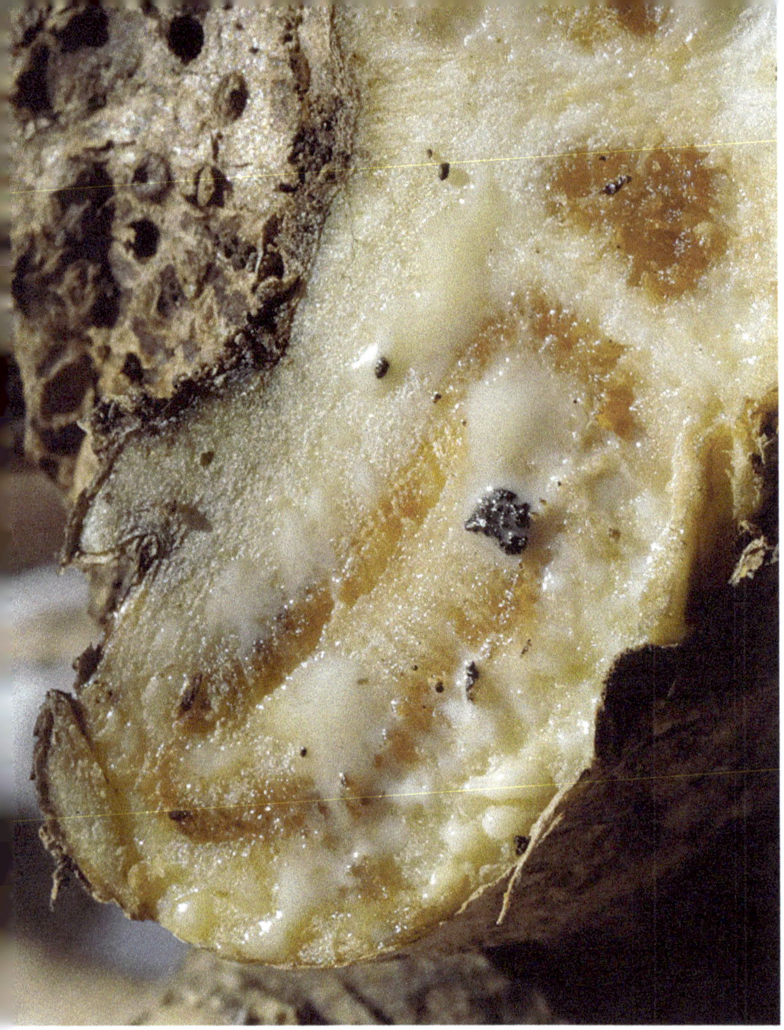

udo; *A. elata* is known as *taranome.* Taranome is a folk medicine for diabetes. Interestingly, three potent antidiabetic compounds identified as elatosides were found in taranome shoots.[1] Antioxidant, anticancer, and cholesterol-lowering effects were identified in *A. elata.*

CONSTITUENTS: *Aralia* contains oleoresins, volatile oil, triterpenoid saponins, diterpenes (pimarenes), polyacetylenes (falcarinone), choline, chlorogenic acid, ursolic acids, β-sitosterol, araloside, oleanic acid glycosides, starch, pectin, tannins, resin, and panaxosides.[1,8-10]

NUTRITIONAL PROPERTIES: *Aralia* berries contain flavonoids.

MEDICINAL PROPERTIES: The roots are an alterative, antibacterial, anti-inflammatory, antitussive, demulcent, diaphoretic, expectorant, emollient, lung tonic, recuperative, and diuretic (mild). The berries are a subtle adaptogen, antidepressant, energizer, and expectorant. The aromatic leaves enhance the absorption of mineral rich herbs in tea.

TEMPERATURE AND FLAVOR: Warm, pungent, sweet, and bitter.

MEDICINAL USES

ARALIA ROOT: *Aralia californica* root is a highly effective expectorant that aids in treating acute or chronic pulmonary conditions. It is a soothing demulcent, antitussive, and antibacterial agent. The falcarinone and open chain polyacetylenes in *Aralia* root have antibacterial actions.[10] *Aralia* root oozes thick, creamy oleoresins with aromatic expectorant properties.[11] When the preparations are consumed, oleoresins pass through the digestive tract unaltered; they enter systemic circulation and are excreted unchanged in the lungs. These aromatic resins stimulate mucous membrane secretions, normalizing and restoring secretions in the lower respiratory tract.[11] The saponins also have expectorant actions.[1,10] *Aralia* root aids in thinning and expelling thick, viscous mucus; it also stimulates respiratory secretions, treating dry, irritated respiratory mucosa.[9,11] It is ideal for the first stage of a head cold because it relieves a dry, scratchy throat, laryngitis, and pharyngitis.[5,9,11] It also addresses a dry, hacking cough, and prevents deeper respiratory infections from developing. When treating a scratchy throat, dry cough, or inflamed respiratory membranes, combine *Aralia* extract with anise seed *(Pimpinella anisum),* thyme *(Thymus officinalis),* hyssop (*Hyssopus officinalis*), gumweed *(Grindelia),* licorice root *(Glycyrrhiza),* and/or balsam root *(Balsamorhiza).*

Aralia aids in treating asthma, bronchitis, pneumonia, and pleurisy.[5,9-12] When treating acute and subacute lower respiratory infections, combine *Aralia* extract with other warming expectorant and antimicrobial herbs such as oshá *(Ligusticum porteri),* lomatium *(Lomatium),* gumweed *(Grindelia),* balsam root *(Balsamorhiza),* thyme *(Thymus),* or pleurisy root *(Asclepias). Note:* Herbal combinations may be less effective in treating an infection when a patient is medicated with steroids or steroid inhalers, or has a compromised immune system.

Aralia root is effective for treating a moist cough or humid asthma aggravated by a cold, damp environment.[5,9,10] It is highly beneficial as a long-term tonic for individuals with wheezing, asthma, emphysema, or allergies that trigger lower respiratory spasms.[5,9,10] It is best consumed one to three times daily as a tonic. Numerous patients have claimed that they use their inhalers much less when consuming *Aralia* regularly. Although *Aralia* does little to alter structural changes in patients with emphysema, the expectorant and antitussive actions enhance breathing. Bronchial bore (the opening in airways) increases as mucus thins and membrane inflammation decreases.

Lung tonics such as *Aralia* root aid in strengthening the lungs and decreasing the potential for serious lung infections. *Aralia* root extract or honey is highly beneficial as a long-term tonic for individuals who smoke frequently, have weak lungs, or are prone to bronchitis and other lung infections.[11] It helps to prevent lower respiratory infections, hastens recovery, and decreases wheezing. It can be used as a preventative lung tonic or recuperative agent following a respiratory infection. *Aralia* root is also useful for individuals exposed to environmental smoke. Many of them develop severe respiratory infections and breathing difficulties such as wheezing or asthma.

Combine extracts of *Aralia* with gumweed (*Grindelia*), elecampane *(Inula)*, anise *(Pimpinella)*, and/or Senega snake root *(Polygala)* to reduce wheezing due to asthma or seasonal allergies, smoking, or emphysema-related breathing difficulties. This combination helps to deepen respiration, open the airways, expel mucus, reduce bronchial spasms, and decrease membrane inflammation. Add antimicrobial agents when infections are the source of breathing problems.

From a Traditional Chinese Medicine perspective, *Aralia* root has lung qi tonifying properties. Lung qi tonics regulate mucous membrane secretions and deepen respiration by enhancing the lungs' ability to "grasp qi." Lung qi tonifying herbs reduce wheezing due to lung deficiency and ease chronic coughing. Lung qi tonics are also useful to increase energy levels and strengthen one's vital force. They can decrease spontaneous sweating in the afternoon, and increase resistance to infections. Combine *Aralia* with jie geng *(Platycodon)*, ling zhi *(Ganoderma)*, wu wei zi *(Schisandra)*, and licorice root *(Glycyrrhiza)* as a lung qi tonifying compound.

Karyn Sanders, a clinical herbalist, recommends *Aralia* root as a parturient to stimulate contractions during labor; she has found that it has a gentler effect than blue cohosh. It is not appropriate if there are complications, including if the baby is posterior or breech, or if the expecting mother has gestational diabetes, hypertension, or other complications. *Aralia* is indicated for healthy women without complications. Make sure to avoid consuming the root during pregnancy, except for several days or up to one week prior to the due date. *Aralia* root can be used as a single extract or alternated with the extract of cotton root bark *(Gossypium)*. Consume 30 – 60 drops every two to three hours, three to five times daily to stimulate contractions and hasten labor. *Note:* Use these extracts up to one week prior to the due date, but not before.

Aralia has mild diuretic actions; some species are more potent than others. The diuretic properties are attributed to the saponins and volatile oil.[10]

Aralia root also has topical antimicrobial and anti-inflammatory actions for treating cuts, abrasions, burns, herpes, shingles, and sores.[5,6,9,10] It warms and moistens skin, and stimulates circulation to tissues. *Note:* Some individuals can develop contact dermatitis, usually resulting from direct contact or topical applications of the roots. In order to ensure that the inflammatory response does not aggravate a condition topically or internally, place a small amount of the root or medicinal preparation in the delicate, inner part of the arm where the elbow creases. If a rash forms in 24 – 48 hours, avoid using this herb topically, use internally with caution, or avoid internal use completely.

ARALIA BERRY: *Aralia* berry extract has mood-elevating actions. It aids in treating mild to moderate depression, Seasonal Affective Disorder (SAD), as well as premenstrual and postpartum depression.[11,12] The berries can also be used to improve the mental outlook of individuals who are depressed as a result of chronic illness or pain.[11,12] Combine *Aralia* with the following herbs as a subtle mood-elevating compound: St. John's wort *(Hypericum)*, lemon balm *(Melissa)*, hawthorn *(Crataegus)*, and damiana (*Turnera)*.

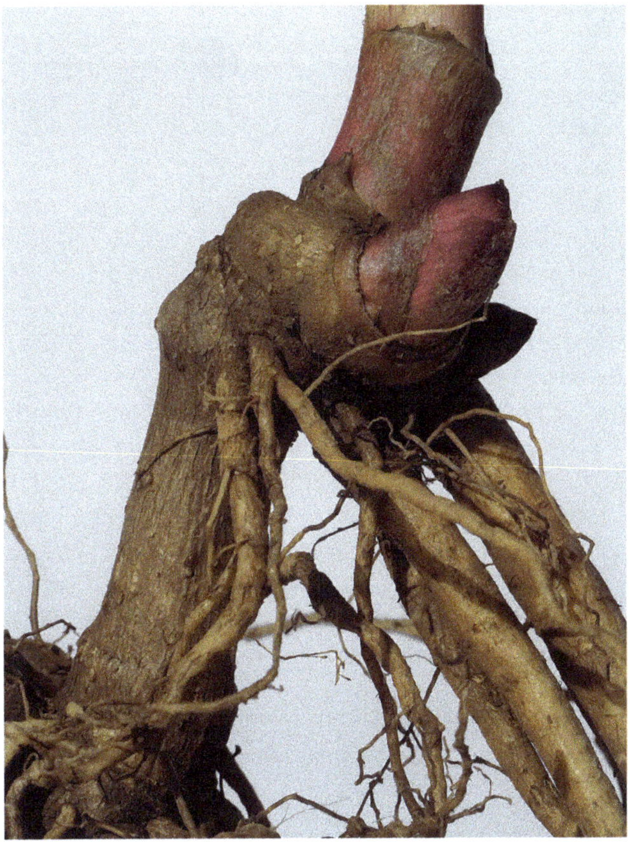

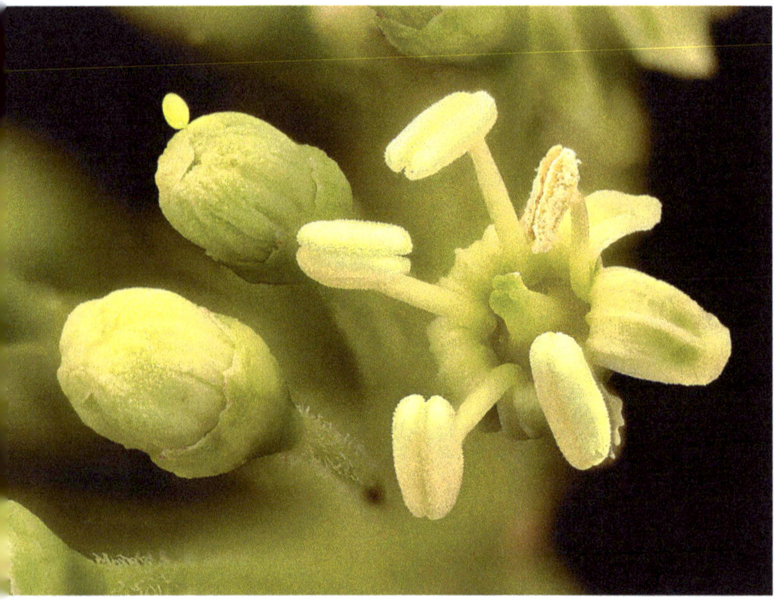

Aralia berries have subtle adaptogenic qualities that modify the body's response to stress.[12] They have a gentle energizing effect, but do not overstimulate the nervous system, like some adaptogen herbs. Combine extracts of *Aralia* berry with reishi *(Ganoderma)*, and smaller amounts of wu wei zi *(Schisandra)* and licorice root (*Glycyrrhiza glabra*) as an adaptogen.

Aralia berries are a sialagogue and have similar but milder aromatic expectorant actions as the roots. Combine *Aralia* berry with elder berry *(Sambucus)*, yerba santa (*Eriodictyon*), and lomatium *(Lomatium)* as an immune stimulant during the first stages of a cold.

CONTRAINDICATIONS

Avoid consuming *Aralia* root and berry during pregnancy, except to induce labor. Individuals with severely compromised liver or kidney function, or liver or kidney disease may want to avoid long-term internal use. Consuming raw ripe berries causes a mildly acrid or tingling sensation in the throat, presumably because the aromatic properties stimulate mucous membranes. In rare cases, topical applications of the root can cause a rash similar to poison oak. Test the oil on the inner portion of the arm; wait 24 - 48 hours to confirm that a rash doesn't develop. If it does, do not use the oil. Exercise caution when working with the fresh root, due to the potential skin sensitizing effects.

PREPARATION AND DOSAGE

TINCTURE: Fresh roots [1:2, 80 - 95% alcohol]; dry roots [1:5, 60% alcohol]; consume 15 - 60 drops, up to four times daily of *Aralia californica*. Fresh berries [1:2, 95% alcohol]; consume 15 - 60 drops up to three times daily of *Aralia californica*. When using extracts of other *Aralia* species, consume 5 - 30 drops, up to three times daily.

GLYCERITE: Fresh roots or berries [1:2, 50% glycerin, 50% alcohol]; consume 10 - 60 drops, up to three times daily.

CAPSULES: Consume 2 - 4 capsules, one to three times daily.

TEA: Prepare a decoction of the roots; consume 8 - 12 ounces, three to four times daily. Prepare the berries as a hot infusion and consume 6 - 8 ounces, one to three times daily. Prepare the leaves as a hot infusion. According to herbalist Michael Moore, the leaves may be added to nutritive tea blends to enhance mineral absorption.[9]

HONEY AND SYRUP: Prepare a fresh root or berry honey [1:4 volume to volume]. Consume 1 tablespoon in hot water or tea, up to four times daily. The honey also can be used as a topical skin soothing preparation if there is no allergy to the root.

Infuse the berries in honey and strain after two to four weeks, or cook the berries with honey in a double boiler. Observe the mixture closely to ensure that the berries do not ferment or mold. Add organic grain alcohol, up to 20 percent of the finished volume, to preserve the honey and prevent the growth of unwanted bacteria. Consume 1 teaspoon, one to three times daily.

TOPICAL USE: Chop *Aralia* root and wilt it one or two days, then cook it in olive oil or a light base oil on low using the double boiler method for three to six hours. Strain, bottle, and apply the oil topically, or make a salve.

ARNICA

DESCRIPTION

BOTANICAL NAMES:
Arnica chamissonis, A. cordifolia, A. latifolia, A. montana, A. mollis, A. acaulis, and A. spp.

COMMON NAMES:
European arnica, heart leaf arnica, leopard's bane, mountain arnica, mountain daisy, mountain tobacco
guldblomme (Danish)
fleurs d'arnica (French)
arnikablüten, berwohlverleih (German)
polmonaria di montagna (Italian)
arnicae flos (Latin)

FAMILY NAME:
Asteraceae (Compositae)

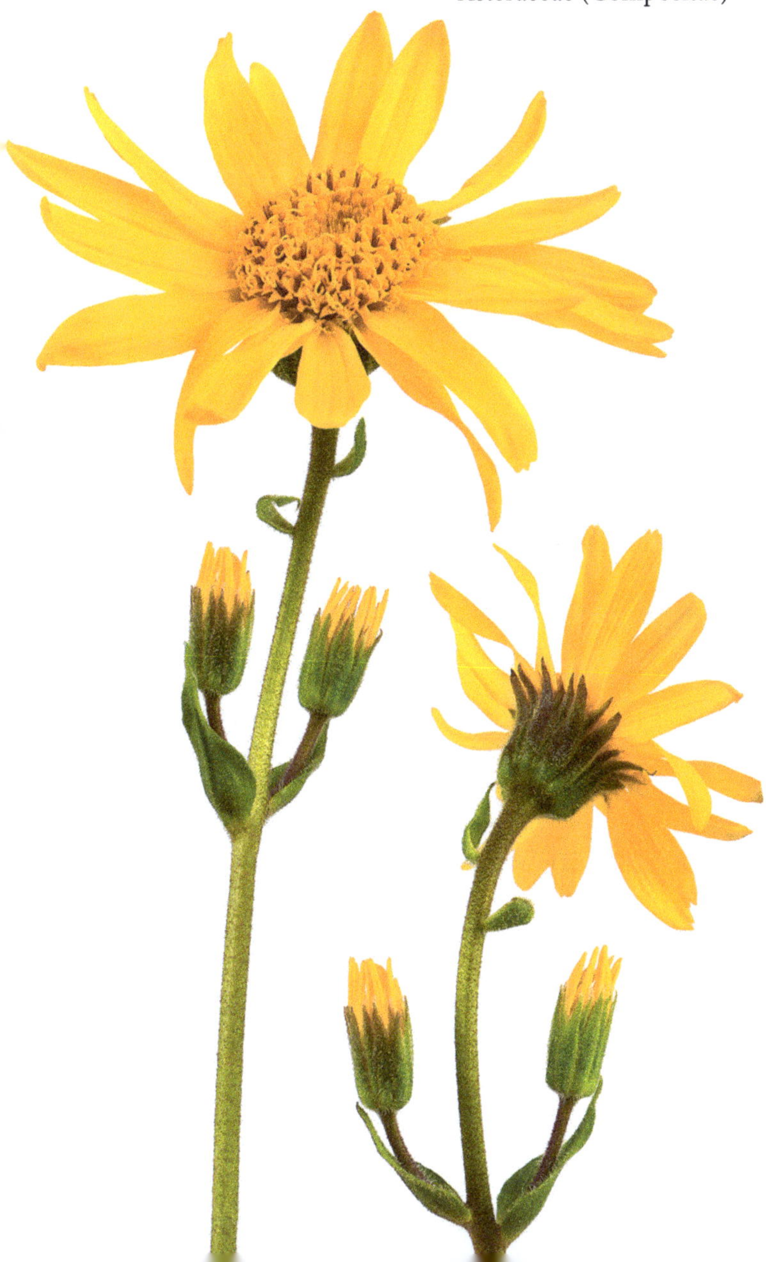

PARTS USED: The flowers and leaves.

BOTANICAL DESCRIPTION AND HABITAT: Arnica is a genus consisting of 29 species of erect, herbaceous perennials that grow in colonies on sunny mountain meadows and slopes.[1] They grow wild in high altitudes from 1,500 – 3,000 meters throughout the Mountain West and circumboreally.[2] Arnica (5 – 100 cm tall), has one to ten pairs of simple, hairy, or glabrous leaves that are predominantly opposite and lance- or heart-shaped, entire or toothed.[2] The leaf morphology between species varies. The horizontal or descending rhizome is beige to light brown. The bright yellow flowering heads grow individually or in clusters. They have 5 – 22 fertile, pistillate ray flowers (though a few species lack them), and many bisexual, fertile disk flowers.[2] The flowers produce a small achene with white or brown bristly pappus.[1]

THE NAME: *Arnica* derives from the Greek *arnikos* ("lamb's skin").[3] The epithet *chamissonis* is named after German botanist, naturalist, and poet Adelbert von Chamisso. The epithet *cordifolia* means "heart-shaped" leaves; *latifolia* ("broad leafed") derives from Latin. The epithet *mollis* means "smooth or soft velvety hair."[4] The epithet *montana* derives from the Latin *mont* ("mountain").[5]

HISTORICAL USES: Eclectic physicians administered arnica internally and topically for sore, strained, or bruised muscles.[6,7] Dr. Finley Ellingwood recommended low, frequent doses to relieve muscular strain and soreness following a difficult labor.[6] Arnica was given for lumbago and weakness in the back muscles. It was also administered to reduce a fever following surgery or a severe injury accompanied by shock, muscular tissue destruction, soreness, or pain.[6] Dr. Harvey Felter prescribed arnica for spinal and vagal enervation due to insufficient nervous response, vascular sluggishness, and depressed nervous system function resulting from exhaustive diseases.[7] He recommended arnica to alleviate "heart strain" resulting from overwork and exertion, severe strain, worry, or excitement.[7] He also reported successfully treating paraplegia and hemiplegia due to acute inflammation from a recent injury.[7] Arnica hastens healing and waste product removal from injured tissues. When muscles were severely lacerated, torn, or bruised, Dr. Ellingwood applied one part arnica with five parts of fresh, warm, sweet milk, changing the

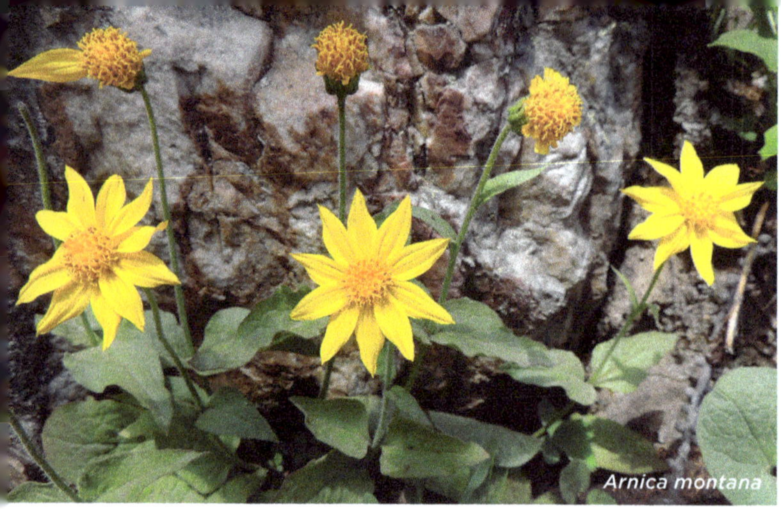

Arnica montana

dressing every two to three hours.[6] This preparation was also administered for slowly healing sores and abscesses.[6]

Native Americans throughout western mountainous regions applied arnica poultices to bruises, swellings, and cuts.[8] They chewed the roots to treat a sore throat, and applied the poultice to toothaches.[8] An infusion was given for tuberculosis.[8]

Arnica montana was used by Europeans topically as an anti-inflammatory for bruises and sprains. Homeopathic preparations were consumed to treat shock and trauma.[8] The recommended dosage of the extract listed in the *British Pharmacopoeia* and *U.S. Pharmacopoeia* is 10 – 30 drops.

CONSTITUENTS: Arnica contains volatile oil (terpenes, thymol, thymol methyl ether, 4-hydroxythymol dimethyl ether, and isobutyric acid thymyl ether), fatty acids (palmitic, linoleic, myristic, and linolenic), resins, a bitter principle (arnicin), sesquiterpene lactones (helenalin, 11,13-dihydrohelenalin, 11,13-dihydrohelenalin esters, 2β-ethoxy-6-O-isobutyryl, 1-2,3-dihydrohelenalin, and 6-O-isobutyryltetrahydrohelanalin), tannin (catechin), sterols (arnisterin, arnidiol, and taraxasterol), carotenoids (α- and β-carotene, cryptoxanthin, and lutein = xanthophyll), flavonoids (betuletol, 6-methoxykaempferol, hispidulin, jaceosidin, pectolinarigenin, isoquercitin, luteolin, glucosides, and astragalin), phenolic acids (*p*-hydroxybenzoic, *p*-coumaric, gentisic, ferulic, vanillic, cynarin, chlorogenic, and caffeic), coumarins (umbelliferone and scopoletin), water-soluble polysaccharides, polyacetylenes, choline, betaine, inulin, arnicolide, loliolide, betuletol, dien-tetrain, en-pentain, eupifolin, faradiol, luteine, arnifolin, trimethylamine, and tridecadiens.[9-12]

NUTRITIONAL PROPERTIES: Although arnica contains flavonoids and carotenoids, it cannot be safely consumed in any appreciable quantities for the nutrient content.

MEDICINAL PROPERTIES: Analgesic, antibacterial, antifungal, anti-inflammatory, circulatory stimulant, diaphoretic, immune stimulant, counterirritant, rubefacient, and vulnerary.

TEMPERATURE AND FLAVOR: Hot, pungent, and bitter.

MEDICINAL USES

Arnica tincture can be consumed in low doses (3 – 10 drops). It has antimicrobial and heating diaphoretic properties. It also contains polysaccharides that stimulate immune function by increasing macrophage activity.[10,11] Consume low doses to treat the first phase of a cold or flu, or gargle with the diluted tincture for chronic tonsillitis or an obstinate sore throat. The sesquiterpene lactones (helanalin, dihydrohelenalin, and their esters) have analgesic, antibiotic, and anti-inflammatory actions.[10] The sesquiterpene lactones helenalin acetate and 11, 13-dihydrohelanalin have antibacterial and antifungal actions *in vitro.*[9] Arnica extracts enhanced phagocytosis of bacteria including *Listeria monocytogenes* and *Salmonella typhimurium* in animal studies.[9]

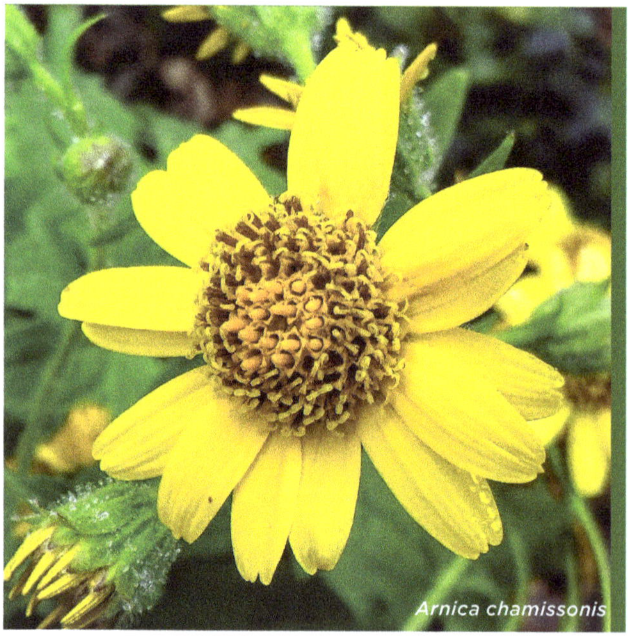

Arnica chamissonis

Arnica is a highly effective first aid remedy. Consuming low doses of arnica extract or homeopathic tablets reduces shock and trauma resulting from an injury or accident. Arnica also reduces inflammation, pain, and swelling caused by a concussion, dental extraction, sprain, broken or fractured bone, or surgery.

The cream, oil, salve, and liniment work efficiently as a counterirritant and anti-inflammatory for bruises, sprains, strains, dislocations, hyperextensions, myalgia, arthritis, bursitis, and bunions. It is specifically indicated for pain worsened from movement, helped by heat, and aggravated by cold.[11] Arnica dilates blood vessels, particularly specialized capillaries that control whether blood is piped into small peripheral capillary beds, or shunted to small veins.[11] It increases blood dispersal, especially when there is stagnation and congestion. Arnica is a counterirritant, increasing circulation in injured or inflamed tissues, hastening healing and waste product removal from injured tissues.[6] Arnica's effects are deeper than many surface counterirritants such as "Tiger Balm," camphor, or mints. Most of the actions are attributed to the sesquiterpene lactones.[12]

Arnica reduces pain and stiffness caused by osteoarthritis, and improves mobility.[3,11] It increases absorption and drainage of hyaline cartilage, and decreases early and chronic congestion that lead to bony cartilage overgrowth.[11] Arnica can be beneficial for rheumatoid arthritis, but should be avoided if it overheats the joints or reddens the skin below the surface. Rheumatoid arthritis is an autoimmune disease; therefore, caution should be exercised when using arnica because of its immune stimulating properties. Discontinue use if it aggravates the condition.

CONTRAINDICATIONS

Internal use of arnica extract is contraindicated during pregnancy or lactation, and in young children (except homeopathic arnica); topical use is acceptable in these cases. Internal and external homeopathic preparations are non-toxic. Consuming large or excessive doses (1 – 2 ounces) of arnica extract can cause a headache, diaphoresis, diuresis, upset stomach, nausea, vomiting, catharsis, mucosa blistering, burning sensations in the stomach, lower digestive inflammation, convulsions, and nervous system disturbance accompanied by abdominal pain.[6,7,10,11] Avoid internal consumption with chronic stomach or intestinal inflammation, overt diseases involving the blood vessels or blood clotting, as well as conditions with impaired heart, liver, or kidney function.[6,7,11]

Topical applications of arnica (salve, oil, liniment, or diluted tincture) should be avoided with broken skin, skin ulcers, or inflamed skin conditions including eczema and dermatitis.[7,8,12] It can cause dermal irritation, pustules, blisters, and eczematous inflammation.[7] Arnica can increase the likelihood of surface inflammation due to its heating and counterirritant qualities. Do not apply near the eyes or mouth. Discontinue topical use if it causes a rash or irritation. Arnica contains sesquiterpenes that can cause topical allergic dermatitis in individuals with hypersensitivity to Asteraceae family plants.[9,12] While it is rare, highly concentrated applications may act as a vesicant, causing blistering if left in contact with the skin for extended periods.[7,12] Individuals with sensitive skin should avoid topical use of undiluted preparations.[7]

PREPARATION AND DOSAGE

TINCTURE: Fresh flowers and/or leaves [1:2 - 1:3, 80 - 95% alcohol]; recently dried flowers and/or leaves [1:5, 70% alcohol]; consume 3 - 15 drops, up to four times daily. The *British Pharmacopoeias* and *U.S. Pharmacopoeias* list a 10 - 30 drop dose range. Dilute the tincture with five parts water for topical use; apply up to four times daily.

TOPICAL USE: Apply a wash, fomentation, or poultice of the hot infusion externally, but do not consume the tea internally. Do not leave a poultice in contact with the skin more than 30 minutes.

Fresh wilted flowers or leaves can be used to prepare infused oils. The alcohol intermediary oil method is preferred for oils and salves because it extracts more of the constituents, though usually only the leaves are used with that method because the flowers go to seed when dried. Arnica can be applied as a fomentation, poultice, or liniment.

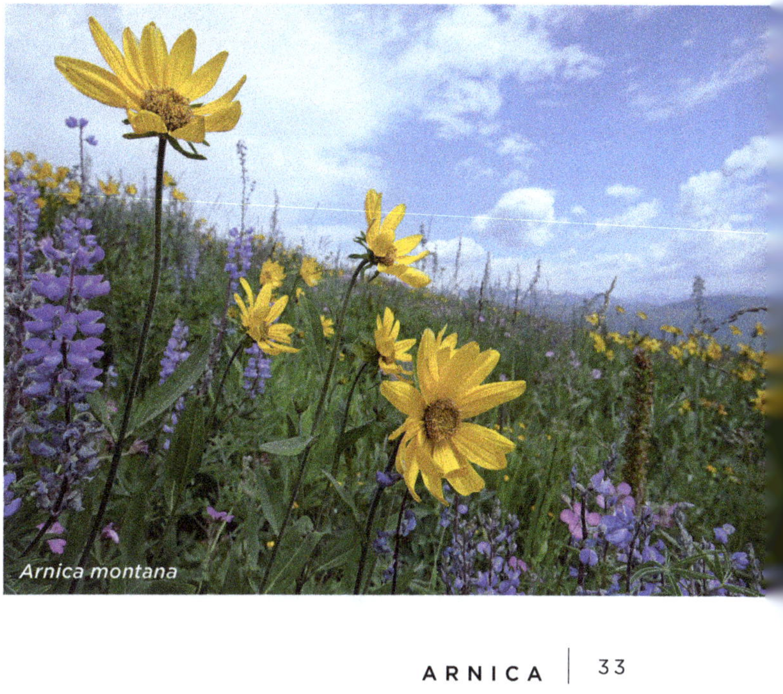

Arnica montana

ARTICHOKE LEAF

DESCRIPTION

BOTANICAL NAMES:
Cynara scolymus
(syn. *C. cardunculus* ssp. *cardunculus*, *C. cardunculus* var. *scolymus*)

COMMON NAMES:
Artichoke, globe artichoke, garden artichoke, French artichoke
artiskok (Danish)
artichaut (French)
artischocke (German)
artiocco, artichiocco, carciofo (Italian)
alcachofra (Portuguese)
alcarchofa (Spanish)

FAMILY NAME:
Asteraceae (Compositae)

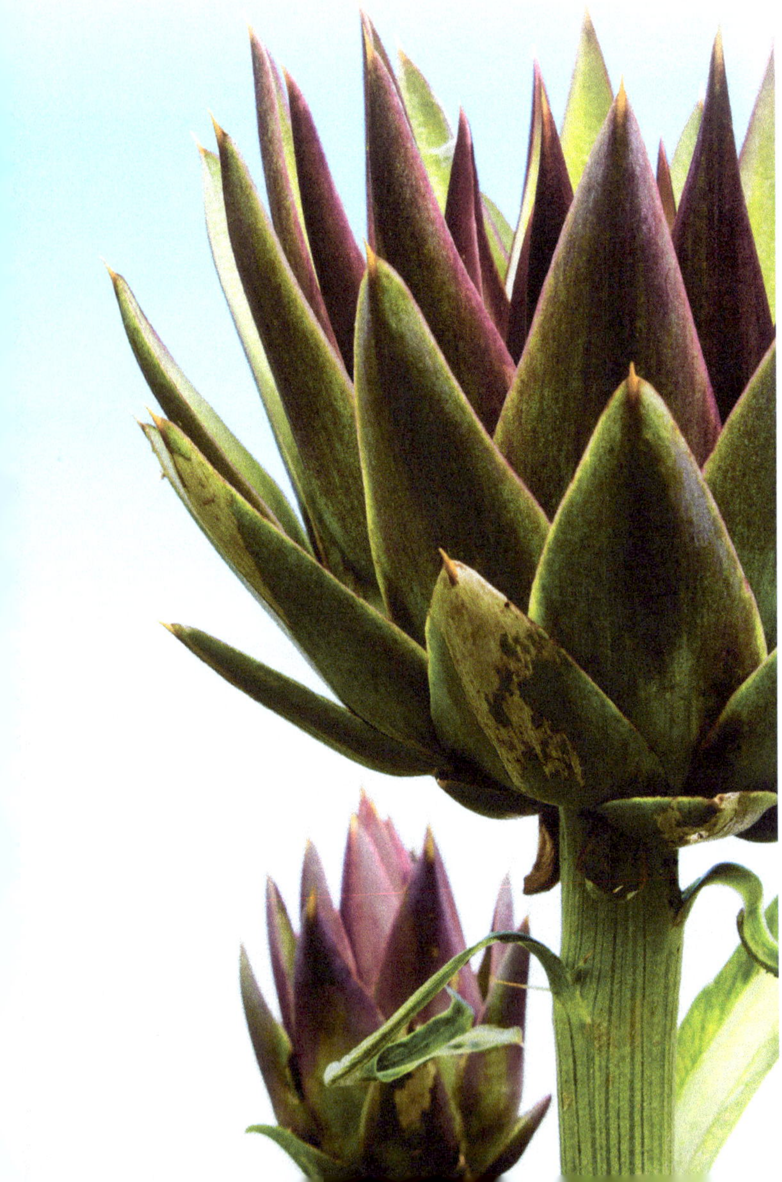

PART USED: The leaves. *Note:* The medicinal properties of the leaves are not contained in the edible portion of the plant, known as globe artichoke.

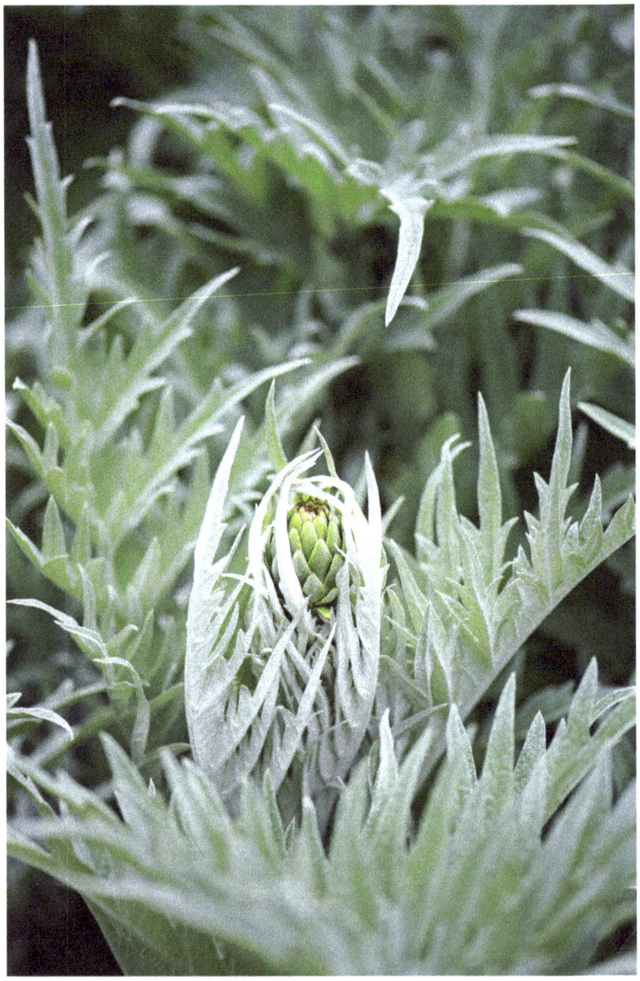

BOTANICAL DESCRIPTION AND HABITAT: *Cynara scolymus* is considered a cultigen of *Cynara cardunculus* (cardoon, wild thistle).[1] Artichoke is native to the Mediterranean; however, it is currently cultivated in temperate regions worldwide. It should not be confused with Jerusalem artichoke *(Helianthus tuberosus)*, a species of sunflower-bearing tuberous roots.

Artichoke is a regal herbaceous perennial with a fleshy taproot. It ranges in height from 50 – 250 cm.[2,3] The large, silver-green, alternate leaves (up to 200 cm long) are oblong, deeply one- to two-pinnately compound, silver-white and woolly underneath.[2,3] The dentate margins of the leaves are often tipped with spines, especially in the wild forms.[3,4] In the first year, artichoke leaves form a basal rosette and grow up to one meter high. The plant bears fruit in the second year.

The immature inflorescence is often consumed as a vegetable. The fleshy, overlapping, leaf-like, lanceolate to ovate involucral bracts, tipped by sharp spines, are mostly tough and leathery.[3] However, their bases have delicate, tender, savory flesh. These bracts surround the cluster of inedible tiny flowers within, also known as the choke, which is cloaked with thin, pale, immature bracts. The choke rests atop the fleshy, firm receptacle, known as the heart, a delectable edible. As the inflorescence matures, it develops into a striking, purplish-blue, thistle-like head, and becomes too fibrous to consume. Each head produces many tiny achenes (4 – 8 mm long), each bearing a long pappus (2 – 4 cm long).[2]

THE NAME: *Cynara,* the botanical name for artichoke, is related to a Greek myth.[5] Cynara was a beautiful woman from the island of Zinari. While the god Zeus was visiting his brother Poseidon on Zinari, he fell in love with Cynara. He transformed her into a goddess in order to bring her to his home on Mount Olympus. Cynara secretly snuck back to earth to visit her mother and home. Enraged when he discovered her visits, Zeus hurled Cynara back to earth and transformed her into the first artichoke.

Another possible origin of the word *Cynara* derives from the Greek *kynára* or *kynaros,* a type of artichoke named after the Aegean island of Kinara. The species name *scolymus* derives from the Greek *skólymus,* originating from *skólop* ("pointed stake"), referring to the plant's pointed thorns.

The spelling of the word artichoke first appeared in 1556, and is likely related to the Latin *coculum* ("cardoon"). It originates from the Arabic *al-harsúf* from which derive names such as alcarchofa (Spanish), alcachofra (Portuguese), artichaut (French), and artiocco and carciofo (Italian).[6] Interestingly, in English, Russian, French, and German, as well as in northern European languages, the name of this plant derives from the Latin and Old Italian *alcocalum, articocalus, articiocco,* or *articoca.* This strongly suggests that Italy was the bridge for distributing artichokes in Europe. Artichoke is known in Greek as Αγγιναρα *(agginara),* which relates to the Ancient Greek Κυον *(kyon),* meaning dog — likening the leaf spines to dog's teeth.

HISTORICAL USES: Artichoke is among the earliest cultivated vegetables, grown by Greeks and Romans as their empires flourished. Greek historian Dioscorides described the large-scale cultivation of artichokes near Carthage. Records from Pliny the Elder, a Roman scholar, mention that artichokes commanded a higher price than any other vegetable.

Catherine de Medici, who became the wife of King Henry II of France, introduced artichokes from Florence into France, where they became an esteemed edible.[7] The Dutch brought artichokes to England, where they grew in Henry VII's garden at Newhall in 1530. Records indicate that Henry VII ate them in generous quantities. Globe artichokes were reserved for members of the European aristocracy who could afford the rare gourmet vegetable. Artichokes were cultivated in Paris from the 16th to 20th centuries.[5]

In Europe during the 16th century, it was considered scandalous for women to consume artichokes, due to the belief that they increased libido and enhanced sexual vitality. Thus, artichokes were often denied to women and reserved for men.[5] Globe artichokes continue to be esteemed aphrodisiacs. The tender, delectable cooked heart and leaves can be dipped in, or stuffed with savory sauces as an amorous appetizer.

French and Spanish explorers introduced artichokes to the U.S. in the 19th century. French immigrants brought artichokes to Louisiana; Spanish immigrants brought them to California.[7] Today, 99% of the artichokes grown in the U.S. are produced in Castroville, California, the self-proclaimed "Artichoke Capital of the World." Most of the world's artichoke cultivation continues in Italy, Spain, and France, followed by Argentina and the U.S.[7]

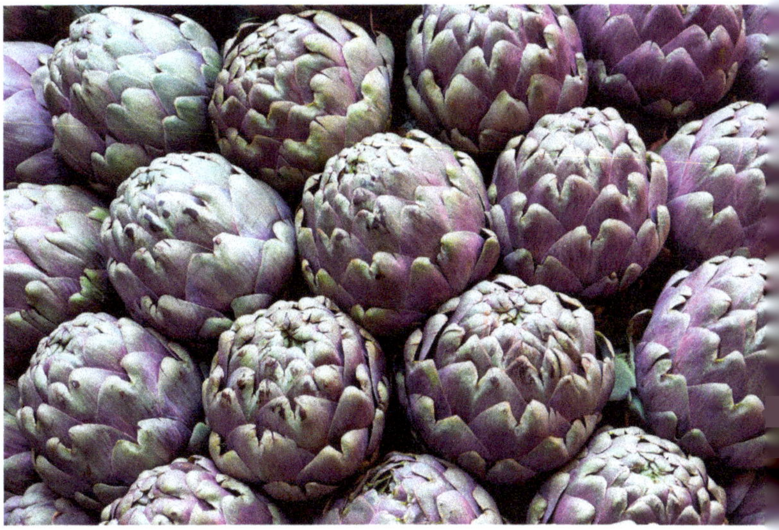

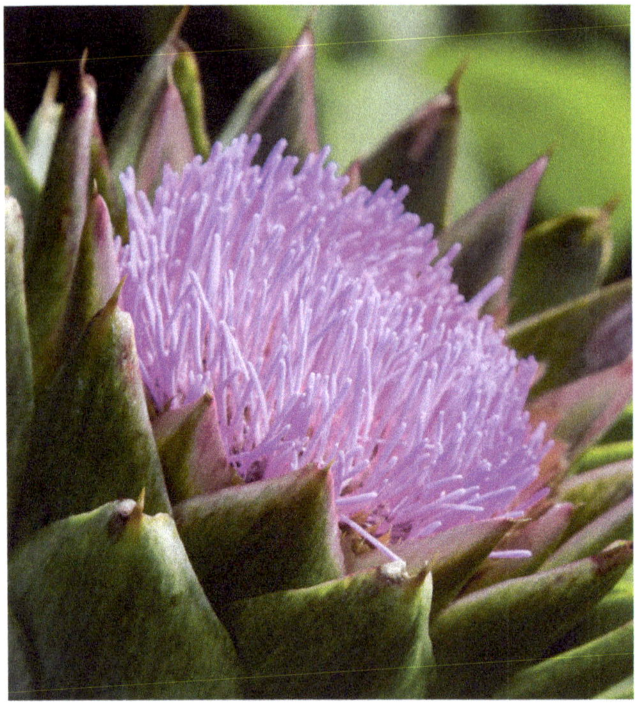

Eclectic physicians used artichoke leaves as a depurative and diuretic medicine to treat jaundice, gout, rheumatism, dropsy, and tic-douloureux. In Europe, the leaves were valued for their choleretic, cholagogue, laxative, and diuretic actions. Extracts and teas were used to clear the complexion, stimulate the appetite, and treat nephrosclerosis, urinary stones, uremia, arthritis, hepatic insufficiency, and hypercholesterolemia.[1,8]

Artichoke is the primary flavor of the Italian liqueur, Cynar. It can be served as an aperitif or cocktail mixed with citrus juice. Cynar is also used to make Cin-cyn, a slightly less bitter version of the Negroni cocktail.

CONSTITUENTS: Artichoke leaf contains *o*-diphenolic derivatives (caffeic acid, 1-, 3-, 4-, and 5-caffeoylquinic acids, 1,5-di-O-caffeoylquinic acid = cynarin, and 1,3-di-O-caffeoylquinic acid), flavonoids (glycosides: luteolin-7-β-rutinoside = scolymoside, luteolin-7-β-D-glucoside, and 4-β-D-glucoside), glycolic and glyceric acids, taraxasterol, ϒ-taraxasterol, inulin, guaianolides (grosheimin, cynaropicrin, and 8-epigrosheimin), cynaratriol, sugars, enzymes, and volatile oil (β-selinene, caryophyllene, α-cadrene, oct-1-en-3-one, hex-1-en-3-one, decanal, non-strans-2-enal, phenylacetaldehyde, and eugenol).[9] The active principles are cynarin, 1,3-dicaffeoylquinic acid, 3-caffeoylquinic acid = chlorogenic acid, and scolymoside.[9] The cynaropicrin content is highest just before the inflorescence appears or the seed matures.[10]

Artichoke leaves provide the highest concentration of active ingredients, such as caffeoylquinic acids = cynarin; however, these compounds are also found in lower concentrations in the bracts and hearts. Globe artichokes also contain inulin (not to be confused with insulin). Inulin is a polysaccharide that encourages the growth of beneficial bacteria in the lower digestive tract. Globe artichokes must be eaten shortly after harvesting, or the inulin will convert to other sugars when the artichokes are stored for any length of time, negating the blood sugar-lowering effects.[7]

NUTRITIONAL PROPERTIES: The nutritional properties of artichoke leaf are unknown; however, fresh globe artichoke contains dietary fiber, magnesium, chromium, vitamin C, folic acid, biotin, and manganese. It also contains moderate amounts of niacin, riboflavin, thiamine, vitamin A, and potassium. Globe artichoke is low calorie, low fat, cholesterol-free, low carbohydrate, and a source of dietary fiber.[7]

MEDICINAL PROPERTIES: Bitter tonic, cholagogue, choleretic, hepatic detoxifier, hepatoprotectant, hepatoregenerative, hypolipidemic, hypotriglyceridemic, laxative, antioxidant, and diuretic (mild).

TEMPERATURE AND FLAVOR: Cool and bitter.

MEDICINAL USES

Artichoke leaf is an impressive medicine for a variety of digestive complaints. The leaves are a bitter tonic that stimulate digestive secretions from the gallbladder and pancreas.[11] Consuming the extract, tea, or expressed juice one-half hour before meals improves the digestion of dietary proteins, fats, and carbohydrates. Artichoke leaf can be used as a bitter tonic for treating sluggish digestion, atonic dyspepsia, belching, nausea, flatulence, bloating, constipation, and fat intolerance.[1,11,12] The bitter principle, cynaropicrin, is a sesquiterpene lactone. The cynaropicrin content is highest just before the plant flowers and after the fruit ripens (globe artichoke). It is rated 11,500 on the *Bitter Index*.[12]

Artichoke leaf supports healthy liver function, enhancing liver detoxification and decreasing liver stagnation. The liver-detoxifying actions aid in treating acne, eczema, and other skin conditions. Artichoke leaf is a long-term treatment for conditions such as hepatitis and jaundice. Tea or capsule preparations are recommended for individuals with compromised liver function or liver disease.

Numerous studies confirm the hepatoprotective and hepatorestorative actions of artichoke leaf. Cynarin was found to be more protective than milk thistle *(Silybum marianum)* against the toxin galactosamine, but less active than milk thistle for carbon tetrachloride (CCl_4) damage. However, cynarin and caffeic acid have significant hepatoprotective actions against CCl_4 *in vivo.* Water-soluble extracts have antioxidant and protective actions against hydroperoxide-induced oxidative stress in the liver (according to rodent studies). Chlorogenic acid and cynarin are the antioxidants, although other unidentified constituents likely contribute to this effect.

Artichoke leaf has choleretic and cholagogue effects that stimulate bile production in the liver and bile excretion from the gallbladder, respectively.[11] It improves biliary excretion of cholesterol, lowering cholesterol levels, and reducing fatty liver.[11] Cynarin is attributed to the cholagogue effects. Artichoke leaf also decreases the hepatic synthesis of cholesterol and inhibits LDL oxidation, lowering hepatic and serum cholesterol and triglyceride levels.[11] Luteolin and cynaroside are the key components inducing these actions.[1,12] Artichoke leaf extracts improve endothelial cell function, enhancing the cells lining the arteries. Endothelial cell dysfunction represents the first stage of atherosclerosis; thus, artichoke leaf exhibits multiple modes of action as an antiatherosclerotic.[7]

The cholagogue actions improve cholesterol elimination, supporting weight loss. They also increase bile secretion, enhancing fat digestion, aiding liver detoxification, and providing gentle laxative effects. The cholagogue effects prevent gallstone formation and aid in eliminating gallstones, treating cholestasis and cholethiasis. The choleretic effects aid digestion and decrease symptoms of nausea, dyspepsia, and bloating in patients who have had their gallbladder removed.

Long-term use of artichoke leaf stimulates intestinal immune function.[10] The caffeoylquinic acids demonstrate activity against the human immunodeficiency virus (HIV). These compounds inhibit the HIV integrase enzyme that is critical for replicating the virus.[1,7]

Artichoke leaf has mild diuretic actions. Folkloric uses as a diuretic aid were confirmed in studies in which cynarin injections stimulated diuresis and the excretion of water or saline load. The leaf also antagonized the action of an antidiuretic hormone contained in a posterior pituitary extract. In a clinical trial, *Cynara* extract stimulated diuresis in patients with ascites caused by portal stasis.[1]

CONTRAINDICATIONS

Artichoke leaf may cause contact dermatitis in individuals hypersensitive to the daisy family (Asteraceae). Due to the cholagogue properties, avoid use with biliary obstruction. When used in the suggested dose range, there are no reported side effects. There are no known drug interactions.

PREPARATION AND DOSAGE

TINCTURE: Fresh leaves [1:2-1:3, 70-95% alcohol]; dry leaves [1:5, 60% alcohol]; consume 30-60 drops, up to three times daily.

ACETUM EXTRACT: Fresh leaves [1:2-1:3, apple cider vinegar]; dry [1:5, apple cider vinegar]; consume 30-60 drops, up to three times daily.

CAPSULES: Consume 2-3 "00" capsules, one to three times daily.

TEA: Prepare a hot infusion; consume 4-8 ounces, up to four times daily.

CULINARY USE: In some countries, artichoke stalks are steamed and consumed. The young leaves may be steamed and consumed in small quantities; they have a buttery, bitter flavor. The leaves and stalks become more fibrous with age.

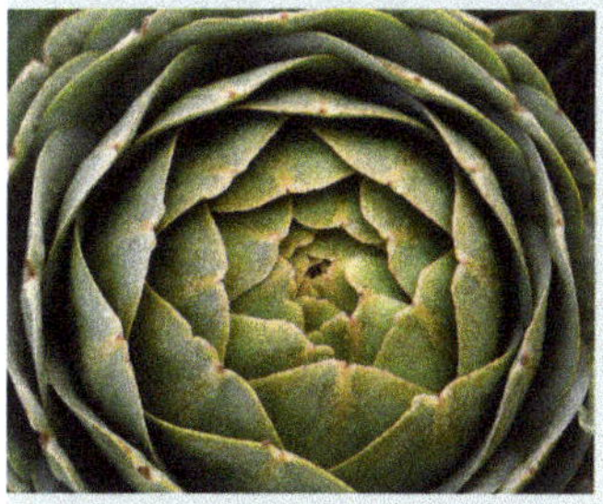

Globe artichokes can be prepared by cutting off the top portion to remove the sharp, inedible leaf tips, and trimming the outer leaves. Before cooking, cut the stem flush at the base. To steam artichokes, stand trimmed artichoke stems down in a vegetable steamer or cook in boiling water. Adding two tablespoons of lemon juice or vinegar to the water prevents darkening of the artichoke. Simmer in a covered pot 30 to 40 minutes, or until some inner leaves can be easily removed. Pressure cooking artichokes reduces the cooking time to 10 to 15 minutes. After they are cooked, invert the artichokes and drain for a few minutes. Dip them in lemon-garlic-butter, a creamy sauce, or stuff and bake them.

ASHWAGANDHA

DESCRIPTION

BOTANICAL NAME:
Withania somnifera

COMMON NAMES:
Ashwagandha, turragi, Indian ginseng, winter cherry
ashvaganda (German)
asgandh, varahakarni, vrisha (Hindi)
asva-gandha (Sanskrit)
ubuvimbha (Zulu)

FAMILY NAME:
Solanaceae

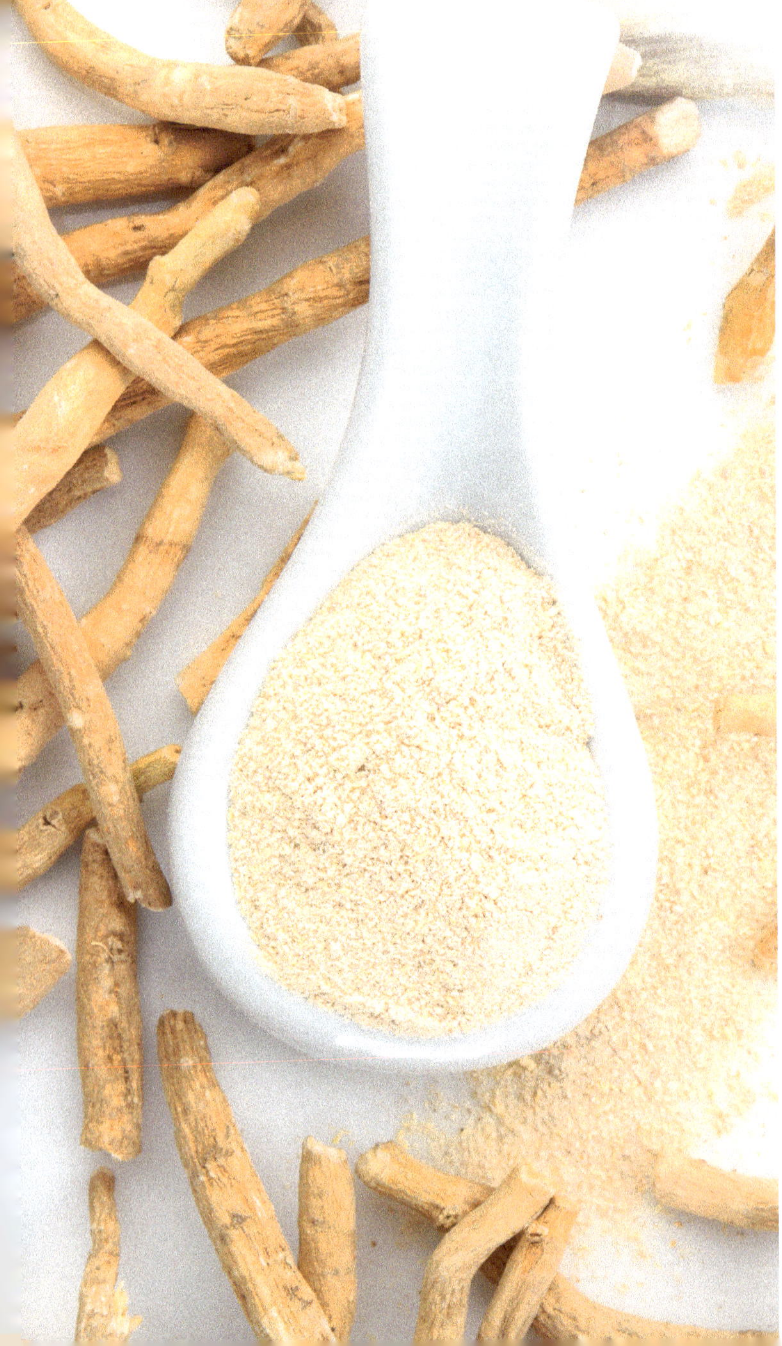

PART USED: The roots.

BOTANICAL DESCRIPTION AND HABITAT: Ashwagandha is a perennial shrub that becomes woody at the base as it ages, while the newer growth remains herbaceous.[1] The erect shrub grows 30 – 150 cm tall.[1] The tomentose stems and branches produce alternate leaves (4 – 12 cm long by 2 – 9 cm wide) on short petioles.[2] The elliptic leaves have a tapering base, an acute apex, and an entire or slightly wavy margin.[2] The upper surface of the leaf is glabrescent, with a somewhat hairier mid-vein; the underside is pubescent.[1]

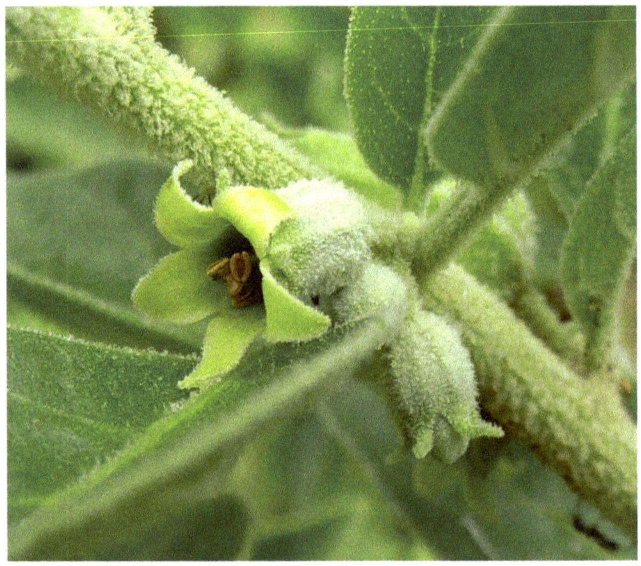

The small sessile, greenish-yellow flowers are arranged in small axillary clusters.[2] The campanulate calyx is densely covered in stellate hairs, and has five acute teeth.[3] The tomentose corolla is more narrowly campanulate with five triangular lobes. Within the corolla are five yellow anthers and two fused carpels with an exserted style.[2] The flower develops into a small scarlet red, globose berry (5 – 8 mm) that is loosely enclosed within the persistent, globose, brown, papery calyx.[3] The berry yields many small yellowish, kidney-shaped seeds.[3,4]

THE NAME: *Withania* is named for Henry Witham (1830), British geologist and fossil botanist. The epithet *somnifera* refers to the sedating qualities of the root. Ashwagandha ("the smell of a horse") refers either to the aroma of the fresh root that resembles the scent of a horse's urine, or because the root increases a horse's sexual stamina.[5] Two

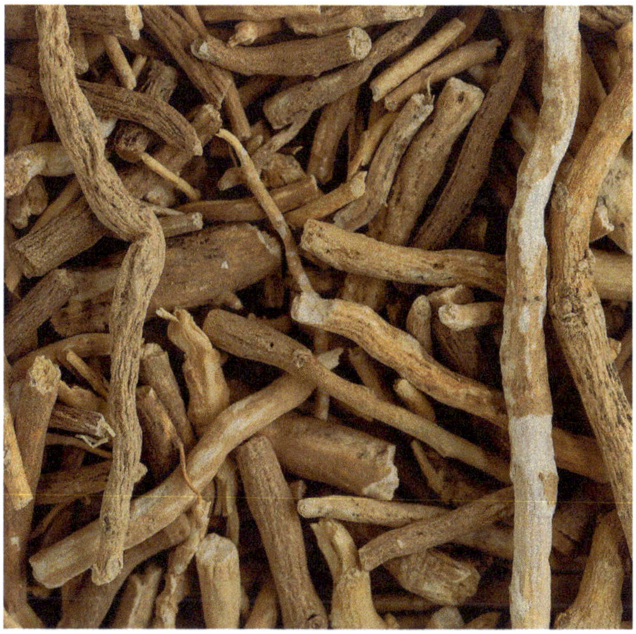

other meanings of the Hindu names include varahakarni ("boar-eared") and vrisha ("amorous").[5]

HISTORICAL USES: Ashwagandha was administered as a nourishing, building, and repleting tonic for weak, emaciated individuals with musculoskeletal or nervous system disorders (high vāta).[5] The herb was given to weak children, and for depletion from nervous exhaustion or insomnia.[6] It also was administered as a uterine tonic during pregnancy. Ashwagandha was used for reproductive concerns including infertility, amenorrhea, and low libido, and to increase sexual potency.[5] Traditionally, the root powder was prepared as ghee or decocted in milk with honey or raw sugar to sweeten.

CONSTITUENTS: Ashwagandha contains alkaloids (ashwagandhine, withanine, withasomnine, isopelieteirine, anaferine, and cuskohygrine), steroidal lactones (withanolides: withaferine A and withanolide E), phytosterols (sitoindosides and β-sitosterol), polyphenolic flavonoids, antioxidant enzymes (superoxide dismutase and glutathione peroxidase), saponins, and iron.[5,7]

NUTRITIONAL PROPERTIES: Ashwagandha contains iron and flavonoids.

MEDICINAL PROPERTIES: Adaptogen, anti-inflammatory, analgesic, antitumor, aphrodisiac, immune modulator, nervine, reproductive tonic, sedative (mild), trophorestorative, and diuretic (mild).

TEMPERATURE AND FLAVOR: Warm, bitter, astringent, and sweet.

MEDICINAL USES

Ashwagandha is an adaptogen that modifies the hypothalamic-pituitary-adrenal axis treating individuals with chronic stress. It is a subtle nervine and trophorestorative agent that restores healthy nervous system function and supports adrenal function. It is highly beneficial for individuals depleted from overwork, lack of sleep, nervous exhaustion, or hypervigilance.[5,7] Ashwagandha has a calming effect, reducing anxiety, palpitations, neurosis, hyperactivity, and attention deficit hyperactivity disorder (ADHD).[5,7] Fatty-based, nourishing preparations such as medicated ghee, milk, or almond milk are the most effective for supporting the nervous, musculoskeletal, and reproductive systems.[5]

Ashwagandha is an anti-inflammatory and mild analgesic, reducing musculoskeletal pain and inflammation.[5] Long-term use aids in treating myalgia, painful joints, rheumatoid arthritis, and osteoarthritis. It is an excellent adjunct therapy for fibromyalgia, chronic muscular fatigue, multiple sclerosis, lupus, and other chronic debilities of the nervous system, muscles, and joints.[5] It enhances anabolic functions, increasing muscle weight and tone for recovering anorexics, weak, convalescing emaciated children or adults, and athletes in training.[5] The withanolides account for the anti-inflammatory effects.[7]

Ashwagandha is an immune modulator, enhancing immune function and suppressing inflammation. It increases vitality and supports immune function in individuals recovering from chemotherapy or chronic illness. Long-term use is recommended as an immune tonic and preventative agent for seasonal allergies, allergic rhinitis, cough, and asthma.[5] Ashwagandha stimulates white blood cell counts. The withanolides exhibit immune modulating, antibacterial, and antitumor effects.[7]

Consumed on a long-term basis, ashwagandha is an aphrodisiac that increases libido, as well as sexual potency and performance.[5,7] It improves circulation to the reproductive organs. In males, this herb improves sperm count and sperm motility.[5] In females, ashwagandha tonifies uterine muscles and warms the womb, treating amenorrhea, dysmenorrhea, and sexual atony.[5] It is also a restorative sexual tonic following a difficult birth.

Ashwagandha is an effective adjunct for treating hypothyroidism.[5] It improves circulation and reduces inflammation of weak muscles and joints. It supports the adrenal glands, as well as the nervous, immune, and reproductive systems.

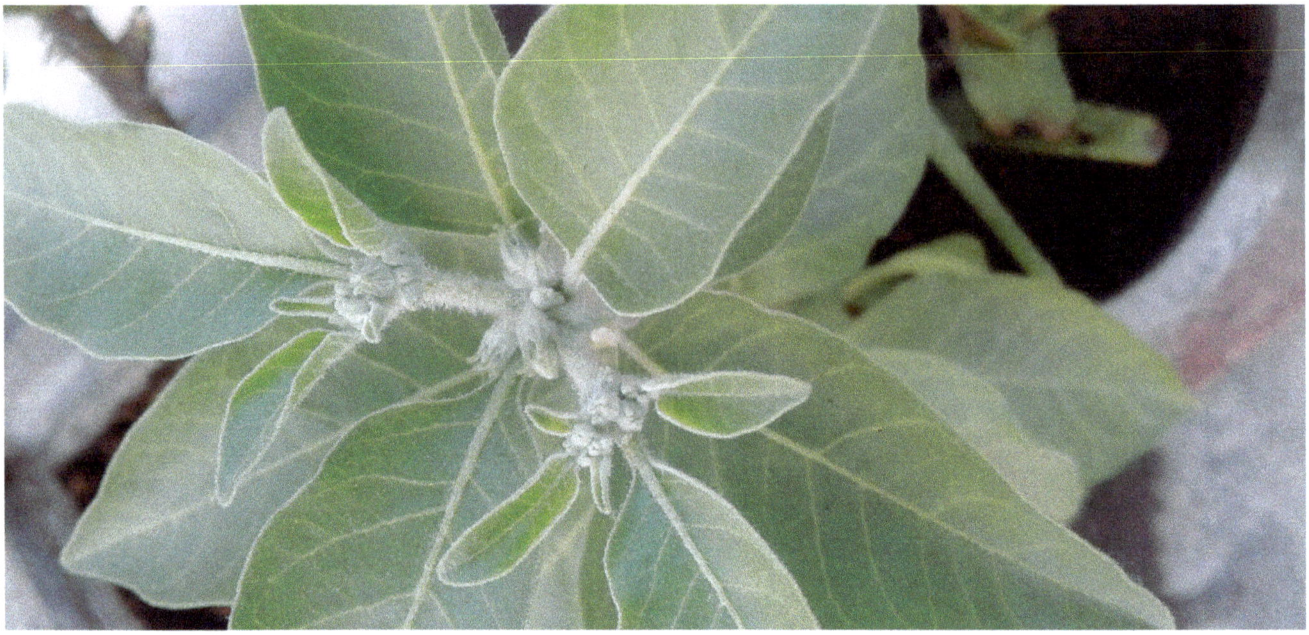

CONTRAINDICATIONS

Although this herb is traditionally administered during pregnancy as a uterine tonic, some sources cautiously affirm its use during pregnancy due to the spasmolytic actions and high iron levels; other sources completely contraindicate use during pregnancy.[5,7] Use caution or avoid in individuals with Solanaceae allergies or sensitivities. Consult a health care practitioner, or avoid use in individuals consuming thyroid hormones, sedatives, or hypnotic medications.[7] Otherwise, there are no known drug-herb interactions.[5,7]

PREPARATION AND DOSAGE

TINCTURE: Fresh roots [1:2, 70-95% alcohol]; dry roots [1:5, 50-60% alcohol]; consume 15-60 drops, up to three times daily.

CAPSULES: Consume 2-4 "00" capsules, one to three times daily.

TEA: Prepare a decoction or cold infusion; consume 8-12 ounces, up to three times daily. Ayurvedic practitioners recommend cooking the powder in diluted milk, or mixing it in hot water.

HONEY AND SYRUP: Prepare a medicated honey and consume 1 tablespoon, one to three times daily.

TOPICAL USE: The plant is applied externally as a poultice for swellings and boils.[7]

CULINARY USE: Consume ½ teaspoon to 1 tablespoon of infused (medicated) ghee or oil, one to three times daily. Consume 4-8 ounces of infused milk, almond milk, or medicated ghee, one to three times daily.

ASPARAGUS

DESCRIPTION

BOTANICAL NAMES:
Asparagus cochinchinensis, A. lucidus, A. racemosus, A. officinalis

COMMON NAMES:
Asparagus tuber, wild asparagus, Chinese asparagus, Indian asparagus, garden asparagus, sparrow grass, hundred-rooted vine, longevity vine
tin dung (Cantonese)
asparge (French)
sahansarmuli, satavar, shatavar, shatavri (Hindi)
tenmendo (Japanese)
chunmundong, chung moon dong (Korean)
tian men dong, tien men dong, tian dong, tien men tong (Mandarin)
satamule, sataavarii (Nepali)
satāvarí, shatavari, sahasravirya, challagadda (Sanskrit)
esparrago (Spanish)
chuang khruea, sam sip (Thai)
mang tay (Vietnamese)

FAMILY NAME:
Liliaceae

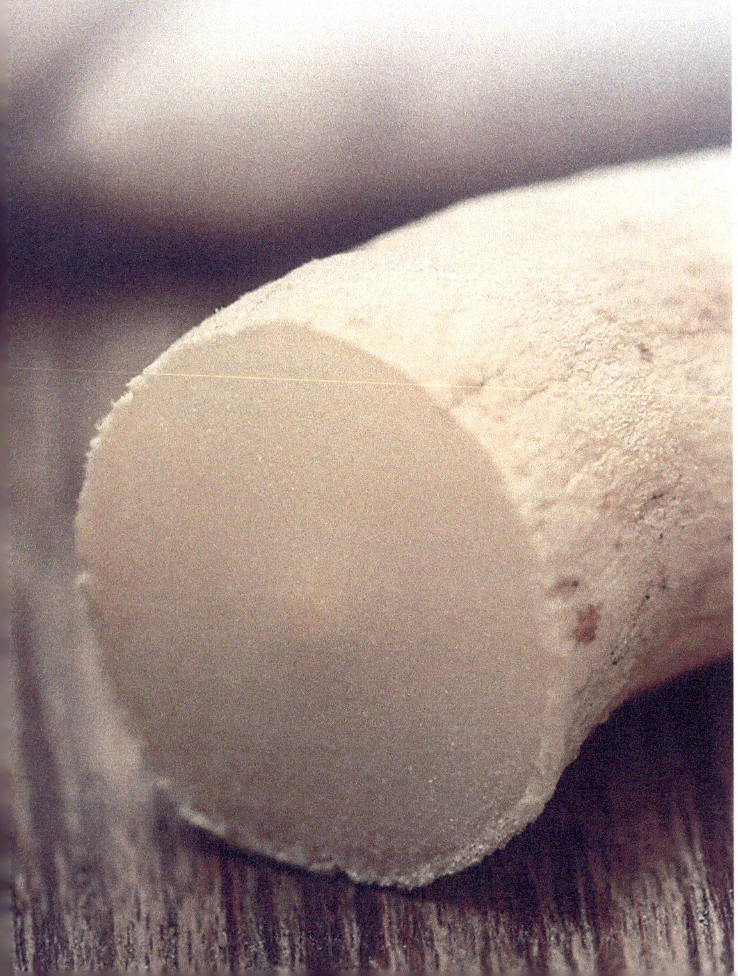

PART USED: The tubers.

BOTANICAL DESCRIPTION AND HABITAT: *Asparagus* is a large genus of perennial herbs (160 – 300 species) with photosynthetic, climbing, or erect branched stems. The plant has rhizomes or fleshy white tubers.[1] Clusters of leaf-like stems (cladodes) grow at branch axils, giving the plant a fluffy appearance.[1] They are narrow, flat, and have spurs at their bases that can be spiny.[2] The true leaves are the small, membranous, scale-like structures pressed along the stem.[3]

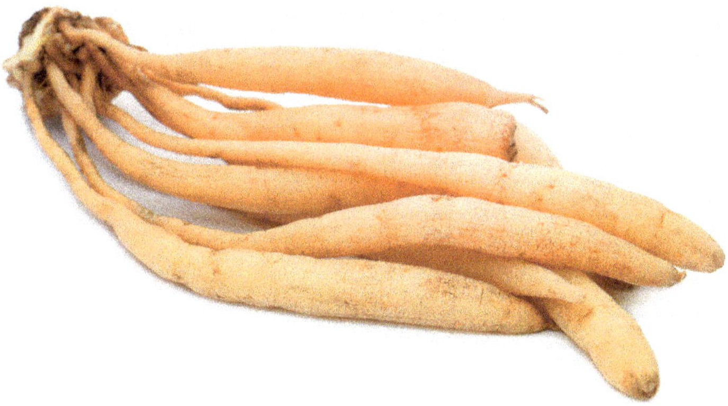

Asparagus species can be dioecious or hermaphroditic.[2] Flowers grow in auxiliary racemes or umbels.[1] The green, yellow, or white campanulate tepals are free or fused at their bases.[1] The perianth contains six epipetalous stamens and three fused carpels, with a single style that splits into three branches.[2] The ovary develops into a red, green, or purple-black berry with one to six black seeds.[1]

Asparagus cochinchinensis is a dioecious herb featuring climbing stems with somewhat woody bases (1 – 2 meters high), and thick, succulent tubers (3 – 5 cm long by 1 – 2 cm wide).[4] The slightly hooked, flat cladodes grow in fascicles of three (0.5 – 8 cm long by 1 – 2 cm wide).[4] The spurs on the leaves are sometimes spiny.[4] The flowers are paired and produce green berries with one to two seeds.[4]

Asparagus racemosus has woody, vining stems (up to 2 meters tall).[5] They die back to the ground each year, and grow clusters of thick, tuberous, whitish-beige roots. The flat, linear cladodes grow in fascicle clusters of three to eight (1 – 2.5 cm long by 1 mm wide).[5] The leaves have a

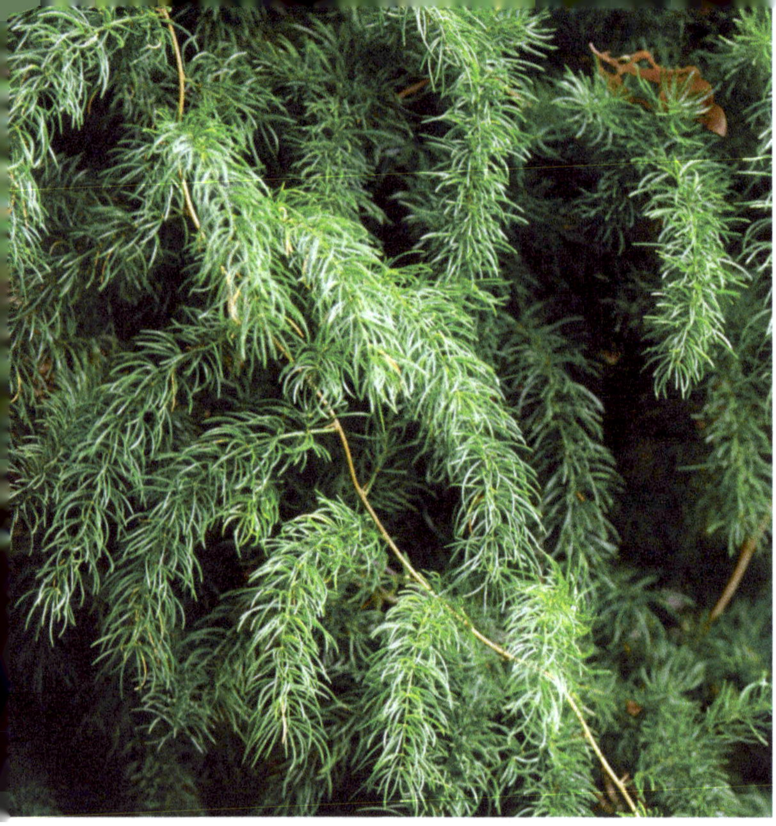

straight, sharp, spiny spur. The inflorescence is a raceme or panicle with many bisexual flowers (1 – 8 cm long).[6] The flowers consist of a white, campanulate perianth with short stamens bearing tiny yellow anthers.[7] The plant produces purple-black berries.[7]

THE NAME: The genus and common name *Asparagus* derives from the Greek *asparagos,* referring to the tender, edible shoots.[8] The epithet *racemosus* refers to plants "with flowers in racemes."[9] The epithet *lucidus* means "glossy, clear, or shiny."[10] The epithet *cochinchinensis* derives from Cochinchina, the former name for a French colony in Vietnam.[11]

The common names of *Asparagus racemosus* include śatāvarí, shatavari, shatavar, and wild asparagus.[12] *A. cochinchinensis* and *A. lucidus* are commonly referred to as tian men dong, tian dong, tien men tong, chung moon dong, and asparagus tuber.[13] Garden asparagus is the common name associated with *A. officinalis.* Tian men dong means "lush winter aerial plant."[13] Shatavari translates as "one hundred roots;" however, because of its use as a reproductive tonic, it is commonly referred to as "the woman who has a hundred husbands."[12]

HISTORICAL USES: In Asia, asparagus tuber *(A. cochinchinensis* and *A. lucidus)* was used by holy men to open the heart, develop unconditional love, and generate shen (spirit).[14] It also was used to strengthen the mind and tonify the kidneys.[14] Asparagus tuber was administered to treat parasitic diseases.[15] The seeds were used as contraceptives. The shoots were incorporated into skin-cleansing preparations to wash the face and dry up pimples and sores.[15]

Asparagus tuber *(A. racemosus)* was first described as a potent rasayana in two important religious texts, the *Rig Veda* and *Atharvaveda.*[16] It was administered to maintain youthfulness, increase physical strength, and improve memory and intelligence.[16] Asparagus tuber was used as a fertility tonic, pregnancy tonic, aphrodisiac, and galactagogue. It was also given to calm the nervous system, reduce spasms and inflammation, and treat liver disease.

A. officinalis tubers were used as diuretics for rheumatism, gravel, and dropsy.[15,17] They were also used as laxatives.[15] The roasted seeds were used as a coffee substitute. [15] Native to the Mediterranean, asparagus tender shoots were prized by the Greeks and Romans as a vegetable.[17] It was cultivated as early as 200 BCE.[17] Nicholas Culpeper recommended decocting the roots in wine to improve vision and nourish sinews "shrunk by cramps and convulsions."[17]

CONSTITUENTS: *Asparagus cochinchinensis* contains asparagines, citruline, serine, threonine, proline, clyccine, β-sitosterol, smilagenin, 5-methoxymethylfurfural, and rhamnose.[13] *A. racemosus* tuber contains alkaloids (asparagamine), saponin steroidal glycosides (shatavarins I-IV, sarasapogenin, and diosgenin), immune stimulating polysaccharides, proteins, tannins, bioflavonoids, B vitamins, calcium, and zinc.[12,16,18] *A. officinalis* tuber contains inulin and eight fructo-oligosaccharides, two bitter glycosides (officinalisnin-I and officinalisnin-II), β-sitosterol, sarsapogenin, nine steroidal glycosides (asparagosides A-I), a phenol glycoside (coniferin), minerals (rich in potassium), amino acids (asparagine), and asparagusic acid.[15,19]

NUTRITIONAL PROPERTIES: Asparagus tuber contains high amounts of chromium, fiber, niacin, phosphorus, potassium, protein, riboflavin, thiamine, bioflavonoids, vitamins A and C, and zinc. It contains low to average amounts of calcium, fat, magnesium, manganese, selenium, and sodium.[18,20]

MEDICINAL PROPERTIES: Adaptogen, anti-inflammatory, aphrodisiac, cardiotonic, demulcent, diuretic, expectorant, female reproductive tonic, galactagogue, immune modulator, laxative, shen tonic, spermatogenic, antibacterial, antihemorrhagic, anticarcinogenic, antipyretic, anthelmintic, and mild smooth muscle relaxant.

TEMPERATURE AND FLAVOR: Cold, sweet, and bitter.

MEDICINAL USES

Asparagus tuber has soothing demulcent properties that reduce inflammation of mucous membranes in the lungs, stomach, intestines, kidneys, and reproductive organs.[21] It aids in treating painful inflammatory conditions in the digestive tract, including acid indigestion, gastric esophageal reflux, gastritis, gastric ulcers, colitis, Crohn's disease, and dysentery with bleeding.[12] The demulcent actions also reduce bleeding caused by inflammation in the digestive tract.[12] Asparagus tuber is used to treat constipation due to yin deficiency. Combine with sheng di huang (unprepared *Rehmannia*), dong quai *(Angelica sinensis),* and huo ma ren *(Cannabis seed)* to treat constipation.[13]

Asparagus tuber has a moistening effect in the lungs. In Traditional Chinese Medicine, it is used to generate fluids, nourishing lung and kidney yin.[13,14] Asparagus tuber aids in treating lung yin deficiency and clearing lung heat. The symptoms of lung yin deficiency with heat signs include: a dry mouth, thirst, thick or blood-streaked mucus that is difficult to swallow or expectorate, and a low grade fever in the afternoon.[13] Asparagus tuber improves the lungs' ability to extract qi from the air; therefore, individuals consuming asparagus long-term experience deepened respiration.[14] It is often combined with mai men dong *(Ophiopogon)* to treat yin deficiency. Asparagus tuber can also be combined with American ginseng *(Panax quinquefolius)* and shu di huang *(Rehmannia glutinosa)* to treat debility and low grade fever resulting from yin deficiency following a febrile disease or severe illness.[13]

In Ayurvedic medicine, asparagus tuber is considered a premier female reproductive and uterine tonic.[12,21] The herb is known as "she who possesses a hundred husbands," and is administered as a fertility tonic to increase reproductive fluids and enhance conception.[12] Ayurvedic practitioner Dr. Vasant Lad claims that it "nourishes the ovum and increases fertility," and increases seminal fluids in men.[21] Asparagus tuber is used to prevent a miscarriage and as a pregnancy tonic.[12] It is administered to regulate menstrual conditions aggravated by excess heat *(pitta),* treating concerns such as dysmenorrhea, menorrhagia, and amenorrhea.[12] Asparagus tuber increases breast milk flow, especially when the mother is dehydrated or depleted following childbirth.[12,21] It is an effective tonic for treating menopausal symptoms, including hot flashes, night sweats, irritability, vaginal dryness, dry skin, and poor memory.[12] In Traditional Chinese Medicine, it nourishes kidney yin, and is a long-term tonic for frigidity and impotence.[13,14] Symptoms of kidney yin deficiency include: dizziness, tinnitus, lower back weakness, low libido, scant urination,

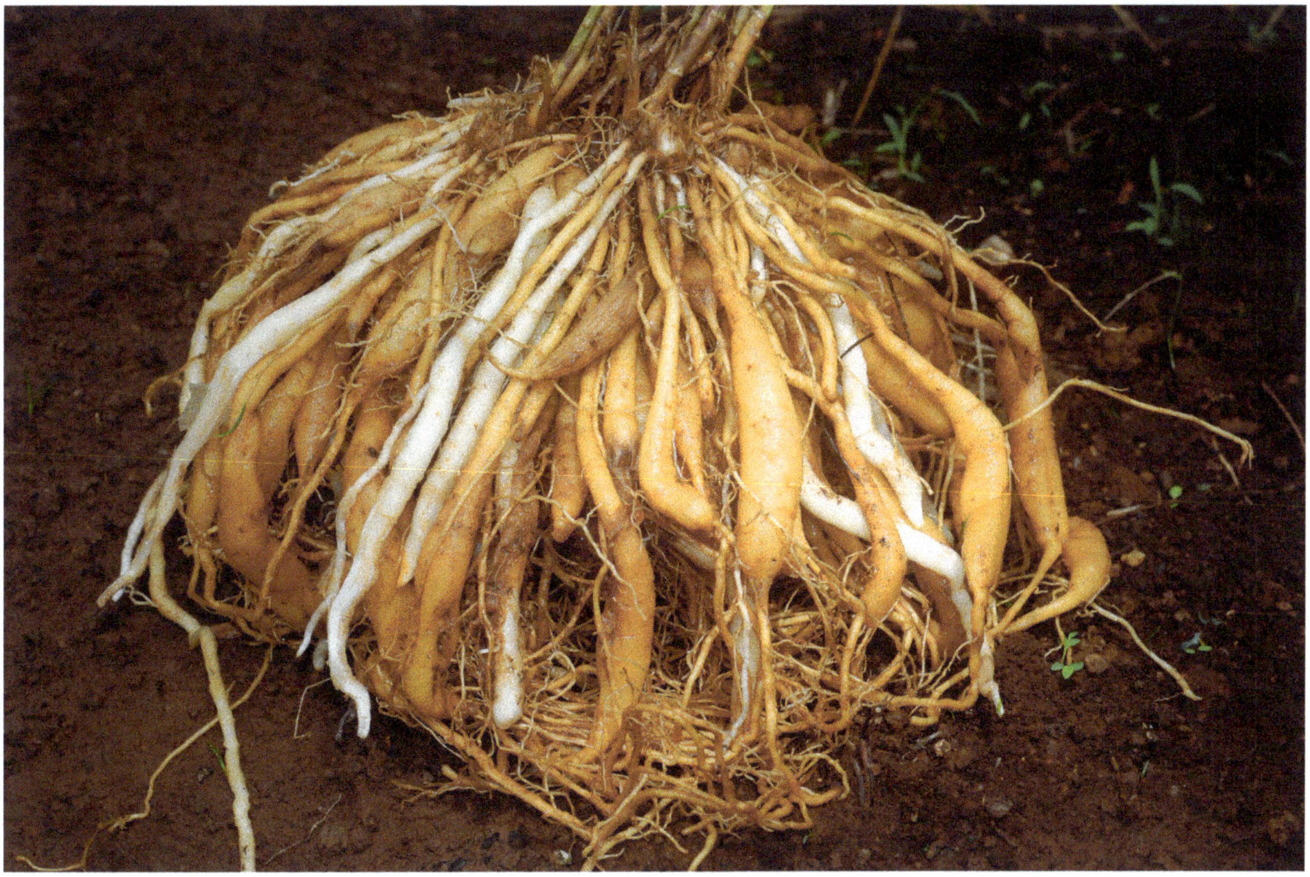

and dry, red tongue.[13] It is also used to treat kidney yin deficiency with heat signs. Indications include symptoms of kidney yin deficiency, as well as dry mouth, red cheeks, red lips, hot palms and soles, palpitations, night sweats, nocturnal emissions, urinary retention, constipation, and rapid, weak pulse.[22]

Asparagus tuber enhances the skin's softness and suppleness.[14] It is moistening and heat-clearing for hot, dry skin conditions such as eczema, psoriasis, and dehydrated or flaky skin. External applications treat dry skin, stiff joints, stiff neck, and muscle spasms.[21]

Asparagus tuber generates shen — the spirit that resides in the heart. Long-term use calms the heart and balances emotions, "allowing love to rule one's nature."[14] It aids in developing peace, strength of mind, and a good memory, in addition to preventing the negative effects of stress. Asparagus tuber calms the nerves, nourishes the brain, and reduces insomnia and spasms.[12] Consuming the herb long-term is said to lead to happiness, encourage a mild manner, and lift the spirits.[14]

Asparagus tuber has immune modulating and anti-inflammatory actions. Research demonstrates that it has antineoplastic effects *in vitro* against the deoxygenase of leukemic cells in acute lymphocytic, chronic granulocytic, and acute mononuclear leukemic cell populations.[13] In animal studies, extracts enhanced Th1 and Th2 immunity.[18] In rodent studies, it inhibited inflammatory cytokines including interleukin 1β and tumor necrosis factor α.[18] Asparagus tuber hastens recovery from chemotherapy, and counters the negative effects of radiation, especially when patterns of yin deficiency prevail.[12]

Asparagus tuber has bacteriostatic effects against *Streptococcus pneumonia, Staphylococcus aureus,* hemolytic *Streptococcus,* and members of the *Bacillus subtilis* group.[13] It is also active against *Entamoeba histolytica.*[12] However, it is not used in Ayurvedic or Traditional Chinese Medicine to treat acute infections.

Asparagus officinalis tuber is primarily a diuretic and laxative with less demulcent (yin tonifying) properties than *A. cochinchinensis* and *A. racemosus.*[15] Drinking the tea flushes the kidneys and aids in passing kidney stones and urinary gravel.[19] A diuretic, it reduces urinary tract inflammation, aids in treating urinary tract infections, and prevents relapses. It aids in treating sodium-related hypertension.[15] The diuretic and antidyscratic properties provide an adjunct therapy for chronic eczema and rheumatic conditions.[19]

CONTRAINDICATIONS

Because asparagus tuber is cooling and moistening, it is generally avoided when excessive mucus or an acute cough or cold is present. It is also contraindicated with an acute digestive infection, acute diarrhea, loss of appetite, or sluggish digestive function (cold from spleen and stomach deficiency). *Asparagus officinalis* should be avoided with obstructive urinary stones, edema due to impaired heart or kidney function, or kidney inflammation.[19]

PREPARATION AND DOSAGE

TINCTURE: Fresh roots [1:2-1:3, 60-70% alcohol]; dry roots [1:5, 50-60% alcohol]; consume 30-90 drops in water, up to three times daily.

FLUID EXTRACT: Dry roots [1:1, 40% alcohol]; consume 30-60 drops, up to three times daily.

CAPSULES: Consume 2-4 capsules, up to three times daily; consume 4-8 tea pills, up to three times daily. Standardized extract: [10:1] >20% saponins; consume 2-3 grams, up to three times daily.

TEA: Prepare a decoction or cold infusion; consume 8-12 ounces, three to four times daily. Add 3 grams of powder to one cup of hot milk; consume 6-8 ounces, up to three times daily.

TOPICAL USE: Apply the poultice, fomentation, or paste, one to three times daily.

CULINARY USE: Add ¼-1 teaspoon in hot water, tea, milk decoctions, or fresh vegetable or fruit juice, one to three times daily. Consume 1 teaspoon of medicated ghee or milk, up to three times daily.

ASTRAGALUS

DESCRIPTION

BOTANICAL NAMES:
Astragalus membranaceous
(syn. *Astragalus propinquus,*
Astragalus membranaceus var. *mongholicus*)

COMMON NAMES:
Astragalus, milk vetch, yellow vetch, goat's thorn
beg kei (Cantonese)
kurjenherne (Finnish)
ōgi (Japanese)
hwanggi (Korean)
huáng qí, meng gu mo (Mandarin)

FAMILY NAME:
Fabaceae (Leguminosae)

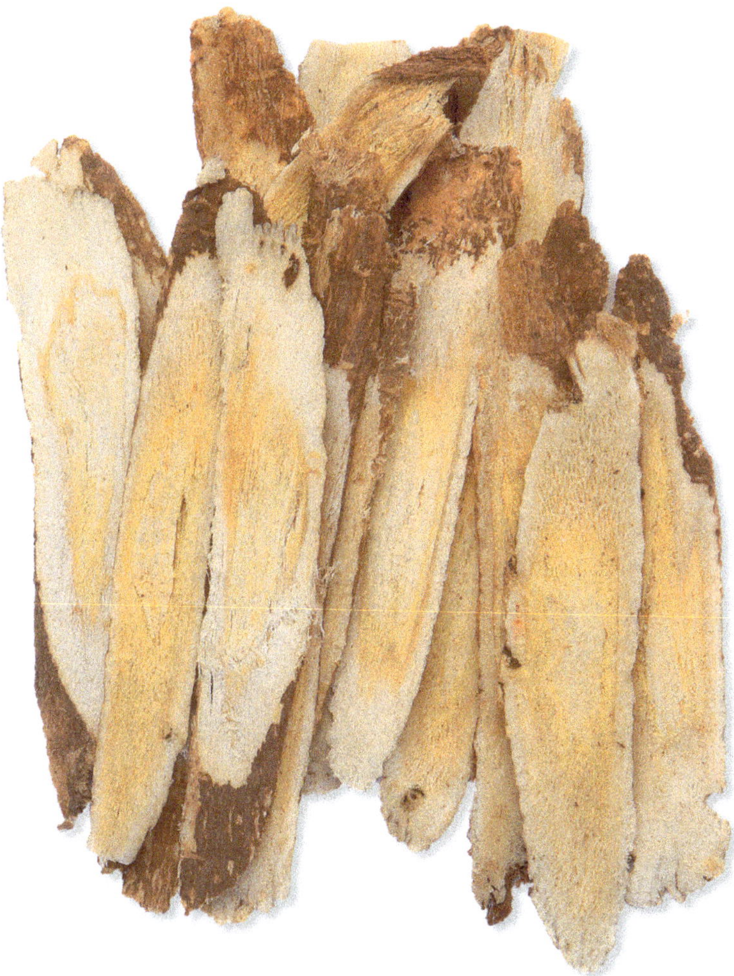

PART USED: The roots.

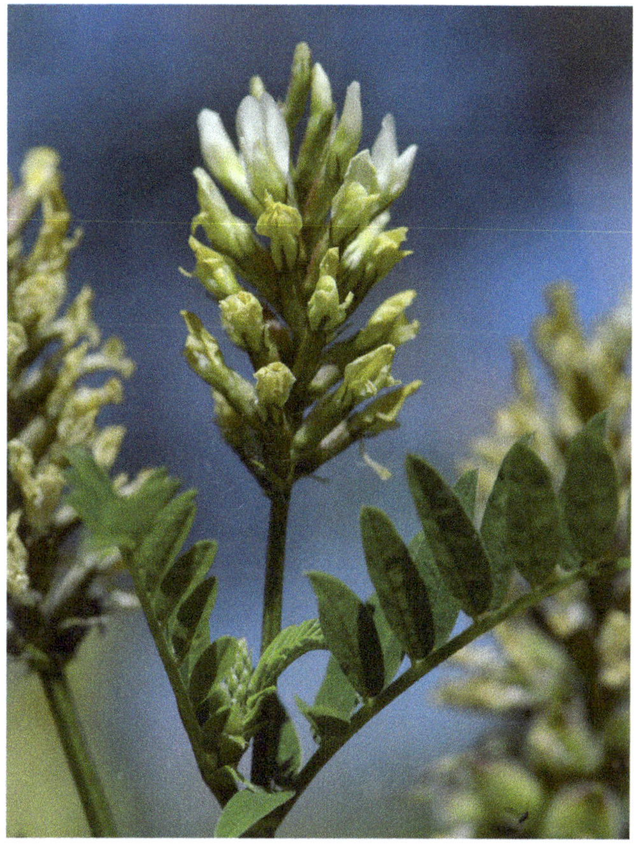

BOTANICAL DESCRIPTION AND HABITAT: *Astragalus membranaceous* grows in meadows and coniferous forests in the mountainous regions and steppes of China, Kazakhstan, Mongolia, and eastern Russia. There are almost 2,000 species of *Astragalus,* many containing indolizine alkaloids that have neurotoxicity in livestock. A common name for many *Astragalus* species is "locoweed."[1,2] *Astragalus membranaceous* does not have this toxicity, and has been safely used in Traditional Chinese Medicine for millennia.[1]

Astragalus is an herbaceous perennial (25 – 60 cm tall.)[3] Most of the plant is covered with long hairs. The deciduous, opposite leaves (6 – 15 cm) are pinnately compound with eight to 12 pairs of narrowly ovate, mostly hairless leaflets (5 – 22 mm long by 3 – 11 mm wide).[3] The nearly sessile leaves have narrowly triangular stipules (up to 1 cm long).[3,4] The racemes, only about 4 – 5 cm long when flowering, can stretch up to 14 cm long when in fruit.[3,4]

They have long peduncles (7 – 13 cm) and bear many yellow, pea-like flowers.[3,4] The bell-shaped calyx (5 – 9 mm) has five lobes and is glabrous or sparsely hairy.[3] The flowers develop into papery legumes (2 – 3 cm long) that can be glabrous or hairy.[3,4]

THE NAME: The genus name *Astragalus* derives from the Greek *Astragalos* ("neck vertebrae"), referring to the vertebrae-like appearance of the flowers. The epithet *membranaceous* means "having a membrane." Huang qi translates as "yellow leader," referring to the roots' use as a superior tonic.[5]

HISTORICAL USES: The medicinal virtues of astragalus, known as huang qi, were recorded more than 2,000 years ago in the *Shen Nong Ben Cao Fing.*[5] Astragalus was combined with *Panax ginseng* to increase vitality and appetite, strengthen resistance, decrease debility, and reduce spontaneous perspiration.[5] It continues to be used as a spleen qi, lung qi, and wei qi tonic. It is also administered to reduce swelling, drain pus, regenerate tissue, and encourage muscle growth.[6]

CONSTITUENTS: Astragalus contains water-soluble polysaccharides (astragalan I- III, AG-1, AG-2, AH-1, and AH-2), D-β-asparagine, 2',4'-dihydroxy-5,6-dimethoxy-isoflavane, triterpene saponins (astragalus saponins I-III, astragalosides I-VIII, acetylastragalosides I, isoastragalosides I and II, astrasieversianin I-XVI, cyclogaleginosides A and B, astramembrannin I and II, and soyasaponin I), amino acids (GABA = gamma-aminobutyric acid), flavonoids (kaempferol, quercetin, isorhamnetin, calycosin, formononetin, rhamnocitrin, kumatakenin, (3R)-2',3'-dihydroxy-7,4-dimethoxy-isoflavone, L-3-hydroxy-9-methoxypterocarpan, (6aR,11aR)-10-hydroxy-3,9-dimethoxypterocarpan, calycosin glucoside, 9,10-dimethoxy-pterocarpan-3-O-β-D-glucoside, and 2'-hydroxy-3',4'dimethoxy-isoflavone-7-O-β-D-glucoside), lignans (lariciresinol and syringaresinol), phytosterols (5-sterol: β-sitosterol), choline, betaine, folic acid, nicotinic acid, glucuronic acid, phenolic acids (ferulic, isoferulic, caffeic, and chlorogenic acids), linoleic and linolenic acids, kumatakenin, sucrose, and coumarins.[6-8]

NUTRITIONAL PROPERTIES: Astragalus contains folic acid, nicotinic acid, choline, betaine, 20 amino acids (asparagine, glutamic acid, canavanine, proline, arginine, β-aminobutyric acid, aspartic acid, alanine, among others), sucrose, linoleic acid, and linolenic acid. The primary trace minerals include iron, magnesium, silicon, and zinc. It contains low to average amounts of chromium, cobalt, copper, molybdenum, phosphorus, potassium, protein, selenium, and sodium.[6,9]

MEDICINAL PROPERTIES: Immune modulator, adaptogen, anti-inflammatory, antioxidant, blood tonic, lung qi tonic, spleen qi tonic, wei qi tonic, hepatoprotectant, cardiotonic, vasodilator, and diuretic (mild).

TEMPERATURE AND FLAVOR: Warm, sweet, and bland.

MEDICINAL USES

Astragalus is an immune modulator that increases resistance to infection.[6,8,10] It can be used as a prophylactic for individuals prone to frequent colds, respiratory infections, or influenza, although it should be discontinued during an acute infection. Astragalus is a restorative agent that repletes the vital force.[5] It increases endurance and stamina, and reduces fatigue and debility.[5,6] Astragalus aids in treating individuals with weakened resistance from

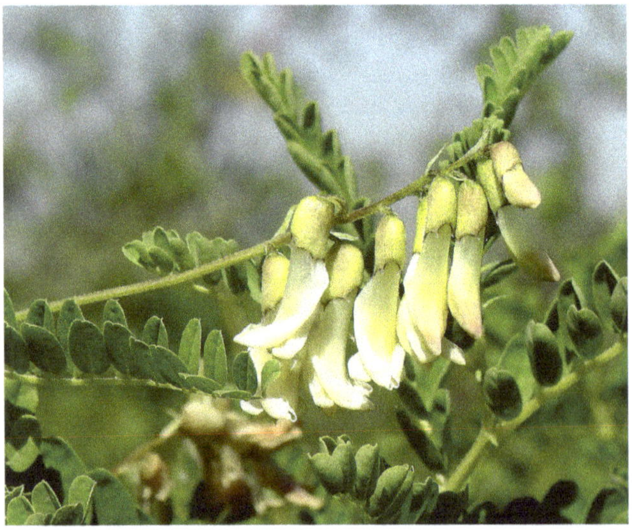

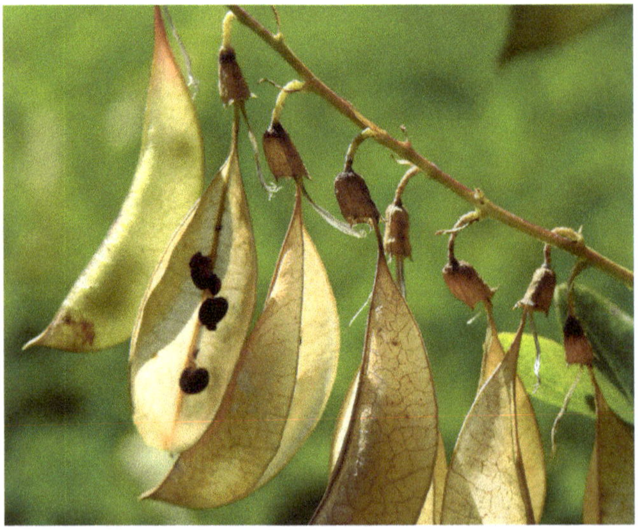

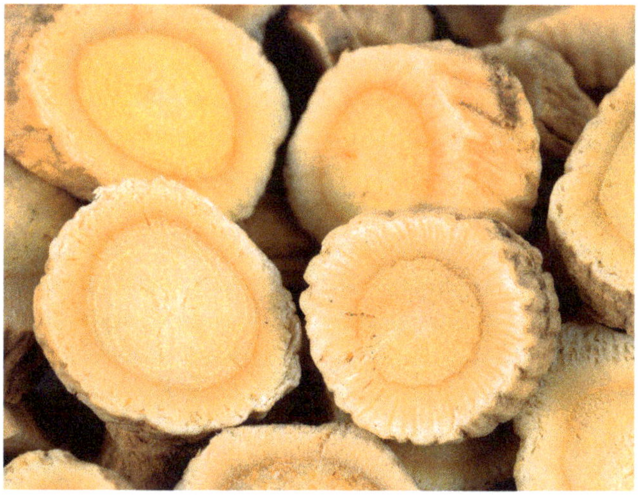

chemotherapy, surgery, lack of sleep, traveling, aging, or a severe infection. It stimulates bone marrow, increasing hematopoiesis and enhancing immune function.[10]

Astragalus is a primary herb included in *fu zheng* therapy — a treatment used to support the immune system in individuals undergoing chemotherapy, radiation, surgery, trauma, or chronic stress.[10] *Fu zheng* therapy improves one's quality of life, enhances overall health and immunity, protects the adrenals, and counteracts the negative side effects of chemotherapy and related medications.[5,10] *Fu zheng* therapy also increases mental clarity, builds the blood, strengthens digestion, and protects the adrenals.

Astragalus has long-term immune supportive properties.[6] It increases natural killer cells (NK), lymphocytes that attack disease-causing organisms.[10] It stimulates macrophages' phagocytic activity, and increases interleukin-2 and interferon production.[8,10] Astragalus stimulates the activity of T-lymphocytes and macrophages, and restores T cell function.[5,8] The immune enhancing actions are attributed to water-soluble polysaccharides.[5,8,10] The lignans contribute to the immune modulating, anti-inflammatory, antibacterial, and antiviral effects.[8]

In Traditional Chinese Medicine, astragalus is known as a superior tonic because it invigorates qi — the vital force. Astragalus strengthens and encourages the movement of wei qi — energy that circulates under the skin and protects the body from the invasion of "pernicious influences" such as wind, heat, cold, and moisture.[7] When the circulation of wei qi is deficient or blocked, environmental influences can penetrate the flesh, causing illness and injury in the blood, flesh, and inner organs. In Western terms, resistance is lowered, increasing susceptibility to infection and environmental allergens.

Astragalus is a qi tonic that aids in treating lung qi, stomach qi, and spleen qi deficiency. Symptoms of lung qi deficiency include: shortness of breath, shallow breathing, dyspnea, pale complexion, and spontaneous sweating.[7] Symptoms of spleen qi deficiency include: lack of appetite, abdominal distention, fatigue, lethargy, weakness in the extremities, loose stools, and diarrhea.[7] Due to the qi tonifying properties, it also helps to restore prolapsed organs, including the uterus, rectum, bladder, and stomach.[7] Astragalus builds qi and blood.[7] To make a blood tonic, combine astragalus with dang shen *(Codonopsis),* fu ling *(Poria),* shu di huang *(Rehmannia),* and dong quai *(Angelica sinensis).*

Astragalus has antioxidant, vasodilating, and mild hypotensive actions in individuals with hypertension.[5,6,8] However, it does not have a blood pressure lowering effect in hypotensive people; instead, it increases circulation and warms the body. Astragalus strengthens contractility of normal heart tissue (positive inotropic effects), and can be combined with dang shen *(Codonopsis)* to support the heart.[5,8] Clinical studies demonstrate that astragalus aids in treating ischemic heart disease and heart conditions including myocardial infarction, heart failure, and angina pain.[11]

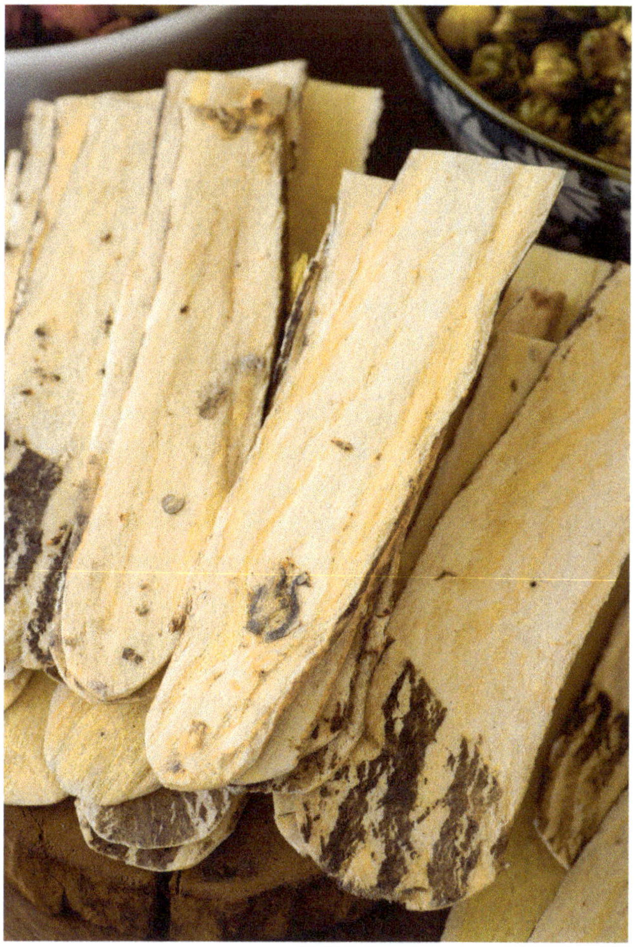

Astragalus hastens the healing of wounds, promotes tissue regeneration, suppurates poisons, drains pus, and reduces swelling.[5,7] It aids in treating abscesses, boils, wounds, ulcers, and slowly healing wounds.[5,7] It is especially helpful in individuals with weakened resistance and qi deficiency who have difficulty in healing wounds. Astragalus helps to heal bones, encourage cartilage growth, and mend connective tissue.[6]

Astragalus has hepatoprotective and hepatorestorative qualities attributed to the lignans.[6,8] It has blood sugar stabilizing effects. It prevents liver glycogen depletion caused by carbon tetrachloride treatments.

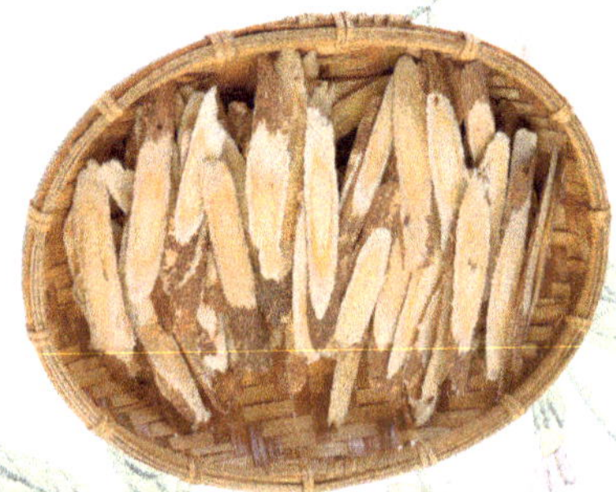

CONTRAINDICATIONS

Avoid consuming astragalus during an infectious illness, fever, or acute inflammation. It should be avoided in individuals with qi stagnation, damp obstruction, and food stagnation, and those with yin deficiency with heat signs (hot flashes or night sweats).[7]

PREPARATION AND DOSAGE

TINCTURE: Fresh roots [1:2-1:3, 70-95% alcohol]; dry roots [1:5-1:6, 60% alcohol]; consume 30-60 drops, up to three times daily.

FLUID EXTRACT: Dry roots [1:1, 55% alcohol]; consume 10-15 drops, up to three times a daily.

GLYCERITE: Dry roots [1:6, 40% alcohol, 30% glycerin, 30% water]; consume 10-40 drops, up to three times daily.

CAPSULES: Consume 3-4 "00" capsules, up to three times daily.

TEA: Prepare a decoction or cold infusion; consume 8-12 ounces, up to three times daily.

HONEY AND SYRUP: Prepare astragalus syrup by simmering a root decoction to one-half the volume; add honey to desired sweetness; consume 1 tablespoon, up to three times daily.

CULINARY USE: Add a bundle of root slices (1-2 inches in diameter) to bone, lamb, beef, or chicken broth. Add 1-2 tablespoons of powdered root to smoothies, vegetable juices, or nut butter.

BAYBERRY

DESCRIPTION

BOTANICAL NAMES:
Morella californica (syn. *Myrica californica, Gale californica*), *M. cerifera* (syn. *Myrica cerifera*), *M. pensylvanica* (syn. *Myrica pensylvanica*)

COMMON NAMES:
Bayberry, wax myrtle, wax berry, California wax myrtle, Pacific wax myrtle, southern wax myrtle, bog myrtle, Pacific bayberry, southern bayberry, candle berry, sweet gale, tallow shrub, tallow tree, northern bayberry, waxberry, tallow bayberry, small waxberry, swamp candleberry, candlewood, candletree
suomyrtti (Finnish)
abre a cire, cirier (French)
gagelstraunch, washgagel, washmyrte (German)
albero della cera, pianta della cera (Italian)
darshishaan, kandula (Persian)
katiphala (Sanskrit)
arrayan, brabantico (Spanish)
pors (Swedish)
mom agaci (Turkish)

FAMILY NAME:
Myricaceae

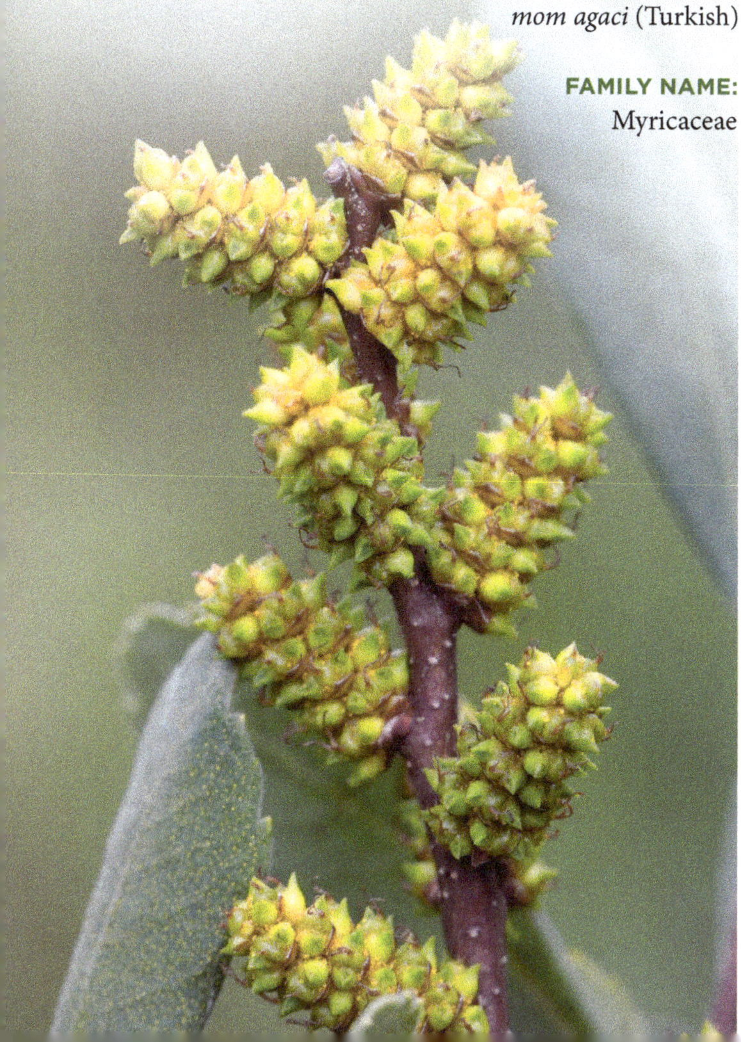

PARTS USED: The root bark (internally and topically) and leaves (topically).

BOTANICAL DESCRIPTION AND HABITAT: *Morella* is a genus of large monecious or dioecious shrubs with aromatic, resinous, alternate leathery leaves. The upper halves of the leaves have serrate margins.[1] The axillary spikes bear small, unisexual flowers that lack a perianth.[1] Male and female flowers are usually found on separate inflorescences.[1] Male flowers produce 3 – 12 stamens.[1] Female flowers have one style with two stigmas atop a superior ovary; each flower produces a small, spheric, waxy drupe.[1]

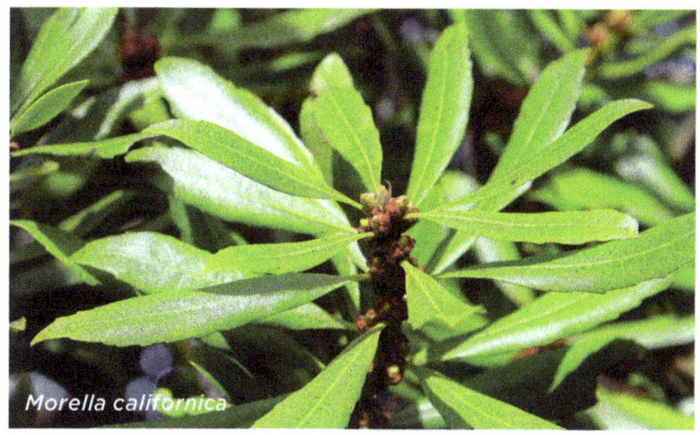
Morella californica

Morella californica is a large monoecious shrub (2 – 10 m tall) growing in dunes, conifer forests, and wetlands along California's Pacific Coast.[1] The densely gland-dotted young branches of *M. californica* are green, and become reddish-brown when mature.[2] The narrowly lanceolate-elliptic, glandular, dark green leaves are shiny on the upper side and pale green underneath.[2] The drupes (4 – 8 mm diameter) of *M. californica* produce less wax than other *Morella* species.[1]

Morella cerifera grows in the southeastern U.S., Mexico, the Caribbean, and Central America, in wetlands, pine and deciduous forests, and sandy areas.[3] It is a large monoecious shrub (up to 14 meters tall) that is sometimes rhizomatous and colony forming.[3] Young branches are spotted with yellow glands, becoming glabrous or softly hairy as they age.[3] The linear-oblanceolate leaves (1 – 13 cm long by 0.5 – 3.5 cm wide) are dotted with yellow glands on both sides.[3] The undersides of the leaves are yellow-green and glabrous (except the midrib); the upper sides are dark green and glabrous to hairy.[3] The round drupes (2 – 4 mm diameter) are covered in a thick layer of blue-white wax.[3]

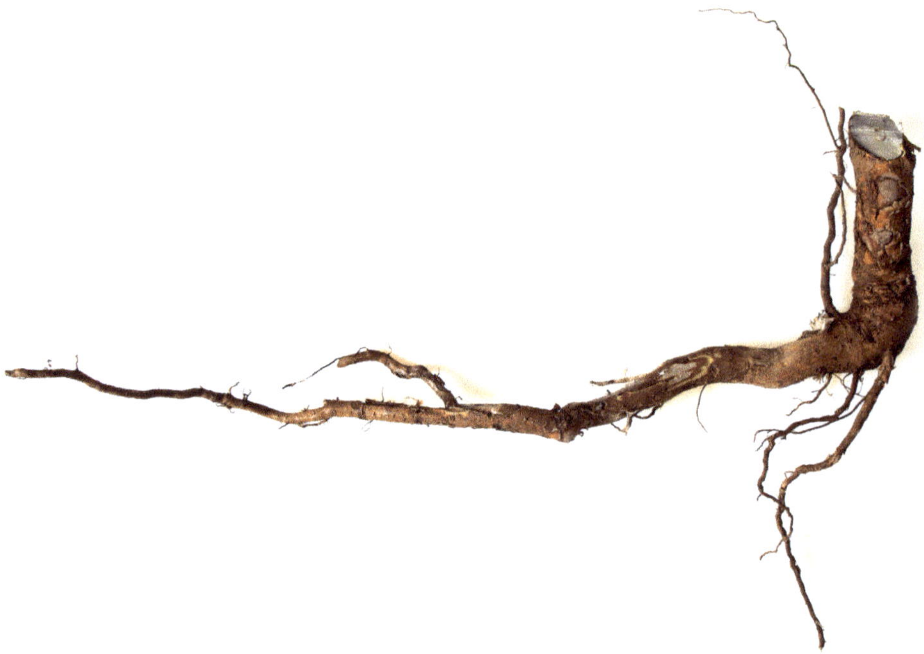

Morella pensylvanica grows in dunes, pine and oak forests, and wetlands in New England, Ohio, and northeastern Canada.[4] It is a dioecious, deciduous, rhizomatous shrub (2 – 4 meters high).[4] The young, glandular branches are reddish-brown, maturing to gray.[4] The oblanceolate leaves (2.5 – 6.5 cm long by 1.5 – 3 cm wide) have pale, glandular undersides and dark green, pubescent upper sides.[4] The male flowers have three to four stamens; the ovaries of the female flowers are mostly glabrous, except for their densely hairy apices.[4] The round fruit (3.5 – 5.5 mm) is also hairy; the hairs are hidden by a thick layer of wax.[4]

THE NAME: The genus synonym *Morella* is a corruption of *Morus* ("mulberry").[5] *Myrica* derives from *myrike,* Greek for tamarisk, a plant with fruit that provides aromatic tallow similar to bayberry candles.[5] The epithets *californica* and *pensylvanica* indicate the plant's origins in California and Pennsylvania (and the East Coast), respectively. The epithet *cerifera* derives from the Greek *keros* ("wax bearing").[6]

The following common names correspond with the Latin binomials: Pacific bayberry and California wax myrtle (*M. californica*); southern bayberry and southern wax myrtle *(M. cerifera);* and northern bayberry, small waxberry, and swamp candleberry *(M. pensylvanica).*

HISTORICAL USES: Eclectic physicians administered *M. cerifera* as a stimulating astringent and alterative.[7] It was used to improve mucous membrane tone, and circulation in congested tissues. Eclectics recommended bayberry to treat chronic stomatitis, mucoenteritis, persistent diarrhea, and typhoid dysentery.[7,8] John Scudder suggested using bayberry for patients with chronic malarial symptoms and jaundice, with "imperfect" liver actions, a dull ache on the right side of the abdomen, and cholestasis.[7] The Eclectics believed that bayberry stimulated digestive processes and enhanced nutrient absorption, improving blood quality and nutrition.[7,8] Ellingwood claimed that it enhanced rapid elimination of mercury from the system when combined with geranium.[7] He recommended bayberry for severe forms of measles and scarlet fever with a persistent sore throat.[7] High doses were prescribed as an emetic.[8]

In northern Europe, *M. gale* leaves were used as substitutes for hops and were featured as an ingredient in gruit, a once popular fermented alcoholic brew.[9] In China, they were also infused and consumed like tea.[9] The leaves and bark were used in tanning and to dye wool yellow.[9] The decocted berries were used as a spice in broths.[9]

The fruit of *M. cerifera* was a source of candle wax.[10] The wax was removed from the fruit by boiling the berries in water; the wax then floated to the surface.[9] These candles were reported to be aromatic, brittle, and smokeless after snuffing.[9] The wax was more brittle than beeswax and could be incorporated into sealing wax.[9]

CONSTITUENTS: Bayberry root bark contains tannins, triterpenes (myricadiol, taraxerol, and taraxerone), a flavonoid glycoside (myricitrin), gum, an acrid resin, and starch.[10,11]

NUTRITIONAL PROPERTIES: Bayberry contains high to average amounts of calcium, chromium, iron, manganese, niacin, selenium, sodium, thiamine, and tin. It contains low amounts of aluminum, cobalt, fiber, fat, magnesium, potassium, and protein, and trace amounts of phosphorus, riboflavin, and silicon.[12] The seeds can be consumed as food, although their nutritional properties are unknown, and they are highly astringent.

MEDICINAL PROPERTIES: Astringent, anti-inflammatory, antibacterial, antiseptic, circulatory stimulant, expectorant, lymphatic, resolvent, styptic, and vulnerary.

TEMPERATURE AND FLAVOR: Bayberry has an initial warming effect, followed by a secondary cooling effect. Bayberry is astringent, pungent, and sour.

MEDICINAL USES

Bayberry contains tannins that have an astringent, anti-inflammatory effect. It is highly beneficial for treating chronically swollen, congested mucous membranes.[7,13] However, the stimulating fresh root bark extract is not appropriate for acute inflammation or flareups of chronic conditions.[8,14] The tannins reduce permeability and tighten capillaries, preventing the leakage of fluids and proteins from the bloodstream into the tissues.[13] Bayberry also contains vasodilating resins that increase circulation into the tissues, improving blood flow, as well as nutrient and oxygen delivery. These resins stimulate macrophage activity in the tissues; however, the tannins ultimately have a constricting action in the tissues that decrease inflammation.[14] Bayberry reduces excessive mucus formation, and can be used to treat seasonal allergies, allergic rhinitis, sinusitis, or a lingering, hypersecretory lung infection.[7,13] Combine extracts of bayberry, yerba mansa *(Anemopsis)*, yerba santa *(Eriodictyon)*, *Ambrosia* and/or goldenrod *(Solidago)* to alleviate respiratory congestion.

Bayberry contains myricitrin that has bactericidal actions.[10] It is a resolvent that hastens the removal of waste products from tissues following an infection. It has subtle lymphatic actions for stagnant, swollen lymphatic tissues or lymph nodes. Gargling with the tea or diluted extract reduces swelling in the throat, and can be helpful for treating a sore throat, swollen glands, strep throat, a cold, or flu. Bayberry was a primary component in Samuel Thomson's "Composition Powder," a formula for the first stages of a cold or flu.[13]

The astringent tannins and acrid resins aid in treating chronic digestive ulcers in the stomach, intestine, or colon.[7,8,11] Internal and topical preparations help to treat hemorrhoids and rectal fissures. Consuming tea and using a sitz bath or enema aids in treating diarrhea, an ulcerated colon, or internal hemorrhoids.

Gargling with tea or diluted tincture is beneficial for treating periodontal diseases. It is highly effective for treating indolent gum sores, gingivitis, and bleeding gums, and as a follow up for gum abscesses.[7,9,11] Bayberry also aids in treating gum conditions resulting from methamphetamine addiction.

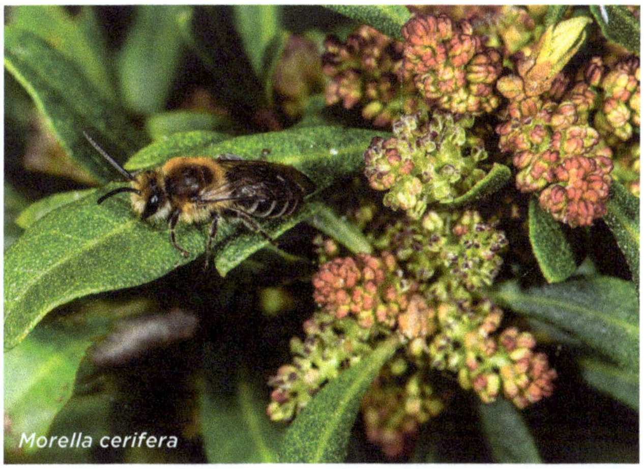
Morella cerifera

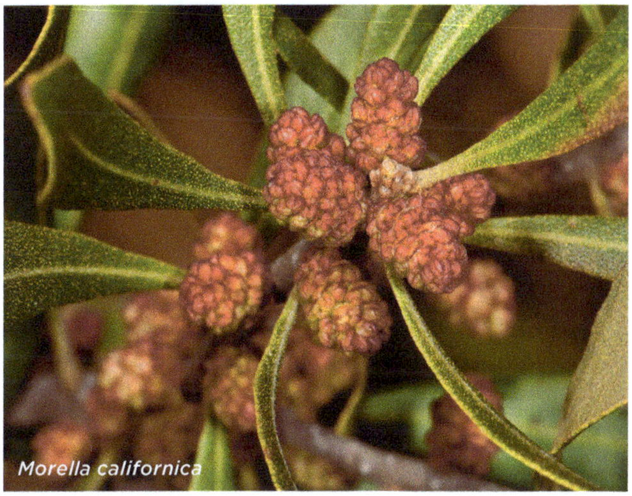
Morella californica

A sitz bath or vaginal irrigation with tea prepared from dried leaves or root bark aids in treating leukorrhea, candida, and vaginitis, as well as perineum, vaginal, or labial tears following childbirth.[11] Topical applications of the leaf tea, fomentation, or poultice hasten the healing of wounds, diabetic ulcers, staph infections, and boils. An oil or salve reduces inflammation and bleeding from hemorrhoids, and aids in treating varicose veins and spider veins.

CONTRAINDICATIONS

There are no known side effects or contraindications when consumed in recommended doses.[11] No toxicity has been reported; however, consuming large quantities can cause an upset stomach, nausea, or vomiting.[11] Some herbalists caution against the internal use of bayberry during pregnancy, because the effects of the acrid resins on the fetus are not yet known.[11]

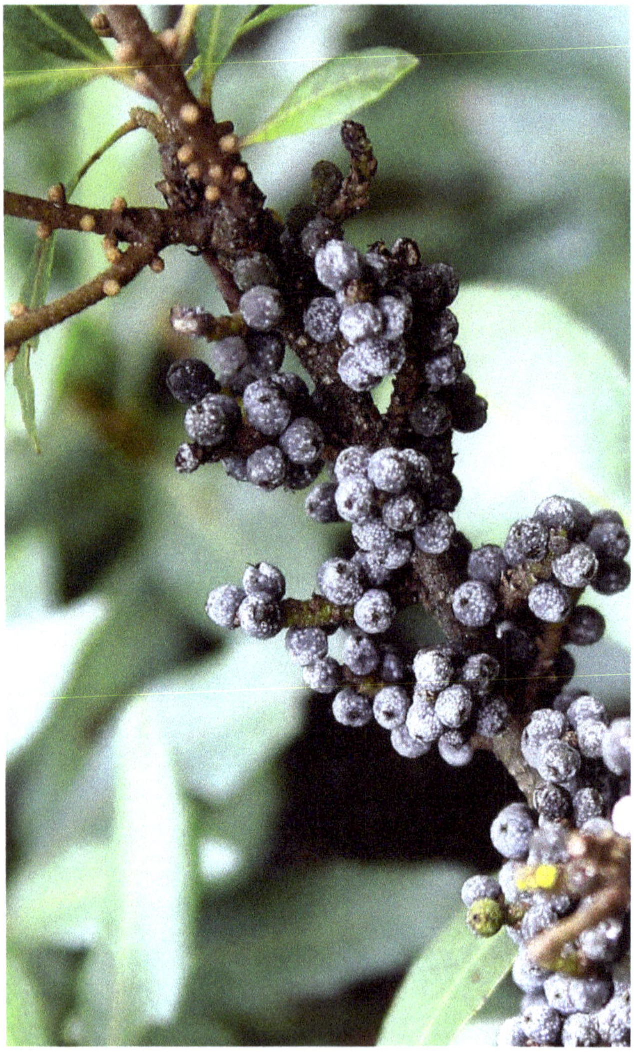

PREPARATION AND DOSAGE

TINCTURE: Fresh root bark [1:2, 70-95% alcohol, or 90% alcohol and 10% glycerin]; dry root bark [1:5, 60% alcohol, or 1:5, 50% alcohol and 10% glycerin]; consume 15-60 drops, up to four times daily. Add 10% glycerin to tannin-rich alcohol extracts to prevent proteins from precipitating out of solution.

CAPSULES: Consume 2-3 capsules, one to three times daily.

TEA: Prepare root bark as a decoction or cold infusion; consume 4-8 ounces, up to four times daily. Prepare the leaves as a hot or cold infusion; consume up to 8 ounces, two to four times daily.

HONEY AND SYRUP: Mix the powdered root with honey and apply topically. Due to the content of particulate matter, open wounds should eventually be flushed.

TOPICAL USE: Prepare a tea of the leaves or roots for a gargle, vaginal irrigation, or sitz bath. Apply a fomentation, poultice, wash, or dust of the leaves or roots. Prepare an oil of the leaves using the alcohol intermediary method.

BERBERIS

DESCRIPTION

BOTANICAL NAMES:
Berberis aquifolium (B. aquifolium var. *aquifolium, Berberis piperiana),* *B. nervosa, B. repens* (syn. *B. aquifolium* var. *repens*), *B. vulgaris, B. fremontii, B.* spp. (syn. *Mahonia* spp.)

COMMON NAMES:
Oregon grape, tall Oregon grape, dull Oregon grape, mountain grape, barberry, European bayberry, holy thorn, mountain holly, odostemon, pipperidge bush, Fremont's barberry
mahonia (Finnish)
mahonie (French)
gewöhnliche (German)
beriberi, berbero (Italian)
yerba de sangre, algerita, palo amarillo (Spanish)
mahonia (Swedish)
diken üzümü (Turkish)

FAMILY NAME:
Berberidaceae

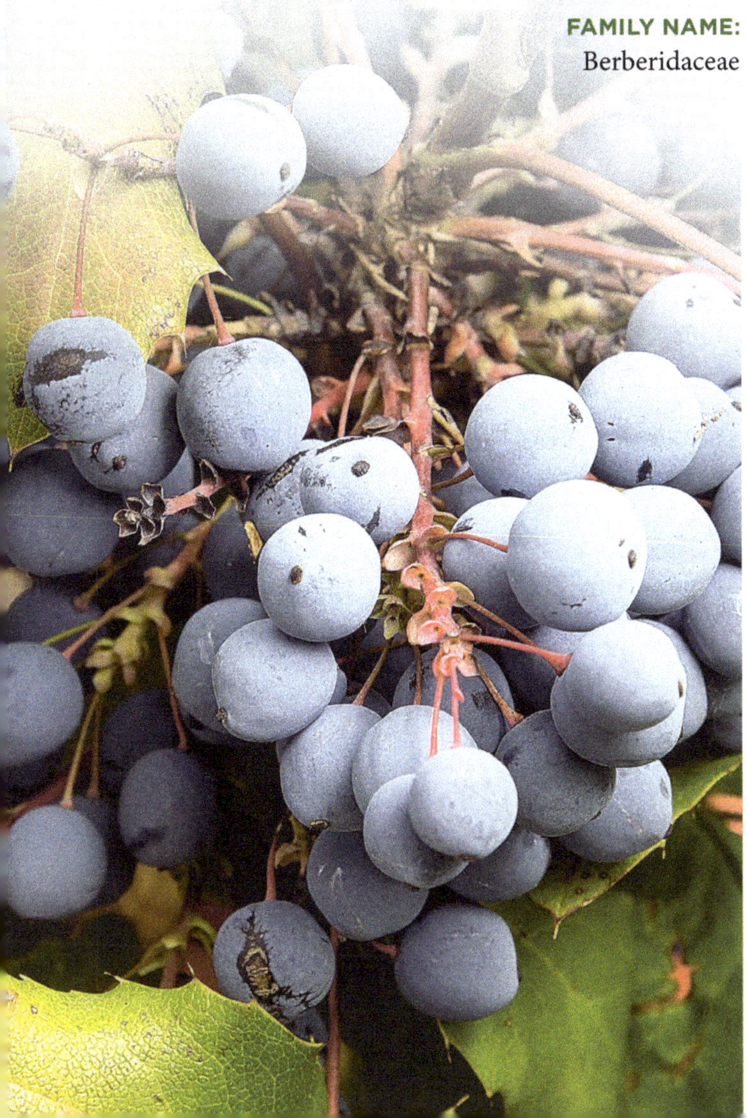

PARTS USED: The roots and root bark; *Berberis vulgaris* stems are also used medicinally. The leaves can be used in topical preparations.

BOTANICAL DESCRIPTION AND HABITAT: *Berberis aquifolium* grows on dry, rocky slopes and is native to the Rocky Mountains. It also extends west, throughout North America and into British Columbia.[1,2] It is a woody peren-

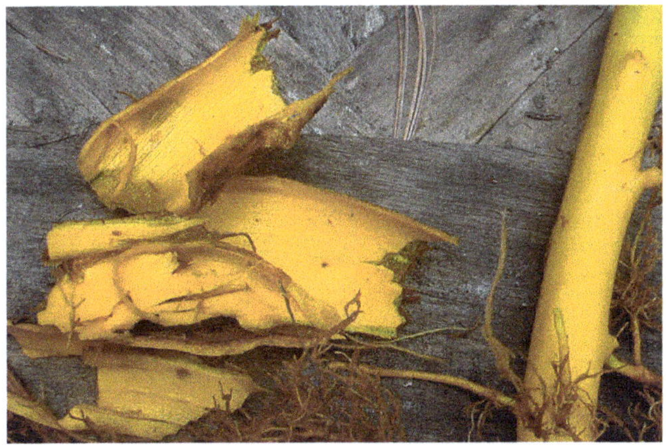

nial (up to two meters high) with an erect habit.[3] The wood and inner bark of the stem and root are bright yellow due to the alkaloid berberine. The hard, rough, branched or knotty rhizomes have a yellowish-brown, wrinkled exterior and yellow interior. Berberis has pinnately compound leaves (10 – 24 cm long) spaced evenly along the branches on petioles (1 – 3 cm long).[3] Each leaf bears five to nine ovate leaflets with serrate margins, and 12 – 24 spine-tipped teeth.[3] Unlike *B. nervosa,* the bud scales are deciduous.[3] The dense inflorescence is 3 – 6 mm long.[3] The yellow flowers have nine sepals, six petals, six stamens, and a spheric stigma.[3] The glaucous dark blue fruit (4 – 7 mm in diameter) is ovoid.[3]

Berberis repens is similar to *Berberis aquifolium,* but with a more spreading habit and much shorter stature (usually less than 80 cm tall).[3] It extends from southern British Columbia to central Oregon.[1] The leaves (8 – 18 cm long) have petioles (1 – 6 cm long) and five to seven leaflets with 11 – 15 marginal teeth.[3]

B. nervosa is found most commonly in second growth, closed canopy fir forests from southern British Columbia to central Oregon.[2] It has an erect habit (10 – 60 cm tall)

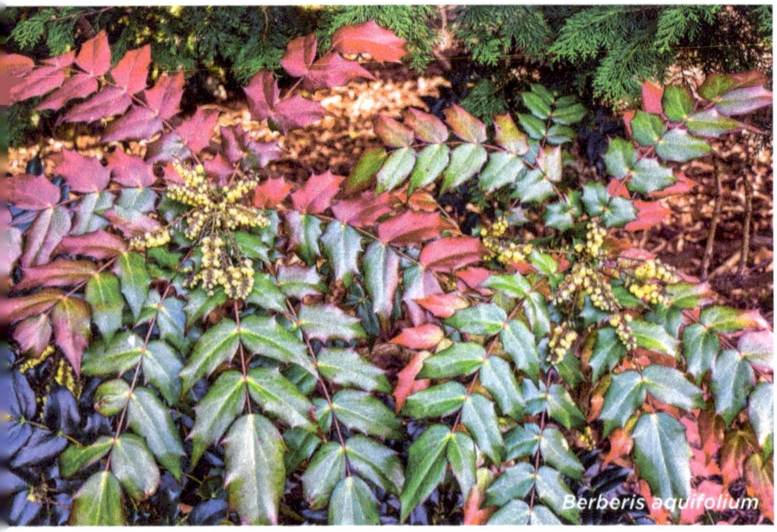

with persistent, lanceolate bud bracts (15 – 45 mm long).[3] The leaves (12 – 45 cm long) are crowded at the top of the plant, with a petiole (2 – 7 cm long).[3] Each leaf has 7 – 23 lanceolate to ovate, flat leaflets (2.5 – 8 cm long) with serrated margins and 10 – 24 bristle tipped teeth.[3] The open inflorescence bears more than 20 flowers.[3] The sub-glaucous, bluish-purple fruits are 8 – 12 mm in diameter.[3]

Berberis vulgaris is native to Europe, but has naturalized throughout eastern North America, North Africa, and temperate Asia.[1,4] A deciduous shrub with 20 – 30 arching dimorphic stems and gray bark, it grows 1 – 3 meters high.[5,6] Spines grow 1 – 2 cm long at nodes along the stem.[6] The plant has an extensive root and rhizome system.[5,6] The simple, alternate leaves are arranged singly on primary branches, or in fascicles on secondary spur shoots emerging from the spine axils.[7] The thin obovate blade (1 – 6 cm long by 1 – 3 cm wide) has finely serrate margins bearing 16 – 30 teeth.[5] The dull leaves have a glaucous coating on the upper sides, and turn shades of red, orange, and purple in the fall.[5] The inflorescence of *B. vulgaris* is a drooping raceme of 10 – 20 flowers borne from the fascicles of leaves (up to 2 – 6 cm long).[5,6] Each long yellow flower (3 – 8 mm) has three deciduous, scale-like sepals, six petals, six stamens, and one pistil, eventually producing red or purple juicy berries.

THE NAME: *Berberis* is a variation of the Latin *barberis* ("barberry") stemming from the Arabic *barbārīs* ("shell"), referring to the glossy leaves resembling the inside of an oyster shell.[4,8,9] *Mahonia,* the genus synonym, was named for Bernard McMahon, a horticulturist and garden mentor to Thomas Jefferson.[10,11] The epithet *aquifolium* originates from the Latin *acrifolium* ("to have holly-like leaves").[12] The botanical term *nervosa* refers to a tree or trunk-like pattern of leaf veins. The epithet *repens* derives from Latin ("creeping"), as does *vulgaris* ("common").[9] The Spanish name palo amarillo means "yellow wood." Yerba de sangre ("herb for the blood") refers to its traditional use as a blood cleanser.

The following common names correspond with the Latin binomials: European barberry, common barberry, mountain grape, holy thorn, pipperidge bush, mahonie, beriberi, berbero, and gewöhnliche, épine-vinette, and berbéris vulgaire *(Berberis vulgaris);* Oregon grape, tall Oregon grape, berberis, trailing mahonia, and mountain holly *(B. aquifolium);* yerba de sangre, algerita, palo amarillo, and Fremont's barberry *(B. fremontii* and *B. fendleri);* creeping barberry *(B. repens);* and dull Oregon grape *(B. nervosa).* Berberis is a common name refering to all medicinal species of the *Berberis* genus.

HISTORICAL USES: Ancient Egyptians combined *Berberis vulgaris* with fennel seed to prevent plagues. Ayurvedic healers administered the herb for dysentery. Throughout the Middle Ages, European herbalists used *Berberis* to treat liver and gallbladder ailments. Russian healers utilized berberis to reduce inflammation, hypertension, and abnormal uterine bleeding.[13] A tart jam was prepared from the scarlet berries for culinary use.[4] The berries were also used as a sweetmeat, and were included in sugarplum jelly and comfit. The berries garnished dishes.[4]

Berberis species have been used medicinally by Native Americans throughout the U.S. The roots were considered a general tonic and blood purifier to treat a variety of ailments, including sore throats, respiratory infections, tuberculosis, and syphilis, as well as liver, gallbladder, digestive, and kidney problems.[2,14] Blackfoot Indians administered berberis root to treat rectal hemorrhage, dysentery, and other stomach problems.[9] The root was applied externally as an antiseptic for wounds, sores, and eye infections, and to relieve itching.[9,14] The Blackfoot also administered a root infusion or fresh berries to open boils.[9] The roots were used as a yellow dye for buckskins, baskets, and fabrics.[2,15]

In New Mexico, the roots and branches of *Berberis fremontii* (palo amarillo) were boiled, then prepared as a bath for tubercular patients.[16] Decoctions were consumed and applied as a bath to treat rheumatism and rib pain.[16] The tea was administered as a remedy for jaundice.[16] Palo amarillo was shaped into two small crosses attached by leather, one worn on the chest, the other on the back; this was believed to protect the wearer from being struck by lightning.[16]

The berries were consumed for kidney problems and constipation.[9,14] Small quantities of tart berries were consumed, and often mixed with salal or other sweet fruits.[2] A tea of berries and crushed juice was administered to treat a coughing horse.[9] Paint comprised of pulverized berries, larkspur flowers *(Delphinium decorum),* and salmon glue decorated bows and arrows.[15]

Eclectic physicians considered berberis to have lymphatic, alterative, and bitter tonic properties that enhanced digestive secretion and excretion, improving digestion and assimilation.[17-19] Extracts of the root were administered for atonic dyspepsia with sluggish hepatic function, chronic gastritis with cholecystitis, and nonobstructive jaundice.[18,19] Topical and internal preparations of berberis were given for chronic dry, scaly skin conditions such as dry eczema, psoriasis, dandruff, and pruritis.[17-19] Berberis also was recommended for moist skin conditions such as moist eczema, acne, and herpes.[17,18] Berberis was commonly administered as an antidyscratic and tonic alterative treatment for syphilis; it was considered a supportive therapy, rather than a direct antisyphilitic.[17-19] Its actions were considered comparable to goldenseal (*Hydrastis*).[17,18] Decoctions were administered as an eye wash for conjunctivitis and sore eyes, and were gargled for mouth ulcers.[19]

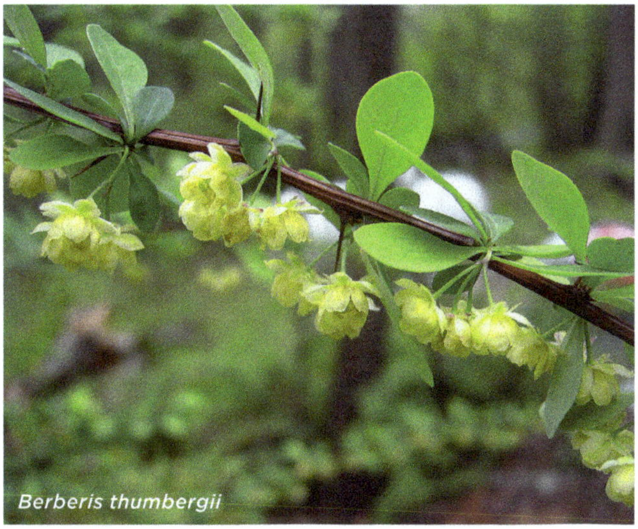
Berberis thumbergii

CONSTITUENTS: Berberis contains a wide spectrum of berberine alkaloids (berberine, berberubine, berbamine, bervulcine, berbamunine, berlambine, oxyberberine, oxyacanthine, jatrorrhizine, columbamine, columbianine, palmatine, vulvracine, yatroricine isotetrandine = berbamine methyl ether, magniflorine, magnoflorine, aromoline, obamegine, canadine, corypalmine, hydrastine, hydroxycanthine, isocorydine, lambertine, mahonine, and yatrorizine). Berberis also contains anthocyanin, flavonoids (quercetin and rutin), zeaxanthin, chlorogenic acid, cheladonic acid, tannin, resin, starch, and minerals (calcium, potassium, and magnesium).[1,13,20-22]

Ripe berberis fruit contains organic acids (citric and malic acid), vitamin C, phenolic acids (cholorogenic acid), anthocyanins, pectin, sugars, and triterpenes (ursolic acid).[4,20]

NUTRITIONAL PROPERTIES: Berberis roots contain calcium, potassium, and magnesium.[21] The berries contain vitamin C, anthocyanins, sugars, and citric and malic acid.[4,20]

MEDICINAL PROPERTIES: Alterative, antibacterial, antifungal, anti-inflammatory, antimicrobial, antiprotozoal, antiseptic, bitter tonic, cholagogue, choleretic, laxative (mild), liver detoxifier, antidyscratic, lymphatic, and refrigerant.

TEMPERATURE AND FLAVOR: Cold, bitter, and astringent.

MEDICINAL USES

Berberis contains bitter berberine alkaloids that stimulate upper and lower digestive secretions. Consumed prior to meals, berberis increases hydrochloric acid and pepsin levels in the stomach, raising gastrin levels.[23] This process initiates the release of gastroenterones (gastric hormones) such as cholecystokinin and pancreatic polypeptide.[24] These hormones influence the gallbladder and pancreas, facilitating the release of bile and pancreatic enzymes, respectively.[24] Bile salts emulsify fats and pancreatic enzymes stimulate the breakdown of fat, protein, and starch in the duodenum.[24] Berberis is an appetite stimulant used for weak, painful, or sluggish digestion. It is beneficial for treating anorexia (loss of appetite), gas, and bloating, and for individuals recovering from a debilitating illness. It is an effective remedy for upper and lower digestive deficiency, as it strengthens secretions throughout the digestive tract.[23,25] Symptoms of digestive deficiency include: poor digestion, gas, bloating, constipation, blood sugar fluctuation, a white or yellow coating on the tongue, as well as gum and tooth problems.[23,25] Because Berberis is classified as a cold herb, it is best used in low doses (10 – 30 drops) as a digestive bitter tonic, and should be combined with warming, aromatic carminative herbs, especially in individuals who are frail, cold-bodied, or prone to loose stools or diarrhea. Combine with other alkaloid-based digestive bitter tonic herbs such as gentian *(Gentiana)* or bogbean *(Menyanthes),* and carminative herbs such as fennel *(Foeniculum),* anise *(Pimpinella),* or licorice *(Glycyrrhiza).*

Berberis aids in treating liver and gallbladder disorders. It increases bile production in the liver (choleretic) and bile secretion from the gallbladder (cholagogue), and decreases bilirubin levels.[22,26] Increasing bile secretion enhances the digestion of fatty foods because bile salts emulsify fats. The choleretic actions can be helpful for reducing nausea associated with poor fat digestion, especially for individuals who have had their gallbladder removed. The cholagogue actions help to liquefy bile, prevent gallstone formation, and aid in passing gallstones (except in cases with a blocked bile duct). Berberis is useful for treating gallbladder disorders such as cholestasis, cholethiasis, cholecystitis, and cholangitis. It is also used for an acute gallbladder attack, in addition to other antispasmodics and cholagogue herbs. Additional smooth muscle antispasmodic and analgesic herbs, such as silk tassel (*Garrya*) or California poppy (*Eschscholzia*) aid in alleviating the pain from passing a stone. Berberis tea or capsules are beneficial for individuals with jaundice, hepatitis, or cirrhosis of the liver. Berberine helps to correct metabolic abnormalities in patients with liver cirrhosis.[22] The cholagogue properties act as a natural laxative, reducing constipation.[23] Berberis also aids in elimination and detoxification because waste products excreted by the liver are released in bile from the gallbladder.

Berberis detoxifies the liver and hastens the removal of waste products from it. Berberine exhibits anti-inflammatory effects attributed to its heat-clearing and liver-detoxifying actions.[27] Berberis can be beneficial for treating skin conditions such as acne, cysts, boils, dandruff, dermatitis, eczema, psoriasis, abscesses, and indolent skin sores.[17-19,27] In Traditional Chinese Medicine, plants containing berberine alkaloids are used to drain damp-heat and cool the liver and gallbladder.[27] Damp-heat in these organs manifests as gallstones, migraines, red eyes, jaundice, hepatitis, and other forms of liver inflammation.[27] Damp-heat of the liver and gallbladder is common in individuals with diets high in refined flour or sugar, alcohol, caffeine, fried food, poor quality fats, processed meats, and other processed foods. Berberis is also useful for alleviating heat toxicity in individuals with reddish complexions who are easily agitated or angered, feel worse due to heat, and have liver-heat rising patterns.[27] In addition, it can be used to reduce migraine headaches resulting from liver-heat rising.[27]

Berberis increases blood flow to the spleen and reduces splenic swelling.[22,26] It has immune modulating activity, stimulating macrophages that engulf and destroy microbes and tumor cells.[22] Berberis can be administered to treat

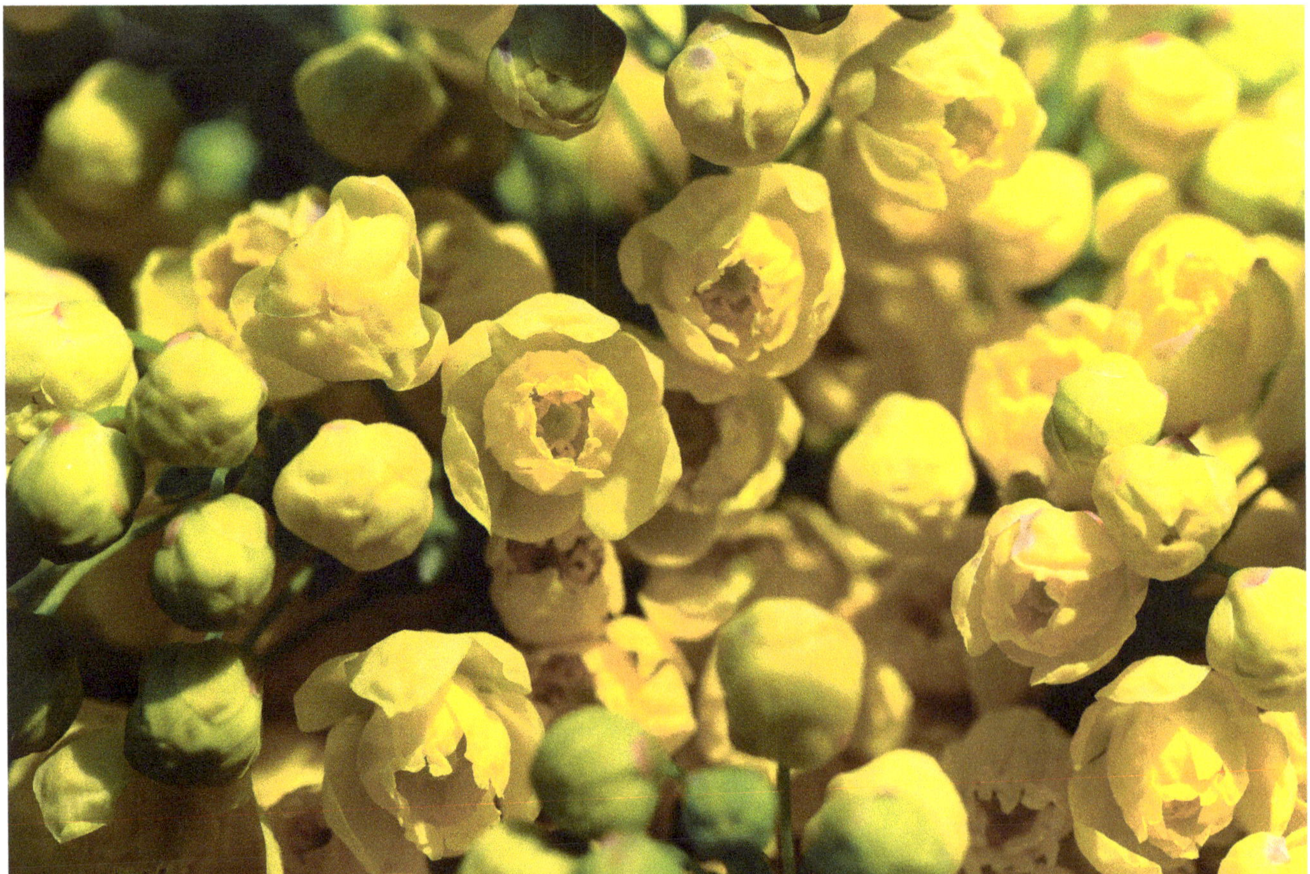

Berberis aquifolium

spleen or liver swelling caused by mononucleosis or other infectious diseases. Current research indicates that berberine increases the blood supply to the spleen, likely potentiating blood filtration.[22] It stimulates macrophages and enhances immune function.[22] These actions, in addition to enhancing liver function, likely account for its traditional use as an antidyscratic, alterative, and lymphatic.

Berberis exhibits wide-spectrum antimicrobial actions. It contains berberine alkaloids, including berberine, oxycanthine, and columbamine that are bactericidal against *Bacillus dysenteriae, Bacillus subtilis, Corynebacterium diphtheria, Staphylococcus epidermidis, Staphylococcus* spp., *Streptomyces* spp., *Neisseria gonorrhoeae, Neisseria meningitidis, Escherichia coli, Salmonella typhi,* and other bacteria.[1,20,22] Berberine also prevents streptococci from adhering to host cells.[22]

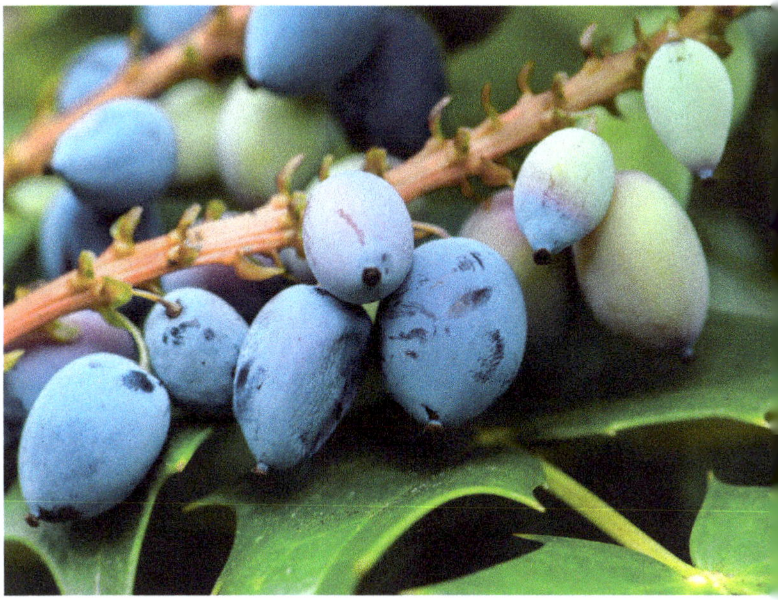

Berberis has pronounced antibacterial effects for treating sinusitis, strep throat, sore throat, bronchitis, and conjunctivitis. It can be consumed internally or applied topically to treat staph infections and infected, slow-healing wounds. It is beneficial for individuals with chronically low immune function, especially when due to poor digestion.

In addition to the antimicrobial effect from stimulating hydrochloric acid secretions, Berberis aids in treating digestive microbes. It can be useful for treating acute digestive episodes, and as a followup to digestive infections and diarrhea resulting from food poisoning *(Salmonella paratyphi),* shigellosis *(Shigella dysenteriae), Klebsiella,* giardiasis *(Giardia lamblia),* or cholera *(Vibrio cholera).*[22,23] Berberine alkaloids are also antiprotozoal against *Colpidium colpoda.* In addition to the antibacterial and antiprotozoal actions, berberine inhibits enterotoxins produced by the microbes.[22]

Berberine has antiprotozoal actions against *Entamoeba histolytica, Giardia lamblia, Leishmania donovani,* and *Trichomonas vaginalis.*[1,20,22] Berberine sulfate is amebicidal and trypanocidal.[1] Berberis is used to restore digestive secretions as a followup treatment for giardia.[23] When treating intestinal parasites, combine berberis with antiparasitics such as chaparro amargosa *(Castela),* huang lian *(Coptis),* wormwood *(Artemesia absinthium)* or sweet Annie *(Artemesia annua),* and/or garlic *(Allium sativum),* as well as soothing carminative herbs such as licorice *(Glycyrrhiza)* and fennel *(Foeniculum).*

Berberis is an antifungal agent for the short- or long-term treatment of intestinal or vaginal candida. It also helps to prevent candida overgrowth following antibiotic consumption.[22] Berberine has antifungal activity against *Candida albicans.* Probiotics are also beneficial for preventing the excessive growth of candida and rebuilding intestinal flora destroyed by antibiotic use.[22] In addition to internal consumption, vaginal irrigation with a well-strained, cooled decoction is beneficial for treating vaginal candida.

Washing the eyes with a well-strained, tepid tea aids in treating eye conditions such as allergic and bacterial conjunctivitis, blepharitis, inflamed eyelids, and hypersensitive eyes.[28] Water-based preparations or poultices reduce inflammation from psoriasis, eczema, boils, and acne.[22] Apply the root topically as a wash, dust, powder, or poultice, or use as the diluted tincture as an antibacterial and antifungal for cuts, scrapes, abrasions, staph, athlete's foot, or ringworm.[23] While berberis' antimicrobial properties are equal to other berberine alkaloid-containing plants such as goldenseal *(Hydrastis canadensis)* or coptis *(Coptis chinensis),* it is less astringent.

Berberis fruits have antiarrhythmic, sedative actions according to Iranian traditional medicine.[13] One study found that *Berberis vulgaris* fruit acted as a hypotensive agent because it opened potassium channels, activating cell membrane depolarization.[13] The alkaloid berbamine was found to have antifibrillatory actions, likely through augmented potassium channel activity and the inhibition of sodium and calcium channel overload.[13,1] In a study using rodents, berbamine, isotetrandine, and hydroxyacanthine exerted hypotensive effects. Berberine also had an antiarrhythmic and hypotensive influence.[1] Berberine counteracts the arrhythmic effect of adrenaline and noradrenaline.[27]

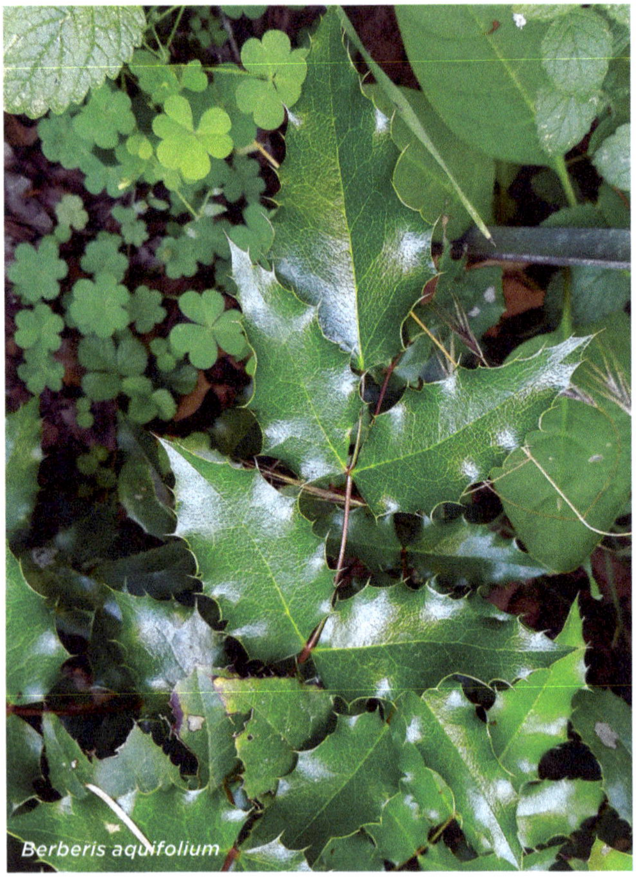

CONTRAINDICATIONS

Pending further studies, avoid internal use during pregnancy and lactation; topical use is acceptable.[13] Berberis is not recommended for children under two years old. A low strength is recommended for individuals over 65 years old.[13] Discontinue use if it causes acid indigestion or heartburn.[23] Berberis is contraindicated with obstructive gallbladder disease.[22] Discontinue use if the herb causes dizziness, fainting, lethargy, nausea, vomiting, convulsions, depressed heart and respiratory rate, nosebleed, skin and eye irritation, or kidney irritation.[13] Individuals with heart disease, chronic respiratory disease, and those medicated for these conditions should avoid consuming large doses of this herb, and consult a health care practitioner before use.[13]

Consumed in excessive amounts, berberis root is potentially too cooling and astringent, contracting the mucous membranes. Combine berberis with marshmallow *(Althaea officinalis)* or a small quantity of licorice *(Glycyrrhiza glabra)* to counteract the over-drying effects on tissues.

PREPARATION AND DOSAGE

TINCTURE: Fresh roots [1:2, 70–95% alcohol]; dry roots [1:5, 60% alcohol]; consume 15–60 drops, up to four times daily.

ACETUM EXTRACT: Fresh roots [1:2–1:3, apple cider vinegar]; dry roots [1:5, apple cider vinegar]; consume 30–90 drops, up to three times daily before meals as a digestive bitter tonic. *Note:* Not all of the constituents can be extracted in a vinegar menstruum.

CAPSULES: Consume 2–4 "00" capsules, up to three times daily.

TEA: Prepare the decoction or cold infusion; consume 6–8 ounces, up to four times daily.

TOPICAL USE: Prepare the leaves using the alcohol intermediary oil method for oils and salves. Topically apply a wash, fomentation, poultice, or finely powdered root or leaf. For an eye wash, use strained tea, or place 4–10 drops of tincture in 2–3 ounces of boiled water, then wait 15 minutes or more for the alcohol to evaporate, and allow the hot water to cool. Place in an eyecup or flush the eyes with the solution to treat eye infections. For vaginal irrigation, allow to cool, then strain the decoction through a paper filter or fine cloth.

CULINARY USE: The berries are tart, but edible in small amounts. Prepare them as a jelly or wine. Herbalist Terry Willard provides the following jelly recipe: two cups of Oregon grape berry juice, 2 cups of salal berry juice, 5 cups of sugar, and 1.75 ounces (49 grams) of pectin. Dissolve the sugar and pectin in the heated berry juice, then pour into sterile canning jars.[9]

BLACK COHOSH

DESCRIPTION

BOTANICAL NAMES:
Actaea racemosa
(syn. *Cimicifuga racemosa, Macrotys racemosa*)

COMMON NAMES:
Black cohosh, black snakeroot, rattleroot, rattleweed, bugwort, bugbane, cohosh bugbane, cimicifuga
sølvyls (Danish)
racine d'actée à grappes, cimicaire (French)
schwarzes wanzenkraut, schwarze schlangenwurzel, traubiges wazenkraut, cimicifugawurzelstock (German)
cimicifuga negra, cohosh negro (Spanish)
spjutsil verax (Swedish)

FAMILY NAME:
Ranunculaceae

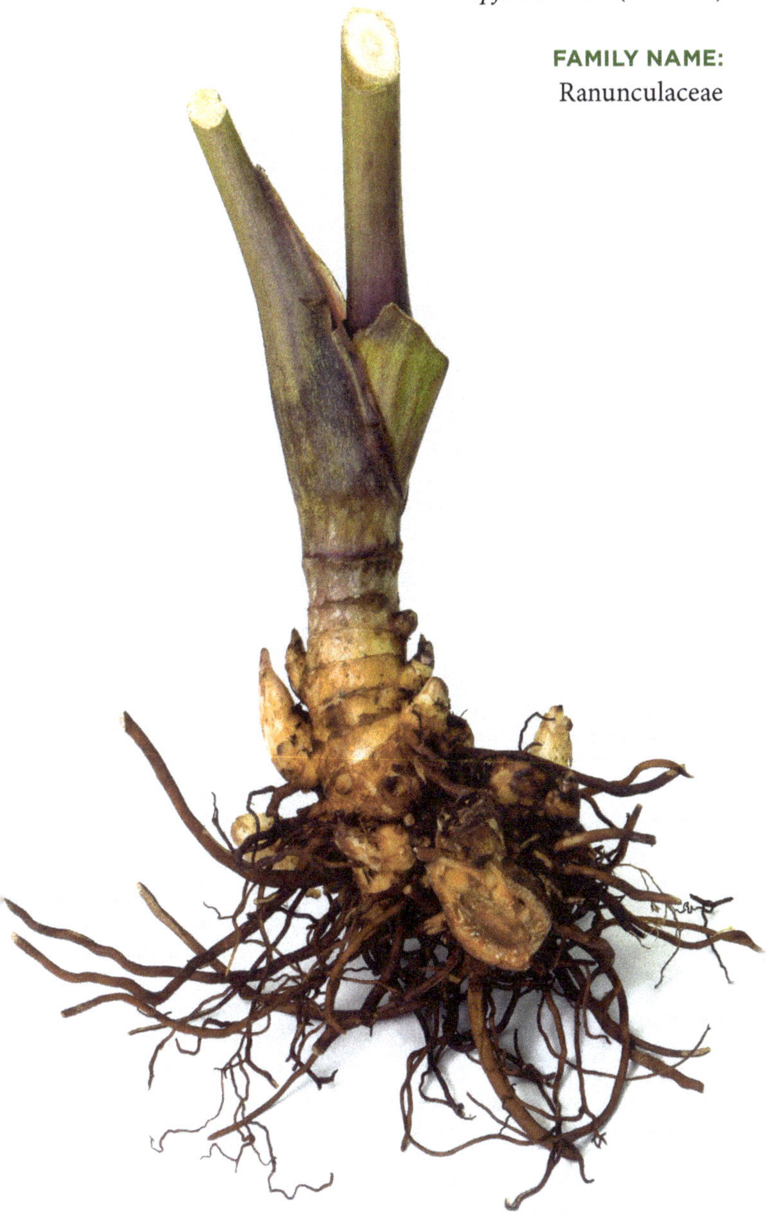

PART USED: The roots.

BOTANICAL DESCRIPTION AND HABITAT: *Actaea racemosa* is a forest-dwelling plant, native to the Ozark and Appalachian mountains in the eastern U.S.[1] Black cohosh grows 75 – 250 cm tall.[2] It has glabrous stems and smooth, dark green leaves (15 – 60 cm long).[2] The two- to three-pinnately compound leaves have 20 – 70 deeply dentate to pinnately-lobed leaflets.[2] The terminal, central leaflet is the largest, with three lobes; it sometimes has hairy veins underneath.[2] In late summer to early fall, a tall terminal panicle on a long peduncle displays four to nine beautiful fluffy branches (10 – 60 cm long).[2] The branches have numerous small flowers on pubescent pedicels.[2] The flowers have four greenish sepals, four inconspicuous white petals, 50 – 100 showy stamens with long filaments (up to 1 cm long), one carpel, and a short, broad style.[2] Each flower creates an ovoid follicle (5 - 10 mm long) that produces several brown seeds.[2]

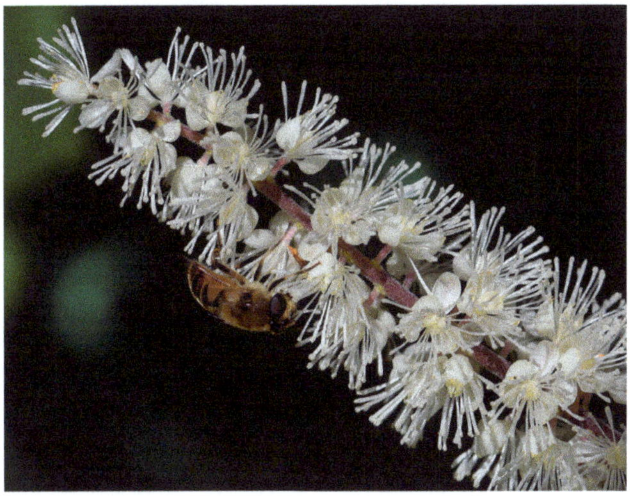

THE NAME: The former genus name, *Cimicifuga,* derives from two Latin words: *cimex* ("bedbug") and *fugare* ("to drive away") because the European species were used to exterminate bugs.[3] The current genus name, *Actaea,* derives from the Greek *acte,* due to its resemblance to elder tree leaves and berries.[4] *Macrotys,* an epithet used by Eclectic physicians, was an erroneous term given by French botanist Augustin De Candolle. The correct term, *macrotrys,* derives from two Greek words meaning "a large bunch," alluding to the large raceme of fruit.[3] The epithet *racemosa* refers to the striking floral racemes. The epithet

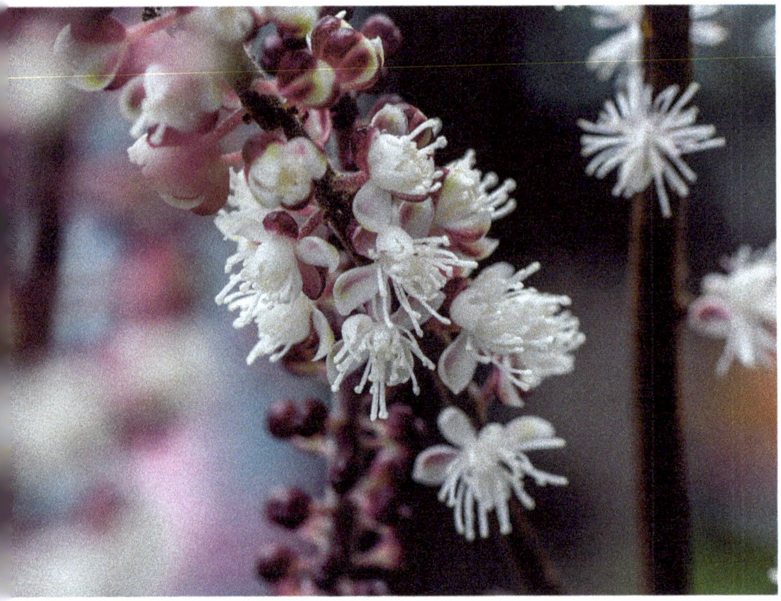

rubra means "red." Black cohosh refers to the dark color of the roots; cohosh is Algonquin for "rough with hairs." Rattleroot, snakeroot, and black snakeroot allude to the plant's use for treating snakebites.[3] Rattleweed refers to the sound of seed pods blowing in the wind.[3]

HISTORICAL USES: Black cohosh was widely used by Native Americans. Numerous northeastern tribes administered a black cohosh decoction to ease childbirth and afterbirth pains, and to treat sore throats, coughs, colds, and debility, as well as female and pediatric conditions.[4,5] As a female tonic, the Delaware tribe administered it in combination with other plants.[6] Algonquin treated kidney problems with black cohosh.[6] Cherokee administered the root as a diuretic or female tonic, and to treat tuberculosis and sore joints.[6] Iroquois used the tea to bathe rheumatic joints.[6] Black cohosh was used as an internal and external remedy for snakebites by Winnebago, Penobscot, and Dakota tribes.[7] In New Mexico, the pulverized roots of *A. rubra* were mixed with powdered leaves of native tobacco *(punche,* a *Nicotiana* species*)* and applied to rheumatic limbs.[8] Quileute applied crushed leaves of *A. rubra* to bring boils to a head.[9] Quinault applied leaf poultices to wounds.[9]

European settlers and Eclectic physicians based their uses of the plant on Native American practices. Early American colonists consumed black cohosh preparations to treat fevers, yellow fever, malaria, bronchitis, and nervous and uterine disorders.[4]

Black cohosh was listed in the *U.S. Pharmacopeia* (1820 to 1926), and the *National Formulary* (1935 to 1950).[7] Dr. John King, a prominent obstetrician, popularized the use of black cohosh among U.S. physicians.[3] The root extract (or resinoid) was used to stimulate spleen, digestive, hepatic, lymphatic, renal, and mucous membrane secretions.[3] Small doses were administered to increase appetite and enhance digestion.[3] Black cohosh was prescribed to treat headaches resulting from cold, neuralgia, dysmenorrhea, or la grippe.[3] It was also used to treat heart disorders, including rheumatic carditis and pericarditis, angina pectoris, and arrhythmia.[10] It was administered as a diaphoretic for intermittent and remittent fevers, rheumatic fever, and febrile cerebral complications, and to decrease bone aches from smallpox.[3,10] Black cohosh aided in alleviating headaches and backaches preceding measles and scarlet fever.[3] It was also used to treat throat muscle stiffness, eye strain, ocular muscle tension, and (internally) for acute conjunctivitis.[3] Due to its nervine, sedative, and antispasmodic actions, black cohosh was administered to treat epilepsy, convulsions, nervous excitement, delirium tremens, and other spasmodic conditions.[3] The extract or liniment was applied as an anodyne and counterirritant to treat rheumatism, nerve inflammation, tic douloureux, spinal cord inflammation, broad ligament spasms, aphthous ulcers, and cricks in the back or side.[3]

Dr. King used black cohosh as a reproductive tonic. He recommended the herb for congestive conditions of the uterus and ovaries characterized by tense, dull, aching, dragging pain.[3] Black cohosh was prescribed to treat irregular menstruation, amenorrhea, dysmenorrhea, menorrhagia, ovarialgia, ovaritis, endometriosis, leukorrhea, and neuralgia.[3,10,11] It was also prescribed for mastitis and mastodynia.[3] Black cohosh was believed to have a sedative influence on "nerves of the womb," and was used to treat premenstrual depression (melancholia), mania, and "hysteria."[10] It was a primary ingredient in Lydia Pinkham's Vegetable Compound, a female reproductive tonic.[5] Black cohosh was administered as a partus preparator several weeks prior to a due date.[3,10,11] The resinoid or fluid extract was valued for stimulating labor and encouraging uterine contractions from suppressed menstruation.[3,10] As an oxytocic parturient (partus accelerator), a dosage of 10–20 drops in hot water was prescribed every 20 minutes until uterine expulsion was induced.[3,11] Dr. King also considered the herb the safest and most effective agent for afterbirth pains.[3] For males, it was administered to treat orchialgia, achy prostate, spermatorrhea, and gonorrhea.[3,10]

CONSTITUENTS: Black cohosh contains a resin (cimicifugin = macrotin), cimigenol, quinolizidine alkaloids (N-methylcytisine, cytisine, and others), triterpene glycosides (actein, racemocide, cimicifugoside = cimigoside, 27-deoxyactein, deoxyacetylacteol, racemoside, and

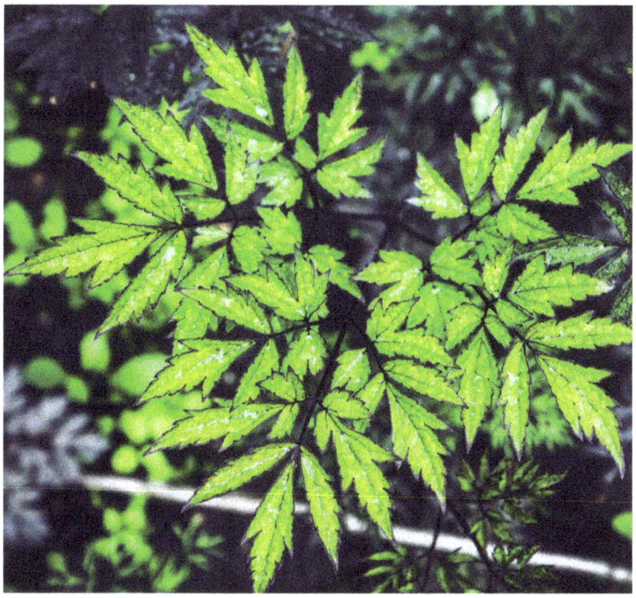

cimiracemosides A-H), free aglycones (actylacteol and cimigenol), isoflavones (formononetin), racemosin, volatile oil, a bitter substance, tannins, and starch, as well as salicylic, isoferulic, gallic, butyric, caffeic, and oleic acids.[3-5,12-16]

NUTRITIONAL PROPERTIES: Black cohosh contains high amounts of chromium, iron, and selenium. It has low to average amounts of aluminum, calcium, cobalt, fiber, fat, magnesium, niacin, phosphorus, potassium, protein, riboflavin, silicon, sodium, and vitamins A and C.[3,7]

MEDICINAL PROPERTIES: Alterative, analgesic, anti-inflammatory, antirheumatic, antispasmodic, antitussive, astringent (mild), emmenagogue, potential estrogen-mimetic, hypoglycemic, hypotensive, nervine, parturient, pelvic decongestant, sedative, subtle antidepressant, uterine tonic, and vasodilator.

TEMPERATURE AND FLAVOR: Warm, sweet, bitter, and mild astringent.

MEDICINAL USES

Black cohosh aids in treating menstrual cycle disturbances, secondary amenorrhea, and symptoms caused by ovarian dysfunction or insufficiency.[12] It decreases the symptoms of premenstrual syndrome (PMS), reducing emotional instability, depression, nervousness, insomnia, headaches, and night sweats.[12,13] It is effective for reducing menstrual cramping (dysmenorrhea), and aids in treating mastodynia (breast pain).[3,10] Black cohosh has uterine-tonifying effects and increases circulation to the reproductive organs, decreasing congestion.[3,17] For best results, consume regularly for two to six months.[17] Black cohosh has emmenagogue effects, especially when menstrual suppression results from nervousness.[11] Administer the extract in hot water every two to four hours until menstruation commences. Eliciting effects on the nervous and reproductive system, the constituent cimicifugoside is speculated to affect the hypothalamic-pituitary system.[13] To enhance the regulation of menstrual cycles, it can be combined with other hormone-balancing agents and reproductive tonics such as vitex berry *(Vitex)*, white peony *(Paeonia)*, and smaller amounts of ashwagandha (*Withania*), dong quai *(Angelica sinensis)*, chai hu (*Bupleurum*), saw palmetto *(Serenoa)*, and/or licorice *(Glycyrrhiza)*.

Based on German studies, black cohosh is believed to have an estrogen-like effect and a luteinizing hormone (LH) inhibiting effect.[12] However, the precise mechanisms of these actions have not been established, and deserve further research. Black cohosh extract reduced serum LH in ovariectomized rats.[12] The follicle stimulating hormone (FSH) and prolactin levels were unaltered.[12] Originally, the isoflavone formononetin, a coumestan derivative, was thought to be the active estrogenic component.[14] It was found to bind with estrogen receptors in the rat uterus.[13] However, formononetin was undetectable in commercially available extracts, and is not present in the dry root.[14]

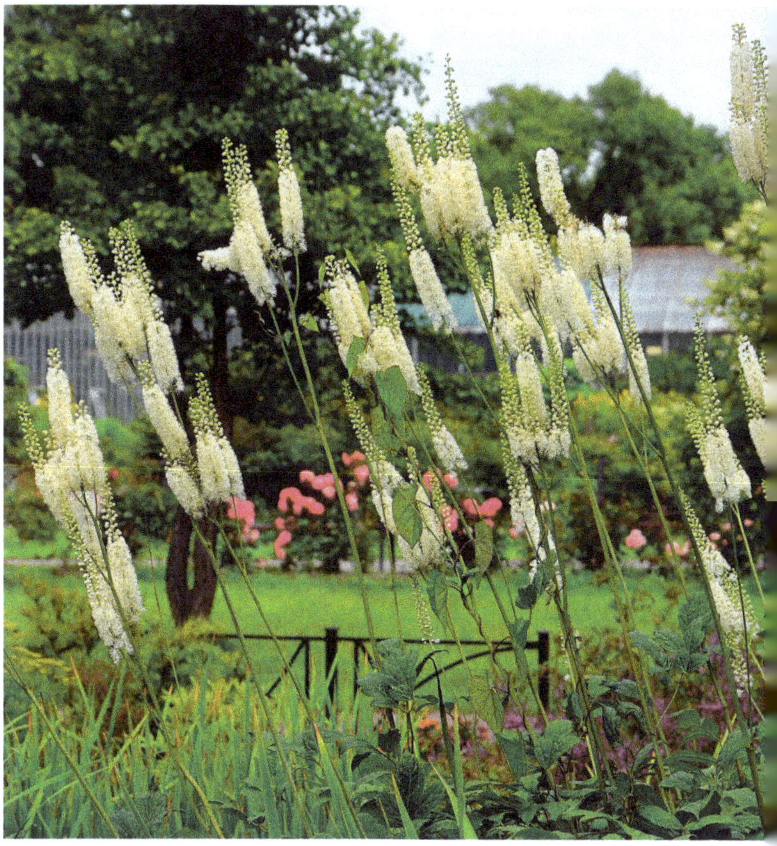

Prolonged injections of black cohosh extract increased the weight of the uterus and established menstrual cycles in rats and mice.[12] The trichloromethane fraction of black cohosh methanolic extract was found to bind with estrogen receptors *in vitro.* When that fraction was separated into three subfractions, two fractions suppressed LH secretion, and the other displaced estrogen *in vitro.*[12] The active component, isoflavone formononetin, did not reduce serum LH levels in ovariectomized rats. Therefore, it is speculated that it may have estradiol antagonist actions (binds to the receptor, but does not produce an effect), as opposed to the estrogen agonist effects (binds to, and activates the receptor).[12] Following three days of intraperitoneal injections of black cohosh methanolic extract in ovariectomized rats, the chloroform fraction had a potent LH-suppressing effect. Further investigation of the chloroform extract found that three mutually synergistic compounds were attributed to the LH-suppressive effect.[12] LH suppression could be due to neurotransmitter interference, or the fact that black cohosh metabolites mimic the effects of estrogen in the hypothalamic-pituitary, without affecting the tissues.[14,17]

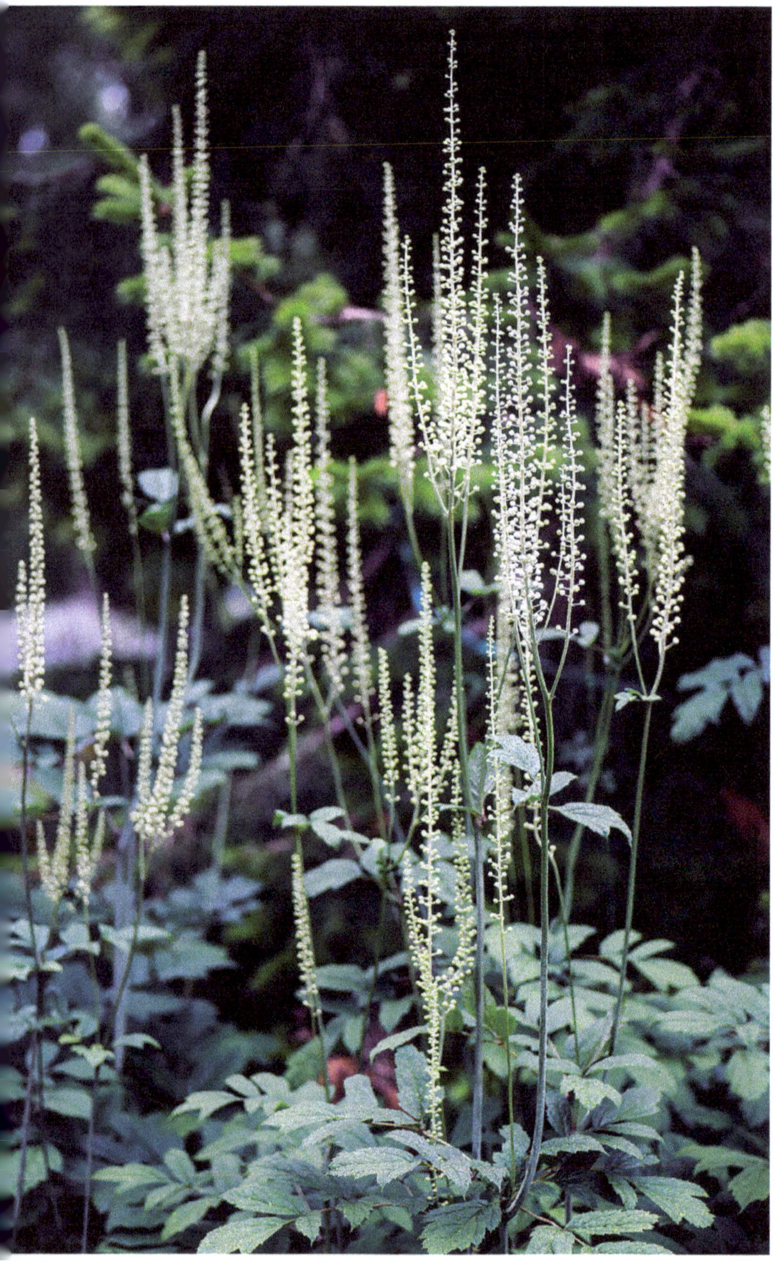

Numerous clinical studies since the 1950s have confirmed the beneficial effects of black cohosh in treating premenopausal, menopausal, and surgically-induced menopausal symptoms.[12,14] It alleviates conditions arising from estrogen deficiency.[17,18] In a controlled study of women with menopausal symptoms, four tablets of standardized black cohosh were administered per day. Following eight weeks of treatment, LH levels were significantly reduced in the black cohosh group.[12] In other experiments, dosages of the standardized extract (30 – 80 drops per day) were administered. The extract was consumed for six weeks to six months, but most women experienced beneficial effects in four weeks.[12] Some women were taking estrogen therapy.[12] Black cohosh successfully reduced hot flashes, night sweats, heart palpitations, anxiety, depression, irritability, mood swings, sleep disturbances, vertigo, short-term memory loss, and to a lesser extent, vaginal atrophy and dryness.[6,11,12,14] In one animal study, black cohosh extract decreased pyridinoline and deoxypyridinoline, two markers of bone metabolism, demonstrating a potential benefit for slowing bone loss.[14] To mitigate the symptoms of perimenopause and menopause, combine black cohosh with vitex berry *(Vitex),* motherwort *(Leonurus),* white peony *(Paeonia),* and smaller amounts of ashwagandha *(Withania),* dong quai *(Angelica sinensis),* and/or licorice *(Glycyrrhiza).*

There is concern about the contraindication of estrogen (or estrogen agonist substances) in individuals with estrogen-sensitive cancer, because estrogen can encourage tumor cell growth. Unlike estradiol, black cohosh extract does not stimulate mammary tumor cells *in vitro,* it inhibits proliferation.[12,14] In one study, it also synergized the effects of tamoxofin (an estrogen antagonist, anticarcinogenic medication used to treat estrogen receptor-positive breast cancer), demonstrating more potent inhibition of tumor cell growth than either substance alone.[12,14] Black cohosh does not exacerbate estrogen-influenced conditions such as breast, uterine, or ovarian cancer, or uterine fibroids.[12,15]

Black cohosh is a smooth muscle antispasmodic.[4,15] It reduces dull, aching cramping, including uterine, fallopian tube, testicular, and prostatic cramps.[15] Black cohosh aids in treating slow-starting, crampy, clotty menses, and afterbirth

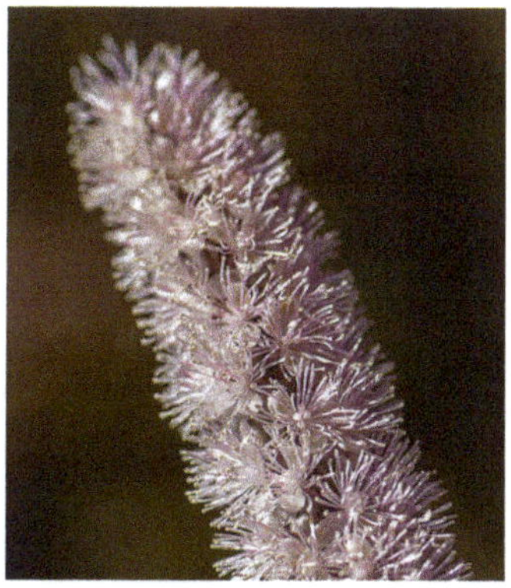

pains, and reduces cramps from extended arousal following lack of ejaculation.[10,11,15] It increases bronchial secretions and is an antitussive, decreasing respiratory spasms. These actions are helpful in treating a dry cough, whooping cough, and asthma.[3,4,10,12] Its mild antispasmodic actions decrease stomach, intestinal, and bladder spasms, as well as pain from passing kidney or gallbladder stones.[15] Contained in the fresh root, the ranunculoside cimicifugin exerts antispasmodic and sedative actions.[7] When the root is cut or bruised, cimicifugin is converted to protoanemonine; when dried, it is oxidized into an anemonic acid with little to no sedative or antispasmodic effects.[7] Therefore, the fresh root extract is preferable medicinally.

Black cohosh has subtle nervine, sedative, analgesic, and anti-inflammatory actions. It reduces throbbing, dull, achy pain known by 18th and 19th century physicians and Eclectics as "rheumatic" pain.[3,10,12,15] It is not recommended for sharp, shooting pain.[15] Black cohosh aids in treating rheumatoid arthritis, osteoarthritis, myalgia, fibromyalgia, neuralgia (not of spinal origin), and tendonitis.[3,10,12,17] It has slow-acting, mild prostaglandin inhibiting effects that reduce chronic inflammation.[17] It also has vasodilating actions that enhance circulation in the microvasculature, and anti-inflammatory properties that aid in treating occipital headaches.[15,19] The anti-inflammatory actions attributed to the actein have been confirmed in animal studies.[4,13] Black cohosh alleviates aches from overworked, strained muscles.[10] The nervine and sedative actions are mild, and most effective for treating insomnia resulting from pain (headaches, cramps, and muscle or joint pain).[15] Combine with valerian *(Valeriana)* to synergize the sedative and analgesic properties.[3] Black cohosh extract or powdered root poultice can be applied topically as an analgesic and anti-inflammatory.[19]

Black cohosh has peripheral vasodilating and subtle hypotensive effects.[13,15] It slows the heart rate, increasing its force and normalizing circulation.[3,4,15] The water insoluble resins are attributed to the vasodilating effects.[13] The triterpene actein demonstrated hypotensive actions in cats and rabbits, and vasodilating actions in humans.[4,5]

Note: Actaea rubra (baneberry) and *A. elata (Cimicifuga elata)* rhizomes can substitute for black cohosh in some cases, as they share black cohosh's anti-inflammatory, antispasmodic, sedative, and peripheral vasodilating actions; however, they do not have a hormonal effect.[15,19] A lower dose range of 5 – 20 drops, up to three times daily is recommended.

Caution: Avoid consuming berries from all species of *Actaea*, as they are toxic.[15] The berries can cause a stomachache, cramping, headache, increased pulse, and circulatory failure.[9] They have emetic and purgative effects; hence, the common name baneberry that derives from the Anglo-Saxon *bana* ("murderous").[9]

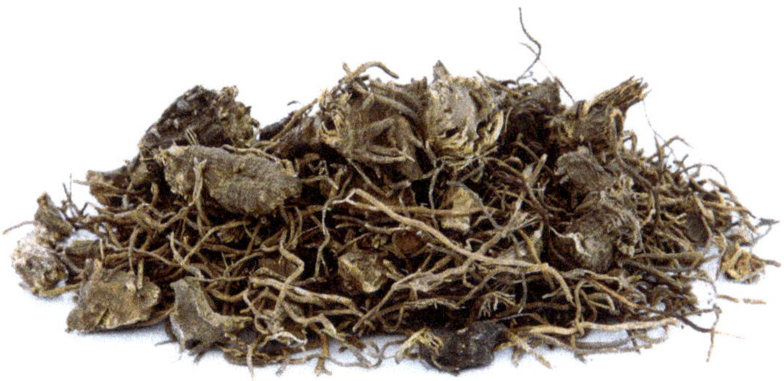

CONTRAINDICATIONS

Avoid use during pregnancy, except to ease labor.[12,14,15] It is contraindicated during lactation unless recommended by a health care practitioner.[12,14,15] Large doses can cause a frontal headache (between and above the eyebrows), intraocular pressure, pupil dilation, dizziness, giddiness, nausea, upset stomach, and gastric discomfort.[3,10,12,15,16] Consult a health care practitioner or avoid long-term use in individuals with hypotension, bradycardia, or those consuming blood pressure-lowering medications or blood thinners.[15]

PREPARATION AND DOSAGE

TINCTURE: Fresh roots [1:2, 70 – 95% alcohol]; dry roots [1:5, 70 – 80% alcohol]; consume 15 – 60 drops, up to four times daily.

CAPSULES: Consume 2 – 4 freeze-dried "00" capsules, up to three times daily. Consume 2 tablets twice daily of the standardized product Remifemin.

BLACK HAW

BOTANICAL NAMES:
Viburnum prunifolium,
V. prunifolium var. *ferrugineum* (syn. *V. rufidulum*)

COMMON NAMES:
Black haw, blackhaw, blackhaw viburnum, smooth blackhaw, smooth blackhaw viburnum, stag bush, sweet haw, American sloe, sloe-leaved viburnum, wayfarer's tree, nanny berry, sheep berry

FAMILY NAME:
Adoxaceae (formerly Caprifoliaceae)

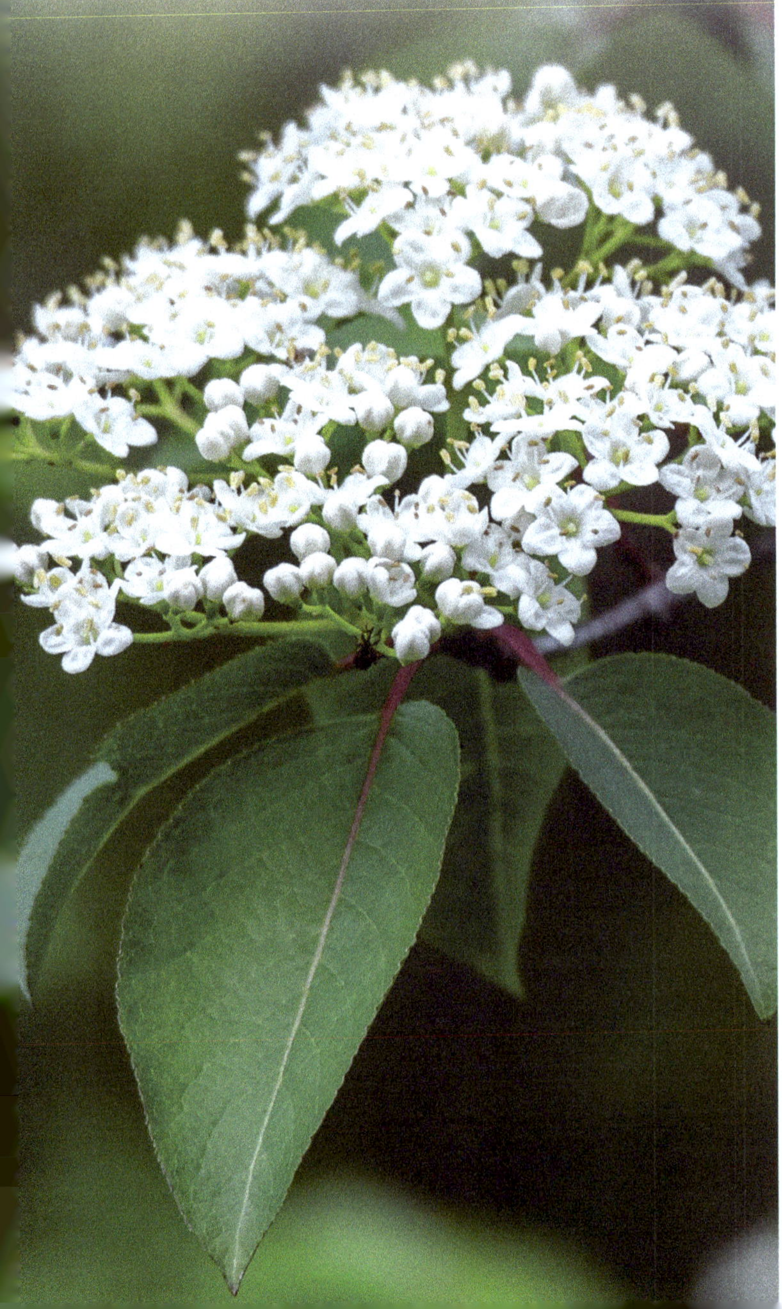

DESCRIPTION

PARTS USED: Bark, stems, and root bark.

BOTANICAL DESCRIPTION AND HABITAT: Black haw grows wild in moist, wooded areas and along stream banks in the northeastern, midwestern, and southeastern U.S. It is a native deciduous plant that grows as a shrub (5 meters tall by 2 to 3.5 meters wide), or a small tree (up to 9 meters

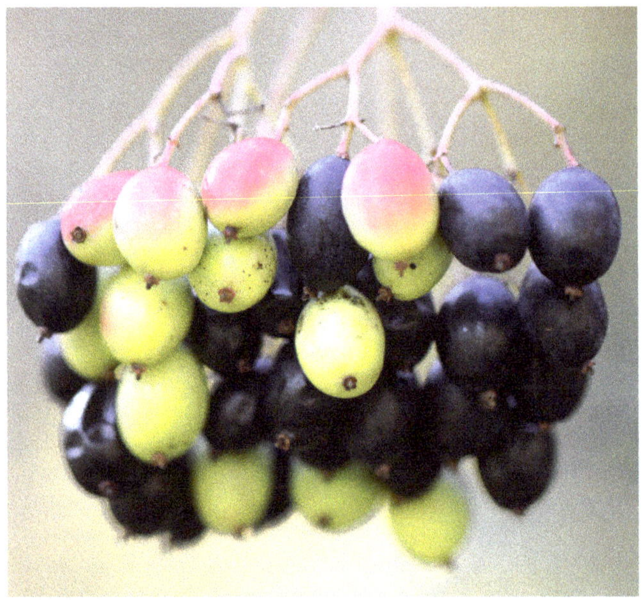

tall).[1] The young twigs are dotted with round lenticels, and the older wood is covered with corky "alligator hide," patterned bark. The opposite, dark green, shiny, ovate leaves (up to 10 cm long) are finely serrated; in fall, they turn rich crimson and purple, adding a dramatic accent to the landscape.[1] The axillary, flat-topped cymes (up to 12 cm in diameter) blossom in the spring. The flowers (about 7 mm across) have five fused sepals, five free white petals, five stamens, and a single pistil comprised of three carpels (though only one carpel matures into fruit).[1,2] The fruits mature into edible, bluish-black, berry-like drupes, and are the largest of this genus.[1]

THE NAME: *Viburnum* ("wayfaring tree") derives from Latin.[3] It acquired the epithet *prunifolium* because the leaves are similar in shape to *Prunus* (wild cherry). The common name black haw refers to the bluish-black berry (haw is another word for berry).[4] The name sweet haw refers to the sweet aroma of the bark, likely caused by the scent of coumarin released after the bark dries.

HISTORICAL USES: Cherokee and other Native American tribes administered black haw tea to treat menstrual cramps and prevent miscarriages, and as a postpartum antispasmodic.[4] Pioneer women and Eclectic physicians adopted most of those uses for gynecological purposes.[4] Other tribes used black haw to strengthen the reproductive organs and reduce muscle spasms, for asthma, and as a diaphoretic.[4,5] A strong black haw tea was consumed as an astringent for chronic diarrhea and dysentery. The Iroquois, Menominee, and Ojibwa consumed the fruits. A mouth rinse was gargled for sore gums.[4]

The Eclectics valued black haw for its calming effects on the nervous system, to treat palpitations, and lower blood pressure.[4-6] In the *American Materia Medica, Therapeutics, and Pharmacognosy,* Ellingwood makes claims about the antiabortive effects:

> Viburnum prunifolium is especially a uterine sedative in threatened miscarriage. It is particularly indicated in habitual abortion, preventing an anticipated occurrence and permanently overcoming the habit. I have had practical experience for over thirty years, and have perfect confidence in the agent based on repeated success. In one of my cases it caused the womb to suspend expulsive action and to retain a dead foetus for months. ... Doses of one dram of the fluid extract every four hours are necessary until the pain subsides and the flow eases. The patient must be kept in recumbent position and perfectly quiet.[5]

However, Felter challenges these claims in *The Eclectic Materia Medica, Pharmacology and Therapeutics*:

> Many practitioners, whose opinions we value and whose experience has been wide, report success with black haw in restraining the expulsion of the product of conception. Our own experience leads us to doubt its reputed value in that condition, but this in no way disparages the statements of others who may have been more successful with it. Rest in bed and quieting agents, such as Dover's powder, may enable the product to be retained; perhaps black haw may aid. But we have utterly failed in every attempt to prevent miscarriage with the agent where there was any considerable hemorrhage or where enforced and prolonged rest was not insisted upon. If any reports are to be expected from it in habitual abortion it must be in cases of functional debility of the reproductive organs, and not in those due to inherited taints or syphilitic infections, or criminal operative influence. We believe however, that much may be done with black haw to strengthen conditions in cases having had a previous miscarriage, and in uneasy, cramp-like sensations during pregnancy, but with no considerable hemorrhage.[6]

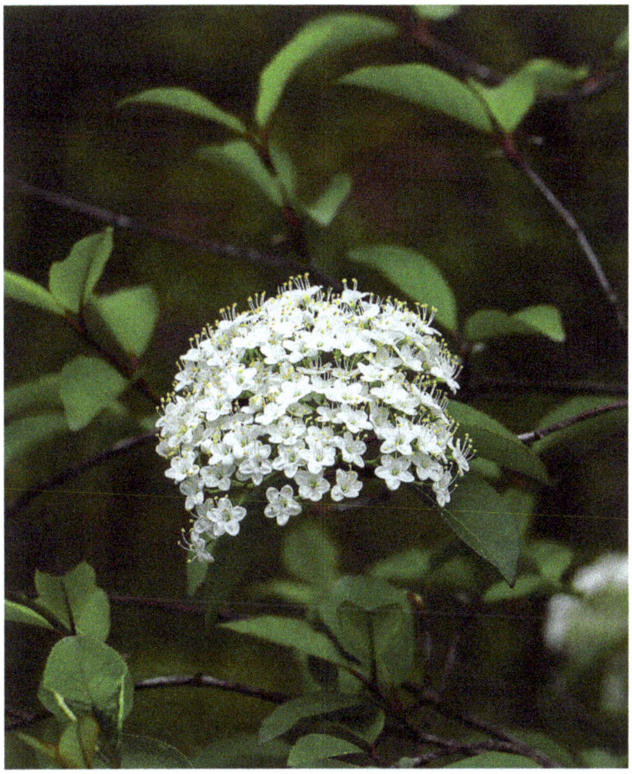

Slaveholders used black haw to prevent miscarriages in raped women slaves in order to increase their slave holdings. Enslaved women consumed cotton root as an abortifacient, but slaveholders forced them to drink black haw daily to prevent a miscarriage, as their offspring were considered valuable assets. The following statement from *Specific Medications and Specific Medicines* describes this practice:

> It is claimed in the Southern States that the Viburnum (prunifolium) is a specific against abortion. I have been told by several parties, that it was a common practice among planters to make their slaves drink an infusion of the Viburnum daily whilst pregnant, to prevent abortion from taking the Cottonroot. A physician from Texas assured me, that from an observation of fifteen years, he was confident that it exerted this influence, and that he had prescribed it in many cases without a failure.[7]

Eclectic physicians administered black haw for nocturnal cramping in leg muscles. In *The Eclectic Materia Medica, Pharmacology, and Therapeutics,* Felter recommended using black haw to withdraw from alcohol:

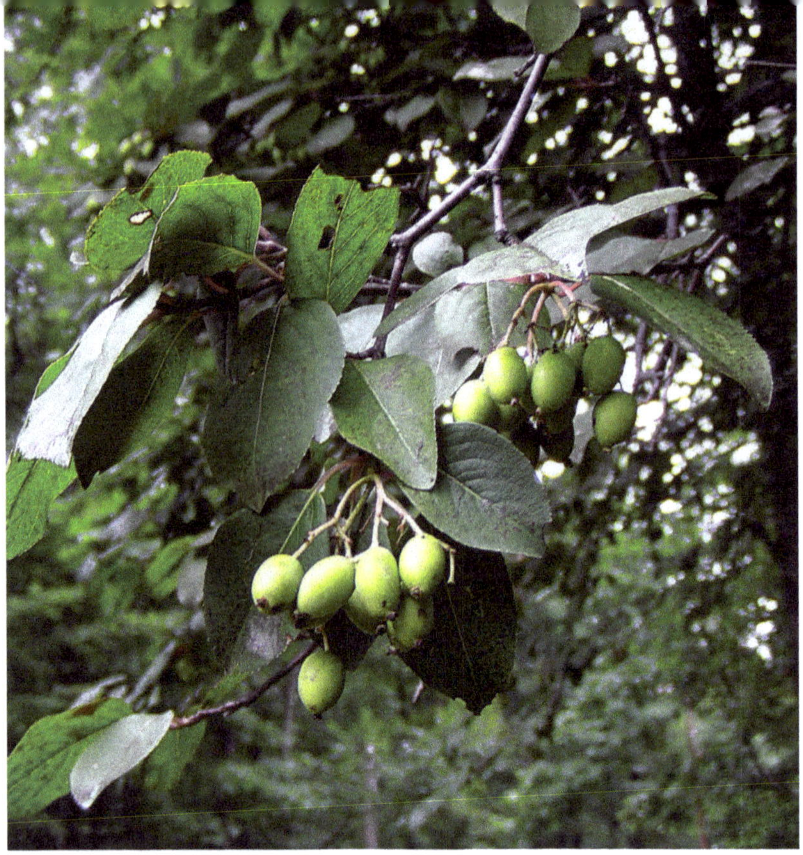

glycerin. This compound was used to relieve menstrual cramping and other menstrual-related disorders. A modified version of the formula contains fluid extracts of cramp bark *(Viburnum opulus)*, black haw *(Viburnum prunifolium)*, wild yam *(Dioscorea villosa)*, skullcap *(Scutellaria)*, cinnamon *(Cinnamomum)*, clove *(Syzygium)*, orange peel *(Citrus sinensis)*, alcohol, and simple syrup or glycerin. In addition, black haw was an ingredient in Howe's Black Haw Cordial, as well as wild cherry, aromatic herbs, brandy, and syrup.[6]

> Black haw is of very great value in treating those having a craving for alcoholic drinks. The specific medicine of black haw with essence of cinnamon or of clove, or preferably 'Howe's Black Haw Cordial' may be given. It relieves discomfort experienced in the throat and the gnawing distress in the stomach, from which these unfortunates suffer.[6]

Black haw was a primary ingredient in Lydia E. Pinkham's Vegetable Compound, a top-selling patent formula for female concerns. Additional ingredients included: pleurisy root *(Asclepias tuberosa)*, life root *(Senecio aureus)*, fenugreek *(Trigonella foenum-graecum)*, unicorn root *(Aletris farinosa)*, black cohosh *(Actaea racemosa)*, and 18% alcohol. A recent version of the formula was adapted by Numark Laboratories of Edison, New Jersey, adding several herbs such as motherwort *(Leonurus cardiaca)*, Jamaican dogwood *(Piscidia erythrina)*, licorice *(Glycyrrhiza glabra)*, gentian *(Gentiana lutea)*, and dandelion *(Taraxacum officinale)*, as well as vitamins E and B_6, magnesium, and zinc. This formula is currently sold in pharmacies as Lydia Pinkham's Herbal Compound.[8]

William Richard Hayden marketed his famous herbal compound, Hayden's Viburnum Compound, in 1866. The original patent compounds contained fluid extracts of black haw *(Viburnum prunifolium)*, cramp bark *(V. opulus)*, beth root *(Trillium)*, unicorn root *(Aletris)*, dandelion *(Taraxacum)*, wild yam *(Dioscorea)*, skullcap *(Scutellaria)*, clove *(Syzygium)*, cinnamon *(Cinnamomum)*, alcohol, and

CONSTITUENTS: Black haw contains coumarins (aesculetin and scopoletin = 7-hydroxy-6-methoxy coumarin), flavonoids (a biflavone: amentoflavone), triterpenes (oleanic and ursolic acids), tannins, phenolic acids (chlorogenic acid), phytosterols (5-sterols: β-sitosterol), a bitter principle (viburnin), salicosides, resin, plant acids (valeric, valerianic, malic, oxalic, and citric acid), arbutin, carbonates, and phosphates. The stem bark contains 1-methyl-2, 3-dibutyl hemimellitate.[4-7,9,11]

NUTRITIONAL PROPERTIES: The bark contains chlorides of calcium, magnesium, potassium, and iron.[6] The berries are considered an antiscorbutic, and contain vitamin C.

MEDICINAL PROPERTIES: Antidiarrheal, antispasmodic, astringent, hemostatic, mild sedative, mild diuretic, parturient, and partus preparator.

TEMPERATURE AND FLAVOR: Warm, sweet, astringent, and bitter.

MEDICINAL USES

Black haw is a smooth muscle antispasmodic useful for treating pelvic cramps.[4-6,9,10,12] Two coumarins, scopoletin and aesculetin, reduce smooth muscle contraction.[4,11] Scopoletin, a constituent of black haw, is a uterine relaxant.[4,9,12] Black haw reduces the pain of dysmenorrhea, endometriosis, fibroids, ovarian cysts, ovaritis, and fallopian tubes.[5,6,9,10,12] It is a primary ingredient in Hayden's Viburnum Compound used to ease uterine cramping. Black haw decreases uterine cramping during pregnancy, including spasms in the womb and digestive system.[4-6,9] It has mild antispasmodic actions for respiratory, stomach, and intestinal cramping, and is useful as a long-term treatment for asthma, irritable bowel syndrome, Crohn's disease, and colitis.[4] It also reduces nocturnal leg cramping.[5,6] The bark and root bark contain small quantities of salicin that can have mild anti-inflammatory actions; this may contribute to its pain relieving effects.[4,12] The astringent tannins decrease swelling in inflamed mucous membranes, reducing pain. Black haw has weaker antispasmodic properties than its cousin, cramp bark.

Black haw enhances blood flow to the pelvic region, subtly reducing stagnation and enhancing nutrient delivery to the womb and intestines.[5,6] It has mild nervine properties, acting as a subtle nervine and relaxant during pregnancy.[4-6]

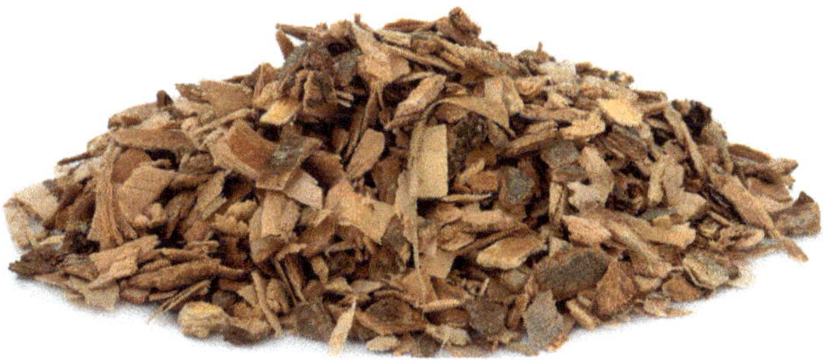

Black haw has astringent and hemostatic actions that diminish spotting and irregular bleeding in the first trimester.[6] It also reduces heavy or irregular bleeding during menstruation and menopause. Black haw alleviates bleeding caused by inflammatory bowel disease and hemorrhoids. It tightens mucous membranes, decreases inflammation, and reduces diarrhea. Topical use of the fomentation or powdered herb acts as a styptic, staunching bleeding.

Black haw has numerous benefits for pregnant women; it aids in preventing miscarriage, and is a partus preparator, and uterine hemostatic. Consuming black haw during the first and second trimester of pregnancy can improve the likelihood of carrying a baby full term.[4,5,7,12] Combine two parts of black haw and wild yam *(Dioscorea villosa)*, and one part of raspberry leaf *(Rubus idaeus)* and partridge berry *(Mitchella repens)* to aid in preventing a miscarriage, abate cramping, and staunch passive uterine bleeding.[6] Black haw can be combined with raspberry *(Rubus)*, partridge berry *(Mitchella)*, and/or white peony *(Paeonia lactiflora)* as a uterine tonic and partus preparator. *Note:* Multiple factors affect the potential for miscarriage, including: progesterone deficiency, hypothyroidism or hyperthyroidism, birth defects, and other serious concerns. Consult a health care practitioner regarding a threatened miscarriage.

Black haw allays afterbirth pains and prevents postpartum hemorrhage.[5] It restores tone to the uterus following a birth, and curbs irregular bleeding that can occur in the weeks following a birth.

CONTRAINDICATIONS

Black haw has no known contraindications, toxicity, or side effects.[10,12] It is safe to consume during pregnancy, while lactating, and for children. However, a health professional should be consulted regarding gynecological conditions before using black haw.[10] Due to the presence of small quantities of salicosides, some herbalists speculate that it should be avoided by individuals with aspirin allergies or Reye's syndrome.

PREPARATION AND DOSAGE

TINCTURE: Fresh bark or root bark [1:2-1:3, 70-95% alcohol, or 1:2-1:3 60% alcohol and 10% glycerin]; dry bark or root bark [1:5, 60% alcohol and 10% glycerin]; consume 30-120 drops, up to four times daily.

FLUID EXTRACT: Dry bark or root bark [1:1; 40% alcohol]; consume 15-60 drops, up to four times daily.

CAPSULES: Consume 2-4 "00" capsules, one to three times daily.

TEA: Prepare a decoction or cold infusion; consume 8-12 ounces, three to five times daily.

HONEY AND SYRUP: Prepare a decoction in distilled water, and add the desired amount of honey or simple syrup to sweeten. Adding 20% alcohol to the blend will increase the shelf life; however, it should be refrigerated. The syrup can last up to one month. Consume 1 teaspoon to 1 tablespoon, three to five times daily.

TOPICAL USE: Prepare a decoction and apply the hot fomentation or poultice to sore muscles or joints, or bathe the affected joints in hot tea.

CULINARY USE: Fresh fruits are edible, or freeze the berries for later use. Add the berries to jams, juices, pies, sauces, liqueurs, wines, cordials, and pemmican.

BLACKBERRY

DESCRIPTION

BOTANICAL NAMES:
Rubus villosus, R. ursinus, R. fructicosus, R. canadensis, R. armeniacus, and *R.* spp.

COMMON NAMES:
Blackberry, dewberry, low-bush blackberry, low blackberry, high blackberry, trailing blackberry, California blackberry, Himalayan blackberry, bramble, bramble-kite, bumble-kite, bly, brummel, brameberry, scaldhead, brambleberry, goutberry
brombaer (Danish)
braam (Dutch)
murier, ronce commune (French)
brombeere (German)
mora, rova (Italian)
amora-preta (Portuguese)
mora, zarzamora, zarza (Spanish)
björnbär (Swedish)

FAMILY NAME:
Rosaceae

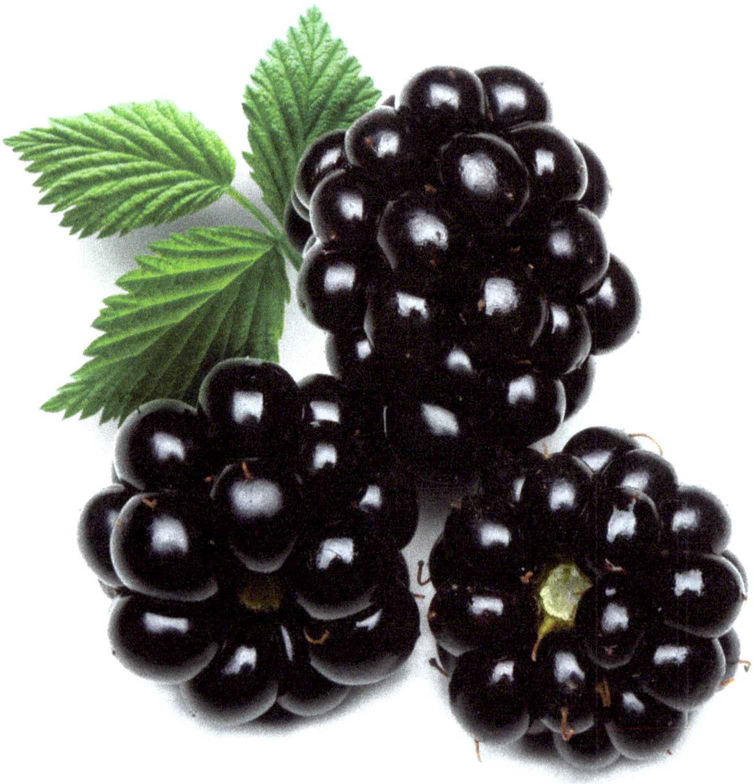

PARTS USED: The roots, leaves, and fruit.

BOTANICAL DESCRIPTION AND HABITAT: Blackberry is a prolific perennial plant that grows in well-drained, sandy soil throughout North America. It often colonizes in vacant lots, ditches, wastelands, woods, hillsides, and hedgerows. Blackberry plants can create impenetrable

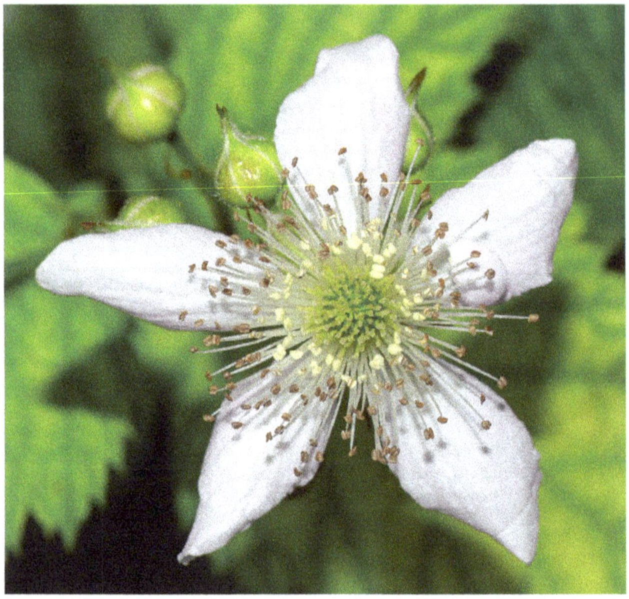

thickets covering wide swaths of land (up to three meters high) in the case of Himalayan blackberry.[1] Blackberry has trailing prostrate or erect stems varying in length among species, featuring sharp prickles. While the roots are perennial, the dense, arching stems are biennial, bearing fruit during their second year. Primocanes, the first-year stems, lack flowers; floricanes, the second-year stems, flower. The branching stems grow adventitious roots where they touch the ground. Each pinnately compound leaf has three to five ovate leaflets that are smooth above and tomentose below, with dentate or doubly serrate leaf margins. Growing in clusters of five to 20, the flower is comprised of five sepals and five whitish-pink petals, as well as many stamens and separate carpels. The flowers mature into delicious edible aggregate fruit comprised of small, deep purple-black drupelets attached to an inner core, the torus. Blackberries are distinguished from raspberries and their relatives by whether the torus stays with the fruit upon harvesting. Blackberry fruit retain the torus; raspberry fruit have a hollow core and do not retain the torus.

THE NAME: *Rubus* ("red") derives from Latin. Also derived from Latin, the epithet *villosus* ("shaggy or hairy") refers to the leaves, and *ursinus* ("of or pertaining to a bear") refers to bears' fondness for the fruit. *Fructicosus* derives from the Latin *fructus,* meaning "fruit, produce, proceeds, crops; an enjoyment, delight, satisfaction." *Canadensis* means "of or referring to Canada." The common name "bramble" originates from the Old English *braembel,* meaning a "prickly or impenetrable shrub." Three possible origins relate to the common name scaldhead: 1) it produces a skin eruption known as scaldhead when children excessively consume the fruit; 2) the leaves and berries cure scalp problems; or 3) in England, the leaves were a household remedy for burns and scalds.[2] It was also believed that creeping under a bramble bush provided a charm against boils, blackheads, and rheumatism. The flowers and fruit were used to treat venomous snakebites.[2]

Rubus villosus is known as American blackberry, bramble, fingerberry, or brombeere. It originated in Europe, but is cultivated in the U.S. where it has naturalized. *R. ursinus* is known as California blackberry, trailing blackberry, bramble, and dewberry. *Rubus armeniacus* (syn. *R. discolor*), or Himalayan blackberry, is the most prevalent on the U.S. West Coast. *Rubus fruticosus* corresponds with the common names European blackberry, bramble, bramble-kite, bumble-kite, bly, brummel, brameberry, scaldhead, and brambleberry. *R. canadensis* is known as smooth blackberry or thornless blackberry; it grows in Canada and the southeastern U.S.

HISTORICAL USES: In Europe, blackberry leaf and root were traditional remedies for diarrhea. The tea was consumed to treat chronic appendicitis, enteritis, leukorrhea, and dropsy.[3] In Ancient Greece, blackberries were consumed as a remedy for gout, and the leaves were chewed for bleeding gums.[3] In Britain, a wash made from the leaves was used to treat skin eruptions.[4] In the U.S., Eclectic physicians had similar applications for blackberry root, but also used it for chronic dysentery and cholera infantum.[5] Physician Harvey Felter described the following uses of blackberry root in *The Eclectic Materia Medica, Pharmacology, and Therapeutics:*

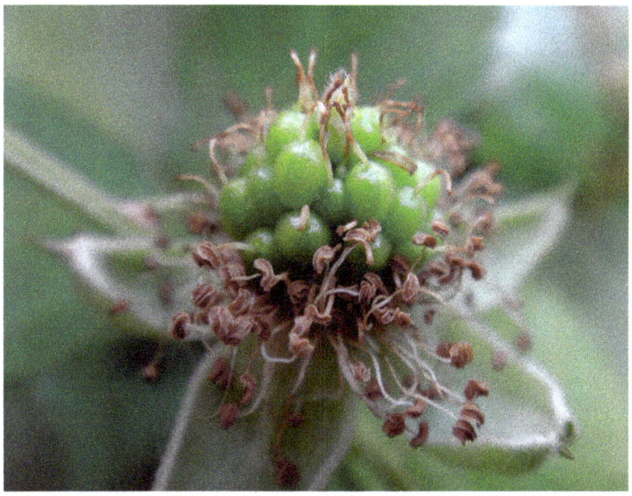

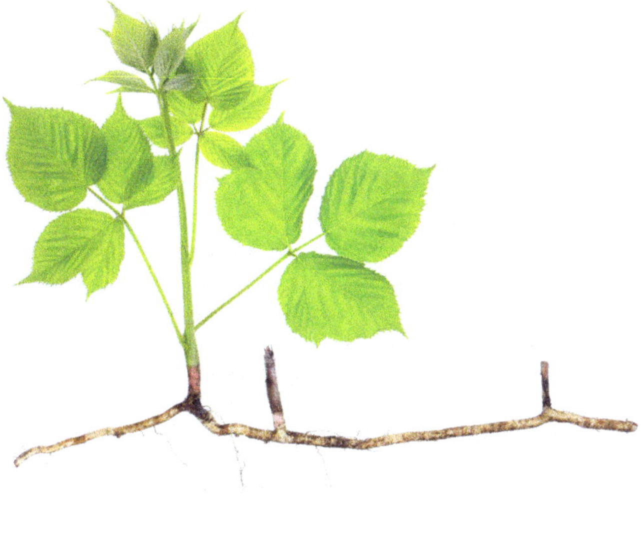

> The decoction of *Rubus* is a mild, agreeable astringent for watery diarrheas, especially in children, when the stools are clay-colored and pale. There is marked enfeeblement of the stomach and a bowel, the child is fretful, has no appetite, and there is marked pallor of the skin.[6]

Finley Ellingwood claimed that the tonic and astringent properties were underestimated, and mentioned similar indications in *American Materia Medica, Therapeutics, and Pharmacognosy.*[7]

Trailing blackberry *(R. ursinus)* is one of the only native blackberry species in the Pacific Northwest. According to a Canadian origin myth from the Stl'al'imx and Coastal Salish, a jealous husband chased his wife up a tree, then her blood fell from the tree and became a blackberry. Before their spirit dance, the Coastal Salish scrubbed blackberry stems across an individual's body in purification ceremonies.[8] Preparations of leaves and roots were consumed to treat diarrhea, dysentery, cholera, excessive menstruation, hemorrhoids, fevers, and mouth sores.[8] Northwest coastal tribes harvested fresh berries for immediate consumption, or dried and stored them.[8]

Early settlers used blackberry brandy as a cure for diarrhea. The West Coast Luiseno used the berries as a black dye for basketry.[9] Picking blackberry fruit was a favorite pastime.

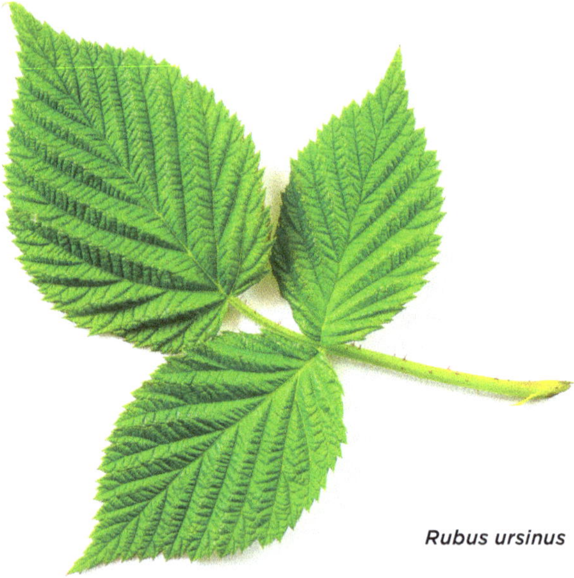

Rubus ursinus

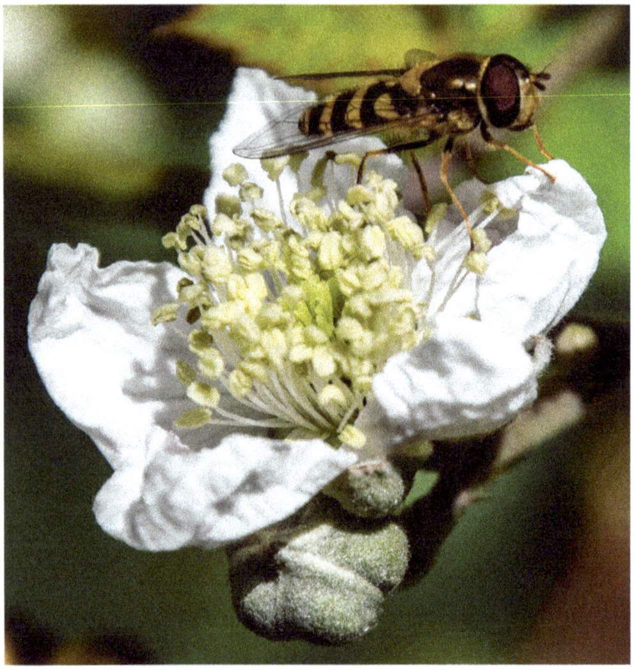

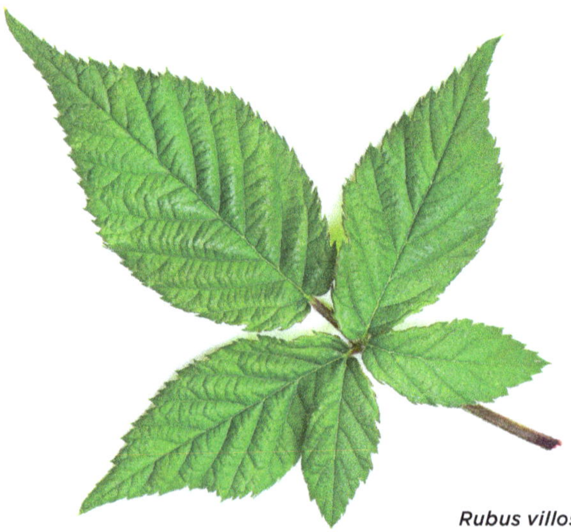

Rubus villosus

CONSTITUENTS

BLACKBERRY ROOT: Blackberry root and root bark contain tannins, gallic acid, villosin, starch, and calcium oxalate.[4,10,11]

BLACKBERRY LEAF: Blackberry leaf contains tannins, flavonoids (flavonols), organic acids (citric and isocitric), triterpenes (ursolic acid), mucilaginous polysaccharides, and traces of volatile oil.[10] According to herbalist Michael Moore, blackberry leaf contains fragarine, a uterine tonic.[12]

BLACKBERRY FRUIT: The fruit is a good source of organic acids (citric, ellegalic, and malic), pectin, polyphenols (quercetin), anthocyanins, cyanidin, flavonoids (lutein), vitamins A, C, and K, folate, choline, calcium, magnesium, manganese, and fiber (soluble and insoluble). Blackberries contain low amounts of vitamin E, sugar, sodium, niacin, pantothenic acid, betaine, copper, iron, potassium, phosphorus, zinc, and selenium.[6,13-15]

NUTRITIONAL PROPERTIES: Blackberry leaf contains flavonoids and organic acids. The nutritional properties of blackberry fruit are listed in the previous paragraph.

MEDICINAL PROPERTIES: Blackberry root is an astringent, antidiarrheal and anti-inflammatory. The leaves are astringent, antidiarrheal and anti-inflammatory, as well as a uterine tonic and uterotropic. The fruit is an antioxidant, blood tonic, laxative, mild diuretic, refrigerant and yin tonic.

TEMPERATURE AND FLAVOR: The roots and leaves are cool, astringent, sour, and bitter. The fruit is cool, sweet, and sour.

MEDICINAL USES

BLACKBERRY ROOT AND LEAF: Like many plants in the rose family, blackberry root, root bark, and leaf astringe the mucous membranes, decreasing inflammation. The root and root bark are significantly more astringent than the leaf. Consuming blackberry root tea or tincture is highly effective for treating diarrhea and dysentery. Additional anti-infective herbs are necessary when treating microbial infections such as giardiasis, stomach flu, or dysentery. When compounding blackberry root extract, it is preferable to combine it with tannin-containing antimicrobial herbs such as black walnut hull *(Juglans nigra)*, yerba mansa *(Anemopsis)*, and cinnamon *(Cinnamomum zeylanicum)*, rather than alkaloid-containing herbs, because alkaloids precipitate tannins out of solution when combined in alcohol-based compounds. Blackberry root and leaf tea reduce acute inflammation from gastritis and enteritis, as well as flareups of irritable bowel syndrome, Crohn's disease, and colitis. The astringent properties of blackberry root and leaf reduce mucus secretion, aiding in the treatment of seasonal allergies and sinus infections.

Gargling with the tea or diluted tincture reduces inflammation in the mouth and throat, and aids in treating bleeding gums, laryngitis, pharyngitis, and strep throat. Preparing an eye wash from the tepid tea alleviates eye inflammation due to conjunctivitis, particulate irritation, or allergies. A sitz bath is useful for treating hemorrhoids and anal fissures, and for healing sore tissues in the vagina and perineum following childbirth. Irrigating the vaginal canal with blackberry leaf or root tea decreases excessive vaginal secretions (leukorrhea), and soothes irritation caused by non-specific vaginitis and yeast infections. Additional antifungal herbs are necessary for the latter condition. An enema astringes rectal tissues, reducing bleeding and inflammation of internal hemorrhoids. Sitz baths and compresses act similarly for hemorrhoids. A bath, wash, fomentation, or compress reduces skin inflammation. *Note:* For all of the aforementioned applications, the tea must be strained through a paper filter or very fine cloth to remove all particulate matter. A fresh batch of tea should be prepared daily to prevent the introduction of microbes.

Blackberry leaf and root have hemostatic properties, and can be consumed during and following a birth to prevent hemorrhaging and reduce excessive bleeding. Blackberry leaf tea can be used following labor to cleanse afterbirth from the uterus and reduce postpartum bleeding. It also reduces uterine bleeding due to a miscarriage or abortion. Blackberry leaves reduce excessive menstrual flow, and mid-cycle and menopausal spotting.

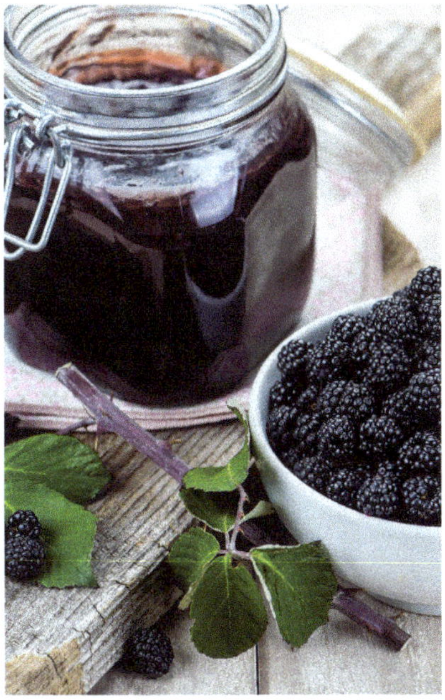

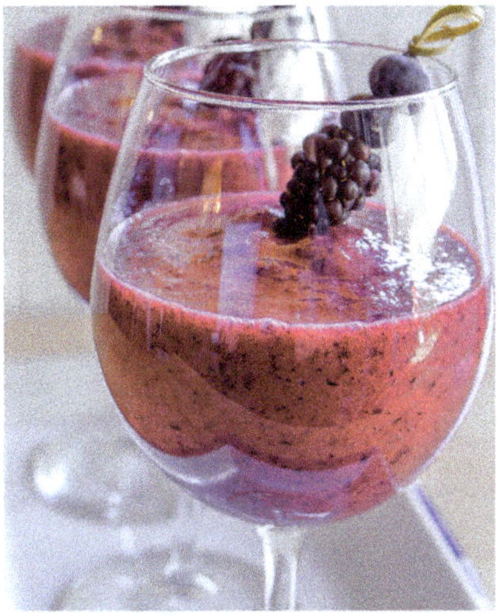

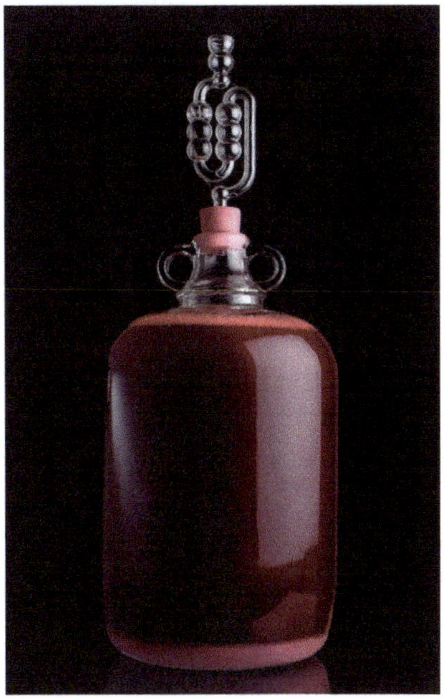

Blackberry leaves are a substitute for raspberry leaves. The leaves contain fragarine, which relaxes and tones the uterine pelvic muscles.[12] Blackberry leaf acts as a female reproductive tonic due to the uterotropic (uterine normalizing) actions and uterine tonic properties. During pregnancy, blackberry leaf tea can be consumed daily to strengthen the uterus and promote a smooth delivery; it also aids in restoring uterine tone after birth. The tea can be beneficial for easing morning sickness during pregnancy. *Note:* In rare cases, blackberry tannins can aggravate the stomach or cause nausea; discontinue use if this occurs.

Blackberry leaf contains vitamins and minerals, and is considered a nutritive and "blood builder." An infusion of the fermented leaves resembles the flavor of black tea and is a caffeine-free substitute. The dried, cut, and sifted leaves can be added to smoking mixtures as a bulking agent.

BLACKBERRY FRUIT: Blackberry fruit has yin and blood tonifying actions according to Traditional Chinese Medicine.[13] The berries are used to treat iron deficiency anemia.[13] They are rich in anthocyanins, flavonoids, and vitamins A, C, E, and K, which have antioxidant actions.[13] Blackberries hydrate the bowels and contain fiber, acting as a gentle laxative. The pectin content thickens preserves and jellies.[14] The sweet, slightly sour fruit is a refrigerant and cooling, moistening, hydrating tonic for consuming in hot weather.

Blackberries provide vitamin C and flavonoids that synergize the effects of vitamin C. The vitamin C content reduces inflammation, enhances the integrity of connective tissue, and counters the body's response to stress. Vitamin C and flavonoids inhibit the

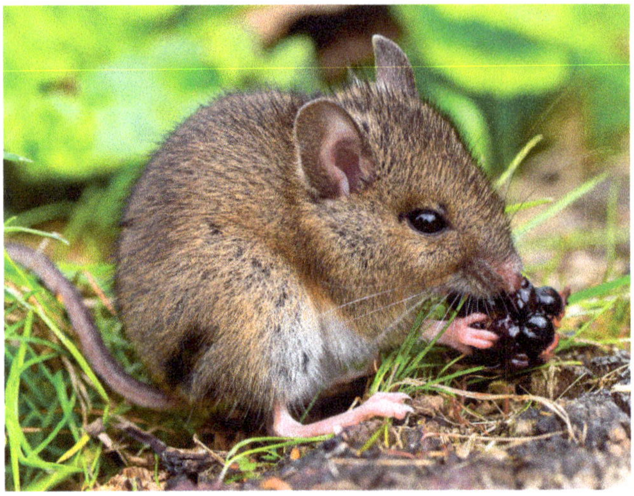

release of histamines that aid in treating allergies, allergy-related asthma attacks, wheezing, respiratory infections, and nasal congestion. Vitamin C and flavonoids are antioxidants that inhibit free radical formation, supporting the cardiovascular and immune systems. They enhance the integrity of the vascular system, and can be consumed as a daily tonic to reduce capillary fragility and permeability. Blackberries also aid in the long-term treatment of varicose veins, atherosclerosis, hypertension, and diabetes. They hasten wound and bruise healing.

Blackberries contain pectin — a highly ionic substance. Pectin draws and binds with heavy metals in the tissues, enhancing detoxification. It also aids in lowering cholesterol.

CONTRAINDICATIONS

Blackberry leaf is drying and may exacerbate dry conditions. Avoid long-term use in individuals with dry mucous membranes. Excessive consumption of blackberries can cause loose stools, diarrhea, or scaldhead.

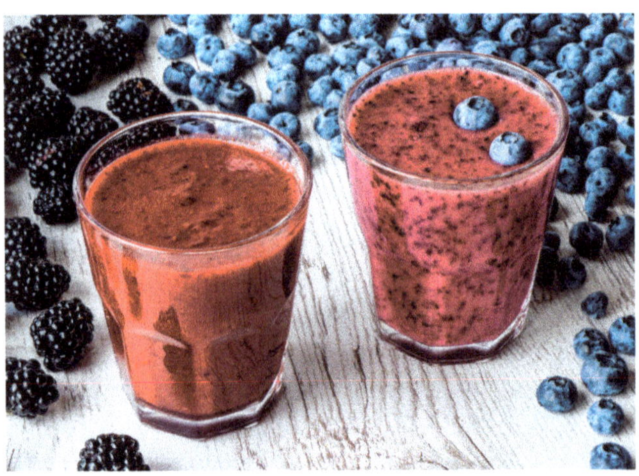

PREPARATION AND DOSAGE

TINCTURE: Fresh roots [1:2-1:3, 60-90% alcohol and 10% glycerin]; dry roots [1:5, 50% alcohol, 40% water, 10% glycerin]; consume 30-90 drops, up to four times daily. Fresh leaves [1:3-1:4, 50-95% alcohol]; dry leaves [1:5, 50-60% alcohol]; consume 15-60 drops, up to four times daily. For cordials and elixirs, use the Simpler's method to infuse the berries in brandy or vodka; after straining, add honey or syrup to desired sweetness.

ACETUM EXTRACT: Prepare the berries using the Simpler's method to infuse them in rice vinegar, champagne vinegar, or balsamic vinegar for culinary use.

CAPSULES: Consume 2-4 "00" capsules of the root, up to four times daily. Consume 2 "00" capsules of the leaf, one to three times daily.

TEA: Prepare a decoction of the root or root bark; consume 8-12 ounces, up to four times daily. Prepare a hot or cold infusion of the leaves; consume 8-12 ounces, up to four times daily. *Note:* As a nutritive, blackberry tea is less bitter and astringent when using hot water that is well below boiling temperature; alternatively, use a cold infusion.

HONEY AND SYRUP: Prepare syrup by placing 2 ounces of dried roots in 32 ounces of distilled water, then decoct to one-half the original volume of water (16 ounces); add honey or simple syrup to desired sweetness. Consume 1 teaspoon to 1 tablespoon, one to three times daily. Refrigerate up to one month.

TOPICAL USE: Cool the leaf or root tea to room or body temperature, then strain through a paper coffee filter. Use as a vaginal irrigation, enema, eye wash, mouthwash, fomentation, or poultice.

CULINARY USE: Blackberry fruit can be consumed raw or cooked in pies, jellies, preserves, and syrups. The fruit is delicious in wines and meads. The young shoots with prickles removed can be sliced and eaten in salads or cooked in soups.

CAUTION: Make sure to pick unsprayed blackberries, and avoid picking them roadside. Individuals have become seriously ill from herbicide poisoning.

BLUE COHOSH

DESCRIPTION

BOTANICAL NAMES:
Caulophyllum thalictroides, C. giganteum (syn. *C. thalictroides* var. *giganteum*)

COMMON NAMES:
Blue cohosh, blue ginseng, yellow ginseng, women's best friend, blueberry root, beechdrops, papoose root, squaw root
cohost bleu (French)
blauer hahnenfuss, frauenwurzel, stengelblett (German)
steblelist moshny (Russian)
caulofilo, cohosh azul (Spanish)

FAMILY NAME:
Berberidaceae

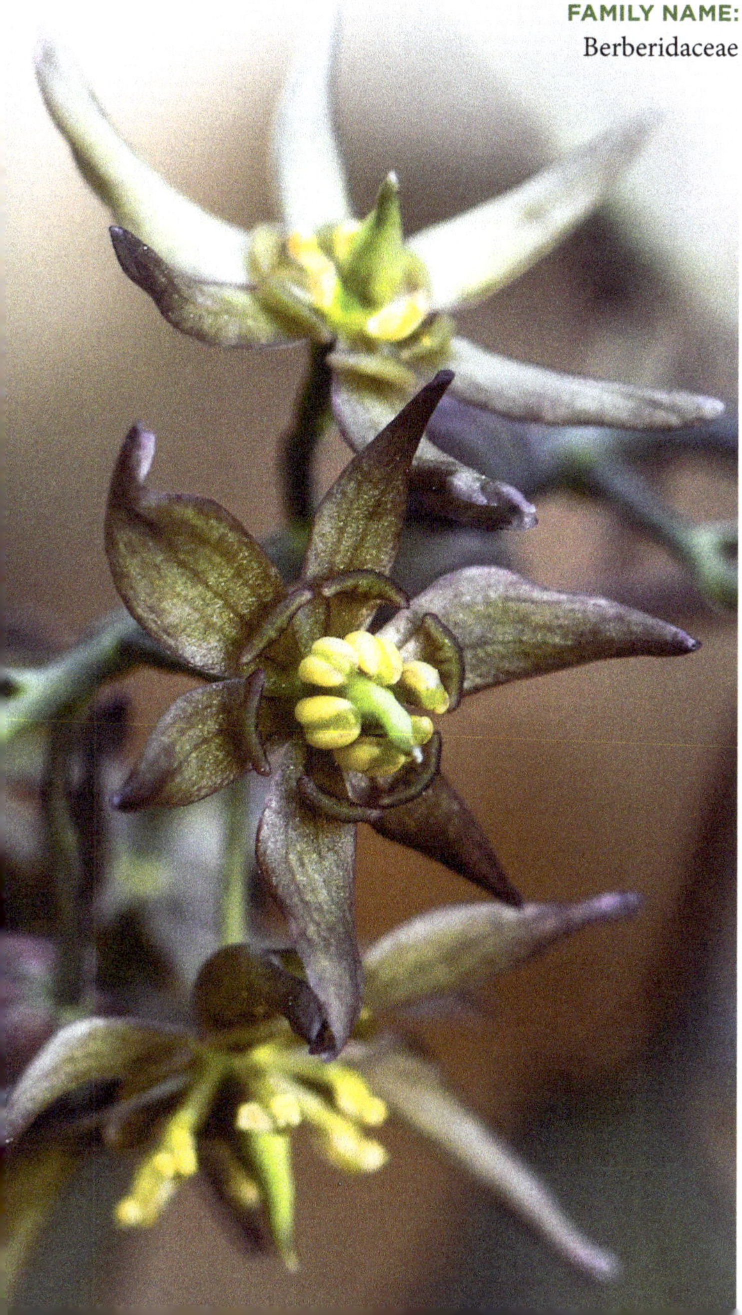

PARTS USED: The roots (rhizomes) or whole fresh plant.

BOTANICAL DESCRIPTION AND HABITAT: Blue cohosh is a glabrous, herbaceous perennial (20 – 90 cm tall) native to the moist, shaded deciduous forests in eastern North America. Only two delicate, light blue-green, 2- to 4-ternately compound leaves emerge from the underground rhizomes annually.[1] The irregularly lobed leaflets

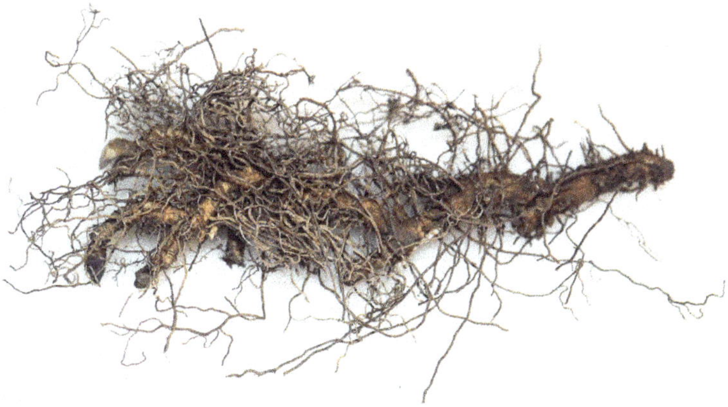

are obovate in shape (3 – 8 cm by 2 – 10 cm).[2] The yellow-green flowers (6 – 20 mm diameter) have six large, petal-like sepals subtended by three or four sepal-like bracts that fall off early. The flowers also have six small, nectar-producing petals, six stamens, and a single, unicarpellate pistil with a superior ovary.[1] The flowers grow in terminal, compound cymes of up to 70 flowers that mature into pairs of naked, globose, berry-like seeds with dark blue, fleshy seed coats.[1-3] The uncooked seeds are inedible and can be poisonous.[4]

THE NAME: *Caulophyllum* derives from two Greek words: *kaulos* ("stem") and *phyllon* ("leaf"), referring to the stem that forms a single stalk for the compound leaf.[5] The epithet *thalictroides* was acquired because the leaves have a similar shape to those of *Thalictrum* (meadow rue). *Cohosh* is an Algonquin word meaning rough, referring to the gnarled appearance of the rhizomes.[5] The common names blue cohosh and blueberry root refer to the berry color. Squaw root and papoose root (pappoose) refer to its use in facilitating childbirth. The plant was called "women's best friend" due to its reputation for aiding childbirth and treating menstrual difficulties.[2]

HISTORICAL USES: Blue cohosh was traditionally used by more than ten Native American tribes.[4] Some tribes consumed the root tea to stimulate labor and menstruation, as well as for uterine inflammation and chronic uterine conditions.[4,7] The Meskwaki and Menominee drank the tea to treat profuse menstruation.[6] The Menominee valued the herb as a female remedy.[6] The Potawatomi used blue cohosh to aid childbirth and treat profuse menstruation.[6] The Ojibwa consumed the tea for stomachaches due to painful menstruation.[6] The Cherokee utilized the herb to stimulate labor, reduce uterine inflammation, and relieve toothaches, rheumatism, and anxiety.[7] The Omaha prized the herb as a fever remedy.[6] The Chippewa used blue cohosh as a remedy for stomach cramps, indigestion, and lung conditions.[7] Various tribes also used the herb to treat urinary tract infections, lung ailments, venereal disease, rheumatism, and fevers.[4-7]

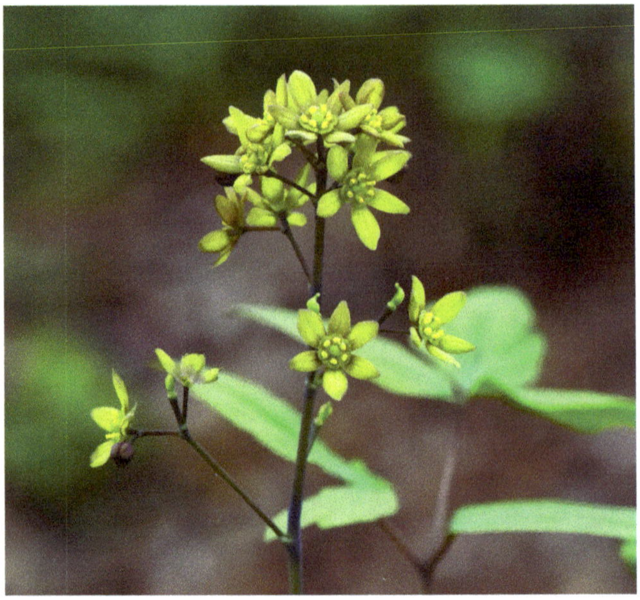

Healer Peter Smith adopted herbal healing approaches from Native Americans, and introduced traditional uses of blue cohosh to Eclectic physicians in 1813, when he published *Medical Facts*.[5] Smith described Native practices using "pappoose root" or "squaw root" two to three weeks before parturition in order to facilitate a smooth delivery.[5] He also described its value as an emmenagogue. Two decades later, Dr. John King began administering blue cohosh, and published his clinical applications and preparations in the *American Dispensatory* (1853). Following his publication, blue cohosh was popularized among the Eclectics and homeopaths.[5] Blue cohosh was an ingredient in Compound Syrup of Mitchella (Mother's Cordial), a formula commonly employed as a partus preparator and uterine tonic by Eclectic physicians and Thomsonians. This compound was also administered as a uterine tonic following labor, and for women with difficulty conceiving.[10] Benjamin Colby lists Dr. P.F. Sweet's recipe for Mother's Cordial in *A Guide to Health:* one pound of partridge berry *(Mitchella repens),* four ounces each of cramp bark *(Viburnum opulus),* unicorn root *(Chamaelirium),* and blue cohosh *(Caulophyllum).* The following are directions for preparation, dosage, and use:

> Boil in two gallons of water to one; strain and add one pound and a half of sugar, and three pints of brandy. Its effects are to shorten and diminish the sufferings of childbirth, and thus place both mother and child in a state of safety. It should be used daily for two weeks immediately preceding confinement as a preparatory. Dose — from half to a wine-glassful two or three times a day, and one at bed-time, in a little hot water.[6]

Blue cohosh root and a more concentrated preparation of its resinoid *(caulophyllin)* were used by numerous Eclectic and Physiomedic practitioners. Harvey Felter prescribed the herb for uterine pain with a sense of weight and fullness in the legs, pelvic congestion, sluggish labor pains, and as a partus preparator.[10] John King and Finley Ellingwood recommended the herb as a partus preparator, for false labor pains, severe afterbirth pains, and subinvolution of the uterus.[5,11] King and Felter offer the following indications for blue cohosh, according to *King's Dispensatory:*

> ...uterine pain with fullness, weight, and pain in the legs; fullness of tissues as if congested; debility (irritability) of the nervous system, with impaired muscular power; epigastric and umbilical colicky pains; dull frontal headache; as an oxytocic; to relieve false pains and uterine irritability; sexual debility with excitability; spasmodic uterine contractions; dysmenorrhea, irregular menstruation; crampy pains in stomach and bowels after eating; pain in toes and fingers not due to tissue changes.[5]

CONSTITUENTS: Blue cohosh roots contain quinolizidine alkaloids (N-methylcytosine = caulophylline, baptifoline, magnoflorine, laburnine, and anagyrine — a lupine alkaloid), triterpene glycosides (caulosaponin), flavonoids (hederagenin and leontin), gum, starch, salts, resins, and traces of volatile oil.[4,5,8,12-14] *C. robustum,* a Russian species, also contains triterpene glycosides (caulosides A – G).[8] The alkaloids anagyrine, baptifoline, and magniflorine are found in the leaves and seeds.[6]

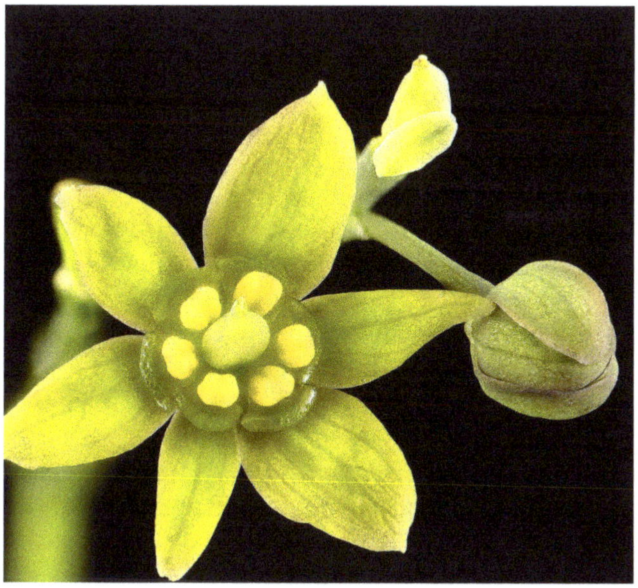

NUTRITIONAL PROPERTIES: While this root contains many nutrients, it is not safe to consume as a nutritive or culinary herb. Blue cohosh root contains the following vitamins and minerals: aluminum, ash, calcium, chromium, cobalt, fiber, fat, iron, magnesium, manganese, niacin, phosphorus, potassium, protein, riboflavin, selenium, silicon, sodium, thiamine, tin, and vitamins A and C.[13]

MEDICINAL PROPERTIES: Anti-inflammatory, antispasmodic, emmenagogue, oxytocic, parturifacient, uterine tonic, and mild diuretic. It was formerly used as an anthelmintic and diaphoretic.

TEMPERATURE AND FLAVOR: Warm, bitter, and sweet.

MEDICINAL USES

Blue cohosh is a nervine and smooth muscle antispasmodic that decreases cramping in the intestines, respiratory tract, urinary tract, and reproductive organs.[5,10,11] It aids in treating dysmenorrhea, menorrhagia, ovarialgia, ovaritis, interstitial cystitis, and spasmodic retention of urine.[5,10] Blue cohosh reduces acute and chronic pain associated with endometriosis, fibroids, and uterine and ovarian cysts. Additional analgesic and smooth muscle antispasmodics such as California poppy *(Eschscholzia)* or opium poppy *(Papaver)*, silk tassel *(Garrya)* or cannabis *(Cannabis)* may be necessary to ease severe spasms and pain. *Note:* It is important to begin treatment with a low dose (5 – 10 drops) of blue cohosh, and increase the dosage incrementally until the desired antispasmodic effects are obtained.

Blue cohosh reduces bronchial spasms such as a dry, irritable cough caused by bronchitis, pneumonia, or asthma.[5,7] Additional anti-infective agents are required when treating bronchitis and pneumonia. When treating asthma, blue cohosh is best used by unmedicated or minimally medicated, healthy adults, and should be avoided in highly medicated adults and children.

Blue cohosh has uterine tonifying actions; it also reduces uterine inflammation.[4,10,15,16] Low doses can be administered daily to improve blood flow to the reproductive organs, and reduce uterine pain due to blood stagnation.[5,10,16] For long-term use, a low dose range is preferable (5 – 15 drops per dose); it works most effectively in a compounded formula. Combine it with additional alkaloid-containing uterine tonics such as black cohosh *(Actaea racemosa)* and yellow pond lily *(Nuphar)*, as well as dong quai *(Angelica sinensis)*, white peony *(Paeonia alba)*, and partridge berry *(Mitchella)*.

Blue cohosh is a parturifacient and oxytocic that hastens delivery and facilitates smooth labor.[5,14-16] It coordinates uterine muscular contractions, increasing their power without inducing spasms (like ergot).[5] Blue cohosh also speeds placenta delivery and alleviates afterbirth pains.[5] Obstetrician Dr. Hale noted that it eased labor and improved recovery in women 10 – 12 days overdue.[5] Blue cohosh also aids in treating stalled labor, especially when the mother experiences nervous exhaustion.[7,15] It was historically used to alleviate false labor and afterbirth pain.[10] The glycosides caulosaponin and caulophyllosaponin stimulate uterine contractions; however, they can have vasoconstrictive effects, elevating blood pressure in the fetus and mother.[6,7] Therefore, the fetal heart rate should be closely monitored.[17] *Warning:* If the fetus or expectant mother's blood pressure becomes elevated, discontinue use immediately. Additional constituents of blue cohosh, including cytisine and N-methylcytosine, stimulate nicotinic receptors, and may potentiate the effects of caulosaponin.[4,14] N-methylcytosine also increases blood pressure and intestinal motility, and elevates blood sugar levels.[7] Water-based preparations, such as Mother's Cordial or a compounded syrup of blue cohosh are considered safer in facilitating delivery than the alcoholic extract. *Note:* Blue cohosh should only be used if there are no fetal complications, and if the expectant mother is healthy, and has no apparent complications such as preeclampsia or gestational diabetes. Prior to administration, it is important to note the fetal and maternal pulse rate, and to retake the pulse 10 – 15 minutes following consumption. If the pulse is elevated, discontinue use.

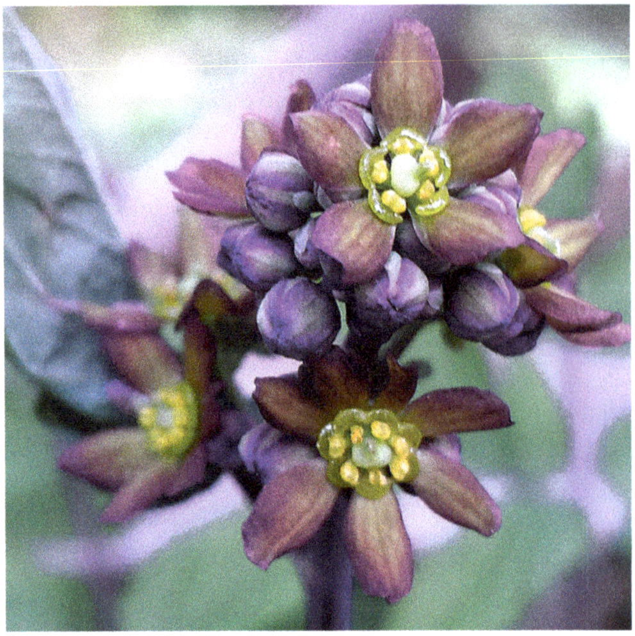

An emmenagogue and oxytocic, blue cohosh stimulates menstruation delayed due to nervous debility, anxiety, or oxytocin deficiency.[10,11,15] It aids in treating slow-starting, crampy menses with a dull, achy sensation in the uterus. It works most effectively to stimulate menstruation when 4 – 6 ounces of hot tea are consumed every two to three hours, or when 10 – 30 drops of the tincture are administered in hot water every two to three hours. Do not exceed four doses daily.

The fresh roots (and sometimes dried powdered roots) have a caustic quality that can irritate mucous membranes and stimulate salivation. This likely explains Eclectics' use of the plant as a glandular stimulant.

Blue cohosh combines with other alkaloid-containing herbs, but should not be combined with tannin-containing herbs in tincture form.

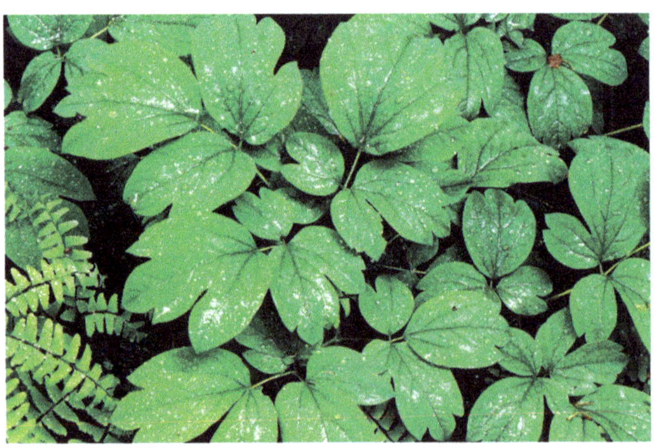

CONTRAINDICATIONS

Blue cohosh is contraindicated during pregnancy, except as a parturifacient. To hasten labor, use only under the care of a health care practitioner or birth attendant.[4] Women with preeclampsia or gestational diabetes should completely avoid use. Blue cohosh is also contraindicated when fetal or gestational concerns are present. Discontinue use with oxytocin stimulating medications, or following administration of an epidural. Avoid use when lactating, unless prescribed by a health care practitioner.[14]

High doses of the root or uncooked berries (three times the normal dose range) can cause nausea, gastric upset, vomiting, dilated pupils, headache, thirst, muscle weakness, or convulsions.[4] The berries are poisonous. Blue cohosh should be avoided by individuals with peptic ulcers, gastroesophageal reflux, hiatal hernia, or acid indigestion.[14] An excessive dose can also cause liver toxicity. Low to moderate dose ranges are recommended.

Due to the methylcytosine content, blue cohosh should be avoided in individuals with cardiovascular disease, especially those with high blood pressure, or individuals consuming blood pressure-lowering medications.[14] It is contraindicated in individuals taking blood thinning agents such as warfarin (Coumadin), insulin, blood sugar regulating medications, steroidal anti-inflammatory agents, pain medications, narcotics, parasympathomimetics, antinauseant medications, birth control, or hormone replacement therapy. When handled, the fresh plant can sometimes cause contact dermatitis and irritate the mucous membranes and skin.[7]

PREPARATION AND DOSAGE

TINCTURE: Fresh whole plant or roots [1:2-1:3, 70-95% alcohol]; dry roots [1:5, 60-70% alcohol]; consume 5-30 drops, up to four times daily. Do not consume more than three times daily for chronic conditions.

CAPSULES: Consume 1-2 "00" capsule, one to three times daily.

TEA: Prepare a decoction of the roots and consume 4-8 ounces, up to four times daily.

BOGBEAN

DESCRIPTION

BOTANICAL NAME:
Menyanthes trifoliata

COMMON NAMES:
Bogbean, buckbean, marsh trefoil, water trefoil, marsh clover, water shamrock, bean trefoil, brook bean, bog myrtle, moon flower
bocks, boonan (Dutch)
raate (Finnish)
herbe à canards, menianthe, menyanthe, trifolie, trefle d'eau (French)
bocksbohne, sharbocks-klee (German)
scarfano, trefoglio d'acqua, trifoglio fibrino (Italian)
vattenklöver (Swedish)
su yoncasi (Turkish)

FAMILY NAME:
Menyanthaceae (formerly Gentianaceae)

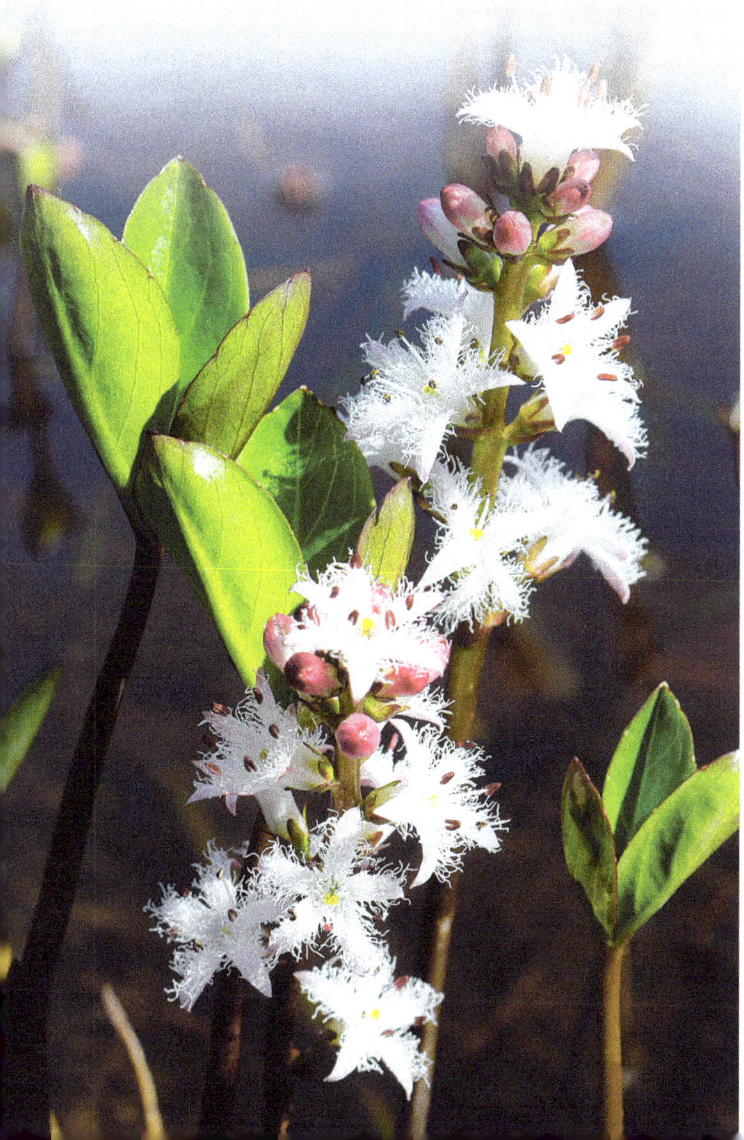

PARTS USED: The leaves, stems, and flowers.

BOTANICAL DESCRIPTION AND HABITAT: Bogbean is a colony-forming, semiaquatic to aquatic perennial plant. It grows in the margins of lakes, ponds, bogs, swamps, marshes, and wet meadows throughout North America,

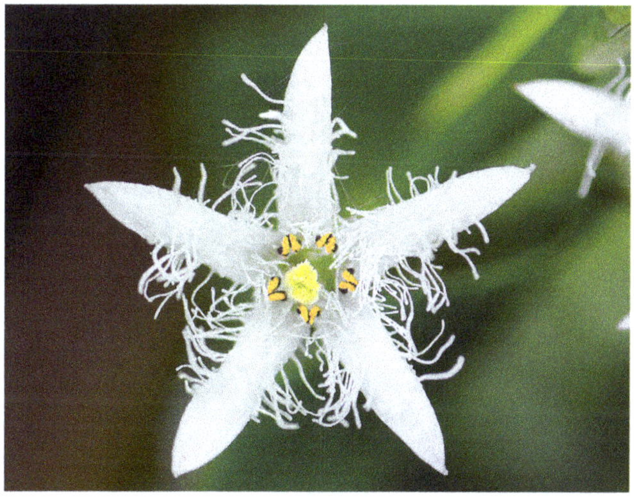

Europe, and central and southwest Asia.[1] The aging leaf bases wrap around the submerged rhizomes. Bogbean has alternate, trifoliate leaves with obovate, entire leaflets (2.5 – 4 cm long), and long, erect petioles (12 – 20 cm long).[1] The white, funnel-shaped flowers have five calyx lobes (4 – 5 mm) and five corolla lobes (about 1.5 cm) that are pinkish-purple when in bud, and bright white and covered with long white hairs when open.[1] Within the distylous flower are five epipetalous stamens (about 6 mm long) and two fused carpels bearing a single style (short styles 6 – 7mm, long styles 10 – 12 mm).[1,2] The flowers grow on naked racemes and mature into an ovate, two-valved capsule.[2] The rank odor of these showy flowers attracts pollinators such as flies, beetles, and nectar- and pollen-feeding bees. The flowers provide egg-laying sites for dragonflies.

THE NAME: *Menyanthes* derives from *menanthos* (Greek), meaning "moon-flower" or "month-flower," respectively referring to the lunar glow of the white flowers, or the plant flowering for a month.[3,4] Another source claims that it derives from two Greek words: *menyein* ("disclosing") and *anthos* ("flower").[5] The epithet *trifoliata* and common name trefoil describe a plant "having three leaflets."[3] Bean, a term used in several common names including bogbean, buckbean, brook bean, and bean trefoil, refers to the resemblance of the trifoliate leaves to bean leaves commonly grown in gardens.[4] Marsh clover, water trefoil, marsh trefoil, and water shamrock refer to the habitat and clover-like appearance of this three-leaf herb. Bogbean and bog myrtle also describe the environment where the plant grows. The common name buckbean comes from the German name "scharbock" that evolved from *scorbutus,* the original Latin term for scurvy.[4]

HISTORICAL USES: Native American tribes used bogbean to treat digestive ailments including gas pains, constipation, and nausea. The tea was consumed as a recuperative agent following severe illness in order to increase appetite and assist in weight gain. Bogbean was used to relieve fevers, headaches, and rheumatism. The stems and rhizomes were ground and decocted, then the tea was consumed three times daily for the spitting of blood.[6] The Kwakwaka'wakw tribe consumed a decoction for stomach ailments.[6] Alaskan tribes used preparations of bogbean when food was scarce. The rhizomes were dried, ground, and washed in several changes of water until the bitterness was removed; they were dried before consumption.[6] A poultice was applied topically to ulcers, wounds, herpes, sore muscles, and glandular swellings.[3,6]

European herbalists used the herb to improve appetite and treat liver-related headaches, biliousness, skin diseases, rheumatoid arthritis, and gout.[7] An infusion of the herb was used to treat scurvy.[6] Juice from the fresh herb was said to cure dropsy; when mixed with whey, it treated gout. A large dose of powdered herb was consumed as a purgative. Topical applications were applied to swollen glands. The leaves were smoked like tobacco.[4]

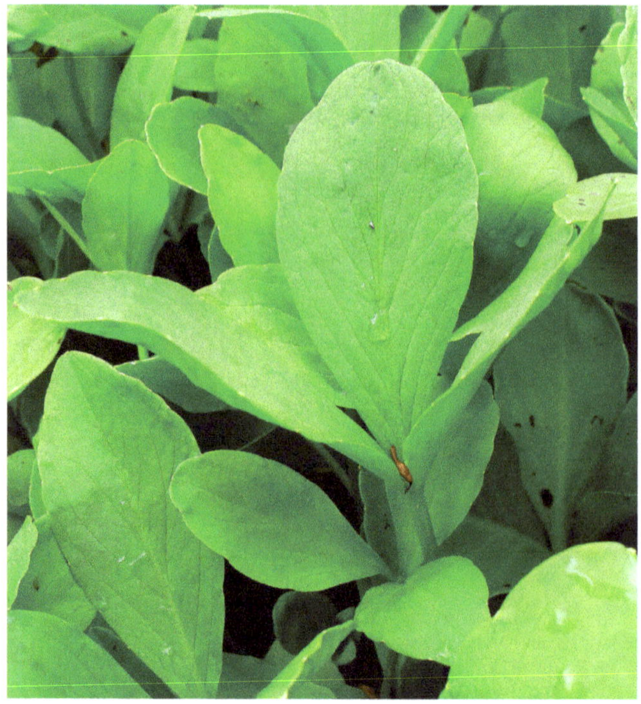

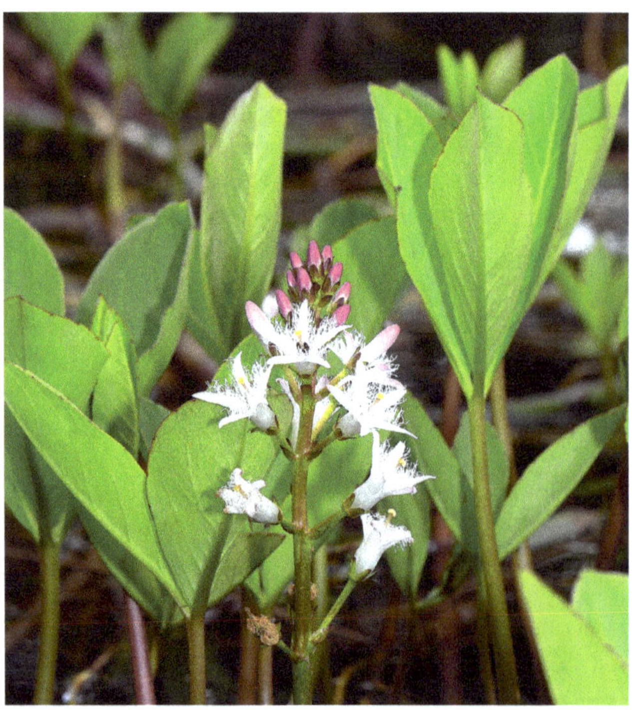

CONSTITUENTS: Bogbean contains menyanthin, dihydrofoliamenthin, menthiafolin, loganin, saponins, bitter principles (secoiridoids: menthiafolin), secoiridoid alkaloids (gentialutine), flavonoids (hyperin), coumarins (scopoletin), phenolic acids (caffeic acid), triterpenes (butulinic acid), small amounts of volatile oil (hexanals, pentenols, and terpene aromatics), and tannins.[8,9]

NUTRITIONAL PROPERTIES: Unknown.

MEDICINAL PROPERTIES: Bitter tonic, cholagogue, choleretic, hepatoprotectant, mild laxative, anti-inflammatory, immune modulator, diuretic, antibacterial, antifungal, and antiviral.

TEMPERATURE AND FLAVOR: Cool, bitter, and astringent (mild).

MEDICINAL USES

Bogbean is a digestive bitter tonic that works most effectively when consumed 15 to 30 minutes before meals.[8-10] It stimulates upper and lower digestive secretions, enhancing fat and protein digestion.[3,8-10] Bogbean is a choleretic and cholagogue that increases bile production and flow, respectively, enhancing the emulsification of fats in the duodenum, and acting as a mild laxative.[8,9] It is a liver protectant.[9] Bogbean is beneficial for individuals with deficient digestive secretions resulting in fullness, belching, gas, bloating, indigestion, sluggish bowels, or constipation.[3,8-10] The iridoids are attributed to the bitter tonic, cholagogue, liver protectant, laxative, anti-inflammatory, antimicrobial, and immune modulating effects.[9] The phenolic acids also contribute to the hepatobiliary effects.[9]

Bogbean reduces congestion in the portal vein, and is helpful in the long-term treatment of hemorrhoids, varicose veins, and spider veins.[8,10] It can also be used to treat symptoms resulting from poor fat metabolism, including dry skin conditions such as psoriasis and eczema.[8,10]

Bogbean has immune modulating effects.[9] It decreases histamines and humeral antibodies.[10] Bogbean also reduces subacute inflammation via the digestive tract, likely by encouraging a more complete breakdown of proteins.[10] Proteins inadequately broken down into amino acids in the duodenum can leak into the bloodstream through inflamed capillaries in the microvilli, causing an autoimmune response and leading to chronic low-grade inflammation. When consumed as a long-term bitter tonic, bogbean is helpful for treating conditions such as rheumatoid arthritis, chronically dull, achy joints or muscles, multiple sclerosis, food sensitivities, candida, chronic allergies, and environmental sensitivity.[8,10] Bogbean can be used as a recuperative agent for individuals exhausted from infectious illness.[11] The iridoids in bogbean also have antifungal, antibacterial, and antiviral properties.[9]

CONTRAINDICATIONS

Avoid use during pregnancy and lactation unless recommended by a health care practitioner.[9] Herbalist Michael Moore describes bogbean as an herb "for cold, deficient, achy conditions...not hot, inflamed, excess states."[8] Bogbean should be avoided when acute digestive inflammation is present.[8,10] Do not consume with excess conditions such as acid indigestion, gastroesophageal reflux, gastric ulcers, ulcerative colitis, diarrhea, or flareups of Crohn's disease or irritable bowel syndrome.[8] Excessive doses can cause nausea, vomiting, or diarrhea.[9] As a cholagogue agent, it should be avoided in individuals with a blocked bile duct. *Note:* This plant is considered at-risk or threatened; please use sparingly.

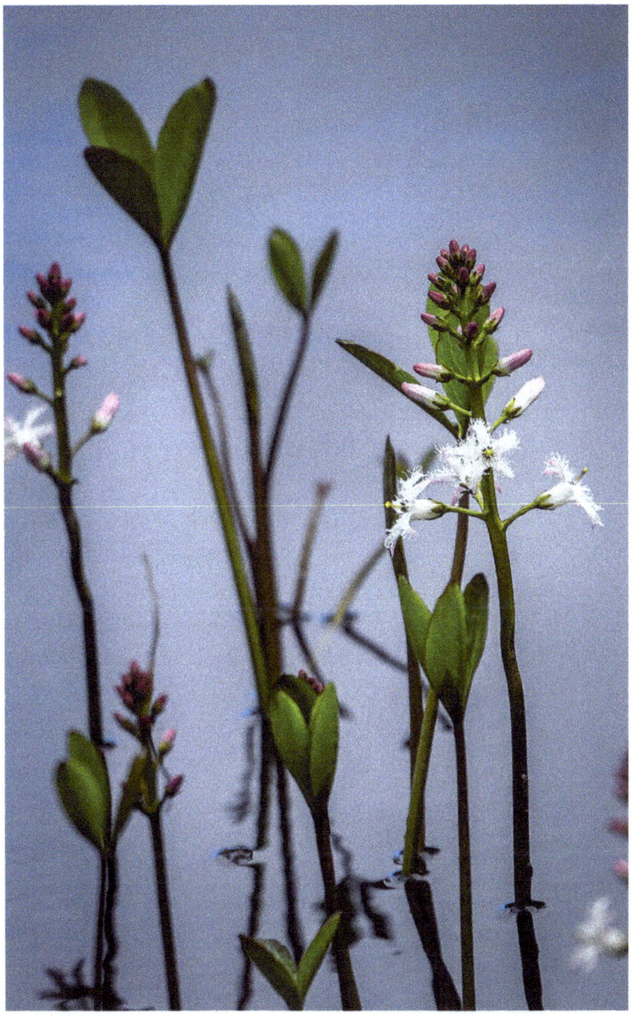

PREPARATION AND DOSAGE

TINCTURE: Fresh aerial portions [1:2-1:3, 70-95% alcohol]; recently dried aerial portions [1:5, 50-60% alcohol]; consume 10-60 drops, up to three times daily.

ACETUM EXTRACT: Fresh aerial portions [1:3, apple cider vinegar]; consume 15-45 drops, up to three times daily.

TEA: Prepare the cold or hot infusion; consume 4-8 ounces before meals, up to three times daily.

TOPICAL USE: Apply the fresh or dry herb poultice or paste.

BONESET

DESCRIPTION

BOTANICAL NAME:
Eupatorium perfoliatum

COMMON NAMES:
Boneset, common boneset, thoroughwort, thoroughstem, agueweed, crosswort, feverwort, Indian sage, sweating plant, teadral, vegetable antimony, wild Isaac, wood boneset
eupatoire perforée, herbe á la fievre, herbe parfaite (French)
durchwachsdost, virginischer walddosten (German)
rompe zaraguey, alba haquilla, hierba de chiva, Santa Maria (Spanish)

FAMILY NAME:
Asteraceae (Compositae)

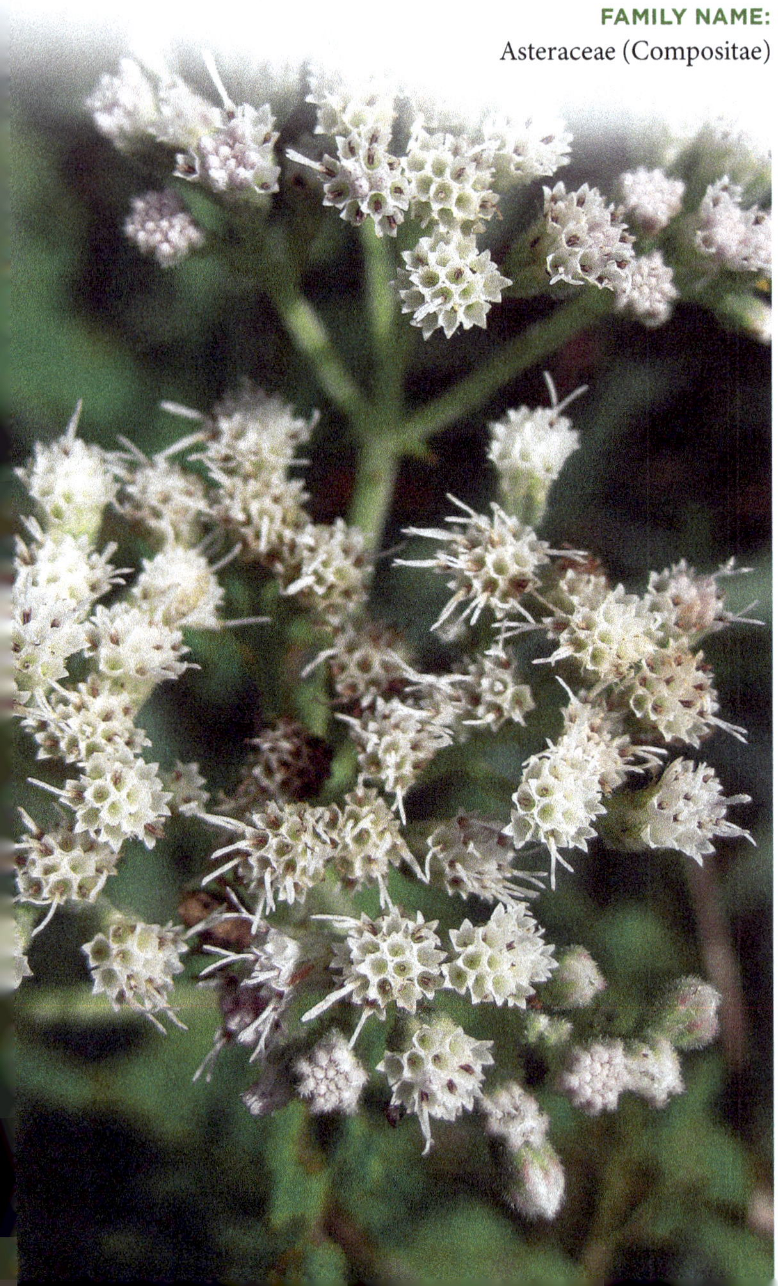

PARTS USED: The leaves and flowering tops.

BOTANICAL DESCRIPTION AND HABITAT: Boneset is a perennial herb with clumps of erect, sturdy, hairy stems (40 – 100 cm tall).[1] Fine hairs cover the entire plant.[1] The pairs of opposite, sessile leaves are joined at their bases and

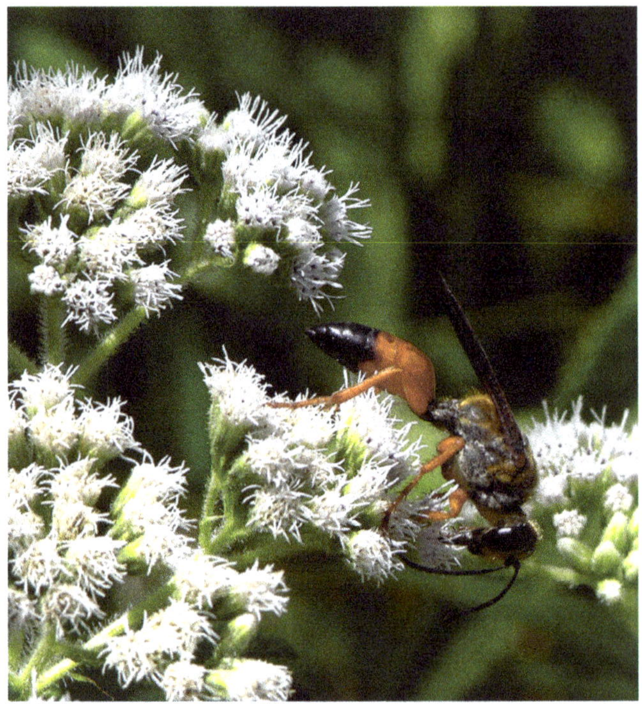

encircle the stem; this gives the appearance of perforation by the stem.[2] The leaves are (50 – 150 mm long by 15 – 40 mm wide) and oblong to lanceolate, with finely dentate margins and acute apices.[1] The undersides are pubescent and covered in glands; the upper sides are glabrous.[1] The terminal inflorescences are compound corymbs of many small, fluffy heads.[2] Each head consists of 7 – 11 tiny white florets with corollas (3 mm long) that bloom August through October.[1] The fruit is an achene with pappus comprised of 20 – 30 bristles.[1]

THE NAME: *Eupatorium* was named after Mithridates Eupator, the 1st century king of Pontus who purportedly found a poison antidote in a species of the *Eupatorium* genus.[3] The epithet *perfoliatum* refers to the leaves perforated by the stem.[4] The common name boneset originated from the herb's use in treating breakbone fever during the early 20th century flu epidemic.[4]

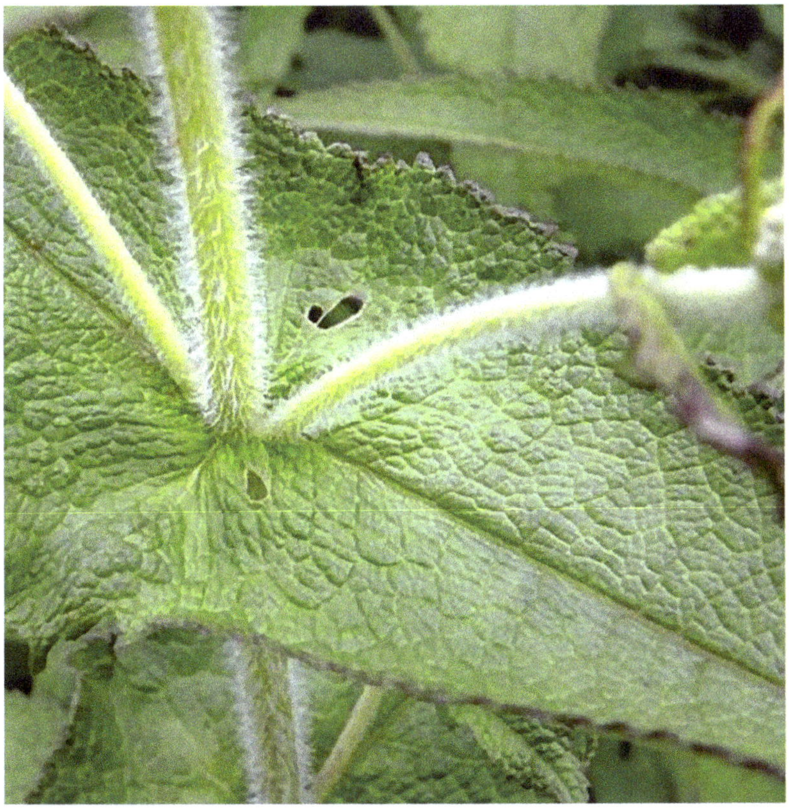

NUTRITIONAL PROPERTIES: Not applicable.

MEDICINAL PROPERTIES: Alterative, analgesic, antibacterial, antipyretic, antiviral, astringent, bitter tonic, cooling diaphoretic, expectorant, febrifuge, and immune stimulant. It is also a cathartic, choleretic, cholagogue, emetic, and laxative.

TEMPERATURE AND FLAVOR: Cool, bitter, and mild astringent.

HISTORICAL USES: More than 12 North American tribes introduced the plant to American settlers.[3,5] Eclectic physicians administered low doses of the cold infusion or extract prior to meals as a stomachic and bitter tonic to treat nonulcer dyspepsia, indigestion, and general debility.[4,6] Large doses of boneset tea were given as an emetic and purgative.[3,4] Hot tea was administered as a febrifuge to treat breakbone fever, typhoid fever, and yellow fever.[3,4] One-half cup of tea was given every 15 minutes until the patient vomited. The patient was then put to bed, and continued ingesting smaller quantities of the tea until they perspired for two to three hours. Low doses of boneset cold infusion were then given as a tonic.[6,7] Boneset was also administered to alleviate hoarseness and a cough, and reduce mucus secretions.[7] Boneset tea was given to expel tapeworms and treat skin disease.[4] It was included in the *U.S. Pharmacopoeia* until the 1950s.[3]

CONSTITUENTS: Boneset contains flavonoids (quercetin, kaempferol, quercetin-3-β-galactoside = hyperoside, kaempferol-3-β-glucoside = astragalin, quercetin-3-rutinoside = rutin, kaempferol-3-rutinoside, and eupatorin), terpenoids (chromenes), sesquiterpene lactones (euperfolin, euperfolitin, eufoliatin, and euperfolide), diterpenes (dendroidinic acid and hebeclinolide), triterpenes (α-amyrin), sterols (sitosterol and stimasterol), hydrocarbons (dotriacontane), volatile oil, a polysaccharide (4-0-methylglucuronoxylan), and resin.[8,9]

MEDICINAL USES

A cooling, anti-inflammatory alterative with immune stimulating effects, boneset increases resistance to bacterial and viral infections.[9] The immune stimulating actions are attributed to the polysaccharide content and bitter principles (sesquiterpene lactones and diterpenes).[8,9] Boneset is specific for influenza; one study using diluted alcohol-based extracts showed *in vitro* that boneset protects cells from influenza-A by inhibiting viral attachment to the host cells. The study stated that polyphenolic compounds were the likely active agents.[10] Paul Bergner reported success in treating West Nile encephalitis and meningitis using boneset as a primary therapy.[11] The following tincture compound aids in treating a cold or flu: four parts echinacea *(Echinacea)* and elder berry *(Sambucus);* two parts propolis resin; one part boneset; and one-half part licorice *(Glycyrrhiza)*. Consume 30 – 90 drops every two hours, up to five times daily.

Administered as a hot tea in small, frequent doses, boneset is a diaphoretic, febrifuge, and analgesic that reduces fever resulting from a cold or flu. Boneset also decreases muscle aches, soreness, and rheumatic pain caused by a fever.[4,9] It reduces inflammation in the upper respiratory tract.[9] Boneset contains sesquiterpene lactones and flavones that have cytotoxic, antineoplastic, and anti-inflammatory actions.[8,10] Although the tea tastes extremely bitter, boneset can be combined with yarrow *(Achillea)*, elder flower *(Sambucus)*, chamomile *(Matricaria)*, and peppermint *(Mentha piperita)* as a sudorific.

Low doses of the extract or tea (cold infusion) act as a bitter tonic, stimulating the appetite.[6,9] It aids in treating nonulcer dyspepsia.[9] Large doses have an emetic and cathartic effect.[8]

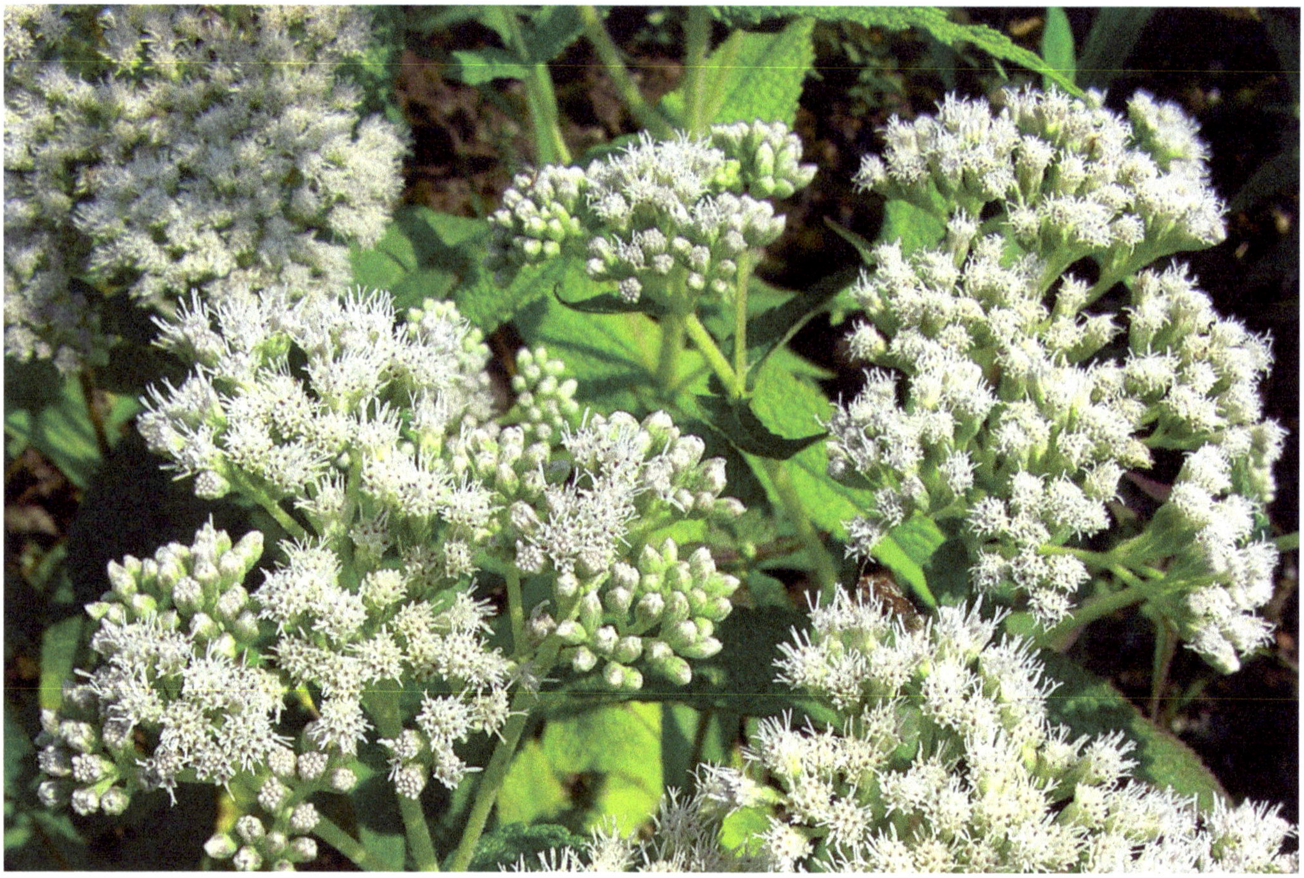

CONTRAINDICATIONS

Boneset contains pyrrolizidine alkaloids (PAs); thus, it is contraindicated during pregnancy and lactation, and in young children and the elderly.[9] Avoid consuming boneset products in high doses and for long periods of time (more than two to six weeks per year), due to the cumulative effects of pyrrolizidine alkaloids. Internal use of boneset is contraindicated in individuals who consume alcoholic beverages regularly, use prescription or over-the-counter medications that compromise liver function or induce liver damage, or individuals with existing liver conditions or liver damage. When used in small amounts in moderation, it is unlikely to cause problems in healthy individuals. For more information on PAs, review the *Safety Concerns* section in the comfrey monograph.

Exceeding the recommended dosage can cause an upset stomach, nausea, vomiting, or diarrhea.[9] Boneset contains sesquiterpene lactones that can cause contact dermatitis.[9]

PREPARATION AND DOSAGE

TINCTURE: Fresh flowering herb [1:2-1:3, 70-95% alcohol]; dry flowering herb [1:5, 60% alcohol]; consume 10-60 drops in hot water, up to four times daily.

TEA: For a tonic, prepare a cold infusion; for a diaphoretic, prepare a hot infusion. Consume 4-6 ounces of either preparation, up to four times daily.

BUGLEWEED

BOTANICAL NAMES:
Lycopus virginicus, L. americanus, L. europaeus

COMMON NAMES:
Bugleweed, Virginia bugleweed, European bugleweed, gypsywort, cut-leaved water horehound, water horehound, sweet bugle, water bugle, Paul's betony
chanvre d'eau, lycope d'Europe, pied de loup (French)
wolfstrapp, wolfsuss (German)
marrobio acquatico (Italian)
menta de lobo (Spanish)

FAMILY NAME:
Lamiaceae (Labiatae)

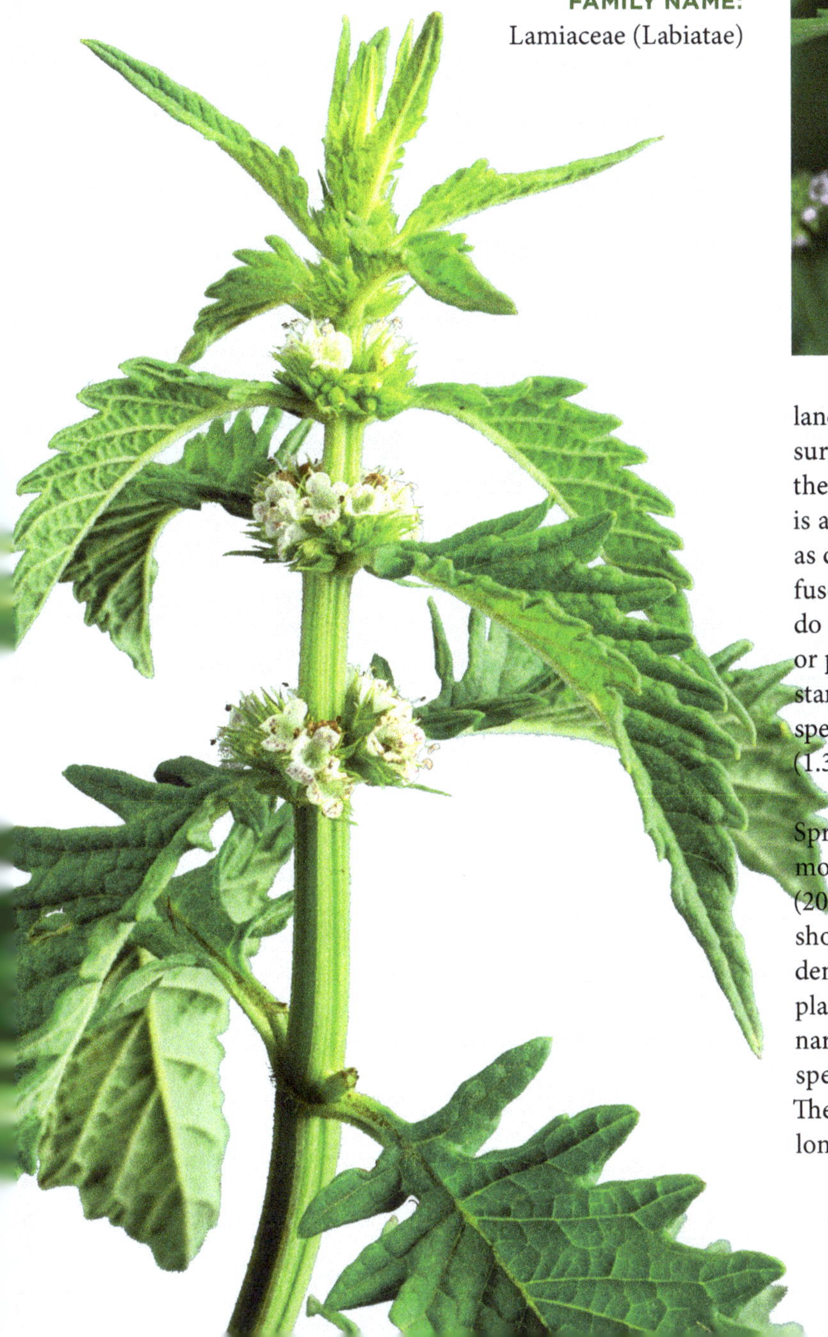

DESCRIPTION

PART USED: The leaves.

BOTANICAL DESCRIPTION AND HABITAT: *Lycopus virginicus* is an herbaceous perennial with fibrous roots that spread from stolons, forming vegetative colonies. The erect, unbranched, sparsely pubescent, light green, square stems (50 – 100 cm tall) bear opposite leaves (9 cm long by 4.5 cm wide).[1,2] Leaves lower on the stems have a short petiole; those higher on the stems are almost sessile. The leaf base tapers toward the petiole; the entire leaf has a

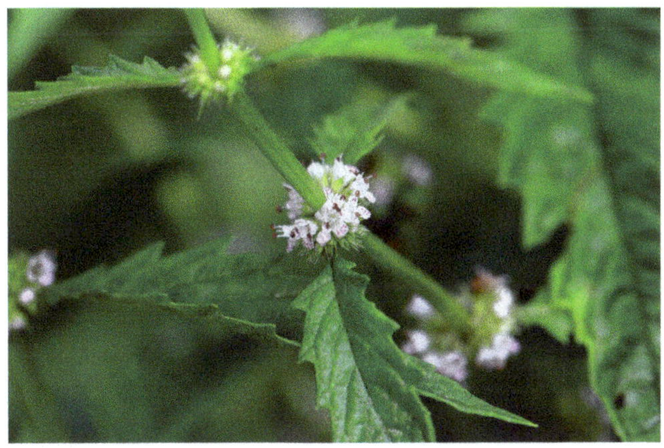

lanceolate-ovate shape with serrated margins. The adaxial surface of the leaf is glabrous; the abaxial surface along the central vein is slightly pubescent. The inflorescence is a verticillaster common to the mint family, appearing as dense clusters in the leaf axils. The tiny flowers have a fused calyx with wide triangular teeth (1 mm long) that do not extend past the mature nutlets.[1,2] The fused white or pinkish bilabiate corolla (0.3 mm across) encloses two stamens that do not protrude past the petals, unlike other species of *Lycopus*.[1,2] The fruit, a schizocarp of four nutlets (1.3 – 2.1 mm long), bears teeth along the apices.[1,2]

Spreading from thin rhizomes, *Lycopus americanus* is a mostly hairless, herbaceous perennial with square stems (20 – 80 cm tall).[3] The opposite leaves (2 – 10 cm long) have short petioles, and vary from oblong to lanceolate, with dentate to lobed margins.[3] Particularly at the base of the plant, the basal lobes of the leaves can be quite deep and narrow, distinguishing *L. americanus* from other *Lycopus* species.[4] Flowers grow in verticillasters at the leaf axils. The four spreading lobes of the white corolla (2 – 3 mm long) barely extend past the narrow, awned lobes of the

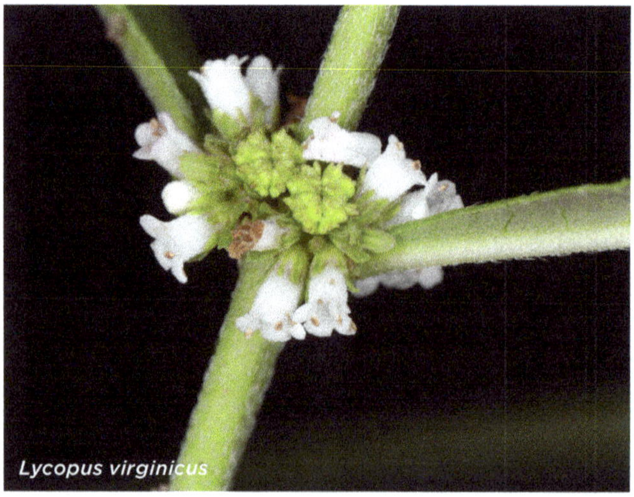
Lycopus virginicus

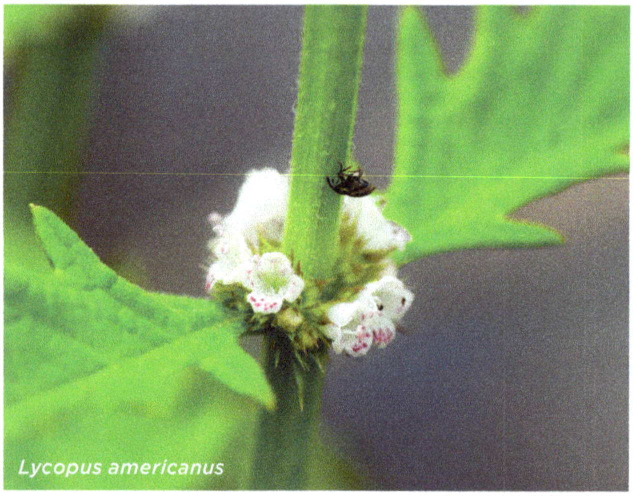
Lycopus americanus

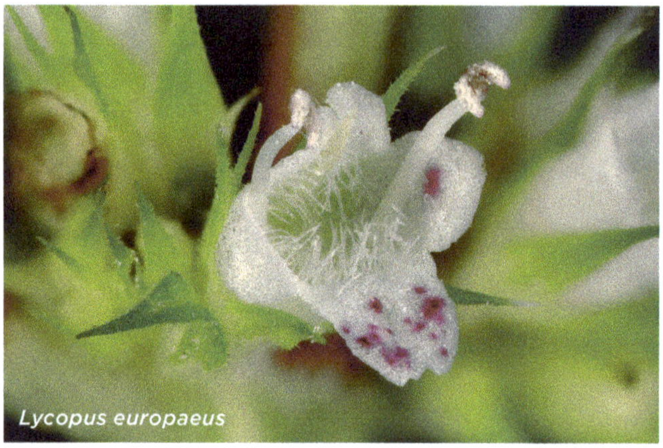
Lycopus europaeus

calyx.[3] Encircled by the perianth are two exserted stamens, a single style, and two fused carpels that mature into four flattened nutlets nested within the persistent calyx.[3]

Lycopus europaeus (20 – 80 cm tall) has pubescent, square stems that are seldom branched, and can be reddish at the base.[5] It spreads vegetatively from long, delicate runners. The opposite, pubescent leaves are lanceolate to narrowly ovate, with large, toothed, pinnate lobes. The bracts subtending the inflorescence appear similar to the rest of the leaves. The inflorescence is a verticillaster like other *Lycopus* species, though the calyx and corolla are almost regular, and less bilabiate than other species. The campanulate calyx has five lobes. The tubular corolla (4 mm long) is white with red spots, with the notched upper lip representing two fused petals, and the lower lip consisting of three distinct petals.[5] Two fertile stamens and sometimes two vestigial stamens grow with two fused carpels. The flowers mature into a schizocarp of four yellowish-brown nutlets.

THE NAME: The genus *Lycopus* derives from two Greek words: *lykos* ("wolf") and *pous* ("foot").[6] The epithets *virginicus* ("from Virginia"), *americanus* ("from America"), and *europaeus* ("from Europe") indicate the plant's origin.[7,8]

HISTORICAL USES: Eclectic physicians administered bugleweed to increase the contraction of nonstriated muscular fibers in the heart and arteries, strengthen the heart, and slow the pulse frequency.[9,10] It was given to treat cardiac palpitations, irregular heartbeat, dyspnea, feelings of oppression in the chest, pericarditis, and endocarditis.[9,10] Bugleweed's actions on the heart were compared to digitalis, although it was regarded as less powerful, nontoxic, and noncumulative.[9,10] Eclectics recommended bugleweed as an antitussive and anti-inflammatory to treat a dry, irritating cough, chest pain, pneumonia, and bloody sputum.[9-11] Bugleweed was given to alleviate passive hemorrhage and treat epistaxis, hematemesis, hematuria, metorrhagia, and intestinal bleeding.[9,10] It was administered as a narcotic sedative to reduce nervous excitement and treat nervous debility, irritability, insomnia, and mental vigilance.[9,11] Ellingwood mentioned using bugleweed to cure exopthalmic goiter.[10] Bugleweed was consumed as a bitter tonic to improve digestive secretion and enhance absorption.[9] It was also used to treat diarrhea, dysenteric diarrhea, and digestive disturbances in alcoholics.[9,10] The infusion and ointment were applied to treat burns and slow healing, irritable ulcers.[11]

CONSTITUENTS: Bugleweed contains volatile oil (α-pinene, β-pinene, β-phellandrine, limonene, β-ourbonene, germacrene-D, caryophyllene, linalool, gamma-muurolene, D-cadinene, 1-ocetn-3-ol, α-terpineol, and pulegone), phenolic acids (caffeic, rosmarinic, chlorogenic, ellagic, lithospermic, and hydroxycinnamic acids), pimeric acid, flavonoids (luteolin 7-glucoside, luteolin 3',7-diglucoside, luteolin 7-glucuronide, and apigenin 7-glucoside), minerals (manganese, magnesium, and zinc), coumarins, and phytosterols.[13-16]

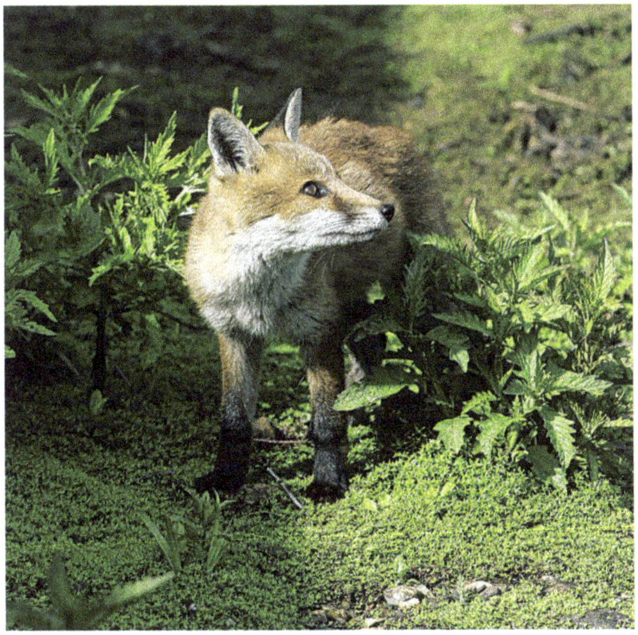

NUTRITIONAL PROPERTIES: Not applicable.

MEDICINAL PROPERTIES: Antithyrotropic, antitussive, anxiolytic, astringent, bitter tonic, cardiotonic, hemostatic, nervine, sedative, styptic, thyrosuppressive, and diuretic (mild).

TEMPERATURE AND FLAVOR: Cool, bitter, and mild astringent.

MEDICINAL USES

Bugleweed is a fascinating herb with moderate antithyrotropic and thyrosuppressive actions in patients with subclinical or mild forms of hyperthyroidism. The symptoms of hyperthyroidism include: anxiety, nervousness, insomnia, palpitations, elevated blood pressure, rapid pulse and heart rate, rapid metabolism, elevated body temperature, increased perspiration, difficulty gaining weight, nervous exhaustion, and in some cases, goiter and exopthalamus (bulging eyes). As a single herb or combined with others, it is often insufficient for treating Grave's disease — an autoimmune-related hyperthyroid condition. Bugleweed can be useful in managing the early stages of Grave's disease; however, its effects are limited.[12] In these patients, the author recommends allopathic treatment using thyrosuppressive medications when the heart is strained, blood pressure is elevated, and the patient is exhausted, or experiencing extreme anxiety or insomnia. It is important for patients with hyperthyroidism or Grave's disease pursuing natural therapies to work with a health care practitioner.

In animal experiments, high doses of *L. europaeus* extract reduced levels of TSH and thyroid hormone.[18] *L. europaeus* extract also lowered body temperature in thyroxine-induced hyperthyroidal rodents; however, TSH and thyroid hormone levels, food intake, and weight gain were unaffected.[18]

The effect of *L. europaeus* was tested in a study of patients with hyperthyroid symptoms and a basal TSH of less than 1.0 mU/l. The results demonstrated that hyperthyroidism symptoms were diminished, and urinary excretion of T4 was significantly increased in patients treated with *L. europaeus* (likely resulting from a glomerular modification or impaired tubular reabsorption).[19] In another study, low doses of *L. europaeus* extract were administered to hyperthyroid patients. The results showed no changes in TSH or thyroid hormone concentration, but marked improvement of cardiac symptoms, including reduced heart rate and blood pressure.[18] Bugleweed was found to lower thyroid-releasing hormone (TRH) levels, thus lowering TSH and thyroid hormone levels.[13] *In vitro* studies showed that bugleweed inhibited TSH, decreasing thyroxin (T4) production.[15] Bugleweed may also interfere with thyroid hormones by blocking the hepatic conversion of T4 to T3.[15] *Note:* T3 is a more biologically active form than T4. The antithyrotropic effects are due to the ester-like derivatives of caffeic and hydroxycinnamic acids.[12]

Based on clinical observation, bugleweed has the most profound effects in individuals with mild or subclinical forms of hyperthyroidism, and those with sympathetic-related heart issues. Its actions are limited in patients with overt clinical hyperthyroidism (Grave's disease); most of them eventually require thyrosuppressive medications, and sometimes, hypotensive agents. Bugleweed is most helpful as a long-term treatment for mild cases of hyperthyroidism. Combine three to four parts of bugleweed *(Lycopus)* extract with one to two parts of motherwort *(Leonurus)* and lemon balm *(Melissa)* extracts to treat many symptoms associated with the early stages of hyperthyroidism.

Bugleweed is a nervine, anxiolytic, and moderate sedative that aids in treating insomnia and hypervigilance.[9-11,13,] It decreases a rapid heart rate, heart palpitations, tachycardia, anxiety, panic attacks, and insomnia caused by patterns of adrenergic and thyroid stress (mild hyperthyroidism).[9-13] Combine bugleweed with motherwort *(Leonurus)*, lemon balm *(Melissa)*, and/or wild oats *(Avena)* to treat the aforementioned conditions.

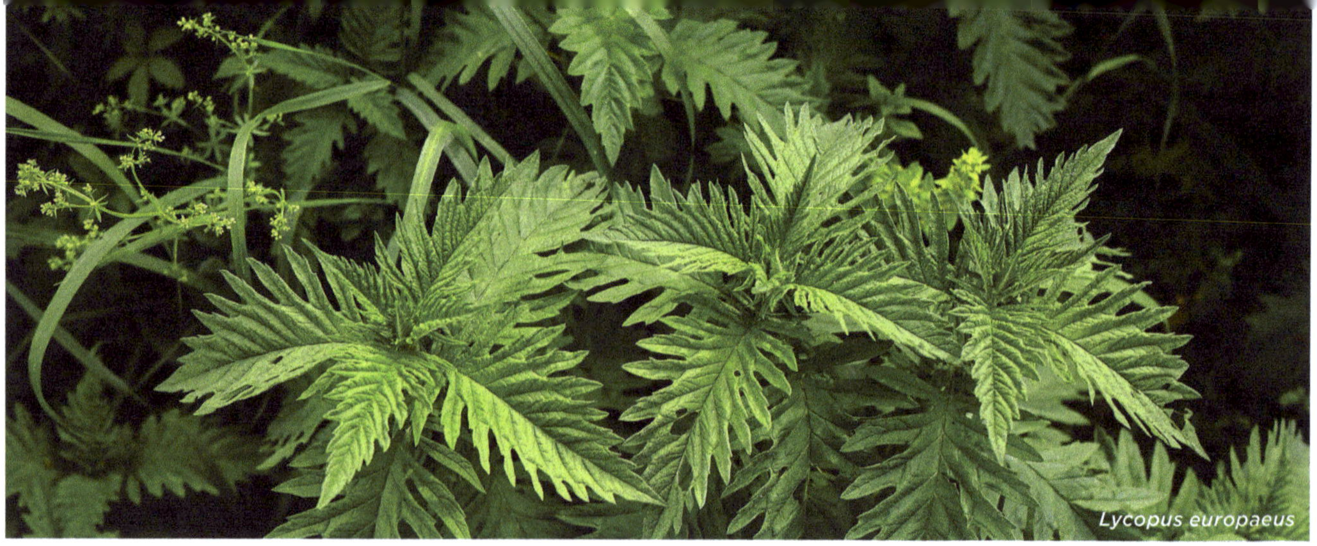

Lycopus europaeus

Bugleweed is a gentle, effective cardiotonic.[9-11] It reduces heart palpitations, slowing a rapid heartbeat and relieving feelings of oppression in the chest.[10,12] Bugleweed slows the heart rate and lowers mild to moderately elevated blood pressure in individuals with stress-induced hypertension or elevated thyroid hormone levels.[18] Combine an alcohol extract of bugleweed with motherwort *(Leonurus)* and hawthorn *(Crataegus)* when treating heart palpitations and stress-induced hypertension. Eclectic physicians administered bugleweed to treat pericarditis, endocarditis, and valvular heart diseases.[9,10] In recent studies, *L. europeaus* extract lowered β-adrenoreceptor density in heart tissue, demonstrating nearly equal effectiveness as the drug atenolol.[18] However, in my practice patients diagnosed with Grave's disease experienced some cardiovascular relief from bugleweed, with more significant reductions in heart rate and blood pressure by using propanolol or atenolol medication.

Bugleweed is a hemostatic that reduces passive hemorrhage.[9,10,13] It aids in treating intestinal bleeding, hematuria, hemoptysis (pulmonary bleeding), and uterine bleeding.[9,10,13,] It reduces nosebleeds and decreases bloody sputum. Combine extracts of bugleweed, cinnamon *(Cinnamomum)*, shepherd's purse *(Capsella)*, and yarrow *(Achillea)* as a hemostatic. Consuming fresh bugleweed extract works most effectively to treat internal bleeding; applying a poultice of the fresh plant also reduces bleeding from cuts and bruises.

Bugleweed is a prolactin-inhibiting substance that prevents milk letdown.[12,13,17] It can be combined with other anti-galactagogue agents such as sage *(Salvia officinale)* and parsley leaf *(Petroselinum)* in the cessation of nursing.[17] Bugleweed also aids in treating mastodynia (breast pain).[12]

Applied topically, bugleweed is an astringent and styptic that reduces wound bleeding. Water-based extracts of *L. europaeus* have topical antibacterial activities against *Staphylococcus aureus*.[20] Rosmarinic acid and luteolin-7-O-glucoronide were attributed to the antibacterial and antioxidant effects.[20]

CONTRAINDICATIONS

Avoid consuming bugleweed during pregnancy or lactation. Due to the prolactin-inhibiting properties, lactating women should avoid consistent use of bugleweed, unless they intend to stop nursing. Long-term use of bugleweed is contraindicated in individuals with depressed thyroid function or hypothyroidism, and those taking thyroid hormones.[12,13] Avoid consuming bugleweed when testing for thyroid hormones, as it can interfere with diagnostic procedures involving radioactive isotopes. High doses consumed for a long period of time or abrupt discontinuation of bugleweed can cause a goiter.[12]

PREPARATION AND DOSAGE

TINCTURE: Fresh leaves [1:2-1:3, 70-95% alcohol]; recently dried leaves [1:5, 60% alcohol]; consume 15-60 drops, up to three times daily. Consume 30-60 drops of standardized extract, or use as directed.

CAPSULES: Consume 2-4 freeze-dried or "00" capsules, one to three times daily.

TEA: Prepare a hot infusion; consume 8-10 ounces, up to three times daily.

TOPICAL USE: Apply a fresh plant poultice as a styptic, or apply the fomentation, wash, salve, or ointment as an antibacterial agent.

BURDOCK

BOTANICAL NAMES:
Arctium lappa, A. minus, A. japonica

COMMON NAMES:
Burdock, great burdock, beggar's buttons, burr seed, cocklebur, thorny burr, clothburr, great bur, clot-bur, hardock, turkey burseed, lappa, lappa minor, fox's clote, happy major, love leaves, philanthropium, personata
níu báng zí (Chinese)
isotakianen (Finnish)
bardane, rhubarb du diable (French)
bardana, lappola (Italian)
gobo, goboshi (Japanese)
ubanja (Korean)
shu nian (Mandarin)
lophuh, repeinick (Russian)
bardana (Spanish)

FAMILY NAME:
Asteraceae
(Compositae)

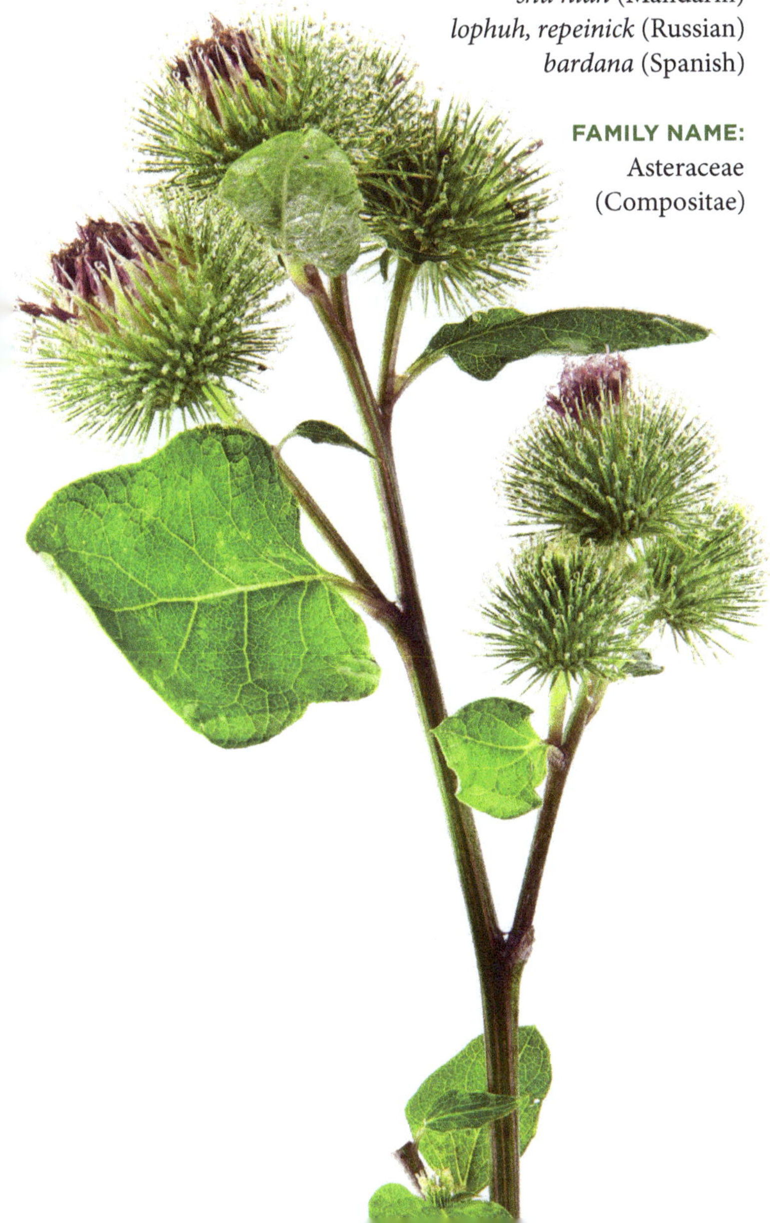

DESCRIPTION

PARTS USED: The roots, seeds (fruits), and leaves. The roots are harvested in the fall of the first year or spring of the second year, though the second-year roots are too fibrous for culinary use.

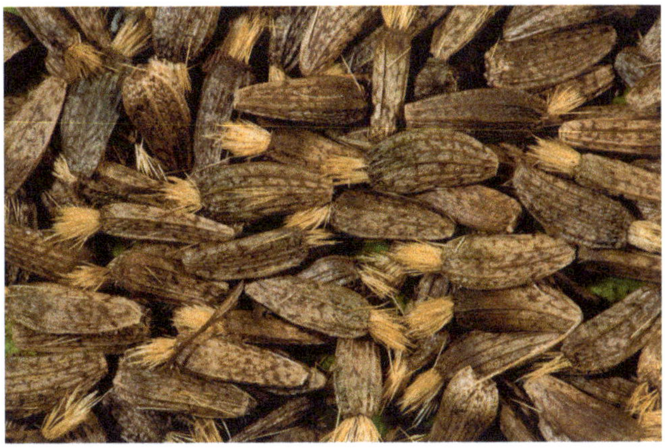

BOTANICAL DESCRIPTION AND HABITAT: A biennial herb native to Europe and Asia, burdock naturalized throughout North America following its introduction by European settlers.[1] Burdock can be cultivated rather easily, although precautionary measures are recommended to prevent the wide spread of seeds, as it is considered an invasive weed. Cut off the flowering heads before the seeds mature, or cover the seed heads with a bag and twist tie it to keep them from spreading.

Burdock is a handsome, vivacious, robust plant. During its first year, it forms a basal rosette (60 to 120 cm tall). In the second year, the plant bolts up to 300 cm tall.[2] Burdock has large, pale green, wavy, alternate leaves. The undersides of the leaves are grayish-green, coated with a fine woolly covering. The thick petioles of the basal leaves reach up to 36 cm long, while the wide, cordate blades measure 25 – 80 cm long and 20 – 70 cm across. The upper leaves are smaller and more ovate.[2] The exterior portions of the lengthy roots have longitudinal light brown to dark brown wrinkles; the inside is creamy white. A transverse cross section of the root shows light brown lines radiating from the center. The rounded, burr-like, purple flower heads (2 – 5 cm in diameter) feature imbricated scales with hooked extremities that adhere to objects.[3] The florets are tubular, with tiny purple corollas (9 – 14 mm long), dark purple stamens, and white styles.[2] The smooth, narrow, ovoid achenes are flattened, and brownish-gray; they are bitter, oily, and inodorous.

THE NAME: *Arctium* derives from the Greek *arktos* ("bear"), referring to the roughness of the burrs.[4] The epithet *lappa* ("to seize") also derives from Greek, referring to the clinging nature of the fruit.[4] The epithet *minus* means "small;" *japonica* refers to a plant originating in Japan. The common name burdock is a contraction of *bur* and *dock*. Bur originates from the Latin *burra* ("a lock of wool") because the flowering heads often entangled with sheeps' wool as herds grazed near the plant.[4] Dock refers to the large leaves.[4]

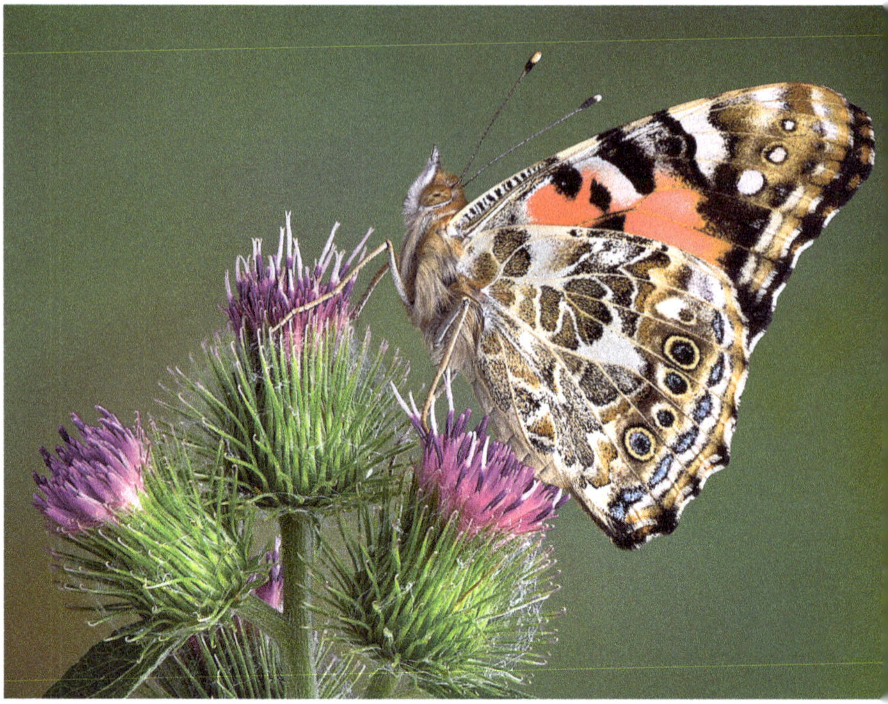

HISTORICAL USES: The dried or roasted fruit, known as *níu báng zí* (Mandarin) and *goboshi* (Japanese), were administered to clear wind-heat and heat, and relieve toxicity.[5] They continue to be used to treat colds, sore throats, tonsillitis, mumps, measles, coughs, sores, and abscesses.[1,5] The fruit was recommended to treat red swellings, carbuncles, erythemas, and acute febrile maculopapular rashes.[5]

In Europe, a decoction of burdock root was consumed as an antiscorbutic agent to treat scurvy and alleviate boils and rheumatic conditions.[4] A wash was applied to ulcers and scaly skin conditions.[4] An infusion of leaves was consumed to tone and strengthen the stomach.[4] A leaf poultice was applied as a resolvent and anti-inflammatory for tumors, gout, bruises, and inflamed skin.[4] Due to their oily nature, the seeds were believed to influence the sebaceous and sudoriferous glands, and restore smoothness to skin. Infusions and decoctions of the seeds were consumed several times daily for kidney afflictions and dropsical complaints.[4]

Eclectic physician Finley Ellingwood recommended burdock as an antidyscratic (blood cleanser), and to regulate mucous membrane and glandular secretions, alleviate irritable coughs, and relieve aphthous ulcerations of membranes.[6] He also recommended burdock for psoriasis and chronic cutaneous eruptions. Ellingwood noted the soothing effects on the urinary system, and emphasized its use in promoting the excretion of urea, uric acids, and urinary solids.[6]

After its introduction in North America, Menominee and Micmac tribes used burdock for skin sores; Cherokees used it to treat numerous conditions.[7] Many tribes used this invasive weed to treat rheumatism, urinary calculi, and scurvy. The seeds were administered for kidney disease, and the leaves were chewed to relieve stomachaches.[8]

CONSTITUENTS

BURDOCK ROOT: Burdock root contains the polysaccharide, inulin (up to 50% by weight), polyacetylenes (1,11-tridecadiene-3,5,7,9,-tetrayne and 1,3,11-tridecatriene-5,7,9-triyne), arctic acid, an acetylenic acid containing volatile acids (acetic, propionic, butyric, isovaleric, 3-hexanoic, 3-octaenoic, and costic acids), nonhydroxy acids (lauric, myristic, stearic, and palmitic acids), flavonoids (quercetin and rutin), theophenes, a crystalline plant hormone, γ-guanidino-*n*-butyric acid, tannin, polyphenolic acids (chlorogenic, caffeoylquinic, and caffeic acids), mucilage, a bitter glycoside (arctiin), lignans (lignaol A and B), resin, sesquiterpene lactones, triterpenes, terpenes, and mucilaginous polysaccharides.[1,4,7,9]

BURDOCK SEED: Burdock seed (fruit) contains fixed oils, a bitter glucoside (arctiin), *l*-arctigenin, isoarctigenin, chlorogenic acid, arachidic acid, globosterin, volatile oil, fatty oils, two lignans, a germacranolide, and others.[1,5]

BURDOCK LEAF: Burdock leaf contains flavonoids (quercetin and rutin), arctiol (8α-hydroxyeudesmol), fukinone (dehydrofukinone), fukinanolide, β-eudesmol, petasitolone, eremophilene, and taraxasterol.[1]

NUTRITIONAL PROPERTIES: Burdock root contains calcium, chromium, cobalt, crude fiber, dietary fiber, fat, iron, magnesium, manganese, niacin, phosphorus, potassium, protein, riboflavin, selenium, silicon, sodium, thiamine, tin, zinc, and vitamins A and C.[7,9]

MEDICINAL PROPERTIES: Burdock root is an alterative, antidyscratic, cholagogue, mild choleretic, demulcent, mild diuretic, laxative, liver detoxifier, lymphatic, nutritive, and mild astringent. Burdock seed is a diaphoretic, diuretic, and kidney detoxifier. The leaf is a mild topical anti-inflammatory and astringent.

TEMPERATURE AND FLAVOR: The roots are cool, bitter, sweet, mildly astringent, and salty. The seeds are cool, bitter, and oily. The leaves are cool and astringent.

MEDICINAL USES

BURDOCK ROOT: Burdock root is a mild cholagogue and choleretic, with gentle liver cleansing properties that facilitate detoxification. It enhances liver metabolism of proteins and fats.[10] In Europe, burdock was consumed as a pot herb for its spring tonifying and antidyscratic actions. Due to the cholagogue actions, mucilage, and fiber content, burdock is a subtle laxative. Combining burdock root with yellow dock *(Rumex crispus)* and dandelion *(Taraxacum officinale)* synergizes the laxative and hepatodetoxifying effects. Because of its beneficial influence on the liver, burdock root also aids in the long-term treatment of skin conditions, including acne, boils, eczema, dermatitis, and psoriasis. [6,9,10] Burdock helps to lower elevated IgE levels, reducing inflammation.[10]

Burdock root strengthens digestion and assimilation. The fresh root has bactericidal and fungicidal properties attributed to the polyacetylenes.[1,7] Burdock is a gentle long-term treatment for individuals with intestinal bacterial or yeast imbalances. It is an effective long-term tonic for individuals with chronic intestinal candida; however, the antifungal properties are not present in the dry root.[1,7] Burdock root exerted antibacterial effects *in vitro* against gram-negative bacteria including: *E. coli, Shigella flexneri,* and *Shigella sonnei.*

Burdock root is a lymphatic-alterative herb, enhancing immune function and strengthening resistance to infections.[7] It contains inulin, which promotes chemotaxis of neutrophils and monocytes by activating the complement cascade.[5,7] (Inulin should not be confused with the hormone, insulin.) Prepare a lymphatic compound by combining the following extracts: three parts of echinacea *(Echinacea);* two parts fresh burdock root, dandelion root (*Taraxacum*), and cleavers *(Galium);* and one part red clover *(Trifolium),* figwort *(Scrophularia),* and red root *(Ceanothus).* Burdock hindered the tumor-promoting activity of Epstein Barr virus. It also exerted cytostatic activity against certain cancer cell lines.

Burdock root is a primary ingredient in Essiac, a formula used as an adjunct therapy to treat cancer. Essiac is water-based and contains burdock root, slippery elm *(Ulmus),* Turkey rhubarb *(Rheum palmatum),* and sheep sorrel *(Rumex acetocella).*

Burdock root is a subtle, soothing diuretic; however, the seed is a more potent diuretic.[6,10] The tannins contribute to the diuretic and mild astringent actions.[11] Prepare a diuretic compound by combining burdock with parsley root *(Petroselinum)* and dandelion leaf *(Taraxacum).*

Burdock root is a nutritive rich in vitamins and alkaline minerals. Add burdock root to nutritive syrups containing nettle leaf *(Urtica),* alfalfa *(Medicago),* oat straw *(Avena),* rose hips *(Rosa),* yellow dock *(Rumex),* and dandelion *(Taraxacum).* Or, prepare a mineral-rich decoction by combining burdock root with dandelion root *(Taraxacum),* fennel *(Feoniculum),* and smaller amounts of yellow dock *(Rumex).* The roasted root can be combined with roasted dandelion and chicory root as a non-caffeinated coffee substitute.

A poultice of fresh grated root has drawing properties used to treat boils, acne, and abscesses. A topical wash or compress soothes inflamed skin conditions such as eczema, psoriasis, and dandruff.

BURDOCK SEED (FRUIT): Burdock seed is a diuretic that reduces edema by enhancing sodium excretion from the kidneys.[10] Consume burdock seed preparations during the luteal phase (two weeks prior to menses) to decrease premenstrual water retention, reduce breast tenderness

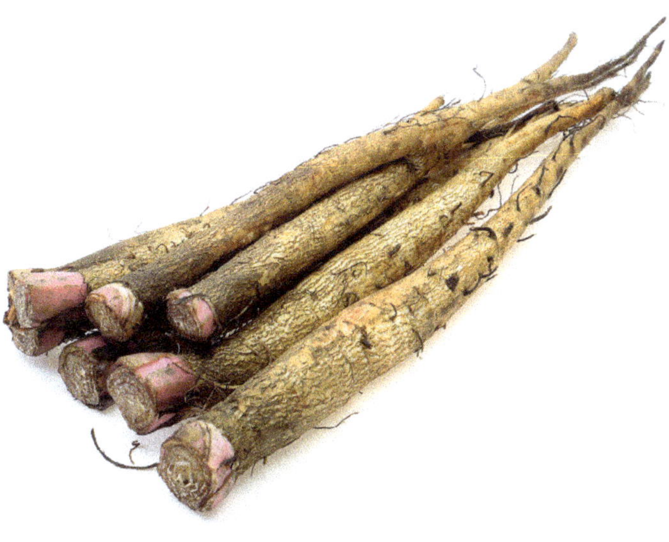

and swelling, and decrease swelling of breast lumps caused by fibrocystic breasts. Consumed in combination with other diuretic herbs such as dandelion leaf *(Taraxacum officinale)* or parsley root or seed *(Petroselinum)*, burdock seed aids in treating sodium-related hypertension.

Burdock seed enhances the filtration of uric acid and other waste products from the kidneys.[6,10] Consume as a long-term tonic to treat gout, arthritis, or kidney stones.[9,10] Due to its diuretic, liver detoxifying, and depurative actions, burdock seed aids in the long-term treatment of moist skin conditions including acne, eczema, dermatitis, and psoriasis.[9,10] Harvest burdock seeds after they have matured, when the flowers turn from purple to brown, and the seeds separate with ease from the calyx.

BURDOCK LEAF: Preparations of burdock leaf are consumed to alleviate digestive inflammation. Topical applications reduce inflammation from a burn, scald, sunburn, skin irritation, rash, poison ivy, or poison oak.[9]

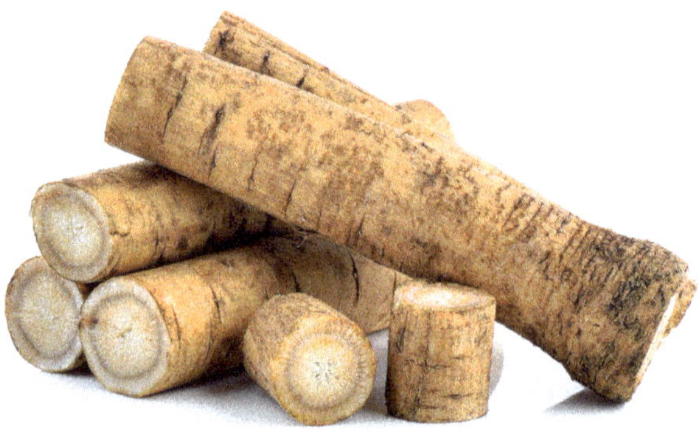

CONTRAINDICATIONS

Burdock root is safe to consume during pregnancy. While the majority of herbal sources do not contraindicate burdock during pregnancy, there is an isolated report of negative side effects. As a cautionary measure, the root and seed are contraindicated during the first two trimesters of pregnancy, but not in the last trimester.[10] Burdock seed is safe for lactating women to consume. According to herbalists Michael Moore and Terry Willard, the seeds may cause spotting, although they have no emmenagogue properties.[7,12] This contraindication is likely attributed to one reported case of atropine poisoning (an alkaloid) that occurred in adulterated batches of commercially prepared burdock. Otherwise, this alkaloid is not present in burdock. Burdock root contains sesquiterpene lactones that can cause allergic contact dermatitis in individuals hypersensitive to Asteraceae family plants.[9] The hairs on the leaves can aggravate skin.

PREPARATION AND DOSAGE

TINCTURE: Fresh roots [1:2, 60-95% alcohol]; dry roots [1:5, 60% alcohol]; consume 30-90 drops, up to three times daily. Fresh seeds [1:2, 70-95% alcohol]; dry seeds [1:5, 60% alcohol]; consume 20-60 drops, up to three times daily.

GLYCERITE: Fresh roots [1:2-1:3, 50% glycerin and 50% alcohol]; consume 15-60 drops, up to three times daily.

ACETUM EXTRACT: Fresh roots [1:2-1:3, apple cider vinegar]; consume 1 teaspoon to 1 tablespoon up to three times daily, or consume the pickled root. Add burdock vinegar to salad dressings or marinades.

SUCCUS: Juice the fresh root and preserve with 20% alcohol; consume up to 1 tablespoon, three times daily. Store in the refrigerator.

CAPSULES: Consume 2-4 "00" capsules, up to three times daily.

TEA: Prepare a decoction of the roots, or a hot infusion or decoction of the seeds. Consume 8-12 ounces, up to three times daily.

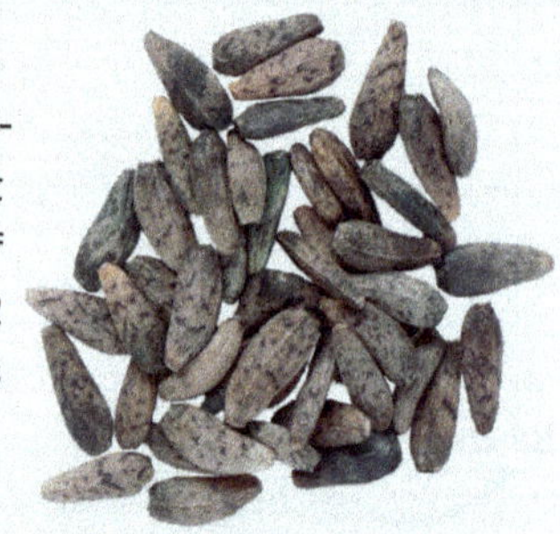

HONEY AND SYRUP: Prepare a decoction of the roots, cooking to one-half the original volume; add honey, molasses, or simple syrup to desired sweetness (at least ⅙ of total volume). Consume up to 1 tablespoon, four times daily. Store in the refrigerator.

TOPICAL USE: Apply fresh roots or leaves as a wash, fomentation, or poultice.

CULINARY USE: Add fresh roots to soups, stir-fries, sautéed vegetables, sauerkraut, and vegetable juices. Roast the roots and prepare as a coffee substitute. Include the young, tender leaves as a pot herb, or they can be steamed or sautéed. Boil the young leaf stalks or eat them raw in a salad with vinegar and oil. Older leaves become more fibrous as they age and taste better steamed or boiled.

CALAMUS

DESCRIPTION

BOTANICAL NAMES:
Acorus calamus, A. calamus var. *americanus* (syn. *A. americanus*), *A. calamus* var. *vulgaris* (syn. *A. calamus* var. *calamus*), *A. calamus* var. *angustatus*, *A. calamus* var. *versus*, and *A. gramineus*

COMMON NAMES:
Acorus, calamus, sweet calamus, kalmus, sweet flag, sweet root, sweet cinnamon, cinnamon sedge, sweet sedge, sweet rush, sweet grass, sweet cane, sweet myrtle, myrtle sedge, gladdon, grass myrtle
acora vrai, jonc odorant, roseau aromatique (French)
ackerwurz, kalmus, magenwurz (German)
calamo aromatico (Italian)
shobu (Japanese)
ch'angp'o (Korean)
shi chang pu, chang pu (Mandarin)
vacha (Sanskrit)
calamo (Spanish)

FAMILY NAME:
Araceae
(formerly Acoraceae)

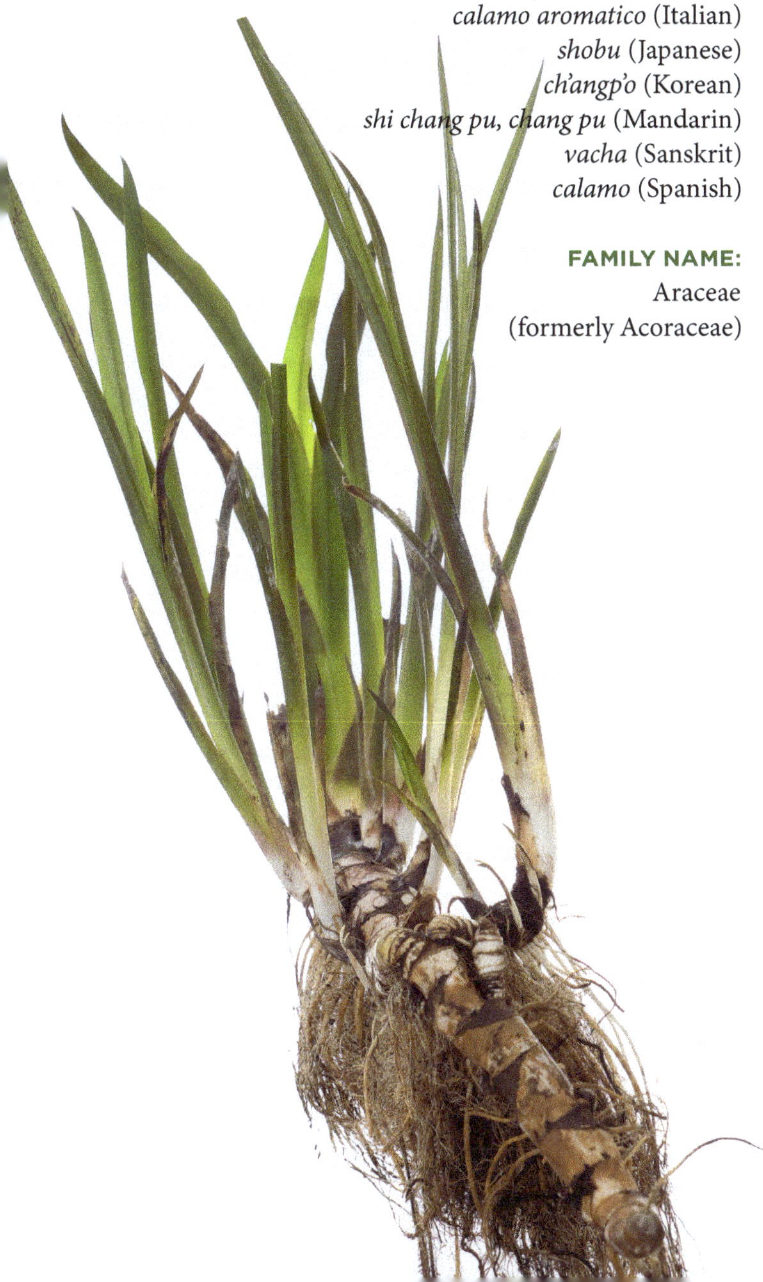

PART USED: The rhizomes.

BOTANICAL DESCRIPTION AND HABITAT: Calamus is a semi-aquatic, perennial plant that grows wild on the margins of freshwater lakes, ponds, swamps, marshes, creeks, and rivers. The reddish-brown, branching rhizomes

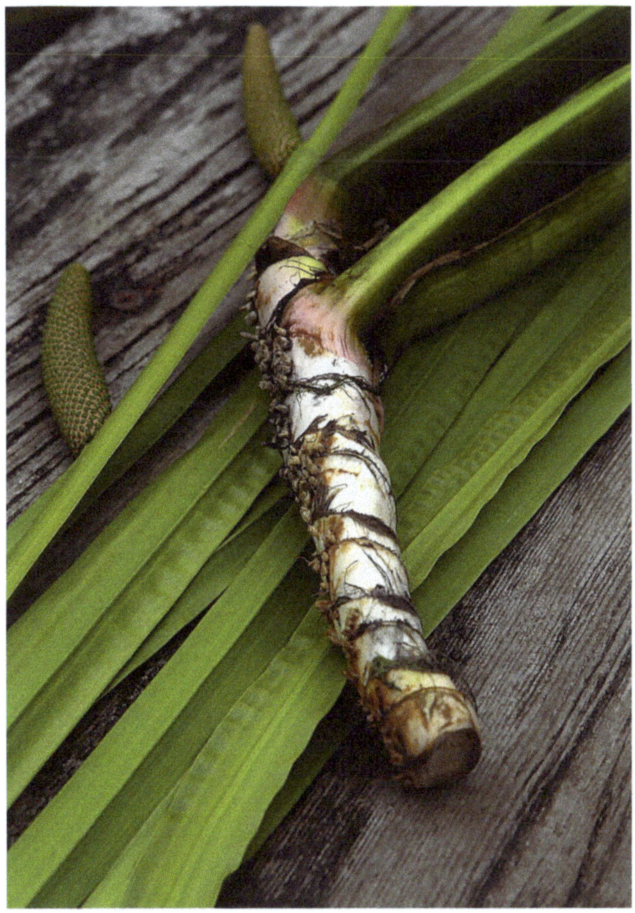

(4 – 10 cm long by 1 – 3 cm diameter) are anchored in the mud from the undersides by abundant, stringy rootlets.[1] The rhizomes have a musky, pungent aroma. The tiny flowers are arranged in crosshatch patterns on a greenish-yellow cylindrical spadix (5 – 10 cm long) emerging at a 45° angle, one-third of the way up the stem. Each flower has six tepals, six stamens, and a single ovary with two or three chambers.[1] The fruit is a minute, leathery berry.[2] The sword-shaped leaves grow up to 180 cm in height. *Acorus calamus* can be distinguished from *Iris* by the fragrance emitted from the leaves when bruised. *A. calamus* var. *americanus* differs from *A. calamus* var. *calamus* because

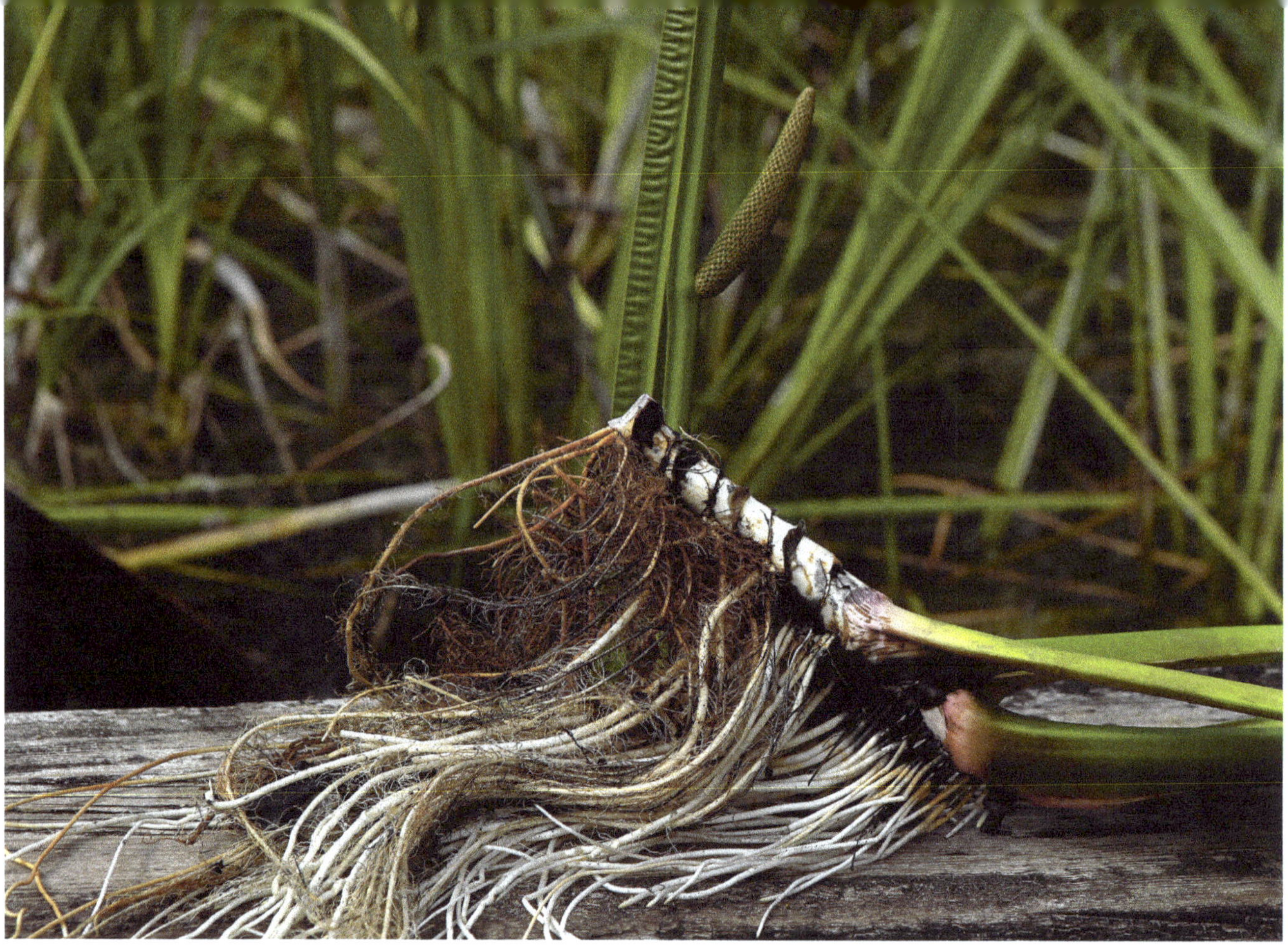

its leaf has a central mid-vein, and one to five additional veins rising above the leaf surface. The leaf of *A. calamus* var. *vulgaris* has only one prominent mid-vein, and the plant does not produce fertile fruits. *A. calamus* var. *americanus* is native to the eastern U.S., but has spread across the country. It can also be propagated from root divisions and cultivated. Other species are native to India and Asia, and naturalized throughout Europe.

THE NAME: *Acorus* derives from the Greek *coreon*, meaning "pupil of the eye." The ancient Greeks traditionally used it to cure eye disease. *Calamus* derives from the Greek *calamos* ("a reed").[3] The name sweet flag was acquired because the leaves resemble yellow flags *(Iris pseudacorus)*, though they are botanically unrelated. Due to the pleasant aroma emitted from the leaves, the adjective "sweet" precedes many of the common names. Sedge refers to a grass-like plant. Villagers in Norfolk where the plant grew in abundance called the herb Gladdon.[3] In Sanskrit, *vacha* translates as "speaking," referring to the power of the word or self-expression stimulated by calamus.[4]

The Latin binomial *Acorus calamus* is often used generically to refer to calamus root; however, it has at least five chemotypes. The American type is *A. calamus* var. *americanus* (syn. *A. americanus*). The European type is *A. calamus* var. *vulgaris* (syn. *A. calamus* var. *calamus*). Asian varieties include *A. gramineus, A. calamus* var. *angustatus*, and *A. calamus* var. *versus. A. calamus* and *A. gramineus* are used interchangeably in China as the medicine *shi chang pu*. Their cultivar named *A. calamus* var. *variegatus* has yellow striped leaves.

HISTORICAL USES: Ancient *Vedic* seers utilized calamus for thousands of years in India. In Ayurvedic medicine, it was believed to revitalize the brain and nervous system, and sharpen memory. It was commonly used for nervous system diseases, and tea was added to baths to calm the nerves and induce tranquility.

Powdered rhizome was traditionally used as an insecticide to kill bedbugs, fleas, lice, moths, and other vermin. An extract of calamus was applied as a parasiticide for lice and scabies infestations. In India, dried rhizome pieces were added to rice to prevent insect infestation. A study conducted by Indian scientist Sexena Marthur confirmed its insecticidal properties. Rice weevils destroy an average 12% of stored grains in tropical countries. According to this study, if chopped calamus root was added to the rice before storing, no pests would be found. Calamus oil can sterilize insects, inhibiting maturation of the ova and impeding copulation. Root pieces can be strained with a sieve before cooking rice.[5,6]

The rhizome has been added to Traditional Chinese Medicine compounds for more than 2,000 years. It was used to treat rheumatoid arthritis and injuries from physical trauma. Calamus detoxifies blood and reduces dampness in the digestive tract (stomach and spleen), treating gastritis, lack of appetite, gas, bloating, and constipation. It is said to clear phlegm that results in deafness, forgetfulness, and strokes. Animal studies have shown that calamus has anticonvulsive actions due to the sesquiterpene aconic acid, confirming its traditional use in treating epilepsy. Additional scientific studies have confirmed its smooth muscle relaxant effects, as well as insecticidal, antifungal, antibacterial, CNS depressant, and hypotensive actions.[8-11]

Calamus was believed to freshen, purify, and sweeten the water where it grew. When Mongolian tribes invaded Asia and the Middle East, they planted calamus in and near water they intended to drink. Thus, the herb became known as "Mongolian poison" among people whose land was invaded.[12]

The earliest records of the uses of calamus (if indeed it was the same plant) were mentioned in the *Bible,* in Exodus, Canticles, and Ezekiel.[3] In Egypt and other ancient cultures, calamus was an ingredient in incense. Remnants of calamus were found in King Tutankhamen's tomb. Ancient Egyptians also regarded calamus as an aphrodisiac.[12]

It was believed that calamus was introduced to Europe from India by the Tartars, who brought it to Poland in the 13th century. In 1588, it was recorded as an abundant plant in Germany. Calamus was first cultivated in Vienna in 1574 by Clusius, a famous botanist who distributed the root to other botanists in Belgium, France, and Germany. Records dating to 1596 indicate that Gerard first cultivated the herb in England, having received roots from Anthony Coline, a practitioner from Lyons. In England, calamus was recommended as a stomachic for dysentery and chronic catarrh. A digestive tonic, "Stockton Bitters," was made from calamus and gentian *(Gentiana campestris).* The volatile oil was used to improve the flavor of gin and lend fragrance to beer. The candied root was widely used throughout Europe, based on a preparation likely borrowed from India. Turks consumed the candied root to prevent contagious diseases. Calamus leaves were strewn on the floors of medieval churches and in private houses because of its sweet odor and effectiveness in repelling insects. The leaves were strewn on the floors of Norwich cathedrals during major festivals.[3]

Calamus was an important trade item among Native Americans, likely leading to its spread throughout the U.S. Great Plains tribes planted calamus near villages and along trails to guarantee easy access to this highly valued medicine.[12] Native Americans chewed calamus roots as a stimulant to increase endurance and stamina when traveling long distances. A tea was consumed for treating digestive complaints, cold, flu, coughs, and fever.[13] The Penobscot tribe made a tea for coughs by combining calamus and wild sarsaparilla *(Aralia nudicaulis).*[14] Calamus roots were chewed to relieve toothaches and clear phlegm. Poultices were applied for cramps, headaches, toothaches, sore chests, and joint pain.[13] Calamus was used in ceremonies because it was believed to have mystical powers.[12] Teton Dakota warriors applied a paste of the root to their foreheads and temples to give them strength, courage, and fearlessness when confronting enemies. Garlands of calamus leaves were worn around the neck by hunters and used for ceremonial purposes. The leaves were burned for their sweet aroma. Various Native American tribes incorporated the leaves, stalks, and rhizomes into food.[7]

Harvey Felter, an Eclectic physician, suggested using the herb as a "breath perfume," and to treat flatulent colic, atonic dyspepsia, and feebleness of the digestive organs. He recommended using the syrup as a digestive aid (30 – 60 drops) and vehicle for unpleasant tasting medicines. He suggested candying the fresh root by slicing it transversely and boiling it in simple syrup.[15] Western cultures valued the herb as a stomachic, carminative, sedative, and febrifuge, among other uses.[8,9]

The root was used in antidandruff and hair tonic preparations.[8,9] The essential oil was added to cosmetics such as creams, lotions, soaps, and perfumes. Calamus rhizome was used in the U.S. as a flavoring agent in a variety of products, including beer, bitter tonics, and tooth powders. However, by the 1960s, it was banned as a flavoring agent, as studies revealed that β-asarone caused malignant tumors in rats.[14] The FDA has banned calamus essential oil in the U.S. due to concerns regarding β-asarone.[8,9] However, they failed to acknowledge that the rhizome grown in the U.S. does not contain β-asarone or toxic phenylpropanoids. Because American calamus does not have the carcinogenic constituent, it is preferred as a medicine.

CONSTITUENTS: Calamus rhizome contains variable amounts of volatile oil (*cis*-methyl isoeugenol, asarone, asarylaldehyde, calamene, linalool, calamol, calameone, eugenol, methyl eugenol, azulene, pinene, cineole, and camphor). Some varieties (Indian and Chinese) also

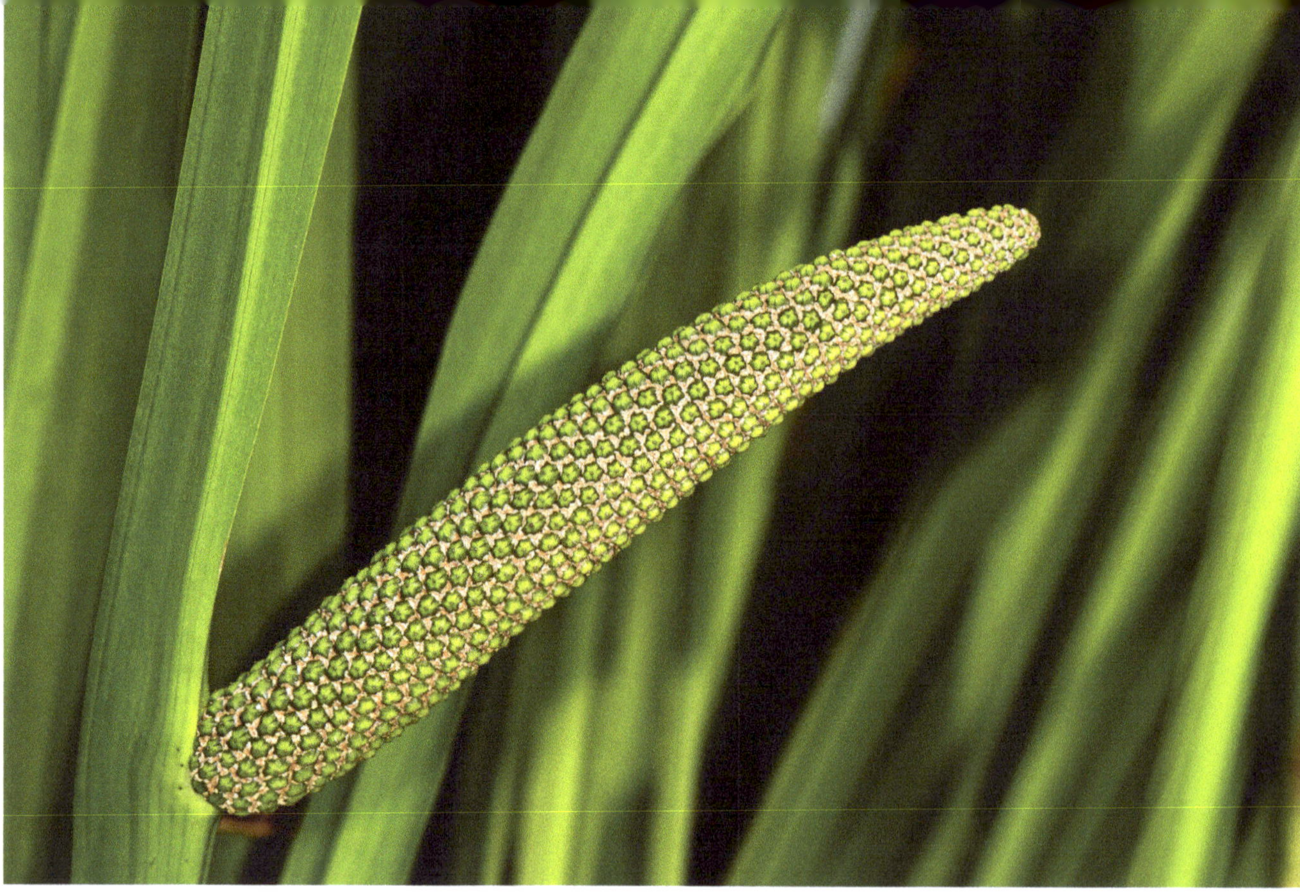

contain the volatile oil β-asarone as a major constituent. β-asarone (= *cis*-isoasarone) has been shown to have mutagenic and carcinogenic effects in animal studies. β-asarone is found in the highest concentration in Asian varieties *(A. calamus* var. *angustatus,* and *A. calamus* var. *versus).* The European variety *(A. calamus* var. *vulgaris,* syn. *A. calamus* var. *calamus)* contains lower amounts of β-asarone and larger amounts of the other beneficial aromatic compounds. The American volatile oil *(A. calamus* L. var. *americanus)* does not contain the carcinogenic β-asarone; it contains sesquiterpene (asarone) as a primary constituent. Calamus rhizome also contains the sesquiterpenes (acoragermacrone, acolamone, and isoacolamone), acoradin, 2,4,5-trimethoxy benzaldehyde, 2,5-dimethoxybenzo-quinone, galangin, sitosterol, acoric acid, a biogenic amine (choline), mucilaginous polysaccharides, starch, sugars, tannins, resin, and others.[8,9]

Note: The carcinogen β-asarone and toxic phenylpropanoids are not found in American calamus *(A. calamus.* var. *americanus).* The Asian varieties *A. calamus* var. *angustatus* and *A. calamus* var. *versus* contain high amounts of β-asarone.

NUTRITIONAL PROPERTIES: Unknown.

MEDICINAL PROPERTIES: Antispasmodic, antitussive, aromatic, astringent, bitter tonic, carminative, expectorant, mild neurocirculatory stimulant, sialagogue, and emetic.

TEMPERATURE AND FLAVOR: Warm, bitter, pungent, astringent, and sweet.

MEDICINAL USES

Calamus rhizome has aromatic, bitter tonic, carminative, and smooth muscle antispasmodic properties. Calamus is incorporated in Indian cuisine, like ginger, as a condiment. It also can be used as a digestive tonic for individuals with deficient digestive secretions, and poor digestion and assimilation. Consume two to four ounces of tea or 5–15 drops of the extract 15 to 30 minutes before a meal to stimulate the appetite. Calamus is beneficial for helping recovering anorexics and bulimics to reduce nausea, quell the gag reflex, and restore proper digestive secretions. It enhances protein and fat digestion, and reduces gas and bloating. The tea can be used to reduce gastritis, heartburn, hyperacidity, nonulcer dyspepsia, and a stomachache. Calamus is also used as an antispasmodic and digestive aid for treating irritable bowel syndrome, Crohn's disease, and colitis. The tannins reduce diarrhea. The cholagogue, choline, and small quantities of mucilage treat constipation. The astringent and demulcent actions reduce inflammation of the mucous membranes that line the digestive tract. The smooth muscle antispasmodic actions are helpful for treating cramps in the respiratory, digestive, and reproductive systems. Calamus speeds recovery and increases the appetite following food poisoning, digestive flu, or other microbial infections in the digestive tract.

Calamus increases mental clarity, and has mild energizing and stimulant actions. This is likely due to its effect on enhancing digestion and increasing cerebral blood flow. It may be used as a digestive bitter tonic for cloudy thinking following a meal. Current Ayurvedic practice asserts that calamus increases cerebral blood flow, enhancing mental clarity and alertness; thus, it is often combined with gotu kola *(Centella asiatica)*.[4] Calamus is also said to counteract the negative effects of smoking marijuana; sometimes, powdered calamus is added to marijuana mixtures. Some herbalists believe that this initiated the use of chewing the rhizome to aid in quitting tobacco.

Calamus has expectorant and subtle antitussive actions beneficial for the respiratory tract. It is used to treat laryngitis, dry cough, spastic bronchitis, asthma, common cold, and fever. Calamus is administered to nasal passages for sinus congestion and polyps.[4] It is also used for convalescing, and to reduce fatigue.

Calamus can be used to reduce cravings for tobacco and cannabis. The combination of chewing the root and smoking tobacco seems to cause mild nausea and illicit a distaste for tobacco.[5] It is speculated that the plant's asarone fills the nicotinic receptors. It may also reduce withdrawal symptoms for recovering alcoholics.

Gargling or consuming diluted extract has a sialagogue effect, reducing mouth and gum inflammation. A poultice can be applied to treat a toothache. Topical applications of calamus have counterirritant properties. Liniments, fomentations, or poultices can be applied for arthritis, joint pain or tenderness, and neuralgic pain. A paste made from the powder may be applied to the forehead for a frontal headache, or to the nape for a tension headache.

CONTRAINDICATIONS

Calamus should be avoided during pregnancy due to its emmenagogue properties. Large doses can act as an emetic and purgative.[4] The Indian variety and to a lesser extent, the European variety, contain potentially carcinogenic compounds. According to Traditional Chinese Medicine, calamus should not be used by individuals with yin deficiency with heat signs, excessive sweating, vomiting blood, or spermatorrhea.

PREPARATION AND DOSAGE

TINCTURE: Fresh rhizomes [1:2, 70-95% alcohol]; dry rhizomes [1:5, 50% alcohol]; consume 5-30 drops, up to three times daily. Fresh rhizome is preferred because it is more aromatic; the dry rhizome is more pungent, and some aromatic oils are lost in the process.

ACETUM EXTRACT: Fresh rhizomes [1:2, apple cider vinegar]; consume 10-30 drops, up to three times daily.

CAPSULES: Consume 1-2 "00" capsules, up to three times daily.

TEA: Prepare a hot infusion or decoction; consume 2-8 ounces, up to three times daily.

HONEY AND SYRUP: Simmer fresh rhizomes in simple syrup 20 to 45 minutes. Strain and refrigerate. The roots may be stored as candied calamus; consume ½-2 grams as a digestive aid. Consume 20-60 drops of the syrup up to three times daily, or use as a base for other compounds. Decoct the fresh roots in honey at a [1:4] ratio.

TOPICAL USE: Apply the poultice or powdered root paste to the affected area.

CULINARY USE: Small quantities of fresh leaves may be added as an aromatic flavoring agent. The root powder is used as a pungent spice in India, but has a slightly bitter taste.

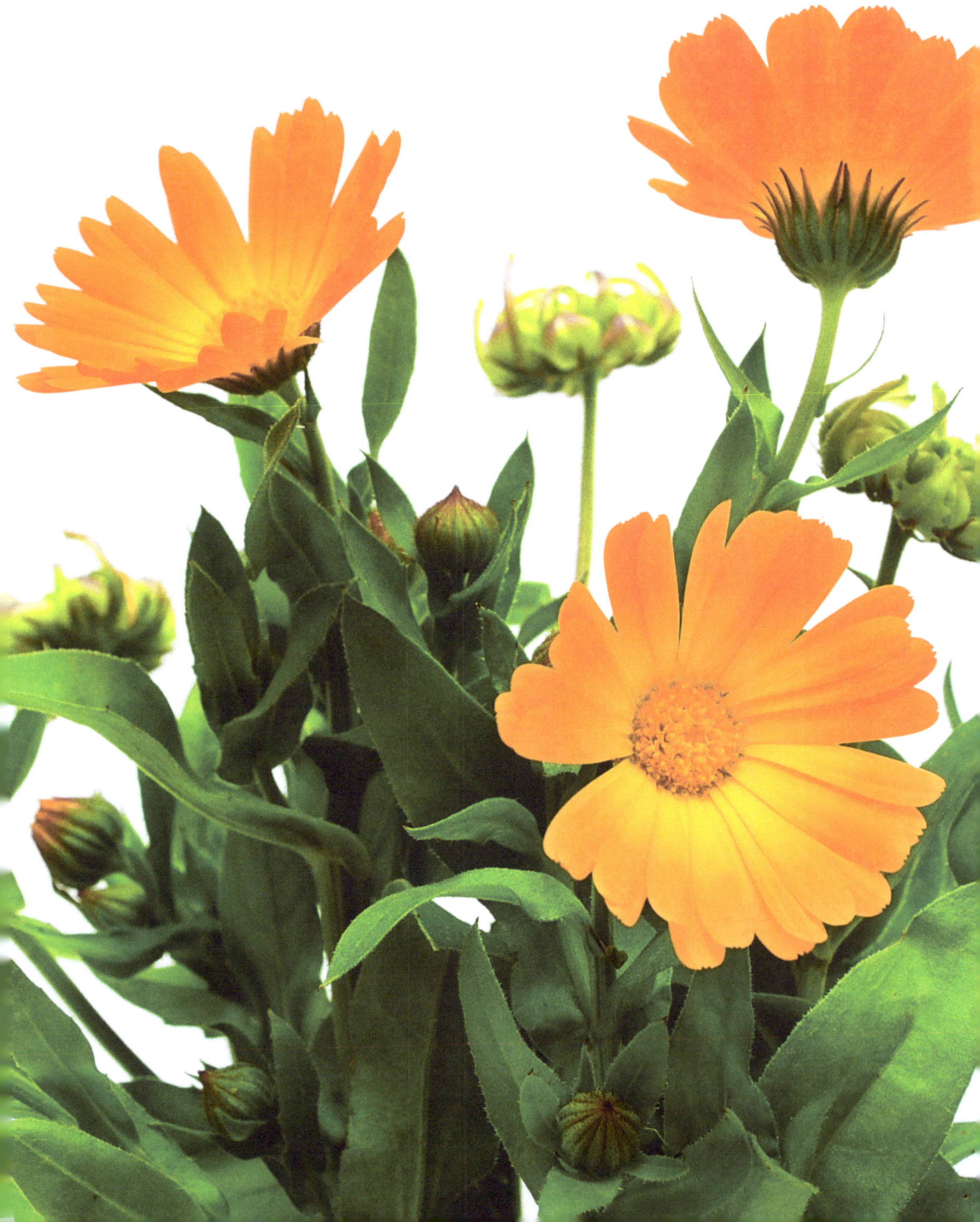

CALENDULA

DESCRIPTION

BOTANICAL NAME:
Calendula officinalis

COMMON NAMES:
Calendula, marigold, European marigold, pot marigold, poet's marigold, garden marigold, bull's eye, poor man's saffron, golds, ruddles, gowan, Mary Gowles, holigold
kehäkukka (Finnish)
fleurs de tous les mois, souci, souci des jardins (French)
goldblume, ringelblume, sonnenwende (German)
fiore d'ogni mese, oculus Christi, solis sponsa, solsequia (Italian)
zergul (Sanskrit)
claveton, flameniquillo (Spanish)
ringblomma, solsocka (Swedish)[1]

FAMILY NAME:
Asteraceae (Compositae)

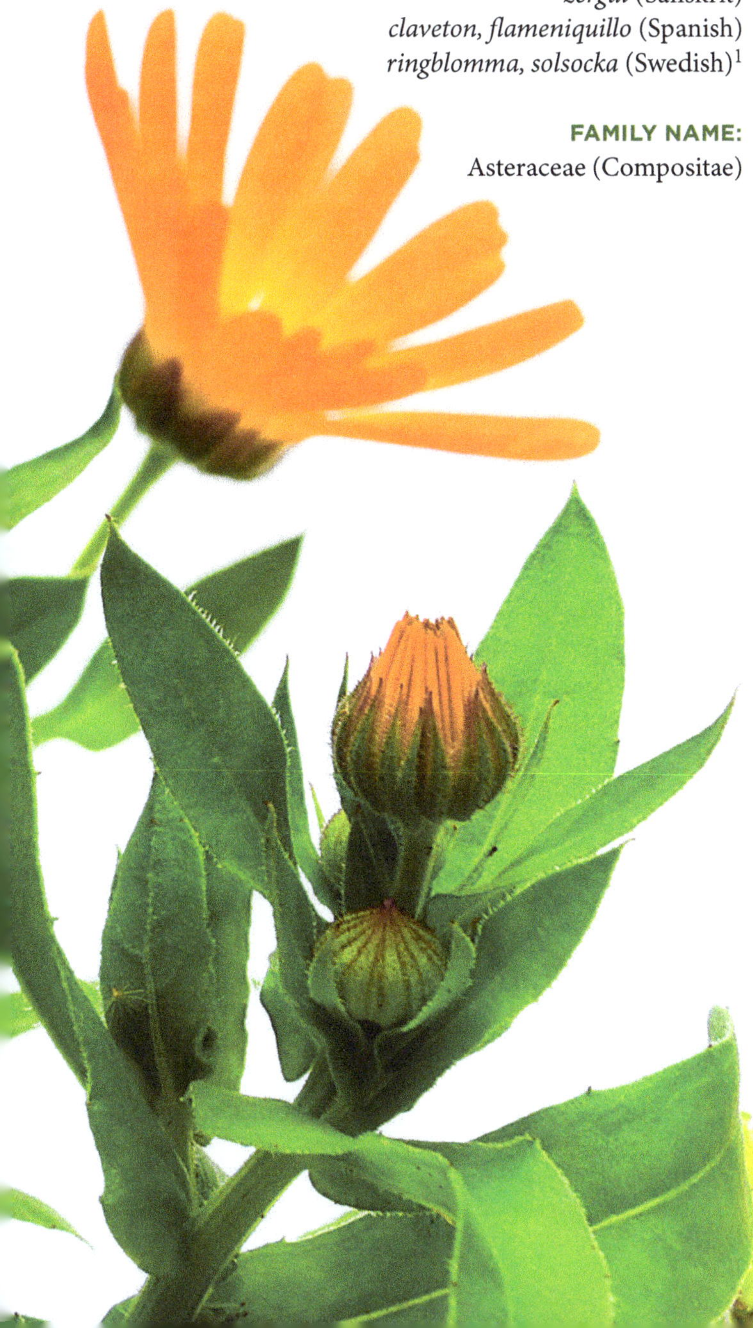

PARTS USED: The flower heads or ray florets.

BOTANICAL DESCRIPTION AND HABITAT: Calendula is native to Mediterranean countries, and is cultivated throughout the U.S. and Europe. A self-seeding annual, it is easily grown, thrives in full sun, and tolerates most types of soil. *Calendula officinalis* is a cultivar with unknown origins.[2] The green stems (20 – 75 cm tall) and leaves are covered with resinous, glandular hairs.[2] The hairy, fleshy leaves are large (15 – 20 cm long) and spatulate or oblong at

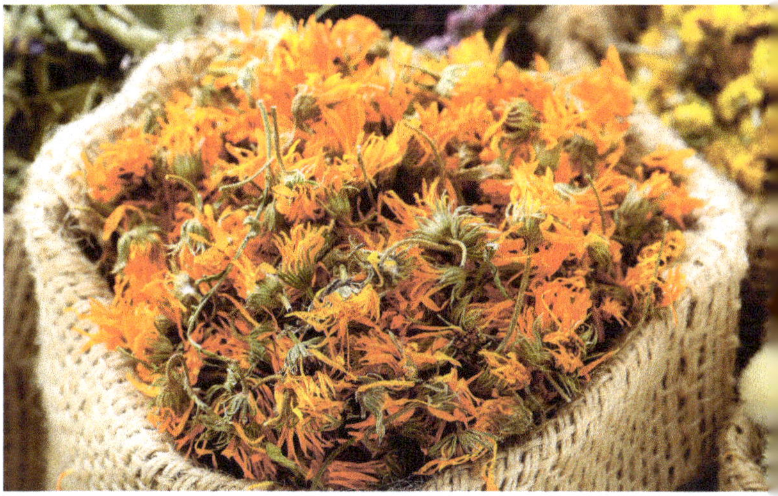

the base of the plant. The stem leaves are oblong to lanceolate (5 – 15 cm long by 1 – 3 cm wide) and clasp the stem.[2] The inflorescence is a radiate head (4 – 5 cm diameter) with glandular, lanceolate phyllaries. Each head has 5 – 50 bright yellow or orange pistillate ray florets (up to 4 – 5 mm wide), and up to 150 or more yellow or orange staminate disk florets.[2,3] The fruits (10 – 20 mm or more) are unique, curved, wrinkled, spiny achenes with a shape reminiscent of larvae or insects.[3]

THE NAME: The genus name *Calendula* derives from the Latin *calendae* ("little calendar" or "little clock"), referring to the frequency of the bloom occurring on the *calends* (first day of the month). The Italian name *fiore d'ogni mese* has a similar meaning, translated as "flower of each month." The species name *officinalis* denotes that this herb was listed as an official drug in European pharmacopoeias. The common name marigold was corrupted from the Anglo-Saxon name for marsh marigold: *merso-meargealla*. Eventually, marigold was associated with traditional

Catholic festivals honoring the Virgin Mary, and in the 17th century, those honoring Queen Mary. Historically, authors writing in Old English referred to the flowers as *golds* or *ruddes.* It acquired the names *solis sponsa* ("the sun's spouse or wife") and *solsequia* ("sunflower") due to the expansion of the blossoms during peak daylight hours, and their contraction as the light waned. It is also known as "poor man's saffron" because the petals were used as a saffron substitute to flavor and color rice and other grain dishes.[1,4]

HISTORICAL USES: Ancient Greeks and Persians garnished and flavored food with the flowers.[4] During the Middle Ages in Europe, the flowers were often added to beverages, soups, and stews.[4] The petals added a gold color to butter and cheese.[1] The fresh flowers were administered as a diaphoretic, and to resolve smallpox and measles eruptions.[1] Calendula was applied to bites, stings, sprains, wounds, and infected or sore eyes.[1] The stem sap and fresh leaf poultice were applied as a folk remedy for warts.[1] Doctors used the leaves to treat burns, superficial wounds, and sores during the Civil War.[4] Calendula was also used by Eclectic physicians as a vulnerary agent for burns, skin ulcers, wounds, varicose veins, sore nipples, conjunctivitis, and a variety of other skin conditions.[1,4]

CONSTITUENTS: Calendula contains salicylic acid, resin, saponins (glycosides A-D, D_2, and F), oleanolic acid 3-O-β-D-glucoronide, and triterpenoids (helinatriol C and F, ursadiol, and 12-ursene-3,16,21-triol), erthrodiol, calenduladiol, and longispoinogenine, calendulosides (A-D, G, and H), α and β-amyrin, taraxasterol, r-taraxasterol, lupeol, carotenoids, β-carotene, calenduline, lycopene, violaxanthin, and other xanthophyls, pentacylic alcohols (farodol, brein, and arnidiol), tocopherols, flavonoids (narcissin, rutin, quercetin, and isorhamnetin), polysaccharides

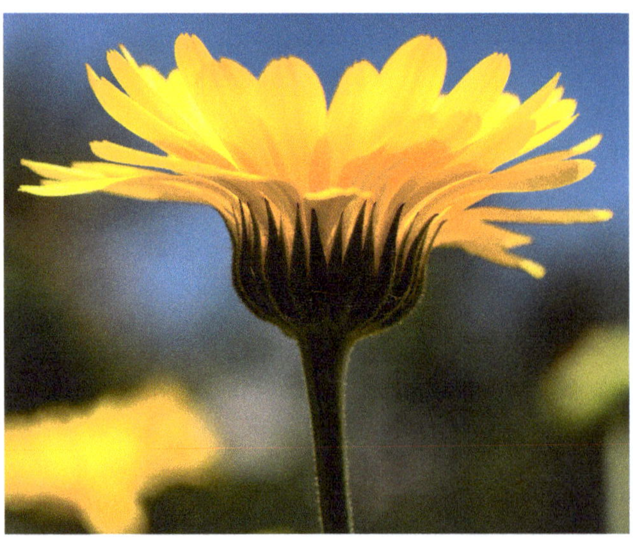

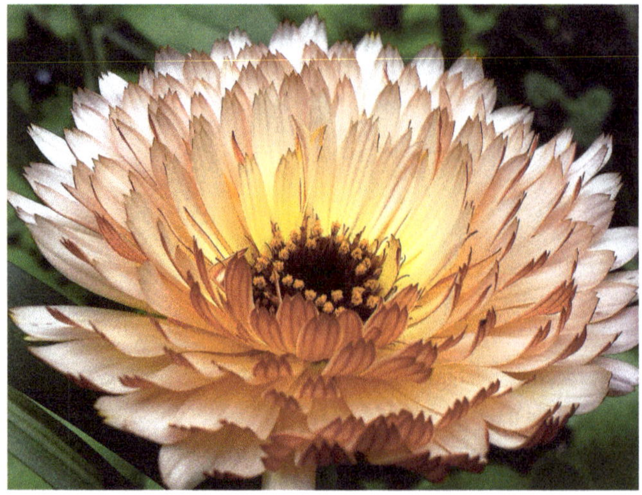

(rhamnoarabinogalactan and arabinogalactans), phytosterols, volatile oil, and chlorogenic acids.[5-7]

NUTRITIONAL PROPERTIES: Calendula contains vitamins A and C, carotenoids, β-carotene, calenduline, lycopene, tocopherols, flavonoids, and polysaccharides.

MEDICINAL PROPERTIES: Antibacterial, antifungal, anti-inflammatory, antimicrobial, astringent, choleretic (mild), demulcent, emollient, immune stimulant, immune modulator, lymphatic, styptic (mild), and vulnerary.

TEMPERATURE AND FLAVOR: Warm, sweet, bitter, and mild astringent.

MEDICINAL USES

Calendula is an antimicrobial, subtle lymphatic immune modulator and immune stimulant that enhances phagocytosis.[4,5,8] It can be consumed short- or long-term for immune and lymphatic support. Calendula is an adjunct for treating a cold, sore throat, swollen glands, post-mastectomy lymphedema, and mononucleosis.[1,4] Internal and topical use hasten the healing of viral infections including: herpes zoster, *Molluscum contagiosum,* shingles, chicken pox, measles, and human papilloma virus (HPV). It also hastens the healing of bacterial infections including: staph, strep, impetigo, and bacterial vaginosis.[1,4] Calendula aids in treating fungal infections, such as *Candida albicans* that causes vaginal infections, intestinal infections, and thrush. Apply topically to treat athlete's foot and ringworm.[4] Prepare an all-purpose antimicrobial and immune supporting compound by combining four parts echinacea *(Echinacea);* two parts calendula, spilanthes *(Acmella),* and usnea *(Usnea);* one part thyme *(Thymus)* and yerba mansa

(Anemopsis); and one-quarter part licorice *(Glycyrrhiza)* and clove (*Syzigium*).

Calendula protects, heals, and regenerates the digestive tract lining.[8] The tea or infused oil can be consumed on an empty stomach to treat mouth, gastric, or duodenal ulcers, chronic gastritis, or ulcerative colitis.[1,5,8] Calendula contains the triterpene esters ψ taraxasterol-3-O-myristate and arnidiol-3-O-myristate that protect the epithelial intestinal barrier.[9] Consume a tea containing mint *(Mentha)*, chickweed *(Stellaria)*, violet *(Viola)*, meadowsweet *(Spiraea)*, calendula, and a pinch of licorice *(Glycyrrhiza)* to heal the digestive tract lining and digestive ulcers. Or combine equal portions of St. John's wort *(Hypericum)* and calendula oil, and consume up to one tablespoon on an empty stomach or between meals.

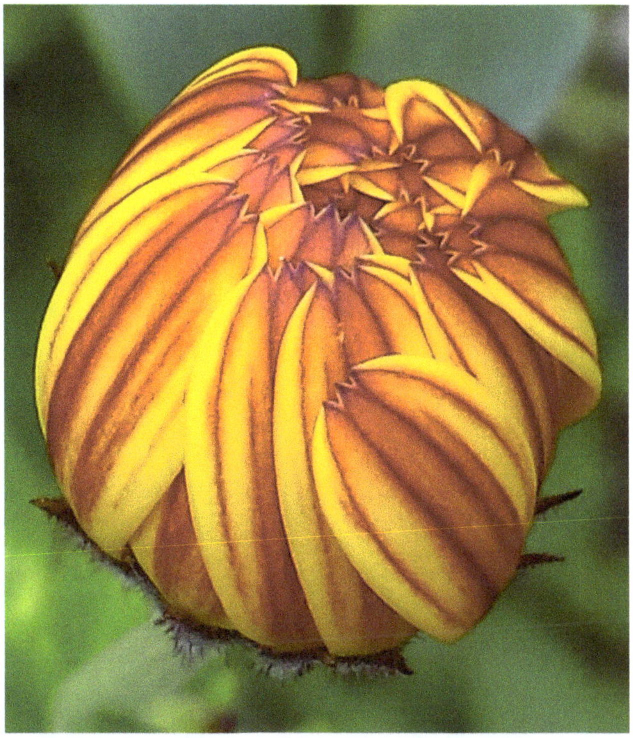

Calendula has astringent, demulcent, emollient, and anti-inflammatory properties.[4] A water-based preparation such as tea, gargle, eye wash, or vaginal irrigation soothes acute or chronic inflammation in the mucous membranes. Gargling with calendula tea or diluted tincture reduces gum, mouth, or throat inflammation or ulcers, and gingivitis.[5] Prepare a mouthwash by combining calendula with extracts of echinacea *(Echinacea)* and yerba mansa *(Anemopsis)*, and smaller amounts of clove *(Syzygium)* and myrrh *(Commiphora)*; dilute in water, and gargle.

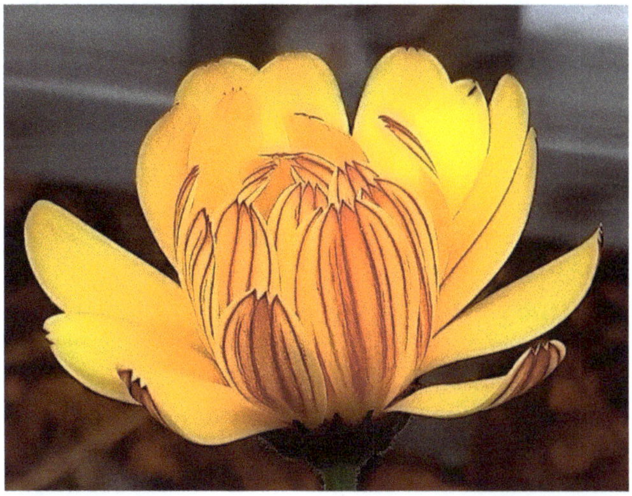

Calendula eye wash aids in treating conjunctivitis, styes, blepharitis, eye wounds, and tired, irritated, bloodshot, or watery eyes. To alleviate eye infections, combine calendula with an antimicrobial herb such as coptis *(Coptis)* or goldenseal *(Hydrastis)*, and an anti-inflammatory such as chamomile *(Matricaria)*, and one-quarter teaspoon of salt per four ounces of tea. Strain the tea through a paper filter to remove particulate matter, and allow it to cool. Flush the eye with an eye cup or tea-saturated cotton ball multiple times daily. Prepare a fresh batch of tea daily, and make sure to wash hands and sterilize the eye cup after use. *Note:* Coptis and goldenseal can cause a temporary yellow stain around the eyes.

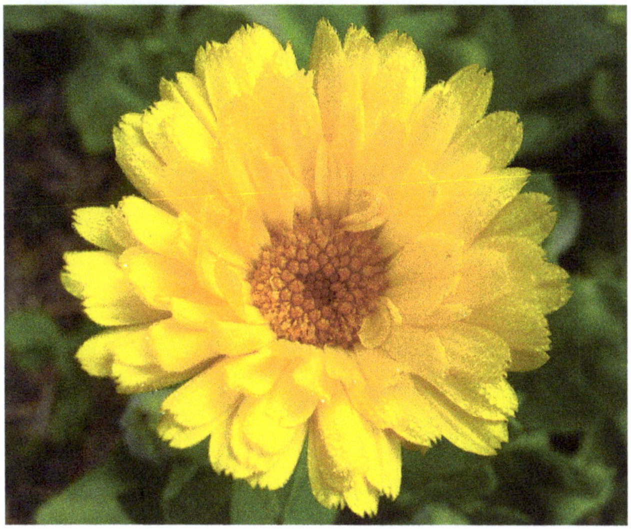

One of the most effective vulnerary agents, calendula hastens skin and wound healing. It stimulates tissue regranulation by increasing glycoprotein, nucleoprotein, and collagen metabolism.[5] Topical applications of calendula stimulate the proliferation and migration of dermal fibroblast cells.[10] *In vitro* studies demonstrate that calendula enhances wound healing and tissue regranulation by up-regulating the expression of two proteins: connective tissue growth factor and α-smooth muscle actin (α-SMA).[10]

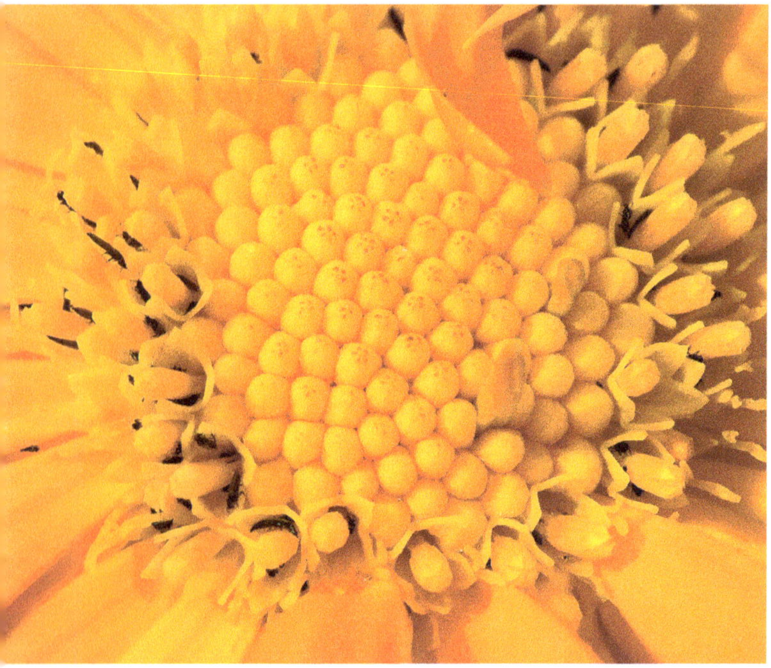

Calendula is highly effective in treating numerous skin conditions. Topical applications hasten the healing of cuts, abrasions, wounds, fissures, burns, sunburn, skin ulcers, pressure ulcers, bruises, sprains, strains, insect bites, wasp or bee stings, and the final stages of poison ivy or poison oak.[1,4,5] It alleviates swelling and pus-filled discharge. Calendula also aids in treating fungal and bacterial skin conditions such as thrush, abscesses, impetigo, boils, and staph infections.[5] Combine it with echinacea *(Echinacea)*, usnea *(Usnea)*, and yerba mansa *(Anemopsis)* or goldenseal *(Hydrastis)*, and apply multiple times daily to treat the aforementioned microbial infections. Calendula is a soothing anti-inflammatory for skin conditions such as diaper rash, eczema, dermatitis, radiation-induced dermatitis, psoriasis, acne, and sore nipples.[1,5] Prepare a poultice or salve by combining it with chickweed *(Stellaria)*, chamomile *(Matricaria)*, comfrey root *(Symphytum)*, St. John's wort *(Hypericum)*, and/or marshmallow *(Althaea)*. As a multipurpose medicinal oil or salve, calendula combines well with St. John's wort *(Hypericum)*, comfrey *(Symphytum)*, and arnica *(Arnica)*. However, arnica should not be applied to broken or severely inflamed skin.

Calendula contains flavonoids that strengthen blood vessels and capillaries. Consume internally in a tea blend with other flavonoid-rich herbs such as hawthorn *(Crataegus)*, rose hips *(Rosa)*, orange peel *(Citrus sinensis)*, lycii berries *(Lycium)*, and/or smaller amounts of wu wei zi *(Schisandra)* and licorice *(Glycyrrhiza)*. Long-term consumption of this tea aids in treating varicose veins, spider veins, and hemorrhoids.[1]

CONTRAINDICATIONS

Consuming the flower calyx may cause throat irritation in some individuals. Otherwise, calendula is a very gentle, non-toxic herb that can be used by most individuals, including children, pregnant women, and the elderly. There are no known contraindications; however, some sources claim that it may have emmenagogue properties, indicating that it should be avoided during pregnancy. These contraindications are likely based on misinterpretations of folkloric uses of the herb that claimed it stimulated menses. These erroneous claims likely confused calendula with *Tagetes*— a flower with emmenagogue actions that looks remotely similar to calendula and is also called marigold. It is true that *Tagetes* should be avoided during pregnancy. However, there is no clinical evidence proving calendula's emmenagogue effects, or demonstrating that it could induce a miscarriage. In fact, the author has administered calendula internally to hundreds of pregnant and non-pregnant patients, and has never seen emmenagogue effects. The author considers internal use of calendula safe during pregnancy and lactation, and in young children.

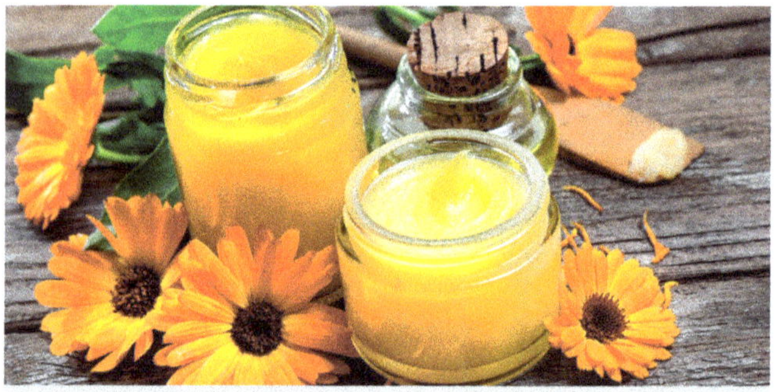

PREPARATION AND DOSAGE

TINCTURE: Fresh flowers or petals [1:3-1:4+, 80-95% alcohol]; recently dried flowers or petals [1:5+, 70-80% alcohol]; consume 10-60 drops, up to three times daily.

TEA: Prepare a hot or cold infusion; consume 8-12 ounces, three to four times daily.

TOPICAL USE: Prepare infused oil using the Simpler's method, double boiler method, or alcohol intermediary oil method. Prepare it as a cream, lotion, ointment, liniment, salve, steam, bath, or aftershave.

CULINARY USE: Add fresh petals to soups, chowders, salads, and desserts.

CALIFORNIA POPPY

DESCRIPTION

BOTANICAL NAMES:
Eschscholzia californica, E. mexicana (E. californica ssp. *mexicana), E. caespitosa, E. glyptosperma, E. lobbii, E. minutiflora*

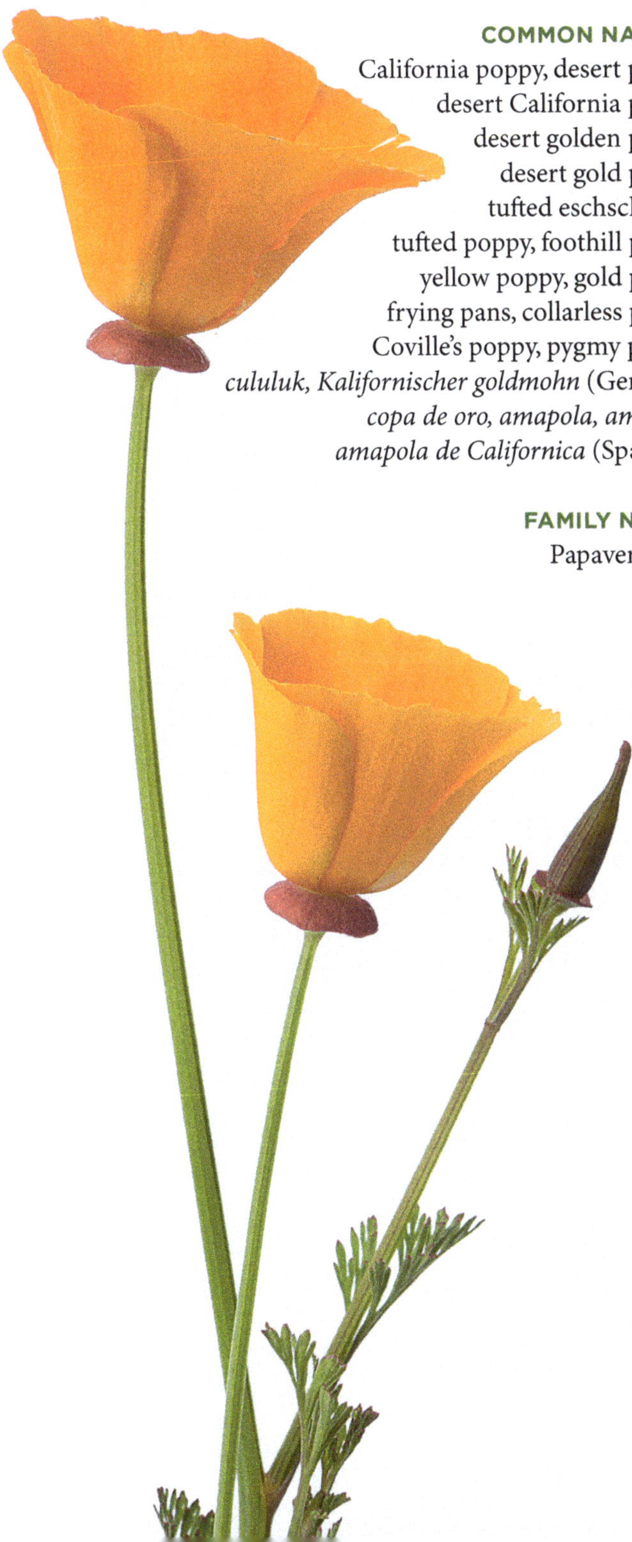

COMMON NAMES:
California poppy, desert poppy, desert California poppy, desert golden poppy, desert gold poppy, tufted eschscholzia, tufted poppy, foothill poppy, yellow poppy, gold poppy, frying pans, collarless poppy, Coville's poppy, pygmy poppy
cululuk, Kalifornischer goldmohn (German)
copa de oro, amapola, amarilla, amapola de Californica (Spanish)

FAMILY NAME:
Papaveraceae

PARTS USED: The whole plant or roots. The aerial parts or whole plant can be collected while flowering; however, the roots are most potent when harvested in the fall after they have gone to seed.

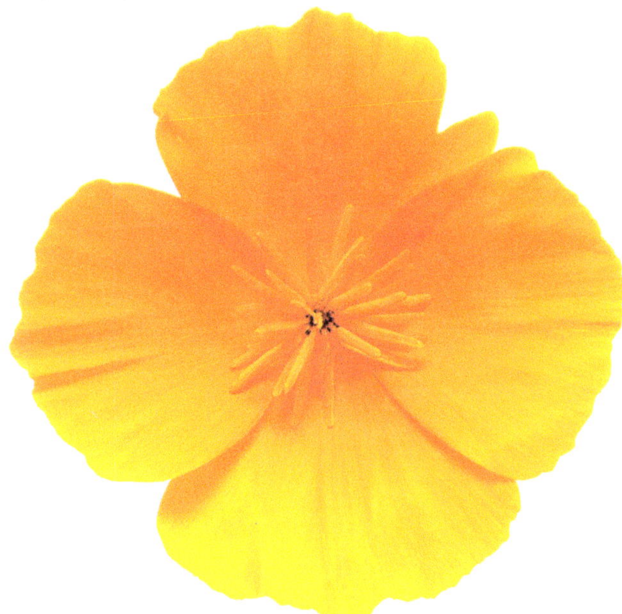

BOTANICAL DESCRIPTION AND HABITAT: California poppy grows wild on roadsides, rocky slopes, grasslands, clearings, and disturbed sites at low elevations. It can be found throughout the U.S., including the West Coast, Mountain West, and Southwest. A self-sowing annual, California poppy is easy to cultivate from seed as an ornamental. The seeds require cold temperatures to germinate most efficiently; therefore, it is best to distribute them in the fall, or combine them with moistened sand in a plastic bag and refrigerate for several weeks before sowing. *Note:* In California, a hefty fine can be imposed from harvesting this herb on public property because it is the state flower.

California poppy forms deep orange, smooth, hairless taproots. The mature roots harvested in fall emit a reddish-orange sap. The plant grows up to 60 cm tall. California poppy has delicate blue-green leaves finely divided into linear leaflets with entire margins.[1] The leaves have a feathery appearance and are mostly basal, though a few grow on the flowering stems. The slender, erect flowering stems bear solitary flowers. When budding, they are entirely closed by two fused sepals that shed as the flower matures. California poppy has four shiny, vibrant orange or yellow-orange obovate petals (2 – 6 cm long) and numerous stamens. The flowers only bloom on sunny days. They are beneficial to native bees and bumblebees.[2] The ovary is comprised of two fused carpels on which the stigma grows; a flattened receptacle rim is located at the ovary base.[1] The ovary matures into a linear, cylindrical, pod-like capsule (3 – 9 cm long) containing numerous round brown or black seeds.[1]

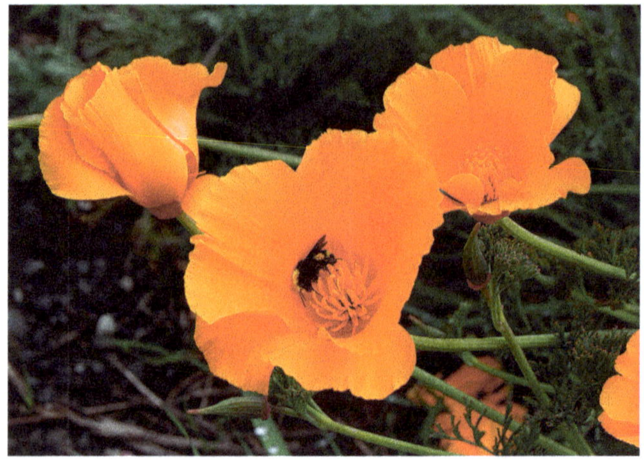

THE NAME: *Eschscholzia* was named after Russian scientist Johann Frederic Von Eschscholtz (1793 – 1831) following his visit to California in 1816.[3] The epithet *californica* indicates the plant's origin. The epithet *caespitosa* derives from the Latin *caespes* ("sod, turf"); botanically, this refers to the plant's growth in dense clumps or tufts.[4] The epithet *glyptosperma* derives from the Greek *glypto* ("to carve") and *sperma* ("seed").[5] The epithet *lobbii* is named after English botanist William Lobb (1809 – 1863). *Minutiflora* translates as "small flower."[6] The common name poppy derives from the Latin *papaver.* The Spanish name copa de oro translates as "cup of gold;" amarilla means "yellow;" amapola means "poppy;" and amapola de Californica translates as "California poppy" or "poppy from California."

The following common names correspond with the following Latin binomials: California poppy, gold poppy, California gold poppy, copa de oro, amapola, amarilla, amapola de Californica, cululuk, and Kalifornischer

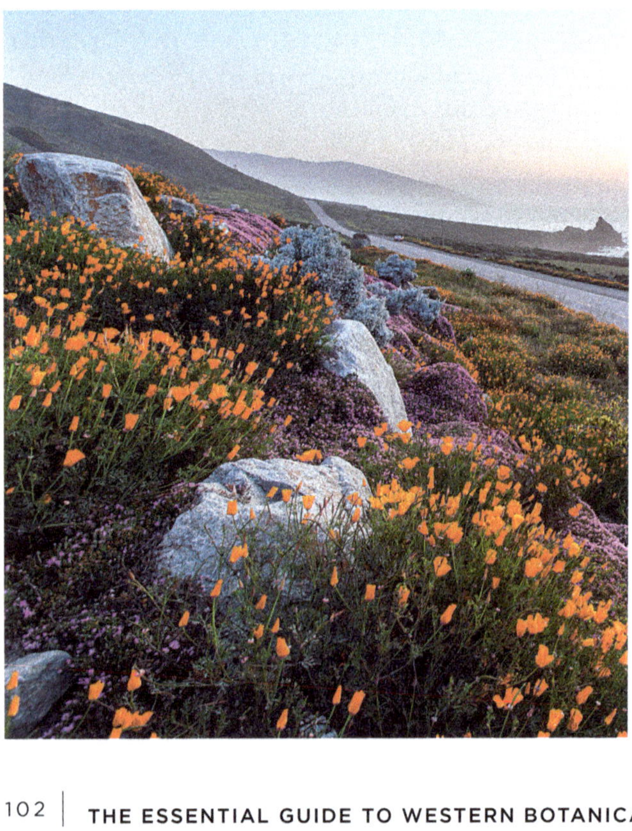

goldmohn *(Eschscholzia californica);* California poppy, desert poppy, and desert California poppy *(E. californica* ssp. *mexicana);* collarless poppy, tufted eschscholzia, tufted poppy, foothill poppy, and yellow poppy *(E. caespitosa);* desert poppy, desert golden poppy, and desert gold poppy *(E. glyptosperma);* frying pans *(E. lobbii);* and Coville's poppy and pygmy poppy *(E. minutiflora).*

HISTORICAL USES: Native American tribes placed the herb under infants' beds and administered it to them as a sedative.[7] A decoction of the flowers was applied to the hair and scalp to kill lice. Crushed leaves were packed around an aching tooth for pain relief.[8] Juice from the roots was consumed to relieve stomachaches and tuberculosis, and was applied as a wash for weeping sores. Pomo Indians applied a poultice of the ground or decocted seed pods to a nursing mother's breast to dry up their milk.[7] The Nisenan of California consumed small amounts of the boiled leaves.[2] Root juice was given as a narcotic to stupefy gambling companions.[7]

CONSTITUENTS: California poppy contains isoquinoline alkaloids (californidine, eschscholtzine, eschscholtzidine, α-canadine, allocryptopine, berberine, bisnorargemonine, chelerythrine, coptisine, cryptocavine, cryptopine, escholine, fumarine, glaucine, lauroscholtzine, protopine, sanguinarine, chelidonine, chelirubine, macarpine, N-methyllaurotetanine, and caryachine), eschscholtzxanthin, xanthophyll, flavone glycosides (rutin — in the flowers), and carotenoids (in the petals).[9-12]

NUTRITIONAL PROPERTIES: The petals contain flavone glycosides (rutin) and carotenoids.[12]

MEDICINAL PROPERTIES: Analgesic, antispasmodic, anodyne, hypnotic, nervine, and sedative.

TEMPERATURE AND FLAVOR: Cool and bitter.

MEDICINAL USES

California poppy is a nervine, hypnotic, and sedative.[9-11] It encourages relaxation and induces a sense of well-being. California poppy calms the central nervous system, reducing feelings of stress, anxiety, and agitation.[10] It is useful for treating hyperactivity and insomnia in children or adults.[10,11] Individuals with mild insomnia may find that consuming 30 – 120 drops before bedtime works effectively. Others with more severe insomnia may require repeated doses, consuming the first dose one to two hours prior to bedtime, and the second right before going to bed. California poppy induces a restful, deep sleep, and rarely causes morning sleepiness. For nervine, sedative, and analgesic effects, combine it with equal parts valerian *(Valeriana),* hops *(Humulus),* and passion flower *(Passiflora).* It also counteracts valerian's heating effects. California poppy contains non-narcotic alkaloids (protopine, cryptopine, and chelidonine) that have hypnotic and sedative effects; the root has the highest content of these alkaloids.[7,11] Studies have confirmed the anxiolytic effects of water-based extracts of California poppy in animals.[11] It also inhibits dopamine-β-hydroxylase.[12]

California poppy is an analgesic and skeletal muscle relaxant, though it is a much milder alternative to *Papaver somniferum* (opium poppy).[9,10] It reduces muscle pain (myalgia), nerve pain (neuralgia), and nerve hypersensitivity. California poppy aids in treating sciatica and muscle spasms. Consume the tincture or tea to relieve pain, or apply topically as an anodyne.

California poppy has smooth muscle antispasmodic actions.[10] While anti-infective agents are also necessary, California poppy is a highly effective respiratory antispasmodic for treating a dry, irritative cough, whooping cough, croup, bronchitis, or pneumonia. It reduces stomach and intestinal spasticity, aiding in managing pain accompanying conditions such as irritable bowel syndrome, Crohn's, and colitis. It also eases menstrual cramps and premenstrual tension. California poppy reduces referred pain caused by passing kidney stones or gallstones. Consuming moderate to high doses (up to one teaspoon) every one to two hours may be necessary to relieve pain and spasms.

California poppy may not work as effectively in individuals with a history of consistently using pharmaceutical or recreational opiates (i.e., oxycodone, methadone, morphine, or heroin). In these cases, it is necessary to administer herbal analgesics other than those in the Papaver family to treat pain or nervous system disorders. Examples of alternative analgesics include: Jamaican dogwood (*Piscidia*), valerian (*Valeriana*), black cohosh (*Actaea*), kava (*Piper methysticum*), passion flower (*Passiflora*), and pedicularis (*Pedicularis*).

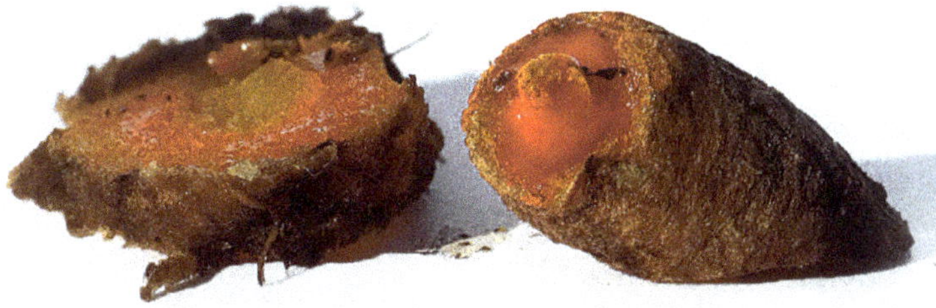

CONTRAINDICATIONS

California poppy is contraindicated during pregnancy due to its alkaloid cryptopine (allocryptopine) content that has a stimulating effect on an animal uterus.[10,13] Avoid operating heavy machinery when consuming California poppy. Consult a medical professional before combining this herb with alcohol or prescription drugs such as sedatives, hypnotics, antidepressants, or analgesics.[10] Naturopathic doctor Joseph Brinker also cautions against concurrent use with phenobarbital.[13] *Note:* Be sure to harvest wild California poppy from unpolluted areas, as it can absorb heavy metals from the soil.

PREPARATION AND DOSAGE

TINCTURE: Fresh whole plant or roots [1:2-1:3, 70-95% alcohol]; consume 15-120 drops, up to four times daily.

GLYCERITE: Fresh roots [1:2-1:3, 50% glycerin and 50% alcohol]; consume 15-60 drops, up to four times daily.

TEA: Prepare a hot infusion or root decoction; consume 4-8 ounces, up to four times daily. The tea tastes bitter. *Note:* Less potent than the fresh plant, the dry plant loses potency 3-12 months after harvesting.

TOPICAL USE: Apply the tincture or glycerite topically as a liniment. Chop the fresh plant or root and apply as a poultice. Prepare recently dried leaves and/or root using the alcohol intermediary oil method; apply oil or salve to the affected area.

CANNABIS

DESCRIPTION

BOTANICAL NAMES:
Cannabis sativa
(syn. *Cannabis sativa* var. *indica, C. indica*)

COMMON NAMES:
Cannabis, marijuana, marihuana, hemp, Indian hemp, true hemp, hemp weed, kief, grass, pot, herb, dope, reefer, muggles, ganja, dagga, Mary Jane, maryjane, weed, ganjah, gunjuh, ganga, guaza, hash, hasish, hasash, hasheeshchurrus, churras, kef, keef, kif (English slang)
al-gnab al-handy, hashish, kayf (Arabic)
chanvre (French)
haschisch (German)
kannabis (Greek)
bhāṅg, ke beej, gā̃jā, charas, caras (Hindi)
mayaku (Japanese)
má, dàmá, taimá (Mandarin)
vijayā, siddhi, bhaṅg, gañjā (Sanskrit)
grifa, hachis, mota, marijuana (Spanish)
bhang, charas (Urdu)

FAMILY NAME:
Cannabaceae

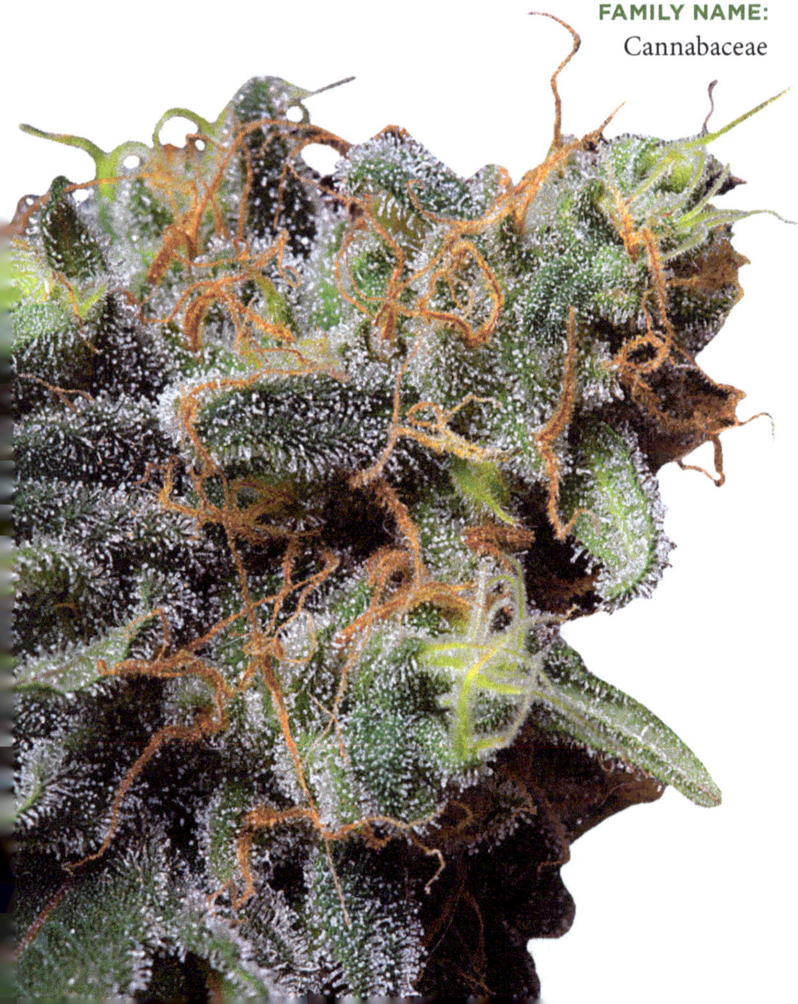

PARTS USED: The flowering tops, leaves, and seeds.

BOTANICAL DESCRIPTION AND HABITAT: *Cannabis sativa* is a dioecious annual, native to central and southern Asia, that has naturalized in Russia, China, India, Pakistan, Iran, and North America, among other places. It is cultivated globally in rich soil.[1,2] Cannabis can reach up to six meters high, but usually grows from 75 cm to 1.5 meters.[1,2] The two most commonly recognized subspecies are *C. sativa* ssp. *sativa,* which is taller and thinner than *C. sativa* ssp. *indica,* which is shorter and bushier.

Angled, fibrous stems are dotted with appressed hairs; the young stems are densely pubescent.[1] The leaves are palmately compound, with long, pubescent petioles (2 – 10 cm long), three to nine narrowly lanceolate leaflets (3 – 15 cm long by 0.5 – 2 cm wide) with tapered apices, serrate margins, and small, thread-like stipules.[1,3] The middle leaflet is the longest, with those growing on either side progressively smaller. The upper sides are rough with stiff hairs, while the lighter colored undersides are densely hairy, and dotted with resinous glands.[1]

Male plants tend to be less robust than females.[2] In males, the green, pendent staminate flowers (4 – 6 mm across) are borne in panicles at leaf axils.[1,4] They sport five elliptic, pubescent, membranous sepals (3 – 5 mm long by 1.5 – 2 mm wide), and no petals.[1,2] Each flower has five banana-shaped anthers. In females, the sessile, green pistillate flowers grow in leaf axils in dense pseudo-spikes at the ends of branches.[5] The female flowers and their subtending leaf-like bracts and bracteoles are densely covered in strongly aromatic, resinous hairs called trichomes.[1] The active constituents of the plant are primarily concentrated in the trichomes. Hermaphrodites are common in cannabis cultivars, although they are usually dioecious.[5] The fruit is a shiny, yellow-brown achene (3 – 4 mm diameter) commonly consumed for its nutritional content.[1]

THE NAME: The genus name *Cannabis* derives from the Greek *kannabis* ("hemp"), which may derive from an ancient Scythian or Thracian word.[6] A widespread, very useful plant thought to have been used since prehistoric times, cannabis has many related common names throughout Indo-European languages. The epithet *indica* is Latin ("of or from India"), referring to the subspecies origin

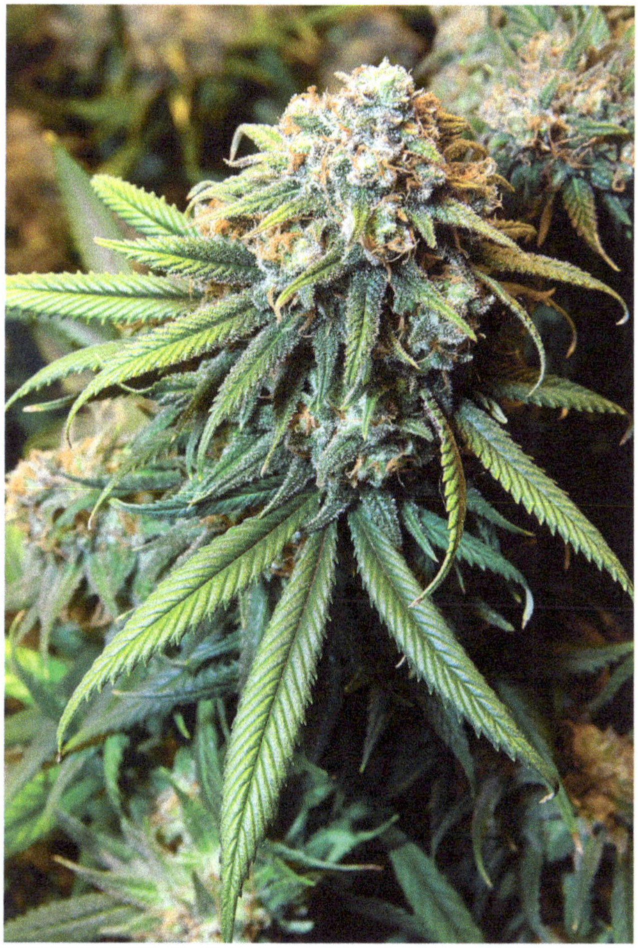

in India. The epithet *sativa* means "cultivated." Hashish derives from the Arabic name for hemp ("green intoxicating liquor") originating from the Hebrew *shesh* ("to be joyous").[7]

HISTORICAL USES: Cannabis is one of the world's oldest cultivated plants. It was used widely in Neolithic China in the Yang Shao period, about 4000 BCE.[5] Cannabis was included in a classical medicine treatise by Chinese Emperor Shen Nung in 2737 BCE. Egyptians cultivated cannabis as a medicine, seed, and fiber.[7] In China, hemp was infused in wine and used as an anesthetic for surgery.[8] In Europe, hemp was used to treat a cough, jaundice, arthritis, gout, lumps, and hard tumors.[8]

Eclectic physicians administered cannabis extract to treat nervous depression, nervous exhaustion, insomnia, pain, spasms, neuralgia, headaches, cerebral anemia, epilepsy, and coughing fits.[9,10] It was also given for digestive pain, and subacute and chronic inflammatory disorders in the urinary tract, such as chronic cystitis, dysuria, and bladder irritation.[9,10] Dr. Finley Ellingwood recommended it for subacute brain inflammation, cerebrospinal meningitis, and delirium tremens.[9]

Dr. Harvey Felter described the effects of cannabis:

> An emotional state of happiness even to ecstasy is experienced, with an endless procession of beautiful visions coming and going, and over which the patient indulges in merriment and even hilarity. So pleasurable becomes his sensations that he may break into boisterous laughter and antics of a ridiculous character...His imagination carries him into ludicrous ideas and strange actions, he has notions of grandeur and greatness, and moments are exaggerated into eons of time. Endless phantasms of beauty and delight pass before his distorted mental vision. He becomes affectionate to the extreme, both to himself and to others, and altogether he is a very happy individual leading to a very full and infinitely extended life. Finally drowsiness overtakes him and he drops into a heavy sleep...from which he awakens...with ravenous hunger.[10]

He also described the effects of hashish:

> It produces a semi-delirium taking on the character of a sense of well-being and exhilaration—a state highly coveted by its devotees, who call it loftily "the increaser of pleasure," "the laughter mover," and "the cementer of friendship"—all indicative of its physiologic influence." These hashish debauches are joyful affairs, and while usually devoid of injurious consequences, may be followed by catalepsy and depressive and maniacal insanity, from which, however, the victim recovers fully in time.[10]

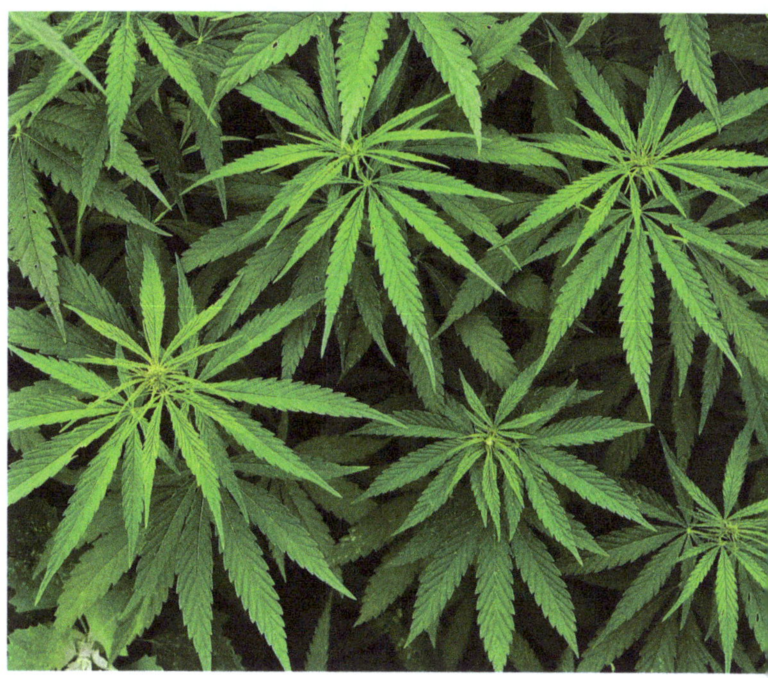

Hemp was grown for fiber to make clothing, cords, sacks, and sail cloths.[7] The first American flag was woven from hemp fibers. Hemp seed was used as a demulcent, birdseed, and varnish.[7]

CONSTITUENTS: Approximately 483 constituents have been identified in cannabis.[8] Cannabinoids are amongst the first constituents identified. There are several subclasses of cannabinoids: cannabigerol (CBG) type and its acid precursor (CBGA) have six related cannabinoid compounds; cannabichromene (CBC) type has five related cannabinoids; cannabidiol (CBD) type has seven related compounds, including CBD acid (CBDA); and Δ^9-tetrahydrocannabinol = tetrahydrocannibinol = Δ^9-THC = THC = dronabinol has nine related cannabinoids, including Δ^9-THC acid (Δ^9-THCA).[8] Additional cannabinoids are: cannabicyclol (CBL) type, cannabielsoin type, cannabitriol type, and a miscellaneous type. The most psychologically active compound is Δ^9-tetrahydrocannabinol (Δ^9-THC). Δ^8-tetrahydrocannabinol (Δ^8-THC) has 80% of the activity of Δ^9-THC.[8] The aromatized derivatives of THC and CBD are cannabinol and cannabinodiol.[8]

Cannabis contains nitrogenous compounds (amides and lignanamides, amines, and two spermidine alkaloids: cannabisativine and anhydrocannabisativine).[8] It contains 18 amino acids, proteins (edestin, zeatin, and zeatinnucleoside), glycoproteins, and enzymes (edestinase, glucosidase, polyphenol oxidase, peptidase, peroxidase, and adenosine-5-phosphatase), sugars (monosaccharides, disaccharides, polysaccharides, cyclitols, and amino sugars), hydrocarbons, alcohols (C1-C16), aldehydes (C2-C13), liphatic ketones (C3-C18), simple acids (aliphatic and aromatic), esters, lactones, steroids (stigmasterol, β-sitosterol, campesterol, and ergosterol), bitter principle, gum, choline, and trigonelline.[7,8,11] Cannabis contains 120 terpenes (linalool, citronellal, α-terpineol, limonene, β-caryophyllene, and α-humulene) that account for the flavor of different cannabis varietals; 25 noncannabinoid phenols (eugenol, dihydrostilbenes, dihydrophenanthrenes, and spiroindans); and 21 flavonoids (O-glycosides of the C-glycosides orientin, vitexoin, and isointexin; and O-glycosides of the flavonoids apigenin, luteolin, quercetin, and kaempferol).[8]

NUTRITIONAL PROPERTIES: Cannabis leaves contain vitamin K, carotene, xanthophyll, chlorophyll, and minerals (mercury, zinc, manganese, copper, iron, magnesium, calcium, potassium, and sodium).[8] Cannabis seeds contain fatty acids (a balanced omega-3, -6, and -9 ratio) and protein.[7,11]

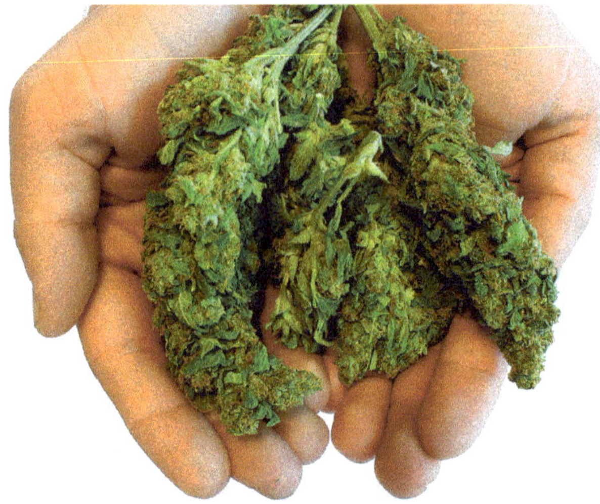

MEDICINAL PROPERTIES: The leaves and flowers are analgesic, anodyne, antidepressant, anti-inflammatory, antioxidant, antispasmodic, euphoric, narcotic, nervine, sedative, and sudorific. The seeds are demulcent, emollient, anti-inflammatory, and hypocholesterolemic.

TEMPERATURE AND FLAVOR: The leaves and flowers are warm, pungent, sweet, and bitter. The seeds are cool and sweet.

MEDICINAL USES

CANNABINOID PHYSIOLOGY

Cannabinoids from cannabis (Δ^9-THC is the most pharmacologically active) interface with the body's endocannabinoid system that includes endocannabinoids produced by the body, and cannabinoid receptors (CB_1, CB_2, CB_3, and others) in the central nervous system, immune cells, and all other organs and tissues.[12,13] Depending on their location and other factors, activation of these receptors can cause effects such as euphoria, anxiety and other emotional states, cognitive impairment, sedation, dry mouth, muscle relaxation, hunger, and pain and inflammation reduction.[12] Cannabinoids from plants (phytocannabinoids) are oxygen-containing, aromatic hydrocarbons; endocannabinoids are fatty acid derivatives.[12] The activation of CB_1 receptors (primarily in the brain, spinal cord, and peripheral nervous system) causes changes in circulation and cognition.[12] Located at the terminals of the central and peripheral nerves, these receptors also act presynaptically as a buffer for the stimulating or inhibiting actions of other neurotransmitters by preventing their release.[12] Overall, the endocannabinoid system is a major mediator of physiological homeostasis, especially in the nervous, endocrine, immune, gastrointestinal, and reproductive

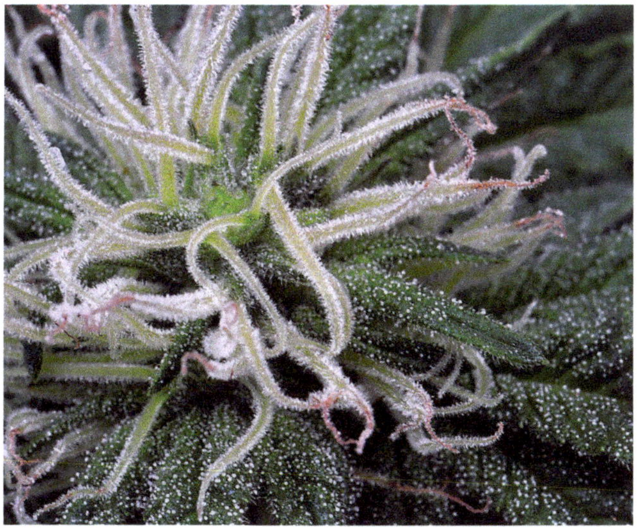

systems.[8,13] Through these important systems, cannabis can affect nearly every organ in the body.

There are relatively few CB_1 receptors in the brain stem, which regulates respiration and cardiac function; this explains why few fatalities are associated with cannabis use. However, these receptors are highly active in the brain regions responsible for movement, memory processing, and pain modulation.[12]

CB_2 receptors found mainly in immune cells modulate cytokine release, and regulate inflammation and immunity.[12] The functions of these receptors are being investigated to further understand their analgesic, anti-inflammatory, and anticancer potential. While not traditionally attributed to the cognitive changes induced by cannabis, CB_2 receptors recently have been found in CNS tissue. Their presence and function in the CNS are not as well established as that of CB_1.[12,14] Although more research is required, evidence shows that CB_2 receptors may help to mediate neuroinflammation in diseases such as multiple sclerosis, traumatic brain injury, Alzheimer's, Parkinson's, and Huntington's disease. They may also have an impact on depression, schizophrenia, and the effects of substance abuse.[14] CB_2 receptors are targeted by some autoimmune diseases; this supports evidence indicating their role in regulating inflammation.[15]

NERVINE AND SEDATIVE EFFECTS

Cannabis is a nervine, anxiolytic, and sedative.[9,10] It aids in treating insomnia and anxiety, as well as premenstrual agitation and depression. The sedative properties are attributed to cannabidiol and the volatile oil (including the monoterpenoids linalool, citronellal, and α-terpineol).[15] Sedative effects vary, based on the user and the strain. Some individuals experience sedative properties from strains higher in Δ^9-THC. In other individuals, cannabis and/or Δ^9-THC have a stimulating effect, producing anxiety, palpitations, and paranoia. Resultant anxiety, and in rare cases, psychotic episodes or schizophrenia, can be due to the Δ^9-THC and 11-OH-THC. However, pesticides, herbicides, and chemicals used in cultivation can also contribute to anxiety and palpitations. The production of 11-OH-THC, the main metabolite of Δ^9-THC, increases in the body when cannabis is ingested, versus when it is smoked. This metabolite may have stronger psychoactive effects than Δ^9-THC, which may indicate why some individuals have more negative and intense cognitive changes when eating cannabis than when smoking it. In contrast, there is evidence that CBD has antipsychotic activity that may benefit those suffering from diseases such as schizophrenia; this activity may balance some of the negative effects of Δ^9-THC.[15]

Dr. Finley Ellingwood prescribed cannabis for "disorders of motility, involuntary, irregular movements, especially of a distressing character."[9] Long-term consumption of cannabis aids in treating epilepsy. In a review of clinical outcomes of epileptic patients consuming cannabis in Washington and California clinics, 55% of patients experienced a 51 – 100% reduction in seizures, while only 14% found no benefit.[16] The majority utilized CBD-enriched artisanal (herbal) formulas.[16] Cannabis reduces the severity and frequency of epileptic seizures, and eases multiple sclerosis symptoms in the early stages. Extracts of cannabis can be combined with skullcap *(Scutellaria),* lemon balm *(Melissa),* milky wild oats *(Avena),* and a small amount of rosemary *(Salvia rosmarinus)* extract to prevent and reduce the frequency and severity of seizures. Cannabis extract can be combined with pedicularis *(Pedicularis),* Jamaican dogwood *(Piscidia),* passion flower *(Passiflora),* and skullcap *(Scutellaria)* to ease the symptoms (or muscle/nerve spasticity) of multiple sclerosis.

ANTIDEPRESSANT EFFECTS

Low doses of cannabis can exert a euphoric and antidepressant effect.[11] The endocannabinoid (EC) system has a role in the neurobiology of depression.[17] Pharmacological manipulations of the EC system have induced antidepressant-like effects. Rats exposed to chronic, unpredictable stress showing signs of depression (indicated by lower sexual motivation) demonstrated decreased CB_1 receptor density in gray matter glial cells, and a significant increase of CB_1 receptor density in the prefrontal cortex.[17] These changes were partially remedied by concurrent treatment with antidepressant medications.[17] In this study, a significant decrease in the endocannabinoid anandamide, named (from the Sanskrit *ananda* "bliss") due to its association with pleasurable feelings, was measured in every part of the brain examined, and it was not reversed by antidepressant treatment.[17] When the coding for CB_1 receptors are erased from rat genomes, the resultant behavioral changes resemble melancholic depression.[17] Conversely, overactive CB_1 receptor signaling may contribute to the development of depression. Increased CB_1 receptor density and activity were found in the prefrontal cortex of depressed individuals who committed suicide.[17] Scientists attempted to reconcile these contradictory findings—positing that the endocannabinoid system "could differentially contribute to the symptomatology of depression in a region-specific manner."[17]

When treating depression with cannabis, it can be helpful initially to use it by itself due to its vastly varying effects on individuals. When beginning treatment, it is also advisable to consult with a health care practitioner. For individuals who do not experience negative effects from cannabis, it can be combined with additional antidepressant, anxiolytic, and nervine herbs including: lemon balm *(Melissa)*, St. John's wort *(Hypericum)*, skullcap *(Scutellaria)*, milky wild oats *(Avena)*, and/or damiana *(Turnera)*. A more uplifting and energizing antidepressant formula can include cannabis, gotu kola *(Centella)*, ginkgo *(Ginkgo)*, rosemary *(Salvia rosmarinus)*, and orange peel or orange flowers *(Citrus sinensis)*.

Some studies suggest that while infrequent cannabis use shows little effect on depression, heavy cannabis use may be associated with a low to modest increase in depressive symptoms in some users.[17] However, the authors of one twin study stated that "comorbidity between cannabis dependence and major depression disorder likely arises through shared genetic and environmental vulnerabilities predisposing to both outcomes," and suggested that cannabis use does not, per se, cause depression.[18]

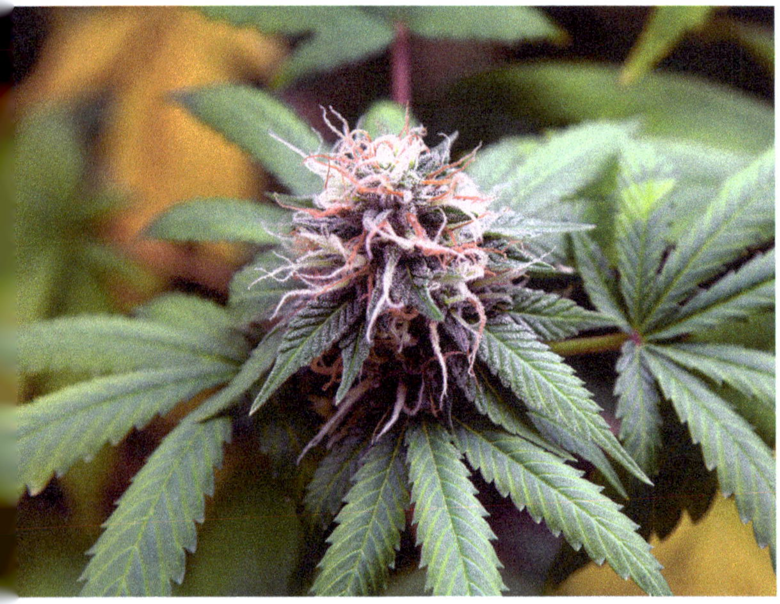

ANTISPASMODIC EFFECTS

Cannabis is a smooth muscle and skeletal muscle antispasmodic. It reduces respiratory, stomach, intestinal, bladder, and uterine cramping.[9,10,19] Cannabis aids in treating nervous gastralgia, gastric neuralgia, gastric ulcer, irritable bowel syndrome, Crohn's disease, enteritis, and colitis.[10] It also eases menstrual cramping, uterine cramping caused by endometriosis, and fallopian tube and afterbirth pain.[9,10,19] Cannabis extract alleviates pain due to cystitis, urethritis, dysuria, interstitial cystitis, and to a lesser extent, referred pain from passing kidney stones.[9,10,19] Consuming the extract, syrup, or edibles can reduce respiratory spasms, easing coughing and asthmatic symptoms. Cannabis is a mild bronchodilator.[8,9] However, inhaling smoke can also elicit respiratory irritation and coughing. Although it can be used alone as an antispasmodic, it also can be combined with kava *(Piper methysticum)*, California poppy *(Eschscholzia)*, or other Papaveraceae family members, and/or Jamaican dogwood *(Piscidia)*.

ANALGESIC EFFECTS

Internal and external use of cannabis eases acute or chronic muscle pain and spasms.[35] THC is a skeletal muscle relaxant.[35] Internal use aids in treating migraines, nervous headaches, and tension headaches.[10,20,35] This is mediated by CB_1, CB_2, and other cannabinoid receptors, possibly including CB_2-like receptors and vanilloid receptors.[21] CB_1 receptors are present on nociceptors, sensory receptors at the end of sensory neuron axons that relay pain signals to the central nervous system. When activated by cannabinoids delivered locally or systemically, these receptors provide analgesia by inhibiting the action of the nociceptor.[22] Activation of these CB_1 receptors in the peripheral nervous system by endocannabinoids is a first defense against pain.[22] Activation of CB_2 receptors also inhibits acute nociception, without cognitive effects.[23] CB_1 receptor activation reduces neuronal excitability by inhibiting the release of glutamate (a stimulatory neurotransmitter), and activating somatic and dendritic potassium channels.[24] In one study, smoking cannabis reduced the perception of pain in multiple sclerosis patients with treatment-resistant spasticity, likely due to the antispasmodic effect of CB_1 and CB_2 receptor activation. CBD inhibits the degradation of anandamide known to reduce inflammatory pain via activation of CB_1, CB_2, and vanilloid receptors.[21]

During acute migraine episodes, Δ^9-THC inhibits the platelet release of serotonin, but this mechanism does little to prevent migraines.[35] Dr. William Courtney, who utilized cannabis to treat more than 7,514 patients with various conditions, states that the best method of delivering cannabis for treating migraines (and other inflammation and immune related conditions) is to consume fresh juice from the leaves and buds in a mature female plant. Using the plant fresh, before drying or heating, improves access to cannabinoid acids and terpenes.[25] Fresh, unheated cannabis has low Δ^9-THC content, as heat is required to transform Δ^9-THC-A (tetrahydrocannabinolic acid) to Δ^9-THC.[25] Because Δ^9-THC-A has very low psychoactivity, utilizing fresh cannabis instead of heated allowed Dr. Courtney to administer a much higher dosage of a wide spectrum of cannabinoids, without overwhelming patients with negative side effects from excessive Δ^9-THC consumption.[25]

External use of cannabis aids in treating myalgia, fibromyalgia, muscle tension, neuralgia, osteoarthritis, and rheumatoid arthritis.[10] Local activation of peripheral CB_2 receptors inhibits inflammation and reduces associated pain.[23] Extracts with terpenes from cannabis will penetrate the skin more effectively, lending greater relief than CO_2 extracts that solely extract cannabinoids.[15] In order to ease muscle spasms and pain, as well as joint pain and inflammation, prepare a salve containing chamomile *(Matricaria)*, St. John's wort *(Hypericum)*, comfrey *(Symphytum)*, figwort *(Scrophularia)*, and/or valerian *(Valariana)*.

ANTI-INFLAMMATORY EFFECTS

Significant anti-inflammatory effects are attributed to cannabis. CBD has been shown to have anti-inflammatory, antioxidant, and other neuroprotective activity that may slow the onset of neurodegenerative diseases.[8,15] Cannabis aids in treating diabetic neuropathy. One mechanism for cannabis' neuroprotective effects is the modulation of excitotoxicity, oxidative stress, and inflammation.[26] These findings support clinical evidence that cannabis benefits arthritis.[15] Endocannabinoid system receptors are likely mediators of colon inflammation.[27] Anandamide induces COX-2 dependent cell death in colon cancer cells, and as mentioned above, CBD can inhibit the degradation of anandamide.[21,27]

Endocannabinoids are derived from, and structurally similar to arachidonic acid, which is transformed into prostaglandins by catalyzing COX-1 and COX-2 enzymes.[27] Endocannabinoids also can act as substrates for COX enzymes, and may compete with arachidonic acid—potentially interfering with the inflammatory process.[27,28]

The inhibition of COX enzymes by CBD and CBD-A has been demonstrated, and results in significant anti-inflammatory activity that may inhibit cancer cell proliferation.[27] In one *in vitro* study, Δ^9-THCA-A, CBDA, CBG, and CBGA showed a more than 30% inhibition of COX-1, and Δ^9-THCA-A, CBG, and CBGA showed a more than 30% inhibition of COX-2.[27] The same researchers evaluated the effect of cannabinoids on prostaglandin production, with a low level of inhibition (less than 10%) shown by THC, THCA-A, CBD, CBG, and CBGA.[27]

IMMUNE EFFECTS

Cannabis has immune stimulating and suppressing effects that aid in treating immune conditions, including autoimmunity. Some of the immune stimulating constituents are: polysaccharides, flavonoids, and terpenoids (quercetin, luteolin, limonene, β-caryophyllene, α-humulene, CBD, CBG, bannabinolic acid, and CBC). CBD, CBG, CBC, cannabinol, and Δ^9-THC have potent antibacterial actions, and are effective against a variety of currently relevant MRSA strains.[29] Incubating herpes simplex viruses with Δ^9-THC decreases their viral potency.[8] However, smoking cannabis regularly appears to compromise the immune function and aggravate respiratory allergies. The immune system depressing effects are due to the presence of THC.[29] Evidence of THC's linkage with immune suppression may be confounded by the fact that cannabis smokers often use other substances with immune compromising potential, such as alcohol, and those using cannabis for medical purposes often have immune-compromised conditions.[30]

The significant anti-inflammatory actions of cannabis demonstrate its potent immune modulating effects, useful with a variety of autoimmune diseases. Cannabis has a wide range of constituents that contribute to its immune modulating capacity. According to Dr. Courtney:

> Cannabis is the sole source of patented lipophilic antioxidants and neuroprotectants, a broad terpenoid profile with complementary immunologic activity as well as altering CB_2 binding affinity through allosteric modulation. In addition cannabis is the unique source of essential cannabinoid acids that aid in down regulation of the inflammatory arm of the immune system, mitigating oxidative associated diseases ranging from diabetes, cancer, CNS and myocardial degenerative and ischemic conditions and autoimmune disorders.[25]

Researchers have attributed most of THC's immune modulating activity to the activation of CB_2 receptors; these receptors are identified as targets of autoimmune diseases, which may further indicate their role in regulating immunity.[15,30] CB_2 receptors are extensively expressed in immune system tissues and cells, and in the central nervous system associated with immune function.[30] B lymphocytes express the highest levels of CB_2 receptors, followed by macrophages, monocytes, NK cells, and polymorphonuclear cells.[30] THC and other CB_2 agonists may suppress T cell proliferation or their maturation into effector/memory cells. These cells may be important in the etiology of autoimmunity due to their potential to target healthy tissues. THC also can inhibit the differentiation of human monocytes into antigen-presenting dendritic cells; these cells are implicated in the pathogenesis of most autoimmune conditions.[30]

ANTICANCER EFFECTS

While significantly more research in this area is necessary, small *in vivo* and *in vitro* studies using various cannabis extracts, THC, and/or CBD show that cannabis has antineoplastic qualities, and can induce apoptosis or reduce cancer cell invasion, angiogenesis, or metastasis in many cancer cell lines, including lung, skin, brain, breast, cervical, colorectal, prostate, and bile duct.[31-34] A small, pioneering clinical study in Spain demonstrated the safety of intracranial injection of THC into glioblastoma tumors, an extremely malignant and deadly brain cancer. They also showed that THC inhibited glioblastoma cells *in vitro*.[35]

Research shows that some cancer cells carry CB_1 and CB_2 receptors, and activation of these receptors may be important mechanisms for the efficacy of cannabis in fighting cancer. Studies of melanoma and bile duct cancer show that the activation of these receptors inhibit growth, proliferation, angiogenesis, and metastasis, and increase apoptosis of cancer cells.[33,36]

Cannabis may be a helpful adjunct during chemotherapy treatment for cancer, reducing pain and nausea, and ameliorating the side effects of conventional cancer treatments. Studies utilizing synthetic and endogenous agonists of the CB_1 or CB_2 receptors demonstrated that concurrent use prevented some of the neuropathy and associated pain induced by use of the common chemotherapy drugs paclitaxel and cisplatin, without compromising their antineoplastic effects.[37,38]

ANTINAUSEANT EFFECTS

Cannabis is an antinauseant and appetite stimulant.[8,10,11,19,39] It can be highly beneficial for easing nausea due to chemotherapy, radiation, food poisoning, or alcohol poisoning.[11,40] It helps to stop dry heaves; an extract or smoke inhalation of the flowers works most effectively for this purpose. If smoking is not possible, it can be combined with extracts or glycerites of ginger *(Zingiber)*, peppermint *(Mentha piperita)*, orange peel *(Citrus sinensis)*, and/or fennel *(Foeniculum)*. It can also be consumed in conjunction with low doses of peppermint spirits *(Mentha piperita)*.

INTRAOCULAR EFFECTS

Cannabis extract reduces intraocular pressure due to glaucoma, hyperthyroidism, or methamphetamine addiction.[8,11,19] It relaxes the eye muscles.[19] In Ayurvedic medicine, a preparation of flowering cannabis known as *bhang* is used to reduce intraocular pressure, spasms, and pain.[39]

Cannabis reduces intraocular pressure through local activation of CB_1 receptors in the eye; this may reduce aqueous humor formation, and improve drainage from the eye.[41] Endocannabinoids are found in all ocular tissues except the lens, and there are CB_1 receptors throughout the eye.[41] The levels of endocannabinoids can vary in different disease states of the eyes, implying their role in maintaining ocular homeostasis.[41] Cannabis has a neuroprotective effect on retinal ganglion cells. As demonstrated *in vitro* and in rat retina, CB_1 agonists such as THC and CBD prevent damage to ganglion cells from glutamate-excitotoxicity and ischemia caused by increased intraocular pressure.[41,42]

The effect on intraocular pressure has a limited duration, necessitating frequent dosing.[43] One small study comparing the effects of THC and CBD on intraocular pressure showed that two hours after administration of THC, intraocular pressure significantly decreased

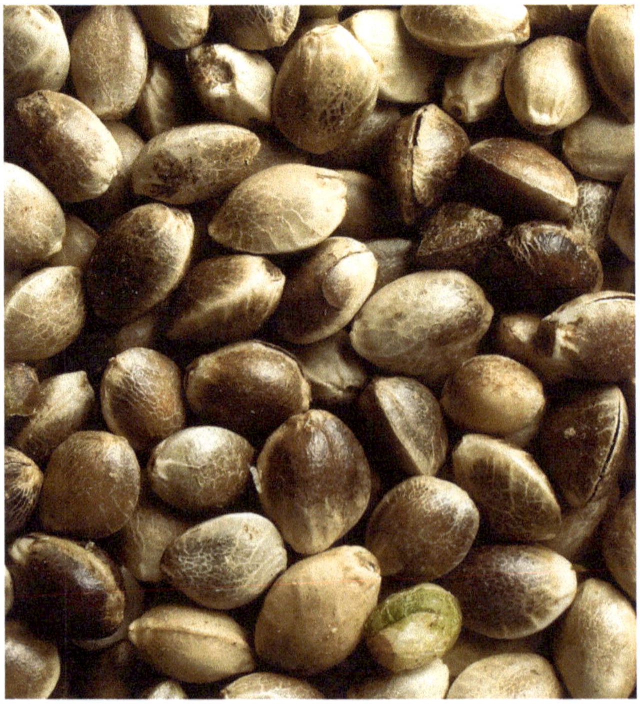

compared to the placebo; however, it returned to baseline within four hours after administration.[44] Interestingly, a lower dose of CBD had no effect on intraocular pressure, while a larger dose of CBD induced a transient increase in pressure at four hours.[44] Other researchers suggest that the side effect of changes in ocular blood flow caused by cannabis may negate the benefits on intraocular pressure.[43] Studies have shown contradictory results regarding whether a tolerance to the beneficial effects develops after continued use of cannabis.[45]

CANNABIS SEED: Cannabis seeds are a highly effective laxative and aperient that aid in treating constipation.[39] The oil extracted from the seeds is anti-inflammatory due to the omega-3, -6, and -9 essential fatty acids.[39] Long-term use aids in treating arthritis, Crohn's disease, and premenstrual syndrome.[39] Consuming the oil daily aids in treating eczema, psoriasis, and acne. It also decreases LDL cholesterol levels, fatty deposits, and blood coagulation.[39] The oil is a lubricating demulcent. Hemp seeds are a complete protein — a source of all essential amino acids. The seeds and seed oil are not narcotic.

CONTRAINDICATIONS

Avoid use during pregnancy and lactation. Youth under the age of 18 should use only under the supervision of a health care practitioner. Individuals with immune suppression, acute or chronic respiratory afflictions, liver or blood sugar conditions, estrogen-related reproductive problems, infertility issues (when trying to conceive), or chronic exhaustion should avoid smoking cannabis. Smoking or consuming cannabis will test positive for drug use. Many states do not have a medical marijuana program, and it is illegal to possess in most states without a medical prescription. Excessive doses can cause paleness, clamminess, a weak pulse, debility, spasms, or convulsions.[9]

Individuals with severe or chronic allergies should avoid exposure to cannabis pollen. Individuals with chronic liver conditions such as jaundice, hepatitis, or cirrhosis, or liver-related skin conditions such as acne, eczema, or psoriasis should limit or avoid use.

Use caution or avoid administering when psychological instability is present. Some evidence indicates that regular or heavy use of cannabis in susceptible individuals can increase the risk of experiencing psychotic symptoms and related disorders, such as hallucinations and delusions.

PREPARATION AND DOSAGE

There are numerous methods of preparing and administering cannabis. The female flowers, known as marijuana, are usually smoked. However, they are also prepared in a variety of other menstrua, including combinations of alcohol, honey, and/or glycerin, as well as oil or butter (using the infused or alcohol intermediary oil method). When consumed orally, the psychoactive effects of cannabis preparations can be much stronger and last much longer than when cannabis is smoked. The resins are soluble in alcohol; however, THC is mostly fat soluble. Another substance called bhang (also known as sidhee, subjee, or siddhi), consists of the budding flowers and leaves ground into a paste with milk, ghee, mangos, spices, and sugar. This can be made into a beverage or rolled into balls to eat. Indians add bhang to their sweetmeat *(majoon)*.[7] A drink containing decocted cannabis flowers and leaves, almonds, pistachio nuts, milk, and sugar is ingested on *Shivaratri*, a festival celebrating Shiva.[39] Charas (churrus) is the pure resin collected from flowering plants; it is more potent than the flowers, and like flowers, it is smoked or ingested.

Another more concentrated preparation of cannabis is hashish, a substance consisting mainly of resinous trichomes. In a 19th century method described by Dr. William Culbreth, hashish was prepared by heating four parts of the flowers and leaves in four parts water and three parts butter until the water dissipated.[7] The strained extract was added to syrup, boiled, and allowed to solidify. Hashish is commonly collected by placing discarded dry, resinous leaves in a framed silk screen and shaking until most of the trichomes have broken off the leaves and fallen through the sieve to be collected. A modern method of preparing hashish involves combining dry or fresh resinous leaves and small flowers with ice water in a sturdy bag with a silk screen bottom, commonly called a bubble bag. This bag should be nested in several more bags, each with silk screens with progressively smaller holes, all contained in a large bucket. The mixture is vigorously stirred, then strained through the bags. The concentrated resin is collected in each bag; smaller particles in the outermost bags are considered the highest grade, as they exclude inert plant matter caught in the inner bags.

Heat treatment (commonly achieved through smoking or cooking) of mature cannabis bud increases Δ^9-THC 1000-fold; it is produced by decarboxylating Δ^9-THC-A. This increases the plant's psychoactive effects exponentially. Drying and extended curing alone will partially decarboxylate the Δ^9-THCA, though to a much lesser extent. Courtney states that by using the plant fresh, before THCA is converted to THC, patients will tolerate much higher doses and can consume more cannabinoids, as they often find they can tolerate no more than 10 mg Δ^9-THC.[25]

Note: When preparing cannabis tincture, glycerite, honey, syrup, or oil, heating the dried flowering tops at 250º for one hour increases the Δ^9-THC content and potency, as well as psychoactive effects. Preparations made from flowering tops are more potent than those made from leaves.

TINCTURE: Fresh leaves or flowering tops [1:2-1:4, 80-95% alcohol]; dry [1:5, 70-95% alcohol]; consume 5-90 drops, up to three times daily.

FLUID EXTRACT: Dry flowering tops [1:1, 60-80% alcohol]; consume 5-30 drops.

GLYCERITE: Fresh leaves (milder) or flowering tops (more potent) [1:2-1:4, 50% glycerin and 50% alcohol]; dry leaves or flowering tops [1:5, 40% alcohol, 30% glycerin, and 30% water]; consume 5-60 drops, up to three times daily.

SUCCUS: Juice the leaves and/or fresh mature buds and consume fresh. To preserve the preparation, measure the volume and add 20% alcohol to the total volume, or add two to six fresh leaves to juice, smoothies, or soup.

CAPSULES: Consume 2-4 "OO" capsules, one to three times daily. Consume 3-4 capsules of hemp seed oil, once daily.

TEA: Prepare a hot or cold infusion of the leaves and/or flowers; consume 6-12 ounces, up to three times daily. Prepare a decoction of ground seeds; consume 8-12 ounces, up to three times daily. Add ground, dried seeds to smoothies, hot cereals, vegetable juice, nut bars, pesto, or paté.

HONEY AND SYRUP: Prepare an infusion of the leaves and/or flowers; blend, strain, add a sufficient quantity of sweetener (simple syrup or honey), and refrigerate. Heat the dried flowers, as noted above, then infuse them in honey [1:4, volume to volume] using the double boiler method, and strain. Consume ¼-1 teaspoon as needed, or apply topically.

TOPICAL USE: Prepare oil using the alcohol intermediary method, infused oil method, double boiler method, or infused ghee. Apply to affected areas. Prepare a liniment [1:4, 70% alcohol, 30% glycerin]; apply topically to the affected area.

CULINARY USE: Consume 5-15 grams of ground seeds, or up to 1 tablespoon of cold pressed oil. Low doses of cannabis-infused ghee, coconut oil, or butter can be consumed internally, but can be very psychoactive, so administer with caution. It takes one to two hours following consumption to absorb oil-based preparations.

CARDAMOM

DESCRIPTION

BOTANICAL NAMES:
Elettaria cardamomum (syn. *Amomum cardamomum, Cardamomum elettaria, Cardamomum officinale*)

COMMON NAMES:
Cardamom, bastard cardamom, Mysore cardamom, Malabar cardamom, green cardamom, Bengal cardamom, grains of paradise
habbahan, hal (Arabic)
cardamome (French)
kardamomom (German)
kakoules, kardamo (Greek)
hel (Hebrew)
elicit, ilaichi, elaichi (Hindi)
amomo (Italian)
byakuzuku shukusha (Japansese)
paektugu (Korean)
yang chun sha, yi jih ren (Mandarin)
elā, sūksmā elā (Sanskrit)
cardamomo (Spanish)
hemame, hiyl, kakule (Turkish)
kardemom (Yiddish)[1]

FAMILY NAME:
Zingiberaceae

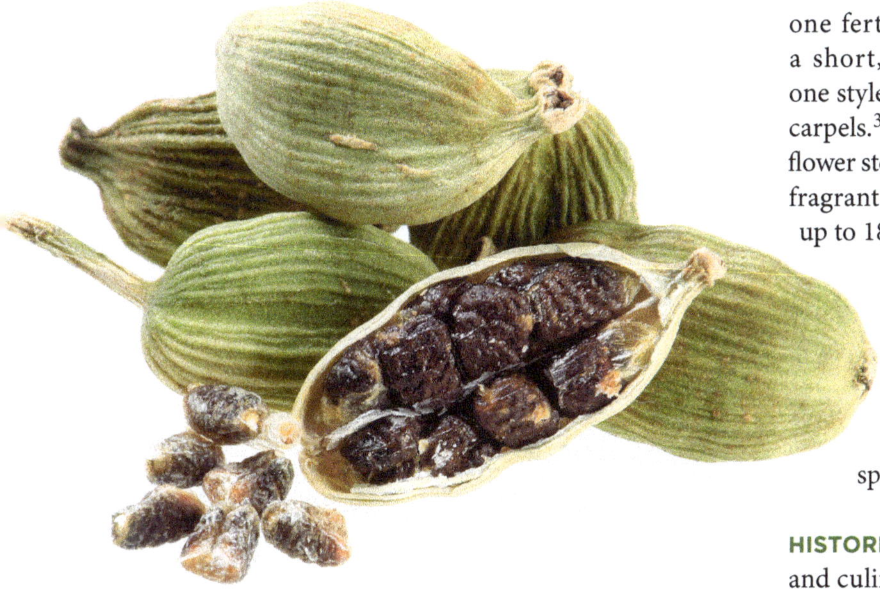

PART USED: The seeds.

BOTANICAL DESCRIPTION AND HABITAT: Cardamom is a perennial plant native to southern India. It is cultivated in India's tropical areas (Malabar Coast), and in Sri Lanka (Ceylon), Laos, Guatemala, and El Salvador.[2]

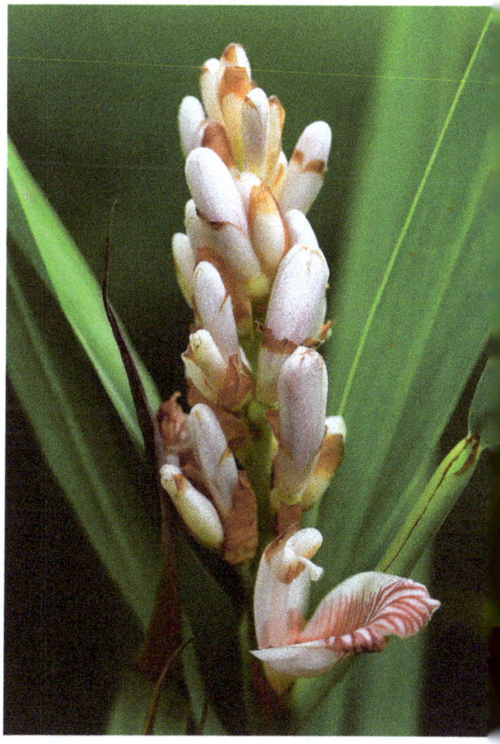

Cardamom is a clumping, herbaceous perennial with branching underground rhizomes from which erect stems grow (2 to 4 meters tall).[3] The dark green lanceolate leaves (26 – 90 cm long by 5 – 15 cm wide) are glabrous above, and lighter colored and hairy underneath.[3] Cardamom has unusual zygomorphic flowers (4 cm long by 1.5 cm wide) consisting of a large white labellum with magenta streaks and three green lobes, one fertile stamen on a short, flat filament, one style, and an inferior ovary comprised of three fused carpels.[3] They grow on loose racemes on erect or prostate flower stems (45 – 120 cm long).[3] The fruit is a small, highly fragrant, ellipsoid capsule (13 mm by 8 mm) containing up to 18 seeds.[4]

THE NAME: The genus *Elettaria* originates from the Hindi *ilaychi* and Punjabi *ilaichi* ("green cardamom").[1] The common name cardamom and the epithet *cardamomum* derive from the Greek *kardamon* ("cress") and *amomon* ("fragrant spice plant or an Indian spice").[5]

HISTORICAL USES: Cardamom has a history of medicinal and culinary use in India, China, and the Mediterranean. It has been used as a carminative and stimulant for weak digestion, gas, bloating, and nausea. The seeds continue to be used to flavor East Indian masala chai tea, as well as coffee in Egypt and Turkey.[6,7] Cardamom was also used to treat urinary tract infections.[2]

Egyptians chewed on cardamom to freshen their breath. Cleopatra burned the crushed seeds as incense prior to visiting Marc Antony.[8] Cardamom seeds were introduced to Europe by Alexander the Great's returning soldiers. Ancient Greeks and Romans valued the herb as a spice, medicine, and perfume.[8]

Cardamom was added as an adjuvant to carminative, stomachic, and laxative preparations.[2,9] The "Compound Cardamom Spirit" was administered by Eclectic physicians as a digestive stimulant and flavoring agent. The essential oil continues to be added as a fragrance to soaps, detergents, creams, lotions, and perfumes.[2]

CONSTITUENTS: Cardamom seed contains volatile oil (α-terpinyl acetate, 1,8-cineole, limonene, sabinene, linalool, linalyl acetate, α-terpinol, α-terpinene, α-terpineol, camphene, myrcene, 1,4-cineole, borneol, α-pinene, nerol, humulene, eucalyptone, and others). The seed also contains acids (acetic, butyric, decanoic, dodecanoic, citronellic, geranic, hexanoic, heptanoic, nerylic, and perillic), minerals (manganese and iron), carbohydrates, fixed oil, and proteins.[2,10-12]

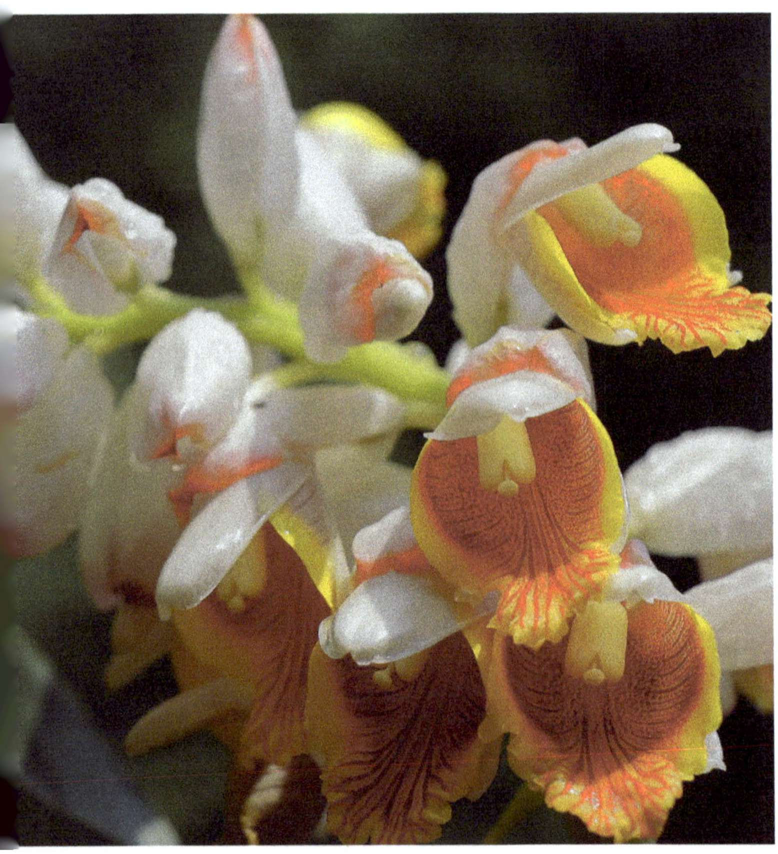

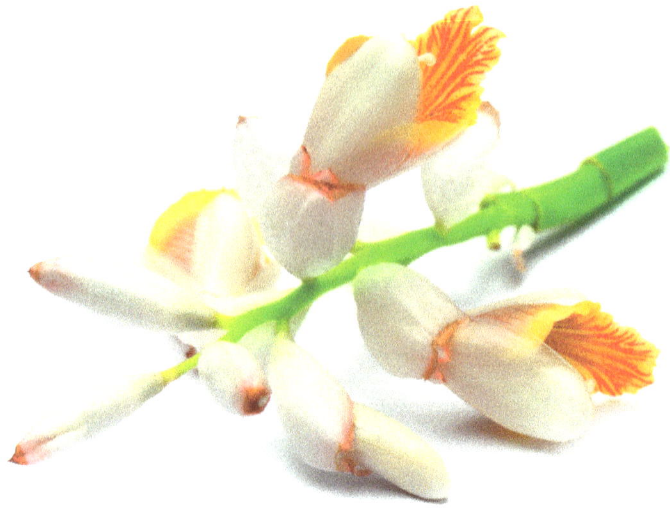

NUTRITIONAL PROPERTIES: Cardamom contains manganese, iron, carbohydrates, and proteins.[12]

MEDICINAL PROPERTIES: Antimicrobial, antinauseant, antispasmodic, aphrodisiac, aromatic, carminative, cholagogue, digestive, diaphoretic, expectorant, mucolytic, stomachic, and adjuvant (harmonizer).

TEMPERATURE AND FLAVOR: Warm, pungent, and sweet.

MEDICINAL USES

Cardamom is a delicious, aromatic carminative and stomachic that increases the appetite, enhances digestion, and stimulates circulation throughout the digestive tract. It eases nausea, vomiting, morning sickness, and belching.[11,13] Cardamom also reduces digestive cramping, and aids in treating nonulcer dyspepsia, gas, bloating, flatulence, indigestion, diarrhea, colic, and digestive headaches.[13] Cooking crushed or powdered cardamom seeds with legumes reduces gas and bloating. It also helps to counter mucus formation and bloating from poor assimilation of dairy products.[11] The antispasmodic properties are attributed to the volatile oil.[2] Cardamom counters the cooling effects of bitter tonics and prevents griping caused by anthraquinone-containing laxative herbs. It is a cholagogue that improves fat digestion, and acts as a mild laxative. Chewing cardamom seeds freshens the breath. A bitter digestive tonic can be prepared by combining extracts of artichoke leaf *(Cynara)* or gentian *(Gentiana)* with cardamom, turmeric *(Curcuma)*, orange peel *(Citrus sinensis)*, ginger *(Zingiber)*, fennel seed *(Feoniculum)*, and/or anise seed *(Pimpinella)*. Prepare a digestive chew by combining two parts of chopped, crystallized ginger with one part each of decorticated cardamom seed, orange peel

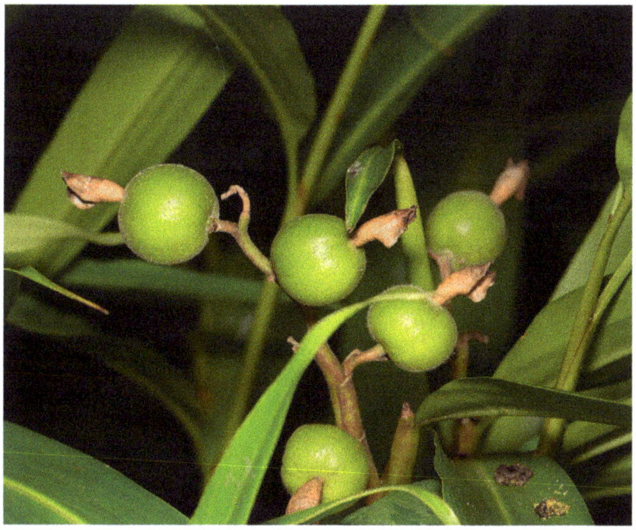

(*Citrus sinensis*), fennel seed (*Feoniculum*), and anise seed (*Pimpinella*).

Cardamom is combined with fresh ginger and dry cinnamon in the spicy, stimulating Indian tea, masala chai. Numerous variations of the tea also include peppercorns, clove, nutmeg, and black tea. After chai has been decocted and strained, milk and honey or sugar are added. Sometimes, a few drops of vanilla extract or nutmeg powder are added to the final blend. Cardamom is also included in five spice blend and curry powder.

The volatile oil in cardamom has antifungal and antibacterial effects. Cardamom also enhances expectoration, and aids in treating upper and lower respiratory tract infections, sore throats, coughs, and asthma with wheezing.[11] Decoctions extract mucilage that coats and soothes the mucous membranes in the respiratory and digestive tracts. Topical applications such as a liniment or diluted essential oil also have antimicrobial actions.

Cardamom is a potentiator (activator) and warming circulatory stimulant. It increases circulation from the core to the extremities, but is not typically overheating. Cardamom has a seductive aroma and is considered an aphrodisiac.[7] It is a flavoring agent (adjuvant) added to cordials, aperitifs, digestifs, and medicines.

CONTRAINDICATIONS

Avoid use in cases of biliary obstruction and severe liver disorders. It is contraindicated for ulcers, excessive heat signs, and aggravated *pitta*.[11] Internal consumption of the essential oil is contraindicated during pregnancy.

PREPARATION AND DOSAGE

TINCTURE: Dry seeds [1:5, 60% alcohol]; consume 10-60 drops, up to three times daily. The crushed, decorticated seeds are preferred in extracts.

GLYCERITE: Dry seeds [1:5, 40% alcohol, 30% water, 30% glycerin]; consume 10-30 drops, up to three times daily.

CAPSULES: Powder the seeds and consume 1-2 capsules, one to three times daily. Fill "0" or "00" capsules with a binding agent such as marshmallow root powder or slippery elm powder, then add 1-2 drops of essential oil into each capsule. Place the tops on the capsules, and store in a zip-lock bag or glass jar in the refrigerator or freezer. Consume 1-2 capsules, one to three times daily.

TEA: Crush the seeds and prepare a decoction, cold infusion, or hot infusion; consume up to 8-12 ounces, one to three times daily. The decoction is recommended, as it is the most potent preparation of the tea.

HONEY AND SYRUP: Decoct the crushed seeds, strain, and sweeten with honey or simple syrup. Add 1-2 drops of essential oil to 1 teaspoon to 1 tablespoon of honey or simple syrup.

TOPICAL USE: Apply the tea, diluted tincture, or essential oil (1-2%) as a wash.

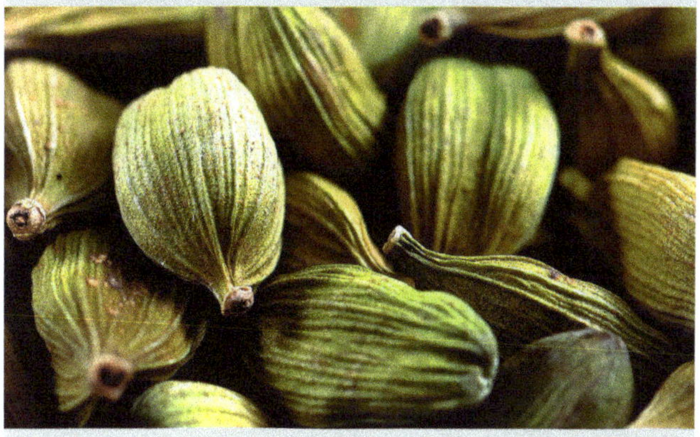

CULINARY USE: Add cardamom to teas, beverages, aperitifs, digestifs, cordials, elixirs, whipped cream, baked goods, desserts, and digestive chews. Add cardamom to five spice or curry blends, or cook with legumes to prevent flatulence.

CARОB

DESCRIPTION

BOTANICAL NAME:
Ceratonia siliqua

COMMON NAMES:
Carob, St. John's bread, locust bean
harrub, hurnub, kharruba, kharub (Arabic)
karoupi (Greek)
algarroba (Spanish)

FAMILY NAME:
Fabaceae (Leguminosae)

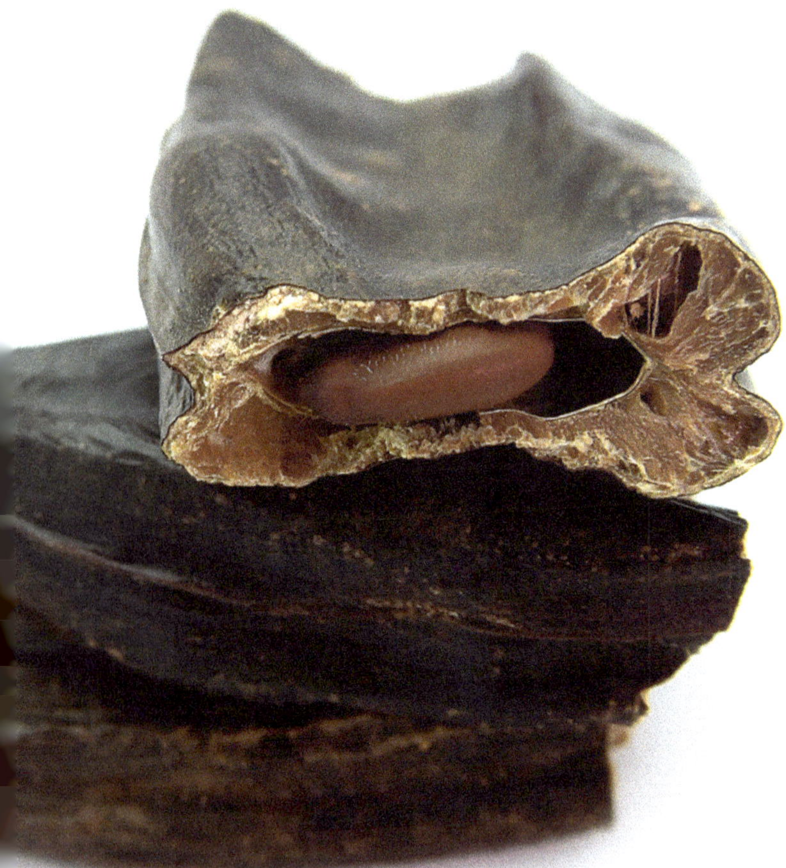

PART USED: The ripe, dried pod.

BOTANICAL DESCRIPTION AND HABITAT: Carob is native to southeastern Europe and western Asia. It is cultivated throughout the Mediterranean region, in Greece, Spain, and Italy.[1] A flowering evergreen, dioecious tree (up to 15 m high), carob has a broad, leafy crown. The glossy and vibrant, pinnately-compound leaves consist of two to five elliptic leaflets (3 – 5 cm long) with notched apices, smooth upper sides, and pubescent undersides.[2]

Racemose inflorescences (5 – 30 cm) are produced from leaf axils.[2] The unisexual flowers have small, disk-shaped calyces, no petals, and five stamens. Carob has a gray, fuzzy ovary with a large stigma.[2] The fruits are curved, flattened, leathery, indehiscent legumes (up to 30 cm long) producing many shiny brown seeds.[2,3] The pods can be used roasted or raw; the pulp and endosperm of the seeds (carob bun) are also utilized.[1]

THE NAME: The common name carob derives from the Arabic *kharrūba*.[4,5] The common name locust bean refers to the pod's supposed resemblance to a locust.[6] It was thought that perhaps the "locusts and wild honey" St. John the Baptist consumed during his biblical journey were carob pods; hence, the common name St. John's bread.[1,7]

The word carat (a gold and fine gem weight measurement) originates from the Greek *keration* ("carob bean"); carob beans were used as a standard for weight in ancient times.[8] *Keration* is a diminutive of *keras* ("animal horn"), referring to carob's curved, horn-like pods, and is the origin of the botanical name *Ceratonia*.[9]

The epithet *siliqua* ("pod, husk") refers to the ancient Roman unit of measure that was the equivalent of the *keration* in actual weight and original inspiration.[9,10] The term silique now refers to a type of fruit exclusive to the mustard family, botanically unrelated to carob.

HISTORICAL USES: Carob flour, syrup, and extracts have been used as nourishment for millenia.[1] The ancient Assyrians called it *eritilla* "Plant of the City of Life," and used it medicinally as early as 500 BCE.[11] It has been theorized that even before the Greeks and Romans, the Assyrians used the carob bean as a unit of weight called the *kisal.*[11] Meanwhile, the *Book of Enoch* (an ancient Jewish religious work circa 300 BCE) identifies the carob as the "Tree of Wisdom."[11] Romans utilized the species at least since Pompeii's volcanic eruption in 79 CE.[12] In *De Materia Medica,* Dioscorides extolled the use of carob as a laxative and diuretic.[7] The *Bible* refers to the prodigal son yearning to eat carob "husks."[13] After the German army invaded Greece during World War II, carob was eaten for subsistence in rural areas.[7]

Carob pods are used in food products to flavor butterscotch, imitation chocolate, and vanilla.[1] Carob continues to be used in desserts, candy, baked goods, gelatins, puddings, imitation dairy products, sweet sauces, and alcoholic and nonalcoholic beverages.[1] A regional alcohol from Sicily was fermented from carob.[7]

The seeds have been employed as rosary beads in Europe.[7] A gum extracted from carob seeds has been used in cosmetics, film, adhesives, inks, paints, and polishes.[12] Carob has been grown as forage for livestock since ancient times.[7]

CONSTITUENTS

CAROB PODS: Carob pods contain sugars (sucrose, fructose, xylose, maltose, dextrose, and glucose), proteins, amino acids (alanine, proline, and valine), gallic acids, fats, starch, absicic acid (a growth inhibitor), cellulose, and starch.[1,14] Carob seeds contain protein, carubin, fats (oleic, linoleic, and palmitic acids), tannins, gum (a galactomannan), and others.[1]

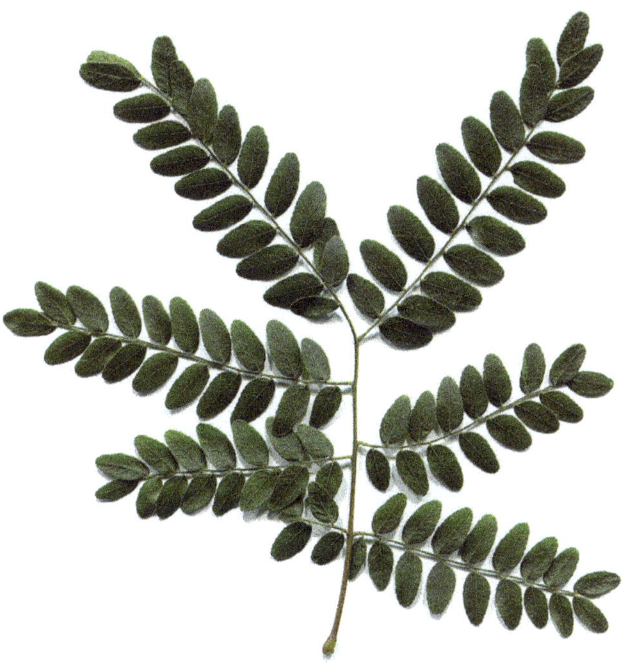

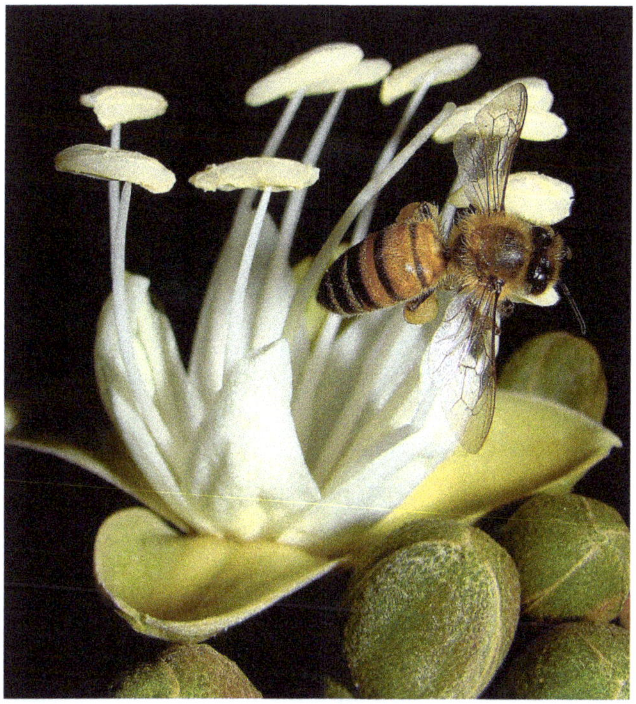

CAROB GUM: Carob bean gum is derived mainly from the endosperm; it is high in mucilaginous polysaccharides (carubin).[1,14]

NUTRITIONAL PROPERTIES: Carob pods contain sugars (sucrose, fructose, xylose, maltose, dextrose, and glucose), proteins, amino acids (alanine, proline, and valine), fats, starch, cellulose, and starch.[1]

MEDICINAL PROPERTIES: Adjuvant, antidiarrheal, astringent (mild), demulcent, and laxative (mild).

TEMPERATURE AND FLAVOR: Carob pods are mildly warming, sweet, and astringent. Carob gum is cooling and sweet.

MEDICINAL USES

CAROB PODS: A carob pod decoction is a soothing demulcent, reducing inflammation in mucous membranes, especially in the digestive tract. It aids in treating gastritis, digestive ulcers, gastroesophageal reflux disease (GERD), gastroenteritis, gluten intolerance, and diarrhea, as well as lower gastrointestinal diseases such as irritable bowel syndrome, Crohn's, and colitis. It is a mild laxative, alleviating constipation. Prepare a demulcent tea by combining four parts of marshmallow root *(Althaea);* two parts of carob pods, fennel seed *(Foeniculum),* and anise seed *(Pimpinella);* and one-quarter part of licorice root *(Glycyrrhiza).*

Carob pods are a delicious adjuvant and harmonizer in decoctions, enhancing the flavor of less pleasant tasting herbal tea blends. Other herbs that taste delicious in tea combined with carob pods are anise seed (*Pimpinella*), fennel seed *(Foeniculum)*, cardamom *(Elettaria)*, marshmallow *(Althaea)*, roasted dandelion root *(Taraxacum)*, cacao nibs *(Theobroma)*, vanilla *(Vanilla)*, and a pinch of licorice root *(Glycyrrhiza)*.

CAROB GUM: Carob gum reduces the levels of blood glucose, insulin, and serum cholesterol.[1] It also increases glucose tolerance. The hypoglycemic and hypoinsulinemic effects can be a useful adjunct for treating diabetes mellitus.[1]

Carob gum contains mucopolysaccharides that are demulcent and used as a thickening agent. It is beneficial for treating diarrhea (especially in infants and children) and vomiting (during pregnancy).

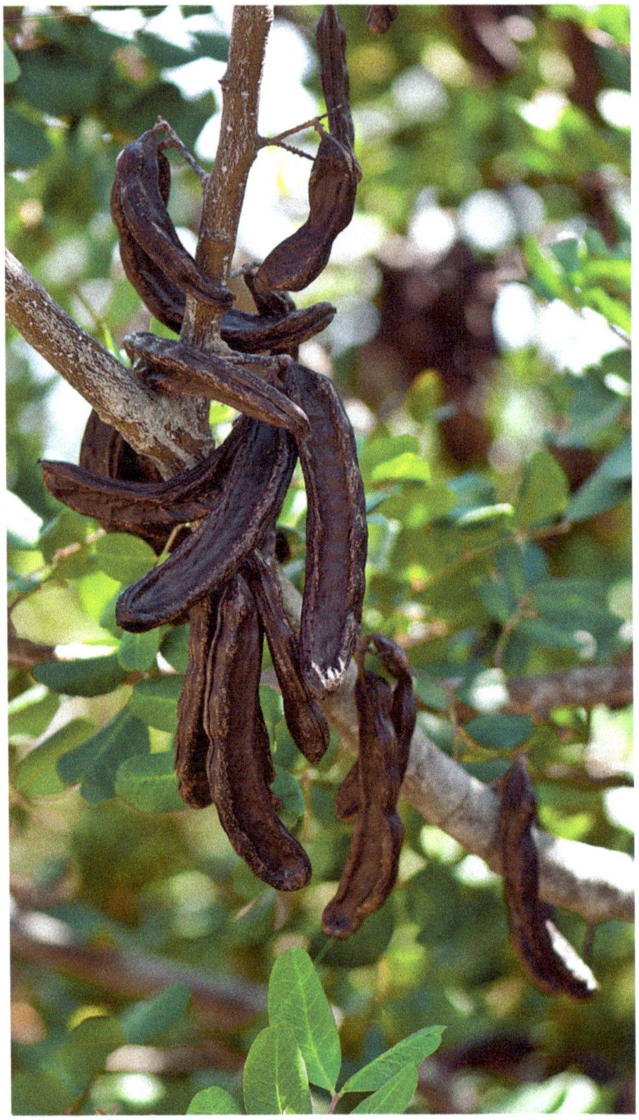

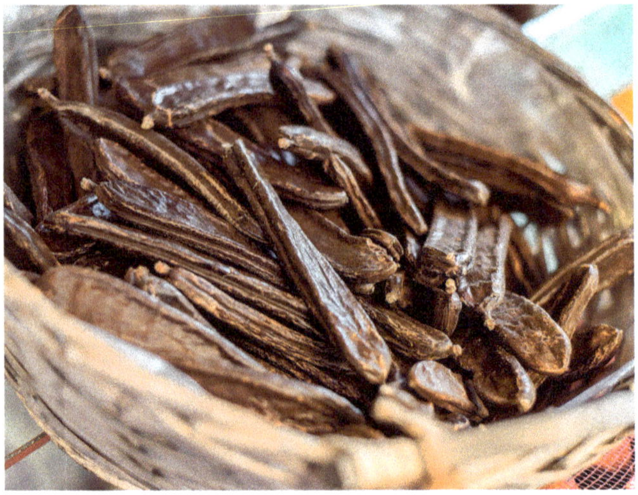

CONTRAINDICATIONS

Consume carob with sufficient amounts of water. Avoid consuming when bowel obstruction is present.[14]

PREPARATION AND DOSAGE

TEA: Prepare carob pods as a decoction; consume 8–12 ounces, two to four times daily.

HONEY AND SYRUP: Combine carob pods with distilled water; decoct to one-half the original volume, then add honey or simple syrup to desired sweetness. Refrigerate up to six months.

CULINARY USE: Add carob flour to desserts, baked goods, imitation chocolate, candy, gelatins, and puddings. Carob pods are a delicious addition to cordials, elixirs, and liqueurs.

CAYENNE

DESCRIPTION

BOTANICAL NAMES:
Capsicum annuum, C. frutescens, C. chinense, C. baccatum var. *pendulum, C. pubescens*

COMMON NAMES:
Cayenne pepper, hot pepper, bird pepper, African bird pepper, African pepper, red pepper, tobacco pepper, chili, chili pepper, habanero pepper, jalapeno pepper
fulful alahmar, fulful haar, shatta, fulaifilah har (Arabic)
aji (Arawak)
gdzoo bghbegh, kcu pghpegh (Armenian)
laaht jiu (Cantonese)
feferon, kajenska paprika (Croatian)
pálivá paprika, pepř cayenský (Czech)
kibe paprika, punapipar, tšili, cayenne'i pipar (Estonian)
chilipippuri (Finnish)
piment-oiseau, piment enragé, poivre rouge (French)
roter pfeffer, chili-pfeffer (German)
piperi kagien, tsili, kafteres pipieres (Greek)
paprika harifa, pilpel adom, pilpel harif, tsili (Hebrew)
lal mirch, mirch (Hindi)
csilipaprika, cayenne bors, igen erős apró (Hungarian)
chilipipar, cayennepipar (Icelandic)
cabé, lombok (Indonesian)
peperone, diavoletto, peperoncino, pepe di caienne, pepe rosso piccante (Italian)
kaienpeppa, tōgarashi (Japanese)
kaien gochu, kochu, gochu (Korean)
kajeno pipirai (Lithuanian)
la jiao (Mandarin)
rato khursani, khorsani (Nepali)
piripíri, pimento de caiena (Portuguese)
ardei iute (Romanian)
kajenskij perets, krasnij perets, chili (Russian)
katurvira, marichiphala ujjvala (Sanskrit)
feferon, karejena-biber (Serbian)
pimento, chile, pimienta picante, ají (Spanish)
pilipili hoho (Swahili)
prik chifa, prik khee nu, pisi hui, prik daeng (Thai)
sipen marpo (Tibetan)
toz biber (Turkish)
ot (Vietnamese)
ferferl, terkish ferferl, shorf ferferl (Yiddish)[1]

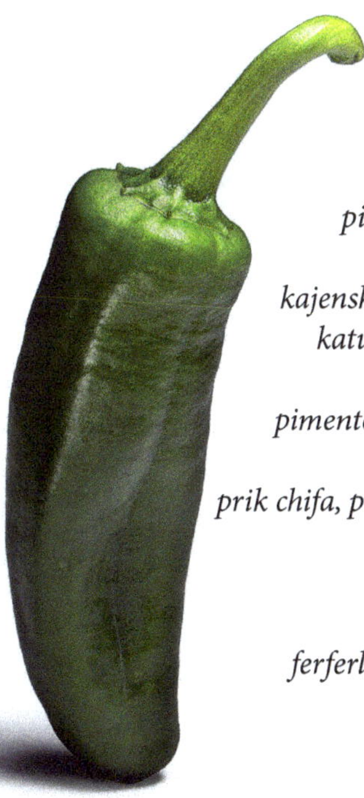

FAMILY NAME:
Solanaceae

PART USED: The fruits.

BOTANICAL DESCRIPTION AND HABITAT: All species and varietals of *Capsicum* peppers are believed to derive from *Capsicum annuum* and *C. frutescens.*[2] *Capsicum annum* originated in southern Brazil and Bolivia, and spread throughout South and Central America. *C chinense* originated in the tropical regions of the Amazon. *C. pubescens* and *C. baccatum*, also known as ají in the Andes, are native to Ecuador, Peru, Bolivia, and Chile. Several

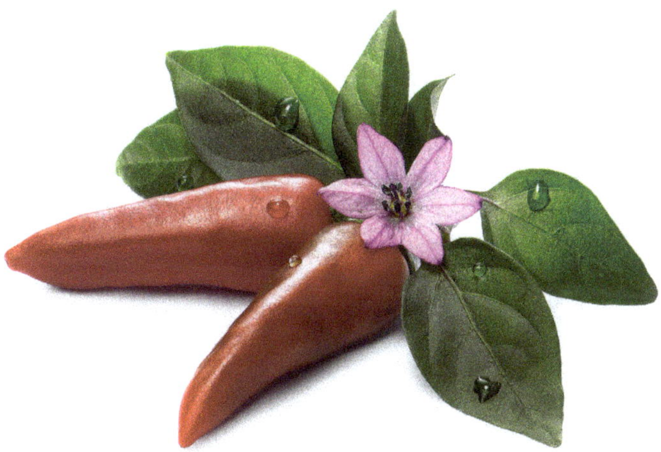

Capsicum varietals have naturalized in southern Texas and Arizona.[3] Cayenne pepper, paprika, chili, pimento, and chili pepper are members of the *Capsicum annuum* species.[3] Tabasco pepper originated from *C. frutescens.*[3]

Capsicum genus consists of 25 species and more than 1,000 varieties.[4] While some species are perennial in tropical climates, they are frost sensitive and grown as annuals in temperate climates.[4] The pubescent plants have solitary or paired leaves that are ovate with a narrowing base and an entire or wavy margin.[4] The flowers are borne singly, or in small, stemless, axillary clusters.[4] The five-lobed calyx varies from bell- to cup-shaped, while the five-lobed corolla is bell-shaped to rotate in tones of white, blue, or violet.[4] Attached to the corolla are five stamens with prominent, ovoid anthers that split open lengthwise to disperse their pollen.[4] The ovary has two carpels, and develops into a berry or capsule that is red, orange, or purple when ripe, and can assume many different shapes and sizes. The fruit contains many small, yellow, discoid seeds. The fruit and seeds are rich in capsaicin.

An annual in any climate, *Capsicum annuum* (20 – 80 cm tall) is distinguished by its white, solitary flowers and fruit that are longer than the pedicels.[5,6] *Capsicum frutescens* is a perennial (in tropical climates) with flowers that grow in small clusters, narrower leaves than *C. annuum*, and fruit that does not exceed the length of the pedicels.[5,7]

THE NAME: The genus name *Capsicum* has two possible origins; the first and most likely is from the Greek *kapsa* ("case, box, or capsule"), referring to the fruit shape.[1] Another possible origin derives from the Greek *kaptein* ("to seize, grasp, or bite"), referring to the fruit's pungency.[1,8] The epithet *annuum* ("a year") derives from Latin, and refers to the plant's life cycle in harsher climates; in milder climates, the plant can survive several seasons.[1] The epithet *frutescens* derives from the Latin *frutex* ("shrub or bush").[1] The epithet *pubescens* ("hairy") describes the surface of the leaves, and *baccatum* ("berry shaped") refers to the fruits that are sometimes globular.[1] The epithet *chinense* ("of or from China") is a misnomer; the plant originated in South American tropics.[1] *Aji* derives from *axi,* the Awarak name for the plant. Chili, chile, and chilli originate from the Náhuatl *chilli* ("red").[1] The common name cayenne (initially spelled *cayan*) was borrowed from the Tupi indigenous people from the Brazilian coast who originally called the spice *kyinha* (also spelled *quiínia*).[1]

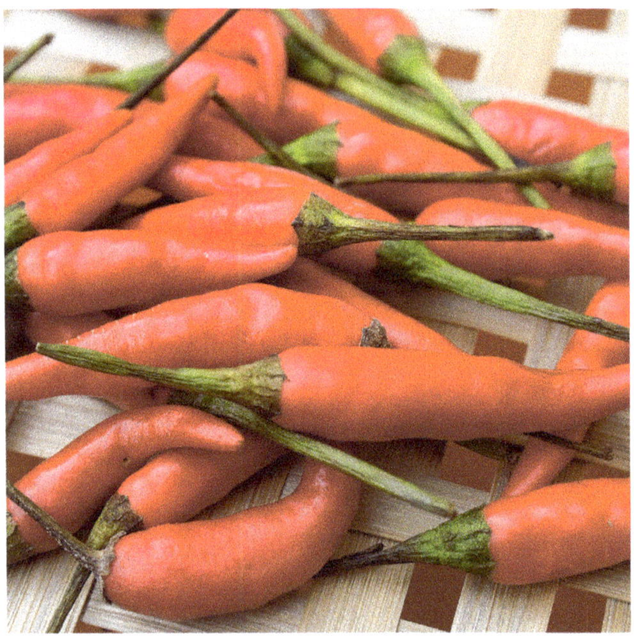

HISTORICAL USES: Chili peppers originated in the Andes and spread throughout the Americas where they were cultivated and diversified into the myriad chilies available today. The Arawak introduced peppers to Europeans when they encountered Columbus as he attempted to discover a new trade route to Indonesia.[3] They served him stews containing pungent cayenne peppers that he later called red peppers and introduced to the Old World.[3] Centuries prior to Columbus' arrival, five species were domesticated.[3] Culinary use eventually spread throughout Europe, Asia, Africa, and America. Today, cayenne is the most widely consumed spice.

In Central America, the Aztecs cultivated and utilized at least seven varieties of *C. frutescens: quauchilli, milchilli, zenalchilli, tlalchilli, tefochilli, chiltecpin,* and *chilocoztli.*[9] It was administered as a purgative and consumed to treat lung afflictions, heart pain, and bad blood, in addition to reducing kidney and brain inflammation.[9] It was included in culinary preparations as a nutritive.[9] Cayenne was applied to tumors, scabies, and toothaches.[10] The Maya administered *C. annuum* to treat infections and sore throats, and referred to the herb as *ic* or *yax-ic.*[9] The Maya also used *C. frutescens* to treat dysentery, and called the herb *max* and *max-ic.*[9]

In the West Indies, a preparation called "mandram" continues to be used to improve appetite and strengthen digestion.[8] Mandram contains thinly sliced, unpeeled cucumbers, shallots, onions or chives, lemon or lime juice, Madeira, and several pods of bird pepper macerated in the liquid.[8]

In the late 1700s and early 1800s, Samuel Thomson popularized the use of cayenne in North America.[3] Today, his simplistic philosophies remain popular among folk herbalists. Following his routinely recommended lobelia purge, Thomson administered cayenne as a stimulant to "retain the internal vital heat of the system and cause free perspiration."[3] The old "Thomsonian number 6" can be prepared by combining 60 ml of myrrh *(Commiphora)* and 15 ml of cayenne *(Capsicum)* diluted in 120 ml of alcohol administered in five-drop doses.[11] Thomson's antispasmodic "Compound Tincture of Lobelia and Capsicum" included equal parts of skunk cabbage, lobelia, and cayenne.[11]

Eclectic physicians administered 1 – 10 drops of *C. frutescens* to warm the stomach, stimulate gastric mucosa, and improve digestive motility.[12] It was used to treat flatulence, diarrhea, dysentery, cholera, constipation, and chronic, non-inflamed hemorrhoids. Small amounts of cayenne, vinegar, and salt were mixed in cold water and administered in low doses as an antiemetic.[12] Large doses were administered as an emetic and purgative.[11,12] Low doses of cayenne were used to treat nervous debility, suppressed digestive secretions, low body temperature, depressed vitality, painful muscles, and stiff joints, especially in the elderly.[11,12] It was prescribed as a stimulant to the heart and circulation, and treated stagnant blood or feeble circulation.[11,12] Cayenne was considered a premier remedy for subacute forms of delirium tremens (alcoholic delirium). It was administered in low doses in hot water, and if well tolerated, in larger doses in strong beef broth to prevent nausea and vomiting, and restore digestion.[11,12] Cayenne was also given for opium, morphine, and cocaine withdrawal.[11] The tincture alone or mixed with glycerin or

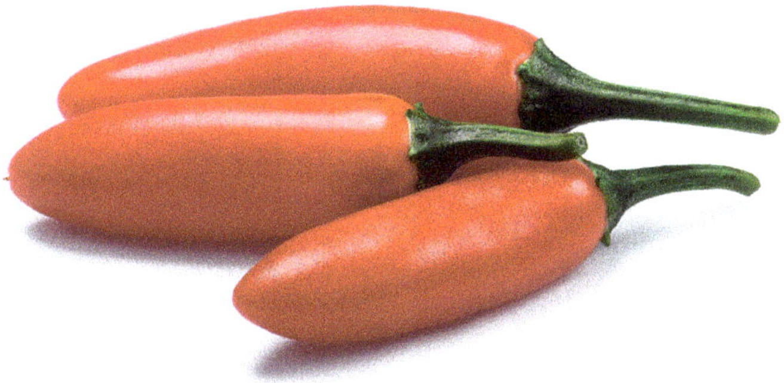

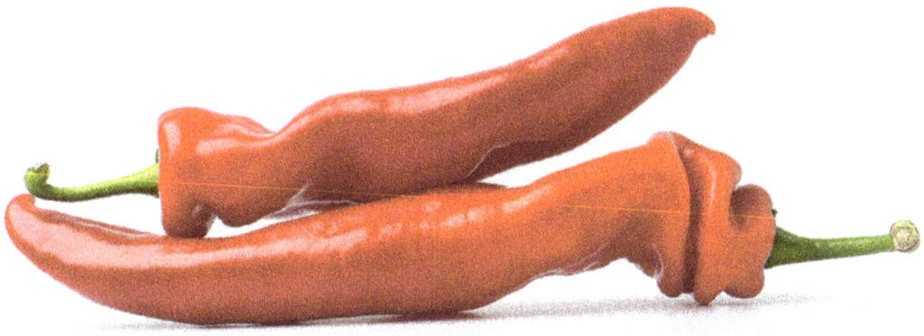

mucilage, was applied topically as a stimulant, rubefacient, and counterirritant to relieve pain.[11,12] It was also applied to the scalp to stimulate hair growth in alopecia.[12]

CONSTITUENTS: Cayenne contains pungent principles, including amides (capsaicin, dihydrocapsaicin, nordihydrocapsaicin, homocapsaicin, and homodihydrocapsaicin), carotenoids (capsanthin, capsorubin, carotenene, and lutein), fats, protein, vitamins A and C, flavonoids (flavones), volatile oil (4-methyl-1-pentyl-2-methyl butyrate, 3-methyl-1-pentyl-3-emthyl butyrate, and isohexyl isocaproate), fixed oil, a liquid alkaloid, a saponin (capsidicin), and a red pigment (capsanthin).[2,13,14] Mild peppers including paprika and bell pepper are similar in composition to other members of *Capsicum*, but with minimal or no pungent principles.[2] Paprika (*Capsicum annuum*) is rich in vitamin C; it also contains carotenoids (capsanthin), flavonoids (flavones), pungent principles (in very low concentrations), and volatile oil.[13]

NUTRITIONAL PROPERTIES: Cayenne pepper is high in vitamins A (β-carotene) and C, cobalt, crude fiber, fat, niacin, and zinc. The vitamin C content doubles when the fruit turns red. It also contains low to average amounts of ash, calcium, dietary fiber, iron, magnesium, phosphorus, potassium, protein, selenium, sodium, thiamine, and tin.[15]

MEDICINAL PROPERTIES: Activator, antioxidant, carminative, carrier, circulatory stimulant, counterirritant, diaphoretic, potentiator, rubefacient, sudorific, stimulant, topical analgesic, and vasodilator.

TEMPERATURE AND FLAVOR: Hot, pungent, and sweet.

MEDICINAL USES

Cayenne has numerous actions that aid in treating cardiovascular disease, including hypertension and atherosclerosis. It dilates the arteries and capillaries, decreasing vascular resistance, and lowering elevated blood pressure. Cayenne also lowers systemic arterial blood pressure by activating cholinergic (parasympathetic) mechanisms, and decreasing sensitivity to the pressor effects of angiotensin II and norepinephrine. Capsaicin, a primary component of cayenne, decreases platelet aggregation and reduces blood viscosity.[10,14,16] It lowers plasma fibrinogen and increases fibrinolytic activity, reducing the potential for thromboem-

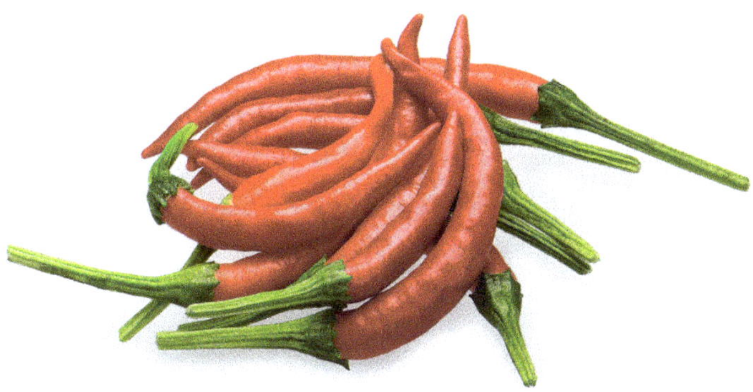

bolism.[16] Capsaicin also lowers thromboxane B2 formation and erythrocyte hemolysis, suggesting a membrane stabilizing action that hinders the activation of phospholipase A2.[14] It works differently from aspirin in thinning the blood.[14] Animal studies demonstrate that capsaicin lowers plasma cholesterol and triglyceride levels, in addition to the low density lipids (LDL) to high density lipids (HDL) ratio.[10,14] Cayenne and capsaicin decrease hepatic cholesterol formation, while increasing biliary excretion of cholesterol.[14] Lastly, cayenne and other peppers contain high amounts of vitamin C, carotenoids, and flavonoids that strengthen the vasculature and have potent antioxidant actions protecting against cardiovascular disease.[10]

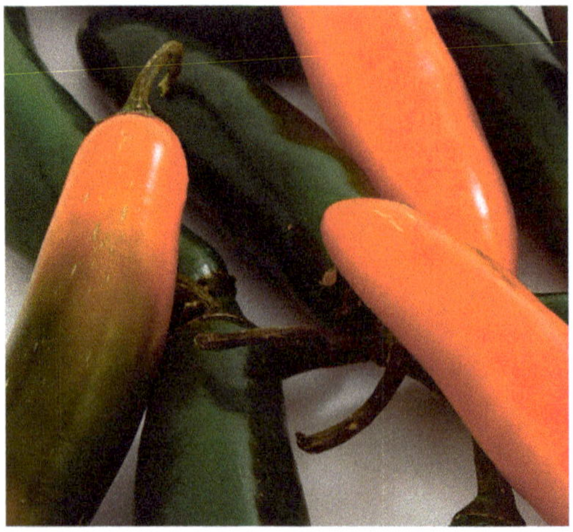

Cayenne is a potent circulatory stimulant, vasodilator, and carrier. It increases blood supply to the periphery, improving circulation in the arterioles, meta-arterioles, and capillaries.[17] Cayenne increases blood flow in the microvasculature, improving tissue oxygenation and hastening waste product removal from tissues. Enhancing blood flow counters the peripheral vasoconstrictive effects of the neurotransmitter and hormone adrenalin, that is released in a flight-or-fight sympathetic nervous system response.[17] The long-term effect of metarteriole and capillary constriction decreases cardiovascular, immune, and renal vitality. Cayenne treats blood vessel constriction by increasing the blood supply to the mucosa and skin in individuals prone to stress.[17]

Cayenne's vasodilating and circulatory stimulant properties aid in treating chronic circulatory deficiency, cold hands and feet, and Raynaud's phenomenon. This herb is especially helpful during cold autumn and winter months for individuals with poor circulation. Adding a very small percentage of the herb (1 – 5%) to a compound formula acts as a carrier agent or catalyst, enhancing the delivery of herbs in a formula and potentiating their actions. Cayenne is also a stimulant and energizing agent that facilitates the release of endorphins.[18]

Cayenne is a heating diaphoretic and vasodilator, alleviating a fever.[10-12] A sudorific, cayenne also reduces body temperature by stimulating the cooling center in the hypothalamus.[16] Consume preparations such as tea, soup, kimchee, or fire cider (cyclone cider) to treat a sore throat, laryngitis, tonsillitis, sinus congestion, or the first stages of a cold or flu.[10-12] Cayenne also encourages expectoration and has mild bronchodilating actions that aid in treating moist respiratory conditions and asthma.[10] Fresh cayenne juice has antibacterial actions *in vitro*.[10]

Cayenne has mild to moderate stomachic, carminative, laxative, and digestive stimulant actions.[11,12,14] It increases salivary and hydrochloric acid secretions, improving the sterilizing capacity of the stomach against potential enteric infections.[11,12] Cayenne stimulates digestion and aids in treating atonic dyspepsia, flatulence, bloating, and poor digestion.[10-12] Adding small quantities of cayenne to kimchee or sauerkraut is a wonderful way to support digestive and immune function.

Topical applications of cayenne and capsaicin-containing products have analgesic, counterirritant, and rubefacient properties that improve circulation in the tissues.[3,10] The analgesic properties are attributed to capsaicin.[2,10] Initially, applications of capsaicin increase the release of substance P — a protein-based neurotransmitter released by nerve endings during the inflammatory response that relays pain messages from the peripheral nerves to the spinal cord, and finally to the brain. However, repeated applications of capsaicin deplete substance P, desensitizing the nerve endings and decreasing the brain's perception of pain.[3] It takes approximately three days of applying the cream two to four times daily to deplete substance P. Capsaicin cream can be applied to alleviate the pain of arthritis, rheumatism, carpel tunnel syndrome, myalgia, lumbago, cluster headaches, surgical trauma, neuralgia, shingles, post-herpetic neuralgia, diabetic neuropathy, and chilblains.[10,14,16]

Pepper pungency is determined by the capsaicin content. Pharmacist Wilbur Scoville established a scale that organoleptically measures the heat of cayenne and other peppers. Based on tests, he determined that one part of pepper heat per one million drops of water was the equivalent of 1.5 Scoville heat unit (SHU). According to the Scoville scale, the heat of peppers ranged from 0 SHU to 16 million SHU. Some examples of peppers and their pungency are: green bell peppers (0 SHU); pimento peppers (100 – 500 SHU); jalapeno peppers (2,500 – 8,000 SHU); serrano peppers (10,000 – 23,000 SHU); cayenne, aji, and tabasco peppers (30,000 – 50,000 SHU); Jamaican hot pepper (100,000 – 200,000); Mexican habanero (350,000 SHU); and pure capsaicin (15 – 16 million SHU).[18]

According to herbalist Michael Moore, the characteristic of a good medicinal cayenne is that its heating response is delayed by seconds and is longer lasting, rather than having an immediate effect; this results from the fixed oils.[17] Medicinal cayenne peppers have more viscous fixed oils; culinary varieties of cayenne have a thinner viscosity.[17] An organoleptic taste test can help to determine the viscosity of the fixed oils; an immediate heating response (occurring in 1 – 2 seconds) that clears rapidly indicates that the peppers are less medicinal. However, when the heat lingers in the mouth for a while, the herb can last in the bloodstream 1 – 4 hours. The viscosity of the fixed oils accounts for the long-lasting effects in the bloodstream.

CONTRAINDICATIONS

Due to its blood thinning properties, avoid internal use of cayenne two weeks prior to, and following surgery or a due date. Consult a health care practitioner or avoid regular consumption of cayenne when taking over-the-counter or prescription blood thinners.

Consult a health care practitioner before consuming cayenne if you have severe hypertension or highly inflammatory reactive conditions. Avoid or limit use when acute inflammatory and heat-aggravated conditions are present. Regular consumption of cayenne can be overheating to warm-bodied individuals and those with patterns of yin deficiency with heat signs (hot flashes and night sweats). Discontinue use if cayenne aggravates heartburn, acid indigestion, gastric or duodenal ulcers, or inflammatory conditions of the upper or lower digestive tract. Excessive or frequent doses can cause mucous membrane irritation, nausea, vomiting, diarrhea, and gastrointestinal and kidney lesions or irritation.[3,14]

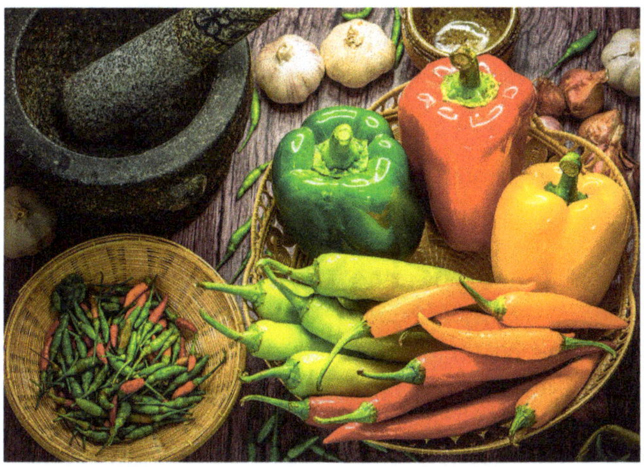

Avoid applying cayenne or capsaicin cream to broken or inflamed skin, the eyes, or mucous membranes.[3,13,14] Exercise caution when applying cayenne preparations topically, as it can cause irritation, blistering, or dermatitis.[3] Short-term use is recommended for topical applications containing a high content of capsaicin.[13]

Warning: Wear gloves when handling hot peppers, and take care not to rub it into the eyes. If delicate membranes or the skin are exposed and irritated by cayenne, apply a fatty-based milk product such as coconut oil, olive oil, yogurt, cream, or whole milk to quell the burning sensation. Consume dairy products to reduce the pungent sensation following ingestion. Capsaicin is not water soluble; washing with water is ineffective in eliminating the burning sensation.

PREPARATION AND DOSAGE

TINCTURE: Fresh fruit [1:2-1:3, 95% alcohol]; dry fruit [1:5, 80% alcohol]; consume 3-15 drops, up to three times daily.

ACETUM EXTRACT: Cayenne is partially extracted in vinegar. Extract the fresh fruit [1:2-1:3, apple cider vinegar]; dry fruit [1:5, apple cider vinegar]; consume 1 teaspoon to 1 tablespoon, up to three times daily.

CAPSULES: Consume 1-2 "0" or "00" capsules, one to three times daily.

TEA: While cayenne has limited water solubility, ¼-1 teaspoon can be infused in one cup of water or milk, consumed one to three times daily. Fat-based mediums such as milk, coconut milk, or chicken broth improve extraction of the fixed oils.

HONEY AND SYRUP: Infuse fresh chopped pepper into honey [1:4] using the double boiler method; consume ½-1 teaspoon, up to three times daily.

TOPICAL USE: Pharmaceutical applications such as capsaicin cream, ointment, gel, lotion, liniment, or plaster can be applied topically as a counterirritant and analgesic, up to four times daily. Powdered fruit can be prepared using the alcohol intermediary method; however, the strength is unpredictable. Topical preparations can cause blistering or ulcers if left in contact with the skin. Use caution with topical applications, and avoid contact with the eyes and mucous membranes.

CULINARY USE: Cayenne is an excellent addition to Latin American, Southern European, African, East Asian, and Indian food. Small to moderate amounts of this spice enrich the flavor of chili, chili con carne, salsa, red sauces, tomato dishes, eggs, egg salad, eggplant, relishes, curry, and kimchee.

CHAMOMILE

DESCRIPTION

BOTANICAL NAMES:
Matricaria recutita (syn. *Matricaria chamomilla, Chamomilla recutita*), *Anthemis nobilis* (syn. *Chamaemelum nobile, Chamomilla nobilis*)

COMMON NAMES:
German chamomile, wild chamomile, pineapple weed, Roman chamomile, English chamomile, true chamomile, common chamomile, camomile, chamomilla, plant's physician
kamille (Danish)
kamomillasaunio (Finnish)
camomile, espargoutte, matricaire, kamille, magdblume, mutterkraut (German)
babuna (Hindi)
camomilla (Italian)
kamille (Norwegian)
babunaj (Persian)
camomila (Portuguese)
romanashka (Russian)
babuna (Sanskrit)
maythen (Saxon)
manzanilla (Spanish)
kamomill (Swedish)
papatye cic (Turkish)
dư̛ờng cam cuc (Vietnamese)

FAMILY NAME:
Asteraceae (Compositae)

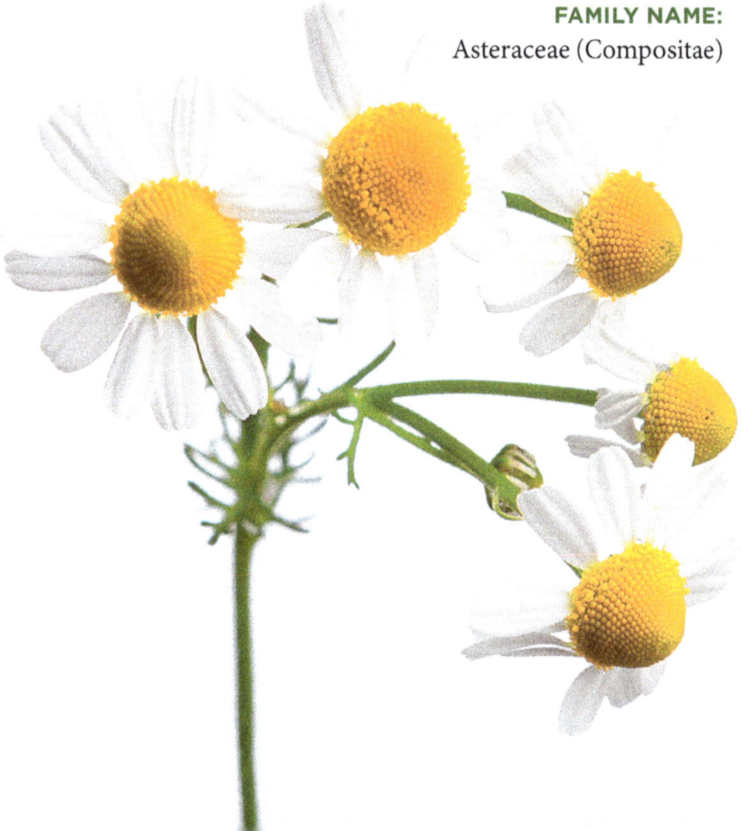

PARTS USED: The entire plant is medicinal; the flowers are the most potent and commonly used parts.

BOTANICAL DESCRIPTION AND HABITAT: Roman chamomile *(Anthemis nobilis)* is native to southern Europe. German chamomile *(Matricaria recutita)* is native to eastern Europe, North Africa, and western Asia, and has naturalized in North America and Australia.[1,2] Essential oil of German chamomile is cultivated in Hungary, Germany, Czech Republic, Slovakia, Argentina, and Egypt. Roman chamomile essential oil is produced in England, France, and Hungary.[3]

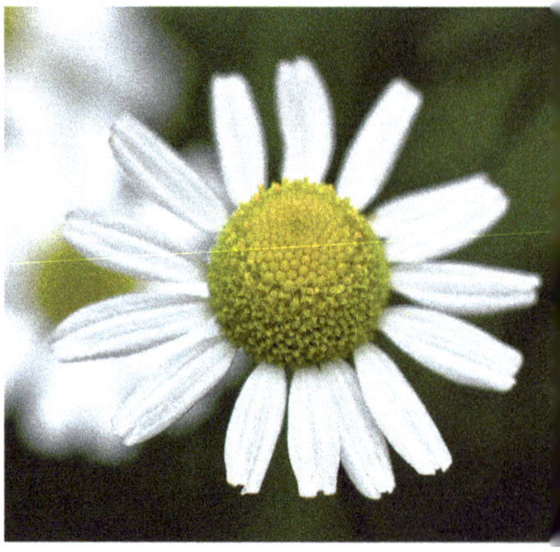

Roman chamomile *(Anthemis nobilis)* is a low-growing perennial. It has branching, prostrate stems (30 cm tall), and tufts of finely divided, twice pinnate, thread-shaped leaflets with a sweet, floral aroma. The erect stalk bears a solitary, daisy-like inflorescence with up to 18 white, strap-shaped, three-toothed ray florets arranged around a conical center (the receptacle). The tiny yellow tubular florets bear five stamens. It has an obovate, inferior ovary, and a slender style with a two-cleft, reflexed stigma. A tiny chaffy scale (bract) grows between each floret. *A. nobilis* is distinguished from other *Anthemis* species by its short, blunt scales.

German chamomile *(Matricaria recutita)* is an annual herb (up to 60 cm tall) with finely divided, feathery leaves that have a mild aroma comparable to Roman chamomile. The small, daisy-like heads display 10 – 20 white, strap-shaped, pistillate ray florets with three-toothed, four-veined corollas. The numerous yellow, tubular disk florets have narrow corolla lobes, a single, hairy, inferior ovary with a two-cleft stigma, nectaries, and four to five stamens. German chamomile differs from Roman chamomile, as it lacks the chaffy scales between florets, and its conical receptacle (or disk) is hollow.

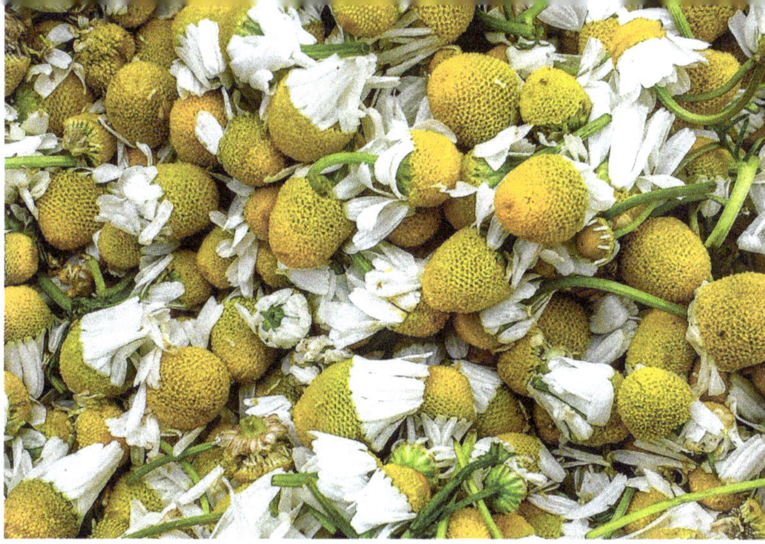

THE NAME: There are two possible related derivations of *Matricaria.* The first derives from the Latin *matrix* ("womb, parent tree, or groundwork"); the second derives from the related *mater* ("mother"). The name chamomile derives from two Greek words: *chamai* ("on the ground") and *melon* ("apple"). The combination of these words translates as "earth apples." Spaniards called the plant manzanilla ("little apple").

Matricaria recutita (syn. *Matricaria chamomilla, Chamomilla recutita*) is the Latin binomial for German or Hungarian chamomile (wild chamomile); *Anthemis nobilis* (syn. *Chamaemelum nobile, Chamomilla nobilis*) is the Latin binomial for Roman chamomile (also known as English chamomile). Additional common names include true or common chamomile, manzanilla, and maythen.

HISTORICAL USES: Chamomile has long been esteemed as a cultivated medicinal herb. Ancient Egyptians believed that chamomile cured ague, so they dedicated it to their gods.[4] Ancient Romans administered chamomile to relieve headaches, in addition to treating bladder, liver, and kidneys conditions.[1] Medieval herbalists believed chamomile dissolved kidney stones and gallstones; they also administered the herb as a diuretic, analgesic, and carminative.[1] Medieval monks grew "healing garden beds" of Roman chamomile where invalids rested in order to alleviate depression.[5] During the Middle Ages, Roman chamomile was often planted along garden paths and strewn as a fragrant, sweet herb to mask unpleasant aromas.[4] It was also considered one of the sacred herbs of Woden, the god of war.[1]

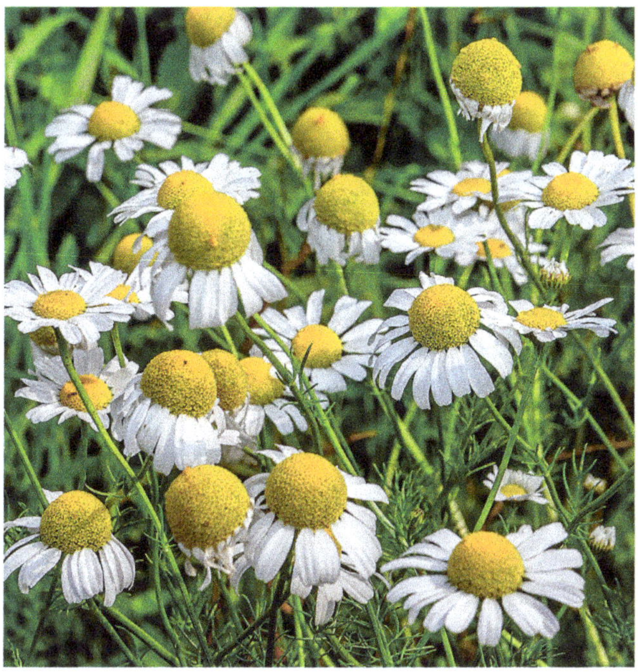

Throughout the European countryside, chamomile was a charm believed to counter the effects of "flying venom" and "loathful things."[1] Nicholas Culpeper recommended chamomile for a variety of concerns, ranging from jaundice to dropsy, and as a topical fomentation for ague, sprains, and strains.[4] Chamomile was combined with purgatives to prevent griping, and was administered in the early stages of delirium tremens.[4] The foliage of Roman chamomile was added to herbal beers. Topical applications of chamomile were applied to treat local or intestinal inflammation, and for a toothache, earache, or neuralgia.[4] Known as the "plant's physician," chamomile was grown near sickly plants.[4] According to Slovakian chamomile specialist Ivan Salamon, "chamomile is the most-favored and most-used medicinal plant in Slovakia. Our folk saying states that an individual should always bow when facing a chamomile plant. The respect results from hundreds of years' experience curing in the folk medicine of the country."[6]

While Eclectic physicians typically used different types of chamomile interchangeably, German chamomile was considered a more specific remedy than Roman chamomile for children. Diluted extracts were given to counteract restlessness and irritability.[7] Chamomile was also administered for *la grippe* and colicky pains.[7] Eclectics prescribed cold infusions of chamomile as a stomachic for gastric debility with flatulence; hot infusions were recommended as diaphoretics to alleviate colds. The hot infusions were administered to treat dysmenorrhea.[8] In *Eclectic Materia Medica, Pharmacology, and Therapeutics,* Harvey Felter suggested the following uses of German chamomile:

> ...it is adapted to the restless, peevish, irritable, discontented and impatient infant, who is only appeased when carried about in order to quiet its nervousness and unrest. In such children it may be equally a remedy for constipation or diarrhea. In the former case, there is usually hepatic tenderness. In the latter, the discharges may be variously

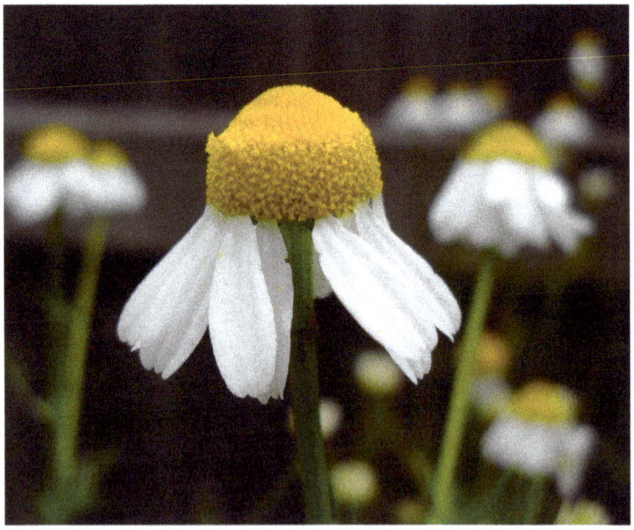

characterized — watery and greenish, slimy, green and slimy, or yellow and white lumps of undigested curds, giving them the known name of 'eggs and greens.' Such stools are passed with difficulty, and there is more or less bloating of the abdomen. Flatulence is marked and the surface is alternately pale and flushed.[8]

Felter valued German chamomile as a nerve sedative during the later months of pregnancy to allay false labor pains, and treat nervous muscular twitching, coughing, and nervousness.[8] He also recommended the herb to treat amenorrhea and dysmenorrhea.[8]

In China, chamomile was administered as a digestive aid, depurative, and poultice for the breasts.[9] Ayurvedic practitioner Dr. Vasant Lad recommends chamomile to alleviate digestive related headaches, blood congestion, jaundice, and biliousness, and as an eye wash.[10] He also suggests that chamomile is beneficial for all constitutions, especially *pitta.* In South Africa, it was used to treat colic, convulsions, croup, hyperacidity, diarrhea, diptheria, gout, hysteria, insomnia, lumbago, rheumatism, sciatica, and sore throat.[9] The Cherokee and Mahuna consumed chamomile tea for colic, bowel complaints, and vomiting.[9]

CONSTITUENTS

GERMAN CHAMOMILE contains volatile oil (chamazulene, farnesene, α-bisabolol oxide A, α-bisabolol oxide B, α-bisabolone oxide A, matricin, and en-yn-dicycloether).[11] It also contains flavonoids (apigenin, apigetrin = apigenin-7-D-glucoside, apigenin-7-acetylglucoside, apiin = apigenin-7-apiosylglucoside, rutin = quercetrin-3-rutinoside, luteolin, quercimeritrin = quercetrin-7-D-gludoside, and some alkylated flavonoids); coumarins (umbelliferone = 7-hydroxycoumarin and its methyl ether-herniarin); proazulenes (matricin and matricarin); phenolic carboxolic acids (vanillic, anisic, syringic, and caffeic acids); fatty acids; mucilaginous polysaccharides (fructane and D-galacturonic acid); choline; amino acids; and others.[11,12]

ROMAN CHAMOMILE contains volatile oil consisting primarily of isoamyl esters of angelic and tiglic acids (butyl, amyl, isoamyl, and hexyl angelates or tiglates). Additional components in the volatile oil include α-pinene, farnesol, nerolidol, chamazulene, α-bisabolol (lesser quantities than German chamomile), *l-trans*-pinocarveol, *l-trans*-pinocarvone, and 1,8-cineole.[3,11] Roman chamomile contains bitter sesquiterpene lactones (germacranolides including nobilin, 3-epinobilin, 1,10-epoxynobilin, and 3-dehydronobilin); flavonoids (apigenin, apigetrin, apiin, quercitrin, and lueteolin-7-glucoside); phenolic carboxolic acids (carboxolic, ferulic, and trans-caffeic); coumarins (scopoletin-7-β-glucoside); choline; fatty acids; and mucilaginous polysaccharides.[11,12]

NUTRITIONAL PROPERTIES: German chamomile contains high amounts of magnesium, niacin, phosphorus, riboflavin, and sodium. It contains low to average amounts of aluminum, ash, calcium, chromium, crude fiber, dietary fiber, iron, manganese, potassium, protein, selenium, silicon, thiamine, tin, and vitamins A and C.[12]

MEDICINAL PROPERTIES: Anti-inflammatory, antispasmodic, anxiolytic, aromatic, astringent, bitter tonic, carminative, demulcent, cooling diaphoretic, nervine, sedative, soporific, sudorific, and vulnerary.

TEMPERATURE AND FLAVOR: Cool, bitter, pungent, sweet, and astringent.

MEDICINAL USES

Chamomile is a nervine, soporific, mild sedative, and anxiolytic that calms the central nervous system, reducing nervousness and anxiety.[1] The anthemic acid, esters, and flavonoids contribute to the nervine and sedative actions.[9,16] Many individuals with chronic insomnia benefit from consuming chamomile tea throughout the day as a calmative agent, or in the early evening to aid relaxation. Prepare a gentle nervine compound by combining extracts of chamomile, wild oats *(Avena),* skullcap *(Scutellaria),* St. John's wort *(Hypericum),* and smaller amounts of lemon balm *(Melissa)* and lavender *(Lavandula).* Combine extracts of chamomile, hops *(Humulus),* passion flower

(Passiflora), and valerian *(Valeriana)* for more potent sedative effects.

Placing a small pillow stuffed with lavender, hops, and chamomile at the head of the bed acts as a soporific agent; the scent is enhanced when blended with roses *(Rosa)*. These "dream pillows" are placed in the beds of children and infants. While chamomile is considered an herb that reduces nightmares, some individuals may notice that their dream state is intensified, while they sleep more deeply.

Chamomile has potent anti-inflammatory actions that reduce pain and inflammation associated with arthritis, tendonitis, carpel tunnel, achy or painful muscles and joints, and hemorrhoids. The anti-inflammatory actions also aid in alleviating muscle tension in the neck, shoulders, and back, as well as treating tension and digestive related headaches. The anti-inflammatory actions are attributed to α-bisabolol, matricin, chamazulene, flavonoids (primarily apigenin), and cyclic ethers (en-yn-dicloether).[16] The flavones interfere with the arachidonic acid pathway, thwarting inflammation by inhibiting phospholipase A, cyclo-oxygenase, and lipoxygenase pathways.[16] Present in the essential oil, chamazulene and α-bisabolol reduce inflammation by blocking the 5-lipoxygenase and cyclo-oxygenase pathway.[16] The essential oil also contains azulenes that have antiallergenic and antianaphylactic actions.[13] Studies reveal that azulene prevents allergic seizures in guinea pigs, likely due to an antihistaminic effect.[13] To quell a fever, prepare hot tea containing chamomile, mint *(Mentha)*, and elder flower *(Sambucus)*, as well as smaller amounts of meadowsweet *(Filipendula)* and yarrow *(Achillea)*. Consume 4 – 8 ounces every one to two hours, until the fever subsides. *Note:* Additional anti-infective herbal extracts that inhibit microbial growth are necessary to address the infection.

An extremely effective herb for the digestive system, chamomile has carminative, stomachic, bitter tonic, demulcent, and astringent properties. Chamomile tea (especially German chamomile) reduces inflammation in digestive tract mucous membranes. It works best when consumed on an empty stomach. Chamomile tea aids in treating colic, heartburn, indigestion, peptic ulcers, nonulcer dyspepsia, loss of appetite, flatulence, and diarrhea.[1,16] It also alleviates inflammation caused by chemotherapy and radiation treatments.[1,16] In animal studies, chamomile was found to prevent and heal peptic ulcers induced by stress, indomethacin, and ethanol; this effect is attributed to α-bisabolol.[13,16] Chamomile is highly beneficial as a long-term tonic for stress-related digestive disorders such as Crohn's disease, ulcerative colitis, and irritable bowel syndrome.[1] It is an antispasmodic that eases digestive and menstrual cramping.[1,11] Numerous constituents antagonize acetylcholine and spinal motor functions, resulting in the antispasmodic actions.[9] The flavonoids apigenin and apigenin-7-O-glucoside, as well as α-bisabolol, chamillin, and chamazulene are attributed to the antispasmodic effects.[9,11] The carminative, relaxant, and antipeptic actions are due to cyclic ethers (en-yn-dicloether), apigenin, chamillin, and chamazulene.[9,11] Combine chamomile with marshmallow *(Althaea)*, peppermint *(Mentha piperita)*, meadowsweet *(Filipendula)*, catnip *(Nepeta)*, and licorice *(Glycyrrhiza)* as a hot or cold infusion to ease gastrointestinal inflammation.

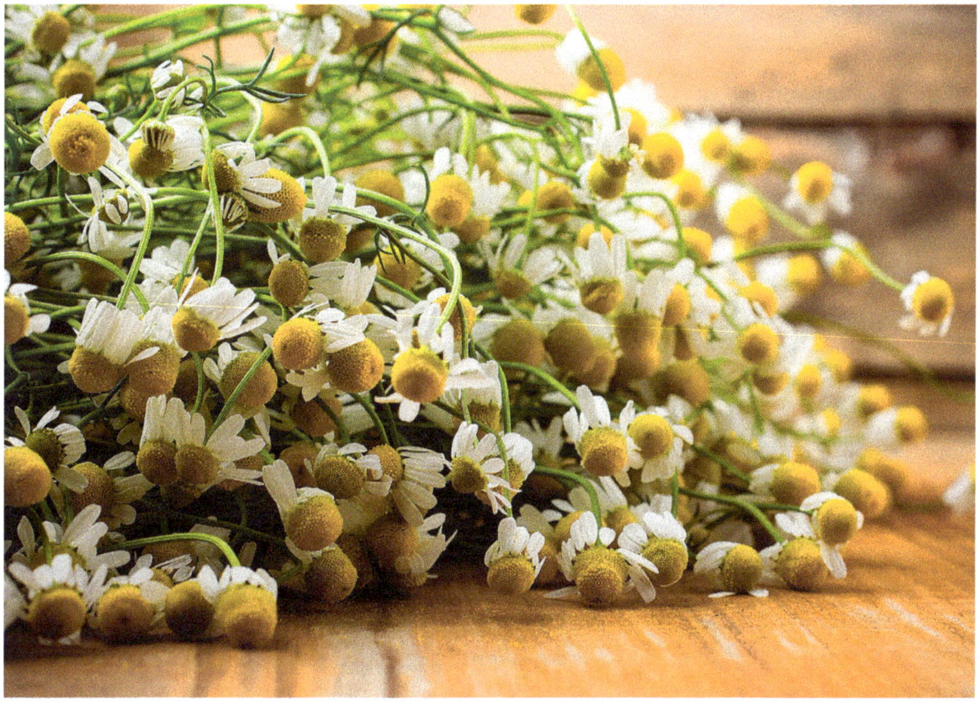

Chamomile is especially helpful for easing the pain of infant teething, colic, and earaches. Consuming chamomile tea or bathing in it acts as a cooling diaphoretic and sudorific, and is excellent for treating children's fevers. It also helps to alleviate children's stomachaches.[1]

Topical applications of chamomile — such as a poultice, salve, or diluted essential oil — have potent anti-inflammatory and antispasmodic actions for treating sore, tense muscles, neuralgia, rheumatic joints, sprains, strains, bruises, earaches, sore gums, and toothaches.[1,5,14,15] A vulnerary, chamomile stimulates tissue regeneration, and hastens healing of cuts, abrasions, cracked nipples, eczema, poison oak, poison ivy, dermatitis, and dermabrasion.[1,11,16] Gargling with chamomile tea reduces mouth and gum inflammation.[1,16] A sitz bath or vaginal irrigation aids in treating hemmorhoids and anogenital inflammation.[16] Chamomile tea also can be applied as a hair rinse for blondes.

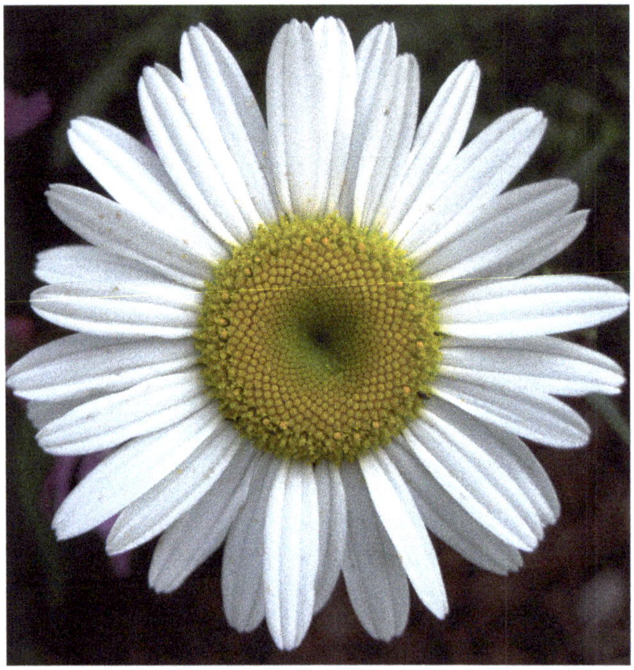

Chamomile eye wash reduces inflammation in the eyes, eyelids, and follicles. It aids in treating conjunctivitis, blepharitis, sties, and eye irritation due to allergies. However, in individuals with Asteraceae family allergies, it can cause allergic conjunctivitis.[16] Be sure to prepare a fresh batch of tea every day in distilled or spring water. Filter the tea through a fine cloth or paper filter to remove all particulate matter. Additional anti-infective agents such as goldthread *(Coptis)* or goldenseal *(Hydrastis)* are necessary when treating bacterial or viral eye infections.

The actions of German chamomile resemble Roman chamomile, with some differences. Consuming German chamomile tea has more soothing demulcent effects in the mucous membranes of the digestive tract. German chamomile is a more potent anti-inflammatory and moderate antispasmodic.[5,14,15] These actions are attributed to the chamazulene, bisabolol and its oxides (en-yn-dicycloether); however, the flavonoids and coumarins are also active principles.[13] Roman chamomile has a distinctive sweet aroma, and surprisingly, a more potent bitter tonic action that stimulates digestive secretions. The nervine and smooth muscle antispasmodic actions of Roman chamomile are slightly more potent than those of German chamomile.

CHAMOMILE ESSENTIAL OILS

GERMAN CHAMOMILE

Essential oil of German chamomile, also known as blue chamomile (especially the (-)α-bisabolol chemotype of German chamomile) has potent anti-inflammatory actions.[5,14,15] Additionally, α-bisabolol has antimicrobial and antipeptic actions.[11] The deep blue color of German chamomile oil is due to the chamazulene content.[5] Chamazulene has analgesic, vulnerary, antispasmodic, anti-inflammatory, and antimicrobial properties.[11] However, α-bisabolol, followed by matricin, has more potent anti-inflammatory effects than chamazulene.[11] German chamomile essential oil contains cyclic ethers that have anti-inflammatory, antianaphylactic, antispasmodic, and antimicrobial properties.[11] It has antibacterial effects against *Staphylococcus aureus, Mycobacterium tuberculosis,* and *Salmonella typhimurium,* and it inhibits bacteriotoxins.[11] The antimicrobial actions are attributed to the chamazulene, α-bisabolol, and cyclic ethers (en- yn-dicloether).[9,11] The flavonoid apigenin inhibits the growth of *Heliobacter pylori in vitro.*[1] German chamomile essential oil has antifungicidal actions against *Candida albicans.*[1,9,11] Umbelliferone also inhibits fungal growth.[9,11]

German chamomile has mild anxiolytic and antidepressant actions.[5] Topically, the anti-inflammatory effects alleviate pain in muscles and joints, as well as arthritis, tendonitis, bruises, sprains, strains, shingles, herpes, and neuralgia.[5] It is highly effective for treating thermal burns, sunburns, allergic rashes, dermatitis, eczema, poison oak, poison ivy, boils, and enlarged capillaries.[5,14] The oil is gentle and nontoxic; therefore, it can be applied directly (neat) or diluted in a base oil or salve.[14] However, it can cause contact dermatitis in some individuals.[11] *Note:* German chamomile should not be confused with Moroccan blue chamomile *(Tanacetum annuum),* a less potent herb that is often falsely marketed as German chamomile.

ROMAN CHAMOMILE

Roman chamomile essential oil mainly contains esters that calm the central nervous system and reduce smooth muscle spasms.[14] Inhaling Roman chamomile is highly effective in reducing nervousness and anxiety, relieving shock, and treating insomnia.[14] Placing one to two drops on the

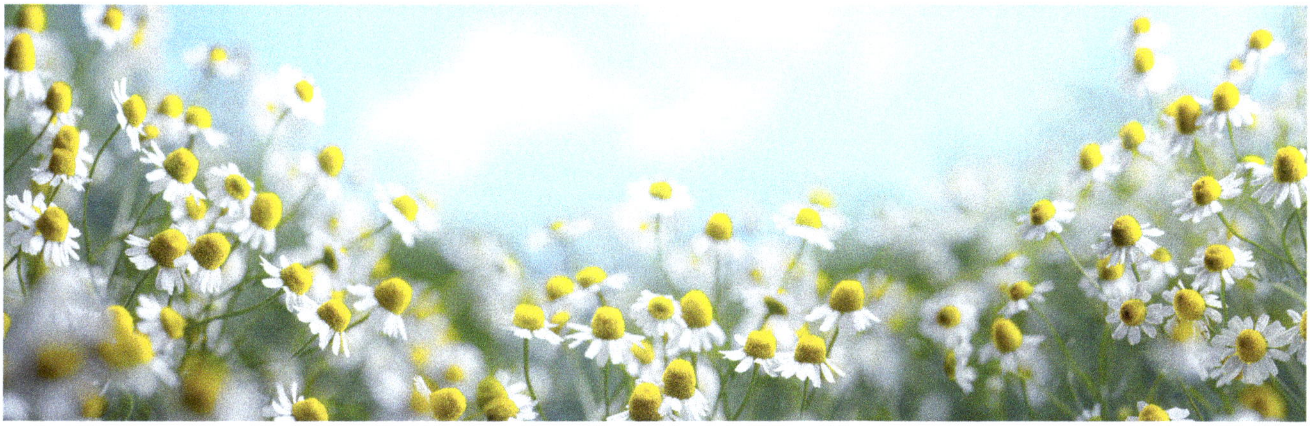

sternum or inhaling the volatile oil reduces asthmatic spasms, especially during emotionally induced asthma attacks.[15] Massaging a few drops of diluted essential oil directly onto the abdomen relieves infant colic, as well as gastrointestinal and menstrual cramping.[14] Roman chamomile contains three sesquiterpene lactones (nonbilin, 1,10-epoxynobilin, and 3-dehydronobilin) that have demonstrated antitumor actions *in vitro* against tumor cells.[11] Roman chamomile essential oil also can be applied directly (neat), or diluted in a base oil or salve. [11]

CONTRAINDICATIONS

Roman and German chamomile can cause contact dermatitis in individuals with Asteraceae family allergies.[11] Large doses of Roman chamomile can act as an emetic.[11]

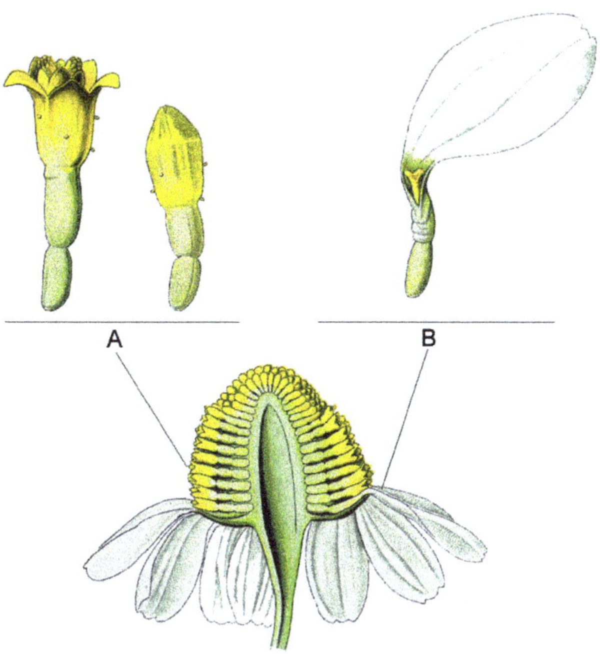

PREPARATION AND DOSAGE

TINCTURE: Fresh flowers or herb [1:3-1:4+, 60-95% alcohol]; dry flowers [1:5-1:6+, 50-60% alcohol]; consume 10-90 drops, up to four times daily.

GLYCERITE: Fresh flowers [1:3+, 60% glycerin, 40% water] or [1:3-1:4+, 50% glycerin and 50% alcohol]; recently dried flowers [1:5-1:10, 40% glycerin, 40% water, 20% alcohol]; consume 10-60 drops, up to four times daily.

CAPSULES: Fill "0" or "00" capsules with a binding agent such as marshmallow root powder or slippery elm powder, then add 1-2 drops of essential oil into each capsule. Place the tops on the capsules, and store in a zip-lock bag or glass jar in the refrigerator or freezer. Consume 1-2 capsules, up to three times daily.

TEA: Prepare a hot or cold infusion; consume 8-12 ounces, up to four times daily. Avoid boiling the herb, as the volatile oil will be destroyed. Keep the lid on the vessel to prevent aromatic oils from evaporating.

HONEY AND SYRUP: Infuse the fresh flowers in honey using the Simpler's method. Cook over low heat in order to liquefy and strain honey. Consume 1 teaspoon to 1 tablespoon in hot water or tea, up to three times daily. Alternatively, mix 1-2 drops of Roman chamomile essential oil to 1 teaspoon honey, and stir into hot water or tea, up to three times daily.

TOPICAL USE: Apply a fomentation, poultice, wash, eye wash, oil, salve, or liniment of chamomile topically. Apply 1-2 drops of Roman or German chamomile essential oil neat, or dilute in a base oil or salve.

CHICKWEED

DESCRIPTION

BOTANICAL NAME:
Stellaria media

COMMON NAMES:
Chickweed, common chickweed, starweed, star chickweed, scarwort, satin flower, stitchwort, chickenwort, adder's mouth, craches, maruns, winterweed, passerina
fuglegrees (Danish)
muur (Dutch)
stellaire, mouron des oiseaux, langue d'oisaux, morgeline, mouron blanc (French)
augentrosgräs, gansekraut, huhnerdarm, mausedarm, sternmiere, vogelmiere (German)
buddelina, centocchio, erba gallina, paperina, stellaria (Italian)
hakobe, hakobera (Japanese)
alsina (Portuguese)
hierba pajarera, pamplina, pamplina de canaries (Spanish)
våtarv (Swedish)
cam out (Turkish)[1]

FAMILY NAME:
Caryophyllaceae

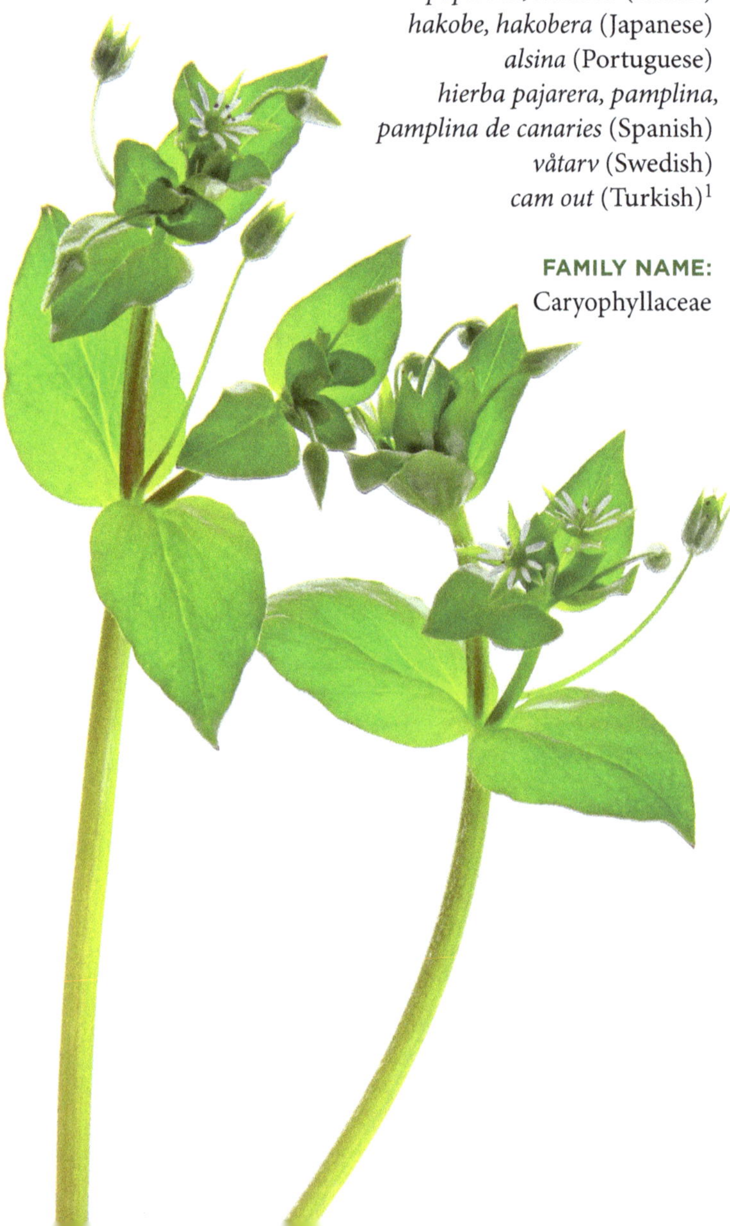

PARTS USED: The leaves and aerial portions.

BOTANICAL DESCRIPTION AND HABITAT: Chickweed is a mat-forming, tender-fleshed, succulent annual herb native to Europe that has naturalized in North America. It grows 7 to 50 cm tall, and is commonly found in gardens and farms where it thrives in cool, moist soils, with growth

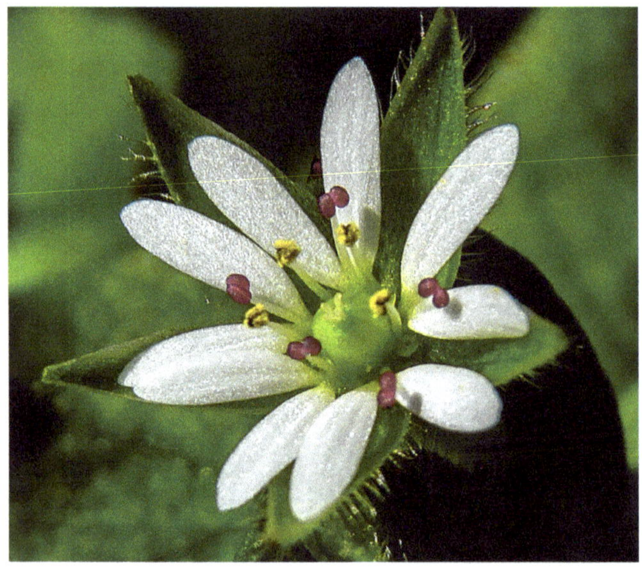

usually peaking in late winter or early spring. A line of fine hairs grows along the pale green, angular stem, distinguishing chickweed from its relatives. The diminutive, pale green leaves (8 – 45 mm long) are ovate and shiny, sometimes sparsely coated with fine hairs.[2] The inflorescences have a few tiny, pretty flowers (2 – 5 mm diameter). Each inflorescence has five lanceolate sepals (3 – 6 mm long) and five white, deeply bilobed petals that are slightly shorter than the sepals.[2,3] Each flower usually has three to eight stamens and three curved styles.[3] Small ovoid capsules produce reddish, kidney-shaped to round seeds.[3] *Note:* Chickweed can be confused with *Cerastium,* a member of the Caryophyllaceae family. *Cerastium* is distinguished by stems completely covered with fine hairs; chickweed has a single line of hair along one side of the stem. *Cerastium* is relatively harmless to consume.

THE NAME: The genus name *Stellaria* derives from the Latin *stella* ("star"), referring to the shape of the flower.[4] The epithet *media* derives from the Latin *medius* ("the

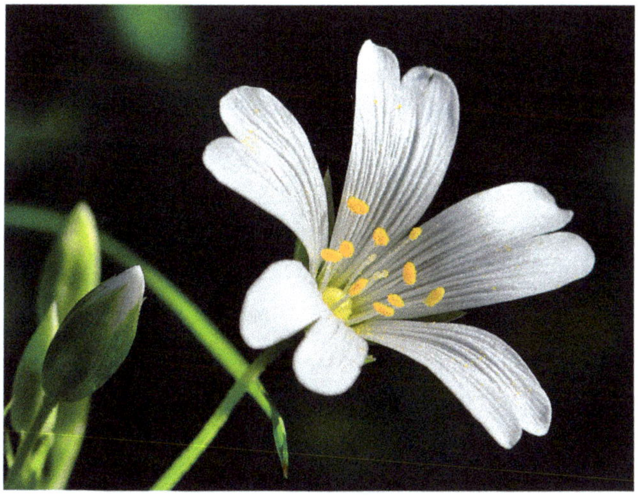

middle").[4] Chickweed and chickenwort refer to wild and domestic birds' fondness of the seeds and aerial portions.

HISTORICAL USES: Chickweed was a common pot herb, eaten as a fresh or steamed green. The juice was consumed as an antiscorbutic and depurative ("blood purifier") for rheumatism.[1] The tea was ingested to alleviate coughs, hoarseness, and constipation.[1] Chickweed was combined with elecampane *(Inula)* for hydrophobia.[1] The fresh herb was infused in lard and applied topically to sores, skin conditions, and hemorrhoids.[1] Nicholas Culpeper applied the bruised herb or juice over the liver area to alleviate heat.[1] The juice and tea were applied to the eyes. Cows, horses, sheep, pigs, chickens, and rabbits feed on chickweed.[1]

CONSTITUENTS: Chickweed contains carboxylic acids, coumarins, hydroxycoumarins, glycosides, flavonoids (rutin), saponins, steroids, triterpene glycosides, vitamins, and minerals.[5,6]

NUTRITIONAL PROPERTIES: Chickweed contains high amounts of aluminum, ash, calcium, cobalt, fat, iron, magnesium, manganese, phosphorus, potassium, protein, silicon, sodium, vitamin A, and zinc. It contains low to average amounts of chromium, crude fiber, dietary fiber, niacin, riboflavin, selenium, thiamine, and vitamin C.[7]

MEDICINAL PROPERTIES: Anti-inflammatory, anti-dyscratic, aperient, demulcent, diuretic, expectorant, laxative, nutritive, refrigerant, emollient, vulnerary, and antirheumatic.

TEMPERATURE AND FLAVOR: Cool, sweet, salty, and bland.

MEDICINAL USES

Chickweed is a highly effective demulcent and emollient.[1,5] It contains mucilage that reduces inflammation in the mucous membranes and skin.[8] The tea, juice, and succus are soothing for upper and lower respiratory tract infections, hoarseness, sore throats, laryngitis, pharyngitis, tracheitis, or colds.[1,6] However, additional anti-infective agents are needed to treat a microbial infection. A mouthwash or gargle reduces mouth or throat inflammation. The mucilage enhances expectoration, and has subtle antitussive properties beneficial for treating dry coughs due to whooping cough or bronchitis.[1,6] Infusing chickweed with calendula *(Calendula)*, anise *(Pimpinella)*, coltsfoot *(Tussilago)*, mullein *(Verbascum)*, and a pinch of licorice root *(Glycyrrhiza glabra)* soothes the respiratory system.

Chickweed aids in treating inflammation and ulceration in the skin, mouth, esophagus, stomach, intestine, and colon.[8] The tea and juice reduce pain and unpleasant sensations resulting from a hiatal hernia, gastritis, gastric reflux, acid indigestion, and peptic or duodenal ulcers. Chickweed reduces chronic inflammation resulting from gastrointestinal conditions, such as irritable bowel syndrome, Crohn's disease, diarrhea, dysentery, and ulcerative colitis. It is best to consume the tea or juice on an empty stomach when treating the aforementioned conditions. Regardless of whether the mucilage has direct or indirect soothing effects on the urinary and respiratory tracts, it is believed to suppress nerve reflexes in the alimentary canal walls, reducing pain in mucous membranes. A well-strained infusion of chickweed tea can be administered as an enema to reduce acute inflammation in the rectum or colon. It combines well with catnip *(Nepeta)* and chamomile *(Matricaria)*. An enema is also beneficial for encouraging elimination when treating severe constipation or impacted bowels.

Chickweed tea soothes kidney and bladder irritation, and has mild diuretic actions. It reduces burning sensations and irritation accompanying cystitis and urethritis. When treating infections in the urinary tract or bladder, additional antibacterial agents are necessary, such as usnea *(Usnea)* and uva ursi *(Arctostaphylos)*. Chickweed tea subtly reduces renal and bladder irritation due to passing kidney stones or kidney inflammation.

Chickweed is a refrigerant and cooling yin tonic. It increases yin fluids and reduces dryness throughout the body. Chickweed can be used as a long-term treatment for yin deficiency or yin deficiency with heat signs (hot flashes and night sweats). It is a restorative tonic that can be consumed following a debilitating illness, childbirth, severe fever, or dehydration, as well as during or after radiation or chemotherapy treatments.

Chickweed tea has gentle laxative properties.[1] It lubricates the stools and contains fiber, a bulking agent. It is a preferred long-term tonic for treating constipation because it does not cause dependency like many cathartic or purgative laxatives.

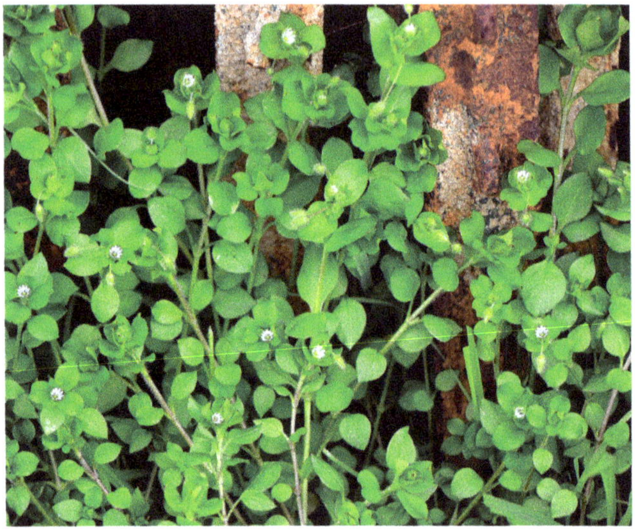

Chickweed is a nutritive tonic with high levels of easily assimilated vitamins and trace minerals. The vitamin A and C content supports immune function. The minerals have an alkalinizing effect on tissues. Chickweed is a gentle long-term tonic that alleviates conditions resulting from hyperacidity in the tissues, such as gout, arthritis, and skin conditions (acne, eczema, or psoriasis).

Topical applications of chickweed (a poultice, wash, fomentation, or bath) reduce inflammation, and are highly effective for treating dry, itchy skin conditions such as eczema, psoriasis, dandruff, poison oak, and poison ivy.[5,6] Apply the fresh plant poultice to insect bites, bee, wasp, or nettle stings, burns, ulcers, bed sores, mastitis, wounds, and hemorrhoids.[5,6,8] Fresh plant poultices have drawing properties that suppurate poisons and infections, promote the healing of abscesses and chronic sores, and reduce necrotic tissue. Hot chickweed compresses aid in treating boils, abscesses, carbuncles, furuncles, benign cysts, and splinters.[1,5] Chickweed applications also soothe abrasions, cradle cap, rashes, and other skin conditions.[8] Strain the fresh juice or an infusion through a coffee filter or fine mesh to create an eye wash, or apply it as a sitz bath to soothe vaginal and rectal tissues.[1]

CONTRAINDICATIONS

Excessive consumption of chickweed may result in loose stools; decrease the dosage or discontinue use if this occurs.

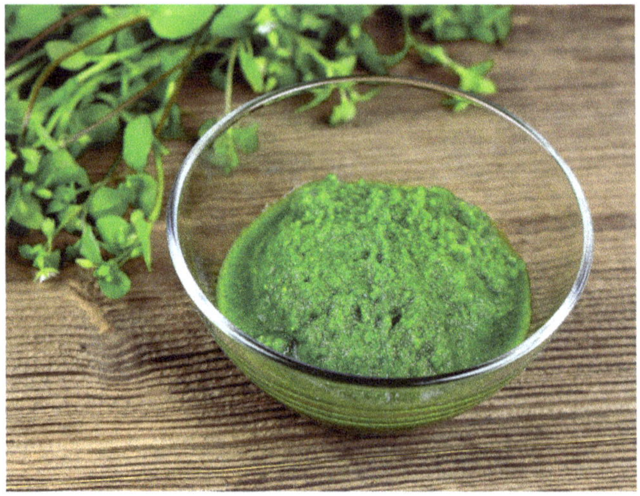

PREPARATION AND DOSAGE

TINCTURE: Fresh aerial portions [1:2-1:3, 80-95% alcohol]; consume 30-90 drops, up to four times daily. *Note:* Succus or tea preparations are preferable for reducing inflammation in mucous membranes.

SUCCUS: Juice the fresh plant, freeze it in small ice cube trays, and store it in a zip-lock bag in the freezer. Alternatively, measure the juice volume and add 15-20% (of 95% alcohol) to the total volume as a preservative. Refrigerate. Consume 1 teaspoon to 1 tablespoon, up to four times daily.

TEA: Prepare a hot infusion; consume 8-12 ounces, up to four times daily.

TOPICAL USE: Apply the ground herb as a fresh poultice, or wilt it for several days and prepare infused oil using the double boiler method.

CULINARY USE: The fresh herb is delicious in salads, pesto, pâté, and soups.

CINNAMON

DESCRIPTION

BOTANICAL NAMES:
Cinnamomum zeylanicum (syn. *C. verum*), *C. burmannii* (syn. *C. pedunculata*), *C. cassia* (syn. *C. aromaticum*)

COMMON NAMES:
Ceylon cinnamon, true cinnamon, Burmese cinnamon, Batavia cassia, Batavia cinnamon, Padang-cassia, Panang cinnamon, Chinese cinnamon, false cinnamon, cassia lignea, cassia
cannelle, casse (French)
kasia (Greek)
cannella, cassia (Italian)
canela (Portuguese)
canela, cassia (Spanish)

FAMILY NAME:
Lauraceae

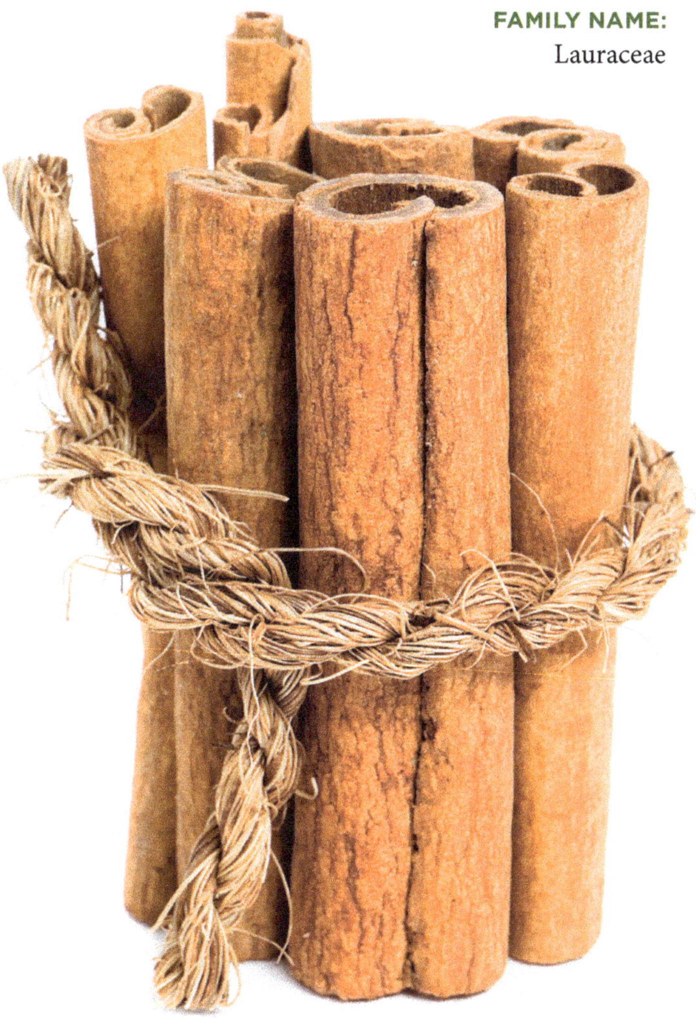

PART USED: The bark.

BOTANICAL DESCRIPTION AND HABITAT: *Cinnamomum* is a genus of strongly scented evergreen trees or shrubs native to the tropical regions of southwestern India and Sri Lanka. *Cinnamomum zeylanicum* is cultivated in Indonesia, the West Indies, the Seychelles, Africa, and South America.[1]

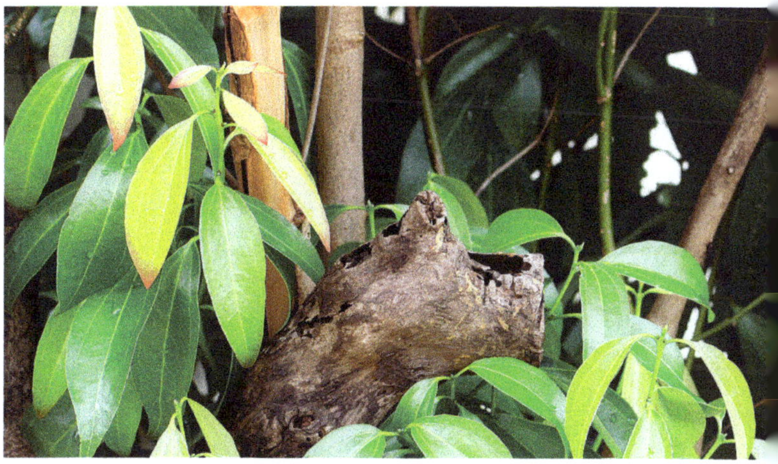

Native to the island of Sri Lanka, *Cinnamomum zeylanicum* is a small evergreen tree with low hanging branches.[2] It grows 8 to 17 meters tall.[2] The tree has thick, gray to dark brown bark; the inner bark contains cinnamic aldehyde, the main chemical giving cinnamon its flavor.[3] When young, the four-sided branches are gray with white blotches.[3] The leaf buds are covered in silky hairs.[3] The variable glabrous, leathery leaves are arranged opposite on the stem and are ovate to elliptic.[2] The young leaves are reddish, but mature to a shiny green on the upper side and a glaucous green on the underside.[2] There are three prominent mid-veins and reticulated transverse veins on both surfaces; the lower surface is dotted with small pits or depressions.[3] The leaves (11 – 16 cm long by 5 cm wide) have entire margins, acute bases, and acuminate apices.[3]

The flowers are found in terminal and axillary panicles (10 – 12 cm long).[3] Silky hairs cover the creamy white peduncle and rachis.[3] The yellow, fetid, apetalous flowers (3 – 6 mm long) have campanulate, pubescent, six-lobed calyces.[2] The androecium consists of nine fertile stamens with hairy filaments, and three stamens that abort during development. The gynoecium consists of a glabrous ovary

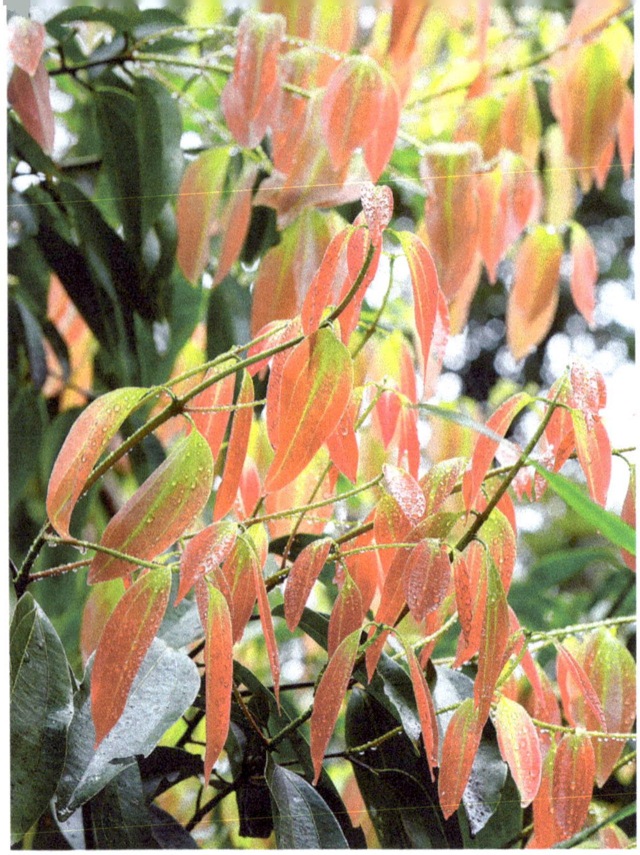

with a short style.[3] The ovary develops into a black, ovoid drupe (1 – 2 cm long) contained by the persistent, enlarged, cup-shaped, toothed calyx at the base.[1,2]

THE NAME: The genus name *Cinnamomum* and the common name cinnamon derive from the Greek word for spice: *kinnamomon*.[4] Cassia, an epithet and common name, derives from the ancient Hebrew *qitsilah* ("spice").[4] The epithet *verum* means "standard or true to type."[5] The epithet *aromaticum* means "fragrant."[6] The epithet *zeylanicum* ("Ceylon") refers to its origin in the country now called Sri Lanka.[4]

The following common names correspond with the Latin names: Ceylon cinnamon or true cinnamon *(Cinnamomum zeylanicum);* Burmese cinnamon, Batavia cassia, Batavia cinnamon, Padang-cassia, and Panang *(C. burmannii);* and Chinese cinnamon, false cinnamon, cassia, and cassia lignea *(C. cassia)*.[7]

HISTORICAL USES: For thousands of years, cinnamon and cassia have been used extensively in Eastern and Western cultures as medicinal and domestic spices.[7] Cinnamon was once worth more than its weight in gold.[1] Cinnamon bark was administered for abdominal pain, chronic diarrhea, nausea, vomiting, colds, flu, respiratory disorders, amenorrhea, menstrual cramping, and heavy menstrual bleeding.[7] Ancient Egyptians considered cinnamon an important ingredient in the embalming process and witchcraft.[1]

Cinnamon was incorporated into religious ceremonies and used as a flavoring agent in Medieval Europe.[1]

Eclectic physicians recommended various preparations of cinnamon as a hemostatic. A decoction was administered to prevent and control postpartum hemorrhage, and for a flaccid womb following delivery.[8] Ellingwood notes that cinnamon restores tone to the uterine muscular structure and induces tonic contraction. A compound used to treat most cases of passive hemorrhage consisted of a dram each of cinnamon and erigeron oils, and enough alcohol to make two ounces; a dosage of 10 – 30 drops was administered.[8] Several Eclectic physicians prescribed cinnamon as a carminative, aromatic, gastric stimulant, antidiarrheal, and antinauseant.[8,9] Felter suggests using cinnamon oil as a germicidal agent for colds, influenza, and la grippe.[9] Ellingwood mentions using cinnamon for diabetes.[9] Several physicians state that long-term use can aggravate the digestive tract, and it should be avoided in cases of mouth or digestive ulcers.[8,9]

Cinnamon continues to be included as a flavoring agent in alcohol (bitters and vermouth), nonalcoholic beverages (tea and soda), baked goods, desserts, candy, condiments, and soups.[7]

CONSTITUENTS: Cinnamon bark contains volatile oil consisting of cinnamaldehyde (60 – 75%), eugenol, eugenol acetate, cinnamyl acetate, cinnamyl alcohol, methyl eugenol, benzaldehyde, cuminacldehyde, benzyl benzoate, linalool, monoterpene hydrocarbons (pinene, phellandrene, and cymene), carophyllene, safrole, and others.[7] Cinnamon bark also contains tannins (polymeric 5,7,3',4'-tetrahydroxyflavin-3,4-diol units), catechins, proanthocyanidins, resins, mucilage, gum, sugars, calcium oxalate, two insecticidal compounds (cinnzelanin and cinnzelanol), and coumarins (smaller quantities in Ceylon cinnamon).[7]

NUTRITIONAL PROPERTIES: Cinnamon bark contains iron, magnesium, and zinc.

MEDICINAL PROPERTIES: Antinauseant, aphrodisiac aromatic, astringent, carminative, circulatory stimulant, demulcent, and hemostatic.

TEMPERATURE AND FLAVOR: Hot, sweet, pungent, astringent, and bitter.

MEDICINAL USES

Cinnamon has aromatic, carminative, and stomachic properties that stimulate and warm the digestive tract. It settles the stomach, quelling nausea and vomiting.[8] Cinnamon aids in treating chronic nonulcer dyspepsia, indigestion, flatulence, diarrhea, dysentery, and abdominal cramping. The volatile oil accounts for the carminative properties.[1] The active principles in cinnamon are 3-(2-hydroxyphenyl)-propanoic acid and its O-glucoside.[7] Eugenol acetate and methyl eugenol have reportedly enhanced trypsin activity *in vitro*.[7] Aqueous extracts of Chinese cinnamon have antiulcerogenic actions in rodents.[7] Cinnamon contains tannins that astringe the mucous membranes. Water-based preparations have demulcent actions that soothe mucous membranes in the digestive tract. Most demulcent herbs are cooling; however, cinnamon can be heating to the tissues. Discontinue use if it aggravates the digestive tract.

Cinnamon is a beloved pungent spice. True cinnamon, also known as Ceylon cinnamon *(Cinnamomum zeylanicum)*, is considered of superior quality to Chinese cinnamon or cassia *(C. cassia)*. Cinnamon is a common ingredient in Mediterranean and Indian dishes, and is added to baked goods, desserts, and candies. The warming qualities improve the digestibility of cooling foods such as dairy products and fruits. Sprinkling cinnamon powder on foods helps to reduce sugar cravings and balance blood sugar. Cinnamon is often added to chai tea.

A hemostatic, cinnamon slows a passive hemorrhage.[8] It reduces uterine bleeding from fibroids, uterine cysts, ovarian cysts, heavy menstrual flow, and postpartum bleeding.[8] Cinnamon also reduces minor pulmonary, intestinal, and rectal bleeding. However, it is very pungent and can be too heating and irritating to inflamed mucous membranes in the digestive tract. Cinnamon can be combined with other hemostatic herbs such as shepherd's purse *(Capsella)*, yarrow *(Achillea)*, or Canadian fleabane *(Erigeron)*. "Compound Spirits of Cinnamon and Erigeron," an Eclectic formula, is an extremely effective hemostatic. Administer the tincture or tea every 15 minutes until bleeding subsides. Topical applications also reduce minor bleeding from cuts or abrasions.

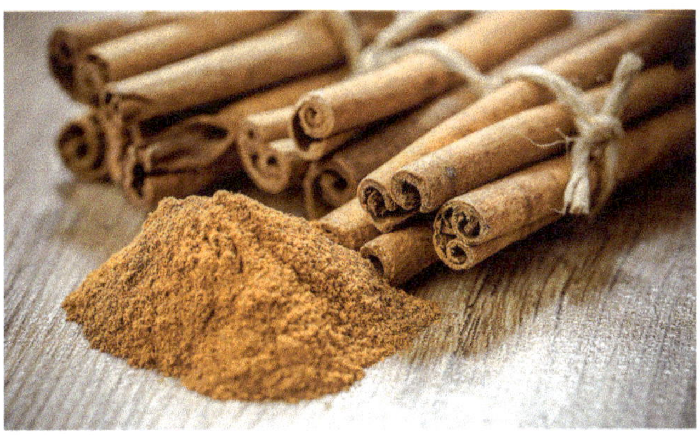

Cinnamon is a circulatory stimulant, improving circulation in the digestive and reproductive tracts, and hands and feet. It aids in treating Raynaud's phenomenon, and joint or muscle pain aggravated by cold. Decoctions or soups are heating diaphoretics during the first stages of a cold or flu. Combining cinnamon with ginger *(Zingiber)*, cardamom *(Elettaria)*, and/or allspice *(Pimenta dioica)* increases circulation and warms the digestive tract. Cinnamon is also an adjuvant and carrier agent in compounds. Topical applications have counterirritant properties.

Cinnamon contains volatile oil that has antifungal, antibacterial, and larvicidal actions.[7] Extracts have been found to suppress the growth of *Escherichia coli*, *Staphylococcus aureus*, and *Candida albicans*.[7] Eugenol has antiseptic, irritant, and anesthetic properties.[7] Volatile oil of cinnamon has been found to inhibit numerous types of oral bacteria and fungus, including oral infections caused by candida.[7]

Cinnamon aids in treating acute upper or lower respiratory infections accompanied by profuse clear or cloudy mucus. It has mild expectorant and astringent actions that dry excessive secretions. Short-term internal use reduces populations of intestinal or vaginal candida, especially when bowel movements contain mucus, or when vaginal secretions are profuse and clear.

CONTRAINDICATIONS

Some sources contraindicate the use of cinnamon during pregnancy because high doses can induce a miscarriage; however, cassia is considered safe during pregnancy.[1] The author hasn't observed problems with moderate internal or culinary use. Discontinue internal use if cinnamon aggravates the digestive tract. Cinnamon can be too heating, aggravating hot flashes, night sweats, and sweating. In rare cases, some individuals may experience an allergic reaction with difficulty breathing.

Note: Cinnamon essential oil is highly concentrated and should never be applied neat. It can be extremely irritating to the skin. If applied topically, it should be diluted at a 1:1,000 ratio (one drop of cinnamon oil to 50 ml of carrier oil).

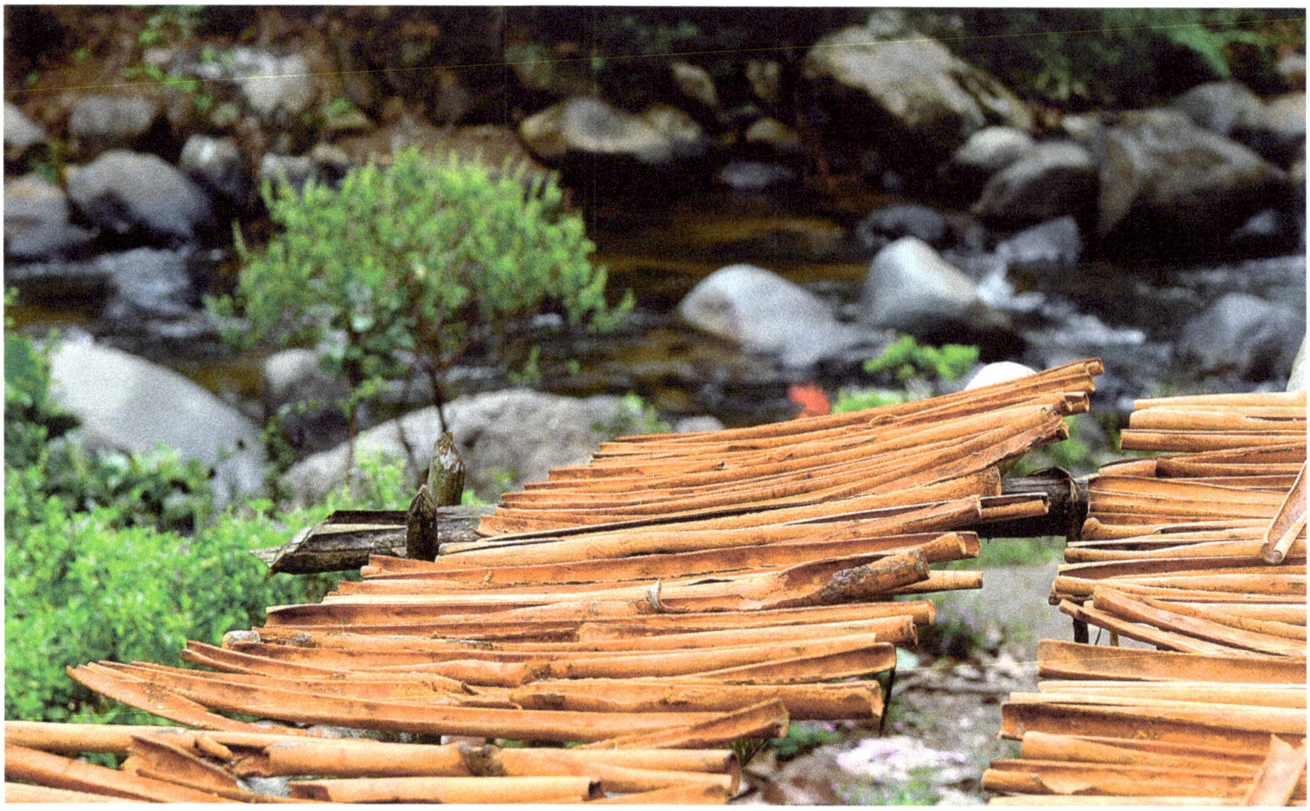

PREPARATION AND DOSAGE

TINCTURE: Dry bark [1:5, 60% alcohol] or [1:5, 50% alcohol, 40% water, and 10% glycerin]: consume 10-60 drops, up to four times daily.

CAPSULES: Consume 2-3 "00" capsules, one to three times daily.

TEA: Prepare a decoction (the most common method), cold infusion, or hot infusion; consume up to 8 ounces, two to four times daily.

TOPICAL USE: Topical applications of the powder can be applied to cuts and abrasions as a hemostatic, or added to clay or arrowroot powder as a topical powder or dust.

CULINARY USE: Cinnamon is a delightful addition to Central American, Mediterranean, East African, Southeast Asian, and Indian dishes, masala chai tea, baked goods, desserts, syrups, cordials, elixirs, aperitifs, and digestifs.

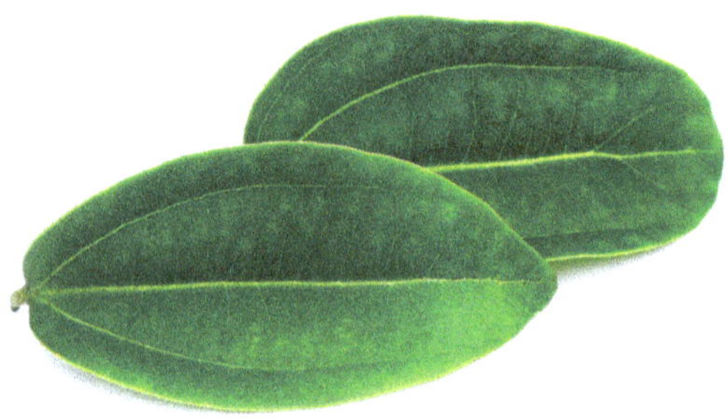

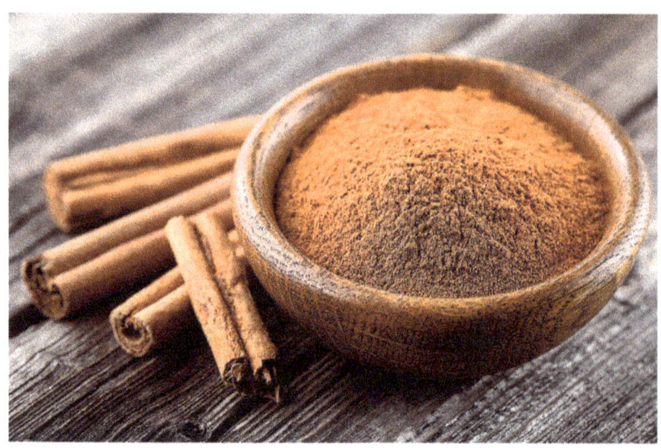

CLEAVERS

DESCRIPTION

BOTANICAL NAMES:
Galium aparine, G. asprellum, G. boreale, G. trifidum, G. triflorum, G. verum, G. spp.

COMMON NAMES:
Cleaver, cleavers, bedstraw, lady's bedstraw, Our Lady's bedstraw, cleaverwort, clivers, goose grass, goose bill, catchweed, sticky willy, hedge-burs, grip-grass, scratweed, mutton chops, robin-run-in-the-grass, poor Robin, maid's hair, loveman, hedgehariffe, hayriffe, eriffe, everlasting friendship
walstroo (Dutch)
aparine, gaillet gratteron, petit muguet (French)
klebenkraut, kletten-labkraut, klimme, vogelheu (German)
aparine, attacca-veste, cappello dei tignosi, gaglio (Italian)
cuaja leche, guaco (Spanish)
coban suzegi (Turkish)[1]

FAMILY NAME:
Rubiaceae

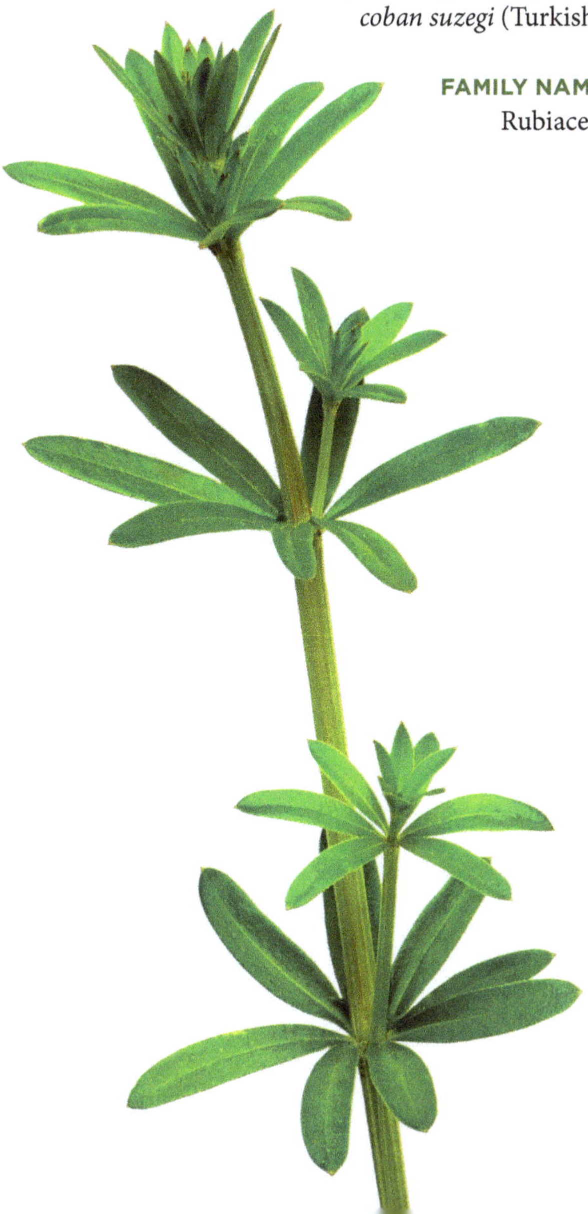

PARTS USED: The foliage or above-ground parts.

BOTANICAL DESCRIPTION: Cleavers is widely distributed in the U.S., although multiple *Galium* species are native to Europe, Asia, and North Africa. It grows in moist, shady, wooded areas next to streams or riverbanks, and thrives in rich, moist, alkaline soils. The origin of cleavers is debated; most sources claim that *Galium* is native to North America.

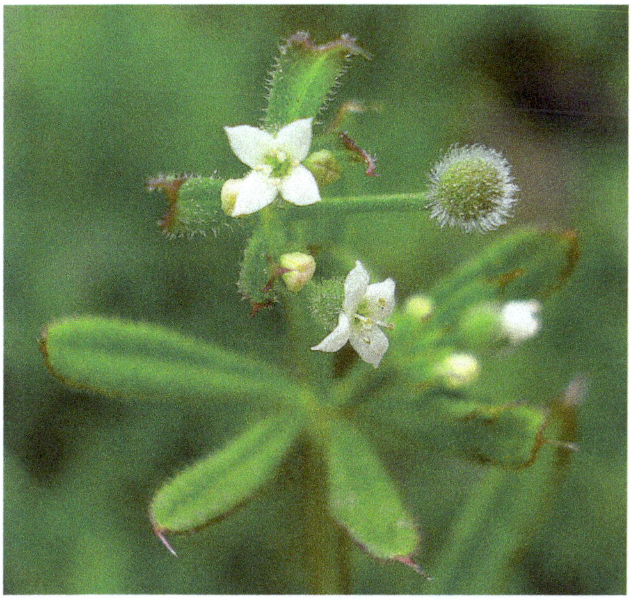

More than 45 species and many subspecies of *Galium* grow in California.[2] *Galium* species range from annuals like *G. aparine,* to perennials like *G. boreale*. Their growth habits range from erect and shrubby, to prostrate or climbing.[2] The plants are glabrous or hairy, and they are often rough to the touch. Many *Galium* species are known for feeling like a cat's tongue when grasped. When young, the stems of *Galium* species are square. The leaves grow in distinctive whorls of four or more, often with leaf-like stipules growing out of the same nodes as the leaves. Some species are dioecious.[2] The inflorescence is a panicle or simply axillary clusters of two or more flowers.[2] The rotate to bell-shaped, asepalous, greenish flowers can be bisexual or unisexual with sterile stamens or pistils.[2] There are generally four lobes in the fused corolla, two lobes in the ovary, and two styles fused at their bases.[2] Depending on the species, the fruit bears two nutlets, or one berry.[2]

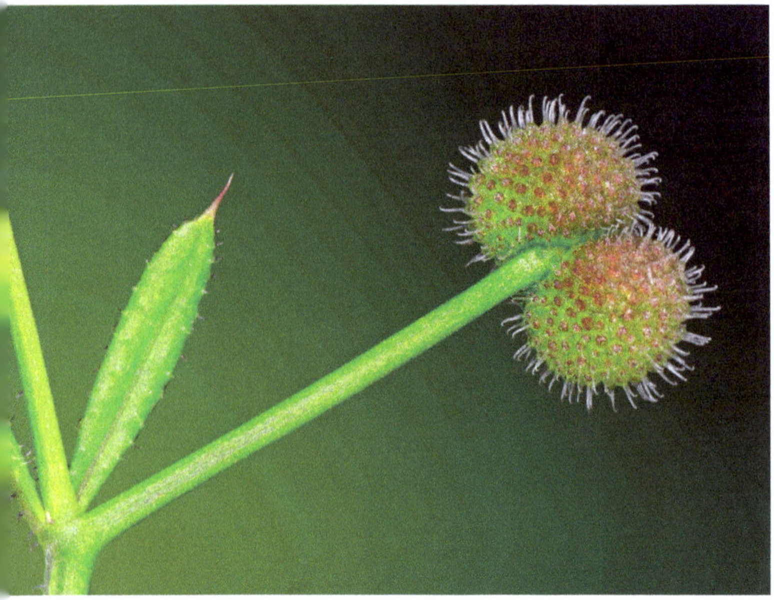

Galium aparine, the species most commonly used in commerce, is a bisexual annual plant that tends to climb or lay prostrate, though it is sometimes low and erect.[2] The small hooked hairs on the plant adhere to surrounding objects and plants, allowing it to climb.[2] The stem grows 30 – 90 cm long, and is brittle and weak.[2] The narrow, oblanceolate leaves grow in whorls of six to eight leaves (10 – 30 mm long).[2] The leaves lower on the stem will be petioled; those higher on the stem are sessile.[2] The flower has a whitish, rotate corolla and bears nutlets.[2]

THE NAME: The genus name *Galium* derives from the Greek *gala* ("milk") because the juice of *G. verum* was used to curdle milk.[3] In Greek, the species name *aparine* means "bedstraw," as the foliage was used to stuff mattresses. A mixture of bracken and bedstraw was believed to have lined the bed of the Virgin and the manger of baby Jesus; thus, *Galium verum* acquired the name "Our Lady's bedstraw."[4] The epithet *boreale* means "of the north."

The common name cleavers *(clivers)* derives from the Anglo-Saxon *clife* and Dutch *kleef-kruid* ("to cleave or cling"). *Clivers* ("claws") derives from Old English. It acquired the common name goose-grass because geese consumed it.

HISTORICAL USES: The tender young greens were consumed as a pot herb. The herb was used traditionally as an antiscorbutic. The Scandinavians used masses of the leaves and stems to filter milk.[4] The roasted seeds of some species are reported to have a coffee-like flavor. Consuming a cold infusion of the herb two to three times daily for two to three months and topical use of the tea were said to remove freckles, according to Old English folklore.[1] Cowichans rubbed cleavers into their hands to remove pitch, and used the dried herb to start fires.[4] Ditidahts applied cleavers hair rinse for lustrous, thick hair.[4] The Cree used dried herb of *Galium triflorum* as a perfume.[5]

CONSTITUENTS: Cleavers contains flavonoids (quercetin and rutin), iridoid glycosides (asperuloside, 10-deacetyl-asperulosidic acid, asperulosidic acid, monotropein, and aucubin), coumarins, a bitter principle, tannins, phenolic acid (caffeic acid derivatives), vitamin C, citric acid and a trace of nicotinic acid.[5-7]

NUTRITIONAL PROPERTIES: Cleavers contains vitamin C and citric acid. It was used traditionally as an antiscorbutic herb.[5-7]

MEDICINAL PROPERTIES: Alterative, anti-inflammatory, diuretic, eliminative, lymphatic, nutritive, and vulnerary.

TEMPERATURE AND FLAVOR: Cool, sweet, salty, and bland.

MEDICINAL USES

Cleavers is a valuable diuretic that reduces edema-related swelling in the hands, feet, eyelids, face, and breasts. Long-term consumption aids in treating dysuria, bladder irritability, benign prostatic hypertrophy, and nephritis.[9] It can be used as a short-term diuretic to treat urinary tract infections. *Note:* Additional anti-infective agents are also necessary to treat bacteria. Cleavers is included in weight loss formulas to reduce water-related weight gain. The flavonoids are attributed to the diuretic effect.[7]

Cleavers supports the kidneys' elimination of metabolic byproducts such as uric acid.[8] Long-term consumption of cleavers tea aids in treating conditions such as gout, arthritis, and kidney stones resulting from uric acid buildup.[6-8] Also, skin conditions, such as eczema, psoriasis, and boils can be aggravated when the kidneys are taxed by excess uric acid.[8,10] Prepare a diuretic tea with cleavers, chickweed *(Stellaria),* couch grass *(Triticum),* nettle leaf *(Urtica),* horsetail *(Equisetum),* and/or dandelion *(Taraxacum)* to enhance uric acid excretion. Consume 8 – 12 ounces, one to two times daily.

Due to its diuretic and lymphatic properties, cleavers is considered a depurative (blood cleanser) and alterative. It is a cooling lymphatic that reduces swelling and tenderness in lymph nodes.[10] Cleavers is not a direct antimicrobial, although it can be combined with other antivirals to treat swollen lymph nodes caused by mononucleosis, cold, flu, or herpes. When lymphatic swelling results from an infection, combine cleavers with extracts of echinacea *(Echinacea)*, red root *(Ceanothus)*, and yerba mansa *(Anemopsis)*. Combine cleavers with lymphatic herbs such as red root *(Ceanothus)*, echinacea *(Echinacea)*, figwort *(Scrophularia)*, violet *(Viola)*, and/or calendula *(Calendula)* for non-infected, hard, swollen lymph nodes.

Internal and external use of cleavers aids in treating tender breasts, fibrocystic breasts, and benign breast lumps. Cleavers is an adjunct that supports individuals receiving conventional treatment for breast cancer as well as breast cancer survivors. Apply the salve or poultices topically, one to two times daily. The following salve recipe has been a very effective topical application for breast tenderness and lymph swelling. This salve contains numerous lymphatic herbs such as figwort *(Scrophularia)*, chickweed *(Stellaria)*, violet *(Viola)*, calendula *(Calendula)*, and cleavers.

Gather the fresh herbs, wilt for one to three days, and cook in a base oil blend containing ⅔ extra virgin olive oil and ⅓ castor oil using the double boiler oil preparation method. Strain the oil and prepare as a salve. Add lymphatic essential oils such as bay laurel *(Laurus nobilis)* to improve the effectiveness of the salve. The salve may be applied one to two times daily to swollen, tender or lumpy breasts, and to swollen lymph in the throat, armpit, or groin.

Apply the fomentation, poultice, salve, or juice of fresh cleavers as a vulnerary and anti-inflammatory.[7,8] Freeze the succus in ice cube trays and apply topically to abrasions, burns, cuts, bites, stings, rashes, dermatitis, eczema, and poison oak to reduce inflammation and itching, and prevent scarring.[7,8] The anti-inflammatory effects are due to the asperuloside.[6]

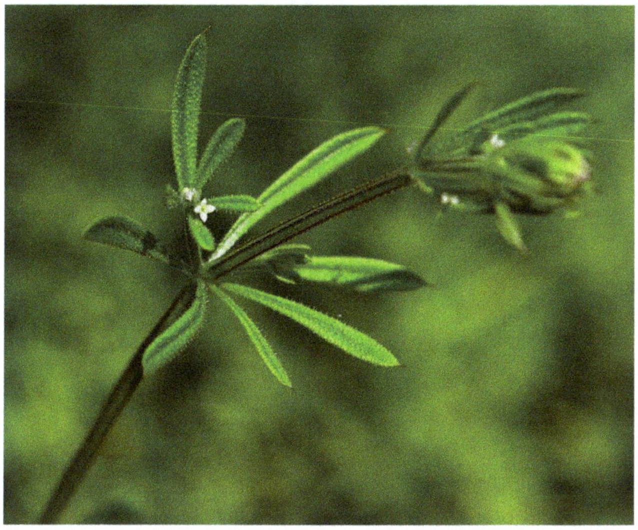

CONTRAINDICATIONS

There are no known contraindications. However, when an individual suffers from chronic edema, it is important to consult with a health care practitioner, as severe edema can be associated with heart, kidney, or thyroid conditions.[7]

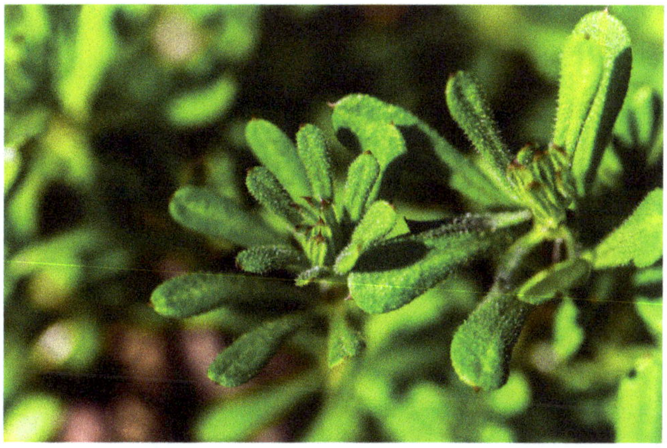

PREPARATION AND DOSAGE

TINCTURE: Fresh foliage [1:2-1:3, 70-95% alcohol]; consume 30-90 drops, up to four times daily.

SUCCUS: Fresh cleavers can be prepared as a succus by juicing the herb, and adding 10-20% alcohol to the total juice volume to preserve it. The low percentage of alcohol can prevent spoilage, but the succus will last longer if it is refrigerated.

ACETUM EXTRACT: Fresh foliage [1:2, apple cider vinegar]; consume 30-90 drops, up to four times daily.

TEA: Prepare a hot or cold infusion of the herb; consume 8-12 ounces, up to four times daily.

TOPICAL USE: Wilt the leaves one to three days and prepare with the oil using the double boiler method. Apply the oil or salve topically, one to three times daily.

CULINARY USE: Fresh leaves or leaf tips can be steamed or added to stews. They are best cooked, because the small, hair-like projections of the fresh herb can irritate the throat. The fresh herb can be juiced for consumption, or poured into ice cube trays and frozen for internal or topical use. After the ice cubes form, freeze them in a sealed container or zip-lock bag.

CLOVE

DESCRIPTION

BOTANICAL NAMES:
Syzygium aromaticum
(syn. *Caryophyllus aromaticum, Eugenia aromatica, E. caryophyllata,* and *E. caryophyllus*)

COMMON NAMES:
Clove, cloves, clove buds, clove tree, Zanzibar red head
kabsn qaranful (Arabic)
kruidnagel (Dutch)
clou de girofle, girofle, giroflier (French)
gewurznelkenbaum (German)
garifalo (Greek)
chiodi de garofano (Italian)
ding xiang, ting hsiang (Mandarin)
cravo (Portuguese)
lavanga (Sanskrit)
clavo, raja (Spanish)

FAMILY NAME:
Myrtaceae

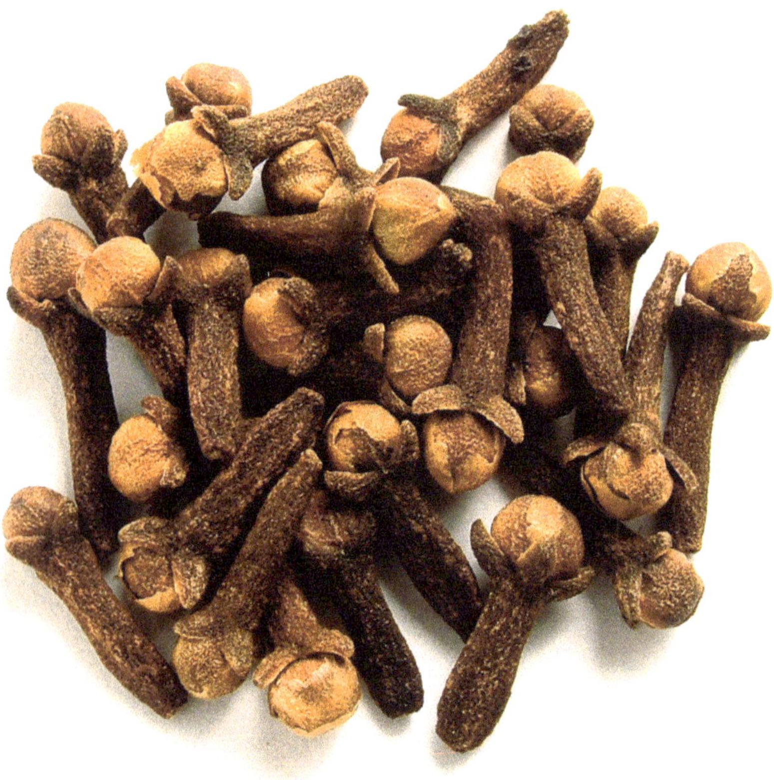

PART USED: Unripe buds.

BOTANICAL DESCRIPTION AND HABITAT: Clove is a perennial, evergreen tree native to Southeast Asia, and cultivated in Asia, Africa, Central America, and South America.[1] It grows 10 – 30 m tall, although it doesn't usually reach its full height under cultivation. It has many

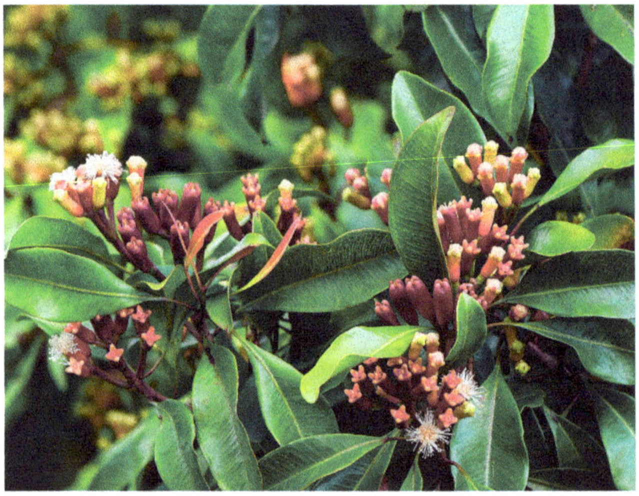

erect branches and a low growing crown.[2,3] The dense root system grows close to the soil surface.[2] The bark, leaves, and flowers are very fragrant.[3] The opposite, ovate to elliptic, glabrous, shiny leaves (up to 13 cm long) bear numerous oil glands underneath.[3] The inflorescence is a terminal cymose cluster; the relatively long flower buds (2 cm long) are initially creamy green, and transition to a dark purplish-red when harvested.[2,3] Each flower is clad with a hypanthium bearing minute triangular sepals and a globose corolla that opens at maturity to reveal many showy stamens.[3,4] The flower produces a single-seeded, dark red berry (2 – 2.5 cm long).[4]

THE NAME: *Syzygium* derives from the Greek *syzygos* ("coupled, joined, jointed"), referring to the calyptrate petals or paired branches and leaves. The genus *synonym Caryophyllus* derives from the Greek *karyo-phyllun* ("nut-leaf"), referring to the appearance of flower buds.[5] *Eugenia* was named for Prince Eugene of Saxony (1663 – 1736).[5] The epithet *aromaticum* ("aromatic, spice-like") derives from Latin. The common name clove derives from the French *clou* ("a nail or spike"), referring to the shape of the buds.[5]

HISTORICAL USES: Records from China's Han dynasty (207 BCE to CE 220) describe how officers of the court were required to hold clove buds in their mouths when speaking. This ensured that their breath would be sweet for the king.[6] Vast clove forests grew wild in Indonesia's Molucca Islands, later known as the Spice Islands. The indigenous people there planted a clove tree when a child was born, ensuring the tree's abundance.[6]

Arab traders introduced clove to Europe in the 4th century. They continued to control the spice trade, bringing in spices such as clove, cinnamon, nutmeg, ginger, and mace until the late 15th century, when the Portuguese ended the monopoly. Spices from China, Japan, and native sources required lengthy, costly transport by land and sea; therefore, Arab traders commanded a high price for them in Europe.[6] Culinary spices were often used as currency because they were valued for their flavoring and food preservation. In 1497, when Vasco de Gama voyaged around Africa to India, Portugal began to dominate the spice trade. The Portuguese entered trade agreements with the Sultan of Ternate (of the Spice Islands) in 1512, creating a clove trade monopoly for 100 years. The Dutch gained control of the trade in the early 17th century. Eventually, larger amounts of spices were cultivated for trade, and the price of spices declined. During the 16th and 17th centuries, these spices became affordable and available to almost everyone, popularizing their culinary and medicinal uses.[6]

Since then, clove has been administered for their antinauseant, antiemetic, carminative, antispasmodic, and anodyne actions.[1,7] Maude Grieves lists clove as "the most stimulating and carminative of all aromatics."[8] Eclectic physicians administered clove extract as a salivary and digestive stimulant. Harvey Felter described clove as a carminative and stimulant of gastric juices that increased peristalsis throughout the digestive tract.[7] He recommended it to prevent griping caused by other herbs, presumably bitters and cholagogues.[7] He administered clove oil externally for dental pain, and clove-containing ointments or liniments as topical anodynes.[7] Clove continues to be included in potpourris and pomanders.

Most of the world's clove production is imported to Indonesia where clove cigarettes are made. They consist of one part powdered clove buds, and two parts tobacco; they produce a crackling sound when smoked.[1]

CONSTITUENTS: Clove contains volatile oil (eugenol, eugenol acetate, β-caryophyllene, and lower amounts of methyl salicylate, methyl eugenol, benzaldehydes, methyl amyl ketones, α-ylangene, and chavicol), glucosides of sterols (sitosterol, stimasterol, and campesterol), triterpenes (oleanolic acid), crataegolic acid, methyl ester, quercetin, eugeniin, kampferol, rhamnetin, tannins (hydrolysable), phenolic acids, protein, lipids, carbohydrates, vitamins, and others.[1,10]

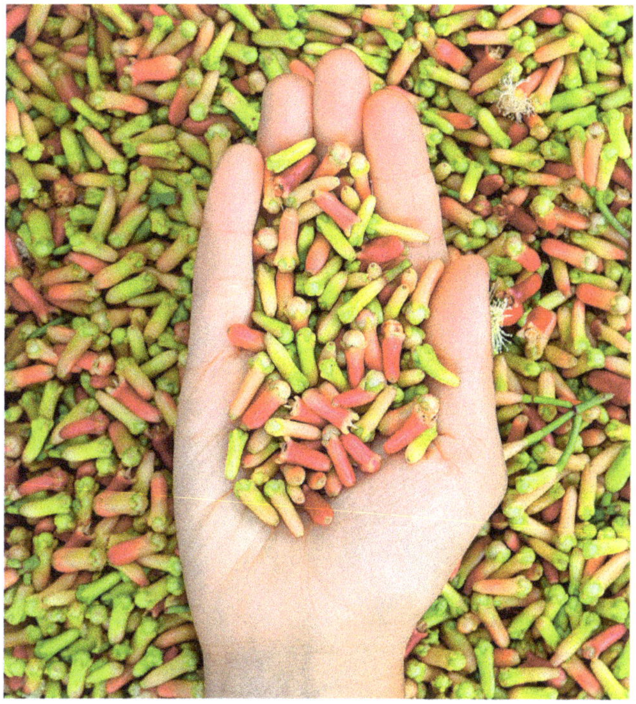

NUTRITIONAL PROPERTIES: Clove contains proteins, lipids, carbohydrates, and vitamins.[1]

MEDICINAL PROPERTIES: Antibacterial, antifungal, antimicrobial, antiparasitic, antiviral, astringent, bitter tonic, carminative, carrier, circulatory stimulant, diaphoretic, local anesthetic, and counterirritant.

TEMPERATURE AND FLAVOR: Hot, pungent, bitter, astringent, and sweet.

MEDICINAL USES

Clove is a potent antimicrobial agent internally and topically. The buds are effective as antibacterial (gram-negative and gram-positive bacteria, and acid-fast bacteria) and antifungal agents for respiratory and digestive microbes.[1,9] Clove extracts aid in treating strep throat, oral bacteria, colds, flu, and digestive microbes (bacterial, viral, and parasitic). Eugeniin has antiviral activity against herpes simplex; it also has potent antioxidant actions.[1] Topical applications of the diluted tincture have antifungal actions for treating athlete's foot.[1]

Clove has potent local anesthetizing actions for throat or gum inflammation.[8,9] Include a small quantity of clove extract in a spray for sore throat, laryngitis, hoarseness, strep throat, cold, influenza, or mononucleosis.[9] Gargling and local applications of the diluted tincture are useful for numbing the gums when treating teething pain, a gum abscess, or other gum problems (until dental work is obtained), dental caries, sub-mandibular irritability with facial nerve irritation, or a lost filling.[8,9] Clove tincture or highly diluted essential oil can be applied to teething children, although undiluted essential oil should never be applied topically.[1] Combine clove tincture with cow parsnip *(Heracleum)*, spilanthes *(Acmella)*, and/or echinacea *(Echinacea)* extracts to mitigate the pain of toothaches and teething. Gargling with clove freshens the breath, and has antibacterial actions against gingivitis.[9]

Clove is a bitter, aromatic herb with carminative actions that reduce gas and bloating.[7-9] It stimulates circulation and warms the digestive tract.[8,9] Consuming extracts or capsules aids in treating acute microbial digestive infections. The astringent properties also aid in treating diarrhea. An infusion of clove has antiemetic actions, although an excessive dose can cause nausea or an upset stomach. Avoid consuming the decocted tea. When treating digestive infections, one can consume one to two drops of essential oil in a capsule with a base such as marshmallow *(Althaea)* powder, one to three times daily for 3 – 14 days. *Note:* Consuming excessively large or frequent doses of clove essential oil can provoke gastroenteritis and irritate the kidneys.[7]

Clove has stomachic and smooth muscle antispasmodic actions for digestive and menstrual cramping due to the eugenyl acetate.[1,9] It also has anti-inflammatory actions inhibiting the biosynthesis of prostaglandins and

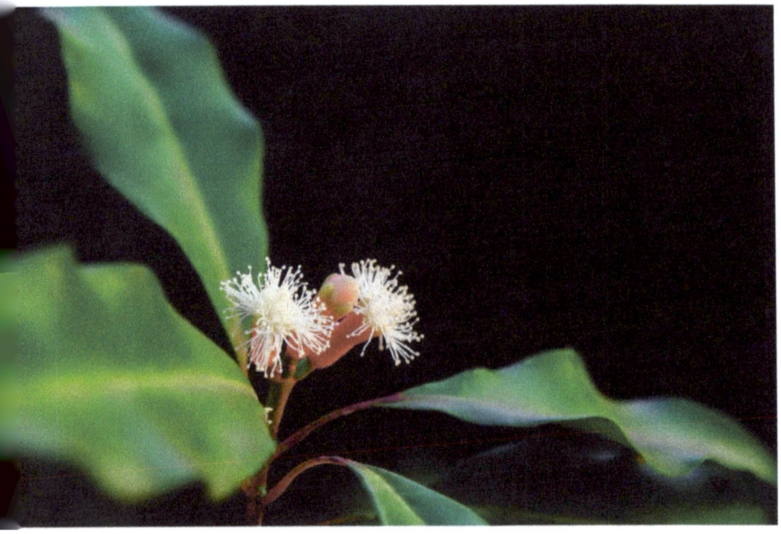

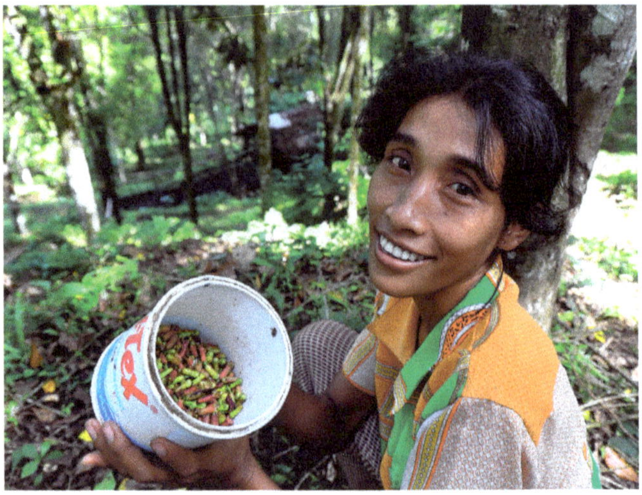

leukotrienes.[9] Consume 24 – 48 hours prior to menses in order to alleviate cramping; clove extract was included in Hayden's Viburnum Compound for this purpose.[9]

Clove is a circulatory stimulant and carrier in compounds for short-term use only, as high doses or long-term use can irritate the kidneys. It is highly potent and should be used only in low doses, as it can easily dominate a formula.

External use of the infused oil (alcohol intermediary oil) or highly diluted essential oil has counterirritant actions. Apply topically as a counterirritant and anesthetic for arthritis, sprains, strains, and muscle or joint aches or pain. The diluted extract or tea is an antibacterial and antifungal; consistent applications eliminate athlete's foot or ringworm.[9]

CONTRAINDICATIONS

Avoid internal use (except light culinary usage) of clove during pregnancy or lactation, or in children under age 10. However, topical use of the tea or extract is not problematic. Clove is contraindicated with stomach or duodenal ulcers, acid indigestion, and gastroesophageal reflux disease. Internal use can also cause kidney irritation and result in a dull lower backache. Avoid consuming clove regularly with any form of kidney irritation or kidney disease, or when consuming over-the-counter or pharmaceutical drugs that irritate or compromise kidney function.

The same contraindications also apply to clove essential oil. Additionally, topical or internal use of the essential oil can be extremely irritating. Due to its skin sensitizing effects, the essential oil should be highly diluted for topical use (recommended use: a 1% dilution, or one drop per 20-milliliters of carrier oil).[10]

PREPARATION AND DOSAGE

TINCTURE: Dry, unripe buds [1:5, 60% alcohol]; consume 5–30 drops, up to three times daily.

GLYCERITE: Dry, unripe buds [1:5, 40% glycerin, 30% alcohol, 30% water]; consume 5–30 drops, up to three times daily.

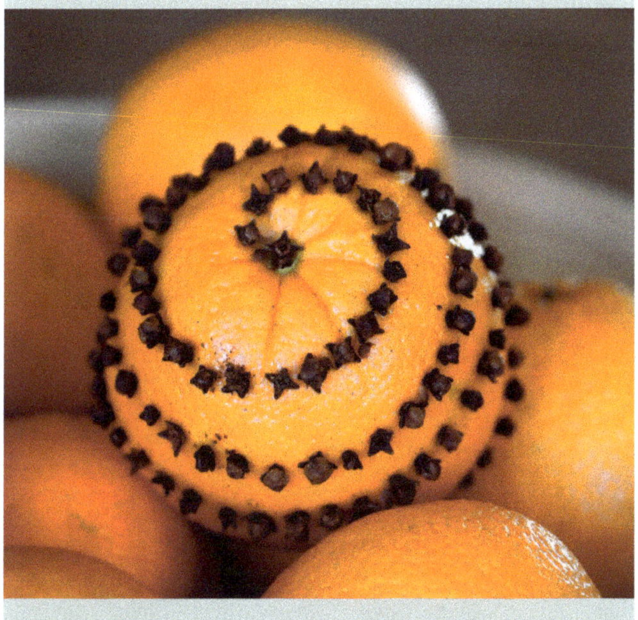

CAPSULES: To prepare clove oil capsules, fill "0" or "00" capsules with a binding agent such as marshmallow root powder or slippery elm powder, then add 1–2 drops of clove essential oil into each capsule. Place the tops on the capsules, and store in a zip-lock bag or glass jar in the refrigerator or freezer. Consume 1–2 capsules, one to three times daily. These are for short-term use only. *Note:* Take care not to drop essential oil onto the walls of the capsules, or they can dissolve.

TEA: Prepare a hot infusion; consume 2–8 ounces, one to three times daily.

TOPICAL USE: Apply tea, diluted extract, glycerite, or highly diluted essential oil as a topical anesthetic or antimicrobial. *Note:* See contraindications listed above for essential oil.

CULINARY USE: Clove powder is used as a spice in Greek cuisine, garam masala, five-spice, curries, ham, mulled wine, fruit dishes, baked goods, and desserts.

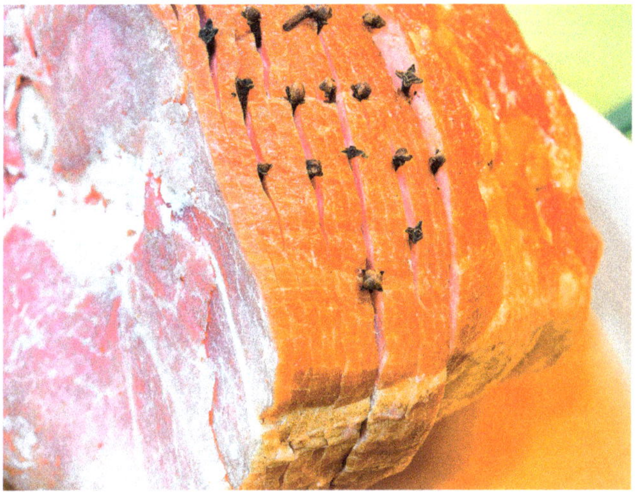

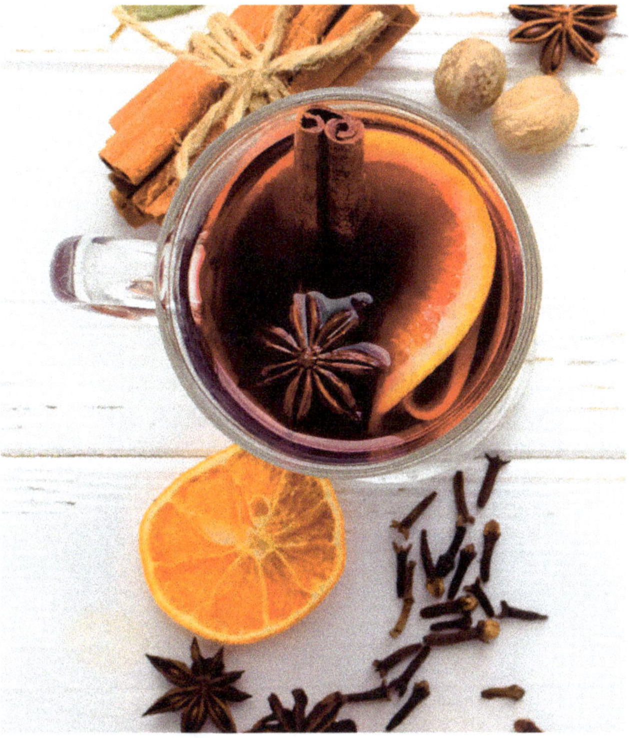

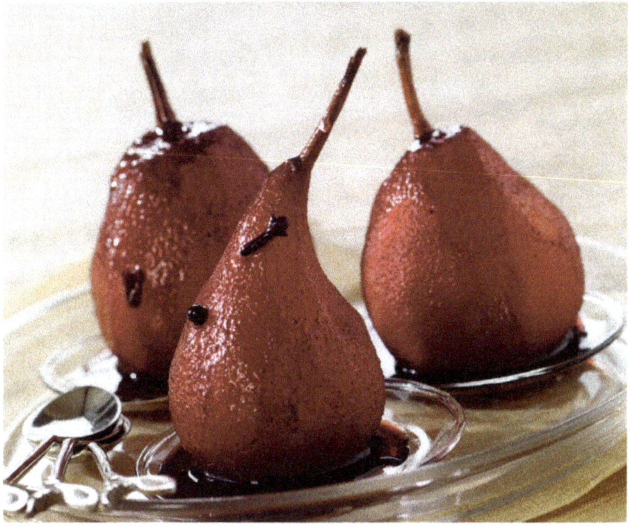

CODONOPSIS

DESCRIPTION

BOTANICAL NAMES:
Codonopsis pilosula, C. lanceolata

COMMON NAMES:
Codonopsis, poor man's ginseng, bastard ginseng, bonnet bell flower, bell flower, woodland bonnet
fong dong sam (Cantonese)
tōjin (Japanese)
tangsam (Korean)
dǎng shēn, dang shen, dangshen, tai dang shen, tang shen, tangshen, shan hai luo (Mandarin)

FAMILY NAME:
Campanulaceae

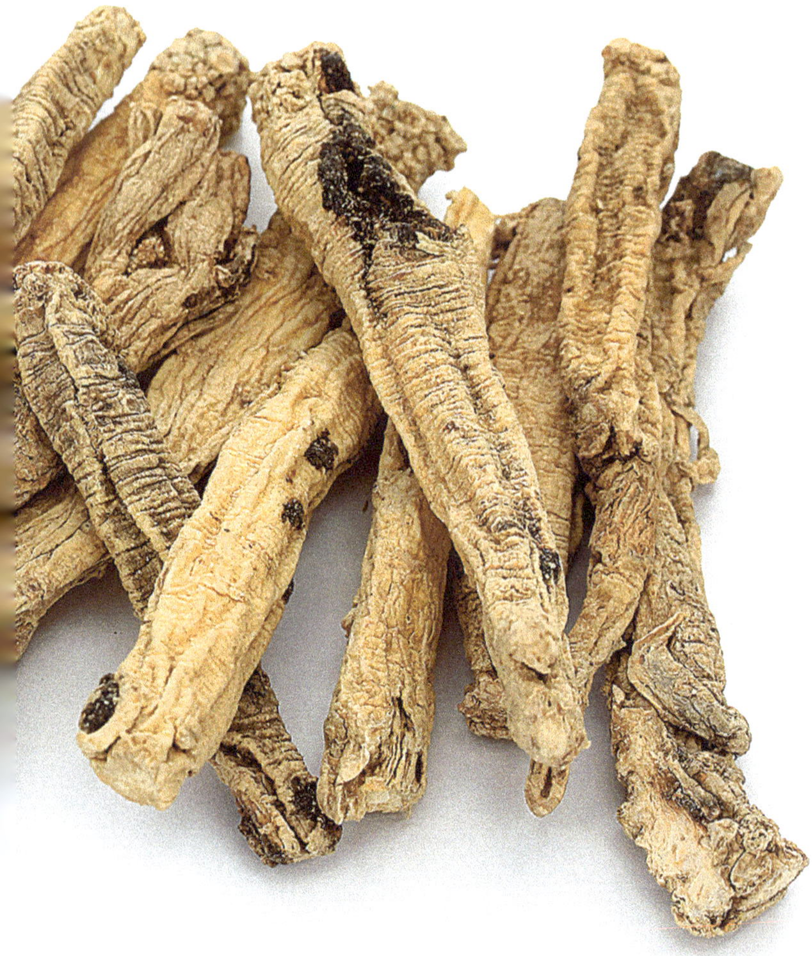

PART USED: The roots.

BOTANICAL DESCRIPTION AND HABITAT: *Codonopsis*, a genus of approximately 40 herbaceous perennial species, grows predominantly in East Asia.[1] The herb has thick, carrot-shaped roots that are usually fleshy, with a whitish

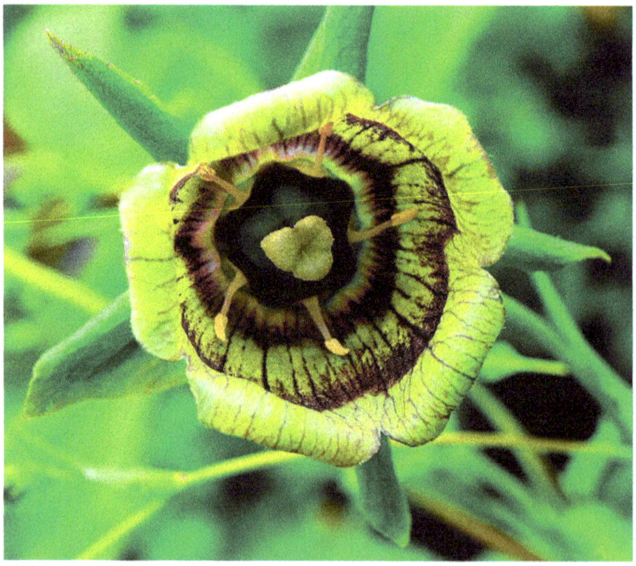

interior.[2,3] *Codonopsis pilosula*, the species used most often in medicine, is a vine that grows over two meters tall. Its cordate leaves (2.5 cm long) are softly pubescent.[3] It has terminal or axillary solitary, pale lavender flowers (2.5 cm long).[3] The perianth consists of a fused, leaf-like calyx and a campanulate corolla with five lobes.[1] It has five stamens with flat filaments, an inferior ovary with three carpels, and three stigmas. The fruit is a many-seeded capsule that is fleshy when young, then dries and hardens with maturity.[1]

THE NAME: The genus *Codonopsis* means "bell-like."[4] The epithet *pilosula* derives from the Latin *pilosus* ("hairy") due to the fine pubescence on the leaves.[5] *Dǎng shēn* is loosely translated as "group root."[6]

HISTORICAL USES: Codonopsis was first described in the *Origin of the Classics of Materia Medica* by Zhang Lu (1670 CE) and *Ben Jing Feng Yuan* (1695 CE) as a lung-clearing *(qing fei)* herb. In 1757, the qi tonifying properties were listed in the *Ben Cao Cong Xin*.[7] Qianlong, the famous Qing Dynasty emperor, credited his longevity to daily consumption of dang shen.[8] It was administered similar to other tonics such as astragalus, ginseng, and jujube date to treat spleen qi, lung qi, and blood deficiencies.[7] In Korea, it was used to treat coughs, palpitations, and anorexia.[8] In Japan, the herb was administered to alleviate shortness of breath and weakness.[8] In India, the powdered roots were used as an edible flour.[4] The roots and leaves were applied as a poultice for wounds and ulcers.[4]

CONSTITUENTS: Codonopsis contains polysaccharides (compounds CP-1, CP-2, CP-3, and CP-4), sugars (inulin, starch, glucose, sucrose, fructose, galactose, arabinose, mannose, xylose, and rhamnose), saponins (tangshenosides I-IV), amino acids, a β-carboline alkaloid (perlolyrine), nitrogen compounds (choline, nicotinic acid, and *n*-butylallophanate), triterpenes (taraxeryl acetate, taraxerol, and friedelin), phytosterols (stigmasterol and α-spinasterol), and their glucosides, atractylenolides II and III, scutellarein glucoside, oroxylin A, a volatile oil, and trace minerals.[7,9]

NUTRITIONAL PROPERTIES: Although a more detailed study of its nutrient content is warranted, codonopsis contains amino acids and minerals (calcium, iron, manganese, and zinc).

MEDICINAL PROPERTIES: Adaptogen, adrenolytic, blood tonic, immune modulator, lung qi tonic, spleen qi tonic, antiulcer, gastroprotective, hypotensive, and peripheral vasodilator.

TEMPERATURE AND FLAVOR: Neutral (slightly warm) and sweet.

MEDICINAL USES

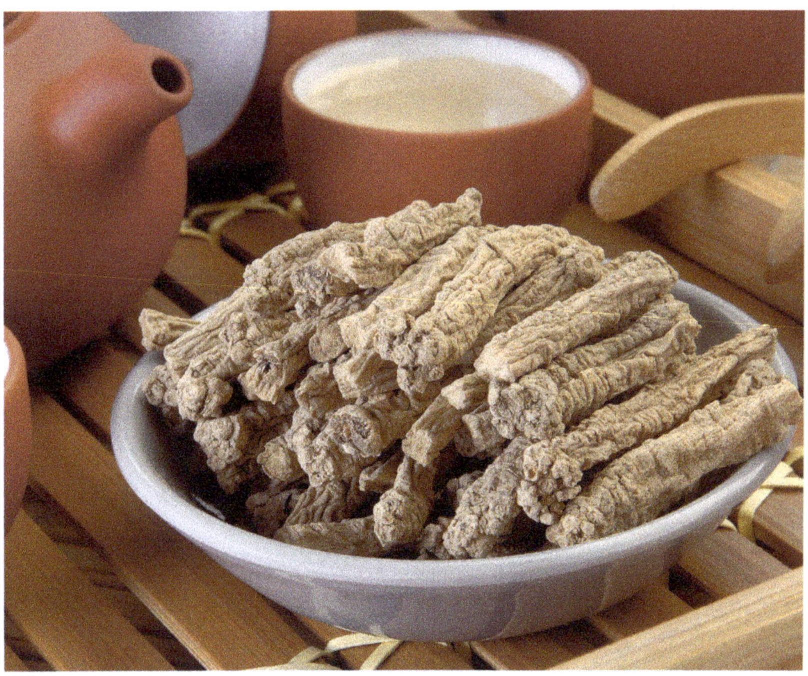

Codonopsis contains immune modulating polysaccharides that strengthen resistance to infection.[7,9] It enhances macrophage phagocytosis, increases neutrophils, and has immune regulating actions.[6,7] Codonopsis stimulates bone marrow, increasing hematopoiesis and enhancing immune function.[10] In rodent studies, codonopsis increased hemoglobin, as well as red and white blood cell counts.[4,6,7]

In Traditional Chinese Medicine, codonopsis is administered as a tonic to aid in treating lung qi deficiency.[6,8] Symptoms of lung qi deficiency include: shortness of breath, shallow breathing, wheezing, chronic cough, dyspnea, copious sputum, pale complexion, and spontaneous sweating.[6,8] Codonopsis deepens respiration, regulates respiratory secretions, and aids in preventing respiratory infections. It is a prophylactic treatment for individuals prone to frequent colds, influenza, and respiratory infections; however, it should be discontinued during an acute infection. It is compounded with huang qi *(Astragalus)*, lycii *(Lycium barbarum)*, and shan yao *(Dioscorea batatas, D. opposita)* in "change of seasons soup" to strengthen resistance during seasonal weather shifts.[10] It can be combined with huang qi *(Astragalus)*, echinacea *(Echinacea)*, and red root *(Ceanothus)* to hasten recovery from mononucleosis.[8]

Codonopsis aids in treating individuals with weakened resistance resulting from chemotherapy, surgery, lack of sleep, travelling, aging, or a severe infection. It also has radioprotective qualities.[7] It is often included in *fu zheng* therapy as an adjunct to chemotherapy, increasing its effectiveness, supporting the immune system, and countering side effects.[8] Administered as a daily tea or soup stock in the fall through the spring, it prevents lower respiratory infections in susceptible individuals.

Codonopsis is an adaptogen and restorative agent that replenishes the vital force.[8,9] It increases endurance and stamina, reducing fatigue and debility.[7-9] Codonopsis improves physical and mental performance, and enhances concentration and mood.[7-9] It has mild central nervous system stimulating effects.[7-9] Codonopsis also exhibits an adrenolytic and antistress effect in mice.[7]

Codonopsis is often substituted for *Panax ginseng* because it is considerably less expensive; however, it is not as potent as ginseng, nor does it contain ginseng saponins.[6,7,10] Codonopsis is a subtle energizer, yet it is not as overheating or overstimulating to the nervous system as *P. ginseng*.[8,10]

A stomach and spleen qi tonic, codonopsis improves digestion and assimilation.[8] Symptoms of spleen qi deficiency include: lack of appetite, abdominal distension, fatigue, lethargy, weakness in the extremities, loose stools, and diarrhea.[6] Consumed as a long-term tonic, codonopsis aids in managing anorexia, chronic fatigue syndrome, digestive ulcers, leaky gut syndrome, irritable bowel syndrome, Crohn's disease, and chronic, non-infectious diarrhea. Attributed to oroxylin A, codonopsis demonstrated antihistaminic effects in isolated guinea pig ileum.[7] In rodent studies, codonopsis prevented ulcer formation.[7] It regulates stomach acid secretions and aids in treating dyspepsia and hyperacidity.[4] Due to the qi tonifying properties, codonopsis also helps to restore prolapsed organs, including the uterus, rectum, bladder, and stomach.[6] It is often combined with bai zhu *(Atractylodes macrocephala)* to treat spleen qi deficiency.[6] Codonopsis is compounded with huang qi *(Astragalus)* to treat lung and spleen qi deficiency.[6]

Due to the spleen qi tonifying and nourishing effects, codonopsis is often included in blood tonifying compounds, because blood tonifying herbs can be dense, cloying, and difficult to digest. Spleen qi tonics build blood and enhance the digestibility of blood tonifying herbs. Symptoms of blood deficiency include: pale lips, face, and tongue, menstrual irregularity, palpitations, dry skin, lethargy, dizziness, and vertigo.[6] Codonopsis is a blood building, restorative agent. It aids in replenishing women who have menorrhagia, anemia, and individuals who feel depleted after menstruation and following childbirth; it is especially helpful for women who have hemorrhaged.[4,10] It also increases breast milk production and the nourishment of breast milk.[10] To optimize the blood tonifying effects, combine codonopsis with spleen qi tonics such as huang qi *(Astragalus)*, fu ling *(Poria)*, and bai zhu *(Atractylodes)*, as well as blood tonifying herbs such as shu di huang *(Rehmannia)* and dong quai *(Angelica sinensis)*.

Codonopsis has hypotensive and peripheral vasodilating effects that aid in treating stress-related hypertension.[6,7] Enhancing blood quality and increasing blood volume improves circulation.

CONTRAINDICATIONS

Codonopsis should be avoided in individuals with a fever, qi stagnation, damp obstruction, bloating, or infectious diarrhea, as well as those with yin deficiency with heat signs (hot flashes or night sweats).[6] Discontinue use with an infectious viral or bacterial infection such as a cold, influenza, or bronchitis.[8] Avoid use in individuals with elevated hemoglobin levels.[8] Traditional sources state that it should not be combined with li lu *(Veratrum)*.[6,7]

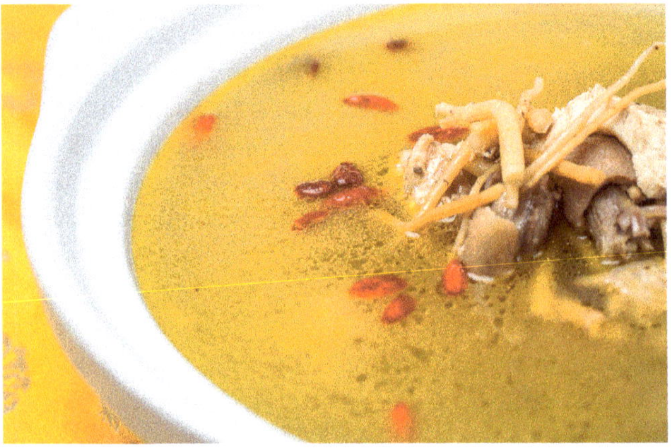

PREPARATION AND DOSAGE

TINCTURE: Fresh roots [1:2, 70-95% alcohol]; dry roots [1:5, 60% alcohol]; consume 20-60 drops, up to three times daily.

CAPSULES: Consume 2-4 "00" capsules, up to three times daily.

TEA: Prepare a decoction or cold infusion; consume 8-12 ounces, up to three times daily.

HONEY AND SYRUP: Prepare syrup by simmering a root decoction to one-half the volume; add honey to desired sweetness; consume 1 tablespoon, up to three times daily.

CULINARY USE: Add a bundle of root slices (one to two inches in diameter) to bone, lamb, beef, or chicken broth or stew, or include while cooking grains or beans. Remove root slices before serving. Add 1-2 tablespoons of the powdered root to smoothies, vegetable juices, or nut butter.

COMFREY

DESCRIPTION

BOTANICAL NAMES:
Symphytum officinale
Additional species include *S. asperum, S. caucasicum, S. grandiflorum, S. orientale, S. tauricum, S. tuberosum,* and *S.* x *uplandicum* (Russian comfrey)

COMMON NAMES:
Comfrey, boneknit, boneset, knitbone, knitback, consound, blackwort, bruisewort, slippery root, yalluc, gum plant, ass ear
rohtoraunioyrtti (Finnish)
consoude, grande consoude, herbe aux coupures, oreille d'ane, sain-foin (French)
beinwell, blutwurz, schmerzwurz, schwarzwurz, wallwurz (German)
consolida maggiore (Italian)
okopnick (Russian)
suelda, consuelda, sinfito (Spanish)
vallört (Swedish)

FAMILY NAME:
Boraginaceae

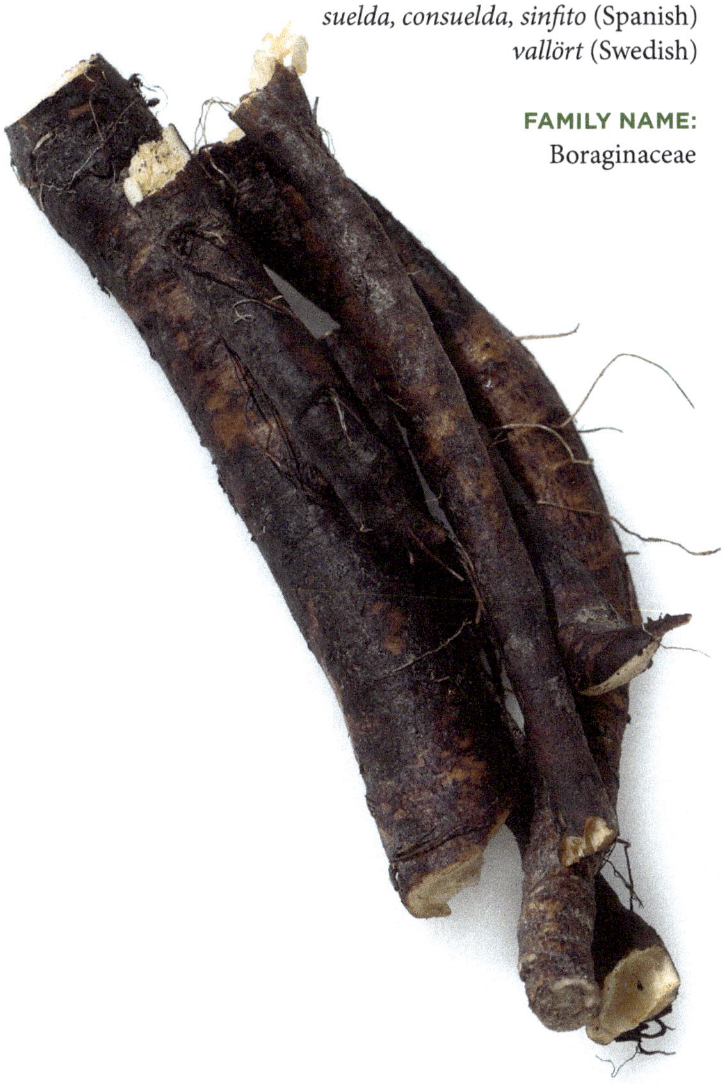

PARTS USED: The leaves and roots.

BOTANICAL DESCRIPTION AND HABITAT: Comfrey is native to Europe and temperate Asia, and was brought to the U.S. by European settlers. A perennial, it is easily cultivated, and when established, grows prolifically. In fact, many gardeners consider comfrey an invasive herb because it spreads easily. After planting, it is almost impossible to eradicate; it will sprout when the smallest root chunks are left in the soil.

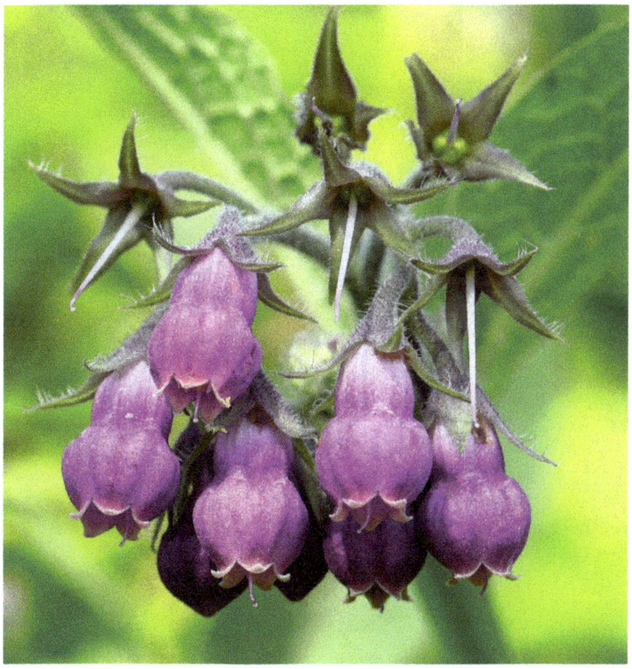

Symphytum officinale is a branching, herbaceous perennial covered in rough, bristly hairs.[1] Hollow stems grow 30 – 90 cm tall.[1,2] Thick roots (up to 30 cm long and 3 cm diameter) have juicy, white flesh and dark skin.[2] The lanceolate to ovate basal leaves (30 – 60 cm long by 10 – 20 cm wide) have acuminate apices and sometimes oblique bases.[1] The progressively smaller leaves on the upper half of the plant are sessile, with decurrent bases.[1] The inflorescence is a scorpioid cyme, bearing clusters of flowers with five-parted calyces.[3] The bell-shaped corollas (1.5 cm) have five tiny revolute lobes, and are light purple, purplish-red, or creamy yellow.[1] The superior ovary has two carpels divided into two more lobes that can develop into as many as four nutlets.[4] Often, only one of four nutlets will mature, as the ovaries are usually sterile.[1]

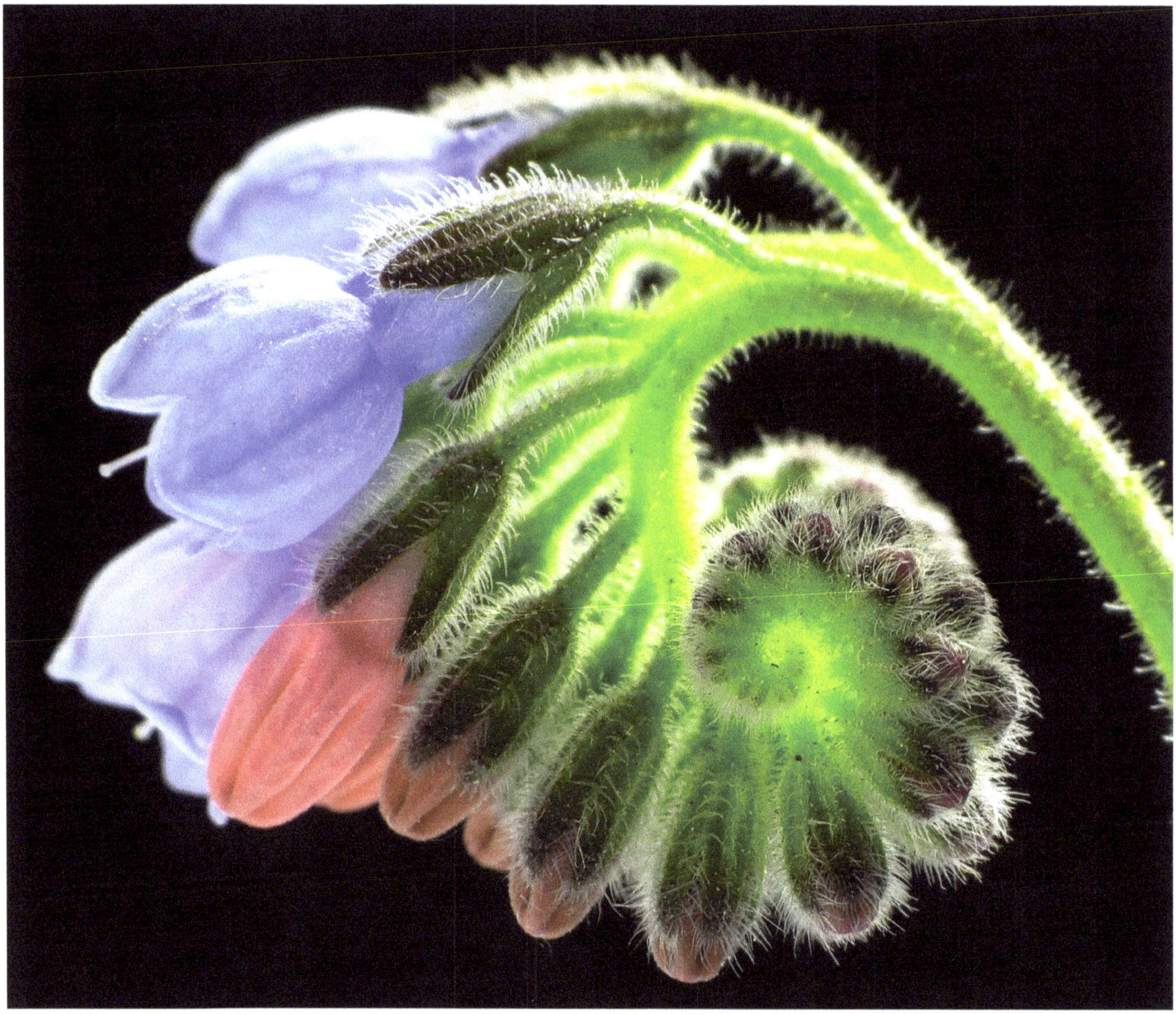

Symphytum officinale is often confused with *S.* x *uplandicum;* there are a few important distinctions. The stem internodes of *S. officinale* are winged, and the leaf bases are decurrent along the stem, while those of *S.* x *uplandicum* are not.[4] The fruit of *S. officinale* are black and shiny, while those of *S.* x *uplandicum* are brown and dull.[4] *S. officinale* flowers range from white to bluish purple; *S.* x *uplandicum* flowers tend to be purplish.

THE NAME: *Symphytum* derives from the Greek *symphyo* ("to unite or united"), referring to the fused corolla.[2] The species name *officinale* indicates its use as an official drug plant in the pharmacopeias. The common name comfrey is a corruption of *con firma,* referring to the uniting of bones, a primary effect of the herb.[2] The common names boneknit, boneset, knitbone, and knitback also allude to its reputation for mending bones.[2] The common name "ass ear" refers to the leaf shape.

HISTORICAL USES: A vulnerary agent, comfrey has a history of folk use — treating broken bones, gout, gangrene, cuts, wounds, bruises, ulcers, boils, abscesses, and hemorrhoids.[2] A root decoction has been used to treat diarrhea, dysentery, whooping cough, pulmonary complaints, and internal hemorrhage, as well as lung and stomach ulcers.[2] Comfrey roots were combined with dandelion and chicory roots as a coffee substitute. The young leaves were included as a pot herb, consumed as a vegetable, a substitute for spinach, and a flavoring for cakes.[2] In Ireland, comfrey was consumed to improve circulation and nourish blood.[2] A leaf poultice or fomentation was applied to sprains, swellings, indolent ulcers, boils, abscesses, cuts, gangrene, and inflamed tissues.[2]

CONSTITUENTS: *S. officinale* contains allantoin, mucopolysaccharides (composed of glucose and fructose), pyrrolizidine alkaloids (symphytine, echimidine, heliosupine, viridiflorine, echinatine, 7-acetyllycopsamine,

7-angelylretronecine, viridiflorate, lasiocarpine, and acetylechimidine), lithospermic acid, a gum consisting of L(-)-xylose, L-rhamnose, L-arabinose, D-mannose, and D-glucuronic acid, pyrocatechol tannins, carotene, isobauerenol, β-sitosterol, stigmasterol, steroidal saponins, triterpenoids, and rosmarinic acid.[5,6]

S. asperum contains the pyrrolizidine alkaloids asperumine, echinatine, heliosupine, and 7-acetyllycopsamine. *S.* x *uplandicum* contains the pyrrolizidine alkaloids symphytine, symlandine, echimidine, 7-acetyllylcopsamine, 7-angelylintermidine, uplandine, lycopsamine, and intermedine.[5]

NUTRITIONAL PROPERTIES: Comfrey leaf was traditionally consumed as a pot herb — a nourishing green added to soups. Dry leaf contains 14 – 35% protein; fresh leaf contains up to 22% protein.[5,7] Additionally, the leaf contains high amounts of vitamins A and C, calcium, chromium, dietary fiber, manganese, niacin, potassium, riboflavin, selenium, and silicon. It contains low to average amounts of aluminum, fat, iron, magnesium, phosphorus, sodium, thiamine, and tin.[5-7] *See Safety Concerns.*

MEDICINAL PROPERTIES: Anti-inflammatory, astringent, demulcent, emollient, expectorant, hemostatic, and vulnerary.

TEMPERATURE AND FLAVOR: Cool, sweet, bland, bitter, and astringent.

MEDICINAL USES

COMFREY ROOTS AND LEAVES: Comfrey is an esteemed vulnerary. As the folk name boneknit suggests, this herb has an impressive ability to mend bones and connective tissue.[2] Due to its allantoin content, it stimulates epithelial tissue regeneration.[2,5,7,10] Consumed internally or applied topically, comfrey hastens the healing of broken bones, fractures, sprains, strains, bruises, cuts, abrasions, skin ulcers, hemorrhoids, varicose veins, and leg ulcers.[2,5,7,9-11] A poultice, fomentation, or salve can be applied topically to alleviate tendonitis, arthritis, gout, joint pain, and back injuries.[2] Comfrey also accelerates post-surgical healing. Topical applications of comfrey root reduce inflammation following radiation treatments. Prepare an all-purpose salve by combining comfrey with calendula *(Calendula)*, St. John's wort *(Hypericum)*, chamomile *(Matricaria)*, lavender *(Lavandula)*, and arnica *(Arnica)*. *Note:* Do not apply arnica to broken skin.

A hemostatic, comfrey staunches bleeding from injuries.[2,5,7] It reduces passive bleeding in the digestive tract due to stomach or duodenal ulcers, ulcerative colitis, or hemorrhoids.[2] A tea that reduces intestinal bleeding is comprised of comfrey, chamomile *(Matricaria)*, and smaller amounts of cinnamon *(Cinnamomum)*, yarrow *(Achillea)*, meadowsweet *(Filipendula)*, and raspberry leaf *(Rubus)*. A sitz bath reduces inflammation and bleeding due to hemorrhoids and vaginitis.

COMFREY ROOTS: Comfrey root has similar properties as the leaf; however, it contains much higher quantities of mucilage. Water-based preparations have demulcent, emollient, and anti-inflammatory actions. Root poultices and fomentations also have emollient properties.[7]

A soothing demulcent, a comfrey root decoction used short-term reduces inflammation, stimulates healing in mucous membranes, and reduces intestinal permeability.[9] It also eases digestive conditions such as acid indigestion, gastroesophageal reflux disease (GERD), gastric and duodenal ulcers, diarrhea, and constipation.[2,5,7,9] Comfrey tea can be consumed following an intestinal infection, or during flareups of Crohn's disease, ulcerative colitis, or irritable bowel syndrome. Administer an enema to reduce rectal or colon inflammation. Combine comfrey root with marshmallow *(Althaea)*, fennel *(Foeniculum)*, cardamom *(Elettaria)*, and a small quantity of licorice *(Glycyrrhiza)* to soothe the digestive tract.

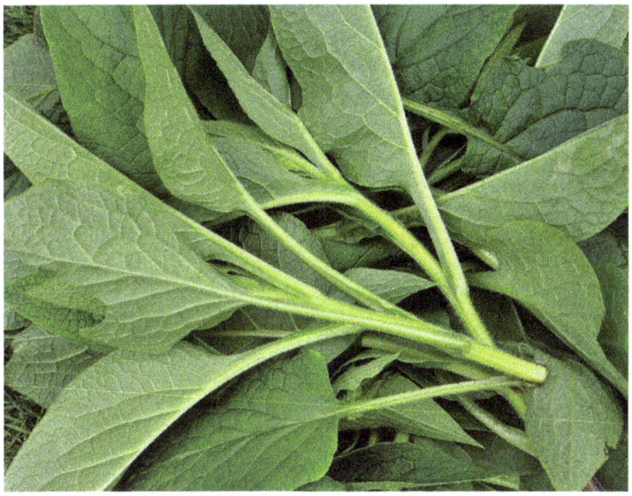

Comfrey root has expectorant and mild astringent properties.[5,7,9] The gargle and tea aid in treating a sore throat, laryngitis, pharyngitis, tonsillitis, and hoarseness, and can be used as a mouthwash for bleeding gums.[2,5] A decoction of the roots is a useful adjunct for treating a dry cough resulting from lung infections, such as bronchitis or whooping cough.[2,5,7,9] Combine it with marshmallow

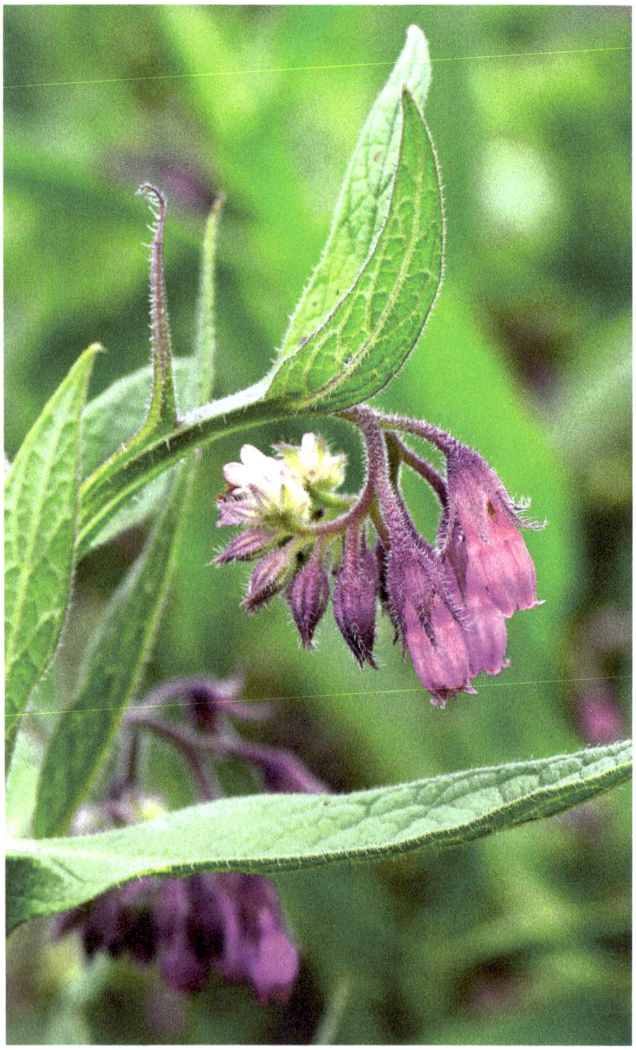

(*Althaea*), anise (*Pimpinella*), cardamom *(Elettaria),* and smaller amounts of licorice (*Glycyrrhiza*).

Comfrey root decoction decreases inflammation in the urinary tract, and discomfort accompanying cystitis, urethritis, and kidney stones. However, it is not an anti-infective; additional antibacterial agents are needed to treat a urinary tract infection.

SAFETY CONCERNS

In recent years, internal use of comfrey has been scrutinized by the FDA. Comfrey has acquired a bad reputation, and concerns have arisen following several studies on the effects of the pyrrolizidine alkaloid (PA) content, as well as PA contamination of grains caused by other plants including *Heliotrope* and *Crotalaria.* The accumulation of PAs caused veno-occlusive liver disease (VOLD), a condition characterized by a restriction of blood flow in the liver due to clotting in the portal veins. The following information summarizes the research that instigated the safety issues regarding the internal use of comfrey.

A 1991 Canadian experiment by Dr. Dennis Awang, head of the Health and Welfare Canada's Natural Products Section, found that Russian comfrey *(S.* x *uplandicum)* and prickly comfrey *(S. asperum)* contain up to eight PAs.[7] These alkaloids include symphytine and echimidine.[7] Echimidine, considered the more toxic of the two, was found in both species; however, it was not found in common comfrey *(S. officinale).*[7,8] The primary alkaloid in *S. officinale* is symphytine.[7]

Questions about comfrey's safety also arose following an experiment by Japanese researchers. In this study, a diet of 0.5 – 8% comfrey root and leaf was fed to rats for 600 days.[7] After 180 days, liver toxicity was recorded, and all groups developed liver tumors.[7] However, the researchers used Russian comfrey *(S.* x *uplandicum)* that contains higher quantities of pyrrolizidine alkaloids and echimidine. Based on this experiment, the FDA concluded that internal consumption of comfrey, regardless of the species, should be banned in the U.S., despite the fact that the comfrey used in the experiment was a different species than the one recommended by herbalists (though sometimes inadvertently dispensed by them). Another issue not considered was that the rats consumed considerably higher quantities of comfrey than normally consumed by humans. It is highly questionable whether it is scientifically accurate to extrapolate to humans, data collected on different *Symphytum* species containing an alkaloid not present in *S. officinale.*[7]

Several occurrences of PA intoxication in humans from internal consumption of comfrey were reported. In one case, a 49-year-old woman displayed symptoms of veno-occlusive liver disease (VOLD) after consuming comfrey tea and comfrey-pepsin pills for four months. Another case of VOLD developed in a 13-year-old boy who consumed comfrey tea for inflammatory bowel disease during a two- to three-year period. A third case of VOLD and death occurred when a 23-year-old, vegetarian, New Zealand male subsisted for weeks on a single dietary item including comfrey leaves.[7] It is unknown which species (and the plants' PA content) these individuals consumed, especially as some comfrey may be mislabeled regarding its true species.

Another situation raising questions about comfrey's safety occurred when a PA-containing plant, *Heliotrope,* contaminated a batch of wheat seeds.[7] The weedy *Heliotrope* commonly grew in the grain fields of Afghanistan during a two-year drought. The heliotrope-contaminated wheat was consumed as a staple diet in a northern Afghanistan population.[7] These individuals ingested approximately three mg of toxic alkaloids per day over a two-year period, resulting in widespread liver impairment and VOLD.[7] A similar situation occurred in Sarguja, India, when commercially produced breakfast cereal was contaminated with the seeds of a PA-containing *Crotalaria.*[7] Nearly 70 people who ate the contaminated cereal became ill with signs of PA poisoning characterized by liver necrosis, and nearly one-half of these patients died.[7]

It is important to understand the difference in PA content of the roots and leaves. Roots contain the highest levels of pyrrolizidine alkaloids, up to ten times higher than leaves.[7] The first spring cutting of leaves contains the second highest levels of pyrrolizidine alkaloids (0.026% or 260 parts per million on a dry weight basis).[7] The second and consecutive cuttings of leaves are much lower in pyrrolizidine alkaloid content (0.005% or five parts per million); therefore, they are safer for internal consumption.[7] Use the first growth of leaves for topical preparations or garden mulch, or make a compost tea to nourish other plants in the garden.[7] As a cautionary measure, internal consumption with the first cutting of leaves should be avoided. Limit internal consumption to the second cutting of leaves in order to minimize PA exposure.

While the effects of PA toxicity are alarming and present concerns about long-term internal use, VOLD is most likely to occur when PAs are consumed in high amounts for long periods of time. Because of the potential cumulative effects of PAs, internal consumption of comfrey root should be limited to six weeks per year. Another option for internal use is to purchase PA-free comfrey, available through several herbal companies. Homeopathic *Symphytum* tablets are another alternative for individuals concerned about PA safety. They can be administered to stimulate bone mending, and do not contain PAs. Topical use of the herb is considered safe.[10]

CONTRAINDICATIONS

Young children, pregnant or lactating women, and the elderly should avoid using comfrey internally.[11] Topical use is acceptable, as are internal uses of homeopathic preparations and PA-free comfrey products.[10] Internal use of comfrey is contraindicated in those who consume alcoholic beverages regularly, use prescription or over-the-counter medications that compromise liver function or induce liver damage, or individuals with existing liver conditions or liver damage. Avoid consuming comfrey products in high doses for long periods of time, due to the cumulative effects of pyrrolizidine alkaloids. Avoid consuming comfrey internally more than six weeks per year.[11] When used in small amounts in moderation, it is unlikely to cause problems in healthy individuals.[7]

Topical applications of comfrey should be used cautiously when treating deep wounds.[11] Comfrey is not an anti-infective herb. Be sure to disinfect the wound before treating with the topical use of comfrey.

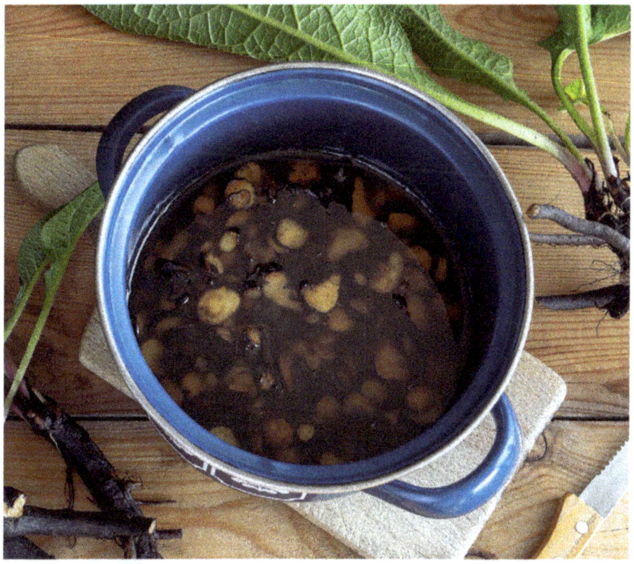

PREPARATION AND DOSAGE

TINCTURE: Fresh roots [1:2, 70-95% alcohol]; second cutting of fresh leaves [1:2-1:3+, 70-95% alcohol]; dry leaves [1:5, 60% alcohol]; consume 5-60 drops, up to three times daily.

TEA: Prepare an infusion of the leaf or decoction of the root; consume 4-8 ounces, up to three times daily.

HONEY: Fresh root honey [1:4]; consume 1 teaspoon, up to three times daily.

TOPICAL PREPARATIONS: Prepare leaf oil using the alcohol intermediary oil method, or infuse the leaves or root using the double boiler method. Apply comfrey topically as a poultice, fomentation, cream, salve, ointment, balm, paste, wash, bath, sitz bath, mouthwash, vaginal irrigation, or enema.

COPTIS

DESCRIPTION

BOTANICAL NAMES:
Coptis chinensis, C. deltoidea, C. japonica, C. laciniata, C. occidentalis, C. quinquefolia var. *trifololiata, C. trifolia* subsp. *groenlandica*

COMMON NAMES:
Coptis, goldthread, canker root, mouth root, yellow root, vegetable gold, coptide, Japanese coptis
huang lian, chuan lian, wei lian (Chinese)
oren (Japanese)
hwangnyon (Korean)
mahmira, tita, mishmi bitter, mishmi tita, hwang-lien, chuen-lien (Sanskrit)

FAMILY NAME:
Ranunculaceae

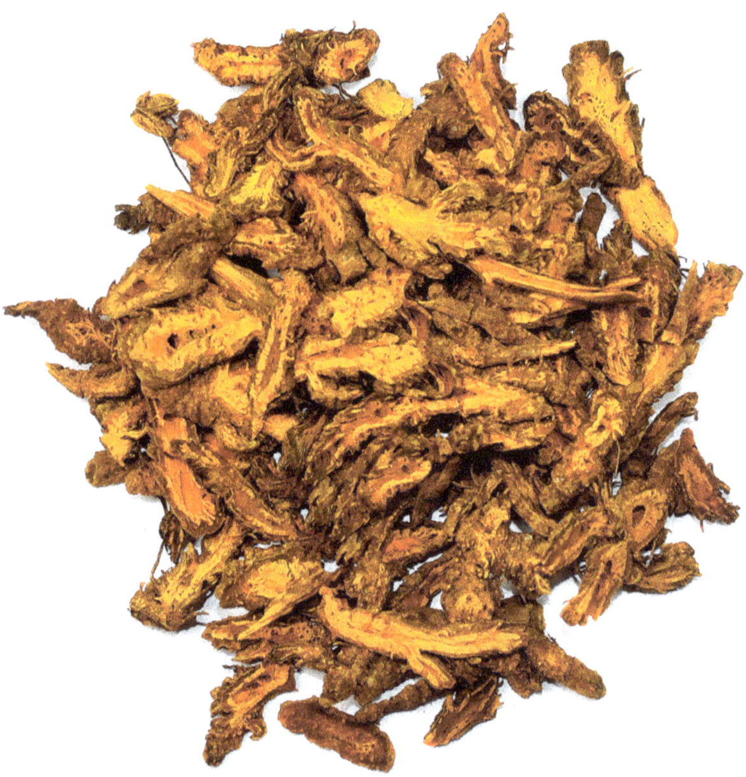

PART USED: The rhizomes.

BOTANICAL DESCRIPTION AND HABITAT: Members of the *Coptis* genus are petite, herbaceous perennials.[1] As indicated by some of their names, they have slender, golden yellow rhizomes. A small basal rosette of leaves with long petioles emerges from the rhizomes.[1] The genus varies according to the leaf structure; depending on the species, it can be ternately or pinnately compound, or simple,

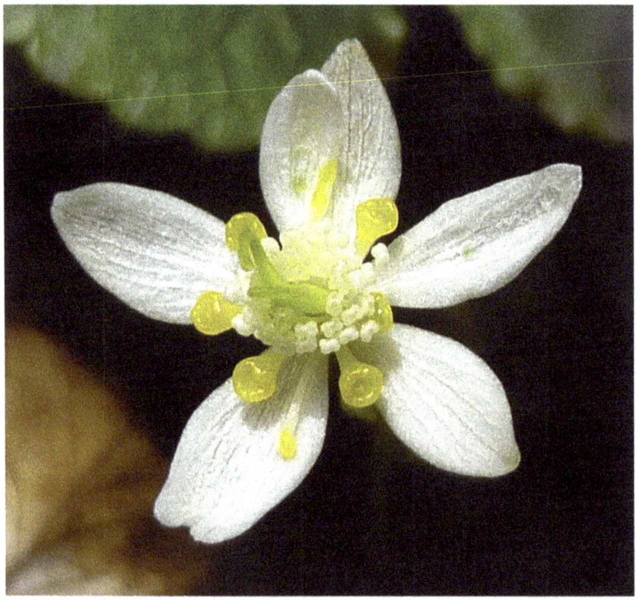

but deeply lobed. Those with compound leaves may have ovate or deltate leaflets with serrate margins.[2] Terminal scapose cymes (up to 3 cm when in flower, 9 cm in fruit) usually bear bisexual, staminate flowers.[2] Each flower consists of five white to greenish yellow, often petal-like sepals, and five to ten or more unusual club-shaped or linear, green, clawed petals (2 – 7 mm long).[1,2] Within are 10 to 60 stamens and 4 to 15 separate pistils on long stalks.[2] The fruits are oblong follicles, also on stalks, with short residual styles.[1]

Coptis chinensis grows in China's Sichuan, Hubei, Shaanxi, and Ganxu provinces; *C. deltoidea* is found in Sichuan.[3] *Coptis occidentalis* grows throughout the western U.S.

THE NAME: The genus *Coptis* derives from the Greek *kopto* ("to cut"), referring to the leaves' lacerated appearance.[4] The finely dissected leaves also explain the origin

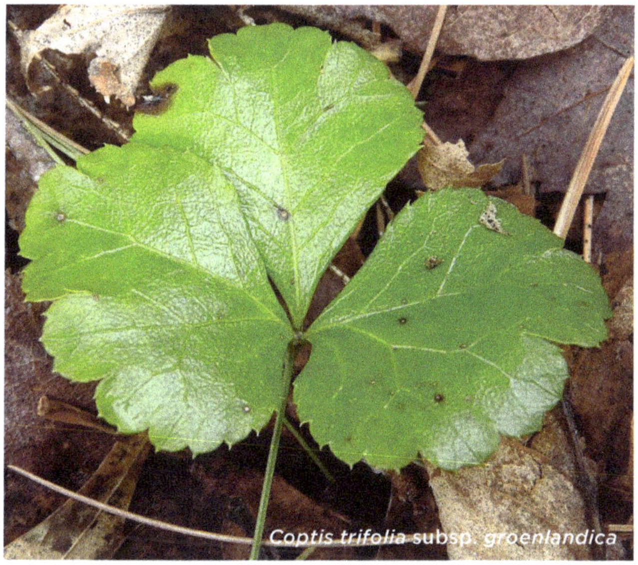
Coptis trifolia subsp. groenlandica

of the epithet *lacinata*, deriving from the Latin *lacerare* ("to lacerate or tear"). The epithet *chinensis* indicates the plant's origin in China. *Deltoidea* ("triangular") refers to the triangular leaf shape, and derives from *delta*, the third letter of the Greek alphabet, depicted by a triangle.[5] The epithet *japonica* refers to the plant's origin in Japan. The epithet Latin *occidentalis* ("of the west") indicates its origin in North America. The pin yin name *huang lian* translates as "yellow links."[3]

HISTORICAL USES: Coptis was first described in the *Shen Nong Ben Cao Jing*, an ancient medical text written during the Han Dynasty. It was noted as an herb for clearing heat and toxins. It was also mentioned later in a classical materia medica from the Ming Dynasty, *Ben Cao Gang Mu*, which described its use for eye diseases and diarrhea.[6]

Rarely growing abundantly, coptis has been a treasured herb. Due to its utility, a closely related species, *Coptis teeta*, was domesticated and has been semi-cultivated in forest settings in Yunnan province for more than 50 years, like American ginseng in the U.S.[7] In the Yunnan province, the whole plant was consumed as a decoction to enhance detoxification, and treat eczema and diarrhea.[7] In Japan, coptis was used to alleviate intestinal catarrh.[8] *Coptis japonica* was traditionally utilized in Japan to create a yellow silk dye.[9] In India, coptis was consumed as a digestive bitter tonic to ease stomach problems.[8] Eclectic physicians administered coptis as a digestive bitter tonic for digestive disorders.[10] They applied the decoction or tincture to treat infant thrush.[10] Coptis was used similarly to golden seal *(Hydrastis)*.[10]

CONSTITUENTS: Coptis contains protoberberine alkaloids (berberine, coptisine, and berberastine) and benzophenanthridine alkaloids (worenine, palmatine, columbamine, obacunone, obaculactone, palmatine, jatorrhizine, magnoflorine, and ferulic acid).[3]

NUTRITIONAL PROPERTIES: Not applicable.

MEDICINAL PROPERTIES: Antibacterial, antifungal, anti-inflammatory, antiprotazoal, antiviral, astringent, bitter tonic, cholagogue, choleretic, and "heat clearing."

TEMPERATURE AND FLAVOR: Cold and bitter.

MEDICINAL USES

Coptis contains berberine, a constituent with broad-spectrum antimicrobial activity.[3] Berberine is bacteriostatic in lower concentrations and bactericidal in higher concentrations.[3] Berberine has been shown to inhibit the growth of hemolytic *Streptococcus pneumonia, Neisseria meningitidis,* and *Staphylococcus aureus.*[3] It also has potent antibacterial effects against *Bacillus dysenteriae, Shigella dysenteriae,* and *S. flexneri,* treating dysentery and traveler's diarrhea.[3] However, berberine is ineffective against *Shigella somnei, Pseudomonas aeruginosa,* and *Salmonella paratyphi.*[3] Coptis was found to be as effective as penicillin, or the combination of penicillin and a sulfa drug for treating scarlet fever.[3] A 10% solution of coptis was administered to 44 patients with scarlet fever, all of whom recovered.[3] In human studies, coptis successfully treated diphtheria.[3] Coptis also aids in treating urinary tract and ear infections.[3,11]

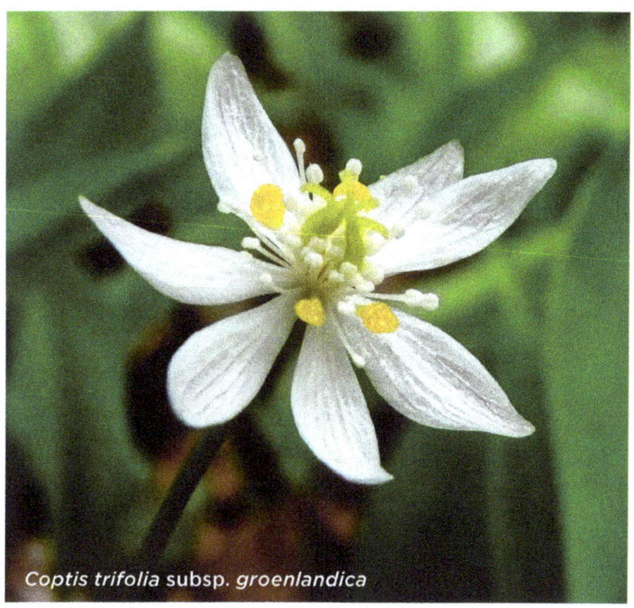
Coptis trifolia subsp. *groenlandica*

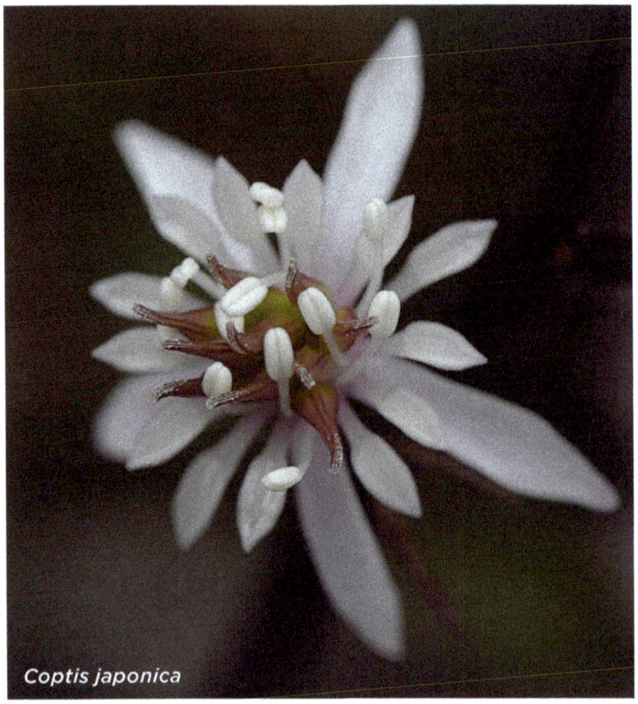

Coptis japonica

Coptis and berberine were found to prevent herpes simplex virus (HSV) cell penetration in HSV-1 and HSV-2.[11,12] Its mechanisms of action included: inactivation of viral particles, inhibition of viral absorption, penetration, and inhibition of viral replication and viral protein synthesis.[11,12] Although it is sometimes used alone, coptis-containing patent formulas such as *Long Dan Xie Gan Wan/Tan/San* and *Ching Wei San* can be administered to treat HSV.[11,12] Numerous patients experience greater success in preventing and/or hastening the resolution of HSV outbreaks with a compound containing coptis, huang qin *(Scutellaria baicalensis),* huang bai *(Phellodendron),* and licorice *(Glycyrrhiza),* than with conventional Acyclovir treatment.

Coptis demonstrated antiviral effects against numerous influenza and Newcastle viruses in experimental studies on chicken embryos.[3] Internal and topical applications (eye washes) of coptis are effective for treating bacterial and viral conjunctivitis.[13] *Note:* When treating eye infections, it is important to make a fresh batch of tea daily to avoid introducing more bacteria, and strain the tea through a coffee filter to prevent the introduction of particulate matter.

Coptis has antifungal actions, and aids in treating *Candida albicans* infections that cause thrush, and intestinal and vaginal candida.[8,10,13] Local applications of coptis aid in treating thrush in infants.[8,10,13] Coptis works most effectively in alleviating a candida infection when consumed internally. Additionally, a local administration, such as vaginal irrigation, sitz bath, or suppositories also aid in treating vaginal candida infections.[13]

Coptis and berberine have antiprotozoal effects against *Entamoeba, Giardia, Leishmania,* and *Trichomonas.*[13] Berberine has potent effects against *Leptospira.*[3] Local applications containing 20% coptis treated vaginal *Trichomonas* (a parasitic infection) with a 95% cure rate.[3] In human subjects, coptis demonstrated effectiveness against typhoid fever.[3]

Short-term use of coptis aids in treating food or alcohol poisoning.[3] Coptis eases vomiting, acid regurgitation, diarrhea, and dysentery resulting from stomach or intestinal inflammation.[3] It also reduces bad breath, putrid-smelling belches, and diarrhea.[3] Due to its cold thermal nature, coptis is cooked in ginger juice *(jiang huang lian)* to stop vomiting and reduce stomach heat.[3] To alleviate damp-heat in the digestion with symptoms including diarrhea, vomiting, and belching, coptis is cooked in yu huang lian *(Evodia),* also known as Evodia fry.[3]

Coptis is a bitter tonic, choleretic, and cholagogue.[3,8,10] Consuming coptis 20 – 30 minutes before meals enhances digestive secretions, treating nonulcer dyspepsia and atonic indigestion.[8,10] Combine it with warming carminatives such as fennel *(Foeniculum)* and ginger *(Zingiber),* and a small quantity of licorice *(Glycyrrhiza).* Coptis reduces gallbladder inflammation, and aids in treating cholecystitis and cholethiasis.[3] It is included in compounds for treating hepatitis, jaundice, and other inflammatory liver conditions. For this purpose, coptis is used alone or combined with other heat-clearing, liver detoxifying herbs such as huang bai *(Phellodendron)* and huang qin *(Scutellaria).* In rodent studies, berberine was found to improve lipid metabolism, lowering serum cholesterol.[3] Berberine also lowered serum triglyceride levels and normalized cholesterol/phosphate ratio in rabbits fed a high cholesterol diet or given a thyroidectomy.[3] The cholagogue actions likely contribute to the cholesterol lowering effects.

In Traditional Chinese Medicine, coptis is used to drain fire and clear damp-heat with symptoms such as high fever, red tongue, rapid full pulse, irritability, disorientation, and delirium.[3] Coptis also reduces excessive heat with toxicity; symptoms include red eyes, sore throat, boils, carbuncles, and abscesses. Coptis has potent detoxifying actions and aids in toxin removal such as alcohol, drugs, or chemicals. Berberine increases the body's anti-inflammatory responses.[3] Coptis is compounded with other herbs to clear heart fire. It reduces irritability and insomnia due to a lack of communication between the heart and kidneys.[3]

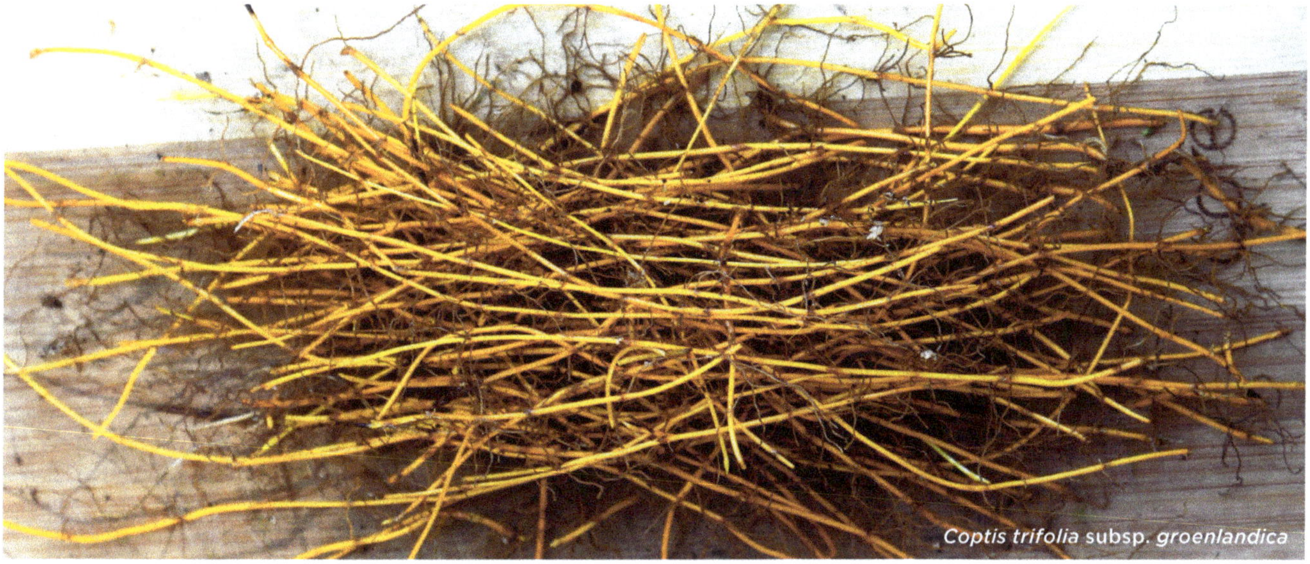

Coptis trifolia subsp. *groenlandica*

Topical preparations of coptis ointment or powder mixed with raw honey aid in healing burns, and decreasing the incidence of infection from second-degree burns. Topical applications of coptis promote healing of anal fissures, and decrease bleeding and itching.

Applying coptis ointment or washing the eyes with a well-strained, tepid tea aids in treating eye conditions such as allergic and bacterial conjunctivitis, blepharitis, inflamed eyelids, and hypersensitive eyes.[3,11] A water-based preparation, fomentation, and/or poultice reduce inflammation of acne, boils, abscesses, psoriasis, eczema, and canker sores.[3,13] Apply coptis topically as a wash, dust, powder, or poultice, or use as a diluted tincture as an antibacterial and antifungal for cuts, scrapes, abrasions, staph, athlete's foot, or ringworm. *Note:* Coptis applications can temporarily discolor the skin yellow and stain clothing.

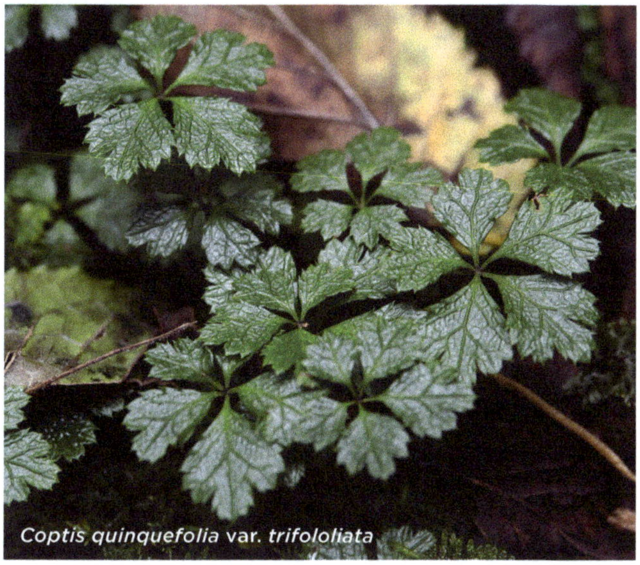

Coptis quinquefolia var. *trifololiata*

CONTRAINDICATIONS

Avoid internal use during pregnancy or lactation, and in infants.[13] Avoid use in cases of obstructive gallstones. Coptis can cause digestive disturbance.[13] High doses can cause gastrointestinal irritation such as nausea, vomiting, or diarrhea.[3,13] Combine coptis with other warming carminative herbs such as ginger to decrease the potential for digestive upset.[3] In Traditional Chinese Medicine, coptis is contraindicated in cases of yin deficiency, nausea or vomiting due to stomach cold from deficiency, or diarrhea due to spleen or kidney deficiency.[3] Avoid long-term internal use, as coptis can injure the stomach or spleen.[3]

PREPARATION AND DOSAGE

TINCTURE: Fresh whole plant or rhizomes [1:2, 70-95% alcohol]; dry rhizomes [1:5, 60% alcohol]; consume 15-60 drops, up to three times daily.

CAPSULES: Consume 2-4 "00" capsules, up to three times daily. Consume 4-8 Chinese herbal tea pills, up to three times daily.

TEA: Prepare a decoction; consume up to 4-8 ounces, up to four times daily.

TOPICAL USE: Apply the powdered root, ointment, oil (alcohol intermediary oil method), salve, wash, fomentation, or poultice. Create a medicated topical paste by adding powdered coptis root to honey.

CORDYCEPS

DESCRIPTION

BOTANICAL NAMES:
Cordyceps sinensis, C. ophioglossoides
(syn. *Ophiocordyceps sinensis*)

COMMON NAMES:
Cordyceps, caterpillar fungus, Chinese caterpillar fungus, deer fungus, deer fungus parasite, summer grass, winter worm, Chinese insect herb, insect herb, club-head fungus
tōchūkasō (Japanese)
tongch'unghach'o (Korean)
chóng cǎo, dōng chóng cǎo, dōng chóng xià cǎo (Mandarin)
yarchagumba, yarsagumba (Nepali)
yartsa gunbu (Tibetan)

FAMILY NAME:
Cordycipitaceae (Clavicipitaceae, Ophiocordycipitaceae)

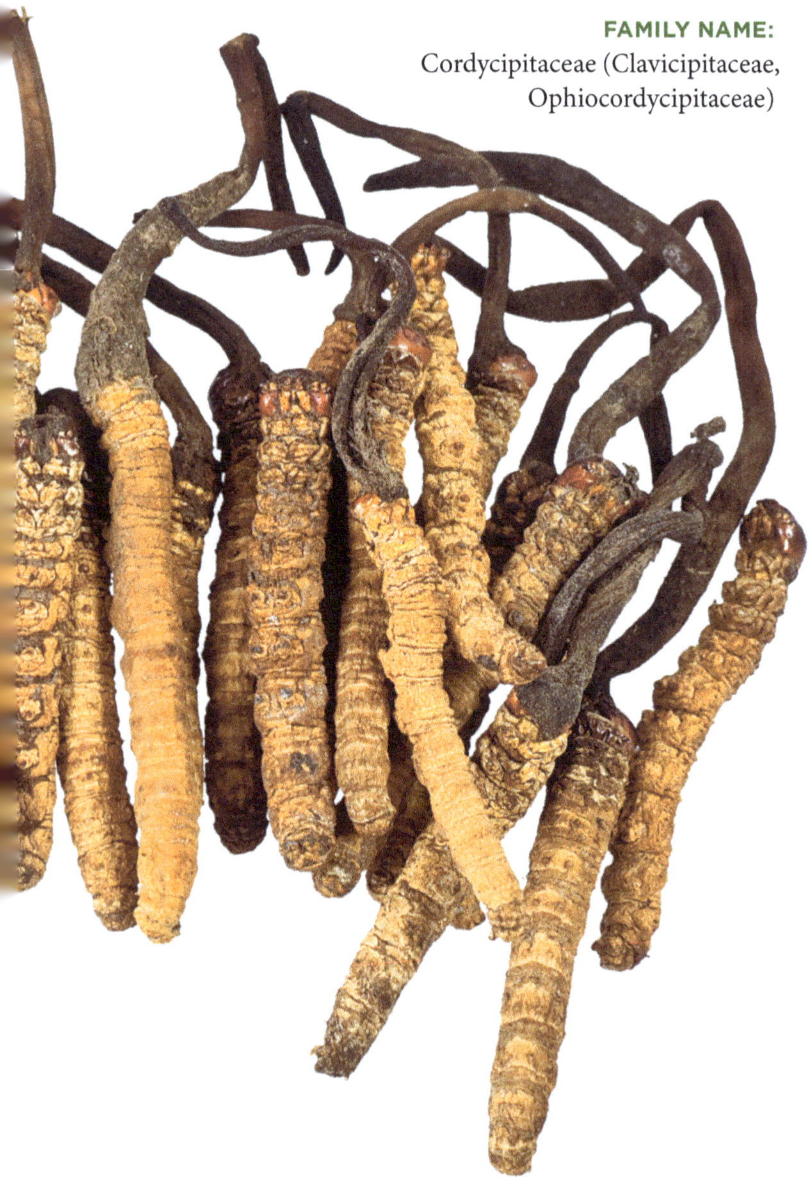

PARTS USED: The stroma, parasitized caterpillar larva, and mycelia. It is harvested in early summer when the fungus has emerged, before the larval body has disintegrated.

BOTANICAL DESCRIPTION AND HABITAT: *Cordyceps* is a genus of parasitic ascomycete fungi. They most commonly parasitize insects and their larvae, but certain North American species parasitize truffles.[1] The most commonly used species, *Cordyceps sinensis,* inhabits the

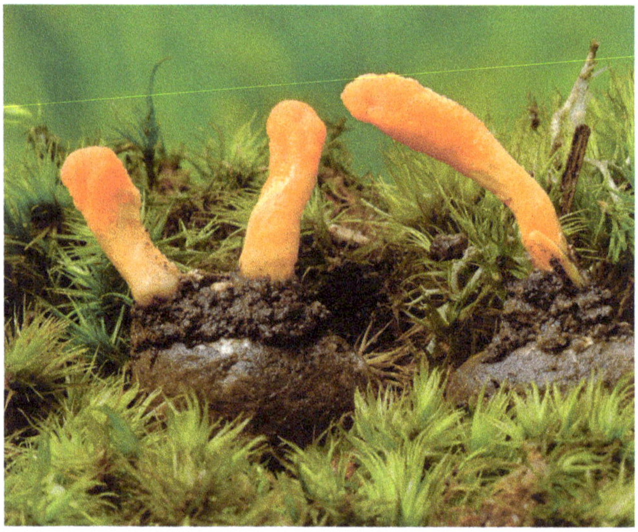

larvae of caterpillars from the genus *Thitarodes.*[2] *C. sinensis* grows in cold, grassy alpine meadows above 3,000 meters in Tibet, China, and other parts of the Himalayas.[2] The two main components of *Cordyceps* fungus are the parasitized larva body and the fungal stroma. In *C. sinensis,* the larva body (3 – 5 cm long, 3 – 8 mm diameter) is yellow-brown with 20 – 30 bands around the body, and eight pairs of feet on the abdomen.[3] The stroma is a black, cylindrical, club-shaped protrusion (4 – 7 cm in length, 3 mm in diameter) from the anterior of the larva body, with an acuminate apex.[3] The stroma bears fruiting bodies that release spores.[2] Cordyceps is commercially cultivated.

THE NAME: *Cordyceps* and *Ophiocordyceps* derive from the Latin *ophi* ("snake"), *cord* ("club"), and *ceps* ("head").[1] The epithet *sinensis* means "of or from China." The epithet *ophioglossoides* derives from *ophi* ("snake") and *gloss* ("tongue").[1] *Dōng chóng xià cǎo* translates as "winter bug, summer herb."[4]

HISTORICAL USES: The earliest records of cordyceps dating back to 200 CE appeared in Pen-ts'ao herbal *Sheng-nung Pan-ts'ao Ching — The Classic Herbal of the Divine Plowman,* and appeared later in 620 CE during the Tang Dynasty.[5,6] Prior to cultivation, cordyceps was rarely found in the wild and was reserved for use by the emperor and the royal family.[1,7] Cordyceps was stuffed into a duck's stomach and slowly roasted over a fire. It was then removed and the duck was consumed twice daily for up to ten days.[1,7] Cordyceps was also cooked with pork or duck and consumed to strengthen the body following depletion, or to treat impotence, neurasthenia, backache, anemia, and opium addiction.[1,7] Food-based preparations were given to nourish individuals recuperating from debilitating illnesses such as tuberculosis and pneumonia.[7] In Traditional Chinese Medicine, it was administered as a kidney yin and yang tonic to treat impotence or a weak lower back, and alleviate pain in the groin and knees.[1,6,8] Cordyceps was also used to treat weak lungs, asthma, and lowered resistance.[1,8] In Tibet, cordyceps was administered to treat heart and kidney problems, and increase libido.[7] In Japan, it was administered to treat impotence.[7]

In 1723, Jesuit priest Father Perennin returned to France bearing samples of cordyceps, and introduced the first medicinal, insect-associated mushroom to the Western world.[6] Soon after, Europeans began using fungi as mycopesticides to control crop pests.[6]

CONSTITUENTS: Cordyceps contains cordycepic acid = D-mannitol, polysaccharides, 18 amino acids, steak acid, mycose, ergosterol, ergosterol 3-O-β-D-glucopyranoside, ergosterol 3-O-β-D-galactopyranoside, uracil, adenine, adenosine, sterols, palmitic acid, cholesterol palmitate, cordycepin, glutamic acid, phenylalanine, proline, histadine, tyrosine, L-tryptophan, valine, oxyvaline, arginine, alanine, and vitamin B_{12}.[1,8]

NUTRITIONAL PROPERTIES: Cordyceps contains protein, fat, fiber, carbohydrates, saturated and unsaturated fatty acids (oleic and linoleic acids), 18 amino acids, uracil, uridine, adenine, adenosine, vitamins, and minerals.[1,8]

MEDICINAL PROPERTIES: Adaptogen, adrenal tonic, antiasthmatic, antiatherosclerotic, anti-inflammatory, antileukemic, antioxidant, antitumor, aphrodisiac, bronchodilator, expectorant, hepatoprotectant, hypocholesterolemic, hypoglycemic, hypolipidemic, immune modulator, immune stimulant, lung qi tonic, lung yin tonic, kidney yin tonic, kidney yang tonic, qi tonic, and nephroprotective.

TEMPERATURE AND FLAVOR: Warm, sweet, and bland.

MEDICINAL USES

Cordyceps is an impressive adaptogen that regulates the hypothalamic-pituitary-adrenal axis, and an adrenal tonic that enhances adrenal cortical function.[6,8] It is highly useful as a long-term tonic for individuals with adrenal insufficiency or adrenal "burnout."[6] Cordyceps is a regenerative agent for individuals with chronic stress, fatigue, or illness.[6] It tonifies qi, strengthening the vital force, and increasing stamina and endurance.[5,8] It counteracts the immune suppressing effects of cortisone and prednisone, and protects the adrenals from drug-induced atrophy. It also has hypnotic and calming actions.[1,6] The sedative actions are attributed to the amino acids: glutamic acid, tyrosine, and L-tryptophan.[1]

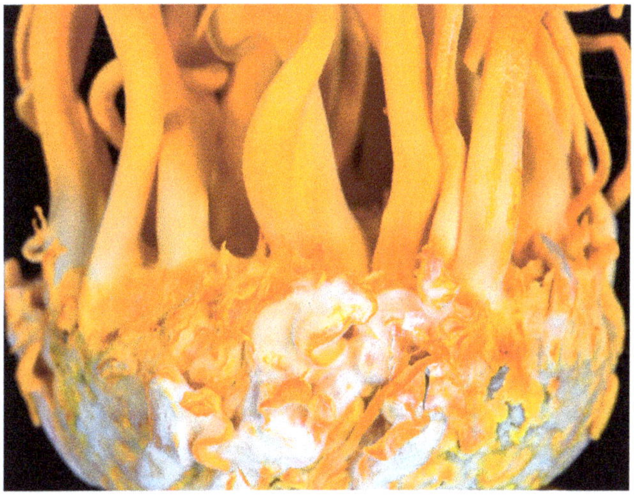

Cordyceps improves kidney function, and protects the kidneys from nephrotoxic drugs and chemical toxicity.[8] It aids in treating degenerative kidney disease, chronic pyelonephritis, glomerulonephritis, and Berger's disease, as well as acute and chronic kidney failure.[1,6,7] However, the previously listed conditions are very serious; consult a health care practitioner before attempting treatment with cordyceps.[6] Cordyceps increases creatinine clearance, decreases blood urea nitrogen (BUN), and decreases protein in the urine, all of which are markers of improved kidney function.[6,8] In a study of chronic renal failure, patients experienced significant improvement after consuming 5 grams of cordyceps for 30 days. Their red blood cell and hemoglobin counts significantly increased, serum creatinine levels improved 39%, BUN levels decreased 34%, proteins in the urine decreased 63%, and arterial blood pressure dropped 15%.[6] Cordyceps also reduces the nephrotoxic side effects of amikacin sulfate, prednisone, gentamicin, and chemotherapy.[5-8] In patients with kidney transplants, cordyceps counteracts the toxic side effects of gentamicin, and protects against the toxicity of cyclosporine — an immune

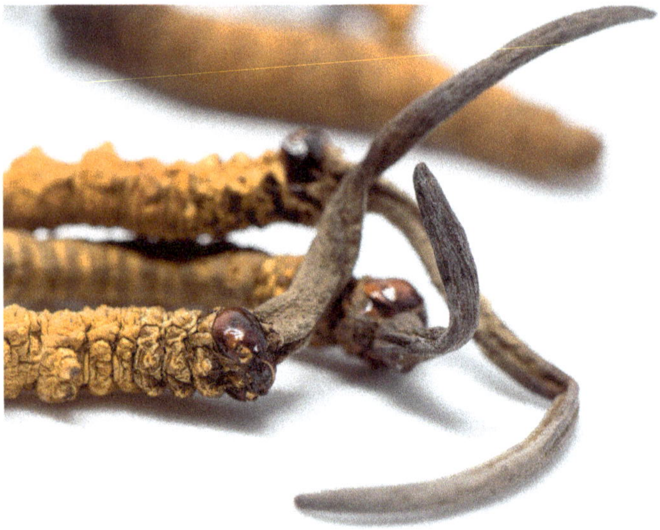

suppressant drug that prevents the immune system from rejecting a newly transplanted organ.[5,6] Cyclosporine can cause acute kidney failure because it constricts blood vessels and damages kidney cells. Cordyceps also helps to restore normal leukocyte levels, enhancing the infection-fighting capacity while one consumes immune suppressant drugs.[6]

Cordyceps is used in Traditional Chinese Medicine to enhance kidney function by strengthening and tonifying kidney yang and yin.[4,6,7] Symptoms of kidney yang deficiency include: exhaustion, fear of cold, cold extremities, sore or weak lower back, weakness in the lower extremities, impotence, spermatorrhea, infertility, enuresis, and dizziness.[4,7] Cordyceps increases libido and sexual vitality. It aids in treating impotence and spermatorrhea, increasing spermatogenesis, and improving sperm count.[1,7,8] Cordyceps improves yang function, warming the body and improving tolerance to the cold; as such, it aids in treating individuals with hypothyroidism.

Cordyceps is a sexual restorative agent that improves sexual and hormonal functions in males and females with low libido.[6] In clinical studies, impotent male subjects consumed one gram of cordyceps three times daily for 80 days. More than half of the subjects reported partial or complete restoration of their sexual function.[5,6] Cordyceps mycelium significantly increases 17-ketosteroid and 17-hydroxycorticosteroid levels that are low in impotent males.[1,6] It normalizes the plasma hormone levels of testosterone, cortisol, and estradiaol.[6]

Cordyceps is an immune amphoteric with immune stimulating and immune modulating actions.[1,7,8] It reduces an overreactive immune response, while increasing immune function when suppressed.[1,7] It contains polysaccharides that stimulate phagocytic functions and macrophage activity, especially in peritoneal macrophages.[1,5,6] Cordyceps stimulates interleukin 2, α- and β-interferon, as well as the IgM and IgG antibody response.[1,8] Additionally, it improves B- and T-lymphocyte production, and increases surface proteins on T-lymphocytes.[1] Cordyceps enhances T cell ratio, natural killer (NK) cell function, immunoglobulin levels, and serum complement levels.[1,7,8] It increases hemoglobin and red blood cell count, and aids in treating anemia.[1] Cordyceps aids in treating conditions with chronic immune suppression, such as chronic fatigue syndrome, HIV, AIDS, cancer, and diabetes. It is helpful with high inflammatory or autoimmune conditions, such as lupus, allergic asthma, and hay fever.[6-8]

Cordyceps is a long-term tonic that enhances respiratory function. It is prescribed in Traditional Chinese Medicine as a lung qi and lung yin tonic.[4] It has bronchodilator and expectorant actions.[1,5] It is a mucolytic that transforms phlegm and reduces bloody sputum.[4] Cordyceps aids in treating a chronic cough, asthma, respiratory weakness, chronic bronchitis, chronic obstructive pulmonary disease, pneumonia, wheezing, and lung cancer.[5-8] It also hastens recovery from lung infections such as pneumonia and bronchitis. Cordyceps has antibacterial actions against *Streptococcus, Burkholderia mallei* (syn. *Bacillus mallei*), *Bacillus anthracis, Pasteurella suiseptica, Staphylococcus, Microsporum gypseum,* and *Microsporum lanosum.*[1] In a promising study conducted at Jiangxi Medical College, patients with chronic bronchitis who consumed three grams of cordyceps three times daily experienced fewer bronchial spasms, coughing spells, and

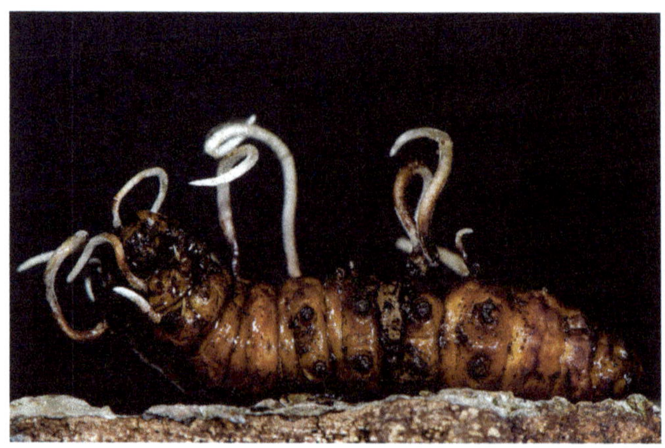

incidences of airway resistance. They also experienced significantly increased maximum breathing capacity and forced expiratory volume.[6] Researchers in the Department of Pulmonary Medicine at Jiang-Su Provincial Hospital found that patients with chronic bronchitis complicated by pulmonary heart disease or emphysema who consumed cordyceps experienced improved expectoration, had fewer asthmatic symptoms, caught fewer colds, and coughed less.[6]

Cordyceps improves the tolerance of chemotherapy and radiation, potentiates the effects, reduces side effects, and hastens recovery.[8] It has bone marrow protective effects, antileukemic activities, and reduces tumor size. Cordyceps is an adjunct therapy for treating lymphoma, B16 melanoma, and cancer in the lungs, breasts, liver, gastrointestinal tract, pancreas, prostate, cervix, and vagina.[1,6,8] Cordyceps also aids in treating precancerous conditions such as cervical dysplasia, and can be used as a preventative cancer treatment.[6] Cordyceps was found to have antitumor effects *in vivo*.[1,8] Protein-bound polysaccharides, CO-N and SN-C, are galactosaminoglycans that stimulate immune function and have a cytocidal action on tumors.[1] As an adjunct to conventional cancer treatment, consume 2 to 3.3 grams, three times daily.[6]

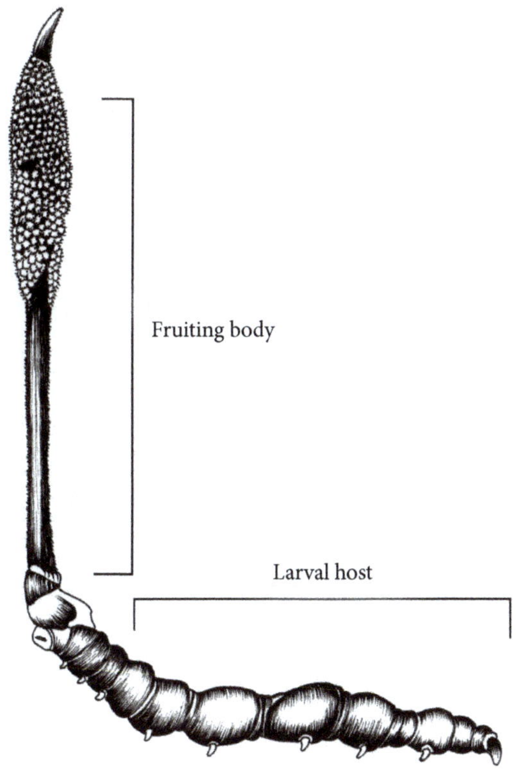

Cordyceps *(Cordyceps sinensis)*

Cordyceps is a cardiotonic and blood pressure normalizing agent.[5,8] It has positive inotropic and negative chronotropic effects.[1] Cordyceps dilates coronary arteries, increasing blood flow to the heart, and reducing myocardial oxygen consumption.[7] It aids in treating cardiac arrhythmia, pulmonary heart disease, and heart failure.[1,6,8] Cordyceps has antiatherosclerotic and hypolipidemic actions.[6,8] It decreases total cholesterol and triglyceride levels, low density lipids (LDL), and very low density lipids (VLDL), as well as increasing high density lipids (HDL).[1,6-8] It also has antioxidant actions that prevent free radical damage.[6-8]

Cordyceps has hepatoprotectant and hepatoregenerative actions.[8] It prevents liver and spleen atrophy, and improves liver function in individuals with hepatitis B or posthepatic cirrhosis.[1,5,6] It also enhances protein metabolism and raises plasma immunoglobulin levels.[6] Cordyceps has antiviral actions that aid in treating viral hepatitis.[5] It also regulates insulin and glucose, and aids in managing diabetes.[8]

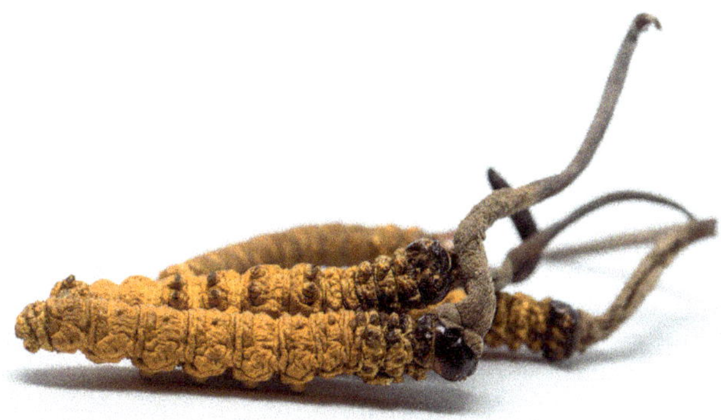

CONTRAINDICATIONS

Cordyceps has no known side effects, and is considered low in toxicity.[1,8]

PREPARATION AND DOSAGE

TINCTURE: Dry stromata and/or mycelia [1:4-1:5, 50% alcohol]; consume 30-120 drops, up to three times daily.

CAPSULES: Consume 3-6 "00" capsules or 3-9 grams of powder, one to two times daily.

TEA: Add ¼-1 teaspoon of powder to 8-10 ounces of hot water. Consume 1-2 cups daily.

CULINARY USE: Add ¼-1 teaspoon of powder to a smoothie, milk, yogurt, broth, or vegetable juice. Cordyceps is traditionally cooked with chicken, duck, pork, or fish stew to treat yin deficiency with heat signs and lowered resistance.[4]

CORN SILK

DESCRIPTION

BOTANICAL NAME:
Zea mays

COMMON NAMES:
Corn silk, maize
maïs (French)
mais (German)
maís (Icelandic)
jagung (Indonesian, Malay)
to-morokoshi (Japanese)
milho (Portuguese)
maíz (Spanish)
maiz (Taíno)

FAMILY NAME:
Poaceae (Gramineae)

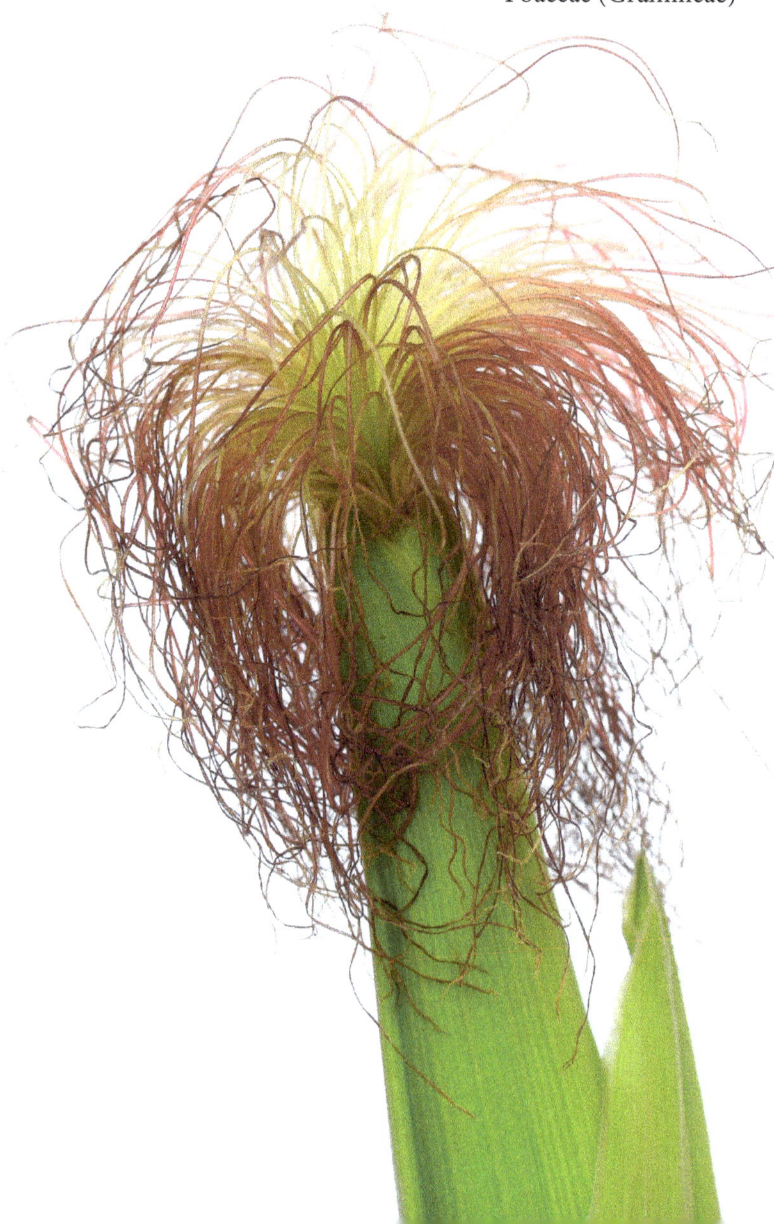

PARTS USED: The pistil stigmata and long styles form fine threads (corn silk) from the female flowers.

BOTANICAL DESCRIPTION AND HABITAT: Corn is an annual grass that thrives in warm climates in full sun with well drained, alkaline soil. It responds optimally in fertilized soil with a high nutrient content. There is one species of corn, *Zea mays,* and many varieties. Scientists believe that corn is autochthonous in the Americas, and is native to the southern U.S.[1] Others postulate that corn was domesticated from the wild plant teosinte, *Zea mexicana,* in Mexico's Tehuacan Valley.[2]

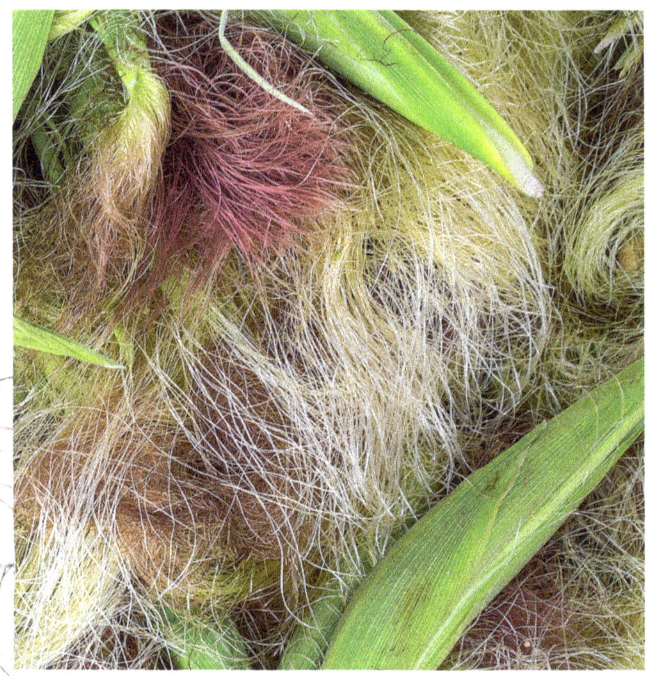

Corn is monoecious and grows approximately eight feet tall. Sessile, sheathing leaves (up to four feet long) grow from each node of the tall stem. Male spikelets bearing two florets each grow in terminal racemes called tassels. Female spikelets are held in inflorescences (ears) in the leaf axils within sheaths of leaves. Each ear has a pithy core (cob) on which the female flowers attach. Each female flower extends a long, silky, filamentous, greenish style (up to seven inches long) known as the corn silk. The silk protrudes out the end of the ear, eventually drying and shriveling up after pollination. The fruit is a caryopsis, or kernel, with a range of colors, including yellow, gray, red, purple, white, and black.[3]

THE NAME: The genus name *Zea* originates from ancient Greek, and is a generic term for cereal and grains. Some scientists believe it also means "sustains life." The species name mays is an adaption of the word maize, derived from the Spanish form of the indigenous Taíno word, maiz, meaning "life giver." The common name maiz originated from several languages, and evolved into the following names: maíz (Spanish), mais (German), maïs (French), and milho (Portuguese). Other common names for corn include jagung (Malaysian or Indonesian) and to-morokoshi (Japanese). In English-speaking countries besides the U.S., Canada, Australia, and New Zealand, the word corn can refer to any cereal, though usually it refers to the predominant cereal in a specific locale.

HISTORICAL USES: Corn is closely associated with the cultures of indigenous Americans for whom it is integral to many aspects of life, including ceremonies, rituals, myths, stories, traditions, and food. It was made into wafer bread known by various names, including *piki* (Hopi), *hewe* (Zuni), *mowa* (Rio Grande Tewa), and *guallabe* (New Mexican Spanish). Corn was also made into *atole,* a kind of gruel, and *posole,* hominy soup. People throughout South and Central America prepared a variety of fermented and non-fermented beverages from corn called *chicha,* and a spirit from corn stalk juice called *pulque de mahis.*[4] Corn flower (corn silk) tea was used to treat stubborn coughs and asthma.[1] It is speculated that corn was developed over 20,000 years, and all varieties developed before the Europeans arrived in the New World. For more accounts of the traditional uses of corn as food and medicine, and its historic and cultural contexts, refer to *Healing Herbs of the Upper Rio Grande.*

CONSTITUENTS: Corn silk contains a fixed oil, volatile oil (carvacrol and thymol), gums, resins, saponins, mucilaginous polysaccharides, sugars, bitter glucosidic substances, a crystallizable acid (maizenic acid), flavonoids (maysin), anthocyanins, allantoin, sterols (β-sitosterol and stigmasterol), an alkaloid (hordenine), hydrocarbons, cryptoxanthin, tannins, plant acids (malic and tartaric), minerals (potassium), and vitamins C and K.[5-7]

NUTRITIONAL PROPERTIES: Corn silk is rich in potassium, and contains vitamins C and K.

MEDICINAL PROPERTIES: Anti-inflammatory, bladder tonic, demulcent, diuretic, and emollient.

TEMPERATURE AND FLAVOR: Neutral, sweet, and bland.

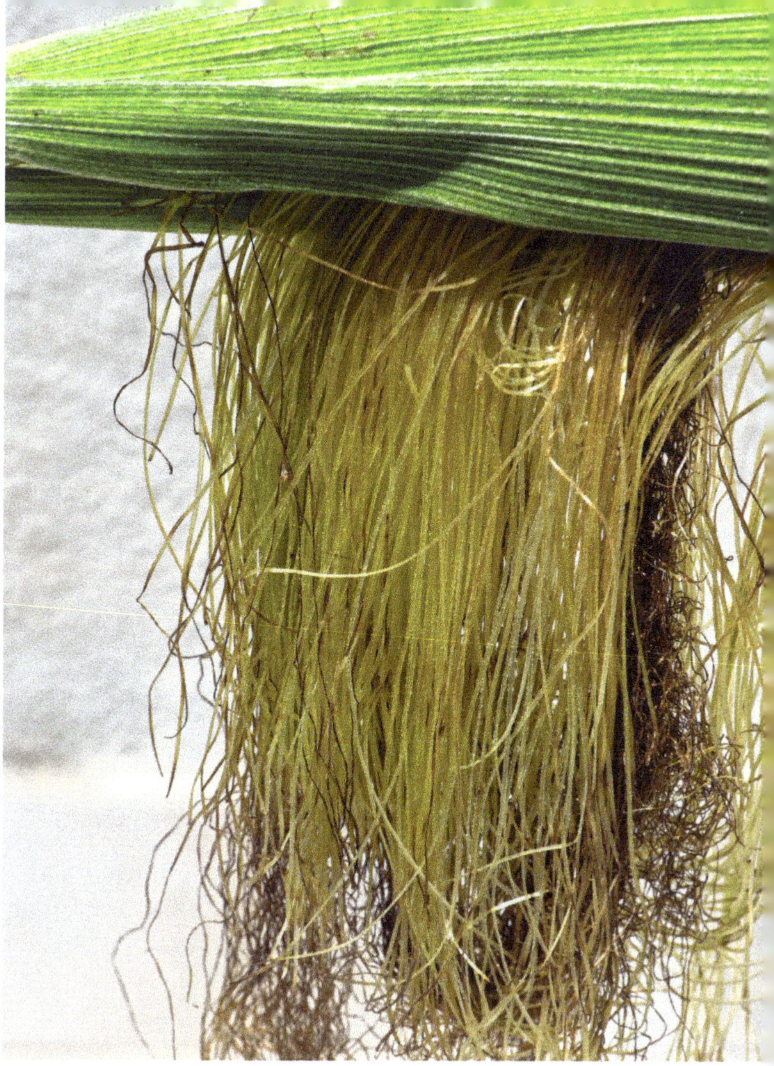

MEDICINAL USES

Corn silk is extremely beneficial for treating urinary conditions. The tea or tincture can be used as an antibacterial to treat cystitis and urethritis. Corn silk contains maizinic acid that is attributed to its antibacterial properties. It has astringent and demulcent properties that reduce inflammation in the mucous membranes lining the bladder and urethra. It eases sensations of pain, burning, and local irritation accompanying urinary tract infections. Corn silk also reduces symptoms such as frequent urination, as well as the sudden urge to urinate. It is most specific for urinary tract infections with alkaline urine. When treating urinary tract infections with herbs, combine corn silk with other diuretic and urinary tract antibacterial herbs such as uva ursi *(Arctostaphylos uva-ursi),* usnea *(Usnea),* and yarrow *(Achillea millefolium).*

Corn silk strengthens and tonifies the trigone muscle at the base of the bladder.[8] It can be used as a long-term treatment for chronic bladder problems. This herb is also highly beneficial for treating frequent bladder infections, pyelitis, and interstitial cystitis. It can be combined with mullein root *(Verbascum thapsus),* horsetail *(Equisetum* spp.), and saw palmetto *(Serenoa repens)* to synergize the bladder tonifying actions. Corn silk helps to treat incontinence resulting from bladder weakness. It works well for children who wet the bed frequently or feel the constant need to urinate when traveling. Corn silk can be used during pregnancy to treat a hyperreactive bladder and bladder weakness. It also strengthens a bladder weakened by pregnancy, childbirth, menopause, or aging. It is beneficial for treating a cystocele. Corn silk can be helpful for the long-term treatment of benign prostatic hypertrophy because it reduces urinary frequency. It can be used as a soothing recuperative agent following antibiotic treatment for prostatitis.

Corn silk is a soothing diuretic that subtly reduces discomfort from passing nonobstructive kidney stones. The tea aids in flushing the stones, and some herbalists claim it is an antilithic.

The mucilaginous polysaccharides have demulcent properties that are beneficial for soothing mucous membranes lining the hollow organs, such as the lungs, digestive tract, and urinary tract. Corn silk tea aids in treating a dry cough and inflammatory conditions of the digestive and urinary tracts.

The poultice and fomentation are effective as emollients, anti-inflammatory agents, and vulneraries. Corn silk contains allantoin, which stimulates the regeneration of connective tissue. Topical applications aid in treating cuts, abrasions, rashes, diaper rash, dermatitis, and hot, dry skin conditions such as eczema or psoriasis.

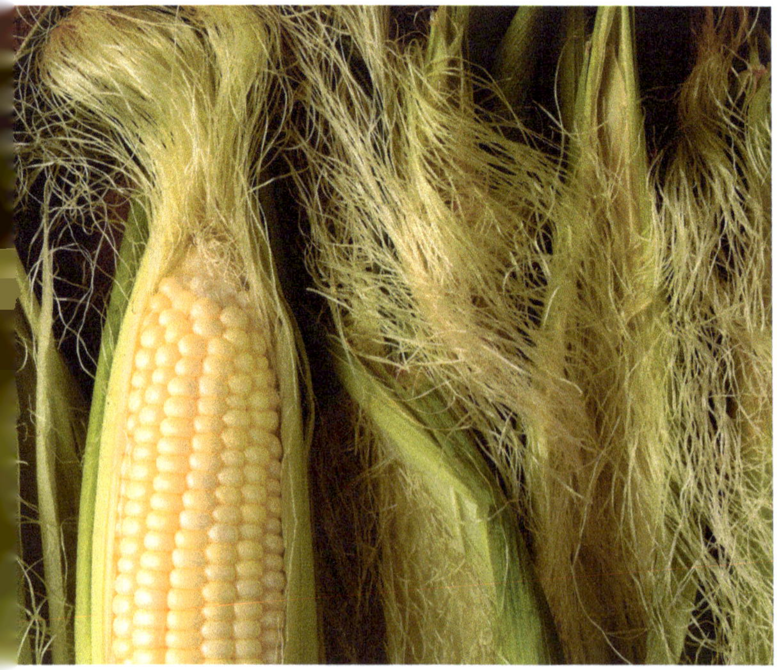

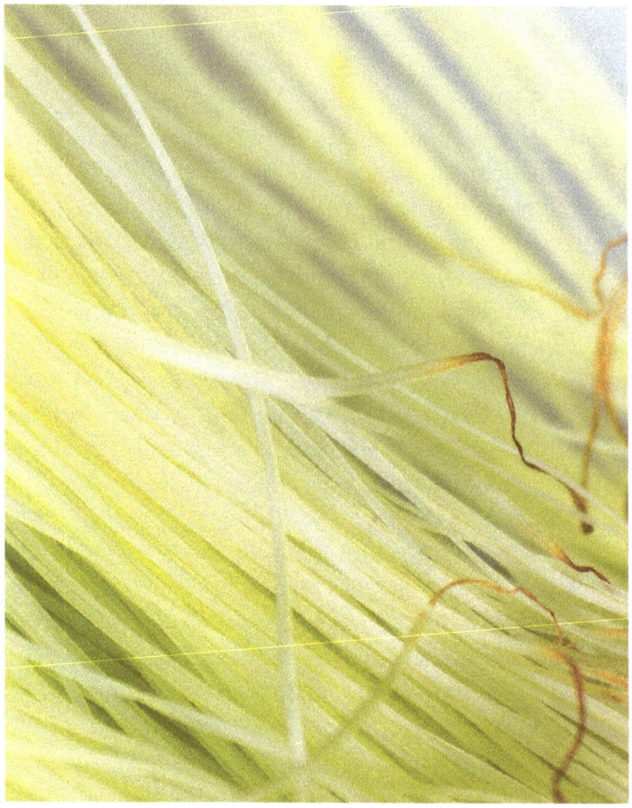

CONTRAINDICATIONS

Corn silk is contraindicated in cases of obstructive kidney stones, edema related to impaired heart or kidney function, or kidney inflammation. Otherwise, corn silk is considered safe for children, pregnant or breastfeeding women, and the elderly. There are no other known contraindications.

PREPARATION AND DOSAGE

Note: Corn silk from organic, non-genetically modified corn is recommended for all medicinal preparations.

TINCTURE: Fresh silk [1:2-1:3, 60-95% alcohol]; recently dried silk [1:5, 50% alcohol]; consume 15-90 drops, up to four times daily.

GLYCERITE: Fresh silk [1:2-1:3, 50% alcohol and 50% glycerin]; consume 15-60 drops, up to four times daily.

TEA: Prepare a hot or cold infusion; consume 8-12 ounces, three to four times daily.

TOPICAL USE: Apply the fomentation or poultice to inflamed skin.

COUCH GRASS

DESCRIPTION

BOTANICAL NAMES:
Agropyron repens (syn. *Elymus repens, Triticum repens, Elytrigia repens*), *A. cristatum, A. desertorum, A. elongatum, A. intermedium, A. mongolicum, A. pectiniforme, A. scabrifolium, A. smithii, A. trachycaulum, A. trichophorum*

COMMON NAMES:
Couch grass, couchgrass, dog grass, quack grass, quick grass, triticum, common couch, triticum, twitch, twitch grass, creeping quackgrass, crested wheatgrass, wheatgrass, cutch, devil's grass, dog's tooth, Scotch grass, Scotch quelch, durfa grass, wheat grass, witch grass
pied de poule, chiendent commun, chiendent rampant (French)
echte quecke, gemeine quecke, grasquecken, kriechende quecke, schiliessgrass (German)
caprinella, dente caprino, gramigna, granaccino (Italian)
pirey polzutchy (Russian)[1,2]

FAMILY NAME:
Poaceae (Graminae)

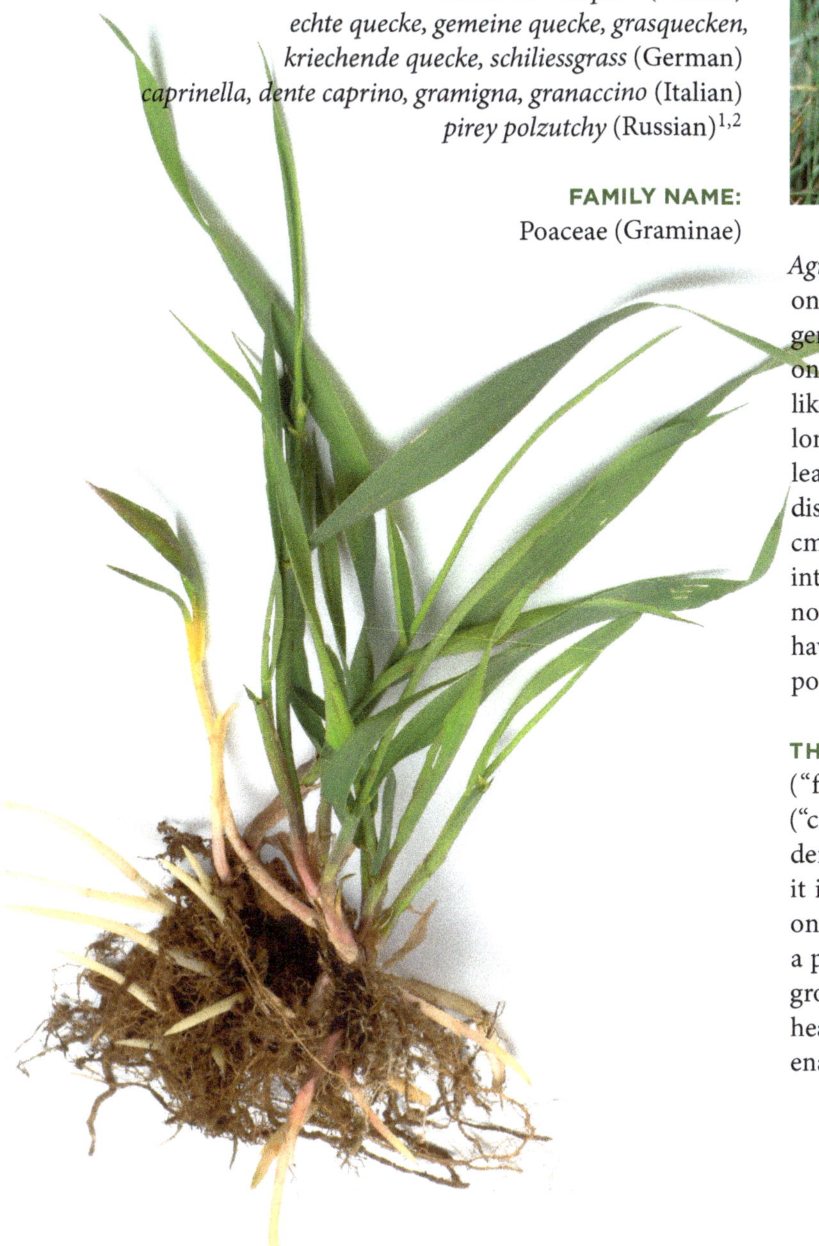

PART USED: The rhizomes.

BOTANICAL DESCRIPTION AND HABITAT: Couch grass is a perennial that grows throughout the western U.S. It is most often found in dry fields, lawns, roadsides, and cultivated areas in Arizona, New Mexico, southern California, and North America.

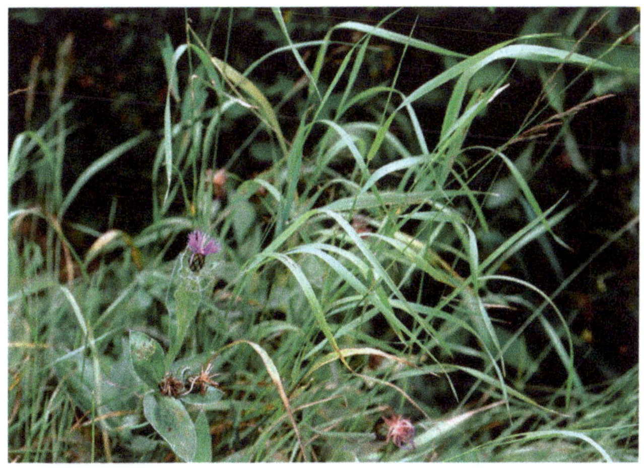

Agropyron repens is a vital perennial grass that grows up to one meter tall from strong, wiry rhizomes.[3] The leaves are generally glabrous, though sometimes they have soft hairs on the sheaths.[4] The flat leaves bear well developed, claw-like auricles (0.3 – 1 mm long), short ligules (0.25 – 1.5 mm long), and blades (6 – 14 mm wide).[4] The widely spaced leaf veins assume two forms — some faint, others more distinctly ribbed.[4] The stiff, erect inflorescence grows 5 – 20 cm long, with overlapping spikelets twice as long as the internodes.[4] The inflorescence produces one spikelet per node, each containing four to seven florets.[4] The glumes have awns (0.5 – 4 mm long); the lemmas come to an acute point, or can bear straight awns (up to 10 mm long).[3,4]

THE NAME: *Agropyron* derives from the Greek *agros* ("field") and *puros* ("wheat").[1] The epithet *repens* ("creeping") derives from Latin. The common name couch derives from the Anglo-Saxon *civice* (vivacious) because it is a persistent weed.[1] In folklore, it is noted that the only way to extirpate couch grass is to avoid cultivating a pasture for years so it can be destroyed by other close-growing grasses. The name "dog grass" refers to its use for healing sick dogs. Dogs search for its rough leaves to chew, enabling them to vomit.[1]

HISTORICAL USES: Dioscorides and numerous other physicians administered a root decoction to treat urinary suppression, kidney stones, and kidney disorders.[1] A decoction was also consumed as a blood purifier and spring tonic.[1] In times of scarcity, dried, ground couch grass roots were used to make bread.[1] Cattle and horses consumed the nutritious roots.

Cherokees consumed couch grass tea to treat incontinence, bedwetting, and kidney stones.[5] The Iroquois used couch grass as a diuretic and to treat worms.[5] A decoction of the roots was ingested to alleviate edema.

CONSTITUENTS: The primary medicinal constituent in couch grass is triticin, a polysaccharide related to inulin. Upon hydrolysis, triticin releases: fructose, mucilage, saponins, sugar alcohols (mannitol and inositol), volatile oil (polyacetylenes and carvone), small amounts of vanilloside (vanillin monoglucoside), phenolcarboxylic acids, silicic acid, and silicates. Lectins are present in the seedlings, leaves, and rhizomes; however, the lectin content of the leaves varies according to season. Additional constituents in couch grass include flavonoids (tricin), agropyrene, thymol, menthol, mucilage, inosite, malate acid, laevulose, iron, silicon, and other minerals.[1,2]

NUTRITIONAL PROPERTIES: Flavonoids (tricin), mucilage, iron, and other minerals.[2]

MEDICINAL PROPERTIES: Demulcent, diuretic, and mild urinary tract antibacterial.

TEMPERATURE AND FLAVOR: Cool, sweet, and bland.

MEDICINAL USES

Couch grass is a soothing diuretic. It contains mucilaginous polysaccharides that reduce urinary tract inflammation and spasms.[2] The diuretic effect is attributed to the presence of mannitol, saponins, and vanillin.[2] Couch grass contains antibacterial volatile oil that aids in treating urinary tract infections.[1,2] It is specific for acid urinary tract infections with dark yellow urine, high specific gravity, and a pH of 5.5 or less.[6] Combine couch grass with usnea *(Usnea)* and other aromatic or resinous antibacterials, such as juniper berry *(Juniperus)*, buchu *(Barosma)*, yerba santa *(Eriodictyon)*, grindelia *(Grindelia)*, red cedar *(Thuja)*, or cypress *(Cyperus)* to treat urinary tract infections. To ease the passing of kidney stones, combine couch grass with other soothing diuretic and antilithic herbs, such as hydrangea *(Hydrangea)*, gravel root *(Eutrochium purpureum)*, parsley root *(Petroselinum)*, and corn silk *(Zea)*.

The diuretic actions enhance renal excretion of sodium and uric acid, alleviating edema, water-related weight gain, and gout.[6] Consume the decoction long-term to treat the aforementioned conditions.

CONTRAINDICATIONS

There are no known contraindications.

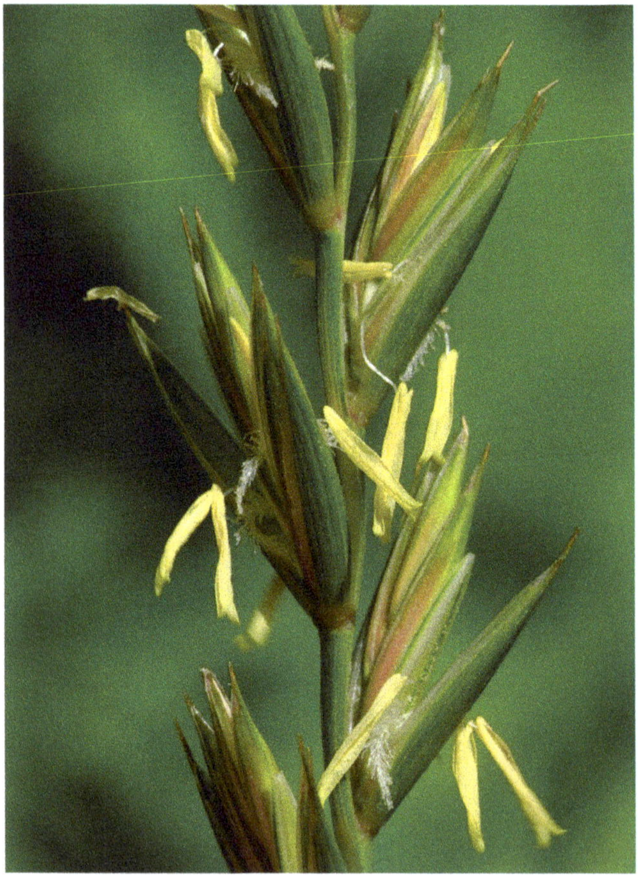

PREPARATION AND DOSAGE

TINCTURE: Fresh rhizomes [1:2, 60-95% alcohol]; dry rhizomes [1:5, 60% alcohol]; consume 30-60 drops of tincture, up to five times daily. Fluid extract [1:1, 40-50% alcohol]; consume 10-30 drops of fluid extract, up to five times daily.

TEA: Prepare a decoction or cold infusion; consume 8-12 ounces, up to four times daily.

COW PARSNIP

BOTANICAL NAMES:
Heracleum lanatum (syn. *H. maximum*), *H. sphondylium*

COMMON NAMES:
Cow parsnip, Indian celery, cow cabbage, American masterwort, woolly parsnip *yerba del oso* (Spanish)

FAMILY NAME:
Apiaceae (Umbelliferae)

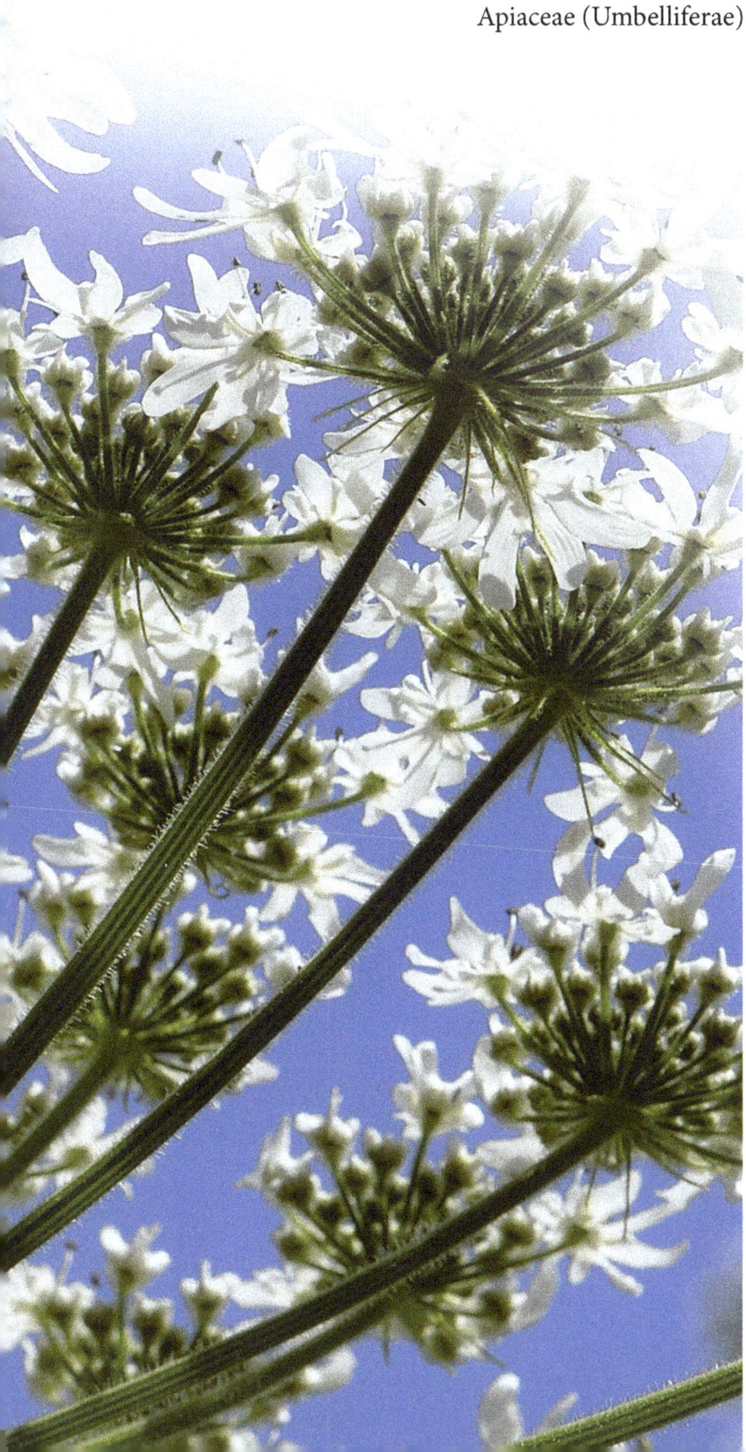

DESCRIPTION

PARTS USED: The seeds and roots are used separately.

BOTANICAL DESCRIPTION AND HABITAT: *Heracleum lanatum* is the primary species of *Heracleum* native to the U.S.[1] Cow parsnip is an herbaceous perennial that grows 1 – 3 meters tall and has a sturdy tap root.[2] The entire plant is covered in stiff hairs and is strongly scented, while the stem base features scattered purple splotches.[2] In the springtime, it emerges from the ground as a basal rosette;

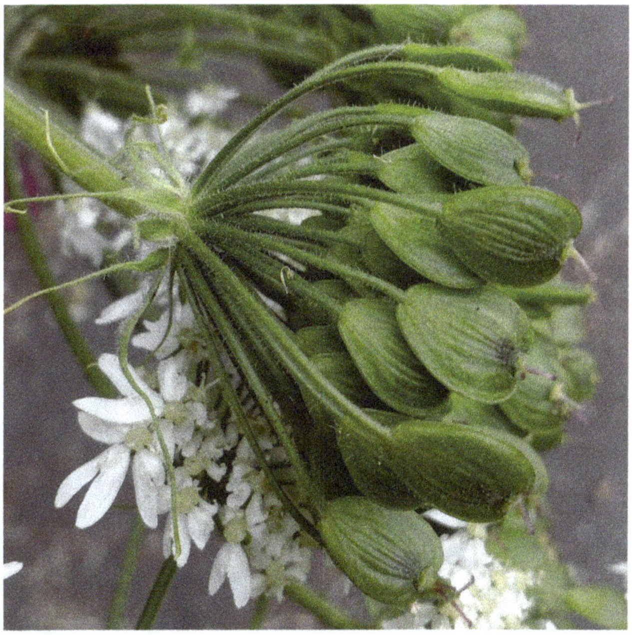

later in the season, it bolts and produces flowers on a tall, leafy stem.[2] Its ternately-compound leaves bear three large, cordate, coarsely serrated, deeply lobed leaflets.[2] The long petioles are thick, succulent, and widely sheathing around the main stem.[2]

The inflorescence lacks obvious involucral bracts, and is enveloped by the uppermost leaves (reduced to enlarged petiole sheaths) until it matures and the peduncle lengthens to full height (5 – 20 cm).[2] The inflorescence is a sizable compound umbel with 15 to 30 rays (5 – 10 cm long and unequal in length).[2] The tiny, asepalous flowers are borne upon pedicels (8 – 20 mm long), and clad with five white, obovate petals, five stamens, and an inferior ovary with two carpels and two styles.[2] The fruit is a schizocarp of two closely appressed, one-seeded halves.[2] The fruit is oblong-ovate, ribbed, and very compressed front-to-back.[2]

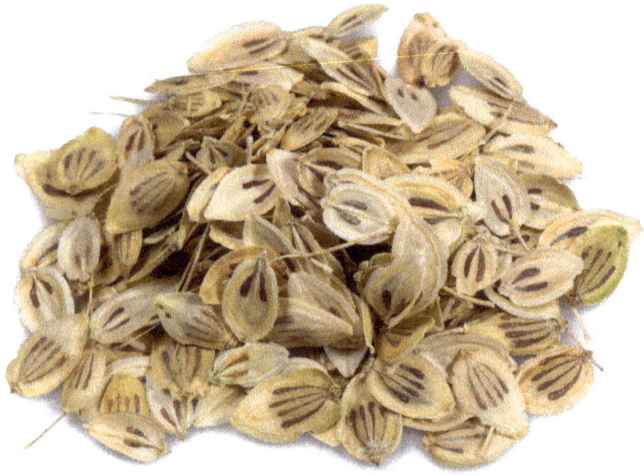

The stems and leaves of *Heracleum lanatum,* as well as other members of this genus contain varying amounts of furanocoumarins that can induce photodermatitis and subsequent hyperpigmentation upon skin contact.[2]

THE NAME: *Heracleum* derives from the Greek *"herákleion,"* referring to the mythological hero Hercules, and the robust size of this plant. The epithet *sphondylium* ("vertebrae") refers to the shape of the segmented stem. The epithet *lanatum* ("woolly") refers to the dense, woolly hairs covering the leaves and stems.[3]

HISTORICAL USES: Many groups of coastal Native Americans consumed cow parsnip as a green vegetable.[4] The young stalks and stems were harvested before the flowers matured, then peeled and consumed raw or boiled.[5,6] Sometimes the plant is referred to as "Indian celery" because the peeled young stems are mild and pleasant tasting. However, some coastal tribes considered this herb poisonous because it caused skin rashes.[4]

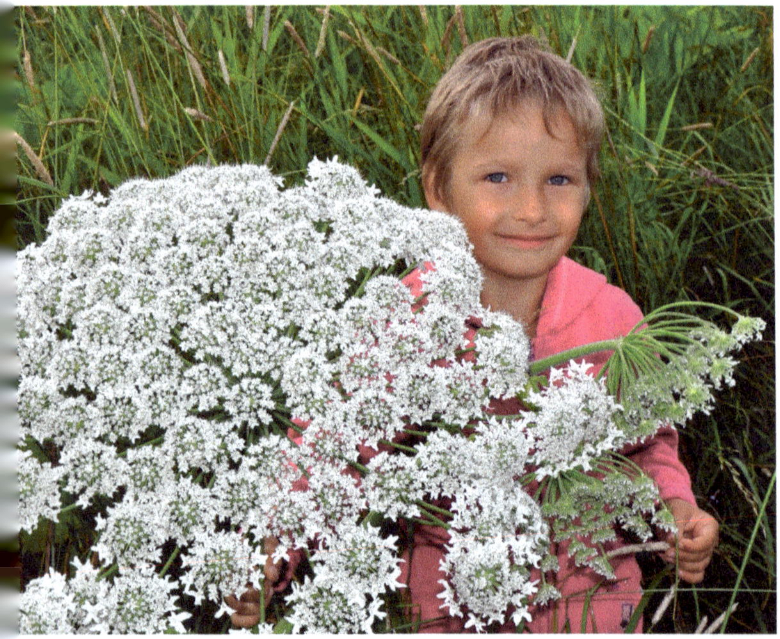

CONSTITUENTS

COW PARSNIP SEED: The whole plant contains angelicin and psoralen. The leaf and seed contain imperatorins. The leaf also contains phellopterin.[5,6]

COW PARSNIP ROOT: The root contains furanocoumarins (pimpinellins, isopimpinellin, bergaptens, isobergapten, and sphondin), coumarins, phenolic acids, *para*-coumaric acid, ferulic acid, phytosterols, apterin, scopoletin, umbelliferone, and 7-(3-methyl-2-butenyloxy)-coumarin.[5,6]

NUTRITIONAL PROPERTIES: Not applicable.

MEDICINAL PROPERTIES: Aromatic, anesthetic, analgesic, antispasmodic, carminative, stomachic, and rubefacient.

TEMPERATURE AND FLAVOR: Warm, bitter, and pungent.

MEDICINAL USES

THE SEEDS: Applying the extract or glycerite of cow parsnip seeds has potent anesthetizing actions that reduce the pain of teething, emerging wisdom teeth, and sore or abscessed teeth.[5] Combine with other anesthetizing and anti-inflammatory agents for gum pain, such as clove *(Syzygium),* spilanthes *(Acmella),* St. John's wort *(Hypericum),* or chamomile *(Matricaria).* The seeds also have mild antimicrobial actions.

Consuming several drops of the seed extract has aromatic carminative, antispasmodic actions that reduce nausea, indigestion, and hiatal hernia pain.[5] It reduces flatulence and intestinal spasms accompanying flareups of lower digestive conditions.[5] The seed also decreases bronchial and menstrual cramping, and stimulates menstrual flow.

The dried, powdered seeds or roots have topical counterirritant and rubefacient effects.[5,6] Apply cow parsnip topically for sore muscles, arthritic joints, rheumatic pain, pain, sprains, strains, bruises, and boils.[5,6] *Note:* Leaving the root in contact with the skin longer than 15–30 minutes can cause blistering. In some individuals, cow parsnip can cause contact dermatitis, so test it on a small area of skin and wait 24 hours before applying. This can cause photosensitivity, so cover the area of application when exposed to sun.[6]

THE ROOTS: The fresh root should not be consumed internally. However, preparations of the dry root are less acrid and caustic, and can be consumed as a tincture, with caution. The root shares similar properties to the seed internally as an antispasmodic for the respiratory, digestive, and reproductive tracts. However, the seeds are just as effective without the potential irritating actions of the root. A dried root poultice can be applied as a counterirritant for sprains, strains, and bruises.

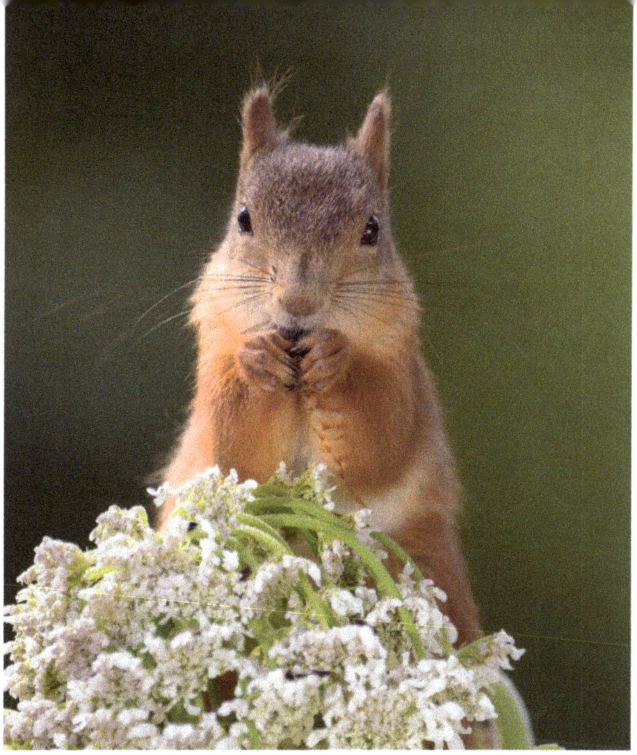

A traditional remedy in New Mexico is to apply a tea of the dried root topically to a recently paralyzed area. Repeat once daily until there are signs of nerve function restoration. Herbalist Michael Moore suggests that the tincture can be applied for similar purposes. The tea is also applied for tic douloureux (trigeminal neuralgia) when there is motor paralysis, and for aigre, a temporary paralysis of the face, neck, or arms attributed to night air or drafts.[5]

CONTRAINDICATIONS

Avoid internal use during pregnancy and while lactating.[5,6] Avoid internal use of the root in children under age 12. The author hasn't observed problems resulting from applying the seed extracts to children's gums. However, as a precaution, when applying to the gums of teething children or infants, protect them from exposure to strong sunlight for the next 24–48 hours following application or consumption. To test for potential allergic sensitivity before using it, apply several drops of the tincture to the inner crease of the elbow. If a rash appears in 24–48 hours, avoid use.

Protect skin from exposure to sunlight when consuming or handling any portion of the plant, as it can cause phototoxic skin irritations.[6] The furocoumarins can cause photodermatitis, contact dermatitis, and permanent, localized pigment changes in the skin.[5,6] This was evidenced in the case of a colleague who applied an extract of the root poultice topically, resulting in permanent discoloration of their skin. In all cases, avoid internal and topical use in individuals with Apiaceae family allergies. Some individuals are highly allergic to this plant.

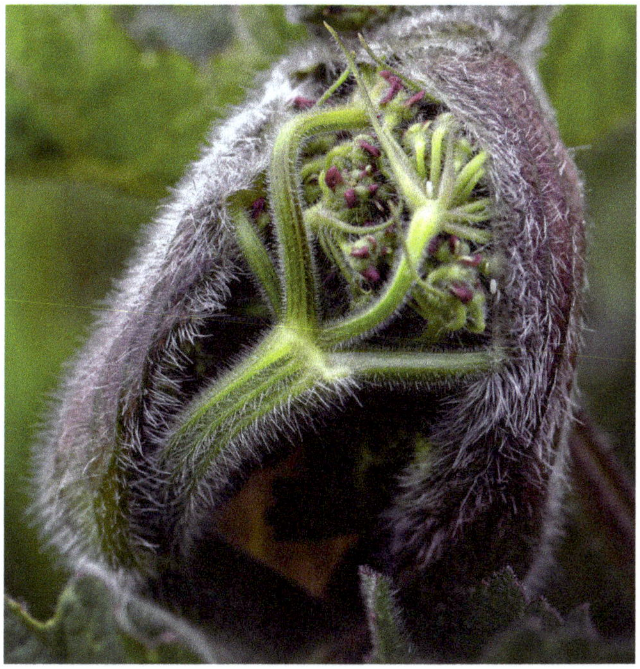

PREPARATION AND DOSAGE

TINCTURE: Fresh seeds [1:2-1:3, 70-95% alcohol]; dry seeds [1:5, 60% alcohol]; apply topically, or adults can consume 5-15 drops, up to four times daily. Dry roots [1:5, 60% alcohol]; apply topically.

GLYCERITE: Fresh seeds [1:2-1:3, 50% glycerin, 50% alcohol]; apply topically. Adults can consume 5-15 drops of tincture internally.

TEA: Prepare a hot infusion of the seeds; consume 4-8 ounces, two to four times daily.

TOPICAL USE: Apply several drops of seed tincture or glycerite to the gums.

CRAMP BARK

DESCRIPTION

BOTANICAL NAMES:
Viburnum opulus, V. edule

COMMON NAMES:
Cramp bark, guelder rose, highbush cranberry, snowball tree, May rose, white sun rose, dog rowan tree, silver bells, mooseberry, squashberry, king's crown, red elder, rose elder, water elder

FAMILY NAME:
Adoxaceae
(formerly Caprifoliaceae)

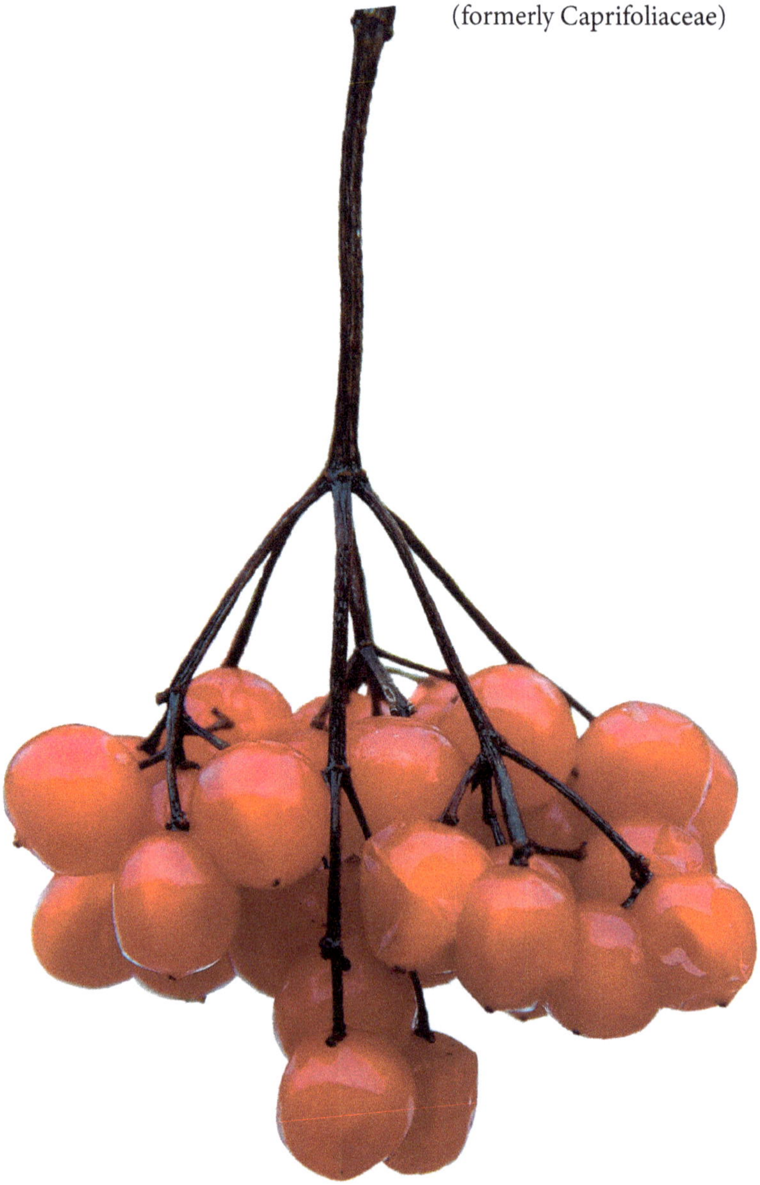

PART USED: The bark.

BOTANICAL DESCRIPTION AND HABITAT: *Viburnum opulus* is a large, deciduous shrub growing up to 6 meters tall.[1] Small, raised lenticels dot the bark.[1] The opposite, three-lobed, broadly ovate leaves (12 cm by 8 cm) have dentate margins and are glabrous on the upper surfaces, but pubescent on the lower surfaces.[1] Two discoid glands grow at the point of attachment with the grooved petiole (2 – 3 cm long); threadlike stipules (1 – 5 mm long) grow at the base of the petioles.[1,2] The attractive umbel-like, terminal flower clusters display an outer ring of five to

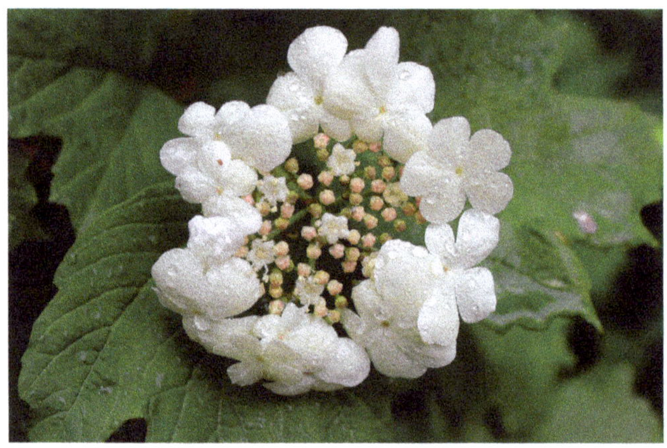

ten showy white sterile flowers (with five-lobed corollas 4 – 5 mm in diameter), and an inner ring of smaller, fertile flowers (corollas 1 – 2.5 mm diameter), each with five exserted stamens and a two-lobed stigma.[1] The bright red berries (8 – 10 mm in diameter) grow in drooping clusters that mature August through October.[1] *V. opulus* was native to Europe, but has naturalized in North America, growing in shaded woods and on riverbanks in the eastern U.S. *V. opulus* grows in northern Idaho and western Montana. *V. edule* grows from northeastern Alaska to Oregon's Central Cascades.

THE NAME: *Viburnum* ("wayfaring tree") derives from Latin.[3] The epithet *opulus* originates from the Latin *opulentus* (n.) and *opulentum* (adj.), meaning wealthy or *op* ("to work, produce in abundance").[3] The epithet *edule* ("edible") also derives from Latin.[4] The name guelder rose originates from the Gueldersland, a Dutch province where *V. opulus* was first cultivated.[5] While cramp bark is completely unrelated to true cranberry *(Vaccinium* *macrocarpon*), its crimson, ripe fruit resembled cranberries, and were sometimes used as a substitute for them; hence, the name highbush cranberry.[5] The name snowball tree was acquired because the broad, bright white flowers resembled snowballs.[5] Due to its resemblance to common elder, the names red elder and rose elder emerged.[5]

HISTORICAL USES: Cramp bark was used to treat convulsions, cramping, and spasms.[5] The Iroquois and other northeastern tribes utilized cramp bark in many ways. It was commonly used for arthritis and joint pain caused by muscle rigidity. The bark was applied topically to the affected joints, relaxing the muscles and restoring blood flow.[6] Eclectic physicians administered the herb as a uterine sedative, tonic, partus preparator, and antispasmodic, and for cramping in the calves, as well as for hysteria and convulsions.[7,8]

The tart berries of *V. edule* were an important food source for people in the Pacific Northwest central and northern coastal regions.[9] The berries were mentioned in numerous Haida myths.[9] They were harvested in late summer and early fall while still hard and green, and stored like wild crabapples — in boxes with water and oil until they softened and sweetened.[9] The berries were served at important feasts; boxes of them were considered a prestigious gift.[9] The Haida prepared an eye wash from the bark.[9] The Nuxalk consumed bark tea to treat lung infections.[9] The Penobscot consumed berry tea for swollen glands and mumps.[4] The fruit was prepared as a dye, and dried berries were used as ink. According to Pojar and Mackinnon, fresh berries make a delicious cranberry sauce when mixed with commercial cranberries.[9]

CONSTITUENTS: Cramp bark contains valerianic acid = viburnic acid, valeric acid, a bitter glucoside (viburnine), vibutnin, bitter resin (viburnin), organic acids, tannins, flavonoids (catechins), salicosides, hydroquinones (arbutin), methylarbutin, coumarins (scopeletin and scopoline), triterpenes (ursolic and oleanolic acids), and calcium oxalate.[5,6,10-12]

NUTRITIONAL PROPERTIES: Limited information is available on the nutritional properties of native *Viburnum* berries, although the presence of large amounts of vitamin C has been confirmed. *Viburnum mullaha* (Indian cranberry) contains vitamins C, B_2, and E, as well as proteins, lipids, carbohydrates, magnesium, copper, iron, zinc, and magnesium.[12]

MEDICINAL PROPERTIES: Antispasmodic, astringent, nervine, and sedative (mild).

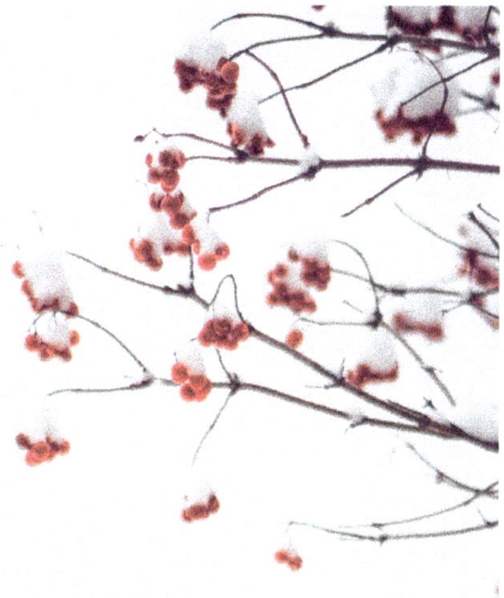

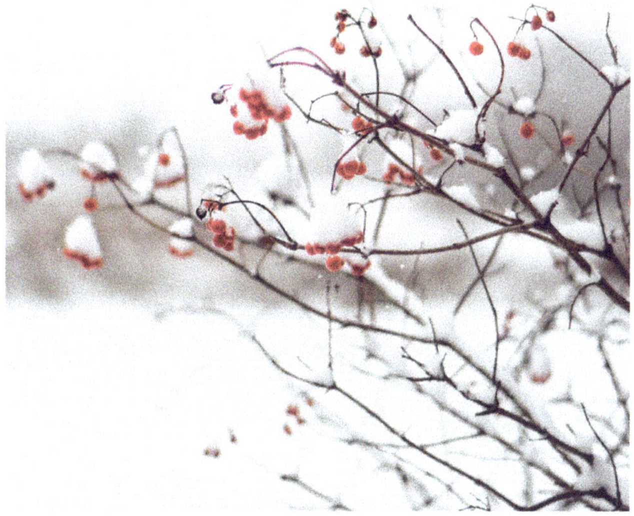

TEMPERATURE AND FLAVOR: Warm, astringent, sweet, and bitter.

MEDICINAL USES

As the name indicates, cramp bark is a smooth muscle antispasmodic that mitigates cramping in the uterus, bladder, and digestive organs.[4-8,10] It alleviates menstrual cramps, mittelschmerz, ovaritis, and fallopian tube pain.[13] It also lessens pain resulting from endometriosis, fibroids, and ovarian cysts. Cramp bark is indicated for pelvic cramping accompanied by pain in the back, extending through the loins and down the thighs.[8] Consume as a single extract or combine with wild yam (*Dioscorea villosa*), black haw (*Viburnum prunifolium*), and ginger (*Zingiber officinalis*) to ease menstrual cramps. Cramp bark tempers irregular spasmodic pain in the uterus and ovaries, and to some extent, intestinal cramping. It has subtle nervine properties, partly due to the constituent valerianic acid also contained in valerian.[10]

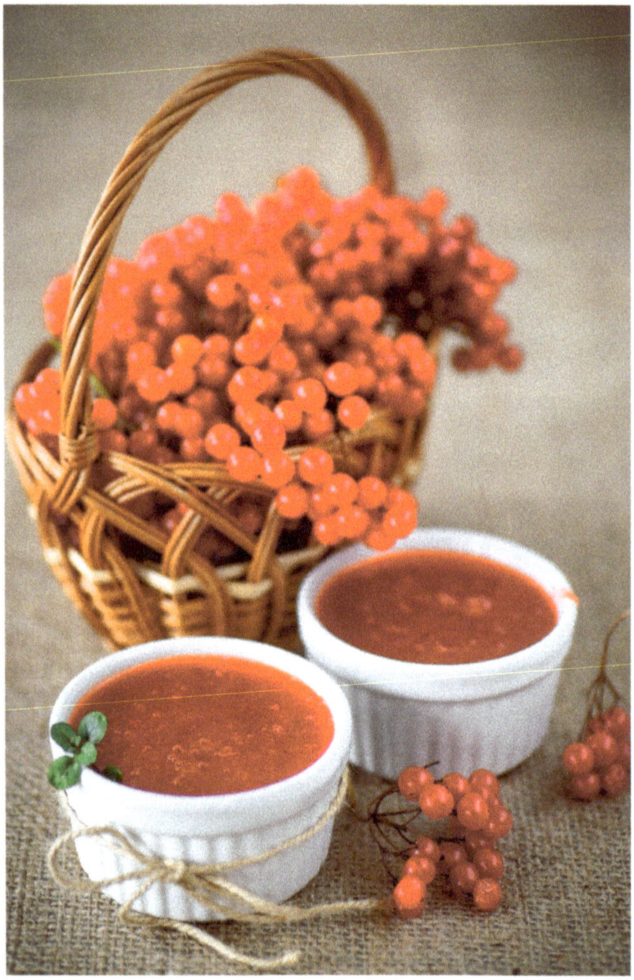

Cramp bark subdues bladder spasms, and helps to manage acute or long-term pain associated with an irritable bladder and interstitial cystitis.[8] When treating interstitial cystitis, cramp bark works more effectively when combined with additional antispasmodics such as wild yam *(Dioscorea villosa)*, as well as bladder tonics such as mullein root *(Verbascum thapsus)* and nettle root *(Urtica dioica)*.

Cramp bark contains high amounts of tannins that astringe tissues. It has hemostatic actions, reducing excessive uterine bleeding, including menorrhagia, postpartum bleeding, and mid-cycle bleeding. Shepherd's purse *(Capsella)*, black haw *(Viburnum prunifolium)*, cinnamon *(Cinnamomum)*, and raspberry leaf *(Rubus)* synergize the hemostatic properties of cramp bark.

Cramp bark is a partus preparator that can be consumed one to two weeks prior to delivery in order to facilitate a smooth labor.[7,8] Consuming cramp bark prior to delivery does not interfere with cervix dilation. It reduces pain after childbirth; however, it should be avoided if a woman is dehydrated, because it can cause nausea and vomiting.[7,8] Cramp bark can be combined with black haw *(Viburnum prunifolium)* and partridge berry *(Mitchella repens)* to attempt to prevent a miscarriage, and as a partus preparator.[7,8]

CONTRAINDICATIONS

Cramp bark has no known toxicity or side effects.[10,11] This herb is considered safe for extended use and does not cause cumulative toxicity; however, consumed in high doses, it can cause nausea, vomiting, and dizziness—likely due to the astringent tannins.[11] Consult a midwife or other health care practitioner before consuming cramp bark during pregnancy.

Some species of *Viburnum* are edible, including *V. edule;* however, consuming too many berries can cause an upset stomach or diarrhea.[5]

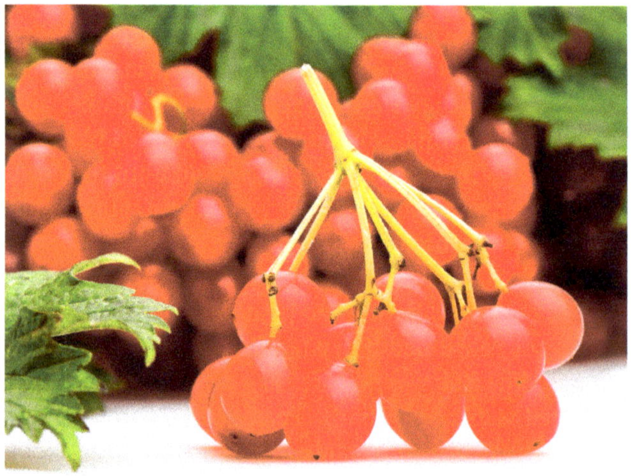

PREPARATION AND DOSAGE

TINCTURE: Fresh bark [1:2-1:3, 70-95% alcohol]; dry bark [1:5, 60% alcohol]; consume 30-120 drops, up to four times daily.

CAPSULES: Consume 2-4 "00" capsules, one to three times daily.

TEA: Prepare a decoction or cold infusion; consume 8-12 ounces, up to four times daily.

CULINARY USE: Add the berries to jams, juices, pies, sauces, liqueurs, wines, cordials, and pemmican. Freeze the berries for later use.

DAMIANA

DESCRIPTION

BOTANICAL NAMES:
Turnera diffusa var. *aphrodisiaca*
(syn. *T. diffusa, T. aphrodisiaca*)

COMMON NAMES:
Damiana, damiane, Mexican damiana, Mexican holly
thé bourrique (French)
grossblä (German)
damiana de Guerrero, oreganillo, aquita de damiana, pasrocita, yerba del pastor (Spanish)

FAMILY NAME:
Passifloraceae
(formerly Turneraceae)

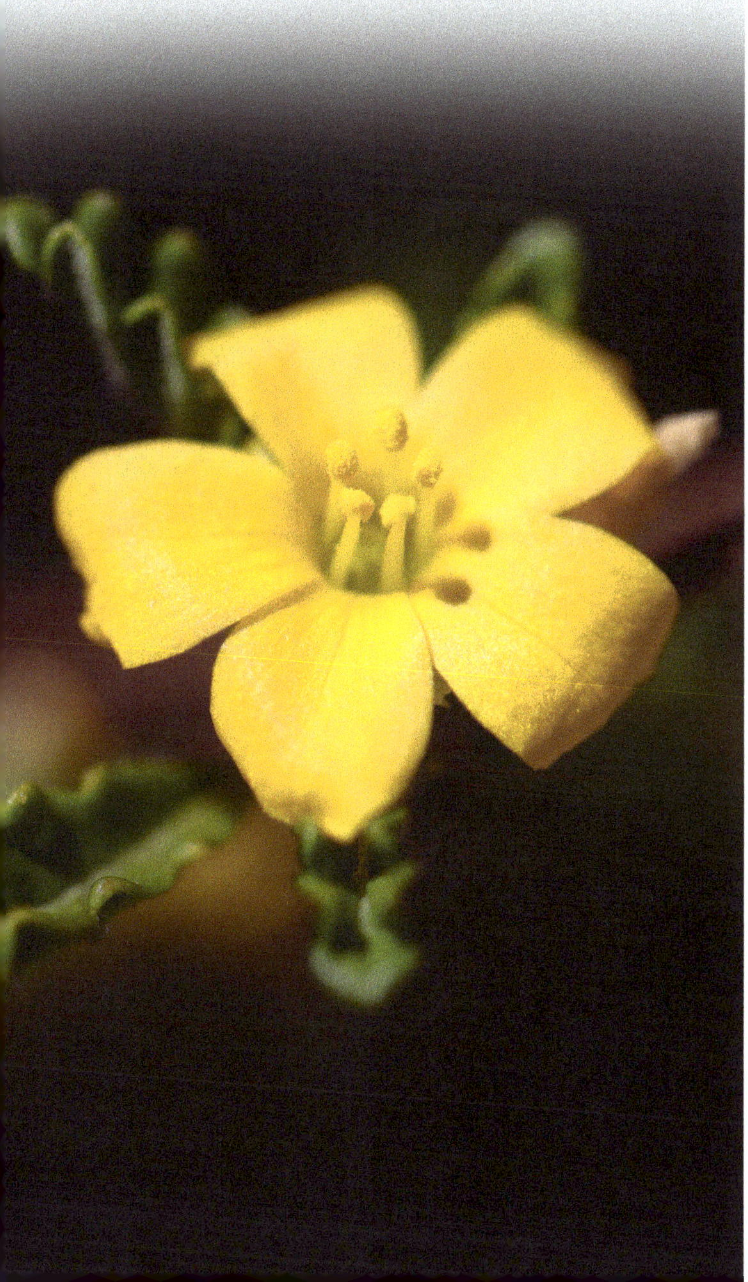

PARTS USED: The leaves and flowers.

BOTANICAL DESCRIPTION AND HABITAT: Damiana is native to hot climates in southern California, Arizona, Texas, western Mexico, Central and South America, and the West Indies. It is a small shrub with reddish stems that are pubescent when young. The stems bear aromatic, pale

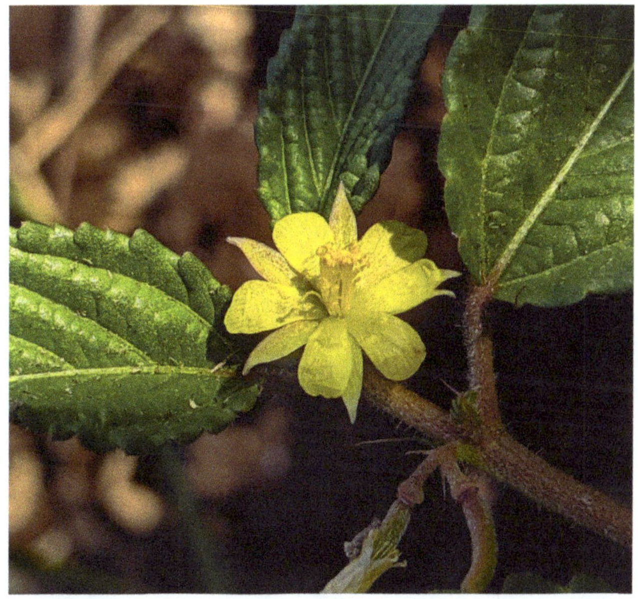

green, serrated, obovate to lanceolate leaves (less than 3 cm long) with distinctive pinnate venation; they are pubescent when young, and glabrous as they age.[1] The axillary flowers have hairy, yellow, tubular calyces with five teeth each, and five yellow petals.[1,2] The fruit is an aromatic, resinous, dry, three-valved capsule; each contains up to six seeds.[1,2]

THE NAME: *Turnera* may have derived from the Anglo-French *tourner* that evolved from the Medieval Latin *tornare,* meaning "to turn" or "to turn on a lathe." It is also possible that the plant was named after Dawson Turner, an English botanist who collected and classified plants. The epithet *diffusa* ("spread out or wide") originates from Latin, referring to the plant's tendency to spread out and cover more horizontal than vertical area. The epithet (and varietal name) *aphrodisiaca* refers to its use as a sexual stimulant. Contrary to claims about the plant's medicinal actions, the common name damiana derives from the Greek root word, *damao* ("to tame").

HISTORICAL USES: Ancient Aztecs and Mayans regarded damiana as a potent aphrodisiac.[3] Mayans also used damiana to treat giddiness and loss of balance.[3] According to reports from a Spanish missionary, Mexican Indians prepared damiana tea with sugar to enhance lovemaking.[3] Damiana liqueur is still produced in Mexico and advertised as an aphrodisiac. Some sources claim that this liqueur was combined with triple sec in the original margarita recipe. Damiana is used as an aphrodisiac in many countries, including Brazil, Cuba, Germany, Haiti, Holland, Mexico, the U.S., and South America.[3] In western Mexico, damiana tea was used to treat colic, stop bedwetting, and stimulate menstruation.[3] A steam inhalation of the tea was said to relieve a headache.[3] In the southwestern U.S., damiana tea was consumed by Hispanic and Native Americans as a sexual stimulant and restorative for sexual debility, and for depression and edema.[4]

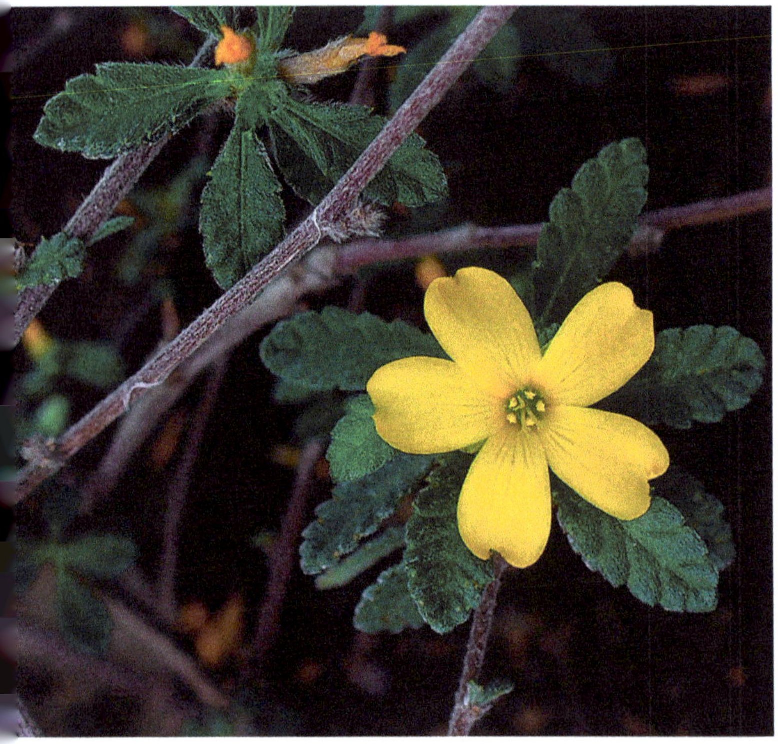

Reports of the use of damiana as an aphrodisiac were recorded in the U.S. more than 100 years ago.[3] *The United States National Formulary* (1888 – 1947) contains information about the use of damiana leaf fluid extract, elixirs, and cordials.[3] Damiana was introduced to American medicine by Dr. F. O. St. Clair, a Washington druggist, in 1874. He sold eight-ounce bottles of the tincture for $2, claiming it was a powerful aphrodisiac "to improve the sexual ability of the enfeebled and aged," and touting that it improved the tone and secretions of the pelvic organs.[5] While Eclectics debated the use of damiana as an aphrodisiac, many employed the herb as a cholagogue and laxative, and for renal and cystic catarrh, or irritated mucous membranes in the respiratory and renal tracts.[6] It was also used as a nerve stimulant for treating lethargy, depression, and debility.[6] Dr. Reid, an Eclectic physician, recommended damiana for dysmenorrhea, headaches, bad complexion, rough or discolored patches on the skin with severe acne, eruptions resembling eczema from insufficient menstruation, and as a tonic for an enfeebled nervous system.[6] Eclectic physician Dr. Watkins recommended damiana for amenorrhea and delayed or suppressed menstruation in young girls, menstrual irregularity, and reducing sensitivities of the sympathetic nervous system caused by disorders of the womb and ovaries.[6] Dr. Ellingwood, another Eclectic physician, stated that "midwives and women of loose morals of western Mexico attribute emmenagogue properties to it."[6] The author disagrees with these outdated Victorian sentiments.

Damiana was used in the Bahamas for childbirth, menstrual irregularities, urinary insufficiency, and headaches. In Germany, the leaves are used to calm the mind, and as a hormonal and nervous system tonic. In Holland, damiana is highly regarded as a tonic for the reproductive organs and an aphrodisiac. The *British Herbal Pharmacopoeia* recommends damiana for "anxiety neurosis with a predominant sexual factor, depression, nervous dyspepsia, atonic constipation, and coital inadequacy."[3]

CONSTITUENTS: Damiana leaves contain volatile oil (1,8-cineole, α- and β-pinene, thymol, *p*-cymene, cymol, thymol, α-copaene, β-cadinene, gamma-cadinene, and calamenene), a bitter amorphus principle (damianin), phenol hydrocarbons (triacontane, etc.), phytosterols (β-sitosterol), glycosides (gonzalitosin I, tetraphyllin B, and arbutin), flavonoids (5-hydroxy-7, 3',4'–trimethoxyflavone), barterin, caoutchouc, quinovopyranosides, chlorophyll, luteolin, resins, tannins, and starch.[3,7-10]

NUTRITIONAL PROPERTIES: Damiana contains aluminum, calcium, chromium, cobalt, fiber, fat, iron, magnesium, manganese, niacin, phosphorus, potassium, protein, selenium, silicon, sodium, thiamine, tin, vitamins A and C, and zinc.[11]

MEDICINAL PROPERTIES: Antidepressant, antitussive (mild), aphrodisiac, aromatic, astringent, bitter tonic, carminative, circulatory stimulant, diuretic, emmenagogue, euphoric, expectorant, laxative (mild), nervine, oxytocic (potential), trophorestorative, and urinary antiseptic.

TEMPERATURE AND FLAVOR: Warm, pungent, bitter, sweet, and astringent (mild).

MEDICINAL USES

Damiana is a soothing diuretic that reduces inflammation in the mucous membranes lining the urinary tract.[3,4,6,8,10] It also contains small quantities of arbutin, a urinary tract antibacterial.[8,10] Damiana tea aids in treating cystitis, urethritis, and interstitial cystitis. More potent antibacterial agents are often necessary for successfully treating urinary tract infections. Damiana tea soothes the urinary tract, and reduces symptoms of benign prostatic hypertrophy in men.

Damiana has a mild nervine effect.[3,6] It can be consumed throughout the day by individuals with nervous excitability or anxiety.[3] Some herbalists consider it a nervous system restorative tonic (trophorestorative) for individuals depleted from stress. For this purpose, it can be combined with extracts of fresh milky oats *(Avena),* skullcap *(Scutellaria),* and St. John's wort *(Hypericum).*[3,6] Damiana can be beneficial for treating women with increased anxiety, irritability, or premenstrual syndrome; consume the tea one to two weeks prior to menstruation.[3,6] In some individuals, damiana can act as a stimulant. Some individuals have difficulty falling asleep when they consume damiana in the evening, or if they consume excessive quantities throughout the day. If this occurs, limit use to earlier in the day, or discontinue use. Other individuals experience a headache or nervous system stimulation when consuming damiana.

Damiana is a mild antidepressant, euphoric, and mood-elevating substance.[3,4] It aids in treating premenstrual depression, seasonal affective disorder, and mild depression due to chronic illness or pain.[3] Drinking the cordial or liqueur can ease social and sexual tension at social gatherings. Some herbalists claim that smoking damiana leaves causes a subtle high with sexual overtones, reminiscent of the effects of marijuana.[5] In 2005, the Louisiana legislature outlawed damiana due to an increase in synthetic cannabis overdoses from a chemically-infused plant formulation containing damiana. Damiana is considered a "prohibited plant" illegal to possess in Louisiana.[12] Damiana also acquired a bad reputation in the United Kingdom. A product called "Black Mamba," erroneously labeled as containing "100% damiana," also contained synthetic cannabis, and was banned because users experienced adverse side effects.[12]

Damiana is an aphrodisiac and sexual stimulant.[3,4,8,10] It increases libido in males and females, and can be used to treat impotence, frigidity, coital inadequacy, and sexual neurasthenia.[3,6] It increases blood flow throughout the pelvic region and to the genitalia, enhancing sexual sensation. Damiana is a gently warming circulatory stimulant and pelvic decongestant. It can be beneficial for some individuals with anorgasmia. In a 1999 laboratory study, Italian researchers administered damiana to sexually potent and impotent rats.[3] While the extract had no effect on sexually potent rats, it increased the percentage achieving ejaculation and enhanced the sexual activity of impotent rats.[3] According to some herbalists, the sexually stimulating actions may be due to a testosteromimetic effect that stimulates and enhances reproductive functions, especially in men.[11]

Based on clinical observations, it is possible that damiana synergizes the hormone oxytocin, and is useful for individuals exhibiting patterns of oxytocin deficiency. Further studies are needed to confirm this theory. Damiana appears to improve oxytocin utilization, which can have many benefits: stimulating menstruation, improving sexual sensation, enhancing orgasm, and hastening labor. Consuming eight ounces of hot damiana tea, extract, or cordial every two to three hours stimulates menses when delayed from stress, pelvic congestion, or oxytocin deficiency.[6] The emmena-

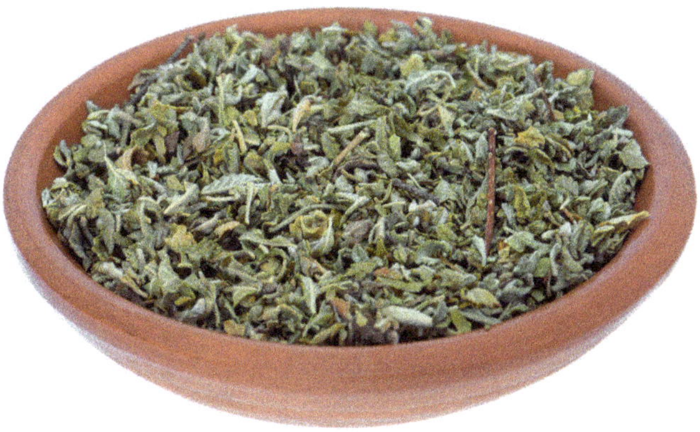

gogue properties are most effective for treating amenorrhea when the hot tea or cordial is consumed one week prior to the expected date of menstruation.[6] Hot tea or extract also can be consumed one week before, or on the due date to gently stimulate uterine contractions and induce labor. Combining damiana with cotton root bark *(Gossypium)* increases the effectiveness of oxytocin utilization by the tissues. Consuming damiana before sexual activity appears to increase circulation and sensitivity of the erogenous zones, improve sexual peak, and intensify or lengthen orgasms.

Damiana reduces respiratory irritation, decreases bronchial spasms, and has expectorant actions.[3,6] Though the antitussive actions are subtle, the tea can be consumed daily to treat asthma or lung problems.[3] Damiana contains copaene

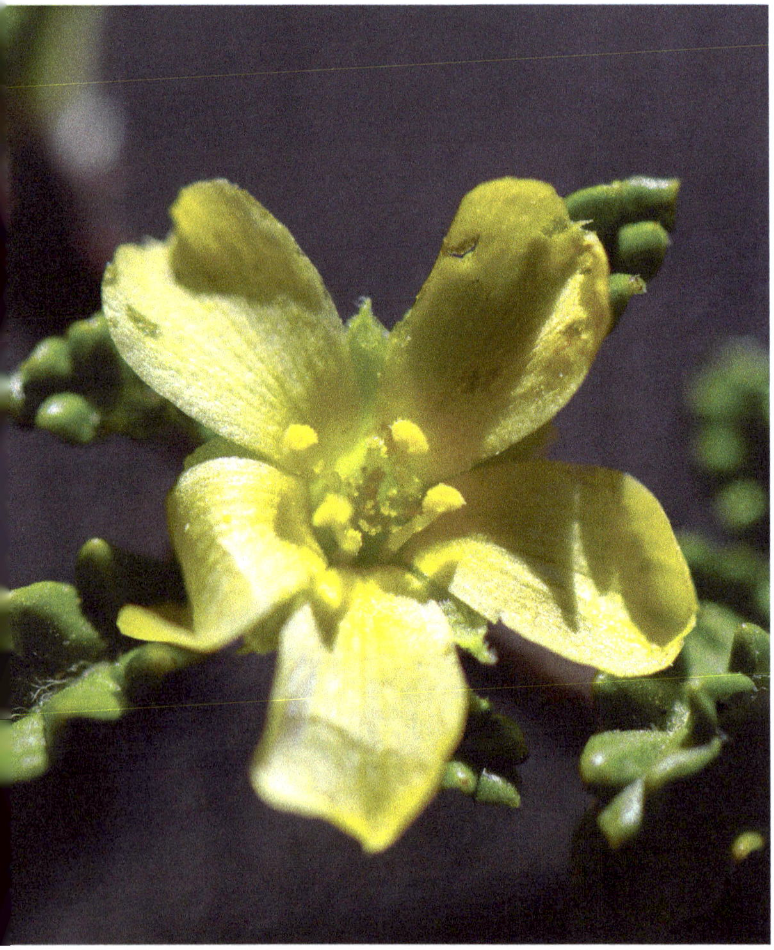

and cadinene that reduce lung inflammation. It is also used in the first stages of a cold or flu to decrease congestion.

Damiana has mild bitter tonic, cholagogue, and carminative actions that aid digestion and reduce gas and bloating.[6,8] It soothes mucous membranes in the digestive tract and aids nerve-related digestive issues. It has a mild laxative effect in some individuals with sluggish bowels or minor constipation.[8,10]

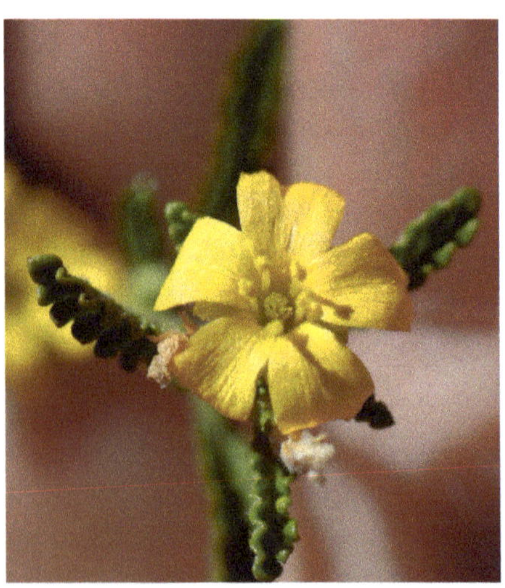

Damiana tea can be beneficial for lowering elevated blood glucose levels.[3] In 1984 Mexican researchers administered damiana tea to diabetic mice, reducing their blood glucose levels.[3] A similar study was performed with the ethanol extract in 2002; however, it did not produce hypoglycemic effects in diabetic mice. Based on these conflicting results, hot infusions, rather than alcohol-based extracts appear to be most effective for reducing blood glucose levels.[3]

CONTRAINDICATIONS

Avoid or discontinue use in individuals with heavy menstrual and uterine bleeding. Avoid consuming damiana during pregnancy, except one week before the due date, or to hasten labor.[3,4,8] Excessive consumption of damiana can cause a headache or insomnia, or act as a stimulant in sensitive individuals. Based on studies showing that damiana tea can lower blood glucose levels, it is important to use caution in individuals with hypoglycemia and those medicated for hyperglycemia, as it may potentiate antidiabetic medications.[3] There is no known toxicity in the literature reviewed.[8]

PREPARATION AND DOSAGE

TINCTURE: Fresh leaves [1:2, 70-95% alcohol]; dry leaves [1:5, 60% alcohol]; consume 15-60 drops, up to four times daily. Dry leaves [1:5, brandy (40% alcohol)]; consume 15-90 drops, up to three times daily.

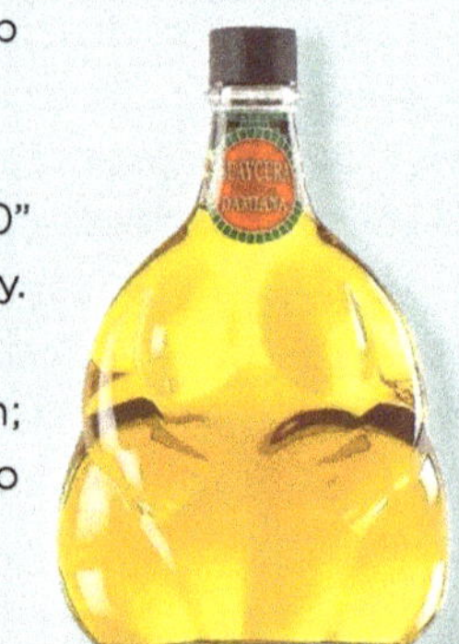

CAPSULES: Consume 2-4 "00" capsules, up to three times daily.

TEA: Prepare a hot infusion; consume 8-12 ounces, up to three times daily.

HONEY AND SYRUP: Consume 1 teaspoon of infused honey or syrup, up to four times daily.

CULINARY USE: Damiana is a delightful addition to cordials, elixirs, aperitifs, and digestifs. It has been used as a flavoring agent in beverages, frozen dairy desserts, baked goods, candy, gelatins, and puddings.[8]

DANDELION

DESCRIPTION

BOTANICAL NAMES:
Taraxacum officinale (syn. *T. campylodes, T. vulgare, T. dens-leonis,* and *Leontodon taraxacum*) and *T.* spp.

COMMON NAMES:
Dandelion, tooth of the lion, lion's tooth, swine's snout, fairy clock, milk gowan, milk witch, monk's head, priest's crown, wild endive, white endive, cankerwort, bitterwort, puff ball, blowball, blow ball, Irish daisy, piddly bed, wet-a-bed
dent de lion, pissenlit (French)
kihblume, löwenzahn (German)
radiki (Greek)
dudhal (Hindi)
diente di lieone, tarasso (Italian)
hokoei (Japanese)
p'ogongyông (Korean)
pú gong ying (Mandarin)
trakhasnkun (Persian)
oduvanchick, pushki (Russian)
dughdapheni (Sanskrit)
hiccoria, consuelda, diente de leon (Spanish)
kara hindiba ootu, yabani (Turkish)
dant y llew (Welsh)

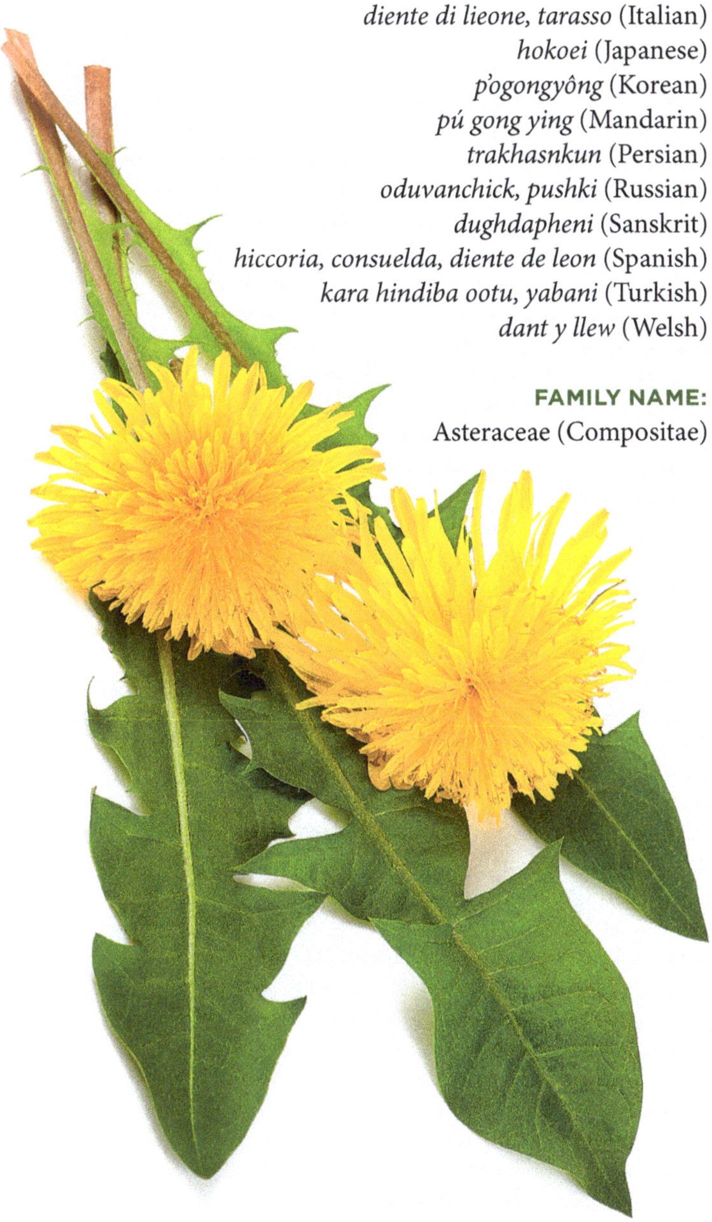

FAMILY NAME:
Asteraceae (Compositae)

PARTS USED: The roots and leaves.

BOTANICAL DESCRIPTION AND HABITAT: Dandelion is a perennial herb native to Greece that spread throughout Europe. It was introduced by European settlers, and has become an endemic weed growing rampantly worldwide.

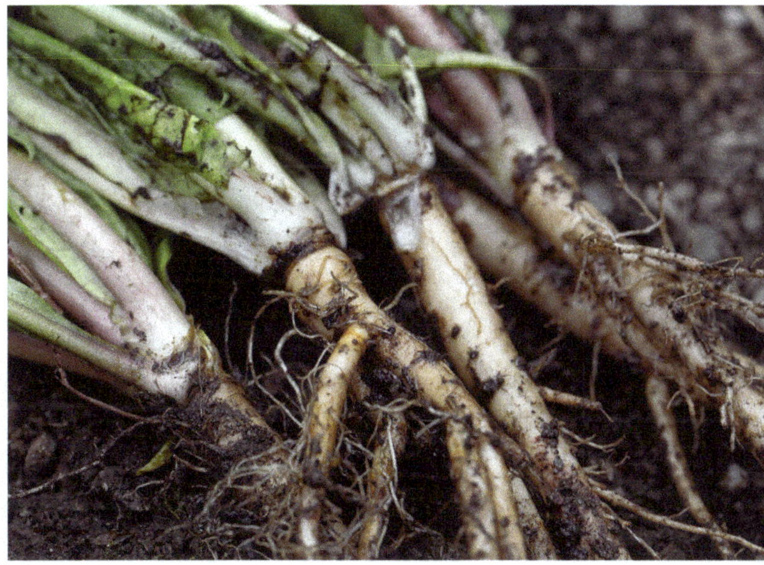

Dandelion has cylindrical, tapering branched roots with a beige to brown exterior and white interior. A cross-section of the root has concentric layers of lactiferous vessels alternating with a whitish, inulin-bearing parenchyma. Often deeply and irregularly toothed, dandelion leaves (4 – 45 cm long by 1 – 10 cm wide) are spatulate in shape, with dentate margins and a prominent green to reddish-purple midrib; they grow in a basal rosette.[1] The vibrant, golden-yellow terminal flower heads grow on a naked stem (up to 40 cm tall) that produces a milky secretion when broken.[1] The flower heads open in sunlight and close at night. The involucre is comprised of two series of lanceolate phyllaries, with the shorter, outer series reflexed, and the inner series appressed to the outer florets. Each head has as many as 100 tiny florets with strap-shaped corollas (up to 22 mm long). The corollas have five teeth; each tooth represents one fused petal.[1] Under each corolla is a narrow, nectar-filled, claw-like tube that rests on a single-chambered ovary containing one ovule. The fruit is a compressed achene with a furry pappus on a stalk for dissemination. The flowers are known to be frequented by at least 93 different types of insects.[2] Plants commonly mistaken for dandelion

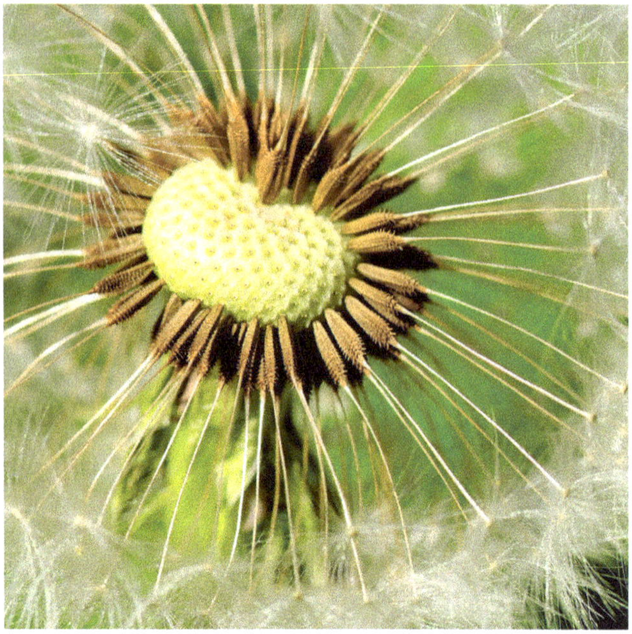

include longleaf hawks beard *(Crepis acuminata),* hawk bit *(Leontodon hispidus),* and common sow thistle *(Sonchus oleraceus).*

THE NAME: The genus name *Taraxacum* originates from two Greek words: *taraxos* ("disorder") and *akos* ("remedy").[3] Another possible derivation is from the Persian-Arabic word *tharakhchakon* ("edible").[4] The epithet *officinale* ("official") derives from the Latin, alluding to the plant's use in the practice of medicine.[4]

The common name dandelion is a corruption of the French dent de lion ("tooth of the lion"), referring to the dentate leaves. Another French name for the plant is pissenlit, translated as "piss the bed," referring to the plant's diuretic actions. The name "white man's foot" alludes to the plant's introduction to North America via European settlers. The name "blow ball' refers to the fluffy spheres of tufted fruit.

HISTORICAL USES: As early as 659 CE, dandelion was described in Chinese materia medicas.[5] It continues to be administered in Traditional Chinese Medicine for lung and breast tumors, mastitis, abscesses, jaundice, hepatitis, and urinary tract infections.[6] During the 10th and 11th centuries, Arabian physicians wrote about dandelion in medical journals.[2,7]

By the 13th century, the use of dandelion was popularized throughout Europe. Raw or blanched dandelion greens were consumed as vegetables; the fresh or dried leaves were fermented in herbal beer.[2] The dried roasted roots were powdered, and either substituted for, or mixed with coffee. Based on their flavor and medicinal actions, they were considered a superior beverage because they lacked the detrimental effects of coffee and black tea on the digestive tract and nervous system.[1] Dandelion flower wine was a popular beverage due to its blood tonifying properties.[2]

American Eclectic physician John Scudder prescribed dandelion root for chronic liver swelling, inflammation, or obstruction; deficient biliary excretion; jaundice; and constipation.[8] He valued dandelion root for its alterative, tonic, stomachic, cholagogue, aperient, and diuretic properties.[8] Finley Ellingwood administered a fluid extract of dandelion root as a cholagogue to enhance liver detoxification, a mild laxative, and to improve uric acid excretion.[9] He combined dandelion root with other herbs to treat chronic jaundice, rheumatism, conditions attributed to autointoxication, and as an alterative for blood disorders. He also recommended dandelion for chronic skin eruptions, skin conditions, as a stimulant to the stomach for chronic catarrhal gastritis, and for aphthous mouth ulcerations.[9] Harvey Felter prescribed dandelion root extract as a bitter tonic and gentle alterative-laxative to treat anorexia, weak digestion, hepatic torpor, constipation, and chronic skin disorders caused by autointoxication.[10]

The *British Herbal Pharmacopoeia* recommended dandelion leaves for treating gallstones, stagnant bile, jaundice, atonic dyspepsia, constipation, and muscular rheumatism.[11] The roots were administered as a gastric stimulant, bitter tonic, anti-inflammatory, anticatarrhal, and antimicrobial.[11] Dr. David Culbreth administered dandelion as a diuretic, tonic, stomachic, aperient, and deobstruent to treat liver congestion, spleen swelling, dyspepsia, constipation, skin conditions, and dropsies.[12]

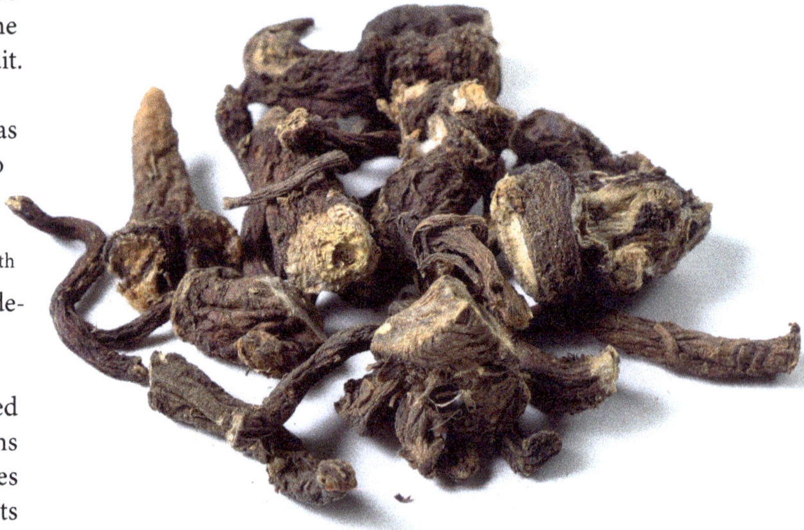

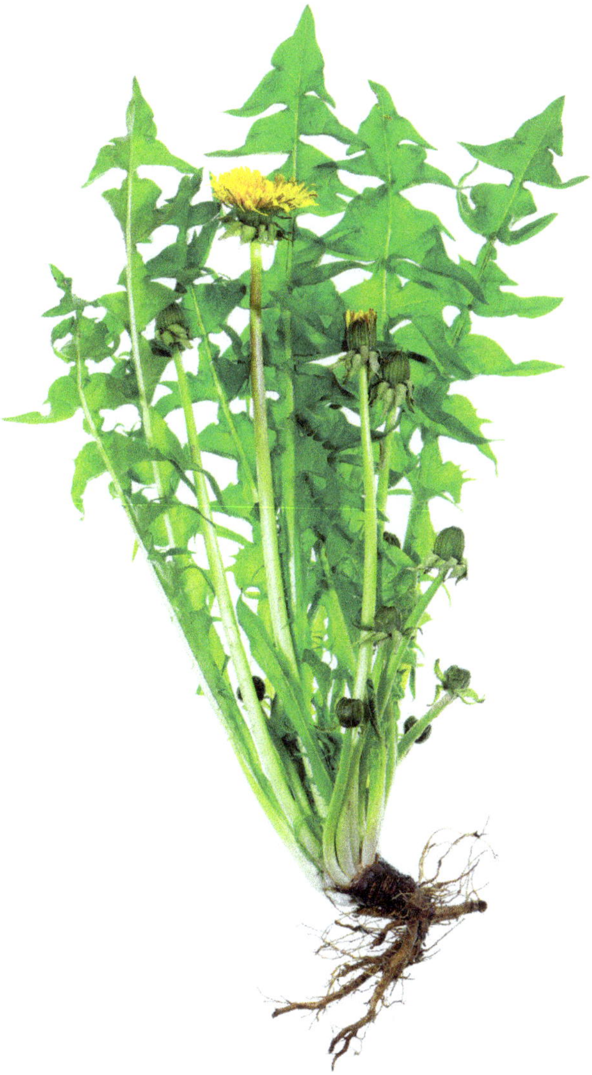

CONSTITUTENTS

DANDELION ROOTS: Dandelion roots contain triterpenes (taraxol, taraxerol, taraxasterol, ψ-taraxasterol, and β-amyrin), phytosterols (stigmasterol and β-sitosterol), inulin, sugars (fructose, glucose, and sucrose), pectin, glucosides, choline, and sesquiterpene lactones (eudesmanolide and germacranolide type), taraxacoside, mannitol, chicoriin, chicoric acid, coumestrol, levulin, luteolines, saponins, tannin, gum, resins, potash, caoutchouc latex, and phenolic acids (caffeic acid and *p*-hydroxyphenylacetic acids).[3,13,14]

DANDELION FLOWERS: Dandelion flowers contain carotenoids (lutein, lutein epoxide, cryptoxanthin, cryptoxanthin epoxide, flavoxanthin, chrysanthemaxanthin, taraxanthin, and violaxanthin), carotenoid monoesters and diesters with fatty acids (mainly myristic, lauric, palmitic, and stearic acids), arnidiol, lecithin, flavoxanthins, lacucerol, levulin, and lutein. The stems contain latex.[13,14]

DANDELION LEAVES: Dandelion leaves contain lutein, violaxanthin, carotenoids, bitter substances, chicoric acid, cichoriin, coumestrol, lactucerol, levulin, luteolins, taraxacosides, and taraxanthin.[12,13]

NUTRITIONAL PROPERTIES: Fresh dandelion leaf contains aluminum, ash, calcium, choline, chromium, cobalt, copper, crude fiber, dietary fiber, fat, iron, magnesium, manganese, niacin, phosphorus, potassium, protein, riboflavin, selenium, silicon, sodium, thiamine, tin, vitamins A, C, and D, and zinc. One raw cup of greens can provide up to 14,000 IU of beta carotene.[4,15]

MEDICINAL PROPERTIES: Dandelion root is an antidyscratic, anti-inflammatory, bitter tonic, cholagogue, choleretic, depurative, hepatic, and mild laxative. The leaf is a bitter tonic, diuretic, hepatic, and cholagogue.

TEMPERATURE AND FLAVOR: Dandelion root is cool, bitter, and mildly sweet. The root is sweeter and less bitter when harvested in winter or spring. Fall harvested dandelion root is more cooling and bitter. Dandelion leaf is cool and bitter.

MEDICINAL USES

DANDELION ROOTS AND LEAVES: Dandelion is a bitter tonic, cholagogue, and mild laxative.[6] It stimulates upper and lower digestive secretions, improving fat and protein digestion.[4,16] Dandelion's bitter tonic actions, attributed to taraxacin, aid in treating a weak appetite, nonulcer dyspepsia, bloating, flatulence, minor constipation, and hemorrhoids.[16,17] The bitter tonic and hepatobiliary effects are attributed to the bitter principles and phenolic acids.[16]

DANDELION ROOTS: Dandelion improves bile production and excretion, reducing liver and gallbladder congestion.[4,13] The high choline content of the root likely contributes to the liver detoxifying and cholagogue effects.[4] Studies of humans and animals have confirmed the cholagogue effects.[4] Rodent studies confirm that the sesquiterpene lactone content of the root increases bile excretion more than 40%, while increasing gastric secretions.[14] Dandelion is a long-term tonic for treating jaundice, hepatitis, and gallbladder-related problems, including cholestasis, cholelithiasis, and cholangitis.[13] It also reduces the propensity to form gallstones. One study demonstrated that dandelion extract successfully treated hepatitis, swelling of the liver, jaundice, and dyspepsia (with deficient bile secretion).[4]

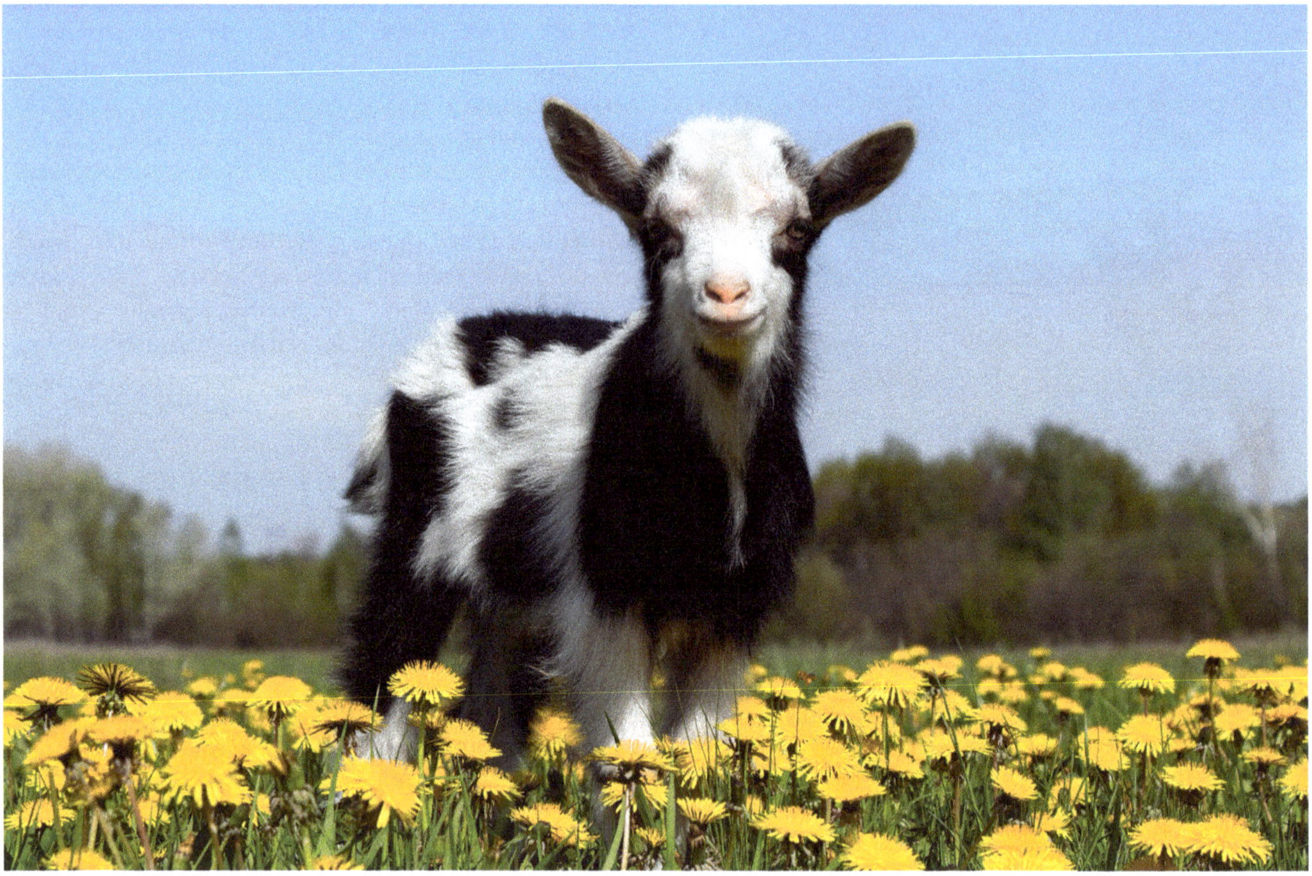

Dandelion root enhances hepatic detoxification of drugs and caffeine, as well as endogenous and exogenous hormones (including birth control pills and hormone replacement therapy). The lipotropic actions of the root may increase biliary excretion of estrogen metabolites, treating liver-related hormone imbalances.[4] Based on clinical observation, the decongestant effects of dandelion in the liver and gallbladder often reduce symptoms of premenstrual syndrome, as well as hormone-related agitation during perimenopausal years. Dandelion improves hepatic and renal filtration of byproducts of cellular metabolism, treating inflammatory skin conditions such as acne, eczema, psoriasis, boils, abscesses, and swellings.

Fresh dandelion root has anti-inflammatory properties that lower elevated IgE levels.[18] Animal studies confirm moderate anti-inflammatory and antioxidant properties.[7] Prepare a decoction with fresh or "pickled" roots, or consume the fresh root or fluid extract to treat inflammatory skin conditions such as hives, urticaria, eczema, dermatitis, psoriasis, and acne.[13] Dandelion root also prevents seasonal allergies and reduces inflammation associated with food sensitivities, hives, rheumatoid arthritis, gout, stiff joints, and fibromyalgia.[13,18]

Dandelion root has anticarcinogenic and antitumor effects.[4,6] It contains immune stimulating inulin that activates macrophages.[6] In a Japanese study, alcohol extracts of dandelion administered to rodents inhibited the growth of inoculated Ehrlich ascites cancer cells within one week after treatment.[4] In 1981, Japanese researchers also isolated the glucose polymer, TOf-CFr, from a freeze-dried, warm water extract of the root that had antitumor properties in rodents.[4] In 1987, a U.S. study found that dandelion consumption produced antibodies to activate polypeptides in tumor-induced mouse ascites fluid.[4] In test tube studies, extracts of dandelion have demonstrated antitumor activity against liver, colon, and melanoma cancer cells.[7]

The latex contained in dandelion has weak antibiotic and antifungal effects; however, it is effective for inhibiting *Saccharomyces cerevisiae* and *Candida albicans*.[6] Some herbalists claim that directly applying the latex two to three times daily enhances wart removal.[6] *Note:* Be cautious when applying the latex topically, as it can have phototoxic effects.[6]

DANDELION LEAVES: Dandelion leaf is a pregnancy-safe diuretic that reduces edema and water-related weight gain. It decreases swelling of the hands, feet, eyelids, and breasts, and alleviates premenstrual edema. Dandelion leaf enhances uric acid elimination, aiding the treatment of gout, arthritis, and kidney stones.[13] Administer the leaves or whole plant to treat gout or kidney stones.

Dandelion leaf facilitates kidney detoxification, improving moist inflammatory skin conditions. Most prescription diuretics such as furosemide (Lasix) leach potassium. However, dandelion is rich in potassium and counters the loss of potassium from diuresis, alleviating concerns of potassium deficiency associated with using prescription diuretics. Consuming dandelion as an alternative to furosemide also prevents exposure to the more serious potential side effects of taking the drug, such as hepatic coma and circulatory collapse.[4] The flavonoids and potassium salts contribute to the diuretic effects.[16] In a study of rodents, consuming eight milliliters of the aqueous fluid extract per kilogram of body weight resulted in a 30% loss of body weight in 30 days.[4] Water-based preparations are best for treating kidney or urinary concerns.

CONTRAINDICATIONS

Dandelion is considered safe during pregnancy and lactation. Avoid use in cases of biliary obstruction and gallbladder empyema.[14,16] Because of the diuretic properties, individuals with frequent urination should avoid dandelion, or consume leaf preparations in moderation. Exercise caution, limit, or avoid use while consuming a prescription diuretic. Dandelion can cause allergic dermatitis in individuals sensitive to the Asteraceae family; avoid consumption if this occurs.[16] Avoid consumption of the leaf if it aggravates conditions such as acid indigestion, gastroesophageal reflux disease, or gastric ulcers.

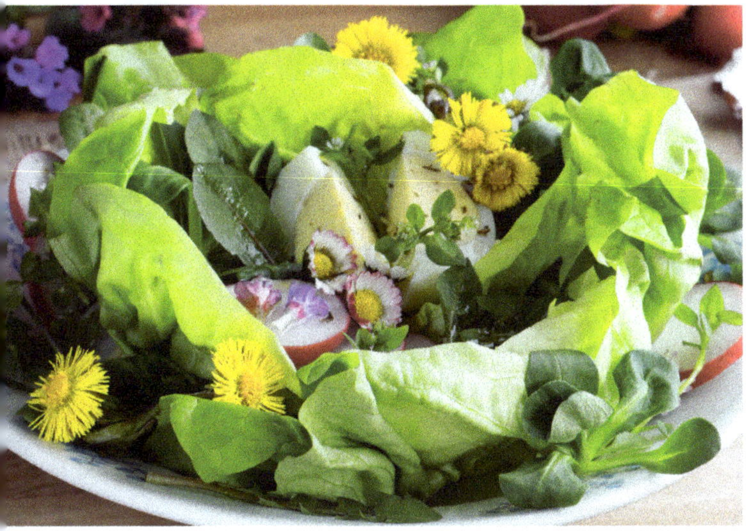

PREPARATION AND DOSAGE

TINCTURE: Fresh whole plant or leaves [1:2-1:3, 60-95% alcohol]; fresh roots [1:2, 60-95% alcohol]; dry roots [1:5, 50-60% alcohol]; consume 30-90 drops, up to four times daily.

FLUID EXTRACT: Dry roots [1:1, 40% alcohol]; consume 30-90 drops, up to four times daily.

GLYCERITE: Fresh roots [1:2-1:3, 60% glycerin and 40% water]; consume 30-60 drops, up to three times daily.

ACETUM EXTRACT: Fresh leaves or whole plant [1:2, apple cider vinegar]; consume 1 teaspoon to 1 tablespoon, up to three times daily.

SUCCUS: Juice the fresh leaves or whole plant and preserve by adding 20% alcohol; consume 1 teaspoon to 1 tablespoon, up to three times daily, and store in the refrigerator.

CAPSULES: Consume 2-4 "00" capsules, up to three times daily.

TEA: Prepare a hot infusion of the leaf or a decoction of the root; consume 8-12 ounces, three to four times daily. Prepare the pickled root by cleaning and chopping the fresh root and placing it in a mason jar; pour enough 95% alcohol to coat the root without drowning it. *Note:* A maximum of one inch of alcohol should remain at the bottom of the jar. Decoct 3-4 tablespoons of the pickled root in 32 ounces of water.

HONEY AND SYRUP: Prepare a decoction of the roots, cooking to one-half the original volume; strain and add molasses, honey, or simple syrup to desired sweetness. Alternatively, infuse the fresh roots in honey [1:4, weight of root to volume of honey]. For either preparation, consume 1 teaspoon to 1 tablespoon, up to three times daily.

TOPICAL USE: Apply a poultice of the leaf or root.

CULINARY USE: Marinate the young tender greens or toss them in olive oil, vinegar, salt, and pepper. Steam, sauté, or add fresh, finely chopped herb to soups.

DONG QUAI

DESCRIPTION

BOTANICAL NAMES:
Angelica sinensis (syn. *A. polymorpha* var. *sinensis*)

COMMON NAMES:
Dang gui, dong quai, dang quai, tang kuei, Chinese angelica
kinesisk kvan (Danish)
tōki (Japanese)
tanggwi (Korean)
dāng guī (Mandarin)

FAMILY NAME:
Apiaceae (Umbelliferae)

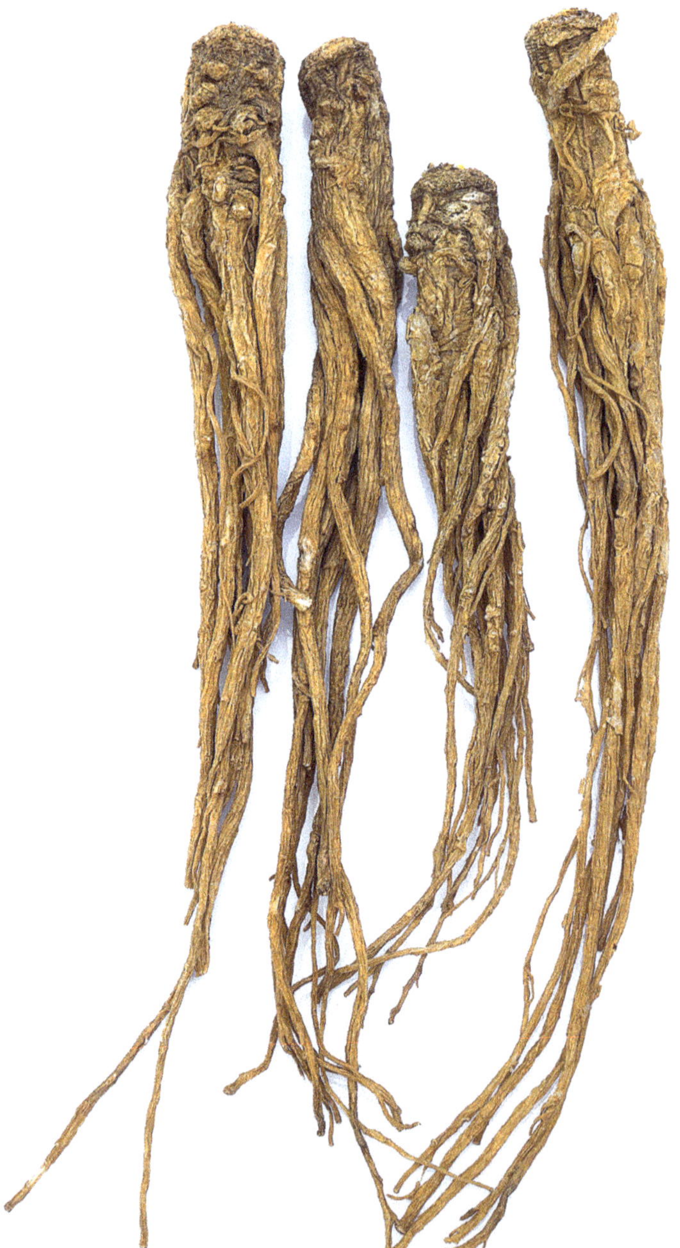

PART USED: The cured roots.

BOTANICAL DESCRIPTION AND HABITAT: A beautiful, feathery, herbaceous perennial (up to one meter tall), *Angelica sinensis* is known for its potent aromatic taproots.[1] The large, two to three ternate-pinnate leaves have succulent, ribbed, purple-green, sheathing petioles (5 – 20 cm long).[1] The ovate leaf blade (10 – 30 cm long by 12 – 25 cm wide) has many lanceolate leaflets with irregularly serrated margins (2 – 3.5 cm long by 0.8 – 2.5 cm wide).[1]

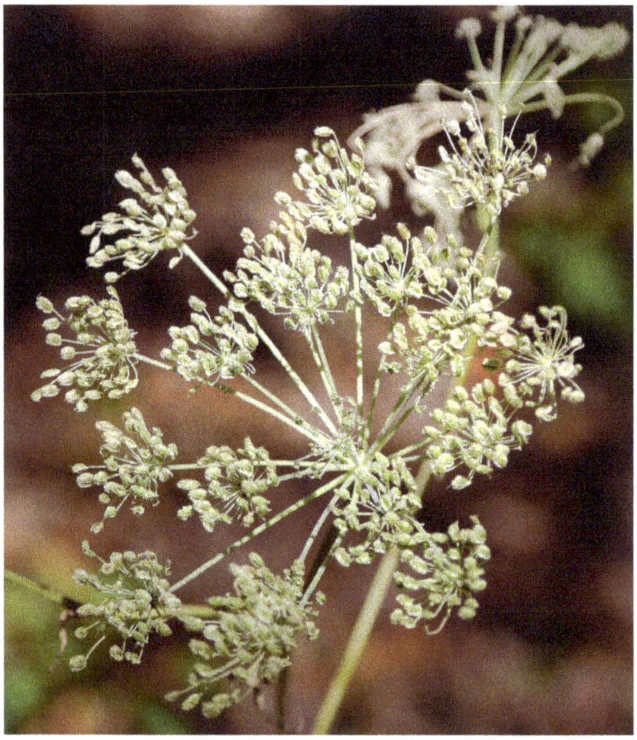

The inflorescence is a compound umbel atop a somewhat hairy peduncle (8 – 20 cm tall).[1] The involucre is either absent, or consists of two linear bracts.[1] Ten to 30 rays of varied lengths bear tiny umbels of 13 – 36 flowers; each umbel is subtended by two to four linear bracteoles.[1] The flowers often lack a calyx, and have five petals that are usually white, or occasionally pink to dark purple.[1,2] An inferior ovary consists of two fused carpels, with two styles emerging from the top.[2] The fruit is an ovoid, ribbed, two-part schizocarp (4 – 6 mm long by 3 – 4 mm wide) with the two lateral ribs expanded into wings.[1,2]

THE NAME: The genus *Angelica* ("angelic") derives from Latin.[3] The epithet *sinensis* indicates the plant's Chinese origin.[3] The epithet *acutiloba* refers to the sharply pointed leaf lobes. *A. acutiloba* (Japanese angelica) is native to Japan, and often substitutes for Chinese angelica.[4]

HISTORICAL USES: Dong quai *(A. sinensis)* has been cultivated and used in China for thousands of years.[5] Its use was first recorded in the *Shen Nong Ben Cao Fing* as a cure for coughs, chills, and fever.[3] Dong quai was used to treat infertility and vaginal infections, as well as painful, abnormal, or absent menstruation.[3,4] It was also administered to promote a healthy pregnancy and smooth delivery.[5] It was applied topically to boils, ulcers, skin diseases, and wounds.[3] Dong quai continues to be one of the most frequently prescribed herbs for women.

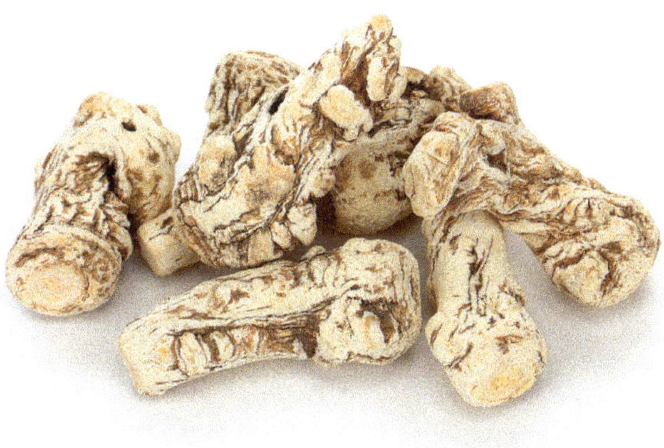

CONSTITUENTS: Dong quai contains volatile oil (n-butylidene phthalide = n-butylphthalide, ligustilide, cadinene, carvacrol, dihydrophthalic anhydride, n-dodecanal, n-tetradecanol, safrole, isosafrole, and sesquiterpenes), phytosterols, β-sitosterol, ferulic acid, linoleic acid, oleic acids, palmitic acid, stearic acid, coumarins (angelol and angelicone), water-soluble polysaccharides, sucrose, carotene, and trace amounts of vitamin B_{12}.[4-7]

NUTRITIONAL PROPERTIES: Dong quai contains high amounts of aluminum, cobalt, crude fiber, iron, magnesium, niacin, and phosphorus. It contains low to average amounts of calcium, chromium, dietary fiber, manganese, silicon, and vitamins A and C.[8]

MEDICINAL PROPERTIES: Analgesic (mild), antianemic, antiarrhythmic, antiatherosclerotic, anti-inflammatory, antispasmodic (mild), bitter tonic, blood thinner, blood tonic, cholagogue, circulatory stimulant, hepatodecongestant, hepatoprotective, hormone balancing agent, hypotensive, immune modulator, laxative, peripheral vasodilator, platelet aggregation inhibitor, reproductive tonic, and uterine tonic.

TEMPERATURE AND FLAVOR: Warm, sweet, pungent, bitter, and salty.

MEDICINAL USES

Dong quai is highly effective for regulating the menstrual cycle. It aids in treating menstrual disorders due to blood deficiency, such as amenorrhea (absent menstruation), oligomenorrhea (irregular menstruation), and dysmenorrhea (painful menstruation).[6,9] Dong quai is a restorative agent, replenishing women who have menorrhagia (heavy menstruation) and anemia, and those who feel depleted after menstruation or childbirth.[3,9-11] It stimulates hematopoiesis in bone marrow, and increases the quantity of red blood cells and platelets.[3,4,10] In Traditional Chinese Medicine, it is classified as a blood tonifying herb.[6] Symptoms of blood deficiency include: pale lips, face, and tongue, menstrual irregularity, palpitations, dry skin, lethargy, dizziness, vertigo, and weakness after menses, birth, or breastfeeding.[6] Dong quai is traditionally combined with these three blood tonifying herbs: bai shao *(Paeonia lactiflora),* chuan xiong *(Ligusticum striatum),* and shu di huang (prepared *Rehmannia glutinosum*). Because blood tonifying herbs can be dense, cloying, and difficult to digest, they can be combined with spleen qi tonifying herbs, such as huang qi *(Astragalus),* fu ling *(Poria),* and bai zhu *(Atractylodes)* to ease digestion and enhance their assimilation.[6]

Dong quai is a uterine tonic with a regulatory effect on uterine contractions.[10] It relaxes uterine muscles and increases uterine tone, strengthening uterine contractions and encouraging more rhythmic, organized contractions.[4-6,10] The subtle emmenagogue effect likely results from increased uterine contractions.[10] Ligustilide and ferulic acid exert smooth muscle antispasmodic effects in the uterus and bronchi.[4,10] Butylidene phthalide also inhibits smooth muscle spasms and reduces uterine contractions.[4] A decoction containing yan hu suo *(Corydalis yanhusuo),* bai shao *(Paeonia lactiflora),* chuan xiong *(Ligusticum striatum),* and dong quai was administered to women with dysmenorrhea five days prior to, and until the cessation of menses, with a 72% cure rate.[4]

Dong quai continues to be used as a hormone balancing agent, and is reputed to have an estrogenic effect.[5,9] Supporting the estrogenic influence, naturopathic physician Michael Murray explains that dong quai contains:

...highly active phytoestrogens, although these compounds are much lower in activity than animal estrogens (1:400 as active). This helps to explain why angelica is used to treat conditions characterized by both high and low estrogen levels. Phytoestrogens demonstrate an alterative effect by competing with estrogen for binding sites on cells. When estrogen levels are low, phytoestrogens exert some estrogenic activity; when estrogen levels are high, phytoestrogens reduce overall estrogenic activity by occupying estrogen receptor sites.[5]

Herbalist Michael Moore suggests that dong quai may enhance the utilization of endogenous estrogen.[12] In order to establish regular menstrual cycles and/or enhance fertility, dong quai is best consumed during the follicular phase of the menstrual cycle, followed by vitex berry *(Vitex)* during the luteal phase.[10,12] I have utilized a similar biphasic protocol effectively in numerous women with amenorrhea, oligomenorrhea, anovulatory cycles, and difficulty conceiving. In order to establish regular menstrual cycles and ovulation, the following combination has been highly effective: bai shao *(Paeonia)*, black cohosh *(Actaea)*, ashwagandha *(Withania)*, wu wei zi *(Schisandra)*, shu di huang *(Rehmannia)*, dong quai, and a small quantity of licorice *(Glycyrrhiza)*. This compound was consumed as a follicular phase formula — post-menstruation until ovulation during days 5 – 14. During ovulation, patients switch to a formula containing higher quantities of vitex berry *(Vitex)*, and smaller quantities of bai shao *(Paeonia)*, dandelion *(Taraxacum)*, turmeric *(Curcuma)*, chuan xiong *(Ligusticum striatum)*, and motherwort *(Leonurus)*. These formulas established regular menstrual cycles, and reduced menstrual cramping, breast tenderness, mood swings, irritability, and hormone-induced inflammation (headaches, migraines, skin conditions, etc.). In Traditional Chinese Medicine, formulas containing liver decongestants, dong quai, and other blood tonifying herbs are consumed two weeks prior to menses or throughout the month (except during menstruation) to balance hormones and reduce PMS symptoms.

Dong quai can be included in formulas to balance hormones as menstrual cycles wane.[5,9] The following compounded herbal extracts have been highly effective in easing the transition during perimenopausal and menopausal years: vitex berry *(Vitex)*, dong quai, black cohosh *(Actaea)*, motherwort *(Leonurus)*, dandelion root *(Taraxacum)*, licorice *(Glycyrrhiza)*, and wild oats *(Avena)*. The formula can be modified to include: American ginseng *(Panax quinquefolius)* to reduce hot flashes; wu wei zi *(Schisandra)*, ashwagandha *(Withania)*, or shatavari *(Asparagus racemosus)* for adrenal support and increased libido; and Chinese ginseng *(Panax ginseng)* or eleuthero *(Eleutherococcus)* for the adaptogen and adrenal tonic effects. Consuming 30 – 90 drops two to three times daily, long-term, is effective for many women in reducing hot flashes and mood swings, and treating decreased libido, depression, and atonic conditions of the urinary and reproductive organs. *Note:* Remove dong quai from the formula if there is heavy bleeding, or if menstruation lasts more than seven days.

According to studies, dong quai has no estrogenic effect.[4,10] In a double-blind, placebo-controlled study of postmenopausal women, it did not exert estrogen-like responses in endometrial thickness or vaginal maturation. Symptoms were reduced in both groups; however, there were no significant differences between dong quai and a placebo.[4]

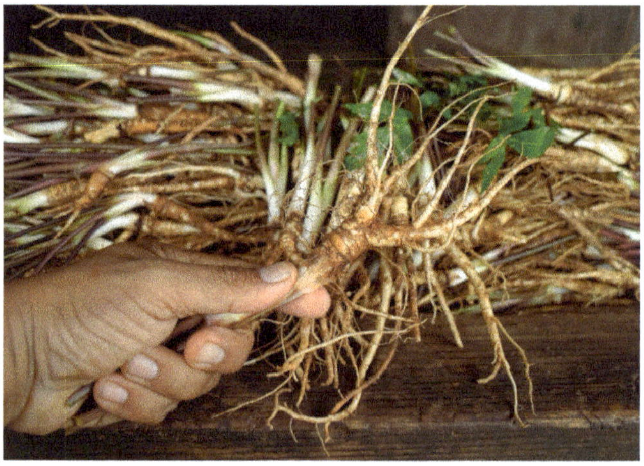

In a study with differing results, the estrogenic influence was evaluated by administering the standardized extract of *A. sinensis* roots to ovariectomized rats.[13] The results demonstrated that the extract stimulated the uterine histoarchitecture, there was significant cornification in the vaginal epithelium, and serum LH levels were reduced, confirming the estrogenic activity of dong quai.[13] In intact female rats, the extract prolonged the estrus stage of the estrous cycle.[13]

A hepatoprotectant, liver decongestant, and cholagogue, dong quai aids in treating liver disorders, including chronic hepatitis and cirrhosis.[4,7] In patients with chronic hepatitis and hepatic cirrhosis, dong quai improved abnormal plasma protein metabolism, and increased plasma protein levels 60% in one to three weeks.[4] Dong quai increased oxygen utilization of the liver (with no effect on nucleic acids), as well as liver metabolism in mice; it also improved glutamic acid and cysteine oxidation.[4,6] Dong quai protects liver cells from carbon tetrachloride, paracetamol, and aflatoxin damage.[10] It has a laxative effect and lubricates the bowels.[6,7,9] Dong quai aids in treating chronic constipation due to blood deficiency.[6]

Dong quai is an anti-inflammatory. It has prostaglandin-regulating effects, inhibiting the synthesis of thromboxane A2, thus reducing blood viscosity and clotting.[10] When consumed regularly, the antiplatelet and smooth muscle antispasmodic effects aid in preventing, and to a lesser extent, treating migraines.[5,9] Dong quai also reduces allergic symptoms to a variety of substances, such as food, pollen, dust, and animal dander.[5] It inhibits the production of immunoglobulin E (IgE) antibodies, lowering their levels.[5] Individuals with allergic conditions have three to ten times the normal level of antibodies; therefore, long-term use of dong quai may help to alleviate allergic sensitivity. To enhance the anti-inflammatory and antiallergenic effects, combine dong quai with reishi mushrooms *(Ganoderma)*, turmeric *(Curcuma)*, dandelion root *(Taraxacum)*, burdock root *(Arctium)*, and/or licorice *(Glycyrrhiza)*.

Dong quai has antiatherosclerotic and cholesterol-lowering effects.[4,6] It lowers blood pressure, dilates coronary vessels, increases coronary flow, and reduces the respiratory rate.[4,6] Dong quai helps to regulate the heart rate and treats arrhythmia.[10] It was found to correct experimentally-induced atrial fibrillation.[4] The ferulic acid in dong quai also inhibits platelet aggregation and serotonin release.[4] It is administered to treat angina, coronary heart disease, strokes, and peripheral vascular disorders.[4,7] It is often combined with dan shen *(Salvia miltiorrhiza)* for the blood-moving, hypocholesterolemic, and antiatherosclerotic effects.[4]

Dong quai is a circulatory stimulant and peripheral vasodilator.[7,10] Consuming the herb regularly improves circulation and aids in treating cold extremities, Raynaud's phenomenon, Buerger's disease, intermittent claudication, and constrictive aortitis.[4,7] Traditionally, it is used to treat congealed blood that presents with abdominal pain, traumatic injuries, swellings, contusions, and bruising.[4] The vasodilating properties aid in reducing elevated blood pressure.

Dong quai is also used to invigorate and harmonize the blood, reducing pain from blood stasis and cold.[6] It aids in treating dysmenorrhea, abdominal pain, and traumatic injury pain.[6,9] It is often combined with yan hu suo *(Corydalis)* and xiang fu *(Cyperus)* to reduce menstrual cramping.[6] It is a subtle analgesic and tranquilizer.[5,7]

Dong quai contains coumarins and polysaccharides (in water-based preparations) that have immune modulating activity.[5] These constituents increase white blood cell activity, and enhance non-specific host defense mechanisms, increasing interferon production and antitumor activity.[5] Extracts have antibacterial actions *in vitro* against hemolytic *Streptococcus* and *Shigella*.[6]

CONTRAINDICATIONS

Dong quai is contraindicated in the first trimester of pregnancy, or throughout pregnancy in women with a tendency to miscarry. Use only under the supervision of a Traditional Chinese Medicine practitioner during the second and third trimesters.[4] Avoid use in individuals with hemorrhagic disease, bleeding tendency, heavy menstrual periods, and those taking blood-thinning medications such as warfarin.[4,7] Discontinue use two weeks prior to, and following surgery. Dong quai should be avoided in individuals with bloating due to damp obstruction, and diarrhea from weak digestion, as well as individuals with yin deficiency with heat signs (hot flashes or night sweats).[6] Discontinue use with an infectious viral or bacterial infection such as a cold, influenza, or bronchitis.[4]

PREPARATION AND DOSAGE

Dong quai is traditionally harvested in the autumn of the third year of growth.[3] After the roots are harvested, the dirt is shaken off rather than washed to avoid bruising and contact with water that can cause decomposition or blackening of the roots.[3] Small root bundles are hung from the ceiling until slightly dried, but soft. The roots are smoked using a fire of wet wood; a light fire is then used to dry the roots 70-80%.[3] The roots are sometimes covered with a damp cloth until they absorb just enough moisture to be sliced, then fully dried.[3]

TINCTURE: Dried, cured roots [1:5, 70% alcohol]; consume 10-60 drops, two to three times daily.

CAPSULES: Consume 2-4 "00" capsules, one to three times daily. Consume 4.5-12 grams of powder daily.

TEA: Prepare a decoction; consume 8 ounces, two to three times daily.

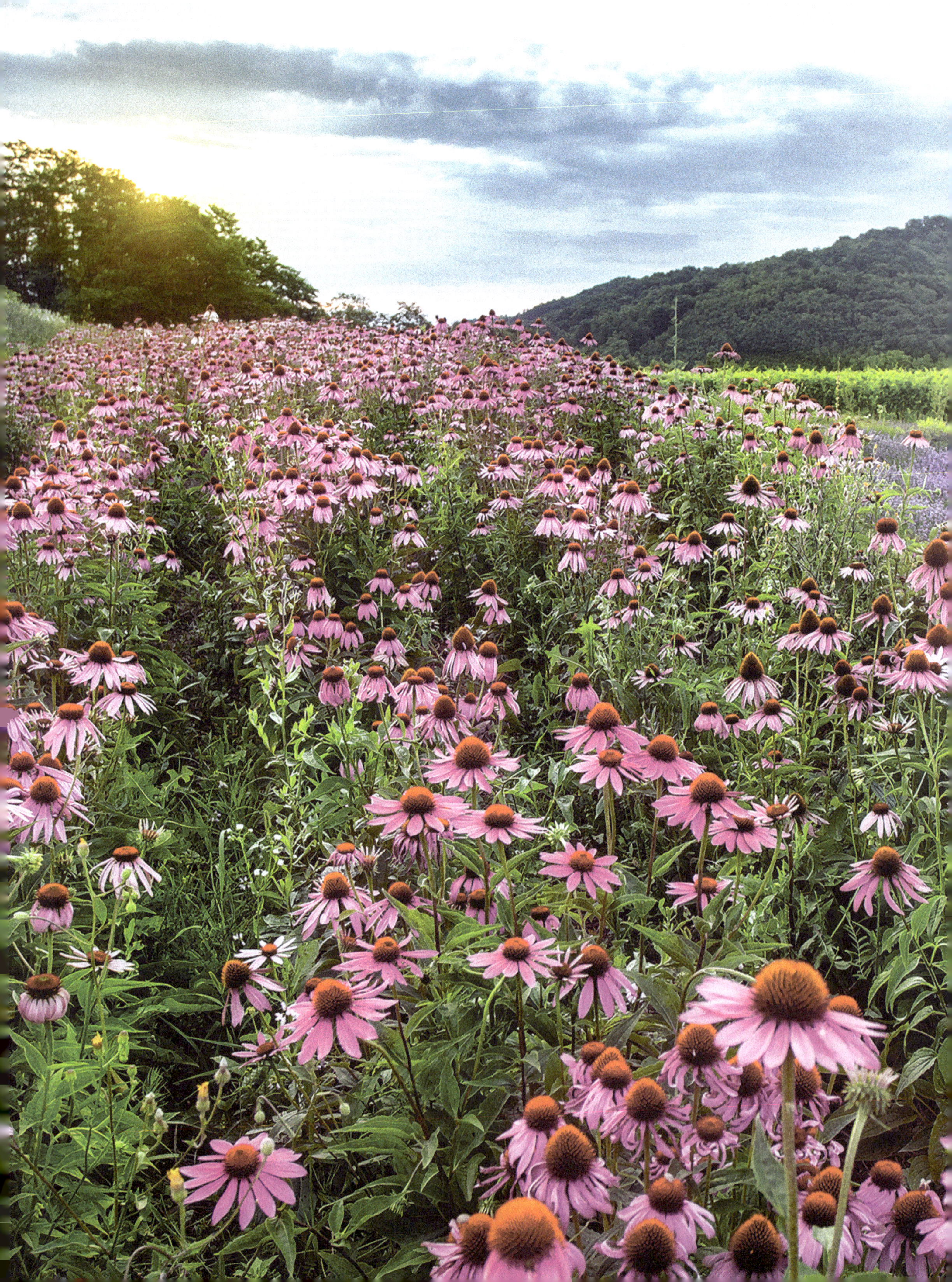

ECHINACEA

BOTANICAL NAMES:
Echinacea purpurea, E. angustifolia, E. pallida (syn. *Rudbeckia*)
Rare or endangered species include *E. atrorubens, E. paradoxa,* and *E. simulata*

COMMON NAMES:
Purple coneflower, coneflower, snakeroot, Kansas snakeroot, narrow-leaf coneflower
smalbladet, solhat (Danish)
kogelbloem (Dutch)
rudbeckie á feuilles étroites, racine d'echinacea (French)
sonnenhut, igelkopf, kegelblume, kupferblume, stachelkopf (German)
sólhattur (Icelandic)
echinacea (Italian)
smalbladet, solhatt (Norwegian)
jezowka (Polish)
equinácea (Spanish)
liten läkerudbeckia (Swedish)

FAMILY NAME:
Asteraceae (Compositae)

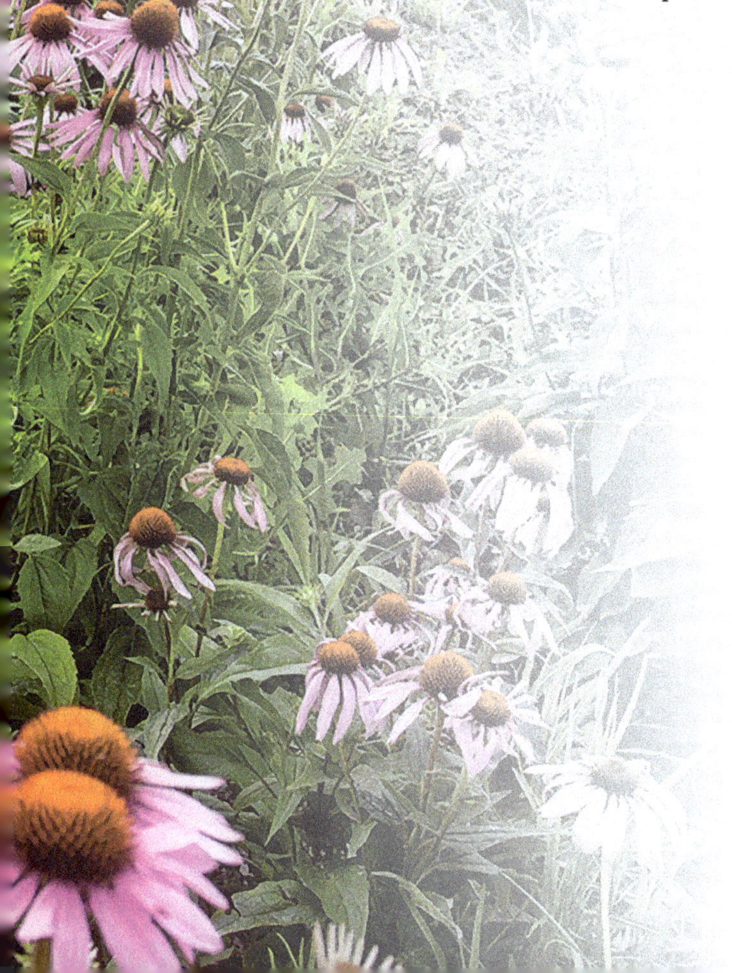

DESCRIPTION

PARTS USED: All parts of the plant, including the roots, flowers, seeds, and leaves.

BOTANICAL DESCRIPTION AND HABITAT: Echinacea grows in well drained, lime-rich soil in the Great Plains, Mountain West, and southeast U.S. It is threatened in the wild due to over-harvesting and the loss of habitat. Avoid purchasing wildcrafted *Echinacea angustifolia* to prevent a negative impact on wild populations; purchase the organically cultivated herb.

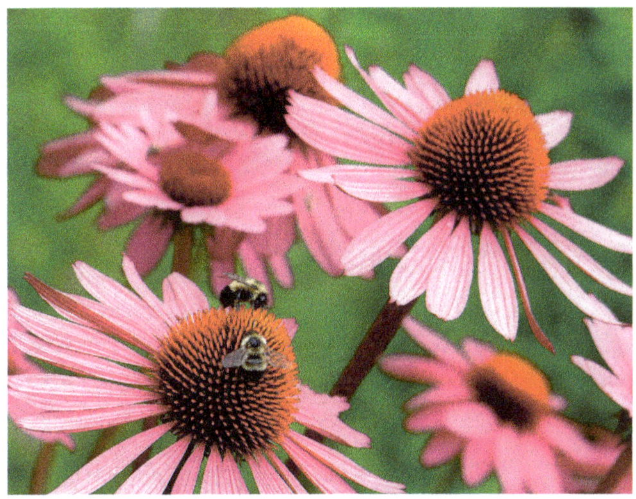

Echinacea angustifolia is an herbaceous perennial (up to 70 cm tall) with a tapering, longitudinally furrowed, cylindrical taproot.[1] The leaves grow basally from the root crown until the plant flowers, when many leaves grow alternately along the flowering stem. The elliptic to lanceolate leaves can have long petioles (2 – 12 cm) and blades (7 – 30 cm), and ciliate margins.[1] The leaves and stems are coarsely hairy. Striking purple flower heads emerge from a tall peduncle (10 – 30 cm), each consisting of up to 40 sterile ray florets with purple, reflexed ligules, and a conical disc bearing many fertile disc florets.[1] Multiple series of overlapping, lanceolate to ovate, densely hairy phyllaries encircle the ray florets, and persist after the fruits develops.[1] The fruit is a bicolored achene: tan proximally, and dark brown distally (4 – 5 mm long).[1]

Echinacea purpurea is a stout, herbaceous perennial (up to 120 cm tall); it is usually hairy.[2] The stems are often brownish green. The plant grows as a basal rosette until it flowers. Its long ovate to narrowly lanceolate leaves have

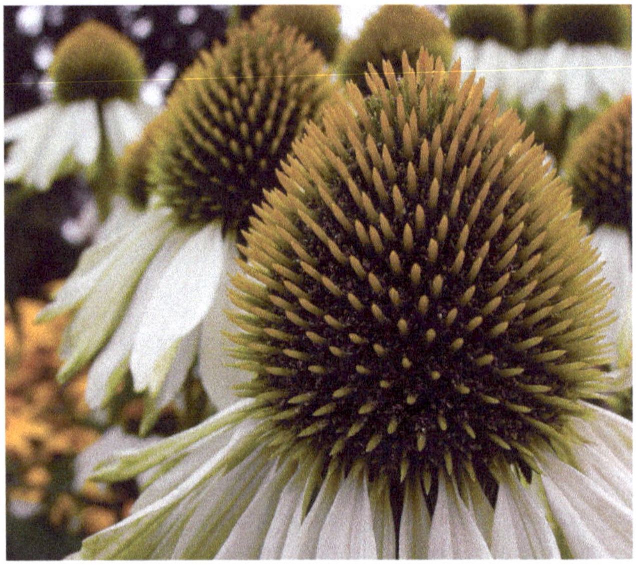

serrate to dentate margins.[2] Basal leaves (5 – 30 cm) have long petioles (0 – 17 cm).[2] The sturdy purple flower heads grow on peduncles (8 – 25 cm long), and consist of 30 – 80 ray florets clad with pink to purple reflexed ligules.[2] The conical disc is 20 – 40 mm long.[2] The glabrous fruit is an off-white achene (3 – 5 mm long).[2]

THE NAME: *Echinacea* derives from the Greek *echinos* ("sea urchin"), referring to the urchin-like flower heads. The epithets have the following meanings: *purpurea* ("purple") referring to the color of the flowers; *angustifolia* ("narrow-leaved'); and *pallida* ("pale").

These common names correspond with the following Latin binomials: purple coneflower and common purple coneflower *(E. purpurea);* pale purple coneflower *(E. pallida);* Kansas snakeroot *(E. angustifolia* or *E. pallida);* and narrow-leaf coneflower, cone flower, and purple cone flower *(E. angustifolia).*

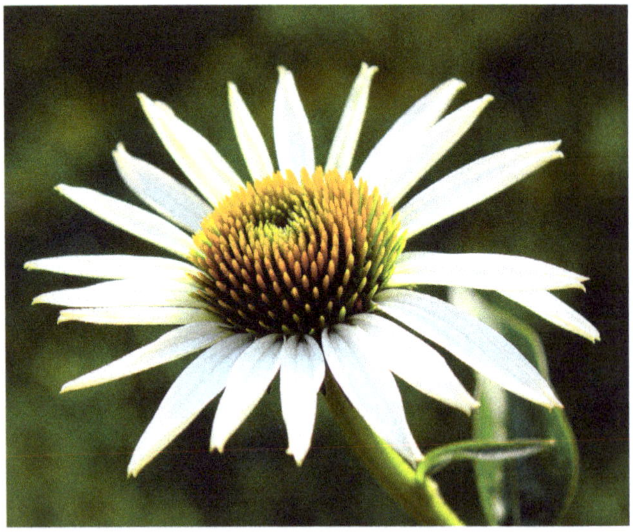

HISTORICAL USES: Echinacea was the plant most widely used by Plains Indians.[3,4] The root was used to treat colds, flu, slowly healing wounds, burns, snakebites, spider bites, and toothaches.[3,4] The Sioux consumed fresh echinacea root to treat snakebites and rabies.[5] The Meskwakis used it to alleviate stomach cramps.[3] The Choctaw administered echinacea to treat a cough and digestive upset.[6] To alleviate a sore throat, the Comanche consumed a root decoction, and applied a poultice for a toothache.[6] The Cheyenne chewed the fresh root prior to their Sun Dance ritual.[3] The herb was smoked to ease headaches.[3]

Eclectic physician Dr. John King introduced the therapeutic uses of echinacea to the Western medical profession in 1852.[6] However, it wasn't until the 1890s that it became popularized in the U.S. following the Lloyd Brothers' pharmaceutical preparation of echinacea.[6] Eclectic physicians extolled the virtues of echinacea's alterative and immune stimulating actions.[5,7] Dr. Victor von Unruh researched echinacea's effects, and concluded that it increased the phagocytic power of leukocytes and normalized neutrophils counts.[5] Echinacea was administered as a depurative to treat septicemia and "bad blood."[5,7] Conditions indicative of "bad blood" included gangrene, boils, abscesses, bed sores, skin or mucosal ulcers, and carcinomatous ulcers with fetid discharge.[5,7] It was commonly administered in high doses to hasten recovery in cases of diphtheria, smallpox, scarlet fever, puerperal fever, cholera infantum, fermentative dyspepsia, typhoid fever, typhoid pneumonia, cerebrospinal meningitis, *la grippe*, and uremia.[5,7] Echinacea was used to alleviate orchitis, epididymitis, and mammitis.[7] A dirty brown or jet-black tongue and a congested purple or bluish hue of the skin or tissues were other indications for using echinacea.[7] The diluted extract (10 – 50% solution) mixed with myrrh extract *(Commiphora)* was applied to gum abscesses, and slowly healing, painful wounds.[7] The same mixture was gargled to alleviate pyorrhea, bleeding gums, mouth ulcers, and herpes eruptions.[7] Echinacea was also applied to treat weepy eczema, chilblains, and poison ivy.[7] Eclectics considered it one of the most effective internal and topical treatments for venomous bites, including snakebites and stings.[5,7] They adopted this practice from Native Americans. Echinacea fell out of demand in the U.S. following the introduction of antibiotics and sulfa drugs in the 1930s, but has since regained popularity.[6]

CONSTITUENTS: Echinacea contains phenolic acids (cichoric acid = 2,3-dicaffeoyl-tartaric acid, verbascoside, carftaric acid, cholorgenic, and isochlorogenic acids), and a closely related phenylethanoid glycoside (echinacoside), alkamides = alkylamides (echinacein, isobutylamide, plus 10 related alkalamides, and related butylamides),

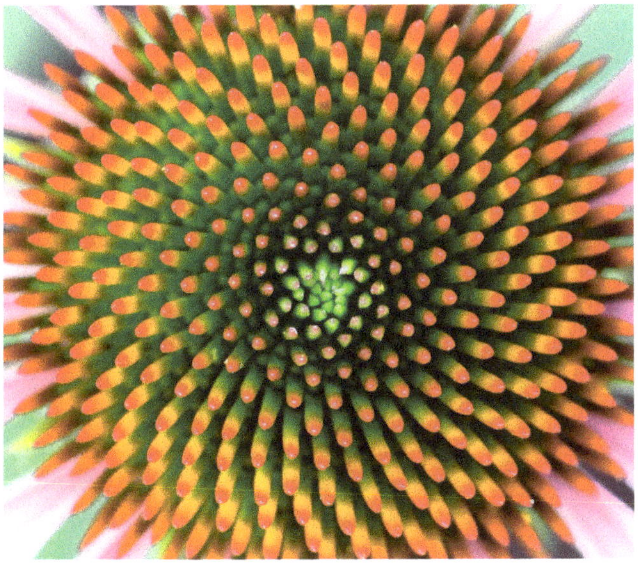

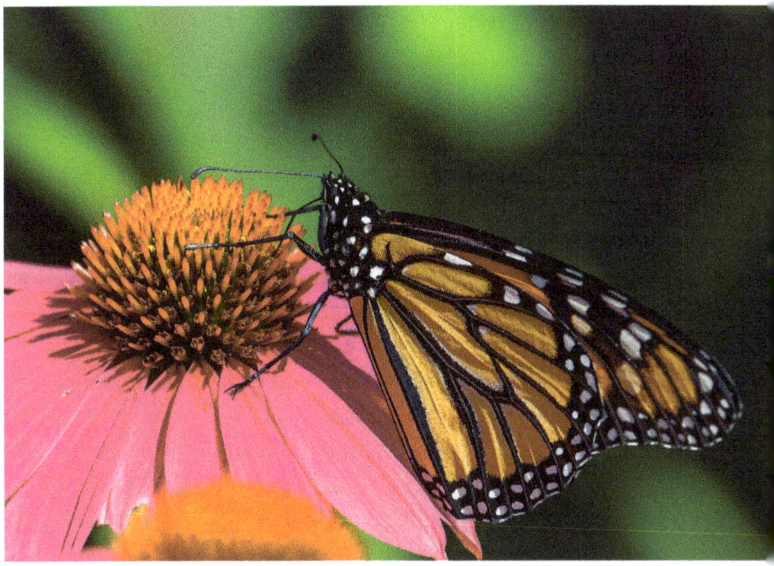

polysaccharides (heteroxylan, rhamnoarabinogalactan, and xyloglucan), acidic arabinogalactan, fucogalactoxyloglucans, polyacetylenes, pyrrolizidine alkaloids (tussilagine: non-toxic), echinacoside, and volatile oil (borneol, bornylacetate, pentadeca-8-en-2-one, germacrene D, caryophellene, caryophyllene epoxide, and palmitic acid). Additionally, the roots of *E. angustifolia* contain cynarin (= 1, 3-dicaffeoyl-quinic acid). The dried roots of *E. angustifolia* and *E. purpurea* contain pyrrolizidine alkaloids (tussilagine and isotussilagine); neither one has a 1, 2-unsaturated necine ring structure associated with hepatotoxicity.[8,9]

The aerial portions of *E. purpurea, E. angustifolia,* and *E. pallida* include borneol, bornylacetate, pentadeca-8-en-2-one, germacrene D, caryophyllene, caryophyllene epoxide, and palmitic acid. Rutoside is the primary flavonoid contained in the leaf of the aforementioned species.

MEDICINAL PROPERTIES: Alterative, antibacterial, antifungal, anti-inflammatory, antinecrotic, antioxidant, antiphlogistic, antiviral, depurative, immune modulator, immune stimulant, lymphatic, and vulnerary.

TEMPERATURE AND FLAVOR: Cool, bitter, salty, sweet, pungent, and mild astringent.

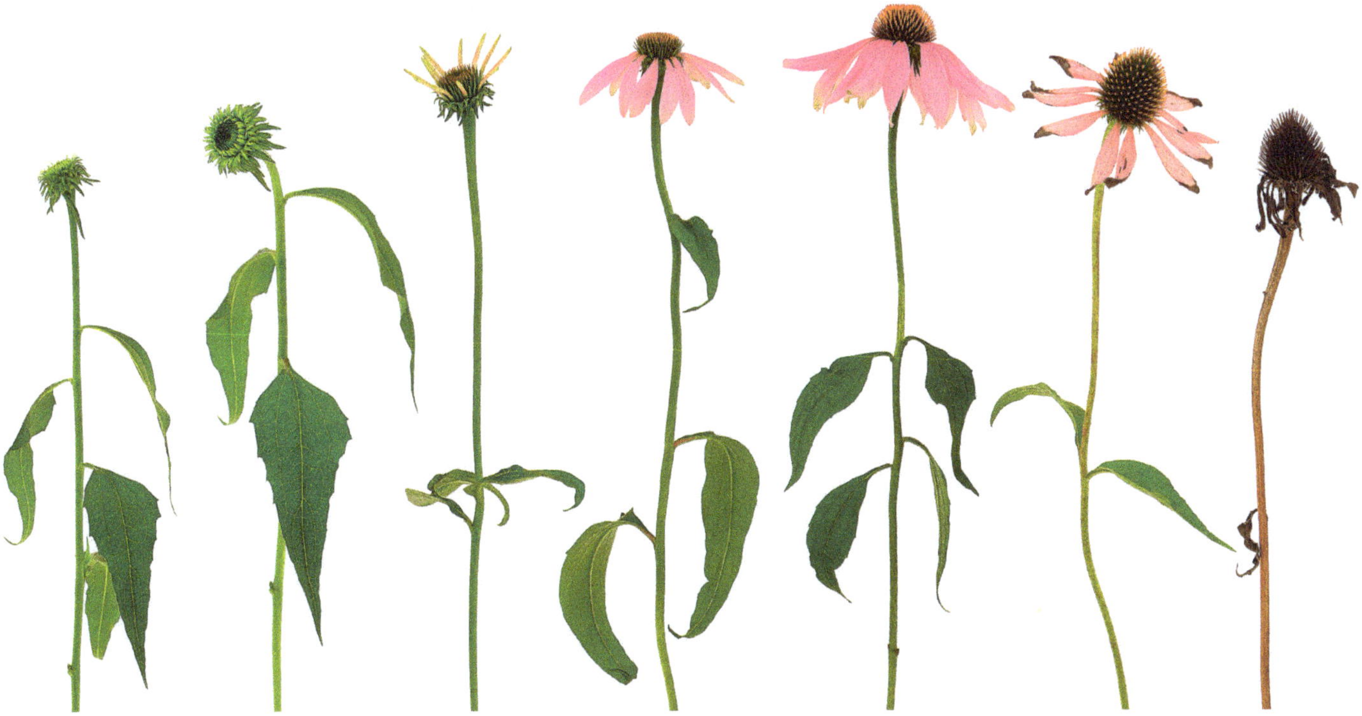

MEDICINAL USES

Echinacea is an immune stimulant that enhances phagocytosis by macrophages and granulocytes.[5,8,13] The polysaccharides, alkylamides, phenolic acid, polyacetylenes, and volatile oil activate the immune response.[7,9,10,13] Two polysaccharides (found in the aqueous extract and expressed juice) increase B- and T-lymphocyte activity, as well as phagocytosis.[8,10,12] Echinacea also stimulates α-1 and α-2 gammaglobulin that prevent viral and bacterial infections. It increases natural killer cell activity and antibody-dependent cellular cytotoxicity.[13] Alcohol extracts the alkylamides and cichoric acid (a derivative of caffeic acid); aqueous extracts and the expressed juice of *E. purpurea* enhance the extraction of the polysaccharides.[8] Therefore, combining the alcoholic and water-based extracts synergizes the immune-enhancing functions.

Echinacea decreases the severity and duration of a cold or flu, especially in immune-compromised individuals.[3,9,10,12] Expressed juice or extracts of echinacea demonstrate interferon-like antiviral activity against vesicular stomatitis, influenza, herpes, and poliovirus.[8,10,12,13] This interferon-like action inhibits the multiplication of RNA- and DNA-containing viruses, as well as some bacteria and protozoa.[10] Echinacea stimulates the properdin-complement system, helping to prevent an infection.[12] It has bacteriostatic and fungistatic actions against *Staphylococcus aureus, Escherichia coli, Pseudomonas aeruginosa, Trichomonas vaginalis,* and *Epidermophyton interdigitale.*[8,13] Echinacoside, a caffeic acid glycoside, has weak antibacterial activity.[8,10] Echinacea has lymphatic, antiphlogistic, and mild antimicrobial actions that reduce glandular swelling and ulceration, enhancing the treatment of strep throat, tonsillitis, mononucleosis, staph infections, chronic fatigue, and mammitis.[7,10] When treating infections, echinacea extracts are most effective if administered frequently in moderate to large doses (60 – 90 drops, every two hours). Fluid extracts can be administered in lower doses (15 – 30 drops, every two hours). Echinacea enhances recovery following an appendectomy, and hastens the dissolution of pus in the abdomen. Combine with huang qi *(Astragalus)* extract to enhance the resolvent effect. It is beneficial as an adjunct treatment for seasonal allergies and hay fever.[6,13] Herbalist Michael Moore recommends using echinacea in the first and final stages of an infection, and to resolve slowly healing infections.[13]

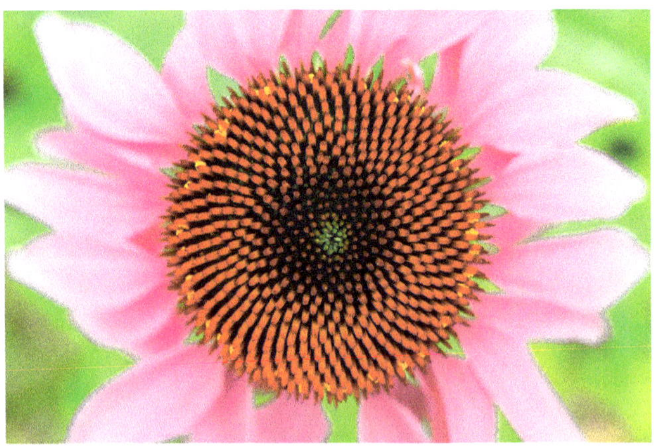

When compounded with additional antibacterial herbs, echinacea aids in treating bacterial vaginosis, pelvic inflammatory disease, cystitis, and urethritis.[6,9] In order to alleviate urinary tract infections, combine extract of echinacea with usnea *(Usnea),* uva ursi *(Arctostaphylos),* yarrow *(Achillea),* and corn silk *(Zea mays).* Consume 60 – 90 drops, every two hours, up to five times daily. Liquid extracts of the fresh root reduce the recurrence of yeast infections and vulvitis caused by *Candida albicans* infections.[13] *E. angustifolia* extract demonstrated weak inhibitory activity against the parasite *Trichomonas vaginalis.*[13] To alleviate bacterial vaginosis and yeast infections, echinacea can be combined with antibacterial and antifungal herbs such as usnea *(Usnea),* berberis *(Berberis)* or yerba mansa *(Anemopsis),* and calendula *(Calendula).* If the tissues are dry and cracked, add a small amount of licorice *(Glycyrrhiza).*

The arabinogalactan content of *Echinacea purpurea* enhances the cytotoxic activity of macrophages against tumor cells and *Leishmania enriettii.*[13] It also increases macrophage production of cytokines, including tumor-necrosis factor (TNF-α) and interleukins (IL-1, IL-6, and IL-10), and increases interferon β_2 and T cell proliferation.[8,13] It has weak activity against Walker carcinoma 256 and P-388 lymphocytic leukemia.[8] Short- or long-term use of echinacea can be helpful for individuals undergoing or recovering from chemotherapy, and those consuming immune-suppressing medications.[13] Combine with other immune modulators such as reishi mushrooms *(Ganoderma),* huang qi *(Astragalus),* dang shen *(Codonopsis),* and smaller amounts of wu wei zi *(Schisandra).*

Echinacea has sialagogue actions that stimulate salivary secretions.[5] Gargling with the diluted alcoholic extract helps to treat a toothache, and mouth or gum infections.[3,5] In order to synergize the anesthetic and antimicrobial properties for oral health, combine echinacea with spilanthes *(Acmella),* yerba mansa *(Anemopsis),* myrrh *(Commiphora),* clove *(Syzygium),* and calendula *(Calendula).*

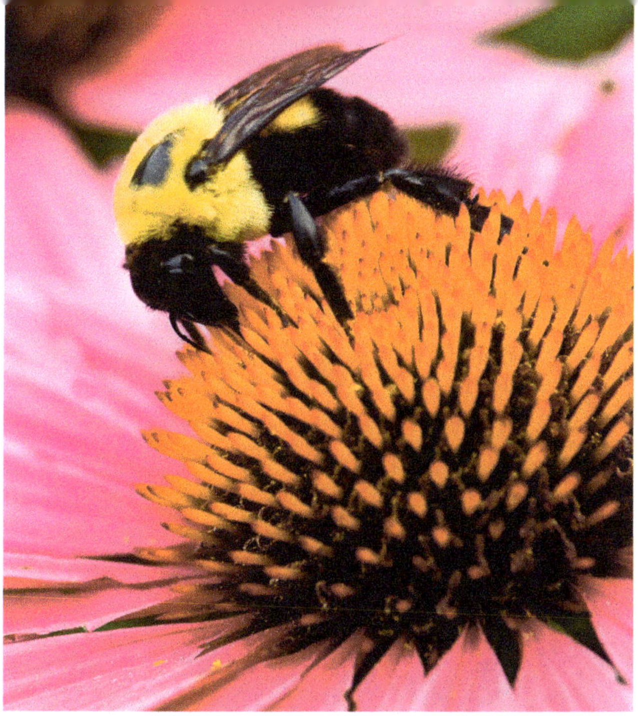

Echinacea is a vulnerary and anti-inflammatory that catalyzes tissue regeneration and wound healing.[10,12,13] Internal use of echinacea strengthens connective tissue and reduces inflammation of tendons, ligaments, and muscle sheaths.[12] Applying expressed juice of fresh flowering echinacea has hyaluronidase-inhibiting actions that protect cells, reduce inflammation and swelling, and prevent the spread of infections.[8,13] This action increases the fibroblasts that stimulate connective tissue regeneration.[13] The antihyaluronidase activity is due to caffeic acid esters.[13] Echinacea contains caffeic acid esters that have antioxidant and collagen protective effects.[13] Topical applications of echinacea help to prevent and treat ultraviolet radiation damage of the skin.[13] They also aid in treating skin ulcers, diabetic ulcers, bed sores, wounds, gangrenous wounds, boils, abscesses, staph infections, infected hair follicles, poison ivy dermatitis, burns, contusions, sprains, eczema, and herpes.[5-7,9,10,12,13] An internal combination for treating boils, abscesses, and infected wounds includes extracts of echinacea, yerba mansa *(Anemopsis)*, red root *(Ceanothus)*, calendula *(Calendula)*, and wild indigo *(Baptisia)*. Consume 30 - 90 drops of this compound, three to five times daily.

Internal and external use of echinacea reduces swelling due to insect bites (spider, bug, and mosquito) and bee stings.[3,5,7,12] Prepare a drawing poultice by combining echinacea extract or glycerite, clay and/or baking soda, with several drops each of lavender and blue chamomile essential oils. Apply a sufficient amount of this poultice to cover two to three times the surface area of the insect sting or bite. Apply two to three times daily until the swelling decreases.

CONTRAINDICATIONS

There are no known contraindications for pregnant or lactating women. In some individuals, high doses of echinacea can cause nausea.[6] Echinacea can cause contact dermatitis in individuals sensitive to Asteraceae family plants. Some people caution against using echinacea long-term in individuals with autoimmune conditions such as lupus erythematosus, multiple sclerosis, rheumatic arthritis, or scleroderma. However, there is a lack of clinical evidence, and as of yet, no case studies prove that echinacea aggravates these conditions.[13]

PREPARATION AND DOSAGE

TINCTURE: Fresh roots [1:2, 70 - 95% alcohol]; fresh flowers or seeds [1:4, 70 - 95% alcohol]; dry roots [1:5, 60 - 70% alcohol]; consume 30 - 100 drops, up to five times daily.

FLUID EXTRACT: Dry roots or seeds [1:1, 60% alcohol]; consume 10 - 30 drops, three to five times daily.

GLYCERITE: Fresh roots [1:2 - 1:3, 50% alcohol, 50% glycerin]; consume 10 - 60 drops, up to five times daily.

TEA: Prepare the root as a decoction or cold infusion, or the flowers or seeds as a hot infusion; consume 8 - 12 ounces, up to four times daily.

HONEY AND SYRUP: Fresh root honey [1:4]; consume 1 teaspoon up to three times daily.

TOPICAL USE: Prepare oil or salve of the leaves, flowers, or seeds using the alcohol intermediary oil method, or apply topically a diluted extract, fomentation, or poultice of the powdered root or ground herb. Alternatively, prepare a paste containing clay, echinacea extract, and essential oils of lavender and blue chamomile. (Refer to the final paragraph in the *Medicinal Uses* section.)

ELDER

DESCRIPTION

BOTANICAL NAMES:
Sambucus nigra ssp. *nigra* (syn. *S. nigra*), *Sambucus nigra* ssp. *canadensis* (syn. *S. canadensis, S. mexicana, S. laciniata*), *Sambucus nigra* ssp. *caerulea* (syn. *S. caerulea, S. mexicana*), *Sambucus racemosa* var. *melanocarpa* (syn. *S. melanocarpa*)

COMMON NAMES:
Elder, elderberry, elder berry, black elder, European elder, American elder, blue elder, Rocky Mountain black elder, Mexican elder, lace leaf elder, cut-leaf elder, blood elder, bour tree, ellhorn, fever tree, danewort, ellanwood, pan pipes, pipe tree, sambu, tree of medicine, tree of music
bozinka (Czech)
hyld (Danish)
vlier (Dutch)
sureau noir (French)
flieder, holunder, schwiztee (German)
bodzafa (Hungarian)
sambreo, sambuco nero (Italian)
chieh-ku mu (Mandarin)
hyll (Norwegian)
bez czarny (Polish)
sabuguiero (Portuguese)
busine (Russian)
flor de sauz, sauco, capulín silvestre (Spanish)
fläder (Swedish)
eirin ysgaw (Welsh)

FAMILY NAME:
Adoxaceae (formerly Caprifoliaceae)

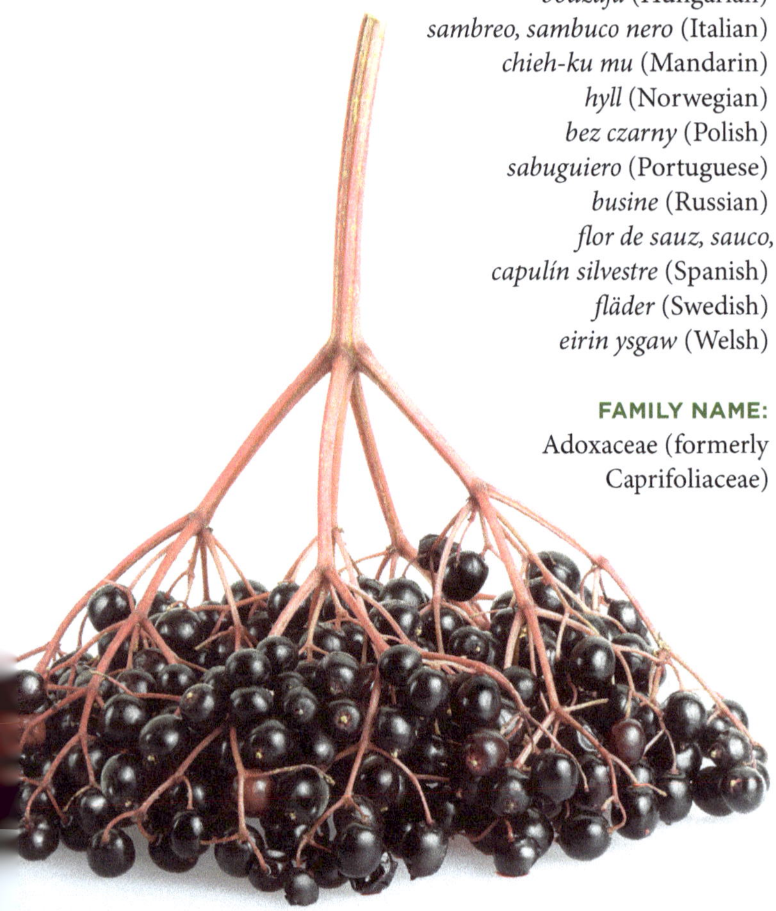

PARTS USED: The flowers and berries.

BOTANICAL DESCRIPTION AND HABITAT: *Sambucus* is a genus of deciduous shrubs and small trees with weak, pithy, arching branches.[1] Younger stems are covered in small pores (lenticels); older stems are covered in thick, furrowed bark. The opposite, pinnate to bipinnate compound leaves have opposite, serrated leaflets with an unpaired terminal

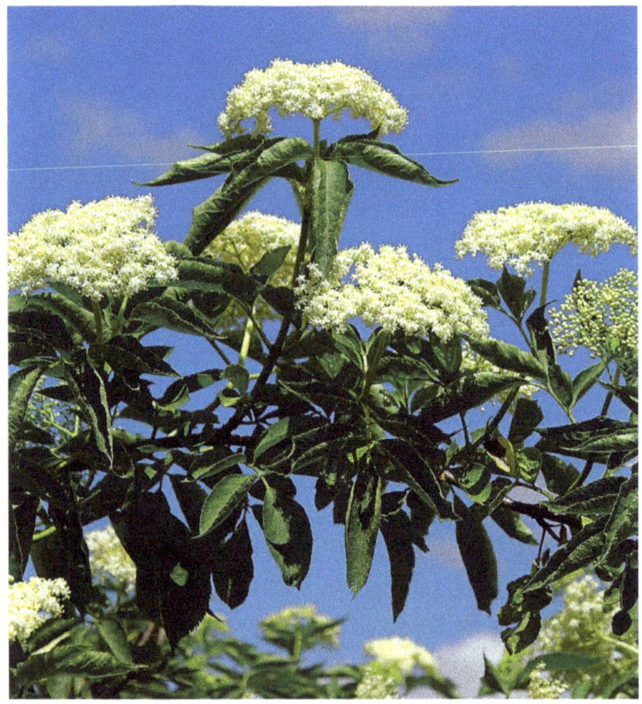

leaflet.[1] The inflorescence is a terminal compound cyme, dome-shaped or flat-topped.[1] The inflorescences bear fluffy clusters of tiny flowers with five calyx lobes, a white rotate corolla with five lobes, five epipetalous stamens, and an inferior ovary with three to five carpels.[1] The fruit is a red, black, or blue fleshy drupe.[1] The blue berries are actually black, with a thick, white, glaucous coating that gives them a blue color.[1] Each drupe contains three to five seeds.[1]

Sambucus nigra grows in temperate areas worldwide. It has as many as six subspecies, including *S. nigra* ssp. *nigra* (European black elder), *S. nigra* ssp. *canadensis* (American black elder), and *S. nigra* ssp. *caerulea* (blue elder).[2] Plants in this species lack stipules, and have flat-topped inflorescences that produce blue or black berries, depending on the subspecies.[3]

Sambucus nigra ssp. *nigra* (European black elder) grows up to 10 meters tall.[3] Each leaf holds five to seven ovate leaflets with acute apices and serrate margins.[3] The leaves can be glabrous, or covered in short, stiff, appressed hair.[3] The inflorescence grows up to 15 cm wide; the flowers eventually produce black drupes.[3]

Sambucus nigra ssp. *caerulea* (blue elder) is a common plant growing by stream banks and forest openings.[4] It grows 2 – 8 meters high, and tends to be as wide as it is tall.[4] Its leaves have three to nine glabrous or hairy, ovate leaflets with acute apices and oblique bases.[4] The flat-topped inflorescence contains flowers with spreading petals that produce a black drupe with a thick glaucous coating, causing it to appear blue.[4] It grows at elevations of less than 3,000 meters throughout the West Coast, as well as Utah and New Mexico, with flowers emerging from March to September, depending on elevation and latitude.[4]

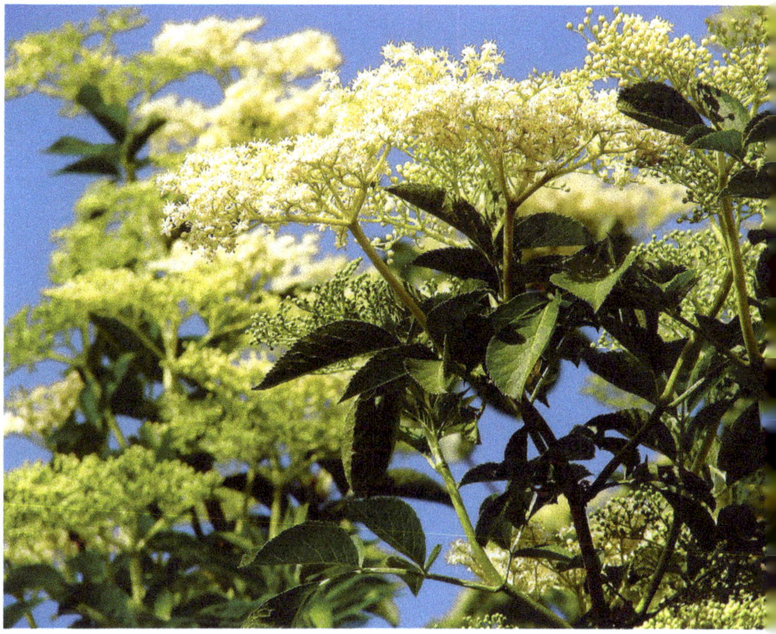

Native to eastern and central North America, *S. nigra* ssp. *canadensis* (American elder) can be a large shrub or small tree (up to 9 meters tall).[5] American elder drops its leaves in cold winter climates, but sometimes retains them year round in warmer areas.[6] There is great variation in its leaf morphology.[6] Leaves are pinnate to bipinnately compound (10 – 45 cm long), with at least four to ten leaflets.[6,7] The ovate to lanceolate leaflets (5 – 20 cm long and 2 – 6.5 cm wide) have acuminate apices and wedge-shaped bases; the underside is lighter in color.[5,6] Large, flat-topped inflorescences (up to 35 cm across) bear up to 200 tiny flowers that develop into black drupes.[5]

Primarily growing in Montana and northern Idaho, *S. racemosa* var. *melanocarpa* (Rocky Mountain black elder) grows along streams and meadows, or in conifer forests in elevations of 1800 – 3600 meters in the Cascades, High Sierras, western Canada, Utah, and New Mexico.[8] It reaches up to six meters tall.[8] The five to seven leaflets have oblique bases and acuminate apices, and are hairless or with hairy veins on the undersides.[8] The inflorescence (4 – 7 cm in diameter) produces flowers with reflexed petals that develop into black drupes.[8]

THE NAME: The genus *Sambucus* derives from the Latin *sanbuke* ("an instrument"), referring to the use of the hollow stems for making reed pipes or "pan pipes."[9] The common name elder, traced to the Old English *aeld* ("fire"), potentially refers to the diaphoretic properties, or the use of hollow stems as smoking tubes.[9] The epithet *nigra* means "black." *Canadensis* means "of or referring to Canada."

The following common names correspond with the Latin binomials: sweet elder, common elder, and American elder berry *(S. nigra* ssp. *canadensis);* and European elder, black elder, elder, elder berry, pipe tree, bore tree, and sambucus *(S. nigra* ssp. *nigra).*

HISTORICAL USES: Throughout European history, there is much folklore, legend, and superstition about elder. It was prized as a medicine in the Egyptian papyri.[10] A recipe for a thick syrup prepared by decocting elder berry fruits (a *rob)* was described in the *Arabian Nights* as a remedy to soothe sleepless hospital patients.[10]

Elder was associated with magic in numerous European countries.[9] The elder tree mother, known as Hylde-Moer, was believed to dwell in the tree and watch over it. Prior to cutting down an elder tree, permission had to be granted by Hylde-Moer. If the tree was made into furniture without Hylde-Moer's consent, it was believed that she haunted the transgressors. If a cradle was fashioned out of an elder tree, Hylde-Moer pulled the child by the legs and lifted them out.[9]

Elder was widely believed to ward off evil and bestow protection from witches. In 17th century England, elder leaves were gathered on April 30, and hung on doors and windows to prevent witches from entering houses. Elder branches were buried in a grave to protect the dead from witches and evil spirits.[9] The Danish believed that if you stood under an elder tree on Midsummer's Eve, you could see the King of Fairyland parading, followed by his entourage.[9] Because of the tree's narcotic scent, it was not

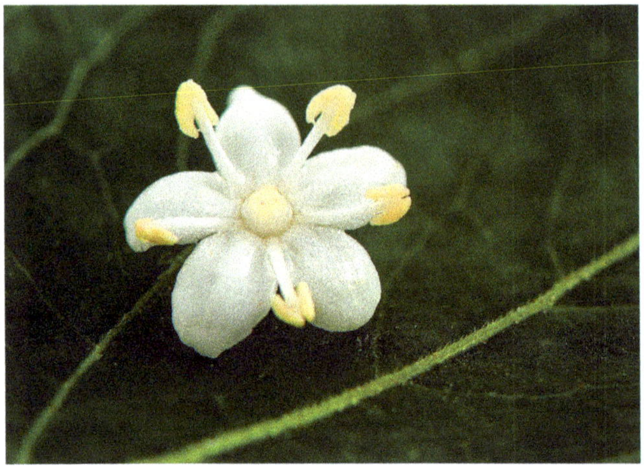

considered wise to sleep under it. In *The Book of Herbs,* Lady Northcote summarizes the folkloric beliefs about elder:

> The Russians believe that Elder-trees drive away evil spirits, and the Bohemians go to it with a spell to take away a fever. The Sicilians think that sticks of its wood will kill serpents and drive away robbers, and the Serbs introduce a stick of Elder into their wedding ceremonies to bring good luck. In England it was thought that Elder was never struck by lightning, and a twig of it tied into three or four knots and carried in the pocket was a charm against rheumatism. A cross made of Elder and fastened to cow-houses and stables was supposed to keep all evil away from the animals.[9]

Elder tree wood was used to make skewers, pegs, and needles for weaving nets, as well as to make mathematical and musical instruments. Elder was planted as a fast-growing fence to protected the garden from wind and beasts.[9] Various parts of the plant were used in dyeing. The bark was an ingredient in black dye, the leaves yielded a bright green dye, and the berries created a blueish-purple dye.[9]

Elder flowers were used to make wine. Elder berries were used in meads, oxymels, wines, cordials, syrups, and chutneys. The berries were a common adulterant in port wine. A drunken American sailor egregiously proclaimed to a Prague physician that getting drunk on port cured his rheumatism. Numerous studies and investigations determined that genuine port had no antineuralgic properties; however, cheap port wine adulterated with elder berries reduced the pain of rheumatism, sciatica, and other forms of neuralgia. Since 1899, prominent Prague physicians have prescribed 30 grams of elder berry juice mixed with 10 grams of port to cure neuralgic complaints.[9]

Elder flower water was applied to remove freckles, and preserve and soften the skin. It was also used in skin lotions and for eye conditions.[9] Elder berries were applied cosmetically as a blush.[9]

North American Indians prized elder *(Sambucus nigra* ssp. *canadensis)* as medicine.[11] Clusters of berries were gathered, dried, and preserved by the Spaniards and Cahuillas.[11] The Cahuillas consumed the fresh berries, and dried berries provided sustenance throughout the winter.[11] In Mexico, syrup prepared from cooked berries was known as *rob de suaco.*[10] A tea prepared from flowers was consumed to treat a cold, bronchitis, sore throat, or fever.[10] The pith and leaves were applied to relieve hemorrhoids.[10] In New Mexico, an infusion of dried flowers was utilized as a bath for a paralytic.[10] Wine was made from fermented berry juice.[10] A bath made from the berries and stems was used to dye elder berry twigs black for basketry.[11] Arrow shafts were fashioned from the branches.[11] Elder was known as the "tree of music;" the stems were hollowed with hot sticks and used to make flutes and whistles.[10] Elder pith of the stem was used as tinder, and the stem was utilized as a twirling stick to start a fire.[11]

Eclectic physicians administered the flowers and inner bark of *Sambucus nigra* ssp. *canadensis.* Harvey Felter recommended a hot infusion of flowers as a diaphoretic, and a cold infusion as a diuretic and alterative.[12] He prescribed two to four ounces of a strong decoction of fresh inner bark to treat edematous conditions with a tendency for ulceration with watery discharge and boggy edges. This preparation was suggested as a diuretic to treat post-scarlatinal dropsy, though the laxative effects were also noted.[12,13] Finley Ellingwood valued elder to aid the excretion of kidney stones accompanied by muscular aching or rheumatic pains.[13] An ointment was applied externally for weeping eczema and indolent, pus-filled ulcers.[12]

CONSTITUENTS

ELDER FLOWER: European elder flower contains a small amount of volatile oil consisting of free fatty acids (palmitic and linolenic acids), alkanes (C_{19}, C_{21}, C_{23}, and C_{25}), triterpenes (α-amyrin and β-amyrin), ursolic acid, 30β-hydroxyursolic acid, oleanolic acid, and sterols (free sterols, esters, and glycosides). It also contains flavonoids, flavone glycosides, and phenolic acids (quercetin, kaempferol, isoquercitrin, rutin, and chlorogenic acid), as well as mucilaginous polysaccharides, pectin, sugar, minerals (rich in potassium), and others.[14,15]

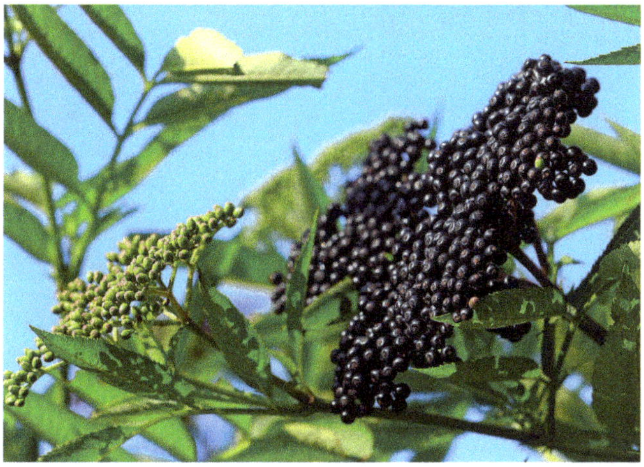

ELDER BERRY: European elder berry contains flavonoids (anthocyanins and rutin), organic acids (citric and malic acid), sugars, vitamins (C and B-complex), cyanogenic glycosides (in the seed), and lectins (in the seed).[15]

NUTRITIONAL PROPERTIES: Elder berry contains flavonoids, as well as vitamin C and B-complex.[15]

MEDICINAL PROPERTIES: Elder flower is an anti-inflammatory, astringent, cooling diaphoretic, demulcent, diuretic (mild), emollient, refrigerant, and sudorific. Elder berry is an antiarthritic, antiscorbutic, antiviral, demulcent, diuretic (mild), laxative (mild), and lymphatic.

TEMPERATURE AND FLAVOR: The flowers are cool, sweet, astringent, and mildly bitter. The berries are neutral, sweet, sour, and mildly bitter.

MEDICINAL USES

ELDER FLOWER: A hot infusion of elder flower has cooling diaphoretic and mild antiseptic actions during the first stages of a cold or flu.[14,15] Elder flower also is a mild expectorant, as well as a subtle astringent and demulcent that reduces inflammation in the mucous membranes.[14,15] Consuming the tea decreases sinus and lung congestion, treating hay fever, allergies, and minor coughs.[15] Gargling with the tea reduces mouth and throat inflammation.[15] Elder flower reduces muscular aching, stiffness, and rheumatic pains accompanying a fever. *Sambucus nigra* flowers were found to have potent antioxidant effects that enhanced free radical-scavenging activity *in vitro.* Flower extracts had a high quercetin and rutin content preventing lipid oxidation.[16] The tea is relatively pleasant tasting and safe for children. A remedy that works effectively to resolve a fever in the first stage of a cold or flu includes two parts of peppermint *(Mentha piperita),* one part elder flower, and one-half part yarrow *(Achillea)* and chamomile *(Matricaria).* Prepare this blend as a strong infusion and consume one cup of tea every hour, up to five times daily; add honey to increase the palatability. *Note:* Make sure to rest, bundle up, and avoid drafts and cold wind or weather when attempting to break a fever.

Elder flower tea has gentle diuretic properties and can be included in tea blends to reduce edema. The tea also aids in decreasing inflammation in the urinary tract. The diuretic properties subtly enhance kidney stone excretion.

Throughout Europe, elder flower water was the most common preparation used topically to reduce tissue swelling and congestion.[9] However, additional preparations such as an infusion, fomentation, poultice, or salve also aid in treating burns, bruises, sore muscles, stiffness, sprains, strains, and rheumatic pain. Water-based preparations help to clear weeping eczema, poison ivy, poison oak, and blisters.[14] An eye wash soothes inflamed, irritated conjunctiva.[14,15]

ELDER BERRY: Elder berry has antiviral, immune modulating, lymphatic, demulcent, and expectorant actions.[15,17-19] It aids in treating a cold, flu, sore or scratchy throat, and mononucleosis, as well as upper and lower respiratory viral infections.[15,17] Elder berry reduces lymphatic swelling and soothes mucous membranes. Standardized elder berry extract was found effective against 10 strains of influenza virus *in vitro.*[17] Randomized, double-blind clinical studies concluded that patients consuming standardized elder berry extract recovered more rapidly from influenza than control groups, and experienced reduced severity of symptoms.[17-19] During convalescence, the group consuming the extract showed higher serum levels of antibodies against the influenza virus than the control group.[18] Elder berry extract improves the integrity of cell membranes, preventing viral penetration. The flavonoid content is believed to inhibit the enzyme neuraminidase contained in viral spikes that penetrate and weaken the cell membrane. Elder berry extract also increases the production of inflammatory cytokines.[18] The immune stimulating and protective effects may be beneficial for healthy individuals, and those with compromised immunity, including cancer and AIDS patients; however, further investigation and *in vivo* studies are necessary.[18] Hydroalcoholic and water-based extracts of elder berry demonstrated dose-dependent, complement-fixating activity and macrophage-stimulating activity.[20] These immune stimulating polysaccharides consisted of pectin-based polymers including homogalacturonan, arabinogalactan-I, and arabinogalactan II.[20] The historical use and current studies continue to confirm elder berry's effectiveness as an antiviral and immune modulator.

Elder berry alcoholic extract has a parasiticidal effect on the parasite *Toxoplasma gondii.*[21] *In vitro* studies demonstrated that concentrations of 5 and 10 mg/ml of elder berry alcohol extract killed 100% of the *T. gondii* tachyzoites and tachyzoite-containing macrophages in 60 to 120 minutes. Higher concentrations (25 – 50 mg/ml) destroyed 100% of the tachyzoites after 30 minutes.[21] Further investigation is warranted to determine the efficacy of the extract *in vivo.*

Elder berry tea has mild laxative actions for treating minor constipation.[15] The berries reportedly contain high amounts of iron, and have been used to treat anemia.[22] They also contain high amounts of vitamin C and flavonoids that support immune function.[22] The berries are used in the food industry as coloring agents.[15]

Note: All parts of red elder *(Sambucus racemosa* var. *racemosa)* including the leaves, bark, twigs, berries, and flowers are considered toxic. They have purgative and cathartic effects.

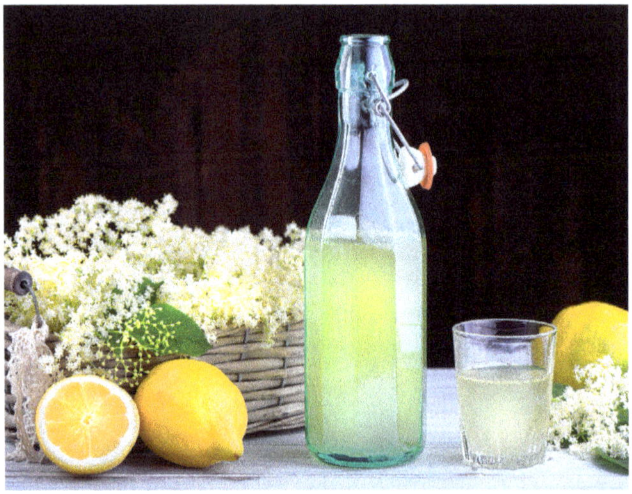

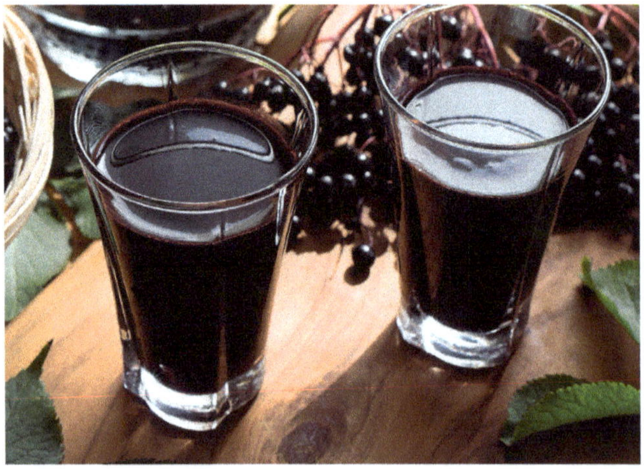

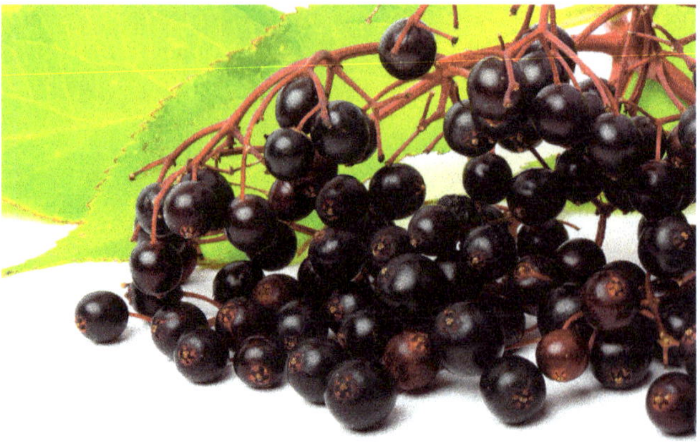

CONTRAINDICATIONS

Elder flower and berry should be processed without the peduncle (stems), as it can cause gastrointestinal irritation.[15] To avoid potential gastrointestinal upset, consider using a well processed, reputable product (peduncle excluded) with a known content of lectins and cyanogenic glycosides.[15] High doses of raw berries, especially those containing the peduncle, can cause nausea or diarrhea, or act as a purgative.[15,22] Cooking the berries reduces gastrointestinal distress, and is preferable for culinary preparations such as jams, wines, pies, muffins, or cupcakes.[22] The inner green bark has cathartic and purgative properties.[22]

PREPARATION AND DOSAGE

TINCTURE: Fresh berries [1:2, 80 - 95% alcohol]; dry berries [1:4, 60% alcohol]; or the standardized berry extract; consume 30 - 90 drops, up to four times daily.

GLYCERITE: Dry berries [1:5, 40% glycerin, 30% alcohol, 30% water] or [1:5, 60% glycerin, 40% water]; consume 30 - 60 drops, up to four times daily.

TEA: Prepare a decoction or hot infusion of the berries; consume 8 - 12 ounces, up to three times daily. Prepare a hot or cold infusion of the flowers; consume 8 - 12 ounces, three to four times daily.

HONEY AND SYRUP: Prepare syrup with the berries, and consume 1 teaspoon to 1 tablespoon, up to four times daily.

CULINARY USE: Elder berry is an ingredient in mead, wine, jam, chutney, pie, muffins, and baked goods. Elder flower is used in liquors.

ELECAMPANE

BOTANICAL NAMES:
Inula helenium (syn. *Helenium grandiflorum, Aster officinalis, A. helenium*), *I. hookeri*

COMMON NAMES:
Elecampane, elecampagne, elfwort, elfdock, scabwort, horseheal, horse elder, velvet dock, wild sunflower, alant, yellow starwort
griekse alant (Dutch)
isohirvenjuuri (Finnish)
grande aunée, heleniaire, herbe d'Hélène, inule aunee, oeil de cheval (French)
alantwurzel, bienerwell, echter alant, lionne, lugenwurz, odenkopf, stickwurz (German)
enula elemie, inula campana (Italian)
senpukuku (Japanese)
sônbokhwa (Korean)
xúan fú hua (Mandarin)
enula-campana (Portugese)
devial sil, de-via-sil, inula (Russian)
enula campana, helopia, raíz del moro (Spanish)
alant, elinsrot (Swedish)[1]

FAMILY NAME:
Asteraceae (Compositae)

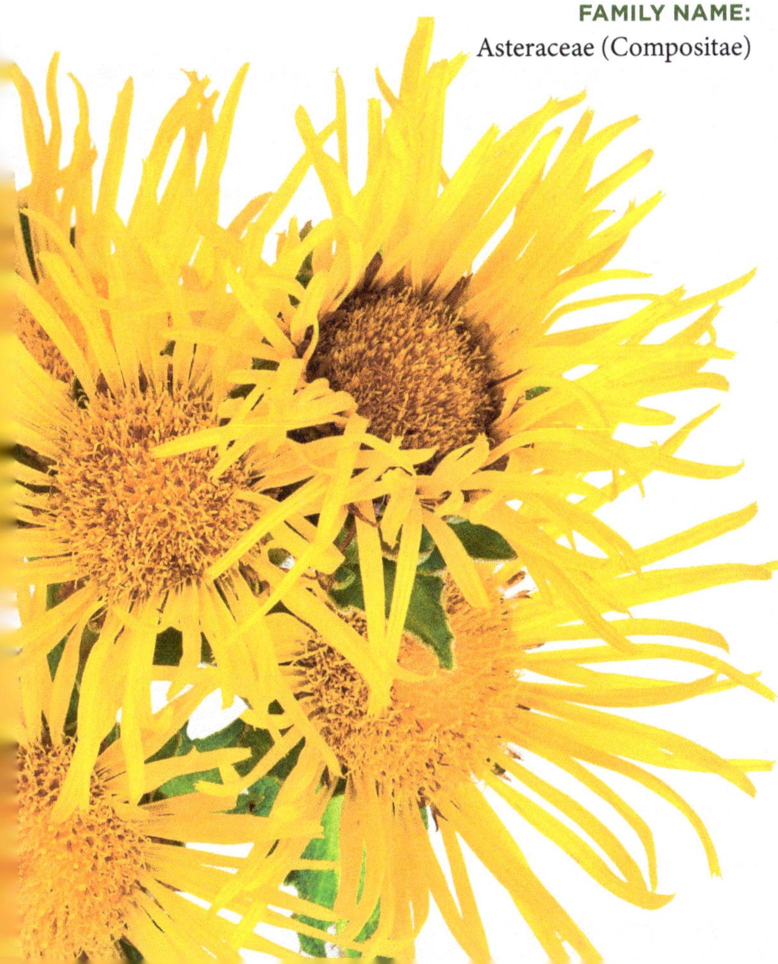

DESCRIPTION

PART USED: The roots.

BOTANICAL DESCRIPTION AND HABITAT: Elecampane is native to southeastern Europe, and has naturalized throughout Europe and eastern Asia. It is cultivated in North America, eastern Europe, and China.[1]

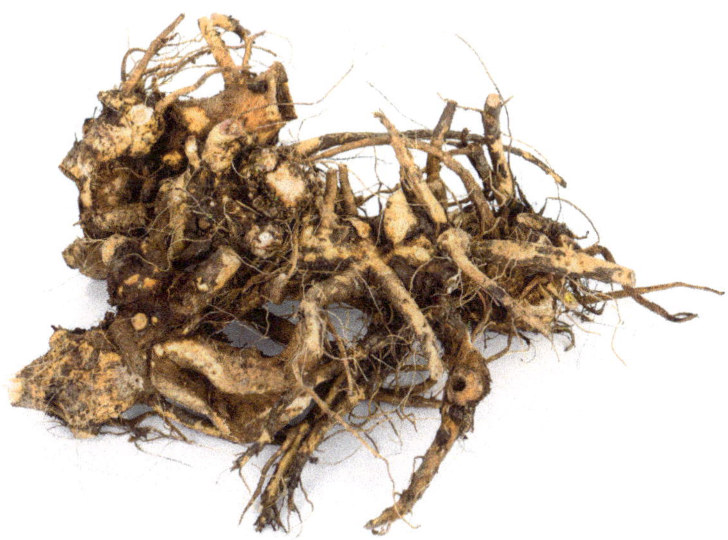

Elecampane is an herbaceous perennial (up to 2 meters tall) with a furrowed, erect stem featuring a coarse, wooly surface.[2] Prior to flowering, elecampane develops a basal rosette, producing large ovate leaves (up to 50 cm long) with petioles (up to 30 cm).[2] The leaves have a bristly upper surface, a densely hairy underside, and irregularly dentate margins. When the plant flowers, the cauline leaves become shorter and broader, and begin to sheathe the stem with their cordate leaf bases. The large, bright yellow heads (7 – 10 cm in diameter) resemble a sunflower, with narrower ray petals.[3] The ray florets, 50 – 100+ per flower, have three lobes at the tips of their petals. The involucre bears multiple layers of phyllaries. The outer bracts are velvety, broad, and leaf-like; the narrower inner bracts are hairless and brittle.[2] The fruit is a narrow, four-angled achene bearing a pale reddish ring of pappus.[2]

THE NAME: The genus name *Inula* is corrupted from the Greek *Helenion.*[1] There are several stories about the origin of the epithet *helenium.* In one legend, Helen of Troy was collecting elecampane when Paris abducted her and brought her to Phrygia. Other tales assert that the plant sprang from Helen's tears, that she used the herb

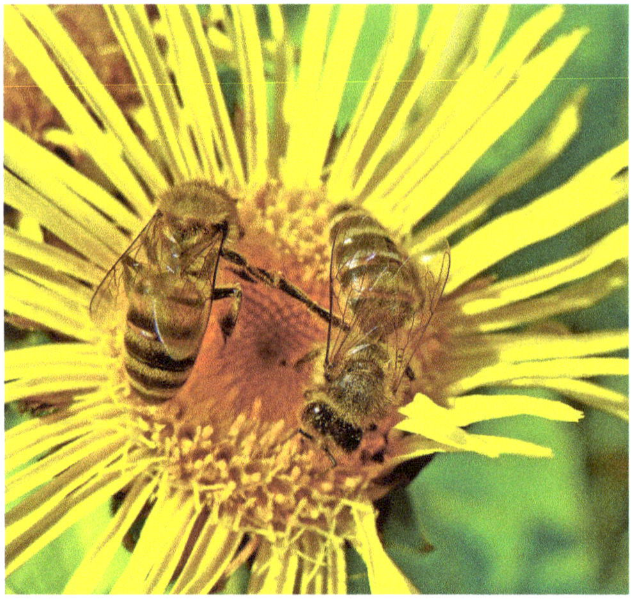

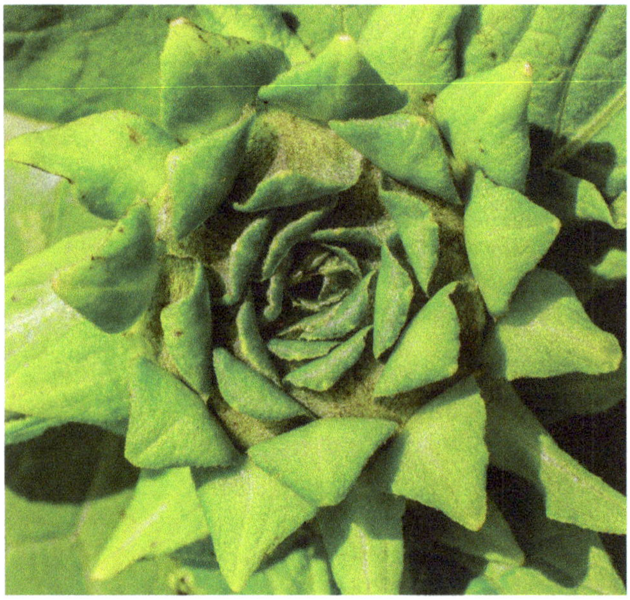

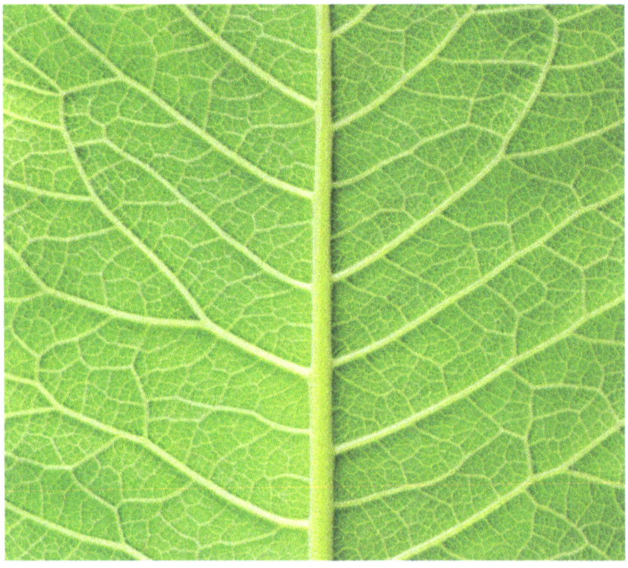

to treat venomous bites, or that the name came from the island Helena, where the plants thrived.[1] The common name elecampane was corrupted from the Medieval Latin name, *enula campana ("Inula* of the field"*)*. The origin of the names scabwort and horseheal refer to the plant's reputation for curing animal wounds. Elfdock and elfwort arose from the belief that it was a favorite plant of the little people.[1]

HISTORICAL USES: Ancient physicians Dioscorides and Pliny described using elecampane to aid digestion and raise the spirits.[1] The herb was also administered to treat dropsy, phthisis, and skin infections, as well as female reproductive infections.[1] In Ayurvedic medicine, *Inula racemosa* is known as pushkaramula; it was administered to strengthen the lungs, and as an analgesic.[4] In southern China, two species related to *Inula* were administered for bronchial conditions and skin infections.[4] For centuries throughout Europe, elecampane was consumed for coughs, consumption, wheezing, asthma, bronchitis, and digestive ailments.[1,4] The root was candied, eaten as sweetmeat, and prepared as a lozenge.[1] One part of powdered root was mixed with two parts of honey and applied to piles.[1] Elecampane was applied as a rubefacient to treat sciatica, neuralgia, and facial neuralgia.[1]

Elecampane was an ingredient in absinthe in France and Switzerland.[1] White port wine was infused with the roots and sweetened with sugar and currants to treat colic.[1] Culpeper suggested that daily consumption of a new ale or beer prepared with macerated elecampane roots cleared and strengthened vision. He also administered the root-infused wine to destroy intestinal worms, and claimed it would prevent losing teeth when gargled. He considered elecampane ointment an excellent remedy for scabs, itching, putrid sores, and cankers.[1]

Eclectic physicians classified elecampane as an aromatic, stimulating expectorant and tonic.[5] It was administered for bronchial irritation with a persistent cough and copious expectorations, as well as for chronic pulmonary disorders with excessive mucus discharge.[5] Elecampane was prescribed for humid asthma and chronic bronchitis, and to promote recovery from respiratory infections. It was given to reduce chronic catarrh of the bronchi, bladder, and vagina.[5,6] Elecampane was valued as a stomach tonic to enhance digestion and assimilation.[5,6] These common uses were followed by more liberal claims. In 1900, the *American Dispensatory* stated that several constituents of *Inula,* including the alkaloid helinin, were fatal to tubercle bacillus. However, most practitioners were skeptical, and this was never proven.[5] German studies in the 1990s concluded that a constituent of the volatile oil alantolactone was effective against tubercle bacilli.[4] Dr. Burd, a German physician, claimed that elecampane cured hydrophobia (rabies). He administered a strong decoction in sweet milk, and gave one-half pint every one-half hour until the patient vomited; the remedy was then discontinued or given in lower quantities.[6]

CONSTITUENTS: Elecampane roots contain up to 44% inulin (a polysaccharide), volatile oil composed predominantly of sesquiterpene lactones (alantolactone and isoalantalactone = helenin, elecampane camphor, alant camphor, dihydroisoalantolactone, dihydroalantolactone, alantic acid, and azulene), resins, mucilage, polyacetylenes, sterols (stigmasterol, β- and y-sitosterol, and damaradienol), friedelin, resin, and pectic substances.[7,8]

NUTRITIONAL PROPERTIES: Elecampane contains high amounts of calcium, crude fiber, magnesium, niacin, protein, thiamine, and zinc.[9] It contains low to average amounts of ash, chromium, cobalt, dietary fiber, fat, iron, manganese, phosphorus, potassium, riboflavin, selenium, silicon, sodium, and vitamins A and C.[9]

MEDICINAL PROPERTIES: Alterative, anthelmintic (mild), antibacterial, antidyscratic, antifungal, antispasmodic, antitussive, aromatic, astringent, bitter tonic, bronchodilator, carminative, cholagogue, choleretic (mild), diaphoretic, diuretic, and stomachic.

TEMPERATURE AND FLAVOR: Warm, pungent, bitter, sweet, and astringent.

MEDICINAL USES

Elecampane is an aromatic expectorant that soothes the respiratory tract.[5,6] It regulates secretions in the respiratory mucosa, drying and expelling excessive mucus caused by moist lung conditions.[5] Elecampane is a bronchialdilator and antitussive that opens the airways and reduces respiratory spasms resulting from asthma or lung infections.[10] An acute or recuperative treatment, it aids in treating lower respiratory infections such as bronchitis, whooping cough, pertussis, pneumonia, and pleurisy.[4-7,10] Elecampane is a long-term tonic that reduces respiratory spasms caused by asthma, chronic bronchitis, emphysema, and smoker's cough.[4-6,8] It has antibacterial and antifungal actions.[4,10] The sesquiterpene lactones alantolactone (also known as helenin and isoalantolactone) have anti-inflammatory, immune stimulating, antibacterial, and antifungal actions.[4,7,8] Elecampane root also

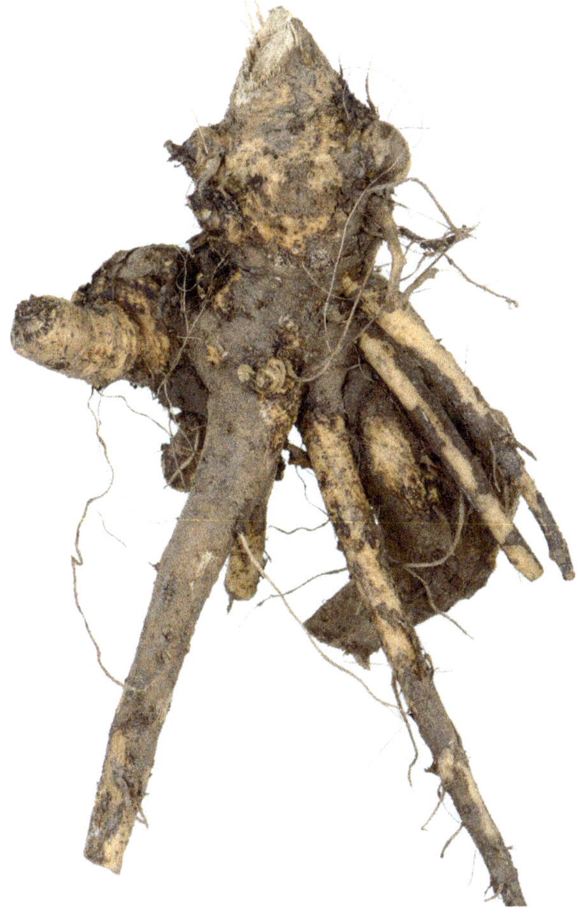

contains the polysaccharide inulin, that has expectorant actions, among other benefits.[4] Combine elecampane with gumweed *(Grindelia)*, aralia *(Aralia californica)*, anise *(Pimpinella anisum)*, Seneca snakeroot *(Polygala)*, and licorice *(Glycyrrhiza glabra)* for the long-term treatment of asthma and lower respiratory disorders.

Elecampane has mild diaphoretic actions, especially when treating respiratory infections.[10] Consuming a hot decoction of the tea every two hours helps to break a fever. Combine with additional heating diaphoretic herbs such as oshá *(Ligusticum)* and angelica *(Angelica archangelica)* to catalyze the diaphoretic properties.

Elecampane enhances digestion by restoring secretions and improving digestive muscle tone.[8] It helps to maintain the balance of beneficial intestinal bacteria, and the astringency reduces intestinal inflammation.[4] The tea and extract are useful for individuals with sluggish digestion, indigestion, or flatulence.[10] Combine elecampane with fennel *(Foeniculum)*, anise *(Pimpinella)*, cardamom *(Elettaria)*, and a pinch of licorice *(Glycyrrhiza glabra)* to treat poor digestion, gas, and bloating. Elecampane also aids in treating nonulcer dyspepsia and hepatobiliary disorders, including cholecystitis, nonobstructive gallstones, and

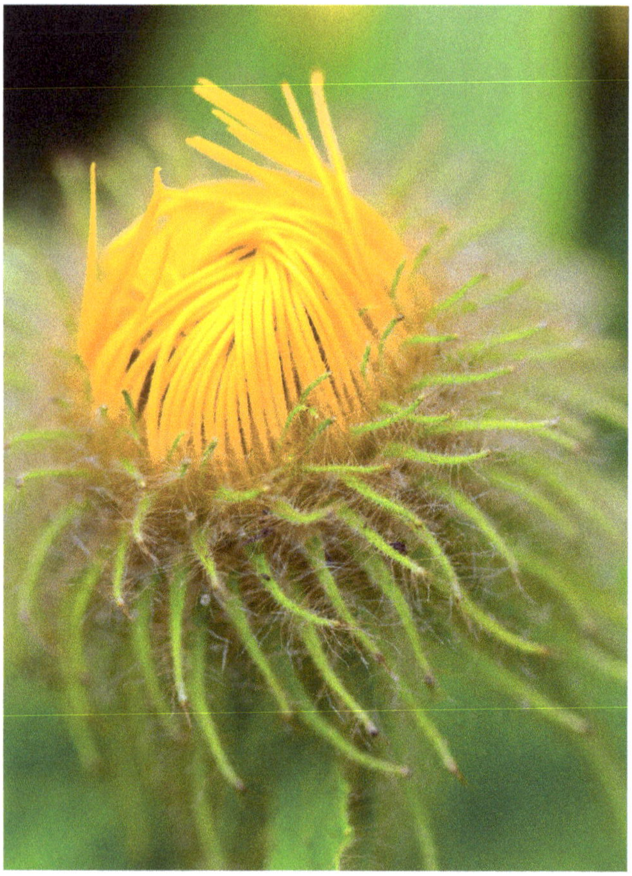

Apply a poultice, paste, fomentation, or topical wash of elecampane to treat skin eruptions and wounds. It is a mild counterirritant with topical antibacterial actions that aid in treating bruises, sprains, and sore muscles.

CONTRAINDICATIONS

Avoid use during pregnancy; limit use during lactation.[8] Exceeding the recommended dose can cause nausea, vomiting, or diarrhea.[8] According to Steven Foster, the lactones in elecampane can be toxic in large doses.[4,5] Elecampane can irritate the mucous membranes in some individuals. Similar to other members of the daisy family, elecampane can cause skin sensitization and allergic dermatitis.[8]

PREPARATION AND DOSAGE

TINCTURE: Fresh roots [1:2, 80-95% alcohol]; dry roots [1:5, 60% alcohol]; consume 10-60 drops, up to four times daily.

GLYCERITE: Fresh roots [1:2, 50% glycerin and 50% alcohol]; consume 10-60 drops, up to four times daily.

CAPSULES: Consume 2-4 "00" capsules, up to four times daily.

TEA: Prepare a decoction; consume 4-8 ounces, up to four times daily.

HONEY AND SYRUP: Prepare fresh root syrup [1:4, volume of root to honey]; consume 1 teaspoon to 1 tablespoon of honey in warm water or tea, up to four times daily. Prepare a decoction and cook liquid until it is one-half the original volume; strain, then add sugar or honey to desired sweetness. Refrigerate. Consume up to 1 tablespoon, up to four times daily.

TOPICAL USE: Apply a poultice, fomentation, wash, or liniment topically.

CULINARY USE: Candy the fresh sliced roots by cooking them in simple syrup, or alternately layer sugar and freshly sliced roots, with sugar as the final layer. Store in a sterile, closed mason jar in a cool, dark place.

impaired bile flow.[8] Alantolactone, a constituent in the volatile oil, has anthelmintic actions that aid in treating intestinal worms, including hookworm, whipworm, and threadworm infections.[7,8]

Elecampane has mild diuretic actions that reduce edema.[4-6] It also reduces excessive discharge from the urinary bladder and vagina.[5,6,8]

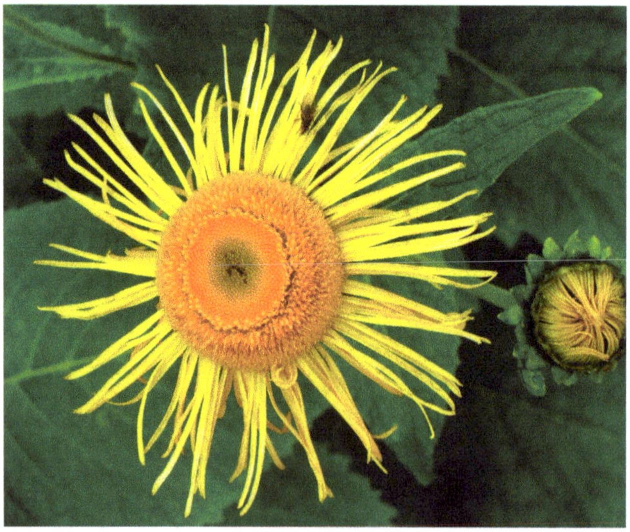

ELEUTHERO

BOTANICAL NAMES:
Eleutherococcus senticosus (syn. *Acanthopanax senticosus*)

COMMON NAMES:
Eleuthero, eleutherococ, Eleuthero ginseng, Siberian ginseng, Devil's shrub, Devil's bush, wild pepper, Ussurian thorny pepperbush, taiga root
ci wu jia, cu wu jia, wu jia pi (Chinese)
Russisk rod (Danish)
Taigawurzel (German)
ezoukogi, gokahi (Japanese)
ogap'I (Korean)
eleuterokokka (Russian)[1]

FAMILY NAME:
Araliaceae

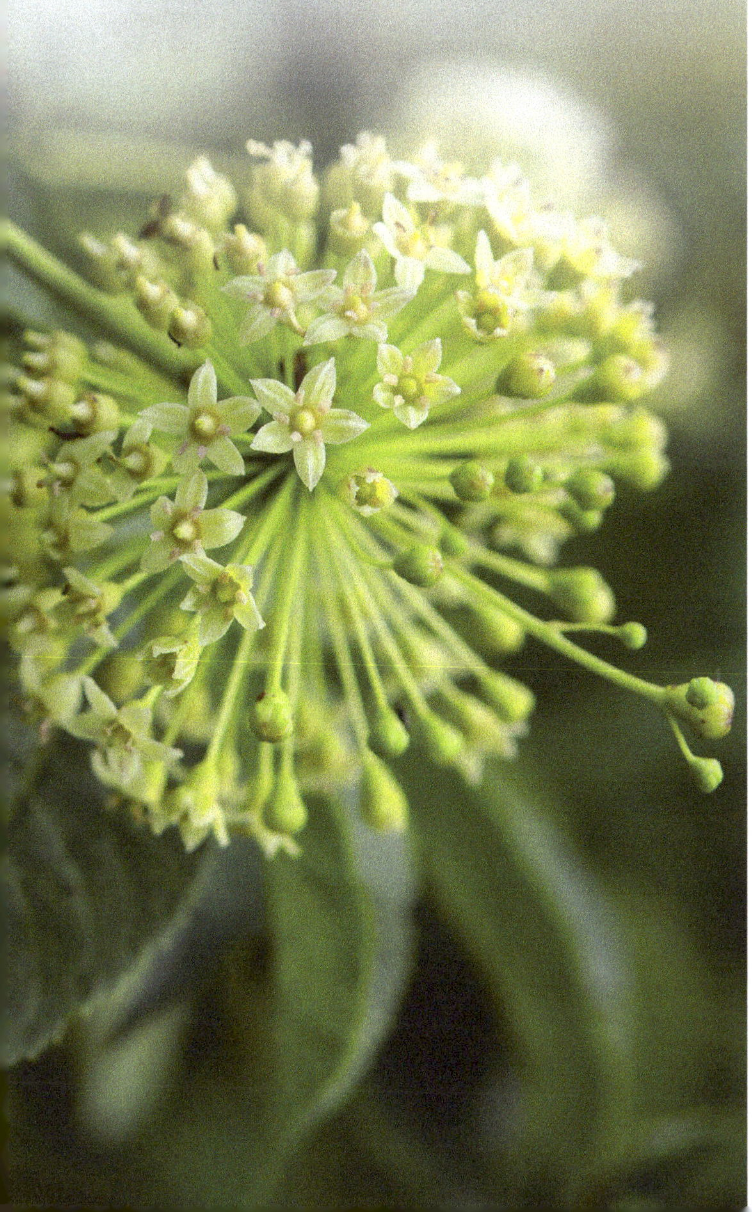

DESCRIPTION

PARTS USED: The roots, and (rarely) the leaves and stems.

BOTANICAL DESCRIPTION AND HABITAT: Eleuthero grows in Russia's arctic sub-tundra, as well as northeast China, Korea, and Japan. It is a perennial, deciduous shrub (2.5 to 6 meters tall). Bristle-like prickles are distributed on the grayish-brown bark of the stems and branches. The root is woody in contrast to the fleshy root of the *Panax*

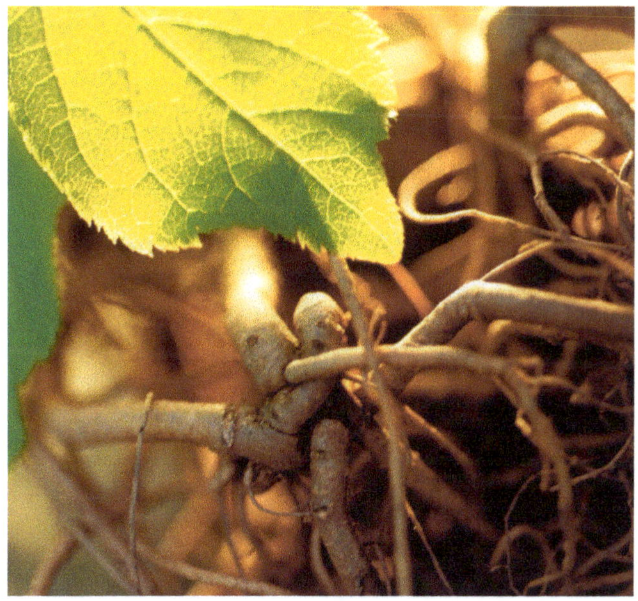

species.[2,3] *Note:* Eleuthero root has minimal odor and a light brown color. If the dried root has an aromatic, spicy, or vanilla scent, it has been adulterated.

The palmately compound leaves have three to five dark green, elliptic to obovate leaflets (5 – 13 cm long by 3 – 7 cm wide). Each leaf has pubescent veins on long petioles (3 – 12 cm long) that bear fine prickles. The leaflets have tapered bases, acuminate apices, and doubly-serrate margins.[2,3]

The inflorescence is a terminal umbel, solitary or compound, with clusters of two to six umbels on glabrous peduncles (5 – 7 cm long). The small flowers are borne on pedicels (1 – 2 cm long); the calyces are fused proximally, and divide into five small teeth distally. The corolla consists of five pink petals with fringes at the apices. Each flower has five short stamens and five fused carpels. The fruit is a purple-black berry bearing a persistent style.[2,3]

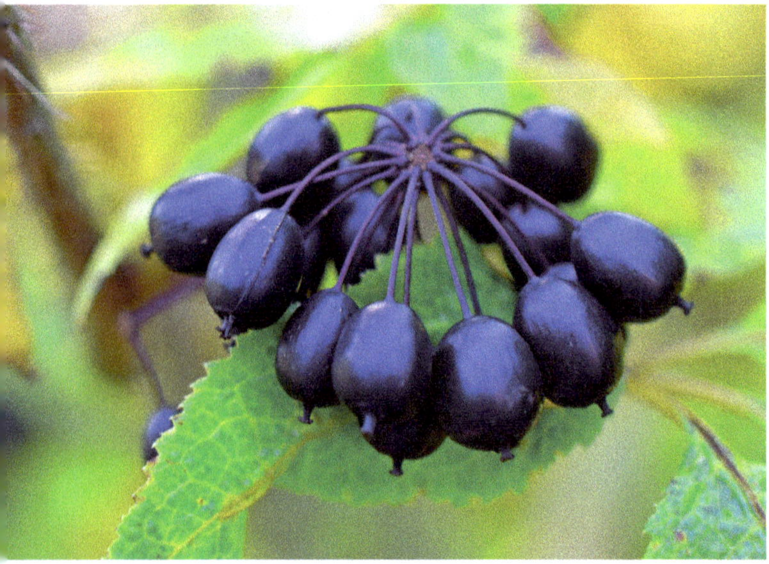

THE NAME: The genus name *Eleutherococcus* means "free-berried shrub." The epithet *senticosus* ("thorny") derives from Latin.[4] Ci wu jia means "five leaves."

HISTORICAL USES: *Eleutherococcus senticosus* was once known as *Acanthopanax senticosus,* a binomial still widely used by Chinese scientists. In China, the medicinal use of *Eleutherococcus,* commonly known as ci wu jia, dates back more than 2,000 years.[5,6] Ci wu jia was administered to prevent colds and flu, respiratory infections, and heart ailments. It was used to strengthen weak tendons and ligaments, as well as for individuals with paralysis and hernias.[1,7] The herb was consumed long-term to improve general health, increase stamina, delay aging, tonify the kidneys, and increase happiness and vigor.[3,6,7] Ci wu jia was combined with other tonic herbs and infused in wine to reduce fatigue, and treat arthritis and lower back pain.[7]

In the 1940s, Russian scientists began studying substances that increased performance; Dr. Nikolai V. Lazarev was among the first of these researchers.[7] He coined the term "adaptogen" to describe a substance that improved the body's response to stress.[7] His colleagues, Israel I. Brekhman and Igor Vasilevich Dardymov, refined their experiments to study natural and tonic substances. Their team of more than 1,200 researchers conducted more than 1,500 studies of adaptogen botanicals.[7,8] O.I. Kiriliov discovered the adaptogenic properties of eleuthero.[8] Between the 1950s and the early 1960s, Brekhman searched for a more affordable, widely available alternative to *Panax ginseng.*[3] He researched *Eleutherococcus senticosus,* and discovered that its adaptogenic actions were comparable to *Panax;* it was more abundant and could be utilized by a wider range of people. By 1960, Brekhman published an article on eleuthero popularizing its use, "A New Medicinal Plant of the Family Araliaceae — The Spiny Eleutherococcus."[7] By the mid 1970s, more than three million people in Russia regularly consumed the extract. In the late 1970s and early 1980s, Russian cosmonauts, Olympic athletes, divers, miners, sailors, pilots, and factory workers consumed eleuthero to increase stamina, focus, and endurance.[7,8] Soon after the Chernobyl nuclear accident, eleuthero was administered to thousands of individuals living in proximity and downwind from ground zero to counter the effects of radiation.[6]

In the late 1960s, eleuthero was referred to as Siberian ginseng as a marketing ploy. In the U.S., it is illegal to market any plant as a ginseng that is not in the *Panax* genus.[5,7]

CONSTITUENTS: Eleuthero contains eleutherosides A – G (eleutheroside A = the sterol daucosterol; eleutheroside B = the phenylpropanoid syringin; eleutheroside B_1 = isofraxidin-7-O-α-L-glucoside = β-calycanthoside; eleutheroside B_2 and B_3 = coumarins; eleutheroside B_4 = sesamin; eleutheroside D = syringaresinol-di-O-β-D-glucoside; and eleutheroside E = acanthoside D are lignans). It contains seven additional triterpenes including eleutherosides I-M (eleutheroside I = mussenin B; eleutheroside M = hederasaponin). It also contains senticosides A – F (oleanolic acid glycosides), additional phenylpropanoids (caffeic acid, caffeic acid ethyl ester, coniferyl aldehyde, and sinapyl alcohol), β-sitosterol, galactose, α- and β-glucose, α- and β-maltose, sucrose, vitamin E, β-carotene, polysaccharides (eleutherans A – G), and two glucose-, galactose- and arabinose-containing polysaccharides. Studies found that eleutherosides B and to a lesser extent, E, had the most potent adaptogenic effects. In Russia, eleuthero was found to contain both eleutherosides; eleuthero *(ci wu jai)* grown in China was far less potent and completely devoid of eleutheroside B. Standardized extracts measure eleutherosides B and E for potency.[4,5,8,9]

NUTRITIONAL PROPERTIES: Eleuthero contains high amounts of magnesium, niacin, phosphorus, and zinc. It contains low to average amounts of ash, calcium, copper, crude fiber, dietary fiber, fat, iron, manganese, potassium, protein, riboflavin, selenium, sodium, and thiamine, as well as vitamins A, C, and E.[8,10]

MEDICINAL PROPERTIES: Adaptogen, immune modulator, immune stimulant, glycemic modulator, anti-inflammatory, antiedemic, diuretic, and gonadotropic.

TEMPERATURE AND FLAVOR: Slightly warming, sweet, bland, and bitter.

MEDICINAL USES

Eleuthero is an adaptogen that increases non-specific resistance, and regulates the hypothalamic-pituitary-adrenal (HPA) axis.[3-5,8] It modifies the body's response to stress by inhibiting the sympathetic nervous system reaction (adrenalin flight or fight response), decreasing adrenal corticoids, and minimizing the loss of vitamin C from the adrenal glands.[3,4,8] Eleuthero also prevents adrenal atrophy and hypertrophy caused by a prolonged stress response.[3] As a long-term tonic, eleuthero supports optimum endocrine system function, and reduces stress-induced damage to the thymus and lymphatic system.[4,5,9] It enhances the body's ability to cope with adverse conditions, such as extreme heat or cold, excessive mental or physical activity, increased workload, trauma, surgery, increased or decreased barometric pressure, and jetlag.[3,4,5,7] It contains eleutherosides, steroidal glycosides attributed to the adaptogenic and anabolic actions.[8] Eleutheroside B has the most profound endocrine system-normalizing actions in the pituitary gland, adrenals, and pancreas.[8] Eleutheroside E prevents gluconeogenesis in the liver and spares creatine phosphate in the muscles.[3,8]

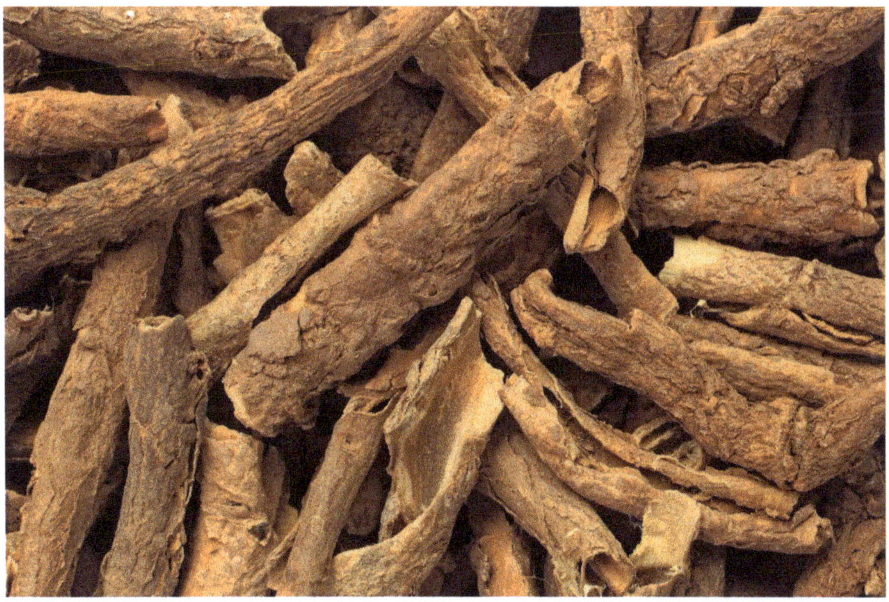

Eleuthero prevents the onset of adrenal "burnout," or adrenal fatigue resulting from chronic stress or the use of steroidal anti-inflammatory medications such as corticosteroids (cortisone and prednisone).[8] Eleuthero also prevents steroid-induced bone loss.[8] Eleuthero extracts demonstrated neuroprotective effects, as well as enhanced neurite regeneration and synapse reconstruction in rodent-cultured cortical neurons with β-amyloid damage.[8]

Eleuthero decreases withdrawal from stimulants such as caffeine, methamphetamines, and cigarettes.[11] It modifies the physical withdrawal effects when tapering from prednisone, barbiturates, heroin, or methadone.[11] It also helps to modify pineal gland stress and organize circadian biorhythms.[8,11]

Eleuthero aids in maintaining female reproductive hormone balance, and reduces perimenopausal hormone imbalances associated with patterns of adrenalin stress (alarm reaction) and adrenal exhaustion (the third phase of Hans Selye's general adaptation syndrome). It modifies menstrual cycle irregularity in females recovering from anorexia, amphetamine use, or prolonged stress.[11] It has subtle gonadotropic actions.[3] Females consuming eleuthero can have increased steroid receptor activation rates in the uterus.[12] Eleuthero binds with progestin, estrogen, mineral corticoids, and glucocorticoid receptors *in vitro*.[5] It helps to synergize the effects of hormone balancing herbs such as vitex berry *(Vitex agnus-castus)*, dong quai *(Angelica sinensis)*, and black cohosh *(Actaea racemosa)*.[13]

Eleuthero is a tonic that increases energy, endurance, stamina, virility, and libido.[9,11,14] Eleutherosides B, D, and E hasten recovery from sexual stress.[12] In rodent studies, eleuthero also strengthened seminal vessels and the prostate.[12] Eleuthero can be combined with ashwagandha *(Withania)*, Chinese white ginseng *(Panax ginseng)*, muira puama *(Ptychopetalum)*, and/or wu wei zi *(Schisandra)* to increase libido, virility, and sexual vitality.

Eleuthero contains immune modulating and immune stimulating polysaccharides that increase non-specific resistance and support acquired immunity.[4,12] It elevates the number of immune competent cells, particularly helper T and natural killer cells, and increases the activity of T-lymphocytes and phagocytic neutrocytes.[3,5,12] Eleuthero increases interferon production, resulting in an antiviral action.[3,8,9] Consuming eleuthero extract long-term (3 – 6 months) aids in treating conditions such as chronic fatigue syndrome, herpes simplex, human immune deficiency virus (HIV), and acquired immune deficiency syndrome (AIDS), and hastens recovery from the Epstein Barr virus.[5-7] Regular use of eleuthero reduces incidence of influenza, cold, and common infectious illnesses.[5-7]

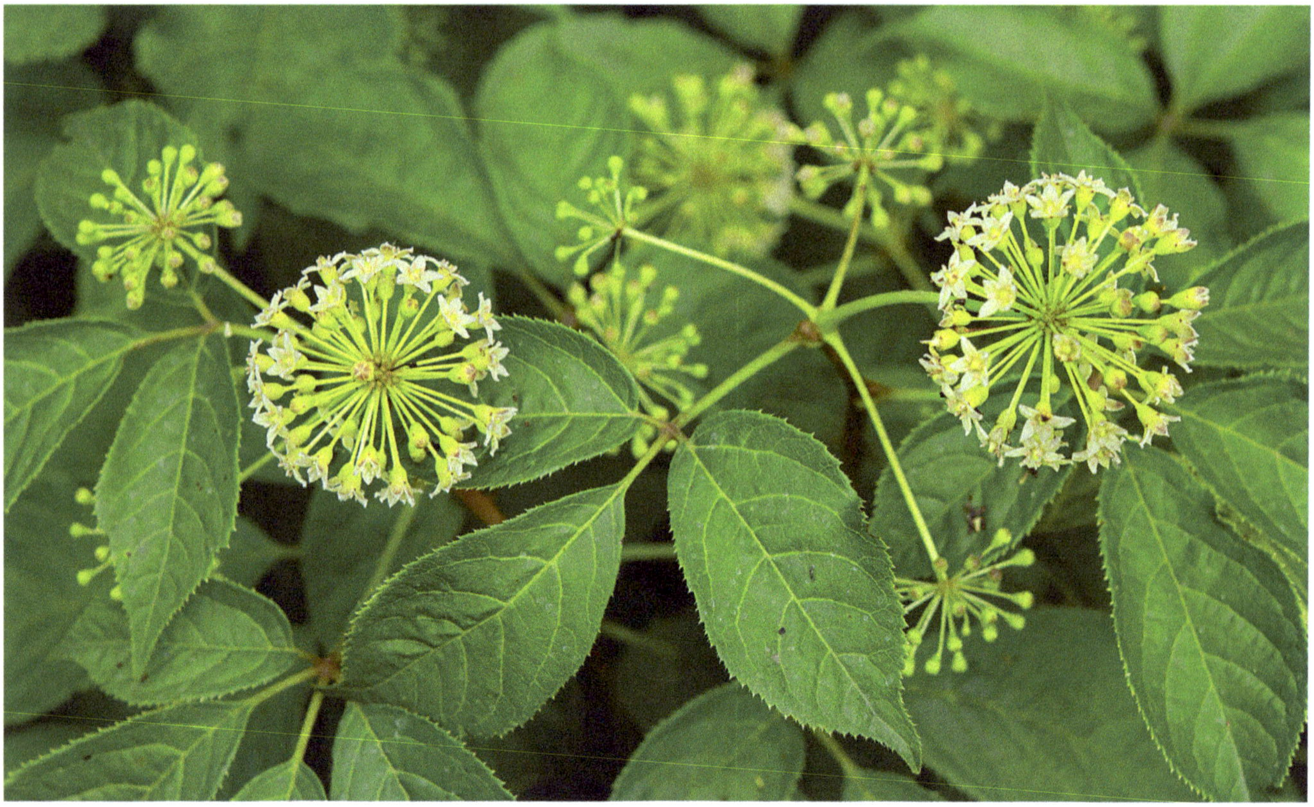

Eleuthero has protective actions for cancer patients receiving radiation and chemotherapy treatment; it minimizes the side effects, and hastens recovery from treatments and surgery.[3,5,8,9] In animal studies, eleuthero demonstrated protection from exposure to X-ray radiation.[4,6,9] It stimulates non-specific immunity following surgery or chemotherapy.[3] Eleuthero has antitumor and carcinostatic effects that inhibit the spread of metastases.[3,9] It has an antiproliferative action on leukemia cells when combined with conventional antimetabolite drugs. Antioxidant actions were also found in animal studies.[4,5,9] Eleuthero has mild anti-inflammatory actions.[9]

As an immune tonic and prophylactic, eleuthero can be combined with other immune modulating herbs such as huang qi *(Astragalus membranaceus)*, reishi *(Ganoderma)*, cordyceps *(Cordyceps)*, dang shen *(Codonopsis)*, and smaller amounts of licorice *(Glycyrrhiza)*, and/or wu wei zi *(Schisandra)*. *Note:* Discontinue use of the compound during an acute infectious illness.

Regular consumption of eleuthero aids in preventing and reducing the frequency of herpes simplex type II outbreaks.[5,6,13] Patients prone to herpes outbreaks from an exacerbated stress response have found that consuming eleuthero in semi-frequent doses (up to four times daily) helps to prevent the sores from erupting if it is taken prodromally.[13] Eleuthero can also reduce the severity, shorten the duration, and hasten the recovery process when an outbreak occurs.[5,6]

Eleuthero has mood elevating and subtle antidepressant actions.[5,14] It is an invigorating herb that increases mental alertness, and improves a sense of well-being.[8,14] Eleuthero also improves visual acuity, color differentiation, hearing, and motor activity.[5,8] It synergizes with antidepressant herbs, and can be combined with extracts of St. John's wort (*Hypericum*), lemon balm *(Melissa officinalis)*, aralia berry *(Aralia californica)*, ginkgo *(Ginkgo biloba)*, and/or fresh milky oats *(Avena sativa)*. Eleuthero extract can aid in treating attention deficit hyperactivity disorder (ADHD), as it increases mental focus.[7]

Due to its adaptogenic properties, eleuthero normalizes blood pressure in hypotensive and hypertensive patients.[8,9] It helps to regulate blood sugar in hyperglycemic and hypoglycemic individuals.[3,8] The leaf has more profound blood insulin and glucose balancing effects than the root.[8] The immune stimulating polysaccharides demonstrate hypoglycemic actions.[9]

Eleuthero adaptogenic qualities are an adjunct for treating individuals with hypothyroidism and adrenal exhaustion. It appears to have mild thyroid stimulating properties, and has slightly decreased requirements for exogenous thyroid hormones in patients. It aids in treating numerous symptoms of hypothyroidism including fatigue, sluggishness, poor concentration, and amenorrhea. It works most effectively with hypothyroidism when combined with iodine-containing seaweeds, as well as extracts of gotu kola *(Centella)*, ashwagandha *(Withania)*, and/or Chinese white ginseng *(Panax ginseng)*. Eleuthero increases the thyroid stimulating hormone (TSH). It increases cyclic AMP levels, and enhances oxygen utilization in working muscles, prolonging the aerobic state.[5] *Note:* It is important for individuals consuming thyroid hormones to work closely with a health care practitioner to monitor thyroid hormone levels, as medication requirements may need adjustment when introducing herbs or iodine-containing seaweeds into their protocol.

Eleuthero has hepatoprotective actions, and enhances liver metabolism and detoxification from drugs.[8] It decreases cholesterol biosynthesis in the liver.[4]

CONTRAINDICATIONS

An excessively high or frequent dose can cause insomnia, anxiety, agitation, irritability, palpitations, tachycardia, headaches, and melancholy.[4,5,14] Individuals with nervousness or anxiety may feel overstimulated when consuming eleuthero; discontinue use if this occurs. Individuals sensitive to stimulants should avoid consuming eleuthero with coffee, caffeinated beverages, chocolate, or other stimulants. Consuming eleuthero after two in the afternoon can cause wakefulness and insomnia.

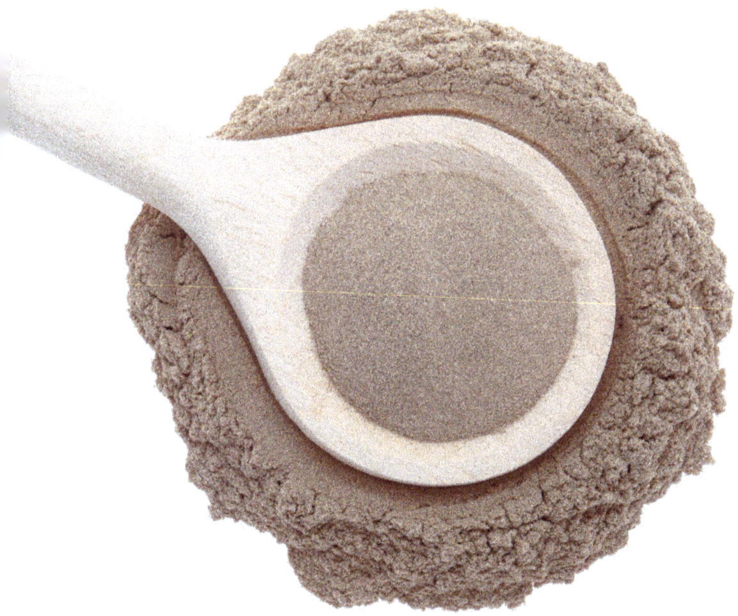

Avoid consumption in individuals with moderate to highly elevated blood pressure, and those consuming prescription hypotensive agents.[14] According to Dr. Michael Murray, individuals with "rheumatic heart disease have reported pericardial pain, headaches, palpitations, and elevations in blood pressure following the administration of Siberian ginseng."[4] Individuals consuming antipsychotic medications should also avoid eleuthero because it potentially aggravates manic behavior.[5] Eleuthero can reduce insulin requirements in diabetics; therefore, patients and medical practitioners should carefully monitor blood sugar and regulate medication dosage.[5]

Avoid consuming this herb during an acute illness or menstruation. There are no known contraindications during pregnancy; however, caution is warranted during lactation, as the stimulating qualities of the herb can be passed through the breast milk to a nursing infant.

Note: Two-month breaks are recommended following two to three months of consistent consumption of eleuthero.[5,7,14] This herb can give a false sense of energy, and cause depletion when consumed consistently, especially in higher doses.

PREPARATION AND DOSAGE

TINCTURE: The dry root tincture is less potent than the fluid extract: dry roots [1:5, 33% alcohol]; or [1:5, 60% alcohol]; consume 15-60 drops, up to three times daily.

FLUID EXTRACT: Dry roots [1:1, 33% alcohol]; consume 15-60 drops, one to three times daily

GLYCERITE: Dry roots [1:5, 50% glycerin and 50% water]; or [1:5, 33% alcohol, 33% glycerin, and 33% water]; consume 30-90 drops, up to three times daily.

CAPSULES: Consume 2-4 capsules, one to two times daily, or consume 2-6 grams of powdered root. Solid extracts prepared from dried, powdered root should contain at least 1% eleutheroside B; consume 100-200 mg, up to three times daily.

TEA: Prepare a cold infusion or decoction; consume 8-12 ounces, up to three times daily.

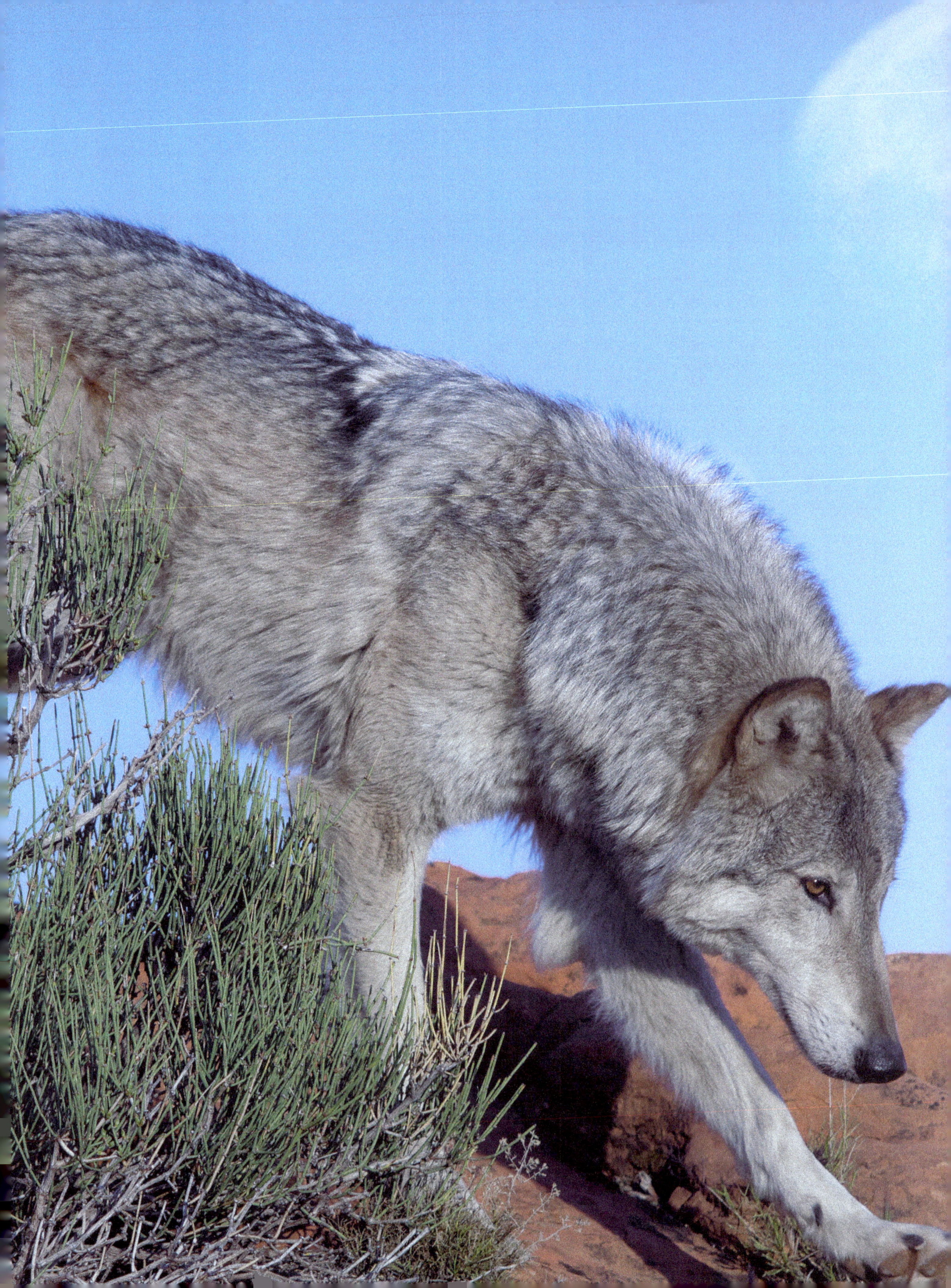

EPHEDRA

DESCRIPTION

BOTANICAL NAMES:
Ephedra sinica, E. monosperma, E. nevadensis, E. viridis, E. torreyana, E. americana

COMMON NAMES:
Ephedra, ma huang, American ephedra, Mormon tea, Brigham tea, Mexican tea, New Jersey tea, cowboy tea, whorehouse tea, desert tea, joint fir, Chinese joint fir
ma wong (Cantonese)
efedra (Finnish)
ephédra du valais (French)
meertäubl (German)
maō (Japanese)
mahwang (Korean)
má húang (Mandarin)
somalata (Sanskrit)
cañutillo, cañutillo del campo, popotillo, tepopote (Spanish)
efedra (Swedish)

FAMILY NAME:
Ephedraceae (formerly Gnetaceae)

PART USED: The herbaceous green stems.

BOTANICAL DESCRIPTION AND HABITAT: *Ephedra* is a unique genus of gymnosperms — a large group of non-flowering plants also including conifer trees. At first glance, *Ephedra* can appear to be a mass of leafless,

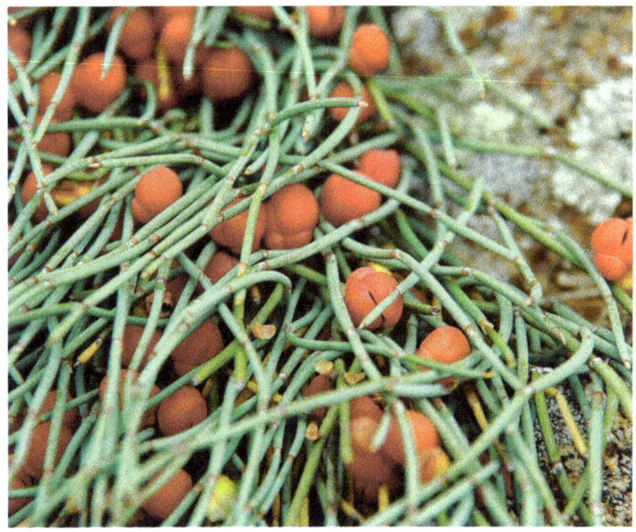

green, brittle stems. Long grooves run along the length of the round, green, photosynthetic stems, and the base can become woody, with gray to reddish-brown fissured bark.[1] The bases of the tiny, scale-like, non-photosynthetic leaves, opposite or whorled, are fused together and sheathe around the stem.[1] *Ephedra* species are usually dioecious, with complex pollen cones or seed cones.[1] Usually, one or two seeds are produced per seed cone; the seeds become red and fleshy when mature.[1,2] It is the sole genus in its family, and grows worldwide, except in Australia.[1]

Ephedra nevadensis grows to 1.5 m tall and has gray bark.[3] It is distinguished by its mostly opposite, deciduous leaves, yellow to light brown pollen cone bracts, and herbaceous inner bracts of the round seed cones that usually bear two seeds.[4] It grows on rocky slopes in the high desert (700 – 1900 meters high) in the Great Basin regions of California, Nevada, Oregon, and Utah, and in Arizona.[3]

Ephedra viridis (approximately 1 m tall) has opposite leaves (2 – 5 mm); the leaf bases persist, becoming hardened and black.[5] The almost sessile, obovoid seed cones have membranous inner bracts and a yellowish center. The

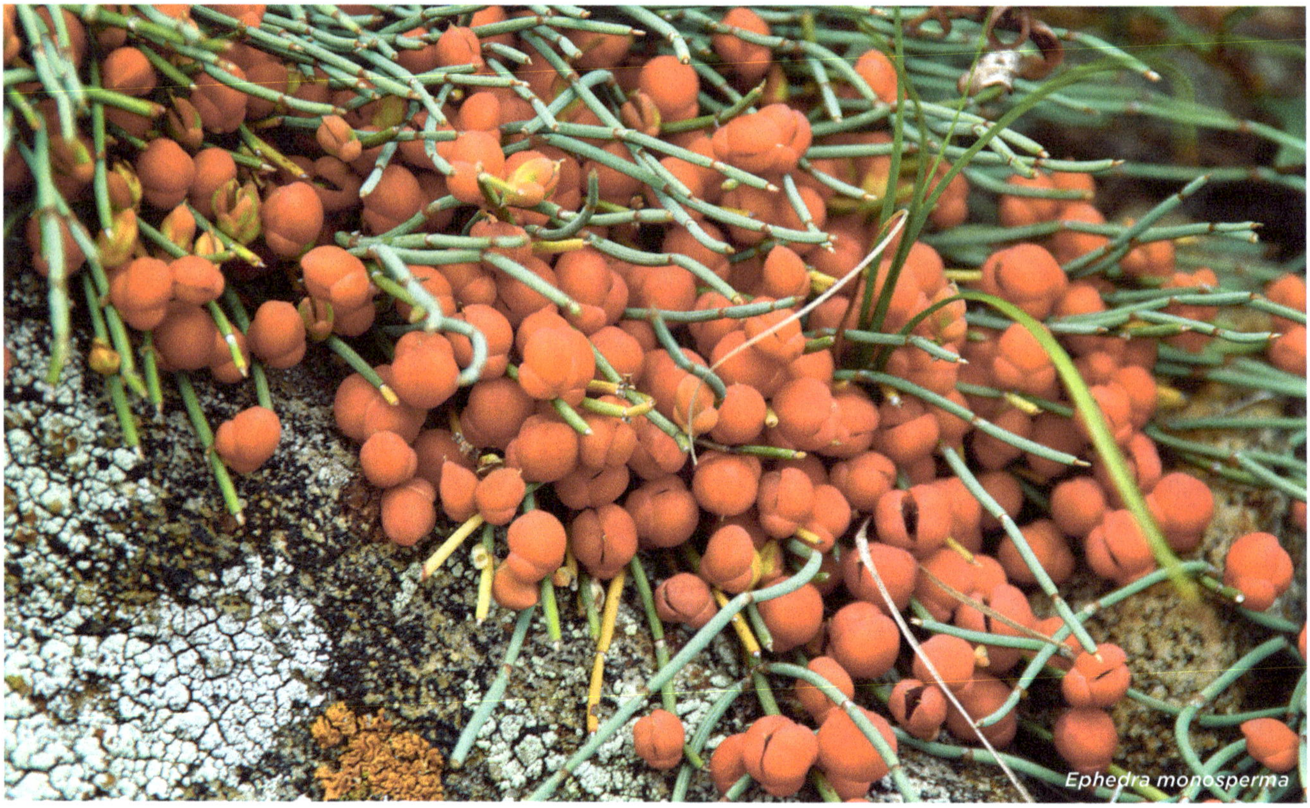
Ephedra monosperma

cones bear two seeds.[4,5] It grows in dry, rocky canyon walls and slopes (800 – 2500 m high) in the high desert of the American West.[5]

Ephedra sinica (up to 40 cm tall) grows on sandy, desolate plains and slopes (700 – 1600 m high) in Mongolia, northeastern China, and parts of southeastern Russia.[6] A notable feature is the opposite, triangular leaf scales with sharply pointed apices.[6] The seed cones usually produce two seeds.[6]

THE NAME: The genus name *Ephedra* was used by Linnaeus, based on Pliny the Elder's name for horsetail, a plant with superficially similar characteristics (although it is not a gymnosperm). It is unknown why Pliny used this name; however, it derives from the Greek *epi* ("upon") and *hedra* ("seat").[7] *Nevadensis* refers to the plant's location in Nevada. *Viridis* ("green, blooming, vigorous") derives from Latin.[8] The common names Mormon tea and Brigham tea highlight the plant's possible use by early Mormon settlers, or its location in the Mormon settlement. Whorehouse tea derives from its purported action against gonorrhea and syphilis, or because it may have affected menses and prevented pregnancy.[9] The name joint fir likely refers to its jointed stems and conifer-like cones.

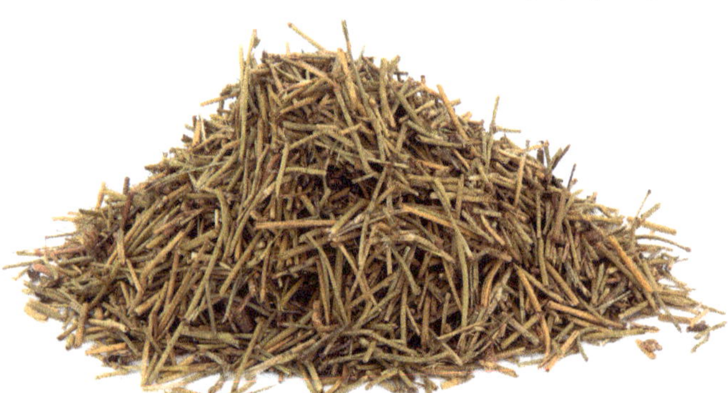
Ephedra sinica

The Spanish name cañutillo means "little tube or pipe."[10] The Chinese name ma huang translates as ma ("astringent" or "hemp") and huang ("yellow"), referring to the plant's action and stem color.[11]

The common names correspond with the following Latin binomials: Chinese ephedra, ma huang, and cao mahuang *(Ephedra sinica);* intermediate ephedra and zhong mahuang *(E. intermedia);* Mongolian ephedra *(E. equisetina);* American ephedra *(E. americana);* Mormon tea, Brigham tea, whorehouse tea, and cowboy tea, *(E. nevadensis);* Mormon tea, cañutillo del campo, popotillo, and tepopote *(E. torreyana);* and desert tea, joint fir, and Mexican tea *(E. viridis).*

HISTORICAL USES: Ma huang *(E. sinica)* has been utilized medicinally in China since 2800 BCE.[12] It was administered in order to open pores and alleviate fevers, chills, and headaches in the first stages of a cold or flu.[11] Ma huang was prescribed to reduce nasal congestion, and treat hay fever, asthma, wheezing, bronchitis, and coughing.[11-13] A decoction of ma huang, apricot, gypsum, and licorice was given to treat asthma.[11] Additionally, ma huang was used as a diuretic to reduce edema.[11,12]

Mormon tea was found in medicine bundles more than 1,000 years old.[14] It was commonly used throughout the U.S. Southwest as a diuretic for urinary disorders, an astringent for diarrhea, and to alleviate respiratory conditions.[14] Navajos prepared tea from the roasted twigs.[10] A decoction was prepared by the Pimas to treat syphilis, and by the Mescaleros to reduce mucus discharge.[10] Desert tribes in southern Californica chewed the stems to prevent thirst when water was scarce on long journeys.[10] In the Southwest, a cup of the decoction was consumed three times daily to treat venereal disease.[10] The decoction was consumed to ease fever and alleviate kidney pain.[10] Frontiersmen used it as a "blood purifier" and diuretic.[10] They also consumed it as an alternative to tea or coffee.[10] Likely due to its reputation for treating syphilis, Mormon tea was commonly served in brothel waiting rooms in Nevada and California.[14]

Ma huang was popularized in the U.S. in 1923, when the alkaloid ephedrine was isolated and found to possess numerous pharmacological effects.[12] Synthesized in 1927, ephedrine was used in allergy and over-the-counter cold medications.[12]

CONSTITUENTS: Ma huang contains alkaloids (l-ephedrine = ephedrine, D-pseudoephedrine = pseudoephedrine, 1-N-methylephedrine, 1-norephedrine, D-norpseudoephedrine = norpseudoephedrine = cathine, ephedine, ephedroxine, pseudoephidroxine, D-N-pseudomethylephedrine, and D-dimethylpseudoephedrine), benzyl-methylamine, 1-α-D-terpineol, tannins (proanthocyanidins), glycans (ephedrans A-E), volatile oil (limonene, caryophyllene, phellandrene, linalool, l-α-terpineol, and 2,3,5,6-tetramethylpyrazine), catechin, gallic acid, flavonoid glycosides, inulin, dextrin, starch, pectin, phenolic acids, plant acids (citric, malic, and oxalic), sugar, and trace minerals.[11,13] The alkaloid content of ma huang can total up to 3.3% (40 – 90% is ephedrine; the rest includes the alkaloids pseudoephedrine and norpseudoephedrine).[12]

Mormon tea contains flavonoids (lucenin 1 and vicenin 2), tannins, syringoside, resin, and vicenin 1 – 3.[14] Mormon tea and American ephedra species do not contain ephedrine.[12] The neopseudoephedrine content is questionable.[14]

NUTRITIONAL PROPERTIES: Mormon tea contains calcium, phosphorus, and protein.[14]

MEDICINAL PROPERTIES: Antiallergenic, antiasthmatic, antibacterial, anti-inflammatory, antitussive, antiviral, appetite suppressant, astringent, bronchodilator, decongestant, diaphoretic, diuretic, expectorant, stimulant, and vasoconstrictor.

TEMPERATURE AND FLAVOR: Warm, astringent, and bitter.

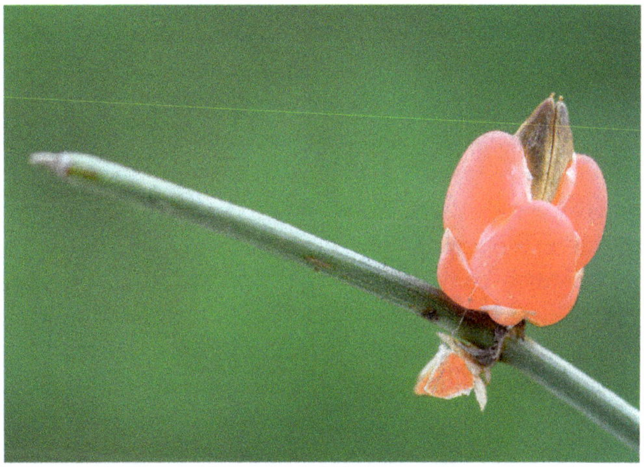

MEDICINAL USES

In this monograph, ma huang or Chinese ephedra *(Ephedra sinica)* and other Asian species of ephedra *(E. intermedia* and *E. equisetina)* are referred to as ma huang. Ephedra species growing throughout the western U.S. *(E. nevadensis, E. viridis, E. torreyana,* and *E. americana)* are referred to as Mormon tea. When the medicinal uses are interchangeable in the Asian and American species, they are called ephedra.

Ma huang contains the alkaloids ephedrine, pseudoephedrine, and norpseudoephedrine that mimic the effects of the neurotransmitters and adrenal medulla hormones, epinephrine and norepinephrine.[12,13] Ephedrine stimulates the sympathetic nervous system (flight or fight response). Therefore, it dilates the bronchioles, dries mucous membranes, stimulates the heart and nervous system, increases blood pressure, and directs blood flow to the muscles and away from the digestive tract and kidneys.[12,13,15] Pseudoephedrine is similar to ephedrine as a bronchodilator; however, it is less stimulating to the heart and central nervous system (CNS), but has more potent diuretic effects.[11-13] Due to having fewer side effects, pseudoephedrine is preferred to ephedrine in treating asthma long-term.[12] Norpseudoephedrine is also a CNS stimulant.[13] To better regulate the pharmacological effects, ma huang products are often standardized to the 10% alkaloid content (ephedrine and pseudoephedrine).[12]

Ma huang contains ephedrine and pseudoephedrine; Mormon tea and western ephedra species *(E. nevadensis, E. viridis, E. torreyana,* and *E. americana)* do not contain ephedrine, but have lower quantities of the weaker pseudoephedrine than ma huang.[16] Therefore, Mormon tea is considerably less stimulating to the central nervous system, and less likely than ma huang to increase blood pressure. It is more appropriate for easily stimulated individuals.

Ma huang, and to a lesser extent Mormon tea, have bronchodilating effects that can be highly effective in treating acute asthma attacks and wheezing.[11,14] The bronchodilating effects are due to the ephedrine and pseudoephedrine content.[11] Few, if any herbs rival ma huang's antiasthmatic actions. Consuming a hot decoction is most effective in opening the airways; however, the extract is an extremely convenient and quick way to administer the herb during an asthma attack.[11] Although ma huang is excellent for the acute treatment of asthma attacks, additional herbs with expectorant, antitussive, and anti-inflammatory actions are better for managing asthma long-term, including: aralia *(Aralia californica)*, gumweed *(Grindelia)*, Seneca snakeroot *(Polygala)*, elecampane *(Inula)*, anise *(Pimpinella)*, and/or licorice *(Glycyrrhiza)*.

If an individual experiences a mild or first-time allergic reaction to bee stings or nut, seafood, or food allergies, and does not have an EpiPen, and is in the presence of a health care practitioner who has ma huang on hand, it can be used temporarily as a bronchodilator until emergency medical care can be obtained. Ma huang extract exerts antiallergenic effects, and the tincture is the easiest to consume in these cases.[13] *Warning:* In case of a severe allergic reaction and bronchiole constriction, ma huang is not a replacement for an EpiPen. Please seek emergency medical assistance.

An astringent and decongestant, ephedra reduces excessive mucus secretion in the sinuses and lungs.[14] It aids in treating allergic rhinitis, sinusitis, and lung congestion.[15] Prepare a decoction of ephedra, cinnamon *(Cinnamomum)*, anise *(Pimpinella)*, marshmallow *(Althaea)*, and licorice *(Glycyrrhiza)* as a decongestant. Additionally, extracts of yerba mansa *(Anemopsis)*, yerba santa *(Eriodictyon)*, and bayberry *(Morella)* alleviate sinus and lung congestion by decreasing mucus production.

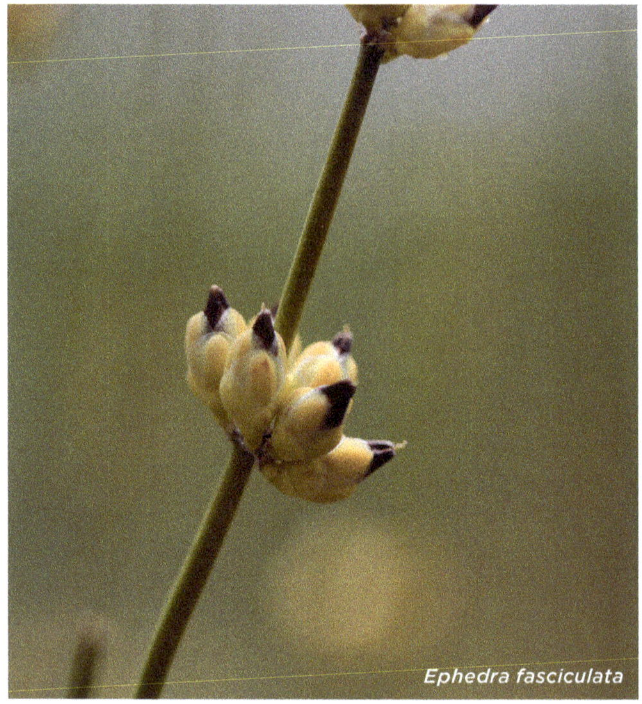

Ephedra fasciculata

Mormon tea can prevent seasonal allergies.[14] Consume one to two cups daily, one month prior to allergy season.[14] These effects are likely due to a combination of tannins, flavonoids, and pseudoephedrine. To alleviate congestion, prepare a decoction by combining one part ephedra, one-half part yerba santa *(Eriodictyon)* and cinnamon *(Cinnamomum)*, and a pinch of licorice *(Glycyrrhiza)*. If the individual can tolerate the flavor, add one-half part yerba mansa *(Anemopsis)*.

When a fever occurs, consume a hot decoction of ma huang to encourage sweating.[11] This action is due to the ephedrine and volatile oil content.[11] The volatile oil content in Ma huang also inhibits the influenza virus.[11]

Ephedrine can elevate blood pressure due to the vasoconstrictive and CNS stimulating effects.[11] It increases systolic pressure more than the diastolic.[11]

Ephedra tea is a diuretic.[11,14] Ma huang and Mormon tea contain pseudoephedrine that stimulates diuresis.[11]

Although there are numerous astringent herbs that do not stimulate the nervous system, ephedra contains tannins that reduce inflammation in the mucous membranes. Gargle with the tea to mitigate a sore throat. Consume the tea to reduce excess mucus secretions and alleviate diarrhea. It is essential to combine ephedra with appropriate antimicrobial herbs if the cause of diarrhea is microbial, as in dysentery. Apply a wash of the tea to wounds, ulcers, skin inflammation, or hemorrhoids.[8]

CONTRAINDICATIONS

Ephedra is contraindicated during pregnancy and lactation. Ma huang and its alkaloids can cause restlessness, anxiety, insomnia, tremors, rapid heartbeat, hypertension, headaches, dry mouth nausea, vomiting, and epigastric pain.[11,12,15] Ephedrine and ma huang should be avoided in individuals with high blood pressure, heart disease, thyroid disease, diabetes, glaucoma, anxiety, insomnia, impaired cerebral circulation, or difficulty urinating due to benign prostatic hypertrophy.[12,13] Individuals who are sensitive to stimulants should avoid consuming ma huang in the late afternoon and evening. Due to the risk of overstimulating the nervous system, avoid consuming ma huang with amphetamines, caffeine, and caffeine-containing plants such as coffee, kola nut, guarana, mate, or black tea.[15] It is contraindicated in individuals taking cardiac glycosides, blood pressure lowering medications, antidepressant drugs or herbs *(Hypericum),* and amphetamines.[11,12,15]

Overuse of ma huang can deplete yin and bodily fluids due to heavy sweating.[11] Discontinue use if this occurs. Roasting the stems with honey reduces this action.[11]

PREPARATION AND DOSAGE

TINCTURE: Fresh aerial parts [1:2-1:3, 90% alcohol, 10% glycerin]; dry aerial parts [1:5, 60% alcohol, 30% water, 10% glycerin]; consume 10-50 drops, up to three times daily. Due to the variation of alkaloid content in ma huang, a standardized extract containing 10% alkaloids can be used. The dosage is 125-250 mg, three times daily.[12]

CAPSULES: Consume 1-3 "00" capsules, up to three times daily.

TEA: Prepare a hot infusion or decoction; consume 4-8 ounces, up to three times daily.

TOPICAL USE: Apply a fomentation as a topical astringent.

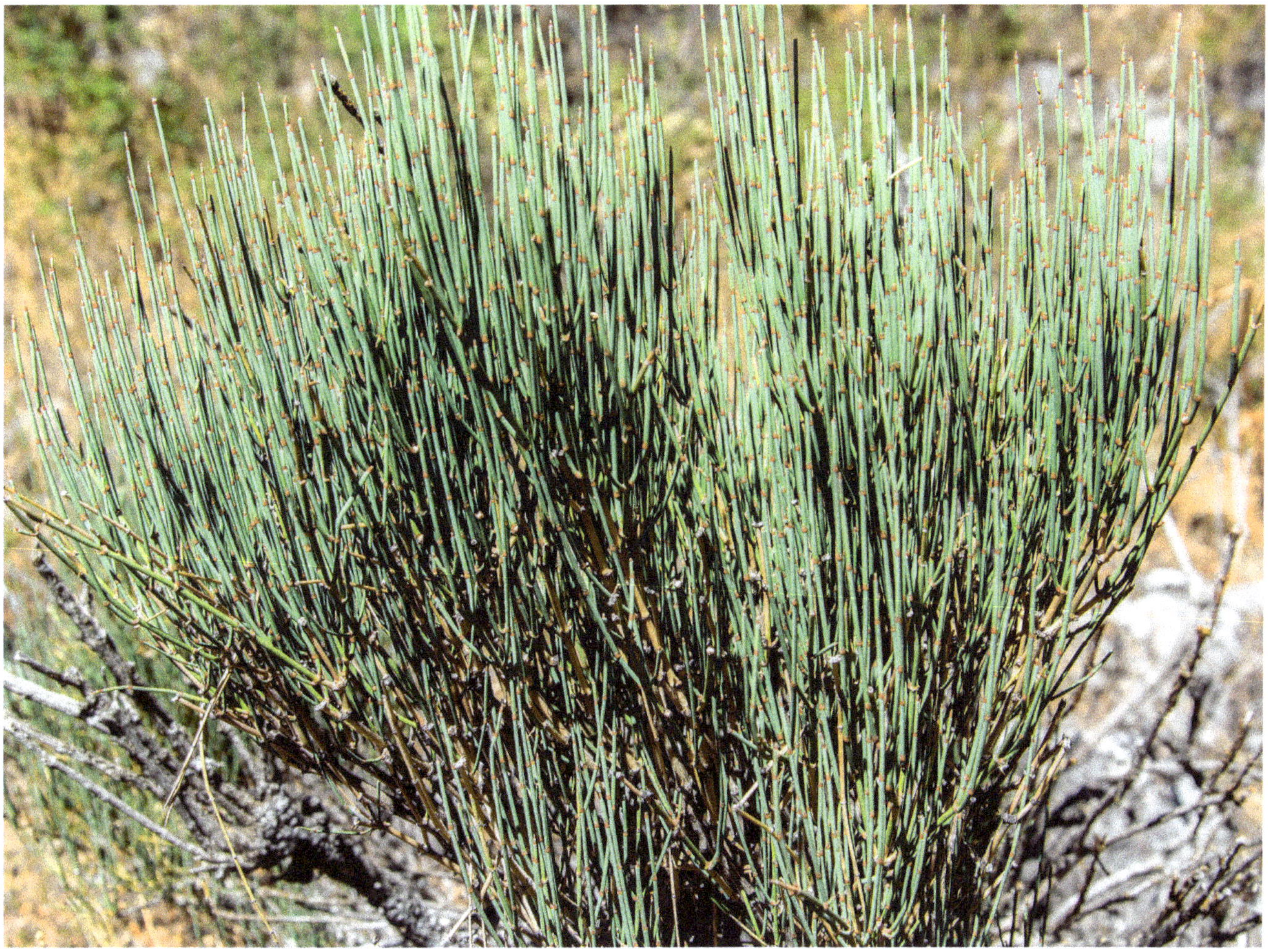

FENNEL

DESCRIPTION

BOTANICAL NAMES:
Foeniculum vulgare, F. vulgare ssp. *vulgare,*
F. vulgare ssp. *vulgare* "rubrum,"
F. vulgare ssp. *vulgare* var. *dulce,*
F. vulgare ssp. *vulgare* var. *azoricum*

COMMON NAMES:
Fennel, bronze fennel, bitter fennel, sweet fennel, Roman fennel
vinkel (Afrikaan)
shamaar (Arabic)
samit (Armenian)
rezene (Bulgarian)
wuih heung (Cantonese)
xiao hui xiang (Chinese)
fenkyl (Czech)
koromac (Croatian)
fennikel (Danish)
venkel (Dutch)
fenkoli (Finnish)
fenouil (French)
fenchel (German)
finkokio (Greek)
shumar (Hebrew)
saunf (Hindi)
jinten manis (Indonesian)
fennika (Icelandic)
finocchio (Italian)
shouikyo, uikyo (Japanese)
hoehyang (Korean)
paprastasis pankolis (Lithuanian)
hú lú bā (Mandarin)
saunf (Nepali)
fennikel (Norwegian)
fenkul (Polish)
funcho (Portuguese)
aptechnyj ukrop (Russian)
madhurika, shatapushpa (Sanskrit)
komorac (Serbian)
fenkel, hinojo (Spanish)
fankal (Swedish)
thian-kaupeluengk (Thai)
rezene (Turkish)

FAMILY NAME:
Apiaceae (Umbelliferae)

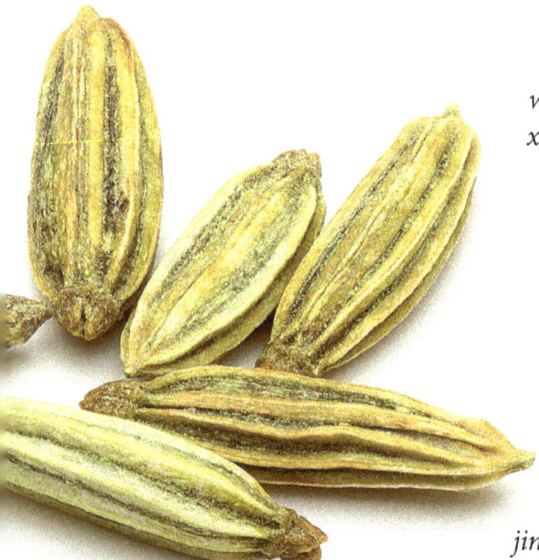

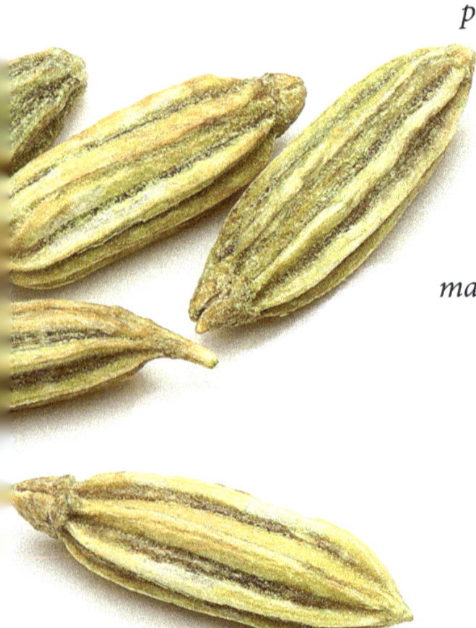

PARTS USED: The seeds are used medicinally and for culinary purposes. The bulb and leaves are consumed for culinary purposes.

BOTANICAL DESCRIPTION AND HABITAT: Fennel is native to the Mediterranean and cultivated throughout Europe, Asia, India, Australia, and North America. It is a biennial or perennial in temperate climates, and an annual in colder climates. It was believed that Italian fishermen

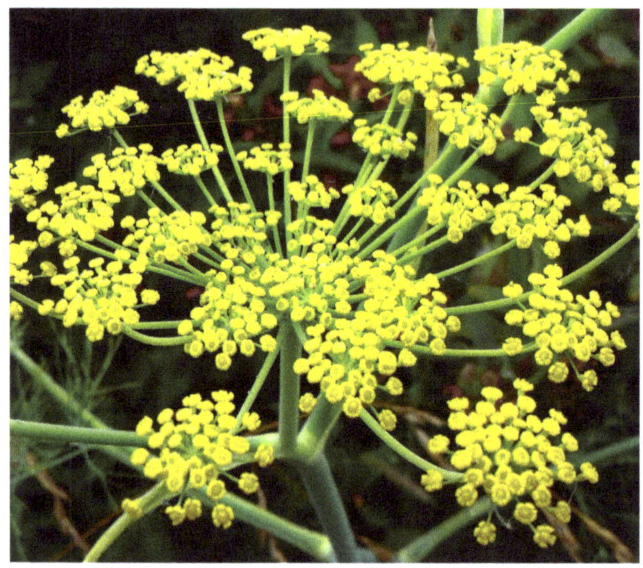

introduced fennel to California where it naturalized or became an invasive weed. Fennel has spread throughout the California and Oregon coasts in dense colonies on roadsides and disturbed sites. It is difficult to eradicate.

Foeniculum vulgare, the only species in the genus *Foeniculum,* is a strongly aromatic, herbaceous perennial (0.9 to 2 meters tall) with a sturdy taproot.[1] The smooth, glaucous, gray-green stem has a solid core.[1] The leaves have widely sheathing petioles up to 15 cm long.[2] The triangular-ovate blade (30 – 40 cm wide) is pinnately dissected with fine linear segments (4 – 40 mm long).[1] A compound umbel (5 – 9 cm diameter) lacking bracts bears 15 to 40 unequal rays (1 – 10 cm long) that grow on a peduncle up to 25 cm in length.[3] Each ray bears 14 to 39 flowers.[3] The flowers lack calyces and have yellow, obovate petals.[2] The oblong, ribbed, glabrous, seed-like fruit, commonly referred to as the seed, is 4 mm long.[1]

THE NAME: *Foeniculum* derives from the Latin *feniculum* or *fenuculum* ("hay"), referring to the sweet odor.[5] The epithet *vulgare* originates from the Latin *vulgaris* ("of or pertaining to the common people, common, or vulgar").[7] In the Middle Ages, *feoniculum* was corrupted to *fanculum,* and evolved into the common name *fenkel.*[5] Ancient Greeks named the plant *marathron,* derived from *mariano* ("to grow thin"), referring to its use as an appetite suppressant for weight loss, or for support during a famine.[5] The Sanskrit shatapushpa means "what possesses a hundred flowers."[6] The following common names correspond with the Latin names: common or wild fennel *(Foeniculum vulgare);* bronze fennel *(F. vulgare* ssp. *vulgare* "rubrum"*);* sweet fennel and Roman fennel *(F. vulgare* ssp. *vulgare* var. *dulce);* bitter fennel *(F. vulgare* ssp. *vulgare* var. *vulgare);* and finocchio or Florence fennel *(F. vulgare* ssp. *vulgare* var. *azoricum).*

HISTORICAL USES: Fennel has been utilized worldwide as a food and medicine. Ancient Romans cultivated it for its succulent, edible shoots and fruit.[8] Pliny, a Roman naturalist and historian, listed the medicinal uses for fennel.[5] Ancient Greeks and Romans believed that fennel bestowed strength, courage, and longevity.[5] In Medieval times, fennel and St. John's wort were hung over doors on Midsummer's Eve to ward off evil spirits and prevent witchcraft.[5] Emperor Charlemagne (742 – 814 CE) was credited with introducing fennel cultivation to central and northern Europe where it was grown on his imperial farms.[5]

Fennel seeds were administered as medicine for conditions of the lungs, kidneys, digestion, liver, spleen, and gallbladder. In Europe, fennel water, also known as *la gripe water,* was a household remedy for infant colic.[5] Fennel leaves or seeds were boiled in barley water and consumed by nursing mothers to increase breast milk flow and impart strength to their infants. Fennel seeds were added to purgatives to prevent griping pain.[5] The seeds continue to be used in cordials and liqueurs as an aperitif or digestif.[5] Europeans commonly boiled fish with fennel leaves to reduce the odor and improve the digestion of fatty fish.[5] Fennel was believed to restore vision and strengthen the eyes. Water-based preparations of fennel were used to treat eye infections.[8] In Traditional Chinese Medicine, fennel was used as a powdered poultice for slowly healing snakebites.[7] Powdered fennel sprinkled throughout kennels and stables was said to ward off fleas.[5]

CONSTITUENTS: Fennel seed contains volatile oil (anethole, D-fenchone, methyl chavicol, anisic aldehyde, anisic acid, D-α-pinene, and diterpene), fixed oil (petroselinic acid, oleic acid, linoleic acid, and tocopherols), phenolic acids (caffeic acid), flavonoids (quercetin-3-glucuronide, rutin, isoquercetin, quercetin-3-arabinoside, and kaempferol-3-glucuronide), saponins (stigmasterol), coumarin (umbelliferone), protein, and sugar, as well as vitamins and minerals (listed below).[7,9,10]

Essential oil of fennel contains volatile oil (transanethole, fenchone, estragole, limonene, camphene, and α-pinene), monoterpene hydrocarbons (β-pinene, α-thujene, α-fenchene, 3-carene, sabinene, α-phellandrine, myrcene, α- and β-terpinene, *cis-* and *trans-*ocimenes, terpinolene, and p-cymene), fenchyl alcohol, anisaldahyde, anisic acid, *trans-*1,8-terpin, myristicin, and apiole (the last two constituents are only present in sweet fennel).[7,11]

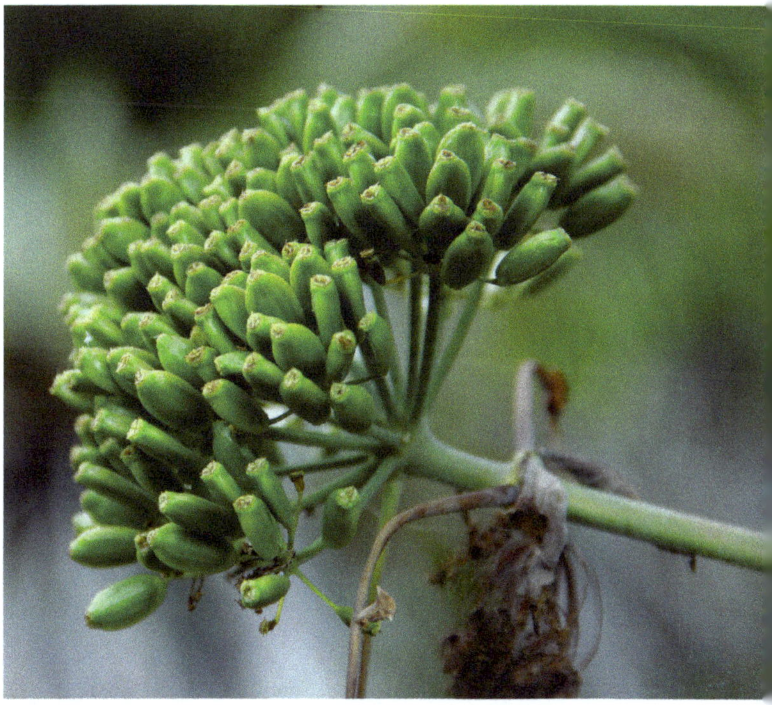

NUTRITIONAL PROPERTIES: Fennel seed contains high amounts of calcium, fiber, fat, magnesium, phosphorus, protein, selenium, sodium, and thiamine.[9] It contains low to average amounts of chromium, iron, manganese, niacin, potassium, riboflavin, and tin.[9,12] Fennel leaf and bulb contain vitamins A and C, calcium, iron, potassium, phosphorus, and protein.[12]

MEDICINAL PROPERTIES: Antibacterial (mild), anti-inflammatory, antispasmodic, antitussive, aromatic, carminative, cholagogue, diuretic, expectorant, galactagogue, harmonizer, and stomachic.

TEMPERATURE AND FLAVOR: Warm, sweet, bitter, and pungent; however, most Ayurvedic practitioners consider the seeds slightly cooling.[6]

MEDICINAL USES

FENNEL SEED: Among the most effective digestive aids, fennel seed has carminative, smooth muscle antispasmodic, and stomachic properties.[5,7-11,14,15] It is highly beneficial for reducing digestive cramping, gas, and bloating.[8,10,11,14,15] Its volatile oil stimulates mucous membranes in the digestive tract, encouraging motility and peristalsis.[8] It also has antibacterial effects against gram-positive and gram-negative bacteria.[11] Anethole, a component of the volatile oil, exerts smooth muscle antispasmodic, carminative, and anti-inflammatory actions.[7,8] Fennel seed tincture and tea are highly effective for treating intestinal spasms resulting from nonulcer dyspepsia, irritable bowel syndrome, ulcerative colitis, Crohn's disease, leaky gut syndrome, celiac disease, intestinal candidiasis, diarrhea, or constipation.[10,14] It combines effectively with wild yam *(Dioscorea)* as an antispasmodic. To enhance the carminative and stomachic effects, combine with anise *(Pimpinella)*, cardamom *(Elettaria)*, ginger *(Zingiber)*, and/or angelica *(Angelica)*. Alternatively, it can be combined with mint *(Mentha)*, chamomile *(Matricaria)*, and catnip *(Nepeta)*.

Fennel seed has antinauseant properties, aiding recovery from stomach flu, food poisoning, digestive infections, and hangovers.[14] Combine with peppermint *(Mentha)*, ginger *(Zingiber)*, and/or cardamom *(Elettaria)* as an antinauseant. Fennel anesthetizes pain from a hiatal hernia or indigestion.[13] Fennel extract has a cholagogue effect.[14] It decongests the liver, and is a useful adjunct for conditions arising from liver stagnation.

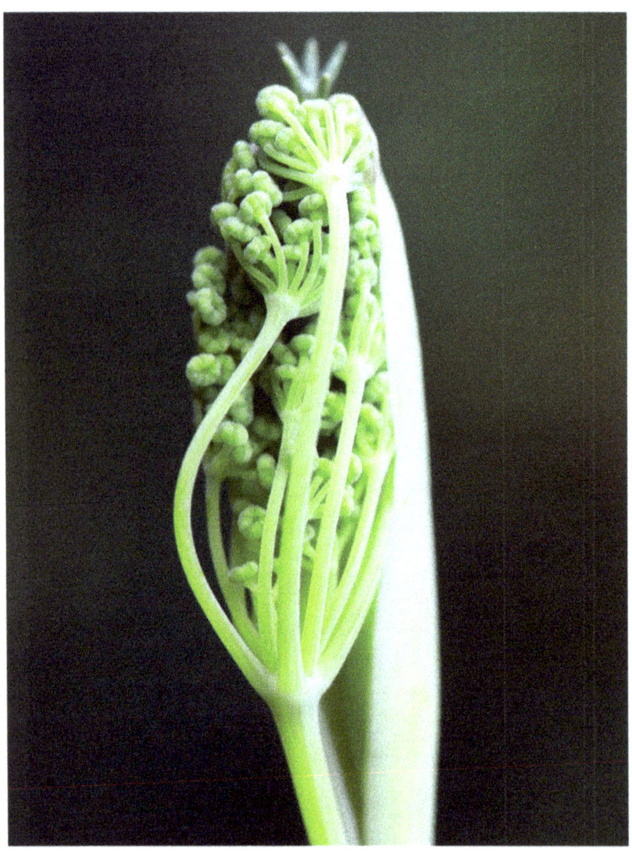

Fennel seed complements cathartic laxative and purgative compounds, as well as digestive bitter tonic and cholagogue formulas.[5,7] It reduces griping caused by more potent purgative and laxative herbs used to treat constipation.[5] It also prevents cramping caused by cooling bitter herbs celandine *(Chelidonium)*, artichoke leaf *(Cynara)*, gentian *(Gentiana)*, or berberis *(Berberis)* that stimulate bile excretion from the gallbladder. Fennel seed tincture can be combined with cooling, bitter, antimicrobial herbs to modify their harshness, or when treating digestive infections such as stomach flu, food poisoning, or giardia.

The seeds have moderate expectorant and antitussive properties.[7,13-15] However, the antitussive actions are not as potent as those of anise, fennel's cousin. Anethole and fenchone stimulate upper respiratory tract secretions.[7,8] While anise seed is preferred for treating respiratory conditions, fennel can be incorporated into compounds to treat a dry, percussive cough, whooping cough, bronchitis, pneumonia, and asthma.[7,8] Fennel also has antioxidant actions.[14] The volatile oil demonstrates antibacterial effects *in vitro*.[7]

Fennel seed has galactagogue actions, increasing breast milk supply.[8,12-14] Additionally, the carminative and antispasmodic qualities pass through breast milk, reducing infant colic.[12,13,15] Fennel seed tea reduces infant dyspepsia, diarrhea, and intestinal spasms. Combine fennel extract with anise *(Pimpinella)*, fenugreek *(Trigonella)*, blessed thistle *(Cnicus)*, and/or alfalfa *(Medicago)* to synergize the galactagogue effects. Prepare a galactagogue tea containing fennel, anise *(Pimpinella)*, fenugreek *(Trigonella)*, alfalfa *(Medicago)*, and spearmint *(Mentha spicata)*.

Fennel seed has subtle diuretic properties, reducing edema.[14] This is probably why it is included in weight loss formulas, although it also was used historically as an appetite suppressant.[5] Fennel extracts promoted diuresis, increasing urinary flow and urinary sodium excretion in mice.[14] Treat urinary tract infections by combining fennel with more potent antibacterial agents such as usnea *(Usnea)*, uva ursi *(Arctostaphylos)*, corn silk *(Zea)*, and yarrow *(Achillea)*. It can be combined with parsley root *(Petroselinum)*, dandelion leaf *(Taraxacum)*, and/or couch grass *(Agropyron)* as a diuretic.

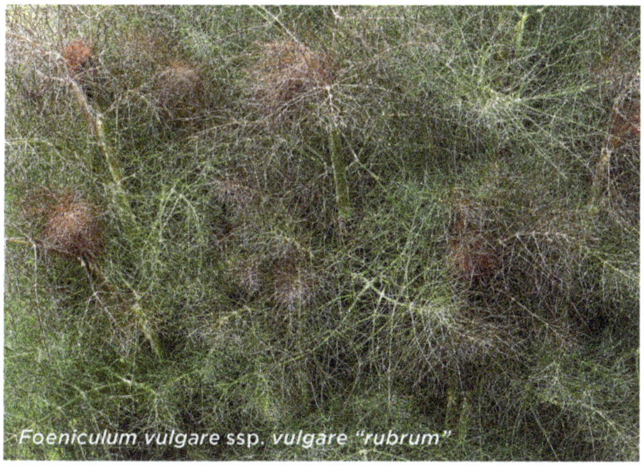

Foeniculum vulgare ssp. vulgare "rubrum"

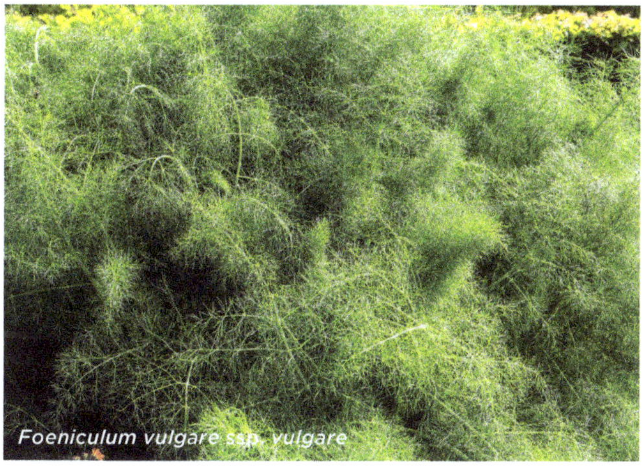

Foeniculum vulgare ssp. vulgare

Fennel is a flavoring agent and harmonizer in blends; however, some patients despise the "licorice-like" flavor. To encourage compliance, it is important to assess whether a patient enjoys the taste before including it in compounds. Fennel essential oil is a flavoring and antimicrobial ingredient in toothpastes and mouthwashes.[14] The sweet taste is attributed to the anethole.[8,10]

A decoction of fennel seed, cooled then strained through a fine cloth or paper filter, may be used as an eye wash. It aids in treating sore, strained, or bloodshot eyes, as well as conjunctivitis and blepharitis (when combined with other anti-infective agents).[8,14,15] Combine fennel with goldthread *(Coptis)* or goldenseal *(Hydrastis)*, chamomile *(Matricaria)*, calendula *(Calendula)*, and licorice *(Glycyrrhiza)* as an antimicrobial and anti-inflammatory agent for eye infections.

FENNEL ESSENTIAL OIL: The essential oil or spirits may be used internally with caution, in one- to two-drop doses. It has spasmolytic actions in the digestive and respiratory tracts.[14] It also reduces nausea, gas, and bloating. Inhaling fennel oil has expectorant and antitussive effects.[14]

Fennel oil has bacteriostatic actions against: *Aerobacter aerogenes, Bacillus subtilis, E. coli, Proteus vulgaris, Pseudomonas aeruginosa, Staphylococcus albus,* and *S. aureus.*[14] In patients with urinary tract infections, it demonstrated antibacterial actions against *E. coli, Streptococcal pyogenes,* and *S. aureus in vitro.*[14]

The sweet aroma of fennel seed essential oil is invigorating. It reduces sluggishness and lethargy, improving energy and motivation.[16] The essential oil is incorporated into face creams as an antiwrinkle and antiaging agent for mature or couperose skin, enhancing the complexion.[14,16] Fennel essential oil has long been included in soaps, detergents, creams, lotions, and perfumes.[14]

CONTRAINDICATIONS

Fennel seeds are considered safe during pregnancy and lactation.[14] In rare cases, they cause allergic reactions in the skin and respiratory tract.[8] Consuming fennel seeds is not considered dangerous; however, the essential oil can be toxic in high doses.[11]

Internal consumption of fennel seed essential oil should be avoided during pregnancy and lactation, and in children under ten years of age. It has been reported to have estrogen-like activities; therefore, it is postulated that internal consumption of the essential oil should be avoided by individuals with estrogen-sensitive conditions (reproductive cancers, tumors, or cysts).[7,8,11,16] The essential oil can overexcite the nervous system, and may cause convulsions

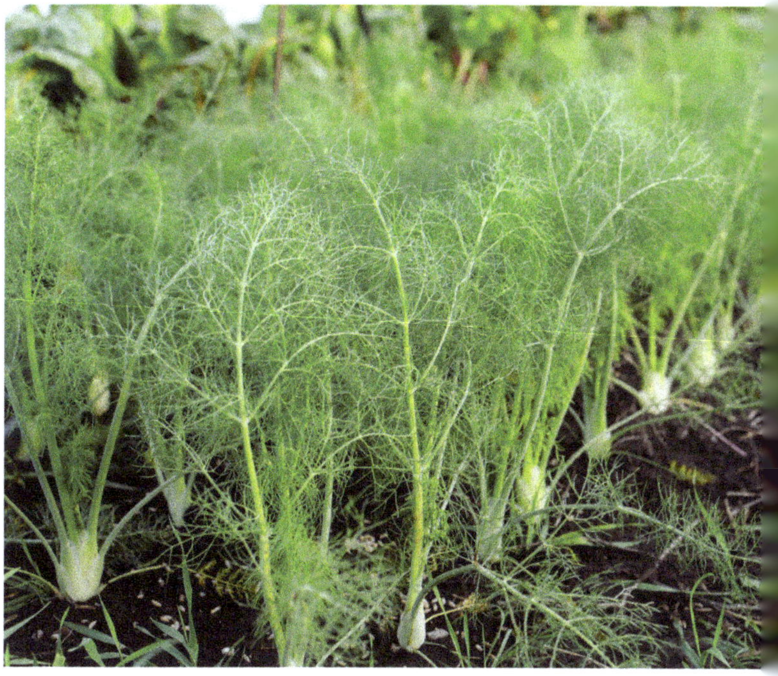

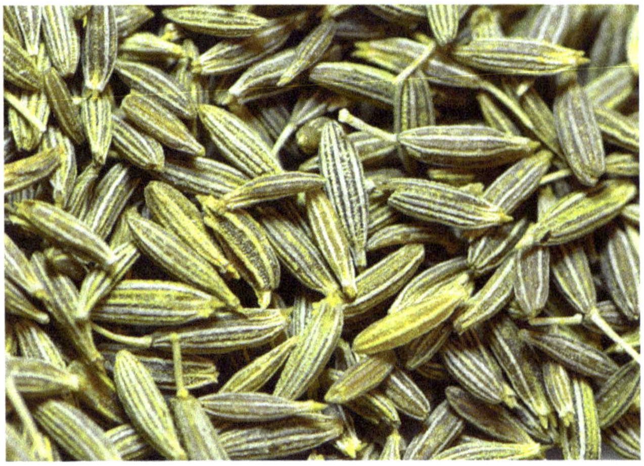

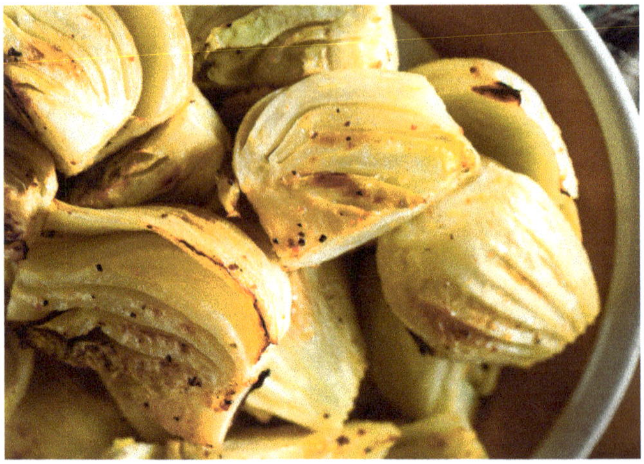

in sensitive individuals.[16] Avoid use with existing nervous system conditions such as epilepsy, Parkinson's disease, or multiple sclerosis.[16] An overdose of the essential oil can cause skin irritation, allergy, nausea, vomiting, seizures, or pulmonary edema.

PREPARATION AND DOSAGE

TINCTURE: Fresh seeds [1:2, 70-95% alcohol]; dry seeds [1:5, 60% alcohol]; consume 15-60 drops, up to three times daily.

GLYCERITE: Fresh seeds [1:2, 50% glycerin and 50% alcohol]; dry seeds [1:5, 40% glycerin, 30% water, 30% alcohol]; consume 15-60 drops, up to three times daily.

ACETUM EXTRACT: Fresh seeds [1:2, apple cider vinegar]; dry seeds [1:5, apple cider vinegar]; consume 30-90 drops, up to three times daily.

CAPSULES: Consume 2-4 "00" capsules, up to three times daily.

TEA: Prepare a hot or cold infusion, or a decoction; consume 8-12 ounces, up to three times daily. Fennel decoction has a richer flavor and creamier consistency than the infusion. A fennel milk decoction can be prepared by simmering the crushed seeds in diluted milk 15 to 20 minutes on a low temperature. Cover the pot while simmering.

HONEY AND SYRUP: To prepare infused syrup, decoct fennel seeds to one-half the original volume, strain the seeds, and sweeten to taste with honey, maple syrup, or simple syrup. Consume 1 teaspoon, up to four times daily. Refrigerate the syrup up to one month. An alternate method is to add 1-2 drops of organic essential oil to 1 teaspoon of honey or simple syrup, and mix thoroughly. Consume the syrup, or add to one cup of hot water or herbal tea.

CULINARY USES: The seeds and essential oil have long been used as flavoring agents in beverages, condiments, and foods. Add the seeds to breads, cookies, and other baked goods. Prepare a delicious digestive chew by combining fennel seed, anise seed, cardamom seed, orange peel, and chopped, crystalized ginger. Or consume the seeds following a meal to enhance digestion and freshen breath. Dry roast the seeds to enhance the aromatics.

Finely chopped, fresh leaves are a lovely addition to salads, root vegetable dishes, vinaigrettes, marinades, soups, herbal butters, cream sauces, and fish or chicken dishes. The tender bulbs are edible in the fall of the first year, but they can become very fibrous later. Fennel bulbs are delicious sautéed with a little butter, cream, sherry, onions, salt, and pepper.

ESSENTIAL OIL: Prepare fennel spirits by adding one part by volume of fennel essential oil to ten parts by volume of organic alcohol. Consume 1-2 drops of spirits, one to three times daily. Place 1-2 drops of fennel seed essential oil on a sugar cube or in 1 teaspoon of honey; dissolve into one cup of warm water, and drink. Place 2-4 drops of essential oil into 1 teaspoon of base oil, and massage into the belly (for adults); for children, use only 1 drop diluted in base oil, and massage into the belly.

FENUGREEK

DESCRIPTION

BOTANICAL NAME:
Trigonella foenum-graecum

COMMON NAMES:
Fenugreek, Greek hay seed, Greek hay, bird's foot, trigonella
hilbeh, hulba (Arabic)
chaiman (Armenian)
sminduh (Bulgarian)
wuh louh ba (Cantonese)
piskavica, pískavice recké, senenka (Croatian)
bukkehornsklover (Danish)
fenegriek (Dutch)
sarviapila (Finnish)
fenugrec, trigonelle (French)
bockshornklee, griechisch heu (German)
trigonella (Greek)
hilbeh (Hebrew)
methi (seed) *sag methi* (leaf) (Hindi)
görögszéna (Hungarian)
kelabet (Indonesian)
fieno greco (Italian)
koroha, henu-guriku (Japanese)
horop'a (Korean)
vaistine ozrage (Lithuanian)
hú lú bā (Mandarin)
methi (Nepali)
bukkehornklover (Norwegian)
kozieradka pospolita (Polish)
feno-grego (Portuguese)
molotru (Romanian)
pazhitinik grecheski (Russian)
methika (Sanskrit)
piskavica (Serbian)
alholva (Spanish)
luk sat (Thai)
cemen (Turkish)
hunba sinna (Ukrainian)
hồ lo ba (Vietnamese)
fenigrekum, khilbe (Yiddish)[1]

FAMILY NAME:
Fabaceae (Leguminosae)

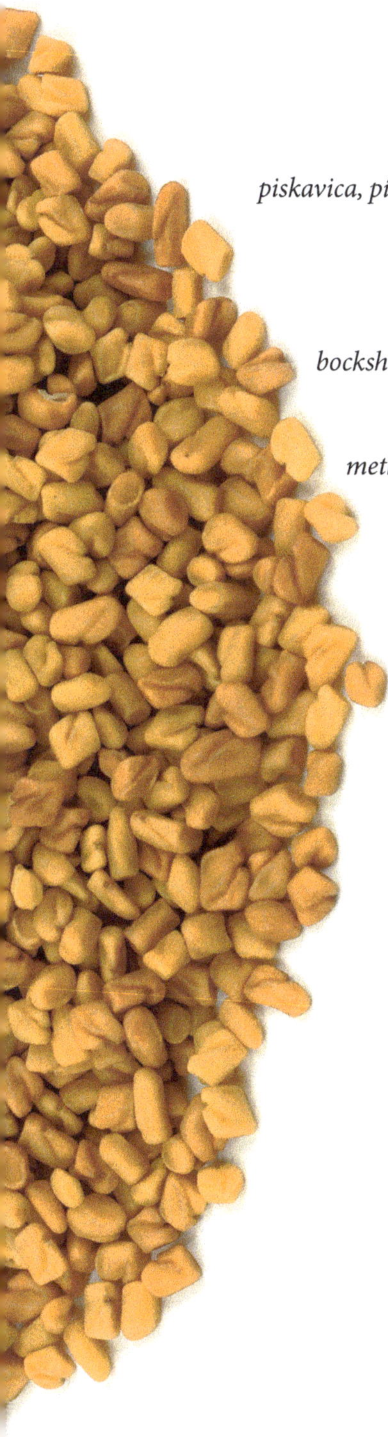

PART USED: The seeds.

BOTANICAL DESCRIPTION AND HABITAT: *Trigonella foenum-graecum* is indigenous to Asia and southeastern Europe. It is cultivated in China, India, Egypt, Morocco, the Himalayas, southwest Asia, southern Europe, and Ethiopia.[2-4] Fenugreek is an annual herb (10 – 80 cm tall) with long taproots (up to 80 cm long).[2,3] The trifoliate leaves have lanceolate stipules and narrowly ovate to oblong leaflets (1 – 3 cm long).[2,3] The upper sides of the leaflets are glabrous; the undersides are sparsely hairy, with dentate leaves on the upper halves.[2]

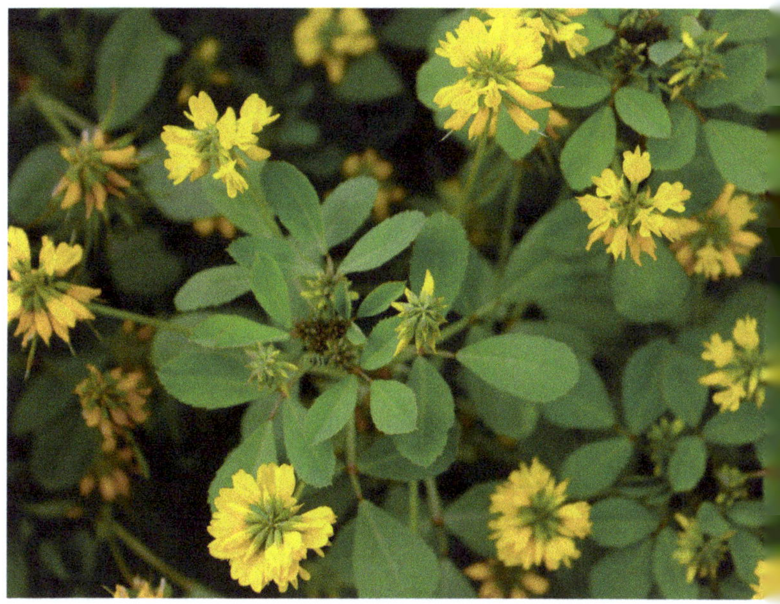

The sessile axillary flowers grow solitary or paired.[2] They consist of a tubular calyx (7– 8 mm long), a light-yellow bilateral, pea-like corolla (12 – 18 mm long), ten stamens, and a unicarpellate, puberulent ovary.[2,3] The thin, curved legume (7–12 by 0.5 cm) has a long, tapered point, and produces 10 – 20 brown, oblong seeds.[2]

THE NAME: The genus *Trigonella* ("three-angled") derives from Greek, describing the corolla form.[4] The epithet *foenum-graecum* translates as "Greek hay."[4]

HISTORICAL USES: Fenugreek has been used as a medicine and seasoning throughout Greece, Italy, India, Egypt, and the Middle East for thousands of years.[4,5] It was found in the tomb of Tutankhamen.[6] Fenugreek was considered the equivalent of quinine in preventing fevers.[4] In India and Egypt, fenugreek was used to treat a chronic cough, bronchitis, mouth ulcers, chapped lips, and digestive problems, and to increase milk production. The soaked seeds were applied as an emollient.[4] The mucilage was used to reduce stomach and intestinal inflammation.[4] The seeds were used as a coffee substitute in Africa.[4] Fenugreek flavored cattle food and rendered moldy hay palatable.[4]

Fenugreek was introduced into Traditional Chinese Medicine during the Sung Dynasty (1057).[5] It was used to dispel wind, cold, and dampness, to tonify kidney yang, and strengthen sinews and bones.[7] Fenugreek was included in Lydia Pinkham's Vegetable Compound — a women's fertility tonic.[8] It continues to be included as a flavoring agent in curries and imitation maple syrup.[5]

CONSTITUENTS: Fenugreek contains mucilage (galactomannan), protein, a fixed oil, volatile oil (n-alkanes, sesquiterpenes, and oxygenated compounds: undecane, hexadecane, elemenes, muurolenes, y-nonalactone, and 5-methyl-D-caprolactone), alkaloids (trigonelline, choline, gentianine, and carpaine), saponins (diosgenin and its isomer yamogenin, tigogenin, and neotigogenin), flavonoids (vitexin, vitexin-7-glucoside, orientin arabinoside, homoorientin, saponaretin = isovitexin, vicenin-1, vicenin-2, quercetin, luteolin, and vitexin cinnamate), amino acids (lysine, tryptophan, leucine, histadine, and arginine), trimethylamine, nurin, betaine, gitogenin, and togogenin.[4,5,7,9] During the roasting process, trigonelline is converted to nicotinic acid, as well as other pyridines and pyrroles.[4,5]

NUTRITIONAL PROPERTIES: Fenugreek contains high amounts of dietary fiber, iron, protein, selenium, and thiamine. It contains low to average amounts of aluminum, calcium, chromium, cobalt, crude fiber, magnesium, manganese, niacin, phosphorus, potassium, riboflavin, sodium, tin, zinc, and vitamins A and C.[10]

MEDICINAL PROPERTIES: Aphrodisiac, aromatic, astringent, bitter tonic, carminative, demulcent, diuretic, emollient, expectorant, galactagogue, hypocholesterolemic, hypoglycemic, kidney yang tonic, laxative, oxytocic, and stomachic.

TEMPERATURE AND FLAVOR: Warm, bitter, sweet, and pungent.

MEDICINAL USES

Fenugreek has hypoglycemic effects that aid in lowering elevated blood glucose levels in type I and type II diabetes.[6,7,11,12] Trigonelline, nicotinic acid, and coumarin are attributed to these effects.[7,12] The high fiber content from consuming the sprouted seeds may also contribute to the hypoglycemic effects.[7] Fenugreek works most effectively for diabetics when consumed as a long-term tonic. Studies demonstrate that daily doses of defatted fenugreek (1.5 – 2 grams per kilogram) lower fasting and postprandial levels of glucose, glucagon, somatostatin, and insulin in diabetic and non-diabetic dogs.[12] In type I diabetics, a 50 mg dose of defatted fenugreek seeds administered twice daily lowered fasting glucose levels, and improved glucose tolerance test results.[12] Urinary glucose excretion decreased more than 50%, and LDL, VLDL, and

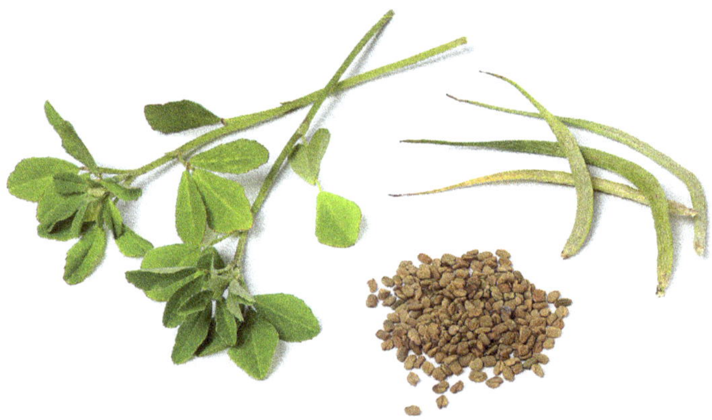

triglyceride levels were significantly reduced.[12] Type II diabetics experienced a significant reduction in postprandial glucose levels after consuming 15 grams of powdered fenugreek seed soaked in water.[12] Rodent studies indicate that trigonelline and fenugreek infusion have hypoglycemic effects and antidiabetic actions.[5] *Note:* Fenugreek is not a replacement for insulin, a medication necessary for all type I diabetics.

Fenugreek has hypocholesterolemic effects.[12] Diosgenin and tigogenin enhance hepatic cholesterol metabolism.[12] The high fiber content of the seeds also prevents intestinal absorption of cholesterol, and enhances the binding of biliary cholesterol subsequently eliminated in the stools.[12] Fenugreek also contains glycosides that enhance the hepatic metabolism of cholesterol. It lowers low density lipid levels (LDLs) and elevates high density lipids (HDLs).[6,12] It is an excellent daily tonic for individuals with elevated cholesterol levels, elevated low density lipids (LDLs), or atherosclerosis. Consume 10 – 20 grams daily to lower LDL levels.[12]

Fenugreek is a soothing demulcent and mild astringent that reduces inflammation in the mucous membranes. The decoction aids in treating a sore throat, laryngitis, pharyngitis, dry cough, and bronchitis. Fenugreek also reduces digestive tract inflammation. It aids in treating acute or chronic conditions in the gastrointestinal tract, including gastritis, dyspepsia, acid indigestion, digestive ulcers, diarrhea, constipation, irritable bowel syndrome, ulcerative colitis, Crohn's disease, and leaky gut syndrome.[11] Fenugreek is an aromatic carminative, reducing gas and bloating.[11,12] It has bitter tonic actions that improve digestion and assimilation.[11] Consuming fenugreek decoction or sprouted seeds aids in treating constipation. Fenugreek contains mucilage and fiber that have a bulk laxative effect.

Fenugreek has kidney yang tonifying properties, enhancing the vitality of reproductive organs. It can be used to treat individuals with kidney yang deficiency manifesting in these symptoms: lower back pain, cold sensation in the lower back, sexual dysfunction, impotence, premature ejaculation, low libido, and spermatorrhea.[9,11] It disperses dampness and cold, and can relieve pain symptoms exacerbated by cold.[9] Fenugreek also aids in treating cold or stagnant qi; patterns include abdominal or flank distention and pain, hernia, soreness or swelling in the legs, and sensations of heaviness in the legs.[9] It increases circulation to the genitalia, and aids in treating dysmenorrhea or cold sensation in the testicles or uterus.[9]

Fenugreek has oxytocic actions.[5,7] It can be used to stimulate uterine contractions one to two weeks prior to a pregnancy due date. Rodent studies demonstrate that fenugreek has a stimulating effect on isolated guinea pig uteri in the last trimester of pregnancy.[5] Fenugreek also can be used following labor for women with hair loss due to depletion from delivering a child. It is beneficial for individuals with iron deficiency anemia. Fenugreek also has demonstrated spermicidal qualities.[7]

Fenugreek is a galactagogue, increasing breast milk production.[6,9,11] Combine with fennel *(Foeniculum)*, anise *(Pimpinella anisum)*, blessed thistle *(Cnicus)*, and/or shatavari *(Asparagus)*.

Fenugreek is a nourishing, repleting herb for debilitated, convalescing individuals. A decoction can be consumed following a lower respiratory or digestive infection, or after radiation and chemotherapy treatment.

Fenugreek enhances bean digestion and improves their flavor. The powdered and dry roasted seeds are often added to curry powder. Sprouted seeds also aid in treating indigestion.

Decocted seeds can be applied as a drawing poultice for abscesses, boils, carbuncles, ulcers, and splinters.[6,11] The emollient qualities are soothing for inflamed skin conditions, such as eczema, psoriasis, dermatitis, and skin rashes.[11,13]

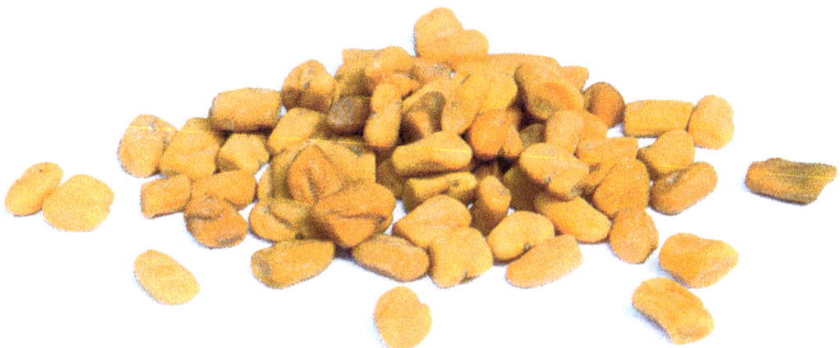

CONTRAINDICATIONS

Fenugreek should be avoided during pregnancy, except to stimulate labor. However, consuming small amounts for culinary use is acceptable. Diabetic individuals may need to modify their medication dosage when taking fenugreek consistently.[6] Individuals with damp-heat or heat resulting from yin deficiency should avoid using fenugreek. Fenugreek may alter the smell of urine.

PREPARATION AND DOSAGE

TINCTURE: Fresh seeds [1:2, 60-95% alcohol]; dry seeds [1:5, 60% alcohol]; consume 15-60 drops, up to three times daily.

CAPSULES: Consume 2-4 "00" capsules, one to three times daily.

TEA: Prepare a hot infusion, cold infusion, or (preferably) decoction; consume 8-12 ounces, up to three times daily.

CULINARY USE: Fenugreek is widely used in Indian and Middle Eastern cuisine.

TOPICAL USE: Prepare a poultice, fomentation, or wash.

FEVERFEW

DESCRIPTION

BOTANICAL NAMES:
Tanacetum parthenium
(syn. *Chrysanthemum parthenium, Leucanthemum parthenium, Pyrethrum parthenium, Matricaria pyrethrum*),
T. parthenium f. *flosculosum* (double flowered)

COMMON NAMES:
Feverfew, feverwort, featherfew, featherfoil, featherfowl, flirtwort, mayweed, midsummer daisy, mother herb, nosebleed, whitewort, wild chamomile, bachelor's buttons, altamisa
espargaoutte, grande camomille (French)
bertram, metram, mutterkraut (German)
chamomilla grande, erba madre, matricale, partenio (Italian)
atasi (Sanskrit)
altamisa mexicana, santa maria, yerba de santa maria (Spanish)
mattram (Swedish)

FAMILY NAME:
Asteraceae (Compositae)

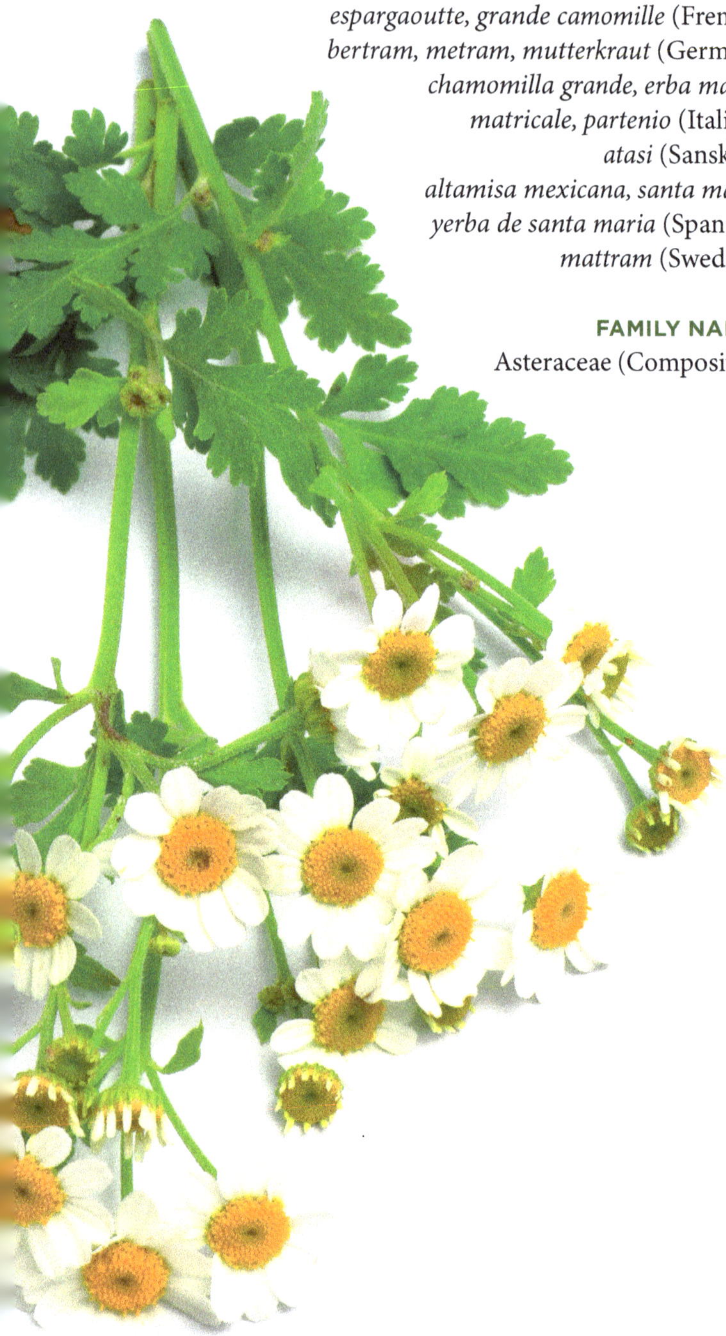

PART USED: Leaves collected when the plant is flowering.

BOTANICAL DESCRIPTION AND HABITAT: Feverfew is easily cultivated and grows prolifically. It has naturalized throughout much of the U.S. in disturbed and urban areas, roadsides, and fields. A companion plant, it contains the insecticide pyrethrin, and protects plants from insect damage.[1]

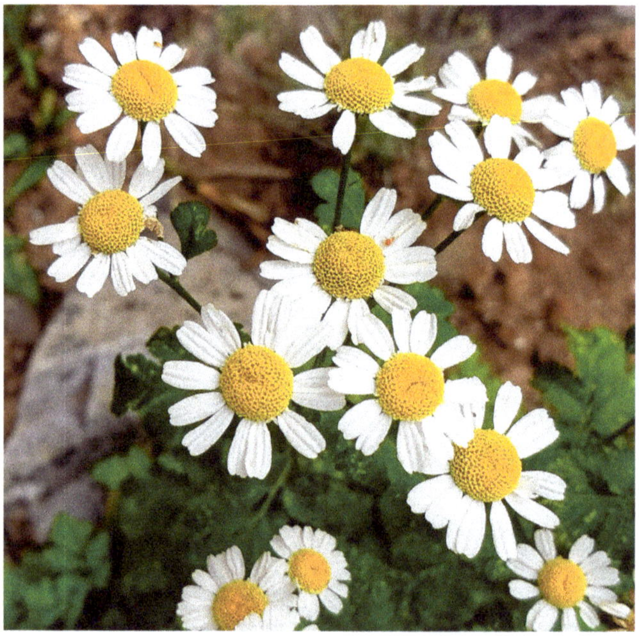

Feverfew is a perennial found in temperate climates. It grows 20 – 80 cm tall with many erect, striate, finely pubescent stems. The branches bear yellow-green, strongly pungent, obovate to oblong leaves, with long petioles that are 1- to 2-pinnately compound with deeply lobed, dentate leaflets. The leaflets are also finely pubescent, predominantly on the lower side. The leaves (4 – 10 cm long by 1.5 – 4 cm wide) and their petioles become smaller as they ascend on the stem. Feverfew has multiple showy, chamomile-like, radiate heads per stem, with two to three series of imbricate phyllaries, and a convex or flat receptacle (unlike chamomile flowers, that have a conical receptacle). They contain many ray florets bearing white petals and numerous tiny, vibrant, yellow disc flowers. Double-flowered varieties have two or more series of ray florets. The fruits are columnar, ribbed achenes (1 – 2 mm long) bearing short, corona-like pappuses. Feverfew blooms from June to November.[2]

THE NAME: *Tanacetum* is modified from the Greek *athanasai (athanatos),* meaning "immortal" or "everlasting," referring to the longlasting dried flowers. The epithet *parthenium* derives from the Greek *parthenos* ("virgin") referring to the plant's ability to alleviate young women's menstrual cramps.[6] The common name feverfew derives from two Latin words: *febris* ("fever") and *fugure* ("to chase away"), based on its use in treating fevers.[3]

HISTORICAL USES: The medicinal uses of feverfew date back to the 1st century when the ancient Greek physician Dioscorides practiced medicine.[4] Feverfew was administered to treat menstrual irregularities and expel the placenta following childbirth.[3,4] Warm infusions were given to treat colds and febrile disease, expel worms, and stimulate menses, and as a choleretic.[5] The herb was also used to treat a stomachache, headache, or toothache, and reduce inflammation.[3] Feverfew tea was consumed at room temperature to treat nervousness, reproductive disorders, and low spirits, and as a tonic.[6] A cold infusion was consumed to reduce a painful earache, as well as for hypersensitive, nervous individuals with rheumatism or dyspepsia.[6] Sweetened tea was consumed to reduce coughing and wheezing.[6] An extract of the herb was diluted with water and applied to alleviate the pain and swelling of insect and vermin bites.[6] Gerard used feverfew as a poultice to treat ague.[6] Culpeper applied the bruised herb to the crown to treat a headache.[6] Eclectic physicians administered the herb as an appetite stimulant, enhancing digestive secretions and assimilation; they also used it to promote renal and cutaneous functions.[5] In Latin America, feverfew was used to stimulate digestion, and treat colic and stomachaches.[7] In Costa Rica, it was consumed to improve digestion, and as an emmenagogue.[4] Feverfew was believed to ward off disease when planted near dwellings.[6]

CONSTITUENTS: Feverfew is rich in sesquiterpenoids (parthenolide, artecanin, canin, chrysanthemolide, chrysanthemonin, 10-epi-canin, 1β-hydroxyarbusculin, 8β-hydroxyreynosin, 3β-hydroxyparthenolide, and magnolide), flavonoids (flavones), reynosin, santamarin, *seco*-tanapartholide A, tanaparthin, tanaparthin-1α-4α-epoxide, tanaparthin-1β,4β-epoxide, and volatile oil (L-camphor, L-borneol, β-farnesene, germacerene, chrysanthenyl acetate, α-pinene derivatives, bornyl acetate, bornyl angelate, terpenes, and miscellaneous esters). The concentration of the parthenolide content varies, depending on the chemotype and geographic location, as well as harvesting, processing, and storage methods.[4,5,7-9]

NUTRITIONAL PROPERTIES: Feverfew contains high amounts of chromium, crude fiber, fat, magnesium, manganese, niacin, phosphorus, potassium, protein, selenium, thiamine, and tin. It contains low to average amounts of calcium, carbohydrates, dietary fiber, riboflavin, silicon, and vitamins A and C. It contains trace amounts of aluminum, ash, cobalt, iron, sodium, and zinc.[10]

MEDICINAL PROPERTIES: Analgesic, anti-inflammatory, antipyretic, antispasmodic, bitter tonic, carminative, cholagogue, emmenagogue, febrifuge, and vermifuge.

TEMPERATURE AND FLAVOR: Cool, bitter, and pungent.

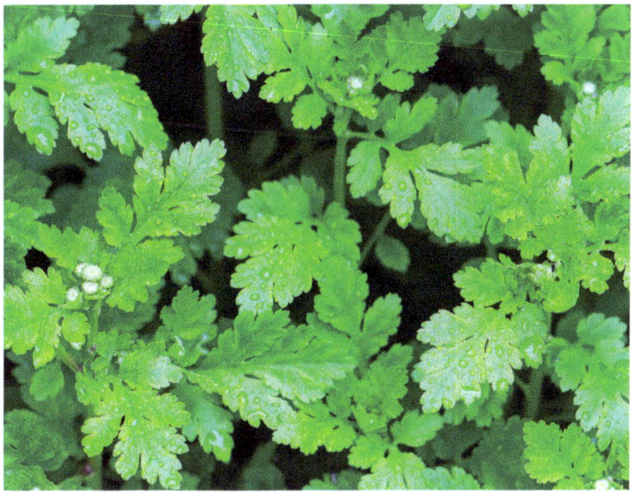

MEDICINAL USES

Daily consumption of feverfew reduces the frequency and severity of migraine headaches, and decreases associated nausea, vomiting, and light and noise sensitivity.[7,8,11] Feverfew also can be effective for the acute treatment of migraines, especially when consumed at the onset. Abnormal behavior of blood platelets triggering spasms in cerebral blood vessel walls is thought to be a cause of migraine headaches. Feverfew inhibits the release of serotonin (5-hydroxytryptamine) from blood platelets induced by aggregating agents, and prevents the spasm and constriction of cerebral blood vessels.[3,8,11] Parthenolide and other sesquiterpene lactones inhibit platelet aggregation and secretory activity in platelets and polymorphonuclear leukocytes.[5,7,11] Feverfew extract was found to inhibit platelet phospholipase A_2; therefore, the antiplatelet activity is likely due to a phospholipase inhibitor that prevents the release of arachidonic acid.[5] The platelets of patients consuming feverfew had normal aggregation to ADP and thrombin, but the platelet aggregation in response to serotonin was reduced. This implies that the biochemical sequence causing a migraine is halted, but

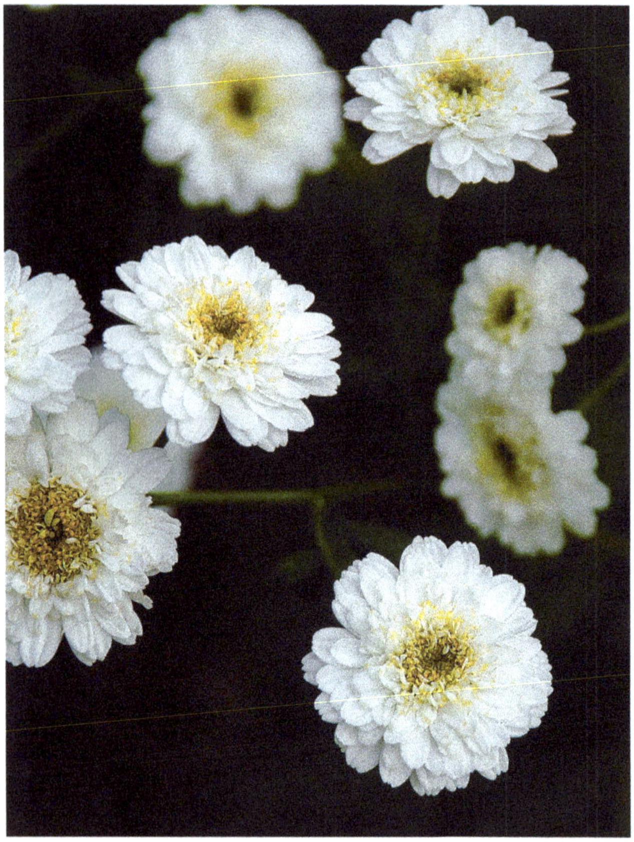

normal clotting mechanisms remain intact.[5] The levels of parthenolide vary widely in commercial preparations. The recommended dose of parthenolide ranges from 0.25 – 0.5 mg for prophylactic treatment of migraine headaches. Higher doses of 1 – 2 grams are recommended for an acute migraine.[11]

Feverfew has anti-inflammatory actions that inhibit the formation of inflammatory prostaglandins, leukotrienes, and thromboxanes.[11,12] The constituents parthenolide, michefuscalide, and chrysanthenyl acetate reduce prostaglandin formation by inhibiting prostaglandin synthetase, which converts arachidonic acid to prostaglandins.[8] Feverfew decreases bronchial constriction by inhibiting phospholipase A_2 activity, aiding in treating asthma and allergy-related bronchial spasms.[8] Sesquiterpene and non-sesquiterpene lactones contribute to the anti-inflammatory effect by inhibiting proinflammatory eicosanoid synthesis, halting 5-lipoxygenase and cyclo-oxygenase in leukocytes.[8] These findings substantiate the herb's historical use for treating fevers, arthritis, and migraines. Feverfew has great potential to aid in the long-term treatment of rheumatoid arthritis and menstrual cramping.[12] Feverfew also reduces inflammation and irritability in the gastrointestinal, vaginal, and urinary tracts.[12]

Feverfew has antipyretic, febrifuge, and diaphoretic properties. Consume the hot tea or tincture in hot water with honey and lemon to stimulate diaphoresis in the first stage of a cold or flu.

Feverfew is an emmenagogue that stimulates menses and decreases menstrual clotting.[3-5] The spasmolytic actions decrease menstrual cramping, especially when consumed several days prior to menses.[12]

CONTRAINDICATIONS

Avoid use during pregnancy or lactation, or in children younger than two.[8,9] Chewing the fresh leaves has been reported to cause mouth ulcers, as well as swelling of the lips and tongue.[3,5,11] This is believed to be caused by the sesquiterpene lactone, parthenolide. In rare cases, feverfew can cause an allergic dermatitis reaction in individuals hypersensitive to the Asteraceae (daisy) family.[9,11]

Feverfew reduces the platelet aggregation factor, and is contraindicated two weeks prior to, and following surgery. Avoid consuming feverfew in individuals with inhibited blood clotting function, bleeding disorders, or a potential hemorrhage. Consult a health care practitioner before combining feverfew with medications that have blood-thinning effects (aspirin, warfarin, etc.).[8]

PREPARATION AND DOSAGE

TINCTURE: Fresh leaves [1:2, 70 - 95% alcohol]; dry leaves (inferior) [1:5, 60% alcohol]; consume 15 - 60 drops, up to three times daily. The fresh leaves are typically more potent; only leaves dried within six to 12 months should be used to make a dry plant extract.

CAPSULES: Consume 2 - 3 capsules, one to two times daily as a prophylactic treatment. For acute treatment of a migraine, consume 2 - 4 freeze-dried capsules, up to three times daily.

TEA: Prepare a hot infusion; consume 4 - 8 ounces, up to four times daily. The bitter and pungent tastes can be difficult to palate; adding honey and fresh lemon juice increase the palatability.

CULINARY USE: Chew 2 - 3 fresh leaves, one to three times daily.

GARLIC

DESCRIPTION

BOTANICAL NAME:
Allium sativum

COMMON NAMES:
Garlic, stinking rose
fum, thoum (Arabic)
skhdor (Armenian)
chesan, chesnov luk (Bulgarian)
syun tauh (Cantonese)
bijeli luk (Croatian)
cesnek (Czech)
hvidlog (Danish)
knofloock (Dutch)
ajlo (Esperanto)
küüslauk (Estonian)
valkosipuli (Finnish)
knoblauch (German)
skordo (Greek)
shum (Hebrew)
iasan (Hindi)
hvítlauker (Icelandic)
bawang putih, kesuna (Indonesian)
aglio (Italian)
garikku, ninniku, taisan (Japanese)
kallik (Korean)
van mahakan (Laotian)
kiploki (Latvian)
da suan (Mandarin)
lasun (Nepali)
hvitlok (Norwegian)
czosnek pospolity (Polish)
usturoi (Russian)
lasuna, laśuna (Sanskrit)
beli luk (Serbian)
ajo (Spanish)
kitunguu sauma (Swahili)
vitlök (Swedish)
gratiem (Thai)
gogpa, sgog pa (Tibetan)
sarmisak (Turkish)
chasnyk (Ukranian)
cây toi (Vietnamese)
knobl (Yiddish)[1]

FAMILY NAME:
Amaryllidaceae (formerly Liliaceae)

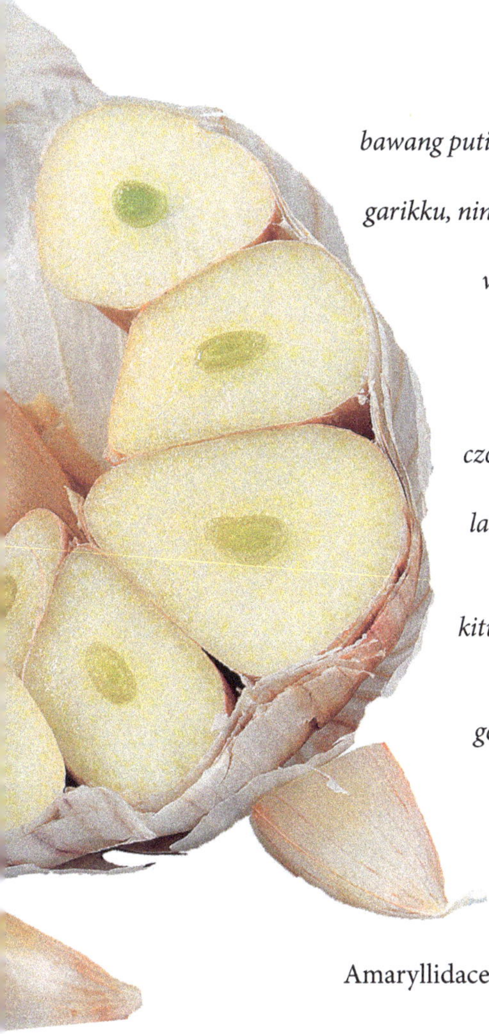

PART USED: The cloves (bulblets).

BOTANICAL DESCRIPTION AND HABITAT: Garlic is a perennial, bulb-forming plant.[2] The globose bulb is an aggregate of six to ten smaller bulblets called cloves. Each clove is wrapped in a thin, white to purple, multi-layered tunic that is membranous when fresh, but brittle and

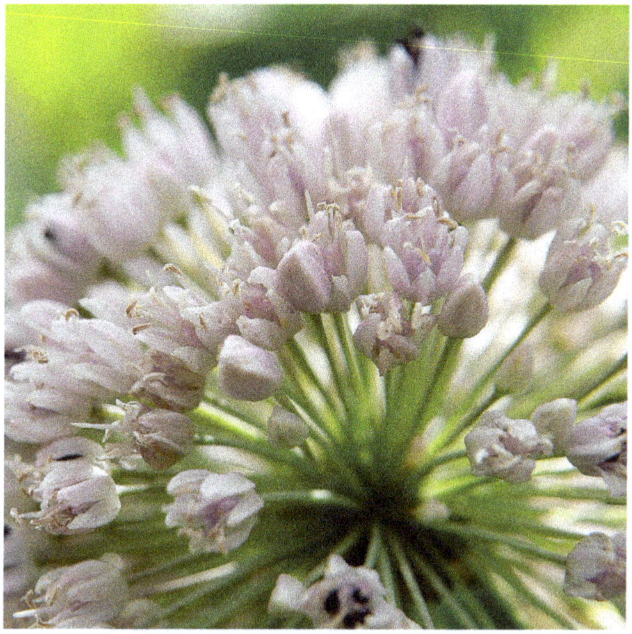

papery when dry.[2] Wide, sheathing, linear leaves (up to 2.5 cm wide) with acuminate apices grow from the base of the bulb.[2] The scape, a tapering, cylindrical, flowering stem (25 – 50 cm tall), extends from the center of the leaves and beyond their tips.[2]

The plant produces an umbel at the apex of the scape. When immature, it is protected by a conical, papery spathe that eventually falls away when the umbel matures.[2] The umbel consists of many acuminate, membranous bracteoles interspersing numerous small, white flowers and tiny bulbs produced as units of asexual reproduction. These bulbs grow and enlarge; as they become heavier, the scape falls to the ground, allowing the bulbs to take root in the soil.[2] The flowers consists of six light red tepals (3 – 4 mm long) surrounding six epipetalous stamens, and a globose ovary consisting of three fused carpels. Cultivated garlic varieties will have sterile flowers or no flowers; wild varieties have fertile flowers.[3]

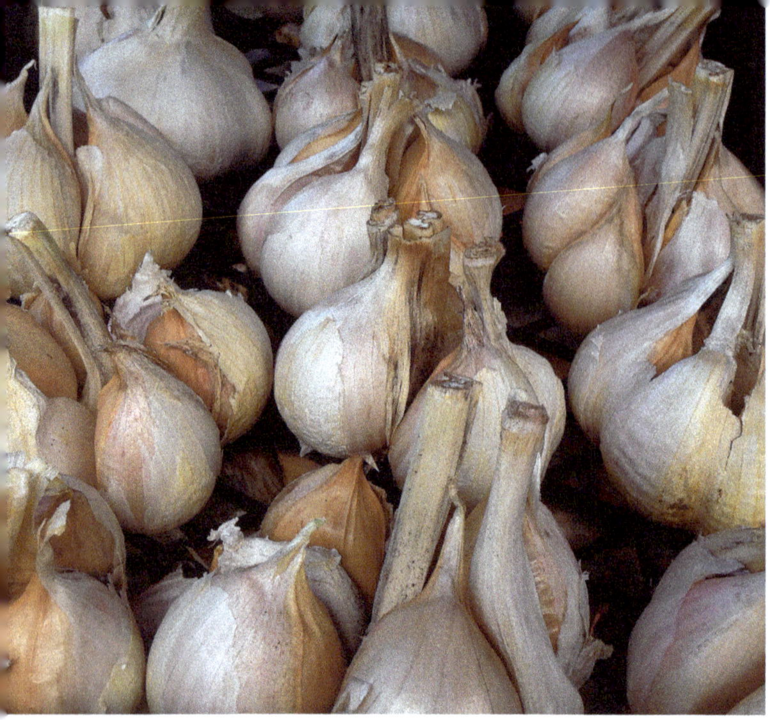

THE NAME: The genus *Allium* is an ancient Latin name for garlic, originating from the Celtic *all* ("hot" or "burning").[4,5] The epithet *sativum* means "cultivated or planted."[4,5] Garlic derives from the Anglo-Saxon *garleac,* also known as "spearplant."[4,5]

HISTORICAL USES: Garlic is believed to have originated in the high plains of west-central Asia.[5] It was cultivated and used medicinally in the Middle East 5,000 years ago.[4,5] Garlic was consumed as a food and medicine during the time of the Egyptian pharaohs and the earliest Chinese dynasties.[5] In Ancient Egypt, records dating to 1550 BCE document the medicinal uses of garlic for treating bites, worms, hypertension, headaches, and tumors.[6] Egyptian characters written on pyramids recorded the quantities of garlic, onions, and radishes consumed by laborers who constructed the pyramids.[5] Garlic was found in the tomb of Tutankhamun.[5]

Ancient Greek and Roman scholars utilized garlic as a cough suppressant for asthma, and an anthelmintic for intestinal parasites.[4] Pliny the Elder administered garlic as an antidote for poisonous snake and shrew bites, and aconite and henbane poisoning.[4] He infused freshly crushed garlic cloves and coriander in wine as an aphrodisiac.[4] Pliny also mentioned that excessive consumption of garlic would injure the stomach and result in flatulence and extreme thirst.[4]

Although garlic was consumed as food and used as folk medicine in China, the first record of medicinal use appears around 510 CE in Tao Hong-Jing's *Ming Yi Bei Lu.*[4] Garlic, also known as da suan, was used to treat the common cold, tuberculosis, dysentery, and digestive ailments.[7] It was applied topically to treat carbuncles, sores, and indolent ulcers, and as an antifungal.[4,7] A cold infusion of freshly crushed garlic bulb was mixed with sugar to treat bacillus dysentery.[4] Garlic enemas were administered to treat pinworm.[4]

CONSTITUENTS: Garlic contains volatile oil consisting of allicin (diallyldisulfide-S-oxide and diallyl thiosulfinate), allylpropyl disulfide, diallyl disulfide, diallyl trisulfide, dimethyl sulfide, dimethyl disulfide, dimethyl trisulfide, allylmethyl sulfide, 2,3,4-trithiapentane, and other sulfur compounds, citral, geraniol, linalool, and α- and β-phellandrene. It also contains alliin = S-allyl-L-cysteine sulfoxide, S-methyl-L-cysteine sulfoxide, enzymes (alliinase, peroxidase, and myrosinase), ajoenes (E,Z-ajoene, E,Z-methylajoene, and dimethylajoene), protein, minerals, vitamins, lipids, and seven amino acids.[8,9]

Garlic contains alliin, a sulfur-containing amino acid that reacts with the enzyme allinase when crushed to produce allicin.[4,9] Garlic's characteristic fragrance and flavor are attributed to the allicin.[4] Ajeone is formed from the combination of allicin and diallyl disulfide.[4] The pungency of garlic directly reflects the amount of sulfur in the soil where it is cultivated. Sulfuric acid is the primary constituent that can aggravate the eyes.

NUTRITIONAL PROPERTIES: Garlic contains high amounts of chromium, phosphorus, protein, selenium, and thiamine. It contains low to average amounts of aluminum, ash, calcium, cobalt, copper, crude fiber, dietary fiber, germanium, iron, magnesium, manganese, niacin, potassium, riboflavin, sodium, tin, and vitamins A.[4,10]

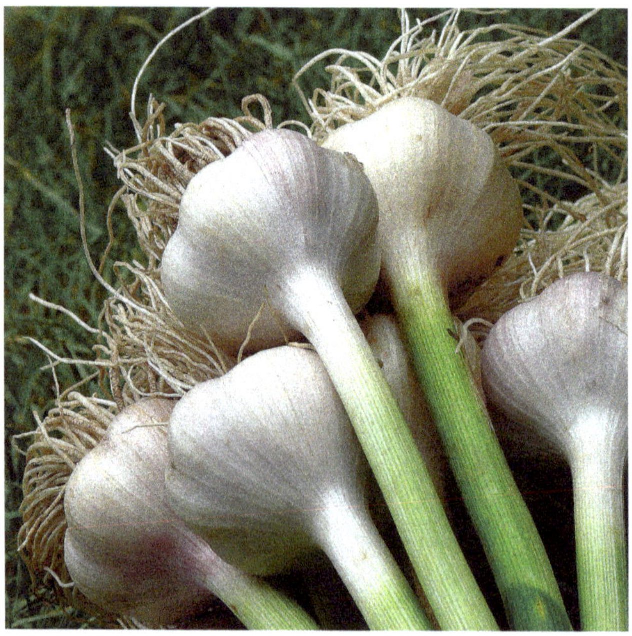

MEDICINAL PROPERTIES: Antiatherosclerotic, antibacterial, antifungal, antioxidant, anthelmintic, antithrombotic, antiviral, carminative, circulatory stimulant, diaphoretic, diuretic, expectorant, hypocholesterolemic, hypoglycemic, hypotensive, vasodilator, and vermifuge.

TEMPERATURE AND FLAVOR: Raw garlic is hot and pungent. Cooked garlic is warm, pungent, and sweet.

MEDICINAL USES

Garlic has impressive actions in the cardiovascular system. It aids in preventing and treating atherosclerosis, reversing atherosclerotic plaque formation, and decreasing the risk of a heart attack or stroke.[5-9,11] Garlic reduces platelet aggregation and thrombus formation by inhibiting the lipoxygenase and cyclo-oxygenase pathways of the arachidonic acid cascade, preventing the formation of prostaglandins (PGE2, PGD2, and PG12) and thromboxanes (TXB2).[9] It exerts fibrinolytic actions, decreasing blood viscosity, and increasing blood coagulation time.[6,8,9,12] High fibrinogen levels contribute to the risk of heart attack and stroke.[6] The component ajoene inhibits the binding of fibrinogen to adenosine diphosphate (ADP) stimulated platelets, preventing platelet aggregation.[9] The antithrombotic actions are attributed to ajoene, diallyl sulfide, and methyl allyl sulfide.[4,5] Garlic also lowers total serum cholesterol levels, decreases phospholipids, triglycerides, and low density lipids (LDL), and increases high density lipoprotein (HDL).[4-9,11,12] LDL oxidation is associated with the development of atherosclerosis; garlic's antioxidant activity protects against LDL oxidation, decreasing the concentration of lipid peroxides in the blood.[6,9] Decreased LDL oxidation is attributed to the component allicin.[6]

Garlic is a hypotensive agent that aids in treating high blood pressure.[4-6,8,9,11] In hypertensive individuals, garlic has lowered systolic blood pressure 20 – 30 mmHg, and diastolic blood pressure 10 – 20 mmHg.[6] The y-glutamylcysteine can impede angiotensin-converting enzyme (ACE), preventing the conversion of angiotensin I to angiotensin II — a vasoconstricting hormone.[9] Garlic dilates peripheral blood vessels, increasing blood volume in the capillaries and lowering blood pressure. The cholesterol and LDL lowering effects, as well as the blood thinning, fibrinolytic, antioxidant, and vasodilating actions contribute to the blood pressure lowering effects. The vasodilating actions increase oxygen and nutrient delivery to the tissues, enhancing cellular vitality.[8] Garlic is a circulatory stimulant that aids in treating cold hands and feet, Raynaud's phenomenon, and varicose veins.[11,12]

Garlic is a potent antiviral agent.[6,8,9] It has virucidal actions against herpes simplex (types 1 and 2), parainfluenza virus (type 3), vaccinia virus, vesicular stomatitis virus, and human rhinovirus (type 2).[6] Fresh garlic has the most effective virucidal effect. The following constituents are listed in order of virucidal potency (strongest to weakest): ajoene, allicin, allyl methyl thiosulfinate, and methyl allyl thiosulfinate.[6] Garlic increases the activity of natural killer cells (NK cells) and improves the helper T to suppressor T cell ratio.[4,8] It is a heating diaphoretic that reduces fever and chills.[5,11] Garlic is an expectorant and decongestant; when cooked, it has mild antitussive actions.[5,8,12] It aids in treating a cold, flu, sinusitis, sinus congestion, bronchitis, pneumonia, pleurisy, whooping cough, strep throat, herpes,

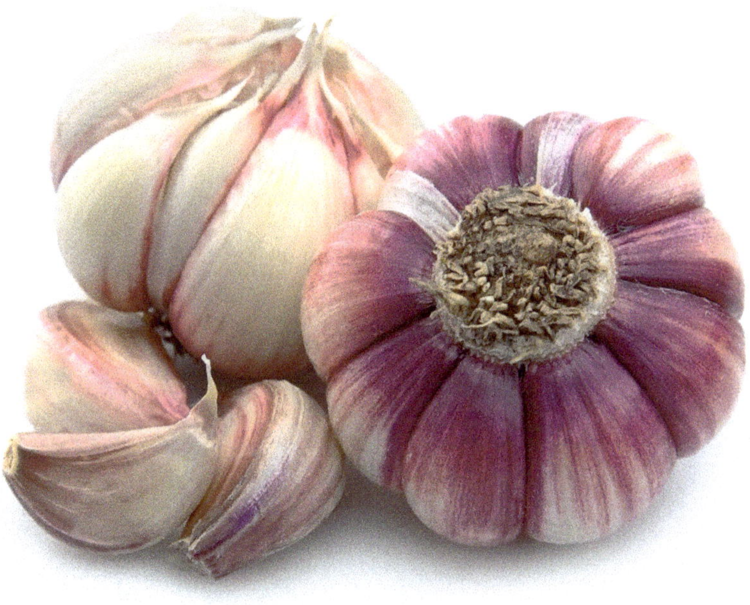

intestinal microbes, and diarrhea.[4,5,7,8,11] *Note:* Due to its heating effects, garlic should be used with caution by individuals with hot infections. If the symptoms of an infection worsen after consuming garlic, discontinue use. This has occurred in individuals with strep throat, lung infections, and some digestive infections. *Note:* If the individual feels worse after consuming garlic, discontinue use.

Garlic is an immune modulator that increases phagocytosis, natural killer cell activity, antibody titer, and lymphocyte counts.[9] Garlic has antiallergenic actions, reducing the release of histamine from mast cells, and decreasing IgE mediated skin reactions *in vitro*.[9] Garlic has potent antitumor effects, and inhibits the formation of nitrosamines (cancer-causing compounds).[6] It may increase the production of cytokines that elicit antitumor responses, including interleukin (IL-2), tumor necrosis factor (TNF), and interferon gamma.[9]

Garlic has impressive broad spectrum antibacterial actions against gram-positive and gram-negative bacteria, including: *Staphylococcus aureus*, α- and β-hemolytic *Streptococcus, Salmonella enteritidis, Mycobacterium tuberculosis, Klebsiella pneumoniae, Escherichia coli, Citrobacter* spp., *Vibrio* spp., *Brucella* spp., *Bacillus* spp., and *Proteus* spp.[4,6,9,11] Studies found that the antibacterial effects of garlic were comparable to antibiotics such as penicillin, streptomycin, chloramphenicol, erythromycin, and tetracycline.[6] Garlic was an effective antibacterial for eight of nine antibiotic resistant bacterial strains.[4,5] The antibacterial and antimutagenic effects are attributed to the allicin.[4,5,8]

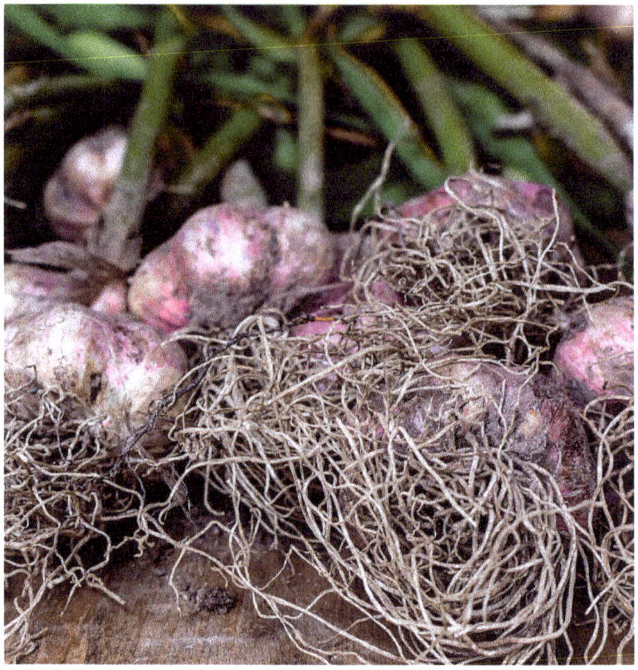

Garlic has carminative, antispasmodic, antifungal, antibacterial, and antiparasitic actions.[4-6,9] It aids in treating food poisoning and bacterial and amoebic dysentery.[4,12] Extracts of garlic have an antiulcer effect, and inhibit *H. pylori* bacteria *in vitro*.[9] Garlic reduces pathogenic bacteria, and has a favorable effect on intestinal microflora, encouraging the growth of lactic acid-producing organisms.[4,5,12] Adding several cloves of fresh garlic to lacto-fermented foods such as kimchee or kraut encourages the growth of beneficial organisms, and inhibits the growth of unwanted organisms. Garlic is also an anthelmintic against *Oxyuris* spp. (pinworms), *Ascaris lumbricoides* (roundworms), and hookworms (*Ancylostoma duodenale* and *Necator americanus*).[6,11]

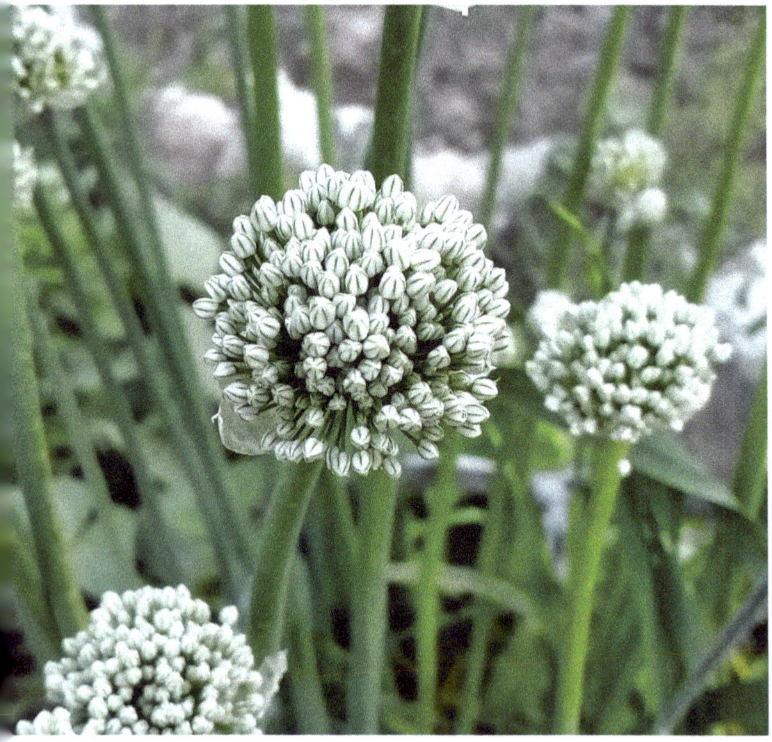

Garlic has antifungal properties against *Candida albicans, Aspergillus* spp., and *Tineas* spp.[6,8,9,11] It is more effective than common antifungal agents such as nystatin and gentian violet.[6] Garlic can be consumed internally to treat intestinal candida, or as a preventative following the intake of antibiotics. Gargling with garlic tea aids in treating thrush.[11] A peeled clove can be inserted into the vaginal canal as an antifungal agent for treating vaginal candida. Make sure to sew a string through the clove to create a tampon-like device, enabling easy removal of the clove. The clove can be dipped in olive oil or yogurt to ease insertion. Change the clove every three to four hours. Individuals with extremely inflamed vaginal tissues may experience discomfort or burning following insertion; remove and discontinue use if this occurs.

Several drops of strained, infused garlic oil can be placed in the ear for the beginning stages of an ear infection, or for irritation of the ear canal caused by exposure to strong winds.[11,12] *Note:* When treating an individual with an ear infection, it is important to consume antibacterial herbs internally. If the bacteria is not properly treated, ear infections can cause damage to the inner ear, resulting in permanent hearing damage. It is especially important to seek proper medical attention for children when treating an ear infection if herbs aren't working effectively.

Garlic and onions contain allicin that has a hypoglycemic action aiding in the treatment of diabetes.[6-8] Garlic may increase hepatic metabolism and/or the release of insulin, and/or have an insulin-sparing effect.[6] It also stimulates a sluggish liver and has hepatoprotectant properties.[8,12]

Topical applications of garlic have counterirritant properties that aid in treating myalgia, neuralgia, sciatica, and rheumatoid arthritis.[11,12] A garlic wash, fomentation, or poultice is an antifungal agent that aids in treating athlete's foot, ringworm, or fungal infections in the scalp.[11,12]

Garlic has insecticidal and larvicidal actions.[8] Garlic-containing preparations kill mosquito larvae, houseflies, and other insects.[4] It is a companion plant that repels cabbage moths, Japanese beetles, and aphids.[5] Prepare garlic as an insecticide by placing one handful of unpeeled cloves into three cups of hot water, steep for several hours until it cools, and spray the mixture onto plants.[5]

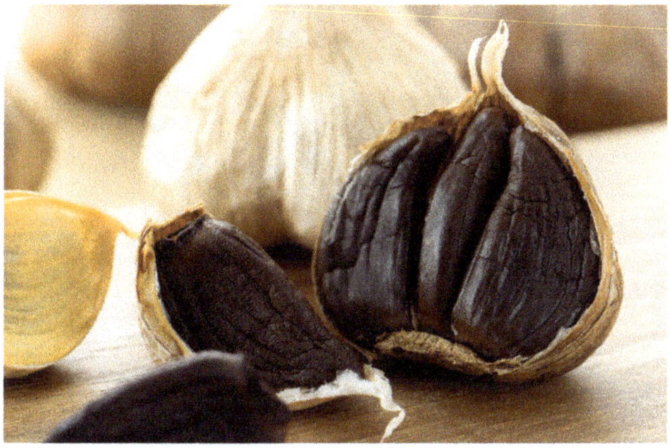

CONTRAINDICATIONS

There are no known contraindications during pregnancy or lactation.[9] However, the pungent qualities of garlic can agitate and stimulate the fetus; therefore, limited use is recommended during pregnancy.[12] The sulfur-containing volatile oil passes through breast milk, and can cause colic and gastric disturbance in nursing infants. Consuming more than three to five cloves of raw garlic daily can cause heartburn, nausea, flatulence, and digestive disturbance.[11] Individuals with gastric ulcers, hiatal hernias, acid indigestion, or active inflammation in the gastrointestinal system should avoid consuming raw garlic.[12] Avoid consuming garlic with hot conditions, or if it aggravates a condition. Cooked or raw garlic can cause flatulence.

Due to its blood thinning properties, avoid internal use of garlic two weeks prior to, and following surgery or the pregnancy due date.[9,12] Consult a health care practitioner or avoid consuming garlic when taking antihypertensives, statins, or over-the-counter or blood thinning agents, such as aspirin or warfarin.[9,11,12] Avoid use in individuals with garlic allergies. Contact dermatitis or blistering upon prolonged contact can occur with the crushed, raw clove.[8]

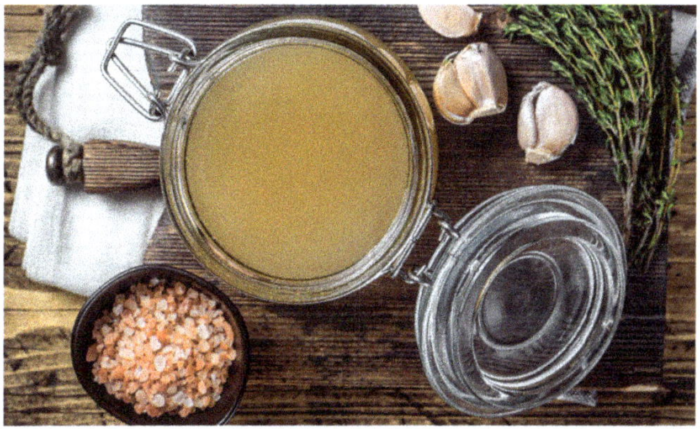

PREPARATION AND DOSAGE

Food-based preparations or broths are preferred methods of administration. Fresh, raw garlic is the most potent.

TINCTURE: Fresh cloves [1:2, 70-95% alcohol]; consume 15-60 drops, up to three times daily.

FLUID EXTRACT: Dry cloves [1:1, 50% alcohol]; consume 15-30 drops, up to three times daily.

ACETUM EXTRACT: Fresh cloves [1:2-1:3, apple cider vinegar]; consume ½ teaspoon to 1 tablespoon, up to four times daily. To improve palatability, garlic vinegar can be mixed with an equal part honey. Or consume 1-3 pickled cloves daily.

SUCCUS: Consume ¼ to 1 teaspoon of the fresh juice. Adding garlic to fresh vegetable juice decreases the intensity of the flavor. The chlorophyll content in fresh green juice helps to reduce garlic breath.

CAPSULES: Consume 2-4 "00" capsules, preferably freeze-dried, up to three times daily.

HONEY: Mince cloves and infuse in honey; add ⅙ to ⅓ parts vinegar to prevent the growth of botulism. Consume 1 teaspoon, up to three times daily.

TOPICAL USE: Mince cloves and infuse in olive oil. Strain well and place 2-3 drops in the ear canal, up to three times daily.

CULINARY USE: Garlic is incorporated in cuisine around the world. It can be added to soups, sauces, salad dressings, meat, fish, poultry, or vegetable dishes.

GENTIAN

BOTANICAL NAMES:
Gentiana lutea, G. acaulis, G. affinis, G. calycosa, G. crinita, G. douglasiana, G. macrophylla, G. pannonicus, G. platypetala, G. punctata, G. purpurea, G. quinquefolia, G. sceptrum, G. scabra, G. triflora, G. rigescens, G. spp.

COMMON NAMES:
Yellow gentian, great yellow gentian, pale gentian, purple gentian, spotted gentian, central European gentian, bitter root, bitterwort, felwort, gallweed, gentian root, king gentian, marsh gentian, swamp gentian, broad-petalled gentian
long dan cao, qin jiao, chin chiu (Chinese)
genciana, racine de gentiane (French)
bitterwurz, enzian, enzianwurzel, gleber enzian, fieberwurzel (German)
jingyo, ryutan (Japanese)
yongcancho'o, chin'gyo (Korean)

FAMILY NAME:
Gentianaceae

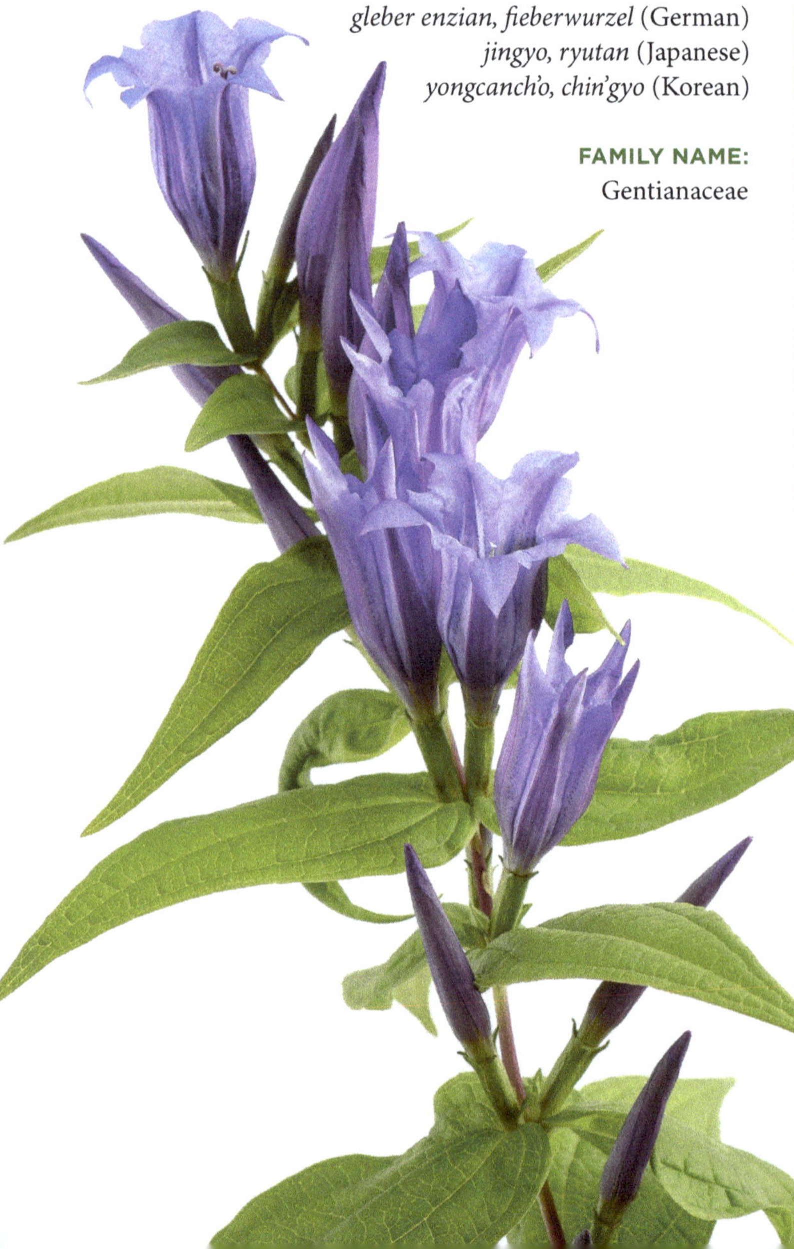

DESCRIPTION

PARTS USED: The roots, above-grounds parts, or whole plant of wild *Gentiana* species.

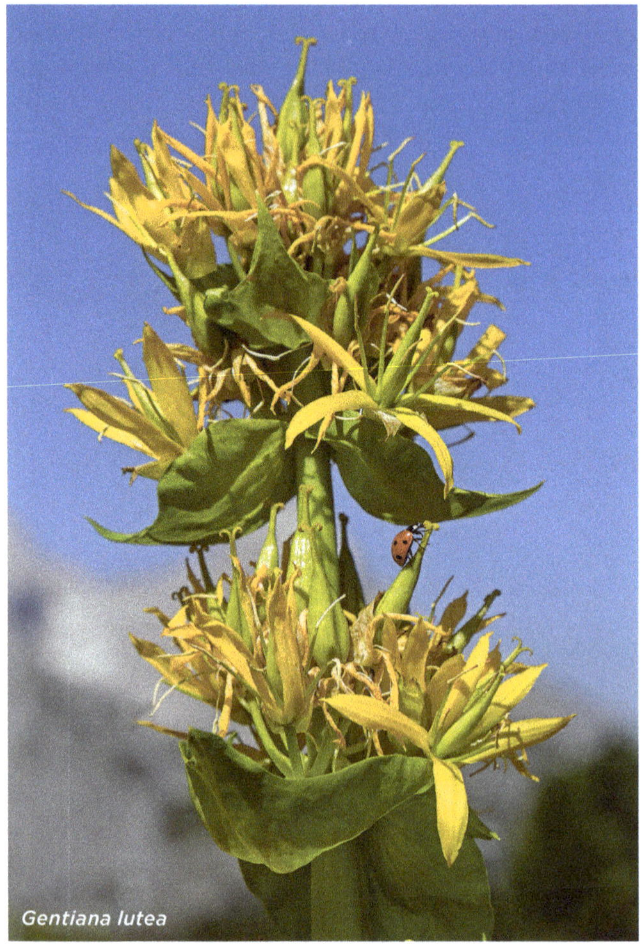

Gentiana lutea

BOTANICAL DESCRIPTION AND HABITAT: Gentian is native to North America, Europe, and Asia Minor. The most widely recognized species, *G. lutea,* is a perennial that grows in Europe and Asia Minor. Gentian thrives in moist mountain meadows, grassy slopes, lake shores, riverbeds, stream banks, swamps, bogs, rocky outcroppings, and slopes. The majority of *Gentiana* species flourish in subalpine to alpine elevations; however, some species tolerate lower elevations. Typically, gentian is an herbaceous perennial, except for a few annual and biennial species.

While the descriptions of gentian vary according to species, the following serves as a generic description of the *Gentiana* genus. Gentian has opposite leaves that are lanceolate-oblong to ovate-oblong with entire margins. The lowest leaves are the largest; the upper leaves are often reduced to bracts. Gentian flowers form clusters; each flower has four to five fused, tubular petals with the same number of sepals as petals. The flowers are bright bluish-purple, though some species are yellow or white. The flowers mature into one superior, single- or double-chambered ovary filled with numerous seeds. *Gentiana lutea* forms a taproot ranging from yellowish-brown to brown; other wild species have smaller brown roots. Refer to more detailed botanical keys for more specific species descriptions.

Note: Wild gentian grows in fragile environments and is subject to overharvesting. It is illegal to harvest many gentian species. Be sure to check the regulatory status of native species before harvesting in the wild, as many species are threatened. Use of the cultivated herb or aerial parts is recommended due to the protected, threatened, or endangered status of numerous gentian species.

THE NAME: *Gentiana* was named after King Gentius, an Illyrian believed to have discovered the plant's medicinal properties. The epithet *lutea* is Latin for "yellow," referring to the flower's vibrant color. *Acaulis* means "stemless;" *affinis* is Latin for "neighboring or adjacent." *Crinita*, of Latin origin, means "with long hair." The epithet *douglasiana* is named after botanist David Douglas. *Macrophylla* derives from two Greek words: *macros* ("large") and *phylla* ("a leaf"). *Pannonicus* originates from the Latin *pannus* ("a cloth or garment"). Three epithets also derived from Latin are: *platypetala* ("broad-petalled"), *punctata* ("a point, dot, or spot"), and *purpurea* ("purple"). *Quinquefolia* derives from two Latin words: *quinque* ("five") and *folia* ("leaves"). *Sceptrum* refers to the scepter-like appearance of the budding flowers; hence, the name "king gentian." *Triflora* is comprised of two Latin words: *tri* ("three") and *flora* ("flower").

The medicinal species classified as long dan cao in Traditional Chinese Medicine include *G. scabra, C. manshurica,* and *G. rigescens.* Additional common names are ryutan (Japanese) and yongcanch'o (Korean). Long dan cao means "dragon gallbladder herb." The species listed as qin jiao utilized in Traditional Chinese Medicine are *G. macrophylla, G. straminea, G. crassicaulis,* and *G. tibetica.* Common names include qin jiao and chin chiu (Chinese), jingyo (Japanese), and chin'gyo (Korean).

The following common names correspond with these Latin binomials: yellow gentian *(G. lutea),* stemless gentian *(G. acaulis),* marsh gentian *(G. affinis),* Rocky Mountain gentian *(G. calycosa),* fringed gentian (*G. crinita*), swamp gentian *(G. douglasiana),* large-leaf gentian, chin chiu *(G. macrophylla),* central European gentian *(G. pannonicus),* broad-petalled gentian *(G. platypetala),* spotted gentian *(G. punctata),* purple gentian *(G. purpurea),* stiff gentian or gallweed *(G. quinquefolia),* Japanese gentian *(G. scabra),* king gentian *(G. sceptrum),* and clustered gentian *(G. triflora).*

HISTORICAL USES: Gentian was first mentioned in the *Divine Husbandman's Classic of Materia Medica* (50 BCE).[1] Ancient Arab and Greek physicians used the herb for stomach and liver complaints, as well as intestinal worms and infectious illness. Gentian is mentioned in the Egyptian papyrus dated 1200 BCE. Pliny, a famous Roman physician, recommended gentian for various digestive afflictions, skin irritations, and infections.[2] Numerous herbalists including Gerard (1597), Rafinesque (1825), and Griffith (1847) described gentian's medicinal virtues.[1]

Gentian was a renowned bitter tonic throughout Europe, where it was cultivated in monastic gardens. It was used to treat fevers, indigestion, and poor appetite, as well as liver and gallbladder disorders. It was considered an antidote to some poisons and a wound antimicrobial. By the 1800s, it was used to stimulate the appetite, improve digestion, enhance circulation, and treat indigestion, diarrhea, jaundice, gout, menstrual problems, hysteria, and chronic disease.[2]

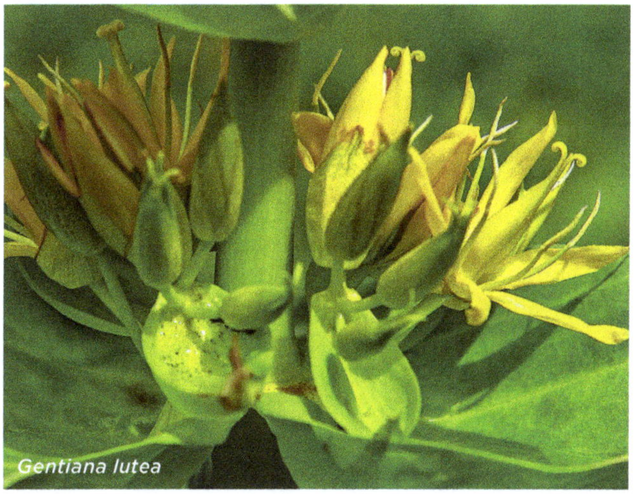
Gentiana lutea

Gentian-based aperitifs were consumed before meals to stimulate the appetite and aid digestion. Many Europeans prepared gentian in bitter tonics and aperitifs. Germans consumed gentian wine before meals as early as the 1700s. Gentian brandy is prepared from distillates of the fresh roots fermented in water.[3] Gentian was included in an Austrian brandy called Enzian schnapps, as well as vermouth, Stockton bitters, and Angostura bitters.

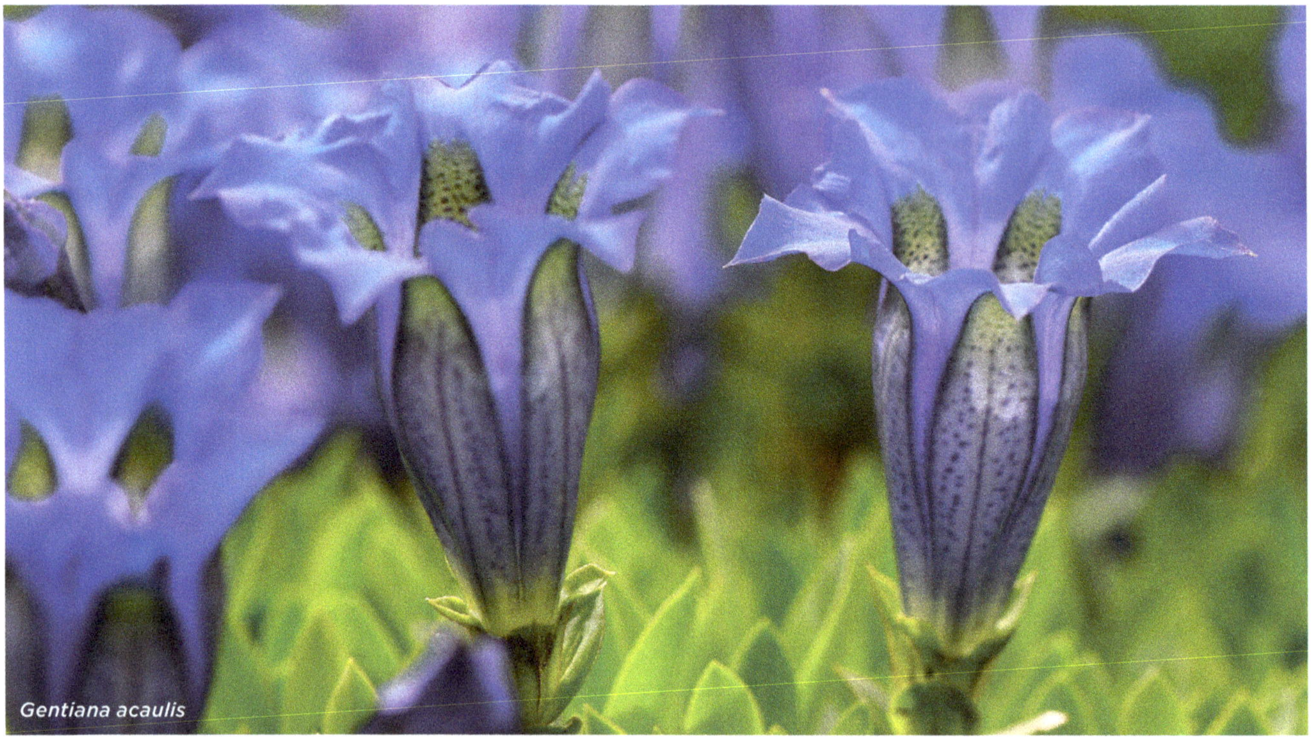

Gentiana acaulis

Angostura bitters were formulated in 1824 by German physician Johann Gottlieb Benjamin Siegert, who successfully treated patients' digestive disorders. This complex blend of bitter and carminative herbs was named after the Venezuelan town of Angostura where Siegert practiced. Angostura bitters has become a famous tonic and flavoring agent sold worldwide.[2] Gentian is used to flavor alcoholic and non-alcoholic bitters. It is widely used in Europe, and is England's most popular digestive stimulant.[4]

In *A Modern Herbal,* author Maude Grieve recommends steeping two ounces of gentian root, one ounce of orange peel, and one-half ounce of bruised cardamom seeds in one quart of brandy. She suggests using this aromatic bitter tonic formula to restore the appetite and promote digestion.[5]

Gentiana scabra (long dan cao) was used in Traditional Chinese Medicine to treat liver and gallbladder-related problems, such as jaundice, pain or swelling in the genital area, foul-smelling vaginal discharge, itching, headache, fever, flank pain, and other symptoms. *G. macrophylla* (qin jiao) was included in formulas to treat muscle pain and cramping, fevers, jaundice, and dry constipation. The aforementioned herbs are currently indicated for the same purposes in Traditional Chinese Medicine.

Navajos considered gentian an antidote for witchcraft. They administered the herb as a snuff to treat headaches and as a stimulant for fainting.[6] Native Americans consumed gentian for snakebites and pain, and as a digestive aid. They also applied a fomentation of blue gentian root to relieve backaches.[7]

Gentian was included in the *U.S. Pharmacopoeia* from 1820 to 1950. Eclectic physicians administered the herb as a tonic to treat chronic debility resulting from poor digestion, prolonged fevers, and infections. They recommended gentian for exhaustive fevers and anemia resulting from malaria; it was administered with a tincture of iron for anemia.[8] Gentian was employed for sinus, digestive, and urinary tract infections. It was also prized as a remedy for liver and gallbladder diseases.[6] The patent medicine, Tobacco Antidote, contained gentian and licorice, and was sold in the U.S. in 1865 to reduce tobacco cravings.[9]

CONSTITUENTS: Gentian contains bitter glycosides (secoiridoids: amarogentin, gentiopicrin = gentiopicroside, swertiamarin = swerocide, gentiin, and gentiamarin), two alkaloids (gentianine and gentialutine), xanthones (gentisein, gentisin, isogentisin, 1,3,7-trimethoxyxanthone, 1-hydroxy-3,7-dimethoxyxanthone, and 2,3',4-6 tetrahydroxybenzophenone), triterpenes (lupeol and β-amyrin), sugars (two bitter sugars: gentiobiose and gentianose), phenolic acids (gentisic, caffeic, protocatechuic, nicotinic, oxycinnamic, synapic, and syringic), and traces of volatile oil. The bitterness is not affected by drying; however, amarogentin and gentiopicroside levels are highest in the spring. *G. acaulis* also contains a xanthose (gentiacauloside) and gentisin.[3,4,10,11]

NUTRITIONAL PROPERTIES: Gentian cannot be consumed in sufficient quantities as a nutritive because it can upset the stomach. However, the root contains low to moderate amounts of aluminum, calcium, chromium, cobalt, fiber, fat, iron, magnesium, manganese, niacin, phosphorus, potassium, protein, riboflavin, selenium, thiamine, tin, vitamins A and C, and zinc, as well as trace amounts of silicon and sodium.[12]

MEDICINAL PROPERTIES: Bitter tonic, cholagogue, choleretic, hepatoprotectant, laxative, anti-inflammatory, antibacterial, antifungal, antiviral, and immune modulator.

TEMPERATURE AND FLAVOR: Cool and bitter.

MEDICINAL USES

Gentian is among the most potent and effective bitter tonics. It is classified as a 'pure' bitter because the bitter taste persists in a dilution of 1:20,000, and secondary constituents such as tannins or aromatics are not present; therefore, the actions of the bitter glycosides are predominant. Bitters stimulate receptors in the taste buds at the back of the tongue. Tasting bitters prior to meals triggers a nerve reflex in the taste buds that stimulates the vagus nerve, initiating a cascade of digestive secretions.[13] Digestive bitter tonics work most effectively when consumed 20 – 30 minutes before meals. They are best used long-term, because they train the vagus nerve to initiate gastrointestinal secretions; even low doses (5 – 10 drops) work effectively.

Gentian contains two extremely bitter secoiridoid glycosides: amarogentin and gentiopicrin that stimulate salivary and digestive secretions. Consumed before meals, gentian increases the stomach's hydrochloric acid and pepsin secretions, raising gastrin levels.[14] This process initiates the release of gastroenterones (gastric hormones) such as cholecystokinin and pancreatic polypeptide. These hormones influence the gallbladder and pancreas, facilitating the release of bile and pancreatic enzymes, respectively. Bile salts emulsify fats and pancreatic enzymes stimulate the breakdown of fat, protein, and starch in the duodenum.[15] Thus, gentian is an appetite stimulant used for weak, painful, or sluggish digestion. It is extremely beneficial for treating anorexia, nonulcer dyspepsia, gas, and bloating, and for convalescing individuals. It is an effective remedy for upper and lower digestive deficiency, as it strengthens secretions throughout the digestive tract. Because gentian is classified as a cold herb, it is best used in low doses (5 – 15 drops), and should be combined with warming, aromatic, carminative herbs, especially in individuals who are cold-bodied or have insufficient digestive secretions. Low doses stimulate the digestive fire; excessively high doses can act as a strong laxative or cause diarrhea.

Gentian has pronounced effects on the liver and gallbladder. It increases bile production in the liver (choleretic) and bile secretion from the gallbladder (cholagogue). The choleretic actions of Gentian can be helpful for individuals who have had their gallbladder removed. It reduces nausea associated with poor fat digestion. This herb aids in preventing the formation of gallstones, and passing gallstones — except in cases with a blocked bile duct. Consuming gentian before breakfast encourages the rehydration of bile that dehydrates in the gallbladder overnight, increasing bile flow in the morning, and decreasing the potential for gallstones to form in non-breakfast eaters. Gentian also enhances the digestion of fatty foods because bile salts emulsify fats. It is useful for treating gallbladder disorders such as cholestasis, cholethiasis, cholecystitis, and cholangitis. Gentian tea or capsules are beneficial for individuals with jaundice, hepatitis, or cirrhosis of the liver.

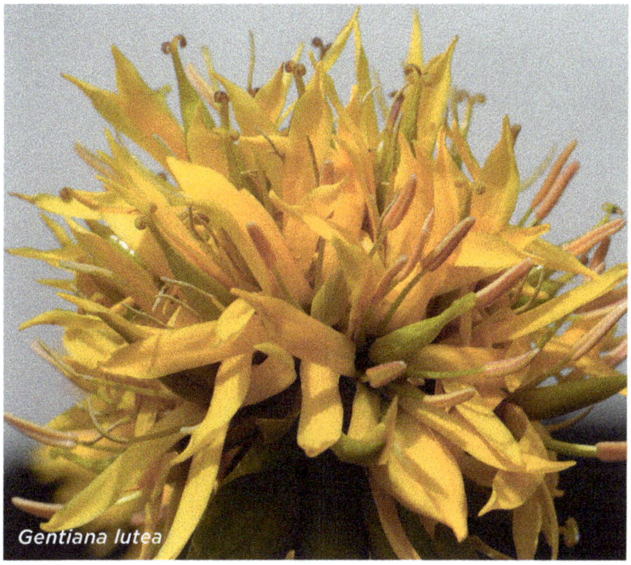
Gentiana lutea

The cholagogue properties act as a natural laxative, reducing constipation. Gentian aids in detoxification, because waste products excreted by the liver are released in bile from the gallbladder. As such, gentian can be beneficial for treating hot, inflamed skin conditions, such as acne, eczema, dermatitis, psoriasis, boils, and abscesses. The alkaloid gentianine exerts anti-inflammatory effects.

In Traditional Chinese Medicine, several species of gentian classified as long dan cao are used to drain damp-heat and cool the liver and gallbladder. Damp-heat in these organs manifests as gallstones, migraines, red eyes, jaundice,

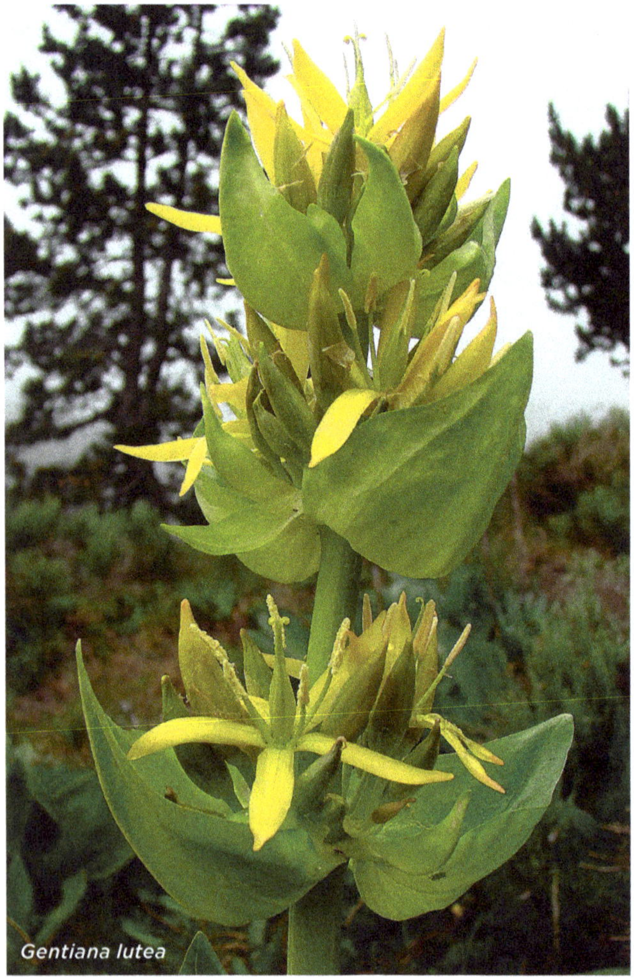

Gentiana lutea

hepatitis, and other conditions. Damp-heat of the liver and gallbladder is common in individuals with diets high in refined flour or sugar, fat, red meat, caffeine, and other processed foods. Gentian is also useful for individuals with reddish complexions who are easily agitated or angered, and feel worse due to heat, as they often have liver stagnation and/or liver heat rising patterns. In addition, it can be used to reduce migraine headaches resulting from liver heat rising.

Laboratory studies have confirmed that extracts of gentian (long dan cao) have antimicrobial and immune stimulating effects.[2] The constituent gentiopicrin exerts mild antipyretic and antimalarial effects.[3] Herbalist Terry Willard states that gentiopicrin is highly poisonous to plasmodium.[16]

CONTRAINDICATIONS

Gentian is contraindicated during pregnancy. It should be avoided by individuals with gastric and peptic ulcers, gastroesophageal reflux disease (GERD), or acid indigestion. Consuming excessive doses (higher than recommended) can cause nausea, vomiting, and diarrhea. Gentian is contraindicated in individuals with a blocked bile duct. In hypersensitive persons, it may cause a headache. Some authors recommend avoiding gentian in individuals with high blood pressure, but it is difficult to find the studies or rationales to support this. In Traditional Chinese Medicine, gentian is contraindicated for those with diarrhea due to spleen and stomach deficiency and cold spleen, or individuals without true damp-heat symptoms.[17,18]

Warning: Proper identification of wild-harvested gentian is critical. *Veratrum album* and *V.* spp. (hellebore) have been found as adulterants in commercial sources of *Gentiana lutea. Veratrum* is a highly toxic plant that grows near *G. lutea* in mountain meadows. Accidental poisonings have occurred in laypersons gathering the herb for home use, and from *Veratrum*-contaminated batches. A factor distinguishing the herbs is that *Veratrum* has alternate leaves, and *G. lutea* has opposite leaves; however, the herbs should be properly identified while in flower. When in question, don't harvest them.

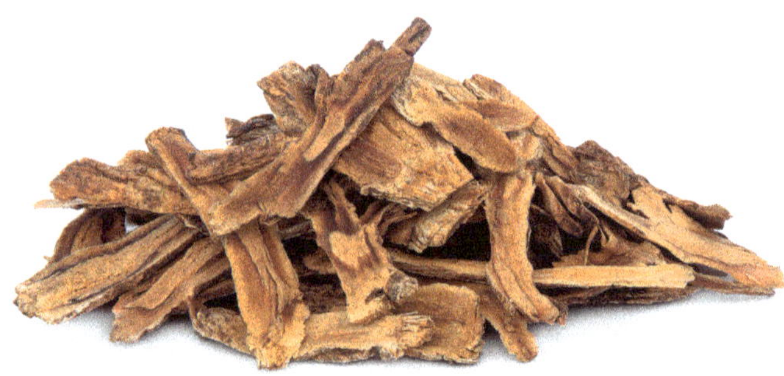

Gentiana macrophylla

PREPARATION AND DOSAGE

TINCTURE: Fresh roots or aerial portions [1:2, 70-95% alcohol]; dry roots [1:5, 50-60% alcohol]; consume 10-30 drops, up to three times daily. Dry roots [1:5, in brandy]; consume 15-30 drops, up to three times daily.

ACETUM EXTRACT: Dry roots [1:5, apple cider vinegar]; consume 1 teaspoon, up to three times daily.

CAPSULES: Consume 2 "00" capsules, up to three times daily.

TEA: Prepare a decoction of the roots; consume 4-8 ounces, 15-30 minutes prior to a meal, up to three times daily.

GINGER

DESCRIPTION

BOTANICAL NAME:
Zingiber officinale

COMMON NAMES:
Ginger
zanjabeel, zanjabil (Arabic)
gojaghbegh, kochapghpegh (Armenian)
dzhindzhifil, isiot (Bulgarian)
geung, saang geung (fresh)(Cantonese)
dumber, ingver (Croatian)
ingefaer (Danish)
gember (Dutch)
inkivääri (Finnish)
gingembre (French)
ingwer (German)
dzinder, piperoriza (Greek)
sangvil (Hebrew)
adi, adrak, adrakh (fresh), *sonth, saunth* (dried) (Hindi)
kai (Hmong)
gyömbér (Hungarian)
engifer (Icelandic)
jahé, lia (Indonesian)
sinséar (Irish), *dinnsear, geinsear* (Gaelic)
zenzero (Italian)
kankyo (dried), *shokyo* (fresh), *jinja, shoga* (Japanese)
kon-gang, kongang, saenggang (Korean)
khing, pidin (Loatian)
jiang, sheng jiang (fresh), *gan jiang* (dried) (Mandarin)
aduwa, sutho (Nepali)
ingefaer (Norwegian)
imbir (Polish)
gengibre (Portuguese)
adraka (fresh), *shunthi* (dried), *shringaveran* (Sanskrit)
ingver (Serbian)
jengibre (Spanish)
tangawizi (Swahili)
ingefära (Swedish)
khing, khing-daen (Thai)
sga smug, sga skya, gakya (Tibetan)
zencefil (Turkish)
imbyr (Ukranian)
can khuong, gung (Vietnamese)
imber, ingber (Yiddish)[1,2]

FAMILY NAME:
Zingiberaceae

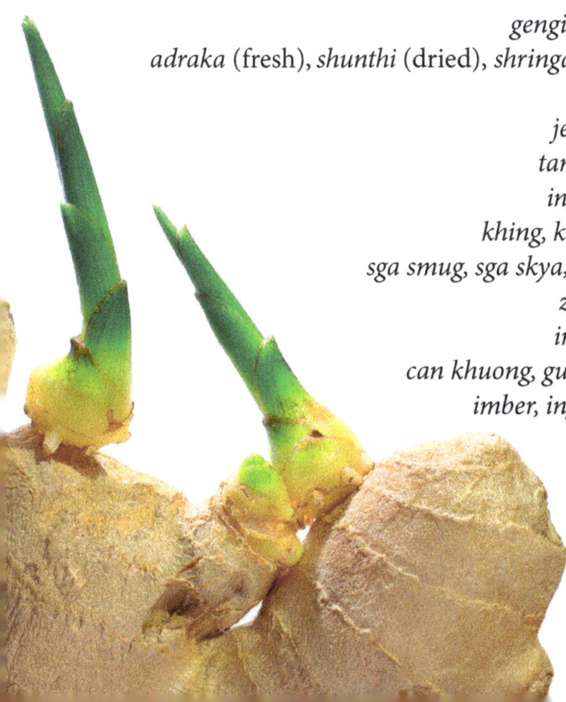

PART USED: The rhizomes.

BOTANICAL DESCRIPTION AND HABITAT: Ginger thrives in tropical climates, and is cultivated in Southeast Asia, Indonesia, India, Jamaica, and Hawaii. It is a rhizomatous, herbaceous perennial. Ginger has thick, branching,

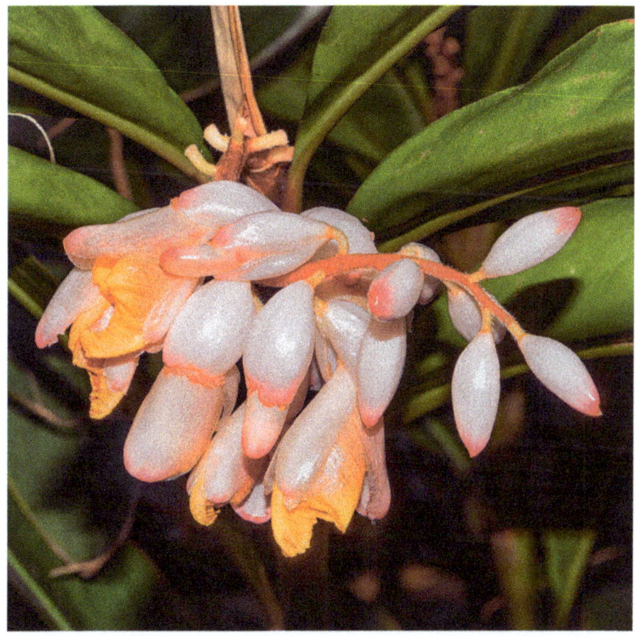

succulent rhizomes with a pale beige, papery skin and strongly scented, fibrous yellow flesh. The shoots (50 – 100 cm tall) and aerial branches of the rhizomes are comprised of long, overlapping sheathes at the bases of the sessile, narrowly lanceolate leaves (15 – 30 cm long by 2 – 2.5 cm wide).[3,4]

Peduncles (up to 25 cm tall) grow straight out of the rhizome.[3] The pale green inflorescence is ovoid (4 – 5 cm long by 1.5 cm wide), and comprised of ovate bracts with mucronate apices in a pine cone-like arrangement.[3] Unique flowers emerge from the bracts. The perianth consists of a minute calyx and a complex corolla comprised of a yellowish tube divided into three long lobes. In the center of the tube, a large, purple-spotted labellum bears two smaller lateral lobes.[3] A large, grooved, purple stamen bears a long, curved appendage from inside the lobes.[3,5] Nestled underneath the stamen along its groove is a cream-colored, funnel-shaped stigma.[5] The inferior ovary consists of three fused carpels.[5]

THE NAME: The genus name *Zingiber* derives from the Sanskrit *singabera* ("shaped like a horn"), alluding to the rhizome shape.[6] The epithet *officinale* denotes a plant included in an official pharmacopoeia.

HISTORICAL USES: Ginger has been utilized as a medicine and spice for thousands of years. Medicinal uses were recorded in ancient Sanskrit, Chinese, Greek, Roman, and Arabic literature.[7] As early as 2000 BCE, the medicinal uses of ginger were recorded in the *Shen Nong Ben Cao Fing.*[8] In Traditional Chinese Medicine, ginger was used to treat an upset stomach, nausea, colic, and diarrhea.[6] Fresh ginger (sheng jiang) was administered to warm the body and expel cold, stimulate digestion, reduce nausea, and alleviate coughing.[2] In addition, it was used to counteract the effects of moderately toxic herbs.[2] Dried ginger (gan jiang)

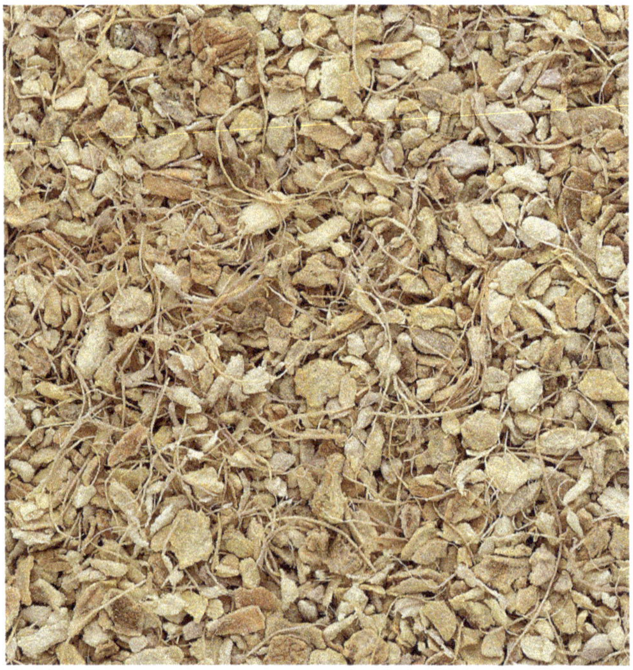

was used to stimulate digestion and allay coughing, stimulate diaphoresis, and disperse exterior cold. It was also administered as a hemostatic to reduce uterine bleeding.[2]

In Ayurvedic medicine, ginger was regarded as "the great or universal medicine."[6] Dry ginger was administered to reduce kapha (cold-dampness), clear ama (digestive toxins), and treat arthritis.[9] Fresh ginger juice was mixed with garlic juice and honey to treat a cough or asthma.[8] Fresh ginger was mixed with honey to treat nausea.[8] A dried ginger poultice was applied to the temples to alleviate a headache.[8] It was used in numerous traditional formulas, including triphala and guggul, as well as curry blends.[9] Fresh ginger was given to increase agni (digestive fire) and treat menstrual cramps.[9]

Ancient Greeks and Romans imported ginger from China and India; they consumed it in order to prevent and eliminate parasites.[6] In Ancient Greece, ginger was an ingredient in specialty breads.[6] It was also applied topically to alleviate muscular and joint pain.[6]

Eclectic physicians administered ginger as a sialagogue, digestive stimulant, antinauseant, carminative, intestinal antispasmodic, and diaphoretic.[10-12] It was prescribed for borborygmus, flatulence, alcoholic gastritis, acute dysentery, diarrhea, cholera morbus, and cholera infantum.[10-12] Ginger tea was given to treat a cold, amenorrhea, dysmenorrhea, and ovarian neuralgia.[10,11] Ginger syrup was a pleasant-tasting adjuvant for stomachic and expectorant compounds.[10] Ginger was applied as a rubefacient and counterirritant.[11]

CONSTITUENTS: Ginger contains an oleoresin comprised of pungent principles (gingerols, shogaols, and zingerone), lipids consisting of triglycerides, phosphatidic acid, lecithins, and free fatty acids (lauric, palmitic, stearic, oleic, and linoleic), protease, protein, starch, vitamin A, niacin, minerals, free amino acids, and resins. Ginger also contains a volatile oil consisting of sesquiterpene hydrocarbons and alcohols (zingiberene, β-bisabolene, arcurcumene, β-sesquiphellandrene, sesquithujene, zingiberol, zingiberenol, *cis*-sesquisabinene hydrate, and *cis*- and *trans*-β-sesquiphellandrol), monoterpene hydrocarbons, aldehydes (phellandrene, camphene, geranial, neral, linalool, and D-borneol), methylheptenone, nonyl aldehyde, gingediacetate, and gingerol.[2,13,14] β-sesquiphellandrene and zingiberene content are highest in fresh ginger; they degrade upon drying or storing.[7] The oleoresins gingerol and shogaol are attributed to the pungency. Shogaol is twice as pungent as gingerol. Gingerol converts to shogaol when heated or dehydrated; this explains why the dried root is more heating and pungent than the fresh root.[13,15] Fresh ginger increases circulation to the periphery; dry ginger increases circulation in the internal organs.[9]

NUTRITIONAL PROPERTIES: Ginger contains high amounts of aluminum, crude fiber, fats, magnesium, manganese, potassium, and silicon. It contains low to average amounts of ash, calcium, chromium, cobalt, dietary fiber, iron, niacin, phosphorus, protein, riboflavin, selenium, sodium, thiamine, and vitamins A and C.[16]

MEDICINAL PROPERTIES: Antibacterial, antiemetic, antifungal, anti-inflammatory, antioxidant, antiparasitic, antiseptic, antispasmodic, antitussive, antiviral, aphrodisiac, aromatic, carminative, cholagogue, choleretic, circulatory stimulant, diaphoretic, expectorant, febrifuge, hepatoprotective, counterirritant, rubefacient, sialagogue, stimulant, stomachic, sudorfic, and yang tonic.

TEMPERATURE AND FLAVOR: Dry ginger root is hot and pungent. Fresh ginger root is warm, pungent, and sweet.

MEDICINAL USES

Ginger is a carminative and stomachic, treating gas, bloating, and abdominal stagnation, cramping, and pain.[10,11,13,17] It stimulates salivary and gastric secretions, increasing the appetite in individuals with weak digestion or anorexia.[2,6,7,10-12,18] Fresh ginger inhibits the development of gastric ulcers.[8,15] Ginger extract and isolated components 6-shogaol and gingerol stimulate intestinal motility.[6,7,14] The pungent principles have an anticathartic action, inhibiting serotonin-induced diarrhea.[6,7] Ginger aids in treating nonulcer dyspepsia, diarrhea, sluggish bowels, digestive cramping, and irritable bowel syndrome.[10,11,15,18] It also treats acute bacterial dysentery and food poisoning.[2,6,10,13]

Ginger is an antinauseant and antiemetic that alleviates nausea, postoperative nausea, morning sickness, seasickness, and motion sickness.[6,7,13-15,18] It also counteracts the gastrointestinal side effects of chemotherapy.[6,7,14] In clinical studies, ginger was as effective as antinauseant and antiemetic drugs.[7] A daily dose of 1 to 2 grams of dried ginger, or 10 grams of fresh ginger is recommended to reduce nausea and vomiting.[15] Ginger works most effectively for seasickness and motion sickness when consumed four hours prior.[7]

Ginger improves circulation to the digestive organs, and counteracts the cooling, constricting effects of cholagogues, digestive bitter tonics, cathartic laxatives, and purgatives.[10,12] In Traditional Chinese Medicine, ginger is administered to warm and tone the stomach and spleen, enhancing digestion and assimilation, and dispelling cold and wind.[2] In Ayurvedic medicine, fresh ginger increases agni (digestive fire); dry ginger clears ama (digestive toxins) and kapha imbalance.[9]

Fresh ginger contains zingibain, a powerful proteolytic, protein-digesting enzyme.[6,15] It contains up to 80 times the amount of proteolytic enzymes by weight than papaya (papain). Consuming ginger with meals facilitates digestion. These enzymes enhance the effectiveness of antibiotics by 50%, and aid in eliminating parasites.[15] The enzymes are attributed to the anti-inflammatory, antibacterial, and anthelmintic effects.

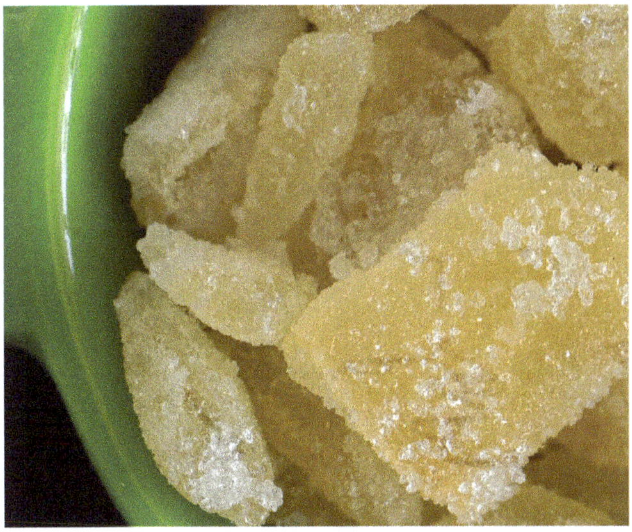

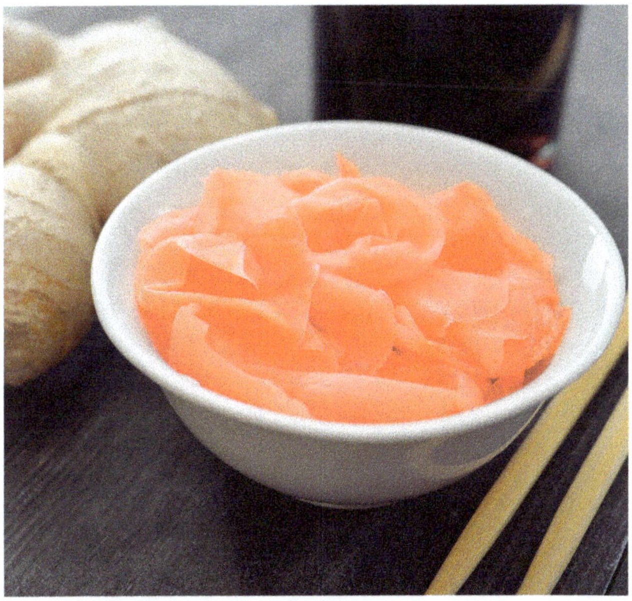

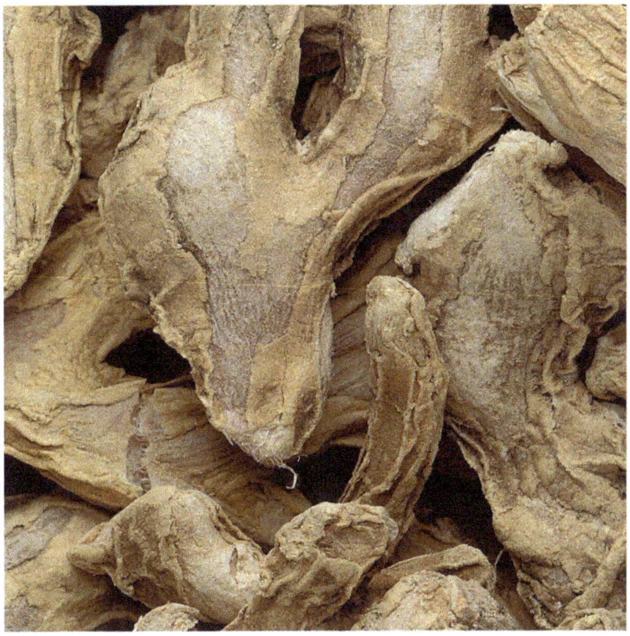

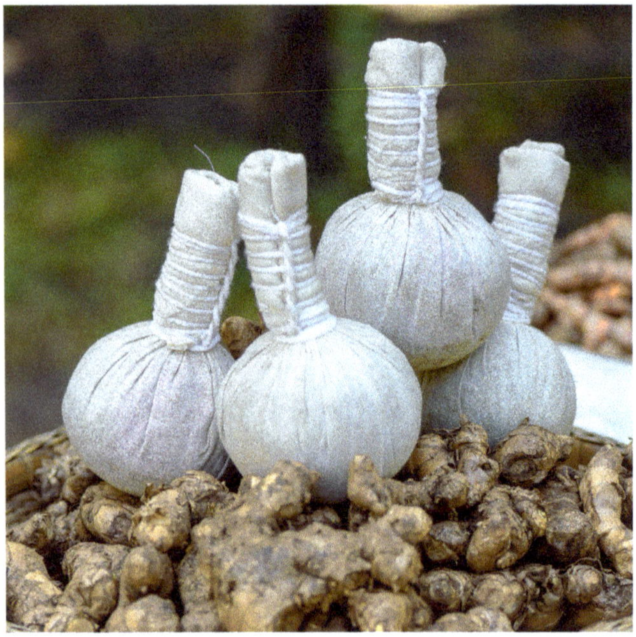

Ginger is a choleretic and cholagogue that increases bile production and secretion, and enhances fat digestion.[6,15,18] It lowers cholesterol absorption and encourages hepatic conversion of cholesterol into bile acids.[7,15] Ginger aids in lowering serum and hepatic cholesterol levels.[7] The active components are 6-gingerol and 10-gingerol.[7] Ginger is also an antihepatotoxic agent, reducing liver toxicity.[7,15] The gingerols and shogaols are attributed to the antihepatotoxic activities.[7]

Fresh ginger is an adjunct for treating heart problems, high blood pressure, and atherosclerosis.[6,14,15,17] It is a cardiotonic that increases contractility of the heart muscle (a positive inotropic agent).[7,15,18] These actions result from increased calcium uptake in the heart muscle, and are attributed to the gingerol.[7,15] Fresh ginger inhibits the conversion of arachidonic acid to thromboxane.[7,14,15] Ginger is an anticoagulant.[7,14,15,18] High doses of ginger reduce platelet aggregation, decreasing blood viscosity and clotting.[6,14,15,17] Ginger has antioxidant effects that protect blood vessels and prevent arterial plaque.[6,7] It decreases platelet lipid peroxide formation.[7,15] The blood thinning and peripheral vasodilating effects help to reduce high blood pressure; however, ginger can be too heating for hot-bodied individuals with hypertension.

Ginger is a potent anti-inflammatory that inhibits the biosynthesis of prostaglandins (PGE2) and leukotrienes (LTB4) by thwarting cyclo-oxygenase and lipo-oxygenase pathways.[7,14,15,18] Due to these properties, fresh ginger tea reduces menstrual and digestive cramping.[9-12,15,17,18] It also aids in treating allergic asthma and reducing respiratory spasms. Consuming ginger has analgesic and anti-inflammatory actions that aid in treating rheumatoid and osteoarthritis, as well as joint and muscle pain.[7]

The anti-inflammatory and analgesic effects are attributed to the protease, volatile oil, and pungent principles (shogaols).[15,18] The shogaols reduce pain by inhibiting the release of substance P, a neurotransmitter released from nerve endings that send pain signals to the brain. They are also attributed to the anti-inflammatory actions.[15] The recommended daily dose for inflammatory conditions is 3 to 4 grams of dried ginger, or 20 grams of fresh ginger.[15]

Ginger is a circulatory stimulant, vasodilator, and carrier.[9] It improves blood flow to the visceral organs and warms the internal organs. Ginger enhances circulation and can be used to treat individuals with cold hands and feet, Raynaud's phenomenon, and other circulatory problems.[10] A hot ginger hand or foot bath warms the extremities for hours, even in very cold weather. Ginger facilitates blood flow to all tissues, increasing oxygen and nutrient delivery, and hastening waste product removal. The circulatory stimulant actions also aid in treating amenorrhea.[7,10,11] Practitioners of Traditional Chinese Medicine use ginger as a yang tonic.

Ginger is an antiviral and highly effective heating diaphoretic.[6,7,9-12,14,15] It aids in treating a cold or flu, digestive infections, and a fever or headache resulting from an infection.[6,9-12] Sesquiterpenes, a component of the volatile oil, demonstrated antirhinoviral activity *in vitro*.[7,14] Consuming a hot infusion of ginger tea with fresh lemon

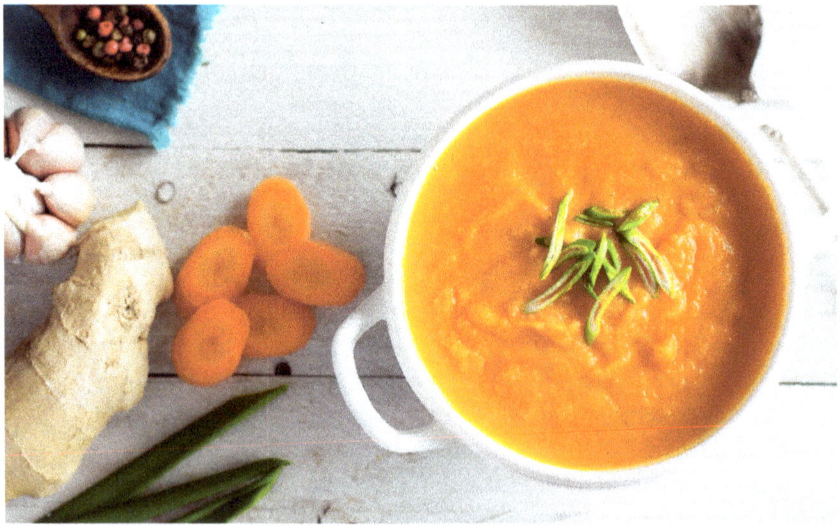

juice and honey aids in treating a cold, flu, fever, or sore throat.[10-12] If an individual is on the verge of getting sick, ginger tea can increase resistance and alleviate discomfort.[11,12] To stimulate diaphoresis, consume the hot infusion frequently, and go to bed wrapped in blankets.[10,11] Ginger has moderate expectorant and antitussive properties that are useful for treating respiratory conditions with clear or white mucus, such as bronchitis or a dry cough.[2,7,18]

Ginger has antibacterial and antifungal effects.[7,14,18] The extract mildly inhibited the growth of gram-positive and gram-negative bacteria, including: *Escherichia coli, Proteus vulgaris, Salmonella typhimurium, Staphylococcus aureus,* and *Streptococcus viridans.*[7] Shogaol and zingerone are attributed to the inhibition of *Salmonella typhi, Vibrio cholera, Trichophyton violaceum,* and *Trichomonas vaginalis.*[15] The antifungal effects are attributed to the pungent principles.[7]

Applying ginger topically has counterirritant and anti-inflammatory actions that aid in treating osteoarthritis, rheumatoid arthritis, muscle or joint pain, tendonitis, bunions, bruising, swelling, muscle cramping, or toothaches.[9-11] A fresh ginger poultice has drawing properties that bring zits, boils, abscesses, and splinters to a head.

CONTRAINDICATIONS

During pregnancy, avoid consuming more than two grams of dry ginger per day, and avoid high or frequent doses of any form of ginger.[9] Some sources contraindicate the use of dry ginger during pregnancy.[14] Low to moderate doses of fresh ginger are not problematic during pregnancy.[14] Ginger should be used with caution by individuals who have yin deficiency with heat signs (hot flashes or night sweats).[2] Individuals with peptic ulcers, acid reflux, or heartburn should avoid consuming ginger, or discontinue use if it aggravates the stomach.[9] Individuals taking anticoagulants (including warfarin) or over-the-counter platelet aggregation inhibitors (i.e., aspirin) should consult a health care practitioner before consuming ginger regularly.[18] Less than 3 to 4 grams daily is recommended for such patients; however, potential interactions are speculative, and no problems have been reported in human clinical trials and documented cases.[7,14] Individuals with a blocked bile duct should avoid consuming ginger.[7,9,14,18] In sensitive individuals, topical applications can cause contact dermatitis.[7]

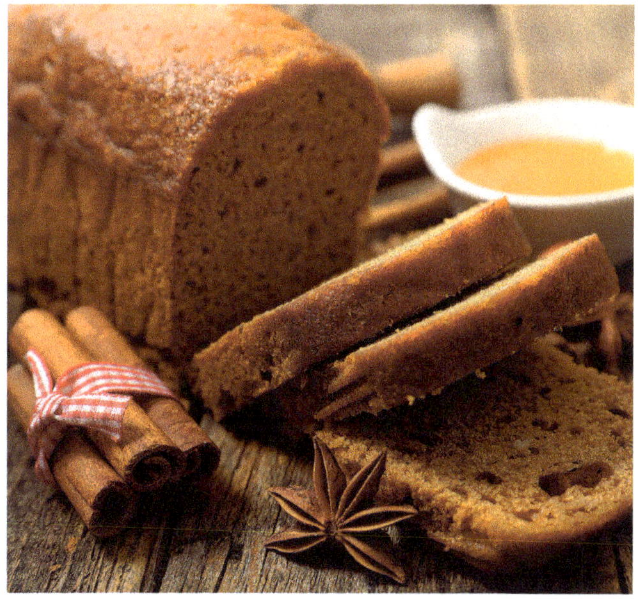

PREPARATION AND DOSAGE

TINCTURE: Fresh rhizomes [1:2, 70-95% alcohol]; consume 10-60 drops, up to three times daily. Dry rhizomes [1:5, 60% alcohol]; consume 5-30 drops, up to three times daily.

GLYCERITE: Fresh rhizomes [1:3, 50% glycerin, 50% alcohol]; consume 10-60 drops, up to three times daily.

SUCCUS: Consume 1-2 ounces of fresh rhizome juice.

CAPSULES: Consume 2-3 freeze-dried or "00" capsules, two to four times daily.

TEA: Prepare a hot or cold infusion or a decoction; consume 8-12 ounces, three to four times daily.

HONEY AND SYRUP: Consume 1-2 ounces of fresh juice mixed with a small amount of honey.

TOPICAL USE: Apply a fresh or dry rhizome poultice or fomentation to the affected area.

CULINARY USE: Ginger continues to be an important culinary spice used in dishes throughout China, Indonesia, Thailand, Japan, India, North Africa, and the Caribbean. Add the fresh root to soups, vegetable, poultry, and meat dishes, salad dressings, or curries.

GINKGO

DESCRIPTION

BOTANICAL NAME:
Ginkgo biloba

COMMON NAMES:
Ginkgo, maidenhair tree, Buddha's fingernails, fossil tree
baak gwat yip, gan hang yip (Cantonese)
jinan dvoulalocny (Czech)
templetree (Danish)
templeboom (Dutch)
neidonhiuspuu, temppelipuu (Finnish)
noyer du japon (French)
ginkgobaum (German)
balkuwari (Hindi)
musteristré (Icelandic)
ginco (Italian)
ginkyō (Japanese)
hangjamok, unhaeng (Korean)
bai guo ye, yin xing ye (leaf), *yin guo* (seed) (Mandarin)
noguiera-do-japão (Portuguese)
arbol de las pagodas, arbol sagrado (Spanish)
tempelträd (Swedish)
cây lá quat (Vietnamese)

FAMILY NAME:
Ginkgoaceae

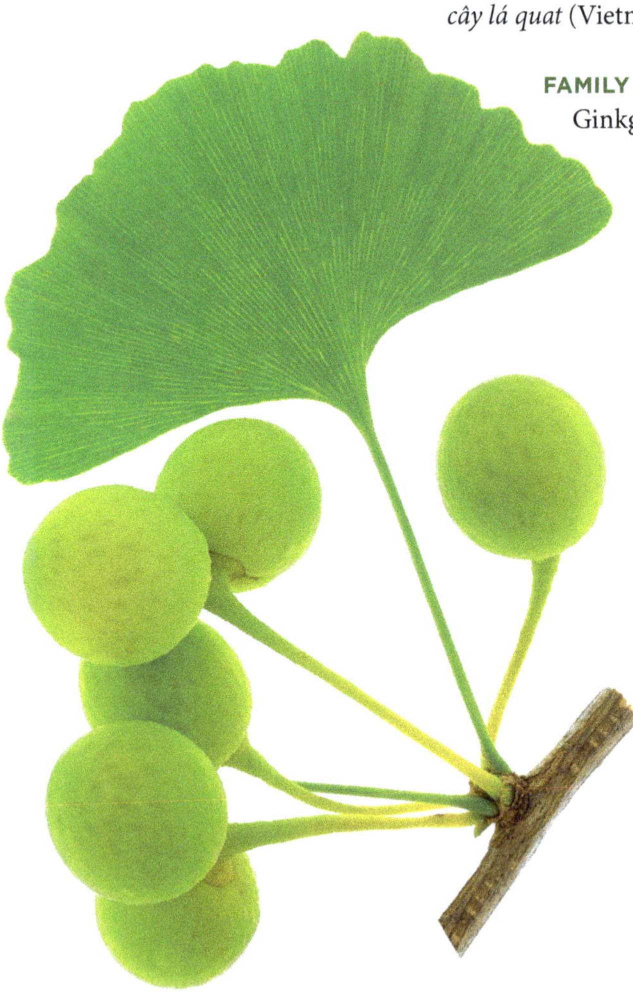

PARTS USED: Green leaves (summer) and yellow leaves (fall). Green leaves are used to make standardized extracts.

BOTANICAL DESCRIPTION AND HABITAT: Ginkgo is a botanically unique, dioecious, broadleaf tree (30 – 40 m tall).[1,2] Its fossil records date back at least 225 million years.[3] It is unknown whether any specimens still grow

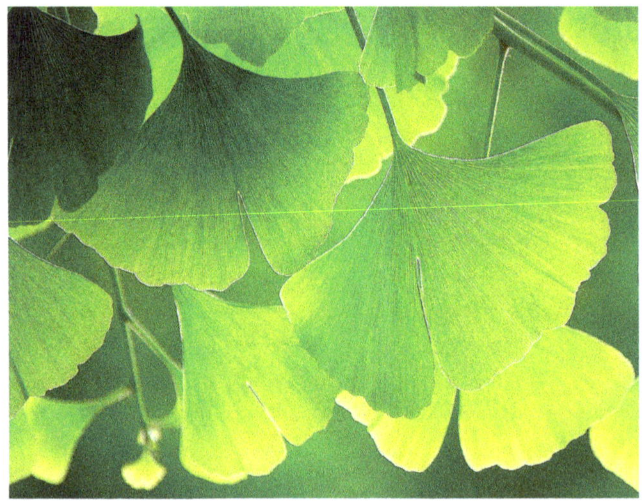

in the wild; it is believed to have been cultivated more than 3,000 years.[2] Ginkgo is the only living species in the botanical division Ginkgophyta; no other members of the division are known to have existed after the Pliocene Epoch.[4] The seeds are not encased by an ovary wall; thus, ginkgo is a member of the gymnosperms and more closely related to conifers than other broadleaf trees. Like other gymnosperms, it does not produce true flowers. They are extremely long-lived trees — possibly more than 2,500 years old.[5]

The crown is conical when young, and broadens as the tree matures. The light gray trunk bark has a corky texture, and is irregularly furrowed. The distinctive fan-shaped leaves (2 – 10 cm long and 2 – 12 cm wide) are always wider than long.[3] They have dichotomous venation, with veins that appear parallel.[3] The glabrous leaves are pale green, fading to bright yellow in the fall. They have an irregularly jagged margin, and can be shallow or deeply divided into two lobes that can further divide. Many leaves are clustered on short spurs that alternate along the branches.

Male trees feature clusters of catkin-like pollen cones (1 – 2 cm long), producing motile sperm.[6] Female trees produce many clusters of female cones consisting of two naked ovules on a short peduncle; usually only one develops into a seed.[1] The large obovoid seeds (2.5 by 2 cm) have yellowish-orange, fleshy outer coverings that smell rancid when ripe.[3]

THE NAME: Ginkgo derives from the Japanese *ginkyō* ("silver apricot"). The epithet *biloba* ("two-lobed") refers to the leaf shape.

HISTORICAL USES: Ginkgo is one of the oldest existing tree species. It has survived more than 225 million years, and is sometimes called a living fossil.[2] The Taoists believe that ginkgo leaves represent "unity within duality" due to the two lobes on each leaf. Ginkgo was one of only 40 tree species that survived in Hiroshima after the atomic bomb was dropped. Ginkgo is highly resistant to fungi and viruses, and filters air pollution; it is often planted along streets for this purpose.

Ginkgo nut has been administered in China for millennia, and was mentioned in the *Shen Nong Ben Cao Jing* dated 2800 BCE.[7] The leaves were not designated for internal use in Chinese texts until 1505 in the *Ben Cao Pin Hue Jing Yaor* by Liu Wen-Tai. Ginkgo nuts were consumed by members of the Chinese royal court to treat senility.[8] The dried nuts were prescribed to reduce mucus discharge, and treat asthma, acute and chronic bronchitis, tuberculosis, leukorrhea, and frequent urination.[11] The leaves were utilized for lung disorders, including excess mucus, asthma, coughs, and bronchitis.[7,8] Ginkgo nut was also used for kidney and bladder problems.[8]

In Asia, the trees were commonly cultivated for their sweet-tasting nuts, similar to the taste of chestnuts. At least 28 varieties have been selected for propagation entirely on nut characteristics.[7] Nut processors were advised to wear gloves or other hand protection to prevent exposure to anacardic acid (also present in poison oak) in the outer coat of the nut, which is removed before consuming. Prior to consumption, the seeds are boiled and roasted.[11] Diners were warned to limit their intake of the nuts (8-10 per day), as eating too many can induce toxic side effects.[7]

CONSTITUENTS

GINKGO LEAVES: Ginkgo leaves contain flavone glycosides (heterosides), flavonoid aglycones (quercetin, quercetin-3-rutinoside = rutin, quercetin-3-glucoside = isoquercitrin, kaempferol, kaempferol-3-rutinoside, kaempferol-3-O-α, isorharmnetin, and 3-O-methylmyricetin-3-rutinoside), glucosic components (glucose and rhamnose), catechins (catechin, epicatechin, gallocatechin, and epigallocatechin), proanthocyanadins (gallocatechin-4,8'-catechin = procyanidin, gallocatechin-4,8'-gallocatechin = prodelphinidin, delphinidine, and cyanidin), several diterpene lactones (ginkgolides A, B, C,

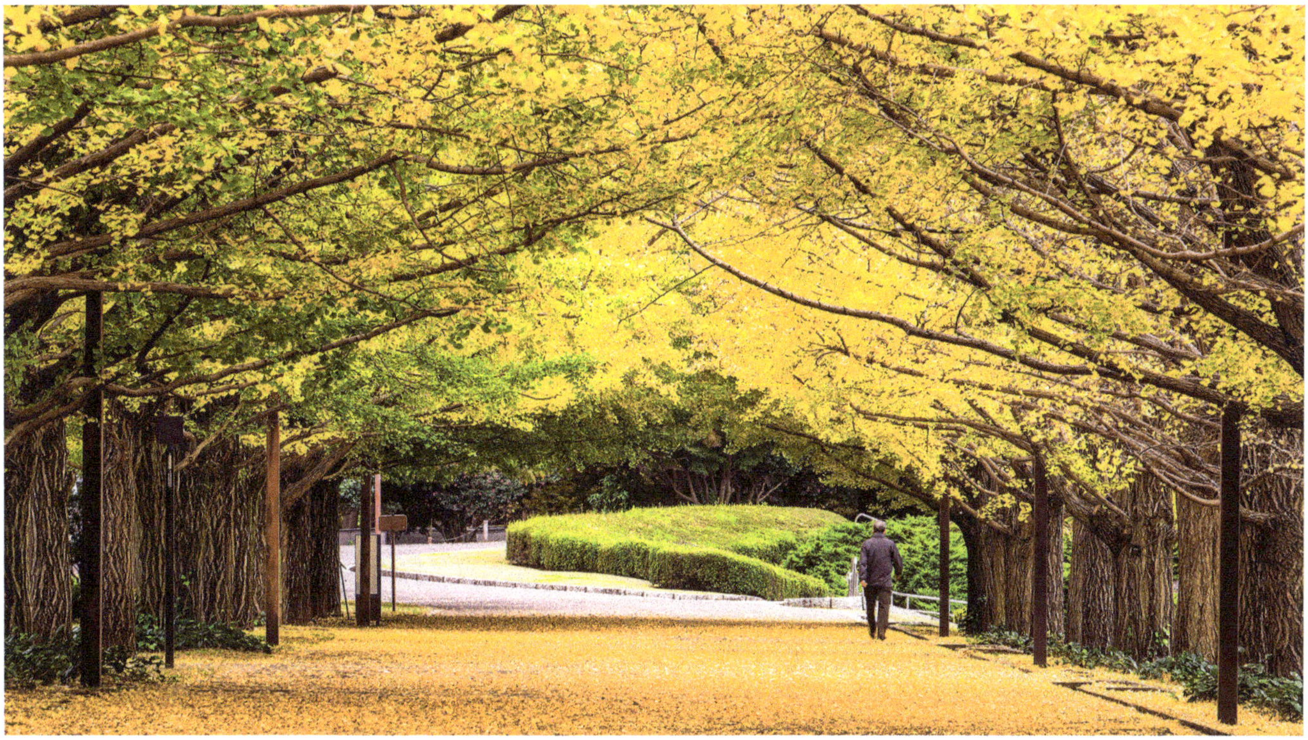

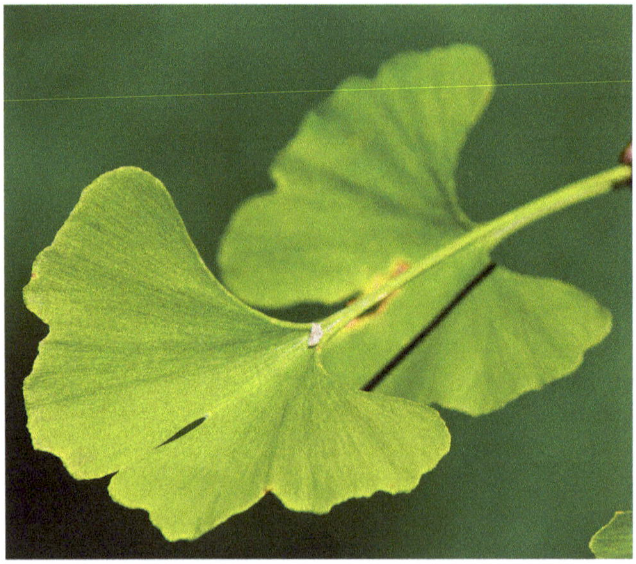

and J), sesquiterpene lactones (bilobalides), lignin, (Z,Z),-4,4'-(1,4-pentadien-1,5-diyl) diphenol, steroids (sitosterol and ipuranol), and organic acids (hydroxykinurenic, kynurenic, protocatechic, and vanillic acid).[9-11]

GINKGO NUTS: Ginkgo nut (seed) contains starch, proteins (globulins, glutelin, and albumins), lipids (linoleic, oleic, palmitic, stearic, linolenic, and α-hydroxypalmitic acids), pentosans, sucrose, glucose, fructose, acids (citric and quinic), and fiber.[11]

NUTRITIONAL PROPERTIES: Ginkgo leaves contain high amounts of calcium, chromium, niacin, phosphorus, and selenium. They contain low to moderate amounts of iron, magnesium, manganese, protein, riboflavin, silicon, sodium, thiamine, vitamin A, and zinc.[12]

MEDICINAL PROPERTIES: Anticoagulant, antidepressant, anti-inflammatory, antioxidant, cardiotonic, circulatory stimulant, neuroprotectant, stimulant, and vasodilator.

TEMPERATURE AND FLAVOR: Warm, bitter, and astringent.

MEDICINAL USES

Most of the research on ginkgo has studied concentrated standardized *Ginkgo biloba* extract (GBE) used in more than 300 clinical and experimental studies.[9] GBE is prepared from the dried, green leaves and is highly concentrated (50:1). It contains 22 – 27% ginkgo flavonol glycosides (quercetin, kaempferol, and isorhamnetin) and 5 – 7% terpene lactones (ginkgolides and bilobalide).[10] Ginkgo is also used clinically as a tincture or tea.

Many uses of ginkgo are attributed to its potent antioxidant effects that enhance free radical scavenging, including hydroxyl, superoxide, and peroxyl radicals.[9,11,15,18] It inhibits lipid peroxidation, improving cell membrane integrity.[9] The free radical scavenging effects are attributed to the flavonoids.[10] Thus, ginkgo is highly beneficial in treating diabetic blindness, diabetic tissue diseases, heart disease, Parkinson's disease, glaucoma, and senile macular degeneration.

Ginkgo is a circulatory stimulant and vasodilator.[11] It improves circulation in the microvasculature, increasing oxygen and nutrient delivery to tissues, and hastening waste product removal. Ginkgo dilates blood vessels by activating the release of the endothelial-derived relaxing factor (EDRF) and prostacyclin in the vascular endothelium.[9] It also strengthens venous tone, and facilitates clearing of toxic metabolites that accumulate in ischemic (oxygen deficient) tissue.[9,18] Long-term use of GBE (at least 8 – 12 weeks) prevents vascular spasms, with positive effects in treating peripheral arterial disease and intermittent claudication (painful cramping of the calf upon exertion).[9,10,18] GBE is most beneficial the longer it is used.[9] It aids in treating peripheral vascular disorders including Raynaud's phenomenon, diabetic peripheral vascular disease, varicose veins, acrocyanosis, post-phlebitis syndrome, cold extremities, and peripheral edema.[10,11] Ginkgo can prevent and treat altitude sickness.[10,18] Combine ginkgo with ginger *(Zingiber)*, gotu kola *(Centella)*, rosemary *(Salvia rosmarinus)*, and/or cinnamon *(Cinnamomum)* to synergize the circulatory effects.

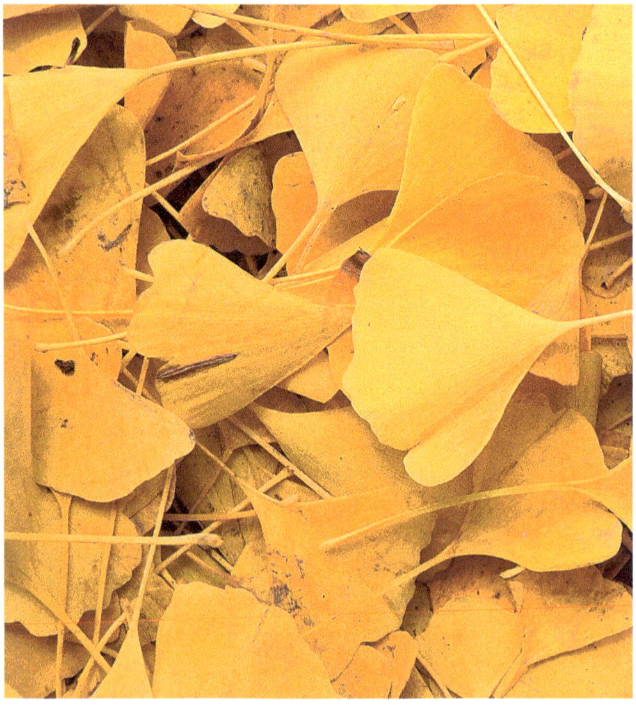

Ginkgo enhances ocular and retinal blood flow. It reduces oxidative stress in the eyes, improving visual acuity, near and far vision, field of vision, and color recognition.[19,20] Improvement in retinal capillary flow benefits patients with diabetic retinopathy.[19] Ginkgo delays the progression of senile macular degeneration and glaucoma (high-tension and normal-tension).[18,19] It improves microcirculation, provides neuroprotection via antioxidant action and its stabilizing effect on mitochondria (possibly allowing the retinal ganglia cells more energy for repair processes), and reduces vasospasms.[19] Ginkgo may be particularly beneficial for individuals with glaucoma progressing despite normal intraocular pressure (IOP) in treated high-tension glaucoma or normal-tension glaucoma. It is often prescribed by glaucoma specialists in these cases, because few other treatments are available.[19] One double-blind study showed that ginkgo improved preexisting visual field damage in normal tension glaucoma patients.[19]

Ginkgo improves coronary blood flow and aortic relaxation, and aids in treating atherosclerosis and high blood pressure.[15] GBE has been shown to prevent LDL oxidation; it also prevents the loss of other antioxidants such as vitamin E and β-carotene.[15] It enhances hepatic metabolism of lipids, having a hypolipidemic and antiatherosclerotic effect.[18] *In vitro,* GBE reduced the cytokine-induced adhesion of monocytes to aortic endothelial tissue, circumventing a key inflammation-driven event that occurs early in the development of atherosclerosis.[16] These actions impede the progress of atherosclerosis and the formation of fatty plaques in vascular tissue.[15,16] For a cardiotonic and antioxidant, combine ginkgo with hawthorn *(Crataegus).*

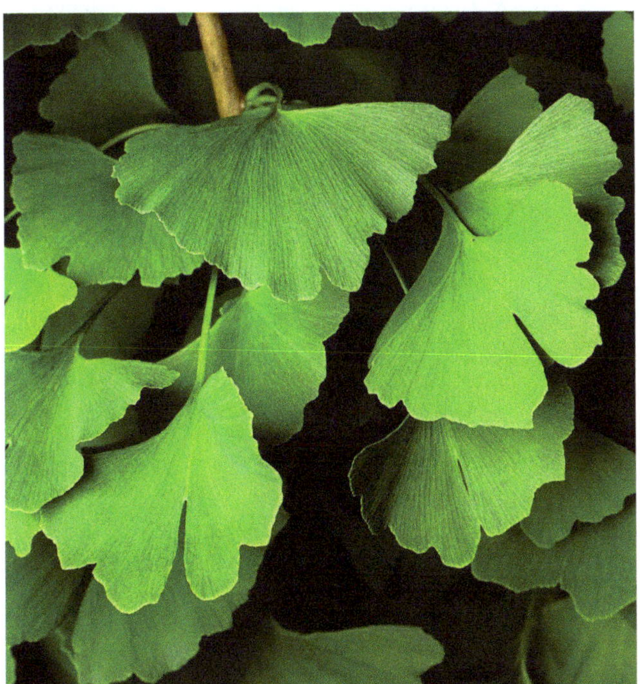

Due to its ability to reduce the platelet aggregation factor (PAF) from binding to platelets, ginkgo reduces blood clotting and thrombus formation, and thins blood.[9,10,18] It hastens recovery from strokes and heart attacks.[18] Animal studies demonstrated that standardized extracts of ginkgo are effective for partially reducing cognitive impairments and hippocampal damage after transient forebrain ischemia.[17]

Involved in numerous inflammatory processes, PAF is also formed by neutrophils, monocytes, and macrophages.[18] Allergic and inflammatory processes including increased neutrophils activation, vascular permeability, bronchoconstriction, and decreased coronary blood flow are also attributed to PAF. GBE and ginkgolides antagonize PAF by binding with PAF binding sites.[9,18] High doses of ginkgolides stabilized mast cell degranulation, and partially countered inflammatory-induced bronchiole constriction.[18] Ginkgolides also hinder eosinophil response to PAF, and reduce IgE-mediated eosinophil cytotoxicity.[18] Ginkgo reduces the wheal response or reagin reaction, decreasing allergic reactions.[9,21] It can be useful for easing inflammatory conditions such as asthma, allergies, and allergic skin reactions.[10]

Ginkgo enhances cerebral blood flow, improving mental clarity, concentration, and working memory.[10,18] It significantly enhances the brain's utilization of oxygen and glucose uptake.[9] It is a neuroprotective that inhibits nitric oxide formation in the brain.[10] GBE is an excellent long-term support for individuals with cerebral anoxia, cerebral insufficiency, poor concentration, global dementia, and Alzheimer's disease.[9-11,14,18] It increases cognitive performance, mental alertness, visual acuity, hearing, and equilibrium, elevates mood, and speeds reaction time.[18] It also enhances membrane polarization by activating sodium-potassium pumps, increasing neural transmission.[9] Ginkgo aids in treating individuals with a short attention span or attention deficit disorder. It enhances short-term memory in individuals with cerebral insufficiency.[10,11] In individuals with dementia, it improves concentration, tinnitus, short-term visual memory, and working memory.[10,11] Combine ginkgo with tulsi basil *(Ocimum sanctum),* gotu kola *(Centella),* red clover *(Trifolium pratense),* and smaller amounts of rosemary *(Salvia rosmarinus)* for the aforementioned conditions.

Ginkgo counters sexual dysfunction symptoms in patients consuming antidepressants (SSRIs, MAOIs, and tricyclics).[9,18] Long-term use counteracts the impotence-inducing side effects of these drugs. As demonstrated by *in vitro* studies, ginkgo extracts may facilitate an erection by improving relaxation of muscles in the penis that allow blood to enter it.[18]

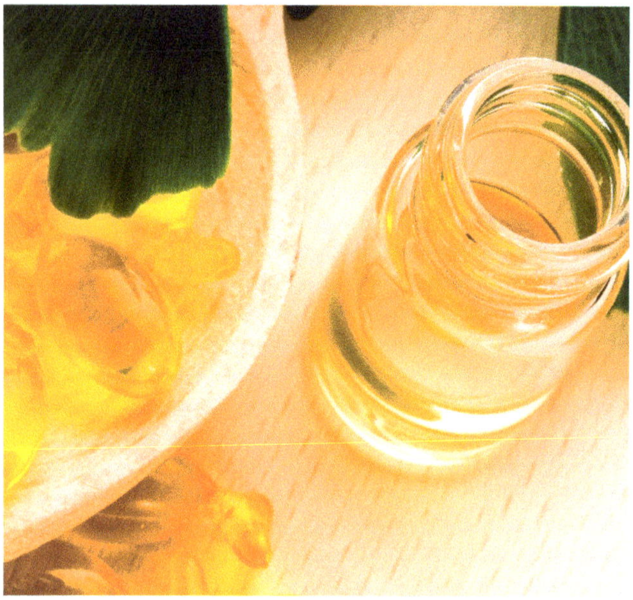

Ginkgo synergizes the effects of antidepressants and has subtle antidepressant actions. It contains flavonoids that increase serotonin release.[10] Prepare an antidepressant compound by combining ginkgo with St. John's wort *(Hypericum)*, tulsi basil *(Ocimum sanctum)*, gotu kola *(Centella)*, lemon balm *(Melissa)*, wild oats *(Avena)*, and smaller amounts of rosemary *(Salvia rosmarinus)* and/or lavender *(Lavandula)*.

Ginkgo also aids in treating migraine headaches. However, it should be avoided by anxiety-prone individuals with heart palpitations or tachycardia. At the onset of a migraine, consume GBE alone, or compounded with equal parts of feverfew *(Tanacetum parthenium)* extract.

CONTRAINDICATIONS

There are no known contraindications in pregnant or lactating women.[10,18] High doses (120 mg) of GBE should be avoided in children younger than 12.[10] Individuals with allergies to ginkgo should avoid its use.[10]

Due to its blood thinning properties, avoid consuming ginkgo at least four weeks prior to, and following surgery or delivery. Ginkgo is contraindicated for individuals with bleeding disorders.[10] Individuals consuming over-the-counter or prescription blood thinners or antiplatelet medication should consult with, and be monitored by a health care practitioner when taking ginkgo.[10,18] However, according to a double-blind, placebo-controlled, crossover study, ginkgo does not interact with warfarin.[10] Another double-blind, placebo-controlled study in which 50 subjects consumed 240 mg of standardized ginkgo with aspirin (500 mg daily dose) found no conclusive evidence of a negative interaction.[10]

Ginkgo can increase sensitivity to epinephrine and norepinephrine. Exercise caution and/or avoid consuming ginkgo with caffeine, as it can be overstimulating. Dizziness and palpitations are side effects of taking ginkgo and GBE.[10] Discontinue use if ginkgo exacerbates anxiety, nervousness, or related disorders. Avoid consumption after noon in individuals with insomnia. Consuming high or repeated doses may cause a headache; discontinue if this occurs.[14]

Similar to poison ivy, the outer coating of ginkgo nuts contains anacardic acid that can cause contact dermatitis. The fresh seeds are toxic and have caused death in children.[10] Ingesting fresh seeds can cause a stomachache, nausea, diarrhea, breathing difficulty, or shock.[10]

PREPARATION AND DOSAGE

TINCTURE: Harvest the green leaves in mid to late summer, and the yellow leaves in fall. Prepare separate tinctures of the green and yellow leaves. Fresh leaves [1:2-1:3, 70-95% alcohol]; dry leaves [1:5, 60% alcohol]; consume 10-60 drops, up to three times daily.

CAPSULES: Consume 2-3 freeze-dried or standardized ginkgo capsules, one to two times daily. Most scientific studies utilize a standardized extract of ginkgo called EGb 761, in this monograph referred to as ginkgo standardized extract (GBE). The dosage of GBE is 120-240 mg, administered in 40-60 mg doses, two to three times daily.[10] Low concentration extracts have minimal scientific validation.[10]

TEA: Prepare a hot infusion; consume 6-12 ounces, one to two times daily.

GINSENG, ASIAN

DESCRIPTION

BOTANICAL NAME:
Panax ginseng

COMMON NAMES:
Asian ginseng, Asiatic ginseng, Chinese ginseng, Korean ginseng, Japanese ginseng, Manchurian ginseng, Oriental ginseng, white kirin ginseng, fine root ginseng, five fingers, human root, red berry, spirit herb, divine herb, essence of man
ginsengrod (Danish)
juuri (Finnish)
panax (French)
ginsengwurzel, koreanischer ginseng (German)
ninjin (Japanese)
insam, sansam (Korean)
jên-shēn, kao-li-sēn, rén shēn, yuan-sēn, yeh-shan-sēng (Mandarin)
jinsão (Portuguese)
lakshmana (Sanskrit)
ginsengrot (Swedish)
sinseng (Turkish)

FAMILY NAME:
Araliaceae

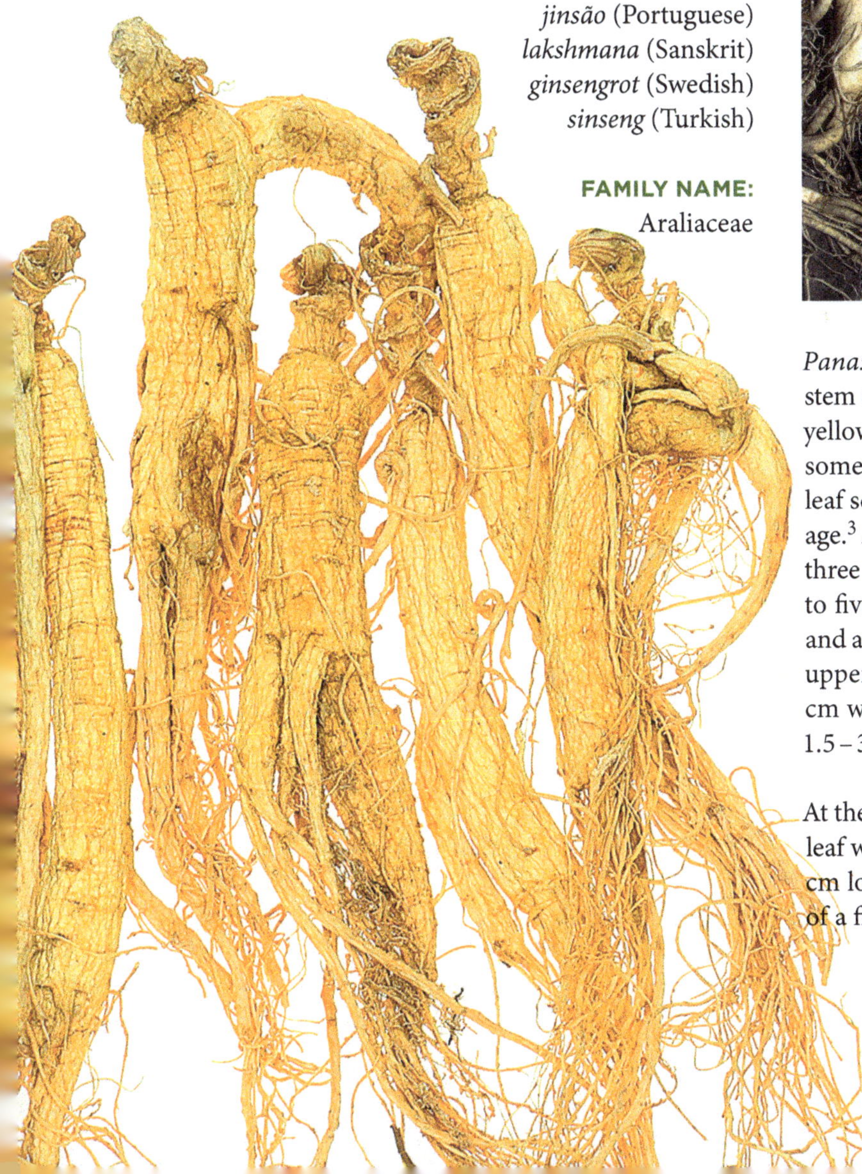

PARTS USED: Roots and rhizomes at least five years old.

BOTANICAL DESCRIPTION AND HABITAT: Ginseng is cultivated in China and Korea. The roots are harvested after 5 – 7 years; however, optimum levels of ginsenosides are obtained by the summer of the fifth year.[1] Cultivated roots are harvested between September and October; wild plants are harvested in late August through September. It is best to use cultivated and woods-grown ginseng, rather than wild ginseng, as it is endangered and currently only persists in a few locations in Russia and China.

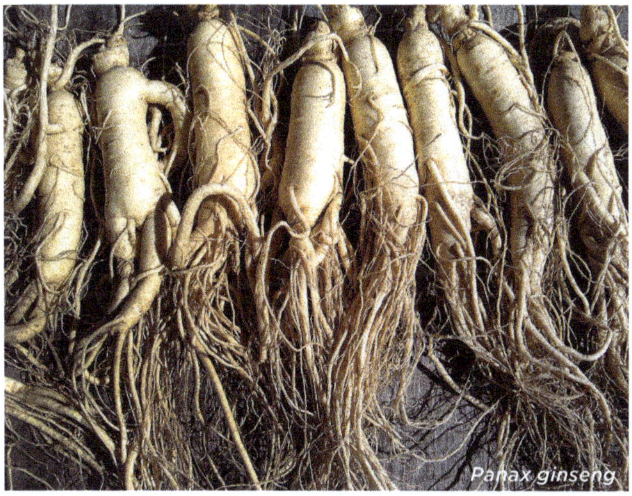

Panax ginseng

Panax ginseng is an herbaceous perennial with a single stem (30 – 60 cm tall).[2] The plant has thick, cylindrical, pale yellow-white tap roots that divide into two to five rootlets, sometimes evoking the shape of the human body.[2,3] The leaf scars on the rhizomatous root crown reveal the plant's age.[3] At the distal end of the main stem is a single whorl of three to six palmately compound leaves, each bearing three to five leaflets.[2,4] The leaflets have finely serrate margins and acuminate apices, with glabrous undersides and bristly upper sides.[2] The central leaflets (8 – 12 cm long by 3 – 5 cm wide) are elliptic; the lateral leaflets (2 – 4 cm long by 1.5 – 3 cm wide) are ovate.[2]

At the end of the main stem and through the middle of the leaf whorl, a single umbel emerges atop a peduncle (15 – 30 cm long).[2] The umbel contains 30 – 50 flowers consisting of a five-toothed calyx, five petals, five stamens, two fused carpels, and two styles.[2,4] The fruit is a small red, globose drupe containing two yellow seeds.[2-4]

THE NAME: *Panax* derives from the Greek words *pan* ("all") and *akos* ("cure"), translated as "cure-all" or "panacea."[5] The name ginseng is a Romanization of the Chinese name jên-shēn, also written rén-shēn, that translates as "man root" or "man essence."[6,7] *Hong shen* specifically refers to steamed red ginseng. The root of cultivated ginseng is called *yuan-sēng;* the wild-harvested roots are *yeh-shan-sēng.*[7] The name human root refers to its resemblance to a human figure.

HISTORICAL USES: Ginseng has been used in Traditional Chinese Medicine for more than 2,000 years.[5] As indicated in the name, often translated as "man root," but also as "man essence," in China, ginseng was highly esteemed. In 1970, Harvard researcher Shiu Ying Hu described an aspect of ginseng's importance in Chinese culture: "According to a conventional Chinese belief, ginseng is the crystallization of the essence of the earth in the form of a man. It represents the vital spirit of earth that dwells in a root. It is the manifestation of the spiritual phase of nature in material form."[7] The importance of the symbolism of the root's human form should not be understated, and roots resembling the human shape were considered most potent and valuable.

Ginseng was believed to promote longevity, imbue wisdom, quiet the spirit, and increase vitality.[5] In China, it wasn't actually applied as a panacea as the name *Panax* suggests, but it was used more judiciously due to its strong action, in order to avoid causing further constitutional imbalances.[7] A qi tonic, ginseng was administered as a recuperative agent following a debilitating illness.[1,5] It has been used to treat fatigue, impotence, dizziness, and cancer.[1] Use in China was based entirely on traditional knowledge until the 1950s, when Chairman Mao Zedong called for the standardization of traditional knowledge, and the canon of knowledge now known as Traditional Chinese Medicine was formed.

Ginseng has been prepared in various ways, including steaming, then drying in the sun or over a low fire (*hung-sēng*, or red ginseng).[7] *Sheng-sai-sēng* (raw sun-dried ginseng) was washed, bleached with sulfur gas, then sun-dried.[7] Ginseng was also bleached with sulfur before it was cooked in boiling water up to seven minutes, then pierced with needles over the surface, soaked in a strong sugar solution, and dried. This sugared ginseng was called *tang-sēng.*

Ginseng was first brought to England in 1740, where it was received enthusiastically and utilized by priests in healing work.[8]

CONSTITUENTS: Ginseng root contains numerous triterpene saponins known as ginsenosides = panaxosides (singsenosides R_0, R_{b-1}, R_{b-2}, R_{b-3}, R_c, R_d, R_e, R_f, R_{f-12}, $R_{20\text{-gluco-}f}$, R_{g-1}, and R_{rg-2}), volatile oil (panacene), sterols (β-sitosterol and β-glucoside), starch, ginseng polysaccharides (panaxans A – U), free sugars (glucose, fructose, sucrose, maltose, and trisaccharides), pectin, vitamins (B_1, B_2, B_{12}, nicotinic acid, pantothenic acid, and biotin), choline, fats, minerals (calcium, iron, manganese, and zinc), polyacetylenes (panaxynol), and a polypeptide.[1]

The volatile oil prepared from the aerial portions of ginseng contains sesquiterpenes (bicyclogermacrene, α- and β-panasinsenes, caryophyllene, α- and β-humulenes, α- and β-neoclovenes, β-farnesene, and α-, β-, and γ-selinenes).[1]

NUTRITIONAL PROPERTIES: Ginseng contains vitamins (niacin, riboflavin, cobalamin, nicotinic acid, pantothenic acid, and biotin), free sugars (glucose, fructose, sucrose, maltose, and trisaccharides), pectin, choline, protein, and fats. It contains small quantities of minerals including calcium, chromium, cobalt, magnesium, manganese, phosphorus, potassium, and selenium.[1,9]

MEDICINAL PROPERTIES: Adaptogen, antiallergenic, anti-inflammatory, antioxidant, aphrodisiac, cardiotonic, hepatoprotective, hypocholesterolemic, hypoglycemic, hypotensive, immune modulator, lung qi tonic, qi tonic, spleen qi tonic, energizer, restorative, stimulant, and vasodilator.

TEMPERATURE AND FLAVOR: White ginseng (uncured) is warm, sweet, and mildly bitter. Red ginseng (cured) is hot, sweet, pungent, and bitter.

MEDICINAL USES

Ginseng has been prized for millennia as a superior tonic that increases qi, energy, stamina, and quality of life. Few herbs have rivaled its popularity and economic importance in world trade. Since 1960, more than 4,000 research articles have been published about ginseng.[13] It is beyond the scope of this book to summarize all of them. The information described below refers to the uses of uncured Asian ginseng *(rén shēn),* not cured red ginseng *(hong shen).*

Ginseng is an adaptogen that regulates the hypothalamic-pituitary-adrenal axis and counters the detrimental effects of stress. It increases physical performance, endurance, and cognitive function.[1,5,12-14] Ginseng is an adrenal tonic that reduces symptoms resulting from adrenal insufficiency (fatigue, compromised immune function, hormone imbalances, low libido, etc.). It increases the efficiency of hypothalamic feedback control during the flight-or-fight response (phase I of general adaptation syndrome — GAS).[14] As stress levels decrease, glucocorticoid levels normalize more rapidly.[14] With prolonged stress (phase II of GAS), ginseng has a glucocorticoid-sparing effect, while adrenal capacity increases.[14] It enhances the body's capacity to adapt to various kinds of stress including: forced exercise, heat and cold stress, food deprivation, radiation exposure, electroshock, and emotional stress.[14] Ginseng increases muscular strength, oxygen utilization, and removal of lactic acid, and has an antifatigue effect.[1,11,14] It has a nootropic effect, increasing mental alertness and well-being.[14] Consumed one to two weeks prior to, and following long flights, it also aids in treating jet lag.

Ginseng aids in treating stomach and spleen qi deficiency, which includes the following symptoms: lethargy, lack of appetite, poor digestion, abdominal distention, chronic diarrhea, and weak, cold limbs.[12] It strengthens heart qi and calms the spirit. Ginseng reduces symptoms of anxiety, restlessness, insomnia, palpitations, and forgetfulness due to qi and blood deficiency.[12]

Ginseng enhances respiratory function and aids in treating chronic respiratory disease.[13] In a single-blind, placebo-controlled study, smokers with chronic bronchitis consumed one 100 mg capsule of ginseng extract for two months. It was concluded that alveolar macrophages' capacity for intracellular killing increased significantly in the ginseng group, but not the control group. Ginseng restored and increased alveolar macrophage activity.[13] In a three month, single-blind, placebo-controlled study, patients with severe chronic respiratory diseases consumed one capsule containing 100 mg of ginseng extract twice daily. Patients in the ginseng group, but not the placebo group, experienced significant improvement in pulmonary function, as well as oxygenation and walking capacity.[13]

Ginseng tonifies lung qi, treating symptoms of lung qi deficiency including shortness of breath, labored breathing, wheezing, asthma, susceptibility to respiratory infections, malor flush, and afternoon sweating.[12] Combine ginseng with wu wei zi *(Schisandra)*, mai men dong *(Ophiopogon japonica)*, shu di huang *(Rehmannia glutinosa)*, and/or tian

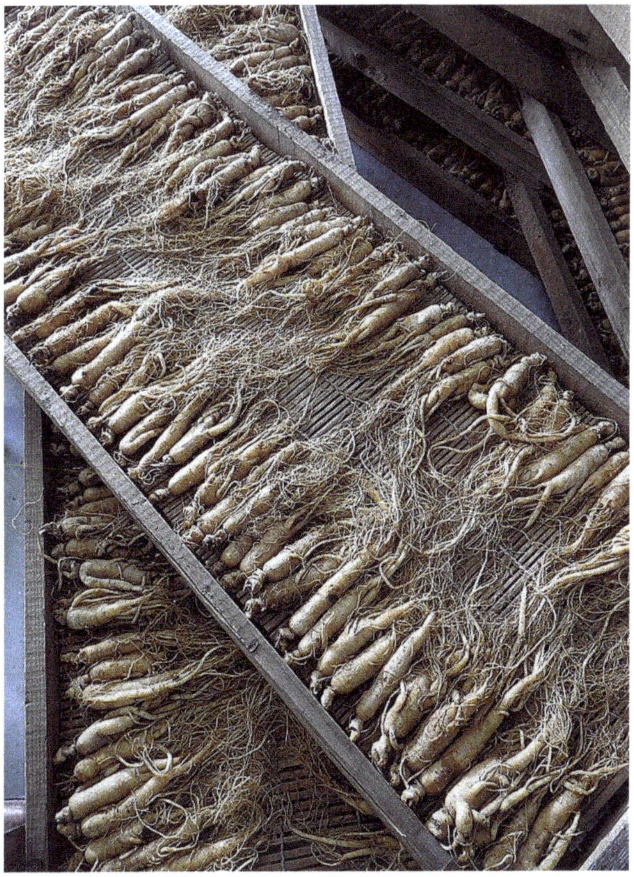

men dong *(Asparagus cochinchinensis)* to treat lung yin and qi deficiency.[12]

Ginseng is an immune modulator that enhances the function of the reticuloendothelial system.[13] It aids in treating immune deficiency due to chronic stress and depletion. Ginseng increases non-specific resistance, including antibody response, T-lymphocyte, natural killer, and lymphokine-activated killer (LAK) cell activity, and interferon production.[11-14] In a double-blind, placebo-controlled study, compared to the control group, both ginseng groups (consuming one 100 mg capsule once or twice daily for eight weeks) showed significant increases in the intracellular killing capacity of polymorphonuclear leukocytes, phagocytosis, and total number of T3 and T4 lymphocytes.[13] The authors concluded that the standardized extract was more effective in stimulating human immunity.[13] Individuals consuming ginseng long-term (up to five years) reduced their risk of getting gastric, lung, ovarian, larynx, esophageal, and pancreatic cancer.[5,13] However, no relevant effects were observed on breast, cervical, bladder, or thyroid cancer.[13] Ginseng reduces the symptoms and side effects of chemotherapy and radiation, and hastens recovery.[1,11] It also contains oleanolic acid that demonstrated antiallergenic actions in animal experiments.[1]

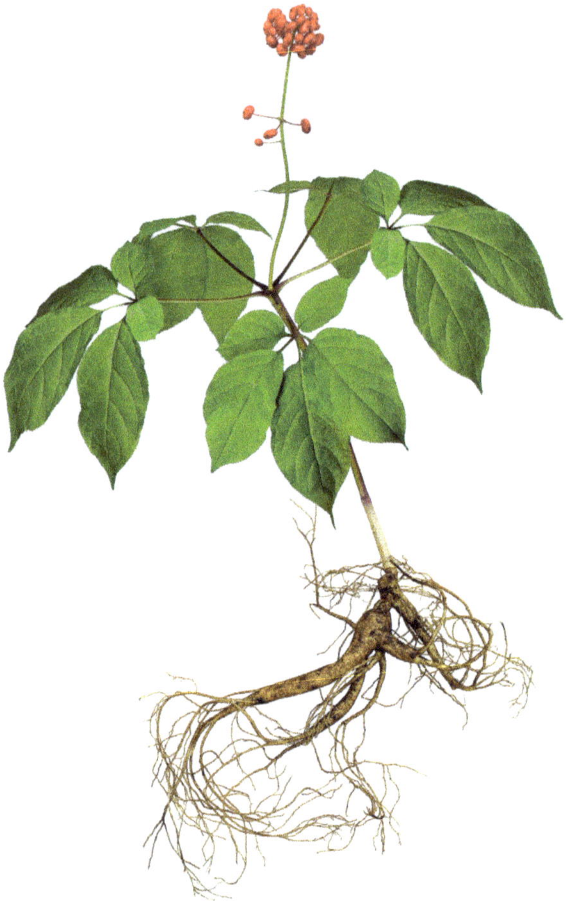

Ginseng exerts blood glucose-stabilizing effects, and appears to synergize insulin's effects. It lowers plasma glucose levels, fasting glucose levels, and hepatic glycogen content, and improves many symptoms associated with Type II diabetes (diabetes mellitus).[1,5,13] In one clinical double-blind study, patients consuming 200 mg of ginseng root daily experienced improved mood and physical performance, decreased fasting glucose levels, and lowered hemoglobin A1c (HbA1c) levels compared to the control group.[13] The polysaccharides and polypeptide were credited with lowering blood glucose levels in animal experiments.[1] In studies of canines with experimentally-induced diabetes mellitus controlled with insulin, ginseng lowered plasma glucose levels and reduced the majority of symptoms.[12] It also lowered epinephrine-induced hyperglycemia in rodents and canines.[12] While ginseng doesn't preclude the necessity for insulin, it enhances its actions, potentially decreasing insulin requirements. Ginseng may also slow the progression of diabetic blindness by dilating the retinal blood vessels, which increases nutrient and oxygen delivery to the retina.

Consuming ginseng four to 12 weeks can have aphrodisiac effects, increasing libido. Ginseng aids in treating impotence in men and increasing sexual desire in women.[13] In an open study, 66 males were treated with 4 g of ginseng extract daily for three months (20 were in control group, 30 had idiopathic low sperm count, and 16 had a varicocele-related low sperm count).[14] After treatment, all groups experienced increased sperm count, total testosterone, sperm motility, free testosterone, and dihydrotestosterone (DHT). More significant increases were noted in both groups with low sperm counts. Ginseng saponins reduce elevated prolactin levels, increasing sperm counts.[13] This aids in treating erectile dysfunction, secondary amenorrhea, and oligomenorrhea.[10] It contains ginsenosides that stimulate sexual responses in male and female animals independently of sex hormones.[1]

Compounding ginseng with hormone-balancing and adaptogen herbs such as vitex *(Vitex)*, dong quai *(Angelica sinensis)*, shu di huang *(Rehmannia)*, ashwagandha *(Withania)*, shatavari *(Asparagus)*, reishi *(Ganoderma)*, wu wei zu *(Schisandra)*, and/or licorice *(Glycyrrhiza)* aids in treating hormone imbalance due to adrenal depletion, deficiency, and stress. Consuming ginseng has adrenal tonifying and hormone balancing actions for depleted women with chronic amenorrhea, as well as perimenopausal and menopausal women. It also can be combined with other herbs to decrease menopause symptoms.[5] Ginseng is a rejuvenating tonic following childbirth, though it can be too stimulating for some nursing mothers and infants. Water-based preparations work best for this purpose, especially when ginseng is combined with spleen qi tonics such as astragalus *(Astragalus)*, codonopsis *(Codonopsis)*, and fu ling *(Poria)*, and blood tonics such as shu di huang *(Rehmannia)*, dong quai *(Angelica sinensis)*, and white peony *(Paeonia lactiflora)*.

It has been beneficial as an adjunct for patients with hypothyroidism. It increases the basic metabolic rate, and aids in weight loss. Ginseng also increases mental clarity, reduces fatigue, and enhances respiration and immune function. Ginseng lowers serum cholesterol and triglyceride levels,

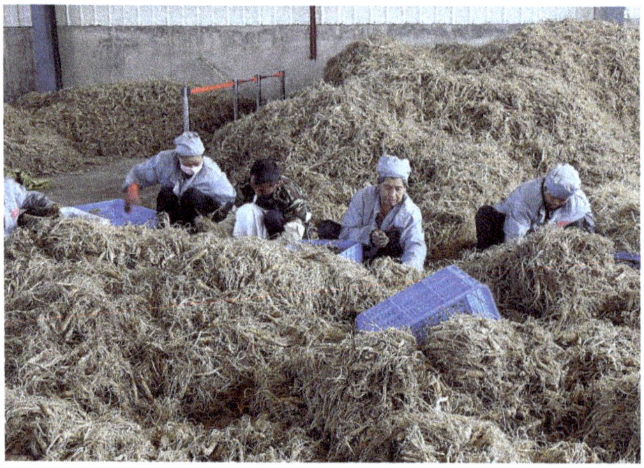

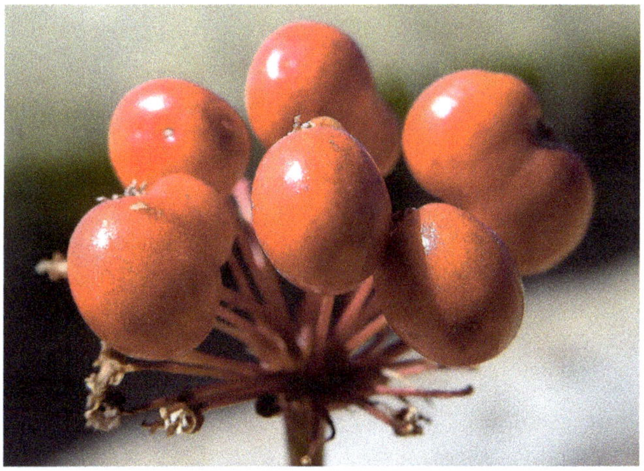

and elevates HDL levels.[13] It protects the liver, improves circulation, and reduces fatigue.[10] However, it can be overstimulating, especially in large doses, and should be avoided when hyperthyroidism is present.

The vast majority of ginseng's properties are attributed to the triterpene saponins and polysaccharides.[1] Uncured white ginseng is less heating and stimulating than cured Asian ginseng (red ginseng); therefore, it has a wider range of applications.

CONTRAINDICATIONS

Ginseng is contraindicated during pregnancy.[5] If prescribed by a health care practitioner, short-term use in lactating mothers may be permissible if they have experienced a hemorrhage or severe depletion from birthing. Because ginseng passes through breast milk, it can be too stimulating for an infant, resulting in restlessness or insomnia; discontinue use if this occurs.

Avoid use during an acute infectious illness, acute asthma attack, or while menstruating.[13,14] Do not consume continuously more than three months.[10,13] However, some herbalists caution against using it continuously for more than six weeks.[5]

Due to the spleen qi tonifying effects, ginseng can lead to a sense of fullness in the chest or diaphragm, or increase heat sensations.[12] In order to prevent this, combine with herbs that reduce qi stagnation, such as citrus peel.

Ginseng can be overstimulating, especially when combined with caffeine or other stimulants.[13] An overdose (up to 15 grams per day) can cause a headache, insomnia, anxiety, palpitations, or elevated blood pressure.[13] Symptoms of overdose (seen in patients who consumed 200 ml of the tincture at one time) include pruritus, vertigo, headache, fever, and in severe cases, hemorrhage.[12] Exercise caution using ginseng in individuals prone to anxiety, depression, or acute inflammatory diseases, as well as patients medicated for the previously listed conditions.[5] Easily stimulated individuals should not consume ginseng after two in the afternoon, as they may experience difficulty falling asleep at night.

Avoid consumption in individuals having yin deficiency with heat signs or heat excess such as night sweats, hot flashes, and dry skin and mucous membranes, unless severe qi deficiency is present.[12] Ginseng is contraindicated in patients with high blood pressure, or hypertensive patients with liver-heat rising which can manifest as flushed face, headache, feeling easily agitated or angry, and inflammation.[12]

Consult a health care practitioner before combining ginseng with other medications. Individuals taking blood pressure medications, phenelzine (an MAO inhibitor), stimulants, amphetamines, warfarin, or zidovudine (an HIV drug) should avoid using ginseng or consult a health care provider.[13,14] Diabetic individuals injecting insulin or consuming medications that affect blood glucose levels may need to alter their medication dosage due to ginseng's blood glucose-lowering effects.[13]

Red ginseng is used to treat patterns of qi and yang deficiency. Red *Panax ginseng* is very heating, and should not be used in cases of yin deficiency with heat signs, heat excess, or the absence of significant qi deficiency.

PREPARATION AND DOSAGE

TINCTURE: Fresh roots [1:2-1:3, 70-95% alcohol]; dry roots [1:5, 60% alcohol]; consume 10-60 drops, one to three times daily. The dosage of standardized ginseng extracts contain 4-7% ginsenosides.

CAPSULES: Consume 2-4 capsules, two to four times daily on an empty stomach before breakfast and lunch.

TEA: Prepare a decoction, preferably in a ginseng cooker; consume 8-12 ounces on an empty stomach before breakfast and lunch. Extended direct boiling may degrade important constituents; ginseng cookers mitigate this.

GOLDENROD

DESCRIPTION

BOTANICAL NAMES:
Solidago canadensis, S. decumbens, S. gigantea, S. epida, S. multiradiata, S. rigida, S. spathulata, S. virgaurea, S. spp. (syn. *Oligoneuron*)

COMMON NAMES:
Golden rod, goldenrod, European goldenrod, Canadian goldenrod, giant goldenrod, sweet goldenrod, sweet scented goldenrod, blue mountain tea, woundwort, Aaron's rod, St. Peter's staff
isopiisku, kanadanpiisku (Finnish)
herbe aux juifs, herbe des juifs, verge'd'or (French)
goldrute, heidnisch wundkraut (German)
piogga d'oro, verga aurea, verga d'oro (Italian)
hsiao pai-lung (Mandarin)
zolotarnik obiknovenny (Russian)
oreja de libre (Spanish)
höstgullris (Swedish)[1]

FAMILY NAME:
Asteraceae (Compositae)

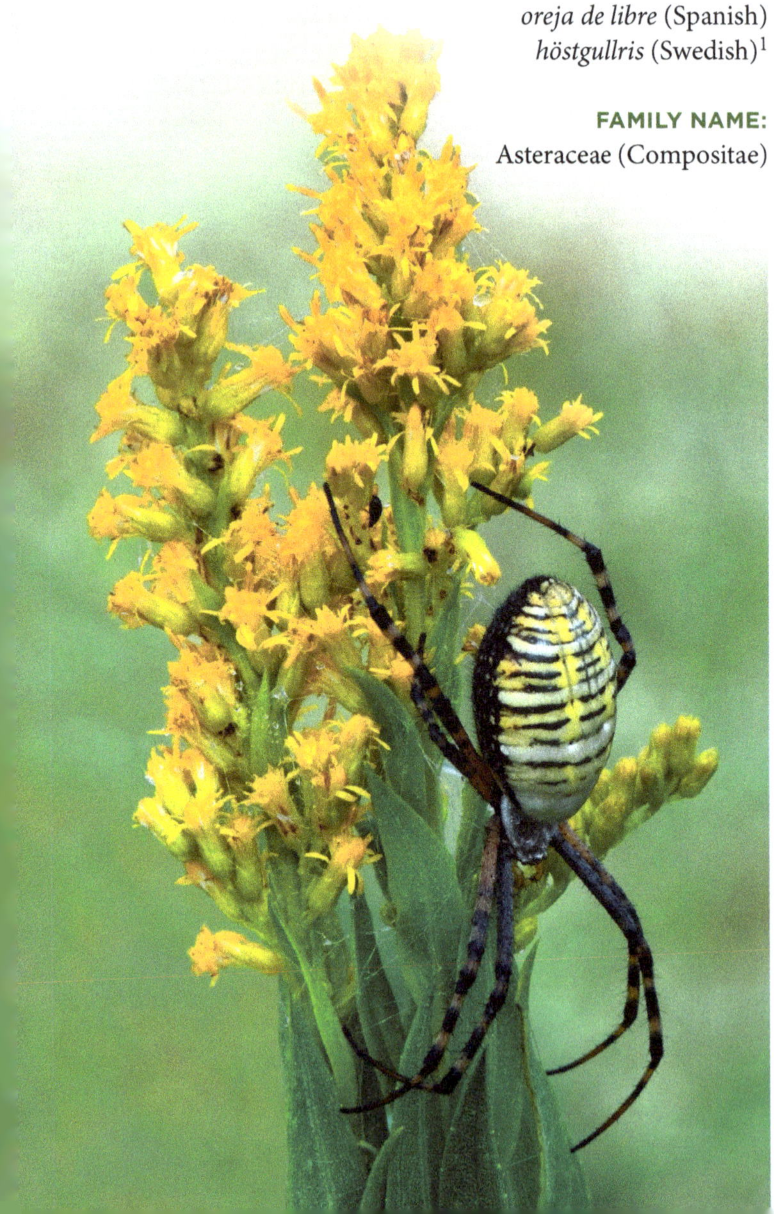

PARTS USED: The leaves and budding or flowering plant.

BOTANICAL DESCRIPTION AND HABITAT: Goldenrod is a perennial that grows in meadows, and on roadsides, thickets, bluffs, forest edges, dunes, riverbanks, gravel bars, and lakeshores.

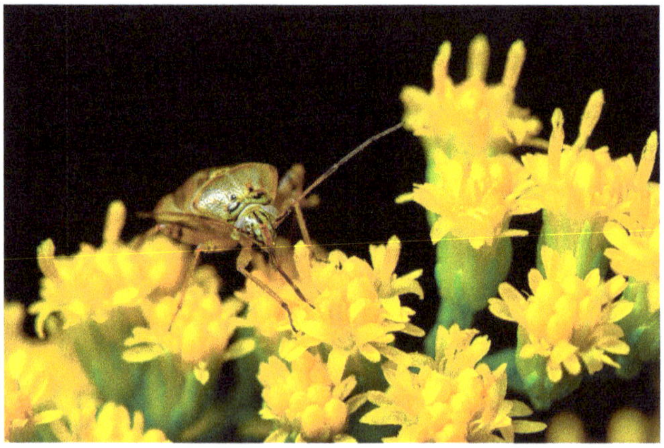

Solidago is a genus with approximately 150 species predominantly native to North America; it also grows in South America and Eurasia.[2] They are herbaceous perennials that reemerge each spring from a woody caudex or rhizome.[2] They have alternate, resinous, and often sessile leaves with a variety of shapes, including lanceolate, oblanceolate, obovate, elliptic, and spatulate.[2] Goldenrods bear radiate heads in flat-topped to panicle-like clusters that are sometimes one-sided.[2] The involucre is cylindrical to bell-shaped, widening when dry, with phyllaries in three to five graduated, overlapping series.[2] Each phyllary has a swollen mid rib and translucent flesh.[2] The yellow, generally glabrous disk flowers have finely hairy style branches bearing a triangular appendage.[2] The fruit is the shape of a compressed, inverted cone, and has pappus of a single series of 25 – 45 long, barbed bristles.[2]

S. canadensis is a rhizomatous plant with sparsely strigose leaves and stems (25 to 150 cm tall).[2] The lanceolate, three-veined, toothed leaves grow 5 to 15 cm long.[2] The panicle-like inflorescence bears many heads and lanceolate phyllaries, with the outer series ¼ to ⅓ the length of the inner series.[2] Each head has 8 – 15 ray flowers with ligules (1.5 – 2 mm long), as well as 5 – 12 disk flowers with corollas (2.5 – 3.5 mm in diameter).[2] The strigose fruit is approximately 1 mm long.[2] This species has many variations, and is considered "one of the most difficult taxonomic problems in North America."[2]

THE NAME: *Solidago* derives from the Latin *solidus* ("whole") and *ago* ("to make"). The genus name means "to make whole," referring to the plant's historical use as a vulnerary.[1] The epithet *canadensis* means "of Canadian origin." *Decumbens* stems from the Latin *decumbent* ("lying down or recumbent"), referring to the stem trailing on the ground, with an extending extremity. *Gigantea* originates from the Latin *gigant* ("very large or giant"). The epithet *multiradiata* derives from two Latin words: *multi* ("many") and *radiata,* stemming from *radiatus* ("to radiate light or shine"), referring to the flowers; *rigida* stems from the Latin *rigidus* ("to be stiff"). *Virgaurea* likely stems from two Latin words: *virga (*"a rod or twig") and *aurea* ("golden"); hence, the name goldenrod.

The following common names correspond with the Latin binomials: Canadian goldenrod *(S. canadensis),* alpine goldenrod *(S. decumbens),* giant early goldenrod *(S. gigantea),* northern goldenrod *(S. multiradiata),* hard-leaved goldenrod *(S. rigida),* and European goldenrod *(S. virgaurea).*

HISTORICAL USES: Native American tribes used topical applications of goldenrod for sores, wounds, burns, and ulcers. A hair rinse was applied to the scalp to prevent balding. The tea was used to wash women following childbirth.[3] Goldenrod tea was substituted for English tea during the American Revolution. The herb was reportedly carried into battle during the Crusades.[4] Germans used the herb for centuries to treat acute and chronic nephritis, as well as kidney diseases.[5] Homeopathic physicians prescribed the herb for referred kidney pain and conditions with dark, scanty urine.[5] The tea and spray were used to treat diptheria.[1] A hot tea was administered as a diaphoretic, and for dysmenorrhea and amenorrhea.[5] The flowers and leaves were used in yellow dye.[6] The leaf poultice was applied to the forehead for headaches.[1] Pioneers consumed goldenrod tea for kidney stones and ulcer pain.[6] Topical applications were used for rheumatism and neuralgia. The ground root was applied to the gums for toothaches.[6]

CONSTITUENTS: Goldenrod contains flavonoids (primarily flavonols: quercetin glycosides), triterpenoid saponins (aglycones), phenol glycosides (leicarposide and virgaureoside), diterpenes (not present in European goldenrod), phenolic acids, tannins, polysaccharides, and volatile oil.[7]

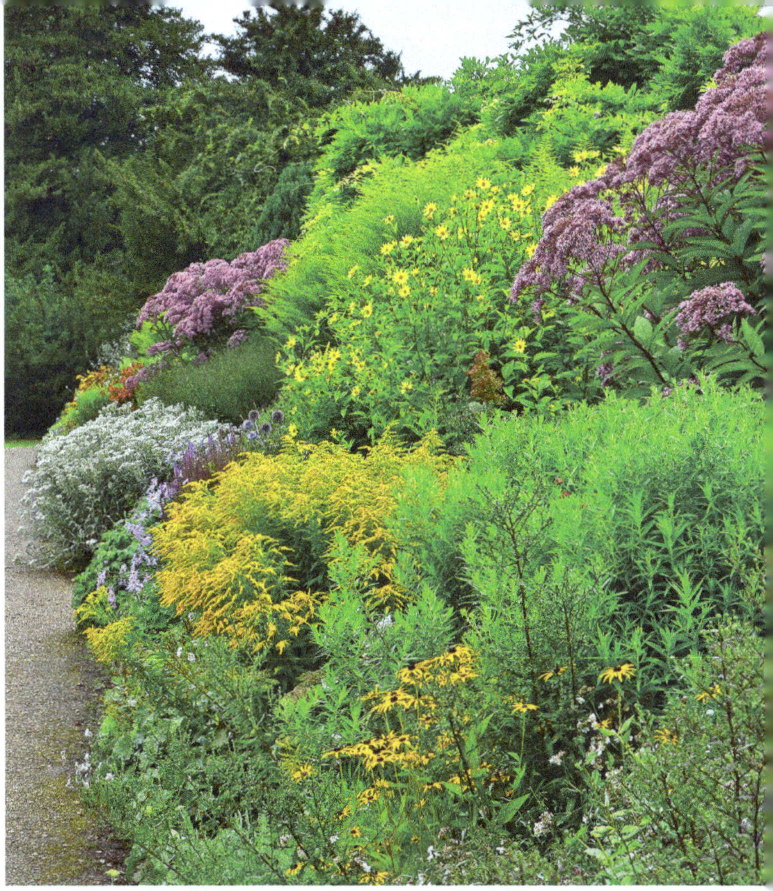

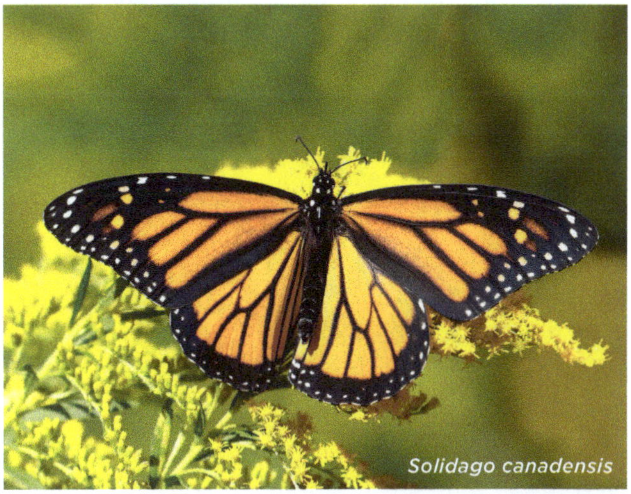

Solidago canadensis

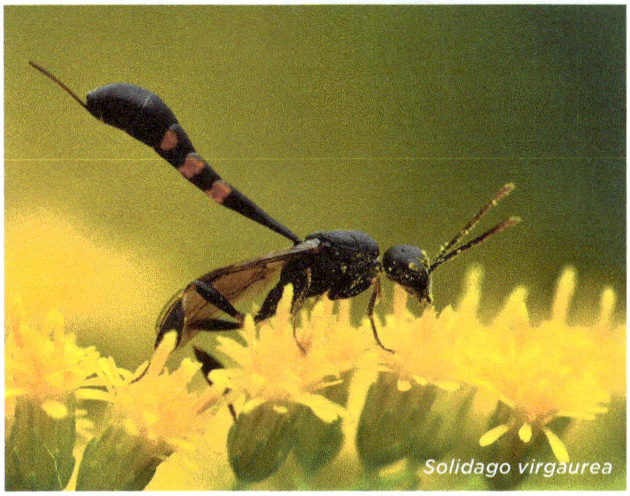

Solidago virgaurea

NUTRITIONAL PROPERTIES: Goldenrod is high in flavonoids (listed above).

MEDICINAL PROPERTIES: Diuretic, antibacterial, anticatarrhal, antifungal, anti-inflammatory, antispasmodic (mild), astringent, styptic, and vulnerary.

TEMPERATURE AND FLAVOR: Warm, pungent, astringent, and bitter.

MEDICINAL USES

A diuretic, goldenrod aids in treating kidney and urinary tract conditions. An infusion alleviates symptoms of cystitis and urethritis; however, more potent anti-infective agents are also necessary to address an infection.[7] Goldenrod is indicated for urinary conditions resulting in difficult or scanty urination, and for suppressed, retained, or concentrated urine.[5] It aids the passing of kidney stones.[5,7] The tea is most effective for kidney and urinary conditions. Combine goldenrod with dandelion leaf *(Taraxacum)*, cleavers *(Galium)*, couch grass *(Agropyron)*, and/or parsley root *(Petroselinum)* to synergize the diuretic actions.

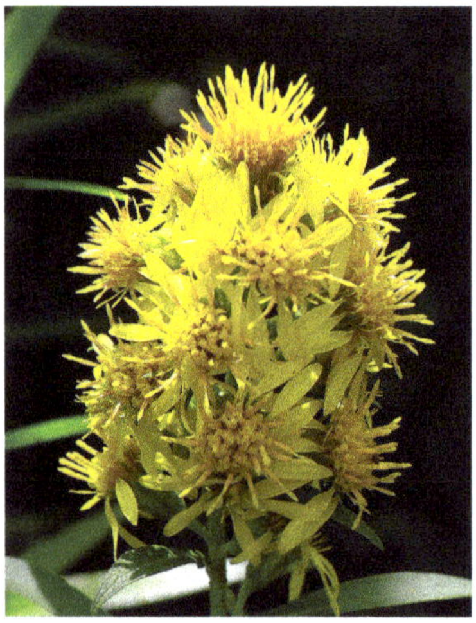

The leaf tea or tincture is useful for treating allergies; however, be sure to extract the herb before it flowers in order to avoid potential pollen exposure. Goldenrod reduces sinus and lung congestion, and sneezing. It is specifically indicated when the eyes water profusely and have a burning sensation. The homeopathic preparation of goldenrod is another effective treatment for individuals with allergies who are concerned that the tea or tincture will aggravate their condition. Combine extracts of yerba santa *(Eriodictyon)*, yerba mansa *(Anemopsis)*, bayberry *(Morella)*, and/or ragweed *(Ambrosia)* to ease seasonal allergies and sinus congestion.

The astringent properties tighten mucous membranes and reduce inflammation. Consume the leaf tea to reduce mucus secretions for moist conditions of the upper or lower respiratory tract.[7] The leaf tea also reduces gastrointestinal inflammation and helps to treat diarrhea, though other anti-infective agents may be required.[5,7] A sitz bath reduces bleeding and pain accompanying hemorrhoids. Gargling with the tea eases a sore throat or tender, bleeding gums.[7]

The leaves, and especially the flowers, are high in flavonoids that improve the integrity of blood vessels, reduce inflammation, and support optimal immune function. Flavonoids reduce inflammation associated with allergies, decrease capillary permeability due to inflammation, and hasten wound healing. Flavonoids also aid in treating varicose veins, as well other degenerative vascular diseases such as atherosclerosis.

Topical applications of goldenrod have vulnerary, antibacterial, antifungal, styptic, and counterirritant actions.[1,7] The leaves have heating properties similar to arnica, but are far less irritating and may be used on open wounds. Poultices, fomentations, washes, oils, and salves aid in treating bruises, sprains, strained muscles, cuts, abrasions, slow-healing ulcers, varicose veins, and arthritis.[6,7]

CONTRAINDICATIONS

Goldenrod pollen can cause allergies. Individuals with goldenrod allergies should use caution when processing the flowering herb. Internal use is contraindicated when the ureters are obstructed, if there is edema due to impaired heart or kidney function, or if the kidney is inflamed.[7]

PREPARATION AND DOSAGE

TINCTURE: Fresh leaves and budding or flowering plant [1:2-1:3, 70-95% alcohol]; consume 10-60 drops, up to five times daily.

CAPSULES: Consume 2-4 "00" capsules, up to three times daily.

TEA: Prepare a hot infusion; consume 8-12 ounces, up to four times daily. Consume every two to four hours to ease acute symptoms.

TOPICAL USE: Prepare the oil using the Simpler's, double boiler, or alcohol intermediary method. The leaves can be applied as a poultice, fomentation, or wash.

GOTU KOLA

BOTANICAL NAMES:
Centella asiatica (syn. *Hydrocotyle asiatica*)

COMMON NAMES:
Gotu kola, Indian pennywort, Indian hydrocotyle, Asian pennywort, Asiatic pennywort, marsh pennywort, marsh penny, marsh pepperwort, water pennywort, sheep rot, white rot, thick-leaved pennywort, elixir of life
man t'ien hsing, ground ivy, arrtaniyal-hindi (Arabic)
gam hok chou (Cantonese)
intianssammakonpukti, makonputk, rohtosammakonputki (Finnish)
ecueille d'eau, hydrocotyle asiatique (French)
wassernabel, wasswenabel (German)
brahmamanduki (Hindi)
idrpcotile, scodella d'acque (Italian)
han ke cao, man t'ien hsing (Mandarin)
brahmi, mandūka-parnī, manduka parn (Sanskrit)

FAMILY NAME:
Apiaceae (Umbelliferae)

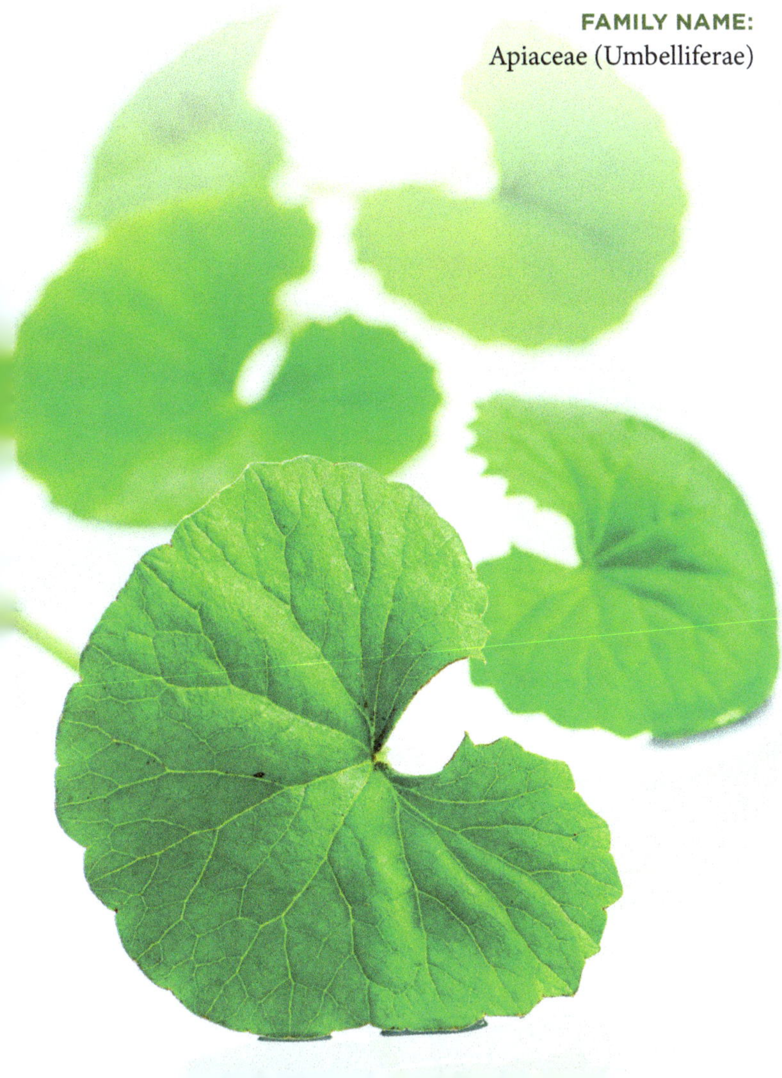

DESCRIPTION

PARTS USED: The leaves and whole plant.

BOTANICAL DESCRIPTION AND HABITAT: *Centella asiatica* is a perennial, herbaceous ground cover (0.5 – 10+ cm tall) with prostrate, creeping stems that root at the

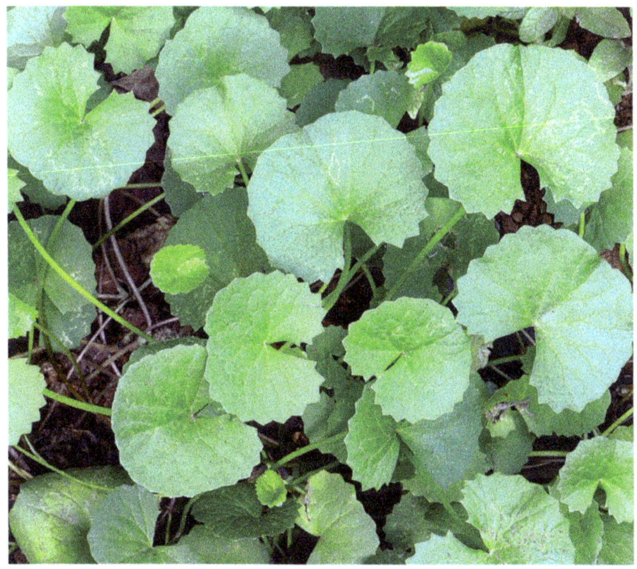

nodes. It grows in shady, moist soil on river edges and grassy areas throughout tropical Asia, Indonesia, Australia, Madagascar, Australia, and southern and central Africa.[1,2] The kidney-shaped, minutely hairy leaves (2 – 3 cm long) are palmately veined with undulating, slightly lobed, or dentate margins.[1,3] The leaf bases sheathe around the stem, like other members of Apiaceae.[4]

The inflorescences are tiny, simple umbels of two to four flowers, each subtended by two involucral bracts on short peduncles (2 – 8 mm long) that grow from leaf axils.[3,4] The almost sessile, minute flowers have five vestigial sepals, five white to pinkish valvate petals, five stamens, two styles, and two fused carpels.[2] The fruit (5 mm long) is a two-parted, ribbed, ovate schizocarp.[3]

THE NAME: The original genus name *Hydrocotyle* derives from two Greek words: *hydro* ("water") and *kotyle* ("plant"). The current genus name, *Centella,* is of unclear origin; it may derive from the Latin *cento* ("patchwork"), centum ("hundred"), centrum ("center"), or from the Greek *kenteo* ("prick, torture, torment").[5] The epithet *asiatica* alludes to the plant's native origin. The Sanskrit name mandūka-parnī refers to the leaves' resemblance to webbed frogs' feet.[6] *Brahmi* is another name for the plant, due to the belief that it increased knowledge of Brahman (the supreme reality).[7] This herb was called pennywort due to the leaves' resemblance to Chinese coins.

HISTORICAL USES: In Ayurvedic medicine, gotu kola continues to be used as a rasayana (rejuvenator) and vayasthapana (brain tonic).[8] It was consumed by yogis to enhance meditation.[7] Gotu kola balances all doshas, and is an important revitalizing agent.[6,7] Ghee medicated with gotu kola was consumed to rejuvenate the spirit.[7] A milk decoction was considered most beneficial for nourishing the nervous system.[7] According to Li Ching Yun, a Chinese herbalist who consumed gotu kola regularly and reportedly lived for 256 years, gotu kola was one of the "miracle elixirs of life."[9] In Chinese folk medicine, gotu kola is administered as an antidote for poisoning from toxic mushrooms, arsenic, or yellow jasmine *(Gelsemium elegans)*.[10] The tea was also consumed to treat tonsillitis, colds, pleurisy, jaundice, infectious hepatitis, and dysentery.[10]

A combination used to treat fevers includes gotu kola, tulsi basil *(Ocimum sanctum)*, and ginger *(Zingiber)*.[6] Gotu kola was administered to ease intermittent fevers from malaria.[7] It was consumed as a blood purifier to treat leprosy and syphilis.[6,7] Gotu kola leaf juice is an energizing beverage served by Indian street vendors.

CONSTITUENTS: Gotu kola contains triterpene saponins (asiaticoside, oxyasiaticoside, madecassoside [Madagascar chemotype], centelloside [Sri Lanka chemotype], isothankunoside [India chemotype], brahmoside, brahminoside, and thankunoside); sapogenins that vary according to chemotype (asiatic, madecassic, centellic, centoic, asiatocentioc, indocentoic, brahmic, thankunic, and isothankunic acids); and volatile oil (*trans*-β-farnesene, germacrene D, β-caryophyllene, camphor, cineole, n-dodecane, *p*-cymol, α- and β-pinene, methanol, allyl mustard, and an unidentified terpene acetate). It also contains sugars (rhamnose, arabinose, glucose, fructose, sucrose, raffinose, and centellose); fatty acids (oleic, linoleic, lignoceric, palmitic, stearic, linolenic, and elaidic acids); phytosterols (β-sitosterol, stigmasterol, campesterol, and sitosterol); amino acids (glutamic acid, serine, and alanine); flavonols (kaempferol, quercetin, 3-glycosylkaempferol, and 3-glycosylquercetin); polyphenols, tannins, resins, a bitter principle (vellarin), and ascorbic acid.[8,10]

NUTRITIONAL PROPERTIES: Gotu kola contains high amounts of aluminum, calcium, fiber, fat, magnesium, manganese, niacin, riboflavin, silicon, sodium, thiamine, vitamin A, and zinc. It contains average to low amounts of chromium, cobalt, iron, phosphorus, potassium, protein, selenium, tin, and vitamin C.[11]

MEDICINAL PROPERTIES: Alterative, analgesic, antiaging, anti-inflammatory, antibacterial, antifungal, antioxidant, connective tissue regenerative, demulcent, depurative, diuretic (mild), gentle stimulant, circulatory stimulant, hypotensive, immune modulator, nervine, rejuvenator, vasodilator, and vulnerary.

TEMPERATURE AND FLAVOR: Cool, salty, and bitter.

MEDICINAL USES

Gotu kola nourishes nerves and brain cells, improving mental clarity, alertness, concentration, and memory.[7,8,10] It is a neuroprotector, increasing oxygenation in the brain and reducing oxidative stress.[8] It aids in treating individuals suffering from memory loss and senility, and delays the progression of Alzheimer's and global dementia.[7,8] Gotu kola inhibits the brain's uptake of glutamate, a contributing factor in dementia.[8] It supports brain and nervous system function in individuals with ADHD, Asperger's syndrome, and autism.[6] It contains xanthines that increase blood flow to the brain, and gently stimulate the nervous system. Gotu kola is an adjunct therapy for epileptics.[7,12] Asiatic acid, a triterpene, decreases the buildup of amyloid plaque, slowing the onset of Alzheimer's.[8] Combine gotu kola with tulsi basil *(Ocimum sanctum)*, reishi *(Ganoderma)*, and smaller amounts of brahmi *(Bacopa)* and rosemary *(Salvia rosmarinus)* to enhance mental clarity and improve concentration.

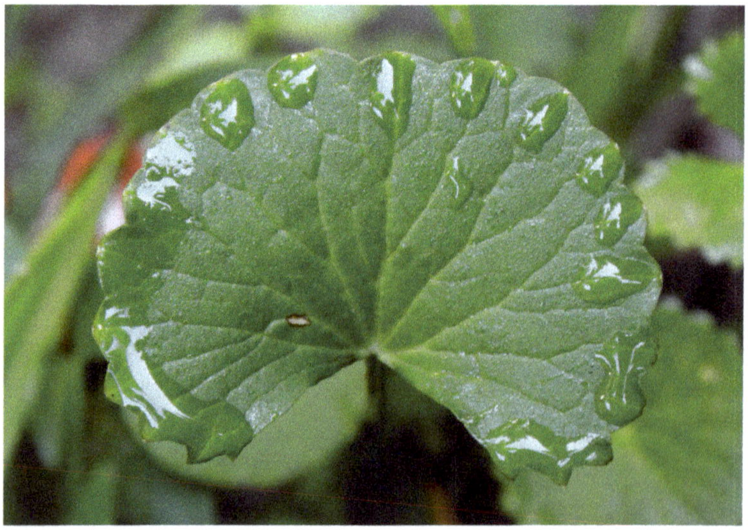

Gotu kola calms the central nervous system and is a gabaminergic agent.[8,12] Its antidepressant qualities aid in treating seasonal affective disorder (SAD), and premenstrual and postpartum depression. Gotu kola is an adjunct for individuals weaning from antidepressant pharmaceuticals.[8] Prepare a mood elevating compound by combining extracts of gotu kola, St. John's wort *(Hypericum)*, lemon balm *(Melissa)*, damiana *(Turnera)*, and/or Siberian ginseng *(Eleutherococcus)*, with smaller amounts of wild oats *(Avena)*, rosemary *(Salvia rosmarinus)*, and/or lavender *(Lavandula)*.

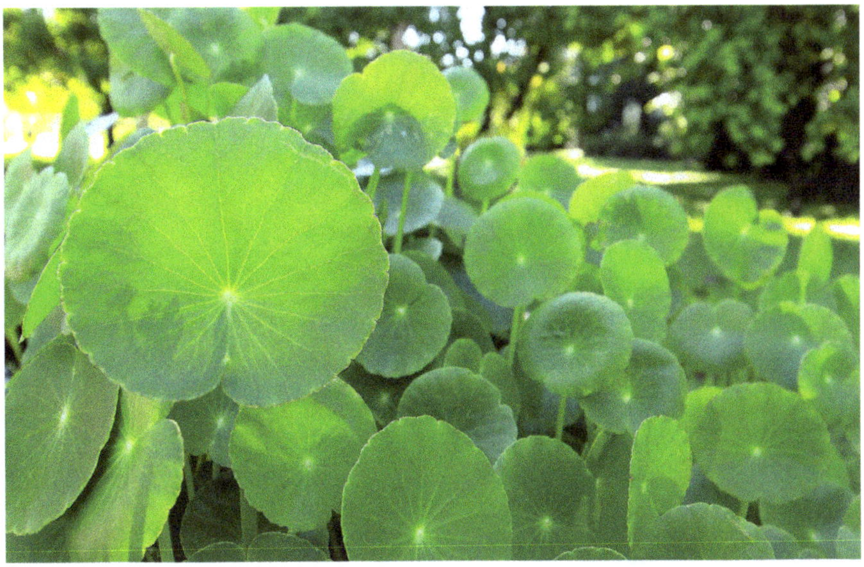

Gotu kola is an impressive connective tissue tonic. It stimulates keratinization of the epidermis, improves tissue tensile strength, increases dermal strength, and decreases tissue fibrosis.[9,10] Gotu kola hastens scar tissue maturation by increasing type 1 collagen production.[8] The standardized extract was found to aid in treating keloids and hypertrophic scars.[9] While scar tissue is forming, it reduces the inflammatory phase, and hastens the scar tissue maturation phase.[9] The development of keloids and hypertrophic scars is due to a prolonged inflammatory phase of healing that fails to progress to the maturation phase.[9] Gotu kola hastens the healing of postsurgical wounds, skin grafts, burns, broken bones, fractures, sprains, strains, and bruises.[8,10] It mends tissue following traumatic injuries, episiotomies, and vaginal and perineal tears from childbirth.[9] Gotu kola speeds the healing of wounds and ulcers.[10] It aids in healing skin conditions such as eczema, psoriasis, acne, and urticaria.[6-8] It improves blood flow to the skin, reduces wrinkling, and delays the aging process. It also is used to decrease cellulite and reduce skin hardening. Gotu kola contains the triterpene asiaticoside that stimulates regeneration of the reticuloendothelial system and hastens wound healing.[9,10] Gotu kola extract was found to reduce hepatic fibrosis in individuals with alcohol-induced cirrhosis.[9] It aids in healing stress-related peptic ulcers.[8,12]

Gotu kola is a circulatory stimulant, and a cardiovascular and venous tonic.[8,9] It improves the integrity of blood vessels, and aids in treating venous insufficiency, varicose veins, venous distention, spider veins, and hemorrhoids.[8,9] Gotu kola enhances the elasticity of blood vessels, which aids in treating hypertension and atherosclerosis.[12] It also reduces edema and venous distention in the lower extremities, especially in the ankles and feet.[8] The flavonoids quercetin and astragalin are attributed to strengthening blood vessels. Alcohol extracts demonstrated cardioprotective function in one study, demonstrating the reduction of ischemic reperfusion-induced myocardial infarction and related injuries in rodents.[8]

Gotu kola aids in treating symptoms of hypothyroidism because it improves clarity and vitality, reduces depression, and via metabolism elevation, supports weight loss. It enhances immune and adrenal function.[7] Combine extracts of gotu kola, Siberian ginseng *(Eleutherococcus)*, Asian ginseng *(Panax ginseng)*, and/or ashwagandha *(Withania)* to support thyroid and adrenal function.

Apply a poultice, fomentation, oil, or salve topically as a vulnerary. Gotu kola aids in treating varicose veins, spider veins, skin ulcers, burns, postsurgical wounds, eczema, acne, and psoriasis.[7] Topical applications also aid in treating hair loss.

CONTRAINDICATIONS

Gotu kola is well tolerated by most individuals; however, excessive doses can cause a headache, dizziness, and vertigo.[6,7] Although it is rare, internal or topical use can aggravate itching, and topical use can cause contact dermatitis.[7,9] Avoid use in individuals with hyperthyroidism, or if it is too stimulating to the nervous system. Consuming gotu kola in the late afternoon or evening can cause insomnia in some individuals. Use only under the guidance of a health care practitioner during pregnancy and lactation, or when being treated for hypothyroidism, hypocholesterolemia, or hypoglycemia.[6,12] Avoid use during an acute illness or menstruation.

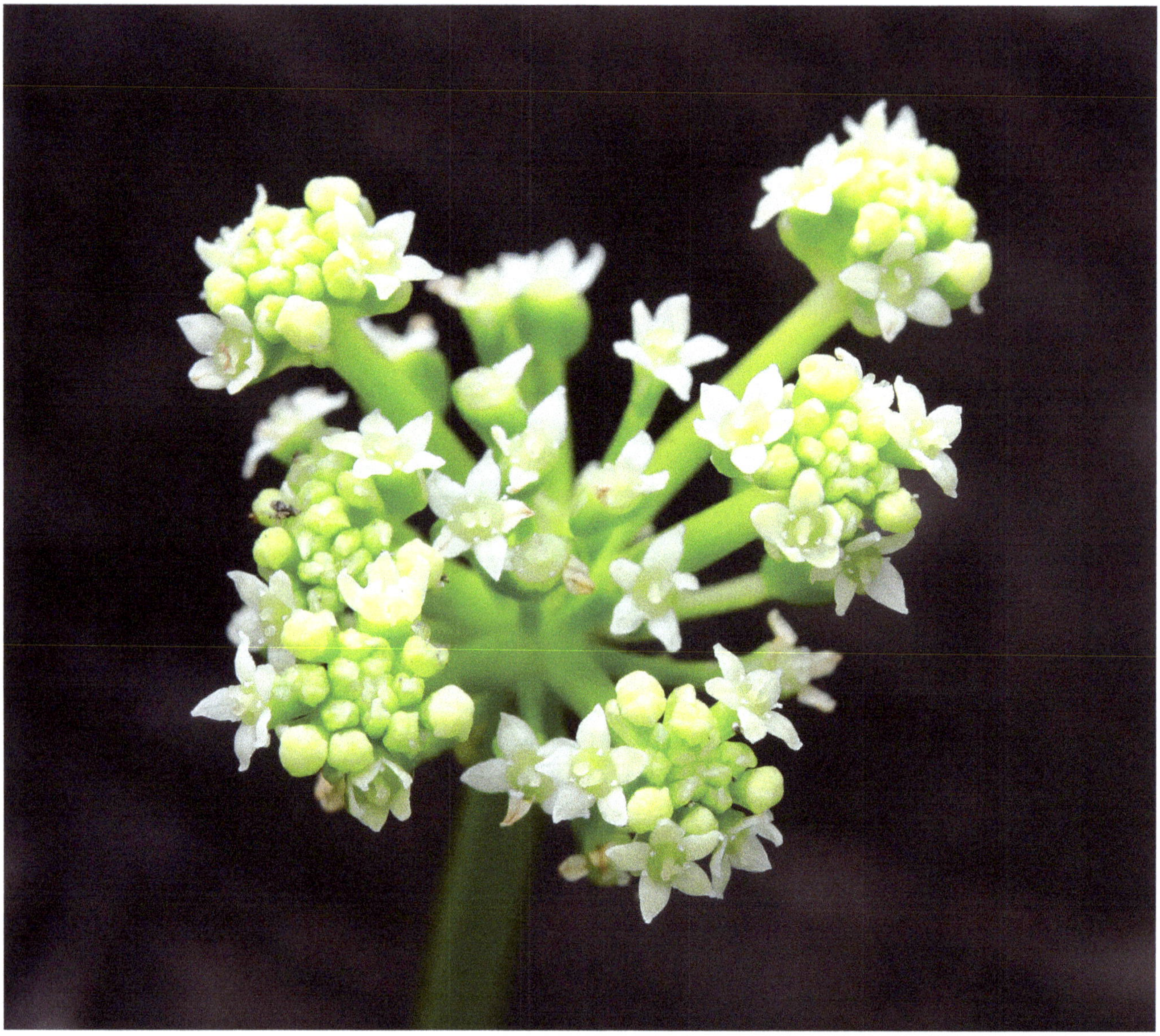

PREPARATION AND DOSAGE

TINCTURE: Fresh herb [1:2-1:3, 70-95% alcohol]; recent dry herb [1:5, 60% alcohol]; consume 15-60 drops, up to three times daily. Consume 200 mg of the standardized extract two to three times daily. Standardized extracts produced from the Madagascar variety commonly yield 29-30% asiatic acid, 40% asiaticoside, and 1-2% madecassoside.[9]

FLUID EXTRACT: Dry herb [1:1, 50% alcohol]; consume 10-60 drops, up to three times daily.

SUCCUS: Consume 10-20 ml of fresh juice in the morning or early afternoon.

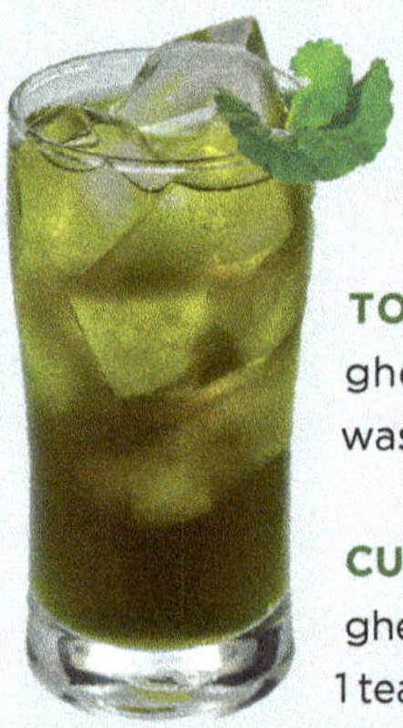

TEA: Prepare a hot or cold infusion; consume 8-12 ounces, up to three times daily.

TOPICAL USE: Apply a medicated ghee, oil, poultice, fomentation, or wash of gotu kola topically.

CULINARY USE: Prepare a medicated ghee or oil of gotu kola, and consume 1 teaspoon to 1 tablespoon, one to three times daily. Infuse gotu kola in milk or almond milk, and consume 6-12 ounces, one to two times daily. Small amounts of gotu kola can be substituted for spinach in a wide variety of dishes.

GRAVEL ROOT

BOTANICAL NAMES:
Eutrochium purpureum (syn. *Eupatorium purpureum, Eupatoriadelphus purpureus*), *E. maculatum, E. ternifolium, E. trifoliatum, E. verticillatum*

COMMON NAMES:
Gravel root, gravel weed, queen of the meadow, Jopi weed, Joe-pye weed, sweet-scented Joe-pye weed, kidney wort, kidney root, purple boneset, trumpet weed, hemp weed, thoroughwort, marsh milkweed
punalatva (Finnish)
eupatoire (French)
purpur-wasseredost (German)
canapa (Italian)
rosenflockel (Swedish)

FAMILY NAME:
Asteraceae (Compositae)

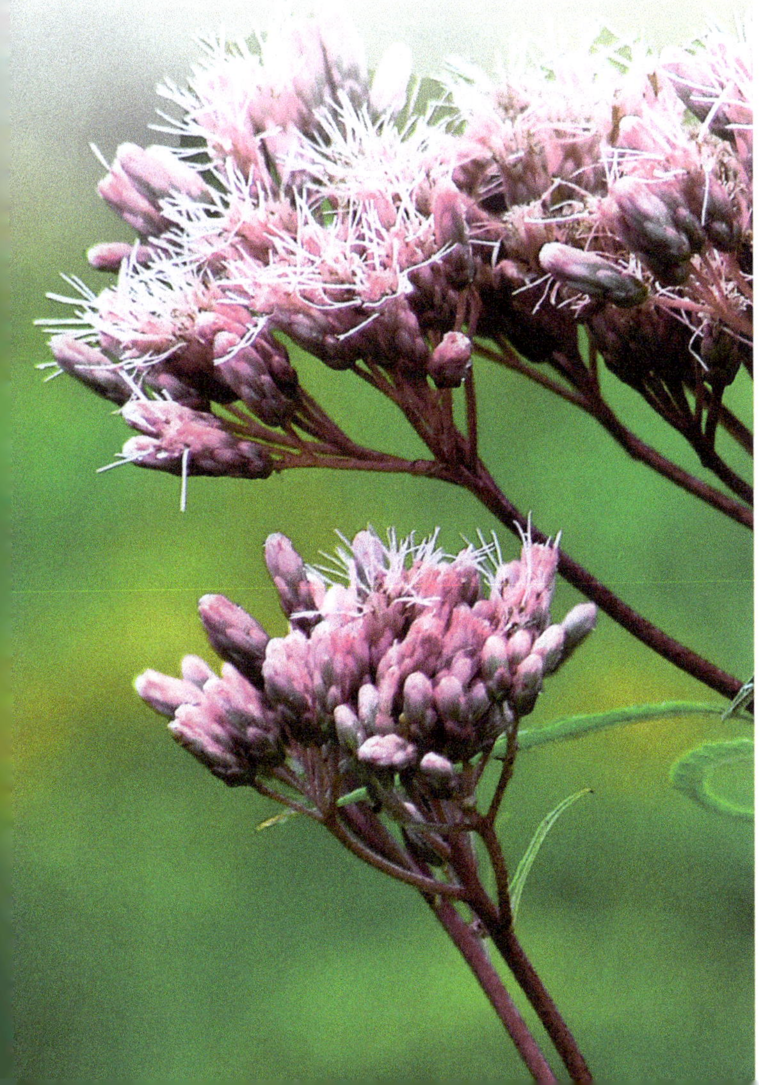

DESCRIPTION

PARTS USED: The roots or whole, fresh plant.

BOTANICAL DESCRIPTION AND HABITAT: Gravel root is native to the Midwest, East Coast, and southeastern U.S. It inhabits moist, swampy areas along ponds, lakes, and streambeds.

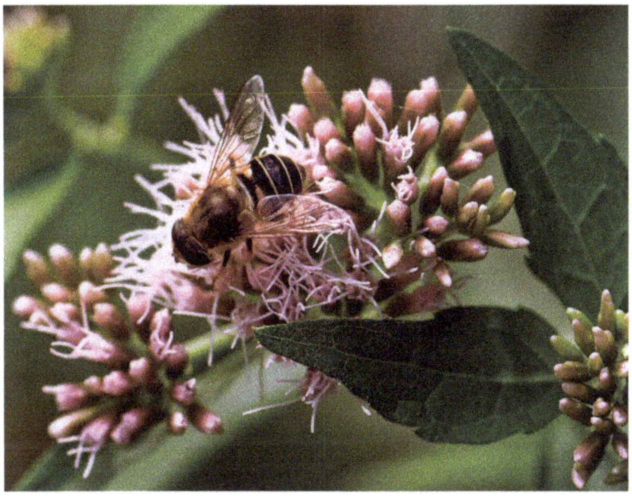

Eutrochium purpureum is an erect, herbaceous perennial growing up to 3 meters tall.[2] The unbranched solid or pithy stems grow in clumps that widen in diameter as the plant matures. The stems are predominantly green, and purple at the nodes; they sometimes feature elongated spots or lines. The lower stems are glabrous; the upper stems can be densely hairy. Whorls of three, four, or five leaves grow at each node. The wrinkly, coarsely serrated, petioled leaves grow up to 26 cm long and have a rough to glabrous upper surface and a hairy, glandular surface underneath.[2,3]

The plant bears a large terminal, corymb-like compound inflorescence atop each stem, contained within an involucre of green bracts. Each inflorescence is comprised of many small, vanilla-scented heads (2 – 5 mm in diameter), with unequal, glabrous or sparsely hairy phyllaries.[2,3] The heads contain five to seven purple or pink flowers that produce brownish-black achenes (4 – 5 mm long).[3] Gravel root blooms from midsummer to fall, and easily hybridizes with other species in the genus.[2,3]

THE NAME: The genus name *Eupatorium* derives from the name Mithridates Eupator, king of Pontus, said to be the first person to use the plant medicinally.[1] The epithet

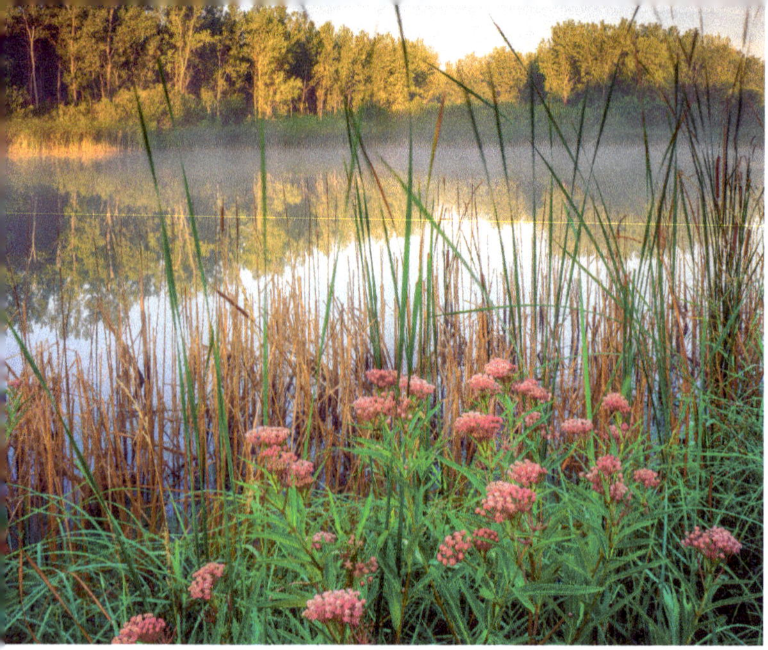

purpureum ("purple") derives from Latin, indicating the color of the flowers. The epithet *maculatum* ("spotted") refers to the purple spots on the stems. The herb acquired the common name "Joe-pye weed" after a Native American healer named Jopi became famous for treating a low form of typhus with this plant.[1] The herb was called "gravel root" and "kidney wort" because it was used to flush kidney stones. The name "trumpet weed" indicates the resemblance of the floral shape to a trumpet.

HISTORICAL USES: Native Americans consumed gravel root tea to ease kidney conditions. Ojibwa bathed their children in gravel root tea to impart strength.

Gravel root was administered by Eclectic physicians to stimulate and impart tone to female reproductive organs. It was used to treat chronic uterine diseases, endometriosis, ovarian and uterine atony, dysmenorrhea, and leukorrhea, and for insufficient labor pains.[4,5] Gravel root was also used to treat dropsy, kidney stones, chronic nephritis, prostatitis, and urinary disorders.[4,5]

CONSTITUENTS: Gravel root contains triterpenoid saponins, bitter principles (sesquiterpene lactones), a benzofuran (euparin), flavonoids (eupatorin), volatile oil, resin, and polyacetylenes.[6]

NUTRITIONAL PROPERTIES: Other than the flavonoid content (eupatorin) and constituents listed above, the nutritional properties have not been studied.

MEDICINAL PROPERTIES: Diuretic, antilithic, antirheumatic, genitourinary tonic, lithotriptic, and uterine tonic.

TEMPERATURE AND FLAVOR: Neutral, sweet, bitter, and mildly astringent.

MEDICINAL USES

Gravel root is a soothing diuretic that reduces urinary symptoms, including a constant desire to urinate, feelings of suppressed urine, burning sensations upon urination, or a dull bladder ache.[4,5] It aids in treating acute cystitis, urethritis, and passive hematuria.[1,4-6] However, additional anti-infective agents are necessary. Gravel root is also a long-term treatment for recurring urinary tract infections, interstitial cystitis, subacute prostatitis, and chronic nephritis.[4,5] The diuretic properties alleviate rheumatic complaints, gout, and edema.[1,4] A decoction is preferable for urinary disorders, although extracts administered in two to four ounces of hot water are also useful.

Gravel root's diuretic action enhances the excretion of calcium oxalate and uric acid stones. It aids in preventing and eliminating urinary stones.[4,5] For this reason, it is considered an antilithic and lithotriptic agent. The diuretic actions also aid in the acute or long-term treatment of kidney stones.[1] Gravel root has mild analgesic effects that ease pain from passing kidney stones; however, more potent analgesics such as valerian *(Valeriana),* California poppy *(Eschscholzia),* poppy *(Papaver),* silk tassel *(Garrya),* or cannabis *(Cannabis)* are often necessary to manage pain. Combine hydrangea *(Hydrangea),* stone root *(Collinsonia),* madder *(Rubia),* and gravel root for acute or long-term treatment of kidney stones.

CONTRAINDICATIONS

Avoid use with obstructive kidney stones, edema due to impaired heart or kidney function, or kidney inflammation. Like other members of the Asteraceae family, it can cause contact dermatitis in hypersensitive individuals due to the sesquiterpene lactones. Avoid use during pregnancy and lactation, although there are no reports of side effects when used properly.

PREPARATION AND DOSAGE

TINCTURE: Fresh root or whole fresh plant [1:2–1:3, 70–95% alcohol]; dry root [1:5, 60% alcohol]; consume 30–90 drops in warm water, up to four times daily.

TEA: Prepare a decoction; consume 8–12 ounces, up to four times daily.

GRINDELIA

BOTANICAL NAMES:
Grindelia camporum, G. robusta, G. squarrosa, G. integrifolia, G. humboldtii, G. hirsuta (syn. *G. humilis*), *G. rigida*

COMMON NAMES:
Gumweed, field gumweed, grindelia, hardy grindelia, scaly grindelia, California gum plant, gum plant, resinweed, rosin weed, tarweed, August flower, Spanish gold
harzkraut, sperriges gummikraut (German)
pte ichi yuha (Lakota)
pezhe wasek (Poncas Omaha)
yerba del buey, boton de oro (Spanish)[1-3]

FAMILY NAME:
Asteraceae (Compositae)

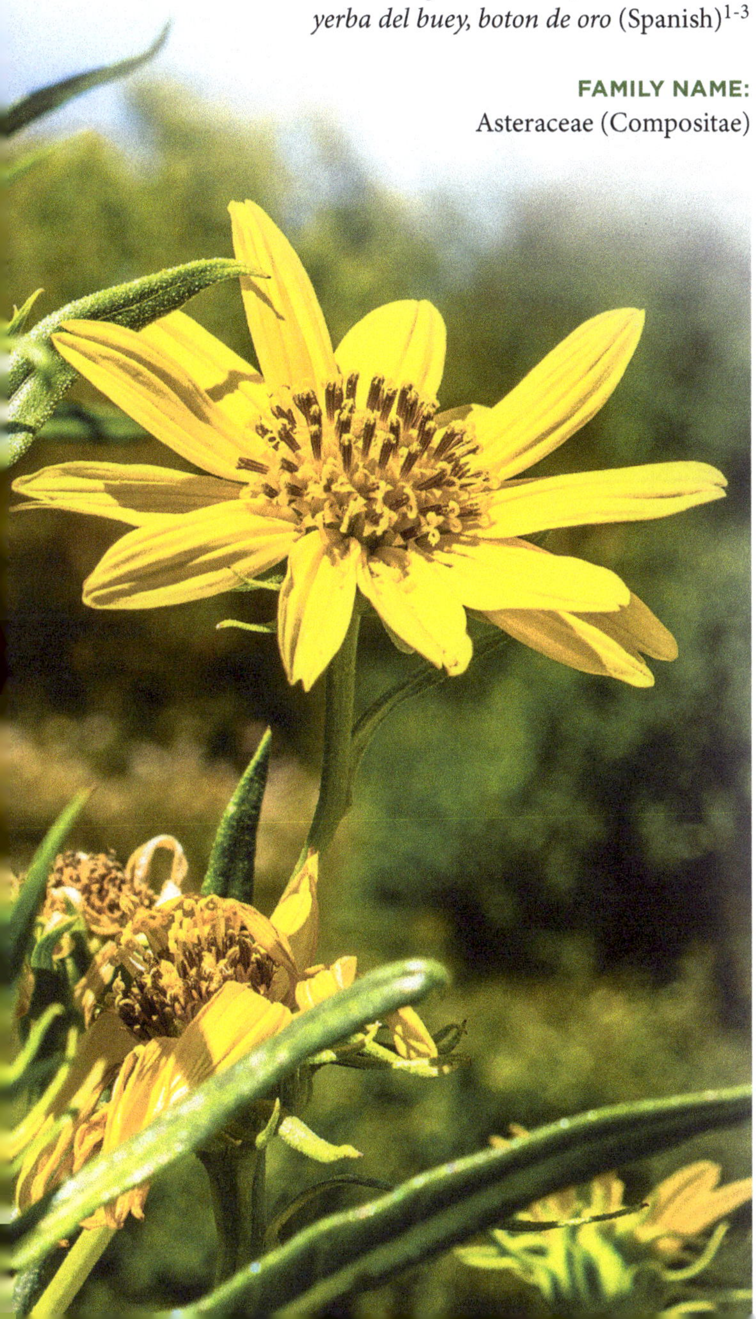

DESCRIPTION

PARTS USED: The resinous buds and flowering tops.

BOTANICAL DESCRIPTION AND HABITAT: *Grindelia* is a varied genus with at least 80 species of tap-rooted perennials and subshrubs native to North and South America.[4] The erect, often resinous stems can be branched, and are hairy or glabrous.[4] The alternate leaves vary in shape, depending on the species, and can be glabrous, hairy, or

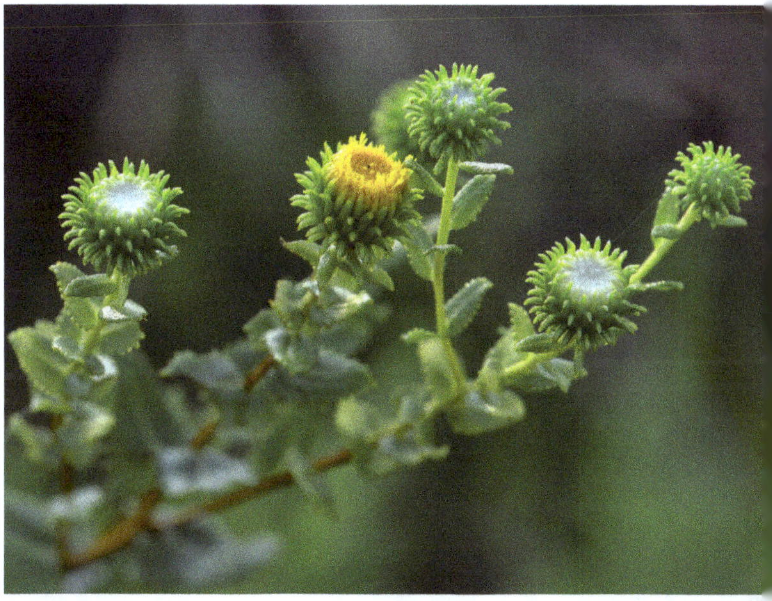

sticky to the touch.[3,4] The lower leaves are petiolate; the upper leaves are stemless, with bases that often clasp the main stem.[6] The inflorescence is found in clusters or singly, and is a radiate or discoid head with a sturdy, globose involucre that exudes a white, sticky gum.[6] There are up to 60 yellow ray flowers, and usually over 100 yellow disk flowers.[6] The fruit is a white to brown, glabrous achene, varying in shape according to species, with a pappus of up to six short, deciduous awns.[5]

THE NAME: *Grindelia* is named for German botanist, David Grindel (1717 – 1783).[3] The epithet *camporum* derives from the Latin *campus* ("plain, field, open country, or level place").[7] The epithet *hirsuta* means "covered with hair;" *integrifolia* ("with entire leaves") describes the uppermost leaves of the plant; *rigida* refers to the stiff leaves.[8-10] *Humboldtii* was named for Friedrich Wilhelm Heinrich Alexander von Humboldt (1769 – 1859), German geographer and naturalist.[8] The epithets *squarrosa* ("rough") and *robusta* ("strong, hard, oaken") derive from Latin.[11] Gumweed, gum plant, and resinweed refer to the bracts that are coated with sticky, resinous latex.

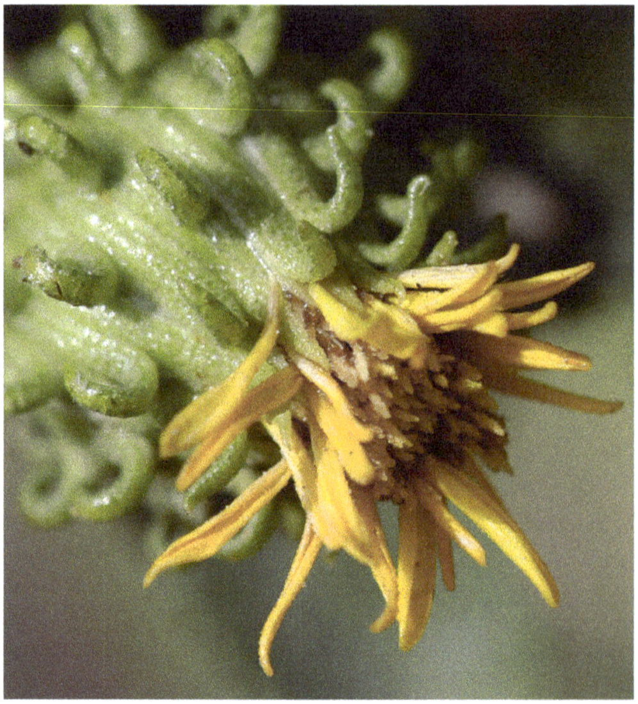

HISTORICAL USES: Grindelia was included in the *U.S. Pharmacopoeia* from 1882 to 1926, and remained in the *U.S. National Formulary* until 1960.[3] Eclectic physicians administered grindelia to alleviate a dry, labored cough, whooping cough, asthmatic breathing, emphysema, and acute and subacute bronchitis.[12,13] They recommended smoking the leaves mixed with other herbs, such as *Lobelia* or *Stramonium* to relieve spasmodic asthma.[12] Grindelia was applied topically to hasten the healing of skin conditions such as wounds, indolent ulcers, insect bites, vesicular eczema, poison oak, and poison ivy rash.[12,13] *G. squarrosa* was administered as an antimalarial to reduce spleen congestion and poor digestive system health.[12,13] In Europe, grindelia was utilized similarly for respiratory complaints; it was also administered to treat cystitis and urinary catarrh.[1]

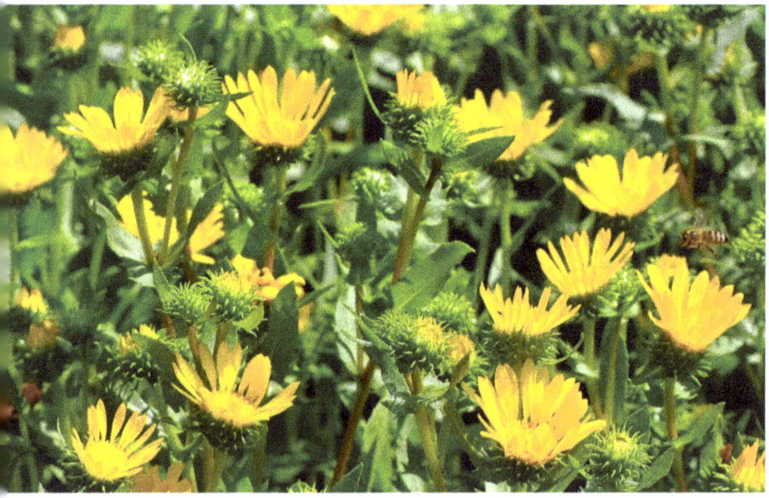

North American Indian tribes utilized grindelia for respiratory, urinary, kidney, digestive, and skin conditions.[14] Southwest Indians consumed grindelia to treat asthma, as well as bladder and kidney problems.[2] Blackfoot Indians consumed a decoction of the dried roots as a spring purge, and for liver problems.[15] Nevada Indians applied a topical wash to measles and smallpox.[14,15] Costanoan Indians bathed the skin with grindelia tea to treat boils, burns, wounds, and poison oak.[14] Southwestern tribes applied warm preparations of grindelia for burns, blisters, skin eruptions, sore joints, paralysis, and "cold in the bones."[2] The resin was rubbed on the eyes to treat snow blindness.[14]

CONSTITUENTS: Grindelia contains resin (grindelin, as well as grindelic acid and its derivatives: 17-acetoxygrindelic acid, 6-oxo-grindelic acid, 13-isogrindelic acid, 7,8-epoxygrindelic acid, and strictanoic acid; and acetylenic compounds such as matricarianol and matricarianol acetate), volatile oil (mono- and sesquiterpenes, borneol, α-pinene, *trans*-pinocarveol, bornyl acetate, limonene, and 3-methylkampferol), an alkaloid (grindeline), flavonoids (luteolol, quercetol, kaempferol-3-methylether, kaempferol-3,7-dimethylether, and various quercetin-methyl-ethers: quercetin-3-methyl-ether and 6-OH-kaempferol-3,6-dimethylether), tannins (hydrolysable), triterpenoid saponins (grindelia sapogenin D, bayogenin and oleanolic acid are the sapogenins), phenolic acids (chlorogenic, *p*-hydrobenzoic, and *p*-coumaric acids), and laevoglucose.[1,3,12,16-18]

NUTRITIONAL PROPERTIES: Unknown.

MEDICINAL PROPERTIES: Anti-inflammatory, antitussive, astringent, bronchodilator, expectorant, diuretic, respiratory and urinary tract antibacterial, and vulnerary.

TEMPERATURE AND FLAVOR: Warm, pungent, bitter, and astringent.

MEDICINAL USES

Grindelia is an aromatic expectorant and antitussive. It aids in treating a dry, irritable cough or sore throat accompanying a cold, flu, laryngitis, bronchitis, hay fever, or whooping cough.[12,13,15-17] It contains aromatic resins that stimulate respiratory secretions.[16] Grindelia is also indicated for a moist cough or humid asthma aggravated by a cold, damp environment. As a long-term tonic, grindelia deepens respiration and reduces respiratory spasms; it also reduces wheezing, asthma, emphysema, and allergies that trigger lower respiratory spasms.[3] When treating an unproductive cough or difficulty breathing, combine grindelia extract with aralia *(Aralia)*, anise seed *(Pimpinella anisum)*, elecampane *(Inula)*, Senega snakeroot *(Polygala)*, thyme *(Thymus officinalis)*, and/or licorice root *(Glycyrrhiza)*. When treating acute and subacute lower respiratory infections, combine grindelia extract with other expectorant and antimicrobial herbs, such as aralia *(Aralia)*, balsam root *(Balsamorhiza)*, lomatium *(Lomatium)*, thyme *(Thymus)*, and/or usnea *(Usnea)*.

Ethanolic extracts of grindelia containing resins, polyphenols, and phenolic acids have been found to inhibit the growth of *Staphylococcus aureus* and *Bacillus subtilis*.[3] Grindelia contains saponins that have had fungistatic effects on *Candida tropicalis, Mucor mucedo, Trichoderma viride*, and *Botrytis cinerea*.[3] Essential oil of grindelia also inhibited the growth of *Penicillium expansum, Aspergillus flavus, Trichoderma viride, Phomopsis* spp., *Monilia fructigena*, and *Fusarium culmorum*.[3]

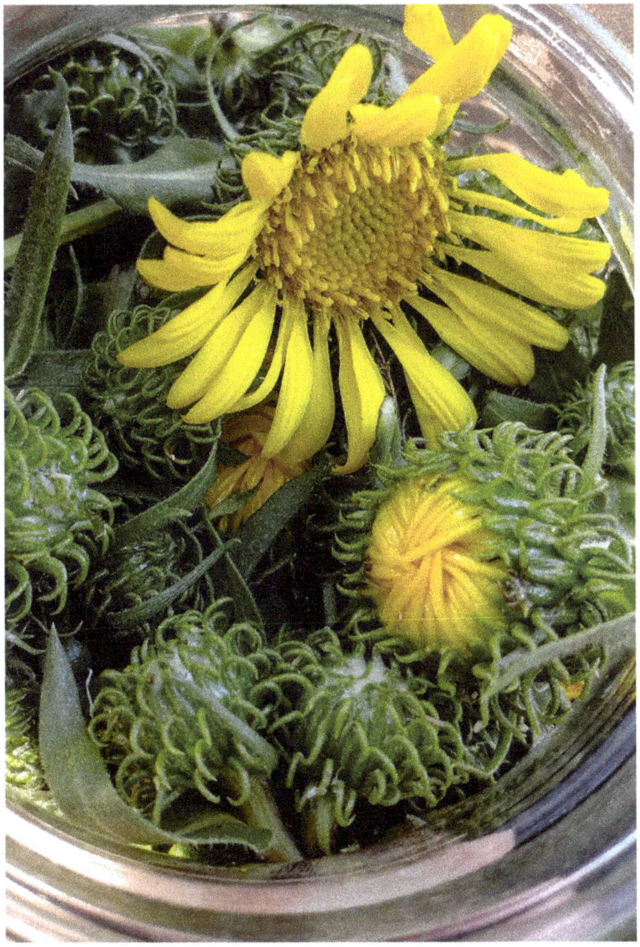

Grindelia extract and/or secondary metabolites demonstrated significant anti-inflammatory actions.[3] It inhibited the secretion of lipopolysaccharide (LPS)-induced secretion of inflammatory mediators, including IL-6, RANTES, MCP-1, and to a lesser degree, PGE(2) and TNF-α, as well as matrix metalloproteinase (MMP-1, -3, -7, -8, -9, and -13) secretion.[3] The flavonoids quercetin-3-methylether and 6-OH-kaempferl-3,6-dimethylether were attributed to the anti-inflammatory actions.[3] Essential oil of grindelia was found to have considerable antioxidant activity.[3]

Grindelia extract aids in treating slowly resolving bladder and urinary tract infections.[3,15,16] It contains aromatic resins excreted in the urinary tract that have antibacterial actions.[1] For this purpose, it combines effectively with extracts of yerba santa *(Eriodictyon)*, yerba mansa *(Anemopsis)*, usnea *(Usnea)*, and/or buchu *(Barosma)*.

Diluted alcoholic extract can be applied to burns, insect bites, sores, wounds, poison oak, or poison ivy.[12,13,15,16] For an all-purpose topical application, grindelia can be used interchangeably with calendula *(Calendula)* as an epithelial regenerative.[16] Grindelia also has mild antimicrobial and rubefacient actions.[16]

CONTRAINDICATIONS

Grindelia has the potential to irritate the urinary and digestive tracts when used in doses higher than recommended.[1,17] In rare circumstances, grindelia can cause allergic reactions in individuals with Asteraceae family allergies.

PREPARATION AND DOSAGE

TINCTURE: Fresh buds and flowering tops [1:2–1:3, 80–95% alcohol]; dry buds [1:5, 70% alcohol]; consume 15–60 drops, up to five times daily.

TEA: Presoak the buds, flowers, and leaves in alcohol prior to preparing tea. Prepare a hot infusion of the flowering tops; consume 8 ounces, up to four times daily.

TOPICAL USE: Prepare oil with the dry plant using the alcohol intermediary method. Dilute the tincture in water and apply as a liniment to the affected area.

GYMNEMA

DESCRIPTION

BOTANICAL NAME:
Gymnema sylvestre

COMMON NAMES:
Gurmar, gymnema, cowplant, Australian cowplant, periploca of the woods, small Indian ipecacuanha, miracle fruit, ram's horn
kharak (Arabic)
meshashrunga (Bengali)
waldschlinge (German)
gudmar (Gujarati)
gurmar (Hindi)
kawli (Konkani)
cakkarakkolli (Malayalam)
bedakicha pala (Marathi)
Lakshmi, mendhasingia, nagapushpi (Oriya)
madjunashini (Sanskrit)
cirukurinca, kokilam (Tamil)
podapatri (Telugu)
sa si nga, sa sri ngi (Urdu)[1]

FAMILY NAME:
Apocynaceae
(formerly Asclepiadaceae)

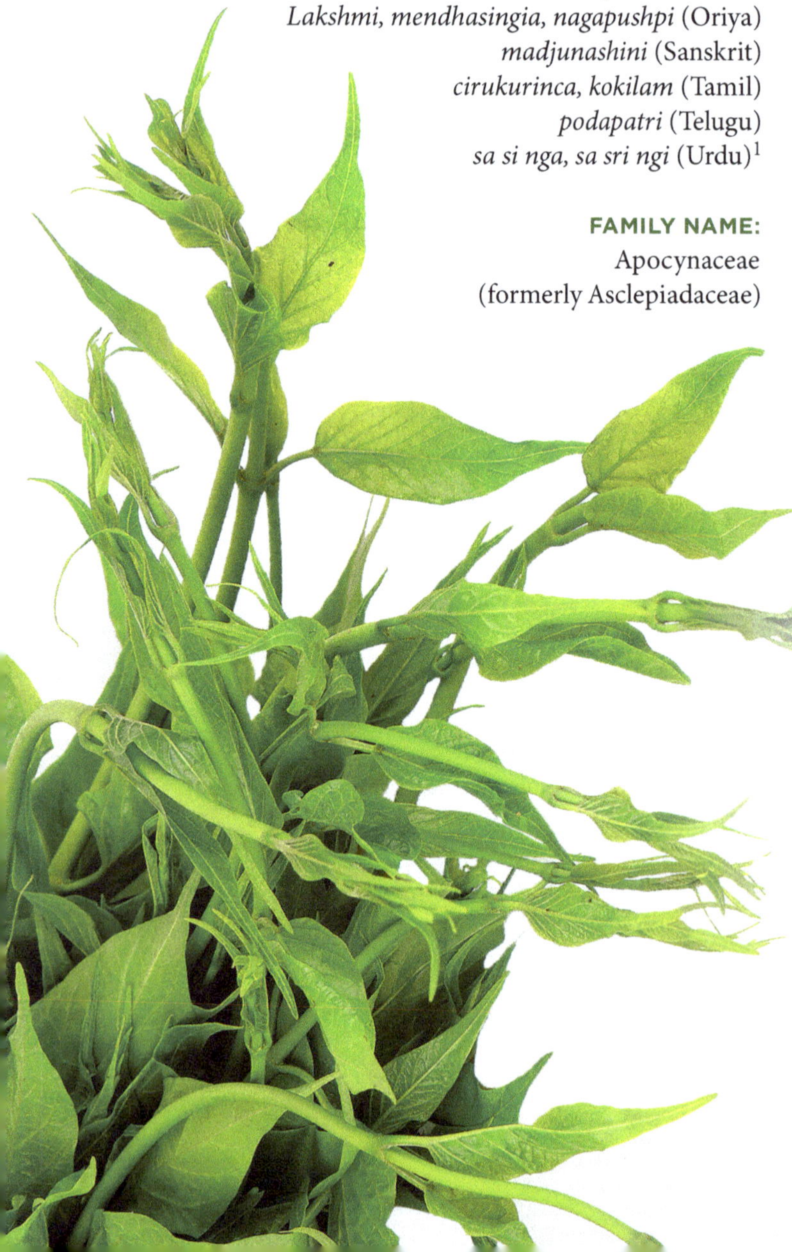

PART USED: The leaves.

BOTANICAL DESCRIPTION AND HABITAT: *Gymnema sylvestre* is a woody vine with stems growing up to 8 meters long. It grows in open woods at elevations of 100 – 1000 m in parts of southeastern China, southern India, Indonesia,

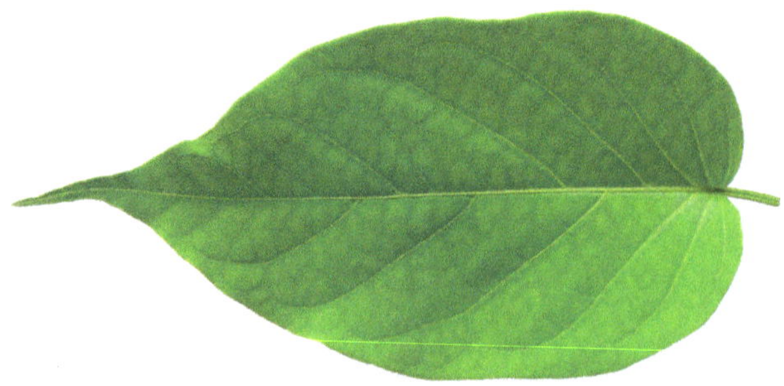

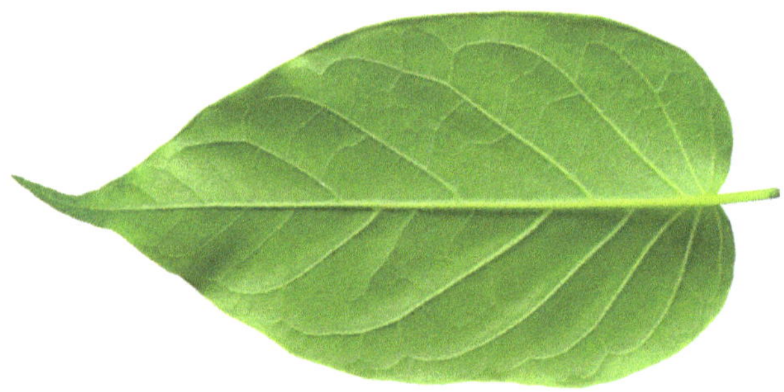

Japan, Malaysia, Sri Lanka, Vietnam, and tropical Africa.[2,3] The young branchlets are covered in thick brown hairs, and the stems exude milky latex when damaged.[3] Simple, opposite, papery ovate leaves (3 – 8.5 cm long by 1.5 – 5.5 cm wide) can be lightly hairy on the upper side and tomentose on the underside.[3] The four to five pairs of veins coalesce at the acute apex of the leaf.[3]

Short, hairy cymes bear inconspicuous, complex, yellow-green flowers.[3] Five ovate sepals covered in long hairs encircle the smooth, fused, five-lobed corolla.[3] Five fused stamens form a tube, and fuse at their bases to the petals and carpels.[4] Pollen is produced in two fused sacs in the anther (pollinia) that are part of the pollinarium, a complex structure involved in pollination.[4] The two carpels of the superior ovary are connected at their apices. They mature into long, conical, green follicles (5 – 9 cm long by 2 cm diameter) with acuminate beaks, sometimes found in pairs fused at their bases.[3] These follicles are filled with many ovate seeds surrounded by silky hairs.[3]

THE NAME: The genus *Gymnema* derives from two Greek words: *gymnos* ("naked") and *nēma* ("thread").[5,6] The epithet *sylvestre* derives from the Latin *sylva* ("wood"), referring to its forest habitat.[7] The common name gurmar means "sugar destroyer."

HISTORICAL USES: Gymnema has been used in India since antiquity for *prameha* (excessive urine) and *madhu meva* (sweet urine).[8] These traditional diagnoses are components of diabetes mellitus.[8] In order to treat diabetes in Tamil Nadu, southern India, gymnema was combined with navalkottai *(Syzygium cumini)* and Bermuda grass *(Cynodon dactylon)*.[9] The leaf powder was sometimes mixed with cow's milk and consumed. The leaf power also was utilized for joint pain, breathing problems, constipation, jaundice, and allergies due to insect bites.[9] The root powder was applied topically and taken internally for snakebites.[10] Central Indians also consumed it for stomach pain.[11]

The ability of gymnema to temporarily block the sense of sweet taste was known throughout India and East Africa.[12] *The British Medical Journal* (1890) reported that during a "Lady's Night" at the Royal Society of England, guests marveled over the plant's capacity for blocking this sense.[13]

CONSTITUENTS: Gymnema contains triterpene saponins (gymnemic acids including gymnemasaponins, gymnemasides, gymnemagenin, 23-hydroxylnogispinogenin, and gymnestrogenin), an alkaloid (gymnamine), a polypeptide (gurmarin), biogenic amines and amino acids (including gamma-aminobutyric acid = GABA), anthraquinones, flavones, hentriacontane, pentatriacontane, phytin, resins, acids (tartaric, formic, and butyric), lupeol, β-amyrin related glycosides, stigmasterol, gymnemanol, D-quercitol, hydroxycinnamic acids, coumarols, and calcium oxalate.[14,15]

NUTRITIONAL PROPERTIES: Gymnema contains calcium oxalate, betaine, and choline.

MEDICINAL PROPERTIES: Antidiabetic, astringent (mild), bitter tonic, cholagogue, diuretic, hypocholesterolemic, hypoglycemic, and stomachic.

TEMPERATURE AND FLAVOR: Cool, bitter, and astringent (mild).

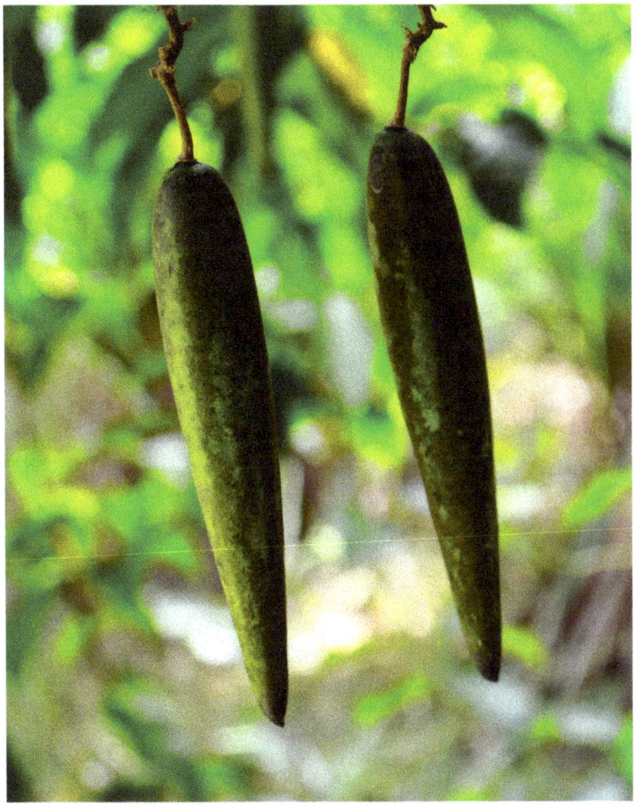

MEDICINAL USES

Gymnema has diverse therapeutic applications for type I and type II diabetes mellitus, as it positively affects blood sugar metabolism, decreases sugar cravings, and may support pancreas healing.[14,16,17] It aids in regulating blood glucose levels and enhancing glucose tolerance.[16,17] Gymnema appears to improve cellular responsiveness to insulin.[17] It also increases endogenous insulin production, possibly by stimulating the regeneration of pancreatic β-cells (insulin-producing cells).[14,16,17] Supporting this proposed mechanism, one study confirmed that it had no effect on diabetic dogs and rabbits with their pancreas removed.[17] Studies of type I and type II diabetic human subjects also appear to support this conclusion.[17] Gymnema extract does not produce a hypoglycemic effect in healthy individuals.[17]

Type II diabetics can consume gymnema to lower elevated blood glucose levels, aid in blood glucose regulation, and reduce sugar cravings.[15] Gymnema can considerably reduce the need for oral hypoglycemic drugs in type II diabetics.[17] In one study, 22 type II diabetics were treated with 400 mg of gymnema extract daily while they continued to consume oral hypoglycemic drugs. All of the patients experienced enhanced blood sugar control; all but one subject considerably reduced their medication dosage, and five subjects discontinued their medication and

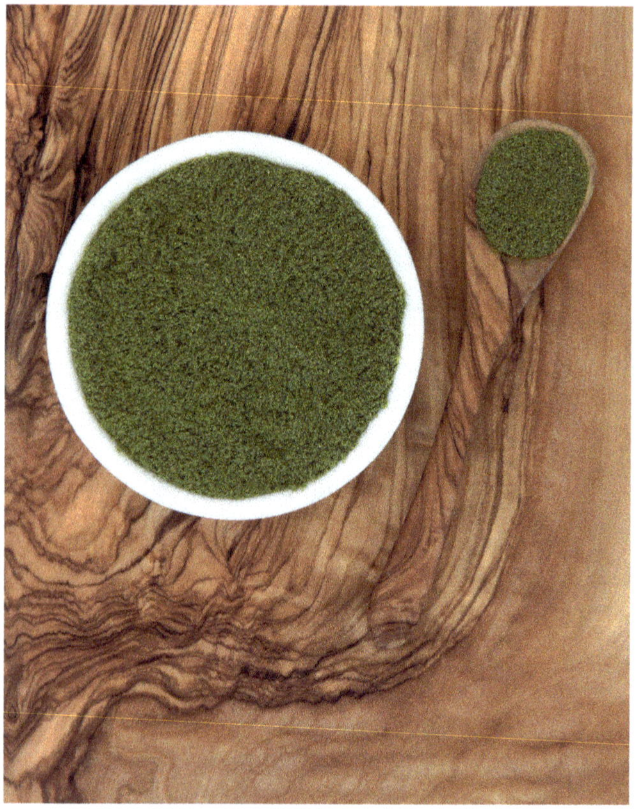

maintained their blood sugar levels solely with gymnema extract.[17]

Type I diabetics may benefit from including gymnema in their regimen. A dosage of 400 mg of gymnema extract was administered daily to 27 type I diabetics already medicated with insulin injections. It reduced insulin requirements and fasting blood sugar levels, and enhanced blood sugar control.[17]

An effective combination for hyperglycemic patients that reduces sugar cravings and stabilizes blood sugar levels includes: gymnema, fenugreek seeds *(Trigonella)*, bitter gourd *(Momordica)*, cinnamon bark *(Cinnamomum)*, Asian ginseng (*Panax ginseng*), and devil's club (*Oplopanax*). In Ayurvedic medicine, gymnema is combined with turmeric *(Curcuma)*, bitter gourd, also known as karella *(Momordica)*, fenugreek seeds *(Trigonella)*, and black pepper *(Piper nigrum)* to normalize blood sugar levels.[16] It is also compounded with guduchi *(Tinospora)*, kutki (*Picrorrhiza*), and gokshura *(Tribulus terrestris)* in order to regulate blood sugar levels and clear kapha.[16]

Applied to the tongue, gymnema aids in controlling sugar cravings by temporarily blocking the capacity to taste sweetness.[17] This effect is due to saponins (such as gymnemic acid), as well as gurmarin, the polypeptide.[14,15] The gymnemic acid fills the sugar taste receptors in the tongue, blocking activation of these receptors by sugar molecules in food.[14] However, it does not block salt and acid tastes.[15] Gurmarin also prevents the taste buds from distinguishing sweet from bitter.[14] Due to these actions, gymnema is an adjunct for enhancing weight loss. A diuretic, it also improves the loss of water weight.[16]

Gymnema stimulates upper and lower digestive secretions, including hydrochloric acid, pancreatic, and gallbladder secretions. Animal studies utilizing gymnemic acid preparations demonstrated significant reductions in serum triglycerides, overall cholesterol, LDL cholesterol, and V-LDL cholesterol; HDL cholesterol increased.[14] *In vitro* studies suggest that gymnema has a hepatoprotective effect.[14] Antiarthritic and anti-inflammatory effects were demonstrated in animal studies in which gymnema potentially protected joint cartilage, prevented bone destruction, and reduced swelling.[14]

Studies showed significant antimicrobial activity against bacteria and other microbes that cause tooth decay *(S. aureus, S. mitis, S. mutans, Candida albicans)* when gymnema extracts were applied topically to dental infections.[14] Gymnema extracts also were effective against *E. coli, P. aeruginosa, B. cereus, B. pumilus,* and *B. subtilis.*[14]

CONTRAINDICATIONS

Individuals medicated for type I or type II diabetes should consult with a health care practitioner, as the medication dosage may need adjustment.[16] Gymnema can stimulate the heart; patients with a rapid heartbeat or hypertension should exercise caution and consult a health care practitioner before using it.[16]

PREPARATION AND DOSAGE

TINCTURE: Fresh herb [1:2, 70-95% alcohol]; dry herb [1:5, 60% alcohol]; consume 15-60 drops, up to three times daily.

CAPSULES: Consume 1-2 capsules (300 mg per capsule), up to three times daily.

TEA: Prepare a hot infusion; consume 8-12 ounces, up to three times daily.

HAWTHORN

DESCRIPTION

BOTANICAL NAMES:
Crataegus laevigata (syn. *C. oxyacantha*), *C. monogyna*

COMMON NAMES:
Hawthorn, common hawthorn, English hawthorn, single-seeded hawthorn, May thorn, May blossom, May bush, May Day flower, quick thorn, quickset, white thorn, haw, hazels, gazels, halves, hagthorn, Ladies' meat, bread and cheese tree, chucky cheese, chastity tree, pixie pears, cuckoo's beads
pyöröliuskaorapihlaja (Finnish)
lépine noble (French)
hagedorn, weissdorn, zweigriffeliger (German)
biancospino (Italian)
sansa (Japanese)
sanza (Korean)
shan zha (Mandarin)
ban-sangli (Sanksrit)
espino (Spanish)
hagtorn, rundhagtorn (Swedish)[1]

FAMILY NAME:
Rosaceae

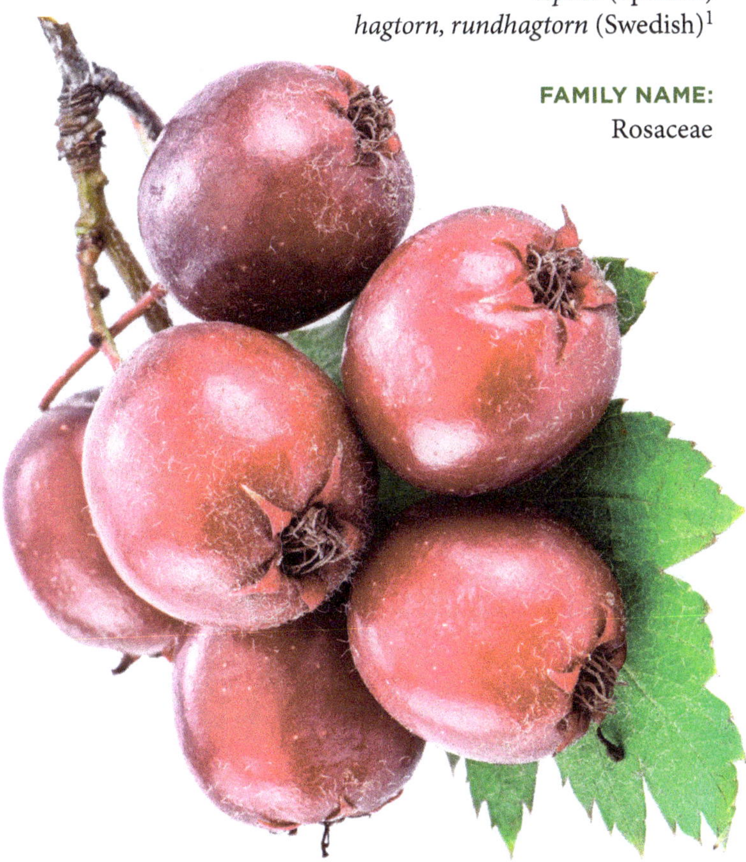

PARTS USED: The fruits (berries), flowers, and leaves.

BOTANICAL DESCRIPTION AND HABITAT: Hawthorn is a small tree or shrub native to the northern temperate regions of Europe, North America, Africa, and Asia.

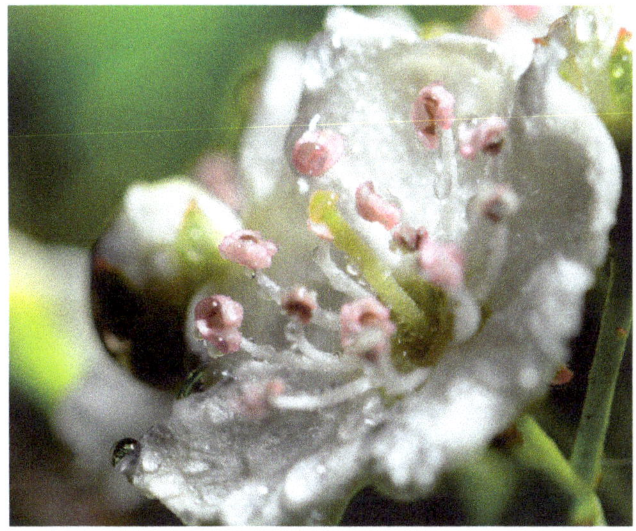

Crataegus monogyna has been naturalized throughout North America, South Africa, and Australia, and is sometimes considered invasive. *C. laevigata* is native to central Europe. Hawthorn grows in the moist soil of wooded areas, and can be planted as a decorative tree or hedge.

Crataegus is a large genus of about 200 species of long-living, deciduous trees and shrubs.[2,3] In the United Kingdom, a specimen of *C. monogyna* is known as the "Hethel Old Thorn." It is at least 700 years old, and is considered Europe's oldest living tree.[4] Thorny branches produce alternate, simple, stipulate leaves with a serrate margin that is usually lobed, though the leaves of some native California species are not lobed.[3,5]

Corymbose racemes at the branch tips bear showy flowers with a cup- or urn-shaped hypanthium that lack the bractlets of other rose family species.[3,5] Each flower has five sepals that reflex as they mature, five white or pinkish petals, 5 – 25 stamens, an inferior ovary with one to five connate carpels, and one to five styles.[3,5] The ovary produces a drupe-like pome, usually red, but sometimes yellow or dark purple, with one to five seeds, and a persistent calyx at the

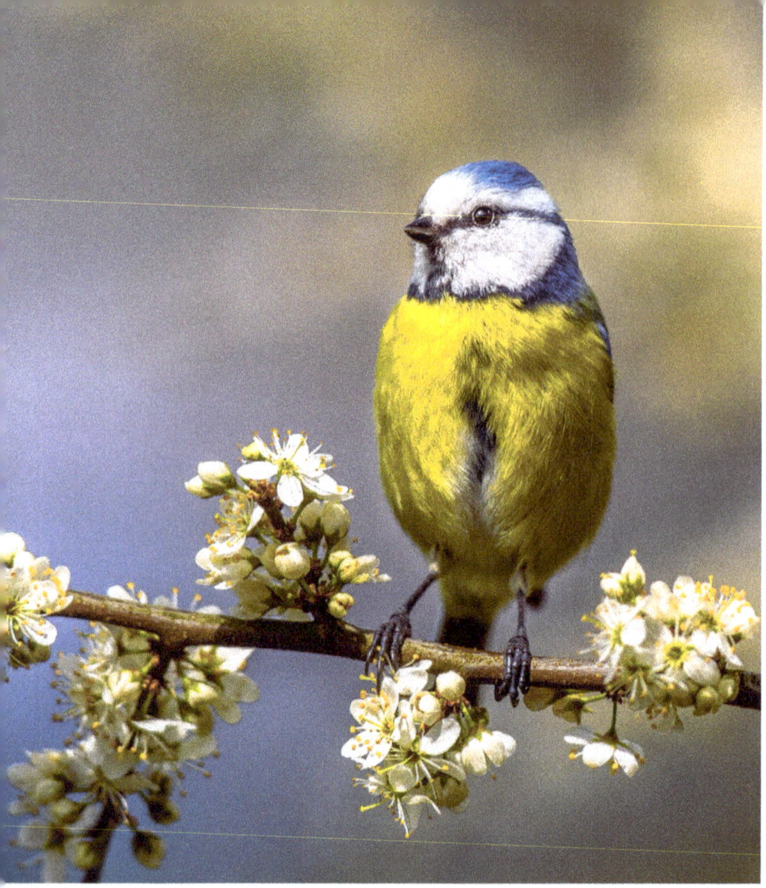

apex.[3,5] Reminiscent of decaying flesh, the aroma emitted by the flowers attracts pollinating carrion insects.[1]

Crataegus monogyna grows 2 – 10 meters tall with leaves that have deep, tripartite lobes pointing outward (2 – 5 cm long and wide).[6] The flower has white petals, one carpel, and one style, and produces a red, globose pome (6 – 11 mm diameter) with a single seed.[6,7]

Crataegus laevigata is similar to *C. monogyna;* the two species often hybridize.[7] It reaches 6 – 8 meters tall and wide, and differs from *C. monogyna* in that its leaves are only shallowly lobed, and the lobes point forward.[8,9] The flowers have white or pink petals, 20 stamens, and two or three styles. They produce a round or cylindric, red pome (6 – 14 mm diameter) with two to three seeds.[8]

THE NAME: The botanical name for *Crataegus* derives from the Greek *kratus* ("hard"), referring to the dense quality of the wood.[1] The epithet *laevigata* means smooth, slippery, lustrous, or shiny.[10] The former epithet, *oxyacantha,* derives from two Greek words: *oxus* ("sharp") and *akantha* ("thorn").[1] The epithet *monogyna* derives from two Latin words: *mono* ("one") and *gyna* ("seed"). There are two possible origins of the common name hawthorn. The first is a corruption of the German *hagedorn* ("hedgethorn"), because it was a dense shrub that formed thickets dividing plots of land in Germany. However, the *Merriam Webster Dictionary* states that hawthorn derives from the Old English *hagathorn,* a combination of *haga* ("hedge") and *thorn* ("thorn"). Haw was the name for a hedge, though it now also refers to the hawthorn berry; it is sometimes borrowed to describe other small fruits, such as black haw *(Viburnum prunifolium).*[1] The name quickset ("formed of living plants") refers to the origin of the word quick ("living, alive, animate"), and describes a hedge that is a living fence.[1,11,12] The common name whitethorn refers to the light-colored bark.

HISTORICAL USES: Since ancient times, hawthorn was used medicinally and for protection. Romans fastened sprigs of hawthorn to cradles in order to protect babies against evil.[13] The branches were hung over doorways to ward off evil spirits in medieval times. Hawthorn branches were believed to be the sources of Christ's crown of thorns, and the tree is often associated with the Virgin Mary and Christ.[1] Hawthorn wood was considered the hottest burning fuel, preferred over oak.[1] The root wood was used to make boxes and combs.[1] The dried fruits were consumed to treat scurvy.[14] The berries and flowers were gargled to treat a sore throat.[1] Hawthorn leaves were used as an adulterant for black tea.[1] Preparations of the fruits, flowers, and leaves were consumed as a cardiotonic and diuretic.[14]

Eclectic physicians administered hawthorn as a heart tonic and restorative to treat various forms of heart disease, including: angina pectoris, valvular deficiency, endocarditis, myocarditis, pericarditis, tachycardia, rheumatic heart, enlarged heart, mitral insufficiency, and cardiac neuralgia.[15] It also treated palpitations, dropsy, and vertigo.[15] Dr. Jennings administered hawthorn fluid extract to successfully treat albuminuria or Bright's disease, as well as diabetes mellitus and diabetes insipidus.[15] In the 1800s, Dr. Clement believed his experiments confirmed that hawthorn helped to dissolve calcareous deposits in arterial lumen.[15] Dr. Ellingwood stated that hawthorn "dispels gloomy forebodings, increases strength, regulates the action of the heart, and causes a general sense of well being." He administered hawthorn for general curative effects in the nervous system.[15] The fruit, bark, and leaves were used as astringents.

Native American tribes utilized hawthorn to treat general debility, a stomachache, and female concerns, as well as a diuretic for kidney or bladder problems.[14,16] Black hawthorn bark *(C. douglasii)* was administered to strengthen the heart, thin the blood, reduce swelling, and treat venereal disease.[17] Black hawthorn thorns were used as rake prongs to catch herring, and as lances for probing skin blisters and boils, and piercing ears.[17] The dense wood of black hawthorn was used for making tool and weapon handles.[17] The fresh and dried fruit were consumed by numerous coastal tribes.[17]

CONSTITUENTS: Hawthorn leaves and flowers are rich in flavonoids (hyperoside = hyperin = quercetin-3-D-galactoside; quercetin-3-rhamnogalactoside = quercetrin; quercetin; vitexin = apigenin-3-C-glucoside; vitexin-2'-O-rhamnoside; acetylvitexin-2'-O-rhamnoside, vitexin-4'-L-rhamno-D-glucoside, vitexin-4'-L-rhamnoside, vitexin-4'-7-di-D-glucoside, luteolin, luteolin-3,7-diglucoside, rutin, and others). They also contain oligomeric proanthocyanidins = OPCs (procyanidin B-2, (+)-catechin, and (-)-epicatechin), triterpenes (oleanolic acid, ursolic acid, acantolic acid, neotegolic acid, and 2-α-hydroxyoleanolic acid = crataegolic acid), amines (dimethylamine, guanine, trimethylamine, isobutylamine, isoamylamine, ethanolamine, β-phenylethylamine, choline, acetylcholine, O-methoxyphenylethylamine, tyramine, adenine, adenosine, and others), β-sitosterol, chlorogenic acid, caffeic acid, amygdalin, pectin, fructose, traces of volatile oil (benzaldehyde, 4-methoxybenzaldehyde, and methyl 4-methoxybenzoate = methyl anisate), and ascorbic acid (vitamin C).[14,18-20,23]

Hawthorn fruits contain flavonoids (hyperoside = hyperin = quercetin-3-D-galactoside, flavone glycosides, C-glycoside, vitexin = apigenin-3-C-glucoside, vitexin-2'-O-rhamnoside, vitexin-4'-rhamnoside, luteolin, and kaemperfol), oligomeric procyanidins = OPCs ((+)-catechin, (-)-epicatechin), polymeric procyanidins, triterpene acids (oleonolic and crategolic acids), ascorbic acid, citric acid, chlorogenic acid, oxalic acid, palmitic acid, pectin, betulin, aesculin, and daucosterol. The fruits also contain cardiotonic amines (phenylethylamine, O-methoxyphenylethylamine, and tyramine), acetylcholine, choline, and purine derivatives (adenosine, adenine, guanine, and caffeic acids).[14,16,18-21]

The most biologically active substances in hawthorn are the flavonoids and procyanidins. The flavonoid levels are highest in the flowers (1.31%), and the OPC levels are highest in the unripe, green berries (3.18%) and spring leaves (3.02%) as the flowers bloom.[23] Compared to the leaves and flowers, the fruits contain lower levels of flavonoids (0.15% in unripe berries and 0.13% in ripe berries) consisting primarily of oligomeric and polymeric procyanidins.[18] *Note:* The terms oligomeric proanthocyanidins, oligomeric procyanidins, procyanidins, procyanidolic oligomers (PCOs), and condensed tannins are synonymous.

Throughout Europe and the U.S., the fruits were used medicinally for hundreds of years. They contain many of the same constituents as the flowers and leaves, but in lower concentrations. Preparations using the flowers and leaves are the subjects of the most recent clinical trials.

NUTRITIONAL PROPERTIES: Hawthorn berry has large amounts of flavonoids and chromium. It contains low to average amounts of aluminum, β-carotene, calcium, cobalt, fiber, glucose, iron, magnesium, manganese, niacin phosphorus, potassium, protein, selenium, silicon, sodium, starch, zinc, and vitamins A, B_1, B_2, and C.[14,22]

MEDICINAL PROPERTIES: Antiarrhythmic, anti-inflammatory, antioxidant, astringent (mild), cardioprotective, cardiotonic, circulatory stimulant, collagen stabilizer, connective tissue stimulant, hypocholesterolemic, hypotensive, vasodilator, vascular tonic, nervine, and shen tonic.

TEMPERATURE AND FLAVOR: The berries are warm, sweet, sour, and salty. The flowers and leaves are neutral, sweet, and astringent.

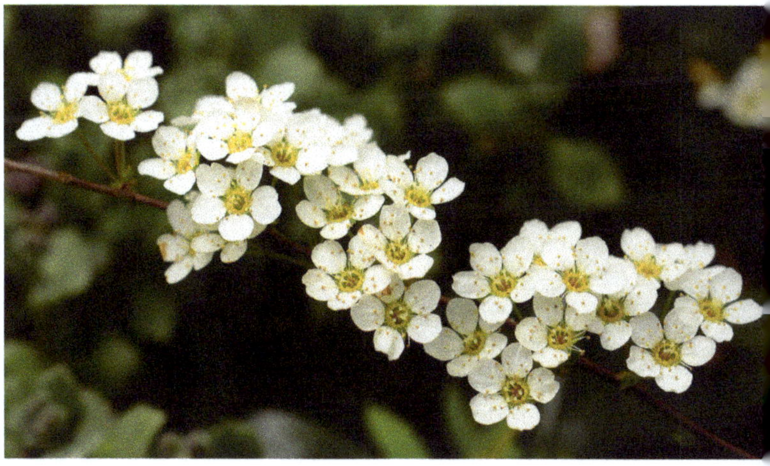

MEDICINAL USES

Hawthorn is a cardiotonic, peripheral vasodilator, and carrier.[14,15,23,24] It supports a poorly functioning, tired, or aging heart, and prevents degenerative, age-related changes in the myocardium.[24,25] Hawthorn flowers and leaves dilate the coronary artery and enhance myocardial perfusion, in addition to improving cardiac performance and output.[14,18,20,24,25] Increasing oxygenation of the heart decreases the potential for angina attacks and hypoxemia.[25] Hawthorn does not have an instant effect on the heart muscle; because it increases intercellular calcium levels, it is slow acting.[25] Consume hawthorn at least two months for optimal results in treating coronary disease.[25]

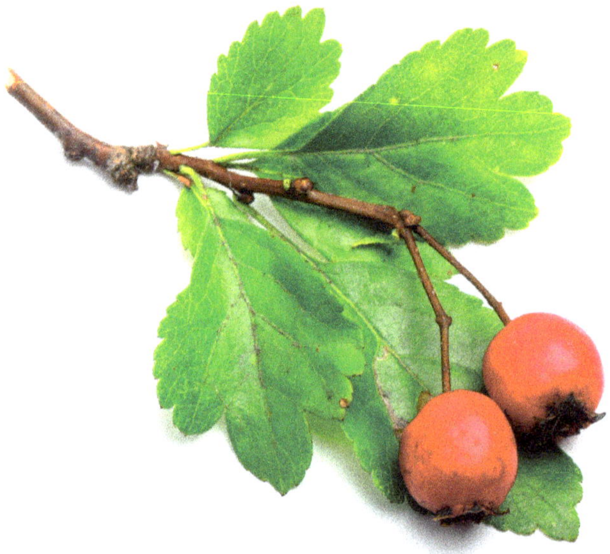

Hawthorn aids in treating numerous heart conditions, including: angina pectoris, cardiac neuralgia, early stages of congestive heart failure, heart murmurs, palpitations, tachycardia, and pericarditis.[13,15,20,24] It strengthens cardiac function by increasing cardiac muscle contractility (positively inotropic) and conductivity (positively dromotropic), and decreasing excitability (negatively bathmotropic), and heart rate (negatively chronotropic).[13,14,18,20,24,25] The crataegolic and ursolic acid increase coronary flow; crataegolic acid is positively inotropic.[24] Vitexin-4'-O-rhamnoside demonstrates positively inotropic and negatively chronotropic effects.[24] Hawthorn stimulates revascularization following myocardial ischemia, and hastens cardiovascular restoration following a myocardial infarction (heart attack).[14,24] Studies demonstrate that hawthorn improves heart function, and alleviates shortness of breath and fatigue in patients with congestive heart failure.[13] It also relieves a sense of pain, pressure, or oppression in the cardiac region by increasing oxygen delivery to the heart.[13,15,18,23] The cardiotonic actions are attributed to the flavonoids (O-glycosides: luteolin-O-glucoside, hyperoside, and rutin; and C-glycosides: vitexin, vitexin-2'-rhamnoside, and monoacetyl-vitexin-rehamnoside), oligomeric procyanidins, and (-)-epicatechin.[14,24,25]

Hawthorn normalizes the heartbeat and aids in treating cardiac arrhythmias (irregular heartbeat), extra systoles, heart murmurs, paroxysmal tachycardia, and tachycardiac attacks.[13-15,20,23-25] It strengthens the heart valves and enhances valvular function, treating heart murmur and arrhythmia with mild valvular trouble.[15,23] Hawthorn slows a rapid heartbeat and decreases palpitations caused by stress or anxiety. It works most effectively when consumed long-term by individuals with valvular insufficiency or palpitations. Hawthorn supports the myocardium following infectious diseases, including influenza, pneumonia, diphtheria, scarlet fever, or streptococcal infections.[25] It also has antibacterial actions against *Escherichia coli, Shigella flexneri, S. sonnei, and Proteus vulgaris.*[14] Intravenous injections of aqueous hawthorn extract are used to stop paroxysmal tachycardia.[25]

Hawthorn reduces heart strain and calms an overexcited nervous system.[15,23] It enhances respiration, and aids in treating dyspnea (difficulty breathing) and persistent sighing caused by extreme nervous tension or exhaustion.[15,23] Hawthorn has very mild nervine and sedative properties, as well as shen tonifying actions.[20] In Traditional Chinese Medicine, shen is the spirit residing in the heart. Symptoms of disturbed shen include anxiety, palpitations, insomnia, dream-disturbed sleep, and restlessness. Consuming hawthorn long-term calms shen and treats stress-related heart issues such as palpitations.[18] Combine hawthorn with bugleweed *(Lycopus),* motherwort *(Leonurus),* lemon balm *(Melissa),* and wild oats *(Avena)* to treat anxiety and palpitations.

Low doses of hawthorn (5–10 drops of fluid extract) aid in treating mild forms of bradycardia (slow heart rate) and bradycardiac arrhythmia.[25] It is best to try this herb alone in lower doses to confirm that it doesn't further lower the pulse. Individuals with bradycardia usually find that it strengthens the pulse, gently increases the heart rate, and improves circulation. However, some hypotensive individuals may find that hawthorn further lowers their pulse rate, and causes dizziness when standing. If this occurs, discontinue use or lower the dose.

Hawthorn is a subtle hypotensive agent that aids in treating mild to moderate hypertension.[24] It helps to maintain a healthy heart muscle when hypertension is present.[14,24] Hawthorn is a less potent hypotensive agent than mistletoe or rauwolfia; however, it increases cardiac function, aiding in normalizing blood pressure.[14,24] Oligomeric procyanidins (OPCs) prevent the conversion of angiotensin I to angiotensin II in the heart by inhibiting the angiotensin-converting enzyme (ACE).[18,19,24] Angiotensin II is a potent vasoconstrictor that elevates blood pressure. Numerous clinical studies used a concentrated hawthorn leaf and flower extract (with a 3:1 or 5:1 ratio, standardized to 2.2% flavonoids or 18.75% OPC) administered to subjects with heart disease in daily doses of 180–900 mg.[24] These studies revealed that hawthorn extracts reduced the heart workload, decreased systolic and diastolic blood pressure, reduced heart rate and pressure rate, decreased shortness of breath, reduced ankle edema, and increased performance.[24] The extracts also decreased total cholesterol levels, and reduced cardiac arrhythmias and tachycardia.[24] Hawthorn berry extract exerted blood pressure lowering effects, reducing mean systolic pressure from 205 mmHg to 148 mmHg, and mean diastolic pressure from 112 mmHg to 83 mmHg.[24]

Hawthorn is a supportive therapy for treating atherosclerosis and arteriosclerosis.[13,24] It has potent antioxidant effects attributed to OPCs, and flavonoids that protect against plaque formation in arterial walls, and decrease the size of existing atherosclerotic plaques.[13,19,24] The most active components are (-)-epi-catechin and procyanidin B-2.[24] Hawthorn has a cholesterol-lowering effect that treats diet-induced hypercholesterolemia.[19,24] Hawthorn lowers low density lipids (LDL) by enhancing their binding to liver plasma membranes and up-regulating hepatic LDL receptors. It also decreases hepatic cholesterol synthesis and increases bile acid secretion.[13,24] Additionally, it is a prophylactic treatment for diabetics prone to circulatory problems and atherosclerosis.

Hawthorn decreases peripheral vascular resistance, improving circulation and increasing oxygen and nutrient delivery to the tissues.[14,24] It contains flavonoids that dilate blood vessels.[13] Hawthorn can be beneficial for individuals with cold hands and feet due to poor circulation.[13] As a carrier, it is less likely to cause sensations of overheating, especially in individuals with excessive heat.

Hawthorn contains oligomeric procyanidins (OPCs) and flavonoids that stabilize collagen, a protein that maintains the integrity of tendons, joints, ligaments, cartilage, bones, skin, and vascular tissue.[19,24] OPCs and flavonoids enhance cross-linking between the polypeptide chains of collagen, reinforcing the collagen matrix of connective tissue, and increasing tensile strength.[19,24] Strengthening connective tissue hastens the healing of bruises, wounds, injuries, and surgeries. OPCs and flavonoids are potent antioxidants that reduce free radical damage. Flavonoids synergize with vitamin C by increasing intracellular vitamin C levels and stabilizing vitamin C.[19] OPCs and flavonoids also prevent and decrease the inflammatory response that destroys collagen. Hawthorn decreases inflammatory mediators such as prostaglandins, serine proteases, histamines, and leukotrienes.[19] The collagen-protecting actions aid in treating inflammatory conditions in the bones, joints, and cartilage, as well as rheumatoid arthritis and periodontal disease.[19] Long-term consumption of flavonoids decreases the accumulation of uric acid in the joints, preventing gout. OPCs and flavonoids also improve the integrity of the vasculature, and decrease capillary permeability and fragility.[19]

CONTRAINDICATIONS

There are no known contraindications or toxic effects from hawthorn; it is considered safe during pregnancy and lactation.[14,18,24,25] Individuals with chronic heart conditions should seek the care of a health care practitioner before combining hawthorn with heart medications.[24] Hawthorn may potentiate the effects of angiotensin converting enzyme (ACE) inhibitors, calcium channel blockers, and digitalis glycosides.[18,24,26] Therefore, it may be necessary to modify the drug dosage, although adverse effects from the interaction are not anticipated.[18,24] Hawthorn can potentially increase the coronary artery dilating effects of substances such as caffeine, theophylline (in tea), and papaverine (in opium-containing products).[18] Individuals with hypotension should consume only lower doses (5 – 15 drops) and proceed cautiously; discontinue use if it causes orthostatic hypotension (dizziness upon standing).

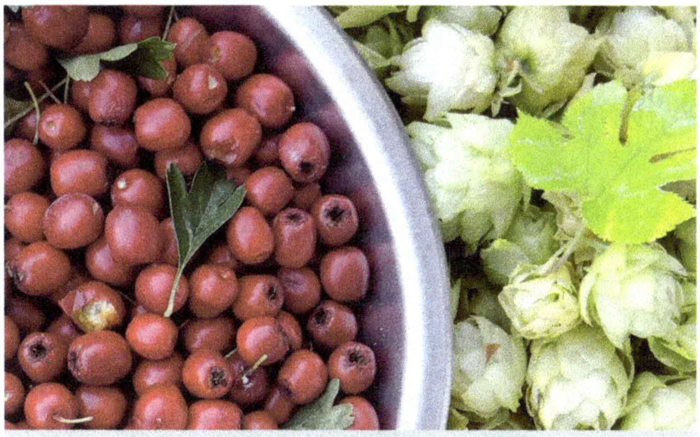

PREPARATION AND DOSAGE

TINCTURE: Fresh flowers and leaves, or berries [1:2, 70 - 95% alcohol]; dry flowers and leaves, or berries [1:5, 60% alcohol]; consume 30 - 120 drops, up to three times daily. Consume 160 - 900 mg daily of the standardized extract of the flowers and leaves (containing 1.8% vitexin-4′-rhamnoside or 20% OPCs).[18,19,24-26]

FLUID EXTRACT: Dry flowers and leaves, or berries [1:1, 25% alcohol]; consume 20 - 60 drops, up to three times daily.

CAPSULES: Consume 2 - 4 freeze-dried berry capsules, one to three times daily.

TEA: Prepare a hot or cold infusion of the flowers and leaves, or an infusion or decoction of the berries; consume 8 - 12 ounces, two to three times daily.

HOPS

DESCRIPTION

BOTANICAL NAMES:
Humulus lupulus, H. lupulus var. *neomexicanus* (syn. *H. americanus*)

COMMON NAMES:
Hops, European hops, common hops, hop plant, hoppe, luplin, lupulus, lupula
humula (Finnish)
houbloùn, houblon grimpant (French)
hopfen, houblon hopfenzapfen, hopfendrusen, zaunhapfen (German)
bruscandoli (Italian for hops shoots), *luppulo, lepone, livertizio, bruscandui, loertis, lòpal, lupari, lupiri, luvertin, orticaccio, reverdixe, ufe, urtizzòn, vartis* (Italian)
ch-ku-ts'aon (Mandarin)
hmel (Russian)
zarza, lúpudos (Castilian Spanish)
lupulo (Spanish)
humle (Swedish)[1-3]

FAMILY NAME:
Cannabaceae

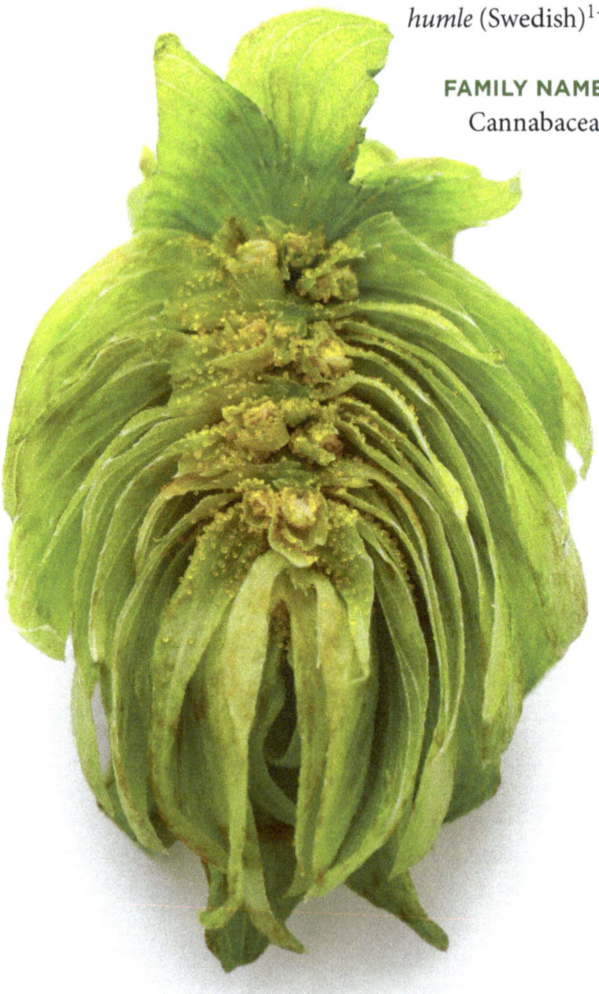

PARTS USED: The female fruits, known as strobiles. Harvest when the green strobiles feel firm and are covered with a yellow, powdery resin. The resin sifted from the strobiles, known as "lupulin" or "lupula," is considered a more potent form of medicine.

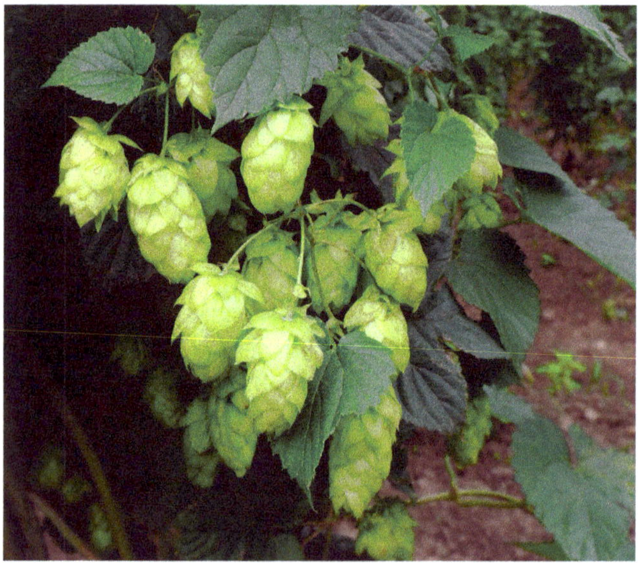

BOTANICAL DESCRIPTION AND HABITAT: Hops are a vining perennial native to Eurasia and North America. In Europe, hops grow wild in swamplands and along moist hedges. Hops are cultivated worldwide, most prominently in the U.S., Germany, and the Czech Republic.[4]

Hops form prolific intertwining vines with hairy stems (up to 6 meters long).[5] The coarse opposite leaves (6 – 12 cm wide) have three to five deeply rounded lobes with serrated margins.[6] Hops are dioecious. Male flowers are found in hanging panicles (7.5 – 10 cm across). Female flowers are held in pale green, cone-like catkins or strobiles (1 – 2 cm long) with papery bracts covering the flowers.[6,7] The strobile axis is studded with small glands bearing yellow, resinous crystals known as *glandulae lupuli* (lupulin). The organs of the creamy white male flowers grow in multiples of five. The perianth of the female flowers is fused into a tube surrounding a superior, unicarpellate ovary.[7,8] The single style divides into two feathery stigmas.[7] The fruit, yellow ovoid achenes, develop in the enlarged strobiles (2 – 6 cm long).[5]

THE NAME: The genus *Humulus* derives from the Latin *humus* ("soil"), referring to the rich, moist ground where the plant grows.[9] The epithet *lupulus* derives from the Latin *lupus* ("wolf"). According to Pliny the Elder, this refers to the stems that strangle shrubbery, similar to a wolf preying on sheep.[9] The common name hops originates from the Anglo-Saxon *hoppan* ("to climb"). The Spanish-speaking people of New Mexico refer to *H. lupulus* var. *neomexicanus (H. americanus)* as *zarza,* a word generically indicating a vine.[2] *Lúpudos* is an 18th century Castilian name for hops.[2]

HISTORICAL USES: The Saxons and Danish created ale liquor prepared from fermented malt. The name ale derives from the Scandinavian *ol,* the Viking's drink.[9] Ales were traditionally prepared with malt, or a mixture of honey, heath tops, ground ivy, and bitter or aromatic herbs (i.e., marjoram, costmary, buckbean, wormwood, yarrow, wood sage, germander, and broom).[9] Hops were not usually added to ale until the 9th century, when brewers included them for their flavor and preservative actions. Fermented beverages retained the name ale for many years after the introduction of hops. However, the German and Dutch only applied the name *bier* or *beer* to ales made with hops.[9] Later, hops were found to have antibacterial actions inhibiting the growth of less desirable microorganisms, and improving the shelf life of beer.

In the 9th and 10th centuries, French and German brewers introduced hops into beer, followed by the Dutch in the 14th century.[9,10] As other European countries incorporated hops into their brews, the British resisted using them until the 16th century, believing they would spoil the taste of traditional ales. In fact, Parliament argued against the use of hops, asserting that they were "a wicked weed that would spoil the taste of the drink and endanger the people."[9] During the reign of Henry VI, hops cultivation was banned in England. Henry VIII forbade brewers from using hops and sulphur in ale; eventually, Edward VI granted permission to cultivate hops.[9]

Hops were recommended as a tonic throughout Europe to treat painful joints, fevers, phlegm, and obstruction of the spleen. They were also administered as a diuretic for urinary stones, and as a sedative, nervine, and anthelmintic.[10] Additionally, hops were given to treat dyspepsia, flatulence, intestinal cramping, diarrhea, jaundice, hysteria, nervous heart conditions, and skin infections.[10] Alcohol-based extracts were used to treat leprosy, pulmonary tuberculosis, and acute bacterial infections.[11] Poultices were applied topically for neuralgia, bruises, and rheumatism.[11]

Native Americans used hops in numerous ways, such as for insomnia and pain.[10] They also brewed hops tea as a blood tonic, sedative, and hypnotic.[2] They prepared a bathing solution that included an infusion of two handfuls of hops to treat swollen limbs resulting from dropsy.[2] A similar bath preparation was made with hops, *coronillo (Gaillardia pinnatifida),* and *yerba del caballo (Senecio filifolius)* to treat rheumatism.[2] Indigenous New Mexican women used wild hops to raise bread.[2]

Hops were a popular remedy among Eclectic physicians. John Scudder recommended using hops as follows: "In cases of nervous irritability attended with wakefulness, hops are anodyne and hypnotic, and are frequently exhibited to alleviate pain, tranquilize the system and procure sleep. In delirium tremens, morbid vigilance, and nervous excitement, they frequently compose the nervous system."[12] He also recommended hopped ale as a tonic and stomachic. He suggested consuming lupulin for stomach or bowel spasms, afterbirth pains, and irritable states of the nervous system.[12] Finley Ellingwood recommended hops and lupulin "in cases of nerve irritation and wakefulness where anxiety and worry are the cause." He prescribed hops "where sexual irritation, spermatorrhoea, and dread of impotence are present, and where there is abnormal or erratic, and at times violent sexual excitement," as well as for "hysteria and in the sexual irritation of females."[13] Ellingwood also recommended applying a hot hops poultice to alleviate pain and encourage sleep, as well as for facial neuralgia, an ulcerated tooth, and children's earaches.[13] Harvey Felter offered similar recommendations, adding that hops would "check fermentation of the stomach contents and prove useful in fermentative dyspepsia with acid eructations." He also stated that hops would "relieve nervous excitability in fevers and induce sleep."[14] The Eclectics believed that the effects of lupulin superseded hops flowers as an internal medicine. More

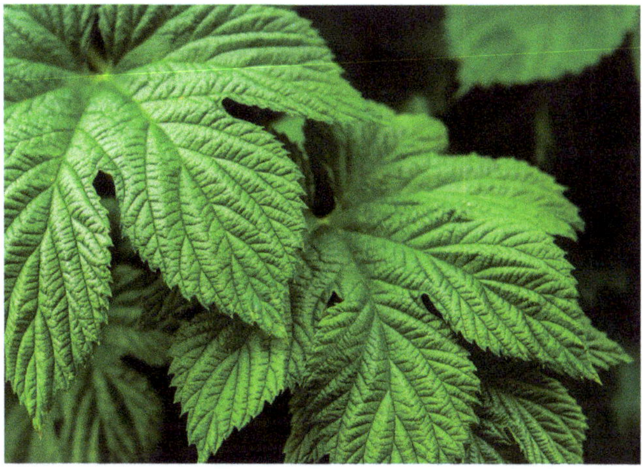

than $2.75 million of a popular patent medicine containing hops, dandelion, buchu, mandrake, and 30% alcohol was sold from 1880 to 1884. Its advertising slogan was "Take hop bitters three times a day, and you will have no doctor bills to pay."[15]

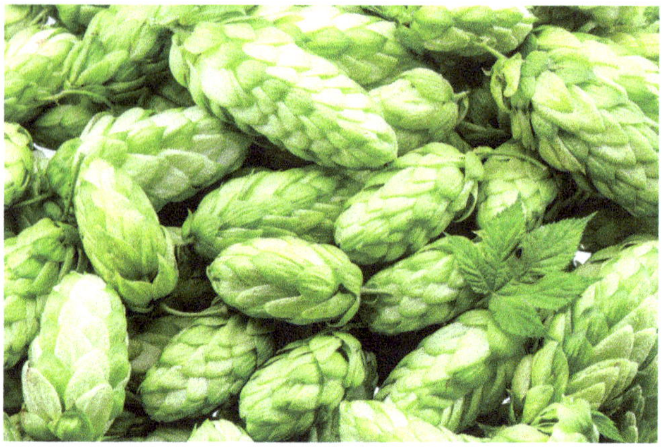

The stalks continue to be used in basket weaving and textiles, including string and yarn produced from the fibrous stems. Pulp made from the stems is used to make paper and cardboard.[16]

CONSTITUENTS: Hops contain a volatile oil consisting of humulene, α-caryophyllene, β-caryophyllene, myrcene, fanesene, lupulin, germacratriene, α- and β-selinenes, selina-3,7(11)-diene, selina-4(14), 7(11)-diene, α-copaene, α- and β-pinenes, limonene, *p*-cymene, linalool, nerol, geraniol, nerolidol, citral, methylnonyl ketone, 2,3,4-trithiapentane, S-methylthio-2-methylbutanoate, S-methylthio-4-methyl-pentananoate, and 4,5-epithiocaryophyllene. They also contain bitter principles composed of α-bitter acids (humulone, cohumulone, adhumulone, prehumulone, and posthumulone) and β-bitter acids (lupulone, colupulone, and adlupulone), resins (some are the oxidative byproducts of α- and β-acids), a chalcone (xanthohumulol), flavonoid glycosides (astragalin, quercitrin, isoquercitrin, rutin, and kaempferol-3-rutinoside), phenolic acids, tannins, lipids (small amounts of gamma-linoleic acid), amino acids, estrogenic substances (of undetermined structure), and numerous other compounds. Upon storage, the bitter acids humulone and lupulone are converted to isovaleric acid.[4,11,17-19]

NUTRITIONAL PROPERTIES: Hops contain high amounts of manganese, niacin, phosphorus, potassium, riboflavin, selenium, tin, and vitamin C. They contain average amounts of ash, calcium, carbohydrates, dietary fiber, fat, magnesium, protein, silicon, and thiamine. Hops also contain low amounts of chromium, cobalt, crude fiber, sodium, and vitamin A.[20]

MEDICINAL PROPERTIES: Antispasmodic, aromatic, bacteriostatic, bitter tonic, carminative, diuretic, fungistatic, hypnotic, nervine, sedative, soporific, stomachic, potential estrogenic, and mild astringent.

TEMPERATURE AND FLAVOR: Cool, bitter, pungent, and astringent.

MEDICINAL USES

Hops are a nervine and sedative that aid in treating insomnia, nervousness, restlessness, and anxiety.[4,10,19] The hypnotic and sedative effects are attributed to the volatile oil (humulene and 2-methyl-3-butene-2-ol) and bitter principles.[4,13] Lupulin, a volatile constituent, calms and soothes the nervous system.[7] The central nervous system depressant effects have been confirmed in animal studies.[7] Consuming 30 – 90 drops one-half hour before retiring is often sufficient to benefit from the sedative effects. Some individuals may notice that their dream state is intensified, and they experience more restful sleep. In order to synergize the sedative, analgesic, and antispasmodic effects, combine hops with equal parts of: valerian *(Valeriana),* California poppy *(Eschscholzia),* and passion flower (*Passiflora*).

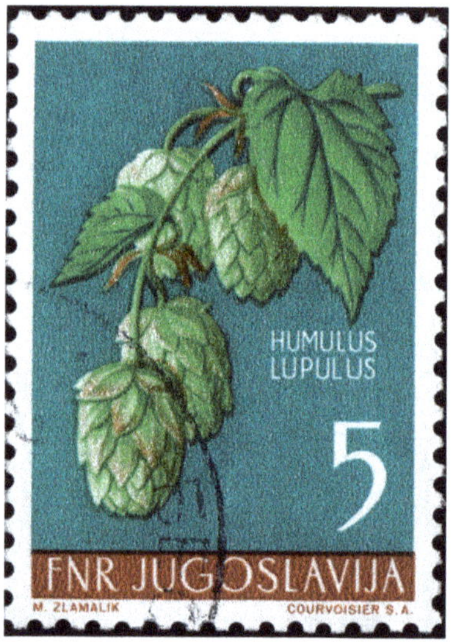

A hops-infused bath is an alternative to internal consumption. Prepare two quarts of a potent hops tea, strain, and pour into a hot bath as a sedative and relaxant. Two to three days prior to experimenting with this method, test for potential (but rare) allergenic dermatitis by applying hops tea or extract to the elbow crease. If a rash forms, avoid bathing in hops. Placing hops in an herb-stuffed pillow also helps to alleviate sleeplessness. If hops' aroma is too pungent, blend it with more pleasant smelling aromatic herbs such as lavender, chamomile, or roses.

Hops are a skeletal and smooth muscle antispasmodic.[4] The tea, tincture, or bath can help to relieve a tension headache or digestive-related headache, as well as neck, shoulder, and back tension. Hops are an excellent smooth muscle

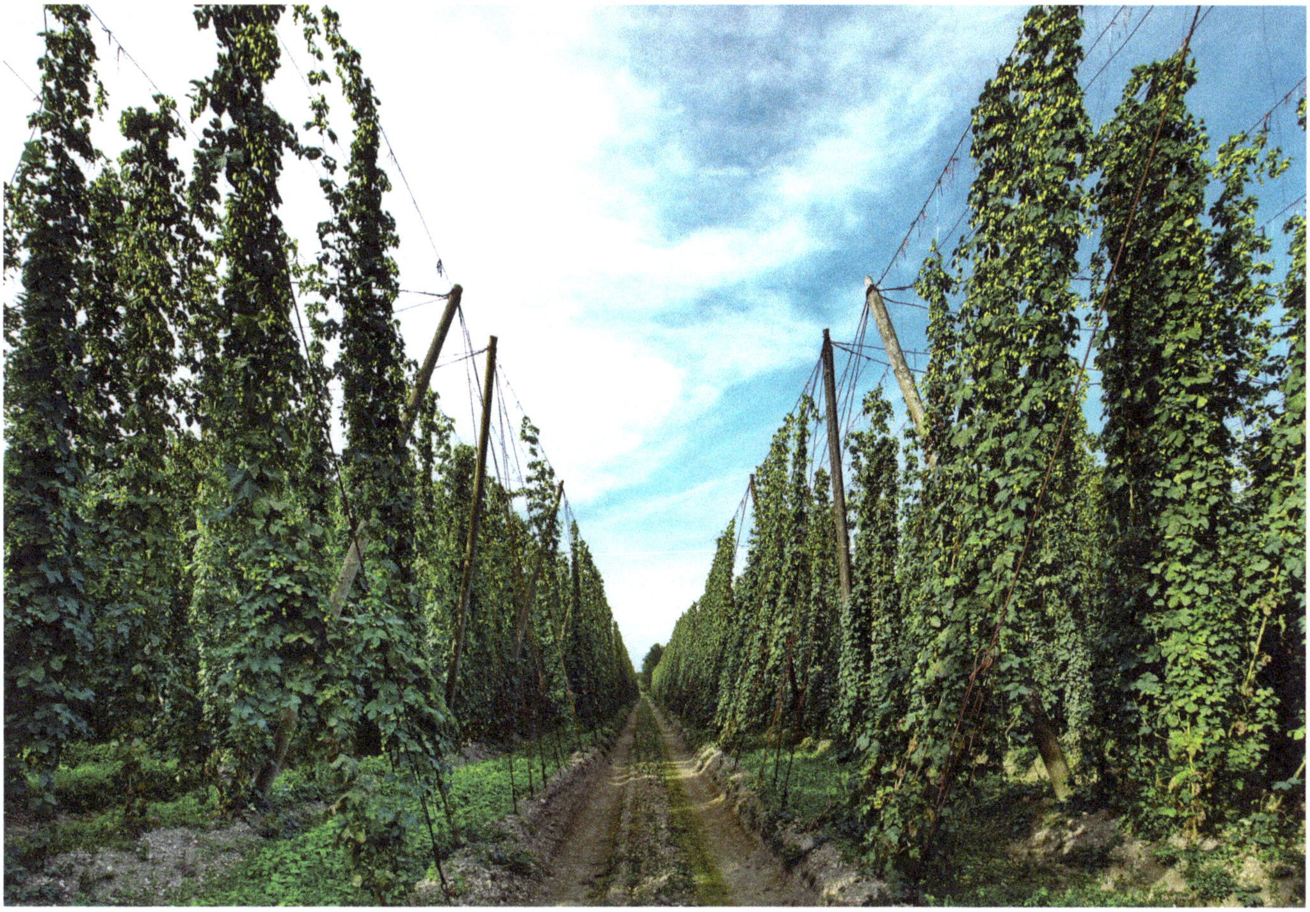

antispasmodic for treating digestive cramps and digestive conditions aggravated by stress, including Crohn's disease, colitis, and irritable bowel syndrome.[10,19] Additionally, hops reduce uterine cramping.[10] Scientific studies have confirmed the smooth muscle antispasmodic effects on the intestines and uterus.[10,11]

Hops have digestive bitter tonic properties that improve the appetite, stimulate gastric secretions, and increase the efficiency of digestion.[4,10,19] They also have carminative properties that reduce gas and bloating. Studies of rodents have confirmed the stimulating effects on gastric secretions.[4,10] The antibacterial properties of hops inhibit upper digestive infections.

Hops have galactagogue actions that enhance milk let-down and increase breast milk production.[21] They are especially helpful for women with delayed milk let-down as a result of a stressful birth. Hops can be consumed as a tincture, tea, or beer for the galactagogue actions. Some midwives recommend consuming a beer after birth to encourage milk let-down.

Hops demonstrate antioxytocic activity, and can be useful as an anaphrodisiac, especially for men.[11,19] They are considered specific for sleep problems caused by sexual excitement (nocturnal emissions, premature ejaculation, and hypersexuality).[19] Fresh hops also have an estrogen-mimetic effect that could contribute to the sexual suppressant effects in men, and perhaps gynecomastia in males who consume excessive amounts of beer.[19] Female hops harvesters have experienced menstrual cycle disruption and amenorrhea; young girls harvesting hops have started their menstrual periods early.[19] This may be attributed to the estrogenic effects of hops; however, the potential hormonal influences require a more thorough investigation.

Topical applications of hops (a poultice, fomentation, salve, or wash) aid in relieving sore muscles, neuralgia, rheumatic joints, sprains, strains, and bruises.[10] Apply the powdered herb or salve as an antifungal agent for athlete's foot, ringworm, or skin tinea, or as a mild antibacterial agent for wounds.[4] The antimicrobial actions are attributed to bitter acids (lupuline and humulene).[4,10,17]

CONTRAINDICATIONS

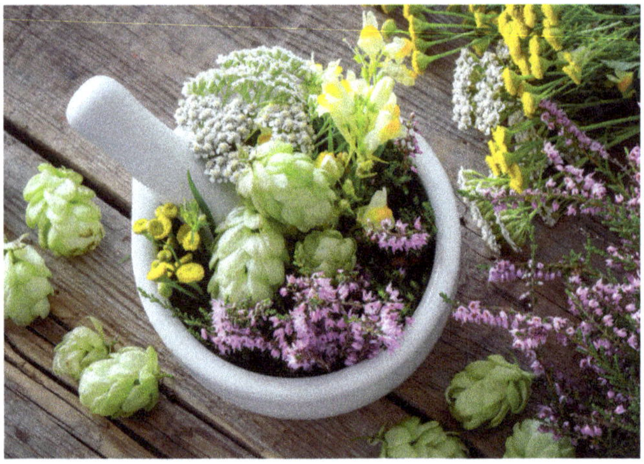

Avoid use during pregnancy.[17] Hops may have estrogenic effects when consumed long-term or in frequent high doses; exercise caution and limit use with estrogen-sensitive conditions. Consult a health care practitioner before combining hops with prescription sedatives, hypnotics, or antidepressants.[17] Hops are best avoided in depressed individuals, due to the sedative effects. They can interact with alcoholic beverages and increase phenobarbital-induced sleeping time.[1,17] In some individuals, hops pollen or leaf hairs have an allergenic effect causing contact dermatitis.[4] Avoid internal consumption or topical applications with allergic sensitivity. Otherwise, there are no reports of contraindications, side effects, or toxicity when used according to directions.[17]

Hops-containing beer has sedative and bitter tonic properties; however, beer also contains yeast, sugar, and fermented grains that can be difficult for some individuals to digest. Individuals with yeast or gluten sensitivities should avoid consuming beer; other medicinal preparations of hops suffice. Beer also has an initial sedative effect, but for some individuals, the starch content can cause nighttime awakening.

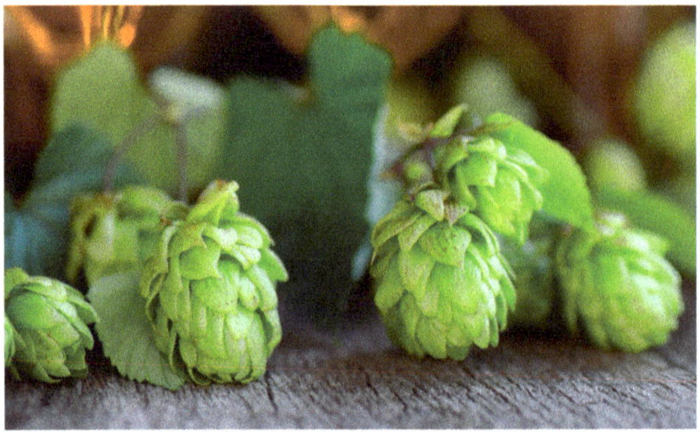

PREPARATION AND DOSAGE

TINCTURE: Fresh strobiles [1:3-1:4, 80-95% alcohol]; dry strobiles [1:5-1:8, 60% alcohol]; the ratio depends on the bulkiness, or prepare as a percolation to obtain the 1:5 ratio. Chopping the fresh herb or grinding the dried herb reduces the bulkiness, allowing for a lower ratio. Consume 15-90 drops, up to three times daily. *Note:* Freeze-dried hops are often higher quality than dried hops.

GLYCERITE: Fresh strobiles [1:4, 50% alcohol and 50% glycerin]; consume 15-60 drops, up to three times daily. The glycerite is easier for children to palate, although it is still bitter.

CAPSULES: Consume 2-4 "00" freeze-dried capsules, up to three times daily.

TEA: Prepare a hot or cold infusion; consume 4-8 ounces, up to four times daily. However, the flavor is very bitter and difficult to mask. The tea can be strained into a bath for children or adults, and the properties are absorbed through the skin.

HONEY AND SYRUP: Prepare fresh strobiles as an infused honey or syrup; add 20% alcohol to the total volume of syrup to increase the shelf life. Consume 1 teaspoon, one to two times daily. Refrigerate the syrup.

TOPICAL USE: Apply the hot poultice or fomentation. Powdered hops can be applied topically as an antimicrobial dust. Prepare medicinal oil using the alcohol intermediary or double boiler method; then apply as an oil or salve. Apply the tincture or glycerite of hops as a liniment.

CULINARY USE: Hops strobiles may be added to beer or herbal fermented beverages. The young spring shoots can be consumed as an asparagus substitute; avoid consuming mature shoots.[12]

HORSETAIL

BOTANICAL NAMES:
Equisetum arvense, E. fluviatile, E. hyemale, E. laevigatum, E. palustre, E. telmateia, E. variegatum

COMMON NAMES:
Field horsetail, shave grass, water horsetail, swamp horsetail, marsh horsetail, long slender horsetail, scouring rush, river horsetail, pipes, common scouring rush, smooth scouring rush, variegated scouring rush, giant horsetail, running club moss, pewterwort, bottlebrush, devil's guts, joint grass, toad pipes
maan chok (Cantonese)
akkerig paardestaart (Dutch)
equisitte, prêles, prêle des champs, prêle fluviatile, prêle panache (French)
ackerschtelhalm, kannenkraut, katzenschwanz, schafteu, zinnkraut (German)
asperella, coda di cavallo, equiseto palustre (Italian)
mokuzoku, tsukushi (Japanese)
mokchok (Korean)
mù zei (Mandarin)
cañutillo del llano (Spanish)

FAMILY NAME:
Equisetaceae

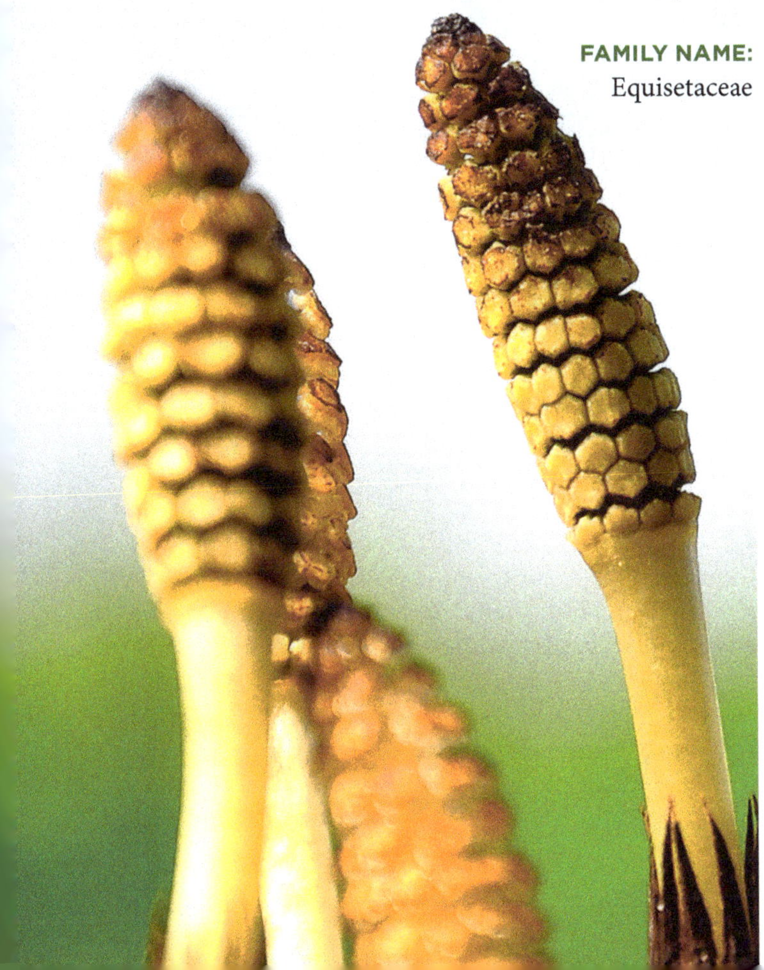

DESCRIPTION

PARTS USED: The thallus or young, infertile stalks (above ground parts). Harvest the plant when it is 6 – 18 inches tall, just as the branches unfold.

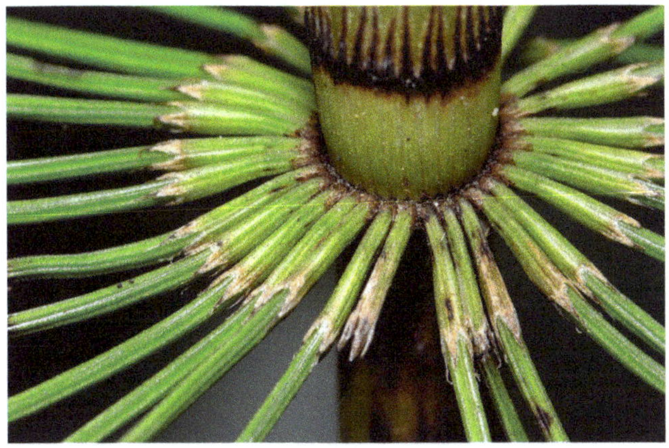

BOTANICAL DESCRIPTION AND HABITAT: Horsetail grows in moist areas worldwide, along the banks of streams or lakes, and in moist forests, swamps, and meadows.

Equisetum is a genus of 15 rhizomatous, perennial, seedless vascular species that occur globally.[1] Resembling reeds, they usually have hollow, grooved, brittle, dimorphic stems. One form is sterile and only provides the vegetative function; the other is fertile.[1] The stems can be perennial or annual, with whorled branches or none at all.[1] The whorled, scale-like leaves are fused into a sheath around the stem.[1] The reproductive organ on the fertile stems is a terminal cone-like strobilus bearing scales with sporangia that produce round, green spores.[1]

Equisetum arvense (common horsetail, prêle des champs) is a native throughout North America, Europe, and Asia.[2] It has annual, dimorphic stems.[2] The green vegetative stems (10 – 60 cm) bear up to 14 sheath teeth (1 – 3.5 mm) and whorled branches.[2,3] The brown, succulent, short-lived fertile stems (11 – 32 cm tall) mature in early spring, lack branches, and have larger sheaths than the sterile stems.[2,3]

E. fluviatile (river horsetail, pipes, prêle fluviatile) has monomorphic green stems that can be branched, with 12 – 24 teeth (2 – 3 mm) on black sheaths (35 – 115 cm).[4] The strobiles mature in summer.[4] *E. fluviatile* grows in standing water in North America and Eurasia.[4]

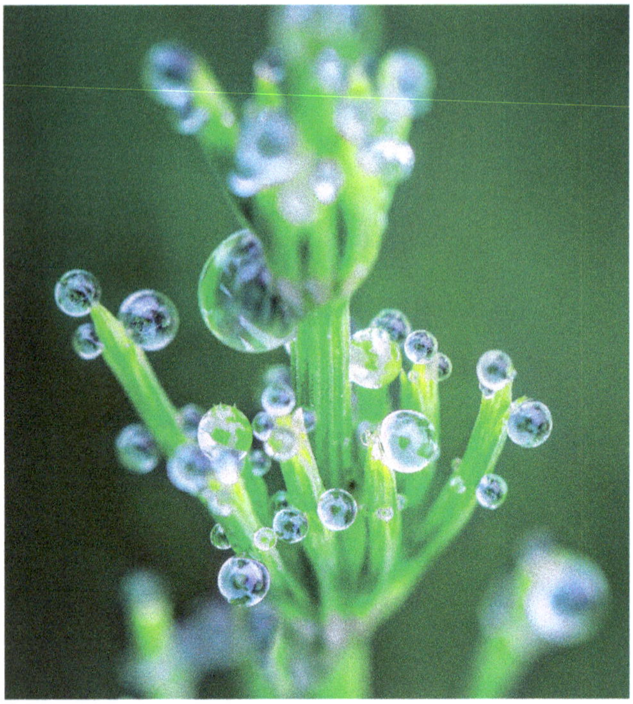

E. hyemale (common scouring rush, mù zei) grows in forests and along stream and riverbanks in Europe, Asia, Central America, and North America.[5] The monomorphic, green, scabrous, perennial stem (up to 2 meters tall) has no branches.[5,6] It generally bears a dark brown sheath (7 – 11 mm wide) with 16 – 50 deciduous, brown teeth (0.3 – 0.5 cm).[5,6] The sessile, ovate strobilus (1 – 1.6 cm by 0.4 – 0.7 cm diameter) has an acute apex.[5,6]

E. laevigatum (smooth scouring rush) has green, monomorphic, non-branching stems (30 – 180 cm tall) that are usually annual, but can be perennial in southern locales.[7] The dark, banded sheath has 10 – 26 deciduous teeth.[7] Smooth scouring rush is found in moist, sandy areas throughout the U.S. and far western Canada.[7]

E. palustre (marsh horsetail, quan wen jing) has narrow, green, monomorphic, annual stems (20 – 80 cm tall) with long hollow branches (up to 20 cm long) bearing green sheath teeth.[8,9] The long sheaths (4 – 9 mm) are half brown and half green, and bear five to ten black teeth (2 – 5 mm long).[8,9] The strobilus (0.6 – 2.5 cm by 4 – 6 mm in diameter) has a blunt tip.[8] Marsh horsetail grows in marshes on both U.S. coasts, and in Asia and Europe.[9]

E. telmateia ssp. *braunii* (giant horsetail) has annual, dimorphic stems.[10,11] The sterile, hollow, branching stems (30 – 100 cm) have sheaths (7 – 18 mm) with up to 28 green teeth (4 – 10 mm).[11] The brown, short-lived, non-branching, fertile stems (up to 45 cm tall) have larger sheaths (15 – 40 mm) with up to 30 teeth (5 – 16 mm).[10,11] *E. telmateia* ssp. *braunii* grows in wet places at elevations less than 1,000 meters, from California to Alaska.[10,11]

E. variegatum (variegated scouring rush, prêle panachée, ban wen mu zei) is shorter (6 – 55 cm tall) and has thinner stems (1 – 1.5 mm diameter) than other horsetails.[12,13] The perennial, monomorphic stems have green sheaths (0.2 cm wide) with a blackish band and six to eight teeth (1 mm).[13] The strobilus (5 – 8 mm long by 2 – 4 mm diameter) has an acute tip.[12] *E. variegatum* grows in forests and meadows, and along roadsides in Asia, Europe, and North America.[12]

THE NAME: The genus name derives from the Latin *equus* ("horse") and *seta* ("bristle").[13] The epithet *arvense* (Latin) means "of the field." *Fluviatile* means "to grow near streams." [13] *Hyemale* (Latin) means "of winter." *Telmateia* means "of muddy waters or marshes."[13] The name scouring rush refers to the use of horsetail for cleaning objects such as dishes, and for polishing pewter and wooden objects, such as arrow shafts, canoes, and gambling sticks.[13] The Spanish name cañutillo means "pipe or little tube" because children made whistles from scouring rush.

HISTORICAL USES: In prehistoric times, giant horsetail *(E. telmateia)* grew as tall as trees (30 – 40 feet).[13] The young spring shoots were consumed in moderation by the Salish and Nuu-chah-multh.[13,14] Native Americans consumed the tea as a diuretic.[14] Women drank the tea to expel afterbirth and treat gonorrhea.[14] A poultice was applied to heal wounds.[14] The powdered, fertile stems were added to horses' water to invigorate them.[14] Horsetail powder was placed in moccasins to prevent foot cramps during long journeys.[14] The Salish applied the roots of *E. arvense* to gums in order to ease teething pain in children.[14] The Tlingit and Salish decorated baskets with *E. hyemale.*[13]

Ancient Romans consumed the young fertile shoots of *E. flutviatile.*[13] They prepared tea and a thickening powder from the shoots.[13] Horsetail was used as an abrasive to polish wooden objects such as canoes, dishes, and arrow shafts. It was also used to decorate baskets and clean dishes.[13] It was the first plant to regrow following the eruption of Mount St. Helens in 1980.[13]

CONSTITUENTS: Horsetail contains minerals (see *Nutritional Properties*), saponins (articulatin, equisetrin, equisetonin, and sitosterol), flavone glycosides (apigenin, flavonols, flavones, galuteolin, gossypitrin, herbacetrin, isoquercetrin, luteolin, kaempferol, and quercetin), phenolic acids (E-caffeoyl-meso-tartaric acid, and methyl esters of protocatechuic and caffeic acids, caffeic acid derivatives, aconitic, oxalic, malic, tannic, arabinoic, and threonic acids), polyacetylenes (equisetolic acid), phytosterols, alkaloids (nicotine, palustrine, and palustrinine), and tannins.[15-17,19]

NUTRITIONAL PROPERTIES: Horsetail contains high amounts of silica (silicon dioxide, free silicic acid, and water-soluble silicates), calcium, chromium, fluorine, iron, magnesium, manganese, potassium, and vitamin A. It contains moderate amounts of aluminum, cobalt, niacin, phosphorus, protein, riboflavin, selenium, sodium, sulfur, tin, and vitamin C. It contains low amounts of PABA, fatty acids, vitamin B_5, and β-carotene.[15-17]

MEDICINAL PROPERTIES: Astringent, diuretic, hemostatic, nutritive, styptic, and vulnerary.

TEMPERATURE AND FLAVOR: Neutral, astringent, salty, bland, and mildly bitter.

MEDICINAL USES

Horsetail contains high amounts of silica (silicon dioxide and silicic acid), an important mineral that strengthens and regenerates connective tissue.[14-16] The silica found in horsetail strengthens bones, and can be used as a tonic to prevent osteoporosis and strengthen teeth.[16,18] A vulnerary agent, silicic acid hastens the healing of broken bones, torn tendons, cartilage, and injured muscles or joints.[15,16,19] Similarly, horsetail is beneficial for accelerating tissue healing after a surgical procedure.[16] Prepare an extract containing gotu kola *(Centella)*, hawthorn *(Crataegus)*, calendula *(Calendula)*, and horsetail to hasten connective tissue healing.

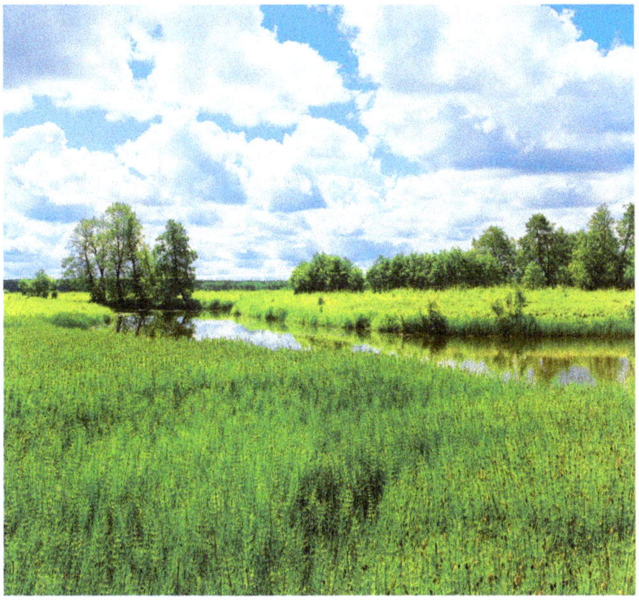

The silica content in horsetail improves the integrity of elastic tissue in the lungs and bladder.[16] Horsetail can be useful as a recuperative agent following respiratory infections such as bronchitis, pneumonia, or pleurisy. It is beneficial for individuals with weak lungs, or those who are susceptible to infections resulting from tissue weakness. Horsetail strengthens the tissues and reduces sensitivity to allergens common in individuals with allergies, asthma, or leaky gut syndrome. It can be used as a tonic to strengthen the mucous membranes in individuals with chronic allergies or chronic sinus infections. In addition to the silica content, the astringent properties reduce mucus secretions and decrease bloody sputum.

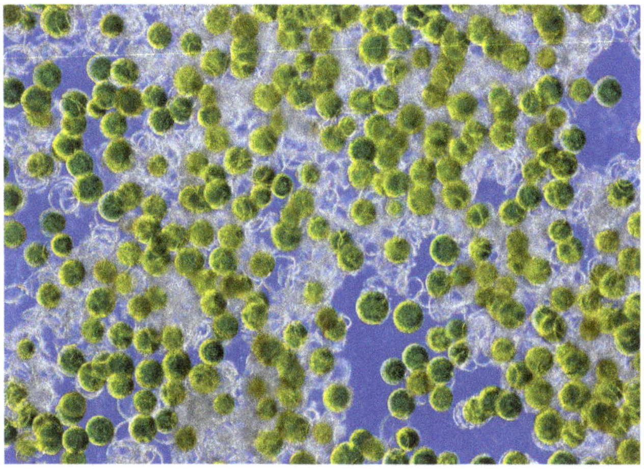

A low dose of horsetail tincture (5 – 10 drops, two to three times daily) aids in strengthening the bladder.[17] It can be very useful for individuals with frequent bladder infections, interstitial cystitis, or childhood enuresis.[17] It is specific for women who have taken antibiotics several times or bladder infections without positive results. The inability of tissues to respond to antibiotics indicates tissue weakness. While horsetail is not effective as an antibacterial agent, it enhances the integrity of tissues, improving their resistance. Combine extracts of mullein root *(Verbascum)*, corn silk *(Zea)*, saw palmetto *(Serenoa)*, and horsetail to strengthen the bladder.

Horsetail tea is a diuretic.[15,18] It reduces edema and premenstrual water retention, and aids in flushing the kidneys and nonobstructive stones.[19] Horsetail tea enhances urinary excretion of sodium, chloride, and potassium.[15] It decreases a burning sensation in the urethra, reduces the concentration of urine, and serves as an adjunct treatment for urinary tract infections (with other anti-infective herbs).[18,17] It contains flavonoids that are attributed to the diuretic properties.[19] Prepare a diuretic compound containing nettle leaf *(Urtica)*, parsley root or seed *(Petroselinum)*, dandelion *(Taraxacum)*, and horsetail.

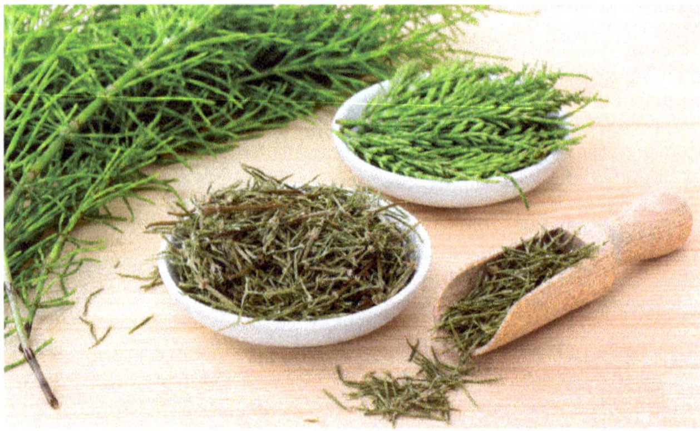

Horsetail's silica and flavonoids improve the integrity of blood vessels.[16,19] Low doses of the tincture can be used to treat varicose veins and bruises. Horsetail can be used as a tonic for individuals with vascular weakness or atherosclerosis.

Horsetail is a hemostatic.[14-16] It is beneficial for reducing excessive menstrual bleeding, as well as mid-cycle or menopausal spotting.[14-16] It is effective for treating nosebleeds, bloody sputum, bleeding ulcers, ulcerative colitis (with bleeding), bleeding hemorrhoids, and small amounts of blood in the urine or mucus.[16] Combine horsetail with shepherd's purse *(Capsella),* nettle leaf *(Urtica),* and raspberry leaf *(Rubus)* to reduce bleeding.

Horsetail tincture or tea used internally or externally can reduce split ends and beautify hair that lacks luster. It strengthens nails that break or split easily, and reduces hangnails. Combine with nettle as a hair tonic.

An effective vulnerary agent, horsetail fomentation or poultice can be applied topically to hasten wound healing.[14-16] Applying a fresh poultice also reduces inflammation and bleeding from cuts, wounds, and ulcers.[16,19] Gargling with horsetail tea or diluted extract reduces mouth and gum inflammation.[14,19]

According to Ayurvedic practitioners Vasant Lad and David Frawley, horsetail clears *pitta* and fiery emotions from the nerves and mind.[18]

CONTRAINDICATIONS

Sensitive individuals (i.e., children and the elderly) should use moderation when taking horsetail internally. It can be drying, and its silica content can irritate the kidneys. If sensitive kidneys are an issue, it is better to consume low doses of the tincture (alcohol evaporated in hot water), rather than the tea. Internal consumption of horsetail should be avoided completely by individuals with obstructive stones, kidney inflammation, or edema due to impaired heart or kidney function.

Consuming excessive amounts of *E. palustre* can cause toxicity in horses and sheep.[15] Toxicity resembling nicotine poisoning has been reported in children who have chewed the stems, likely due to the alkaloid palustrine.[15] Horsetail has been shown to have potential antithiamine action (destroys vitamin B_1) when ingested by horses, and in the stomachs of monogastric animals (including humans).[15] Some commercial preparations of *E. arvense* are free of thiaminase-like activity. According to herbalist Terry Willard, consuming B vitamins will reverse the major side effects of the antithiamine action.[14]

It has been speculated that the diuretic actions of horsetail could lower potassium levels, contributing to hypokalemia (low potassium levels). Regular use of horsetail should be avoided by individuals with hypokalemia or heart arrhythmia, and by those consuming heart medications such as digoxin (Lanoxin), or diuretic medications.

Caution: Avoid harvesting horsetail near polluted streams, or when toxic minerals or chemicals are present in the soil.[15] Heavy metals and chemicals can concentrate in the plant.

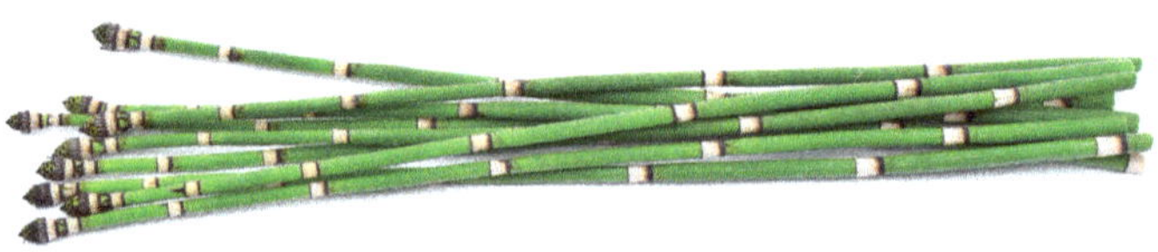

PREPARATION AND DOSAGE

TINCTURE: Fresh infertile stalks [1:2-1:3, 60-95% alcohol]; consume 5-60 drops, up to three times daily.

ACETUM EXTRACT: Fresh infertile stalks [1:3-1:4, apple cider vinegar]; consume ½ to 1 teaspoon, one to two times daily, or apply topically.

TEA: Prepare a hot infusion; consume 4-8 ounces, three to four times daily.

TOPICAL USE: Apply the fomentation, poultice, wash, oil (alcohol intermediary method), or salve.

HYDRANGEA

DESCRIPTION

BOTANICAL NAMES:
Hydrangea arborescens, H. quercifolia, H. macrophylla, H. paniculata

COMMON NAMES:
Stone root, seven barks, hydrangea, wild hydrangea, smooth hydrangea, mountain hydrangea, tree hydrangea
pallohortensia (Finnish)
hortensie, hydragelle de Virginie (French)
baumartige hydrangie, grosser wasserstrauch, hortensie, kehlopf (German)
vidjehortensia (Swedish)

FAMILY NAME:
Hydrangeaceae
(formerly Saxifragaceae)

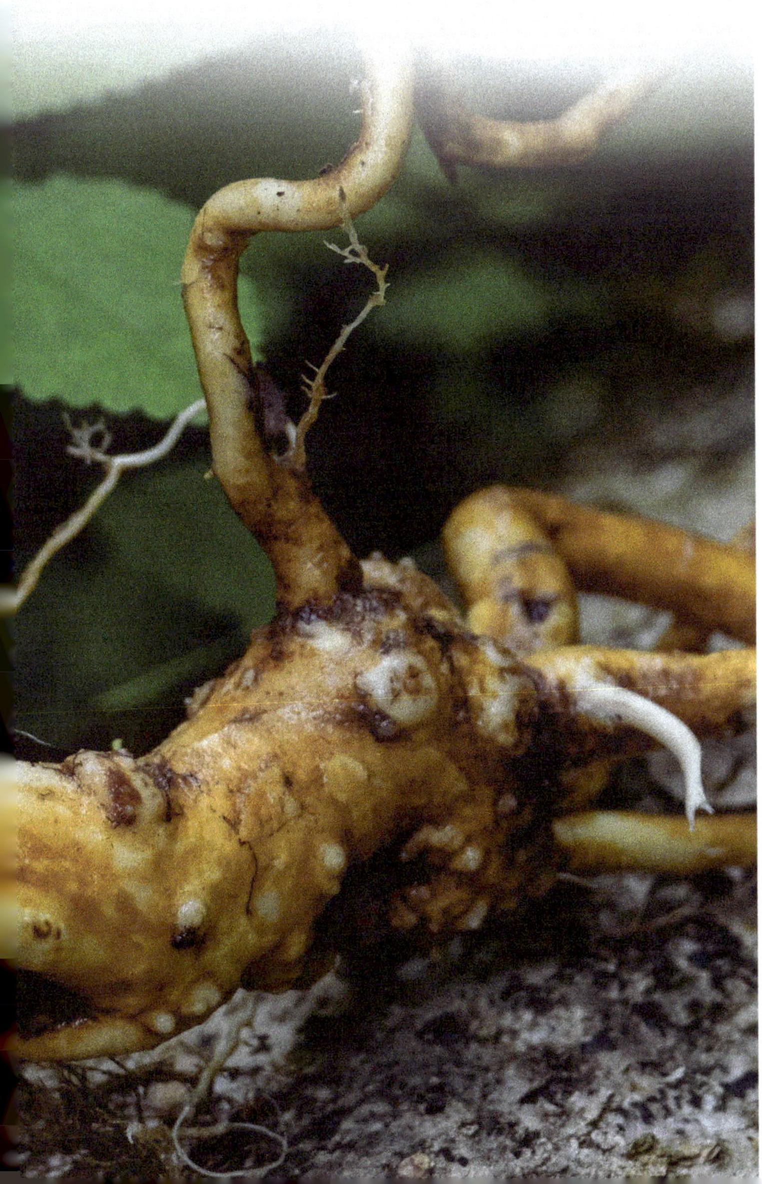

PARTS USED: The roots and rhizomes.

BOTANICAL DESCRIPTION AND HABITAT: Hydrangeas are shrubs that grow an average of ten feet tall. *Hydrangea arborescens* and *H. quercifolia* can be found in woodlands and stream banks in North America, from the northern to southeastern states. *H. macrophylla* and *H. paniculata* are of Asian origin.

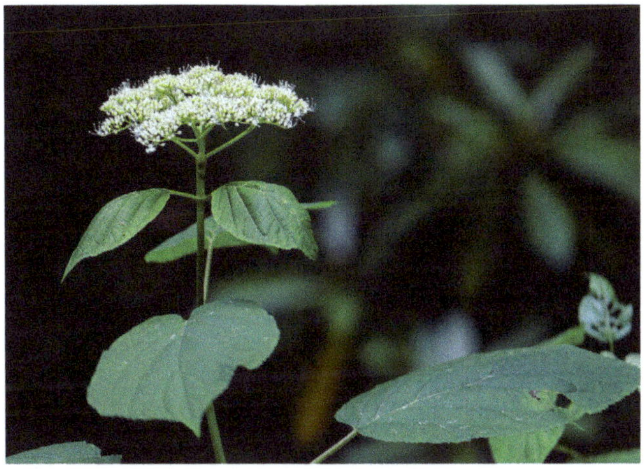

Hydrangea arborescens is a deciduous shrub that usually grows up to 2 meters tall, though it can get larger.[1] It has glabrous, brownish-gray bark that peels off in thin, multicolored layers.[2] The ovate to cordate, dark green, dentate, opposite leaves have acuminate apices and long, purplish petioles (up to 15 cm long).[3] The leaves turn yellow in autumn before falling off the slender, flexible branches. It has loose, broad cymes of tiny greenish-white, fertile, partially inferior flowers that bloom in late spring to early summer.[2] Each flower has five petals, ten stamens, two carpels, and two styles.[3] Along the margins of the corymb there are also a few larger false flowers with showy white bracts up to one centimeter in diameter. The flowers turn into dry, dehiscent capsules in the fall.[3]

THE NAME: The genus name *Hydrangea* derives from two Greek words: *hydror* ("water") and *agneion* ("vessel or capsule"), referring to the shrub's cup-shaped seed pods.[4] The epithet *arborescens* derives from the Middle English *arbor* ("tree"). Native Americans called it "stone root," as they used it to treat kidney stones, and because the root was dense and hard like a stone. "Seven barks" refers to the multiple colors of peeling bark.[4]

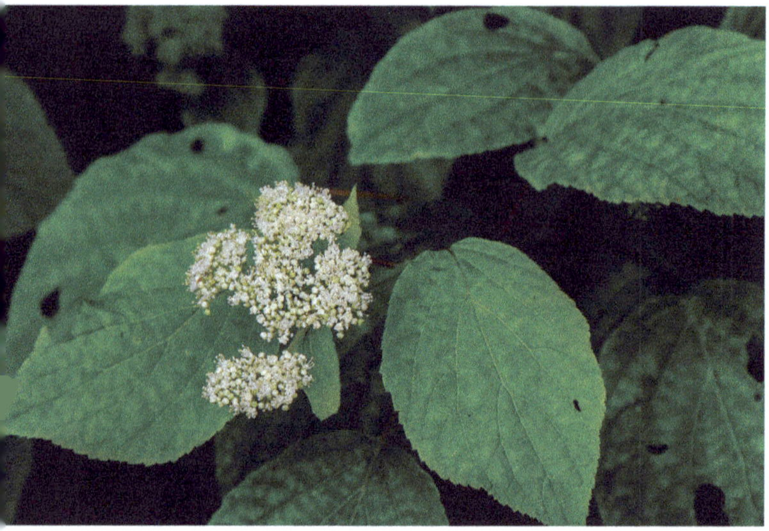

MEDICINAL PROPERTIES: Diuretic, urinary analgesic, antilithic, lithotriptic, and anti-inflammatory.

TEMPERATURE AND FLAVOR: Cool, sweet, bitter, and bland.

MEDICINAL USES

Hydrangea has soothing diuretic actions and strengthens the genitourinary organs.[6] It reduces inflammation in urinary tract mucous membranes, decreasing bladder and urethra pain, and minimizing sharp, burning sensations upon urination.[6] Hydrangea aids in treating acute cystitis and urethritis.[9] Although umbelliferone and hydrangenol have antimicrobial actions, additional anti-infective agents are necessary to treat urinary tract infections.[9] Hydrangea is also a long-term tonic for frequently recurring urinary tract infections, interstitial cystitis, and benign prostatic hypertrophy (B.P.H.).[9] Combine saw palmetto *(Serenoa repens),* yellow pond lily *(Nuphar),* mullein root *(Verbascum),* corn silk *(Zea),* and horsetail *(Equisetum)* to treat interstitial cystitis. Hydrangea eases the symptoms of B.P.H. in combination with saw palmetto *(Serenoa),* stone root *(Collinsonia),* nettle root *(Urtica dioica),* poria *(Poria)* and/or yellow pond lily *(Nuphar).*

Hydrangea can be consumed as an acute and long-term treatment for kidney stones. Short-term use of it reduces referred pain patterns in the mid to lower back caused by the passing of kidney stones.[6] Long-term use prevents

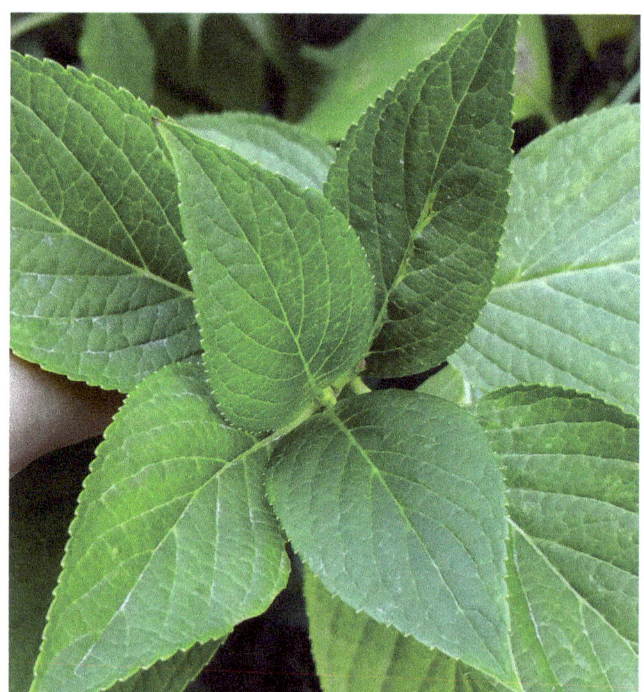

HISTORICAL USES: In Traditional Chinese Medicine, the roots, leaves, and flowers of *H. macrophylla* are used as a diuretic and antitussive, and to treat malaria.[5] Cherokees consumed a decoction of the roots to ease the passing of kidney stones and relieve pain. The bark was applied externally to treat wounds, burns, sore muscles, and sprains. American settlers and Eclectic physicians adopted these practices.

Eclectic physicians administered hydrangea as a soothing diuretic.[6] It was used to reduce sharp, burning urethral pain, to ease pain from passing stones, and partial suppression of urine.[6] Dr. Finley Ellingwood stated, "I am convinced after a lifetime of experience that it is more specifically, more universally a sedative to pain and distress in the kidneys and urinary bladder than any other one remedy." Hydrangea was also administered to treat acute nephritis when combined with yellow jasmine *(Gelsemium)* and black cohosh *(Actaea).*[6,7]

CONSTITUENTS: Hydrangea contains glucosides (hydrangin), saponins, gum, starch, sugars, flavonoids (rutin, quercetin, and kaempferol), resins, stilbenoids (hydrangenol), a quinazoline alkaloid (febrifugine), volatile oil, fixed oil, and acids (sulphuric and phosphoric). *H. macrophylla* and *H. paniculata* contain hydrangenol, hydrangeic acid, phyllodulcin, lunularic acid, glycosides (lunularin and 3,4'-dihydroxystilbene), a mucilaginous polysaccharide (paniculatan), hydrangetin (7-hydroxy-8-methoxycoumarin), rutin, umbelliferone, an alkaloid (febrifugine), gum, and resin.[5-9]

NUTRITIONAL PROPERTIES: *Hydrangea arborescens* root contains aluminum, ash, calcium, chromium, cobalt, fiber, iron, magnesium, manganese, niacin, phosphorus, potassium, protein, selenium, silicon, and tin.

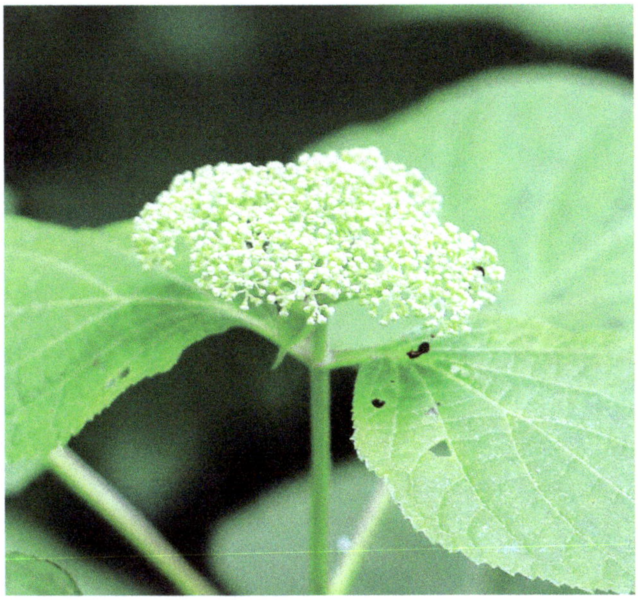

PREPARATION AND DOSAGE

TINCTURE: Fresh roots [1:2, 60-95% alcohol]; dry roots [1:5, 60% alcohol]: consume 20-60 drops, three to four times daily.

FLUID EXTRACT: Dry roots [1:1, 50% alcohol]; consume 5-30 drops, three to four times daily.

CAPSULES: Consume 2-4 "00" capsules, up to three times daily.

TEA: Prepare a cold infusion or decoction; consume 8-12 ounces, up to three times daily.

uric acid and phosphate deposits from accumulating in the kidneys, reducing the potential formation of kidney stones.[6] Some herbalists claim that it has antilithic and lithotriptic actions that break up stones, although this has not been scientifically validated. In order to prevent the buildup of kidney stones and ease their passing, drink ample water and consume three to four cups daily of a tea blend containing stone root *(Collinsonia)*, gravel root *(Eutrochium purpureum)*, parsley root *(Petroselinum)*, fennel *(Foeniculum)*, and hydrangea *(Hydrangea)*. Additional demulcents such as marshmallow *(Althaea)* can be added to the tea formula to soothe the kidneys and urinary tract. Frequent dosing of potent analgesics extracts are often necessary to reduce the severe pain of passing stones. The most effective herb extracts for pain relief include: California poppy *(Eschscholzia)*, opium poppy *(Papaver)*, cannabis *(Cannabis)*, silk tassel *(Garrya)*, and valerian *(Valeriana)*. Moderate to high doses every one to two hours are often needed to manage pain.

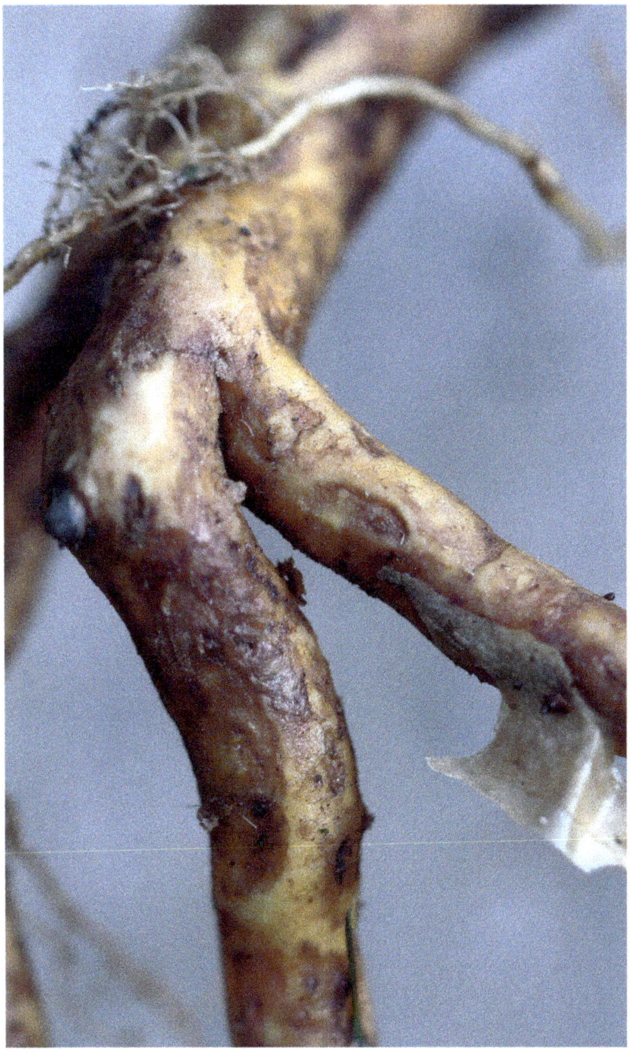

CONTRAINDICATIONS

Avoid use during pregnancy and lactation.[9] Hydrangea is contraindicated in cases of obstructive kidney stones or kidney disease.[9] Individuals with edema related to impaired heart or kidney function should consult a health care practitioner before consuming hydrangea. An excessively high dose may cause vertigo, oppression in the chest, or gastrointestinal disturbance.[9]

JAMAICAN DOGWOOD

DESCRIPTION

BOTANICAL NAMES:
Piscidia piscipula (syn. *P. erythrina, P. communis, Erythrina piscipula, Ichthyomethia piscipula, I. communis*)[1]

COMMON NAMES:
Jamaican dogwood, West Indian dogwood, fish poison tree, Florida fish poison tree, fish fuddle, fish catching coral tree
malungú, marungú, guana hediondia (Cuba)
palo de zope, zopilocuave (El Salvador)
flor de papagallo, cocinte, javín, haabí, haabin, jabín, chijol (México)
ventura (Puerto Rico)
barbasco (Venezuela)[2,3]

FAMILY NAME:
Fabaceae (Leguminosae)

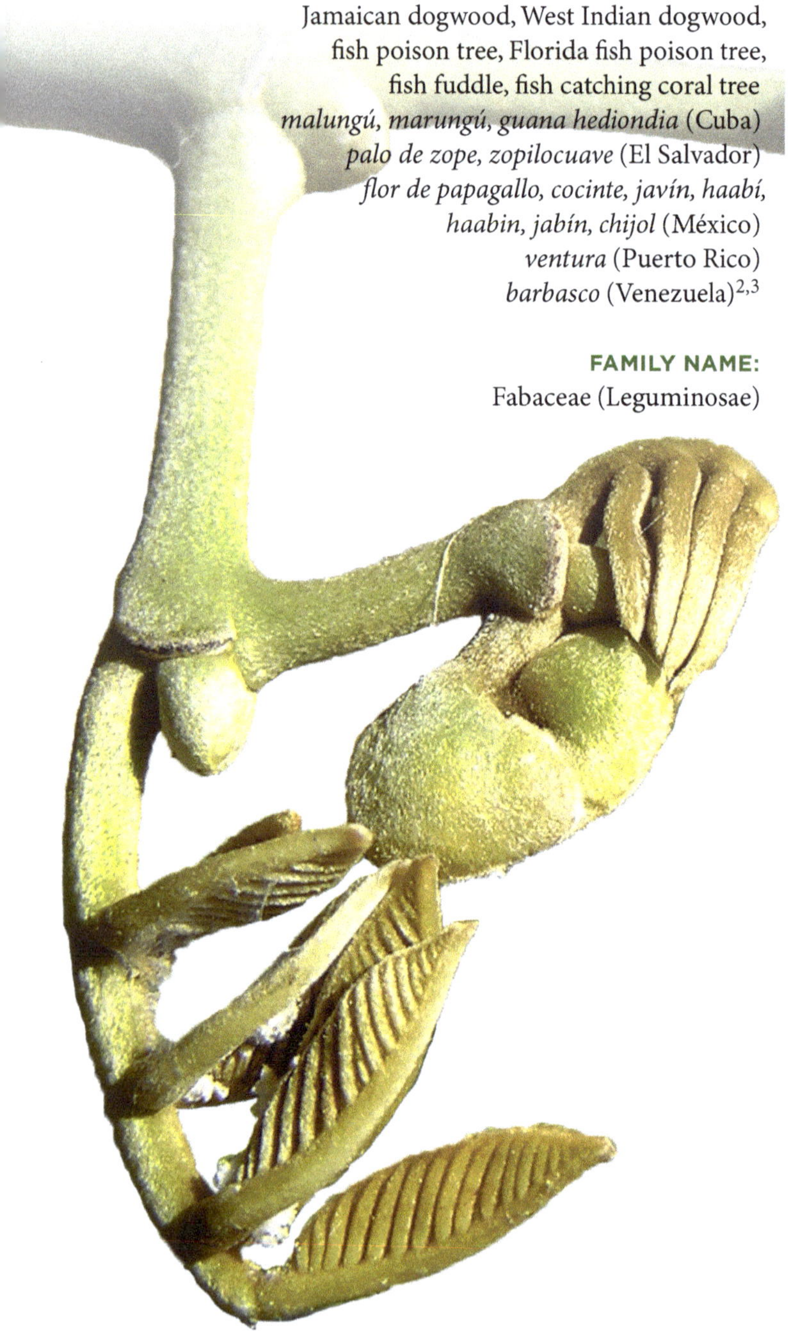

PARTS USED: The stems, tree bark, root bark, and roots.

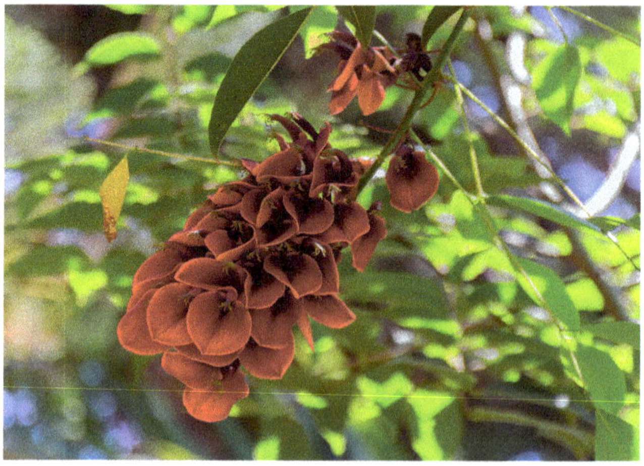

BOTANICAL DESCRIPTION AND HABITAT: *Piscidia piscipula* is a medium-size deciduous tree that grows along the coast of Florida, Texas, Jamaica, Martinique, and northern South America. The light olive-gray bark displays irregular dark patches and small scales. The alternate pinnately compound leaves have five to eleven leaflets (4 – 8 cm long). The deep green leaflets have prominent veins and are glabrous above, with a pale green color and pubescence below. The attractive flowers grow in pea-like clusters, and are lavender, pink, or white, tinged with red or pink. The light brown fruit develops into a pea-like pod with four longitudinal papery wings containing reddish-brown, oval fruit. This tree is a larval host for cassius blue butterflies *(Leptotes cassius)*, hammock skipper butterflies *(Polygonus leo)*, and non-native fulvous hairstreak butterflies *(Electrostrymon angelia)*.[4]

THE NAME: *Piscidia* derives from two Latin words: *piscis* ("fish") and *caedo* ("to kill"). The epithet *piscipula* is Latin for "little fish."[5] Florida fish poison tree, fish poison tree, and fish fuddle refer to the traditional use of the herb in which Native South Americans pounded the leaves, young tree branches, and root bark, tossed them into water, and temporarily paralyzed fish for an easy catch.[2] Fortunately for humans, the constituents causing paralysis are only poisonous to cold-blooded creatures.

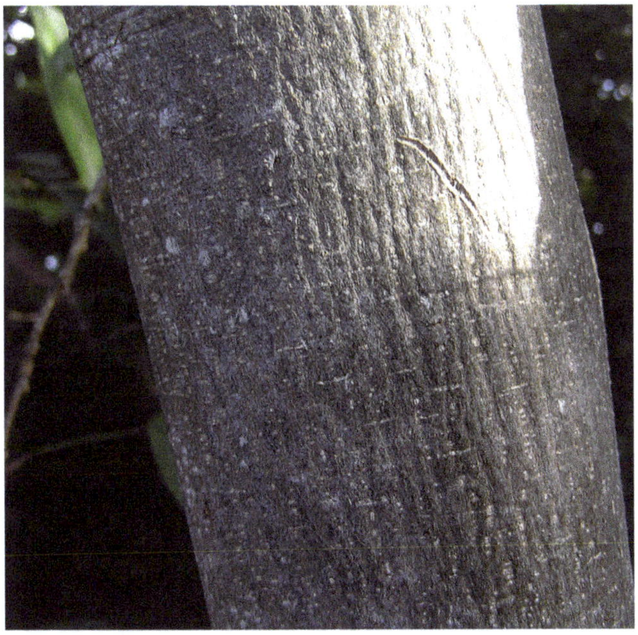

HISTORICAL USES: The indigenous people of Antilles used Jamaican dogwood as an analgesic and to paralyze fish. They wrapped a poultice of pulverized leaves around their heads to treat headaches. Poultices also were applied to sprains in order to reduce inflammation and pain.

The plant's use as an analgesic and sudorific was popularized in the Western world in 1844.[2] Eclectic physicians employed Jamaican dogwood to treat toothaches, anxiety, insomnia, neuralgia, and arthritis.[6] It was also administered as an antispasmodic for whooping cough, asthma, birthing pains, and dysmenorrhea.[2] When patients couldn't tolerate morphine or opium, Jamaican dogwood was used as a substitute, although its analgesic properties were considered inferior.[6]

CONSTITUENTS: Jamaican dogwood contains glycosides (piscidin and piscidone) and flavonoids (flavones: glabranin; isoflavones: ichthynone jamaicin and lisetin), rotenonoids (rotenone, milletone, isomilletone, and dehydromilletone), organic acids (piscidic, fukiic, malic, 3'-O-methylfukiic, oxalic, succinic, tartaric, and *p*-hydroxy=benzyltartaric), a saponin (β-sitosterol), tannins, resins, an alkaloid, and others.[6-10]

NUTRITIONAL PROPERTIES: Not applicable.

MEDICINAL PROPERTIES: Analgesic, anti-inflammatory, antispasmodic, antitussive, hypnotic, sedative, and sudorific.

TEMPERATURE AND FLAVOR: Cool, bitter, astringent, and mildly sweet.

MEDICINAL USES

Jamaican dogwood is a potent anti-inflammatory and analgesic. It reduces pain, muscle spasms, and inflammation caused by tension headaches and muscle tension. Its anti-inflammatory properties act as a sudorific, lowering fevers and reducing fever-related aches and pains. Jamaican dogwood is one of the few herbs comparable in action to over-the-counter anti-inflammatory agents such as ibuprofen. It is beneficial for treating flareups of tendonitis, carpal tunnel, rheumatoid arthritis, and osteoarthritis, and for alleviating the pain of fibromyalgia and chronic fatigue syndrome (CFS). Other mild anti-inflammatory herbs such as turmeric *(Curcuma)*, chamomile *(Matricaria)*, meadowsweet *(Filipendula)*, and black cohosh *(Actaea)* can be consumed long-term to prevent flareups of the aforementioned conditions. Jamaican dogwood reduces pain and inflammation caused by toothaches until dental help can be obtained. *Note:* Gum abscesses require medical attention and can result in serious health problems when not properly treated.

The effects of Jamaican dogwood are synergized when combined with other anti-inflammatory and analgesic herbs such as St. John's wort *(Hypericum)*, meadowsweet *(Filipendula)*, and white willow *(Salix)*. When compounded with a vasodilating agent such as feverfew *(Tanacetum parthenium)* and very small quantities of pulsatilla *(Anemone)*, it can effectively treat migraine headaches. Combined with pedicularis *(Pedicularis)*, it enhances skeletal muscle antispasmodic actions.

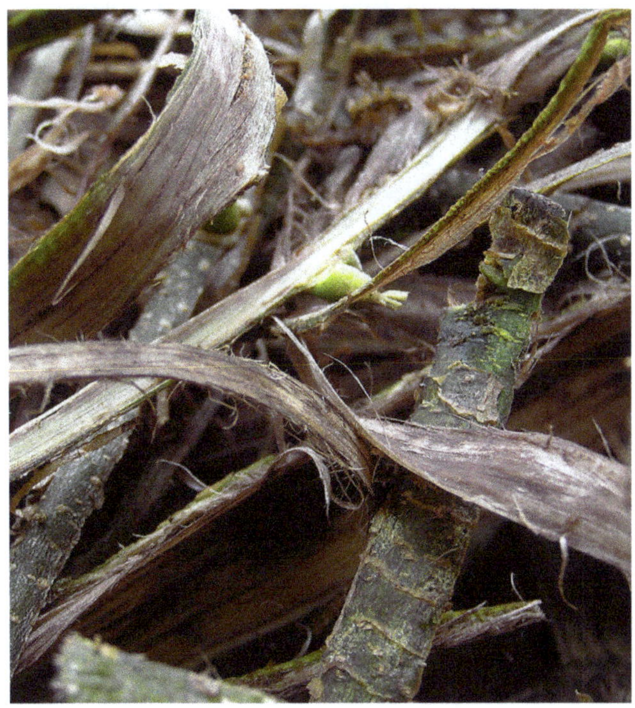

Jamaican dogwood is a nerve sedative and hypnotic useful for treating neuralgia and insomnia resulting from nervous excitement, anxiety, or pain. It can be helpful when weaning off conventional prescription sedatives. Jamaican dogwood also eases symptoms of opium withdrawal.[9] It reduces pain resulting from an impinged nerve or sciatica. Jamaican dogwood also has musculoskeletal antispasmodic properties that relieve myalgia. It alleviates neck and jaw tension, and aids in the treatment of trigeminal neuralgia. The constituents in Jamaican dogwood, rotenone and isoflavones (ichthyone, piscidone, and piscerythrone), have potent neural depressant effects.[11]

Jamaican dogwood is a powerful smooth muscle antispasmodic. The tea or tincture reduces tracheal spasms, painful breathing, and a spastic cough resulting from bronchitis, whooping cough, or croup. It induces restful sleep that has been interrupted by coughing fits. Additional anti-infective herbs may also be necessary. Jamaican dogwood reduces menstrual cramping and labor pain without interfering with uterine contractions. It combines harmoniously with wild yam *(Dioscorea villosa)*, cramp bark *(Viburnum opulus)*, and black haw *(Viburnum prunifolium)* for gynecological pain. Jamaican dogwood decreases referred pain patterns caused by passing a gallstone or kidney stone. It has a limited effect on digestive cramping compared to angelica *(Angelica)*, wild yam *(Dioscorea villosa)*, or silk tassel *(Garrya)*.

Jamaican dogwood is an anodyne. Apply the poultice or tincture topically to relieve the pain of toothaches, burns, bruises, sprains, strained muscles, fractured bones, local neuralgia, hemorrhoids, and boils.

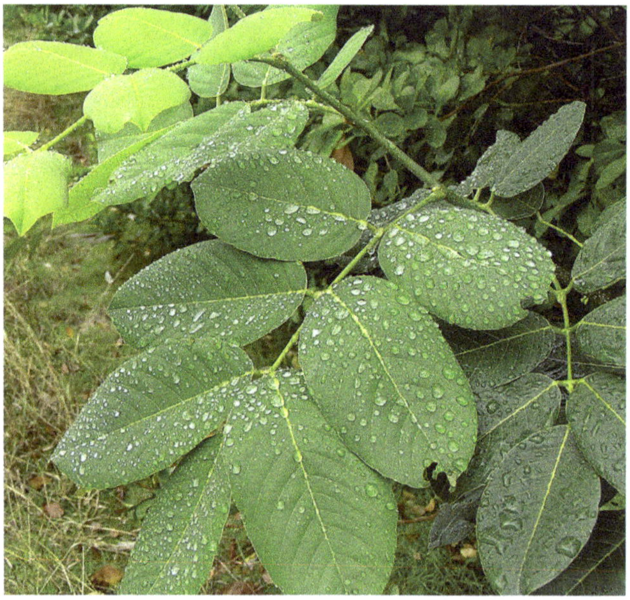

CONTRAINDICATIONS

Consume Jamaican dogwood with care. Unless recommended by a health care practitioner, avoid use during pregnancy or lactation. Use caution when administering to children and the elderly. It is contraindicated in individuals with heart problems.[9] Jamaican dogwood can potentiate the effects of alcohol, recreational drugs, and over-the-counter drugs, as well as analgesic, anti-inflammatory, hypnotic, and sedative medications. An overdose of the herb can result in gastric distress, nausea, dizziness, dilation of the pupils, difficulty breathing, or a decrease in heart rate and respiration.[2,6]

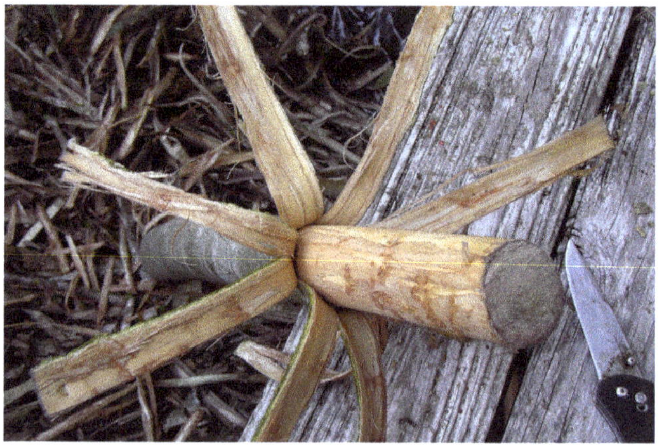

PREPARATION AND DOSAGE

TINCTURE: Fresh bark or root bark [1:2-1:3, 70-95% alcohol]; dry bark or root bark [1:5, 60% alcohol]; consume 10-90 drops, up to four times daily. Start with a low dose (20 drops) and increase in 10-drop increments; do not exceed 90 drops per dose. When treating pain, consume moderate doses (30-60 drops) every hour or higher doses (60-90 drops) every two hours.

CAPSULES: Consume 2-4 "00" capsules, up to four times daily. Start with the lowest dosage and work up to three capsules if necessary.

TEA: Prepare a decoction using 1 teaspoon to 1 tablespoon of herb per cup of water. The dose range for tea is 4-12 ounces, up to three times daily.

TOPICAL USE: Apply the poultice topically; the tincture can be used as a liniment.

KAVA

BOTANICAL NAMES:
Piper methysticum (syn. *P. methysticum* var. *methysticum*), *P. methysticum* var. *wichmannii* (syn. *P. wichmannii*)

COMMON NAMES:
Kava, kava kava, pepper, kava pepper, inebriating pepper, intoxicating pepper, intoxicating long pepper, inebriating pepper
kavarod (Danish)
waka, yoqona, yangona (Fijiani)
kawa, poivier (French)
kawa pfeffer, rauschpfeffer (German)
'awa (Hawaii)
pepe kava (Italian)
lawena, bari, wati, tigwa (Papua New Guinea)
'ava (Samoa)
kavaka (Spanish)
kava kava (Tonga)
kava biberi (Turkish)

FAMILY NAME:
Piperaceae

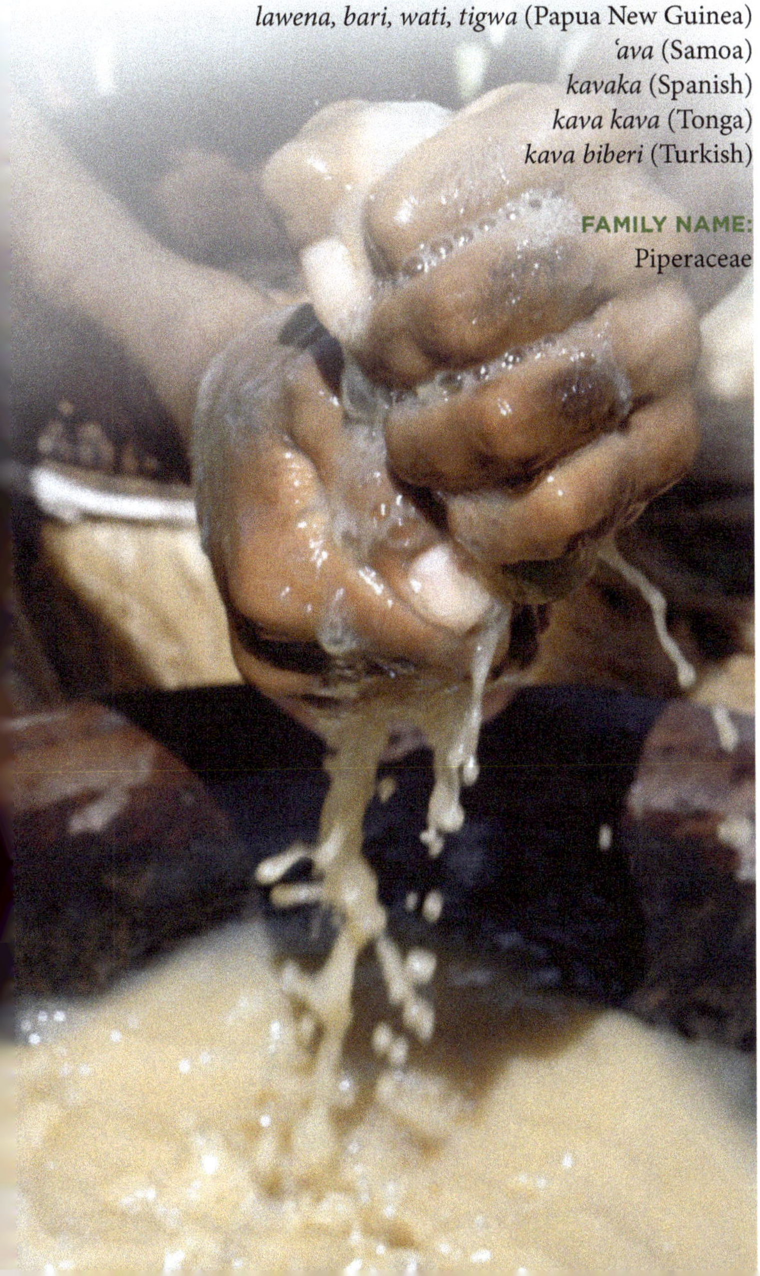

DESCRIPTION

PARTS USED: The central and lateral roots.

BOTANICAL DESCRIPTION AND HABITAT: Kava is indigenous to Polynesia, Melanesia, and the tropical islands of Oceania. It is a woody perennial shrub with a large root crown from which the shoots grow (2 – 4 meters tall).[1,2] The erect green, reddish-brown, or dark purple shoots (1 – 3 cm in diameter) have swollen nodes and prominent leaf scars.[1,2] The alternate, deciduous cordate leaves (10 – 30 cm long and 8 – 25 cm wide) are palmately veined, with entire margins and a glabrous to finely pubescent surface.[1,2]

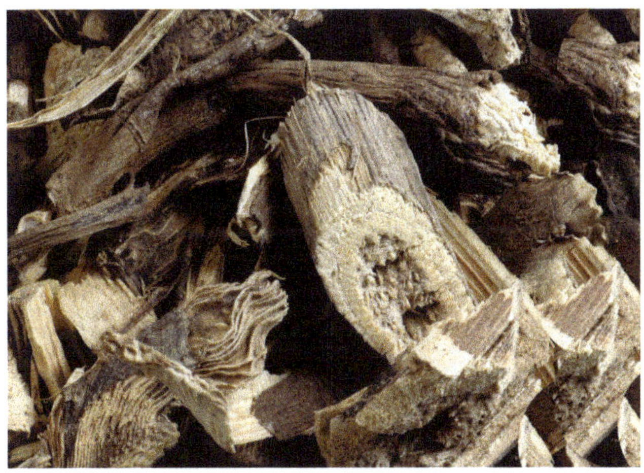

Kava is dioecious, although it rarely flowers and does not fruit.[1,2] The plant is sterile and propagates asexually.[1,2] Female plants are particularly rare.[1,2] When it flowers, kava produces narrow, yellow-green spikes (3 – 9 cm long) on a short peduncle that grows axillary or opposite the leaves.[1,2] Both male and female flowers lack sepals or petals.[1,2] The male flowers have two stamens; females have one carpel.[1,2]

The Latin name *P. methysticum*, sometimes called *P. methysticum* var. *methysticum*, refers to the group of sterile cultivars known as kava that are found only in cultivation.[3] *P. methysticum* var. *wichmannii* is the fertile, wild plant from which *P. methysticum* var. *methysticum* originated.[3] *P. methysticum* var. *wichmannii* is differentiated by its spadix, which is as long as the leaf lamina, while the spadix of *P. methysticum* var. *methysticum* is always shorter than the lamina.[3] *P. methysticum* var. *wichmannii* is more erect, with fewer stems, and has harder, more lignified roots than *P. methysticum* var. *methysticum*.[3]

THE NAME: The genus name *Piper* derives from the Greek *peperi* ("pepper"). The epithet *methysticum* ("intoxicating") derives from Latin.

HISTORICAL USES: The indigenous peoples of Micronesia, Polynesia, and Melanesia believed that kava improved access to the spirit world, and facilitated connections with the gods and ancestors.[4] Kava has been used in Pacific Islander ceremonies for thousands of years.[5] It was originally reserved for chiefs, priests, elders, and nobles in South Pacific islands.[4] Kava ceremonies were enacted on formal occasions, during village meetings with respected tribe members, and at informal social gatherings.[5] Oceanic people used kava for rites of passage, such as observing births, marriages, deaths, initiations, and naming ceremonies.[4] Kava was also consumed to restore goodwill, for peacekeeping ceremonies, social bonding, and public atonement.[4] Warring tribes consumed kava in ceremonies to amend their differences and make peace. Kava was also consumed as a relaxant and to combat fatigue.[4]

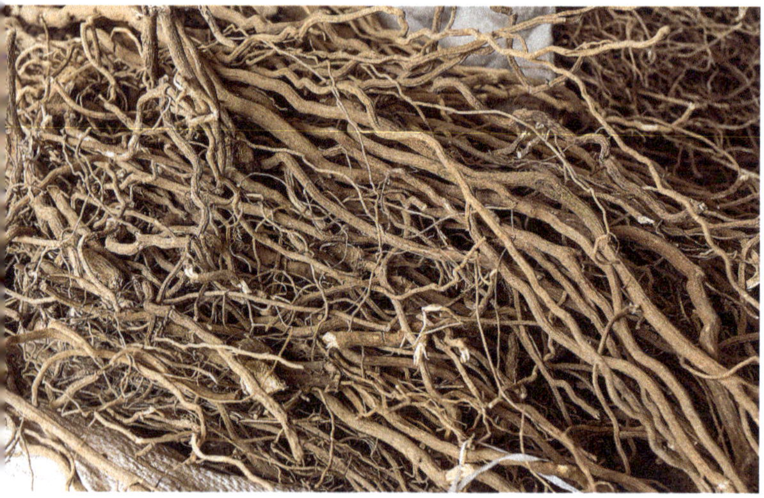

In the 1760s, Captain James Cook voyaged to the Pacific Islands, and was introduced to a kava ceremony by the indigenous people.[5] Kava roots were chewed, spat into a bowl, mixed with coconut water, and strained. The liquid was then presented in a coconut shell to the main guest who consumed the contents; the shell was refilled and presented to the next person by rank.[5]

Saliva breaks down starch and facilitates the suspension of fat soluble resins.[6] Missionaries were disturbed by the practice they considered unsanitary, and pressured the islanders to alter their preparation by grating or pounding the herb.[4] Kava was then prepared by placing the ground root in a cloth, and pounding it to produce a thick, milky white beverage.

Kava was consumed in low doses as a strengthening tonic and stimulant.[7] It was administered to treat nervous exhaustion and weakness, and reduce chills from head colds.[4] Moderate or higher doses were administered as a calmative and relaxant.[4,7] Kava was administered to treat gonorrhea, syphilis, chronic cystitis, urogenital infections, migraine headaches, difficulty sleeping, cramps, muscle pain, asthma, tuberculosis, and difficulty breathing.[4,8] It was used to treat gout and rheumatic ailments.[4,7] It also was applied to skin diseases such as leprosy.[8] Children chewed kava buds as a general restorative.[4]

Eclectic physicians borrowed from traditional native uses. They administered kava as a diuretic, and to alleviate bladder and urethra pain, in addition to treating dysuria, strangury, acute urethritis, nocturnal enuresis, prostatic troubles, and catarrh of the bladder.[9,10] Kava was given to cure gonorrhea and gleet.[9,10] It was recommended to stimulate digestion, improve assimilation, and overcome constipation.[9,10] Diluted extracts of kava were applied to reduce itching in the vulva and anus caused by an infection or poison ivy.[9]

CONSTITUENTS: Kava root contains starch, fiber, water, sugars, proteins, and minerals. The pharmacological actions are primarily due to the kavalactones (kavapyrones or kava α-pyrones) contained in the root's fat-soluble resin. The kavalactones include kavain, 5,6-dihydrokavain, 7,8-dihydrokavain, yangonin, 5,6,7,8-tetrahydroyangonin, methysticin, dihydromethysticin, 5,6-dehydromethysticin, 5,6-dihydroyangonin, 7,8-dihydroyangonin, 10-methoxy-yangonin, 11-methoxy-yangonin, 11-hydroxy-yangonin, hydroxykavain, and 11-methoxy-12-hydroxy-dehydrokavain.[8] Kava root also contains flavokavins A, B, and C, the alkaloid pipermethystin, cepharadione A, ketones (cinnamalaketone and methylene dioxy-3,4-cinnamalaketone), and alcohol (dihydrokavain-5-ol).[5,7,8,11,12]

NUTRITIONAL PROPERTIES: The roots contain minerals including potassium, calcium, magnesium, sodium, aluminum, iron, and silica, as well as sugars (saccharose, maltose, fructose, and glucose), and 15 amino acids.[8,12]

MEDICINAL PROPERTIES: Analgesic, anesthetic (local), antibacterial, antidepressant, antifungal, antiseptic, antispasmodic, anxiolytic, anodyne, diuretic, euphoric, hypnotic, nervine, relaxant, sedative, sialagogue, soporific, aphrodisiac, and expectorant.

TEMPERATURE AND FLAVOR: Warm, pungent, and bitter.

MEDICINAL USES

Kava is an analgesic, and a skeletal and smooth muscle antispasmodic that reduces pain and muscle tension.[4,6,8,11] It aids in treating tight or injured muscles, including muscle spasms, tension headaches, and fibromyalgia.[6] Kava reduces nerve pain, easing trigeminal neuralgia, sciatica, impinged nerve, and carpal tunnel flareups. Additionally, it is effective in reducing bladder and uterine cramping.[9,10] Consume the extract or tea, or apply the extract, salve, or poultice topically to relieve pain. Kava is a direct muscle relaxant that does not inhibit neuromuscular transmission, or depress the central nervous system.[4,11] The analgesic, antispasmodic, and sedative effects are attributed to the dihydrokavain and dihydromethysticin.[8] It synergizes the effects of aspirin, and in one study, it was considered superior to propanediol, benzazoles, and benzodiazepines as a muscle relaxant.[6,8] Additionally, kava reduces withdrawals from benzodiazepines.[6]

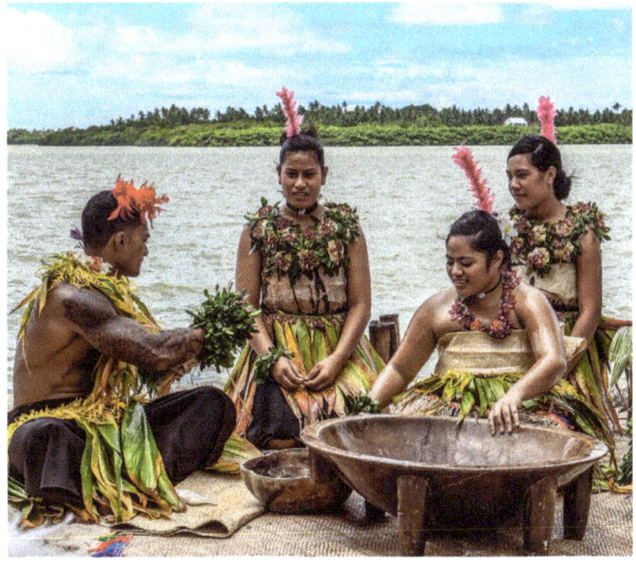

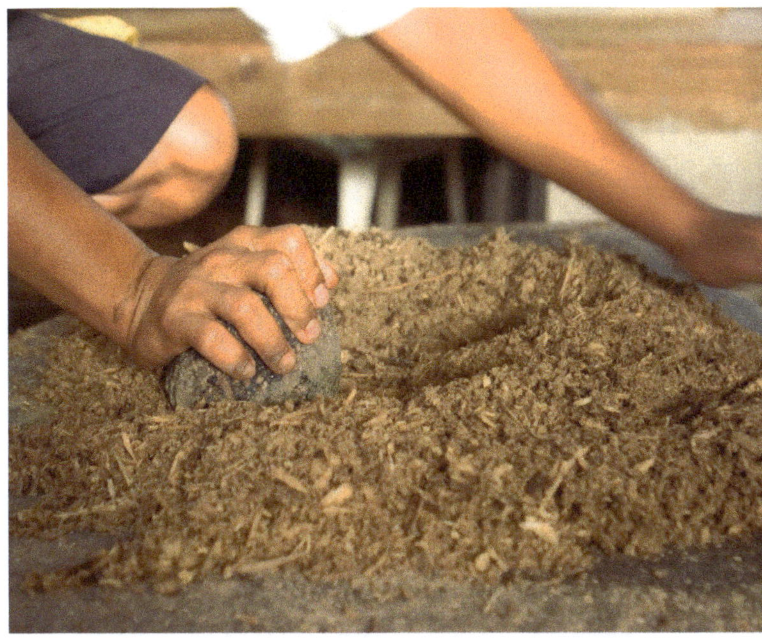

Kava is an anxiolytic, nervine, hypnotic, and sedative that reduces stress, nervousness, anxiety, premenstrual anxiety, and emotional tension.[4,11] It is a nonaddictive relaxant with minimal stupefying or hallucinogenic actions.[4] Numerous studies have confirmed kava's effectiveness in treating anxiety, tension, and agitation.[4,5] Kavalactones and kavain act on the limbic system, in particular the amygdala.[5,6] Kavalactones bind to various neuroreceptors in the brain, including dopamine and possibly GABA-A receptors, explaining the euphoric, analgesic, sedative, tranquilizing, and muscle relaxing effects.[4,6,11] Further studies are necessary to confirm the GABA-A receptor binding actions. Kava was also found to inhibit [3H]-noradrenalin (norepinephrine) uptake, contributing to its psychotropic properties.[6,11] In one double-blind study, individuals consuming kava experienced a substantial reduction in anxiety and nervousness, as well as associated symptoms, including heart palpitations, chest pains, headache, dizziness, and gastric irritation.[5] In another study, women with menopausal symptoms took kava and experienced a significant reduction of stress and anxiety, as well as improvement in mood, well-being, and hot flashes.[5] Kava is as effective in treating anxiety as diazepam (a prescription tranquilizer); however, it has fewer negative side effects, is nonaddictive, and doesn't lose effectiveness over time.[4,5] Kava increases delta, theta (daydreaming), and slow alpha brain wave activity; it also decreases fast alpha and beta (concentrating) activity in a dose-dependent manner.[11] This herb can be highly beneficial for treating pain-induced insomnia. It improves the ability to sleep, reduces wakefulness, shortens the light sleep phase, and lengthens the deep sleep phase.[6] Kava works effectively when combined

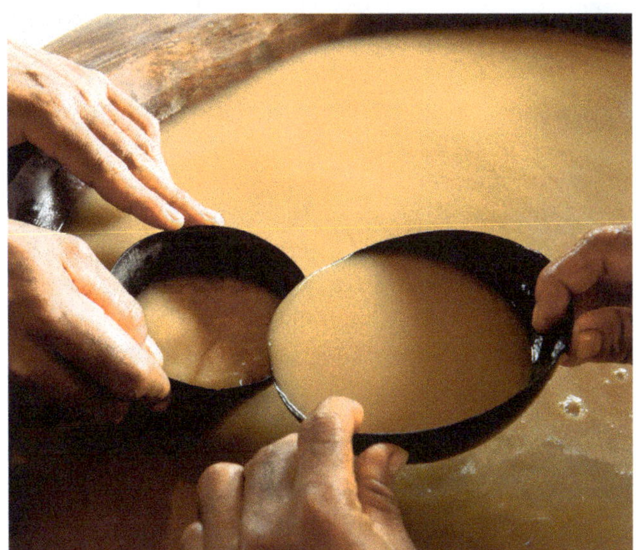

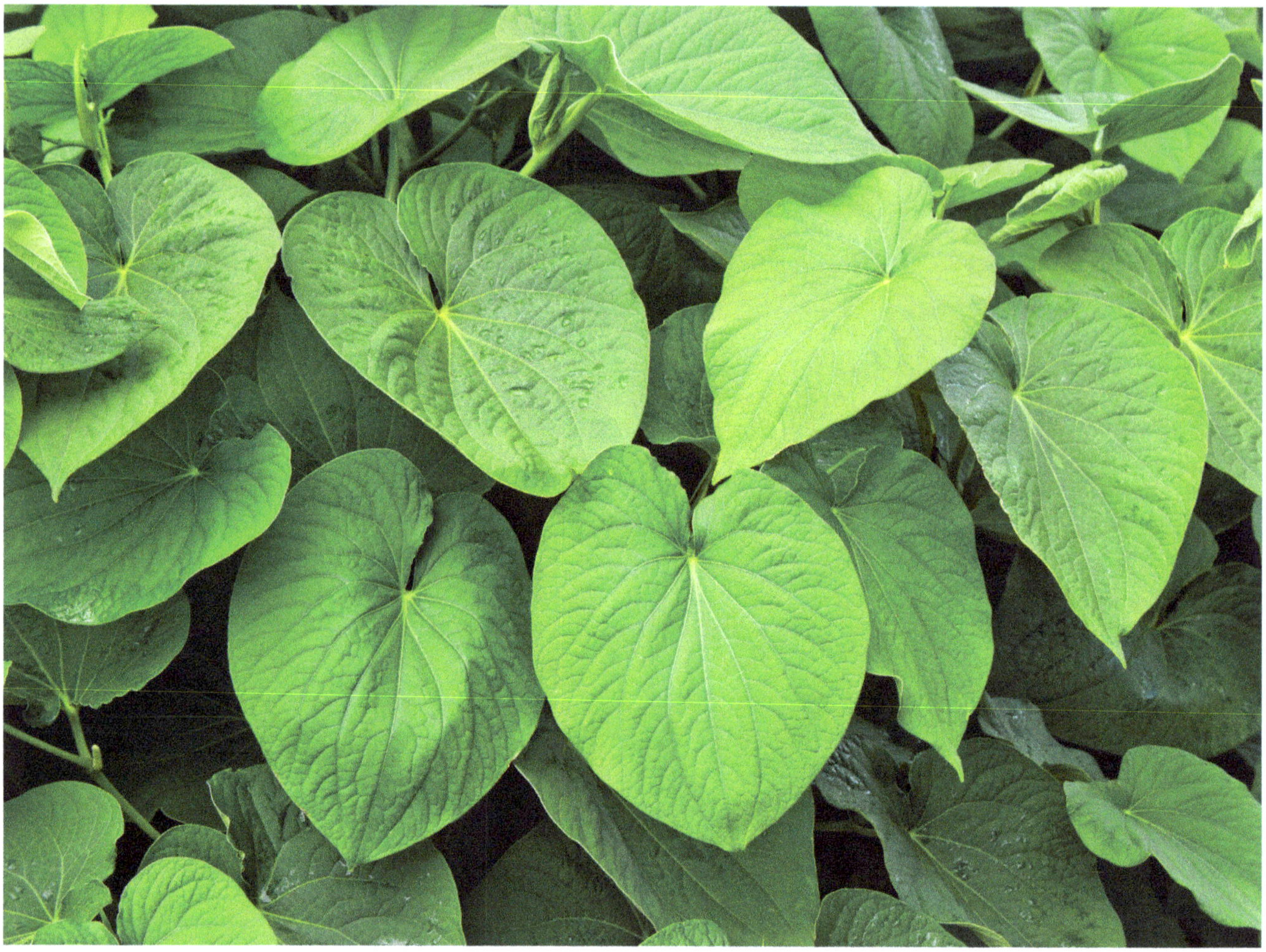

with passion flower *(Passiflora incarnata)* for the anxiolytic, nervine, and sedative actions. *Note:* Kava can be mildly stimulating or relaxing; therefore, the dosage must be determined on an individual basis. Because of potential sedative properties, kava is best consumed in the evening and throughout the night to reduce pain and alleviate sleeplessness; however, some individuals are not sedated from daytime consumption.

Kava is an anesthetic, analgesic, and sialagogue.[4,6] Applying it topically or chewing the root numbs the gums, alleviating the pain of gum abscesses and emerging wisdom teeth until dental work can be obtained. The lactone kavain produces the local anesthetic effect.[4] Kava sedates the nerves, relaxes the jaws, and reduces nerve sensitivity. Consume the tincture and/or apply kava topically prior to a dental visit to reduce gum sensitivity. It alleviates some of the pain and tension of having braces tightened. Avoid use in teething infants and young children, as it is too potent.

Kava has antidepressant and euphoric actions. It induces a sense of tranquility, peace, and contentment, especially in individuals with depression caused by stress or depletion. Kava works most effectively in treating mild to moderately depressed individuals prone to anxiety, nervousness, and nervous depletion. It blocks monoamine uptake resulting in the elevation of serotonin and dopamine levels.[11] Kava lactones have cellular actions similar to mood-stabilizing agents.[11] Kava can be beneficial for treating premenstrual or perimenopausal anxiety, agitation, depression, and mood swings.[5] In one study, kavain, a purified lactone, was administered for anxiety and improved reaction time, vigilance, and memory.[5] Kava is a mild mental stimulant.[13]

Kava helps to decrease social barriers, and can have aphrodisiac effects for individuals who experience stress-related sexual tension. It works most effectively as an aphrodisiac for nervous, high-strung females, not for those who tend to be calm. Kava can have an anaphrodisiac effect in males.[11] It produces a wide range of physical and social responses; experimentation is recommended prior to utilization in social or sexual encounters. Kava can be sedating or stupefying in some individuals, and can cause social discomfort or sedation, negating the beneficial effects.

Kava has mild antibacterial properties that aid in treating urinary tract infections.[6] Kava lactones are metabolized and excreted in urine, which may have antibacterial actions.[6] It has antispasmodic and analgesic actions that alleviate urinary pain associated with irritable bladder, interstitial cystitis, urethritis, passing kidney stones, pyelitis, and urinary incontinence.[4,7,12] It also reduces painful urination in males with prostate swelling.[9,10] Kava pyrones have an endoanesthetic effect in the bladder and gastric mucosa, easing pain in the mucous membranes.[7]

Kavalactones exhibit antifungal actions against *Candida albicans;* however, internal consumption can be sedating in moderate doses.[6] Kava aids in treating sleeplessness resulting from a severe yeast infection. Consume kava before bedtime; use internal antifungal herbs such as usnea *(Usnea)*, spilanthes *(Acmella)*, black walnut hull *(Juglans nigra)*, thyme *(Thymus vulgaris)*, and/or oregano *(Origanum vulgare)* throughout the day. The root powder, diluted tincture, oil, or salve prepared using the alcohol intermediary method can be applied topically to treat *Candida albicans*, athlete's foot, ringworm, and skin tinea. Topical applications of diluted kava extract reduce the pain and itching of spider bites, bee stings, and mosquito bites, as well as poison oak and poison ivy.

CONTRAINDICATIONS

Avoid internal consumption during pregnancy or lactation, and in endogenous depression; topical use is permissible.[4,12] Kava should not be used with children or individuals under the age of 18.[11] Avoid operating heavy machinery or vehicles when using kava.[4]

Consult a health care practitioner or avoid consuming kava with prescription medications, including antidepressant, anxiolytic, hypnotic, analgesic, sedative, or psychopharmaceutic drugs.[4,12] Individuals consuming a dopamine antagonist medication to treat Parkinson's disease should avoid consuming kava because of the possible dopamine antagonism.[6,11] In rare cases, excessive consumption of kava can result in photophobia, diplopia, and temporary oculomotor paralysis.[8]

Do not consume kava more than three to six consecutive months unless advised by a health care practitioner.[12] Alcoholic beverages may interact with kava and impair liver function.[4,12] Consuming large, frequent doses (400 mg or more of kavalactones per day) long-term can potentially alter liver function, and cause liver-related skin disorders such as skin lesions and epidermal dryness (known as kava dermopathy) characterized by urticarial patches with itching.[6,8,11] The skin conditions resolve when kava use is discontinued.[11] Continuous use of kava may result in liver disorders; symptoms to watch for include yellow discoloration of the skin, hair, and nails, nausea, vomiting, light-colored stools, unusual fatigue or weakness, loss of appetite, and stomach or abdominal pain.[8,11] Avoid using kava with individuals who consume high quantities of alcohol or hepatotoxic medications, as well as those with compromised liver function or liver disease (hepatitis, cirrhosis, or liver failure).[4,11] According to herbalist Mark Blumenthal of the American Botanical Council, "Current research does not provide clear evidence of any scientific rationale that kava use is associated with liver damage; nonetheless, consumers and patients are advised to heed the above cautions. A detailed review of the chronology of the events related to kava and its alleged association with hepatotoxicity can be found on the American Botanical Council website."[11]

PREPARATION AND DOSAGE

TINCTURE: Fresh roots [1:2, 95% alcohol]; dry roots [1:5, 70% alcohol]; consume 10-90 drops, up to three times daily.

FLUID EXTRACT: Dry roots [1:1, 50% alcohol]; consume 5-60 drops, up to three times daily.

CAPSULES: Consume 1-3 capsules, one to three times daily, or consume 60-180 mg of kavalactones per day via powdered extract (not less than 30% kavalactones) or semisolid (paste) extract (not less than 50% kavalactones).[6,11]

TEA: Prepare a cold infusion or decoction; consume 8-12 ounces, one to three times daily. Infusing the root in coconut milk or coconut water with ½-1 teaspoon of lecithin enhances the extraction of fat-soluble components.

TOPICAL USE: Apply the diluted tincture or alcohol-infused oil topically. The powder can be applied as an antimicrobial dust.

KELP AND BLADDERWRACK

DESCRIPTION

BOTANICAL NAMES:
Laminaria digitata, L. spp.
Fucus vesiculosus, F. spp.

COMMON NAMES:
Kelp, sugar wrack, kombu, oarweed, devil's apron, sea colander, and tangle; fucus, bladder fucus, bladderwrack, seawrack, rock rack, black tang, tangleweed, oarweed, cutweed, dyer's fucus, red fucus, vraic
rakkolevä (Finnish)
fucus, laminaires (French)
blasentang (German)
quercia marina (Italian)
encina de mar, fuco verigoso (Spanish)
blåstång (Swedish)

FAMILY NAMES:
Laminariaceae (*Laminaria* spp.) and Fucaceae (*Fucus* spp.)

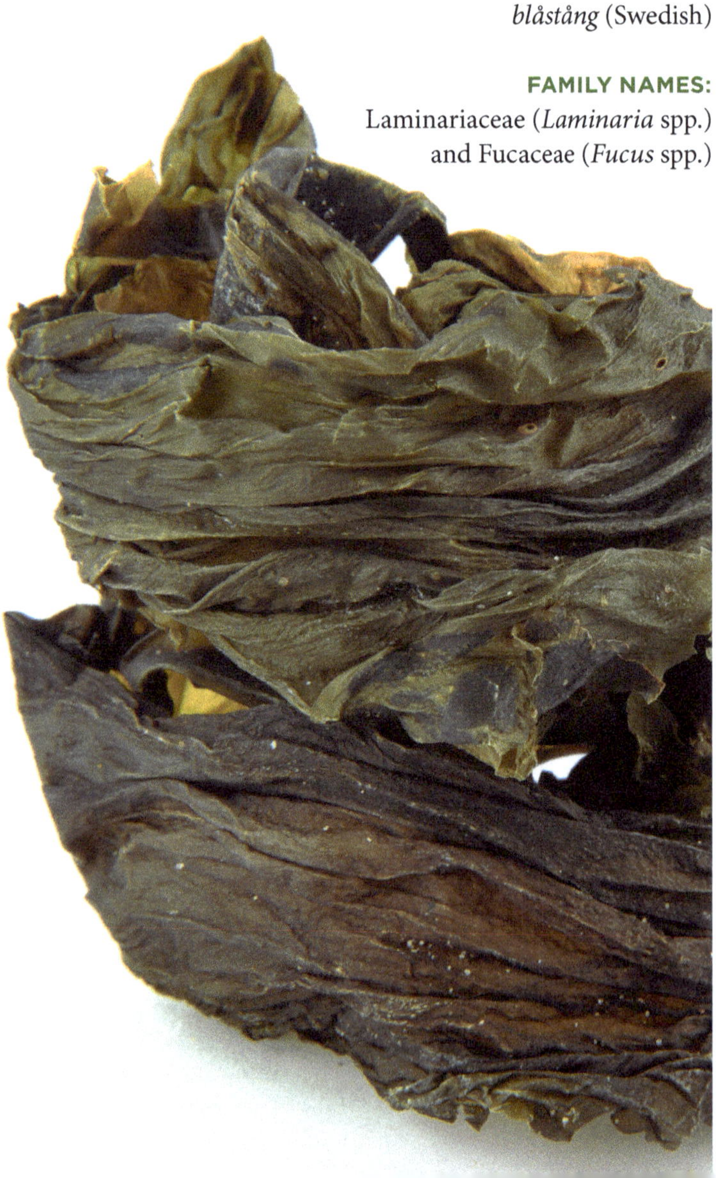

PARTS USED: The blades (fronds) and sodium alginate.

BOTANICAL DESCRIPTION AND HABITAT: *Laminaria* (kelp) is a brown algae found in the North Atlantic and North Pacific Oceans. It grows in the subtidal zone to depths of 8 – 30 meters, or in intertidal zones on rocky shores where it forms dense colonies.[1] *Laminaria* species

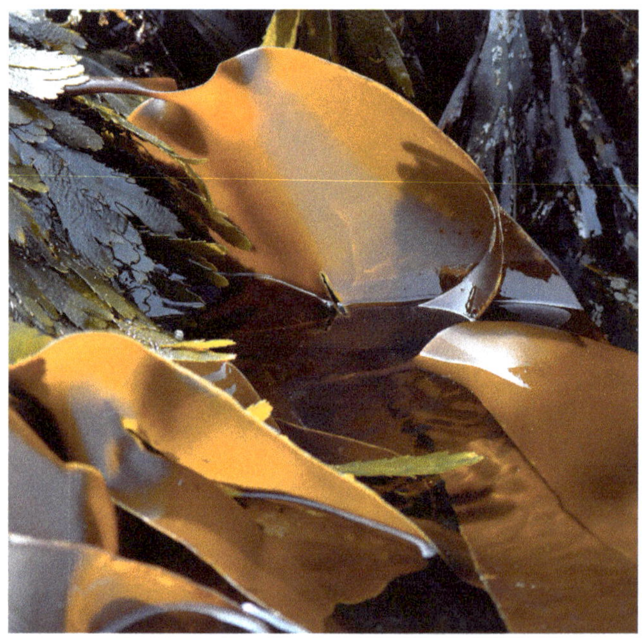

are olive green to dark brown and grow 30 – 200 cm long.[2] The branched holdfast resembles a cluster of roots.[2] Some species have long, thin, cordlike stipes. The thallus can be unbranched and straplike; the main branch can divide into a fan shape. The laminas are often corrugated.[2]

Fucus (bladderwrack) is a brown algae found in the intertidal zones of oceans worldwide. It attaches to rocks with a sturdy branching, discoid holdfast.[3] The brownish-green to light yellow, erect thallus has a leathery texture, often with a distinctive midrib; most species have entire margins. *Fucus* exhibits a dichotomous branching pattern and grows up to four feet long.[3] At the branching tips, fertile reproductive receptacles balloon out when mature. In *F. vesiculosus,* pairs of spherical air vesicles develop on either side of the midrib and at the branch forks.[3,4]

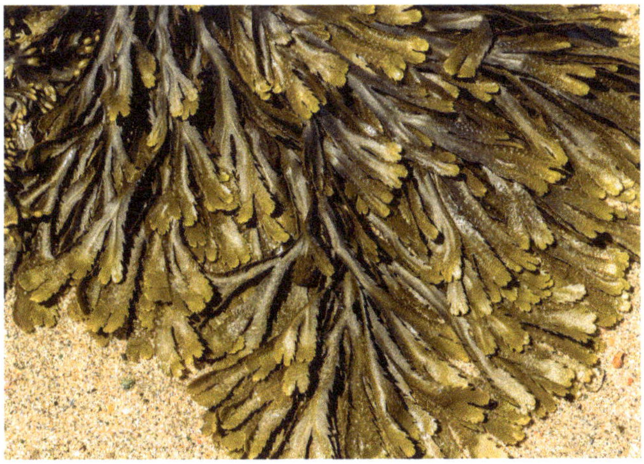

THE NAME: The genus *Laminaria* ("plate") derives from Latin.[5] The epithet *digitata* means "finger-like," referring to the branch tips.[6] The common names oarweed and tangleweed refer to the plant's dense, floating, tangled mass.[6] The genus *Fucus* originates from the Greek *phykos,* a derivative of *phytein* ("to grow").[7] The epithet *vesiculosus* derives from the Latin *vescicula* ("vescicle"), referring to the bulbous frond tips.[7]

The following common names correspond with the genus names: kelp, horsetail kelp, Iceland kelp, Atlantic kelp, seawand, tangleweed, sea colander, oarweed, sea staff, and devil's apron *(Laminaria);* bladderwrack, black tang, seawrack, toothed wrack, rockweed, bladder fucus, sea oak, dyer's focus, red focus, rockwrack, cut weed, and tangle weed *(Fucus);* rockweed, knotted wrack, knotted kelp, egg wrack, and Norwegian kelp *(Ascophyllum nodosum = Fucus scorphioides);* and giant kelp and giant Pacific kelp *(Macrocystis).*

Laminaria and *Macrocystis pyrifera* are in the Laminariaceae family. *Fucus* and *Ascophyllum* are in the Fucaceae family.

HISTORICAL USES: Sea vegetables have been consumed in Japan since 8000 BCE, and for thousands of years in China and Korea.[6,8] In China, sea vegetables were a delicacy served to royals and other honorable guests.[8] Kombu was the only soup stock base consumed by Buddhist priests.[2] In East Asia, it continues to be used as an ingredient in soup and sushi. Kelp was used as a folk medicine to treat thyroid disorders, goiters, and low blood pressure.[6] In Japan, bathing in kelp-infused baths was believed to alleviate nervous disorders.[6]

In Europe, dried red wrack was heated with sulfuric acid, then cooled, fermented with brewers' yeast, and distilled into alcohol.[3] *Fucus helminthocorton* (Corsican moss) was used in Europe as an anthelmintic primarily to expel the lumbricoid worm.[9] An expressed kelp juice and decoction was consumed to treat rheumatism.[3] Kelp preparations were applied topically to sprains and bruises, and to strengthen the limbs of children with rickets.[3] Due to a lack of chemical fertilizers during the war, kelp was applied to the soil as an agricultural fertilizer.[3]

Eclectic physicians administered kelp as an alterative and diuretic, and to reduce adipose tissue in healthy individuals.[10,11] It was given to soothe acute nephritis, and for bladder irritation and inflammation.[10-12] Kelp was used to treat scrophula, as well as exophthalmos and simple goiters.[3,10] It was administered to remove tissue hypertrophies, as well as benign and malignant tumors.[12] Kelp also treated fatty degeneration of the heart.[10-12] It was prescribed for women with menorrhagia and leukorrhea resulting from poor uterine muscle tone.[10] In North America, this highly nutrient seaweed continues to be included in cattle and horse feed, and in plant fertilizer.[12]

CONSTITUENTS: *Fucus* contains iodine, bromine, polysaccharides (fucoidan = fucan = fucosan = sulfated fucan; laminarin; and alginic acid), saturated fatty acids (palmitic, stearic, myristic, and squalane), unsaturated fatty acids (olein and arachidonic), mucilaginous compounds (salts of alginic acid, including sodium alginate), protein, amino acids, vitamins, and minerals (see *Nutritional Properties*), β-sitosterol, and fucosterol.[7]

Laminaria contains alginic acid, laminarin, fucoidan, mannitol, carrageenan, D-glucose, D-galactose, kainic acid, laminine, xeaxanthin, protein, amino acids, vitamins, and minerals (see *Nutritional Properties*).[2,6]

Algin refers to the hydrophilic colloidal substance isolated from the members of brown algae.[13] Algin is produced by pre-washing the seaweed and extracting the alginic acid with an alkaline solution. The unctuous, gelatinous mass is clarified, and the alginic acid is obtained following mineral acid treatment. Alginic acid can then be converted to sodium alginate, the primary form of algin.[13]

NUTRITIONAL PROPERTIES: *Fucus* contains high amounts of aluminum, ash, calcium, dietary fiber, iodine, magnesium, manganese, potassium, selenium, silicon, sodium, tin, and vitamin A.[7] It also contains low to average amounts of chromium, cobalt, crude fiber, iron, phosphorus, potassium, protein, vitamins B_2, B_3, B_{12}, C, and E, and zinc.[2,7]

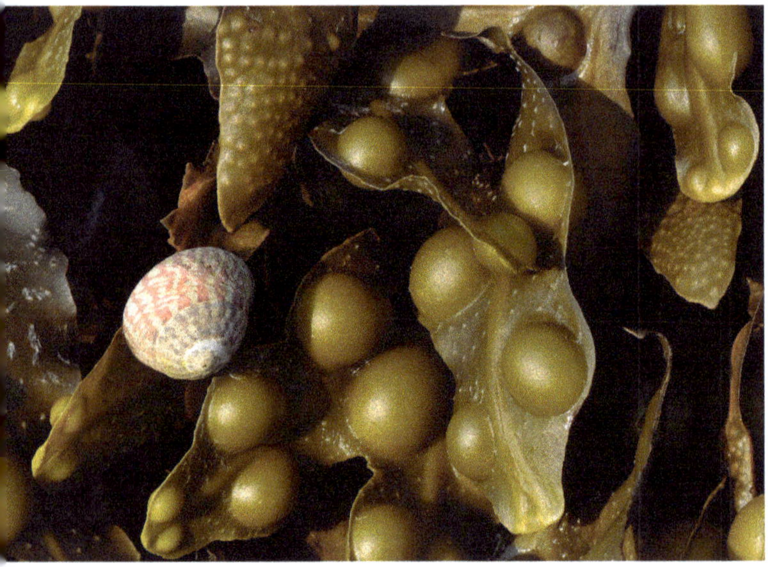

Laminaria contains high amounts of iodine, calcium, and potassium.[2,6] It also contains β-carotene, vitamins B_1, B_2, B_3, B_5, B_9, B_{12}, and C, iron, magnesium, phosphorus, protein, and sodium.[2,6]

MEDICINAL PROPERTIES: Alterative, antibacterial, anticarcinogenic, antidyscratic, antioxidant, demulcent, diuretic, emollient, expectorant, hepatic, hypocholesterolemic, immune modulator, laxative, nutritive, stomachic, and thyroid stimulant.

TEMPERATURE AND FLAVOR: Cool, salty, and sweet.

MEDICINAL USES

In this document, kelp refers to brown seaweed or algae in the Phaeophyceae class, including kelp *(Laminaria)*, bladderwrack *(Fucus)*, Japanese wakame *(Alaria)*, rockweed *(Ascophyllum)*, and kombu *(Saccharina japonica)*. Kelp and other iodine-containing seaweeds have a thyroid-stimulating effect.[14] Due to the iodine content, kelp increases thyroid hormone levels, which aids in treating iodine-deficient hypothyroidism.[7] Kelp supports symptoms of hypothyroidism by gently increasing metabolism and enhancing weight loss.[7,14] It decreases fatigue, lethargy, joint tenderness and swelling, and arthritis.[3] The thyroid-stimulating actions support related conditions, such as amenorrhea, menstrual irregularity, and infertility resulting from hypothyroidism.[15]

Kelp contains iodine 127, a natural isotope that is absorbed and stored almost exclusively in the thyroid and used to manufacture thyroid hormones.[16] Iodine 131, a hazardous decay product of nuclear explosions, is continually released into the atmosphere by all nuclear weapons, bombs, reactor fuel rods, and nuclear facilities.[16] There is no way to selectively excrete it. In the absence of sufficient dietary levels of iodine 127, iodine 131 is absorbed into the thyroid, causing thyroid disease and cancer.[16] Consuming sufficient amounts of natural iodine 127 daily (150 mcg or 5 – 10 grams of seaweed) prevents iodine deficiency and the absorption of hazardous iodine 131 into the thyroid and other tissues.[16] Consuming kelp before, during, or after exposure to X-rays, CT scans, radiation, barium shakes, barium enemas, or other radioactivity aids in detoxifying radioactive substances and preventing their absorption.[16]

The iodine content of kelp varies among species and habitats; consequently, the iodine content of a kelp preparation should be stated on the label. When addressing hypothyroid symptoms, the minimum suggested daily intake of iodine is 150 micrograms, although 150 – 750 mcg of iodine is often recommended. Some practitioners recommend maintaining daily supplemental iodine levels below 600 mcg, while others suggest a daily maximum of 750 mcg.[17] To be cautious, begin by consuming 150 mcg daily; increase the dosage in 150 mcg increments every two to four weeks until the symptoms of hypothyroidism decrease. *Note:* Do not exceed 750 mcg per day unless recommended by a health care practitioner. Decrease the dosage or discontinue if signs of excess iodine intake are experienced, such as altered thyroid function, rapid heart rate, anxiety, sweating, acne, or skin rash.[16]

Kelp is an adjunct treatment for fibrocystic breast disease (FBD), especially with concurrent symptoms of hypothyroidism or iodine deficiency.[17] A higher incidence of breast cancer is correlated with iodine deficiency and/or hypothyroidism.[17] The breast cancer preventative effects are attributed to the iodine, algin, and fiber content.[14,17] According to naturopathic doctors Michael Murray and Joseph Pizzorno, iodine (iodine caseinate) may be an effective treatment of FBD. It is theorized that an absence of iodine renders the breast cells more sensitive to estrogen stimulation. Also, oral iodine supplementation is known to have significant anti-inflammatory and antifibrotic effects in acute and chronic experimental models. This hypersensitivity to estrogen in iodine deficiency leads the breast ducts to produce small cysts, and later fibrosis.[17]

Kelp contains sodium alginate, a high molecular weight polysaccharide.[13] Sodium alginate protects the body from heavy metal contamination, and aids in detoxifying heavy metals.[16] Sodium alginate binds with other radioactive divalent metal ions, including barium, tin, cadmium, manganese, zinc, mercury, lead, and iron.[13,16] It then transforms the ions into an insoluble, gel-like salt that is eliminated in the feces.[13]

Sodium alginate decreases plasma and liver cholesterol by enhancing the biliary excretion of cholesterol in rats.[13] Laminine dioxalate, a component of *Laminaria* species, has hypotensive activity.[13] Sodium alginate also enhances steroid hormone binding that eliminates estrogen and reduces symptoms of estrogen excess.

The alginates have immune modulating actions.[14] The alginates and additional polysaccharides potentially stimulate T cells.[14] Fucoidan stimulates cellular production of antiviral cytokines that hinder viral attachment and penetration to cells.[16] Fucoidin and alginates also prevent viral infections, including influenza, herpes simplex, and HIV.[6] Kelp has been shown to be active against many pathogenic organisms, including *Staphylococcus, Streptococcus, Brucella, Klebsiella, Proteus, E. coli,* and *Salmonella.*[14]

Glands in kelp fronds produce profuse quantities of mucilage.[6] This helps the algae to prevent water loss at low tide when exposed to air.[6] The mucilage contains algin, a substance with soothing demulcent and emollient effects.[7] Water-based preparations such as a decoction, cold infusion, or kelp-containing soup stock decrease inflammation of the mucous membranes in the throat, lungs, stomach, intestines, and urinary tract. The demulcent properties are beneficial for treating a sore throat, laryngitis, dry cough, and whooping cough. It also alleviates heat-induced phlegm (yellow or green mucus).[18] As a long-term tonic, it aids in treating inflammatory conditions in the upper and lower gastrointestinal tract, including gastric ulcers, gastritis, leaky gut syndrome, irritable bowel syndrome, ulcerative colitis, and Crohn's disease. Kelp is best consumed on an empty stomach to heal the digestive tract lining. The mucilaginous and demulcent properties have yin tonifying actions.[18] Water-based preparations also serve as recuperative agents following a febrile disease and to treat summer-heat symptoms. Kelp contains fucans that reduce inflammation.[8,16]

A demulcent, kelp lubricates the stools, reducing constipation.[14] Due to its soluble fiber content, kelp also serves as a bulk-forming laxative. Kelp inhibits carcinogenic fecal flora, which may aid in preventing cancer in the colon and rectum. It reduces fungal and candida yeast overgrowth.[18] A kelp-containing soup, a rehydrated sea vegetable salad, or water-based preparations are ideal as laxatives. Add 3 – 6 inches of dried kombu in cooking water for each cup of dried beans in order to enhance their digestibility, reduce flatulence, and hasten the cooking process.[8]

Kelp contains numerous minerals, vitamins, amino acids, and proteins that increase vitality and reduce fatigue.[6,7,16] Because stress depletes B vitamins, kelp is beneficial for individuals who experience high stress or anxiety levels.[8] Folic acid and magnesium aid in protecting the heart and cardiovascular system.[8] Regular consumption of kelp aids in treating anemia and blood deficiency following a heavy

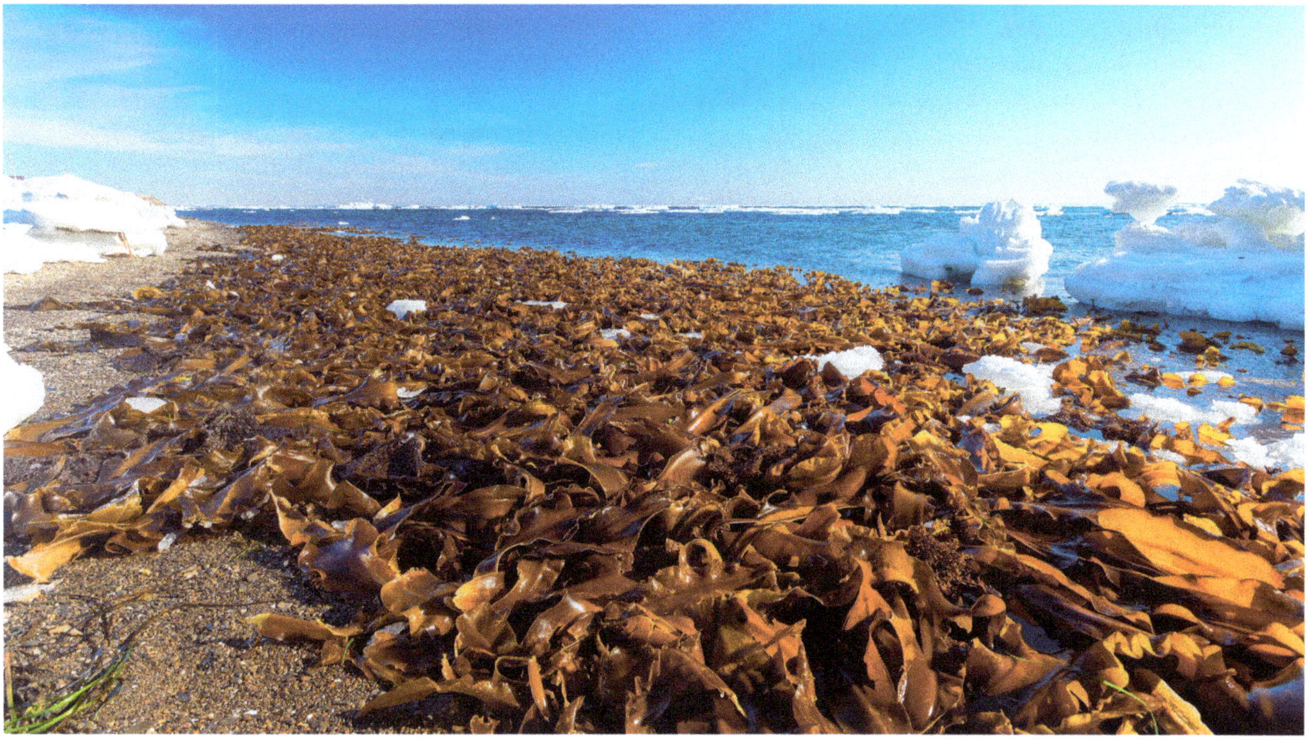

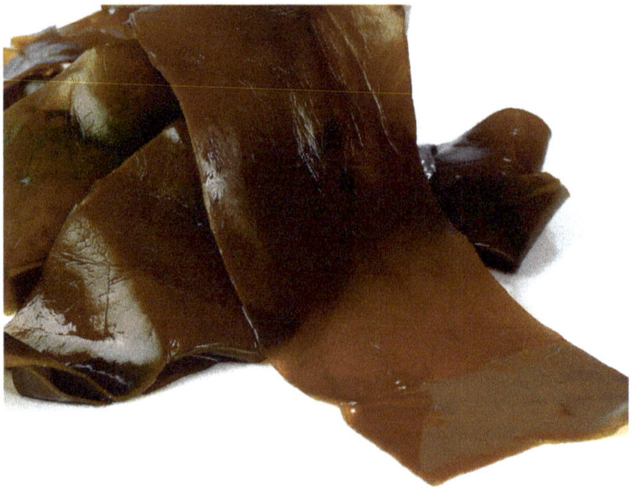

menstrual period, childbirth, or irregular menopausal bleeding. The magnesium and lignans aid in reducing menopausal symptoms.[8] Kelp, especially its ash, is a good alternative to salt, due to its high proportion of potassium to sodium.[16,18] An excellent fertilizer, add kelp to garden soil and spray plant foliage with kelp tea.[16]

Sodium alginate is used as a thickening agent in various products, including gelatins, puddings, condiments, frozen dairy products, baked goods, soups, and beverages.[13] It is also used in cosmetic products (gels, creams, and lotions), and is a stabilizing agent in oil-in-water emulsions.[13]

Topical water-based applications of kelp have emollient properties that reduce inflammation.[16] Apply tea, baths, fomentations, or poultices to dry, cracked skin, wrinkles, dry eczema, fissures, rashes, the dry stages of poison oak or poison ivy, dandruff, or hangnails.[16] Water-based preparations of kelp lubricate vaginal tissues and are added to natural lubricants.

Midwives recommend using pre-moistened kelp to ripen the cervix. Topical applications of kelp help to heal vaginal and labial tears following childbirth. Presoak the seaweed and apply it to inflamed or torn tissues.

CONTRAINDICATIONS

Avoid collecting kelp in polluted water. Kelp is contraindicated in individuals with loose, watery stools.[18] Individuals consuming supplemental thyroid hormones should consult a health care practitioner before taking kelp daily. Individuals medicated for Hashimoto's thyroiditis should consult a health care practitioner before consuming kelp. Kelp can be less effective as a thyroid stimulant in individuals with a partially removed thyroid. It has no effect on thyroid gland function if the thyroid has been removed or irradiated. Kelp supplementation is contraindicated for individuals with clinical hyperthyroidism or Grave's disease, and those consuming thyrosuppressive medications. Additionally, recent studies indicate that iodine (particularly iodized salt) can aggravate autoimmune thyroid disease, including Hashimoto's thyroiditis and Grave's disease.[19] *Note:* Iodide exerts a stronger effect on thyroid function than iodine.

Excessive iodine consumption can inhibit thyroid gland synthesis.[17] Although the recommended levels are disputed, some sources advise not exceeding 750 mcg per day; others suggest a maximum 600 mcg dosage.[16,17] An overdose of dietary intake of iodine is associated with acne-like skin eruptions.[6] *Note:* Iodized salt contains 70 mcg of iodine per gram of salt, which should be factored into a thyroid-stimulating regimen. Soaking seaweed and discarding the water dramatically decreases the sodium content for sodium sensitive individuals and those with sodium-related hypertension.[8,16]

PREPARATION AND DOSAGE

FLUID EXTRACT: Dry seaweed [1:1, 50% alcohol]; consume 30-60 drops, up to three times daily.

CAPSULES: Consume 2-4 tablets or capsules, up to three times daily. The minimum recommended dosage of iodine for individuals 11 and older is 150 mcg, 175 mcg for pregnant women, and up to 200 mcg for lactating women.

TEA: Prepare a cold infusion or decoction; consume 4-8 ounces, up to four times daily.

TOPICAL USE: Prepare a decoction and apply as a poultice or fomentation, or add the strained tea into bath water.

CULINARY USE: Consume 1-3 teaspoons daily. Add chopped seaweed or granules to vegetable or bone broths, soup stock, miso soup, bean dishes, and lacto-fermented vegetables. Prepare a seaweed food sprinkle by combining kelp or bladderwrack granules with ground, toasted sesame seeds and other seaweeds of choice, such as sea lettuce, dulse, or nori. If the flavor is palatable, add ⅓-2 teaspoons of powdered herb or granules to smoothies.

LADY'S MANTLE

DESCRIPTION

BOTANICAL NAMES:
Alchemilla vulgaris (syn. *A. xanthochlora*), *A. mollis, A. alpina, A. arvensis*

COMMON NAMES:
Lady's mantle, Our Lady's mantle, common lady's mantle, silvery lady's mantle, dewcup, lion's foot, bear's foot, nine hooks, great sanicle, stellaria
leeuvenvoet (Dutch)
poimulehti (Finnish)
alchémille, manteau de Notre Dame, patte de lapin, pinou, porte-rosé, pied de lion (French)
frauenmantle, grosser sanikel, mutterkraut, ohmkraut, sinnau, taumantel (German)
alchemilla commune, pie di lione (Italian)
Leontopodium (Medieval Latin)
alquimila (Spanish)
daggkapa (Swedish)[1]

FAMILY NAME:
Rosaceae

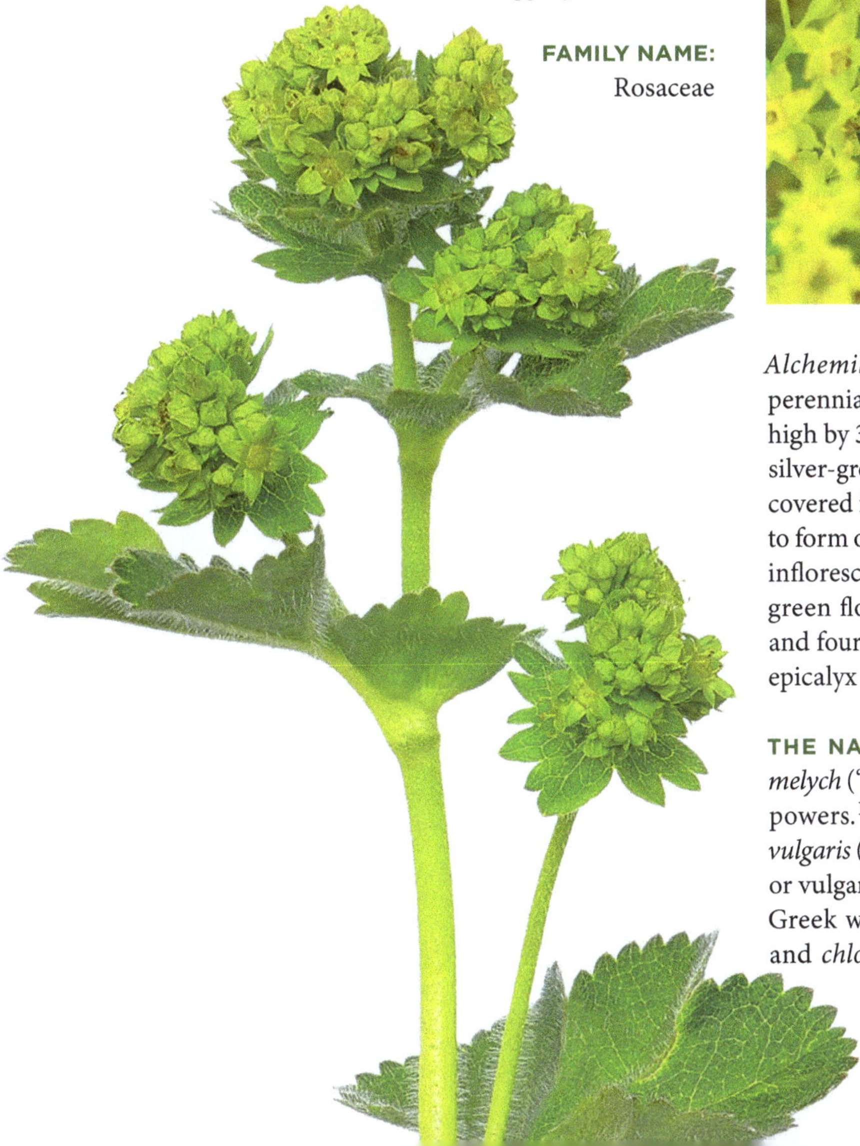

PARTS USED: The aerial portions, including the leaves and flowers; roots are used as an astringent.

BOTANICAL DESCRIPTION AND HABITAT: Lady's mantle is a lovely herbaceous perennial native to western and central Europe; its range has extended to Sweden, Latvia, Greece, Greenland, and northern Asia. A few species have naturalized in damp or dry, shady wooded areas of eastern North America.

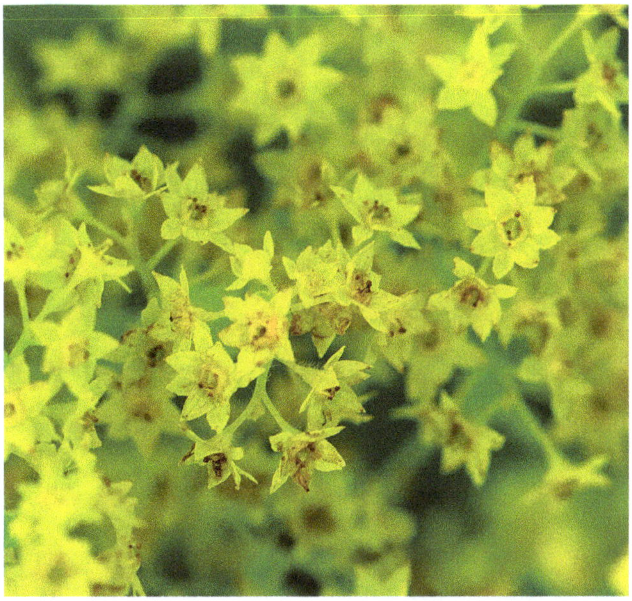

Alchemilla vulgaris is a mound-forming, herbaceous perennial with decumbent stems. It grows up to 14 inches high by 30 inches wide.[2] The palmately-lobed, fan-shaped, silver-green leaves have serrated margins, and are densely covered in hairs on both surfaces, allowing beads of water to form on the upper surface and along the margins.[2,3] The inflorescence is a loose corymb of numerous tiny, yellow-green flowers that lack petals, each bearing four sepals and four stamens upon a hypanthium.[2,3] Segments of the epicalyx alternate the sepals.[2,3] The fruit is an achene.[2,3]

THE NAME: *Alchemilla* derives from the Arabic *alkemelych* ("alchemy"), referring to the plant's versatile healing powers.[1] The epithet *vulgaris* originates from the Latin *vulgaris* ("of or pertaining to the common people, common, or vulgar").[4] The epithet *xanthochlora* is composed of two Greek words: *xantho,* derived from *xanthos* ("yellow"), and *chlora,* derived from *khloros* ("pale green"), likely

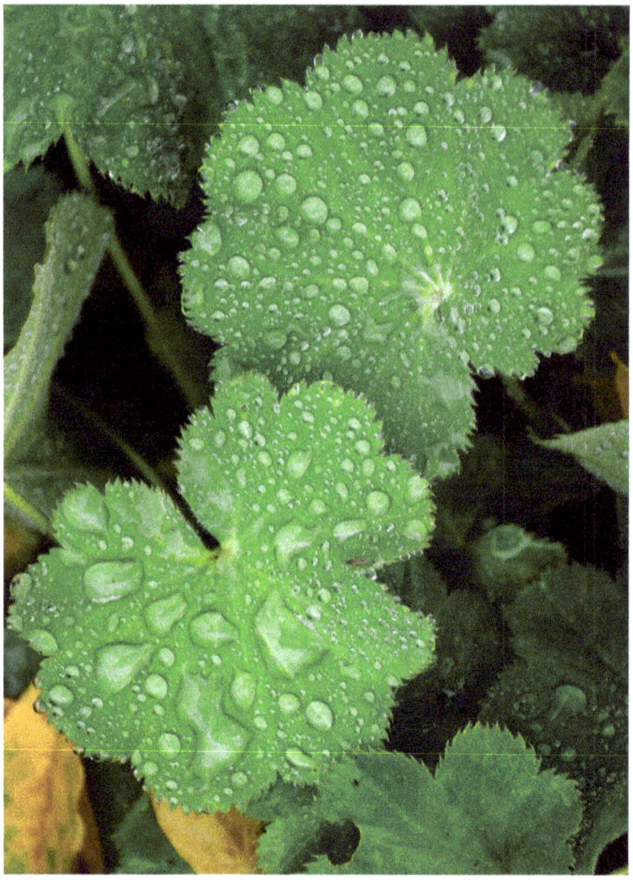

referring to the yellow-green color of the flowers, or the yellow flowers and pale green leaves. The Latin origin of the epithet *arvensis* means "of the field, meadow, or grassland." The epithet *mollis* refers to the earlier Proto-Indo-European *molduis* ("soft or weak"), presumably named for the leaves' softness.[4] In the Middle Ages, the herb acquired the name lady's mantle due to its association with the Virgin Mary. The lobes of the leaves were said to resemble the scalloped edge of a mantle.[1] Jerome Bock, 16th century botanist, named the herb *frauenmantle* (German for lady's mantle).[1] The name "nine hooks" was given because of the herb's nine broad, shallow lobes of leaves with finely toothed edges.[1] The medieval name *Leontopodium* and French name pied-de-lion mean "lion's foot," likely referring to the paw-like shape of the leaves.[1] Referring to the star-like flowers, the herb was called *Stellaria,* not to be confused with *Stellaria media* (chickweed).[1]

HISTORICAL USES: Lady's mantle was used for centuries throughout northern Europe and the Middle East.[5] Alchemists revered it as a magical plant because the leaves collected dew drops. In fact, dew was considered a holy water that could cleanse and purify all illnesses, so it was used as a base in many alchemical formulas.[5] Arabs have administered this plant for centuries to ensure fertility.[5] In Switzerland, it was revered as a woman's herb, and is still commonly grown. Today, women continue the tradition of applying a poultice of lady's mantle in order to firm and tone breast tissue.[5] In Sweden, the tincture was employed for spasmodic or convulsive diseases, and a leaf placed under the pillow was said to promote restful sleep.[1] Culpeper prized the herb as a vulnerary for slowly healing, inflamed wounds, and indolent sores.[1] Sheep, horses, and cattle graze on the leaves after the moisture dissipates.[1]

CONSTITUENTS: Lady's mantle contains tannins (ellagitannins and gallotannins), flavonoids (flavonols and leucoanthocyanidins), glycosides, triterpenes (oleanolic and ursolic acids), agrimoniin, pendunculagin, and a trace of salicylic acid.[7,8]

NUTRITIONAL PROPERTIES: Lady's mantle contains flavonoids; additional nutritional properties have not been identified.

MEDICINAL PROPERTIES: Astringent, anti-inflammatory, hemostatic, styptic, vulnerary, and mild febrifuge.

TEMPERATURE AND FLAVOR: Cool, astringent, mildly sweet, and bitter.

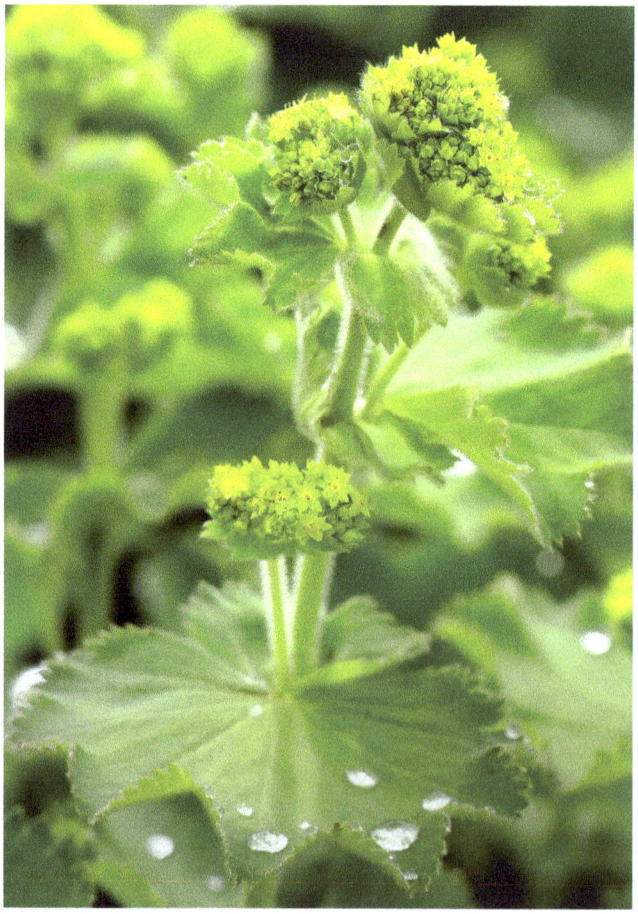

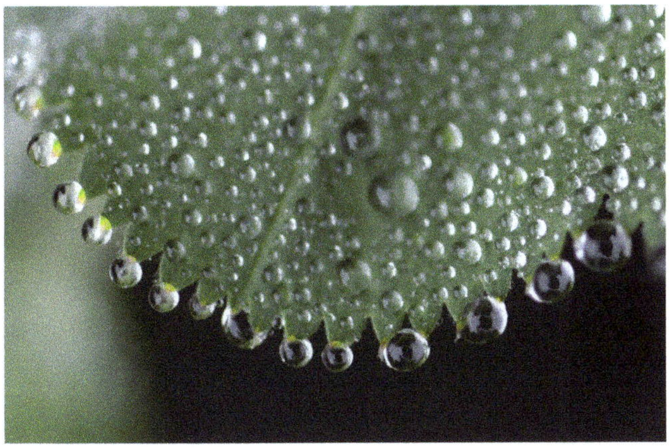

MEDICINAL USES

Like many members of the rose family, lady's mantle contains tannins that tighten and astringe the tissues, reducing inflammation in the mucous membranes and epidermis.[1] Consuming the tea is effective for treating gastritis, enteritis, or diarrhea; however, additional anti-infective agents are required when inflammation is caused by a microbial infection.[8] While the leaves suffice as an astringent and hemostatic, the roots are a more potent astringent for treating more persistent diarrhea or bleeding.[7,8] Gargling with the tea or a diluted tincture reduces mouth and throat inflammation.[8] Vaginal irrigation aids in treating leukorrhea and vaginitis.[5] An eye wash prepared from well-strained, cooled tea reduces irritation and discharge caused by conjunctivitis or blepharitis. *Note:* Prepare a fresh batch of tea daily when treating eye infections. A sitz bath reduces inflammation in the labia, perineum, and rectum resulting from birthing, yeast infections, or hemorrhoids.[8]

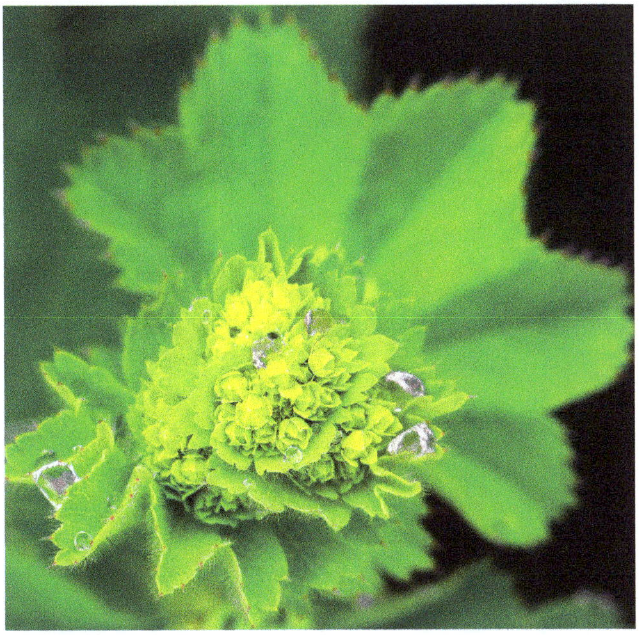

The astringent tannins are hemostatic and reduce excessive menstrual blood flow. Lady's mantle reduces mid-cycle, breakthrough, postpartum, and perimenopausal bleeding, and bleeding due to conditions such as fibroids, cysts, and endometriosis.[1,5-8] Apply the leaf poultice topically as a styptic to staunch bleeding from cuts, abrasions, or bruises.[1,8]

Lady's mantle contains small amounts of salicylic acid, which has anti-inflammatory actions similar to aspirin.[5] Although its actions are very subtle, it can be helpful in alleviating menstrual cramps, mild joint inflammation, headaches, or a mild fever. Other herbs such as meadowsweet *(Filipendula)* and Jamaican dogwood *(Piscidia)* are more potent analgesics.

CONTRAINDICATIONS

There are no known side effects or contraindications.[5,8]

PREPARATION AND DOSAGE

TINCTURE: Fresh leaves and flowers [1:2-1:3, 60-95% alcohol]; dry leaves and flowers [1:5, 60% alcohol and 10% glycerin]; consume 15-60 drops, up to four times daily.

CAPSULES: Consume 2-4 "00" capsules, up to three times daily.

TEA: Prepare a hot or cold infusion; consume 8-12 ounces, up to three times daily.

TOPICAL USE: Strain the hot infusion through a coffee filter and allow it to cool. Use in applications such as an eye wash, mouthwash, vaginal irrigation, enema, sitz bath, fomentation, or poultice. Apply the freshly ground herb as a poultice.

CULINARY USE: Use fresh flowers as a garnish; individual flowers can be lightly sprinkled on soup or salad. Fresh leaves make a lovely display for holding goat cheese or other rounded molds of cheese.

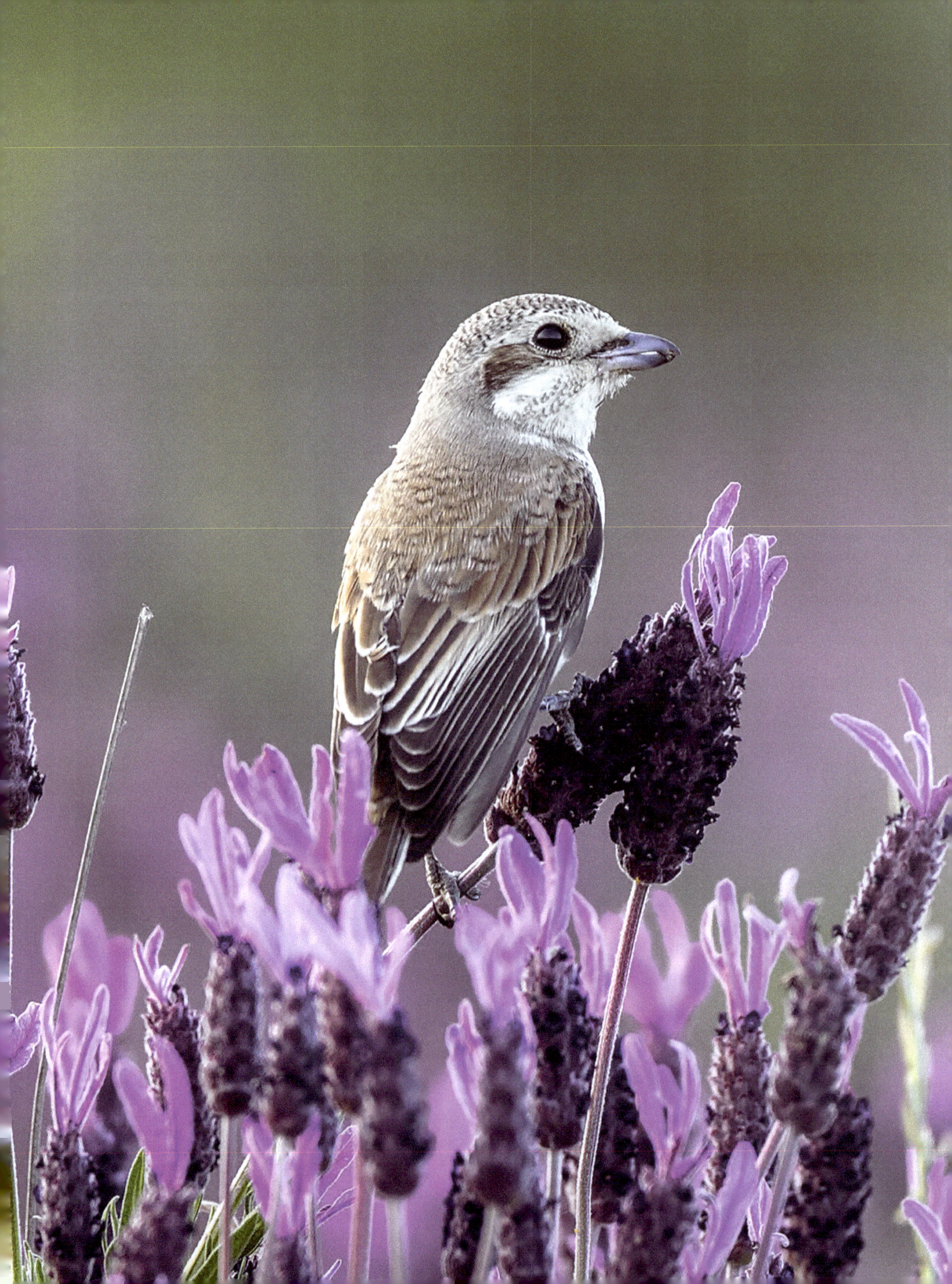

LAVENDER

BOTANICAL NAMES:
Lavandula angustifolia (syn. *L. vera*, *L. officinale*), *L. latifolia*, *L. stoechas*, *L. dentata*, *L.* × *intermedia* (syn. *L.* × *hybrida*)
Note: Unless otherwise specified, this monograph refers to the uses of *L. angustifolia* (English lavender)

COMMON NAMES:
English lavender, true lavender, lavender fine, spike lavender, lavandin, stoechas lavender, French lavender, Portuguese lavender, Spanish lavender, stickadove, elf lead, lavers, nard, spike
khuzaama, lafand (Arabic)
hoosam (Armenian)
lavandula (Bulgarian)
ljekovita lavanda (Croatian)
levandule (Czech)
lavendel (Danish)
lavendel (Dutch)
tupsupäälaventeli (Finnish)
lavende (French)
kopwehblume, lavendel, tabakblumen (German)
lavanta (Greek)
levendula (Hungarian)
lofnarblóm (Icelandic)
lavanda, nardo, spigot (Italian)
rabenda (Japanese)
rabandin (Korean)
xun yi cao (Mandarin)
lavendel (Norwegian)
lawenda waskolistna (Polish)
alfazema (Portuguese)
lavanda (Russian)
dharu (Sanskrit)
espliego, lavanda alhuccema (Spanish)
lavendel (Swedish)
lawendeort (Thai)
lavânta cicegi (Turkish)
hoa oai huong (Vietnamese)
lavendl (Yiddish)

FAMILY NAME:
Lamiaceae (Labiatae)

DESCRIPTION

PART USED: The flowers.

BOTANICAL DESCRIPTION AND HABITAT: Lavender is native to the Mediterranean. It is cultivated commercially in France, southern Europe, and India, and in gardens throughout the U.S. and other temperate regions. Harvest the buds when the flowers are open, preferably on a warm, dry, sunny day.

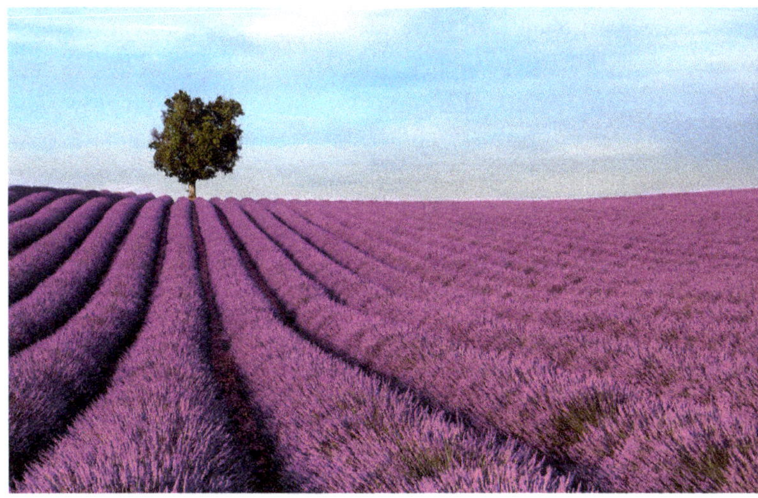

English lavender *(Lavandula angustifolia)* is a woody, evergreen perennial (30 – 90 cm tall and 60 – 90 cm wide).[1,2] It has an upright, spreading habit with many short, crooked, branches that become woody with age. Younger branches are herbaceous, square-stemmed, finely pubescent, and aromatic. The stems have many opposite, sessile, lanceolate to linear leaves that are somewhat tomentose on both surfaces, especially when young; they are also quite fragrant.[2] The inflorescences are spike-like verticillasters with many compact whorls of small bilabiate, perfect flowers arranged along a tall stem. The color of the connate, five-petalled corolla ranges from blue to violet to lavender, with strongly fragrant connate calyx ranging from purple to gray. Most essential oil produced by the flower comes from oil glands on the calyx.[1] When mature, the flowers produce fruit common to the mint family, consisting of four small nutlets nestled in the persistent calyx.[1,2]

Spike lavender *(Lavandula latifolia)*, also known as Portuguese lavender (50 – 100 cm tall), has broader, more spatulate leaves, and a more compressed inflorescence than *L. angustifolia*.[3] It yields three times more essential oil than *L. angustifolia,* with a higher camphor and menthol content.[3] The aroma is sharper and lacks the delicate floral scent of *L. angustifolia.*[1] The inflorescence stalk is branched, often forming a trident shape (up to 25 cm tall).[3] The spike (5 – 8 cm long) is often interrupted.[3] Similar to *L. × intermedia* and *L. angustifolia,* the corolla is bilaterally symmetrical, with upper corolla lobes larger than the lateral lobes; inside is a bilobed stigma.

Lavandin *(Lavandula × intermedia* or *L. × hybrida)* is a naturally occurring, sterile hybrid of *L. angustifolia* and *L. latifolia.*[3] It is much larger than *L. angustifolia,* growing 60 – 150 cm tall.[3] The leaves average 7 cm long and 0.5 cm wide.[5] The inflorescence stalk is branched, and the spike is occasionally interrupted. Ovate bracts subtend the flowers. The corolla is lilac-purple to white and bilaterally symmetrical, with upper lobes larger than lateral lobes. The variety *Lavandula × intermedia* 'Grosso' is most often grown for essential oil production.[3,4] The volatile oil content is highly variable.[3]

Stoechas lavender *(Lavandula stoechas),* also known as Spanish lavender, French lavender, or topped lavender, grows 30 – 100 cm tall.[3] The linear to narrowly oblong leaves (1 – 4 cm long) are covered with a fine, gray down.[3,6] The corolla has blue to mauve lobes of similar size. The pink to dark purple flowers (6 – 8 mm long) are produced on short, compact spikes (2 – 3 cm long) with violet cordate-shaped bracts subtending each flower (4 – 8 mm).[3,6] At the apex of the spike are distinctive, long, purple bracts (10 – 50 mm long) arranged into an attractive corona.[3] Inflorescence stalks are 10 – 30 cm long.[3] This species is native to southwestern and south-central Europe, growing up to an elevation of 1,000 meters.[3] The essential oil is of low quality and very camphorous.[3]

THE NAME: *Lavandula* and lavender derive from the Latin *lavare* ("to wash"). The epithets have the following meanings: *angustifolia* ("narrow leaves"), *latifolia* ("broad leaves"), and *vera* ("true"). Two etymological origins have been identified for the epithet *stoechas.* First, *stoechas* was Dioscorides' name for lavender that grew on islands off the coast of France, now called the Ile de Hyeres.[7] Secondly, the Greeks named those islands *Stoichades,* meaning "the rows," due to the lavender rows seen by sailors when they entered the island. The epithet *dentata* refers to the dentate leaves.

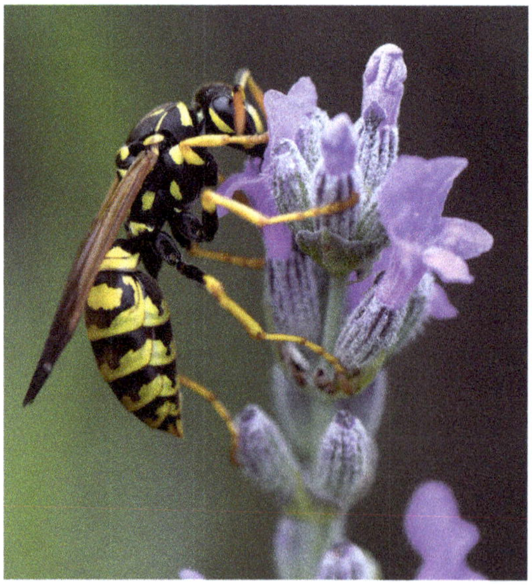

The following common names correspond with the Latin binomials: English lavender, true lavender, and lavender fine *(Lavandula angustifolia,* syn. *L. vera, L. officinale);* Portuguese lavender and spike lavender *(L. latifolia);* Lavandin (syn. *L. × intermedia* or *L. × hybrida*); stoechas lavender, Spanish lavender, French lavender, and stickadove *(L. stoechas);* French lavender is also a common name for *L. dentata.*

HISTORICAL USES: Lavender has been used extensively throughout Europe and the Mediterranean. Romans and Libyans scented their bathwaters with lavender (likely *L. stoechas).*[1] On festive occasions, lavender flowers were strewn on the floors of Portuguese and Spanish churches and homes.[1] Lavender flowers were burned in bonfires on St. John's Day for protection from evil spirits.[1] *Lavandula stoechas* was one of four ingredients in "four thieves' vinegar" used in the Middle Ages as protection from the plague.[1] The rural French and Spanish applied an infused oil of lavender flowers to wounds.[1] Arabs administered lavender flowers as an antispasmodic and expectorant.[1] Lavender sachets were placed in dresser drawers and closets to scent linens, apparel, gloves, and feathers, and protect them from moth and insect damage.[1] Bees frequent lavender flowers providing a good source of nectar for honey.[1]

Eclectic physicians administered essential oil of *Lavandula angustifolia,* spirits of lavender, and compound spirit of lavender as a carminative and antispasmodic for the digestive tract.[8,9] Lavender was also used for pectoral conditions, nervous debility, hysteria, seizures, and fainting.[9] The delicious "Compound Spirit of Lavender" consisted of lavender and rosemary essential oils, clove, nutmeg, Saigon cinnamon, and red saunders in a base of alcohol and water. This compound was administered as a carminative and digestive tonic to treat nausea, flatulence, and stomach and intestinal pain.[8,9] It was also added as a coloring and flavoring agent for unpleasant tasting medicines.[9] Creams and ointments containing lavender spirits or volatile oil were applied topically for headaches caused by fevers and debility.[8,9]

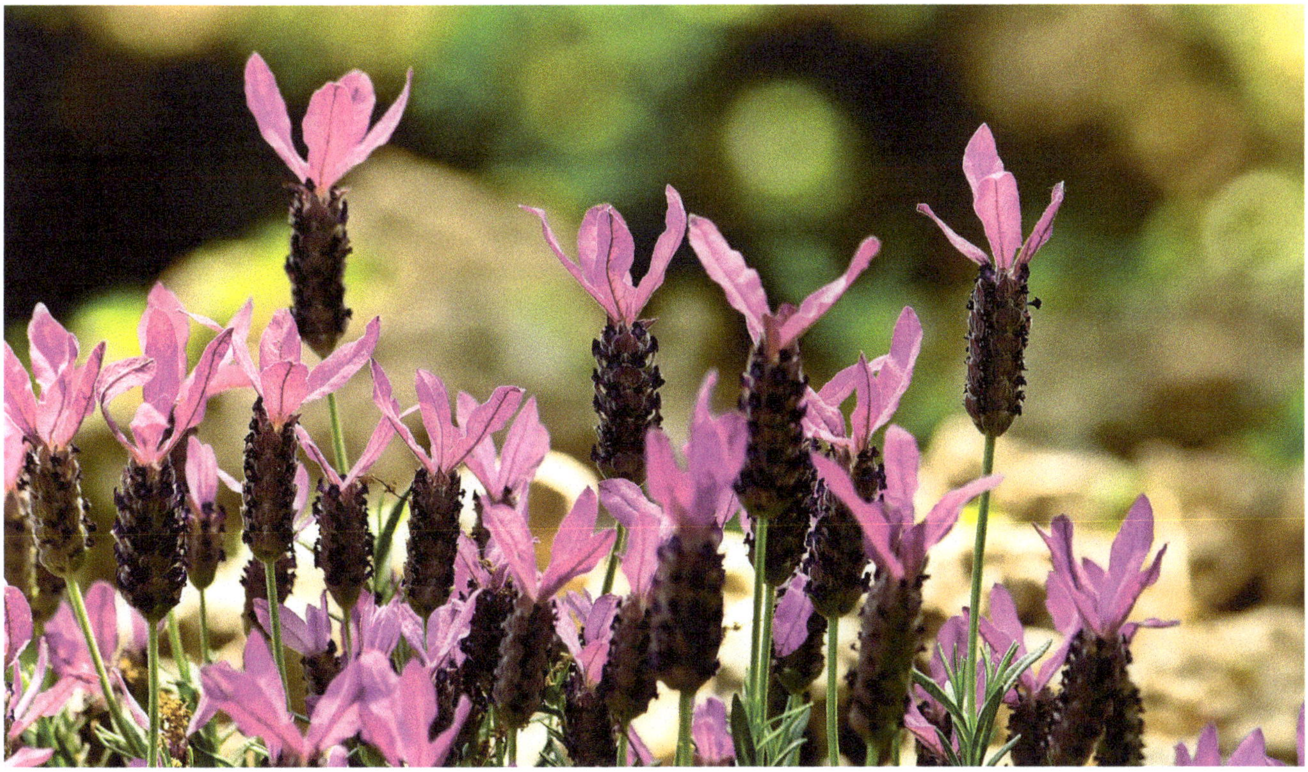

All types of lavender essential oils continue to be included as fragrances and antiseptics in perfumes, creams, lotions, ointments, oils, salves, soaps, detergents, and insect repellants.[10] Lavender oil and herb are also incorporated into food products, such as beverages, desserts, candies, baked goods, gelatins, syrups, honeys, and aromatic vinegars.[10]

CONSTITUENTS

ENGLISH LAVENDER: English lavender contains up to 1.5% volatile oil (linalool, linalyl acetate, lavandulyl acetate, 1,8-cineole, terpinenol-4-ol, camphor, borneol, pinene, cymene, and limonene), tannins (rosmarinic acid and other caffeic acid derivatives), coumarins (coumarin, umbelliferone, and herniarin), flavonoids (luteolin), and triterpenoids (ursolic acid).[10]

ENGLISH LAVENDER ESSENTIAL OIL: English lavender essential oil contains linalool, linalyl acetate, lavandulyl acetate, terpinen-1-ol-4, 1,8-cineole, camphor, β-phellandrene, terpinolene, α-thujene, *n*-hexanol, *n*-heptanal, methyl amyl ketone, ethyl amyl ketone, perillaldehyde, perillyl alcohol, D-borneol, α-terpineol, α-pinene, limonene, lactones (4-butanolide, dihydrocoumarin, 4-methyl-4-vinyl-4-butanolide, 5-pentyl-5-pentanolide, and 4,4-dimethyl-2-buten-4-olide), sesquiterpenes (caryophyllene and cadinene), fatty acids (propionic acid, isobutyric acid, caproic acid, and *p*-coumaric acid), and others.[10]

SPIKE LAVENDER ESSENTIAL OIL: Spike lavender and lavandin essential oil contain many constituents similar to English lavender; their difference is based on their relative content of linalool, 1,8-cinole, terpene ketone (camphor), and linalyl acetate. For more information, review the descriptions of essential oils in the *Medicinal Uses* section.

NUTRITIONAL PROPERTIES: English lavender flowers contain vitamin A, calcium, and iron.

MEDICINAL PROPERTIES: Lavender is an anti-inflammatory, antimicrobial, anxiolytic, aromatic, astringent, bitter tonic, carminative, cholagogue, choleretic, nervine, mild sedative, stomachic, smooth muscle antispasmodic, and mild counterirritant.

TEMPERATURE AND FLAVOR: Cool, bitter, pungent, and astringent. Some sources classify lavender as warm.

MEDICINAL USES

English lavender has nervine, anxiolytic, and mild sedative actions that calm the central nervous system. It aids in treating nervous tension, anxiety, stress, insomnia, and irritability. Lavender also has mood elevating properties, and is beneficial for treating depression, melancholy, and mood swings. In some cases, lavender aids in relieving headaches, migraines, and neuralgia. Lavender can be uplifting and refreshing, with a stimulating, restorative, and regenerative effect on the nervous system. It aids in treating hormone-related nervous system imbalances, and reduces irritability associated with premenstrual syndrome and perimenopause. Extracts of chamomile *(Matricaria)*, lemon balm *(Melissa)*, wild oats *(Avena)*, and/or St. John's wort *(Hypericum)* can be combined with small quantities of lavender for their calming and antidepressant effects.

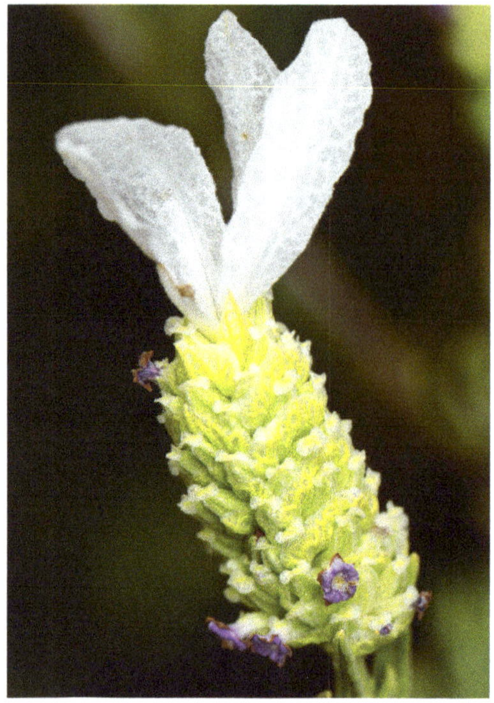

Lavender has smooth muscle antispasmodic and carminative properties that relieve flatulence, upper and lower gastrointestinal spasms, and menstrual cramping. It also aids in treating nerve-related digestive conditions, including Crohn's disease, colitis, and irritable bowel syndrome. It is mildly astringent and drying to the mucous membranes. Aromatic herbs such as orange peel *(Citrus sinensis)*, lemon grass *(Cymbopogon)*, lemon balm *(Melissa)*, chamomile *(Matricaria)*, and spearmint *(Mentha spicata)* can be combined with small amounts of lavender to ease digestive cramping.

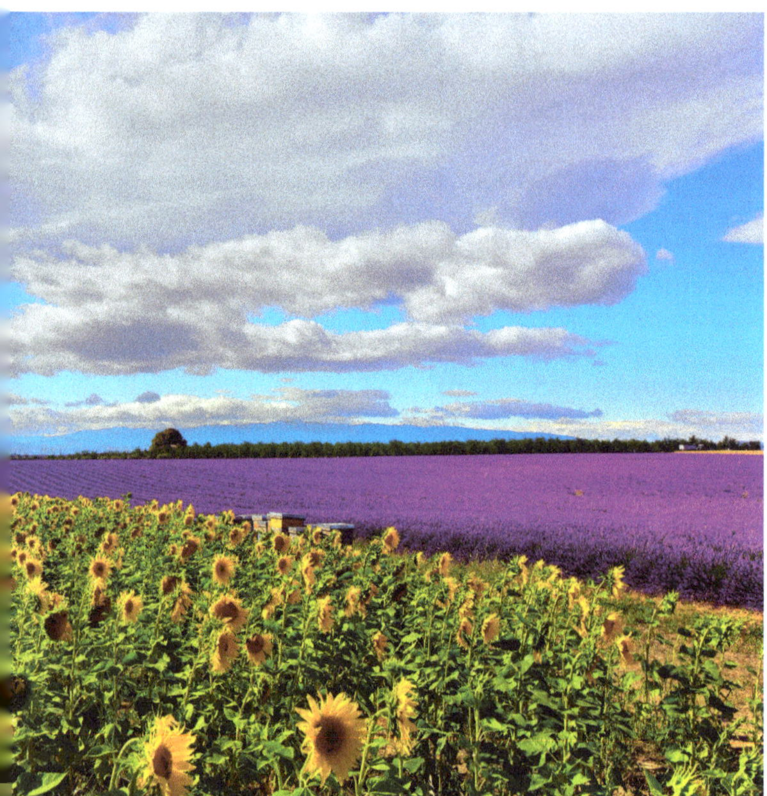

Lavender stimulates digestive secretions, increasing the efficiency of digestion. It has choleretic and cholagogue effects primarily attributed to the caffeic acid derivatives.[11]

Apply lavender poultices, fomentations, essential oils, or salves topically to treat sore muscles, neuralgia, rheumatic joints, sprains, strains, and bruises. Lavender reduces irritation and itching associated with poison oak, eczema, dermatitis, and psoriasis. For more information about topical uses, review the information on essential oils below.

LAVENDER ESSENTIAL OIL: While there are many similarities in essential oils of various lavender species, there also are important differences.

ENGLISH LAVENDER (LAVANDULA ANGUSTIFOLIA)

Essential oil of English lavender is superior to essential oils of other lavender species for medicines and perfumes. Lavender acts as a harmonizer in essential oil blends. It contains a higher linalool and linalyl acetate content than other *Lavandula* species.[10] Linalool, and to a lesser extent, linalyl acetate are the components with sedative actions.[12] Lavender has calming, spasmolytic, and restorative properties. In rodent studies, lavender oil had CNS-depressant effects.[10]

Consuming one to two drops of lavender spirits (lavender essential oil diluted in alcohol) 15 – 30 minutes prior to a meal reduces appetite and decreases colic, gas, and bloating.[12] It also helps to normalize hepatic blood sugar output.[12]

Lavender oil is a vulnerary agent that promotes cell regeneration.[13] Apply lavender essential oil neat (directly) or diluted as a first-aid remedy for bee stings, wasp stings, spider bites, mosquito bites, poison oak, poison ivy, cuts, and abrasions. Topical applications are excellent for reducing pain and inflammation from thermal burns and sunburns.[12] Combine lavender with peppermint essential oil to increase the anti-inflammatory and cooling effect that relieves burns. Apply lavender cream, diluted essential oil, or hydrosol to treat sun-damaged skin or to delay wrinkle formation.[13] Lavender oil also prevents scarring and stretch marks.[13]

Lavender essential oil has antimicrobial properties that can benefit the healing of wounds, acne, boils, and infected hair follicles.[10] Inhaling essential oil aids in treating sinus and lung congestion.[13] Topical applications have counterirritant effects that help to reduce muscle pain. Suppositories containing lavender aid in treating vaginal infections including candida and bacterial vaginosis.[13]

SPIKE LAVENDER (LAVANDULA LATIFOLIA)

Spike lavender or aspic oil contains higher amounts of 1,8-cineole, terpene ketone (camphor), and terpene alcohols, with smaller amounts of linalyl acetate than English lavender.[10,12] However, the quantity of linalool is higher in spike lavender than in true lavender.[10] Spike lavender has antiviral and expectorant actions for colds and respiratory infections.[12] The pungent camphorous compounds act as a mucolytic, alleviating congestion. In laboratory animals, spike lavender has spasmolytic effects on smooth muscles.[10,12] Apply spike lavender essential oil as a mild antiseptic for acne, pimples, blackheads, boils, infected hair follicles, and wounds. The camphor also aids in repelling insects and moths. Most spike lavender essential oil is produced in Spain.[13] *Note:* Due to the potential neurotoxic effects of the terpene ketone (camphor), epileptics, small children, and pregnant or nursing women should completely avoid internal use, and consult an aromatherapist before applying externally.[12,14]

LAVANDIN (LAVANDULA × INTERMEDIA)

Lavandin essential oil is obtained from *Lavandula × intermedia* (syn. *L. × hybrida*), a naturally occurring hybrid of *L. angustifolia* and *L. latifolia.* The chemotype of lavandin grown in Croatia has similar antimicrobial properties; however, it is higher in borneol and terpenes.[12]

There are numerous strains of lavandin, including Abrial, Super, Grosso, Standard, and Maime Epis Tête.[13] Lavandin yields much higher volatile oil content than lavender and spike lavender; therefore, it is less expensive than English lavender, although it is considered a lower quality. It is also used to dilute English lavender and spike lavender essential oils.[10]

Lavandin contains linalool (20 – 60%), linalyl acetate (15 – 50%), 1,8-cineole (5 – 25%), and terpene ketone (camphor)(5 – 15%) ranging between those of English lavender and spike lavender.[10,14] Because the content of cineole and camphor is higher than lavender, lavandin is a more potent counterirritant, antimicrobial, and deodorant. *Note:* Due to the potential neurotoxic effects of the terpene ketone (camphor), epileptics, small children, and pregnant or nursing women should completely avoid internal use, and consult an aromatherapist before applying externally.[12,14]

STOECHAS LAVENDER (LAVANDULA STOECHAS)

Stoechas lavender contains high amounts of the terpene ketone, camphor (15 – 30%) and fenchone (45 – 50%). The camphor content of stoechas lavender is higher than English lavender; therefore, the essential oil should only be applied topically. It has counterirritant, vulnerary, and anti-inflammatory properties.[13,14] *Note:* Due to the potential neurotoxic effects of the terpene ketone (camphor), epileptics, small children, and pregnant or nursing women should completely avoid internal use of stoechas lavender essential oil, and consult an aromatherapist before applying externally.[12,14]

CONTRAINDICATIONS

Internal and topical uses of *Lavandula angustifolia* are considered safe during pregnancy and lactation, and in small children. However, due to the potential neurotoxic effects of the terpene ketone (camphor), avoid internal consumption of spike lavender, stoechas lavender, and lavandin in epileptics, small children, and pregnant or nursing women.[12,14] Consult an aromatherapist before applying those oils externally. Spike lavender, lavandin oil, and lavender absolute are generally non-irritating and non-sensitizing to human skin; however, one source reported lavender absolute to be skin sensitizing.[10] In rare cases, lavender essential oil can cause contact dermatitis.[10]

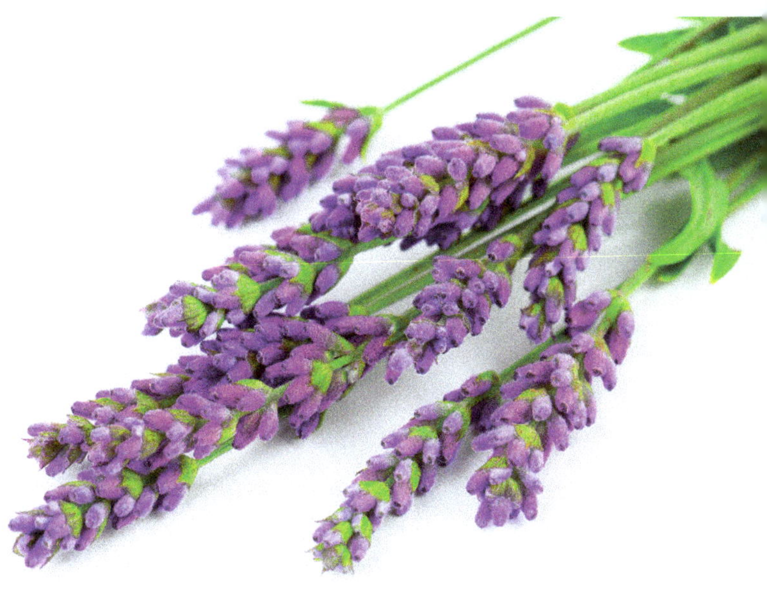

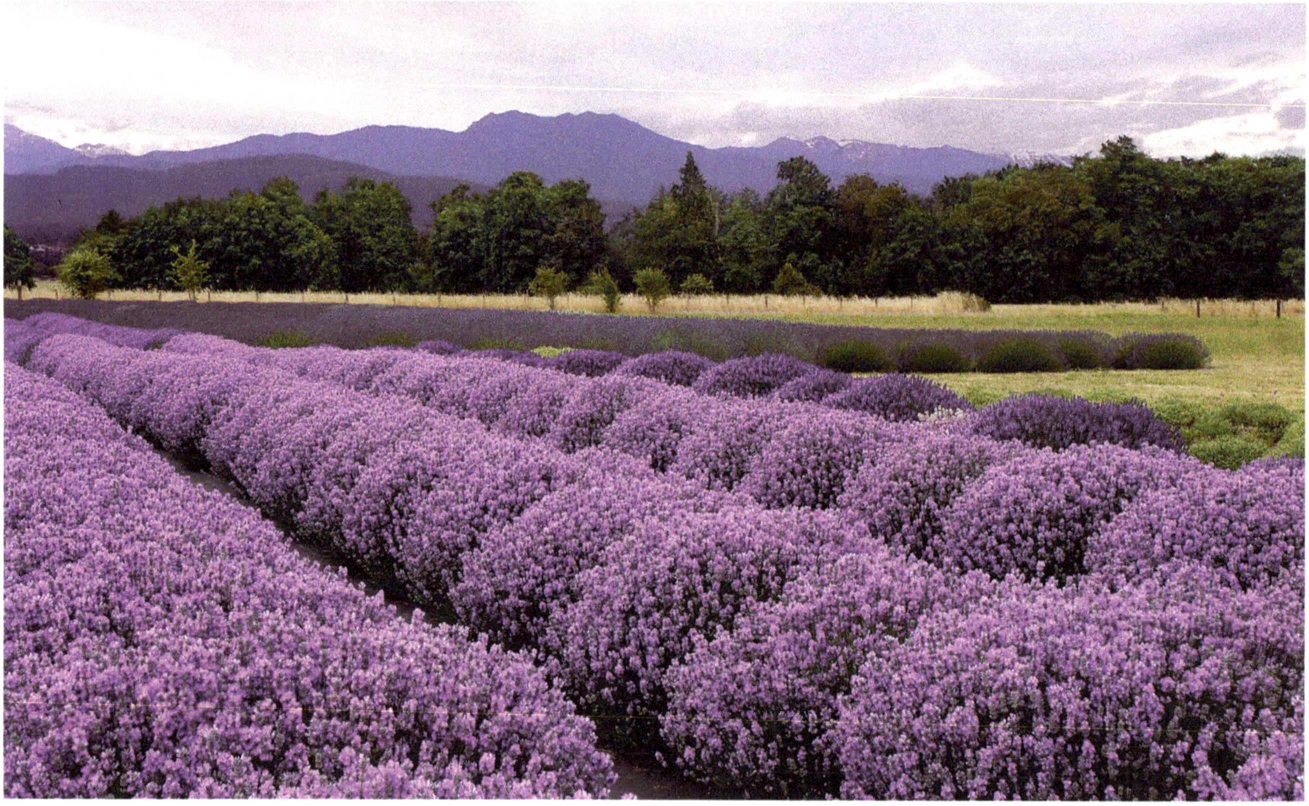

PREPARATION AND DOSAGE

TINCTURE: Fresh flowers [1:2–1:3+, 60–95% alcohol]; dry flowers [1:5–1:6+, 50–60% alcohol]; 10–60 drops, up to three times daily.

GLYCERITE: Fresh flowers [1:2–1:3+, 50% glycerin and 50% alcohol]; dry flowers [1:5–1:6+, 40% glycerin, 30% water, and 30% alcohol]; consume 5–30 drops, up to three times daily.

ACETUM EXTRACT: Infuse fresh or dry lavender into vinegar; use sparingly in culinary preparations and for digestive properties.

CAPSULES: Consume 1–3 drops of *L. angustifolia* essential oil in a capsule with a binder such as powdered marshmallow or kudzu, up to three times daily.

TEA: Prepare a hot or cold infusion; consume 6–12 ounces, up to four times daily.

HONEY AND SYRUP: Infuse fresh or dry lavender flowers in honey, then strain and consume one teaspoon in hot water or tea. Stir 1–2 drops of *L. angustifolia* essential oil into 1 teaspoon to 1 tablespoon of honey, and add to hot water or tea. Apply the essential oil neat or lavender honey topically for burns.

TOPICAL USE: Apply the poultice or fomentation topically. Apply the hydrosol or essential oil neat, or add to creams, salves, massage oils, baths, soaps, perfumes, and aftershaves. Add essential oil to a spritzer or diffuser, or in hot water when inhaling steam.

CULINARY USE: Layer lavender flowers in coarse salt and drizzle with olive oil; use a pinch in culinary preparations. Lavender flowers can be incorporated into a variety of recipes, including scones, biscuits, cookies, and other confections. Infuse lavender flowers in oil or butter, and use sparingly in cooking.

ESSENTIAL OIL: Place 1–3 drops of essential oil on a sugar cube, then dissolve in hot water and consume. Consume 1–3 drops of *L. angustifolia* essential oil in a capsule with a binder such as powdered marshmallow or kudzu, up to three times daily. To prepare lavender spirits, combine one part *L. angustifolia* essential oil with ten parts alcohol [1:10]; consume 1–3 drops.

LEMON BALM

DESCRIPTION

PART USED: The leaves, preferably fresh.

BOTANICAL NAME:
Melissa officinalis

COMMON NAMES:
Lemon balm, balm, sweet balm, blue balm, garden balm, English balm, common balm, heart's delight, honey plant, cure-all, sweet melissa, sweet mary, balm mint, dropsy plant
sitruunamelissa (Finnish)
mélisse (French)
melisse, zitronenmelisse (German)
melissophyllon (Greek)
melissa (Hebrew and Italian)
remonbamu, seiyo-yamahakka (Japanese)
xiang feng cao (Mandarin)
sitronmelisse (Norwegian)
erva-cidreira (Portuguese)
roinita (Romanian)
melissa limonnaya, limonnik (Russian)
balsamita major, toronjil (Spanish)
melise (Yiddish)

FAMILY NAME:
Lamiaceae (Labiatae)

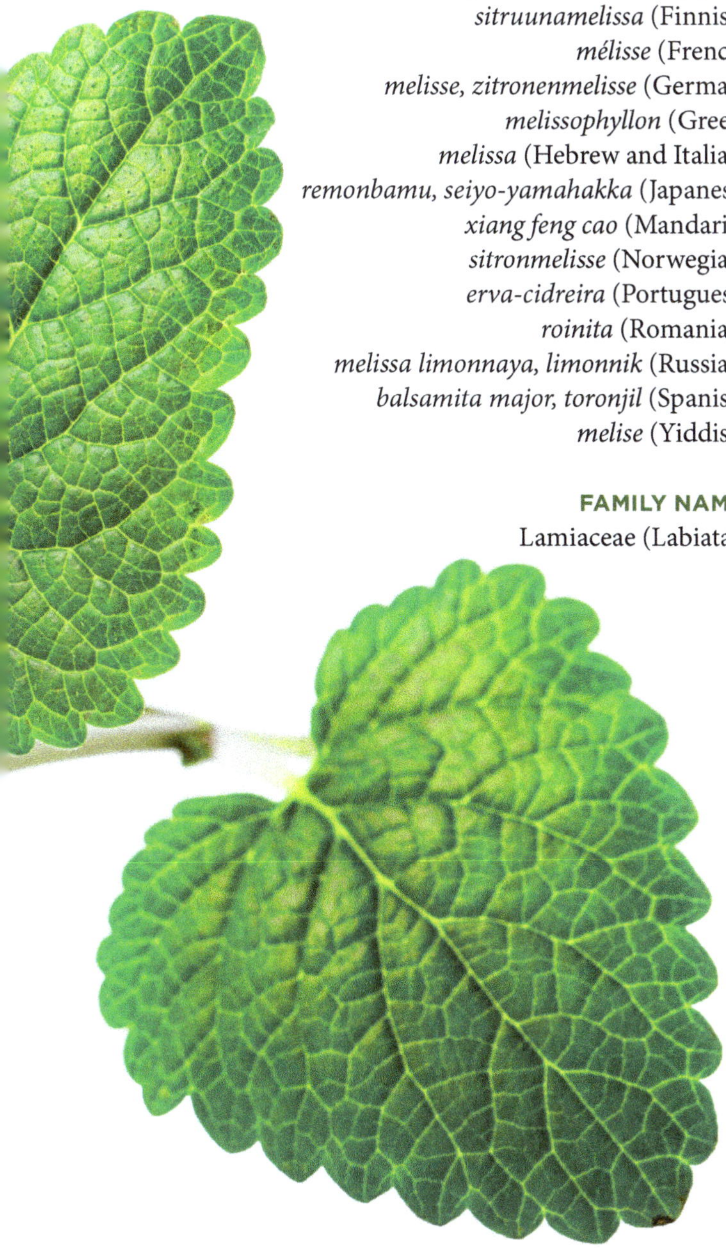

BOTANICAL DESCRIPTION AND HABITAT: Lemon balm is an herbaceous perennial originating in southern Europe. It has naturalized throughout Europe, western Asia, southwestern Siberia, northern Africa, and the U.S. It thrives in moist, but well drained, loamy soil, in partial light. Overexposure to sunlight turns the leaves a pale, yellow-green color and can wilt them. Like other members of the mint family, lemon balm spreads rapidly. It proliferates by seed. To prevent the plant from spreading, cut it back to the base before it seeds. If lacking ample room to spread, plant it in a container.

Lemon balm has a bushy appearance, averaging 20 – 150 cm tall and 30 – 60 cm wide.[1] It has erect, quadrangular, branching stems with opposite ovate or cordate, pubescent, wrinkled leaves (2 – 14 cm long and 1.5 – 7 cm wide) that have dentate margins.[1] The leaves release a pleasant lemon aroma when bruised. The tiny pinkish-white, tubular flowers have a pubescent, five-toothed calyx (7 – 9 mm long), a bilabiate corolla (8 – 15 mm long), and four stamens.[1] They grow in whorled clusters of four to 12 flowers.[1] Like other members of the mint family, the four-lobed ovary yields four tiny, one-seeded nutlets.

THE NAME: *Melissa* ("bee") derives from Greek, signifying the attraction of the insect to its flowers.[2] The epithet *officinalis* describes an herb listed as an official drug plant in European and U.S. Pharmacopoeias. Balm is an abbreviation of balsam, a term used to describe an aromatic plant.[2] The common names lemon balm and sweet balm refer to the sweet, citronella-lemony aroma of the crushed leaves.[2]

HISTORICAL USES: Pliny and Dioscorides applied lemon balm to wounds in order to prevent infections and promote healing. They also used a topical application of the leaves steeped in wine to cure bites from venomous beasts and scorpion stings.[2] Pliny recommended planting lemon balm near beehives and rubbing the hives with lemon balm leaves to encourage the bees' return and keep them from straying.[2]

Spirits of lemon balm, a preparation made from steeping the herb in wine, was consumed as a remedy for fevers, nervous system disorders, to improve memory, and lift the spirit.[2] During the Middle Ages, lemon balm was used for nervous system and digestive disorders.[3] Avicenna, Muslim physician and philosopher (980 – 1037), administered lemon balm to treat wounds and ulcers.[3] Paracelsus, 16th century Swiss physician and alchemist, regarded lemon balm as the "elixir of life."[4] He believed the plant could revive someone close to death, and cure all nervous system disorders.[2,3]

During the 16th century, Carmelite nuns produced the alcoholic beverage, Carmelite Water, also known as *Eau de Melisse de Carmes* that popularized lemon balm. Carmelite Water contained two pounds of fresh lemon balm leaves steeped for two weeks in one-half gallon of orange blossom water, and one gallon of alcoholic spirits. Warming aromatic herbs such as cinnamon, coriander, clove, lemon peel, nutmeg, and angelica root were then added. This beverage was considered a cure for nervous headaches and neuralgic afflictions. Carmelite Water was also applied as an after-bath rub, and incorporated in alcohol-based perfume.[2,3] English herbal physician, John Evelyn writes that spirits of lemon balm "comforts the heart and driveth away melancholy and sadness."[2] Seventeenth century herbalist Nicholas Culpeper writes that lemon balm "causeth the Mind and Heart to become merry...and driveth away troublesome cares."[3] Lemon balm was also included in the alcoholic beverages Benedictine and Chartreuse.[4] It was a common strewing herb and ingredient in potpourri.[2] Lemon balm oil was used to polish furniture.[4]

Lemon balm was listed in the *U.S. Pharmacopoeia* in the 1840s – 1890s.[5] However, it was eventually removed because it was considered too mild.[6] Lemon balm was substituted for lemons in jams and jellies when the fruit was scarce.[3] Thomas Jefferson grew lemon balm in his gardens.[3] Cherokees consumed lemon balm tea to treat chills, fever, colds, and typhus. Costanoan Indians drank the tea as a digestive aid.[3]

CONSTITUENTS: Lemon balm contains volatile oil (citral A = geranial, citral B = neral, caryophyllene oxide, citronellal, eugenol acetate, geraniol, linalool, and limonene, plus small amounts of terpene hydrocarbons, such as *trans*- and *cis*-β-ocimine, caryophyllene, α-cubenene, copaene, and β-bourbonene), polyphenols (rosmarinic acid, protocatechuic acid, a tannin composed of caffeic acid and other caffeic acid derivatives), triterpenes (ursolic, pomolic, and oleanolic acids), flavonoids (luteolin-7-glucoside and rhamnazin), and glucosides (nerol, benzyl alcohol, β-phenylethyl alcohol, neric acid, and geranic acid).[7-10]

NUTRITIONAL PROPERTIES: Lemon balm contains vitamin C and thiamine (a B vitamin), and is high in flavonoids.[4]

MEDICINAL PROPERTIES: Antibacterial, antidepressant, antispasmodic, antiviral, anxiolytic, astringent, cooling diaphoretic, nervine, sedative, stomachic, sudorific, and potential hypothyroidal agent.

TEMPERATURE AND FLAVOR: Cool, astringent, pungent, sour, and sweet.

MEDICINAL USES

Lemon balm is a nervine, mild sedative, and relaxant. It soothes the nervous system, reducing stress, anxiety, and anxiety-induced palpitations. Lemon balm reduces premenstrual irritability and anxiety. According to medical herbalist David Hoffman, lemon balm has a tonic effect on the heart and circulatory system, and acts as a mild vasodilator.[9] Lemon balm calms an overactive mind, and aids in treating insomnia and stress-related headaches. Professor Holm at Heidelberg University conducted animal studies and found that lemon balm's volatile oil affected the limbic brain, and had a gentle, tranquilizing effect on the autonomic nervous system.[11] The sedative actions are attributed primarily to the terpene citronellal and citral (neral and geranial).[3,12] Prepare a stress and anxiety relief compound by combining lemon balm with other nervine herbs, such as chamomile *(Matricaria),* skullcap *(Scutellaria),* wild oats *(Avena),* St. John's wort *(Hypericum),* and a smaller amount of lavender *(Lavandula).* One or more of the following herbs can be combined with lemon balm to make a sedative compound that aids sleep: hops *(Humulus),* Jamaican dogwood *(Piscidia),* chamomile *(Matricaria),* and skullcap *(Scutellaria).* Avoid compounding lemon balm extract with herbs high in alkaloids such as passion flower *(Passiflora),* because the alkaloids precipitate the tannins out of solution.

Alchemists and herbalists revere lemon balm for its mood elevating and antidepressant actions. It is beneficial for children, teenagers, and adults with mild to moderate forms of depression. Lemon balm can be used to lift the spirits in melancholic individuals with seasonal affective disorder, as well as premenstrual and menopausal depression.

When administered in conjunction with making lifestyle and dietary changes, lemon balm has been helpful for hyperactive children and individuals with attention deficit hyperactivity disorder (ADHD). Making these changes prior to beginning medication facilitates the herb's effectiveness. The herb has a calming effect and aids with mental focus. The glycerin extract or glycerin/alcohol combination is most palatable for children; the dose ranges from 15–60 drops, two to three times daily. Start with the lowest dose, and increase until the desired effect is reached. Combine two parts of lemon balm extract with one part gotu kola *(Centella)* and one-half or one-quarter part rosemary *(Salvia rosmarinus)* to enhance focus.

Lemon balm has mild carminative, stomachic, and smooth muscle antispasmodic effects, although it is most suited for nerve-related digestive complaints such as nervous dyspepsia. The effects on the digestive tract are milder than peppermint *(Mentha piperita)* or fennel *(Foeniculum vulgare)*; however, it is a useful adjunct for treating digestive cramping, colic, flatulence, stomach cramps, or intestinal cramps. Lemon balm has mild antispasmodic actions for the respiratory system and menstrual cramps. Studies have demonstrated that eugenol contributes to the antispasmodic and carminative properties.[7,8] In order to enhance its digestive, carminative, and antispasmodic actions, combine lemon balm with aromatic herbs including orange peel *(Citrus sinensis)*, fennel *(Foeniculum)*, anise *(Pimpinella)*, and/or other members of the mint family, such as spearmint *(Mentha spicata)* or peppermint *(Mentha piperita)*.

Hot water extracts of lemon balm demonstrated potent antiviral properties against herpes simplex, mumps, Newcastle disease, vaccinia *(Orthopoxvirus)*, and other viruses.[10] Essential oil of lemon balm has antibacterial actions against *Mycobacterium phlei* and *Streptococcus hemolyticus*, as well as antifungal activities.[10] The polyphenols (rosmarinic acid and other caffeic acid derivatives) and tannins contribute to the antiviral, antibacterial, and astringent effects.[7,8,10]

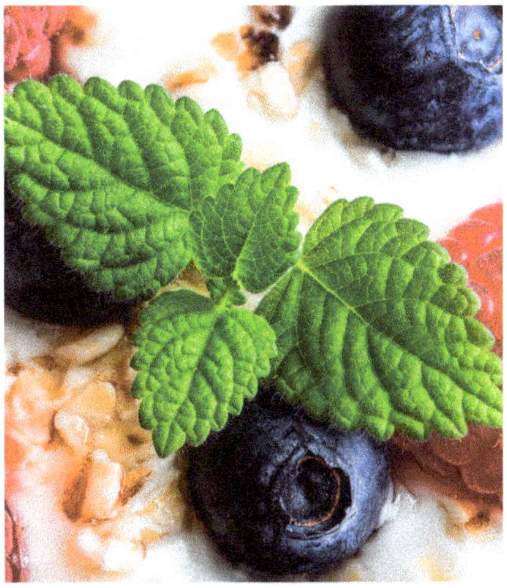

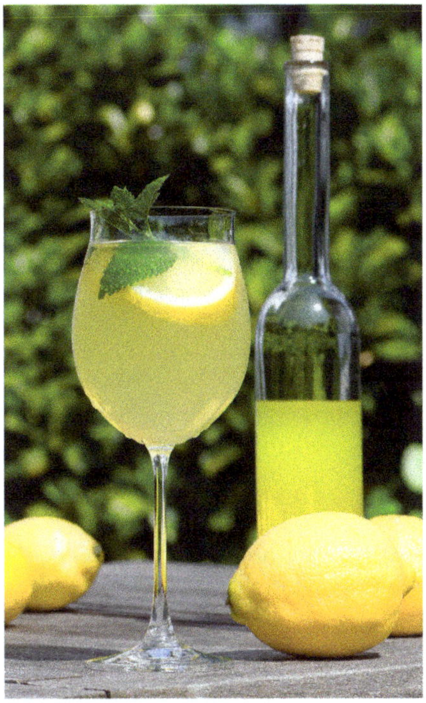

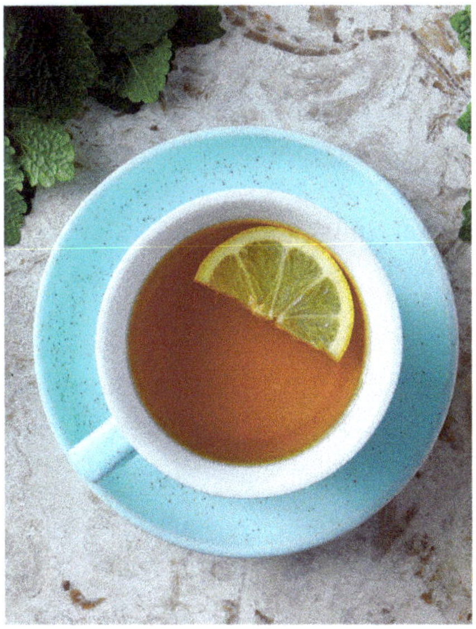

Consuming lemon balm extract and applying a fresh lemon balm leaf poultice, cream, or essential oil speeds the healing of herpes sores and reduces the rate of recurrence. Topical applications are most effective when applied within one or two days of the sore eruption. The antiviral effects on herpes have been confirmed in animal and human studies.[9] The speculated modes of action are that lemon balm inhibits protein synthesis and blocks viral receptors in the host cells.[3]

Consuming a hot tea of lemon balm is a cooling diaphoretic to reduce a fever in the first phase of a cold or flu. Lemon balm is an ideal remedy to calm the nerves of children who become hyper or restless in the early stages of a cold or flu. It encourages restful sleep during an illness. Lemon balm tea with fresh squeezed lemon juice, a dollop of honey (or sugar), and muddled cucumber and spearmint is a refreshing beverage and refrigerant in hot weather.

Lemon balm has demonstrated a hypothyroidal effect, and aids in treating symptoms in the early stages of hyperthyroidism. Freeze-dried aqueous extracts have inhibitory effects of the thyroid stimulating hormone (TSH) on the thyroid gland.[9] *In vitro* laboratory studies showed that lemon balm prevented the binding of TSH to plasma membranes, and inhibited the enzyme iodothyronine deiodinase. It also prevents biological activity of immunoglobulins in the blood, and inhibits receptor binding in patients with Grave's disease, a condition that causes hyperthyroidism.[9] Daily consumption of the extract or freeze-dried aqueous extract is recommended to reduce symptoms associated with elevated thyroid hormone levels, such as anxiety attacks, palpitations, and many excess nervous system symptoms. It also has been helpful for some individuals in the early stages of Grave's disease. For treating hyperthyroidism and symptomatic relief, lemon balm works most effectively when combined with bugleweed *(Lycopus)* and motherwort *(Leonurus).*

Note: It is important for patients with Graves' disease or other thyroid disorders to consult a health care practitioner in addition to using natural treatments. It is critical to monitor blood levels of thyroid hormones and antibody levels. Herbal support and natural therapies are not always adequate for treating hyperthyroidism.

Topical applications of lemon balm act as an astringent anti-inflammatory agent and mild antimicrobial. The tannins reduce bleeding and encourage wound sealing. The tannins and volatile oil help to prevent infections from wounds. Apply a lemon balm compress or poultice to weeping sores, cuts, abrasions, bruises, sprains, strains, bites, or skin ulcers.

CONTRAINDICATIONS

Lemon balm can potentially interfere with the actions of thyroid hormones.[9] Consult a health care practitioner before frequently consuming lemon balm with thyroid conditions or before combining lemon balm with medications that affect thyroid function. Individuals with hypothyroidism should avoid long-term, daily consumption of lemon balm. Several authors warn against consuming lemon balm during pregnancy or lactation.[3] However, this author has never observed problems resulting from occasional consumption of small to moderate amounts of the tea or tincture during pregnancy or lactation for stress and anxiety relief. Individuals with mint family allergies should avoid contact with the leaves; in rare cases, they can cause contact dermatitis.

PREPARATION AND DOSAGE

TINCTURE: Fresh leaves [1:2-1:3, 60-95% alcohol]; recently dried leaves [1:5, 50-60% alcohol]. Consume 10-90 drops, up to four times daily. The volatile oils in lemon balm dissipate quickly upon drying; store the herb in a tightly sealed container. If making the tincture with dried leaves, prepare an extract with them one to six months after harvesting.

GLYCERITE: Fresh leaves [1:3-1:4, 50% glycerin and 50% alcohol] or [1:3-1:4, 60% glycerin and 40% distilled water]; consume 10-60 drops, up to four times daily.

ACETUM EXTRACT: Infuse lemon balm leaves in rice vinegar or champagne vinegar for culinary use.

SUCCUS: Juice the fresh herb and preserve with 20% alcohol. Consume 1 teaspoon, up to three times daily.

CAPSULES: Consume 2-4 "00" capsules of the freeze dried or recently dried powdered herb, up to three times daily.

TEA: Prepare a hot or cold infusion with the fresh or recently dried herb; consume 8-12 ounces, three to four times daily. Use hot water well below boiling temperature to make the most effective, flavorful tea. Boiled water dissipates the volatile oil more rapidly and extracts more of the tannins, increasing the astringency. It is important to ensure that the vessel is tightly sealed so the volatile oil does not dissipate from the hot water.

HONEY AND SYRUP: Infuse the fresh, cleaned, macerated leaves in honey; steep two to four weeks, and strain. Add 1 teaspoon of infused honey to hot water or tea. Infuse the leaves in simple syrup one to three days; strain and refrigerate. The syrup lasts up to one month.

ESSENTIAL OIL AND HYDROSOL: Apply the essential oil neat or diluted. Lemon balm essential oil is expensive and often cut with other essential oils. Lemon grass or palmarosa essential oils are less expensive alternatives to lemon balm, with similar properties and uses. Consume 1-2 tablespoons of lemon balm hydrosol *(Melissa* water), up to four times daily.

TOPICAL USE: Apply the fomentation, poultice, oil (alcohol intermediary or infused oil method), or salve.

CULINARY USE: Add fresh chopped leaves sparingly to fruit or vegetable salads, herbal vinegars, dressings, marinades, stuffing, punch, wine, beer, soups, compound butters, cheese, fish, egg dishes, jams, jellies, sorbets, ice cream, cookies, and other desserts or baked goods.

LICORICE

DESCRIPTION

BOTANICAL NAMES:
Glycyrrhiza glabra (G. glabra var. *typica, G. glabra* var. *violacea,* and *G. glabra* var. *glandulifera),* and *G. uralensis*

COMMON NAMES:
Licorice, liquorice, sweet root, the great detoxifier, the great adjunct
madoodag (Armenian)
sladnik (Bulgarian)
gam chou (Cantonese)
lakrids (Danish)
zoethout (Dutch)
lakritsikasvi (Finnish)
réglisse (French)
lakritze (German)
glykoriza (Greek)
shush, shush kireah (Hebrew)
mulhathi (Hindi)
lakkrís (Icelandic)
liquirizia, regolizia (Italian)
kanzō, rikorisu (Japanese)
kamch'o (Korean)
gan cao (Mandarin)
lakrisrot (Norwegian)
alcacuz (Portuguese)
lakrichnik, lakrista (Russian)
yashimadhu, madhuuka (Sanskrit)
lakrits (Swedish)
cam thao (Vietnamese)
lakrets (Yiddish)

FAMILY NAME:
Fabaceae (Leguminosae)

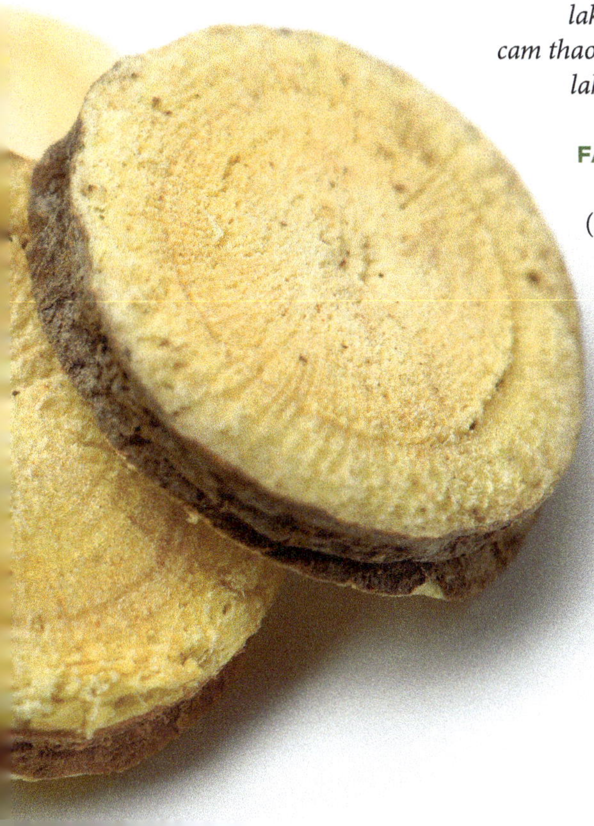

PARTS USED: The roots and rhizomes after the third or fourth year of growth.

BOTANICAL DESCRIPTION AND HABITAT: *Glycyrrhiza glabra* is native to Eurasia and northern Africa, and has naturalized in Australia and North America.[1] It often grows along roadsides, in saline areas, or on the edges of farms, preferably in alkaline, sandy, moist soil.[1] Reaching 30 – 150 cm tall, licorice is a glabrous to finely pubescent, herbaceous perennial that can become woody at the base.[1,2] The pinnate leaves (5 – 14 cm long) have deciduous,

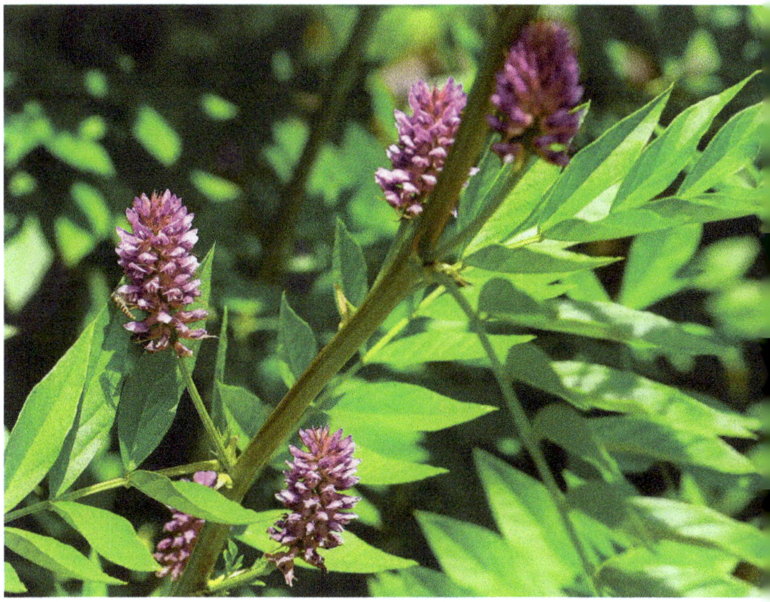

linear stipules, and 9 – 17 widely ovate, gland-dotted leaflets with rounded bases and apices.[1,3] The inflorescence is an open, axillary, spike-like raceme (up to 20 cm long). It bears many small, bluish to purple pea-like flowers (9 – 12 mm).[3] The tubular calyx has five unequal lobes (3 mm long); the upper two lobes are mostly joined.[2] The nine filaments of the androecium are fused, but sometimes accompanied by one non-fused filament. The narrow, oblong, glandular fruit is an indehiscent legume (12 – 30 mm long).[3] It persists on the plant, and produces 2 – 8 dark green seeds.[1]

Glycyrrhiza uralensis is native in parts of north-central China, Russia, Inner Mongolia, and Pakistan.[4] It thrives in sandy, alkaline soils near stream and river banks, but can also be found in dry, hot climates.[4] This herbaceous perennial has sturdy roots and rhizomes, as well as

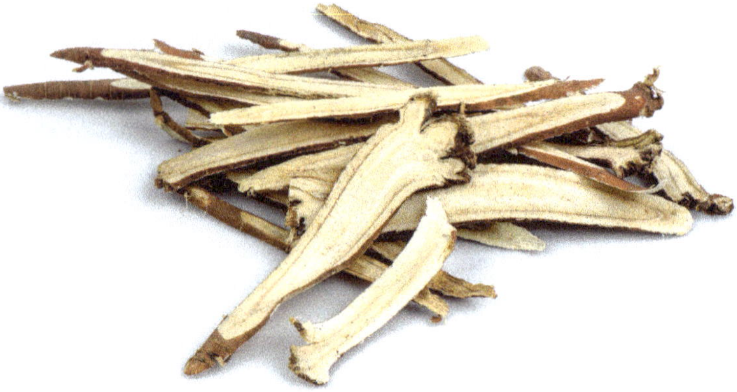

tomentose, gland-dotted stems (up to 120 cm long) that bear pinnately compound leaves.[5] The leaves have 5 – 17 hairy, gland-dotted, ovate leaflets (1.5 – 5 cm by 0.8 – 3 cm) with rounded, mucronate apices.[5] Dense axillary racemes have brown, oblong bracts (3 – 4 mm long) subtending the flowers.[5] The long, narrow flower has a bell-shaped, five-lobed calyx (up to 14 mm long) and a purple, white, or yellow corolla with specialized petals characteristic of the pea family. The petals have a long, narrow banner, short wings, and an even shorter keel. The glandular ovary matures into a hairy, glandular, strongly curved legume (6 – 7 mm broad) densely covered with hard, spiny projections and bearing 3 – 11 seeds.[4,5]

THE NAME: The genus *Glycyrrhiza* derives from two Greek words: *glukos* ("sweet") and *rhiza* ("root").[6] The epithet *glabra* means "smooth." The Mandarin pinyin name, gan cao, translates as "sweet herb."[6] Greeks called the plant "sweet herb."[6] The following common names correspond with the Latin names: Spanish licorice and Italian licorice *(G. glabra* var. *typica);* Persian licorice and Turkish licorice *(G. glabra* var. *violacea);* Russian licorice *(G. glabra* var. *glandulifera);* and Chinese licorice *(G. uralensis).*

HISTORICAL USES: Licorice has been used extensively in Eastern and Western cultures for thousands of years. It continues to be used in Traditional Chinese Medicine to strengthen digestion, alleviate coughing, moisten the lungs, and reduce inflammation and fire toxicity (sores, carbuncles, and sore throats).[7] In Ayurvedic medicine, licorice continues to be used to treat sore throats, respiratory ailments, food poisoning, and snake and scorpion bites.[6] Theophrastus, a Greek philosopher, prescribed licorice to alleviate thirst and coughs.[6] Pliny the Elder utilized licorice as an antitussive; Dioscorides prescribed it to treat laryngitis and soothe the nervous system.[6] Licorice was utilized throughout Europe to treat digestive discomfort, hoarseness, sore throats, bronchial irritation, and infections.[6] Brewers added licorice to porter and stout beers as a thickening and darkening agent. Native Americans consumed licorice tea to alleviate fevers, soothe throat and chest pain, and treat coughs, digestive upsets, and diarrhea.[6]

Eclectic physicians added licorice fluid extract or syrup to conceal unpleasant tasting medicines such as quinine *(Cinchona),* cascara sagrada *(Rhamnus purshiana),* aloe *(Aloe),* and quassia *(Picrasma excelsa, Quassia armara).*[8] Syrup was prepared by adding two parts of licorice fluid extract with 14 parts of simple syrup.[9] Eclectics also administered licorice as a demulcent, expectorant, and laxative.[8,9] Licorice powder was used to solidify pills, and as a dusting powder to prevent adhesion of pills.[8] It was an ingredient in "Compound Licorice Powder," a laxative formula containing senna *(Senna)* and fennel *(Foeniculum).*

CONSTITUENTS: Licorice contains a triterpene glycoside glycyrrhizin (also known as glycyrrhizic or glycyrrhizinic acid). The intestinal flora hydrolyze glycyrrhizin yielding glycyrrhetinic (or glycyrrhetic) acid and glucoronic acid.[10,11] Licorice contains flavonoids and isoflavonoids (licoflavonol, kumatakenin, licoricone, glabrol, glabrone, glyzarin, licioflavones A and B, licoisoflavone, glycyrol, formononetin, liquiritigenin, isoliquiritigenin, liquiritin, neoliquiritin, rhamnoliquiritin, glyzaglabrin, 7-hydroxy-2-methylisoflavone, 4',7-dihydroxyflavone,

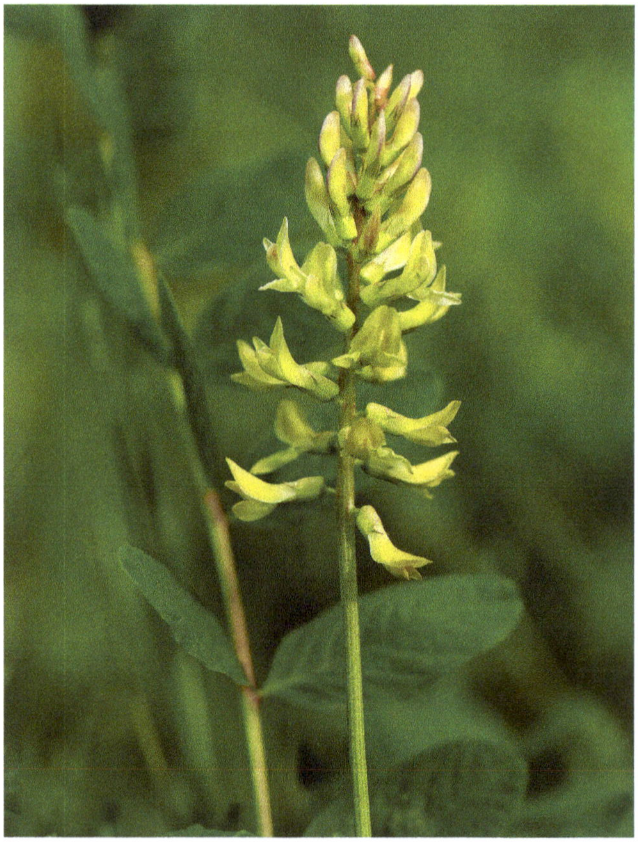

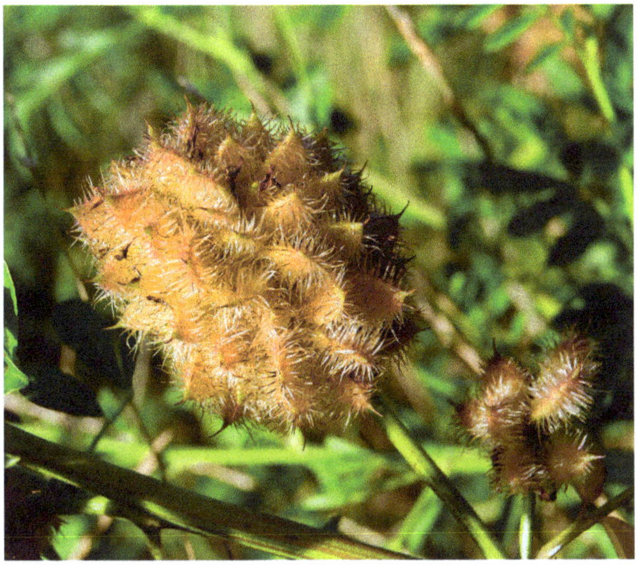

quercetin, and glabranine), chalcones (isoliquiritigenin, isoliquiritin, neoisoliquiritin, licuraside, rhamnoisoliquiritin, echinatin, licochalcones A and B, and 4-hydroxychalcone), coumarins (umbelliferone, herniarin, liqcoumarin, and glycyrin), triterpenoids (liquiritic acid, glycyrrhetol, glabrolide, isoglabrolide, licoric acid, β-amyrin, and 18-β-glycyrrhetinic acid), sterols (β-sterol, stigmasterol, and 22,23-dihydrostigmasterol), phenolic compounds (glicophenone and glicoisoflavanone), starch, glucose, sucrose, lignin, amino acids (proline, serine, and aspartic acid), amines (asparagines, betaine, and choline), gums, and wax.[7,10-12] Licorice also contains a volatile oil consisting of acetol, 2-acetylfuran, propionic acid, 2-acetylpyrrole, furfuryl alcohol, benzaldehyde, pentanol, hexanol, *trans*-hex-3-en-1-ol, oct-1-en-3-ol, linalool, linalyl oxide, α-terpineol, butyrolactone, thujone, and fenchone.[11]

NUTRITIONAL PROPERTIES: Licorice contains low to average amounts of aluminum, calcium, fiber, fat, manganese, phosphorus, potassium, protein, thiamine, and vitamin C. It contains high amounts of ash, chromium, cobalt, iron, magnesium, niacin, silicon, sodium, and tin.[13]

MEDICINAL PROPERTIES: Adrenal tonic, antiallergenic, antiangiogenic, antibacterial, anticarcinogenic, antifungal, antihepatotoxic, anti-inflammatory, antioxidant, antispasmodic, antitussive, antiulcer, antiviral, aperient, choleretic, demulcent, emollient, estrogenic, expectorant, hepatoprotectant, hypertensive, mild laxative, mineral corticoid mimetic, mucoprotective, and pseudoaldosteronic.

TEMPERATURE AND FLAVOR: Neutral, sweet, bitter, and acrid. Dry-fried or honey-fried licorice is warm and sweet.

MEDICINAL USES

Licorice substantially influences the endocrine system, primarily as an adaptogen that enhances adrenal cortical hormone function. It aids in treating individuals with adrenal hypofunction ("adrenal burnout") due to prolonged stress. It counteracts the drying effects of adrenergic hormones (epinephrine and norepinephrine) in mucous membranes. It also has multisystem effects, enhancing digestive, liver, kidney, respiratory, and immune function, and counteracting the detrimental effects of stress in those systems.

Licorice supports adrenal function due to its cortisol- and aldosterone-like effects. A glucocorticoid, cortisol is a potent anti-inflammatory hormone produced by the adrenal cortex in response to an injury or stress.[6,10,14] Licorice has cortisol-like, anti-inflammatory and antiallergenic effects. It contains glycyrrhizin (GL) and glycyrrhetinic acid (GA) that bind to glucocorticoid receptors. GL and GA also reduce the enzyme 5-β-reductase that inactivates cortisol and aldosterone, potentiating their effects; it also restores DHEA.[10,15] Glycyrrhetinic acid inhibits 11-β-hydroxysteroid dehydrogenase in rats, and synergizes hydrocortisone in humans.[11] According to Michael Murray, "Licorice's major cortisol-like effect relates to its ability to inhibit phospholipase A_2. This enzyme cleaves lipids from cellular membranes, thus beginning the manufacture of inflammatory prostaglandins and leukotrienes. In addition to this effect, glycyrrhizin also inhibits prostaglandin formation."[10] These actions play an important role in preventing inflammation.

Although licorice is less potent than steroidal anti-inflammatory pharmaceuticals such as hydrocortisone (the synthetic form of cortisol) or prednisone (a related synthetic corticosteroid), it has significantly fewer side effects.[10,14] Similar to cortisol, glycyrrhizin inhibits antibody formation, suppressing a hyperimmune response.[10] Unlike cortisol, licorice counters adrenal and thymus

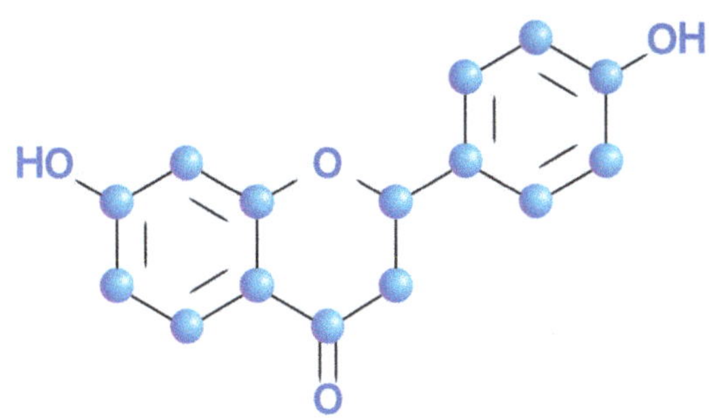

Liquiritigenin

atrophy, and inhibits hepatic cholesterol formation.[10] According to phytotherapists Simon Mills and Kerry Bones, "Glycyrrhetinic acid (GA) inhibits the enzyme that inactivates cortisol (to cortisone), leading to a high level of cortisol in the kidney, that in turn activates type 1 mineralocorticoid receptors to cause sodium retention."[15]

Licorice has aldosterone-like (pseudoaldosterone) effects.[7,10,15] Aldosterone is a mineral corticoid hormone produced by the adrenal cortex that stimulates sodium reabsorption and increases potassium excretion by the kidneys. Sodium causes water retention, increasing blood volume and blood pressure, while decreasing urine output. In healthy individuals, aldosterone is secreted when sodium levels are low. Glycyrrhetinic acid inhibits the breakdown of aldosterone in the liver, intensifying aldosterone's actions.[10,11]

The Western medical perspective on blood pressure is often simplistic; high blood pressure is bad, low blood pressure is good. The potential for high blood pressure leading to a life-threatening or debilitating condition such as a heart attack or stroke is a serious concern. Blood pressure medications are also among the top selling medications in the U.S., and often have side effects. Low blood pressure is rarely addressed by Western medical professionals, likely because there are few medications for treating it. Although the symptoms are more subtle, individuals with hypotension may experience dizziness upon standing, frequent urination (with dilute urine), and nighttime urination. These conditions are affected by dehydration and salt consumption; however, they are also caused by deficient renin secretion by the kidneys, and deficient aldosterone secretion by the adrenal cortex. Herbalist Michael Moore classifies these symptoms as "kidney deficiency." Although hypotension is not usually serious, it is not conducive to optimal health. Decreased blood volume and blood pressure reduce fluid transport in the kidneys, lungs, digestive system, and skin, decreasing oxygen and nutrient delivery to the tissues. Consuming small quantities of licorice is ideal for treating individuals with hypotension and kidney deficiency due to its aldosterone-like actions. *Note:* Deglycyrrhinized licorice (DGL) does not affect the adrenals or adrenal hormones.

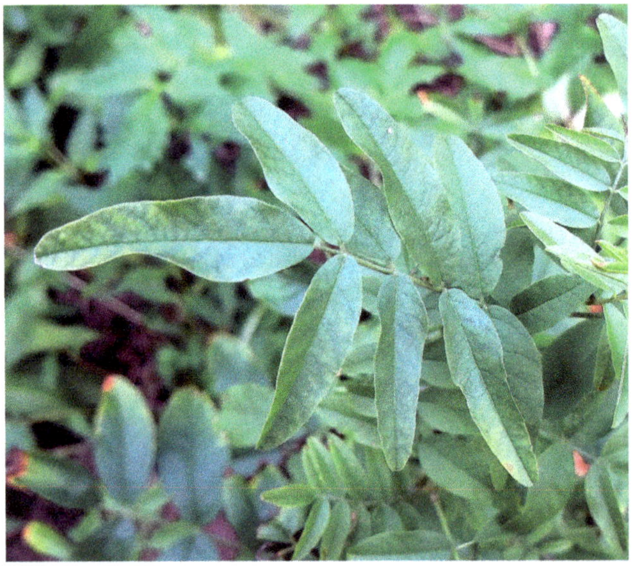

Due to the glycyrrhizin, licorice has an antiallergenic effect, inhibiting the formation of prostaglandins and phospholipase A2.[11,12,15] Consuming licorice or glycyrrhizin-containing products reduces allergic skin reactions, and aids in treating hives, contact dermatitis, allergic eczema, psoriasis, rashes, carbuncles, sores, and the dry stages of poison oak or poison ivy.[10,11] Consume licorice internally and apply water-based preparations to treat the aforementioned conditions. Licorice also decreases allergic respiratory responses, and aids in treating lower respiratory spasms due to allergies or asthma.[10] Glycyrrhizin reduces minor anaphylactic and skin reactions.[7] Glycyrrhetinic acid prevents histamines from causing capillary permeability, reducing excess swelling associated with the inflammatory response.[7] *Note:* Anaphylaxis requires prompt medical attention. Combine extracts of dandelion root *(Taraxacum),* turmeric *(Curcuma),* burdock root *(Arctium),* and licorice to reduce inflammation.

Licorice is highly effective for healing gastric and duodenal ulcers, and soothing the digestive lining.[15] It contains GL and GA that promote ulcer healing; glycyrrhetinic acid also reduces local inflammation.[15] Unfortunately, glycyrrhizin causes undesirable side effects including edema and hypertension, though it is not as important as GA for ulcer healing; therefore, DGL is often used to treat gastric and duodenal ulcers.[15] DGL is a concentrated extract of licorice containing no more than 3% GL, but it is not completely glycyrrhizin-free.[15] The mucoprotective effects are also attributed to licorice's high flavonoid content.[11,15] DGL prevents ulcers, reduces gastric acid secretion, and has mucoprotective effects against aspirin and bile-induced damage to the GI tract lining.[15] DGL and GA decrease the number and size of ulcers.[15] DGL is most effective for treating ulcers when it is chewed and swallowed 20 minutes before meals.[10] It is as effective in treating gastric ulcers as Zantac and Tagamet, and it is more effective in protecting the mucosa and preventing a recurrence.[10] As an alternative to antacids, consume DGL after a meal to alleviate heartburn. A decoction of licorice consumed on an empty stomach reduces inflammation related to lower gastrointestinal conditions such as irritable bowel syndrome, Crohn's disease, ulcerative colitis, and some cases of diverticulosis. Prepare a tea containing marshmallow *(Althaea)*, chamomile *(Matricaria)*, fennel *(Foeniculum)*, meadowsweet *(Filipendula)*, and licorice daily to reduce stomach and intestinal inflammation and spasms.

In Traditional Chinese Medicine, licorice (especially honey-fried) is administered as a spleen qi tonic. It alleviates symptoms of spleen qi deficiency, such as fatigue, poor digestion and assimilation, gas and bloating, loose stools and diarrhea, and extremity weakness.[7] As previously mentioned, licorice has potent demulcent properties that soothe the digestive tract and help to heal the above symptoms.

Licorice enhances liver function; it is a choleretic, cholagogue, detoxifier, and hepatoprotective agent.[6,7] It inhibits liver cell injury, but does not reverse protein synthesis.[10] GL and GA are hepatoprotective.[15] Glycyrrhetinic acid prevents free radical formation, and reduces free radical and liver damage.[10] Licorice lowers LDL cholesterol levels, and inhibits the progression of atherosclerotic lesions.[7] It contains the antioxidants isoflavones and chalcones that prevent LDL cholesterol against peroxidation.[15] Glycyrrhizin lowers cholesterol levels.[7] In Traditional Chinese Medicine, licorice is used as a poison antidote, indicating its hepatoprotective function. Decoctions of *G. uralensis* reduce the toxicity of numerous substances, including cocaine, arsenobenzol, and urethane. The decoctions also have mild to moderate detoxifying effects on caffeine, acetylcholine, pilocarpine, and nicotine.[7] Licorice aids in treating chronic, active viral hepatitis, and helps to prevent post-transfusion hepatitis.[6]

Licorice is a potent antimicrobial agent. It has antiviral effects against herpes, shingles, viral hepatitis, and HIV.[6,10,11] It also aids in treating a cold and influenza.[10] The antiviral effects are due to glycyrrhizin, which stimulates interferon production.[10] Interferon binds to cellular surfaces, stimulating the synthesis of intracellular proteins that inhibit viral DNA infection.[10] Interferon also has immune stimulating effects, activating macrophages and natural killer cells.[10] Licorice increases interleukins. Glycyrrhizin impedes the growth of cultured DNA and RNA viruses, including herpes simplex, herpes zoster, vaccinia, Newcastle disease, and vesicular stomatitis.[10,15] Diprenylated bibenzyl isolated from licorice extract has moderate anti-HIV-1 activity.[16] Topical preparations of glycyrrhetinic acid aid in treating herpes.[10] Alcohol-based extracts of licorice have antibacterial activity *in vitro* against *Staphylococcus aureus, Streptococcus mutans,* and *Mycobacterium smegmatis,* as well as antifungal effects

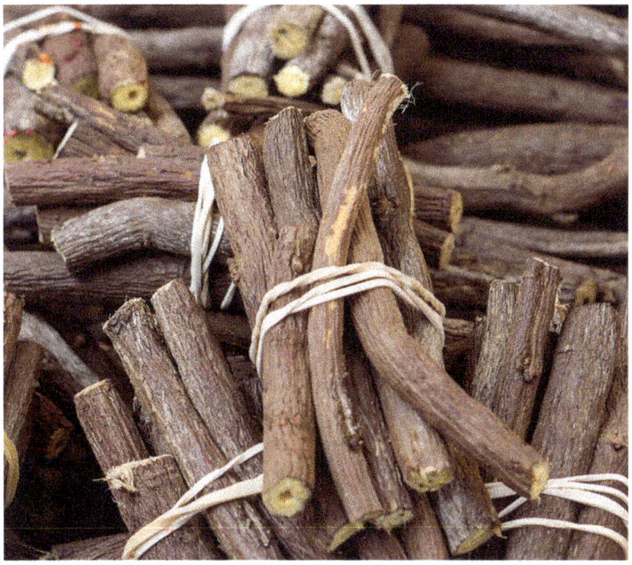

against *Candida albicans.*[10] Licorice also inhibits the growth of *Trichomonas,* a parasitic protozoa.[11]

Licorice is a soothing expectorant, antitussive, and demulcent, reducing inflammation in respiratory mucosa. Due to its moistening effects on tissues, it is best used for dry respiratory conditions. The antitussive effects are due to a derivative of 18-β-glycyrrhetinic acid.[11] Licorice is highly effective in treating upper and lower respiratory conditions, including a sore throat, pharyngitis, laryngitis, tracheitis, strep throat, a dry, hacking cough, bronchitis, wheezing, and whooping cough. To soothe upper or lower respiratory irritation, prepare a decoction of marshmallow root *(Althaea)*, anise *(Pimpinella)*, and carob pod *(Ceratonia)* with smaller amounts of licorice. Alternatively, prepare an infusion containing mullein leaf *(Verbascum)*, coltsfoot *(Tussilago)*, hyssop *(Hyssopus)*, peppermint *(Mentha piperita)*, and a pinch of licorice. Combine extracts of echinacea *(Echinacea)*, spilanthes *(Acmella)*, propolis resin, red root *(Ceanothus)*, and licorice as a throat spray or gargle in order to treat a sore throat or laryngitis. Combine extracts of aralia *(Aralia californica)*, anise *(Pimpinella)*, gumweed *(Grindelia)*, Senega snakeweed *(Polygala)*, and licorice to alleviate asthma, wheezing, or a dry cough.

Licorice extract, powder bolus, and DGL aid in treating canker sores.[10,11] In fact, 75% of patients using a mouthwash (containing 200 mg of powdered DGL dissolved in 200 ml of warm water) four times daily experienced significant improvement in one day (50 – 75%), and complete healing by the third day.[10]

Licorice has anticancerous, antitumorigenic, and antiangiogenic effects.[7,15,16] Licorice extract has cancer-suppressive effects in breast, endometrial, lung, gastric, pancreatic, and

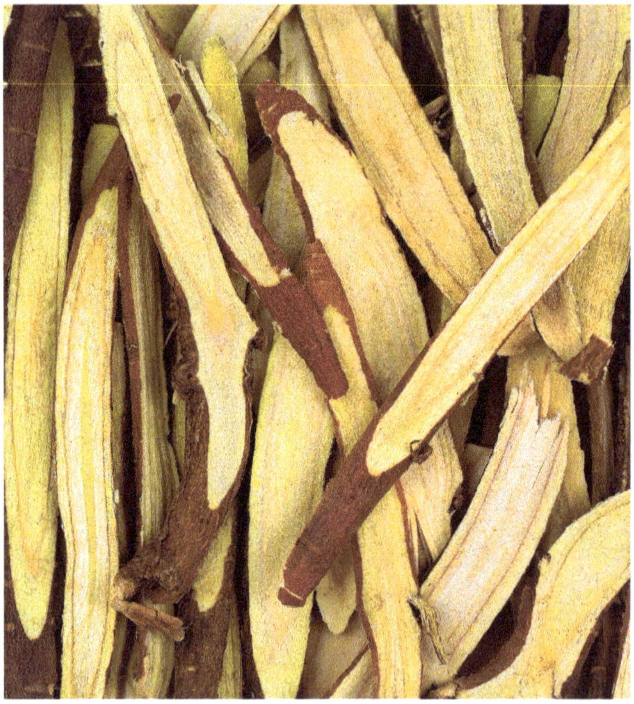

prostate cancers.[16] Licorice extract and GA inhibit 5-lipoxygenase (5-LOX), and cyclooxygenase-2 (COX-2) enzymes that form proinflammatory eicosanoids from arachidonic acid.[16] GA prevents the binding of tumor promoters in test cells, possibly due to protein kinase C inhibition.[15] These actions are highly sought in anticancer drugs. Glycyrrhizin inhibits hepatitis-induced liver cancer.[16] It also aids in treating ascitic hepatic cancer with granuloma and ascites.[7] GA inhibits tumor growth of sarcoma 45 and Ehrlich ascites cells.[11] In rodents, GA also inhibits Oberling-Guerin myeloma.[7] The oral administration of licorice water extract (1%) has protective effects against chemical carcinogen-induced lung and stomach cancer in mice.[15] In patients undergoing radiation and chemotherapy, DGL reduces inflammation and ulceration of oral mucosa.[16] It improves cellular immunity, and total leukocyte and lymphocyte counts in irradiated mice.[15]

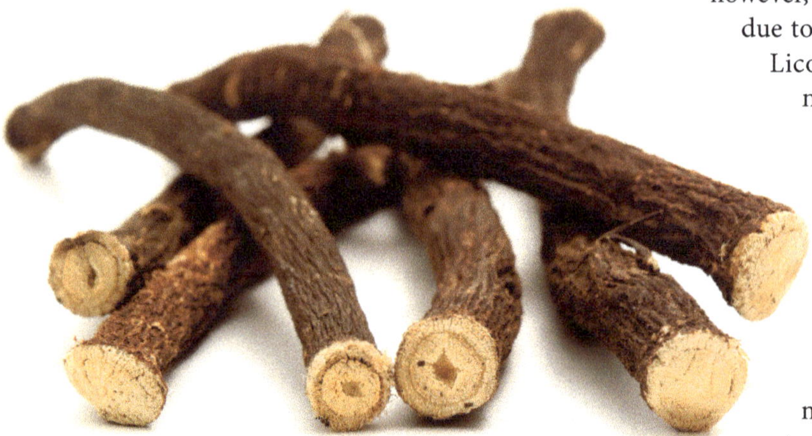

Licorice contains phytosterols (β-sitosterol, formononetin, coumarins, and others) that exert weak estrogen activity.[18] It has minor effects in treating hormonal imbalances; however, the hormone-balancing effects are more likely due to its adaptogenic influence on the HPA axis.[17] Licorice may have alterative actions on estrogen metabolism, inhibiting estrogen when levels are too high, and potentiating estrogen when levels are too low.[10] Compared to estradiol, β-sitosterol has a weak affinity for estrogen receptors (¼00th).[18] GL also has weak influence in estrogen and androgen receptors.[17] Isoflavone components exert weak estrogenic activity in laboratory animals.[10,11] However, GA antagonizes the effects of exogenous estrogens.[10] It inhibited estrodiol's effects on uterine growth in ovariectomized animals.[18] Adding small amounts of licorice to compounds harmonizes hormone-balancing formulas during reproductive years, and is especially helpful for women with hypofunctioning adrenals.[17] For easing menopausal symptoms, small amounts of licorice work well when combined with extracts of vitex *(Vitex agnus-castus)*, Eleuthero *(Eleutherococcus)* or ginseng *(Panax)*, black cohosh *(Actaea)*, motherwort *(Leonurus)*, and peony *(Paeonia lactiflora)*.

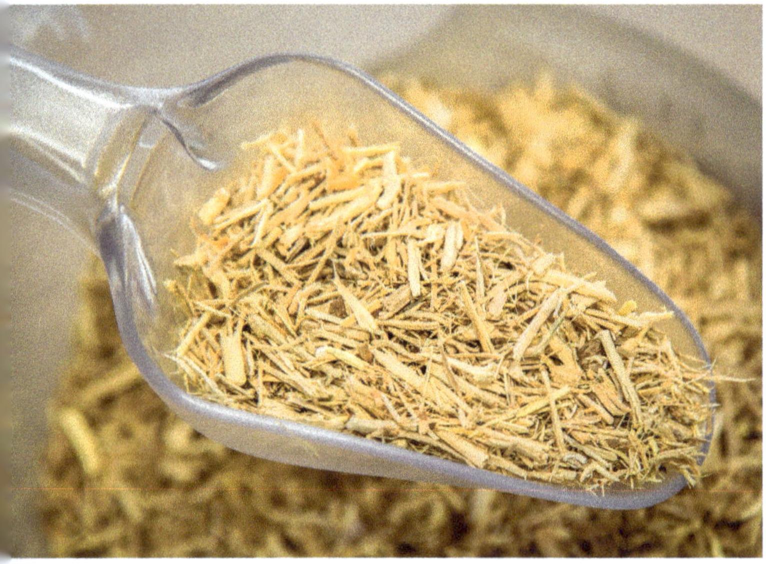

A combination containing *G. glabra* and *Paeonia lactiflora* (or peaoniflorin, a component of *P. lactiflora*) was successfully used to treat polycystic ovarian disease (PCOD). GA decreases testosterone synthesis from androstenedione.[17] Licorice lowers prolactin secretion.[17] These hormonal effects enhance ovulation rates and increase fertility.[17] In one study, infertile, hyperandrogenic and oligomenorrheic women consumed 5 – 10 g of the formula daily for

2–8 weeks; serum testosterone levels and ovulation were normalized.[15] In another study, a combination of 7.5 g of *Paeonia* and *G. glabra* was administered to women with PCOD for 24 weeks. After four weeks, serum testosterone and free testosterone levels were decreased; however, after 12 weeks, testosterone was only lower in patients who became pregnant. Following 24 weeks of treatment, the LH to FSH ratio was lower.[15] Overall, this two-herb formula decreases the excessive production of ovarian androgens, reducing testosterone levels and increasing the rate of androgens' conversion to estrogens.[17] On a similar note, women with PCOD treated with spirinolactone (a hypotensive diuretic that also has antiandrogenic activity) experienced fewer side effects from consuming 3.5 grams of licorice extract per day.[16]

Licorice is an effective harmonizing and flavoring agent. It contains glycyrrhizin, which is 50–100 times sweeter than sucrose.[10] Adding small amounts to tea blends (¼ to ½ teaspoon per liter) or tincture compounds (5–15 ml per 120 ml) enhances the flavor, reduces the harshness of acrid and astringent herbs, and masks bitter herbs. Numerous Chinese herbal formulas contain licorice as a harmonizer.

CONTRAINDICATIONS

Due to the aldosterone-like effects, licorice is contraindicated in individuals with edema, hypertension, hypokalemia, or renal failure.[10] Avoid use in individuals consuming blood pressure-lowering and digitalis-based medications, and/or diuretics. Consuming more than 3 grams per day for more than six weeks, or more than 100 milligrams per day of glycyrrhizin daily can cause hypertension, edema, and hypokalemia. Increasing potassium intake and minimizing sodium consumption aid in preventing undesired side effects in healthy individuals. Discontinue use if licorice consumption causes palpitations. Individuals medicated with prednisone or cortisone should consult a health professional before consuming licorice.[16]

Pregnant women should limit their use of licorice by consuming no more than 3 g daily.[15] GL and GA have the slight potential of counteracting the contraceptive pill; high doses and prolonged use of licorice should be avoided.[15]

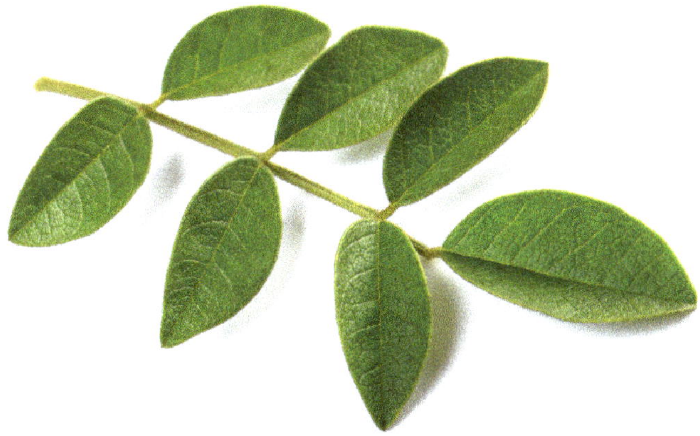

PREPARATION AND DOSAGE

TINCTURE: Fresh roots [1:2, 60–95% alcohol]; dry roots [1:5, 50–60% alcohol]; consume 15–60 drops, up to four times daily.

FLUID EXTRACT: Dry roots [1:1, 50% alcohol]; consume 10–30 drops, up to three times daily. Or consume 250–500 mg daily of the standardized extract (containing 25% glycyrrhizic acid).

CAPSULES: Consume 1–2 capsules, two to three times daily. Chew 2 tablets of deglycyrrhinized licorice before or two hours after a meal, up to three times daily.

TEA: Consume 8–12 ounces of the decoction, or less preferably, the cold or hot infusion, one to four times daily. When treating digestive ulcers, consume the decoction on an empty stomach up to one hour before meals, or two hours after meals.

HONEY AND SYRUP: Add licorice to herbal pills, cough drops, herb-infused honey, syrups, or pastes.

TOPICAL USE: Apply a water-based preparation such as a fomentation or poultice of the decocted root, or apply a paste of root powder mixed with water or honey.

LOBELIA

DESCRIPTION

BOTANICAL NAMES:
Lobelia inflata, L. cardinalis, L. siphilitica

COMMON NAMES:
Great blue lobelia, cardinal flower, Indian tobacco, wild tobacco, asthma weed, bladder pod, puke weed, emetic weed, emetic herb, vomit weed, vomit wort, gag weed, gag root
rohtolobelia (Finnish)
lobélie enflée, tabac Indien (French)
aufgeblasene lobelie (German)
hanpenren (Japanese)
dhavala (Sanskrit)
läkelobelia (Swedish)

FAMILY NAME:
Campanulaceae
(formerly Lobeliaceae)

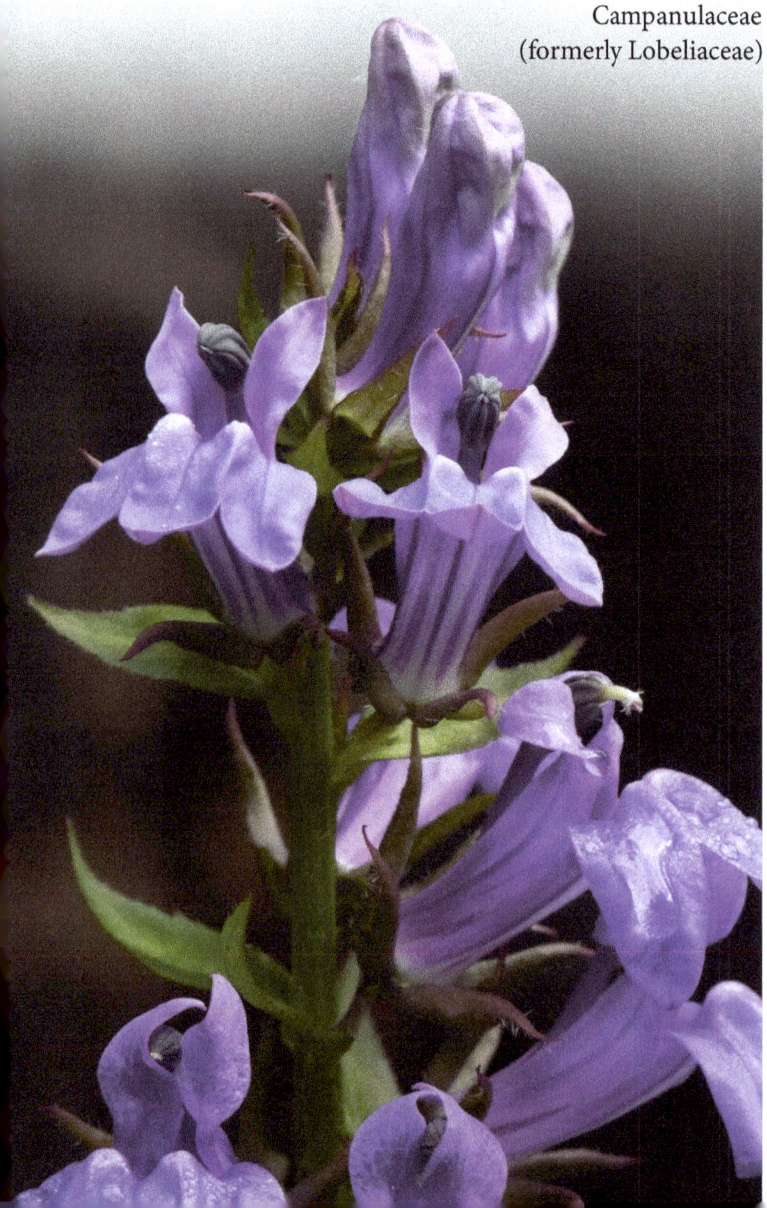

PARTS USED: The leaves and flowering tops. The seeds are also used, but are more likely to induce nausea in moderate doses.

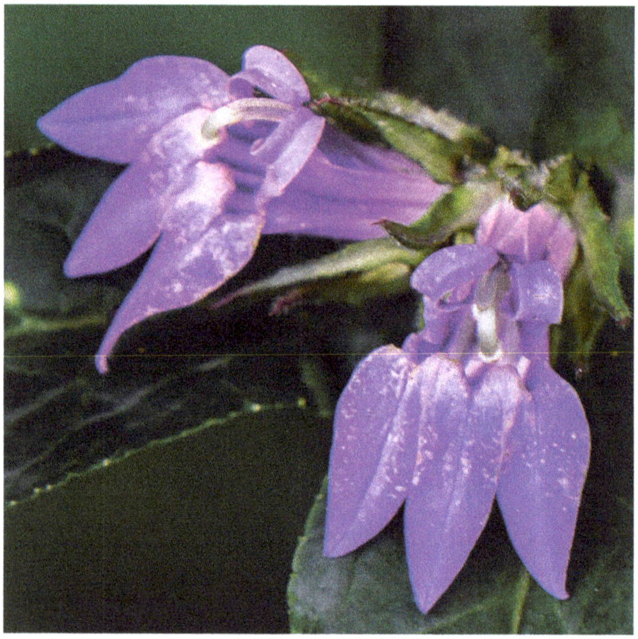

BOTANICAL DESCRIPTION AND HABITAT: Lobelia belongs to a large genus of plants growing mostly in the tropical and subtropical areas of Africa and the Americas, although the species described in this monograph are found in temperate North America. Lobelia species are usually herbaceous perennials with stems that exude milky latex.[1] The linear to elliptic leaves (0.5 – 1.5 cm wide) are basal or alternate on the stem.[2] Inflorescences are usually racemes with bilaterally symmetric flowers on twisted pedicels, resulting in upside down flowers.[2] The calyces and corollas have tubular bases with five narrow, often outspread lobes. The bilabiate corolla is red, blue, or white; the upper lip has two lobes, and the lower lip has three.[1] The connate stamens enclose the style and extend past the corolla.[1] The usually inferior, two-chambered ovary develops into a many-seeded, two-valved capsule, or a berry enclosed within the persistent calyx.[1]

Lobelia inflata grows in moist, often poor soil in woods and fields, and along roads throughout southern Canada and the eastern U.S.[3] A diminutive plant, the pubescent, herbaceous stems (75 cm tall) bear alternate, elliptic to ovate, sessile leaves (up to 7 cm long by 3 cm wide) with irregular, whitish-tipped teeth.[3,4] The tiny, indigo-tinged white flowers (7 mm) grow in terminal, sparse, leafy racemes.[3] The fruit (8 mm long, 5 – 6 mm diameter) is an inflated capsule.[4]

Lobelia cardinalis is a gorgeous herbaceous perennial growing from eastern Canada through northern to southern South America.[5] Occupying wet places in rich, alkaline soil at the edge of woods, stream banks, roadsides, open meadows and pastures, and swamps, the population has been diminished due to wildflower lovers excessively picking the flowers.[5] The cardinal flower has smooth, unbranched stems (30 – 120 cm tall).[5] The lanceolate, finely dentate leaves (up to 20 cm) have acuminate apices and wavy margins.[5,7] The plant is known for its terminal racemes (up to 20 cm long) of showy, cardinal red flowers.

Lobelia siphilitica (60 – 100 cm tall) is an herbaceous perennial growing in wet areas in woods and meadows, and along ponds in eastern North America.[8] It has angular stems with few hairs.[9] Alternate, sessile, pubescent leaves are lanceolate to oblong (up to 15 cm long by 2 – 3 cm wide), with irregularly dentate margins.[9] The leafy racemes of lavender-blue flowers (2 – 3 cm long) have pubescent calyces (1.5 cm long) with lobes that lay flat along the corolla tube.[9]

THE NAME: *Lobelia* was named for Flemish botanist Matthias de Lobel.[10] The epithet *cardinalis* refers to the vibrant red flowers. The epithet *siphilitica* derives from the Iroquois practice of using the root to treat syphilis. The epithet *inflata* ("inflate") derives from the Latin *inflatus* referring to the inflated seed pods. Numerous common names refer to its use as an emetic, including: puke weed, vomit weed, vomit wort, gag weed, and emetic weed.

HISTORICAL USES: A classic American herb with a colorful history, lobelia was a favorite of Samuel Thomson, a prominent herbalist who practiced in the early 1800s. Thomson idolized this plant, and regarded it as the core agent in his practice. He used it to remove "canker" or wastes from the body (a concept analogous to "ama" in Ayurveda), as a relaxant, and a diffusive agent to move the vital force from the body's core to the surface, removing obstacles along the way.[11] Thomson valued the emetic quality of lobelia, and employed the plant in large doses until it caused repeated episodes of vomiting. Over the years, it was used in smaller doses.[11]

An integral agent in Thomson's patented "Course of Medicine," lobelia was frequently combined with cayenne *(Capsicum)*, bayberry *(Morella cerifera)*, and myrrh *(Commiphora)*. His system of medicine spread throughout the U.S. and Europe, partly due to Dr. Albert Isaiah Coffin's work.[12] While mainstream physicians of the day were using the method of excessive bloodletting and administering mineral agents such as concentrated mercury, Thomson and aligned physicians were accused of murder, and prosecuted for using lobelia. This was likely because they spoke out against the standard medical practice, and drew clients away from "regular" physicians.[12]

In 1846, Dr. Benjamin Colby, a student of Thomson, described lobelia as "the most powerful, certain, and harmless relaxant that has ever been discovered," and cited other physicians' use of it as an antispasmodic for cramps, spasms, lock-jaw, and contracted sinews.[13] The antispasmodic properties were attributed to lobelia's cholagogue, diaphoretic, and diuretic actions that relaxed the bile ducts, blood vessels, skin pores, and ureters, respectively.[13] It was also applied topically to boils, skin cancer, hernias, dislocations, and fractures (to relax the muscles).[13] Eclectics administered lobelia during labor to help relax the mother's musculature, reduce resistance in the body, and ease labor.[13-15]

Samuel Thomson introduced lobelia to the Eclectics, who lauded it as one of the most valued vital stimulants.[14,15] Dr. Finley Ellingwood employed lobelia as a nauseating expectorant and respiratory sedative.[14] Lobelia was used to relieve respiratory conditions such as asthma, croup,

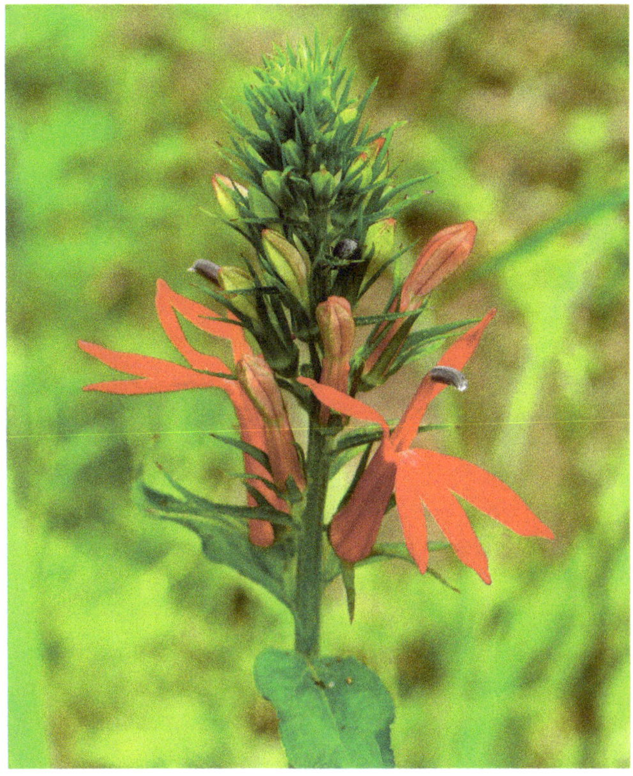

tuberculosis symptoms, pleurisy, whooping cough, measles, colds, laryngitis, and fevers.[13-15] It was administered as an emetic for chronic, atonic stomach disorders with intermittent fever.[15] However, it was never administered as an emetic to children, the elderly, or weak individuals.[15] The "Compound Powder of Lobelia," also known as "emetic powder," contained six parts lobelia, four parts ipecac, three parts blood root and skunk cabbage, and one part cayenne. As an emetic, two drams were administered in ¼ to ½ dram doses in warm water, every 15 minutes.[15] Although internal use of the powder waned, it was applied topically to the chest for bronchopulmonary afflictions such as bronchitis, pleurisy, pneumonia, and pectoral wall soreness.[15] The powder was sprinkled on a warm cloth suffused with lard and applied to the chest.[15]

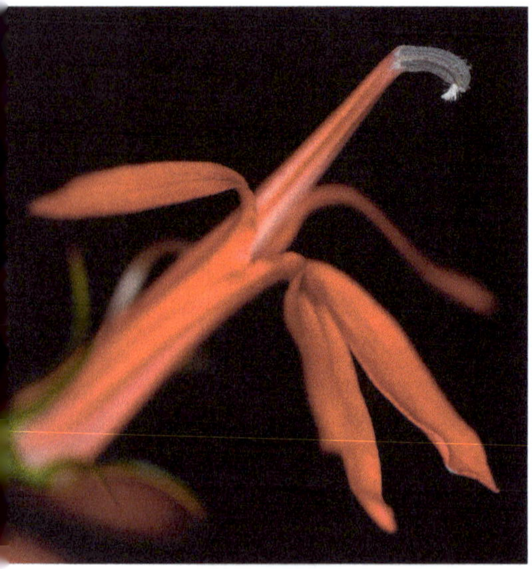

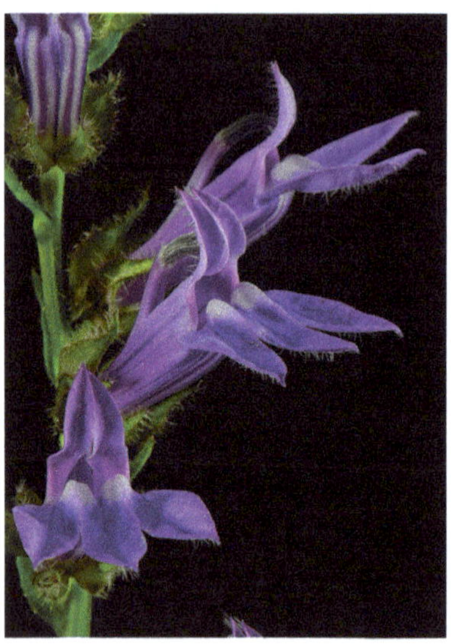

Eclectics administered lobelia to treat angina pectoris, heart neuralgia, and pulmonary apoplexy.[14,15] A 20-drop dosage was administered, and sometimes repeated as needed.[15] It was given in low doses as a cardiac stimulant when the pulse was "full, sluggish, oppressed, and doughy."[15] Another indication for lobelia was nausea with a full, pale, broad, flabby, heavily coated tongue (at the base), engorged tissue, difficulty breathing, and a bruised, oppressive feeling in the chest.[15] Low doses were administered for atonic dyspepsia, indigestion, la grippe, and habitual constipation.[14,15] Dr. John King recommended lobelia applications to ease herpes, eczema, and nettle rash.[16] He recommended a liniment combining ½ ounce of oils of sassafras and amber, 1 dram of oil of lobelia, and a ½ dram of oil of capsicum applied in order to ease neuralgic and rheumatic pain.[16]

CONSTITUENTS: Lobelia contains pyridine (piperidine) alkaloids, including lobeline, lobelanine, lobelanidine, norlobelanine (isolobelanine), lelobanidine, norlelobanidine, norlobelanidine, lobinine, isolobinine, lobinanidine, isolobinanidine, 8-methyl-10-ethyllobelidiol, and 8-methyl-10-phenyllobelidiol. It also contains resin, gum, fats, lobelic acid, chelidonic acid, and fixed and pungent volatile oil (inflatin and lebelacrin).[14,15,17]

NUTRITIONAL PROPERTIES: Not applicable.

MEDICINAL PROPERTIES: Analgesic, anodyne, antiasthmatic, antispasmodic, antitussive, anxiolytic, diaphoretic, expectorant, nauseant, nervine, relaxant, sedative, sialagogue, and counterirritant. High doses have emetic and purgative actions.

TEMPERATURE AND FLAVOR: Hot, acrid, bitter, and astringent.

MEDICINAL USES

Lobelia has potent medicinal actions. It should be used with caution, and consumed in very small quantities (5 – 30 drops), diluted in 4 ounces of water. Begin by consuming a 5-drop dose in 2 – 4 ounces of water. If necessary, increase in 5-drop increments until the desired effect is achieved. It contains lobeline that has an expectorant action, but large doses can have emetic, purgative, and diuretic actions.

Lobelia is a potent smooth muscle antispasmodic, effective for respiratory spasms.[14,15] It alleviates a dry, hacking, unproductive cough with difficult expectoration and dyspnea.[14,15] Lobelia is a somewhat irritating expectorant that stimulates salivation and mucous membrane secretions.[14,15] For respiratory applications, it aids in treating a cough, cold, dry bronchitis, pleurisy, croup, whooping cough, pneumonia, and dyspnea.[14-16,18] Lobelia aids in treating respiratory conditions that worsen when an individual reclines and has difficulty sleeping.[15] Consuming a low dose before sleep reduces insomnia-related respiratory spasms. It also is useful for easing digestive spasms when gentler remedies have been exhausted.[14,15]

Lobelia is effective for treating acute spasmodic asthma attacks, especially when consumed at the onset.[14,15] Consuming 5 – 15 drops of lobelia as needed has reduced inhaler use in numerous patients. Some patients have consumed up to 30 drops during an acute asthmatic attack without a nauseant or emetic effect. *Note:* Although lobelia is helpful for symptomatic relief, it is also necessary to address food and environmental sensitivities in asthmatic individuals.

Lobelia is a skeletal muscle antispasmodic; internal and topical applications of it aid in treating muscle spasms and rigidity, myalgia, and neuralgia.[14,16] It has multifaceted benefits for individuals suffering from an extended acute or chronic cough (days or weeks), who may experience serious muscle tension in the neck, shoulders, or upper back. Some patients have thrown their ribs or vertebrae out of alignment due to excessive coughing. A lobelia compress can be applied topically to the affected area.

Lobelia is a potent nervine and central nervous system sedative that affects the sympathetic nerve ganglia.[14,15] It should be used as a last resort, only when gentler nervine herbs are ineffective. Lobelia calms the nervous system in individuals with more severe anxiety, insomnia, multiple sclerosis, tremors, or seizures. Use it alone, or alternate it with California poppy *(Eschscholzia)*, valerian *(Valeriana)*, or Jamaican dogwood *(Piscidia)* extracts.

Lobelia slows the heart rate, deepens respiration, and lowers elevated blood pressure.[14,15] It also reduces a sense of pain and oppression in the chest.[14,15] Lobelia improves circulation by relaxing blood vessels.[15] Although there are safer alternatives, low doses of lobelia (1 – 10 drops) reduce symptoms of nicotine withdrawal. This is due to its lobeline content that fills the nicotinic receptors.

An anodyne, a lobelia poultice eases pain and inflammation due to insect bites and stings, bruises, sprains, strains, swelling, arthritis, swollen joints, tendonitis, carpel tunnel, boils, and bunions.[15-17] A frequently applied compress eases itching due to poison oak or poison ivy.[15,16] It also eases neuralgia, neuritis, and myalgia.[15,16] Trace a spastic nerve with a lobelia extract. For insect bites, combine the powdered herb with clay and water, and apply to the inflamed area.

CONTRAINDICATIONS

Avoid use during pregnancy or lactation, and in children under the age of ten.[18] It should be used cautiously with asthma medications. Lobelia is contraindicated with prescription narcotics, analgesics, sedatives, and steroids. Excessive doses of lobelia, especially the seeds or dry plant, can cause nausea, vomiting, dizziness, cold sweats, headaches, respiratory depression, convulsions, and collapse.[14,15,17,18] Lobelia will cause emesis before a poisonous amount can been ingested; therefore, it will not cause fatal results.[15] Limit topical application to a small, localized region. Do not consume while operating heavy machinery. Lobelia is eliminated by the kidneys.[15]

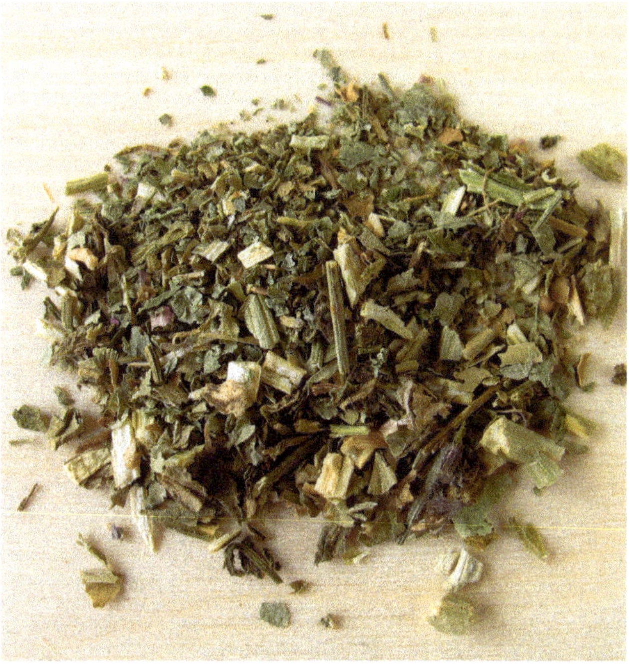

PREPARATION AND DOSAGE

Note: Exercise caution when processing lobelia. Use in well ventilated areas and wear protective gloves to prevent nausea or vomiting from overexposure.

TINCTURE: Fresh flowering herb [1:4, 70 - 95% alcohol]; recently dried herb [1:5, 50% alcohol]; consume 5 - 30 drops in 2 - 4 ounces of water, up to four times daily for acute conditions. Dry seeds [1:5, 50 - 60% alcohol]; consume 5 - 15 drops in 2 - 4 ounces of water, up to four times daily for acute conditions. Use the seed extract cautiously, as an excessive dose can cause vomiting.

ACETUM EXTRACT: Dry herb [1:5, apple cider vinegar]; apply topically.

TEA: It is difficult to regulate the dosage of lobelia; therefore, tea consumption is not recommended.

TOPICAL USE: Prepare lobelia oil using the alcohol intermediary, infused oil, or double boiler method. Apply the tincture undiluted or diluted with water as a liniment. Or apply the fresh plant poultice.

LOMATIUM

DESCRIPTION

BOTANICAL NAMES:
Lomatium dissectum, L. nudicaule, L. californicum, L. utriculatum, L. spp. (syn. *Leptotaenia*)

COMMON NAMES:
Lomatium, biscuit root, Indian balsam, Indian consumption plant, spring gold, fine-leaved desert parsley, barestem desert parsley, western wild parsley, mountain wild parsley

FAMILY NAME:
Apiaceae (Umbelliferae)

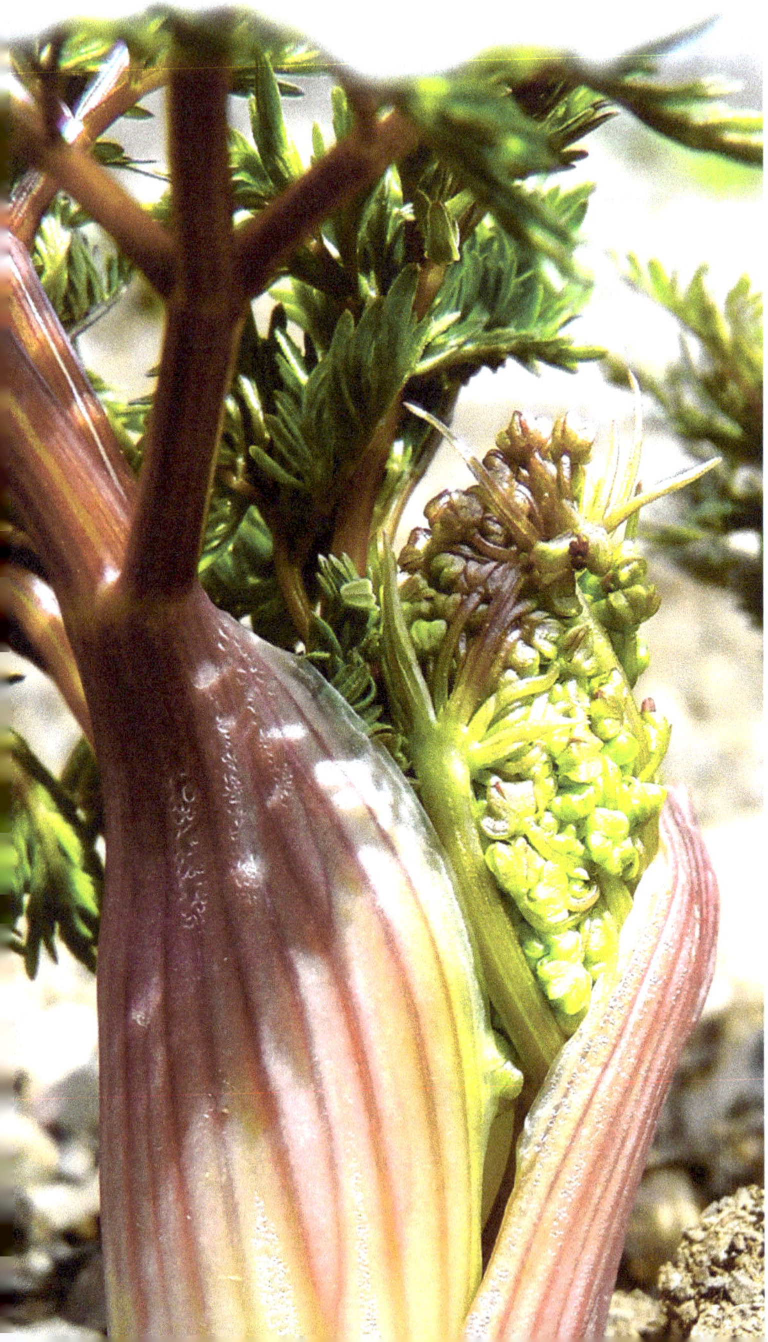

PARTS USED: The roots are used medicinally; the leaves for culinary purposes.

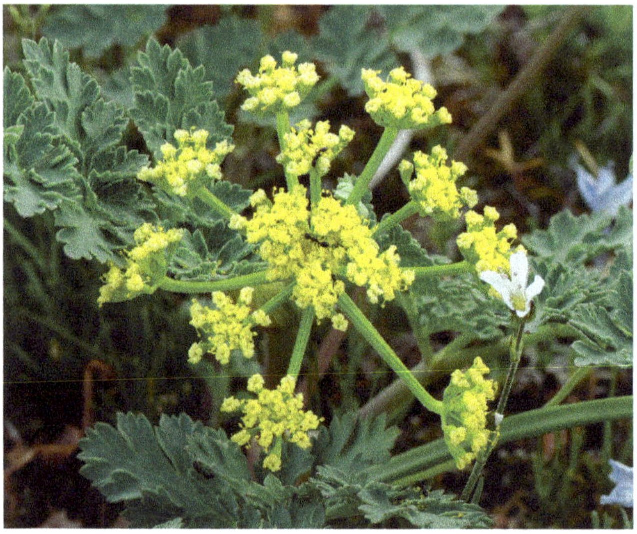

BOTANICAL DESCRIPTION AND HABITAT: *Lomatium dissectum* is a striking plant known for its thick, strongly scented, resinous taproot. It is an herbaceous perennial growing up to 140 cm high, and is the tallest member of the genus.[1,2] Its surface ranges from glabrous to minutely hairy, and is often covered with a bluish-white, waxy coating.[1] The bulk of the plant is a basal rosette with extremely feathery, rounded to triangular, fern-like leaves with sheathing bases.[1] The ternate-pinnate compound leaves have linear leaflets (up to 2 cm long).[1] The leaves are quite large; petioles reach up to 30 cm long, and the blades grow up to 35 cm wide.[1]

The inflorescence is a compound umbel with a smooth peduncle (up to 60 cm long), subtended by linear bractlets.[1] There are 10 to 30 rays (3 – 10 cm long) bearing dense clusters of flowers on short pedicels (up to 2 cm long).[1] The tiny asepalous flowers have five chocolate-red to yellow petals, five stamens, one inferior ovary consisting of two fused carpels, and two styles.[1] The fruit is a two-parted, glabrous, elliptic schizocarp with thickened wings.[1] *Note:* It is crucial to correctly identify this plant, as it can be mistaken for toxic members of the Apiaceae family.

Lomatium dissectum grows in sagebrush and pinyon-juniper woodlands at 500- to 10,000-foot elevations throughout the western U.S. and Canada.[2]

THE NAME: The genus *Lomatium* derives from the Latin *loma* ("winged or ribbed"), referring to the fruit.[3] The epithet *dissectum* means "cut into many deep lobes," referring to the leaflets.[4] *Lomatium dissectum* was known as *Leptotaenia dissecta* until 1942. *Leptotaenia* derives from the Latin *lepto* ("slender").[4]

HISTORICAL USES: Lomatium is often recommended as an antiviral agent, likely stemming from Dr. Earnest Krebs' *Bulletin of the Nevada State Board of Health, No. 1.* He reported that during the 1918 influenza epidemic, no deaths were recorded among the Washoe Indians in Nevada's Great Basin where they treated patients with a root decoction. He mentioned that Native Americans living in other regions of Nevada with no access to the roots died in large numbers. The roots were gathered in the fall, fresh or dry roots were decocted in water, and the tops were skimmed. Large doses of the tea were administered. An average one pound of roots was administered throughout three days to resolve fevers from influenza or pulmonary disease. Dr. Krebs borrowed from Native American practices, and studied the roots and their effects. He administered the herb to non-Native people, successfully treating hundreds of cases of virulent influenza, and reducing related complications. He considered lomatium the most effective agent for treating influenza pneumonia and lobar pneumonia. Dr. Krebs described lomatium as a diaphoretic, a stimulating expectorant, a tonic to the respiratory mucosa, and an antiseptic for bronchial, intestinal, and urinary systems. Other physicians administered lomatium with positive results.[5]

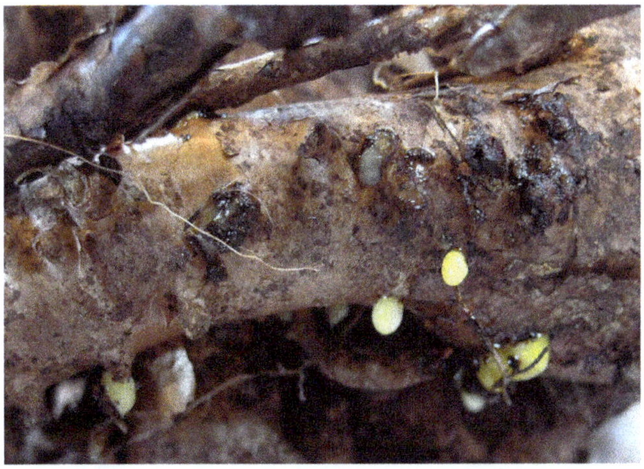

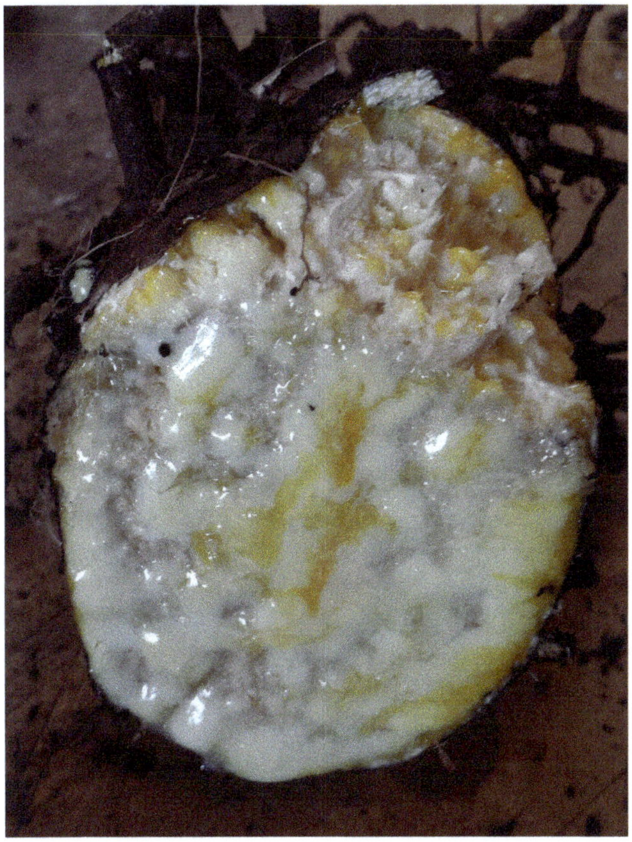

In 1941, Percy Train, James R. Henrichs, and W. Andrew Archer published *Medicinal Uses of Plants by Indian Tribes of Nevada.* In 1959, Edith Murphey recorded the tribes' medicinal uses of the plant in *Indian Uses of Native Plants.* The Washoe, Paiute, and Shoshone regarded lomatium as an extremely important medicine. A decoction of lomatium was consumed to alleviate a cold, influenza, or cough. The tea was also consumed to treat respiratory afflictions, including hay fever, bronchitis, pneumonia, and tuberculosis. The roots were chewed to alleviate a sore throat; they were also placed on coals and inhaled to relieve asthma and respiratory congestion.[5,6] The decoction was applied as an antiseptic to cuts, sores, skin rashes, and smallpox sores. The fresh root sap was applied to open wounds and sores. The roots were carried to ward off illness and rattlesnakes.[6]

The roots of certain *Lomatium* species were peeled, dried, and ground into flour.[4] The flour was then mixed with water, kneaded into pie-like crusts, and flattened into cakes.[4] The Blackfoot prepared large loaves of lomatium flour (2 by 1 feet); a hole was carved in the center to fasten the loaves onto a pack for long journeys.[4] The seeds were consumed raw, roasted, or dried, and prepared as flour; the common name "biscuit root" stems from these uses. Lomatium seeds were also used to flavor stews, soups, teas, and smoking mixtures.[4]

In Canada, Ditidaht, Coast Salish, and Kwakwaka'wakw regarded lomatium as an important medicine.[3] The Saanich, Songish, and Cowichan consumed the seeds to treat sore throats, colds, and tuberculosis.[3] The Salish consumed lomatium leaves raw, or as a pot herb.[3] The leaves were consumed as a fresh spring vegetable.[3] The

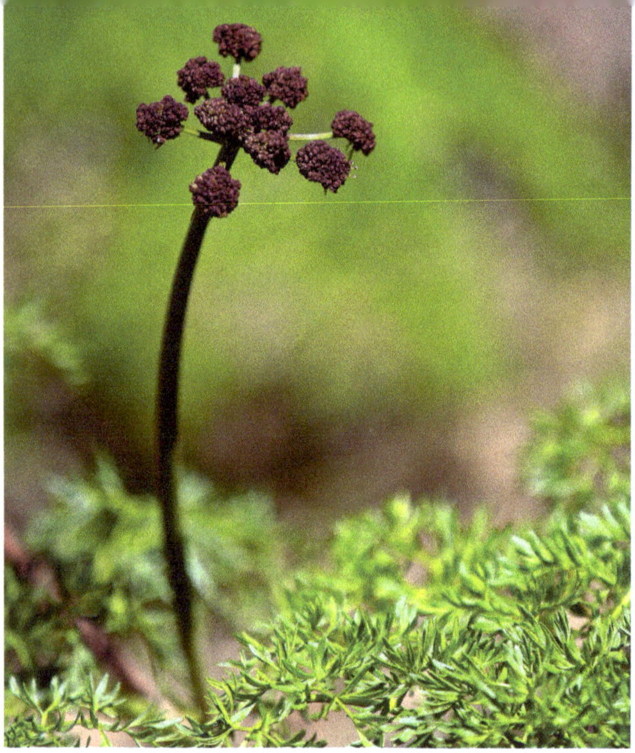

seeds are an important flavoring for stews, soups, teas, and tobacco.[3] The seeds were also consumed to alleviate a cold, sore throat, or tuberculosis.[3]

The root wash was applied to heal severed umbilical cords.[4,6] A wash was applied to treat slowly healing wounds, as well as sores, burns, bruises, sprains, cuts, broken bones, sore muscles, and rheumatic complaints.[6] A root poultice was applied topically to treat sprains, strains, and rheumatism.[4,6]

Lomatium smoke fumes were blown into the nostrils of distempered horses after they ran vigorously.[4] A piece of root was strung on a mare's neck, based on the belief that an exceptionally strong foal would be born in the spring.[4]

CONSTITUENTS: Lomatium contains volatile and fixed oils, resins, resinoids, gums, tetronic acids, (+)-falcarindiol, coniferyl ferulate, ferulic acid, (Z)-ligustilide, a flavonoid (luteolin), an alkaloid, coumarin glycosides (columbianin, luvangetin, and apiose), and one furanocoumarin.[5,7,8]

NUTRITIONAL PROPERTIES: The leaves are rich in vitamin C.[3] Some *Lomatium* species have roots rich in carbohydrates.

MEDICINAL PROPERTIES: Antibacterial, antiviral, diaphoretic, expectorant, and immune stimulant.

TEMPERATURE AND FLAVOR: Warm, acrid, bitter, and sweet.

MEDICINAL USES

Lomatium root is an immune stimulant, and an effective adjunct for treating respiratory infections, such as a cold, flu, bronchitis, or pneumonia.[6,7] It contains coumarin-based glycosides and furan-based acids that stimulate white blood cells and increase phagocytosis.[7] Lomatium also contains aromatic oleoresins that are excreted unchanged in the bronchial mucosa, enhancing expectoration and inhibiting bronchial microbe growth.[7] These resins limit viral replication, shorten the duration of viral infections, and prevent the spread of infections through respiratory mucosa.[7] The tetronic acids and a glucoside of luteolin are also attributed to the potential antiviral effects.[9] For best results in treating respiratory infections, combine small quantities of lomatium with other aromatic expectorant and antimicrobial herbs, such as oshá *(Ligusticum)*, aralia *(Aralia)*, gumweed *(Grindelia)*, usnea *(Usnea)*, and/or licorice *(Glycyrrhiza)*. In order to reduce its potential to cause a rash, when treating acute respiratory conditions, compound it with these herbs that improve elimination via diaphoresis: oshá *(Ligusticum)*, lovage *(Levisticum)*, or ginger *(Zingiber)*.

Lomatium demonstrated antibacterial effects *in vitro* against the gram-positive bacteria *Staphylococcus aureus* and *Bacillus subtilis*.[8] These actions were attributed to (+)-falcarindiol, coniferyl ferulate, ferulic acid, and (Z)-ligustilide.[8] Lomatium aids in treating sinus infections, strep throat, staph infections, and mouth sores.[7] When treating sinus infections, combine it with yerba mansa *(Anemopsis)*, yerba santa *(Eriodictyon)*, bayberry *(Morella)*, and/or usnea *(Usnea)*. When treating a sore throat, combine lomatium with propolis resin, elder berry *(Sambucus)*, echinacea *(Echinacea)*, and licorice *(Glycyrrhiza)*; add usnea *(Usnea)* for strep throat.

Although further clinical studies are necessary, lomatium could be a beneficial adjunct for HIV patients taking nucleoside reverse transcriptase inhibitors (NRTIs). Lomatium fruit contains suksdorfin that was found to inhibit HIV-1 replication in T cells.[10] Suksdorfin had HIV suppressive effects in peripheral blood mononucleocytes, monocyte/macrophages, and promonocytes.[10] It also synergized the effects of anti-HIV nucleosides (ddI and ddC) inhibiting HIV-1 replication (not viral inhibition); however, it was not synergistic with AZT (Azidothymidine).[10] *In vitro* studies demonstrated that lomatium root extract completely inhibited rotavirus' cytopathic effects, but no antiviral effects were demonstrated in six other viruses tested.[11]

Lomatium is a topical antimicrobial agent. Herbalist Michael Moore states that irrigating the vaginal canal with a cold infusion of lomatium warmed to body temperature aids in treating vaginal infections, such as *Candida albicans* and *Gardnerella vaginitis* (bacterial vaginosis).[7]

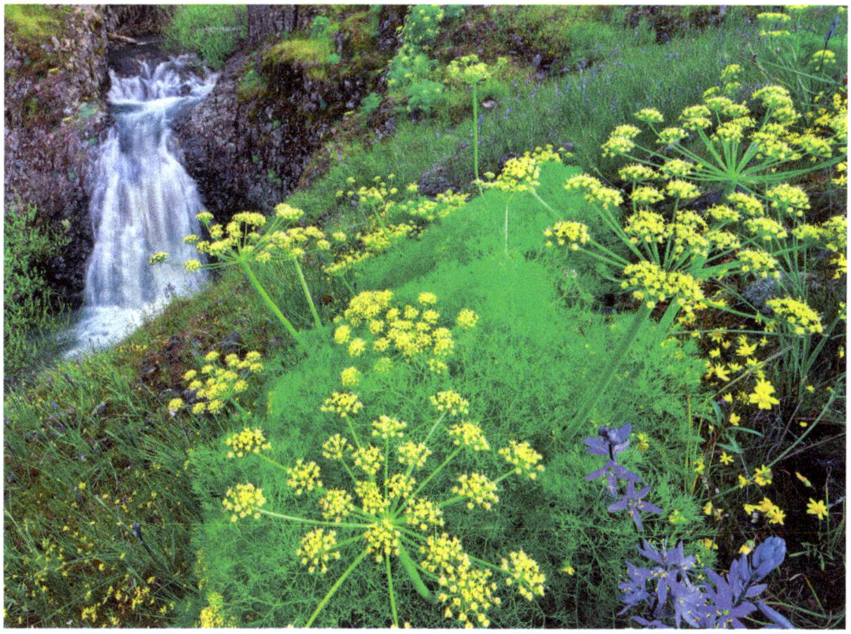

The diluted extract or root-infused oil can be applied as a first aid antimicrobial.[7] Lomatium is an emollient, moisturizing the skin.[7] *Note:* Lomatium contains photosensitizing coumarins that may increase sun sensitivity when used topically or internally. Some individuals are highly sensitive to the oleoresins that can cause a rash. Make sure to test lomatium on a small area of skin and wait 48 hours before applying it to a larger area. Avoid topical use on infants, young children, and individuals with sensitive skin.

CONTRAINDICATIONS

Internal or topical applications can cause a skin rash or hives in some individuals.[6,7] The rash may be caused by resins or coumarins.[9] Discontinue use if this occurs. Herbalist Michael Moore postulates that the rash may result from "a short-term nitrogenous waste product overload from immunologic stimulation, cytokine excess, or the waste products of viral die-off."[7] He recommends countering this effect by supporting systems that enhance waste product metabolism and excretion.[7] For long-term use, combine lomatium with other herbs that hasten liver and kidney elimination and detoxification, such as burdock root *(Arctium)* and dandelion root *(Taraxacum)*.

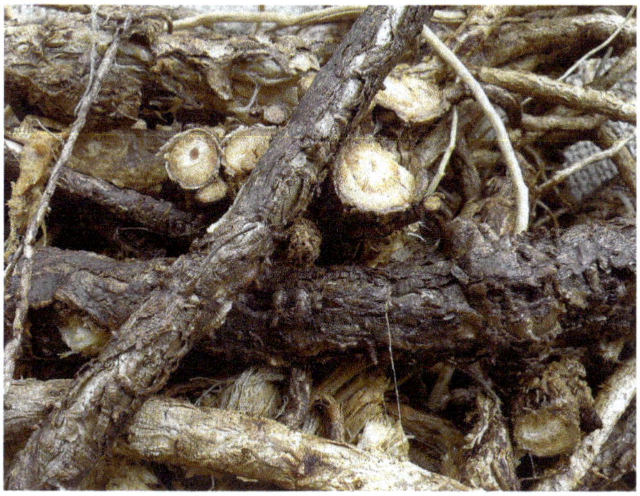

Until lomatium is more thoroughly investigated, avoid use during pregnancy and lactation. Compounds containing lomatium can be administered in low doses (5 – 10 drops) to children five years of age and older. Discontinue use if a rash occurs. The furanocoumarins can cause phototoxicity.

PREPARATION AND DOSAGE

TINCTURE: Fresh roots [1:2, 80 - 95% alcohol]; dry roots [1:5, 70% alcohol]; consume 10 - 30 drops, up to four times daily.

CAPSULES: Consume 2 - 4 capsules, one to three times daily.

TEA: Prepare a cold infusion or decoction; consume 4 - 8 ounces, up to four times daily. Prepare the leaves as a hot infusion.

HONEY AND SYRUP: Fresh root honey [1:4]; consume 1 teaspoon, up to four times daily.

TOPICAL USE: Cook freshly chopped, wilted roots in oil (allow them to wilt a few days before adding the oil). Prepare the oil using the double boiler method.

CULINARY USE: The young leaves are edible, with a celery-like taste; the fresh, spring leaves are more tender than mature summer leaves.[4] The leaves can be consumed in small quantities or cooked in soups.

MARJORAM

DESCRIPTION

BOTANICAL NAMES:
Origanum majorana (syn. *Majorana hortensis*)

COMMON NAMES:
Marjoram, knotted marjoram, sweet marjoram
khezama, mardaqoush, mardaqush, marzanjush (Arabic)
marjolaine (French)
majoran, wurstkraut, maigram, mairan (German)
matzourana (Greek)
mayoran (Hebrew)
maggiorana, persa (Italian)
amaracum (Latin)
mairūnas (Lithuanian)
merian (Norwegian)
măghiran (Romanian)
mažuran (Serbo-Croatian)[1]

FAMILY NAME:
Lamiaceae (Labiatae)

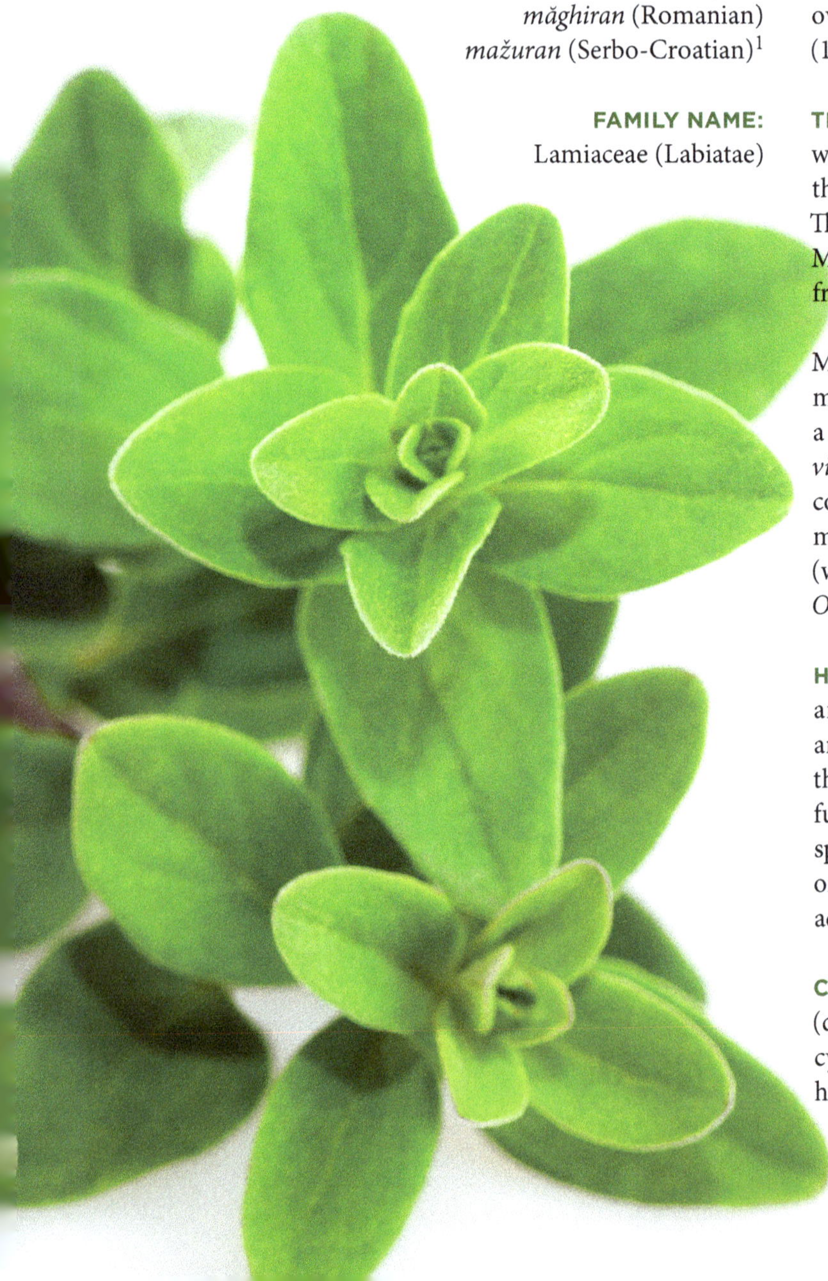

PART USED: The leaves.

BOTANICAL DESCRIPTION AND HABITAT: Marjoram is native to Cyprus. It has naturalized in southern Europe, and is cultivated in the U.S., Egypt, France, Greece, and Hungary.[2] Growing up to 80 cm tall, marjoram is a perennial herb with stems that become woody with age.[3] The opposite, gray-green, oblong, pubescent leaves (25 mm wide and long) have a spicy, sweet aroma.[3] Blooming in the summertime, the flowers are held in dense, rounded spikes interspersed with small, hairy, green bracts. The flowers consist of hairy, tubular calyces (2 mm long) that contain a tiny, white, bilabiate corolla (3 – 7 mm long), four stamens, a single style with a two-lobed stigma, and an ovary of two carpels.[3] The ovary produces four nutlets (1 mm wide and long).[3]

THE NAME: The genus *Origanum* derives from two Greek words: *oros* ("mountain") and *ganos* ("joy"), referring to the native mountainous habitat where the plant thrives.[4] The epithet *majorana* means "greater, larger, or bigger."[5] Marjoram was formerly called amaracum in Latin, derived from the Greek *amarakos* ("a fragrant flower").[1]

Marjoram is sometimes confused with hardy sweet marjoram or Italian oregano *(Origanum × majoricum),* a hybrid between *O. majorana* and *O. vulgare* subsp. *virens.*[2] The following Latin binomials correspond with the common names: *O. majorana* (sweet marjoram or knotted marjoram), *O. onites* (pot marjoram), *O. heracleoticum* (winter marjoram), dittany of Crete *(O. dictamnus),* and *O. sipyleum* (hop plants).[4,6]

HISTORICAL USES: Sweet marjoram sachets, powders, and washing water were used to enhance the body's aroma.[4] The herb was strewn in chambers to improve the scent of living quarters, and was used to scour wood furniture. Marjoram infusions were consumed to relieve spasms, colic, dyspepsia, and whooping cough.[4] A poultice or essential oil was applied to reduce the pain of a toothache, sprain, or bruise.[4]

CONSTITUENTS: Sweet marjoram contains a volatile oil (α-terpinene, γ-terpinene, terpinen-4-ol, α-terpineol, *p*-cymene, sabinene, linalool, borneol, carvacrol, *cis*-sabinene hydrate, *trans*-sabinene hydrate, linalyl acetate, ocimene, cadinene, geranyl acetate, citral, estragole, eugenol, and 3-carene). It also contains flavonoid glycosides (luteolin-7-diglucoside, apigenin-7-glucoside, and diosmetin-7-glucoronide), arbutin, methylarbutin, Lamiaceae tannins (rosmarinic acid, labiatic acid, and other caffeic acid derivatives), bitter principles, triterpenes (oleanolic acid and ursolic acid), β-sitosterol, paraffins (η-triacontane), protein, vitamins, and minerals.[6-8] *Cis*-sabinene hydrate creates the characteristic aroma of sweet marjoram.[6,7]

Pot marjoram *(O. onites)* contains volatile oil consisting of carvacrol, thymol, borneol, *p*-cymene, γ-terpinene, β-phellandrene, *trans*-thujanol, *cis*-thujanol, linalool, linalyl acetate, and α-muurolene.[7]

NUTRITIONAL PROPERTIES: Marjoram contains protein, vitamins A and C, calcium, phosphorus, iron, magnesium, and trace amounts of manganese.[6]

MEDICINAL PROPERTIES: Antibacterial, antifungal, antioxidant, antispasmodic, antitussive, antiviral, aromatic, carminative, diaphoretic, diuretic, and counterirritant.

TEMPERATURE AND FLAVOR: Warm, pungent, and sweet.

MEDICINAL USES

Marjoram has antimicrobial properties similar to oregano; however, it is gentler, and less pungent and heating. Its antibacterial properties aid in treating laryngitis, strep throat, bronchitis, and staph infections.[8,9] Marjoram is a subtle antifungal agent, reducing *Candida albicans* overgrowth in the digestive and vaginal tracts.[9] It has antiviral actions that aid in treating herpes simplex, as well as a cold or stomach flu.[7,8] Consume hot marjoram, thyme, and oregano tea, or infuse the herbs in chicken broth as a diaphoretic.[7] Marjoram contains less rosmarinic acid and carvacrol than thyme or oregano; nevertheless, these constituents are attributed to the antifungal, antibacterial, and antiviral properties.[7,8] The terpene alcohol (terpinene-4-ol) also contributes to the antibacterial and antifungal effects.[9]

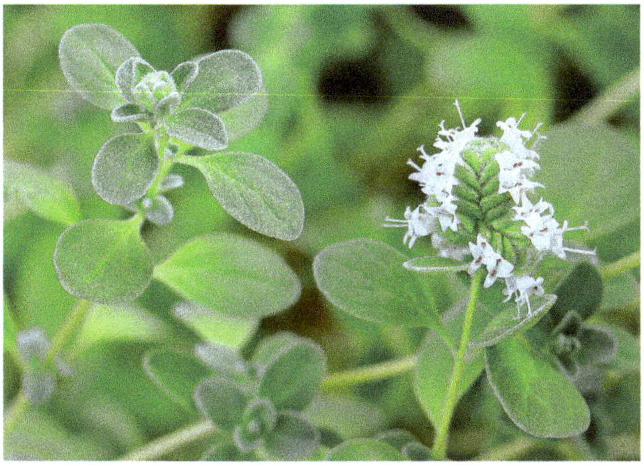

Marjoram is an aromatic carminative and stomachic.[2,7,8] It aids in treating sluggish digestion, nonulcer dyspepsia, flatulence, colic, and diarrhea.[2,8] Marjoram has antispasmodic properties that affect smooth muscles. A hot poultice, fomentation, or diluted essential oil can be applied over the belly or womb as an antispasmodic for digestive or menstrual cramps.[4,9]

Marjoram has a unique pungent, sweet, woody aroma. It enhances the flavor and facilitates digestion of meat, poultry, fish, eggs, beans, sauces, tomato dishes, vegetable dishes, salads, and vinaigrettes. It combines well with tarragon, basil, or oregano.

Marjoram is an antioxidant.[2] It can be combined with other Mediterranean herbs to cure and preserve meat.[4,11] The antioxidant effects are attributed to the labiatic acid and flavonoids.[7]

Marjoram has subtle nervous system calming effects.[8] It is used to treat nervous headaches and exhaustion.[8]

MARJORAM ESSENTIAL OIL (ORIGANUM MAJORANA)

Marjoram oil contains terpene alcohol (terpinene-4-ol) which has antiseptic properties. It also contains terpene esters with spasmolytic and calming properties.[9] It is a potent antibacterial and antifungal agent. Aromatherapist Kurt Schnaubelt considers marjoram gentle enough for older children.[10]

Marjoram oil alleviates menstrual cramps, stomach cramps, a dry cough, and muscle spasms.[9,11] Add several drops of essential oil to a base oil or salve, and apply to the affected area; cover with a hot cloth, heating pad, or hot water bottle. Consume one drop of essential oil in one teaspoon of syrup, inhale the oil, or apply a marjoram-based chest rub as an antitussive, expectorant and antimicrobial for a dry cough, bronchitis, whooping cough, laryngitis, cold, or flu.[9,11] Marjoram has a calming effect on the nervous system, easing stress, anxiety, nervous tension, and premenstrual irritability.[9-11] Marjoram oil has antiviral properties that aid in treating herpes simplex.[2]

Marjoram essential oil helps to ease toothache pain.[2] Apply neat or diluted oil to the gums surrounding the tooth pain. Marjoram oil can be applied (neat or diluted) topically to reduce pain and spasms. It is an effective adjunct for treating bruises, sprains, strains, sore muscles, and rheumatic and arthritic joints.[2,4,11]

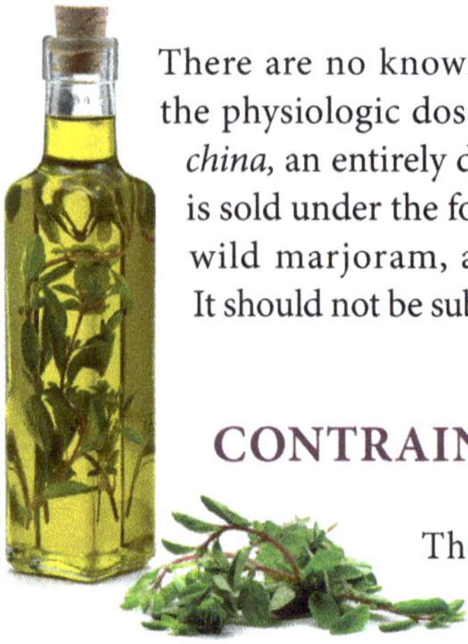

There are no known contraindications with the physiologic dosage.[9] *Note: Thymus mastichina,* an entirely different genus and species, is sold under the following names: marjoram, wild marjoram, and Spanish marjoram.[9] It should not be substituted for true marjoram.

CONTRAINDICATIONS

There are no reported side effects or contraindications when used in the recommended doses.[8] According to herbalist Gazmend Skenderi, marjoram should not be applied externally on babies or young children due to the hydroquinone content.[8] Although it is rare, fresh sweet marjoram can cause skin or eye irritation.[7]

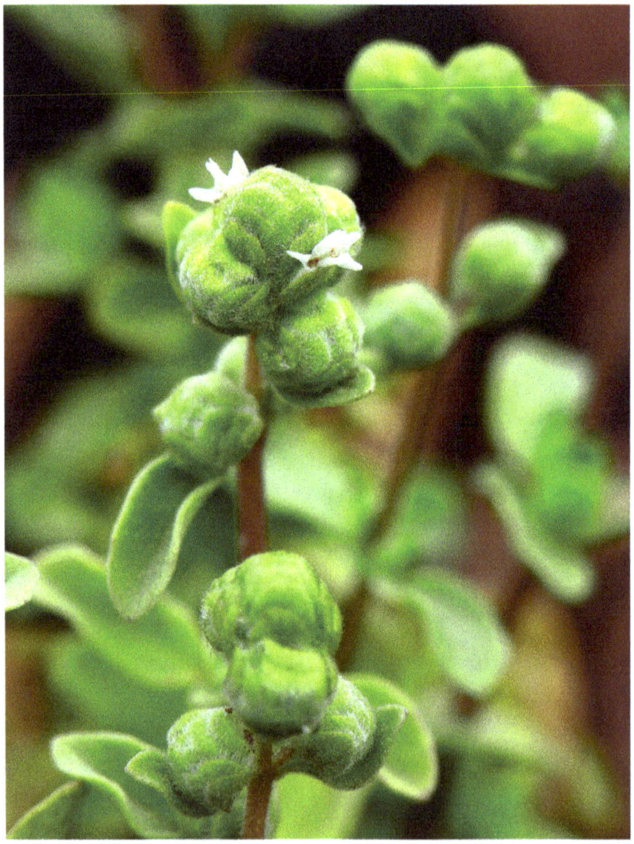

PREPARATION AND DOSAGE

TINCTURE: Fresh leaves [1:2-1:3, 70-95% alcohol]; dry leaves [1:5-1:7, 60% alcohol]; consume 15-60 drops, three to four times daily.

ACETUM EXTRACT: Fresh or wilted leaves [1:2-1:3, apple cider vinegar]; consume in food preparations such as vinaigrettes.

CAPSULES: Consume 1-2 capsules of enteric coated marjoram oil capsules, one to three times daily. Add 1-3 drops of marjoram essential oil to a charcoal tablet, or a capsule containing a binding agent; consume 1-2 capsules, one to three times daily.

TEA: Prepare a hot infusion; consume 8-12 ounces, one to three times daily.

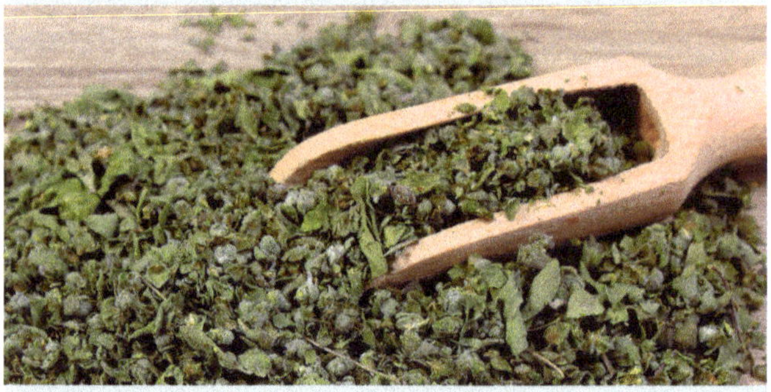

HONEY AND SYRUP: Simple syrup can be prepared in two ways: dissolve one part by volume of sugar into one part of a strained marjoram infusion, or infuse marjoram directly into prepared simple syrup. Add 1-2 drops of marjoram essential oil to 1 teaspoon of simple syrup or honey, then mix with a toothpick. Add the honey to one cup of tea or hot water; consume up to four times daily.

TOPICAL USE: Apply the poultice or fomentation. Prepare culinary oil by wilting the fresh herb, then chopping and infusing it in olive oil. Prepare medicinal oil using the infused oil or alcohol intermediary method. Dilute the essential oil in cream, oil, salve, or liniment.

CULINARY USE: Freshly chopped or ground dried marjoram is a seasoning for meat, poultry, soups, sauces, potatoes, bean, tomato, and root vegetable dishes, vinaigrettes, and salads.

MARSHMALLOW

DESCRIPTION

BOTANICAL NAMES:
Althaea officinalis, Althaea rosea (syn. *Alcea rosea*), *Malva neglecta, M. rotundifolia, M. sylvestris, M. parviflora,* and other *Malva* species

COMMON NAMES:
Althaea officinalis:
Marshmallow, marsh mallow, sweet weed, mortification root, cheese plant, wymote, mallards, mauls, schloss tea
racine de guimauve, guimauve (French)
eibischwurzel, eibisch, radix Althaea (German)

Althaea rosea (syn. *Alcea rosea*):
Hollyhock

Malva spp.:
mallow, dwarf mallow, low mallow, little mallow, malva, cheese plant
groot kaasjeskruid (Dutch)
grande mauve, mauve sylvestre, mauve des bois (French)
kultur-käsepappel (German)
apotekerkattost (Norwegian)
malva común, malva silvestre (Spanish)
rödmalva (Swedish)
büyük ebegümeci (Turkish)

FAMILY NAME:
Malvaceae

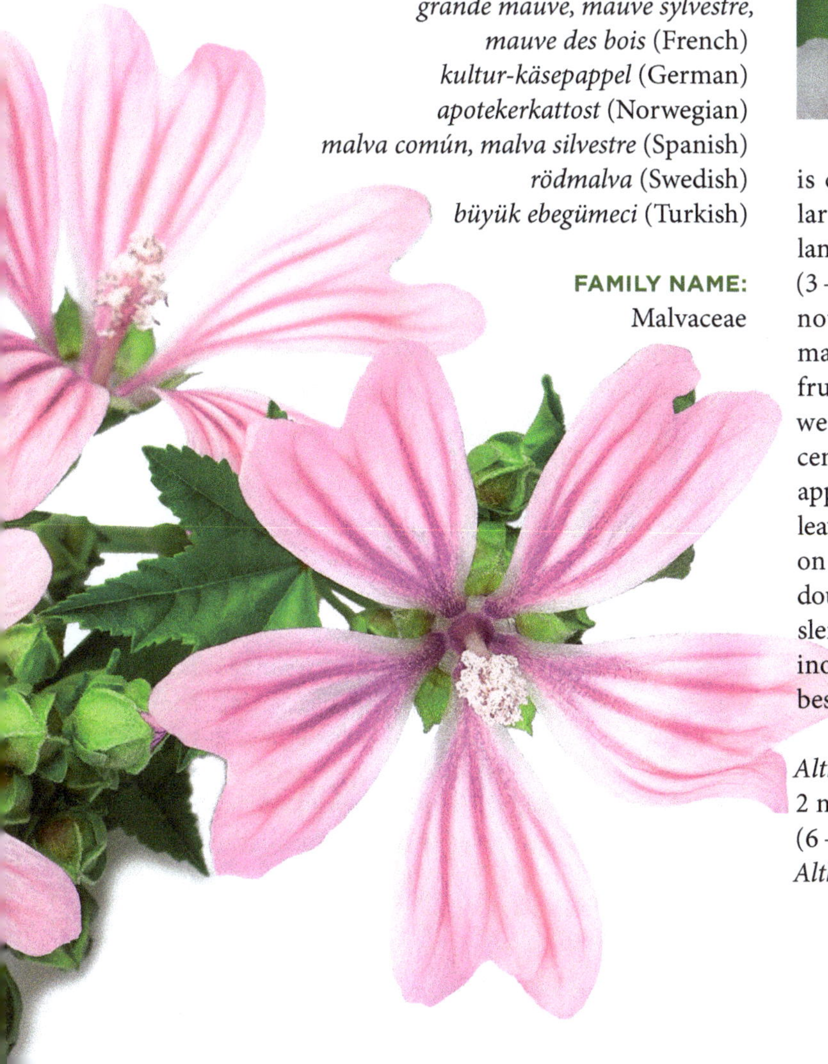

PARTS USED: The roots are the most potent medicinally; the leaves, flowers, and whole plant have milder properties, and can be used interchangeably.

BOTANICAL DESCRIPTION AND HABITAT: Marshmallow *(Althaea officinalis)* is a shrub-like perennial growing up to two meters tall.[1] Indigenous to Europe, it grows wild in moist meadows, bogs, salt marshes, and on riverbanks. Marshmallow thrives in rich and well-drained soil, and

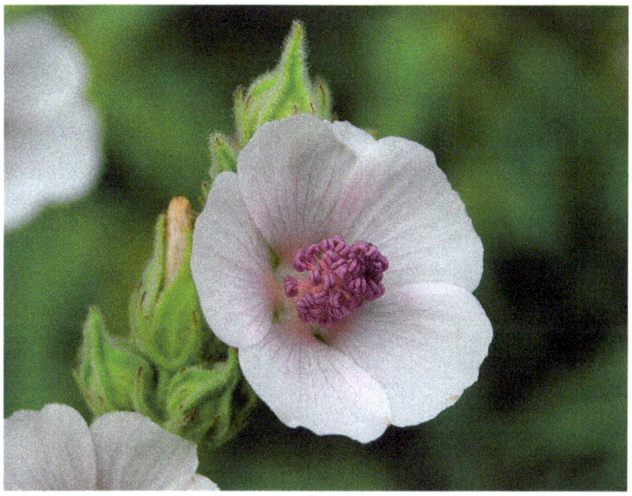

is cultivated in the U.S. and Europe. The showy, axillary flower has a fused calyx (6 – 10 mm long) with five lanceolate lobes, subtended by 8 – 12 short epicalyx lobes (3 – 5 mm long).[1] The light pink corolla consists of five notched petals (1 – 2 cm long).[1] The perianth contains many stamens arranged in a tube around the ovary. The fruit is a disk-shaped schizocarp that breaks into many wedge-shaped pieces. The plant has numerous pubescent stems that branch from the base, with a more woody appearance in early fall. The palmately-lobed, light green leaves (3 – 5 cm long by 2 – 4 cm wide) are finely tomentose on both sides, and have a rounded triangular shape with doubly-serrated margins.[1] Marshmallow has whitish-beige, slender, tapering roots that have a sweet-tasting, mucilaginous quality when chewed or macerated. The roots are best harvested in the fall or early winter of the third year.

Althaea rosea, a biennial with rough, hairy stems (up to 2 meters tall), has rounded, palmately-lobed, hairy leaves (6 – 16 cm in diameter) with doubly serrate margins.[2] *Althaea rosea* is often grown for its large, beautiful flowers

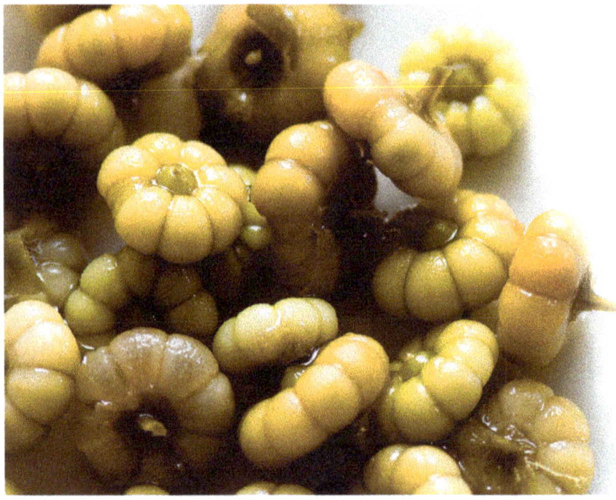

on long, terminal spike-like inflorescences. The flowers have a densely hairy, cup-like epicalyx with six or seven lobes enclosing a hairy, bell-shaped calyx (2 – 3 cm diameter) with five lobes.[2] The notched, triangular petals grow in shades of red, purple, pink, yellow, or white, with the entire corolla reaching up to 10 cm in diameter.[2] Similar to *Althaea officinalis,* the many stamens form a tube around the ovary that produces a pubescent, disk-shaped schizocarp.[2]

A genus of common tap-rooted weeds, mallows *(Malva* spp.*)* grow from sea level to 7,000-foot altitudes throughout the U.S. However, they are most prominent in the western states and can be found in vacant lots and gardens, along roadsides, and in disturbed soil. *Malva* species are often hairy, with erect or prostrate stems bearing stipulate, round to kidney-shaped, palmately-lobed leaves with serrate margins.[3] The beige taproots emit mucilage when crushed. The inflorescences are racemes with showy flowers that have five-lobed, tubular calyces subtended by three linear bractlets, and five pink, purple, or white petals with notched tips.[4] Within the perianth are five or more stamens forming a tube, five staminodes, and up to 15 pistils with linear stigma.[3,4] Like the other species described in this monograph, the fruit, a schizocarp, is shaped like a wheel of cheese, and breaks into 6 – 15 pieces.[3]

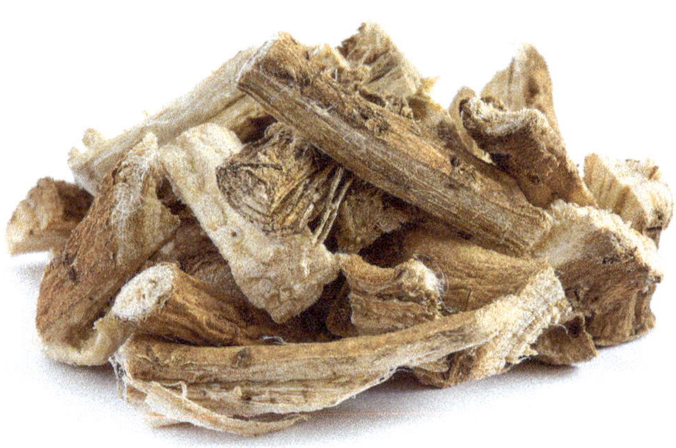

Malva sylvestris is native to Europe and central Russia, but has naturalized in North America, eastern Australia, and Mexico. The pinkish-purple flowers of *M. sylvestris* are large, with inversely cordate petals displaying prominent burgundy to purple veins. The many stamens are fused at the base. *M. neglecta* is also native to Europe, and has become endemic in the U.S. It has smaller, pinkish-white or lavender cup-shaped flowers.

THE NAME: *Althaea* derives from the Greek *altho* ("to cure"). The epithet *officinalis* derives from the Latin "official," referring to the plant's medicinal use.[5] The epithet *rosea* ("red") derives from Latin, and refers to the flower's color. The family name Malvaceae and genus *Malva* derive from the Greek *malake* ("soft"). The origin of the epithet *neglecta* ("overlooked, disregarded, and neglected") is Latin. The Latin origins of the following epithets are: *parviflora* ("small-flowered"), *rotundifolia* ("round-leaved"), and *sylvestris* ("of the forest"). The common name marshmallow refers to the plant's salt marsh habitat. People from the British countryside coined the common name *mallowsky,* from which marshmallow and mallow derived. The common name "cheese plant" originates from the seed heads' resemblance to small wheels of cheese.

HISTORICAL USES: Ancient Greeks described the medicinal virtues of marshmallow as early as the 9th century BCE. Hippocrates, the renowned Greek physician (4th century BCE), prescribed marshmallow to treat wounds.[6] Early Greek physicians also recommended marshmallow infusions for toothaches, and to soothe insect bites. During Dioscorides' era (1st century CE), mallow was valued as a medicine and used to decorate graves.[7] The following quote from Pliny the Elder demonstrates his reverence for marshmallow: "Whosoever shall take a spoonful of the Mallows shall that day be free from all diseases that may come to him."[7] He also recommended preparing a drawing poultice from fresh leaves to remove thorns and prickles embedded in the flesh.[7] Arab physicians applied leaf poultices to inflamed skin.[6] Romans utilized the herb as a laxative, and prized the young cooked leaves as a delicacy.[6,7] Mallow was consumed as a nutritious food when crops failed and food was scarce.[6,7] During famines, poor Chinese, Egyptians, Greeks, Armenians, and Fellas subsisted on marshmallow and other herbs for weeks.[7] Regardless of famine, the tender leaves and shoots were considered delicacies and consumed as early spring greens. The leaves were often incorporated as a pot herb in soups and stews. The green, unripe seed capsules were known as "cheeses" and consumed as a salad topping.

The most common folkloric uses of marshmallow since the Middle Ages include: lung and chest ailments, coughs, upset stomach, ulcers, diarrhea, bladder infections, and insomnia. In addition, marshmallow tea was gargled to relieve mouth and gum infections. Poultices of fresh roots or leaves were applied as a first aid treatment.[6] Throughout Europe, mallow leaves *(Malva sylvestris)* and flowers were applied topically to reduce acute inflammatory skin conditions, such as eczema. The tea was gargled to relieve a sore throat.[13]

A confection was prepared with powdered marshmallow root, water, and sugar, and cooked to form a thick paste. This recipe was the origin of the spongy white confection roasted over campfires, known today as marshmallow.[6] In France, a soothing lozenge prepared from powdered marshmallow roots, *pâté de guimauve*, was used to treat sore throats and coughs.[8]

In Ayurvedic medicine, marshmallow root is used to tonify *vata* and reduce *pitta*. It is believed to increase *kapha*. It is considered a rejuvenator of the lungs and kidneys.[9]

Eclectic physicians administered marshmallow root for its soothing demulcent and emollient effects. Dr. Finley Ellingwood recommended consuming marshmallow tea to reduce pain and irritation in the urinary tract and bladder due to cystitis, ammoniacal urine, and bladder spasms, and to treat kidney stones resulting from uric acid crystals.[10] Dr. Harvey Felter suggested using marshmallow as a soothing drink for a sore throat, hoarseness, cough, gastrointestinal inflammation, renal inflammation accompanying cystitis, or gravel.[11] He recommended vaginal irrigation for acute vaginitis and gonorrhea, and an enema for dysentery.[11] He prescribed a compress for painful piles (hemorrhoids).[11]

Marshmallow has been used in beverages, desserts, candies, baked goods, gelatins, and puddings.[6] Marshmallow root has been used as a source of fiber for rope and coarse fabrics. The pulp also has been used to make bags and wrapping papers.[12]

Spanish New Mexicans believed that mallow was the remedy for "All the ills that men endure."[11] They consumed the tea to reduce fever and induce perspiration in sweat lodges. In New Mexico, mallow tea *(Malva neglecta)* was consumed to facilitate labor and wash infants. A leaf decoction strained and mixed with sugar was consumed to cleanse afterbirth. Using a more complicated method, 15 – 25 leaves were simmered for an hour with one-third cup of raisins in one cup of water. This brew was prepared at night and placed outside to collect dew, then consumed in the morning on the first, second, and third days after childbirth.[15] A wash was prepared from decoctions for a variety of skin diseases. A poultice containing mallow leaves, salt, and vinegar was applied to the temples to treat headaches. A powder of the dry leaves was blown into the throat to relieve swollen glands. Southwest Native American tribes observed that mallow was an indicator of materials for hard-pan and clay suitable for pottery making.[15] Young mallow shoots and leaves were consumed as a pot herb and a thickening agent in soups.[16] Herbalist Michael Moore mentions that range-fed chickens lay eggs with pink whites when eating mallow.[14]

CONSTITUENTS: Marshmallow root contains mucilaginous polysaccharides (L-rhamnose, D-galactose, D-galacturonic acid, D-glucuronic acid, L-arabinose, arabinose, glucose, and exulose), starch, sucrose, pectin, asparagine, choline, gossypin-3-sulfate, hypoletin-8-O-β-D-gluoside-3'-sulfate, malvinic acid, malvidin, malvin, octacosane, calcium phosphate, calcium oxalate, fixed oil, quercetin, kaempferol, and polyphenolic acids (chlorogenic acid, caffeic acid, and *p*-coumaric acid). The mucilage content of the root is 18 – 35%, and is reportedly highest in the fall.[6,12,14,17-20]

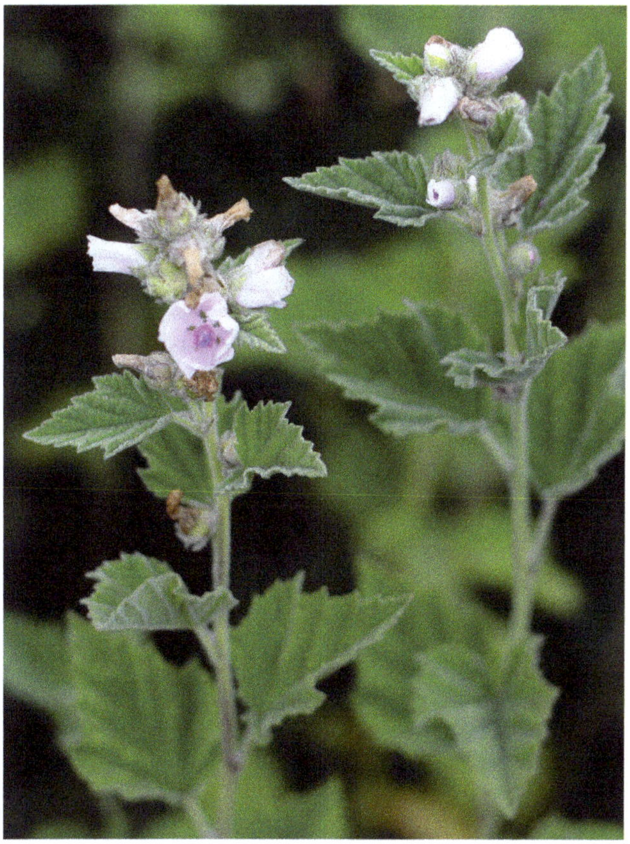

The leaves contain mucilaginous polysaccharides (up to 16%), kaempferol, quercetin, diosmetin glucosides, and polyphenolic acids (9-syringic, caffeic, salicylic, vanillic, and *p*-coumaric). The polysaccharides develop their mucilaginous content after the flowers develop. The flowers contain anthocyanins.[14,18-20]

Malva neglecta and *M. silvestre* contain mucilaginous polysaccharides (arabinose, L-arabinose, D-galactose, D-galacturonic acid, D-glucoronic acid, and 1-rhamnose), gossypin-3-sulfate, hypoletin-8-O-β-D-gluoside-3'-sulfate, malvinic acid, malvidin, malvin, octacosane, calcium, phosphorus (leaf), β-carotene (leaf), and choline.[14,21]

NUTRITIONAL PROPERTIES: Marshmallow leaf *(Althaea* spp.*)* contains calcium, phosphorus, β-carotene, and asparagine. Mallow leaf *(Malva* spp.*)* contains calcium, phosphorus, β-carotene, and choline.[14,21]

MEDICINAL PROPERTIES: Anti-inflammatory, antitussive, demulcent, diuretic, emollient, expectorant, immune modulating, laxative, nutritive, vulnerary, and mild antimicrobial properties.

TEMPERATURE AND FLAVOR: Cool, sweet, salty, and bland.

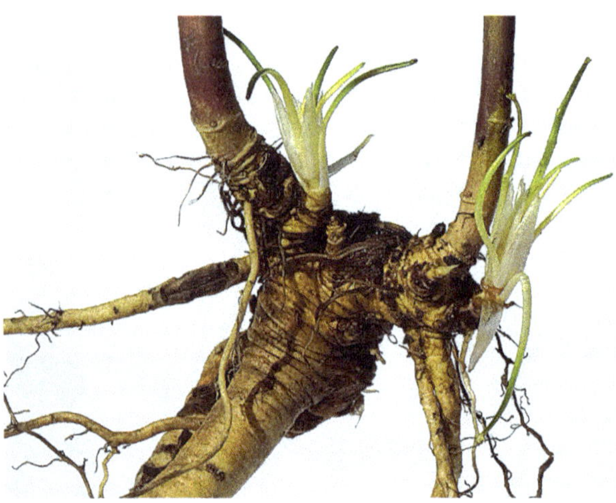

MEDICINAL USES

While *Althaea* (marshmallow) and *Malva* (mallow) species can be used interchangeably, marshmallow root contains the highest quantity of mucilaginous polysaccharides. The potency is highest in marshmallow root, followed by hollyhock and *Malva* root, then the leaves and flowers of marshmallow, hollyhock, and other *Malva* species. However, the name marshmallow refers to all of the related herbs throughout the *Medicinal Uses* section.

Marshmallow is an effective demulcent and emollient. It contains mucilaginous polysaccharides that reduce inflammation in the mucous membranes and skin. The polysaccharides stimulate leukocytes (white blood cells) that increase phagocytosis, enhance immune function, and have a mild immune modulating effect.[12,14,18] According to several sources, cold water extracts (cold infusions) are preferable for extracting mucilage, and hot water extracts more of the starch.[9,13] From a clinical perspective, hot decoctions and cold infusions are equally effective, and recommending that patients drink cold, slimy tea results in limited compliance. However, cold infusions can be heated (but not boiled), or hot water can be added in order to increase compliance. Marshmallow has antimicrobial activity against *Pseudomonas aeruginosa, Proteus vulgaris,* and *Staphylococcus aureus.*[20]

Marshmallow tea and syrup are very soothing for upper and lower respiratory tract infections, such as a sore throat, strep throat, laryngitis, pharyngitis, tracheitis, cold, or flu. A mouthwash or gargle reduces inflammation in the mouth or throat. The mucilage enhances expectoration, and has antitussive properties beneficial for treating dry coughs related to whooping cough or bronchitis. Decocting marshmallow root with anise *(Pimpinella anisum)* and licorice root *(Glycyrrhiza glabra)* soothes the upper and lower respiratory systems. Marshmallow can be substituted for slippery elm bark, which is threatened in the wild.

Marshmallow is helpful for treating inflammation and ulceration in the skin, mouth, esophagus, stomach, intestines, or colon. The tea reduces pain and unpleasant sensations resulting from a hiatal hernia, gastritis, gastric reflux, and acid indigestion, as well as peptic and duodenal ulcers. Marshmallow can be very helpful for reducing chronic inflammation caused by gastrointestinal conditions such as irritable bowel syndrome, Crohn's disease, and ulcerative colitis, as well as diarrhea and dysentery. It is best to consume marshmallow tea on an empty stomach when treating the aforementioned conditions. Regardless of whether the mucilage has direct or indirect soothing effects on the urinary and respiratory tracts, it is believed to suppress nerve reflexes in the alimentary canal walls, reducing pain in mucous membranes throughout the body.[22] A well strained, lukewarm decoction of marshmallow tea can be administered as an enema to reduce acute rectal or colon inflammation. An enema also encourages elimination, alleviating severe constipation and impacted bowels.

Marshmallow tea soothes kidney and bladder irritation. It contains asparagine that has mild diuretic actions.[22] Marshmallow tea reduces burning sensations and irritation accompanying cystitis and urethritis. When treating infections in the urinary tract or bladder, additional antibacterial agents are necessary, such as usnea *(Usnea)*, uva ursi *(Arctostaphylos uva-ursi)*, or manzanita *(Arctostaphylos* spp.*)*. Marshmallow tea reduces renal and bladder irritation due to passing kidney stones or kidney inflammation.

Marshmallow root is a cooling yin tonic. It increases yin fluids and reduces dryness throughout the body and mucous membranes. Marshmallow root can be used as a long-term treatment for yin deficiency or yin deficiency with heat signs (hot flashes, night sweats, etc.). It is a highly beneficial replenishing and nourishing recuperative tonic that can be consumed following a debilitating illness, severe fever, childbirth, or dehydration, as well as during or after radiation or chemotherapy treatments.

Marshmallow tea has gentle laxative properties and lubricates the stools. It is a preferred long-term tonic for treating constipation because it does not cause laxative dependency like many cathartic or purgative laxatives.

Topical applications of the root (such as a fomentation, poultice, wash, or bath) reduce inflammation, treating dry skin conditions such as poison oak, poison ivy, eczema, psoriasis, or dandruff. Poultices can be applied to burns, bedsores, and wounds. It is believed to have strong drawing properties, suppurating poisons and infections, promoting healing of abscesses and chronic sores, and reducing necrotic tissue. Marshmallow root compresses can be used to treat boils, abscesses, carbuncles, and furuncles, and to remove splinters. Marshmallow root applications also soothe diaper rash, abrasions, cradle cap, rashes, and other irritated skin conditions. Well strained decoctions of the root applied as a sitz bath help to soothe vaginal and rectal tissues. They also provide an effective eye wash for irritated conjunctiva. Dried leaves can be added as a bulking agent to herbal smoking mixtures.

CONTRAINDICATIONS

Excessive consumption of marshmallow can result in loose stools; decrease the dosage or discontinue use if this occurs. Some sources claim that marshmallow can slow or inhibit the absorption of some prescription drugs due to its mucilaginous properties. While this contraindication is mentioned in numerous sources, the author has never observed this in clinical practice, and has yet to find the original source of this claim. She has treated thousands of patients who consumed this herb while taking various medications, and has never observed a decrease in the effectiveness of medications, or changes in blood levels of medications.

PREPARATION AND DOSAGE

TINCTURE: Fresh roots [1:2, 60% alcohol]; dry roots [1:5, 30-50% alcohol] or [1:5, 30% alcohol]; the latter preparation extracts a higher mucilage content; consume 15-60 drops, up to four times daily.

GLYCERITE: Dry roots [1:5, 40% water, 30% glycerin, and 30% alcohol]; consume 15-60 drops, up to four times daily.

CAPSULES: Consume 2-4 "00" capsules, up to four times daily. The powder can be incorporated into capsules, lozenges, cough drops, or pills.

TEA: Consume 8-12 ounces of the root decoction, cold infusion, or infusion of leaves or flowers, three to four times daily.

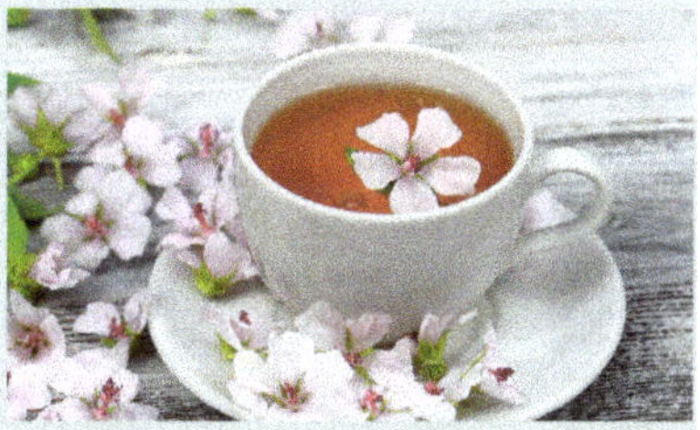

HONEY AND SYRUP: Prepare fresh root honey [1:4, root volume to honey volume]; consume 1 teaspoon, up to five times daily. Prepare syrup by simmering a root decoction [1:4, volume to volume] to half the volume; add honey to desired sweetness; consume 1 teaspoon, up to five times daily. Refrigerate this preparation. Add 20% alcohol to the total volume of syrup to increase shelf life.

TOPICAL USE: A wash, fomentation, poultice, cream, or medicinal oil can be used topically to soothe the skin.

CULINARY USE: Young marshmallow shoots, leaves, flowers, or roots can be added to soups, sauces, or gravies for nutritional value, and as a thickening agent. The young leaves can be steamed, sautéed, or added sparingly to salads. The fresh flowers decorate confections and salads. Fresh, young roots can be sliced and sautéed with onions and garlic.

MEADOWSWEET

DESCRIPTION

BOTANICAL NAMES:
Filipendula ulmaria (syn. *Spiraea ulmaria*), *Spiraea lucidum* (syn. *Spiraea altaica*), *Spiraea* spp.

COMMON NAMES:
Meadowsweet, queen of the meadow, lady of the meadow, bridewort, meadow queen, spirea, pride of the meadow, medwort, meadwort, honey-wine herb, dropwort, dulloff, goat's beard
herbe aux abeilles, reine des près, spiraea, ulmaire, vignette (French)
geissleitern, moorspierstuade, wiesenkonigin, echtes mädesüss (German)
filipendula, olmaria, regina dei prati, pie di becco (Italian)
barbe de carbra, ulmaria (Spanish)[1]

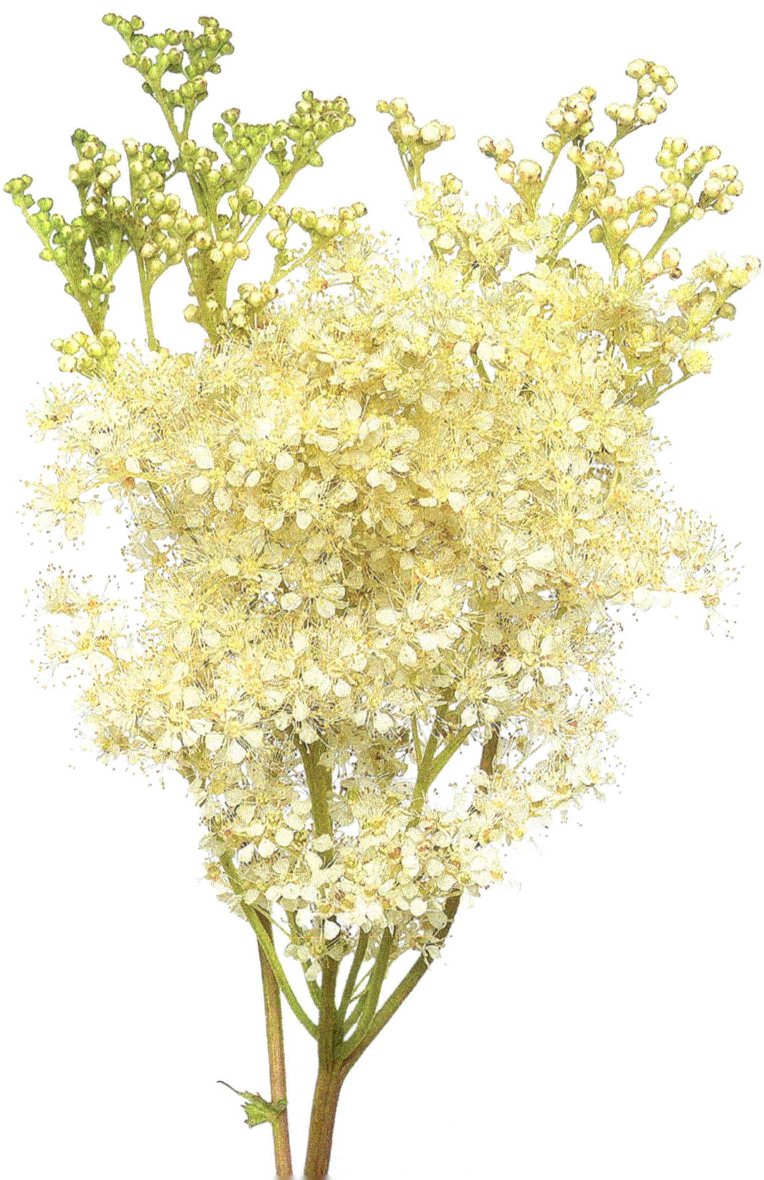

PARTS USED: The leaves and flowers.

BOTANICAL DESCRIPTION AND HABITAT: *Filipendula ulmaria* is a rhizomatous perennial herb commonly found in moist, boggy meadows, and on the edges of river banks and ponds in China, Mongolia, Russia, Central Asia, Southwest Asia, and Europe.[2] Species of *Spiraea* can be found in wooded areas, such as pine and aspen forests at

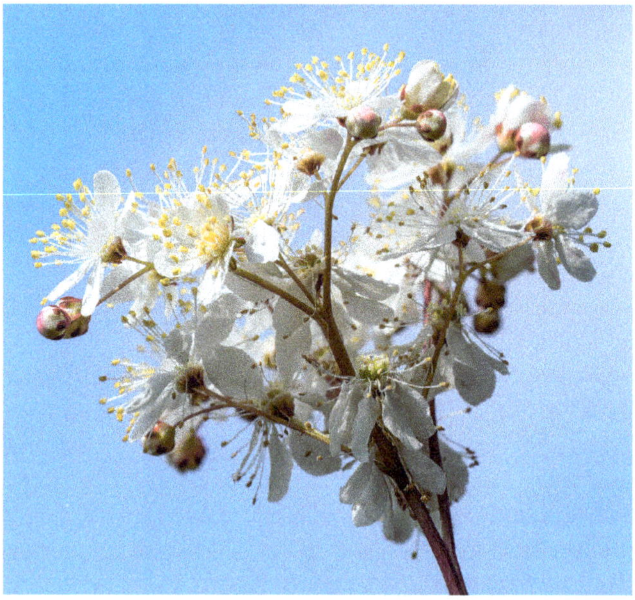

moderate to high elevations. Various *Spiraea* species grow throughout North America and Europe. Flanked by green, semicordate, leaf-like stipules, the pinnate leaves have two to five pairs of rough, wrinkled leaflets with acuminate apices and doubly-serrate margins. The terminal leaflet has three to five oblong-lanceolate lobes.[2] Underneath, the leaflets are densely covered in white hairs, while their upper sides are glabrous.[2] The terminal panicle-like inflorescence is showy with many tiny white flowers (about 5 mm diameter). These flowers have five ovate sepals with pubescent undersides, five overlapping, obovate petals, 20 to 40 stamens, and five to 15 separate carpels.[2,3] The fruit is an achene.[3]

THE NAME: The plant was called *Filipendula* in Holland, and *Spiraea* throughout the rest of Europe. *Filipendula* derives from *filum* ("thread") and *pendulus* ("hanging"). The genus name *Spiraea* derives from the Greek *speiraia* ("a coil").[5] Theophrastus used this name because the plant

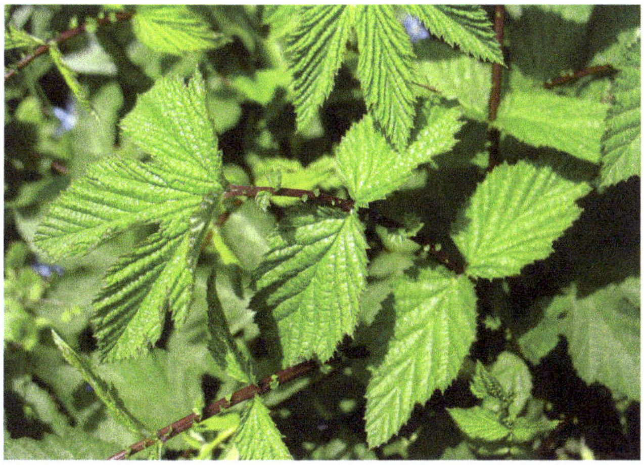

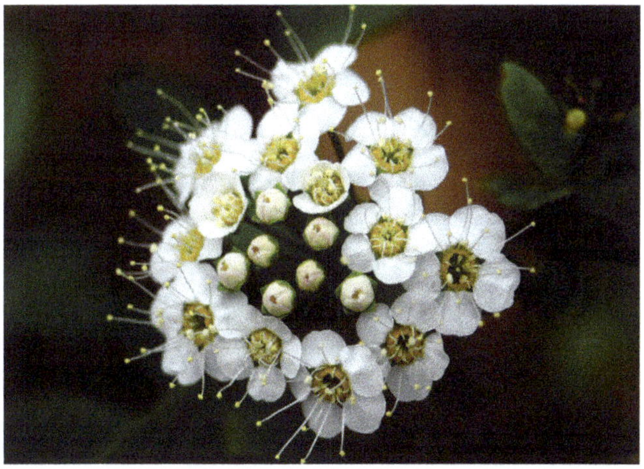

was incorporated into garlands.[5] The word aspirin derived from the genus name *Spiraea,* based on the plant's salicylate content that was isolated and used to make aspirin. The species name *ulmaria* was given to the plant because the leaves resembled wrinkled elm leaves *(Ulmus).*

Because the flowers were often ingredients in wine or beer, the plant acquired the names medwort, meadwort, or honey-wine herb. It acquired the common name "bridewort" because it was made into bridal garlands and strewn at weddings and festivals. The name "queen of the meadow" refers to its growth in moist meadows.[1]

HISTORICAL USES: The Druids considered meadowsweet one of three most sacred herbs, in addition to verbena and water mint. Meadowsweet was an ingredient in a drink called "save" in Chaucer's *The Knights Tale.* Queen Elizabeth I favored this herb above all others in her chambers.[1] Meadowsweet was administered to treat diarrhea, stomach disorders, and gastric ulcers.[4]

Blackfoot Native Americans prepared a tea of the root, and administered it as an enema or applied it topically.[5] *Spiraea* was also used by indigenous people to treat venereal disease; they consumed three cups of the tea daily, and also used it for vaginal irrigation.[5] A decoction of the roots was used to treat diarrhea.[5]

CONSTITUENTS: Meadowsweet contains phenolic glycosides (monotropitin, gaultherin, and spiraein; aglycones salicylic aldehydes and methyl-salicylate), spiroaic acid (salicylic acid), volatile oil (salicylic aldehyde = salicylaldehyde, phenylethyl alcohol, benzyl alcohol, and others), small amounts of spiraeoside, isosalicin, heliotropin, tannins (gallotannins, ellagitannins, and rugosin-D), mucilage, flavonoids (flavonols: quercetin and kaempferol glycosides), vitamin C, and sugar.[5-7]

NUTRITIONAL PROPERTIES: Meadowsweet contains flavonoids (flavonols: rutin, quercetin, and kaempferol glycosides), vitamin C, and sugar.[7]

MEDICINAL PROPERTIES: Anti-inflammatory, astringent, demulcent, diaphoretic, diuretic, and stomachic.

TEMPERATURE AND FLAVOR: Cool, astringent, bitter, and sweet.

MEDICINAL USES

Meadowsweet soothes and heals the digestive tract lining. The leaves and flowers contain small quantities of mucilage and large quantities of tannins; both are beneficial for reducing inflammation in the digestive tract. The mucilage coats and soothes mucous membranes lining the digestive tract. The astringency also reduces diarrhea, although additional anti-infective agents are necessary.[5,7] Meadowsweet tea can be consumed as a long-term mucous membrane anti-inflammatory treatment for individuals with irritable bowel syndrome, Crohn's disease, or colitis. A water-based preparation (infusion) is the best means of reducing mucous membrane inflammation. Prepare a soothing digestive tea by combining equal parts of mint *(Mentha),* chamomile *(Matricaria),* marshmallow root *(Althaea),* and fennel *(Foeniculum)* with smaller portions of meadowsweet and licorice *(Glycyrrhiza);* consume on an empty stomach.

In the stomach, meadowsweet regulates parietal cell secretion of hydrochloric acid, and reduces excess acidity.[8] It is effective for treating stomach or duodenal ulcers, gastric reflux, gastritis, and indigestion.

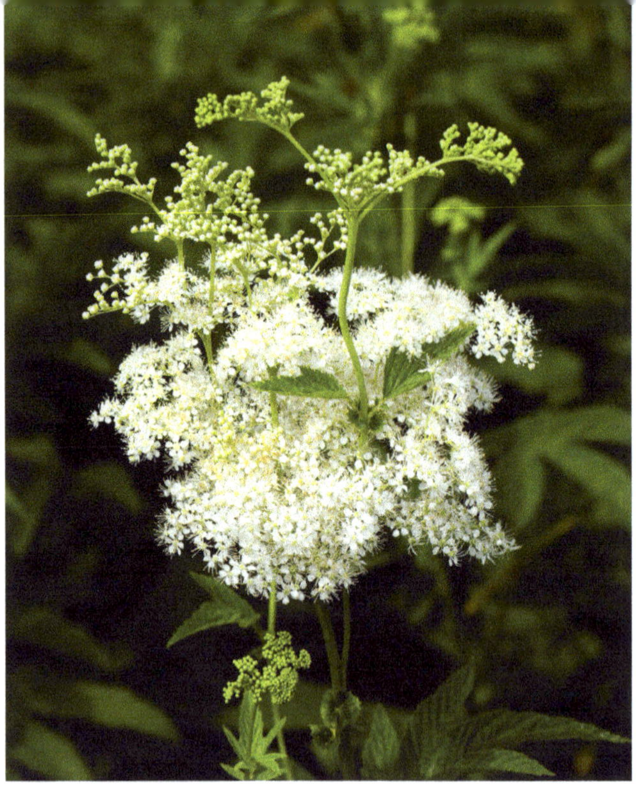

Meadowsweet has another mode of subtle anti-inflammatory action. [7] The glycosides are converted in the liver to the active principle salicylic acid.[7] Salicylic acid is the active principle in aspirin that inhibits prostaglandins and reduces the inflammatory response. The anti-inflammatory actions can be useful for reducing acute or chronic muscle and joint pain, fevers, and headaches. Meadowsweet aids in treating fibromyalgia, arthritis, rheumatic pain, and other inflammatory conditions of the muscles or joints.[7] Combine extracts of meadowsweet with Jamaican dogwood *(Piscidia)*, willow bark *(Salix)*, and/or feverfew *(Tanacetum parthenium)* to ease painful inflammation or headaches. Combine extracts of meadowsweet with turmeric *(Curcuma)*, chamomile *(Matricaria)*, or St. John's wort *(Hypericum)*, and/or licorice root *(Glycyrrhiza)* to reduce acute or chronic inflammation.

Meadowsweet is a cooling diaphoretic and sudorific. It helps to reduce a fever in the first stages of a cold or flu, and mild fevers related to chronic fatigue syndrome.[5,7] Prepare a tea containing peppermint *(Mentha piperita)* and elder flower *(Sambucus)* with smaller amounts of meadowsweet *(Filipendula)* and yarrow *(Achillea)*. Consume eight ounces up to four times daily. *In vitro* studies have demonstrated antimicrobial actions against *Staphylococcus aureus, Streptococcus pyrogenes, Escherichia coli, Shigella flexneri, Klebsiella pneumoniae,* and *Bacillus subtilis.*[6]

According to herbalists Simon Mills and Kerry Bones, in one study the "local administration of the decoction of the flowers resulted in a 39% drop in the frequency of squamous cell carcinoma of the cervix and vagina."[6] An ointment of meadowsweet produced positive results in 32 of 48 cases of cervical dysplasia.[6] Studies have also demonstrated that the flowers have anticoagulant activity, thought to be due to a heparin-like anticoagulant.[6]

Meadowsweet is a mild diuretic that enhances the excretion of uric acid and other nitrogenous waste products. When combined with other diuretics such as parsley seed *(Petroselinum)*, nettle *(Urtica)*, and cleavers *(Galium)*, it is beneficial as a gentle long-term treatment for arthritis, gout, and kidney stones. It has a soothing effect on the genitourinary tract, and aids in treating cystitis and urethritis.[7]

The fomentation or poultice can be applied topically to reduce skin inflammation.[7] It is soothing for cuts, abrasions, scrapes, bruises, contusions, sprains, strains, and sore muscles or joints.[7]

CONTRAINDICATIONS

Use caution or avoid in individuals with sensitivities to salicylates or allergies to aspirin. Exercise caution in patients taking warfarin (Coumadin) or other blood-thinning agents, such as aspirin. Avoid consuming meadowsweet two weeks prior to, and two weeks following surgery. Excessive consumption of the plant's tannins may aggravate the kidneys.

PREPARATION AND DOSAGE

TINCTURE: Fresh leaves and flowers [1:2-1:3, 70-95% alcohol]; dry leaves and flowers [1:5, 60% alcohol]; consume 30-120 drops, up to four times daily.

TEA: Prepare a cold or hot infusion; consume 4-8 ounces, three to four times daily.

SYRUP: Consume 1 teaspoon to 1 tablespoon of syrup, up to four times daily.

TOPICAL USE: Apply the fomentation, poultice, or oil topically. Use well-strained tea as an eye wash, vaginal irrigation, or enema.

CULINARY USE: Small amounts of tender, fresh greens can be incorporated into soup stock. The flowers can be added to alcoholic beverages such as mead, herbal beer, cordials, elixirs, and wine.

MILK THISTLE

BOTANICAL NAMES:
Silybum marianum (syn. *Carduus marianus*)

COMMON NAMES:
Milk thistle, Mary's thistle, St. Mary's thistle, Our Lady's holy thistle, Lady's holy thistle, holy thistle, Venus thistle, Mediterranean thistle, variegated thistle
marietidsel (Danish)
Maarianohdake (Finnish)
chardon béni, chardon Marie, lait de Notre Dame (French)
benedikten distel, Mariendistel, Mariendistelfrüchte, Marienkörner (German)
cardo beneditto, carduo Mariano, cardo santo (Italian)
cardo lechoso, cardo Mariano (Spanish)
Mariatistel (Swedish)
mubarek dikeni (Turkish)

FAMILY NAME:
Asteraceae (Compositae)

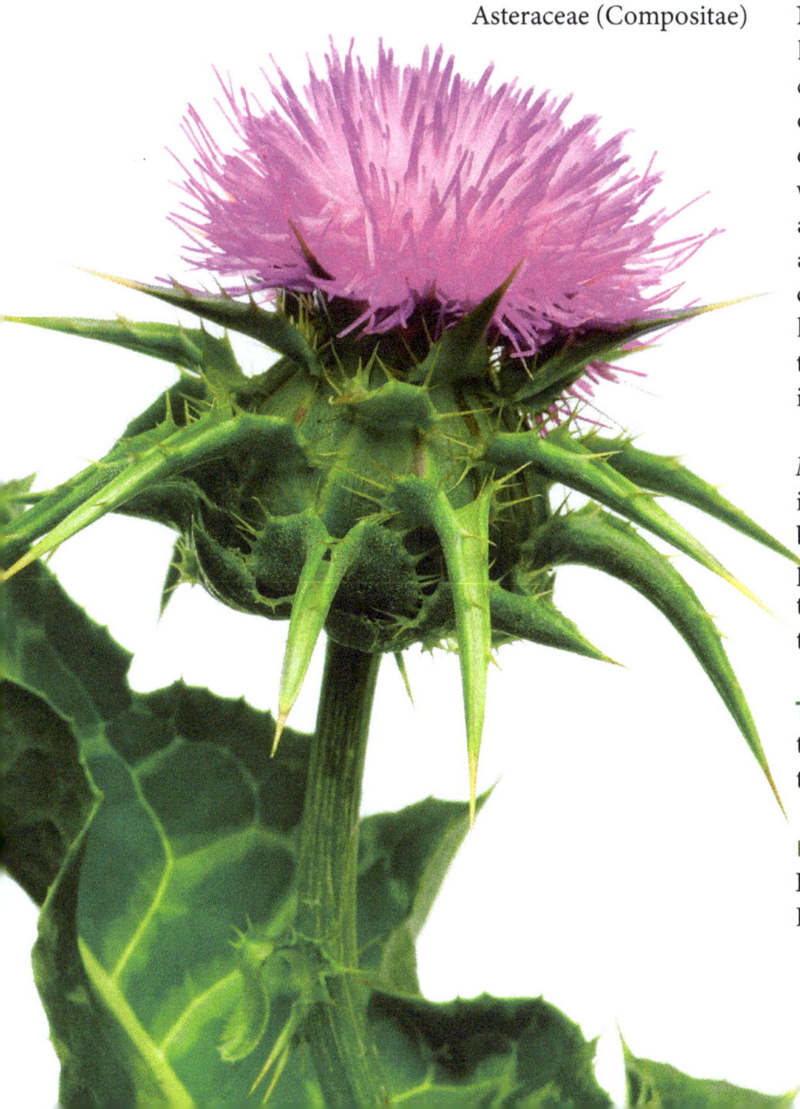

DESCRIPTION

PARTS USED: The fruits (seeds).

BOTANICAL DESCRIPTION AND HABITAT: Milk thistle is a tenacious, weedy thistle that grows wild in pastures, large fields, and disturbed areas, and along roadsides; it is sometimes cultivated.[1] It is native to southern Europe and parts of Asia, but has invaded areas throughout North America.

Milk thistle is an herbaceous, tap rooted biennial or winter annual (20 – 300 cm tall).[2] Initially taking the form of a basal rosette, the alternate, glossy to slightly tomentose leaves are often pinnately lobed with dentate margins; each lobe and tooth is tipped with a sharp spine. The variegated leaves are dark green with white mottling. The basal leaves have a winged petiole (15 – 60 cm long).[1] Becoming cauline as the plant produces flowers, the progressively smaller leaves clasp the stems.

Numerous large, discoid heads are borne terminally on long, bracted peduncles; each has a spheric involucre consisting of four to six series of overlapping bracts.[3] The outer bracts are spiny fringed with spiny tips that spread outward.[1] Each head contains many pink to purple flowers with long tubular corollas that have fused linear lobes, and an abruptly widening throat.[3] The ovoid, glabrous, black and brown spotted fruit are 6 – 8 mm long.[1,2] The fruit is crowned by a ring of barbed, bristly pappus (15 – 20 mm long) that falls off as a single unit.[1] In milder climates, milk thistle blooms February to June; in colder, northern locales, it blooms July to September.[1]

Note: Milk thistle is very difficult to eradicate after it drops its seed, so beware of planting it in the garden. Cinch paper bags around the flowering heads to capture the seeds and prevent it from spreading. It can be painful and laborious to harvest the seed by hand, as they must be removed from the spiny flowering heads.

THE NAME: *Silybum* derives from the name for an edible thistle *("silybum")*.[4] The epithet *marianum* is named for the Virgin Mary.[5]

HISTORICAL USES: During the 1st century, Pliny the Elder espoused the use of milk thistle. In ancient Greece, Dioscorides administered milk thistle as an antidote for

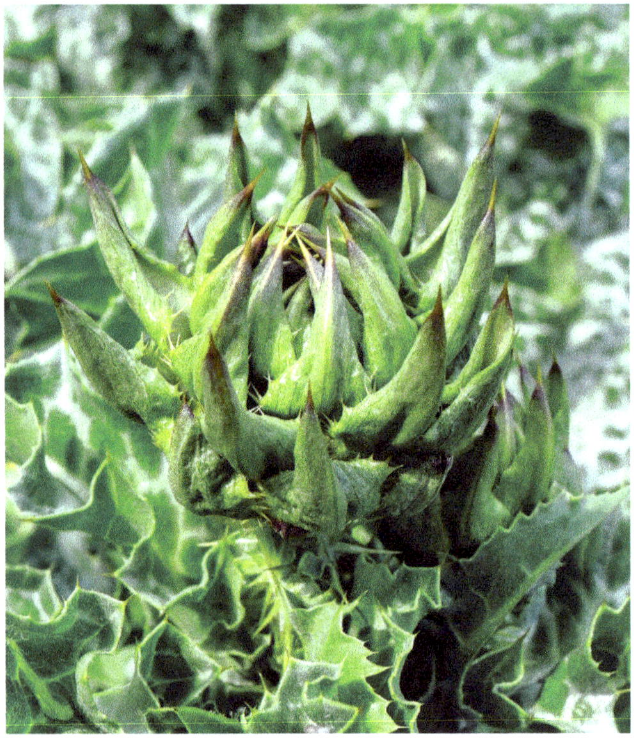

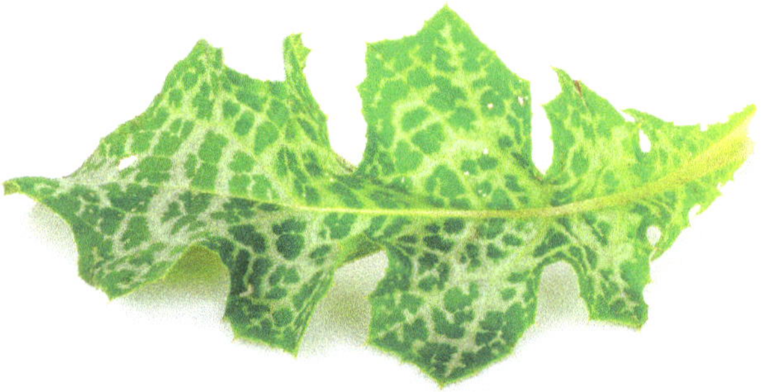

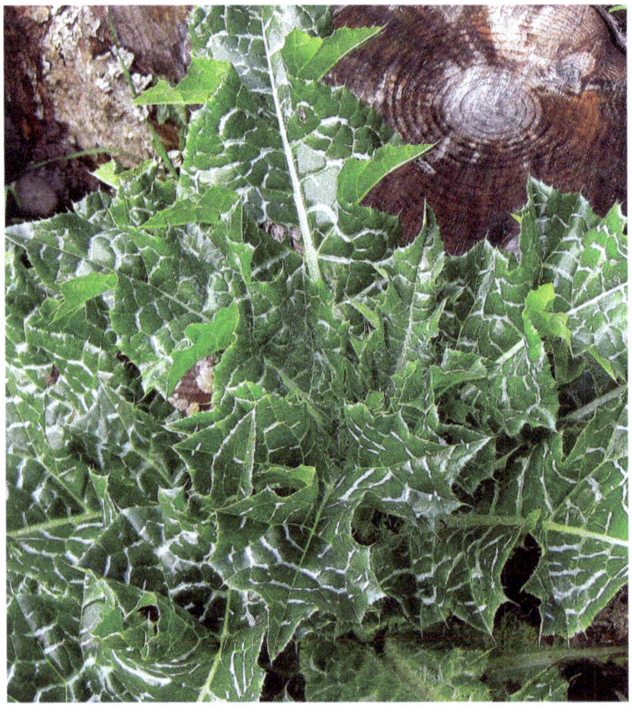

snakebites.[6,7] The herb was widely used in folk medicine to increase breast milk production.[8] During the Middle Ages, milk thistle was revered as a liver protectant.[9] Gerard recommended milk thistle for melancholy disease (liver and gallbladder disorders) in the late 1600s.[7] Culpeper administered the herb for liver and spleen obstruction.[7] Rademacher, a mid-19th century German physician, popularized milk thistle as a cure for liver and gallbladder disorders, as well as jaundice.[8,9]

A concentrated extract of milk thistle was administered by Eclectic physicians for liver and spleen swelling.[10] Ellingwood used milk thistle for pelvic congestion and venous stasis causing varicose veins, hemorrhoids, and chronic reproductive or urinary tissue stagnation.[10] Chronic pelvic stagnation can result in dysmenorrhea, amenorrhea, or passive uterine hemorrhage.[10]

CONSTITUENTS: Milk thistle seed contains three flavanolignans — silybin (silibinin), silychristin (silichristin), and silydianin — collectively referred to as silymarin. Additional flavanolignans include dehydrosilybin, 3-desoxysilichristin, doxysilydianin = silymonin, siliandrin, silybinome, silyhermin, and deosilyhermin. A flavonol, taxifolin, is the structural basis of these flavanolignans: flavonols (quercetin and kaempferol), flavones (apigenin and chrysoeriol), and lignans (coniferyl alcohol dimmers). Milk thistle seed also contains fixed oils (linoleic acid, oleic acid, and palmitic acid), biogenic amines (tyramine and betaine), protein, tocopherol, sterols (cholesterol, campesterol, stigmasterol, and sitosterol), mucilage, and starch.[8,9,11,12]

NUTRITIONAL PROPERTIES: Milk thistle leaf contains high amounts of chromium, iron, magnesium, manganese, phosphorus, selenium, tin, and zinc. It contains low to average amounts of calcium, cobalt, fiber, niacin, potassium, silicon, sodium, thiamine, and vitamins A and C.[13]

MEDICINAL PROPERTIES: Anti-inflammatory, antioxidant, cholagogue, choleretic, hepatodetoxifier, hepatoprotectant, hepatoregenerative, and mild laxative.

TEMPERATURE AND FLAVOR: Cool, bitter, and sweet.

MEDICINAL USES

Milk thistle is a very important herb for treating liver and gallbladder disorders. It contains silymarin, which refers to a group of three flavanolignans: silybin = silibinin, silychrystin = silichristin, and silydianin = siliadin. Silymarin mainly accounts for milk thistle's hepatoprotectant, hepatodetoxifying, and hepatoregenerative actions.[8,9,11] It works most effectively for chronic liver conditions when taken over an extended period of time. Although most of the studies utilize standardized silymarin, consuming capsules, powder, or extract of recently ground seeds is effective for the conditions listed below, though these forms are less concentrated. Alcoholic extracts should be avoided in individuals with liver disease.

Silymarin aids in treating numerous liver conditions, including infectious and drug-induced hepatitis, fatty infiltration of the liver (alcohol-, chemical-, or chemotherapy-induced liver damage), and cirrhosis.[8,11,12] It counteracts alcohol damage to the liver by preventing ethanol-induced mitochondrial changes.[7,8,14] Silymarin also aids in reducing hepatotoxicity from pharmaceutical, over-the-counter, psychotropic, and recreational drugs, as well as chemotherapy. Consuming silymarin before and after an operation reduces liver toxicity caused by the accompanying narcotics.[11] Improving metabolic liver functions, silymarin reduces serum alanine transaminase (ALT), aspartate transaminase (AST), gamma glutamyl transpeptidase (GGT), total bilirubin, and triglycerides.[11] It has antifibrotic actions that hinder collagen infiltration of hepatocytes resulting from inflammation due to chronic viral hepatitis and alcohol abuse.[11] Nineteen percent of patients consuming silymarin (140 mg three times daily for three months) experienced a significant reduction in amino terminal procollagen III peptide (a marker of fibrosis).[11]

Diabetic patients with cirrhosis experienced substantial improvement from consuming 420 mg of silymarin daily. Fasting blood glucose levels, mean daily blood glucose levels, daily glucosuria, and HbA1c levels were significantly reduced.[11] Type II diabetics consuming silybin (231 mg per day for four weeks) had appreciably reduced red blood cell sorbitol levels, demonstrating great potential for preventing and treating diabetic complications.

Silymarin aids in treating liver damage caused by exposure to chemical toxins, including heavy metals, solvents, paints, glues, halogenated hydrocarbons, and environmental pollutants.[14] It reduces liver damage resulting from praseodymium nitrate, indium, and cerium that cause necrosis and fatty degeneration of the liver.[8] In animal studies, silymarin inhibited and reversed liver cell damage induced by chemical toxins, such as carbon tetrachloride, galactosamine, thioacetamide, paracetamol, lanthanides, and ethanol.[7,8,11,14] It is postulated that silymarin does one or more of the following: accelerates elimination of metals from the body; stimulates the formation of metal binding proteins that detoxify metals; inhibits the binding of metals with cellular receptors.[14]

A hepatoregenerative, silymarin stimulates protein synthesis in the liver, increasing production of new liver cells (hepatocytes) and replacing damaged cells.[7,11] This action is catalyzed by increasing the activity of ribosomal RNA that results from the stimulation of nucleolar polymerase A. Silymarin also stimulates DNA and ribosomal RNA synthesis; however, it does not have a stimulating effect on malignant liver tissue.[8,9]

A potent antioxidant (ten times more potent than vitamin E), silymarin prevents free radical cellular damage by increasing glutathione production in the liver, intestines, and stomach.[8,11] Free radicals increase inflammation that damages blood vessels, leading to atherosclerosis. They also compromise immune function, contributing to cancerous and precancerous conditions. In addition to having antiperoxidative activity, silymarin blocks the release of malonyldialdehyde.[8,9]

Milk thistle aids in treating psoriasis, a condition exacerbated by elevated leukotrienes. Silymarin prevents the formation of liver-damaging leukotrienes by Kupffer cells.[8,14] It inhibits lipoxygenase, an enzyme that catalyzes the formation of leukotrienes when an oxygen molecule is transferred to polyunsaturated fatty acids.[7,8,14] Psoriasis is also linked to increased levels of chemical toxins and circulating endotoxins in the cell walls of gut bacteria. When the liver is bombarded with excessive amounts of endotoxins,

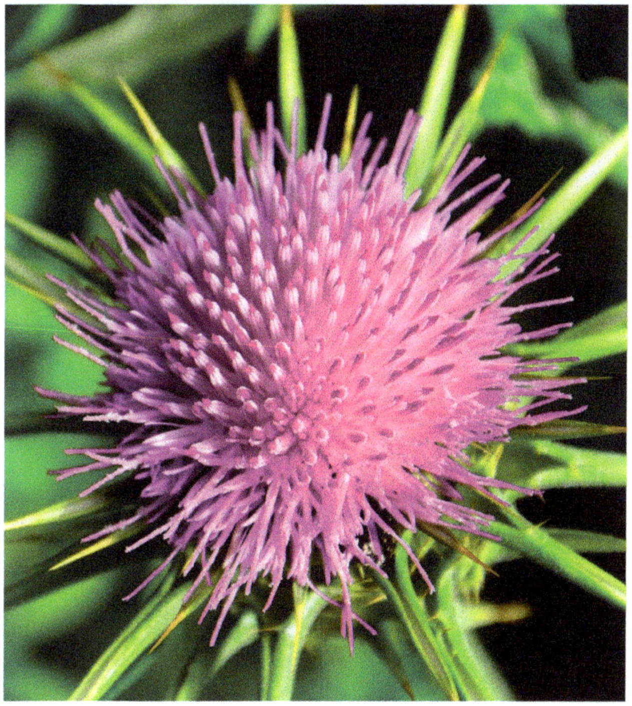

filtration of blood and hepatic detoxification are compromised.[8] Silymarin reduces circulating levels of endotoxins, treating a root cause of psoriasis.[8]

Silymarin also aids in treating psoriasis by regulating cellular replication through the normalization of the ratio of cyclic AMP (cAMP) to cyclic GMP (cGMP). Cellular replication is regulated by the ratio of cAMP to cGMP in skin cells. Patients with psoriasis often have relatively high cGMP levels to cAMP levels; silymarin lowers cGMP levels, and raises cAMP levels.[8] Combine milk thistle with turmeric *(Curcuma)*, berberis *(Berberis)*, dandelion *(Taraxacum)*, burdock *(Arctium)*, and/or smaller quantities of licorice *(Glycyrrhiza)* to ease symptoms of psoriasis.

Silymarin protects against potentially fatal poisoning resulting from deathcap mushroom *(Amanita phalloides)*.[8,14] *Amanita* contains the peptides amanitin and phalloidin, two of the most potent liver-damaging substances. In animals (dogs, rabbits, rats, and mice), a dose of 15 mg/kg silymarin was 100% effective in preventing phalloidine toxicity when administered 60 minutes prior to poisoning.[15] A dose of 100 mg/kg of silymarin injected 10 minutes after phalloidine poisoning also provided total protection in every animal.[15] In another study, intravenous infusions of silibinin demonstrated hepatoprotective and curative effects against *Amanita poisoning*.[9] Administering 50 mg/kg of silibinin (5 and 24 hours after) to beagles intoxicated with *Amanita phalloides* (85 mg/kg) suppressed changes in serum transaminase, alkaline phosphatase, and bilirubin, and the fall in prothrombin time. It significantly reduced hemorrhagic liver necrosis, and none of the silibinin-treated dogs died.[16]

Silymarin is a choleretic and cholagogue.[11] It also increases the solubility of bile, inducing positive effects on stagnant or inflammatory gallbladder conditions such as cholestasis, cholangitis, and pericholangitis.[8,9] Silymarin aids in treating pregnancy- and hormone-related cholestasis.[8] Due to the liver decongesting effects, silymarin aids in treating varicose veins, hemorrhoids, pelvic congestion, and menstrual difficulties.[10]

CONTRAINDICATIONS

There is no record of milk thistle toxicity in human or animal studies.[7,8] It is important to consume adequate amounts of fiber to ensure that the toxins released in the bile are carried out of the body. Due to its bile thinning capacity, silymarin can have laxative effects.[8,12]

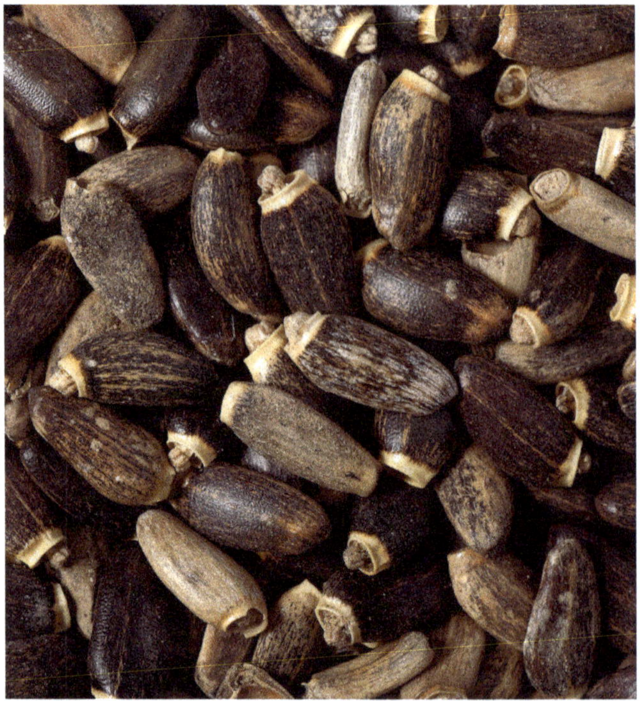

PREPARATION AND DOSAGE

TINCTURE: Dry seeds [1:3, 70% alcohol]; consume 15 - 90 drops, up to three times daily. This preparation is less potent than the standardized extract.

CAPSULES: Standardized milk thistle [40:1 - 70:1, containing 70 - 80% silymarin]; consume the equivalent of 200 - 400 mg divided into three doses. The recommended dose of standardized silymarin is 70 - 210 mg, three times daily. Consume 2 - 3 standardized capsules, up to three times daily. Or consume 2 - 4 "00" capsules, one to three times daily.

TEA: Consume 8 - 12 ounces of the decoction or infusion to treat minor dyspepsia. *Note:* Silymarin is poorly water-soluble; therefore, tea is not effective for treating liver diseases.

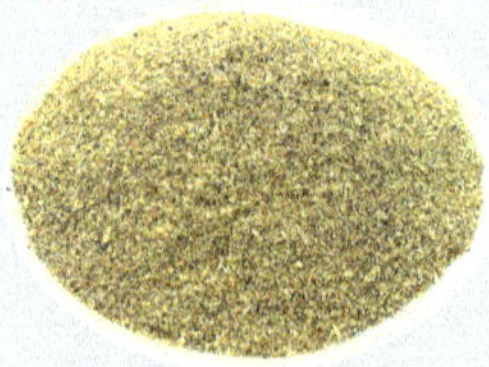

CULINARY USE: Remove the spines from young tender leaves or stalks, and consume raw or cooked. The roots are also edible. Powder the seeds, and sprinkle 1 teaspoon to 1 tablespoon onto food, or add to a smoothie or juice.

MINT

(PEPPERMINT, SPEARMINT, AND BROOK MINT)

DESCRIPTION

BOTANICAL NAMES:
Mentha × piperita, M. arvensis (syn. *M. canadensis, M. arvensis* var. *canadensis*), *M. spicata, M. aquatica*

COMMON NAMES:
Mentha × piperita:
Peppermint, brandy mint
eqama, nana (Arabic)
paprena metvica (Croatian)
pebermynte (Danish)
pepermunt (Dutch)
piparminttu (Finnish)
menthe poivrée, menthe a epis (French)
pfefferminze gruene minze, roemische minze (German)
menta (Greek)
menta (Hebrew)
podina (Hindi)
menta pepe, menta peprina (Italian)
kakka, minto, pepaminto (Japanese)
hobu, mintu (Korean)
hu jiao bo he (Mandarin)
hortelá-pimenta (Portuguese)
piperita (Spanish)
nane (Turkish)
rau tho'm (Vietnamese)

M. spicata:
Spearmint, menthol mint, silver mint
menthe vertebaume vert (French)
ackerminze, katzenkraut (German)
dyosmos (Greek)
supeaminto (Japanese)
spio-minto (Korean)
yerba buena, menta, menta romana (Spanish)
grönmynta (Swedish)

M. arvensis and *M. aquatica*:
Brook mint, water mint, field mint, wild mint, corn mint, Japanese menthol plant, poleo

FAMILY NAME:
Lamiaceae (Labiatae)

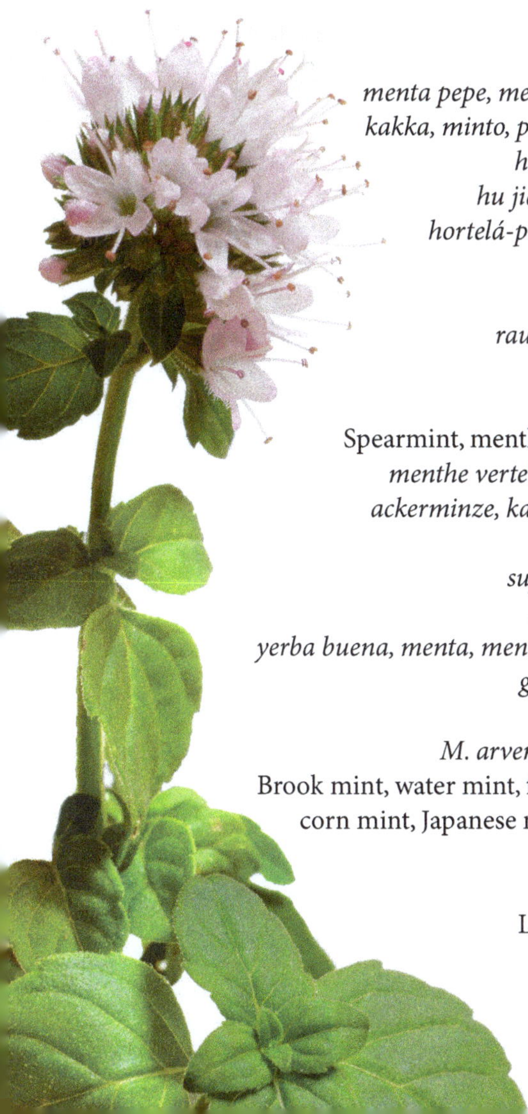

PARTS USED: The leaves or aerial portions. Collect as the flowers appear, or harvest for essential oil after the flowers expand.

BOTANICAL DESCRIPTION AND HABITAT: The perennials peppermint, brook mint, spearmint, and water mint thrive in moist areas along stream banks, lake shores,

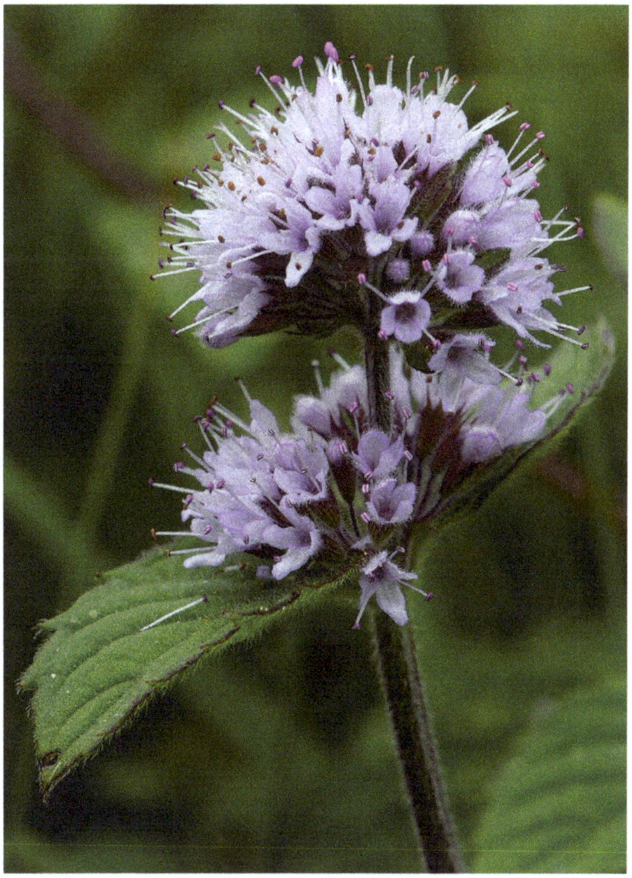

springs, boggy meadows, and sloughs, and in wastelands. *Mentha × piperita* is native to Europe, and is believed to be a hybrid of watermint *(M. aquatica)* and spearmint *(M. spicata). M. arvensis* is native to Europe, temperate areas of western and central Asia, the Himalayas, and eastern Siberia. Peppermint is cultivated worldwide. Brook mint has a circumboreal distribution. Spearmint is native to Europe and cultivated globally.

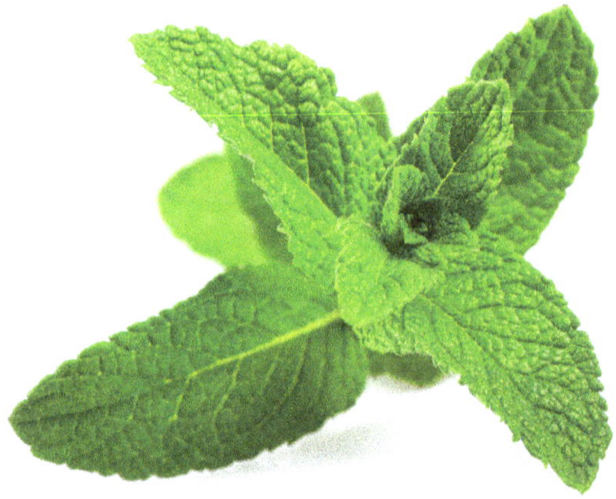

Mentha spicata

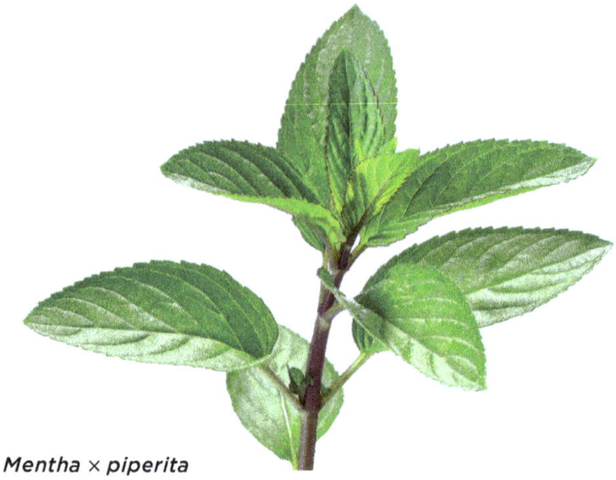

Mentha × piperita

Mint has erect, green or purple quadrangular stems, and opposite lanceolate to oval leaves with short petioles and finely toothed margins. When crushed, the leaves release a pungent menthol odor. The tiny, pale, pinkish-purple flowers in peppermint, and reddish to pinkish-purple flowers in brook mint grow in dense, whorled clusters in upper leaf axils resembling terminal spikes. Peppermint has linear-lanceolate bracts subtending the clusters. Brook mint stamens are exserted beyond the lobes of the corolla; peppermint has included stamens. Brook mint has backward-bending hairs on the stems, calyces, and undersides of the leaves. Peppermint is generally hairless. Mint spreads prolifically from creeping rhizomes. Peppermint grows 30 – 120 cm tall; brook mint grows 10 – 75 cm tall.[1]

Spearmint grows 30 – 120 cm tall; unlike brook mint, it is somewhat hairless, and has sessile leaves with an acute to acuminate apex. The inflorescences are densely clustered and appear more spike-like than brook mint or peppermint, with linear to lanceolate bracts subtending the clusters. Spearmint flowers range from white, pink, or lavender with exserted stamens.[1]

THE NAME: Theophrastus, the ancient Greek philosopher and botanist who succeeded Aristotle, originally applied the genus name *Mentha,* derived from Greek mythology. Pluto fell in love with a nymph named Menthe. In a fit of jealous rage, his wife, Proserpine, metamorphosed Menthe into the plant now called mint.[2]

The epithet *piperita* ("pepper") refers to mint's pungent, spicy flavor.[2] The epithet *aquatica* ("water") derives from Latin, in reference to its moist habitat. The epithet *arvensis* ("of the fields" or "of ploughed fields") originates from Latin. *Canadensis* indicates its origin in Canada. The epithet *spicata* ("like a spire") derives from Latin, in reference to the terminal flowering spikes.

The following common names correspond with the Latin binomials: peppermint *(Mentha × piperita);* water mint *(M. aquatica);* field mint, wild mint, brook mint, corn mint, Japanese menthol plant, poleo, and pudīna *(M. arvensis);* and spearmint *(M. spicata).* The common name spearmint is based on the spear-like shape of the leaves. *Pudīna* is the Sanskrit name for brook mint used throughout India and the Himalayas.

HISTORICAL USES: In ancient literature, several plants are described as mint, although the most common species is spearmint *(Mentha spicata).* Mint was such a highly prized plant that tithes of mint, as well as anise and cumin were accepted as payments to the Pharisees. Records indicate that mint was cultivated by the ancient Egyptians. The medicinal uses of peppermint have been described in Chinese medical literature since the *Tang Pen Tsao* (659 CE).[3] Ancient Greeks and Romans hosted elaborate feasts in which they crowned themselves with mint and adorned their tables with mint sprays. Their cooks flavored wines and sauces with essence of mint. Mint was strewn on banquet chamber floors, perhaps because mice and rats were so averse to its smell that they left food untouched where it was scattered.[2] Ancients also scented bathwater with mint as a restorative.[2] Mint and balm baths were believed to comfort and strengthen the nerves and sinews.[2] Mint tea was consumed for stomachaches. Mint was believed to prevent milk fermentation and coagulation.[2]

As early as the 13th century, *Mentha × piperita* was mentioned in *Icelandic Pharmacopeias,* although it was not differentiated from *M. spicata* in western Europe until the mid-18th century. It was first included in the *London Pharmacopeia* in 1721.[2] Although earlier records from Chinese and Egyptian literature describe the uses of peppermint, other records indicate that it first sprouted from a field of spearmint in England in 1696.[3] Peppermint was first cultivated in England in 1750 and throughout

Europe by 1771.[4] English physician Nicholas Culpeper described more than 40 uses of mint. He suggested gargling with the tea for mouth and gum sores, applying a wash for children's head sores, smelling mint to aid memory, and applying a poultice of mint and rose to encourage sleep.[2] Herbalist and physician Bernard Gerard recommended applying a mint poultice for wasp and bee stings. He also combined mint with salt for bites inflicted by mad dogs.[2]

Volatile oils of mint were believed to improve the digestion of tough meat fibers and prevent intestinal septic changes.[2] Finely chopped spearmint was prepared as a sauce with sweetened vinegar, and served with lamb to improve digestion.[2] In England, fresh mint sprigs were added to flavor green peas, potatoes, and fowl stuffing; powdered mint was added to pea soup and seasonings.[2] In Germany, powdered spearmint was dusted on bean and pea purees, as well as gravies.[2]

In the 14th century, mint was used as a tooth-whitening agent and to freshen the breath. Peppermint oil was administered for puerperal fevers. It was believed that English pilgrims introduced spearmint when they landed in America.[2]

Eclectic physicians employed peppermint for a variety of reasons, including: toothaches, fevers, stomachaches, flatulent colic, nausea, vomiting, cholera morbus, cholera infantum, spasmodic cholera, dysentery, diarrhea with abdominal pain, bowel spasms, palpitations from indigestion, nervous headaches, and painful gonorrhea.[6] Finley Ellingwood recommended using peppermint to induce perspiration, alleviating fevers accompanied by nausea and vomiting resulting from exposure to cold and damp.[6] He also suggested using topical applications of peppermint essential oil for localized relief of rheumatic pain, and as a spray for throat inflammation.[6] Ellingwood recommended inhaling peppermint oil to relieve asthma and bronchitis in the elderly. He suggested peppermint as a digestive and antiseptic to prevent food fermentation in the stomach and bowels.[6]

Peppermint essential oil continues to be used to flavor toothpaste and dental products, chewing gum, and confections. It is also used to scent soap and deodorant.

Native Americans consumed wild mint tea *(Mentha arvensis, M. aquatica, and M. canadensis)* to treat colds, flus, sore throats, coughs, fevers, nausea, colic, gas, digestive pain, kidney problems, and body aches. Steam baths and leaf poultices were used to treat arthritis, rheumatism, pain, and swelling. The fresh herb was strewn in dwellings to discourage bedbugs and other insects.[7] The Cheyenne prepared brook mint tea to prevent vomiting and soothe the stomach.[9] Missouri tribe members drank the tea as a carminative. The Ojibwa used brook mint as a blood purifier, diaphoretic, and stimulant.[9] The Menomonee combined wild mint and catnip in tea, and applied the herb as a chest poultice for pneumonia.[9]

In Canada, the Nuxalk made a tea of *Mentha arvensis* to treat stomach pain.[8] The Quileute used field mint as a "smelling and rubbing" medicine. The Chehalis and Upper Cowlitz drank the tea as a cold remedy.[8]

In China, brook mint was called corn mint *(bo he)*. It was used as an aromatic, antinauseant, stomachic, stimulant, antiseptic, and local anesthetic. Brook mint also was administered as an antispasmodic to treat indigestion, cramps, and diarrhea, as well as for toothaches, sore throats, colds, and headaches. It is used to treat earaches, tumors, and sores.[10]

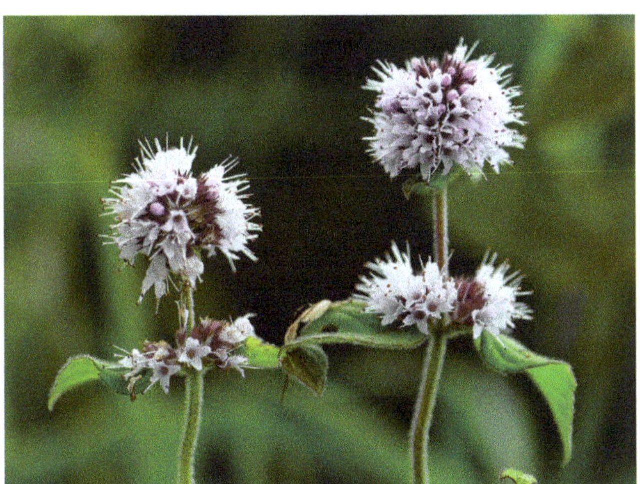

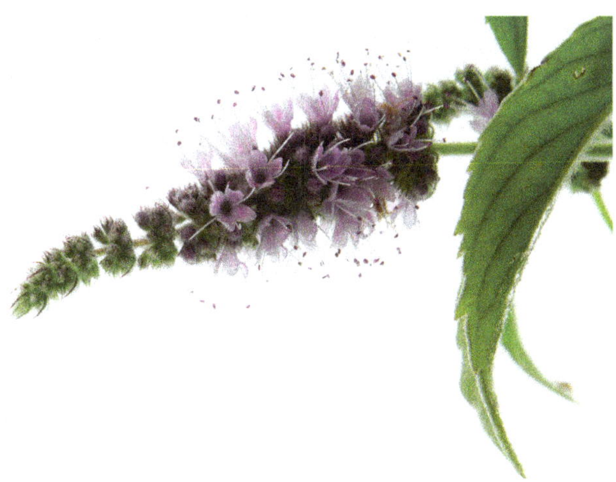

The menthol crystals obtained from *Mentha arvensis* are incorporated into cough drops, breath fresheners, toothpastes, chewing gum, candies, perfumes, confections, tobacco products, lip balms, shampoos, medicated oils, lotions, liniments, and analgesic balms.

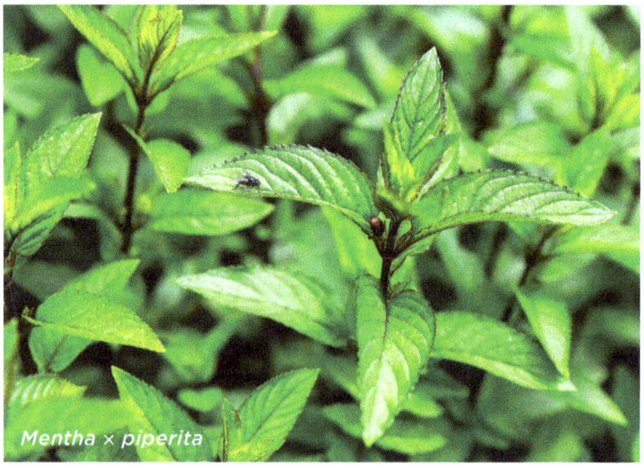

Mentha × piperita

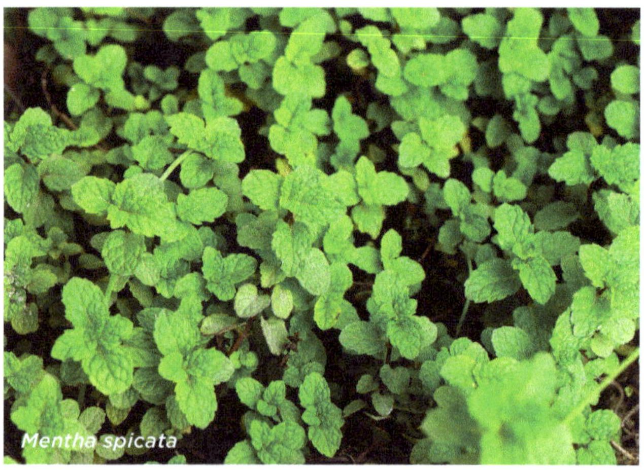

Mentha spicata

CONSTITUENTS

PEPPERMINT: Peppermint contains volatile oil (menthol, menthone, menthyl acetate, menthofuran, limonene, pulegone, 1,8-cineole, piperitone, caryophyllene, bisabolene, isomenthone, isomenthol, α- and β-pinenes, neomenthol, ledol, D-*trans*-sabinene hydrate, and bicycloelemene). It also contains flavonoids (menthoside, isohiofolin, hesperetin, eriodictyol-7-O-rutinoside, eriocitrin, luteolin-7-O-rutinoside, and rutin), phytol, tocopherols (α and γ), carotenoids (α- and β-carotenes), betaine, choline, azulenes, and tannins (rosmarinic acid and caffeic acid derivatives).[10,12]

PEPPERMINT ESSENTIAL OIL: Peppermint essential oil contains 40% menthol (free and esterified), menthone, menthyl acetate, menthofuran, limonene, pulegone, 1,8-cineole, piperitone, caryophyllene, bisabolene, isomenthone, isomenthol, α- and β-pinenes, neomenthol, ledol, D-*trans*-sabinene hydrate, and bicycloelemene.[10,12]

BROOK MINT ESSENTIAL OIL: Brook mint essential oil contains menthol, L-menthol, menthone methyl acetate, isomenthone, thujone, α-pinene, phellandrene, piperitone, menthofuran, (+)-octan-3-one, carvone, (+)-pulegone, octan-3-ol, isopulegone, linalool-acetate, *p*-cymol, ketones, oligosaccharides (raffinose and stachyose), resins, tannins, and rosmarinic acid.[10-12]

SPEARMINT ESSENTIAL OIL: Spearmint essential oil contains carvone, limonene, α-pinene, β-pinene, carvone, 1,8-cineole, linalool, myrcene, caryophyllene, and menthol (0.5% compared to 40% in peppermint).[13]

NUTRITIONAL PROPERTIES: Peppermint contains calcium, iron, magnesium, niacin, phosphorus, potassium, protein, riboflavin, sodium, thiamine, and vitamins A and C. It contains lower amounts of cobalt, crude fiber, dietary fiber, manganese, selenium, and tin.[4] The nutritional properties of brook mint have not been analyzed, but are likely similar to peppermint.

Spearmint contains vitamins A and C, folate, calcium, iron, magnesium phosphorus, potassium, sodium, and small amounts of omega-3 and omega-6 fatty acids, zinc, manganese, and niacin.[14]

MEDICINAL PROPERTIES: Peppermint is an antibacterial (mild), antinauseant, antispasmodic, aromatic, astringent (mild), bronchodilator, carminative, cholagogue, choleretic, counterirritant, diaphoretic, expectorant, stimulant, and anesthetic. Brook mint is an antispasmodic, carminative, cholagogue, diaphoretic, and astringent (mild). Spearmint is an antiseptic (mild), antispasmodic (mild), aromatic, carminative, choleretic, expectorant, and counterirritant.

TEMPERATURE AND FLAVOR: Cool, pungent, and mildly astringent.

MEDICINAL USES

Mint is highly beneficial for treating digestive issues. It has antinauseant, carminative, stomachic, and antispasmodic effects.[9,12,16] Peppermint tea alleviates morning sickness.[19] Preparations of peppermint essential oil are the most effective herbal treatments for nausea resulting from motion sickness, sea sickness, stomach flu, food poisoning, alcohol poisoning, or chemotherapy.[18,19] The tea of any aforementioned mint species will also help to allay these complaints.

Mint tea reduces stomach and intestinal cramping, as well as discomfort associated with indigestion, colic, gas, bloating, and diarrhea.[12,16-19] It provides rapid relief for digestive cramping associated with being bed-bound, and for flareups of irritable bowel syndrome, Crohn's disease, and ulcerative colitis.[12,16,19] Mint has anesthetic effects on the superficial nerves in the stomach and digestive tract, reducing pain associated with heartburn, hiatal hernia, and gastric reflux.[16,19] However, in some individuals, peppermint can aggravate heartburn or gastric reflux. Discontinue use if this occurs.

Research confirms the spasmolytic properties of peppermint essential oil.[9] Enteric coated capsules containing peppermint essential oil bypass the stomach and affect the lower digestive tract. Capsules provide the most effective treatment for flareups of irritable bowel syndrome, Crohn's disease, and ulcerative colitis.[9,12]

Mint is a gentle, pleasant remedy for colds, flus, seasonal allergies, and sinus infections.[9,12] Drinking a hot tea of mint leaf or inhaling the steam aids breathing by decongesting the sinuses and dilating the bronchioles. A throat spray or gargle containing one to two drops of the spirits or essential oil relieves a sore throat and laryngitis.[9] Drinking tea made with equal parts peppermint, mullein leaf *(Verbascum thapsus),* and coltsfoot *(Tussilago farfara)* deepens respiration, and has expectorant and antitussive actions that relieve lower respiratory conditions. Additional antimicrobial agents are necessary for treating respiratory tract infections.

Mint is a cooling diaphoretic, and sudorific, reducing mild fever in the early stages of a cold or flu.[16] Drink 4 – 8 ounces of the hot infusion of mint leaf, yarrow *(Achillea millefolium),* boneset *(Eupatorium perfoliatum),* and elder flower *(Sambucus nigra)* every hour until the fever breaks. If the tea tastes too bitter, reduce the quantity of boneset and yarrow. Make sure to serve the tea hot, and wrap the patient in blankets. If the tea is too difficult to palate, strain it into a hot bath or footbath, and soak. Dry the body and hair quickly, taking care not to get chilled, then wrap the patient in blankets until diaphoresis has commenced. Mint volatile oils have mild vasodilating effects, accounting for its traditional use as a diaphoretic and headache remedy. Mint tea and peppermint spirits are subtle treatments for frontal headaches caused by sinus congestion, or temporal and occipital headaches caused by liver or gallbladder congestion. More potent vasodilators or anti-inflammatory agents are sometimes necessary.

Mint is a gentle, refreshing stimulant with an uplifting, energizing quality. It increases mental alertness and reduces fatigue. Mint is a flavoring and harmonizing agent for tea, modifying harsh or bitter herbs.

THE ESSENTIAL OIL: While there are many similarities between essential oils of the various mint species mentioned, there are some important differences.

PEPPERMINT (MENTHA X PIPERITA)

Peppermint essential oil is obtained by steam distillation. It is an antinauseant, carminative, and spasmolytic. It is also a choleretic and cholagogue that increases bile secretion up to nine-fold.[16] The flavonoids were found to have choleretic actions in canines, possibly by stimulating the vagus nerve, although the exact mechanism has yet to be determined.[3,9] French aromatherapists regard peppermint essential oil as a liver regenerative.[18]

Peppermint oil is a decongestant, expectorant, and bronchodilator. It has antiviral, antifungal, and antibacterial properties *in vitro.*[12] The antiviral properties have been effective against herpes simplex and Newcastle disease.[3,9]

Apply one to two drops of mint essential oil to the temples or occipital region for headaches, but make sure not to touch the eyes with the oil.[12] The essential oil and menthol crystals can be used as smelling salts to revive individuals after a seizure or fainting.

Peppermint essential oil (diluted) can be applied to the gums to relieve pain from emerging wisdom teeth, an abscessed tooth, or cavities. Prepare a 1:10 solution by adding ten drops of peppermint essential oil to 100 drops of cow parsnip seed tincture *(Heracleum lanatum).* This solution is highly effective as a topical application, providing temporary relief for gum pain until dental work is obtained. (Refer to the contraindications before administering to children.)

BROOK MINT (MENTHA ARVENSIS)

Essential oil of brook mint (also known as corn mint) is obtained through steam distillation. Brazil, Japan, China, and Taiwan are the main producers of the essential oil.[15] A varietal of corn mint, *Mentha arvensis* var. *piperascens,* contains particularly high amounts of menthol (70% free menthol and 3 – 20% menthol in esterified form) compared to peppermint. Apply neat or diluted essential oil directly to the affected area to reduce pain and create a cooling, anesthetic effect on the tissues. For sunburns, incorporate essential oil into a spray with a base of aloe gel, rose or lavender hydrosol, and witch hazel. Peppermint

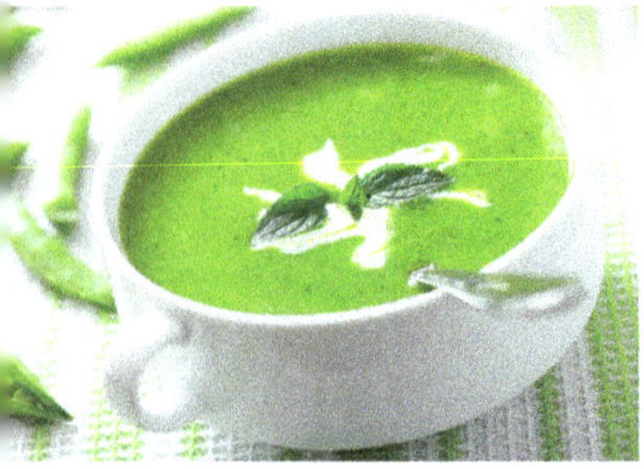

and brook mint essential oils have anti-inflammatory properties.[9] Peppermint essential oil contains azulene, which has anti-inflammatory and antiulcer properties.[3,9]

Brook mint essential oil (neat or diluted) also can be applied to the gums to relieve pain from an abscessed tooth or cavity. However, it should not be applied to the gums of infants or young children; peppermint is safer for children.

CONTRAINDICATIONS

Avoid with mint family allergies. Mint can aggravate acid indigestion and heartburn; discontinue use if this occurs. Avoid use in cases of biliary obstruction, gallbladder inflammation, or severe liver disorders.[12]

Peppermint, brook mint, and spearmint essential oils are highly concentrated, and can cause contact dermatitis or an allergic reaction in some individuals.[3,9] Avoid use in children less than 30 months old, and avoid direct application of the oil in the nostrils of infants and children.[9,18] Internal or external use of the essential oil can cause menthol toxicity in infants or adults with a deficiency of the enzyme glucose-6-phosphate dehydrogenase (G6PD).[15] Avoid consuming essential oil preparations of *Mentha arvensis* and *M. aquatica* during pregnancy or lactation. However, aromatherapist Robert Tisserand explains that the pulegone levels in *M.* × *piperita* are not high enough to cause concern.[15] Consuming peppermint or brook mint essential oil consistently can cause relaxation of the esophageal (cardiac) sphincter.[4] High doses of essential oil consumed over long periods of time can irritate mucous membranes.[3] Contacting the eyes with the essential oil can cause irritation to the conjunctiva. Mint essential oil should be avoided in individuals who have a history of cardiac fibrillation.[15]

PREPARATION AND DOSAGE

TINCTURE: Fresh leaves [1:2-1:3, 70-95% alcohol]; dry leaves [1:5, 50% alcohol]; consume 30-60 drops, up to four times daily.

GLYCERITE: Fresh leaves [1:2-1:3, 50% glycerin, 50% alcohol]; dry leaves [1:5, 70-100% glycerin]; consume 10-60 drops, up to three times daily.

ACETUM EXTRACT: Fresh leaves [1:2, apple cider vinegar]; dry leaves [1:5, apple cider vinegar]; consume 30-90 drops, up to three times daily.

SUCCUS: Juice the fresh leaves and measure the volume, then add 20% alcohol (190 proof) to the total volume. Consume up to 1 tablespoon, three times daily. Storing in the refrigerator improves the shelf life.

CAPSULES: To prepare mint essential oil capsules, fill "0" or "00" capsules with a binding agent such as marshmallow root powder or slippery elm powder, then add 1-2 drops of peppermint essential oil into each capsule. Close the capsules, and store in a zip-lock bag in the refrigerator or freezer. Consume 1-2 capsules, up to three times daily. *Note:* Take care not to add any essential oil into the capsules without a binder, or the capsules will dissolve.

TEA: Prepare a hot or cold infusion; consume 8-12 ounces, up to four times daily.

HONEY AND SYRUP: Infuse fresh leaves in honey and steep in a warm place two to four weeks. Or infuse the leaves in simple syrup one to three days; strain and refrigerate. The syrup lasts up to one month. Consume 1 teaspoon in 8 ounces of tea, up to four times daily.

TOPICAL USE: Apply essential oil (diluted or neat) to the affected area. Include essential oil or menthol crystals in topical preparations such as liniments, oils, and salves.

CULINARY USE: Fresh peppermint and brook mint are more pungent than spearmint; however, they have similar culinary uses. Brook mint tastes slightly more bitter than peppermint or spearmint. Mint can be added to mint jelly or jam, vinaigrette, soup, poultry, lamb, candy, or desserts.

ESSENTIAL OIL: Mint spirits are made by combining one part by volume of organic essential oil with ten parts by volume of ethanol alcohol (190 proof). Consume only 1-2 drops, as the spirits are highly concentrated. Alternately, place 1-2 drops of the essential oil on a sugar cube, dissolve in hot water or tea, and drink.

MOTHERWORT

DESCRIPTION

BOTANICAL NAME:
Leonurus cardiaca

COMMON NAMES:
Motherwort, European motherwort,
Roman motherwort, lion's ear, lion's tail, throwwort
almindelig, hjertespand (Danish)
aartgespan, hartgespan (Dutch)
nukula (Finnish)
agripaume, herbe battudo (French)
Echtes herzgespann, Echtes lövenschwanz (German)
agripalma (Italian)
lovehale (Norwegian)
Scerdecznik pospolity (Polish)
agripalma, marihuanilla (Spanish)
hjärtstilla, bonässla, äkta hjärtstilla (Swedish)[1]

FAMILY NAME:
Lamiaceae (Labiatae)

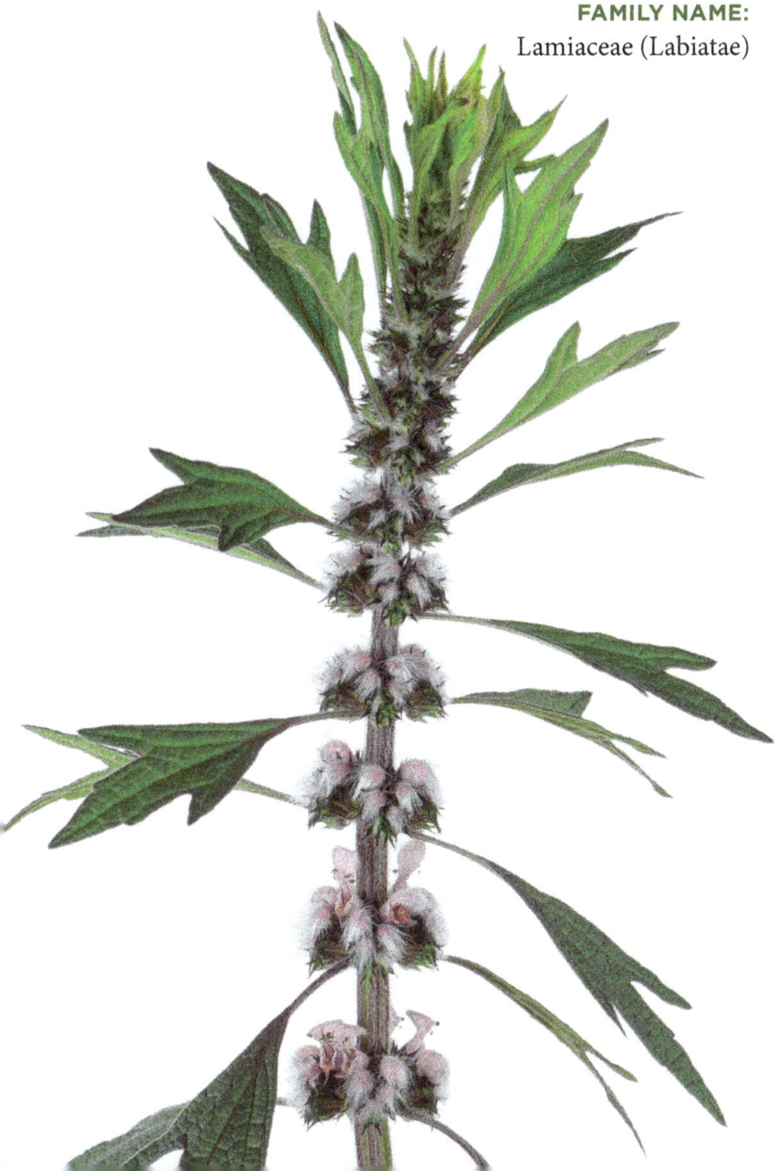

PARTS USED: The leaves and flowers. Harvest while the plant is in flower; wear gloves when stripping the leaves and flowers off the stems. The beneficial chemical constituents are most profuse when the plant is in full bloom.[2]

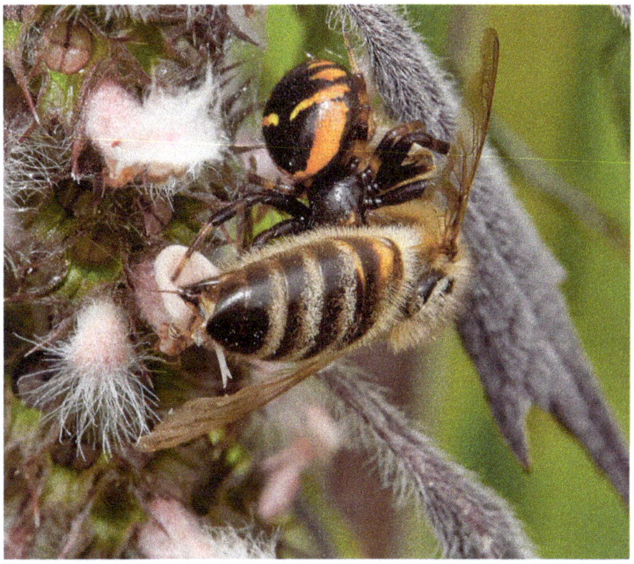

BOTANICAL DESCRIPTION AND HABITAT: Motherwort is a perennial herb found throughout Europe, and has naturalized in the northern U.S. and Canada. It grows wild in well drained, rich, moist soil along creek beds, rivers, lakes, bogs, meadows, and forest outskirts. It prefers full sun, but tolerates partial shade.

Motherwort has deep greenish-purple, erect, quadrangular, hollow, hairy stems (50 – 100 cm tall).[3] The opposite leaves are pubescent, dark green above, and pale green below. The leaves are polymorphous (3 – 8 cm long by 2.5 – 8 cm wide) and variously palmately lobed; those on lower portions of the plant are wider, and consist of three to five deeply cut lobes with deeply dentate margins.[3] The ovate, uppermost leaves are slender with a large, acute-tipped tooth on each side. The pinkish-white flowers appear in densely whorled clusters (10 – 15 mm diameter) in upper leaf axils.[3] The fused calyx (5 mm long) has five sharp, rigid teeth.[3] The upper lip of the bilabiate corolla (12 mm long) has dense, woolly hairs on the backside; the lower lip has three downward-angled lobes. There is a ring of hairs in the floral tubes. Motherwort has four stamens — two longer, and two shorter. The anthers have firm, shiny points. The ovary produces tiny, one-seeded, tetrahedral nutlets.

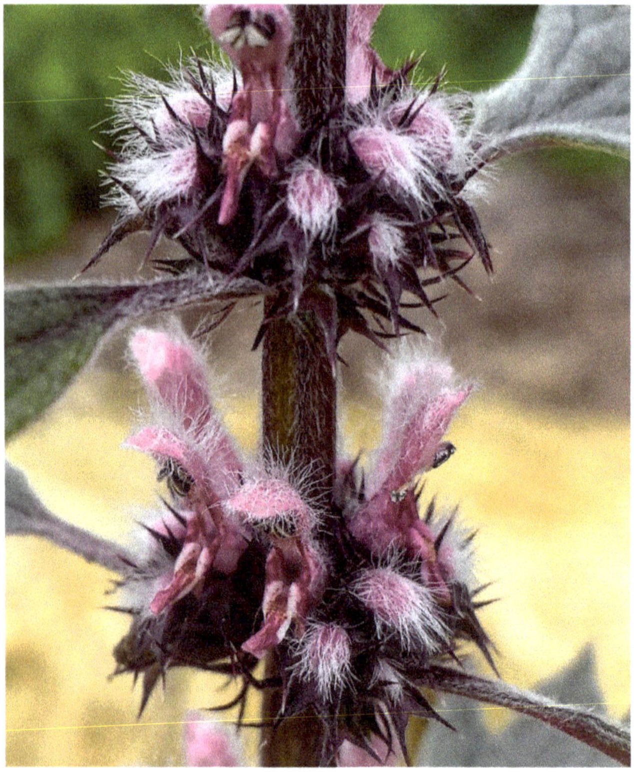

THE NAME: *Leonurus* ("lion's tail") derives from Greek.[4] The epithet *cardiaca* derives from the Greek *kardiakós* ("of or pertaining to the heart").[5] The term *wort* means "herb or root;" therefore, the common name motherwort means "mother's herb." The resemblance of the plant to a lion's tail accounts for its common and genus names.

HISTORICAL USES: Motherwort was used in Europe as a nervine, antispasmodic, emmenagogue, tonic, and diaphoretic. In *A Modern Herbal,* English herbalist Maude Grieve wrote: "there is no better herb for strengthening and gladdening the heart…it is good against hysterical complaints and especially for palpitations of the heart when they arise from hysteric causes, and when made into syrup, will allay inward tremors (and) faintings."[4]

Nicholas Culpeper stated: "There is no better herb to drive melancholy vapours from the heart, to strengthen it and make the mind cheerful, blithe and merry." He described additional uses for motherwort: relieving cramps and convulsions, clearing the chest of cold phlegm, killing digestive worms, and dispersing cold that settles in the veins, joints, and sinews.[4] Herbalist John Gerard also recommended the herb for treating heart infirmities, gangrene, and coughs.[4]

Eclectic physicians administered motherwort for a variety of gynecological conditions including amenorrhea and nervousness from irregular menstruation. Dr. Finley Ellingwood utilized motherwort for "dysmenorrhea with morbid nervous excitability and hysteria," and "pain in the pelvic and lumbar regions in females."[6] John King, Eclectic physician, considered motherwort superior to all remedies for suppressed lochia — the discharge of blood and mucus from the uterus after childbirth. He recommended consuming the herb, and applying a fomentation over the lower abdominal region.[6] Dr. Harvey Felter recommended motherwort as an emmenagogue and antispasmodic.[7] Dr. John Scudder prescribed hot infusions of motherwort as follows:

> Its antispasmodic and nervine powers render it an appropriate and valuable agent in hysteria, chorea, convulsions, and other derangements of the nervous system, associated with uterine irregularity or obstruction.[8]

Motherwort was used to treat a broad range of conditions, including delirium tremens, fevers in a typhoid state, chronic wakefulness, restlessness, disturbed sleep, spinal irritation, heart palpitations, convulsions, feeble digestion, general debility, stomachaches, and headaches.[6]

Following its introduction by European settlers, Native Americans adopted motherwort as a medicine. Many tribes, including the Delaware, Micmac, Moehegan, and Shinnecock consumed motherwort tea for gynecological ailments. The Cherokee valued the herb as a sedative.[2]

CONSTITUENTS: Motherwort contains iridoids (leonuride = ajugoside, and ajugal), volatile oil (caryophyllene, α-pinene, linalool, limonene, β-pinene, and benzaldehyde), α-humulene, ascorbic acid, 3-octanol, 8-β-acetoxy-9-α, 13-α, 15, 16-biepoxy labdanolide, bufenolide, phenolic acids (caffeic-acid-4-rutinoside), flavonoid glycosides (rutin, quinqueloside, genkwanin, quercetin, quercetrin, isoquercetrin, hyperoside, apigenin, and kaempferol), pheylethanoid glycosides (verbascoside = aceteoside), proline-betaines (stachydrine and betonicine), diterpenes (leocardin), triterpenes (ursolic acid), gluridosude, tannins, alkaloids (tachydrine, betonicine, turicin, leonurine, and leonuridine), marrubiin, and stachyose.[9-11]

NUTRITIONAL PROPERTIES: Motherwort contains flavonoid glycosides; however, it is difficult to palate.

MEDICINAL PROPERTIES: Antispasmodic, anxiolytic, bitter tonic, cardiotonic, deobstruent, emmenagogue, hypotensive, nervine, sedative, and stomachic.

TEMPERATURE AND FLAVOR: Cool and bitter.

MEDICINAL USES

Motherwort is a nervine, anxiolytic, and moderate sedative. It is effective for reducing symptoms of autonomic stress and hyperthyroidism, such as hypertension, anxiety, panic attacks, and insomnia. However, further research is necessary to determine whether the effects predominantly influence the autonomic nervous system, or are mildly thyrosuppressive. Herbalist Michael Moore suggests that motherwort's "real effects on the heart derive from a subtle but distinct suppression of thyroid function, helpful in stress-induced thyroid elevation, with little or no effect from simple adrenalin-induced palpitation."[9] However, it decreases heart rate, heart palpitations, and anxiety levels due to patterns of adrenergic stress, as well as thyroid stress.

Motherwort aids in treating patients with chronic anxiety commonly resulting from hyperthyroidism, and from Hashimoto's, an autoimmune hypothyroid disease. Unlike its mint family relative, bugleweed *(Lycopus)*, motherwort does not directly lower thyroid hormone levels in patients with mild forms of hyperthyroidism or Graves' disease; nor does it appear to lower thyroid hormone levels in patients with Hashimoto's or other forms of hypothyroidism. However, motherwort is most helpful for long-term treatment of mild cases of hyperthyroidism.[15] Combining three parts of bugleweed *(Lycopus)* with one and one-half parts motherwort and lemon balm *(Melissa)* has aided in treating many symptoms associated with the early stages of hyperthyroidism and anxiety. Two parts motherwort and kava *(Piper methysticum)* can be combined with one part wild oats *(Avena)* and passion flower *(Passiflora)*, and ¼ to ½ part pasque flower *(Anemone)* (omit if not available) to alleviate anxiety and panic attacks.

Motherwort is a mild cardiotonic with an affinity for the heart. It reduces heart palpitations, slowing a rapid heartbeat and relieving feelings of oppression in the chest.[15] Motherwort lowers mild to moderately elevated blood pressure in individuals with stress-induced hypertension. Alcohol extracts have direct inhibitory effects on myocardial cells that exert antagonistic actions against calcium chloride and stimulated α- and β-adrenoceptors.[11] The blood pressure lowering effect (negative chronotropic effect) are due to glycosides.[9,10] Combine extracts of motherwort, passion flower *(Passiflora incarnata)*, and night blooming cereus *(Cereus grandiflorus)* to treat heart palpitations and stress-induced hypertension. Motherwort also can ease depression due to stress or grief.

Motherwort aids in treating hormone imbalances resulting from premenstrual syndrome (PMS) and perimenopause. It can be helpful in reducing night sweats, hot flashes, irritation, rage, and hormone-related emotional and physical hypersensitivity. During the reproductive years, it is highly beneficial to consume during the luteal phase (post-ovulation to menses), or the week prior to menses for treating PMS and sensations of a stagnant, boggy uterus.

Motherwort has emmenagogue properties that aid in treating suppressed or slow-starting, crampy menses. This herb moves stagnant blood, reducing menstrual clotting and painful menstruation. It contains leonurine and stachydrine that promote uterine contractions and have vasodilating effects.[9,12,13] Motherwort has been helpful in stimulating contractions and hastening delivery.[12,14] For stimulating the onset of labor, consume 10 – 30 drops, one to three times daily, up to one week prior to, or later than the due date. When labor begins, consume up to 30 drops, every two to three hours, up to five times daily. Motherwort aids expulsion of the placenta and lochia; however, if employed directly after birth, it can contribute to uterine bleeding. *Note:* Use caution with women who experience heavy uterine bleeding during menses, after birth, or during perimenopause.

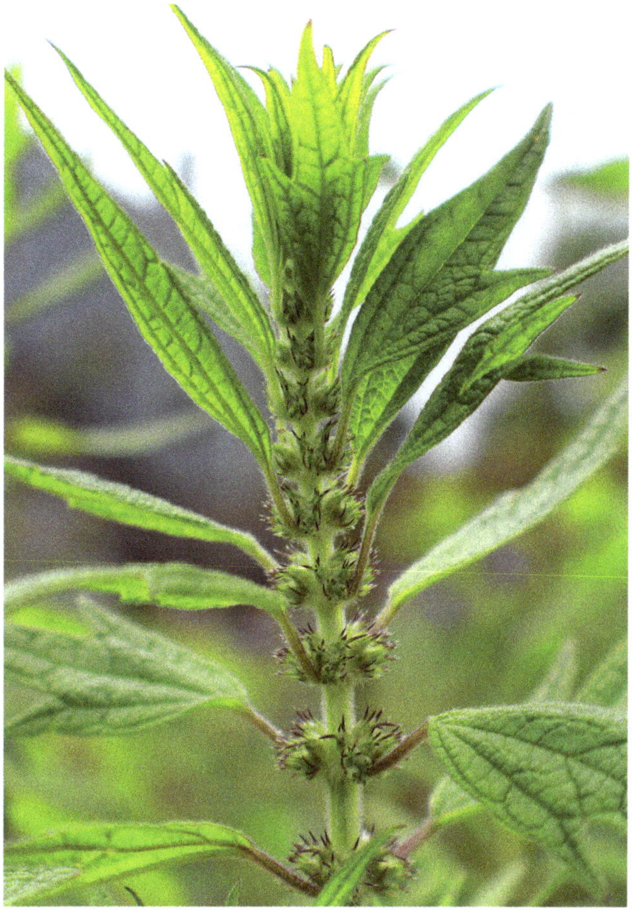

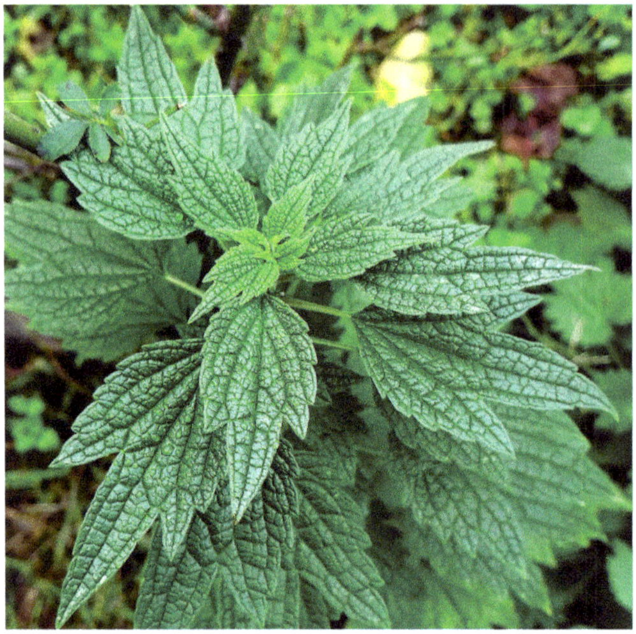

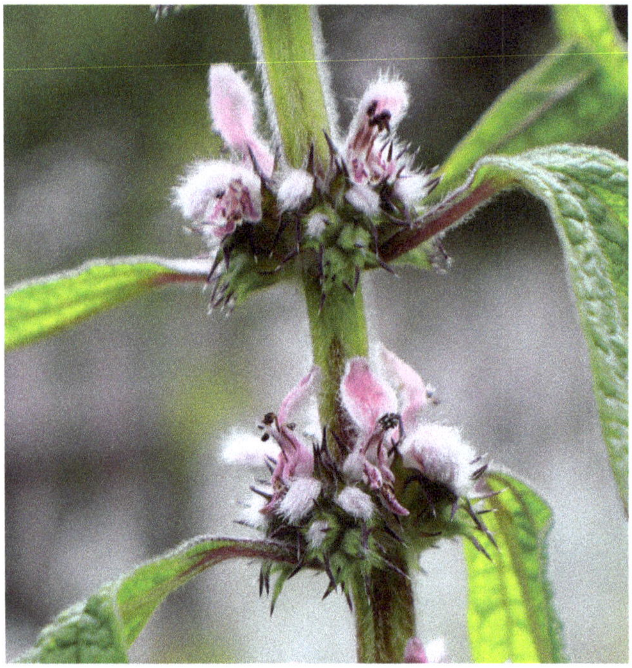

Motherwort is a smooth muscle antispasmodic that works most effectively for menstrual and intestinal cramping. It has mild digestive bitter tonic, cholagogue, and laxative actions. It reduces gas and bloating, especially when combined with aromatic carminatives such as chamomile *(Matricaria)*, lemon balm *(Melissa)*, fennel *(Foeniculum)*, and/or cardamom *(Elettaria cardamomum)*. A compound combining motherwort with one or more of the following herbs works very effectively for menstrual cramps: kava *(Piper methysticum)*, angelica *(Angelica)*, black cohosh *(Actaea racemosa)*, and valerian *(Valeriana)*.

Motherwort stimulates prolactin hormone secretion, facilitating milk letdown. In addition, it reduces postpartum depression, heart palpitations, and anxiety. It has earned its title as the "mother's herb."

Motherwort decreases nerve hypersensitivity.[15] It aids in reducing neuralgia, neuritis, and the pain of herpes and shingles eruptions.[15]

CONTRAINDICATIONS

Avoid use during pregnancy, except to facilitate labor. Discontinue consuming motherwort if it causes heavy uterine bleeding. Individuals with hypothyroidism should consult a health care practitioner before consuming motherwort daily. The plant can cause contact dermatitis in sensitive individuals.

PREPARATION AND DOSAGE

TINCTURE: Fresh leaves and flowers [1:2-1:3, 60-95% alcohol]; recently dried leaves and flowers [1:5, 50-60% alcohol]; consume 30-60 drops, up to four times daily.

ACETUM EXTRACT: Fresh leaves and flowers [1:2, apple cider vinegar]; dry leaves and flowers [1:5, apple cider vinegar]; consume 30-90 drops, up to three times daily. (Less potent than alcohol-based tinctures.)

CAPSULES: Consume 2-4 "00" capsules, up to three times daily.

TEA: Prepare a hot or cold infusion; consume 4-8 ounces, up to four times daily. Motherwort tea tastes bitter; add honey to improve palatability.

HONEY AND SYRUP: To prepare syrup, infuse one ounce of recently dried motherwort in 16 ounces of water, and steep four to eight hours. Strain and sweeten to taste with honey, maple syrup, or simple syrup. Consume 1 teaspoon to 1 tablespoon, up to four times daily. Refrigerate up to one month.

TOPICAL: Apply the hot fomentation to the lower abdominal region to stimulate menses, reduce menstrual cramping, or facilitate expulsion of suppressed lochia.

MULLEIN

DESCRIPTION

BOTANICAL NAMES:
Verbascum thapsus, V. bombyciferum

COMMON NAMES:
Mullein, great mullein, white mullein, woolly mullein, woolen blanket herb, blanket leaf, beggar's blanket, flannel flower, Adam's flannel, feltwort, velvet dock, velvet plant, candlewick, witches candle, hag's taper, Our Lady's candle, torches, Quaker's rouge, hare's beard, Jupiter's staff, Jacob's staff, Aaron's rod, cuddy lungs, duffle, shepherd's club, clown's lungwort
molène (French)
kleinblütige, königskerze (German)
aflego (Greek)
barbasco, verbasco (Portugese)
punchon, gordolobo (Spanish)
kungsljus (Swedish)[1]

FAMILY NAME:
Scrophulariaceae

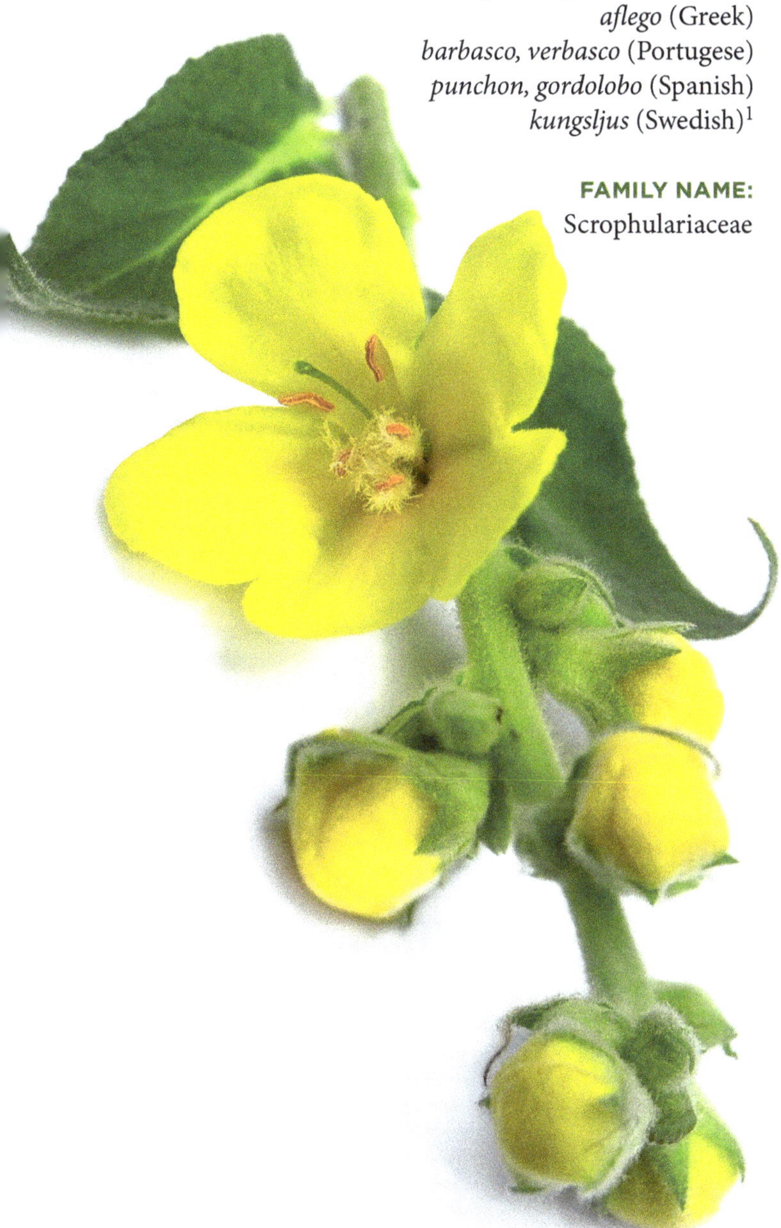

PARTS USED: The flowers, leaves, and roots prepared separately.

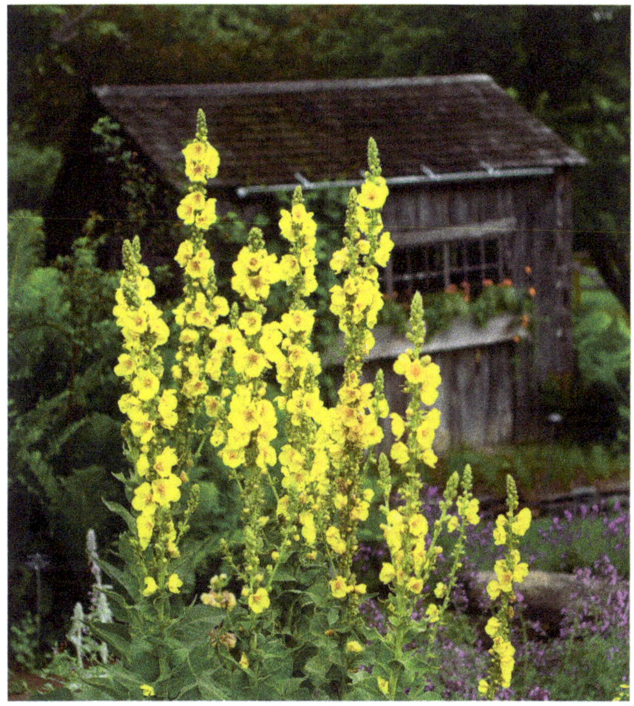

BOTANICAL DESCRIPTION AND HABITAT: *Verbascum* is a large genus containing up to 360 species of herbaceous annuals, biennials, and perennials with erect stems and simple, alternate leaves.[2] The leaves grow in basal rosettes until the second year when the plant blooms and some cauline leaves climb the flowering stem. The terminal inflorescence is a dense spike, raceme, or panicle that can grow quite large in some species.[2] The flowers have a radial, five-lobed calyx and a five-lobed, rotate corolla that is yellow in most species, but sometimes purple or white.[3] There are five hairy stamens, two longer than the other three, as well as two fused carpels, and a round stigma.[2] The fruit is a capsule containing many small seeds.[2]

Verbascum thapsus is a striking biennial plant, with the inflorescence growing up to 200 cm tall with few to no branches (in contrast to *V. bombyciferum,* whose branching inflorescence often resembles a candelabra).[4] The plant is covered with dense, gray hairs, giving the leaves and branches a fuzzy texture.[5] The oblanceolate, petiolate basal leaves have entire margins, and grow up to 50 cm long.[4] The lanceolate, sessile cauline leaves are smaller (up

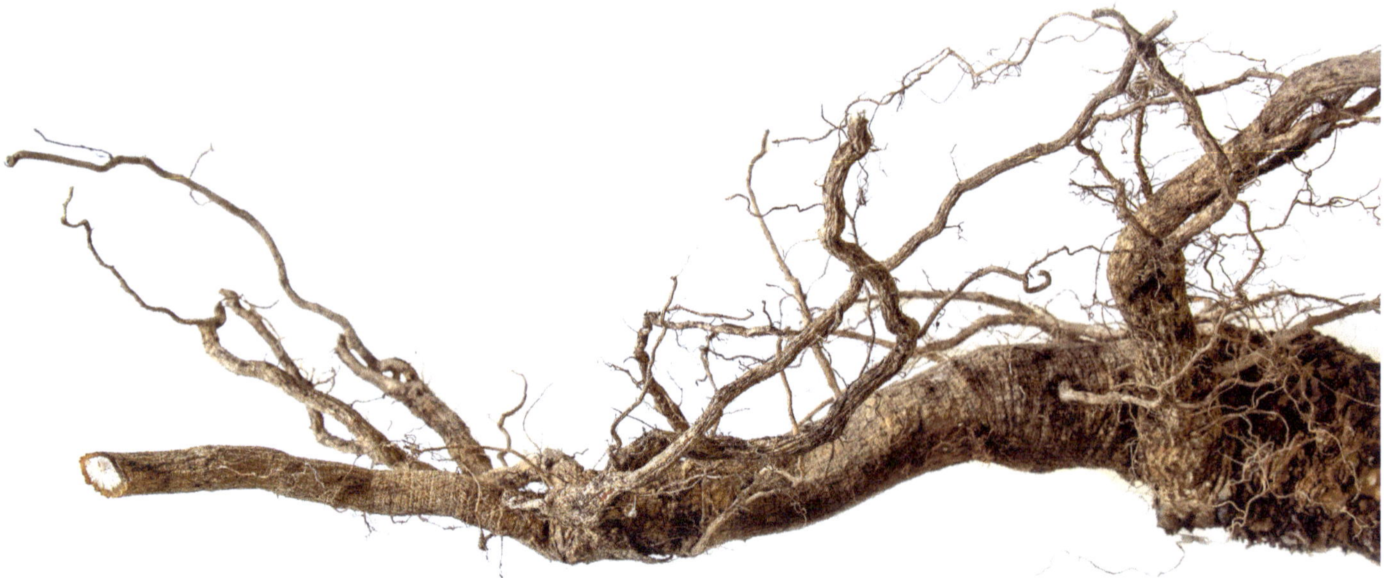

to 30 cm long), with bases that fuse to the stem, forming wing-like structures along it.[4] The inflorescence is a stately, terminal panicle with long, dense, spike-like branches, bearing bright yellow flowers.[4]

V. bombyciferum is extremely woolly, with a shimmery silver color. It grows up to 150 cm high with few to no branches.[6] The blades of the ovate leaves (up to 40 cm high and 20 cm wide) have crenate margins.[6] The fuzzy white, terminal raceme bears bright yellow flowers that are not glandular, unlike other *Verbascum* species.

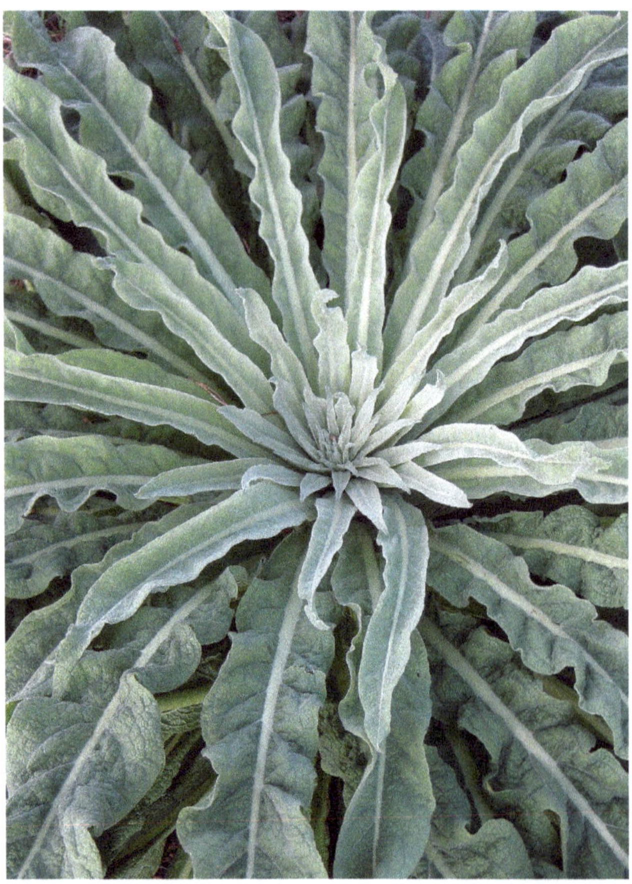

THE NAME: The genus name *Verbascum* derives from the Latin *barbascum* ("a beard").[1] The epithet *thapsus* was named after an ancient town in Tunisia. The common name mullein derives from the Anglo-Saxon *moleyne,* corrupted from the Latin *malandrium* — a term applied to cattle lung diseases, for which mullein was used.[1] Aaron's rod, Jupiter's staff, and Jacob's staff allude to the stem's upright quality. Candlewick, hag's taper, witches candle, and Our Lady's candle refer to the plant's use as a lamp wick. Dry down from the leaves and stems ignited with ease.[1] The common names blanket herb, blanket leaf, beggar's blanket, flannel flower, Adam's flannel, feltwort, velvet dock, and velvet plant refer to the leaves' soothing, soft texture.[1]

HISTORICAL USES: Europeans and Asians believed mullein had protective properties that repelled evil spirits.[1] Mullein stalks were immersed in suet or tallow, and burned as torches on special occasions and funerals.[1] Roman women rinsed their hair with mullein flower tea as a golden dye.[1] In ancient Greece, mullein seeds were thrown into water to intoxicate and stun fish so they could be caught more easily.[1]

Mullein leaves were administered as a pectoral and expectorant for lung problems, including consumption and bleeding. The leaves were smoked for spasmodic coughs and asthma.[1] The leaves also were worn in stockings to stimulate circulation and warm the feet.[1] Fomentations and poultices of leaves were applied to alleviate hemorrhoids.

A decoction of the root was administered to alleviate toothaches, cramps, or convulsions. An application of mullein leaf juice and root powder was believed to remove rough warts.[1] A poultice prepared by boiling the seeds and leaves in wine was applied to draw out splinters and thorns.[1]

Mullein oil was prepared by macerating and steeping mullein flowers in oil for approximately three weeks, in the sun or near a fire.[1] However, Eclectic physicians Harvey Felter and Finley Ellingwood mention that a truer preparation was made by placing mullein blossoms alone in a lidded, glass bottle in the sun for several days. The mass was strained through muslin and stored. Both preparations were referred to as mulleined or mulleinized oil.[7,8]

The oil was then applied topically to reduce inflammation of the mucous membranes, frostbite, bruises, or hemorrhoids.[1] Mullein oil was administered in the ear canal to relieve an earache or discharge; it was also applied to eczema surrounding the ear.[1] The oil was considered a valuable bactericide.[1]

CONSTITUENTS

MULLEIN ROOTS: Mullein roots contain aucubin, heptaose, nonaose, octaose, and verbascose.[11] Mullein seeds contain mucilage and oleic acid.[11]

MULLEIN LEAVES: Mullein leaves contain calcium, magnesium, iron, β-carotene, mucilaginous polysaccharides, iridoids (acubin), triterpene saponins (verbascosaponin), phenylethanoid glycosides (verbascoside = acteoside), flavonoids (rutin), catalpol, verbasterol, and rotenone.[9-11]

MULLEIN FLOWERS: Mullein flowers contain triterpene saponins (verbascosaponin), mucilaginous polysaccharides, flavonoids (rutin), iridoids (aucubin), phenylethanoid glycosides (verbascoside = acteoside), thapsic acid, crocetin, phenylethanoid glycosides (verbascoside = acteoside), gum, resin, and mineral salts.[1,9-11]

NUTRITIONAL PROPERTIES: Mullein leaves contain high amounts of aluminum, calcium, chromium, cobalt, iron, magnesium, manganese, niacin, phosphorus, silicon, sodium, and vitamins A and C. They also contain low to average amounts of fiber, fat, potassium, protein, riboflavin, selenium, thiamine, and zinc.[11,12] The flowers contain flavonoids (rutin).[10,12]

MEDICINAL PROPERTIES: Mullein root is a bladder tonic, diuretic, expectorant, and antitussive. Mullein leaf has soothing expectorant, antitussive, spasmolytic, mucilaginous, and astringent actions. Mullein flower has soothing expectorant, antitussive, spasmolytic, anti-inflammatory, antimicrobial, and diuretic actions.

TEMPERATURE AND FLAVOR: Mullein root is warm, mildly astringent, and slightly bitter. Mullein flowers are neutral, bitter, and sweet. Mullein leaves are cool, astringent, and bitter.

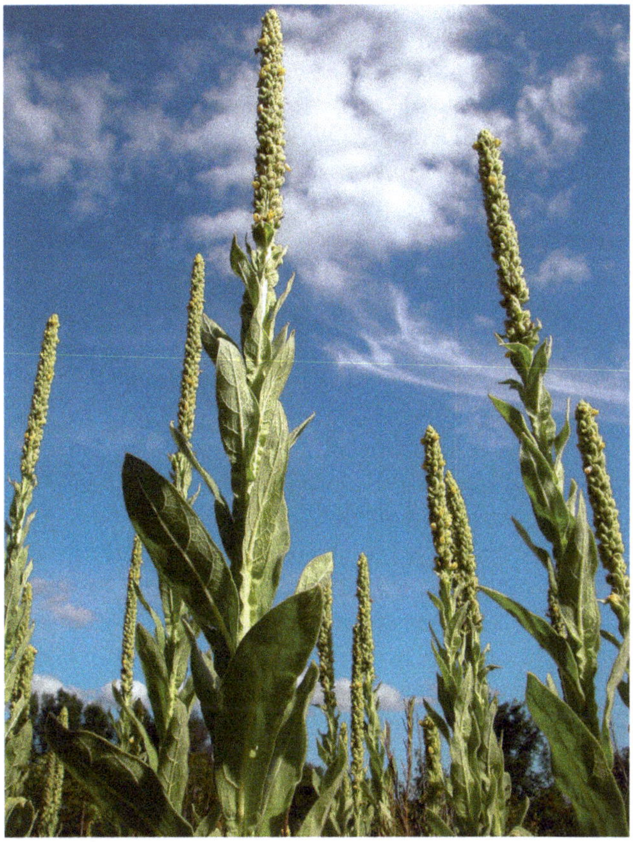

MEDICINAL USES

MULLEIN ROOT: Mullein root is a valuable diuretic, urinary tract astringent, and bladder tonifying agent that aids in treating urinary incontinence (loss of urine without warning).[11] It strengthens and improves the tone of the trigone muscle (a triangular muscle at the base of the bladder), and significantly enhances bladder function.[11,13] Mullein root has soothing diuretic properties; it increases the volume and decreases the frequency of urination. It also has mild astringent properties that reduce inflammation in the bladder mucosa; however, it does not irritate the bladder or kidneys. The flavonoids have a mild diuretic effect; the glycosides reduce inflammation.[9] Mullein root can be consumed as a long-term tonic for individuals with urinary incontinence, recurring bladder infections, interstitial cystitis, or benign prostatic hypertrophy.[11,13]

Mullein root is one of the most effective herbal treatments for stress incontinence caused by coughing, heavy lifting, laughing, running, or aging, in addition to pregnancy- or birth-related incontinence and leakage. Stress incontinence is associated with aging or a cystocele (a bladder hernia protruding into the vagina) resulting from injuries related to childbirth. Mullein root reduces the frequency of urination, decreasing leakage and dribbling. It also improves the integrity of bladder tissues, and restores the tone of a prolapsed bladder.[13] Although a single extract of mullein root works well, combinations containing saw palmetto *(Serenoa* — liposterolic extract*)*, yellow pond lily *(Nuphar)*, and corn silk *(Zea mays)* work effectively for treating a prolapsed bladder and cystocele. However, relief during the latter half of the third trimester of gestation may be limited, due to the constant pressure of the fetus on the bladder. Combine the following herbs for a pregnancy- and nursing-safe bladder compound containing mullein root *(Verbascum)*, corn silk *(Zea mays)*, saw palmetto *(Serenoa* — liposterolic extract*)*, yellow pond lily *(Nuphar)*, and nettle root *(Urtica)*.

Mullein aids in treating urinary incontinence in children, including enuresis (nighttime bedwetting). It is appropriate for children four years or older who continue to have bedwetting problems. Children can experience a significant decrease in bedwetting frequency when consuming mullein root daily; in this case, the cause of bedwetting must be primarily physical, rather than emotional. Prepare a children's bladder strengthening compound using alcohol or glycerin as the menstruum. Combine equal parts of mullein root *(Verbascum)* and corn silk *(Zea mays)*; consume 30 – 60 drops in 2 – 4 ounces of water, two to three times daily. Additionally, limit or discontinue the child's consumption of beverages two to three hours before bedtime. *Note:* It is important for parents or guardians to understand that children should not hold back urine too long, because a urinary tract infection can occur. Also, young children have small bladders and need to urinate more frequently than adults.

Mullein root is a long-term tonic for individuals with recurring bladder infections and interstitial cystitis (chronic bladder inflammation and irritation). It aids in treating symptoms of a urinary tract infection when test results are negative for bacteria. Mullein reduces lingering inflammation in the bladder that can cause a sense of urgency, urinary tenesmus (painful straining), and dysuria (painful urination). Combine the following herbal extracts as a long-term treatment for interstitial cystitis, and to reduce bladder weakness: mullein root *(Verbascum root)*, fresh corn silk *(Zea mays)*, yellow pond lily *(Nuphar)*, saw palmetto *(Serenoa* — liposterolic extract*)*, and horsetail *(Equisetum)*. The following tea formula soothes the urinary system: three parts marshmallow root *(Althaea officinalis)*, two parts mullein root *(Verbascum)*, one part gravel root

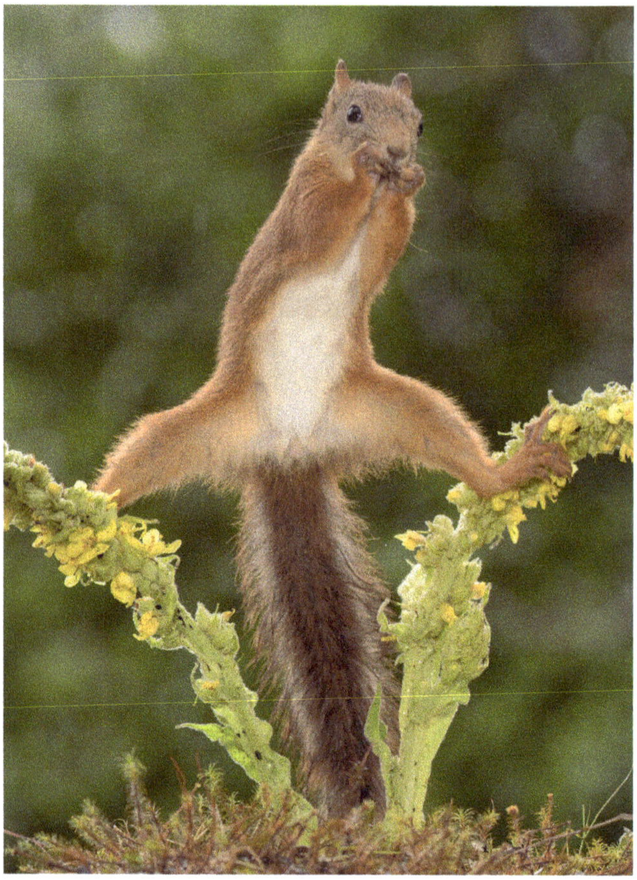

(Eutrochium purpureum), and one-quarter part licorice root *(Glycyrrhiza glabra)*.

Mullein root reduces prostate swelling and inflammation, and can be useful for treating benign prostatic hypertrophy (BPH).[11] The diuretic and astringent actions have a soothing and anti-inflammatory effect on the bladder, prostate, and urethra.[13] The root decreases dribbling and the sensation of a dull ache in the prostate gland. Use the root alone, or in combination, as a long-term tonic to address BPH symptoms. Mullein root can be combined with the following herbs to treat BPH: nettle root *(Urtica)*, yellow pond lily *(Nuphar)*, pygeum *(Prunus africanus)*, and saw palmetto *(Serenoa repens* — liposterolic extract*)*.

When treating patients with urinary incontinence, a cystocele, or benign prostatic hypertrophy, practicing Kegel exercises at frequent intervals throughout the day is important for strengthening the bladder. Patients are also encouraged to practice Kegel exercises during urination by starting and stopping the urinary stream intermittently. Kegel exercises strengthen the pubococcygeal muscles.

In addition, patients with chronic bladder and prostate problems experience a faster recovery when they avoid consuming bladder irritants such as coffee, chocolate, alcohol, citrus, soda, carbonated beverages, refined or processed foods, and foods and beverages containing sulfites. It is also important to identify food allergies, as they can sometimes cause irritation and bladder inflammation.

MULLEIN LEAF AND FLOWER: Mullein leaf and flower have expectorant, antitussive, and soothing demulcent actions in the respiratory tract.[1,9-11] Consuming a tea of mullein leaf or flower aids in treating a sore throat, laryngitis, tracheitis, hoarseness, a dry cough, whooping cough, asthma, a cold, or flu.[10] Mullein leaves and flowers contain triterpene saponins and mucilage that cause the demulcent, antitussive, and emollient actions.[9,10,12] The saponins are likely responsible for the expectorant actions.[9] Additional anti-infective agents are necessary; however, mullein leaves reduce respiratory tract inflammation.[11,13] The anti-inflammatory actions of the flowers are due to verbascoside, which inhibits the biosynthesis of leukotrienes.[11] The flowers also contain aucubin and other irodoids that have mild antimicrobial actions.[11] Water-based preparations have demulcent and mild astringent actions that reduce inflammation in the digestive tract.[1]

Mullein leaf is an expectorant, antitussive, and bulking agent for smoking blends. Smoking the herb has mild expectorant and antitussive actions; however, smoking can irritate respiratory tissue.[1,11,13] To prepare a smoking blend, combine mullein leaf with coltsfoot *(Tussilago or Petasites)*, raspberry leaf *(Rubus idaeus)*, pearly everlasting leaf *(Anaphalis)*, and smaller amounts of damiana *(Turnera)* and/or mint *(Mentha)*.

A water-based poultice prepared from the leaves has topical anti-inflammatory actions. The poultice aids in treating abrasions, wounds, bruises, ulcers, and hemorrhoids.[9,10]

The infused oil or a glycerin-alcohol based extract of mullein flower aids in treating an earache or the early stages of an ear infection.[8,9] It can be combined with more potent antibacterial and anti-inflammatory agents for increased effectiveness. For example, combine equal parts of echinacea *(Echinacea)*, St. John's wort *(Hypericum)*, and mullein flower glycerin extracts (fresh plant extracts containing 50% glycerin and 50% alcohol), then place two to five drops in the ear canal, three times daily. Another option is to combine equal parts of infused oils of mullein and St. John's wort, then infuse the blend with fresh chopped garlic 8 – 12 hours before straining the mixture. Place three to five drops of finished oil in the ear canal. Add 1 – 2 drops of blue chamomile essential oil *(Matricaria recutita)* per 1 – 2 ounces of the blend to further reduce pain and inflammation.

CONTRAINDICATIONS

The entire plant is non-toxic; however, the wooly hairs on the leaves can irritate the skin, and may cause a rash in sensitive individuals. The hairs from the leaves and flowers can irritate the mucous membranes in the throat, causing a slight tickle. Consider wearing a mask and gloves when processing mullein leaves. When preparing tea, strain the leaves and flowers through a fine cloth or paper coffee filter before consuming. Otherwise, there are no known side effects of mullein.[10] Consumption is considered safe during pregnancy and lactation, as well as in small children and the elderly.[10]

PREPARATION AND DOSAGE

TINCTURE: Fresh leaves or flowers [1:2-1:4, 70-95% alcohol]; dry leaves or flowers [1:5, 60% alcohol]; consume 15-90 drops, up to four times daily. Fresh roots [1:2, 70-95% alcohol]; dry roots [1:5, 60-70% alcohol]; consume 10-60 drops, up to three times daily.

GLYCERITE: Fresh leaves or flowers [1:3, 50% glycerin, 50% alcohol]; consume 10-60 drops, up to four times daily, or place 2-5 drops in the ear canal.

TEA: Prepare the leaves or flowers as a hot infusion; consume 8-12 ounces, up to four times daily. Prepare a decoction of the root; consume 8-12 ounces, three to four times daily.

TOPICAL USE: Infuse wilted mullein flowers in olive oil, steep up to three weeks, and strain. Or prepare dry flowers as an infused oil using the alcohol intermediary method. Before administering compounded oil or extract in the ear, the patient should be reclining, lying on the side opposite the affected ear. Place several drops of compound in the ear, then cover with a warm cloth or a garlic and onion poultice, and recline 15 to 30 minutes. Many patients find relief from this application. Consuming an antimicrobial compound also aids in fighting an ear infection. Dilute the tincture in water and apply as a liniment to the affected area. *Note:* The *Historical Uses* section refers to the Eclectic method of preparing the medicinal oil.

MYRRH

DESCRIPTION

BOTANICAL NAMES:
Commiphora myrrha, C. molmol, C. madagascariensis, C. habessinica

COMMON NAMES:
Myrrh, myrrh gum, myrrh resin, myrrh pitch, hirabol myrrh, gum tree, karan
mo yao shu, mo yao (Chinese)
mirhami (Finnish)
myrrhe (French)
myrrhe (German)
mirra (Italian)
motsuyaku (Japanese)
molyak (Korean)
bola (Sanskrit)
bissa bol, molmol (Somali)
mirra (Spanish)

FAMILY NAME:
Burseraceae

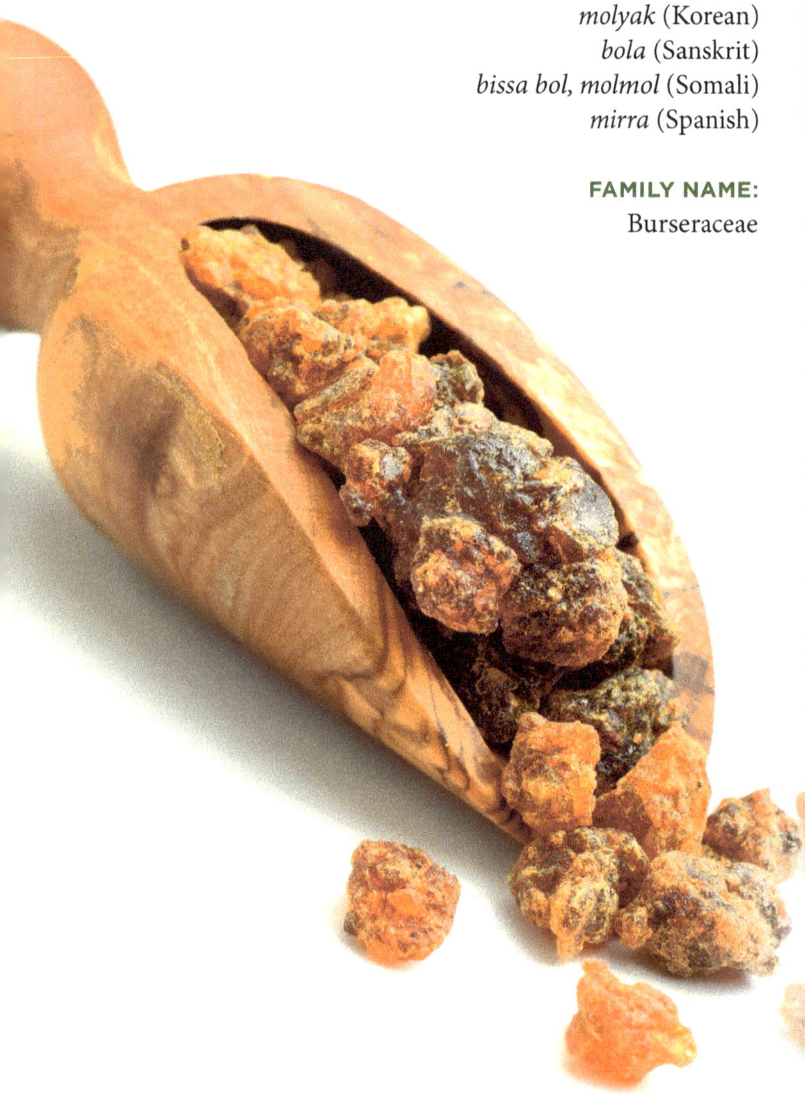

PART USED: The hardened oleo-gum-resin (pitch or gum) exuded from the tree.

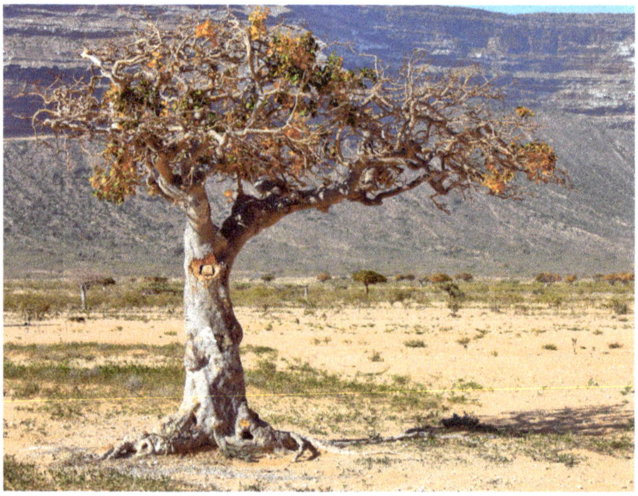

BOTANICAL DESCRIPTION AND HABITAT: *Commiphora* is a genus of aromatic, often spiny, dioecious trees and shrubs native to Ethiopia, Somalia, and the Arabian Peninsula.[1-3] The resin collected from these trees is cultivated commercially throughout North Africa, the Middle East, and western Asia.[2] Myrrh thrives in hot, arid conditions in well-drained soil.[2]

Many species of *Commiphora* have stout trunks with smooth or papery bark. The green inner bark is capable of photosynthesis.[1,4] When the bark is cut or damaged, a fragrant yellow, oleo-gum-resin is secreted that hardens and clarifies as it dries. The compound leaves grow alternate along the branches, or are found in fascicles.[4] The unisexual flowers have a fused calyx and four petals; male flowers have eight unequal stamens. The female flowers have a short stigma and a two- to four-chambered, ovoid ovary that matures into a fleshy, resinous drupe.[1,4]

Commiphora myrrha is the species most often utilized medicinally in the U.S. It is a spiny shrub or small tree native to the Arabian Peninsula and northeastern Africa. It grows up to four meters tall and has pale, papery bark and trifoliate light green leaves (6 – 44 mm long by 3 – 20 mm wide) varied in shape.[5]

THE NAME: The genus name *Commiphora* derives from two Greek words: *kommi* ("gum") and *phoros* ("carrier"). The epithet *myrrha* and the common name myrrh derive from the Arabic *mur* ("bitter").[2] The epithet *madagascariensis* indicates its Madagascar origin.

These common names correspond with the following Latin binomials: African and Somali myrrh *(Commiphora myrrha)*, Arabian and Yemen myrrh *(C. madagascariensis)*, and myrrh *(C. molmol)*.

HISTORICAL USES: Myrrh has been a precious commodity since ancient times.[2] Ancient Egyptians utilized myrrh as medicine and in the embalming process.[2,3] Northeast Africa and Arabian cultures prized the herb as a slow-burning incense and holy oil in religious rituals.[2] Myrrh was an important ingredient in incense and perfumes.[2] Myrrh, frankincense, and gold were among the offerings of the Wise Men at Christ's birth.[2] In biblical times, myrrh was used to treat mouth sores, infected wounds, and respiratory and digestive concerns.[2] The resin was utilized in Ayurvedic medicine to treat mouth sores, gum disease, sore throats, and skin ulcers.[2] Myrrh was introduced to China in 600 CE, and continues to be used for similar purposes.[2]

Eclectic physicians administered myrrh extract as an antiseptic, sialagogue, and expectorant.[6] It was believed to stimulate the mucous membranes, as well as the respiratory and circulatory systems. Myrrh was given as an astringent to suppress excessive respiratory secretions, and enhance circulation in inactive mucous membranes, encouraging expectoration and diaphoresis.[6] Myrrh was administered to treat gum sores and mouth or throat ulcers, as well as catarrh of the leukorrhea and bladder.[6] Physician Finley Ellingwood recommended using myrrh to stimulate digestive secretions and enhance nutrient digestion and assimilation.[6] He also recommended myrrh to treat apepsia and inactivity of the stomach in alcoholics.[6] Myrrh was administered with aloe and iron as an emmenagogue for amenorrhea with a dragging sensation in the pelvis.[6,7] A mouth rinse of myrrh was recommended to treat mercurial salivation.[6,7]

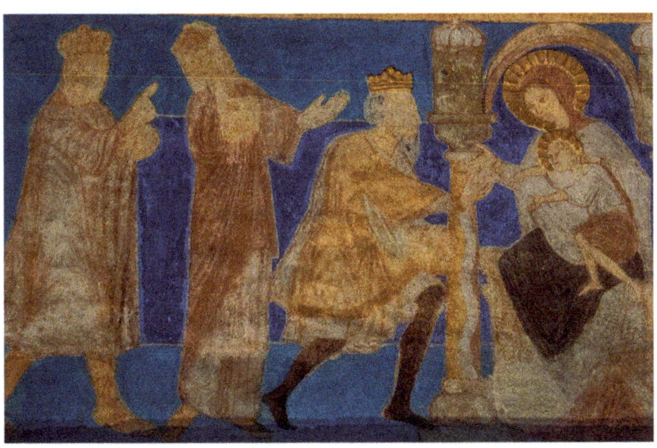

Myrrh continues to be incorporated into perfumes, cosmetics, dentifrices, and soaps.[3,8] Burn myrrh resin to cleanse a meditation space.

CONSTITUENTS: Myrrh contains volatile oil (heerabolene, limonene, dipentene, pinene, eugenol, cinnamaldehyde, cuminaldehyde, cumic alcohol, m-cresol, cadinene, curzerene, curzerenone, dihydropyrocurzerenone, furnoeudesma-1,3-diene, 1,10(15)-furanodiene-6-one, and lindestrene), resin (α-, β-, and γ-commiphoric acids, commiphorinic acid, α- and β-heerabomyrrhols, heeraboresene, commiferin, campesterol, β-sitosterol, cholesterol, α-amyrone, and 3-epi-α-amyrin), and gum (which on hydrolysis yields arabinose, galactose, xylose, and 4-O-methylglucuronic acid).[8,9]

NUTRITIONAL PROPERTIES: Not applicable.

MEDICINAL PROPERTIES: Antibacterial, anticatarrhal, antifungal, anti-inflammatory, antiviral, astringent, bitter tonic, carminative, expectorant, hemostatic, immune stimulant, stomachic, and vulnerary.

TEMPERATURE AND FLAVOR: Warm, bitter, pungent, and astringent.

MEDICINAL USES

Myrrh is a potent antimicrobial, immune stimulant, and astringent.[6-8] It has antibacterial, antifungal, antiviral, and expectorant properties.[6,7,9] The sesquiterpenes have antibacterial and antifungal effects.[11] *In vitro* studies of two sesquiterpenes (furanodiene-6-one and methoxyfuranoguaia-9-ene-8-one) demonstrated antibacterial activity against *Pseudomonas aeruginosa, Staphylococcus aureus,* and *Escherichia coli,* as well as antifungal activity against *Candida albicans.*[11] It contains oleoresins (oleo-gum-resin) that are excreted unchanged in the respiratory and urinary tracts; they disinfect and stimulate the mucous membranes.[12] Myrrh aids in treating a common cold, sinusitis, pharyngitis, laryngitis, tonsillitis, strep throat, mononucleosis, bronchitis (moist), chronic mucus, candida, and diarrhea.[9] Consuming small quantities of myrrh extract (5 – 10 drops) enhances immunity by increasing the number and quality of white blood cells and their scavenging capacity.[12] However, it is best used as a short-term, acute immune stimulant to increase

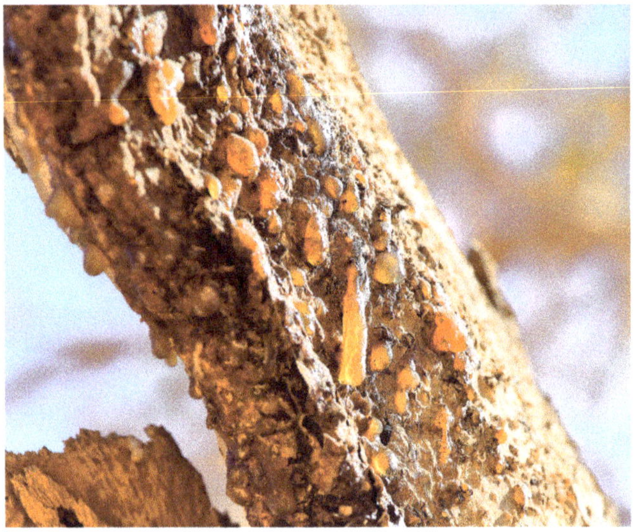

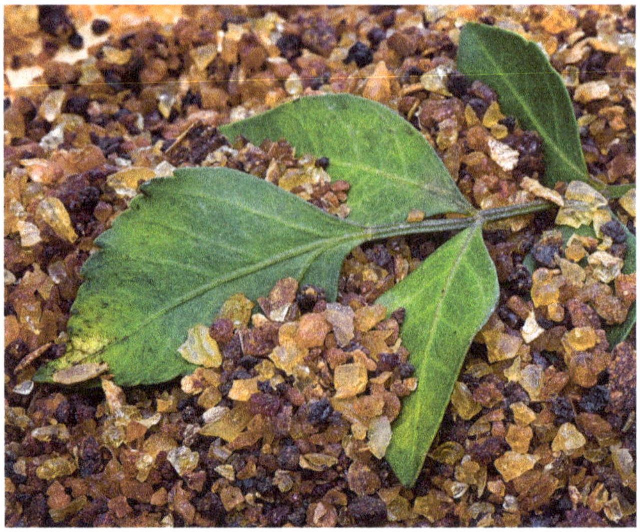

resistance to infection. Myrrh is also a urinary tract antibacterial; however, it should be consumed no more than 7 – 10 consecutive days.[12]

Myrrh has carminative, stomachic, and bitter tonic properties that stimulate the appetite, especially following an acute digestive infection.[6,7] Low doses (5 – 10 drops) aid in treating dyspepsia and chronic gastritis.[6-8] It is an intestinal antiseptic and astringent that reduces diarrhea.[7,10] It has antiparasitic effects against various schistosome species, including *Schistosoma mansoni, S. haematobium,* and *S. japonicum.*[11] Myrrh stimulates smooth muscles and may stimulate peristalsis.[11] While further clinical studies are warranted, rodent studies demonstrated that myrrh lowered blood glucose levels and reduced hepatic gluconeogenesis. [11] Myrrh could be of interest in treating diabetes mellitus, pending future studies on humans.

Myrrh extract is extremely effective for treating dental and oral conditions.[3,6-10] Gargling with a mouthwash or diluted tincture aids in treating thrush, gingivitis, pyorrhea, canker sores, denture sores, gum infections, and abscessed teeth.[7-9] Combine with echinacea *(Echinacea),* calendula *(Calendula),* spilanthes *(Acmella),* yerba mansa *(Anemopsis),* bayberry *(Morella),* and/or clove *(Syzygium)* as a mouthwash for the aforementioned conditions. *Note:* The resin does not dissolve in water; when myrrh extract is combined with water, the solution will become cloudy.

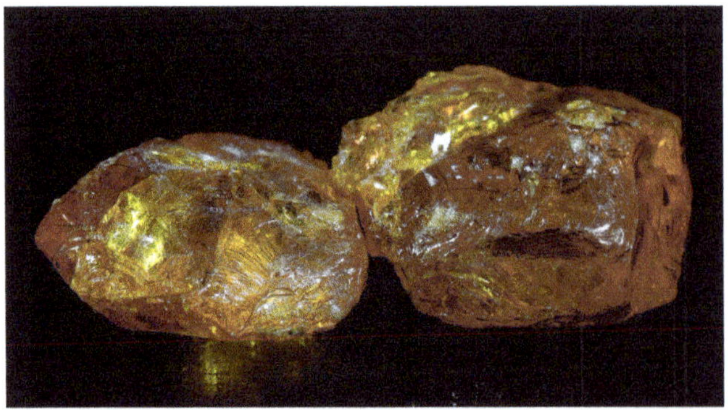

Topical preparations (i.e., liniment, tincture, salve, or diluted essential oil) have antimicrobial, astringent, anti-inflammatory, hemostatic, and vulnerary actions. Employ myrrh preparations to treat indolent ulcers, bedsores, herpes, shingles, cuts, bruises, wounds, hemorrhoids, bacterial infections (including staph), and fungal infections (athlete's foot, ringworm, tinea, and thrush).[3,9-11] Myrrh also reduces minor bleeding of the skin. It can be combined with usnea *(Usnea),* calendula *(Calendula),* echinacea *(Echinacea),* yerba mansa *(Anemopsis),* and/or chaparral *(Larrea)* for topical use as an antimicrobial. Or add 2 – 5 drops of myrrh essential oil per one ounce of salve.

CONTRAINDICATIONS

Avoid consuming myrrh during pregnancy or lactation.[7-9] Administer with caution in children under the age of 12. Myrrh is contraindicated with existing kidney weakness, inflammation, or disease.[12] Excessive doses can cause gastric burning, diaphoresis, vomiting, or purgation.[6,7] The resins in myrrh can aggravate the kidneys; discontinue use if a dull ache in the mid to lower back occurs.[12] Due to the potential hypoglycemic effects, exercise caution with individuals using Type II diabetes hypoglycemic medications.[11] Use caution with individuals consuming blood thinning medications such as warfarin (Coumadin), as well as one to two weeks prior to, and following surgery, because it can increase hepatic enzymes that encourage metabolism of this medication.[11]

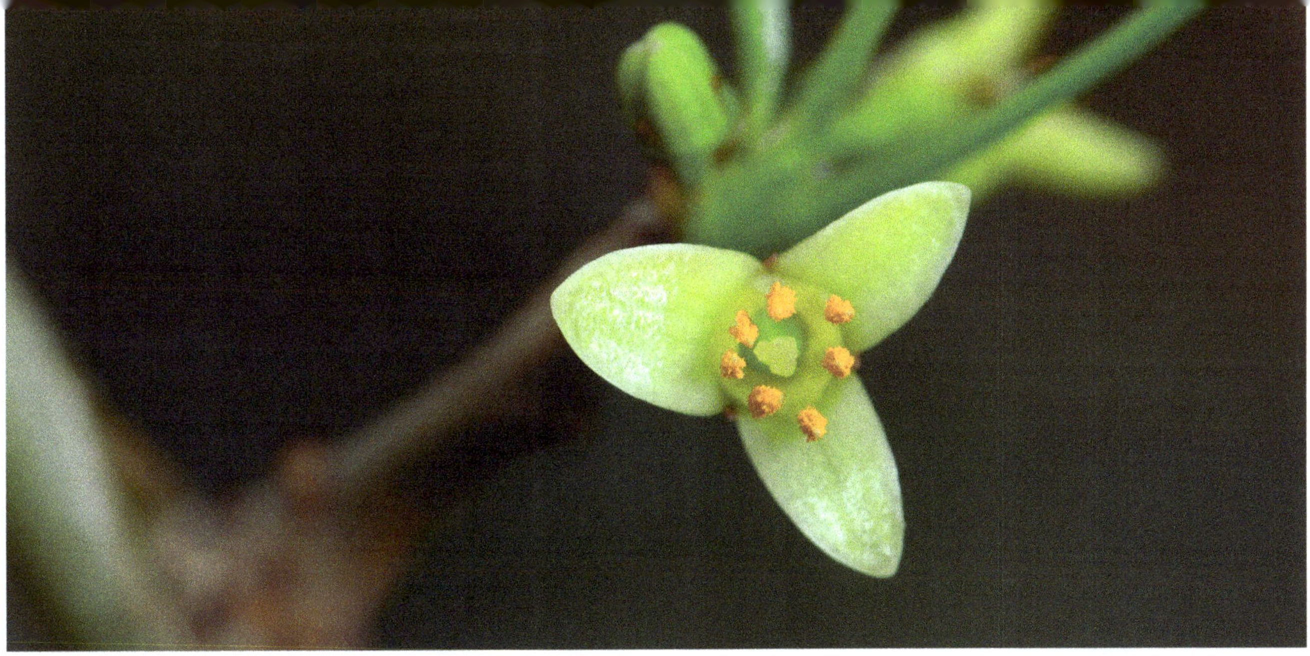

PREPARATION AND DOSAGE

TINCTURE: Resin [1:5, 95% alcohol]; consume 5–30 drops, up to three times daily. Dilute the tincture in water, or add to a salve for topical use.

CAPSULES: Consume 2–3 capsules, up to three times daily. To prepare myrrh essential oil capsules, fill "0" or "00" capsules with a binding agent such as marshmallow root powder or slippery elm powder, then add 2 drops of essential oil into each capsule. Close the capsules, and store in a zip-lock bag in the refrigerator or freezer. Consume 1 capsule, up to three times daily. *Note:* Take care not to drop essential oil into the capsules without a binder, or the capsules will dissolve.

TEA: Not advisable, as the only water-soluble portion of myrrh is the gum. The resinous portion does not extract in water.

HONEY AND SYRUP: Add 1–3 drops of essential oil to 1 tablespoon of honey; apply topically or dissolve in hot water or tea for internal consumption.

TOPICAL USE: Add the tincture to a salve, or prepare an oil using the alcohol oil method, infused oil method, powder, dust, or diluted essential oil. Myrrh powder can be added to dentifrices. The resin can be burned on coal as incense.

ESSENTIAL OIL: Dilute 2–4 drops of essential oil in a carrier oil and apply topically as needed.

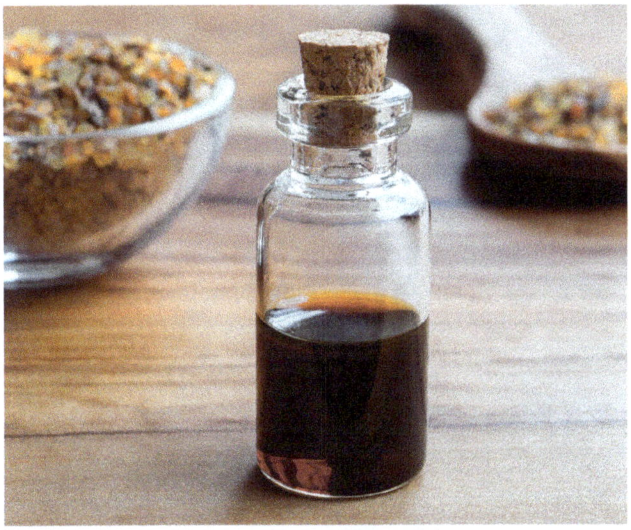

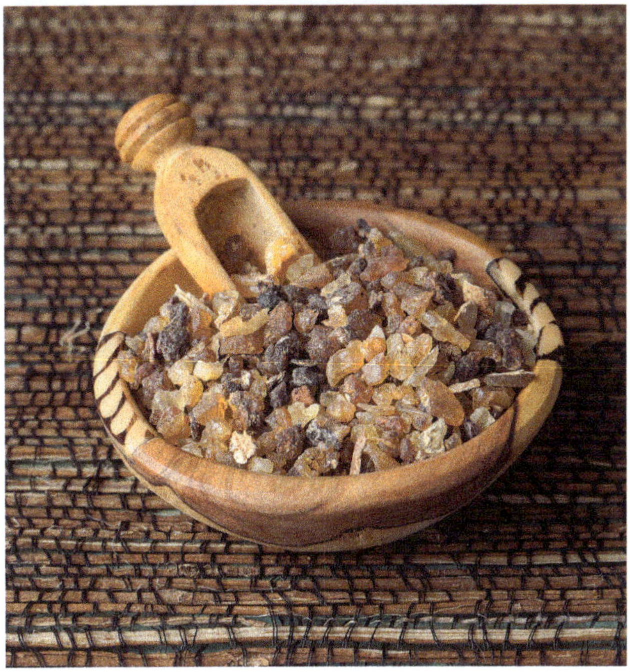

NETTLE

DESCRIPTION

BOTANICAL NAMES:
Urtica dioica, U. urens, U. gracilis

COMMON NAMES:
Nettle, stinging nettle, Indian spinach, wild spinach, devil's leaf, devil's plaything
kopriva (Bulgarian)
naelde, braendenaelde (Danish)
braunetel (Dutch)
buluhan (Filipino)
nokkonen (Finnish)
ortie, herbe d'ortie, racine d'ortie (French)
brennessel, brennesselkraut, brennesselwurzel, haarnesselkraut, haarnesselwurzel (German)
horreig, sorbei (Greek)
sirpad (Hebrew)
bichu (Hindi)
ortica (Italian)
nesle (Norwegian)
pokrzywa (Polish)
krapiva (Russian)
bichu (Sanskrit)
ortiga (Spanish)
brännässla, nässla (Swedish)

FAMILY NAME:
Urticaceae

PARTS USED: The leaves, roots, and seeds.

BOTANICAL DESCRIPTION AND HABITAT: Nettle grows in colonies, usually in shaded, woody areas. It thrives in moist soil, often near a water source. Do not harvest nettle from polluted areas, as it can absorb heavy metals,

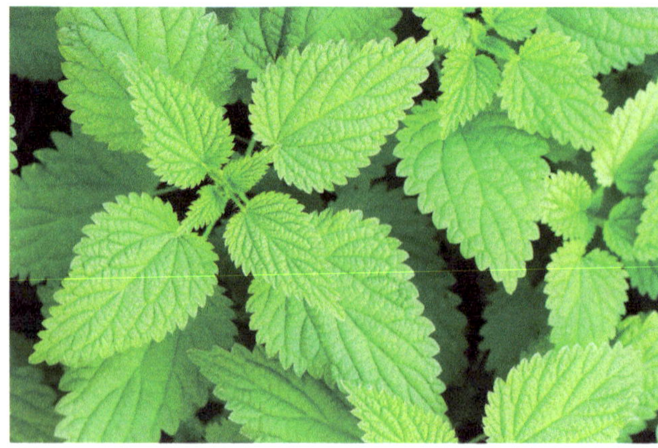

pesticides, and toxins from the soil. Nettle grows wild throughout North America. The roots colonize and spread prolifically, becoming quite invasive in the garden; cultivate with caution.

Urtica dioica is an erect, herbaceous perennial (1 – 3 meters high) dying back each year to its dense system of rhizomes.[1] The entire plant is covered with stinging hairs that dispense irritating chemicals, immediately causing contact dermatitis when touched. The weak stems contain long, coarse bast fibers. The opposite, narrowly lanceolate to widely ovate, dark green leaves (3 – 15 cm long) have prominent veins, serrate margins, and obvious stipules.[1] Their bases may be cordate or simply narrow toward the petiole.[1]

The plant bears dense, pendant, axillary clusters (1 – 7 cm long) of tiny green, unisexual, apetalous flowers.[1] Each flower has four opposite sepals; staminate flowers have four stamens. In pistillate flowers, the outer two sepals are smaller than the inner two, which surround a superior ovary with a single carpel.[1] The fruit is an ovate achene.[1]

Urtica dioica ssp. *dioica* (European stinging nettle) is native to Europe, and while naturalized in other parts of North America. It is dioecious.[2]

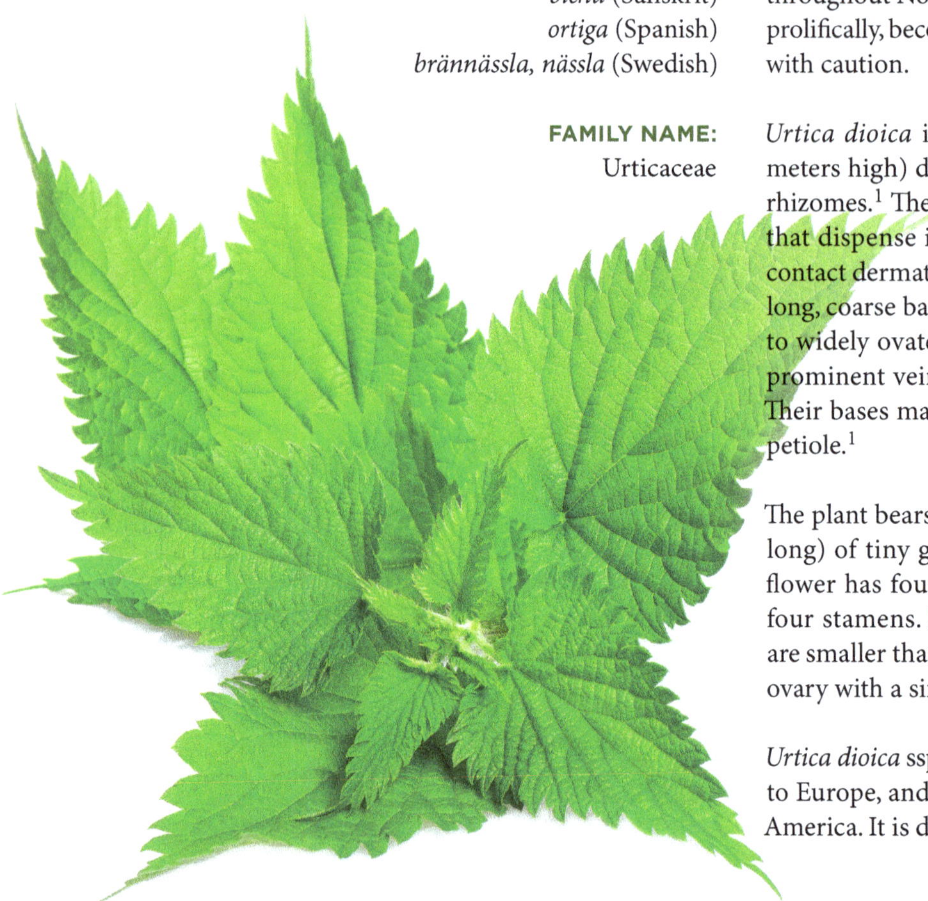

U. dioica ssp. *gracilis* (American stinging nettle) is native to North America. It is monoecious, with a green stem. The quantity of non-stinging hairs on the stem and undersides of the leaves can vary; in some plants there is a moderate amount, while others lack them.[3]

U. dioica ssp. *holosericea* (hoary nettle) is usually monoecious.[4] Native to the western U.S., it usually grows in wetlands. The stem is grayish, due to the moderate to dense non-stinging hairs on the stem and leaf undersides.[4]

U. urens (dwarf nettle) is a closely related, monoecious, annual species of stinging nettle.[5] Generally smaller than *U. dioica,* this species (up to 80 cm tall) bears smaller, smoother, elliptic leaves (2 – 9 cm long by 1 – 4.5 cm wide) with lobe-like serrations on the margins.[5] This species also differs from *U. dioica,* as its inflorescences are more spike- or panicle-like and smaller. It is native to Eurasia, but grows throughout North America, especially in cultivated areas and roadsides.

THE NAME: *Urtica* ("sting") derives from Latin.[6] The epithet *dioica* means "two houses," referring to the fact that there are male flowers on some plants, and female flowers on others. The epithet *urens* also means stinging or burning; *gracilis* means slender or graceful.[6] Nettle comes from the Anglo-Saxon and Dutch synonym *netel* that derives from *noedl* (a needle), referring to the sharp sting.[7] The names wild spinach and Indian spinach refer to its use as a wild, nutritious food.[8]

HISTORICAL USES: Native Americans and Europeans consumed nettle as food and medicine.[8] Fresh leaves were often included in soups.[7] In Scotland, it was combined with leeks and broccoli to make nettle pudding.[7] Nettle, dandelion, and cleavers beer was a folk remedy used to treat arthritis and gout.[7] A decoction of nettle leaf mixed with salt was used as a rennet substitute to curdle milk.[7] A hemostatic, nettle tea or tincture was consumed to staunch bleeding.[7] Young, fresh shoots were consumed as a spring tonic, blood purifier, and alterative.[7] The seed or leaf tea eased consumption.[7] Nettle leaf tea mixed with leaf juice was applied to heal burns and alleviate nettle rashes.[7] Nettle seeds were consumed to ease spider bites and insect stings, and as an antidote for hemlock, henbane, or nightshade poisoning.[7] Eclectic physicians administered nettle to treat diarrhea, dysentery, colon disease, hemorrhoids, bleeding, nephritis, kidney stones, and chronic skin eruptions.[9] Nettle seeds were used to treat consumption and goiter.[9] The seeds and flowers were combined to ease ague.[9]

Native Americans and Romans practiced urtication (flogging with nettle) in order to provoke inflammation, and reduce arthritic pain through counterirritant action.[6,7] Roman soldiers rubbed nettle on their limbs to stimulate circulation and reduce stiffness or numbness when travelling in cold northern European climates.[7] European herbalists stimulated hair growth by applying nettle juice mixed with nettle tea to the scalp.[7]

Nettle was used by Nevada Indians to fumigate sweat lodges when treating a flu or pneumonia.[6] The Salish administered nettle to relax women's muscles during birth.[6] It was also used to improve breast milk flow.[6] Nettle fiber was used to make fish nets, snares, and tumplines.[8]

Early farmers fed livestock dried nettle leaves mixed with hay because they believed it enabled cows to produce more milk.[7] Malnourished horses thrived from consuming nettle-enriched fodder, and their coats improved.[7] Powdered nettle added to chicken feed increased egg production and fattened fowls.[7]

Nettle fiber was used to make durable for clothing, stockings, sacking, sailcloth, cord, and fishing net twine.[7] When Germany and Austria ran out of cotton during World War

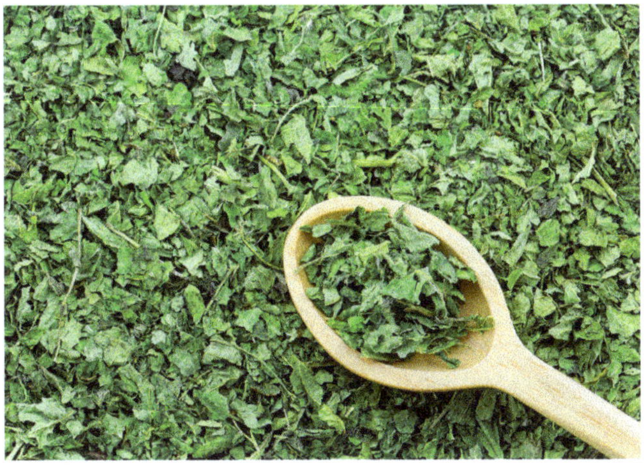

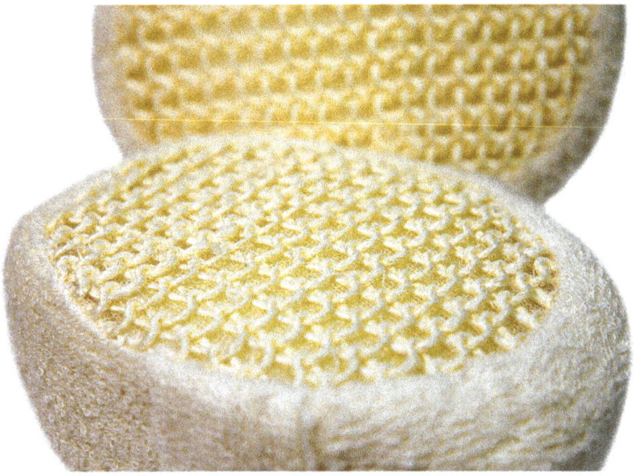

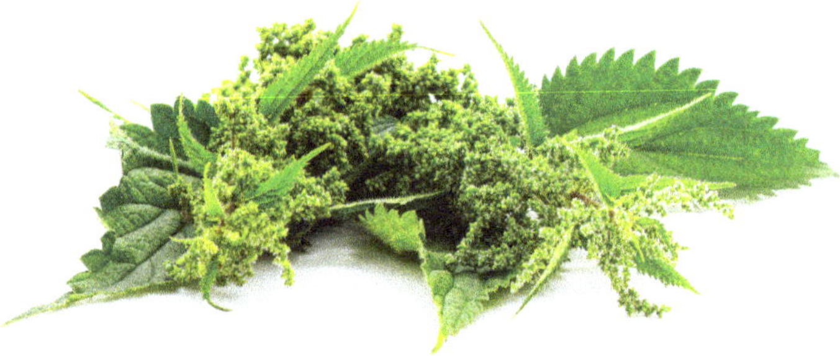

II, nettle fiber was substituted.[7] A decoction of nettle leaves was used to dye wool. Nettle fiber was used to produce paper.[7]

The adage "nettle in, dock out" refers to using fresh yellow dock *(Rumex crispus)* leaf poultice to remedy a nettle sting. Plantain or other astringent herbs may be substituted.

CONSTITUENTS

NETTLE LEAVES: Nettle leaves contain amines (histamine, serotonin, 5-hydroxytryptamine, and acetylcholine), flavonoids (isoquercitrin, rutin, kaempferol, and isorhamnetin), a lectin *(Urtica dioica* agglutinin*)*, acetophenone, butyric acid, phenolic acid, caffeic acid, formic acid, silicic acid, citric acid, vitamin C, triterpenes, β-sitosterol, chlorophyll, carotenoids, calcium, and potassium.[9-12]

NETTLE ROOTS: Nettle roots contain phytosterols (β-sitosterol and β-sitosterolin = β-sitosterol-glucoside), coumarins (scopoletin), lignans (secoisolariciresinol, (-)-3,4-divanillyltetrahydrofuran, and (-)-pinoresinol neo-olivil), a lectin (*Urtica dioica* agglutinin = UDA), polysaccharides, phenylpropanes, polyphenols, triterpenes (oleanolic acid), minerals (silicic acid), 13-trihydroxy-10-octadecenoic acid, oisalariciresinol, stigmast-4-en-3-one, and ceramides.[9,11,12]

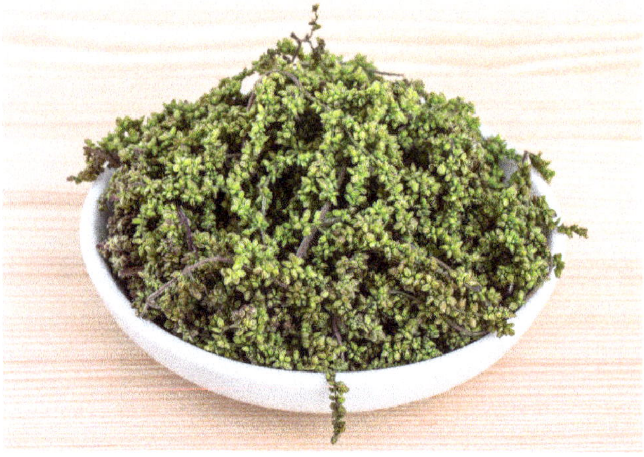

NETTLE SEEDS: Nettle seeds contain linoleic acid, linolenic acid, and palmitic acid.[11,13]

NUTRITIONAL PROPERTIES: Nettle leaf is rich in minerals, including calcium, chromium, cobalt, iron, magnesium, manganese, potassium, phosphorus, selenium, silicon, sodium, sulfur, and zinc. It also contains nutrients such as protein, chlorophyll, α-tocopherol, β-carotene, and vitamins C and K. Nettle contains some B vitamins, including niacin, pantothenic acid, riboflavin, and thiamine. It is a highly nutritious herb that can be consumed in tea or food.[10,11,14,15] Nettle tea contains nitrogen that nourishes plants.

MEDICINAL PROPERTIES: Nettle leaf is an alterative, antiallergenic, anticatarrhal, anti-inflammatory, antidyscratic, antioxidant, antirheumatic, antiscorbutic, astringent, blood tonic, decongestant, depurative, diuretic, expectorant, galactagogue, hemostatic, mucolytic, nutritive, recuperative, and styptic. Nettle root inhibits cell proliferation in benign prostatic hypertrophy and inhibits sex hormone-binding globulin. Nettle seed is a kidney trophorestorative.

TEMPERATURE AND FLAVOR: Nettle leaf is neutral, salty, astringent, and mildly bitter. Nettle root is neutral, sweet, salty, and bland. Nettle seed is neutral, mildly bitter, and astringent.

MEDICINAL USES

NETTLE LEAVES: An effective anti-inflammatory, antiallergenic, decongestant, and astringent, nettle aids in treating allergies, allergic rhinitis, food sensitivities, and congestion due to sinus or lung infections.[6,9] It also reduces wheezing and coughing.[6,7] Due to its astringent qualities, nettle reduces inflammation in mucous membranes and tissues.[11] Nettle reduces the allergic response by inhibiting prostaglandin and leukotriene biosynthesis.[12] Nettle leaf extract reduces the release of inflammatory cytokines, and stimulated interleukin-6 (IL-6) secretion.[9] IL-6 antagonizes the actions of IL-1-β in reducing prostaglandin E_2 synthesis, and stimulates inhibitors of proteinases, reducing inflammation.[9] The anti-inflammatory effects are attributed to caffeic malic acid and other related phenolic acid derivatives that inhibit arachidonic acid metabolites, including cyclooxygenase and 5-lipoxygenase-derived reactions.[9,12] However, there may be additional components involved that are not yet known.[9] As a preventative, consume two 300 mg freeze-dried nettle leaf capsules daily, one to two months prior to allergy season. For acute treatment of allergies, consume 2 – 6 freeze-dried capsules daily (300 mg

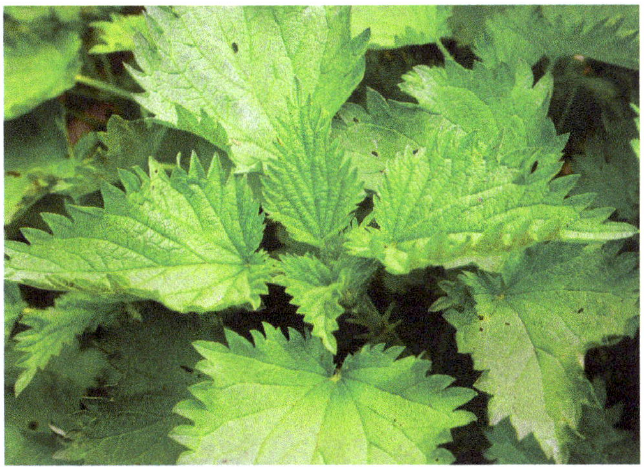

each).[10] Combinations containing quercetin and freeze-dried nettle work more effectively than nettle alone. Nettle has antibacterial activity against *Staphylococcus aureus* and *S. albus, in vitro.*[9,10]

Nettle leaf aids in treating and slowing the progression of rheumatoid arthritis and osteoarthritis. In these conditions, activated monocytes and macrophages produce the cytokines TNF-α and IL-1-β that destroy bone and cartilage, catalyzing the disease process. Nettle leaf prevents joint and bone destruction by inhibiting cytokine-induced destruction of cartilage and bone. In contrast, prostaglandin-inhibiting medications solely reduce the inflammatory process, but not disease progression.[9] In a three-week clinical study, rheumatoid arthritis patients found nettle leaf extract as effective as NSAID therapy in reducing pain and increasing motility.[9] In another comparative two-week trial, patients with acute arthritis consumed 50 g of stewed, fresh young leaves and a 50 mg dose of diclofenac, or a 200 mg of diclofenac daily. Both groups experienced notable improvement in C-reactive protein levels, and total joint scores improved an average 70%. Stewed nettle leaf significantly improved the antirheumatic effectiveness of the NSAID.[9] Another three-week trial was conducted with 8,955 patients suffering from osteoarthritis or rheumatoid arthritis. Based on a self-rated scale, 82% of patients experienced symptom relief, 38% could reduce NSAID therapy, and 26% no longer required NSAID therapy.[9]

Nettle leaf tea and fresh juice are diuretics that aid in treating edema and water-related weight gain.[10,11] Nettle eases pregnancy-related edema, and premenstrual and diabetic water retention.[11] It has mild hypotensive effects in individuals with sodium-related hypertension.[10] Nettle reduces mild cardiac edema and venous insufficiency.[11] It enhances kidney elimination of sodium, uric acid, and other byproducts of protein metabolism.[11] Nettle eases the passing of kidney stones.[9] Consuming the tea or juice long-term prevents the buildup of solids in the kidneys.[6,9-12] Prepare a diuretic tea by combining nettle, parsley root or seeds *(Petroselinum),* cleavers *(Galium)* or chickweed *(Stellaria),* dandelion leaf *(Taraxacum),* and peppermint *(Mentha piperita)* for flavor. To encourage diuresis, consume 15 ml of fresh or defrosted juice in 4–6 ounces of water, three times daily.[11] Potassium salts are attributed to the diuretic effect.[12] *Note:* It is important to include other antispasmodic, analgesic, and diuretic herbs to ease the passing of kidney stones.

A hemostatic, nettle reduces passive hemorrhage and nourishes individuals who have bled excessively.[6,10,11] The hemostatic actions are likely due to the vitamin K content and the astringency.[9] Nettle decreases excessive menstrual bleeding, and mid-cycle and menopausal spotting.[6] It reduces minor bleeding in the sputum, urine, and stools.[6] Due to the hemostatic and astringent properties, it aids in treating gastrointestinal inflammation and conditions such as diarrhea, ulcerative colitis, and hemorrhoids.[12] Prepare a hemostatic compound by combining extracts of nettle leaf, shepherd's purse *(Capsella),* cinnamon *(Cinnamomum),* and yarrow *(Achillea).* A hemostatic tea blend includes the same herbs listed above, in addition to a rose family plant such as raspberry leaves *(Rubus idaeus)* or rose *(Rosa)* petals. Omit shepherd's purse in tea, as the dry herb is ineffective. *Caution:* Seek immediate medical attention in case of a severe hemorrhage.

A nutritive tonic, nettle is rich in easily assimilated vitamins and trace minerals. Regular consumption of nettle sustains energy levels and reduces fatigue. Nettle contains relatively high amounts of iron (a nonheme source) that aids in treating iron deficiency anemia. Combining it with vitamin C enhances the assimilation of nonheme iron. However,

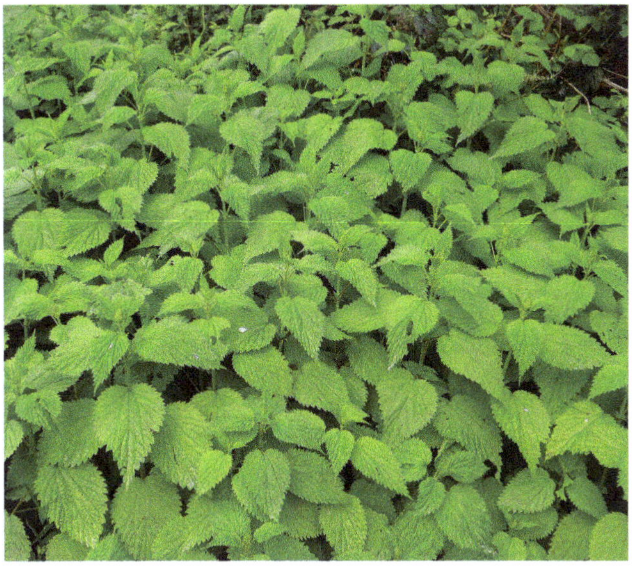

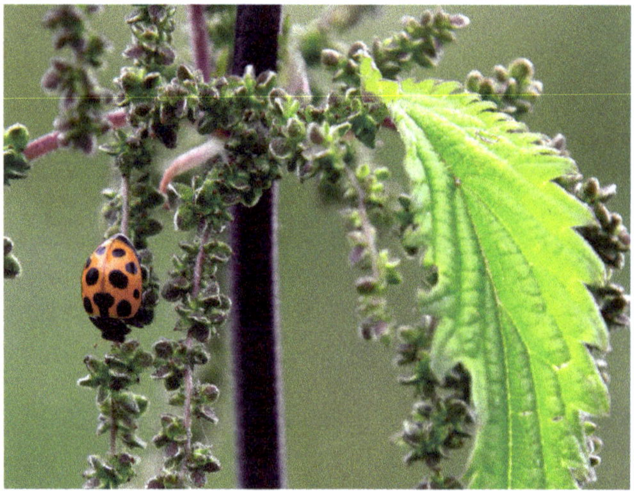

heme sources of iron are significantly more bioavailable; therefore, they are more effective in treating iron deficiency anemia. Due to its mineral content, nettle has subtle blood sugar stabilizing effects and helps to reduce sugar cravings.

Nettle contains high amounts of silica (silicic acid and silicon dioxide), an important mineral that improves the integrity of connective tissues and hastens tissue repair. Silica strengthens bones; thus, nettle can be used as a tonic to prevent osteoporosis and strengthen teeth. Ensuring sufficient silicic acid in the bloodstream hastens the healing of broken bones, torn tendons, cartilage, and injured muscles or joints. It also accelerates tissue healing after a surgical procedure.

Silica is an important component in the protein elastin, which lends elasticity to connective tissues. Silica also strengthens connective tissues throughout the body, including the lungs, bladder, and vasculature. In the respiratory system, silica hastens recovery from infections, and is useful for treating bronchitis, pneumonia, or pleurisy. It is beneficial for individuals with weak lungs, or those who are susceptible to infections resulting from tissue weakness. By improving tissue integrity, sensitivity to allergens common in individuals with allergies, asthma, or leaky gut syndrome is reduced.

Long-term consumption of nettle strengthens the bladder and can prevent relapsing urinary tract infections. Nettle is specific for women who have taken antibiotics several times for bladder infections, without positive results. The inability of the tissues to respond to antibiotics indicates tissue weakness. While nettle is not effective as an antibacterial agent, it enhances the integrity of tissues, improving their resistance. It can be very useful for individuals with frequent bladder infections, interstitial cystitis, or childhood enuresis.[12] Combine extracts of nettle, mullein root *(Verbascum)*, corn silk *(Zea)*, horsetail *(Equisetum)*, and/or yellow pond lily *(Nuphar)* as a long-term bladder tonic. The liposterolic extract of saw palmetto also strengthens the bladder.

The minerals in nettle have an alkalinizing effect on tissues. Due to the high levels of calcium, magnesium, and silica, nettle supports the skeletal system and prevents osteoporosis.[11] Long-term consumption aids in treating many conditions aggravated by hyperacidity in the tissues, including gout, rheumatoid arthritis, and skin conditions (acne, eczema, or psoriasis).[6,10,11] The vitamin A and C content supports immune function. Nettle is a gentle tonic for treating chronic immune conditions.

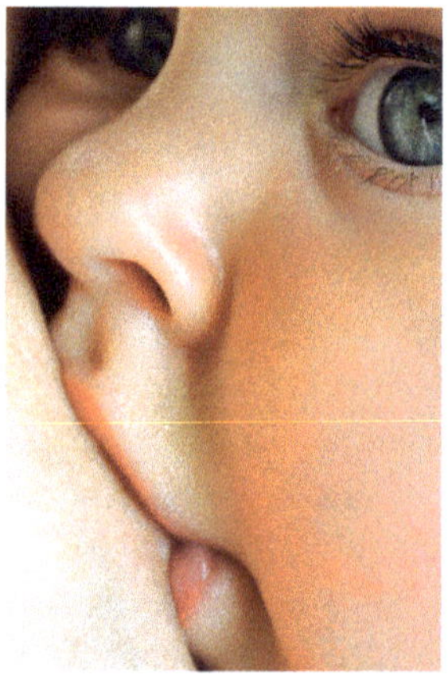

A galactagogue, nettle increases breast milk flow and nourishment.[6,15] It is a recuperative for women depleted from childbirth or nursing.[15] A nourishing, blood-building infusion helpful throughout pregnancy includes: oat straw *(Avena)*, alfalfa *(Medicago)*, raspberry *(Rubus)*, and peppermint or spearmint *(Mentha* spp.*)*.

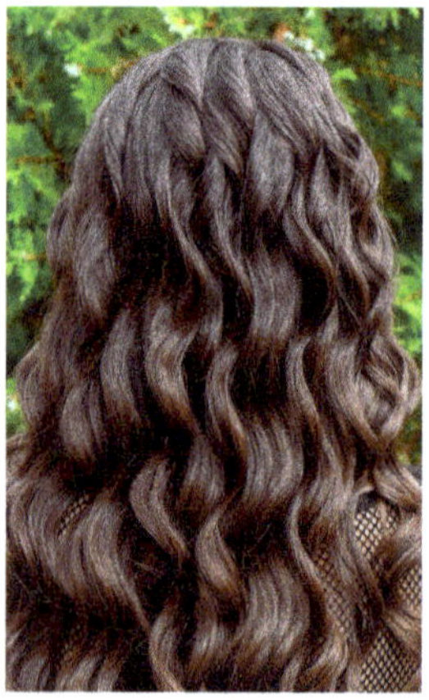

Nettle improves hair luster and strength, encourages hair growth, and reduces dandruff.[7] Daily applications of nettle leaf tea, vinegar, and/or oil strengthen hair. Although the treatment can be used for all hair colors, nettle is typically used with dark hair. Prepare a hair rinse using tea containing nettle, horsetail *(Equisetum)*, and rosemary *(Salvia rosmarinus)*.

Fresh nettle applications produce a counterirritant effect, stimulating circulation into local tissues. This action aids in treating tendonitis, arthritis, lumbago, sciatica, and neuralgia. Upon contact, amines (histamines), acetylcholine, and formic acid contained in the vessel-like base of the stinging hairs are released into the skin, producing burning, itching, blistering, or contact dermatitis.[9,10] However, the lingering stinging effects are likely due to the release of other mediators or substances that are toxic to the nerves.[9]

NETTLE ROOTS: Nettle root aids in treating benign prostatic hypertrophy (BPH). It decreases the frequency of urination and residual urine, and increases urinary flow and volume.[9] *Urtica dioica* agglutinin (UDA) was found to bind to the cell membranes of smooth muscle and epithelial cells in BPH tissue.[9] Nettle root contains several lignans, including secoisolariciresinol and (-)-3,4-divanillyltetrahydrofuran that reduce human sex hormone-binding globulin (SHBG) *in vitro.*[9] The metabolites of secoisolariciresinol (enterodiol and enterolactone), and to a greater extent, (-)-3,4-divanillyltetrahydrofuran (entorofuran), demonstrated an affinity for binding with SHBG.[9] Nettle root lignans may also competitively inhibit SHBG-5-α-dihydrotestosterone receptor interaction in human prostatic membranes.[9]

Nettle root extracts reduced prostate enlargement in animal studies. Methanolic extracts of nettle root administered to mice with experimentally induced BPH inhibited prostate growth 51% compared to control groups.[9] In animals suffering from BPH, nettle root extract (5 : 1) reduced prostate volume 30%, and plasma testosterone levels were slightly lower following a 100-day treatment with 90 mg/kg.[9] Nettle root extract (5 : 1, 1200 mg per day) was administered to human BPH patients for 20 weeks, and was found to inhibit the excessive growth of prostate cells.[9] In an uncontrolled clinical study, nettle root extract (5 : 1, 1200 mg per day) reduced nocturia in one-half of BPH patients in 8 – 9 weeks. In a similar trial using the same dosage, 78% of patients experienced improvement within three months, and 91% improved within six months.[9] More than 50% of BPH patients consuming nettle root extract for 8 – 10 years did not require surgery, and the usual prostate enlargement was not evident.[9] Nettle root extracts reduced nocturia in men over age 60 with prostatic adenoma.[10] To increase the efficacy of BPH treatment, consume nettle root extract, pygeum *(Prunus a-fricanum)* extract, and liposterolic extract (LSE) of saw palmetto *(Serenoa).*

NETTLE SEEDS: Nettle seed extract is a kidney trophorestorative. It aids in treating patients with glomerulonephritis and chronic nephritis with degeneration. It also helps to protect the kidneys from nephrotoxic medication.[16] Nettle seed extract reduces serum creatinine levels by improving renal glomerular function.[13] Herbalist David Winston first proposed using the seeds for this purpose.[16] He administered nettle seed extract in more than 30 cases of degenerative kidney disease, with impressive results. Herbalist Jonathan Treasure confirmed that nettle extract lowered serum creatinine levels.[13] Considering the lack of botanicals with kidney-restorative effects, nettle seed fills an important gap in managing kidney disease. *Note:* It is important for individuals with these conditions to consult a health care practitioner.

CONTRAINDICATIONS

Although it is rare, some individuals are allergic to nettle. Hypersensitive individuals or those with a history of anaphylactic response should avoid nettle stings. Some individuals have eaten raw nettle, but it is not recommended because it can cause an anaphylactic reaction. Prior to ingesting, nettle leaves should be thoroughly steamed or cooked to eliminate the sting. Nettle can cause contact dermatitis. High quality, dried nettle can still sting. *Caution:* Wear thick gloves and protective clothing when harvesting fresh nettle.

Discontinue using nettle leaf in cases of obstructive urinary stones, edema due to impaired heart or kidney function, or kidney inflammation.[12] Individuals with extreme kidney deficiency (frequent urination) or yin deficiency (dryness in the tissues and mucous membranes) may find nettle leaf too potent as a diuretic or astringent. Discontinue use if this occurs, or add a pinch or two of licorice root to counter this effect. In rare cases, nettle root can cause mild gastrointestinal upset.[9]

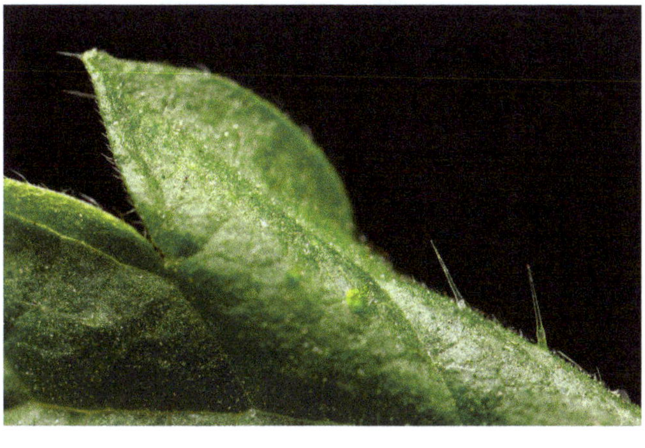

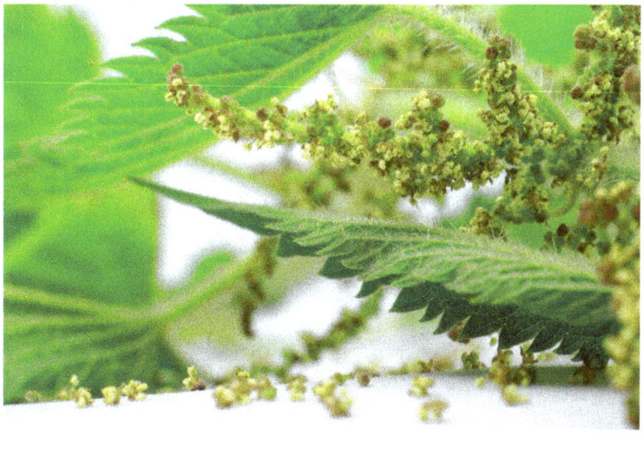

PREPARATION AND DOSAGE

TINCTURE: Fresh leaves or roots [1:2-1:4, 60-95% alcohol]; dry leaves or roots [1:5, 50% alcohol]; consume 30-90 drops, up to three times daily. Fresh seeds [1:5, 30% alcohol]; consume 30-90 drops, twice daily.

GLYCERITE: Fresh leaves [1:2-1:4, 40% glycerin, 30% alcohol, and 30% water]; consume 30-60 drops, up to three times daily.

ACETUM EXTRACT: Fresh leaves [1:2-1:4, apple cider vinegar] or use the Simpler's method (pack a jar with the leaves and pour vinegar over them). Consume 1 teaspoon, one to three times daily before meals.

SUCCUS: Fresh nettle leaves can be juiced and preserved with 10-20% alcohol, or juiced and frozen in ice cube trays. Consume 15 ml of nettle juice in 4-6 ounces of water, up to three times daily.

TEA: Prepare a hot or cold infusion of the leaves; consume 8-12 ounces, three to four times daily. Prepare a decoction of the root; consume 8-12 ounces, two to three times daily.

TOPICAL USE: Dilute acetum extract with water, and use the vinegar as a hair rinse. Wilt fresh nettle leaves one or two days, and infuse them in olive, almond, or jojoba oil for two weeks, or cook the leaves in olive oil using the double boiler method. Apply infused nettle oil topically to hair and scalp as a hair conditioner.

CULINARY USE: Substitute nettle leaf oil for vegetable oils in most savory food recipes. Use nettle leaf acetum extract to replace vinegar in recipes. Add fresh steamed or frozen nettle to soup, spaghetti sauce, pizza, calzone, or lasagna. *Note:* The fresh leaves must be cooked or steamed until the sting is no longer present.

Dried nettle can be cooked in soups or sprinkled on salads. The powder can be added to smoothies. Dried nettle also can be added to a sea mineral sprinkle as a nutritive.

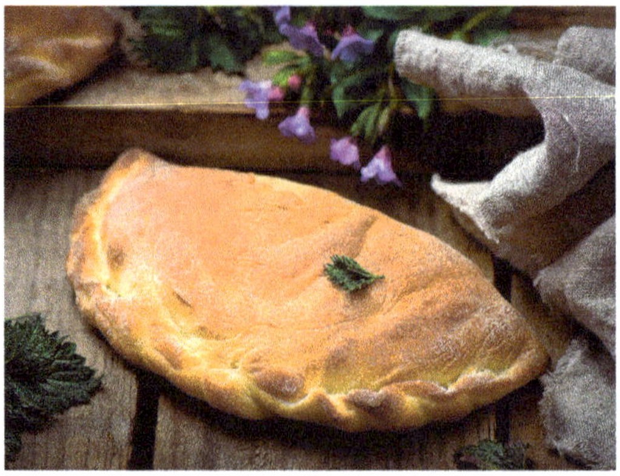

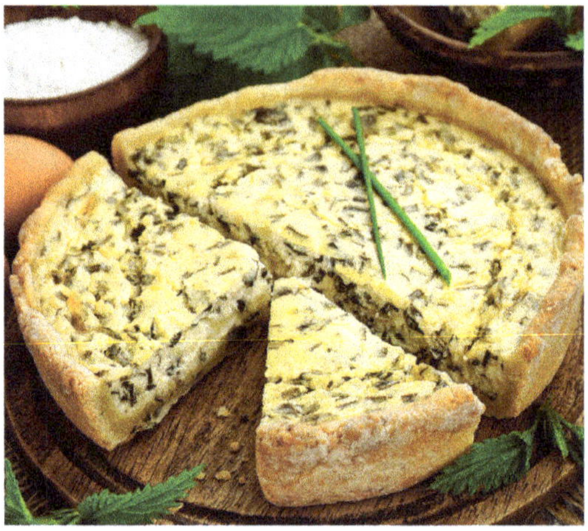

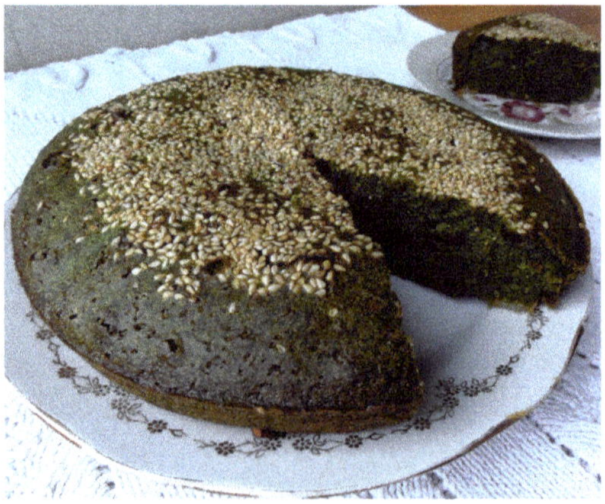

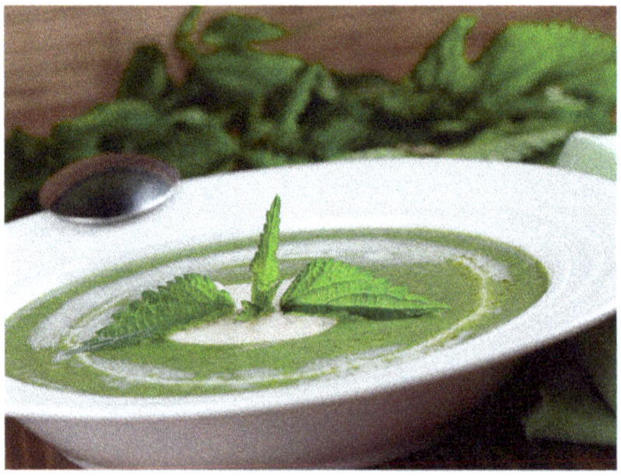

OATS

DESCRIPTION

BOTANICAL NAMES:
Avena fatua, A. sativa

COMMON NAMES:
Wild oats, cultivated oats, milky oat, oat straw, common wild oat, spring wild oat, black oat, wheat oat, oatgrass, red oat, side oat, tree oat, shaufan
zamyr (Arabic)
cugula (Catalan)
avoine, avoine cultivee, folle avoine (French)
flughafer, hafer, windhafer (German)
shibolet, shaul, kvaker (Hebrew)
karasu-mugi, ma-karasu-mugi (Japanese)
aveia, aveia-selvagem (Portuguese)
oves (Russian)
avena comun, avena loca, avena silvestre, ballueca (Spanish)
flyghavre, havre, vipphavre (Swedish)[1]

FAMILY NAME:
Poaceae (Gramineae)

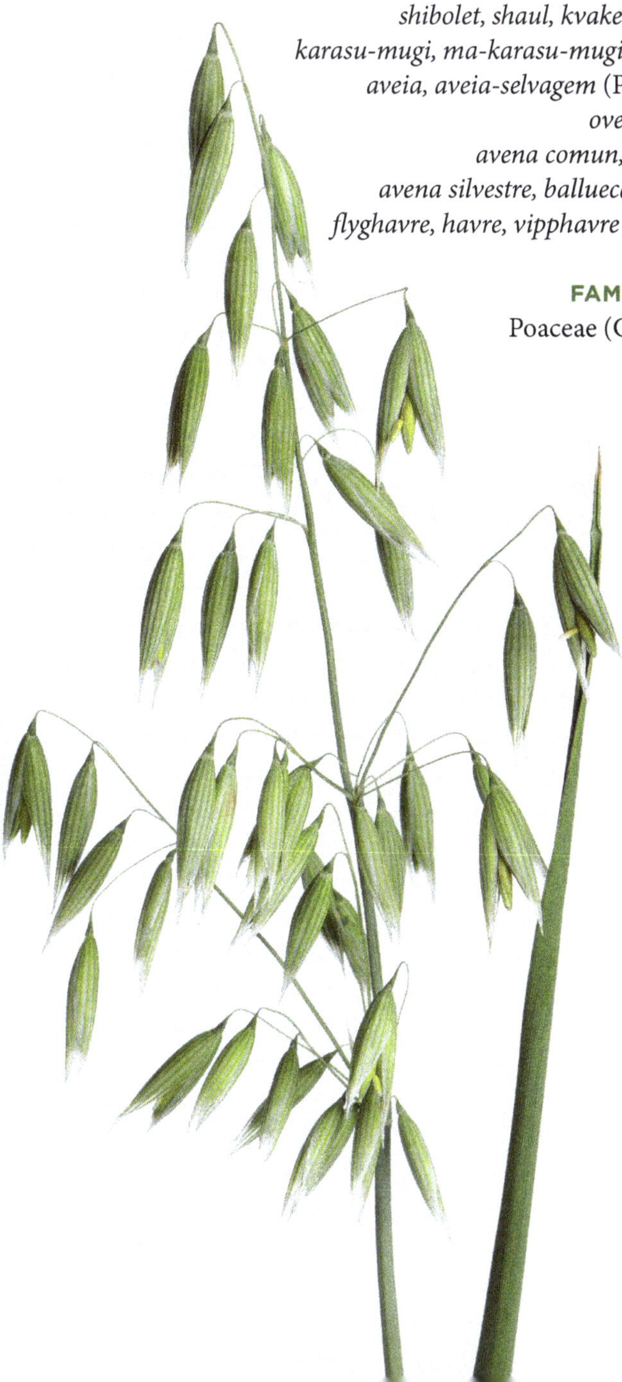

PARTS USED: Fresh milky, unripe seeds for tincture preparations, and the dry stem and unripe seeds for tea (oat straw).

BOTANICAL DESCRIPTION AND HABITAT: Wild oats grows in sunny meadows throughout the U.S. It is commonly found with legumes as a winter cover crop to protect the soil and improve soil fertility. It adds organic matter to the soil when the cover crop is tilled in the spring.

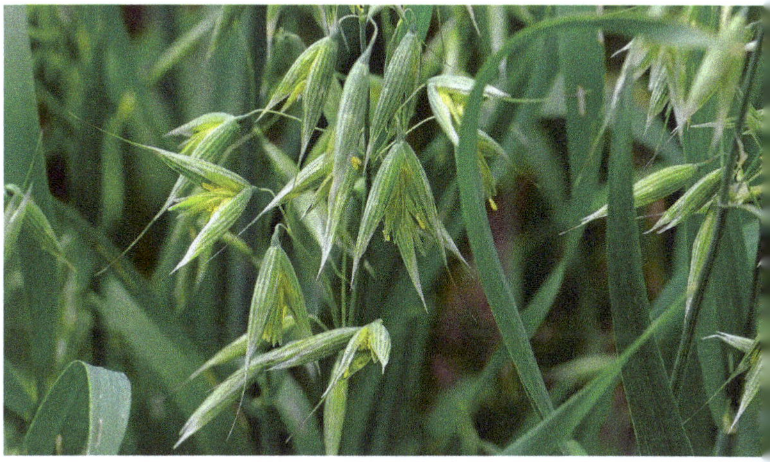

Avena is a genus of about 25 species of annual grasses with erect stems and linear, flat blades.[2,3] The leaves grow basally and on the stem, and have membranous ligules.[2,3] The inflorescence is a large panicle bearing large, pendent, laterally compressed spikelets (15 – 50 mm long).[2,3] There are two or more florets per spikelet, some reduced.[2,3] In wild species, the glabrous or pilose rachilla breaks apart between florets.[2,3] The lanceolate, glabrous glumes are usually as long as the spikelet, and about equal in size to each other, with rounded backs and acuminate apices.[2,3] The apices of the leathery to papery lemmas are acute or minutely forked, sometimes becoming bristles.[2,3] A stiff, often bent awn emerges from the middle of the lemma, and is variably coiled and sometimes absent in cultivated species.[2,3] The palea is generally shorter than the lemma, and has hairy keels.[2,3] There are three anthers and a hairy, unicarpellate ovary that eventually produce a single-seeded, pubescent fruit that is spindle-like in shape.[2,3]

Avena sativa grows 40 – 180 cm high, with stems growing in tufts or individually.[4,5] The glabrous leaves grow 8 – 45 cm long and 3 – 16 mm wide, with ligules (3 – 6 mm) that

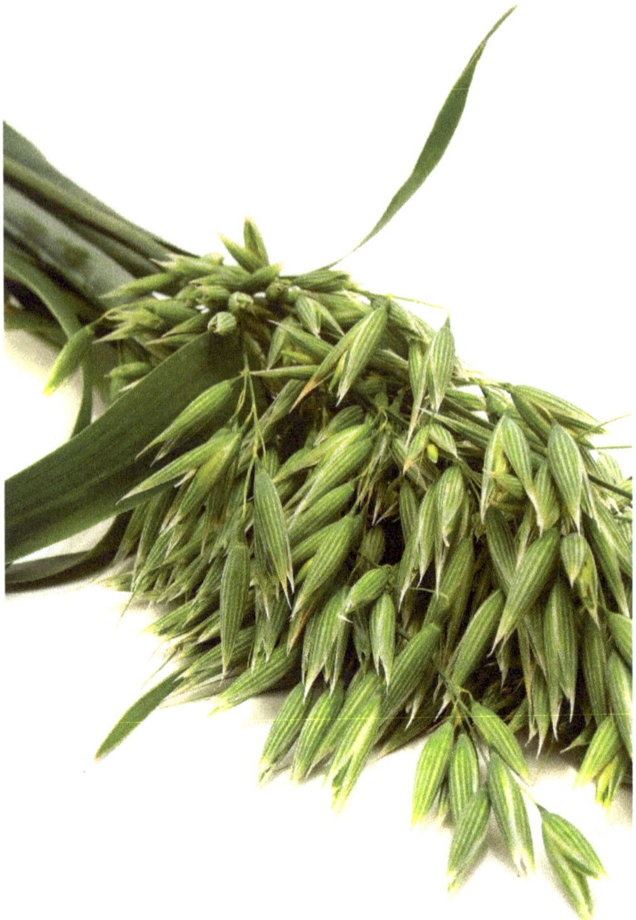

sometimes feature rough margins.[4,5] The panicles (20 – 40 cm long) do not break up at the joints below each spikelet when mature, as occurs in *A. fatua*.[4,5] The spikelets (2 – 3 cm long) usually contain two florets.[4,5] The glumes are equal in length to the spikelet.[4,5] The leathery lemma (12 – 25 mm long) is glabrous on the back, and sometimes hairy at the base.[4,5] The florets of *A. sativa* usually lack awns, but when they are present, those of the upper floret are 15 – 30 mm, and those of the lower floret are generally less than 15 mm.[4,5] *A. sativa* hybridizes with *A. fatua* and *A. sterilis*.[4,5]

Avena fatua (30 – 160 cm tall) have scabrid or pilose green blades (10 – 45 cm long and 4 – 15 mm wide).[6,7] Each floret of the spikelets (17 – 25 mm long) has a bearded callous.[6,7] The herbaceous glumes are 18 – 32 mm long, while the lemmas lack bristles at their apices, and bear awns (25 – 40 mm long).[6,7] The main features distinguishing *A. fatua* from *A. sativa* are the long awns that are not present in *A. sativa*.[5] Other differences are that *A. fatua* produces much smaller grains than *A. sativa,* and the leaves of *A. fatua* are often pubescent; *A. sativa* has glabrous leaves.[6]

THE NAME: *Avena* ("straw or reed") derives from Latin. The epithet *fatua* means fool; *sativa* derives from the Latin *sativus* ("sown"). The name milky oats refers to the fresh, immature seeds that exude a milky fluid when crushed.

HISTORICAL USES: Oats have nourished humans and livestock since ancient times. The earliest records of oat grains were found in Egypt in about 2,000 BCE. The earliest records of oat cultivation were found in Swiss caves dating from the Bronze Age. Oats were first brought to the U.S. with other grains in the early 1600s.[8]

Oat flour was incorporated into breakfast cereals and bread. Oat products have been used as an antioxidant and stabilizer in ice cream and other dairy products. Gruel from oatmeal continues to be used as an emollient to soothe dry, inflamed skin conditions and poison oak.

Eclectic physicians administered an extract of fresh milky oats to treat nervous exhaustion, cardiac weakness or irregularity due to nervous debility, neurasthenia, nervous dyspepsia, tremors, and occipital headaches.[9,10] It also was used to treat impotence, sexual neurasthenia, and debility caused by masturbation or excessive sexual indulgence.[9,10] Dr. Finley Ellingwood administered the extract to ease amenorrhea due to a feeble nervous system, painful and congestive dysmenorrhea with cold skin and extremities, and the condition formerly known as "hysteria."[9]

The term "sowing wild oats" is a common phrase dating back to the 16th century. Farmers considered wild oats *(A. fatua)* a nuisance weed that self-seeded in oat fields. It resembled cultivated oats *(A. sativa),* but yielded little grain, and required tedious hand weeding when the plant was in flower, before the seeds ripened. The saying "sowing wild oats" became a way of describing unprofitable activities. Because of the reputed invigorating properties of oat seed, and the implicit correlation between the plant and human "seed," the phrase came to refer to the sexual liaisons of an unmarried young male resulting in unwanted children born out of wedlock.

CONSTITUENTS: Wild oats contains avenin, avenacines A and B, avenacosides, ergothioneine, histamine, hordenine, trigonelline, and flavonoids (chiefly the flavones vitexin and apigenin).[9,10]

NUTRITIONAL PROPERTIES: Oat straw contains vitamins A, C, E, and K, as well as many B vitamins, including folic acid, niacin, pyridoxine, riboflavin, and thiamine. It is rich in minerals such as calcium, chromium, iron, magnesium, phosphorus, silicon, and sodium. It contains low to average amounts of cobalt, potassium, selenium, and tin. Additionally, oat straw contains protein and some amino acids, such as argenine, histadine, leucine, lysine, phenylalanine, and tryptophan.[11,12]

MEDICINAL PROPERTIES: Fresh milky oats extract is a nervine and trophorestorative. Oat straw tea is nutritive.

TEMPERATURE AND FLAVOR: Neutral, bland, salty, and sweet.

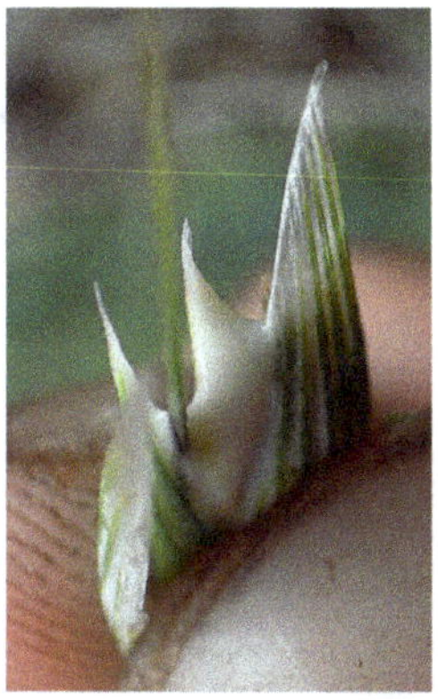

MEDICINAL USES

FRESH MILKY OATS EXTRACT: There is a short window of time between late spring and early summer for harvesting the fresh, unripe seeds. When pressed between the fingers, the unripe seed heads exude a milky substance to which the nervine properties are attributed. The seeds can be stripped from the stem and tinctured fresh immediately. Blending the seeds and alcohol in a Vitamix (or other powerful blender) reduces their bulkiness, and produces a vibrant green extract. The stems can be dried for tea (see oat straw tea below). According to Eclectic physician Finley Ellingwood, the extract works most effectively and rapidly when it is administered in hot water. When administered in cold water before bed, it has a more prolonged calmative effect.[9] *Note:* After the seed heads are dried or produce the mature oat seed (used to make oat meal), they no longer exert an influence on the nervous system.

Long-term use of fresh, milky oats extract is a phenomenal trophorestorative, nervine, and subtle mood elevator that nourishes the nervous system.[9,13] It is highly effective in treating nervous exhaustion (burnout from excessive excitement of the sympathetic nerves).[9] Under stressful circumstances, the adrenal medulla and sympathetic-adrenergic post-synaptic neurons secrete high amounts of adrenalin (epinephrine) and noradrenalin (norepinephrine) into the tissues and bloodstream, affecting every organ and skeletal muscle. Frequent or long-term secretion of these hormones and neurotransmitters tax the adrenals and nervous system, leaving a feeling of depletion, restlessness, and (sometimes) depression. Chronic stress can lead to numerous physical imbalances. Although wild oats extract is not an adaptogen, it can be added to adrenal-supporting formulas for the trophorestorative actions.

Milky oats extract is a gently calming, restorative nervine that is not sedating. It can be consumed throughout the day by insomnia-prone individuals who become nervous, and have difficulty relaxing. Milky oats extract reduces anxiety, agitation, heart palpitations, and restlessness.[9,10] Combine it with hawthorn *(Crataegus),* lemon balm *(Melissa),* and bugleweed *(Lycopus)* for a weak heart, irregular heartbeat, or palpitations. It also can be combined with motherwort *(Leonurus)* to calm the heart. Milky oats extract eases nervous headaches, as well as premenstrual and menopausal anxiety and irritability.[9,10,13] It also aids in treating mild depression and irritation due to physical exhaustion or withdrawal from drugs (i.e., methamphetamines, cocaine, and opiates), as well as caffeine and tobacco.[9,13-15] Combine extracts of milky oats and skullcap *(Scutellaria)* to ease withdrawal; you can also add extracts of lemon balm *(Melissa)* and St. John's wort *(Hypericum)* to strengthen the effects.

Fresh milky oats extract helps to reduce nervous jitters, nerve tremors, eye twitches, leg cramps, and cold cramps.[9] Epileptics can consume the extract as a seizure preventative in times of stress, but it does not replace seizure medication.[9] Combine extracts of milky oats with skullcap *(Scutellaria),* lemon balm *(Melissa),* and in some cases, a high CBD, low THC, extract of cannabis *(Cannabis sativa).*

OAT STRAW TEA: Oat straw tea contains numerous minerals that aid in developing and maintaining healthy bones, teeth, hair, and nails. The easily assimilated calcium and magnesium help to prevent osteoporosis, and support the nervous system. Oat straw nutrients support women during their reproductive years, especially during pregnancy and lactation. The magnesium content reduces premenstrual syndrome, decreases sugar and chocolate cravings, and aids in balancing blood glucose levels.

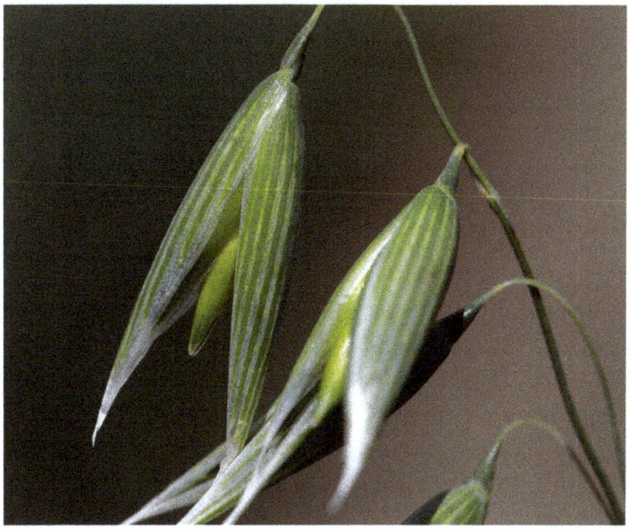

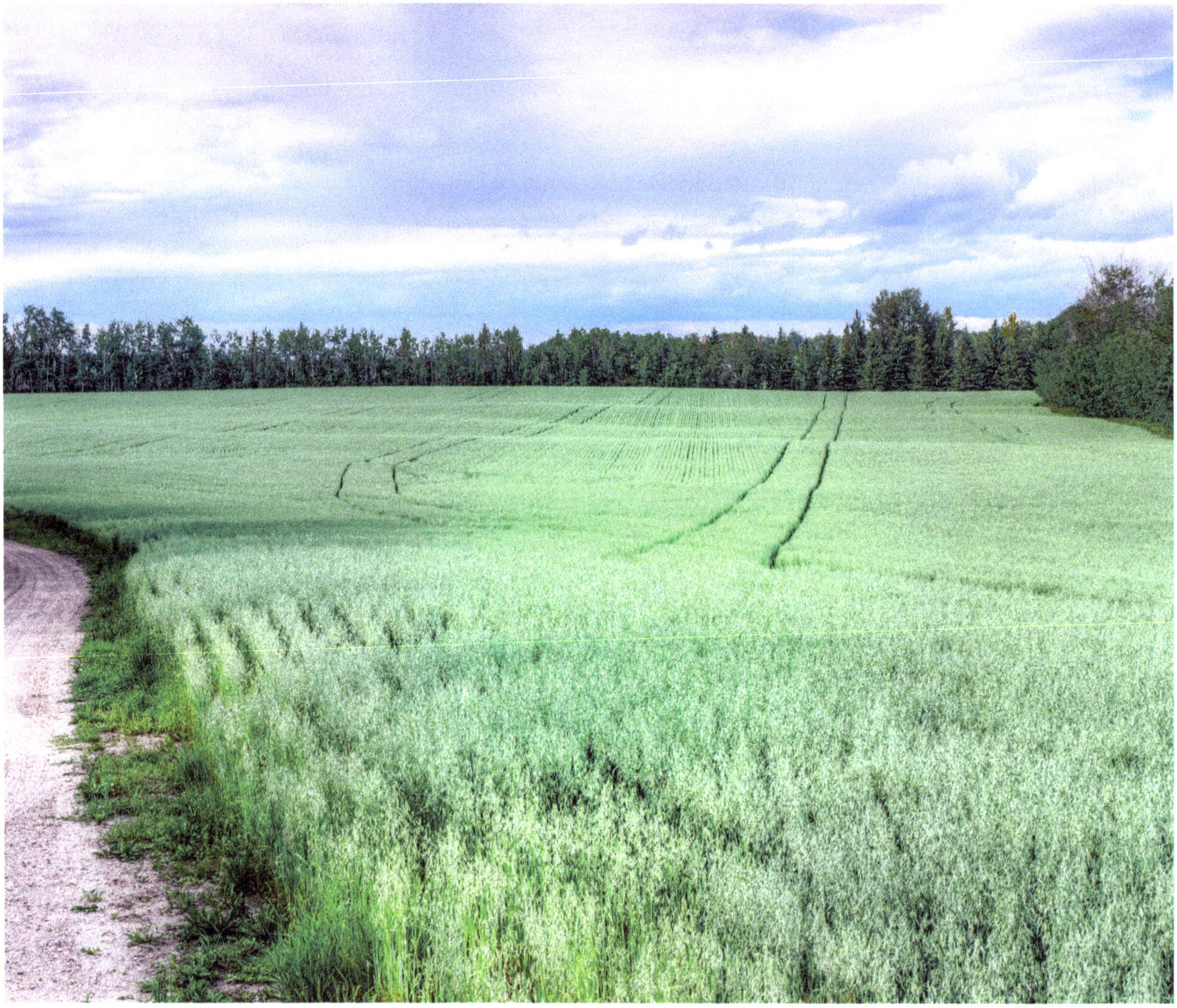

Oat straw tea provides readily available alkaline minerals that are easily depleted from the body due to the consumption of coffee, other caffeine-containing beverages, and predominantly acidic foods. The brain is constantly maintaining homeostasis; blood alkalinity must be balanced, and is essential for enzyme function. As one ages, mineral depletion from the tissues and bones can contribute to osteoporosis and other problems.

CONTRAINDICATIONS

When the tincture is consumed in excessive doses, it can induce a third eye headache.[9,15] Individuals with gluten sensitivity may want to avoid consuming the tea or tincture. However, the protein (gliadin) that triggers allergic sensitivity is denatured in alcohol-based extracts; thus, the tincture is very unlikely to aggravate gluten-sensitive individuals.

PREPARATION AND DOSAGE

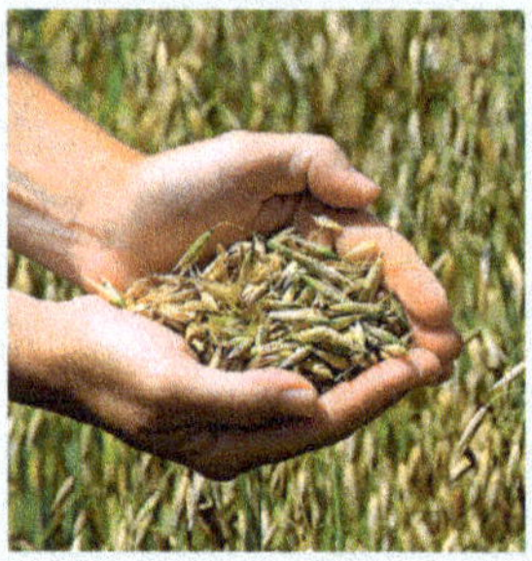

TINCTURE: Fresh, milky, unripe seeds [1:3-1:4+, 70-95% alcohol]; consume 10-60 drops, up to four times daily.

GLYCERITE: Fresh, milky, unripe seeds [1:3-1:4, 50% glycerin, 50% alcohol]; consume 10-60 drops, up to four times daily.

TEA: Prepare a standard or cold infusion of oat straw or dry, unripe seeds; consume 8-12 ounces, three to four times daily.

ORANGE

DESCRIPTION

BOTANICAL NAMES:
Citrus sinensis (syn. *C. aurantium* var. *sinensis* or *C. aurantium* var. *dulcis*), *C. aurantium* (syn. *C. aurantium* var. *amara, C. bigaradia*), and *C. reticulata*

COMMON NAMES:
Orange, Seville orange, sweet orange, bitter orange, sour orange, tangerine, mandarin
naranj (Arabic)
chen pi (Mandarin for aged fruit)
qing pi (Mandarin for immature peel)
zhi shi (Mandarin for immature fruit)
neratzi (Greek for bitter orange)
portokali (Greek for sweet orange)
nagaranga (Sanskrit)

FAMILY NAME:
Rutaceae

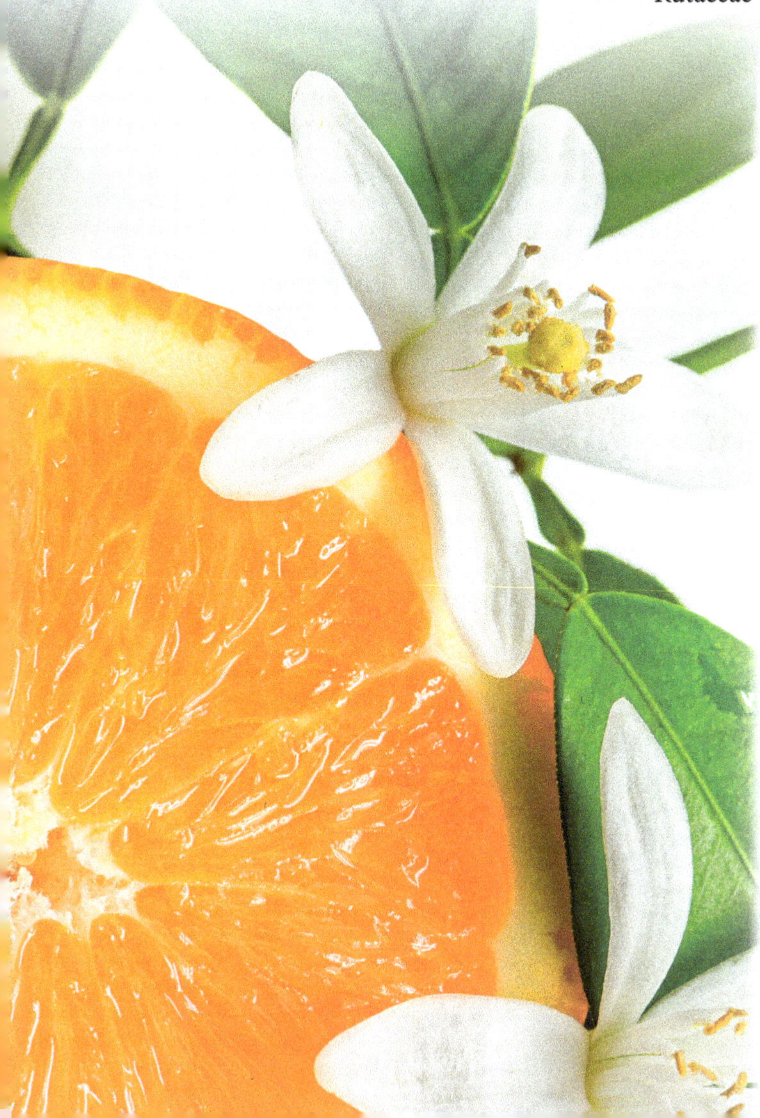

PARTS USED: The unripe, ripe, and mature peel (pericarp), flowers, and pulp. Essential oils are made with ripe peel, flowers, twigs, and leaves.

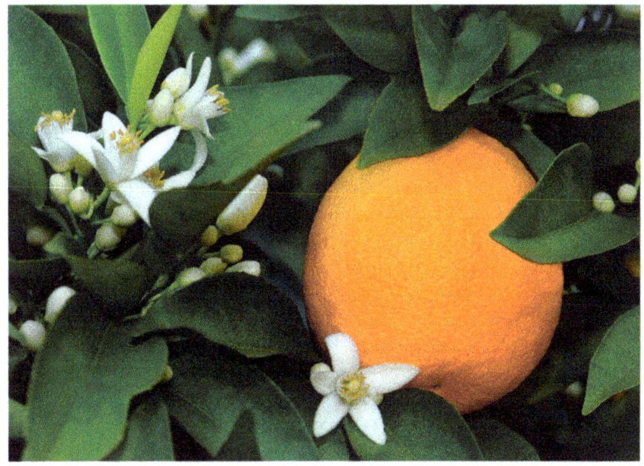

BOTANICAL DESCRIPTION AND HABITAT: *Citrus* is a genus of evergreen trees and shrubs native to Southeast Asia. Most species are domesticated and only known in cultivation.[1] The plants have smooth, grayish-brown bark. Many species have spines at the axils of alternate leaves. These shiny leaves have a leathery texture, and usually feature wide, winged petioles with wavy margins.[1,2] The sweetly fragrant flowers are solitary or axillary racemes, or clusters.[1,2] Inside the flower is a cup-shaped calyx with three to five lobes and four or five white petals.[1] Orange flowers have 16–80 stamens and a prominent stigma atop an ovary consisting of 5–14 chambers.[1,2] The distinctive fruit is a specialized berry known as a hesperidium, and can be globose, oblong, or oblate.[1] The rind can be loosely or tightly appressed to the segments, and is covered in essential oil glands. Many seeds are embedded in each pulpy segment.[1]

Recent molecular studies suggest that of all the *Citrus* species, only mandarins *(C. reticulata),* pomelo *(C. maxima),* and citron *(C. medica)* are considered true species; the rest are naturally occurring or artificially created hybrids of those three species.[3]

Sweet orange (*C. sinensis*) likely originated in Asia, near the border of China and Vietnam. In the U.S., it is commercially cultivated in Florida, southern California, and Texas. It is also cultivated in Sicily, Cyprus, Guinea, Spain, Israel, and

Brazil, among other countries. There are numerous varietals of sweet orange, including navel, Jaffa, and Valencia. Sweet orange trees grow up to 10 meters tall, and bear a few slender spines.[4] Fragrant ovate leaves (7.5 – 11 cm long) are attached to the stems via narrowly winged petioles.[4] The clusters of flowers are borne in leaf axils.[4] They contain 20 stamens, and produce an oblate fruit (6 – 9 cm diameter) with a yellow to orange-red rind, and yellow-orange to reddish sweet flesh.[4]

Bitter orange *(C. aurantium)* is native to southern China and northeast India. It is a small tree (7 to 8 meters tall) cultivated in China, Spain, Italy, Guinea, Brazil, the West Indies, and the U.S.[5] Bitter orange branches have many long, sharp, axillary spines (up to 8 cm long).[5] The flowers have 20 – 24 fused stamens.[5] Bitter orange globe-shaped fruit (7.5 cm diameter) has a rougher peel than sweet orange. Bitter orange pulp is very bitter and sour.

Mandarin *(C. reticulata)* is a small tree (4 – 6 meters tall) with only a few or no spines.[6,7] The lanceolate to ovate leaves (6 – 8 cm long) have serrate margins.[7] One to three flowers grow per cluster, bearing 20 – 25 fused stamens and a long, thin style.[6] The fruit rind is pale yellow to scarlet and loosely attached to the inner flesh, which is plump with sweet to acidic juice.[6]

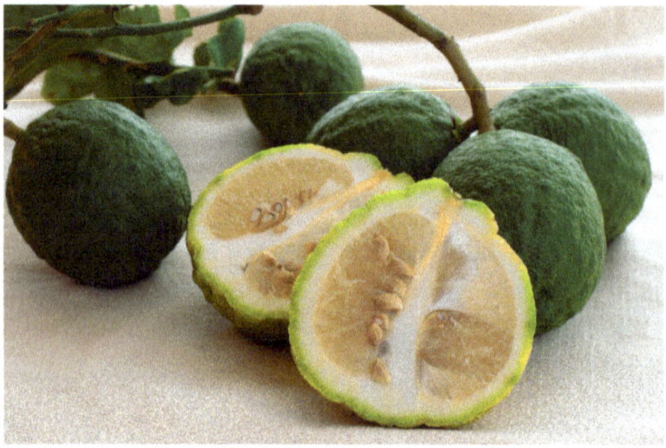

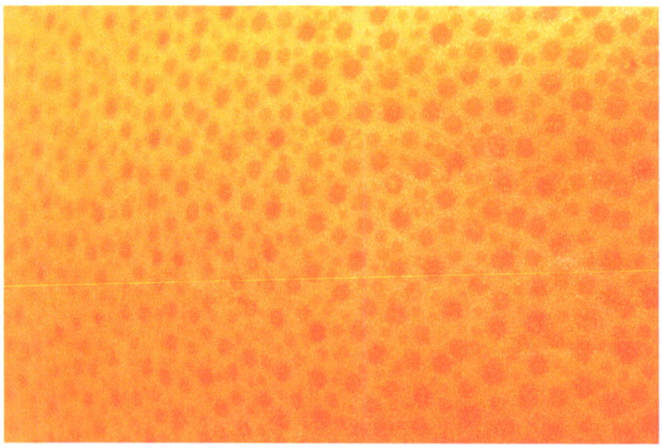

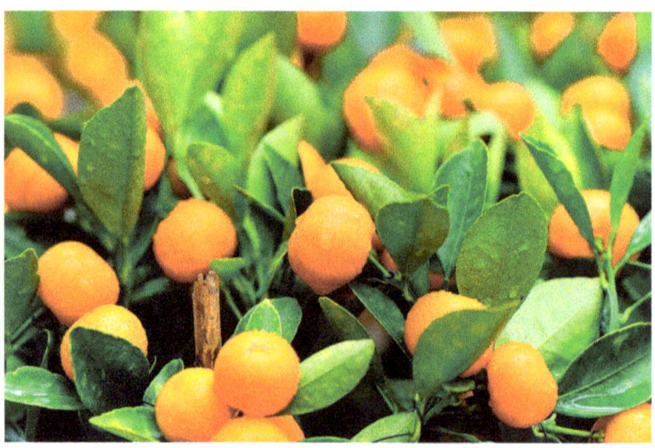

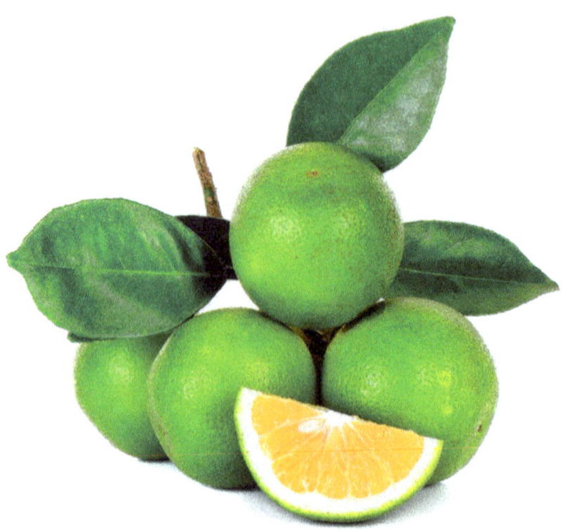

THE NAME: Derived from Latin, the word *Citrus* ("citron tree") is named after the African tree with aromatic wood and lemon-like fruit. The citron tree provided the first citrus fruit in western Europe. The epithet *sinensis* refers to the plant's origin in China. The epithet *bigaradia* refers to France's Bigerade region where bitter orange was extensively cultivated. *Reticulata* derives from the Latin *reticularis* ("little net").[8] The common name orange derives from naga-ranga (Sanskrit) and naranj (Arabic).[9]

Citrus sinensis is the Latin binomial for the sweet orange cultivated for eating. *C. aurantium* is known as bitter orange; the fruit is not consumed fresh—it is prepared in marmalade. The flowers from this species yield neroli oil; the twigs yield petitgrain oil. *Citrus reticulata* is the binomial for mandarin or tangerine orange.

HISTORICAL USES: Arab traders introduced the Asian bitter orange tree to Europe. Arab physician Avicenna described the uses of bitter orange juice in the 10th century.[10] The first shipment of bitter oranges reached England on a Spanish ship in 1290.[10] Europeans began drinking the juice to quench thirst, especially resulting from fevers and inflammatory conditions. The peel was used to treat digestive disorders and malaria. As a gift to their prime minister,

Portuguese sailors introduced the first sweet orange tree to Europe in the 15th century.[10] Spanish explorers transported the first orange trees to Florida in the 16th century, and Spanish missionaries brought them to California in the 18th century.[11]

The oldest reference to oranges appeared in the second book of *The Five Classics* in China in 500 BCE.[11] Approximately 2,000 years ago, the uses of citrus peels (*zhu pi*) were first mentioned in the *Shen Nong Ben Cao Jing*. In 1178 CE, a monograph describing the uses of citruses was published in China.[12] Dried bitter and sweet orange peels were used as carminatives for dyspepsia and to improve the appetite. They continue to be used in Traditional Chinese Medicine to reduce phlegm related to coughs, colds, or flu, to strengthen the spleen, and regulate energy. They are also administered to treat vomiting, diarrhea, blood in feces, and uterine or rectal prolapse.[13]

The antiscorbutic actions of oranges were known several centuries earlier than the discovery of their vitamin C content in the 20th century. Many British sailors died from scurvy on long voyages without access to fresh food. In the 18th century, British naval surgeon James Lind began prescribing citrus fruits to curb scurvy, and British sailors became known as "limeys."[10]

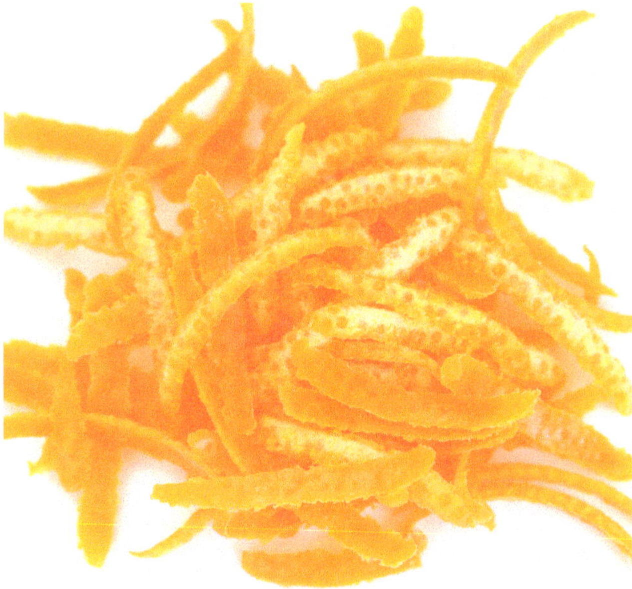

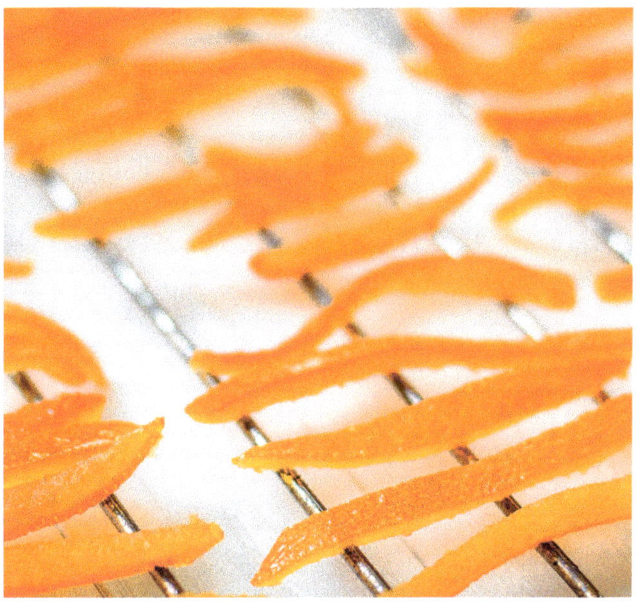

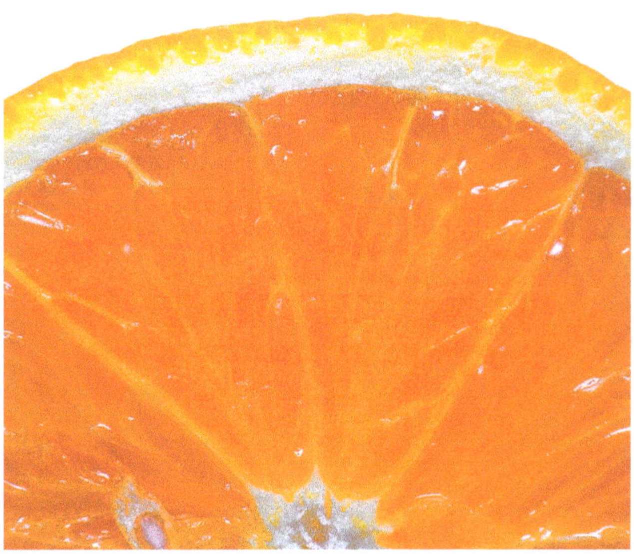

Oranges have long been used in cooking, food products, perfumes, and medicines. Orange peel syrup and elixir are flavoring agents in medicines. Orange peel and flower syrup enhance the flavor of compounds, and are added to sedative formulas. A hot infusion of bitter orange tea is used as a mild sedative, and can be combined with other sedative herbs. In Europe, an evening sedative consisted of a cup of bitter orange tea with up to one teaspoon of valerian extract.[14] Orange-flavored wine was combined with the intoxicating drink absinthium to mitigate the bitter flavor.[9]

Orange flowers have adorned brides and bridal bouquets throughout southern Europe. Orange blossoms were candied in Grasse, France. Orange flower water is used by French biscuit makers for added crispness. Essential oil of orange blossoms (neroli) is a primary ingredient in eau-de-cologne, the classic toilet water that also includes essential oils of lavender, bergamot, lemon, and rosemary.[9,15]

Bitter orange fruit has been used historically for many culinary applications, and is still used today in the following preparations. Bitter orange fruit is an ingredient in marmalade. Bitter orange zest (or essential oil) is used as a flavoring agent in triple sec, Grand Marnier, Cointreau, and other liqueurs. The immature fruit of bitter orange (orange berries) is used to flavor Curacao.[9]

Bitter orange essential oil is used as a flavoring in non-alcoholic beverages, candy, baked goods, gelatins, puddings, meat products, frozen dairy desserts, condiments, and relishes.[13] Sweet orange essential oil is used in food products such as jams, jellies, gravies, sweet sauces, breakfast cereals, and processed vegetables. Essential oils of bitter and sweet orange, neroli, and petitgrain are used as fragrances in lotions, creams, cosmetics, soaps, detergents, and cleaning products.[13]

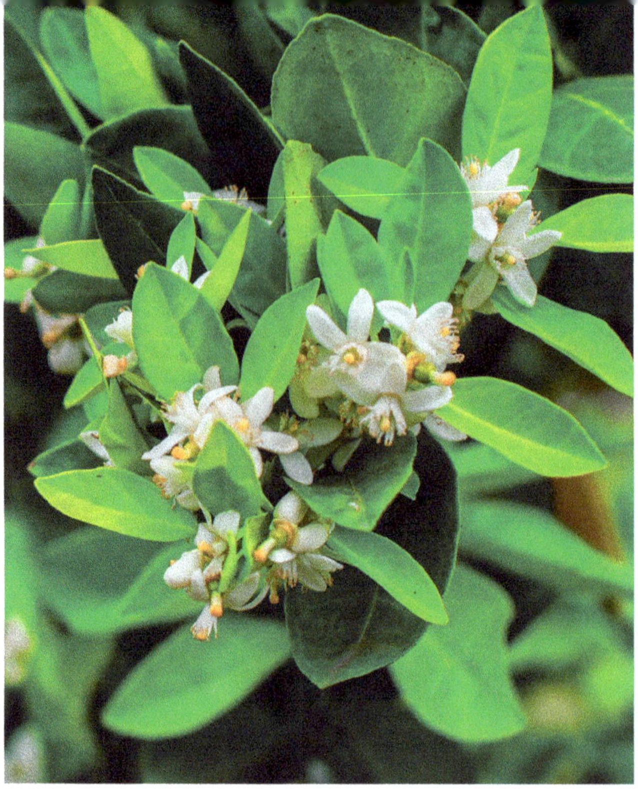

CONSTITUENTS

SWEET ORANGE PEEL: Sweet orange peel contains volatile oil (refer to the essential oil below), flavonoids (neohesperidin, hesperidin, naringin, tangeretin, auranetin, and nobiletin), vitamins (B_1, C, and E), limonin, coumarins (6,7-dimethoxycoumarin), carotenoids, pectin, citrantin, and constituents similar to bitter orange peel.[13,16]

SWEET ORANGE ESSENTIAL OIL: Sweet orange volatile oil is similar to bitter orange oil (refer to the following paragraph). It contains similar monoterpenes, alcohols, aldehydes (mostly decanal and octanal), ketones, free acids, and esters. Cold-pressed orange oil also contains coumarins (bergaptene and auaptenol), valencene, and α-ylangene.[13]

BITTER ORANGE PEEL: Bitter orange peel contains volatile oil (refer to the essential oil below), flavonoids (neohesperidin, hesperidin, naringin, rhoifolin, lonicerin, tangeretin, nobiletin, sinensetin, auranetin, and rutin), vitamins (A, B_1, and C), coumarins (6,7-dimethoxycoumarin and umbelliferone), carotenoid pigments (citraurin, violaxanthin, and cryptoxanthin), pectin, citrantin, and others. The white part of the peel contains limonoid-type triterpenes and flavonoids (hesperidin, nargingin, and neohesperidin).[13,16]

BITTER ORANGE ESSENTIAL OIL: The volatile oil of bitter orange contains monoterpenes (D-limonene, myrcene, camphene, pinene, ocimene, and *p*-cymene), small amounts of alcohols (linalool, terpineol, nerol, farnesol, nerolidol, and octanol), aldehydes (decanal, nonanal, dodecanal, citronellal, neral, acetaldehyde, and formaldehyde), ketones (carvone, α-ionine, and jasmone), free acids (octadecadienoic, pelargonic, cinnamic, and acetic), esters (linalyl acetate, decyl pelargonate, octylacetate, and geranyl acetate), coumarins (osthole and auraptenol), and others.[13]

NEROLI (ORANGE FLOWER) ESSENTIAL OIL: Neroli oil contains linalool, linalyl acetate, limonene, β-pinene, nerolidol, geraniol, nerol, methyl anthranilate, indole, jasmone, citral, nonanal, *cis*-8-heptadecene, 2,5-dimethyl-2-vinyl-4-hexenal, neryl acetate, valeric acid, and others.[13]

PETITGRAIN ESSENTIAL OIL: Petitgrain oil contains esters (linalyl acetate and geranyl acetate), linalool, nerol, α-terpineol, geraniol, nerolidol, farnesol, and limonene.[13]

NUTRITIONAL PROPERTIES: Orange peel contains flavonoids, carotenoids, and vitamins B_1, C, and E. For the nutritional properties of oranges, refer to the pulp under *Medicinal Uses* below.[13]

MEDICINAL PROPERTIES: Antinauseant, astringent, bitter tonic, carminative, circulatory stimulant, cholagogue, detoxifier, expectorant, and stomachic.

TEMPERATURE AND FLAVOR: Warm, pungent, bitter, sweet, and astringent.

MEDICINAL USES

RIPE PEEL: The ripe peel of sweet and bitter orange enhance digestion due to their carminative, cholagogue, and bitter tonic properties. The peel contains two intensely bitter flavonoid glycosides, naringin and neohesperidin. Orange peel stimulates digestive secretions, and can be used to treat appetite loss. It reduces a sense of fullness, belching, hiccups, dyspepsia, gas, and bloating. The volatile oil in the peel reduces nausea and vomiting. Orange peel increases circulation, especially in the digestive tract. It is often combined with other bitter and carminative herbs in digestive bitter tonic compounds and cordials, including bitter herbs such as artichoke leaf *(Cynara)*, gentian *(Gentiana)*, or berberis *(Berberis)*, and carminative herbs such as cardamom *(Elettaria)*, coriander *(Coriandrum)*, fennel *(Foeniculum)*, and ginger *(Zingiber)*. According to Traditional Chinese Medicine, orange peel warms the spleen, enhances digestion, and regulates the middle burner. It is combined with qi tonifying herbs such as ginseng *(Panax ginseng)*, codonopsis *(Codonopsis)*, or astragalus *(Astragalus)* to reduce qi stagnation.

An expectorant, orange peel thins and expels mucus, and reduces copious watery phlegm. It is beneficial for treating moist lung conditions, including asthma, chronic bronchitis, a productive cough, or a cold. The volatile oil has antiseptic and lymphatic actions. The flavonoids and pectin are antibacterial and antifungal. Orange peel astringes mucous membranes, especially in the respiratory and digestive tracts. The astringent actions aid in treating loose stools and diarrhea. According to Traditional Chinese Medicine, orange peel dries and disperses dampness in the chest and abdomen.

Orange peel, pulp, and juice are excellent sources of vitamin C and flavonoids that synergize the vitamin's effects. The vitamin C content reduces inflammation, enhances the integrity of connective tissue, and counters the body's response to stress. Vitamin C and flavonoids inhibit the release of histamines, and are highly beneficial for reducing allergies and allergy-related asthma attacks, wheezing, respiratory infections, and nasal congestion. Vitamin C and flavonoids are antioxidants that inhibit free radical formation, supporting the cardiovascular and immune systems. They enhance the integrity of the vascular system, and can be used as a daily tonic to reduce capillary fragility and permeability. Orange peel also can be used for the long-term treatment of varicose veins, degenerative vascular diseases such as atherosclerosis and hypertension, and diabetes. It facilitates the healing of bruises and wounds.

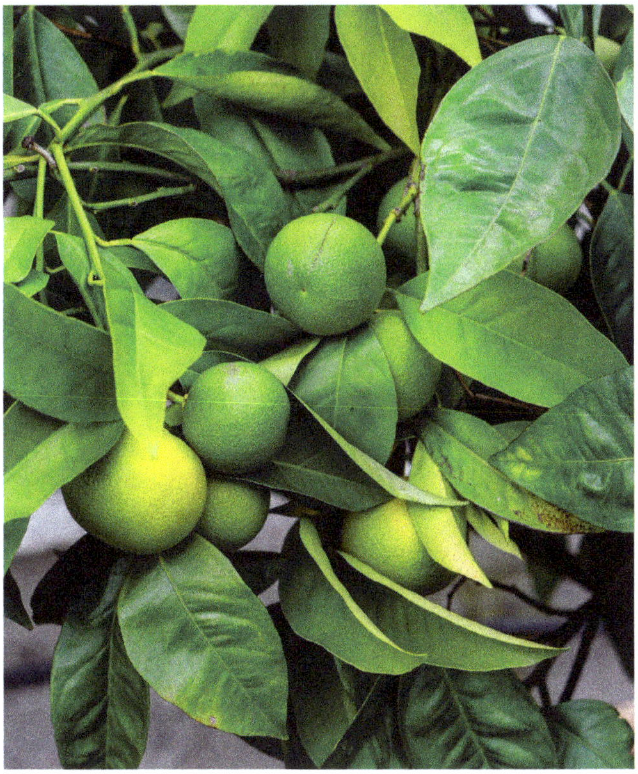

Orange peel enhances detoxification. It contains pectin which is highly ionic, drawing from the tissues and binding with environmental toxins and heavy metals. The pectin and cholagogue actions also help to lower cholesterol.

UNRIPE PEEL: The green peel from the immature fruit of *C. reticulata* (syn. *C. reticulata viride*) is known as green tangerine, blue citrus, or qing pi. Green tangerine peel has the same actions as orange peel in the digestive, respiratory, and cardiovascular systems, and in its energetic properties (warm, bitter, and acrid). However, it is used specifically in Traditional Chinese Medicine as a liver decongestant. It encourages the smooth flow of liver qi and breaks up qi stagnation, treating symptoms such as distension and pain in the chest, breast, or hypochondriac regions. It alleviates food stagnation, easing abdominal pain and distension. It is often combined with chai hu *(Bupleurum)* and turmeric *(Curcuma)* for pain and distension in the chest and flanks due to liver and stomach disharmonies. It is combined with xiang fu *(Cyperus)* for chest and flank pain associated with liver qi stagnation.[17]

The immature fruit of bitter orange *(C. aurantium)* is known as zhi shi (Chinese), kijitsu (Japanese), or chisel (Korean). While it shares some energetic properties of other citrus peels (bitter and acrid), it is also slightly cooling. Zhi shi shares the same expectorant, bitter, carminative, and laxative actions, but is most specific to direct qi downward, unblocking the bowels and treating abdominal pain, constipation, and dysenteric diarrhea.[17] Small doses relax the intestines; large doses increase peristalsis. Zhi shi is a carminative that reduces food stagnation, indigestion, gas, and bloating.[17] It can be combined with other qi tonifying herbs to treat organ prolapse. It is used to treat prolapsed hollow organs such as the uterus, rectum, or stomach. Zhi shi also prevents qi stagnation when combined with qi tonifying herbs. It has expectorant actions and reduces sensations of fullness in the chest.[17] It is contraindicated during pregnancy, and for individuals with deficient qi or cold in the stomach due to deficiency.[17]

AGED CITRUS PEEL: Aged or mature tangerine peel *(C. reticulata)* is known as chen pi (Mandarin), or "aged peel." Additional names include chinpi (Japanese) and chinp'i (Korean). Western herbalists prefer the fresh aromatic qualities of recently dried citrus peel; aged citrus peel is equally valued in Traditional Chinese Medicine. The energetic properties are warm, bitter, acrid, and aromatic.

Like ripe citrus peel, chen pi is used for the digestive and respiratory systems, and to regulate qi.[17] It warms the spleen and regulates the middle burner. Chen pi is a carminative; it reduces a sense of fullness, belching, hiccups, gas, bloating, nausea, and vomiting.[17] It enhances spleen transforming and transporting functions, improving digestion and assimilation. It also can be used to treat loss of appetite. Chen pi reduces potential stagnation that can result from tonifying herbs, and is often used in combination with qi tonifying herbs. It dries and disperses dampness in the chest or abdomen, reducing phlegm in the lungs and treating loose stools.[17] It is contraindicated for hot conditions, including a red tongue, yellow or orange phlegm, dry cough, or spitting of blood.[17]

THE PULP: The fleshy part of orange fruit can be consumed raw or juiced. It contains vitamin C and flavonoids. For more information on vitamin C and flavonoids, refer to the second to last paragraph in the section on the ripe peel. Orange also contains several B vitamins (B_1, B_2, B_6, folic acid, and pantothenic acid), carotenes, pectin, and potassium. The fruit is a good source of fiber, and is hydrating on hot days.[14] The sour flavor of the fruit, especially with the pith, stimulates digestion, and is a natural bile stimulant and mild laxative.

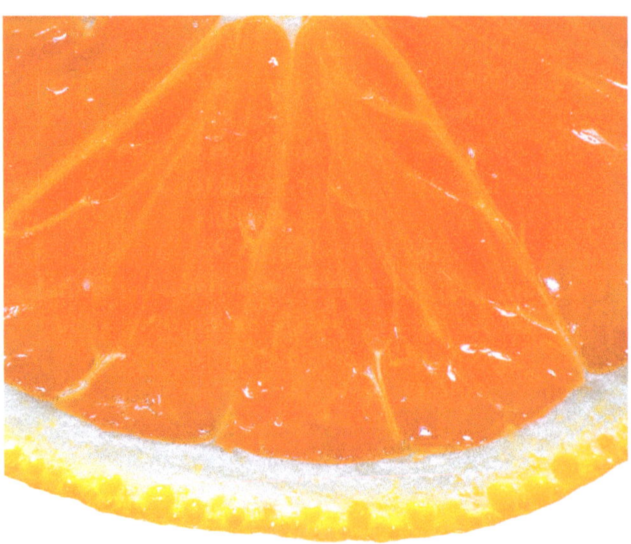

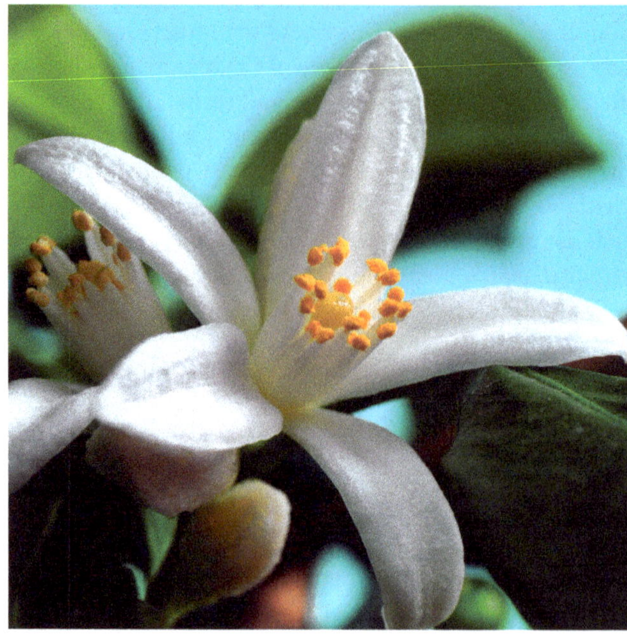

THE FLOWERS: Bitter orange flowers are consumed primarily in tea, syrup, or honey. They have calming effects, and can be used to treat nervousness, anxiety, and insomnia. They are also added to cordials and elixirs as an aphrodisiac, and are employed as a harmonizer.

THE ESSENTIAL OIL: Varied essential oils are produced from different species of orange and numerous parts of the plants.

ORANGE FLOWER, NEROLI (CITRUS AURANTIUM VAR. AMARA)

Neroli was named in honor of Anne-Marie, the 16th century princess of Nerola who loved the scent. She used neroli to perfume her gloves and bath water. Her glove perfume became so popular, it was known as *guanti di Neroli*.[15] The white flowers of bitter orange *(C. aurantium* var. *amara)* are used to produce the exotic, prized essential oil of neroli. Bitter orange spring flowers are considered superior to fall and sweet orange flowers. The aqueous byproduct of distillation is called orange flower hydrosol, or orange flower water. Three methods used to extract the essential oil are distillation, concrete, and absolute.

Neroli has calming and mildly sedating actions.[18] The essential oil and hydrosol are used to treat anxiety, insomnia, nervous tension, and shock.[12] Neroli decreases the amplitude of heart muscle contraction, and is beneficial for alleviating palpitations, cardiac spasms, and anxiety attacks. It is an antidepressant and mood elevator.[12,18] Neroli oil and hydrosol have aphrodisiac actions and can be used in perfume. Blending neroli with sandalwood, rose, and jasmine essential oil produces an exotic perfume. Neroli

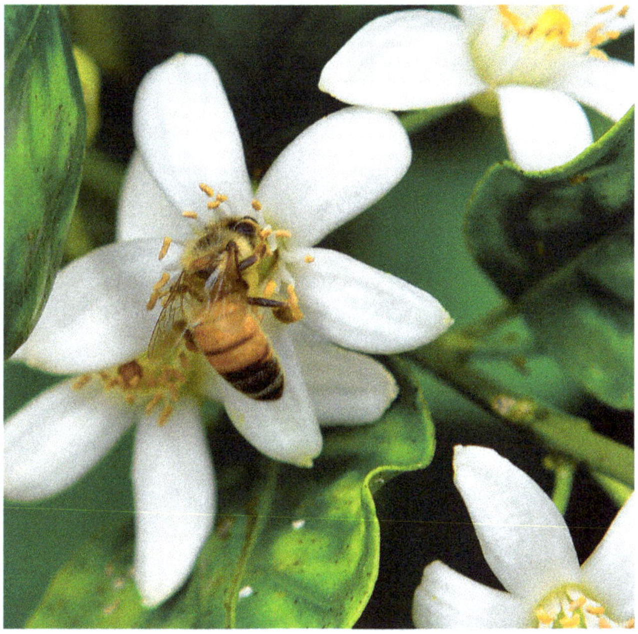

is beneficial for all skin types, and can be added to facial serums, creams, and lotions. It stimulates cellular regeneration in skin, and reduces irritation, relieving redness, broken skin and veins, and couperose skin.[12] Orange hydrosol soothes the digestive tract, acting as a carminative and stomachic. It is useful for treating infant colic and as a sedative for children. There are no known contraindications with the physiological dosage.[18]

DIRECTIONS: Apply one to two drops of neroli essential oil topically (neat or diluted) or add to a diffuser. Orange flower hydrosol can be consumed internally (one teaspoon, up to five times daily) or applied topically.

PETITGRAIN (CITRUS AURANTIUM VAR. AMARA)

The name *petitgrain* means "little fruit," and originated from essential oil produced from the unripe, small fruit.[12] A distillation of twigs and young shoots of bitter orange *(C. aurantium* var. *amara)* is used to produce petitgrain essential oil. Benjamin Balansa, 19th century French botanist, first distilled the leaves.[12] Petitgrain has a distinctly bitter, earthy aroma. It has antidepressant and anxiolytic actions. It can be used to decrease anxiety, nervousness, insomnia, and depression, and stabilize the nervous system.[18] Aromatherapist Kathy Keville recommends using petitgrain to increase perception and awareness, and reestablish trust and self-confidence.[12] Petitgrain combines well with other sweet-smelling essential oils such as ylang ylang and palmarosa. An excellent lip balm contains small amounts of palmarosa, a citrus peel oil such as orange, grapefruit or bergamot, and one or two drops of petitgrain. There are no known contraindications with the physiological dosage.

DIRECTIONS: Apply 1 – 2 drops topically (neat or diluted), or place 1 – 3 drops in the diffuser.

SWEET ORANGE (CITRUS SINENSIS) BITTER ORANGE (CITRUS AURANTIUM)

The essential oils of sweet and bitter orange are commonly prepared by cold-pressing the peel. However, essential oil of fresh orange peel (from expressed or unexpressed fruits) is also steam distilled or distilled from byproducts in the manufacture of orange juice concentrates. The latter preparation produces oils inferior to the other methods. Terpeneless orange oils (bitter and sweet) are obtained from vacuum distillation or extraction with dilute ethyl alcohol. Only organic or biodynamic sources of orange essential oil should be used therapeutically because orange peels are heavily sprayed, and contain the concentrated chemical residue of pesticides and herbicides.

Sweet and bitter orange peel have calming and antidepressant qualities. They are mildly sedative for treating nervousness, anxiety, insomnia, depression, hysteria, and shock.[12] They also have a joyful, uplifting quality. Orange oil has antimicrobial and lymphatic actions that aid in treating a cold or flu.[12,18] The limonene in citrus peel has potential cancer-preventative properties and antineoplastic actions in pancreatic and breast cancer. It also has the potential to dissolve gallstones.[19] Orange peel combines well with floral scents such as ylang ylang, jasmine, and neroli. It also harmonizes with more earthy oils such as vetiver, patchouli, and spikenard oil, or sharper, piercing evergreen oils such as pine and fir. Orange peel oil (bitter and sweet) is phototoxic, and should not be applied to the skin less than 12 hours before exposure to strong sun.

DIRECTIONS: Apply topically (diluted), or place 1 – 3 drops in the diffuser.

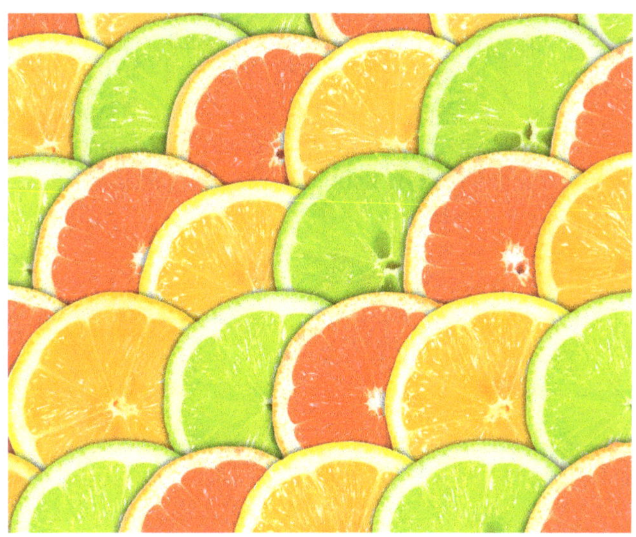

CONTRAINDICATIONS

Orange peel contains limonene that can cause contact dermatitis and phototoxicity. Avoid handling the peel excessively, or applying products containing orange essential oil less than 12 hours before exposure to strong sun. Oranges are a food allergen for some individuals. Individuals with migraines or arthritis should avoid oranges if they aggravate their symptoms.[20] Consuming excessive quantities of bitter or sweet orange peel has been reported to cause intestinal colic, convulsions, and even death in children.[13] Orange peel contains oxalates; thus, individuals with calcium oxalate-containing kidney stones should limit consumption, although peel is rarely consumed in enough quantities to cause problems.[11] Orange peel should be avoided with a dry cough or bloody sputum — a symptom of yin or qi deficiency.[17] It also should be avoided with sticky, yellow phlegm. Avoid with deficient qi, blood, or yin.[17]

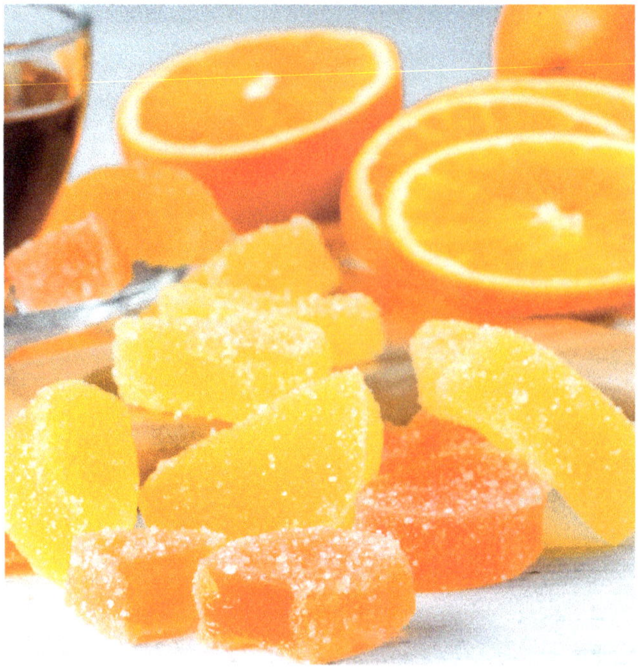

PREPARATION AND DOSAGE

TINCTURE: Fresh peels [1:2-1:3, 70-95% alcohol]; dry peels [1:5, 60% alcohol]; consume 10-30 drops, up to three times daily. Dry peels [1:5, in brandy or vodka]; consume 15-30 drops, up to three times daily.

GLYCERITE: Dry peels [1:5, 40% alcohol, 30% glycerin, 30% distilled water]; consume 10-30 drops, up to three times daily.

ACETUM EXTRACT: Dry peels [1:5, apple cider vinegar]; consume 1 teaspoon, one to three times daily before meals.

TEA: Prepare a standard or cold infusion, or decoction of orange peel; consume 8-12 ounces, three to four times daily. Do not decoct orange peel more than 10-15 minutes. The aromatic oils dissipate rapidly; make sure to use a lid when making tea. Prepare orange flowers with a standard or cold infusion; consume 4-8 ounces, up to four times daily.

HONEY AND SYRUP: Infuse fresh, wilted peel in honey up to one month and strain; consume 1 teaspoon, up to three times daily. Prepare orange peel or orange flower syrup and consume 1 teaspoon, up to three times daily, or add to herbal formulas as a harmonizer. Add the syrup to confections.

TOPICAL USE: Refer to the essential oil use listed below.

CULINARY USE: Orange zest (the orange part of the peel) can be added to salad dressings, sauces, olives, cocktails, syrups, desserts, confections, and fish or meat dishes. Make sure to use only organic oranges for the zest, due to the pesticide residue and artificial coloring in commercial oranges. Orange flower water can be added to candy, confections, frosting, liqueur, and simple syrup, as well as lighter protein dishes, such as scallops, white fish, and chicken.

ESSENTIAL OIL: Add up to 10 drops of orange essential oil to 1 ounce of base oil for topical or culinary use. Add 1-3 drops of orange or neroli essential oil to simple syrup, honey, whipped cream, desserts, etc. Add 1-4 drops of neroli to facial serum, cream, lotion, massage oil, or perfume blends.

OREGANO

DESCRIPTION

BOTANICAL NAME:
Origanum vulgare subsp. *hirtum*

COMMON NAMES:
Oregano, Greek oregano, Turkish oregano, European oregano, wild marjoram, mountain mint, winter marjoram, wintersweet
rigon (Albanian)
anrar, satar barri (Arabic)
rigan (Bulgarian)
ngou lahk gong (Cantonese)
orenga (Catalan)
origano (Croatian)
oregáno (Czech)
oregano (Danish)
origano (Esperanto)
harilik pune (Estonian)
mäkimeirami (Finnish)
marjolaine sauvage, marjolaine bâtarde, origan, pelevoué, penevoué, doste, thym de berger, thé rouge (French)
dost, wilder majoran (German)
rigani, diktamos (Greek)
oregano (Hebrew)
vadmajoránna, oregánó (Hungarian)
oreganó (Icelandic)
oragán (Irish Gaelic)
erba accuiga, origano (Italian)
hana-hakka (Japanese)
bergmynte, kung (Norwegian)
dziki majeranek (Polish)
orégão, orégano (Portuguese)
oregano (Romanian)
dushitsa (Russian)
origano (Serbian)
orégano (Spanish)
kungsmynta (Swedish)
origano (Thai)
kekik otu, kekikotu, güvey otu (Turkish)
materynka (Ukrainian)
origan (Yiddish)[1,2]

FAMILY NAME:
Lamiaceae (Labiatae)

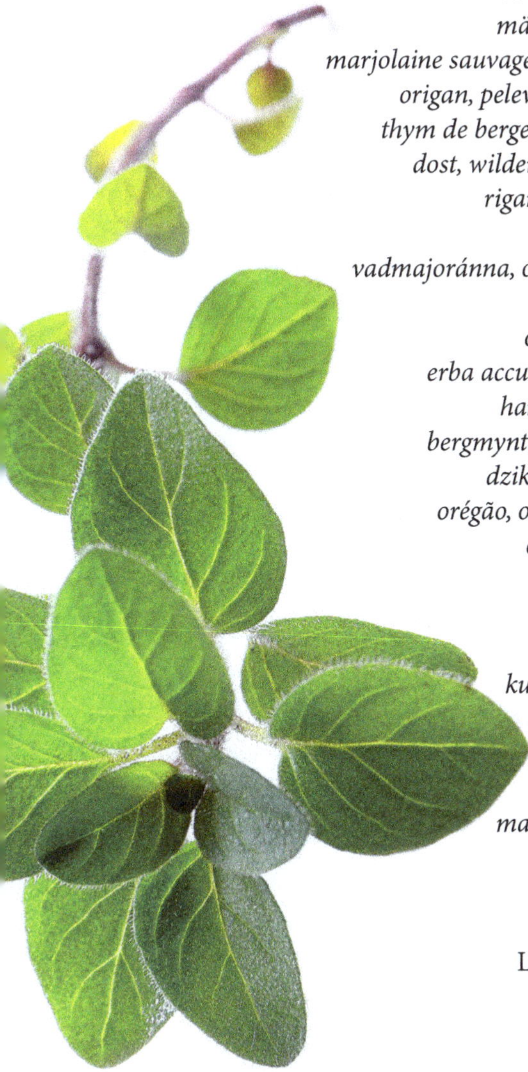

PART USED: The leaves.

BOTANICAL DESCRIPTION AND HABITAT: Oregano *(Origanum vulgare)*, native to the sunny habitats of grasslands and open scrub surrounding the Mediterranean, has two commonly utilized subspecies: Greek oregano *(O. vulgare* subsp. *hirtum)* and wild oregano *(O. vulgare* subsp. *vulgare)*.

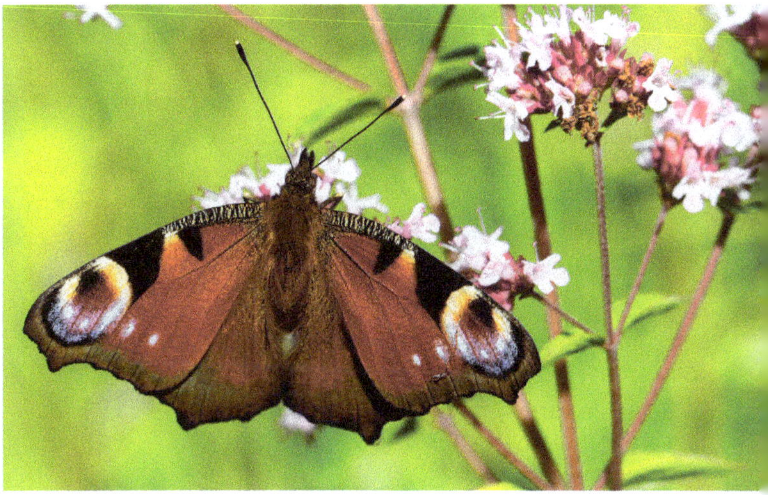

Greek oregano *(O. vulgare* subsp. *hirtum)* is a rhizomatous, colony-forming plant. The pubescent, greenish-purplish stems reach 25 – 60 cm tall.[3] The ovate, glandular, strongly scented, purple-tinged leaves (1 – 4 cm by 0.5 – 1.5 cm) are densely hairy on the undersides, and sparsely hairy on the upper sides.[3] It has an obtuse apex, an entire margin, and a rounded to wedge-shaped base.[3] The spike-like inflorescences bear flowers with calyces (2 – 4 mm long) that have tiny triangular teeth. The lower lip of the white, tubular, bilabiate corolla (5 – 7 mm long) has three lobes; the upper lobe is entire.[4] Four stamens and a four-lobed ovary consisting of two carpels comprise the inner whorls.[4] The tiny fruits have four brown nutlets.[3]

Wild oregano *(O. vulgare* subsp. *vulgare)* is only distinguished from Greek oregano *(O. vulgare* subsp. *hirtum)* by a few characteristics. Wild oregano leaves and calyces lack the glandular hairs of Greek oregano, the corollas are pinkish-purple (not white), and the bracts subtending the flowers are purple.[5] More importantly, wild oregano lacks the strong, pungent aroma of Greek oregano, and is an inferior medicinal and culinary herb.[5]

THE NAME: The genus *Origanum* derives from two Greek words: *oros* ("mountain") and *ganos* ("joy"), referring to the native mountainous habitat in which the plant thrives.[2] The epithet *vulgare* ("common") derives from Latin.[6] The subspecies name, *hirtum* ("hairy, covered with hair, shaggy"), derives from Latin, and refers to the fine hairs covering the leaves and stems.[7]

Oregano is sometimes called "wild marjoram."[2] The following common names correspond with the Latin binomials: true Greek oregano, Greek oregano, Turkish oregano (*O. vulgare* subsp. *hirtum*); wild oregano (*O. vulgare* subsp. *vulgare*); pot marjoram (*O. onites*); and dittany of Crete (*O. dictamnus*).[5] Wild oregano (*O. vulgare* subsp. *vulgare*) has reddish-pink, purple flowers

HISTORICAL USES: In ancient Greek mythology, Aphrodite was credited for creating oregano. After the Greek philosopher Aristotle observed that tortoises consumed oregano leaves after ingesting a snake, he began using oregano as an antidote to poison. Ancient Greeks used oregano to treat convulsions and dropsy.[2] They also planted oregano over graves to ensure that the departed would be content.[2] Oregano was planted around homes to protect against evil. In marriage ceremonies, ancient Greeks and Romans crowned couples with oregano.[2] It was carried as a charm for health and good luck. Oregano was used in spells to bring happiness, health, and good luck, and to aid in letting go of a loved one.

Oregano was given as a diaphoretic, stimulant, carminative, and tonic.[2] A hot infusion was administered to encourage perspiration and elicit the eruption of measles.[2] Topically, the hot fomentation or poultice was applied to rheumatic joints and painful swelling as a rubefacient.[2] Prior to the introduction of hops, oregano was included as a flavoring and preservative in beer and ale.[2,5]

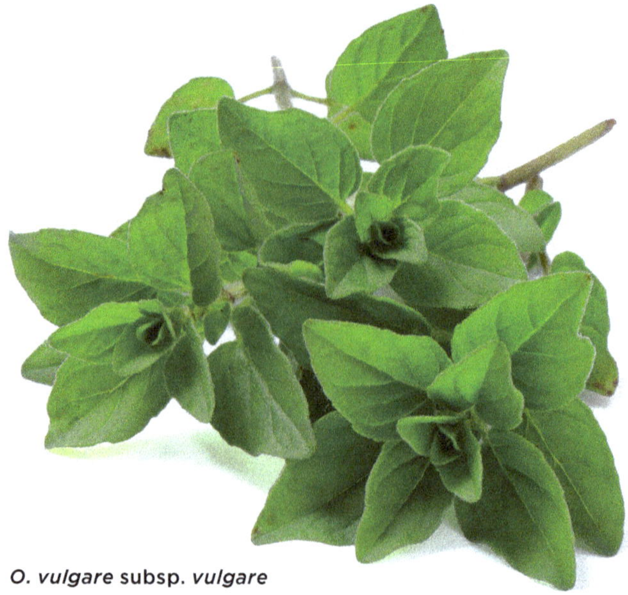

O. vulgare subsp. *vulgare*

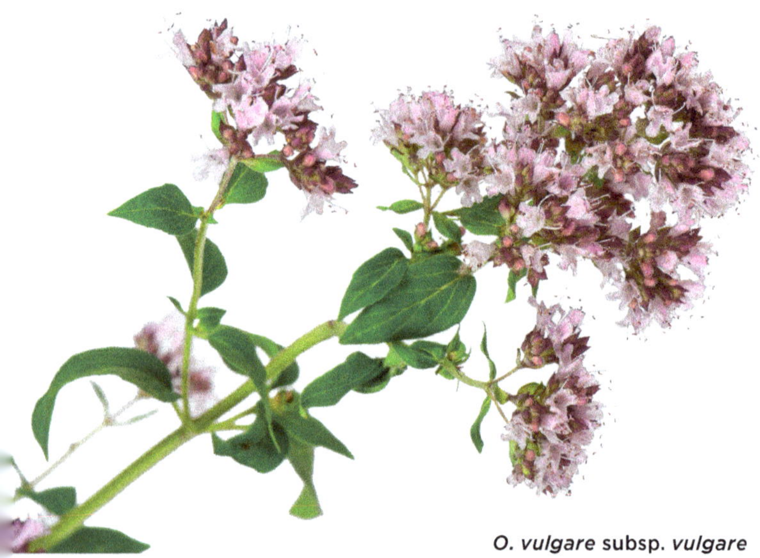

O. vulgare subsp. *vulgare*

CONSTITUENTS

OREGANO LEAVES: *Origanum vulgare* contains volatile oil consisting of thymol, carvacrol, β-bisabolene, caryophyllene, *p*-cymene, borneol, linalool, linalyl acetate geranyl acetate, α-pinene, β-pinene, and α-terpene. It also contains a bitter principle (a flavanone neohesperidoside: naringin), flavonoids (luteolin), apigenin, diosmetin, Lamiaceae tannins (caffeic and rosmarinic acid), triterpeneoids (ursolic and oleanolic acid), phenolic acids (vanillic and syringic acid), protein, vitamins, and minerals.[8,9]

OREGANO ESSENTIAL OIL: Essential oil of *O. vulgare* contains thymol, carvacrol, γ-terpinene, *p*-cymene, β-bisabolene, caryophyllene, borneol, linalool, linalyl acetate geranyl acetate, α-pinene, β-pinene, and α-terpene.[8,9]

NUTRITIONAL PROPERTIES: Oregano contains β-carotene, niacin, phosphorus, potassium, iron, calcium, magnesium, and traces of zinc.[5]

MEDICINAL PROPERTIES: Anti-inflammatory, antibacterial, antifungal, antioxidant, antispasmodic, anthelmintic, antiviral, aromatic, carminative, choleretic, diaphoretic, expectorant, stimulant, and diuretic.

TEMPERATURE AND FLAVOR: Hot and pungent.

MEDICINAL USES

The medicinal properties of oregano described below refer solely to Greek oregano *(O. vulgare* subsp. *hirtum),* not wild oregano (*O. vulgare* subsp. *vulgare).* For more information on other *Origanum* species, refer to the monograph on marjoram.

Oregano is an extremely effective antimicrobial agent.[10] It has antibacterial and expectorant properties that aid in treating sinusitis, laryngitis, strep throat, bronchitis, and staph infections.[9,10] Oregano has antiviral actions that aid in treating a cold, flu, and mononucleosis.[9] Consume hot thyme and oregano tea, or infuse the herbs in chicken broth as a diaphoretic, and to reduce respiratory congestion.[9] Oregano inhibits the biosynthesis of prostaglandins and leukotrienes, reducing inflammation.[9] It contains rosmarinic acid and phenols (thymol and carvacrol) that contribute to the potent antifungal, antibacterial, antiviral, and anthelmintic properties, as well as the anti-inflammatory and choleretic effects.[5,9,10,] Combine extracts of oregano, usnea *(Usnea),* and thyme *(Thymus)* with smaller quantities of orange peel *(Citrus sinensis),* cinnamon *(Cinnamomum),* clove *(Syzygium),* licorice *(Glycyrrhiza),* and rosemary *(Salvia rosmarinus)* as a broad spectrum, warming antimicrobial, and diaphoretic compound for respiratory or digestive infections. Consume 30 – 90 drops, four to five times daily.

Oregano is an antifungal agent that aids in treating *Candida albicans* overgrowth in the digestive and vaginal tracts.[8,10,11] It is an adjunct antibacterial agent that treats bacterial vaginosis. Combine extracts of oregano with usnea *(Usnea),* berberis *(Berberis),* calendula *(Calendula),* spilanthes *(Acmella),* and/or thyme *(Thymus)* to treat candida or bacterial vaginosis. Consume 30 – 90 drops, up to four times daily.

Oregano and its essential oil also have antiparasitic and anthelmintic properties that aid in treating giardia, hookworms, and pinworms.[11] Carvacrol is attributed to the fungicidal, bactericidal, and anthelmintic properties.[8,9]

Oregano is an aromatic carminative, stomachic, and choleretic, supporting healthy digestive function.[5,8,9] It aids in treating sluggish digestion, nonulcer dyspepsia, indigestion, colic, flatulence, and diarrhea.[5,9] Oregano has very mild antispasmodic properties that affect the smooth muscles in the digestive tract. The stomachic and choleretic actions are attributed to the bitter principles and phenolic acids.[9]

Oregano is a delicious, pungent culinary herb that enhances flavor and facilitates the digestion of lamb, mutton, goat, veal, most red gamey meats, pork, poultry, fish, eggs, gravy, stuffing, tomato dishes, pizza, beans, potatoes, vegetable dishes, and vinaigrettes. Greeks often use oregano to season grilled meats, such as gyros and souvlaki. Dried oregano is often sprinkled on Greek salads with lettuce, cucumber, tomato, red onions, feta, and olives. Oregano is used in the cuisine of southern Mediterranean countries including Italy, France, and Spain. Due to its potent antioxidant properties, it is combined with other Mediterranean herbs to cure and preserve meat.[2]

Oregano mouthwash, tea and fresh herb have antimicrobial properties that aid in treating gingivitis and halitosis. A topical antimicrobial, oregano inhibits fungal and bacterial growth; it disinfects wounds and treats athlete's foot, ringworm, skin tinea, and staph.[9] It has counterirritant and rubefacient actions that improve circulation, treating bruises, sprains, strains, muscle pain and spasms, arthritis, and rheumatic pain. Adding dried oregano leaves to medicinal oils or salves prevents rancidity.

OREGANO ESSENTIAL OIL (ORIGANUM VULGARE OR ORIGANUM COMPACTUM)

Essential oil of oregano contains high concentrations of the phenol carvacrol, a potent antibacterial agent.[10] However, it can irritate the mucous membranes and is highly irritating to the skin.[10,12] The essential oil also contains stimulating terpene hydrocarbons.[10] For internal use, it is best to consume oregano essential oil in a carrier oil (containing no more than 1 – 2% of essential oil); the recommended dosage is 50 mg (1 – 2 drops) per application, up to four times daily.[10]

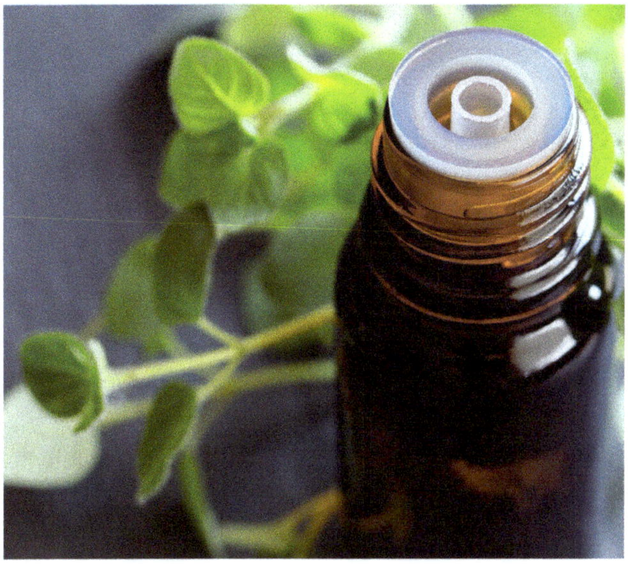

Essential oil of oregano has expectorant, antibacterial, antifungal, antiparasitic, spasmolytic, and choleretic actions.[8,11] An antimicrobial agent, it aids in treating acute respiratory infections, such as a cold, flu, laryngitis, pharyngitis, strep throat, mononucleosis, bronchitis, and pneumonia.[9,10] Oregano essential oil also aids in treating: urinary tract infections (cystitis and urethritis); digestive infections such as intestinal candida, hookworms, pinworms, and giardia; and bacterial and viral gastrointestinal infections.[9-11] The essential oil is one of the most potent antimicrobial agents against *Proteus, Enterococcus, Staphylococcus, Streptococcus, Pneumococcus, Escherichia coli, Neisseria, Corynebacterium xerosis,* and *Candida.*[10] *Note:* Do not apply oregano oil topically, as it is extremely irritating to the skin.[10] Avoid internal use during pregnancy or lactation, and in children under 10 years old. Individuals with inflammatory bowel disease should avoid ingesting oregano oil. Due to the high phenol content, oregano oil should not be consumed more than 10 consecutive days; long-term use can negatively affect liver metabolism.[10]

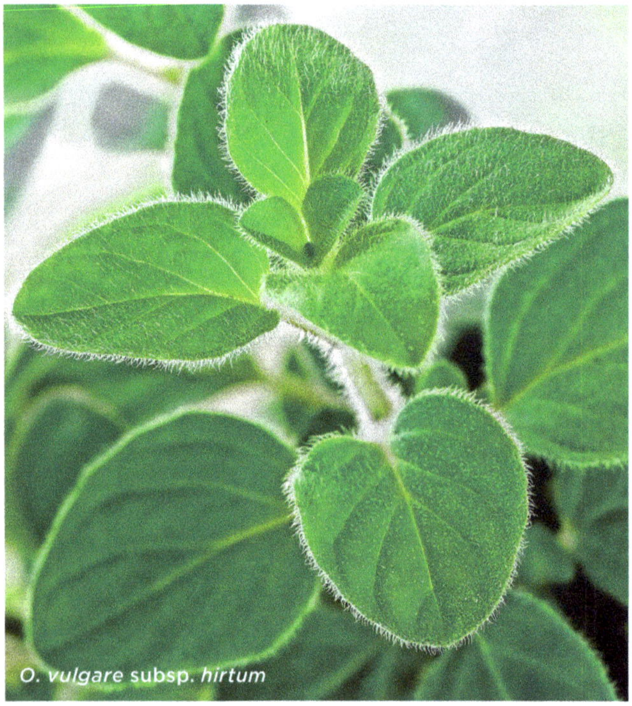

O. vulgare subsp. *hirtum*

CONTRAINDICATIONS

There are no side effects when used in the recommended doses.[9] Avoid consuming essential oil or excessive amounts of oregano during pregnancy, lactation, and in cases of biliary obstruction.[9] Topical application of the essential oil can cause skin irritation; do not apply unless it is diluted.[9] More contraindications are listed in the essential oil section.

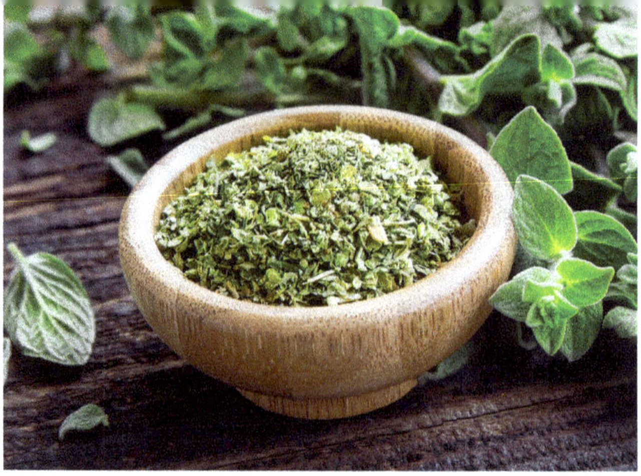

PREPARATION AND DOSAGE

TINCTURE: Fresh leaves [1:2-1:3, 70-95% alcohol]; dry leaves [1:5-1:6, 60% alcohol]; consume 15-60 drops, three to four times daily.

ACETUM EXTRACT: Fresh leaves [1:3-1:4, apple cider vinegar]; consume in food preparations such as vinaigrettes, or apply diluted oregano acetum topically.

CAPSULES: Consume 1-2 capsules of enteric coated oregano oil capsules, one to three times daily. Add 1-2 drops of essential oil to a charcoal tablet, or a capsule containing a powdered binding agent; consume 1-2 capsules, one to three times daily.

TEA: Prepare the hot infusion; consume 8-12 ounces, one to three times daily.

HONEY AND SYRUP: Simple syrup can be prepared by dissolving one part by volume of sugar into one part of a strained oregano infusion, or infusing oregano directly into prepared simple syrup. Add 1-2 drops of oregano essential oil to 1 teaspoon to 1 tablespoon of honey, and mix with a toothpick. Add the honey to one cup of tea or hot water; consume up to four times daily.

TOPICAL USE: Apply the tea as a fomentation, poultice, or foot bath. Prepare the oil using the infused oil or alcohol intermediary method. Dilute the essential oil in cream, oil, salve, or liniment.

CULINARY USE: Freshly chopped or ground, dried oregano is a seasoning for beef, lamb, veal, venison, rabbit, poultry, soup, gravy, sauces, potatoes, root vegetable dishes, and vinaigrettes.

OSHÁ

BOTANICAL NAMES:
Ligusticum apiifolium, L. caldera, L. canbyi, L. grayi, L. porteri, L. scoticum

COMMON NAMES:
Oshá, oshala, bear medicine, Porter's lovage, Gray's lovage, wild lovage, Gray's licorice root, love parsley, cough root, Colorado cough root, Indian root, kishwoof *chuchupáte, hierba del cochino* (Spanish)

FAMILY NAME:
Apiaceae (Umbelliferae)

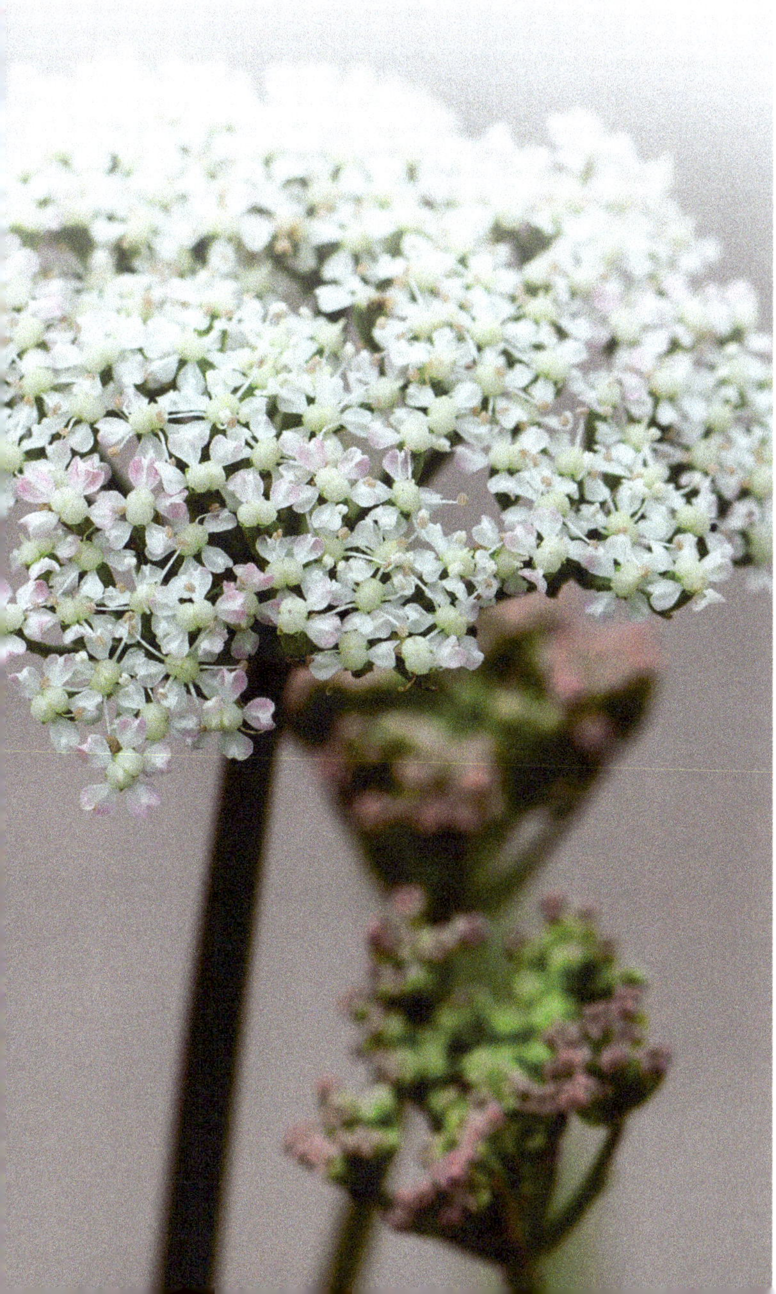

DESCRIPTION

PARTS USED: The roots (medicinal) and leaves (culinary).

BOTANICAL DESCRIPTION AND HABITAT: *Ligusticum* grows at high elevations in moist mountain meadows. It is a poorly defined genus with a complex taxonomy that

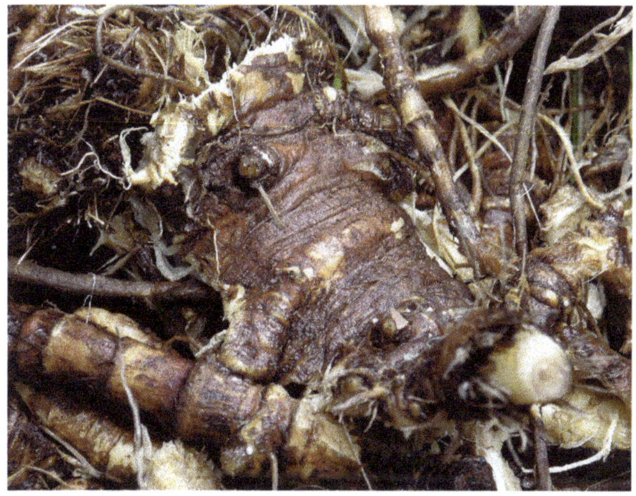

may soon be redefined.[1] *Ligusticum* is a genus of up to 60 perennial, herbaceous species with erect, striated stems.[2] The root crowns are sheathed in brown fibrous remains from prior years' leaves.[2,3] The roots are thick, resinous, and fusiform.[1] Depending on the species, the plants range from glabrous, to scabrous, to pubescent.[3] The leaves are oblong to round, and ternately and/or one to four times pinnately compound.[3] The leaflets are entire to deeply pinnately lobed. The leaves are reduced in size or absent as they ascend the branching flowering stem.[1] The umbels are either terminal or terminal and axial with a minimal involucre consisting of few linear involucels.[2] The number of rays and flowers varies according to species. The flowers have diminished to absent calyx lobes and five petals ranging from white to pink to purple.[1] The oblong to ovoid schizocarp is compressed, with prominent or enlarged lateral ridges forming wings.[1]

Warning: All members of the Apiaceae family should be properly identified before using them medicinally because some are severely toxic. Some distinguishing characteristics are listed here, but further research is strongly recommended for accurate identification. Oshá can be confused with poison hemlock *(Conium maculatum)* or water hemlock *(Cicuta* spp.*)*. Be sure to identify the plants when

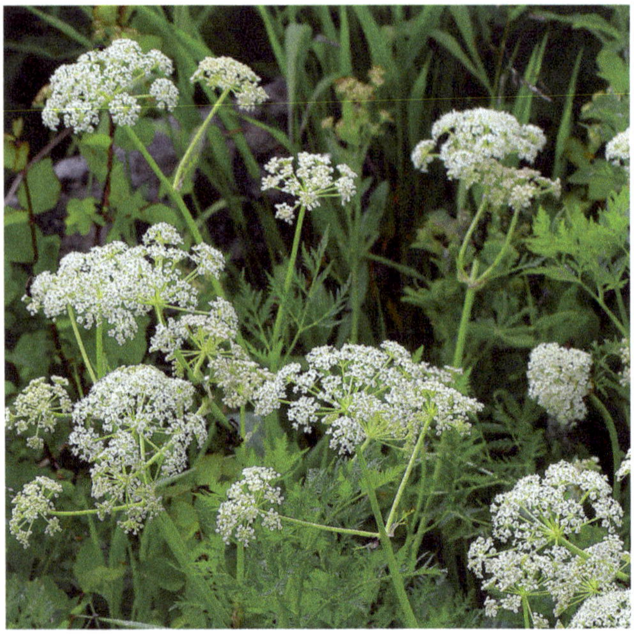

flowers and fruit are present, as they contain distinctive features. Some species of oshá only grow at high elevations, outside the range of *Conium* or *Cicuta* that grow in mid to lower elevations. However, other species of oshá may overlap the elevation range of poisonous look a likes, so elevation is not a sufficient distinction in most cases. Oshá forms taproots with a pungent, celery-like aroma, and a root crown surrounded by fibers from the previous year's leaf growth. Water hemlock root also has a celery-like scent. Poison hemlock does not have a hairy root crown; the roots are lighter brown inside with an acrid scent. When poison hemlock root is cut lengthwise, it has horizontal pith. Water hemlock roots have divided chambers, while oshá and poison hemlock roots do not. Poison hemlock has seeds with downward, reflexed bracts. The idiom "vein to the tip, pretty hip, vein to the cut, pain in the butt" refers to water hemlock's leaf veins that end in side notches of the marginal teeth; the leaf veins of oshá and poison hemlock end at the tips of the teeth.

THE NAME: The genus name *Ligusticum* was used by Dioscorides to describe a plant in Liguria, Italy. The epithet *caldera* was named for Jim Calder, Canadian botanist.[4] The epithet *grayi* and the common name Gray's lovage were named either for Asa Gray (1810 – 1888), a Harvard botany professor, or S.F. Gray (1766 – 1836), a British botanist.[4] The epithet *scoticum* means "from Scotland."[4] The common name oshá is a Native American term for "bear." The Blackfoot and Salish referred to this herb as "bear medicine."[5] Other tribes refer to the plant as "chuchupate" or "oshá."[5,6] The common name "lovage" derives from *love-ache* ("love parsley"), included in Pliny the Elder's translation.[4]

HISTORICAL USES: Southwest Native Americans and Spanish Americans considered oshá an essential medicinal herb. The roots were chewed, or tea was prepared with the powdered roots as a stomachic to treat gas and bloating.[6] The Cochiti chewed a bean-sized piece of root with a pinch of salt, then washed it down with warm water to treat a cough.[6] The powdered root mixed with hot water, sugar, and whiskey was consumed for a cold, flu, chronic cough, pneumonia, and consumption.[6] An oil or salve of oshá was applied to rheumatic joints, bruises, cuts, and sores.[6] A paste of water and powdered root was applied to snakebites to draw out the poison. Shepherds carried bits of root in their pockets to protect against venomous snakes, and sprinkled the powder on the ground around their bedrolls to ward off reptiles.[6] The Apache smoked the dried, hollow stems, and Spanish settlers eventually adopted this practice to replace cigarettes.[6] Oshá leaves seasoned soups and other dishes.[6]

The Atsugewi chewed or decocted oshá root *(L. grayi)* tea to treat a cold, cough, stomachache, and pain, and as a panacea.[7] Steam inhalations of root shavings were used to treat sinus infections.[8] Flathead Indians believed the roots should never be washed in streams where they were gathered, or it would cause a rainstorm.[8] The Zuni used oshá *(L. porteri)* to alleviate body aches and sore throats.[7] Hispanic Americans administered oshá to treat a cold, sore throat, fever, or stomachache.[7] Oshá was carried in medicine bags to prevent sickness.[7]

CONSTITUENTS: Oshá root contains volatile oil (α-pinene, β-pinene, umbelliferone, limonene, timolols, and triterpenoids), alkyl-pthalides (diligustilide, ligustilide,

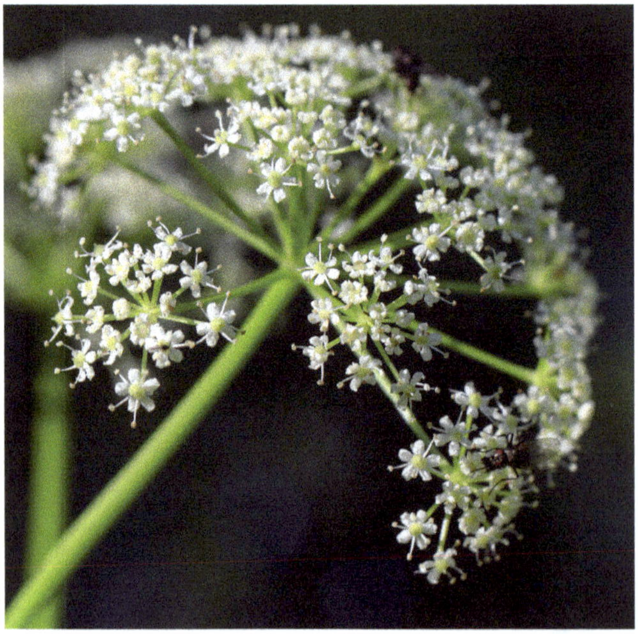

(Z)-ligustilide, and riligustilide), ferulic acid, flavonoids, tannins, and tetramethylpyrazine.[9,10] Additional constituents may include coumarins, furanocoumarins, polyacetylenes, and phenolic acids.[10]

NUTRITIONAL PROPERTIES: Unknown.

MEDICINAL PROPERTIES: Antibacterial, antitussive, antiviral, aromatic, bitter tonic, bronchodilator, carrier, diaphoretic, expectorant, and immune stimulant.

TEMPERATURE AND FLAVOR: Warm, pungent, bitter, and sweet.

MEDICINAL USES

Oshá has antibacterial, antiviral, and immune stimulant actions.[8,9] It anesthetizes mucous membranes in the throat.[9] Oshá aids in treating a cold, flu, sinusitis, laryngitis, sore throat, and strep throat. Combine extracts of propolis resin, elder berry *(Sambucus),* red root *(Ceanothus),* echinacea *(Echinacea),* and/or spilanthes *(Acmella)* with smaller amounts of oshá and licorice *(Glycyrrhiza)* to alleviate a sore throat, laryngitis, or cold. Oshá is a heating herb. If lymph swelling or throat pain occur following consumption, discontinue use and substitute with cooling antimicrobial herbs.

Oshá has warming, soothing, expectorant actions that deepen respiration and reduce respiratory spasms. Consume as an adjunct treatment for bronchitis, pneumonia, whooping cough, or smoker's cough. Because this herb is heating, it can eventually be too drying to the mucous membranes; therefore, it is helpful to combine it with other demulcent herbs such as marshmallow root *(Althaea)* and a pinch of licorice *(Glycyrrhiza).* Oshá helps to increase respiratory volume and aids in adapting to altitude changes.[9] Combine extracts of usnea *(Usnea),* aralia *(Aralia),* gumweed *(Grindelia),* anise *(Pimpinella),* and smaller amounts of oshá, lomatium *(Lomatium),* and/or licorice *(Glycyrrhiza)* to treat lower respiratory infections.

Oshá is a heating diaphoretic that aids in resolving a fever. Consume small, frequent doses (4 – 8 ounces) of the hot decoction, or add the tincture in hot water every two to three hours, up to five times daily. Oshá stimulates circulation and acts as a carrier herb in formulas, especially when treating acute upper or lower respiratory infections. It also has mild emmenagogue actions that stimulate menses delayed from overexposure to cold. Combine with angelica *(Angelica)* to alleviate a fever or stimulate menstruation.

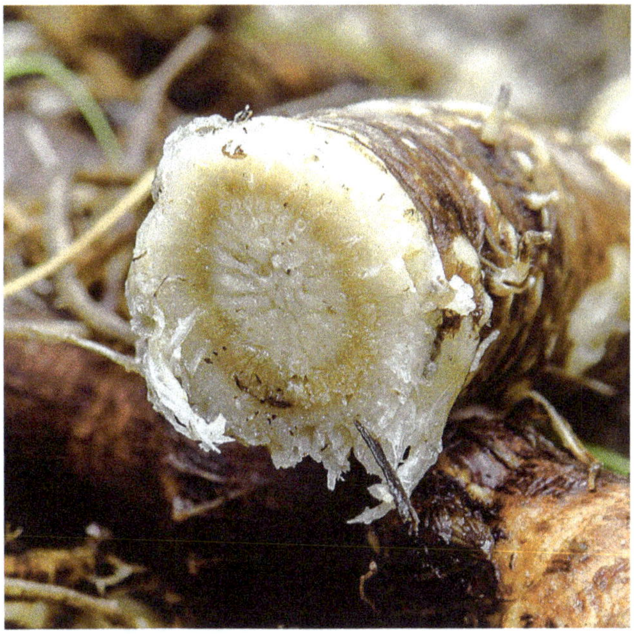

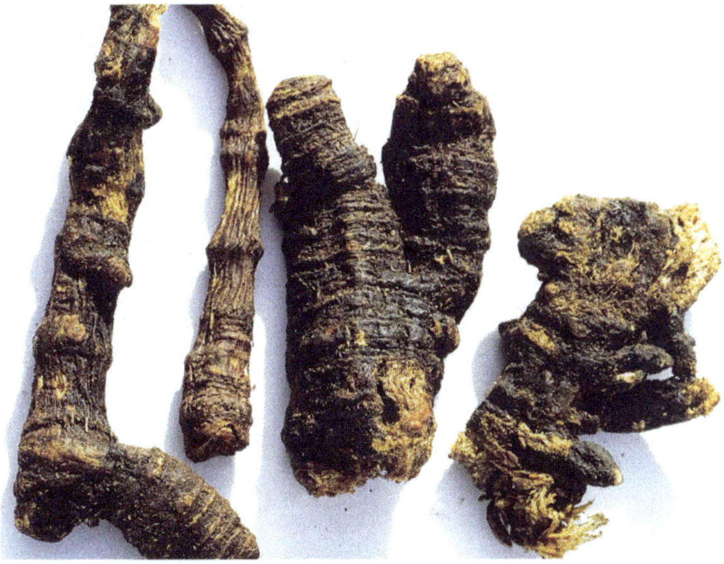

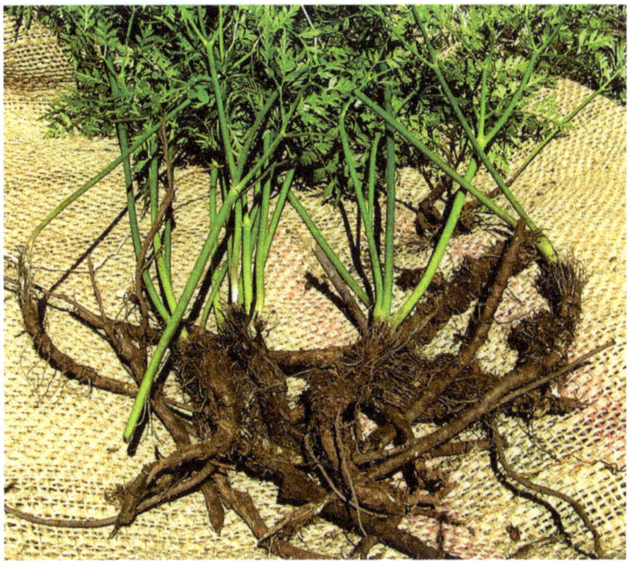

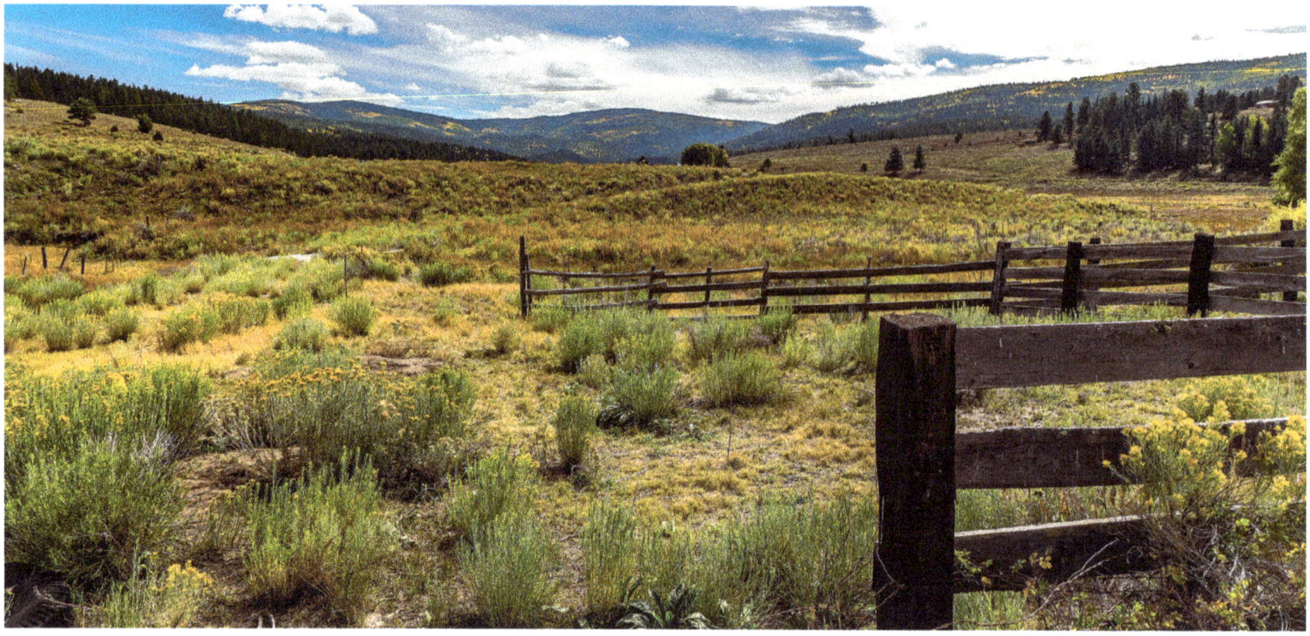

Oshá is an aromatic, warming, bitter digestive tonic. It encourages digestive secretions, and can be used as a recuperative agent following a digestive infection. It stimulates appetite after a stomach flu or vomiting.[9]

Applications of the infused oil, salve, or hot fomentation improve circulation in local tissues, reducing the pain of arthritis, bruises, and sore or strained muscles.[6] A topical wash of the tea can be applied as a antimicrobial for cuts and abrasions.[9]

CONTRAINDICATIONS

According to herbalist Michael Moore, moderate use of the dry plant is safe during pregnancy, but not the fresh root.[9] However, the author cautions against using any form of the root during pregnancy, especially if there are complications. Oshá is contraindicated during menses in women with heavy menstrual flow. Avoid consumption with yin deficiency with heat signs (night sweats and hot flashes). Avoid use or exercise caution in individuals with Apiaceae family allergies.[10] Like other members of the Apiaceae family, it may contain furanocoumarins that can cause phototoxicity.[10] The leaf is safe to consume during pregnancy.[9]

Warning: Always be careful to properly identify oshá and other members of the umbel family before harvesting; misidentification can be fatal. Oshá can be mistaken for poisonous members of the same family, such as poison hemlock *(Conium maculatum)* and water hemlock *(Cicuta maculata, Cicuta douglasii, C.* spp.*)*. Water hemlock is the most poisonous plant in North America; consuming ¼ teaspoon of the root can be fatal within 15 minutes. Accurate identification of the seeds, flowers, and leaves is critical!

PREPARATION AND DOSAGE

TINCTURE: Fresh roots [1:2, 80-95% alcohol]; dry roots [1:5, 70% alcohol]; consume 10-60 drops, up to four times daily.

CAPSULES: Consume 2-4 capsules, one to three times daily.

TEA: Prepare a decoction of the roots; consume 4-8 ounces, up to four times daily.

HONEY AND SYRUP: Prepare fresh root honey [1:4]; consume up to 1 teaspoon, up to four times daily. Prepare a decoction, simmer to half the volume, and add syrup to desired sweetness. Consume 1 teaspoon, up to four times daily.

TOPICAL USE: Apply powdered root as a topical antimicrobial. The infused oil or salve acts as a counterirritant and circulatory stimulant.

CULINARY USE: Add the seeds or leaves sparingly as a flavoring substitute for celery leaves in soups, salad dressings, and meat and vegetable dishes.

PARSLEY

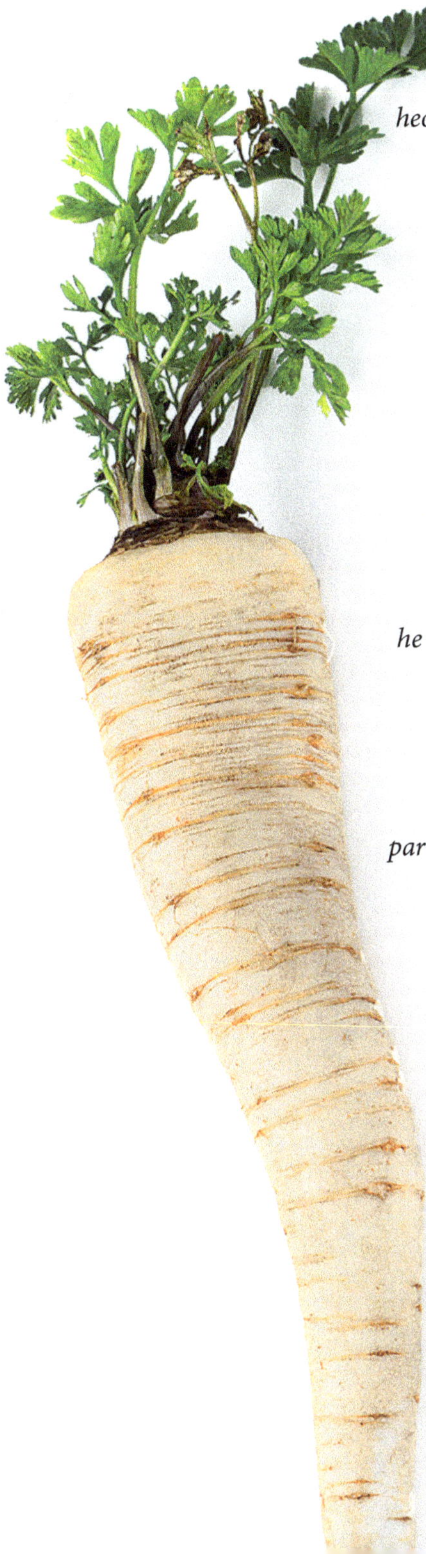

BOTANICAL NAMES:
Petroselinum crispum (syn. *P. sativum, P. italicum*)

COMMON NAMES:
Curly parsley, Italian parsley, flat leaf parsley, garden parsley, rock parsley, petersylinge
baqdounis (Arabic)
azadkegh (Armenian)
magdanoz (Bulgarian)
heong choi, yihn sai (Cantonese)
persin (Cratian)
petrzel (Czech)
persille (Danish)
peterselie (Dutch)
persilja (Finnish)
persil (French)
petersilie (German)
maïntano, persemolo (Greek)
petrosilia (Hebrew)
petreselyem (Hungarian)
peterseli, seledri (Indonesian)
prezzemolo (Italian)
paseri (Japanese)
minari (Korean)
he lan qin, xiang cai (Mandarin)
persille (Norwegian)
salsa (Portuguese)
petrushka (Russian)
perejil (Spanish)
persilja (Swedish)
partasliyat, phakchi farang (Thai)
maydanoz (Turkish)
petreshke (Yiddish)

FAMILY NAME:
Apiaceae (Umbelliferae)

DESCRIPTION

PARTS USED: The leaves, seeds, and roots. The roots are collected in the fall of the second year after the plant has flowered.

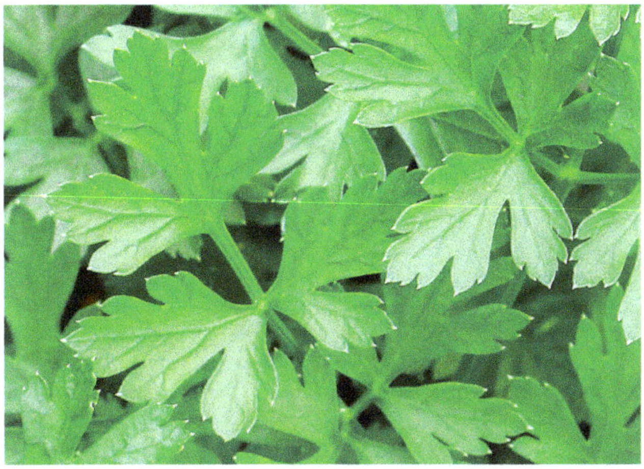

BOTANICAL DESCRIPTION AND HABITAT: Parsley is native to the eastern Mediterranean regions of Turkey, Algeria, and Lebanon. Depending on the climate, this cultivated herb grows as an annual or biennial. The earliest recorded year of parsley cultivation was 1548 in England. Following the introduction of the plant to the British Isles, it naturalized in England and Scotland in the 1600s.

The cultivars of parsley include *P. crispum* var. *crispum* (curly leaf parsley), and *P. crispum* var. *neapolitanum* (flat leaf or Italian parsley), which resembles the wild form of parsley. Parsley is a low growing, erect, glabrous plant (30 – 130 cm tall) with a sturdy taproot.[2] During the first year, it forms a basal rosette that bolts in the second year into a branched cauline plant that flowers and seeds. The leaves change shape after they diverge from the basal rosette to the cauline form. The basal leaves bear petioles (10 – 20 cm long) with ovate, one- to three-pinnate blades (3 – 10 cm long).[2] The first degree leaflets are obovate to ovate-lanceolate, toothed, and lobed. Conversely, cauline leaves are primarily sessile and arranged in a once-ternate pattern, with linear to lanceolate, entire or three-lobed leaflets.[2] A peduncle (3 – 8 cm long) bears a compound umbel with 10 to 20 rays (1 – 5 cm long) of nearly equal length.[2] The pedicels range from 2 – 5 mm in length.[2] The calyx lobes of the flowers are tiny, and the greenish-yellow or white petals are wide.[2] The oblong to ovate, compressed fruit (2 – 4 mm long) has thread-like ribs.[2]

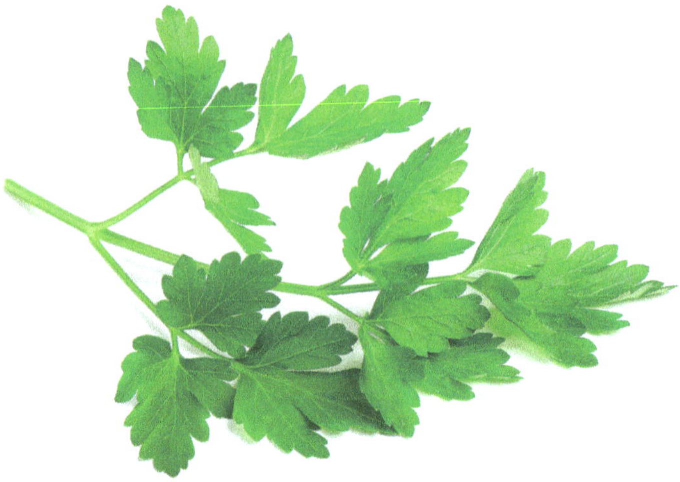

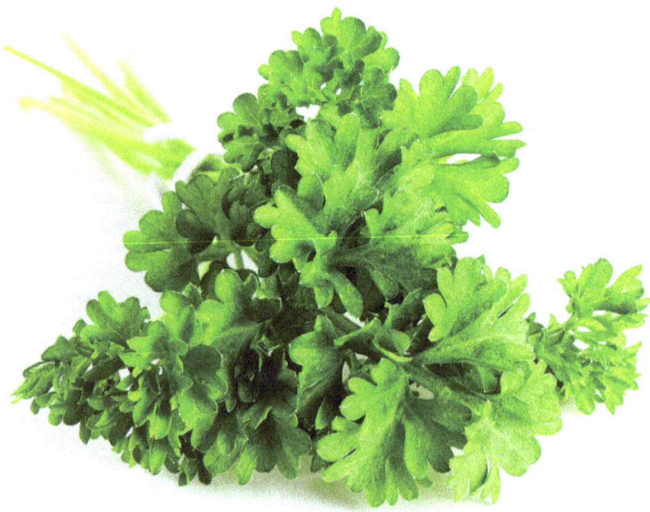

THE NAME: Dioscorides, the Greek physician and botanist, designated the botanical name *Petroselinum*.[1] This name originated from the word *selinon,* used by ancient Greeks to describe two plants: *Heleioselinon* (marsh selinon), the name for celery, and *Oreoselinon* (mountain selinon), the name for parsley. These names evolved into the term *Petroselinum* (rock selinon). During the Middle Ages, *Petroselinum* evolved into *Petrocilium,* later anglicized to the common names petersylinge, persele, persely, and parsley.[1] The epithet *crispum* derives from the Latin *crispus* meaning "curled, wrinkled, or having curly hair." *Italicum* derives from the Latin *italicus* meaning "Italian."[3] *Sativum* means "cultivated." *Petroselinum crispum* is the binomial for curly parsley, and *P. sativum* or *P. italicum* refers to Italian or flat-leaf parsley.

HISTORICAL USES: The ancient Greeks esteemed parsley, and many traditions and myths are associated with it. Legend has it that parsley emerged from the blood of Archemorus, a Greek hero associated with death.[1] This herb was also associated with Persephone and funeral rites.[1] Parsley wreaths adorned tombs.[1] Parsley was never brought to the table, as it was held sacred to the realm of the dead. Victors at the Isthmian games were crowned with parsley.[1] It was planted with rue as a border in Greek gardens.[1] Ancient Greeks and Romans administered parsley as an antidyscratic (blood cleanser) for rheumatic complaints.

Parsley leaves have been used in France topically for dermatological conditions such as fissures, abrasions, chapped skin, and insect bites. A leaf poultice was applied to ease bites and stings from poisonous insects.[1] Parsley leaf hydrosol was administered to colicky children. The leaves and stems were used in dyes and for culinary coloring.[1] A decoction of seeds was used to fight the plague and alleviate intermittent fever.[1] Preparations of the roots were administered for a range of kidney complaints, dropsy, and jaundice.[1,4]

CONSTITUENTS

PARSLEY ROOT: Parsley root contains flavonoids (apiin), volatile oil (apiole, myristicin, and furanocoumarins), polyacetylenes, starch, sugar, and mucilage.[1,4]

PARSLEY SEED: Parsley seed contains volatile oil (apiole, apiolin, myristicin, tetramethoxyallybenzene, and α-pinene), fixed oils (petroselinic acid = *cis*-6-octadecenoic acid, 7-octadecenoic acid, and smaller amounts of palmitic,

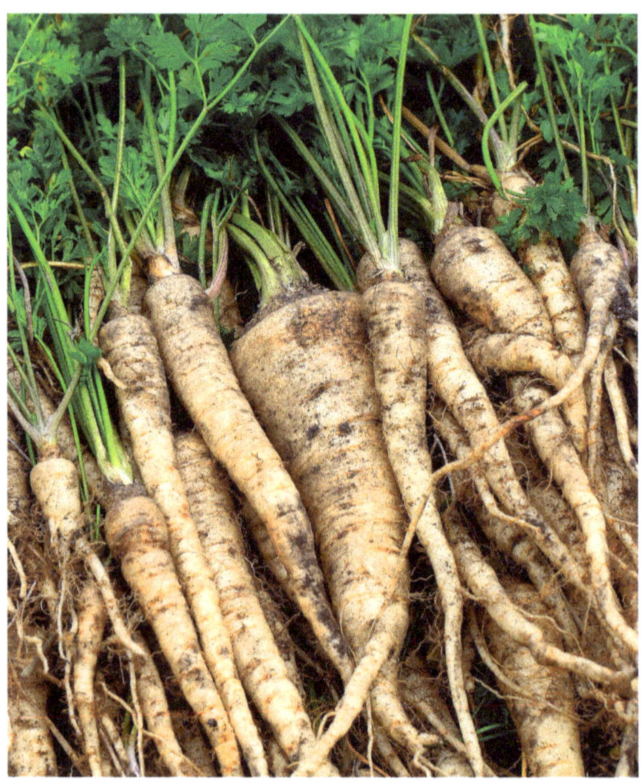

myristic, stearic, oleic, linoleic, and myristolic acids), flavonoids (apiin and apigenin-7-apiosylglucoside), traces of bergapten, and flavonoids.[1,4]

PARSLEY LEAF: Parsley leaf contains an oleoresin (apiole) and volatile oil (myristicin, β-phellandrene, 1,3,8-*p*-menthatriene, myrcene, terpinolene, and 1-methyl-4-isopropenylbenzene). Additional compounds include α- and β-pinenes, trans-β-ocimene, γ-terpinene, methyl disulfide, α-terpineol, α-copaene, caryophyllene, carotol, and furocoumarins (bergapten, xanthotoxin, and isopimpinellin), flavonoids (apiin, luteolin-7-apiosylglucoside, apigenin-7-glucoside, and luteolin-7-diglucoside), protein, fats, vitamins, minerals, and sugars.[4,5]

NUTRITIONAL PROPERTIES: Parsley leaves contain high amounts of protein (up to 22% by weight), vitamins (A, B_1, B_2, B_3, and C), fiber, calcium, chromium, cobalt, fiber, iron, magnesium, manganese, phosphorus, potassium, selenium, silicon, sodium, tin, zinc, and chlorophyll.[6,7]

MEDICINAL PROPERTIES: Diuretic, antidyscratic, antigalactagogue, antioxidant, antiseptic, antispasmodic, aperient, carminative, emmenagogue, expectorant, hypotensive, mild uterine tonic, parturient, and sudoriphic.

TEMPERATURE AND FLAVOR: The roots are warm, salty, sweet, and bland. The seeds are warm, pungent, sweet, bitter, and mildly astringent. The leaves are warm, pungent, salty, and sweet.

MEDICINAL USES

PARSLEY ROOT: Parsley root is a soothing diuretic that alleviates edema.[1] It reduces premenstrual water retention and aids in treating sodium-related hypertension. It is often included in weight loss remedies due to its diuretic actions. It enhances uric acid excretion via the kidneys, easing conditions such as gout, arthritis, and kidney stones.[1,4,5] Short-term use of the tea aids in treating acute urinary tract infections; long-term use eases symptoms of benign prostatic hypertrophy. Flavonoids are attributed to the diuretic effect.[5] To enhance the diuretic actions, prepare a decoction containing parsley root, dandelion root *(Taraxacum)*, burdock *(Arctium)*, gravel root *(Eutrochium)*, and fennel *(Foeniculum)*.

PARSLEY SEED: Parsley seed is a diuretic that can be used interchangeably with the roots; however, it is less soothing to the kidneys than the roots.[10] Long-term consumption of the infusion aids in treating gout, rheumatism, and arthritis.[9] Parsley seed also increases the kidneys' excretion of sodium, reducing edema. The seed contains apiole, a urinary tract antibacterial that alleviates cystitis.[9]

Parsley seed is a carminative, stomachic, and cholagogue.[8] Combine it with seeds from other members of the Apiaceae family such as fennel *(Foeniculum)*, lovage *(Levisticum)*, caraway *(Carum)*, cumin *(Cuminum)*, and/or coriander *(Coriandrum)* to support digestive function. Parsley seed is also an antipyretic and expectorant that eases coughing and asthma.[8]

Parsley seed alcohol extract and parsley seed oil had cytotoxic activity against MCF-7 human breast cancer cells. It significantly reduced cell viability and altered cellular morphology.[11]

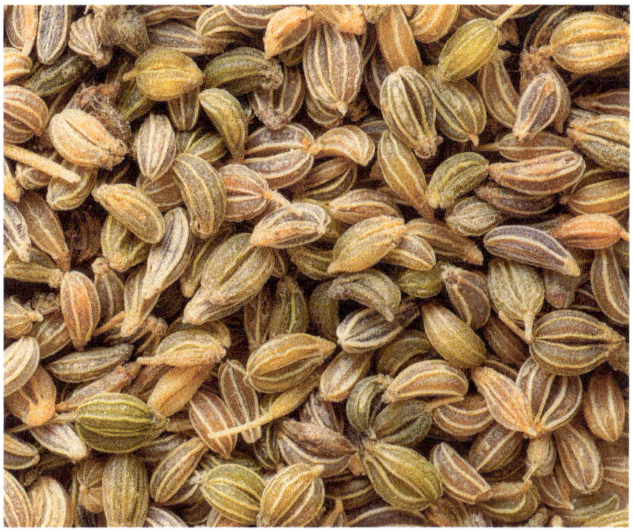

Due to the apiole (also listed as apiol), parsley seed stimulates uterine muscles and has potential emmenagogue actions.[9] Apiole stimulates contraction of the bladder, intestine, and uterus. Apiole refers to the oleoresins contained in the seed (apiole, apiolin, and myristicin).

PARSLEY LEAF: Parsley leaf is rich in easily assimilated, nourishing vitamins and minerals.[4,8,9] Due to its iron and chlorophyll content, it supports individuals with anemia; however, it is not ideal for treating postpartum anemia, due to the antigalactagogue effects. Rich in minerals, long-term consumption of the leaf encourages an alkaline environment in tissues, and aids in treating conditions such as gout and rheumatoid arthritis. To optimize the nutritional and alkalinizing effects, consume fresh parsley leaf and tea containing nettle *(Urtica)*, alfalfa *(Medicago)*, and oat straw *(Avena)* daily.

Parsley leaf is a potent antioxidant and antiallergenic (due to apiin).[9] Short- and long-term consumption of the fresh leaf juice aids in treating inflammatory conditions such as allergies, eczema, dermatitis, atherosclerosis, and asthma. Parsley leaf protects against oxidative damage from heavy metals, especially cadmium.[12] When parsley leaf juice was administered to pregnant mice, it significantly decreased the deleterious effects of cadmium in newborns exposed during pregnancy. It neutralized and reduced cadmium-induced neuronal degeneration as measured by behavioral activities, neurotransmitter, oxidative stress, and brain neuron morphology.[12]

Parsley leaf has potent antioxidant and antidiabetic effects with excellent potential for treating diabetes mellitus (Type I and II) and reducing related complications. For example, it demonstrated hepatoprotective effects in diabetic rats, preventing degenerative changes in hepatocytes. It also significantly reduced levels of blood glucose, alanine transaminase, and alkaline phosphatase.[13] In one study, rats ate a fructose-enriched diet that produced dislipidemia, hepatic steatosis, infiltration of inflammatory cells in the liver, and elevated plasma hepatic markers. *Petroselinum crispum* extract was used to treat hepatic steatosis, reversing chronic metabolic changes in rats with fructose-enriched, diet-induced, nonalcoholic fatty liver disease.[14] Another study confirmed the antidiabetic and antioxidant effects of *Petroselinum sativum* leaf and *Balanites aegyptiaca* extracts in streptozotocin-induced diabetic (Type I) and normal rats. The herbal extracts significantly reduced mean plasma glucose and malondialdehyde levels, and increased mean plasma insulin, liver-pyruvate kinase, and total antioxidant capacity levels in the treated diabetic groups compared to the untreated diabetic control group. Comparatively, the treated group experienced an increase in pancreatic weight and the size of the Islets of Langerhans (insulin producing cells).[15]

Parsley leaf stimulates gastric secretions, enhancing digestion. It has carminative and stomachic properties that alleviate gas and bloating.[8,9] Parsley leaf also has mild cholagogue and laxative actions. Served as a garnish, parsley leaf freshens the breath and is an antidote for garlic breath.[9] This is likely due to the chlorophyll content that enhances the absorption of odors, neutralizing the breath.[9]

Parsley leaf is an antigalactagogue that reduces breast milk flow. Combining parsley leaf with garden sage *(Salvia officinalis)* enhances the antigalactagogue effects. Excessive or regular consumption of parsley leaf should be avoided by women with low volumes of breast milk, although it can be consumed infrequently in small amounts by women with an abundant milk supply. The leaf also has gentle uterine tonifying properties.[5]

When pregnant women have passed their due date, some midwives and doulas recommend applying parsley juice to the cervix in order to encourage labor. Before employing this technique, filter the juice to ensure it is free of particulate matter.

An antibacterial, parsley leaf juice and seed tea ease urinary tract infections.[9] Parsley leaf tea or soup has mild diaphoretic actions that encourage sweating during the first stage of a cold. The vasodilating actions are due to the apiole. Dilute parsley leaf juice with saline solution as an eye wash for conjunctivitis or blepharitis.[9] Additional anti-infective agents such as goldenseal *(Hydrastis)* or goldthread *(Coptis)* are often necessary.

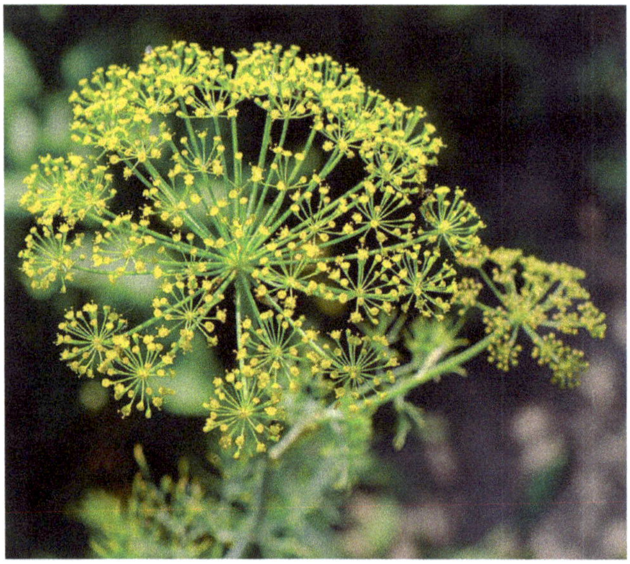

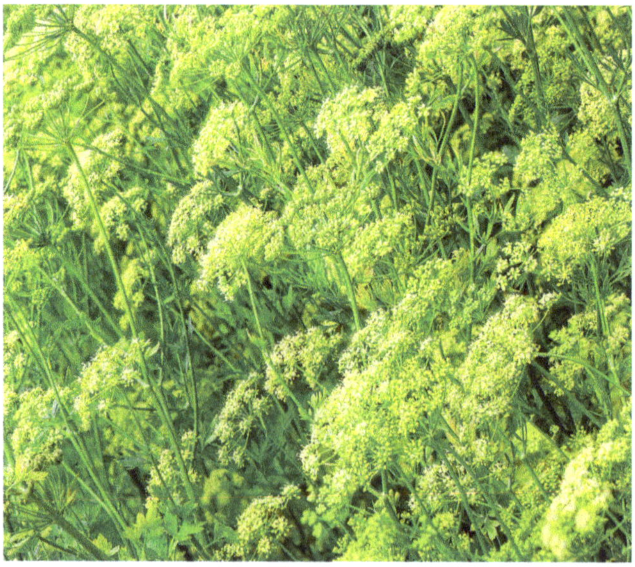

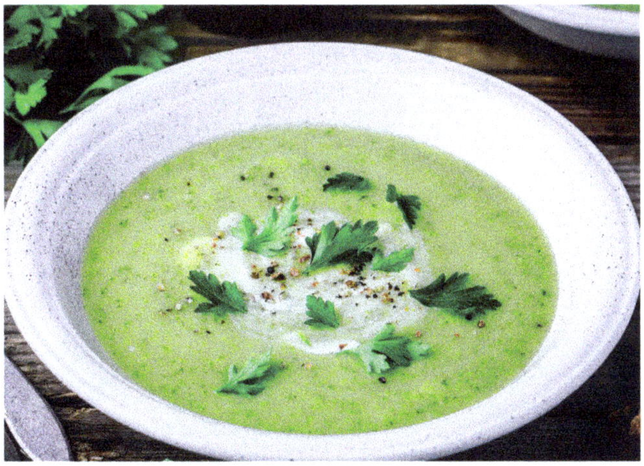

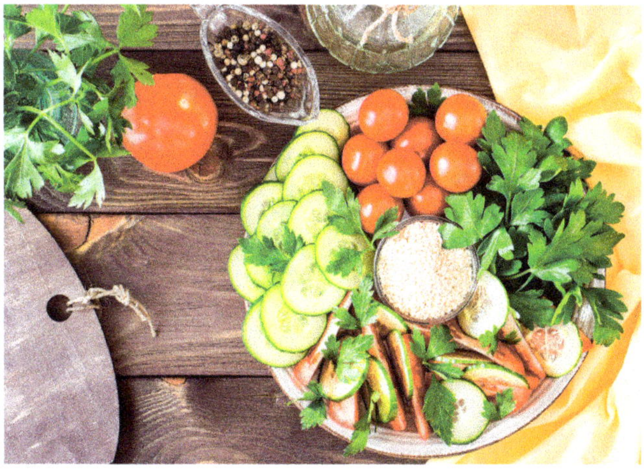

Apply the fresh leaf poultice to sprains, swellings, and insect bites.[9] A leaf or seed tea can be applied as a hair rinse to treat a dry scalp or dandruff. To prepare a hair rinse, make a tea containing nettle leaf *(Urtica)*, horsetail *(Equisetum)*, rosemary *(Salvia rosmarinus)*, and parsley leaf.

CONTRAINDICATIONS

Pregnant and lactating women should limit parsley leaf consumption to occasional culinary use, and avoid other medicinal preparations of parsley.[5] Some sources recommend the complete avoidance of parsley leaf during pregnancy.[5] Parsley root and seed are contraindicated during pregnancy. Avoid consuming parsley leaf in cases of a threatened miscarriage, or in nursing mothers with scant milk.[5]

Parsley seed is contraindicated in individuals with inflammatory kidney disease.[5] Use of the root and seed are contraindicated in cases of obstructive kidney stones, edema related to impaired heart or kidney function, or kidney inflammation.[5]

Handling the plant has caused contact dermatitis in some individuals.[4,5] The plant — especially the root — contains furanocoumarins that cause phototoxicity upon exposure to strong sun rays.[4]

Internal consumption of essential oil of parsley is contraindicated. The concentrated apiole in the seed oil has been found to damage epithelial tissues in the kidneys and cause heart arrhythmia.[4] It can also cause a fatty liver and gastrointestinal tract bleeding.[4] Apiole is contraindicated during pregnancy and lactation, and in individuals with liver, kidney, or digestive disorders. The essential oil has the greatest potential to cause contact dermatitis and photosensitivity.

PREPARATION AND DOSAGE

TINCTURE: Fresh roots or seeds [1:2, 70-95% alcohol]; dry roots or seeds [1:5, 60% alcohol]; consume 15-60 drops, up to three times daily.

ACETUM EXTRACT: Fresh leaves [1:2-1:3, apple cider vinegar]; consume 1 teaspoon to 1 tablespoon, up to three times daily.

SUCCUS: Juice the fresh leaves and consume ½-1 ounce, up to three times daily. Alternatively, preserve the fresh leaf juice by adding 15-20% alcohol, and consume 1-3 tablespoons, up to three times daily. Freeze the juice in ice cube trays and store in a zip-lock bag; consume 1-3 ice cubes daily.

CAPSULES: Consume 2-3 capsules of powdered root, up to three times daily.

TEA: Prepare the leaves and seeds as a hot or cold infusion; consume 4-8 ounces, up to four times daily. Prepare the roots as a decoction or cold infusion; consume 8 ounces, up to four times daily.

TOPICAL USE: Apply the leaf poultice, tea, or juice topically.

CULINARY USE: Parsley leaf is primarily used for culinary purposes, for nourishment. It can be added to fresh vegetable juices, soups, salads, salad dressings, pickles, sauces, pesto, potato and egg dishes, stuffing, minces, fish, sausage, meat, pizza, and spice blends. Parsley root can be added to soup or root vegetable dishes; its flavor resembles parsnips.

PARTRIDGE BERRY

BOTANICAL NAME:
Mitchella repens

COMMON NAMES:
Partridge berry, partridgeberry, running fox, deer berry, madder berry, oneberry, two-eyed berry, checker berry, twin flower, winter clove, squaw vine, and squaw berry[1]

FAMILY NAME:
Rubiaceae

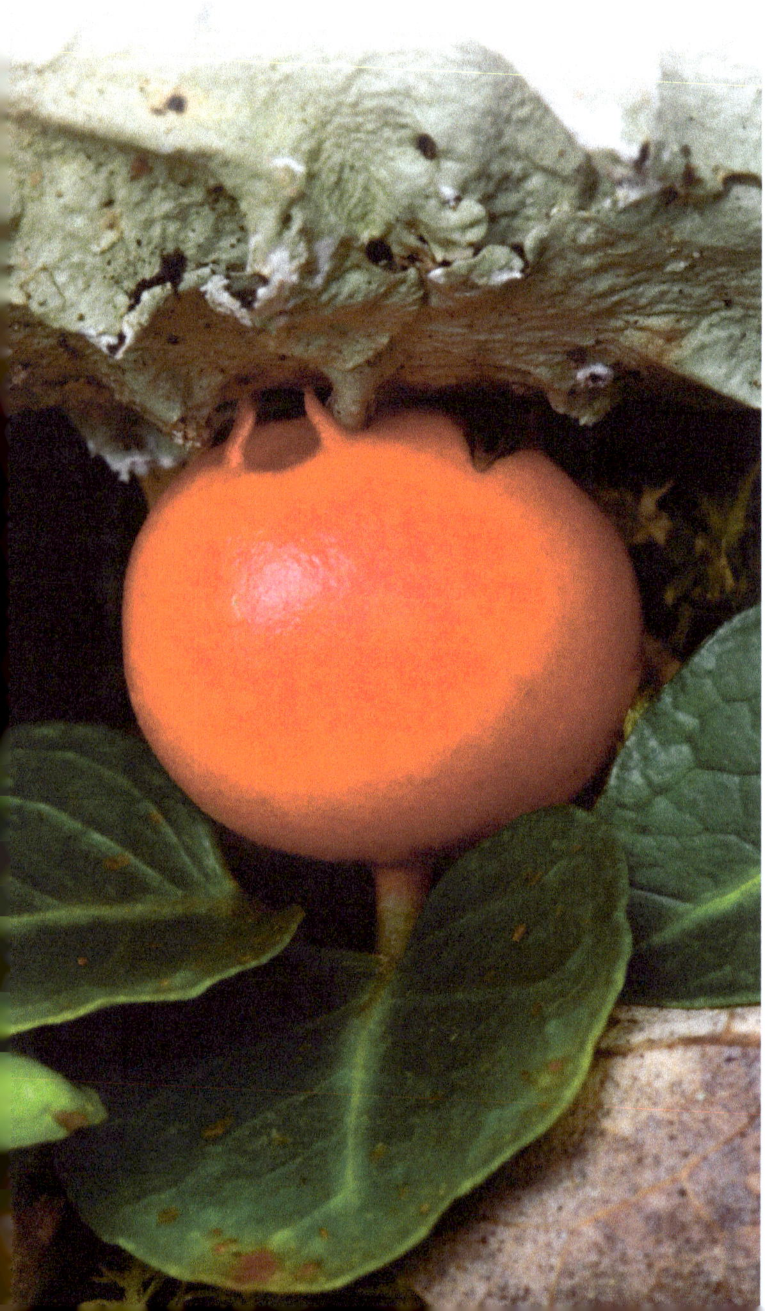

DESCRIPTION

PARTS USED: The leaves are the primary medicinal portions of the plant, although the stems and flowers can be incorporated into medicinal preparations. The berries are edible.

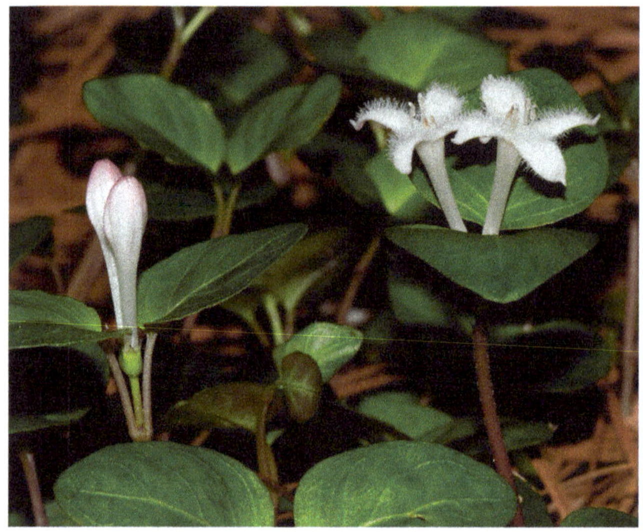

BOTANICAL DESCRIPTION AND HABITAT: Partridge berry is a perennial herb found in moist or dry, shaded forest areas ranging from the northeastern to southeastern U.S., as well as the midwestern states and Canada. Partridge berry is relatively easy to cultivate, and prefers moist, well drained, slightly acidic soil and partial shade.

Partridge berry is a low-growing, mat-forming, evergreen vine with prostrate stems (up to 30 cm long).[2] These stems root at the ends, forming mats reaching several meters across, but only 5 cm high.[3] The opposite shiny, dark green, ovate leaves (1.5 cm across) have a leathery texture and a distinctive whitish-yellow midrib.[4] This delicate herb grows pairs of white, pubescent, trumpet-shaped flowers, each with four petals, four stamens, and one pistil.[4] The plant is dimorphic; individual plants have flowers with short pistils relative to the stamen, or long pistils.[3] This prevents self-fertilization, and fertilization between like individuals, encouraging genetic diversity within a population.[3] Furthermore, both flowers must be pollinated to form fruit, as two flowers within a pair share a calyx, and as they develop, their pistils merge and form a single scarlet berry with two characteristic dimples.[3]

THE NAME: *Mitchella* was named in honor of John Mitchell (1711 – 1768), Virginia botanist.[5] While it may not be relevant since the plant was named after a person, it is interesting to note that both words in the Latin binomial indicate creeping, lurking, and hiding. *Mitchella* originates from the Old French *muchier* or *mucier* ("to hide or lurk"). The epithet *repens* ("creeping") derives from Latin.[5] Partridge berry acquired its name because partridges and other birds, such as ruffed grouse, sharp-tailed grouse, northern bobwhite, and wild turkey relished eating the berries.[7] The names "running fox" and "deer berry" originated because the berries were consumed by foxes, raccoons, and deer. The common name two-eyed berry refers to the two "dimples" in the berries that resemble eyes. The names squaw vine and squaw berry were given to the herb by early English colonists because they observed that Native American women used it medicinally. Squaw derives from *squa* or *ussqua,* the Algonquin term for a woman or young woman. There are numerous offensive associations with the term squaw; thus, the common herbal names incorporating that word are no longer used.

HISTORICAL USES: Partridge berry tea was consumed by Native Americans to regulate menstruation, promote fertility, and encourage a smooth delivery. Eclectic herbalists administered the herb to prevent a miscarriage, for various female reproductive issues, and as a nervous system calming agent.[8] They also used the herb to treat dropsy, suppressed urination, and diarrhea.[8] In *The Modern Herbal,* author Maude Grieve recommends the following cure for sore nipples:

> Two ounces of the herb (fresh, if possible), 1 pint of water. Make a strong decoction, strain, and add an equal quantity of good cream. Boil the whole down to the consistency of a soft salve, and when cool, anoint the nipple every time the child is removed from the breast.[1]

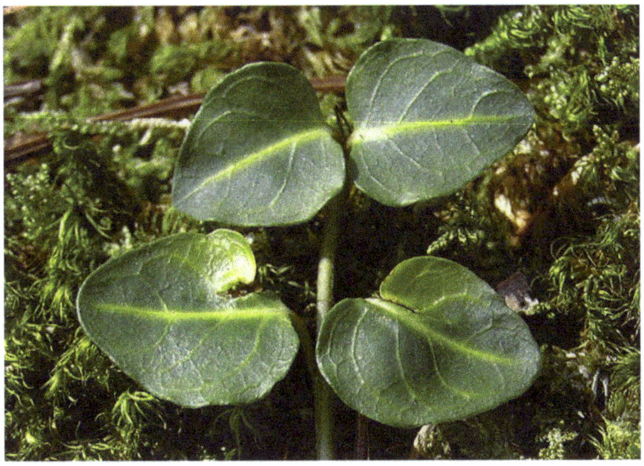

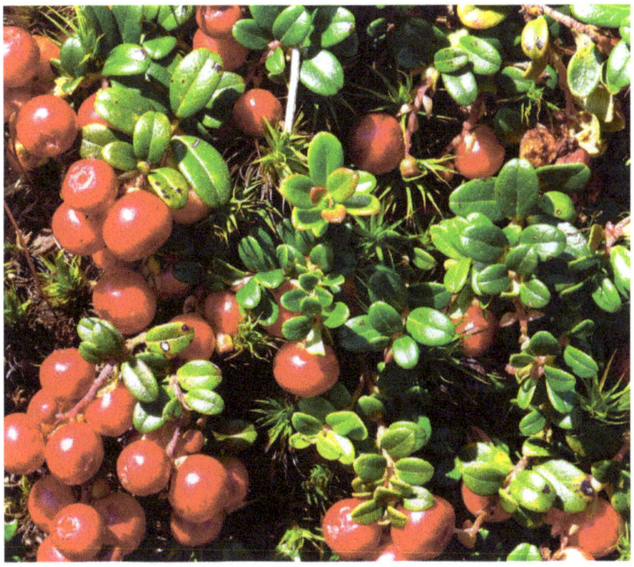

CONSTITUENTS: Partridge berry leaves contain glycosides (iridoids and triterpene saponins), tannins (proanthocyanidins), resin, wax, mucilage, and dextrin.[1,10] Reports assert that the plant contains alkaloids, though this is not verified; further research is needed.[10]

NUTRITIONAL PROPERTIES: The berries are edible; information is unavailable regarding the nutrient content.

MEDICINAL PROPERTIES: Astringent, demulcent, diuretic, parturient, partus preparator, and uterine tonic.

TEMPERATURE AND FLAVOR: Neutral, bitter, astringent, and sweet.

MEDICINAL USES

A gentle but effective herb, partridge berry improves circulation and tones female reproductive organs.[9,10] Consumed in tea or tinctures as a long-term tonic, it aids in treating conditions such as uterine or ovarian cysts, fibroids, endometriosis, amenorrhea, and dysmenorrhea.[9,10] It works most effectively when consumed daily for a minimum of three to six months.

Partridge berry is a partus preparator and parturient that aids in facilitating a smooth labor, hastening delivery, and regulating contractions.[9] It also strengthens and tones the uterus following delivery, and aids in treating uterine prolapse. Under the supervision of a health care practitioner, it can be consumed daily as a uterine tonic to prevent a threatened miscarriage, especially in women with a history of miscarriage.[9] The following compounded herbs have been very effective as a pregnancy tonic, and to

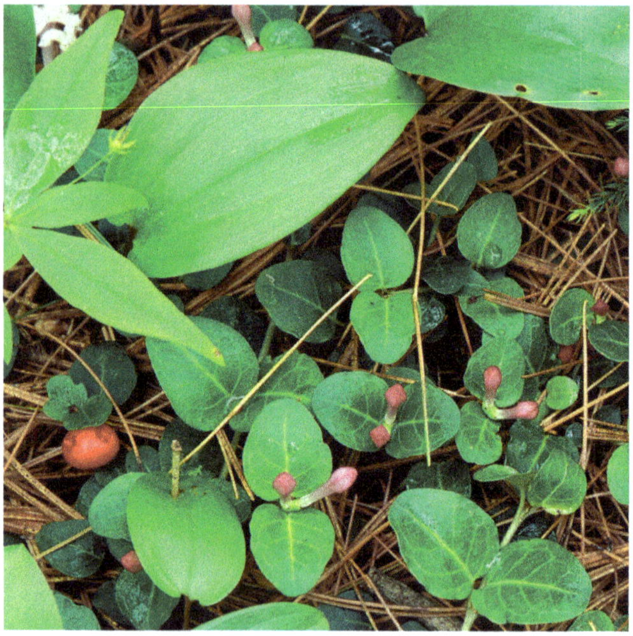

calm the uterus in case of a threatened miscarriage: black haw *(Viburnum prunifolium),* partridge berry *(Mitchella repens),* white peony *(Paeonia alba),* and raspberry leaf *(Rubus idaeus).* This formula also prevents hemorrhage, and facilitates a smooth recovery following an abortion. Additional hemostatics such as shepherd's purse *(Capsella),* cinnamon *(Cinnamomum zeylanicum),* and yarrow *(Achillea)* reduce uterine bleeding and prevent hemorrhage during and after a birth, miscarriage, or abortion.

Eclectic physicians borrowed their use of partridge berry from Native Americans.[8] This passage from the *American Materia Medica, Therapeutics, and Pharmacognosy* by Eclectic physician Finley Ellingwood summarizes his judicious claims of using partridge berry as a partus preparator:

> I have observed this influence in so many cases that doubt is impossible. Erratic pains and unsatisfied longings are removed, the nervous system assumes a tranquil condition, reflex symptoms abate, urinary function is preformed normally, the bowels become regular, imperfect digestion is improved, and the appetite becomes natural. Labor approaches, devoid of the irritating, aggravating complications, the preparatory stage is simple, the dilation is completed quickly, the expulsive contractions are strong, unirritating, and effectual, and are much less painful than without the remedy; involution is rapid and perfect and there are no subsequent complicating conditions to contend with, the patient's strength is not abated, and the function of lactation is in its best condition. This has been proven in very many cases.[8]

Partridge berry use is not limited to women. It also improves circulation to male reproductive organs, and decreases congestion in the prostate gland. It can be incorporated into male reproductive tonics. Herbalist Rosemary Gladstar recommends the herb for men to improve fertility and increase sperm count.[9]

An infusion has mild diuretic activity that aids in treating scant or suppressed urine.[1,10] The subtle astringent and diuretic properties are an adjunct for cystitis; however, additional anti-infective agents are necessary.

Partridge berry is a mild astringent and demulcent that reduces inflammation in mucous membranes and skin.[10] Consuming the tea aids in treating inflammatory conditions in the gastrointestinal tract, although it is not a primary remedy.[10]

CONTRAINDICATIONS

There are no known contraindications.[9] Based on the author's clinical observations, having used this in low doses with hundreds of women as a pregnancy tonic, this plant has never caused complications during pregnancy, and has never induced a miscarriage. However, unverified, controversial reports stating that the plant potentially contains alkaloids and iridoid glycosides have raised concerns regarding use during pregnancy.[10] At this time, there is a lack of research backing these claims. The author considers the herb safe to use during pregnancy.

PREPARATION AND DOSAGE

TINCTURE: Fresh leaves [1:2, 70 - 95% alcohol]; recently dried leaves [1:5, 60% alcohol]; consume 10 - 60 drops, up to three times daily.

CAPSULES: Consume 2 - 4 "00" capsules, one to three times daily.

TEA: Prepare a hot infusion; consume 8 - 12 ounces, up to three times daily.

CULINARY USE: The berries are edible, with a mild flavor and mealy texture. They can be incorporated into jams, sauces, pies, and pemmican, or used as a colorful garnish in salads, meat dishes, or beverages.

PASSION FLOWER

DESCRIPTION

BOTANICAL NAMES:
Passiflora incarnata, P. lutea, P. caerulea, P. quadrangularis, P. serrulata

COMMON NAMES:
Passion flower, passionflower, maypop, purple passion flower, apricot vine, wild passion flower, passion vine, flower of the five wounds, snake tongue
granadita, passiflore (French)
leiden christi, muttergottes-schuzchen, passionblume, passionskraut (German)
lilikoi (passion fruit) (Hawaiian)
mukkopira (Sanskrit)
espina de Cristo, maracuja, passionaria (Spanish)
kärsimyskukka (Swedish)

FAMILY NAME:
Passifloraceae

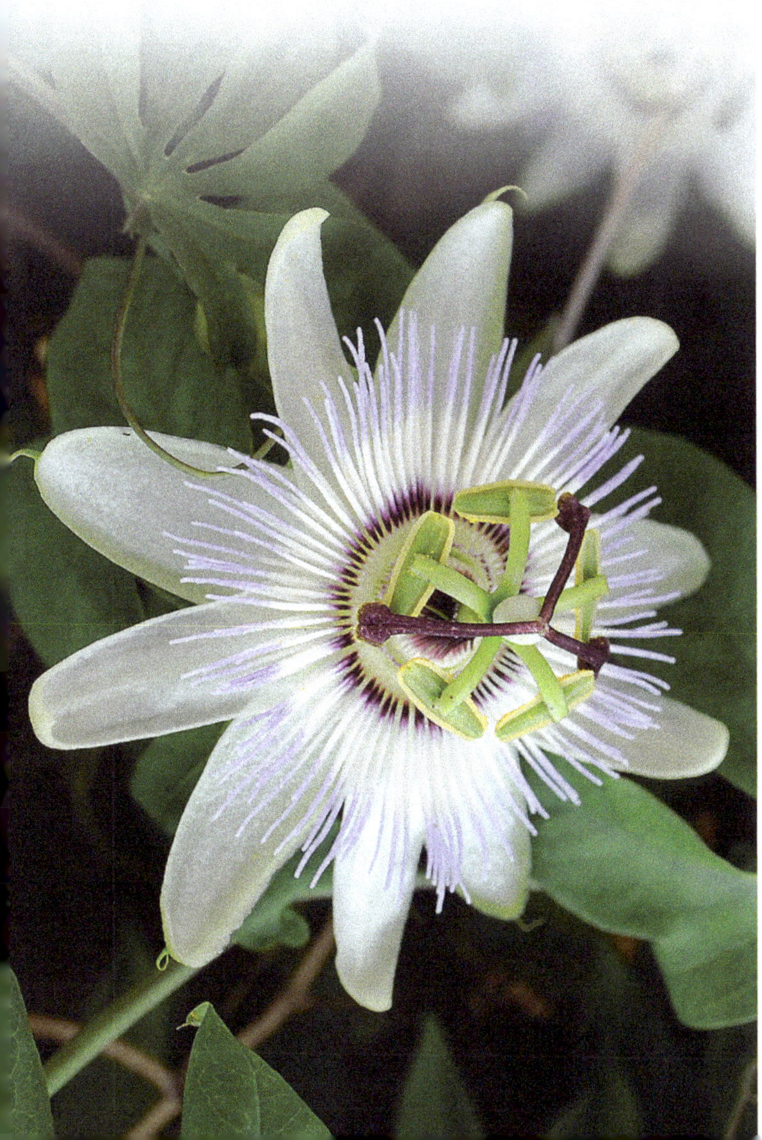

PARTS USED: The leaves are the most potent parts of the plant; the flowers and stem tips also can be used. It is best to harvest the plant in full bloom. The fruits are edible.

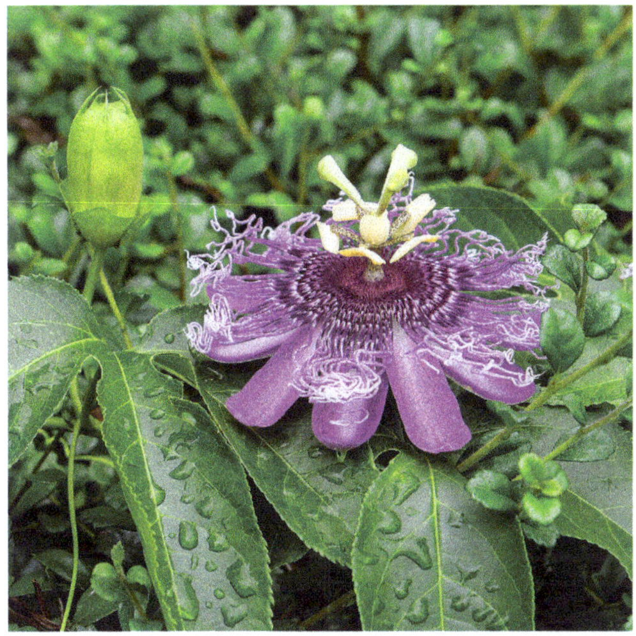

BOTANICAL DESCRIPTION AND HABITAT: *Passiflora incarnata* is native to the southeastern U.S., but is cultivated worldwide.[1] The herbaceous, perennial vines have woody bases that grow prolifically (8 – 12 feet tall), using tendrils to grasp adjacent objects or plants for support.[2] *P. incarnata* is unique among *Passiflora* species, as it is a deciduous, cold-hardy species; other species are frost-tender, tropical evergreens.[2] *Passiflora incarnata* is the primary species used as medicine. *P. lutea, P. caerulea, P. quadrangularis, P. serrulata,* and other species are used traditionally as medicine, but are not as well researched.

Passion flower's alternate, deeply three-lobed leaves (13 – 15 cm) have pubescent petioles (1 – 2 cm long) and minutely pubescent blades (8 – 9 cm long, 7 – 8 cm broad).[1,2] The elliptic-lanceolate lobes have serrate margins and acute apices.[1] Blooming June through August, the solitary flowers (3 – 5 cm across) grow atop a pubescent peduncle at the leaf axil.[1] The stunning flowers sport ten oblong, pale pink tepals (2 – 3 cm long by 8 – 10 mm wide), and a complex, purplish-blue corona. The five stamens have spotted filaments (8 mm long) and large anthers (8 mm long) on the long gynophore (12 – 15 mm long), directly below the pubescent, ovoid, three-chambered ovary (5 mm long) and three styles.[1] The ovary matures into a yellow, ovoid fruit (5 cm long) sometimes called a maypop.[1]

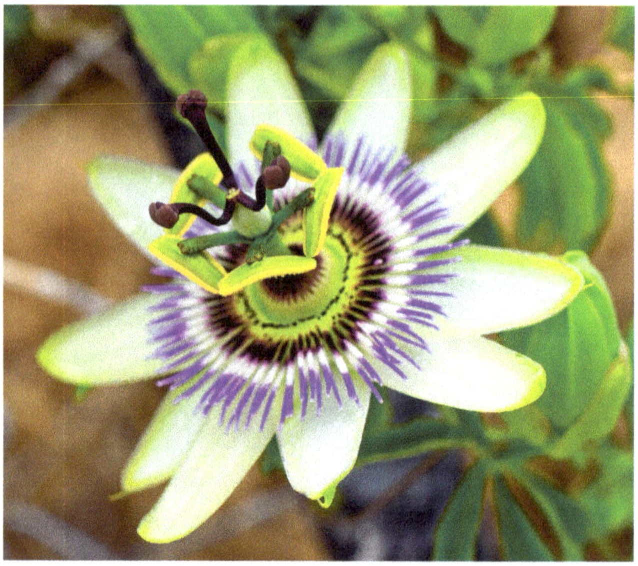

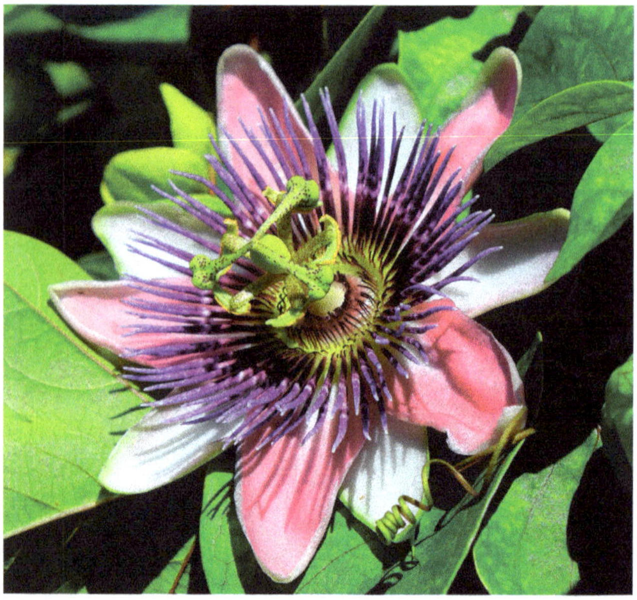

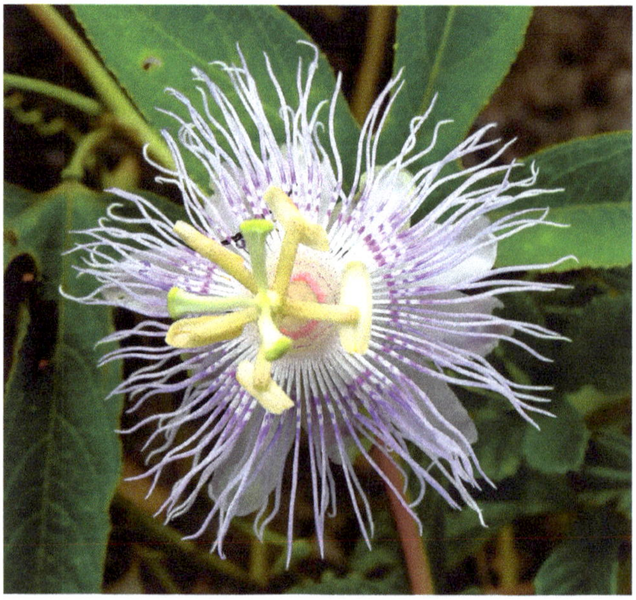

THE NAME: *Passiflora* derives from the Latin words *passio* ("passion") and *flos* ("flower").[5] The epithet *incarnata* means "flesh colored."[6] The epithet *lutea* ("yellow") derives from Latin. In the *Desk Reference to Nature's Medicine,* Steven Foster and Rebecca Johnson describe the origin of the common name passion flower:

> Jesuit missionaries working in South America professed to see symbols of the crucifixion in the plant's blossoms. The three styles of the pistil so prominent in the center of the flower were said to represent the three nails used to attach Christ to the cross. The five anthers on the stamens stood for the five wounds in his body. The dramatic corona of white and purple threadlike filaments that surrounds these plant parts was thought to resemble the legendary crown of thorns. The five sepals and five similar petals beneath this corona were said to symbolize the ten apostles — leaving out Peter and Judas Iscariot, who both betrayed Christ. The lobed leaves and tendrils symbolized the hand and whips of his tormentors. Even the flower's colors, white and purple, symbolized purity and heaven.[7]

HISTORICAL USES: Approximately 5,000 year-old maypop seeds were found at Native American campsites.[8] The Algonquians harvested maypop fruits from corn fields.[8] Native Americans in the northeastern U.S. applied poultices of passion flower to treat earaches, inflammation, bruises, wounds, and boils.[9] They also consumed the tea as a calmative agent.[7] African Americans applied a poultice of bruised leaves to the forehead to treat headaches; they also applied it to bruises as an analgesic.[10] A poultice prepared from a decoction was wrapped around rheumatic joints, or bound to a woman's abdomen for cramps.[10]

Eclectic physicians administered passion flower as a hypnotic, nervine, and antispasmodic.[10,11] It was used to treat sleeplessness resulting from worry, overwork, exhaustion, cerebral fullness, or nervous excitement.[10,11] Passion flower was particularly suited for wakefulness in feeble children and the elderly, but not for insomnia resulting from pain, or in robust individuals.[10,11] It was given to treat a headache due to debility, la grippe, whooping cough, and spasmodic asthma, and to control coughing from tuberculosis.[10,11] Passion flower was given alone, or in conjunction with black cohosh *(Actaea racemosa),* pulsatilla *(Anemone pulsatilla),* or yellow jasmine *(Gelsemium)*

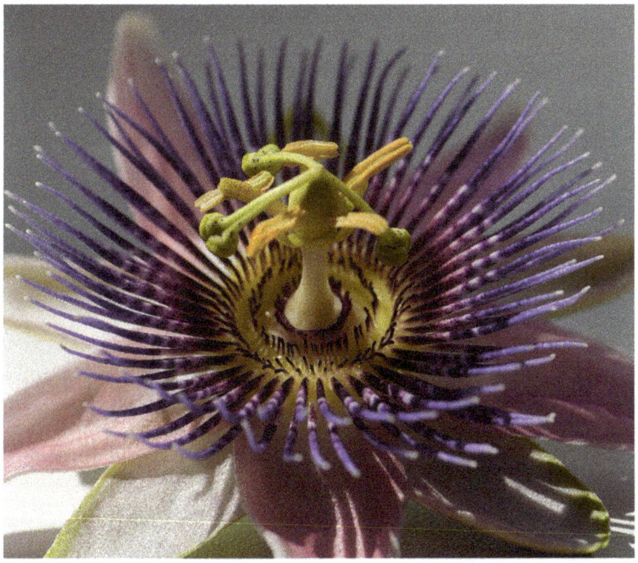

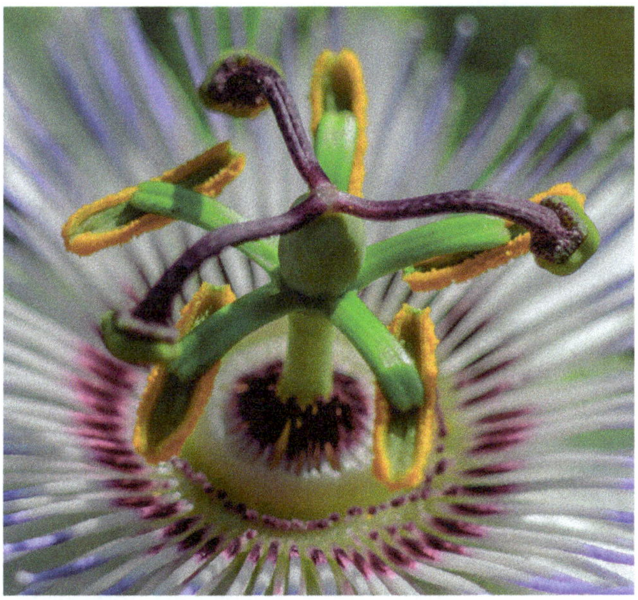

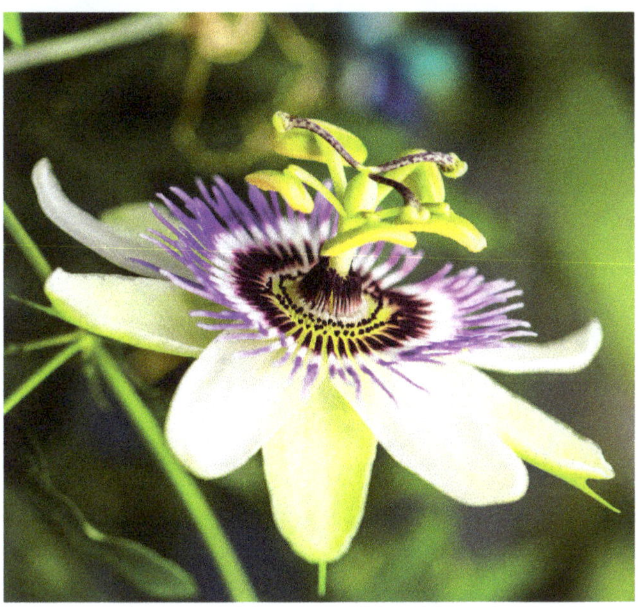

to treat menstrual anxiety and pain.[10] It was combined with Jamaican dogwood *(Piscidia)* and *Cannabis indica* for menstrual pain and anxiety.[10] Passion flower was administered as soon as pre-seizure symptoms were felt in order to ward off an epileptic attack and convulsions.[10,11]

CONSTITUENTS: Passion flower contains flavonoids (isovitexin 2"O-β-D-glucoside, isoorientin 2"O-β-D-glucoside, apigenin, luteolin, quercetin, kaempferol, schaftoside, isoschaftoside, sapanaretin, saponarin, vitexin, orientin, and rutin), a γ-pyrone derivative (maltol = laricinic acid), variable amounts of indole alkaloids (harman, harmol, harmaline, harmine, and harmalol), gynocardin, sugars (raffinose and sucrose), glycoproteins, sterols (stimagsterol and sitosterol), η-nonacosane, phenolic acids, coumarins, and gum.[12,13] Studies question the presence of harmol, harmaline, harmine, and harmalol.[12]

NUTRITIONAL PROPERTIES: Passion flower contains high amounts of chromium, fat, magnesium, niacin, phosphorus, and potassium. It has low to average amounts of calcium, cobalt, fiber, iron, manganese, protein, riboflavin, selenium, silicon, thiamine, vitamins A and C, and zinc.[14] The fruit contains calcium, iron, and phosphorus.[8]

MEDICINAL PROPERTIES: Analgesic, antidepressant, antispasmodic, antitussive, anxiolytic, calmative, hypnotic, hypotensive, nervine, and sedative.

TEMPERATURE AND FLAVOR: The aerial portions are cool and bitter. The fruit is cool, sweet, and sour.

MEDICINAL USES

Passion flower is a nervine, anxiolytic, tranquilizer, and gentle sedative.[7,8,12,13] It is a subtle nervine when consumed in low to moderate doses (30 – 60 drops) during waking hours. Passion flower calms the nervous system, reducing anxiety and treating panic attacks.[8] It can be helpful for reducing symptoms of hyperthyroidism, such as anxiety attacks, although it has no known effect on thyroid hormones. Passion flower reduces premenstrual and menopausal anxiety and agitation. It decreases anxiety and cravings during withdrawal from substances such as alcohol, tobacco, cannabis, benzodiazepine, and opiates.[12,13] Combine passion flower with kava *(Piper methysticum),* motherwort *(Leonurus cardiaca),* and/or wild oats *(Avena)* for anxiolytic effects. Passion flower is an effective nervine for hyperactive children, and may be helpful for treating attention deficit hyperactivity disorder.[7] When treating insomnia, some individuals may require

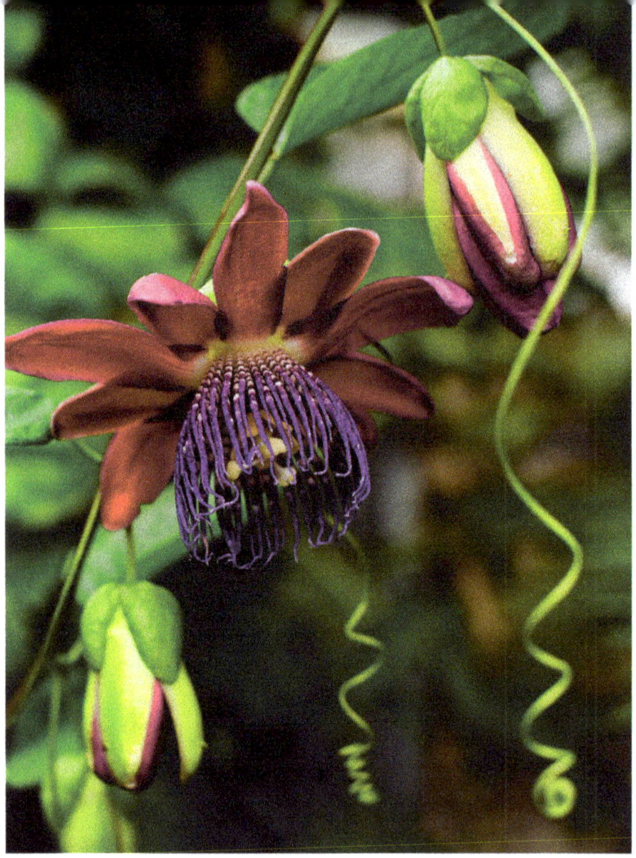

repeated doses of passion flower several hours before retiring. Others may experience immediate sedative effects, and require a larger dose (one teaspoon) one-half to one hour prior to retiring. Passion flower can be combined with kava *(Piper methysticum)*, hops *(Humulus)*, California poppy *(Eschscholzia)*, or valerian *(Valeriana)* as a sedative. The flavonoids (C-glycosylflavones), γ-pyrone (maltol), and possibly the indole alkaloids and coumarins have sedative, antispasmodic, and muscle relaxant effects.[13] The combination of flavonoids and alkaloids has sedative effects.[8]

Passion flower has antispasmodic actions on smooth and skeletal muscles, and is a motor depressant.[8,10-13,15] It is a respiratory antispasmodic for treating a dry, irritable cough or whooping cough, as well as stress- or emotionally-induced asthma in children and adults.[11,16] Passion flower has a moderate antispasmodic influence on the intestinal tract and uterus, treating digestive or menstrual cramping.[11,13,15] In addition, it reduces skeletal muscle spasms and has mild analgesic properties.[12,13] Passion flower relieves general muscle tension and tics, and can be beneficial for treating tension headaches. It aids in reducing pain and tension associated with sciatica, neuralgia, trigeminal neuralgia, and back pain. The antispasmodic and analgesic effects are synergized by combining passion flower with California poppy *(Eschscholzia)*, valerian *(Valeriana)*, and/or kava *(Piper methysticum)*.

Passion flower has hypotensive actions for individuals with stress-induced hypertension.[12,15] It is an arterial sedative that slows the heart rate and lowers blood pressure.[10,13] Combine passion flower with motherwort (*Leonurus cardiaca*) and/or very low doses of pulsatilla (*Anemone pulsatilla*) to treat hypertension, heart palpitations, and tachycardia. It does not elicit hypotensive effects in hypotensive individuals.

Passion flower has mild antidepressant effects, and acts as a mild monoamine oxidase (MAO) inhibitor. It can enhance the effectiveness of other antidepressant herbs when used in combination. Passion flower is specific for stress-induced depression, as well as depression resulting from nervous exhaustion. Both harmine and harmaline are known as potentially hallucinogenic alkaloids when combined with MAO inhibiting drugs.[7,17]

CONTRAINDICATIONS

Avoid use during pregnancy. Consult a health care practitioner before consuming while lactating. Consult a health professional before consuming passion flower with pharmaceutical antidepressant, analgesic, hypnotic, sedative, or blood pressure lowering medications.[13]

PREPARATION AND DOSAGE

TINCTURE: Fresh leaves and flowers [1:2, 70-95% alcohol]; or recently dried leaves and flowers (harvested within six to twelve months) [1:5, 60% alcohol]; consume 15-90 drops, up to three times daily.

FLUID EXTRACT: Dry leaves and flowers [1:1, 50% alcohol]; consume 30-60 drops, up to three times daily.

CAPSULES: Consume 2-4 "00" capsules, up to three times daily. Freeze-dried capsules are preferable.

TEA: Prepare a hot or cold infusion; consume 4-8 ounces, up to four times daily.

CULINARY USE: The fruit is edible.

PEDICULARIS

DESCRIPTION

BOTANICAL NAMES:
Pedicularis bracteosa, P. densiflora, P. groenlandica, P. oederi, P. racemosa, P. spp.

COMMON NAMES:
Pedicularis, lousewort, bracted lousewort, ram's horn pedicularis, elephant's head, betony, wood betony, Indian warrior, parrot's beak, sickletop, cobra's head

FAMILY NAME:
Orobanchaceae (formerly Scrophulariaceae)

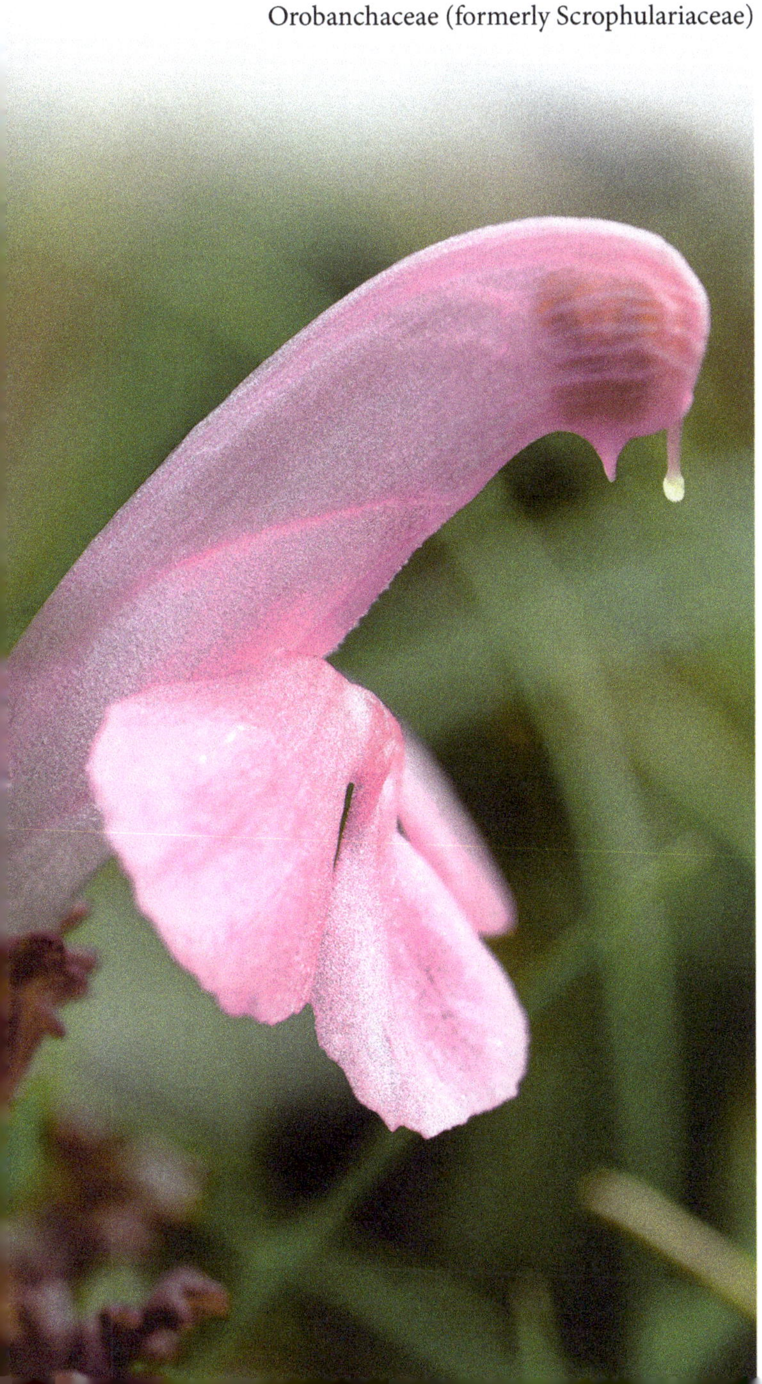

PARTS USED: The aerial portions, including foliage and flowers.

BOTANICAL DESCRIPTION AND HABITAT: *Pedicularis* is a semi-parasitic, perennial herb that grows throughout the circumboreal temperate zones and South America. It is a

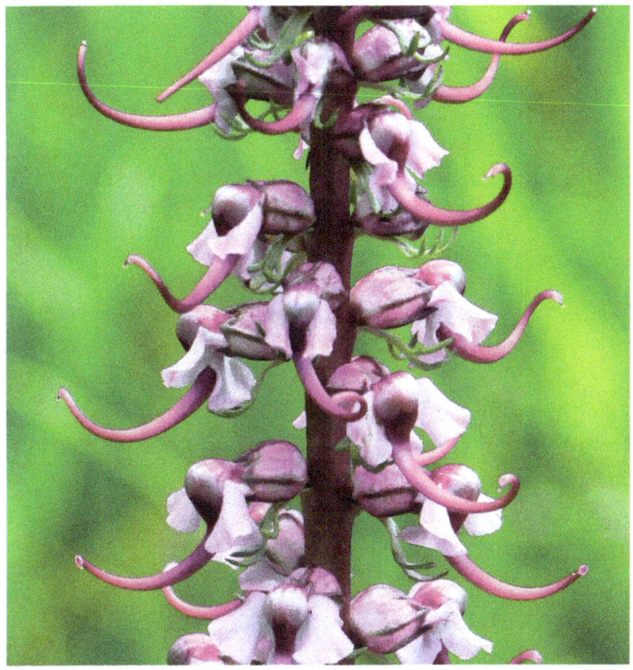

highly diverse genus, with as many as 352 species in China alone.[1] Some species grow in shaded forested areas; others grow in mountain meadows or bogs, or along streams. Many *Pedicularis* species are used interchangeably; this monograph refers to the most common species growing throughout western North America.

Pedicularis bracteosa grows up to one meter tall, with fern-like leaves (1 – 7 cm long) that are finely divided, deeply dentate, with short or non-existent petioles on the flowering stems.[2] The yellow, red, or purple corollas (13 – 21 mm long) are bilaterally symmetrical, with a fused tube featuring a hooded upper lip, and a lower lip consisting of three smaller lobes.[2] The flowers grow in dense, elongated terminal spikes (5 – 18 cm long) with several hairy, leafy bracts.[3] The sepals are fused with five teeth, and four stamens are attached to the petal tube. *P. bracteosa* thrives in moist meadows, open forests, and mountain clearings in subalpine to alpine elevations.

Pedicularis densiflora reaches 15 – 60 cm in height. The plant has lush, deep green, fern-like leaves (50 – 28 cm long) that are finely divided, pinnate, dentate, primarily growing basally, with smaller leaves alternating upward along the stem.[4] The striking dense spikes (4 – 12 cm long) bear crimson flowers. Each flower has four stamens and a fused, hooded corolla (23 – 36 mm long) with a prominent lower three-lobed petal one-fourth the size of the upper petal and surrounded by hairy bracts.[4] *P. densiflora* grows in shaded deciduous or evergreen forests in lower elevations.

Pedicularis groenlandica grows 20 – 70 cm tall.[5] It has reddish-purple, mostly basal, fern-like leaves (3 – 25 cm long) pinnately divided into oblong, toothed segments.[5] The leaves ascending the stem are progressively smaller.[5] The ornate pale pink to purple flowers grow in dense terminal spikes (1 – 30 cm long); each flower resembles an elephant's head.[5] The corolla reaches 8 – 15 mm long.[5] The upper petal is elongated and curved upward (forming the head and trunk); the lower three-lobed petal flares out, resembling elephant ears. The sepals (3 – 6 mm long) are fused into a tube with five teeth.[5] This species is pollinated by bumblebees. *P. groenlandica* grows in moist mountain meadows and bogs, and along streams in middle to high elevations.

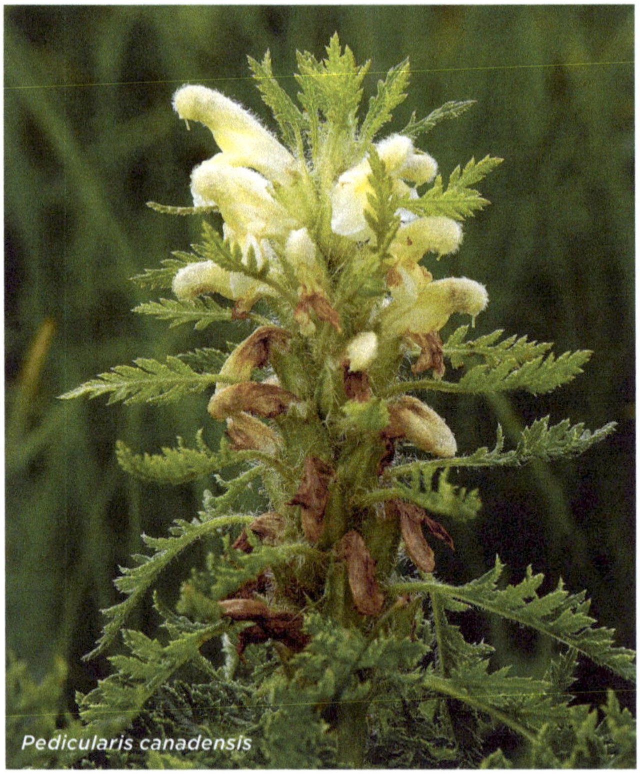
Pedicularis canadensis

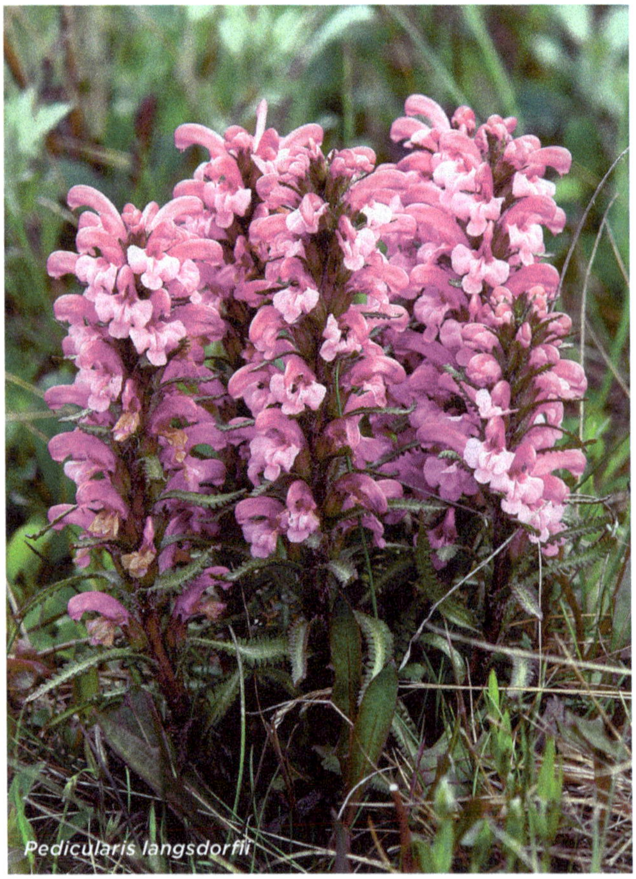
Pedicularis langsdorfii

Pedicularis oederi has a stout, woody stemmed base with thick, hairy stems (5 – 25 cm). The thick, dark green stalked leaves (1.5 – 7 cm long) are very finely, pinnately lobed, and have up to 30 pairs of segments per leaf, with sharp teeth growing mainly at the base. There are only one to two alternating leaves ascending the stem that become progressively smaller than the basal leaves.[6] The bilaterally symmetrical, vibrant yellow flowers are beakless, with a brownish tip featuring two red spots. The flowers grow in dense spikes, (5 – 10 cm long). They have leaf-like bracts and four stamens grouped into two pairs. Each stamen bears long hairs protruding from the filament.[6] *P. oederi* grows on high elevation rocky slopes and cliffs.

Pedicularis racemosa is a perennial growing 15 – 50 cm tall. It has a woody stem base with clusters of lanceolate to narrow, oblong, undivided dentate leaves. The lanceolate leaves (2 – 10 cm long) alternate along the stem, progressively decreasing in size as they near the flowering heads (1 – 5 cm long).[7] The corollas (10 – 16 mm long) are bilaterally symmetrical, ranging in color from white, to pinkish-purple, to scarlet.[7] Emerging from a fused tube, the upper lobe is strongly arched, tapering into the shape of a sickle or ram's horn. The downward curving beak reaches a prominent three-lobed lower platform. The sepals (4.5 – 8 mm) are fused; the four stamens are fused to the petals.[7] *P. racemosa* grows in dry meadows, open coniferous forests, or rocky slopes in middle to subalpine elevations.

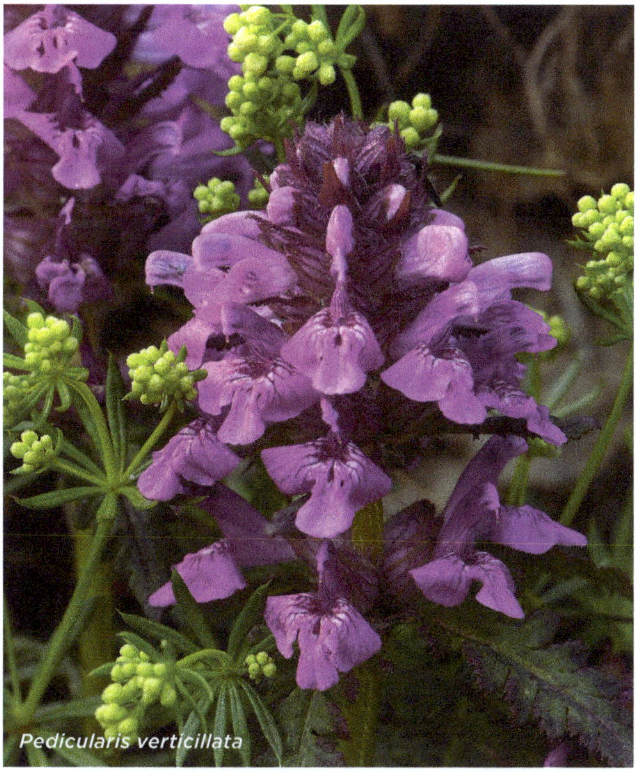

Pedicularis verticillata

THE NAME: The genus name *Pedicularis* means "of lice." The epithet *bracteosa* refers to the leafy bracts surrounding the flowering heads. The epithet *densiflora* describes the dense terminal clusters of flowers. *P. groenlandica* ("Greenland") was first described in 1795 by Swedish natural history professor, Anders Jahan Retzius (1742 – 1821). Retzius did not discover the specimen; it was originally harvested by an unnamed collector in Greenland during the 1700s.[8] The epithet *oederi* was named after Georg Christian von Oeder (1728 – 1791), a botany professor in Copenhagen, and the first editor of *Flora Danica.*[9] *Racemosa* refers to the floral clusters that grow as racemes.

Betony derives from an old Gallic word meaning "medicinal plant."[9] *Pedicularis* and *Stachys betonica* are commonly termed wood betony or betony; however, they have different medicinal properties. Lousewort, a common name applied to many *Pedicularis* species, dates to the 17th century. Cattle grazing in fields where pedicularis grew abundantly became infested with lice.[9]

The following common names correspond with the Latin binomials: bracted lousewort, wood betony, cobra's head, and fernleaf *(Pedicularis bracteosa);* Indian warrior *(Pedicularis densiflora);* elephant's head and lousewort *(P. groenlandica);* Oeder's lousewort *(P. oederi);* and horn pedicularis, sickletop lousewort, or parrot's beak *(P. racemosa).* The common name pedicularis refers to any medicinal species within the genus.

HISTORICAL USES: Infusions of lousewort roots were consumed by numerous tribes in North America to alleviate stomach pain, ulcers, sore throats, and coughs, as a blood tonic, and to reduce blood in stools.[10] A tea prepared from the stems and leaves was consumed as an expectorant and antitussive.[10] *P. canadensis* infusions were consumed to treat internal swelling.[11] The Washoe applied a poultice of lousewort to cuts, sores, and swellings; they also consumed the tea as a general tonic.[10] Inuit children sucked the nectar from flowers.[11] The Ojibwa believed lousewort was an aphrodisiac.[11] The pulverized or cooked root, or finely diced herb was added to food as a love charm to reunite estranged couples.[10,11] According to legend, a *Pedicularis densiflora* plant grows where an Indian warrior has fallen in battle.[12]

Canadian herbalist Terry Willard notes that the fresh, fleshy root can be eaten raw or cooked like carrots, and the fleshy stems were consumed as a pot herb. However, exercise caution because the safety of consumption is questionable due to the varying levels of alkaloids and the semi-parasitic nature of pedicularis.[11] *Note:* Review the *Contraindications* section before collecting, preparing, or using pedicularis. In India, the leaves of *P. pectinata* are used as a diuretic and hemostatic for blood in the sputum.[10]

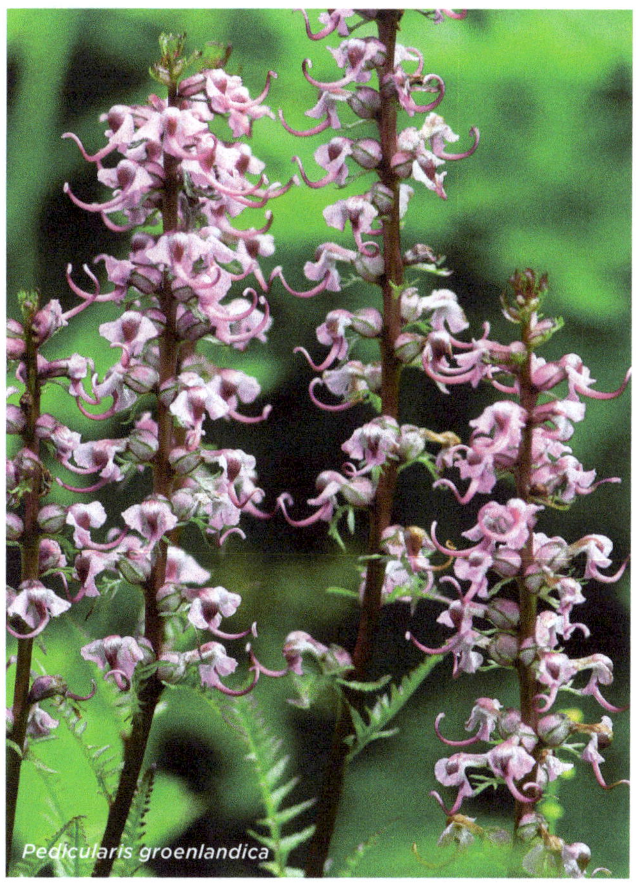

Pedicularis groenlandica

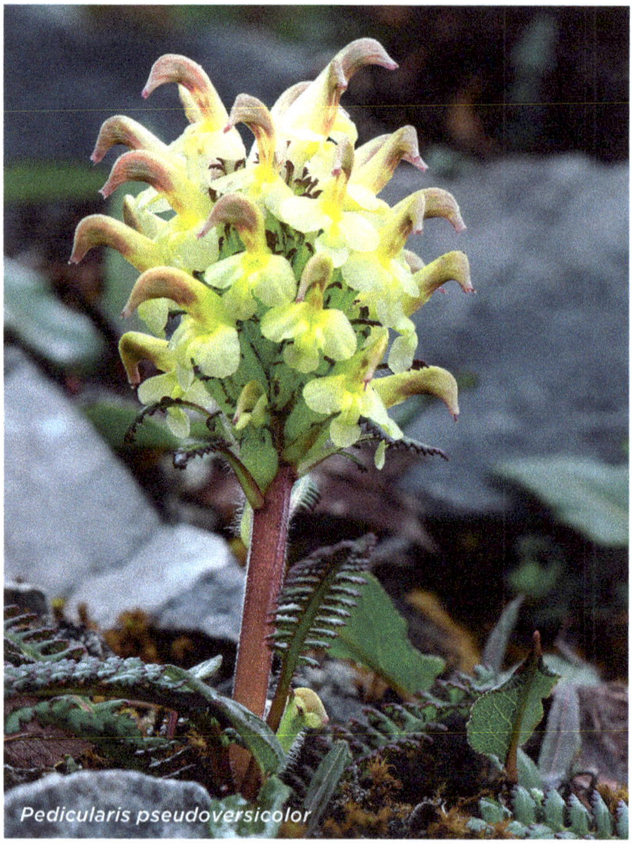
Pedicularis pseudoversicolor

CONSTITUENTS: Pedicularis contains verbascosides, euphroside, geniposidic acid, plantarenaloside, iridoids (aucubins), forsythoside B, leucosceptoside A, martynoside, iridolactone, mussaenoside, echinacoside, shanzhiside methyl ester, cistanoside D, saponins, tannins, monoterpenoid alkaloids (pedicularine, boschniakine, and others), and pedicularioside.[13,14] Antioxidant pheylpropanoids have been extracted from *Pedicularis* species.[10]

NUTRITIONAL PROPERTIES: Unknown.

MEDICINAL PROPERTIES: Smooth and skeletal muscle antispasmodic, and mild nervine.

TEMPERATURE AND FLAVOR: Neutral and bitter.

MEDICINAL USES

Pedicularis is a skeletal muscle antispasmodic that decreases muscle rigidity.[15,16] It can be consumed by adults or children with tight, sore muscles.[15,16] It aids in treating tension headaches, as well as trigeminal pain and tension. Pedicularis relaxes muscle tension and spasms resulting from excessive physical activity such as hiking, gardening, and athletic training. This herb also eases muscle tension resulting from remaining stationary for long periods of time. Some patients with multiple sclerosis have experienced a decrease in muscle spasms.

Pedicularis is very beneficial in managing chronic pain and tension. It relieves muscular guarding, especially in individuals receiving various forms of therapeutic deep tissue massage, Heller work, or Rolfing.[15,16] Pedicularis is effective for loosening muscles before a chiropractic adjustment.[15] A birthing mother can consume the herb as a relaxant with no negative effects on uterine contractions. This herb also can be consumed or applied topically following a birth in order to reduce muscle tension and pain resulting from muscle contractions. Pedicularis alleviates muscle spasms in individuals with sciatica, damage to the spinal cord or discs, chronic back pain, or muscle pain following an injury or accident. It has no known effect on nerve pain, so other nerve sedatives are needed to manage pain; however, it helps to relax the muscles. When consumed in low to moderate doses during the day, it rarely affects mental clarity or acts as a sedative. However, some individuals experience mild sedative or stupefying actions when consuming the herb in higher doses.

Pedicularis has subtle nervine effects, and acts as a sedative in some individuals. It has mild smooth muscle relaxant properties, primarily decreasing menstrual cramping. Pedicularis has little effect on digestive cramping or respiratory spasms, although it will ease skeletal muscle tension resulting from spastic coughing. It can be dried and smoked to obtain gentle euphoric and nervine effects.

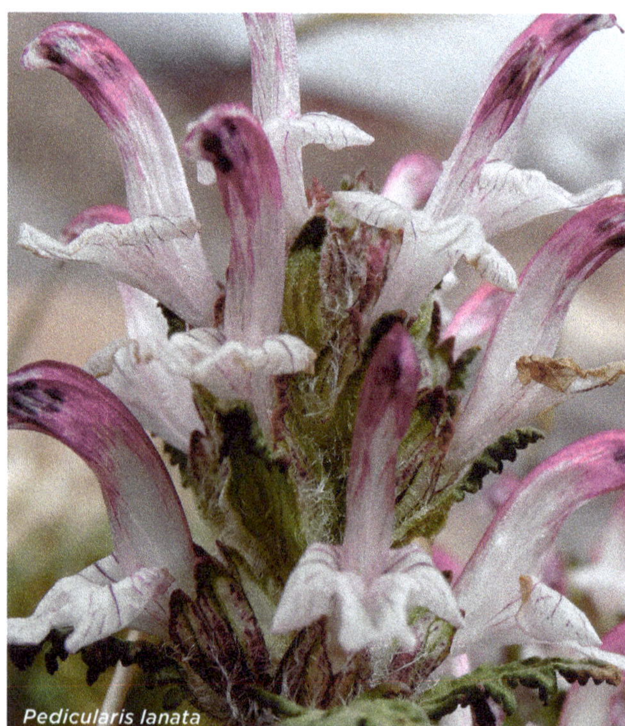
Pedicularis lanata

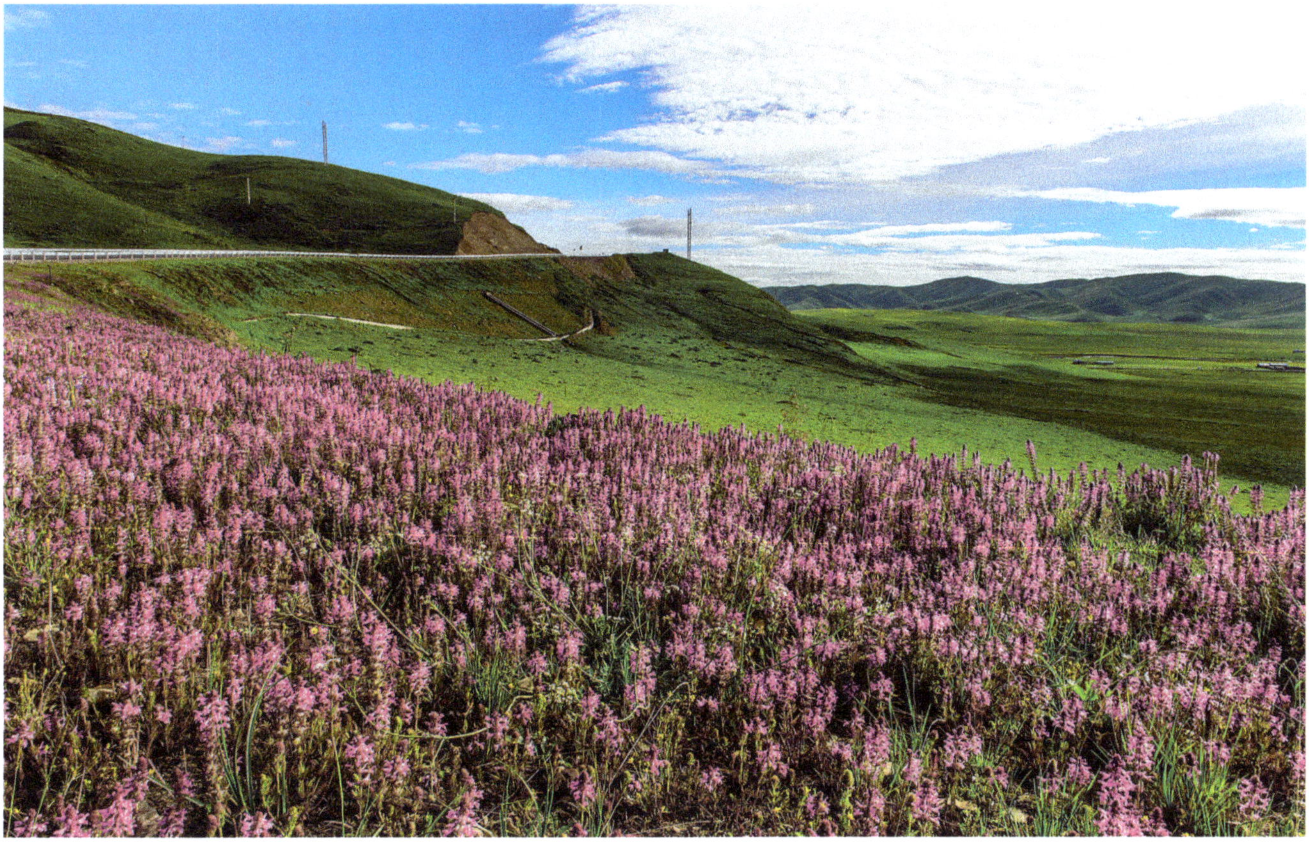

CONTRAINDICATIONS

Excessive doses of the tea or tincture can cause over relaxation of the muscles, and drowsiness or incoherence. Individuals sensitive to the effects of pedicularis should exercise caution or avoid operating heavy machinery. Consume only a low to moderate dose range during pregnancy and lactation until this herb is more thoroughly researched.

According to herbalist Michael Moore, pedicularis is a semi-parasitic plant that may be able to pick up the secondary compounds of plants growing near it.[15] Avoid harvesting pedicularis plants growing alongside alkaloid-containing plants such as *Senecio* (ragwort), *Lupinus* (lupine), or *Thermopsis* (mountain pea).[15] Those plants contain alkaloids that can strain the liver and other organs when administered in high doses. Some species grow around oaks, and may pick up tannins. Other species grow on pine and spruce trees, and may pick up the aromatics that warm the skin and stimulate urination.[15] Having harvested numerous species of *Pedicularis* growing with oaks, spruce, and pines, the author has not noticed that the tinctures are strongly astringent or aromatic. However, due to the plant's potential absorption of toxic alkaloids contained in neighboring plants, take care to identify all plants surrounding pedicularis before harvesting.

PREPARATION AND DOSAGE

TINCTURE: Fresh plant [1:2-1:3, 70-95% alcohol]; recently dried plant [1:5, 50-60% alcohol]; consume 20-120 drops, up to four times daily. Apply topically as a liniment.

GLYCERITE: Fresh plant [1:2, 60% glycerin and 40% distilled water] or [1:2, 50% glycerin and 50% alcohol]; consume 20-90 drops, up to four times daily. Apply topically as a liniment.

CAPSULES: Consume 2-4 "00" capsules of recently dried, ground herb, up to three times daily.

TEA: Prepare a hot infusion; consume 4-8 ounces, up to four times daily.

TOPICAL USE: Apply a liniment, glycerite, fomentation, or poultice to the affected area. Infuse the fresh wilted herb in oil using the double boiler method, or dry the herb and prepare oil using the alcohol intermediary method.

PENNYROYAL

DESCRIPTION

BOTANICAL NAMES:
Mentha pulegium, Hedeoma pulegioides

COMMON NAMES:
European pennyroyal, American pennyroyal, American false pennyroyal, American mock pennyroyal, mock pennyroyal, pulegium, run-by-the-ground, lurk-in-the-ditch, pudding grass, piliolerial, mosquito plant, squaw balm, squawmint, tickweed
puolanminttu (Finnish)
menthe pouliot, puce (French)
flohkraut, herminze, hirschminze, kleiner balsam, polei-minze (German)
menta puleggio, pulce (Italian)
polejmynta (Swedish)[1,4]

FAMILY NAME:
Lamiaceae (Labiatae)

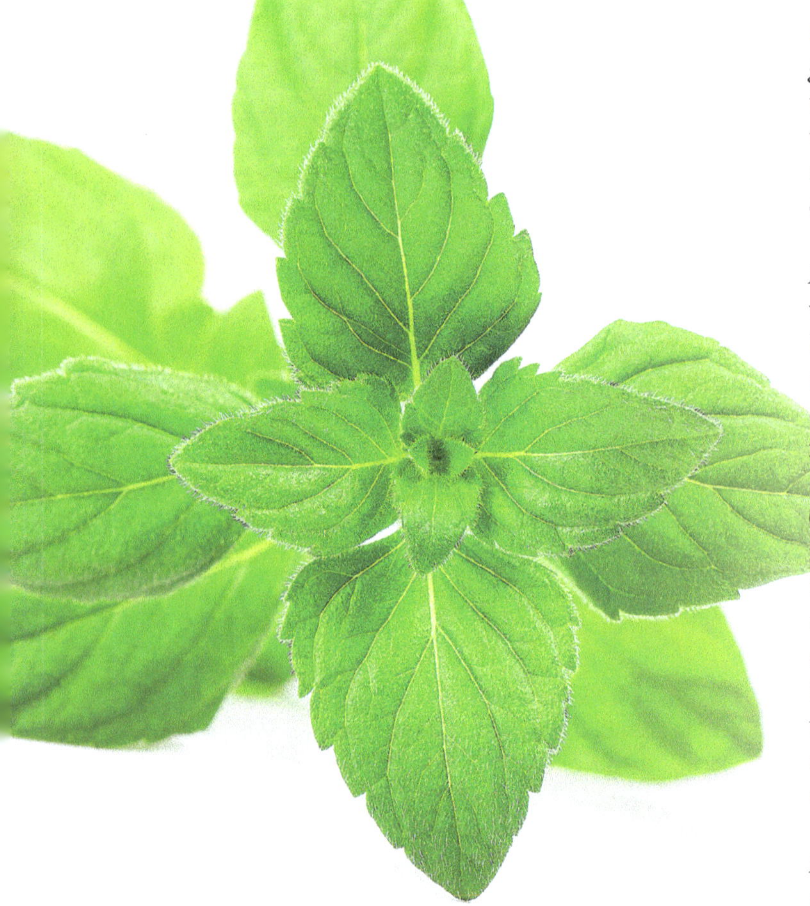

PARTS USED: The foliage or aerial portions in flower.

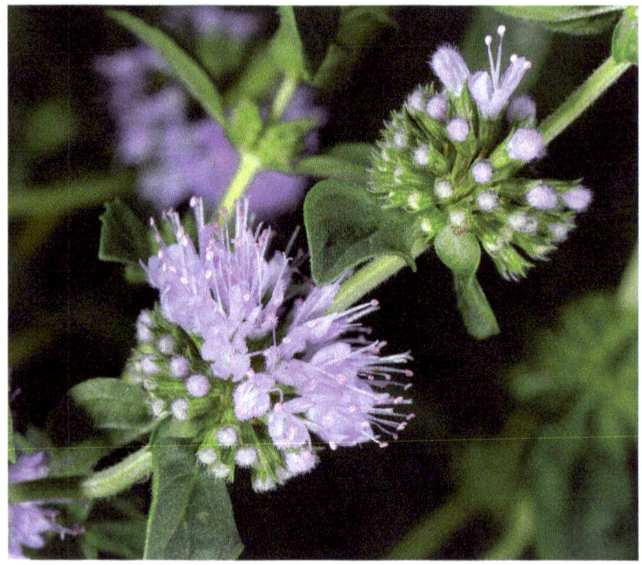

BOTANICAL DESCRIPTION AND HABITAT: *Mentha pulegium* (European pennyroyal) is a perennial herb native to southern and western Europe that has naturalized in the U.S. *Hedeoma pulegioides* (American pennyroyal) is native to the eastern U.S. It grows perennially in temperate climates, and annually in cold climates with harsh winters.

Mentha pulegium is a low-growing mint (10 – 30 cm tall) with square, pubescent stems and opposite, narrowly ovate leaves (0.5 – 2.5 cm long).[2] The strongly scented leaves have smooth to serrate margins, rounded apices, and pubescent undersides.[2] The axillary clusters of lavender to purple flowers are subtended by reflexed bracts.[2] The flowers have small, hairy calyces (2.5 – 4 mm) and bilabiate corollas (5 – 8 mm) shorter than the four stamens.[2] The fruit, like in other mints, is a collection of four nutlets developed from an ovary with two carpels. This herb grows in moist soil along riverbanks, edges of ponds and lakes, drainage ditches, and disturbed sites. European pennyroyal tolerates full sun or partial shade, and is easily cultivated. It spreads with underground runners, and like many members of the mint family, becomes invasive easily. If there is concern about the herb spreading, plant it in a container.

Hedeoma pulegioides is an annual (10 – 30 cm tall) with pubescent stems bearing opposite, elliptic to oblong lanceolate, fragrant leaves (2.5 cm long by 0.5 cm wide) with mostly smooth margins and short petioles.[3] Small axillary inflorescences of one to four flowers bear tiny flowers (5 mm long by 2.5 mm wide) with five-toothed, tubular calyces, and white to indigo bilabiate, tubular corollas.[3] Within are two stamens (unique for a mint family plant) and an ovary of two fused carpels.[3] Each flower is subtended by two leaf-like bracts equivalent in length to the flower.[3] American pennyroyal prefers drier, rocky soils and light shade to full sun in locations with less competition from taller plants.[3]

THE NAME: Theophrastus, the ancient Greek philosopher and botanist who succeeded Aristotle, originally applied the genus name *Mentha,* derived from Greek mythology. Pluto fell in love with a nymph named Menthe. In a fit of jealous rage, his wife, Proserpine, metamorphosed Menthe into the plant now called mint.[1]

Hedeoma originates from two Greek words: *hedys* ("sweet") and *osme* ("odor"), referring to the leaves' scent. The epithets *pulegium* and *pulegioides* derive from the Latin *pulex* ("flea"), as does the French term *puce,* and the Italian *pulce.* These names refer to its historic use as an insect repellent. Romans called the plant *pulegium.* Pennyroyal was a corruption of the folk names pulioll-royal and piloile-rial. Due to its growth habit, European country folk referred to the herb as run-by-the-ground and lurk-in-the-ditch. It acquired the name pudding grass, as it was combined with pepper and honey to flavor stuffing in hog's pudding.[1,5]

HISTORICAL USES: Native Americans consumed the hot tea to warm themselves in cold weather, and to treat fever, chills, congestion, coughs, whooping cough, headaches, stomach pain, indigestion, dysentery, menstrual cramps, and suppressed menstruation.[7] The Iroquois valued pennyroyal tea as a headache remedy and a beverage with winter meals. The Delaware consumed the hot tea to relieve a stomachache.[6] Navajo utilized pennyroyal as an analgesic.[7] A leaf poultice was applied to the gums for toothaches, and to the forehead for headaches.[6,7]

Pliny the Elder recommended hanging the herb in sleeping rooms.[1] Gerard suggested consuming pennyroyal tea and honey to cleanse the lungs from "gross and thick humours." English folk herbalists suggested wearing a garland of pennyroyal around the head for "swimming in the head and pains and giddiness thereof."[1] The herb was widely used in folk medicine as a contraceptive agent, from classical times through the Middle Ages.[1,6]

Culpeper described pennyroyal medicinal uses:

> Drank with wine, it is good for venomous bite, and applied to nostril with vinegar revives those who faint and swoon. Dried and burnt, it strengthens the gums, helps the gout, if applied of itself to the place until it is red, and applied in a plaster, it takes away spots or marks on the face; applied with salt it profits those that are splenic or liver-grown. The green herb bruised and put into vinegar, cleanses foul ulcers and takes away the marks of bruises. One spoonful of the juice sweetened with sugar-candy is a cure for whooping-cough.[1]

CONSTITUENTS: American pennyroyal contains volatile oil (pulegone, menthone, and isomenthone), flavonoids (diosmin), tannins, and organic acids. European pennyroyal contains volatile oil (pulegone, piperitenone or piperitone, isomenthone, menthone, carvacol, isopulegone, α-pinene, β-pinene, and limonene), flavonoids (diosmin), and tannins.[6,8,9]

NUTRITIONAL PROPERTIES: Pennyroyal contains flavonoids, but no other nutrients have been identified.

MEDICINAL PROPERTIES: Abortifacient, antispasmodic, carminative, diaphoretic, emmenagogue, insect repellent, stomachic, and topical counterirritant.

TEMPERATURE AND FLAVOR: Warm, pungent, bitter, and sweet.

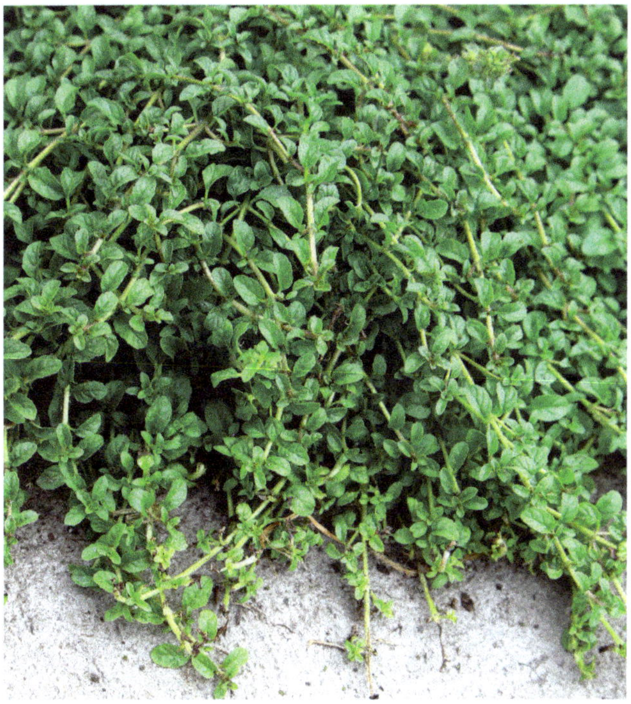

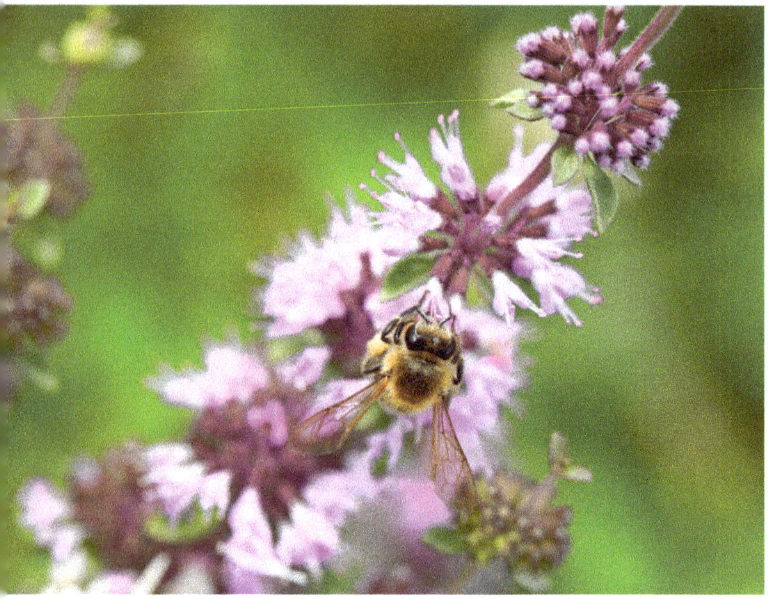

citronella as an insect repellent. *Note:* Review the contraindications before applying.

While the tea has been used medicinally for centuries, concerns about the use of pennyroyal arose from internal consumption of the toxic essential oil. In 1978, a woman died after ingesting one ounce of pennyroyal essential oil to induce an abortion, although apparently, she wasn't actually pregnant.[6] Many articles condemning the use of pennyroyal ensued, and unfortunately, the herb acquired a bad reputation. Dr. Norman Farnsworth of the University of Illinois stated that one would have to ingest about 75 gallons of strong pennyroyal tea within a short time to equal the effect of a one-ounce dose of pennyroyal oil.[6] He also asserted that consuming one ounce of nearly any essential oil could be fatal.[6] Since 1980, six cases of toxicity have occurred from ingesting the essential oil.[6,7]

MEDICINAL USES

American pennyroyal *(Hedeoma)* and European pennyroyal *(Mentha pulegium)* can be used interchangeably as medicine. However, dried American pennyroyal leaf contains 2% pulegone, while dried European pennyroyal leaf contains 1% pulegone.[6,7,11] Pennyroyal is a potent emmenagogue and uterine diaphoretic that encourages shedding of the uterine lining.[6,10,11] It aids in treating amenorrhea, dysmenorrhea, and slow starting, crampy menses.[6,8,10,11] Pennyroyal decreases uterine stagnation, reducing menstrual cramps with a dull, achy character.[11]

Pennyroyal is a smooth muscle antispasmodic that relieves menstrual and digestive cramping.[8,11] It is a stomachic and carminative, relieving nausea, gas, bloating, and stomach and intestinal cramping resulting from poor digestion, poor food combining, and overeating.[6,8,10,11] Combine pennyroyal with peppermint *(Mentha piperita)* and catnip *(Nepeta cataria)* to ease digestive cramping.

Consuming the hot tea has diaphoretic and expectorant actions.[6,8,10,11] It induces sweating in the first stages of a cold or flu, or upon exposure to cold weather.[8,11] Frequently consume small amounts (4 – 6 ounces) of a hot infusion containing peppermint *(Mentha piperita)*, yarrow *(Achillea)*, elder flower *(Sambucus)*, and pennyroyal to encourage diaphoresis.

The infused oil or a spray containing a highly-diluted solution of pennyroyal essential oil has insect repellent properties.[6,10] Apply the spray, oil, or salve topically to repel mosquitoes, tics, mites, and chiggers.[6,10] Blend with essential oils of lemon grass, eucalyptus, lavender, and/or

Consuming the essential oil of pennyroyal is toxic, even in small quantities.[7] It contains a concentrated amount of the ketone pulegone. When consumed, it is known to cause a variety of side effects, such as convulsions, coma, choking, vomiting, elevated blood pressure, irreversible kidney and liver damage, and death due to respiratory failure. The essential oil averages 80 – 94% of pulegone, the dried leaf of European pennyroyal yields about 1% pulegone, and American pennyroyal contains up to 2%.[6]

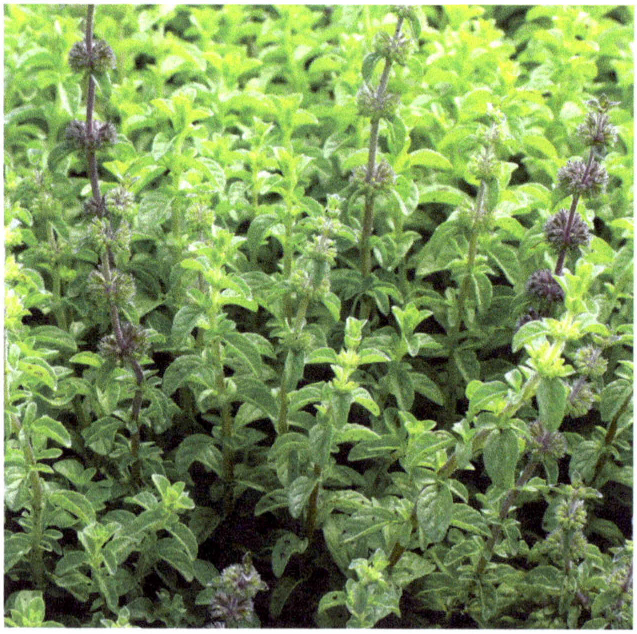

Consuming pennyroyal essential oil is considered hepatotoxic due to its concentration of pulegone. Exercise caution with topical use, and apply the essential oil only when it is highly diluted. *Note:* Review the *Topical Use* section below for recommended dilution.

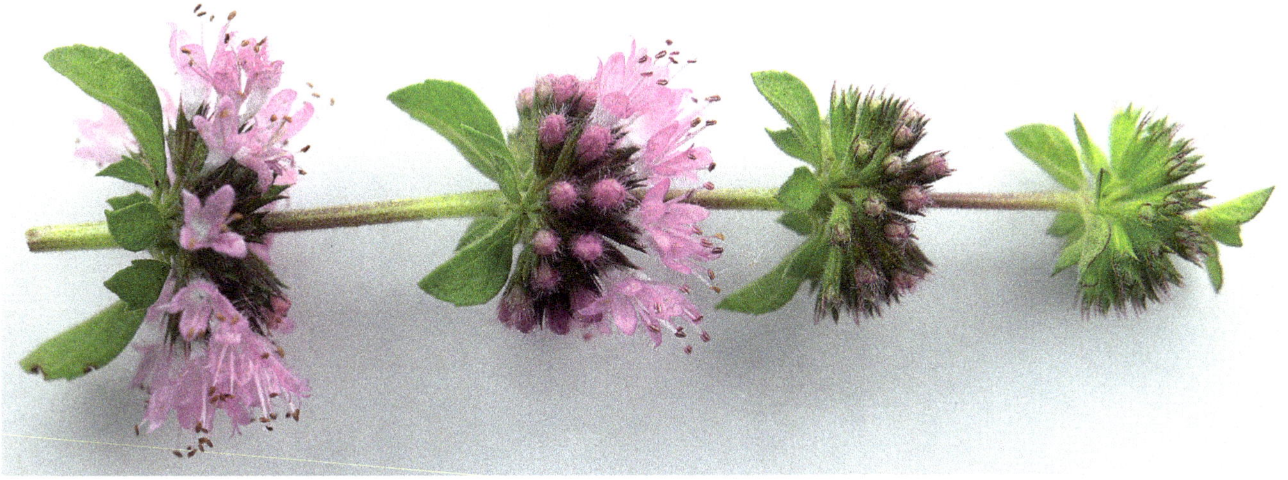

CONTRAINDICATIONS

Due to the emmenagogue and potential abortifacient actions, all forms of pennyroyal should be avoided during pregnancy, and in women with heavy menstruation or uterine bleeding.[6,8-10] Pregnant women should avoid processing pennyroyal herb or herbal products. Topical products containing pennyroyal should also be avoided during pregnancy. Pennyroyal contains ketones; therefore, it should be avoided by infants, children, lactating women, individuals with kidney, liver, or seizure disorders, or those taking antiseizure medications.[8]

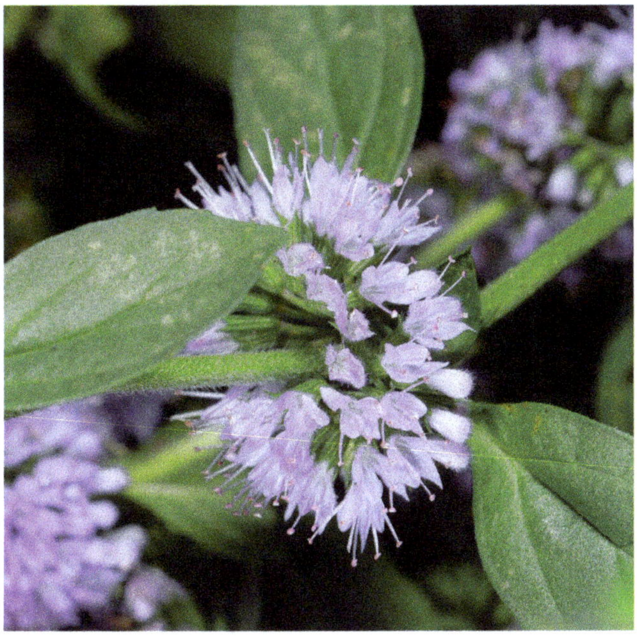

Warning: Never, under any circumstances, should the essential oil be consumed by humans or animals![7] The ketones (pulegone, etc.) concentrated in the essential oil can cause severe headaches, convulsions, coma, choking, nausea, vomiting, abdominal pains, elevated blood pressure, semiparalysis of the limbs, death due to respiratory failure, and irreversible kidney and liver damage.[9] Consuming 4 ml of the essential oil has caused convulsions and severe CNS depression.[9] However, the highly diluted essential oil may be applied topically to humans or pets as an insect repellent, except during pregnancy, lactation, in infants or children, or those with seizure or CNS disorders. Topical applications of the essential oil can cause contact dermatitis.[7,10]

PREPARATION AND DOSAGE

TINCTURE: Fresh aerial parts [1:2-1:3, 70-95% alcohol]; recently dried aerial parts [1:5, 60% alcohol]; consume 10-60 drops, up to three times daily.

GLYCERITE: Fresh aerial parts [1:2-1:3, 50% glycerin and 50% alcohol]; recently dried aerial parts [1:5, 40% glycerin, 30% alcohol, and 30% water]; consume 10-60 drops, up to three times daily.

CAPSULES: Consume 1-2 "00" capsules, one to three times daily.

TEA: Prepare a hot infusion; consume 4-8 ounces, up to three times daily.

TOPICAL USE: Infuse the leaves in base oil using the Simpler's or alcohol intermediary method. Prepare the oil or salve as an insect repellent, or apply topically to the lower pelvic region to relieve menstrual cramps. Dilute 1-10 drops of pennyroyal essential oil per ounce of base liquid containing 20% alcohol and 80% distilled water solution or one ounce of base oil, and apply topically as a flea and insect repellent.

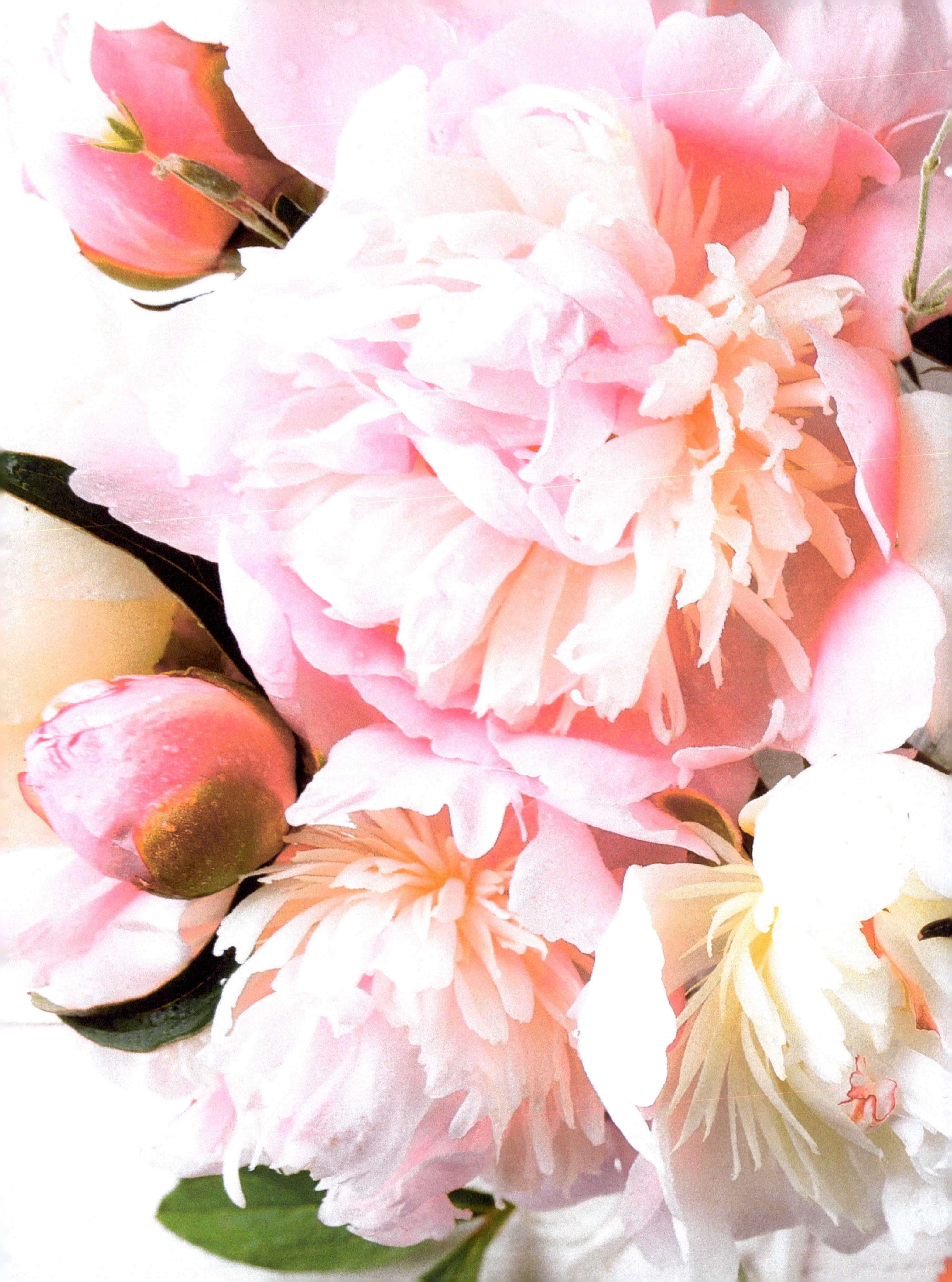

PEONY

BOTANICAL NAMES:
Paeonia lactiflora (syn. *P. albiflora*), *P. officinalis, P. corallina, P. brownii, P. californica*

COMMON NAMES:
White peony root, Chinese peony, European peony, western peony, California peony, male peony, peony, common peony, common garden peony, fragrant peony
byakushaku (Japanese)
paekchak (Korean)
bai shao, pai-shao (Mandarin)

FAMILY NAME:
Ranunculaceae
(formerly Paeoniaceae)

DESCRIPTION

PART USED: The roots.

BOTANICAL DESCRIPTION AND HABITAT: *Paeonia* is a genus of about 30 species growing in the western U.S., northwest Mexico, and Eurasia; many horticultural varieties are commonly found in gardens.[1] *P. lactiflora* (syn. *P. albiflora*) is a perennial herb native to China and Siberia

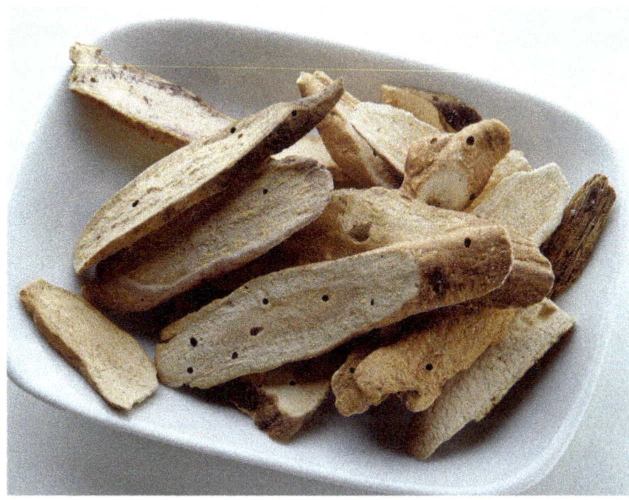

that can be cultivated as an ornamental. It thrives in moist, loamy soil with full to partial shade. *P. officinalis* is native to southern Europe, and is also cultivated in gardens. *P. corallina,* sometimes referred to as "male peony" (no reference to the sex of the flower), is native to Europe and cultivated for its roots. *P. brownii* is native to the dry, mountainous slopes of the western U.S. *P. californica* is found in chaparral and coastal scrub along the coast of southern California.[2]

Paeonia lactiflora grows up to 70 cm tall. It is a robust plant with large, smooth, dark green, ternately compound leaves comprised of large, lanceolate leaflets with decurrent bases, acuminate apices, and sparsely hairy undersides.[3] Encircled by three to four ovate sepals (1 – 1.5 cm long by 1 – 1.7 cm wide), the petals (3.5 – 6 cm long by 1.5 – 4.5 cm wide) of the large, fragrant flowers of *P. lactiflora* range from pinkish-white to reddish-purple; many cultivars have double flowers.[3] The flowers contain many large yellow stamens and two to five separate green or purple carpels that produce large, oblong follicles (3 cm long by 1.5 cm wide).[3] The thick, tuberous *P. lactiflora* roots have brown skin and a pale pinkish-white or yellowish-white inner core. *P. lactiflora* is the source of white peony and red

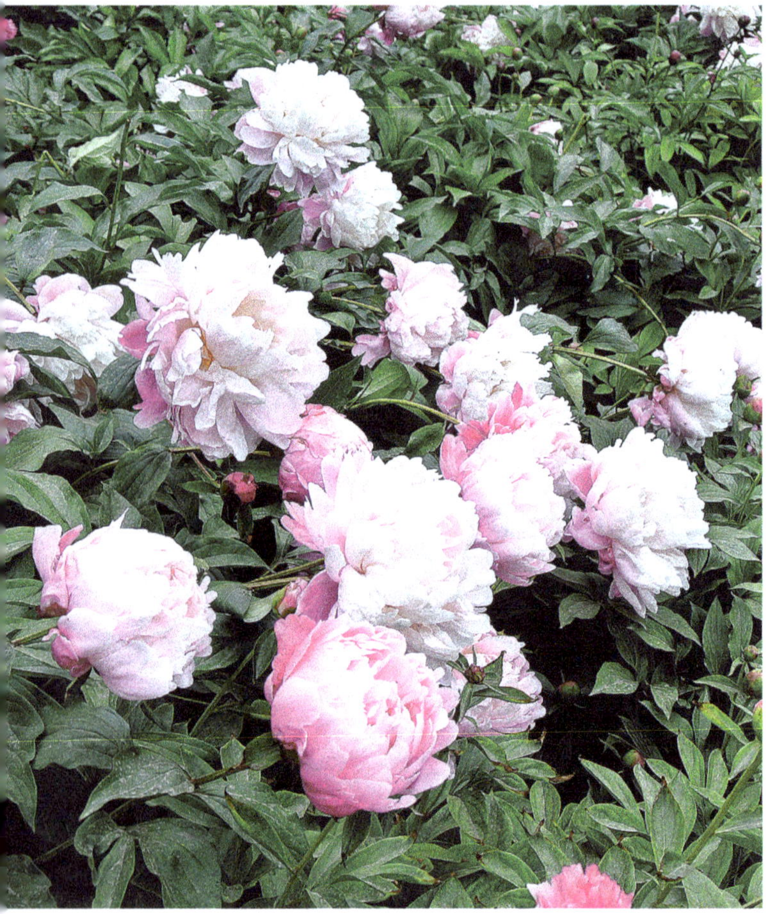

peony — the difference is in how the herbs are prepared. This monograph refers solely to the use of white peony when describing *P. lactiflora.*

The branched stem of *Paeonia officinalis* (up to 70 cm tall) bears ternately compound leaves that are bright green on the upper side, and paler underneath.[4] This species only produces one flower per stem. The pink to scarlet petals are fragrant and single in wild species, but can be double in cultivated varieties.[5] Within are many yellow stamens and two to five separate carpels that develop into large follicles (2 – 3.5 cm long).[1,4]

P. brownii (20 – 40 cm tall) generally grows unbranched stems, each bearing five to eight grayish-green, ternately compound leaves with glaucous coatings and rounded apices.[6,7] Blooming in late spring, the mildly fragrant, nodding flowers of *P. brownii* have five to six large green sepals, five to six reddish-maroon to bronze petals (8 – 13 mm long) with yellowish-green margins, and many stamens.[6,7] Within are two to five separate carpels that develop into large, thick follicles (2 – 4 cm long).[1,6,7] The tubers of *P. brownii* have a pinkish-purple inner core.

Reaching 35 – 75 cm tall, *P. californica* produces branching stems, each bearing 7 – 12 ternately compound leaves that lack the glaucous coating of *P. brownii* and have more acute apices.[8] The flowers bloom December through April. They display dark reddish-purple petals with pink margins (15 – 25 mm long), many stamens, and two to five separate carpels that mature into large, thick follicles (3 – 4 cm long).[8]

P. officinalis roots are harvested from two year-old plants in Europe. In China, the roots are harvested from three to five year-old plants, August through October. Traditionally, the fresh roots are boiled in water 5 – 15 minutes, peeled, then sun dried.

THE NAME: The genus name *Paeonia* derives from Paeon, a pupil of Asclepius, the god of medicine, and a mythical physician to the Greek gods. Leto, Apollo's mother, gave a peony to Paeon, who planted it on Mount Olympus. Paeon used it to cure Pluto, who was wounded during the Trojan War by Hercules. Asclepius became so jealous of Paeon that he plotted to kill him. However, Pluto heard of the plot, and because he was grateful for Paeon's service, prevented his murder by transforming Paeon into the plant that has since borne his name. Linnaeus established the genus *Paeonia* (1753).[9]

After extensive exploration of the Russian Empire, Peter Simon Pallas, German botanist, coined the epithet *P. lactiflora* (1776), and later created the synonym *P. albiflora* (1788). The epithet *lactiflora* means "milky flower;" *albiflora* means "white flower" referring to the light-colored flowers. The epithet *officinalis* implies that the herb was included in the official pharmacopoeia. The pin yin name *bai shao* translates as "white peony."[11]

The following common names correspond with the Latin binomials: Chinese white peony, common garden peony, cultivated peony, bai shao, pai shao *(Paeonia lactiflora* syn. *P. albiflora);* European peony *(P. officinalis);* male peony *(P. corallina);* western peony, Brown's peony *(P. brownii);* and California peony *(P. californica).*

HISTORICAL USES: In ancient times, Europeans believed peony was divine, having emanated from the moon. It was thought to protect the harvest, shepherds, and flocks, and to drive away evil spirits. It was also considered a cure for lunacy. The seeds were strung in necklaces to charm against evil spirits. Pliny the Elder and Theophrastus stressed the importance of harvesting the roots at night:

> That of necessity it must be gathered in the night, for, if any man shall pluck of the fruit in the daytime, being seen of the woodpecker, he is in danger to lose his eyes.

Gerard considered these claims ridiculous, but recommended the herb for treating nightmares and melancholic dreams. Other European herbalists employed peony for treating convulsions and curing epilepsy.[12] The tea was consumed for gout, asthmatic spasms, and eclampsia. A wine extract of peony root was used to treat jaundice, as well as kidney and bladder problems.[13] *P. officinalis* was used to flavor roast pork in 14th and 15th century England. The seeds were also used as flavoring.[9] *P. corallina* roots were used for disorders of the head and nerves.[12]

White and red peony root *(P. lactiflora)* were administered for thousands of years in Chinese folk medicine and Traditional Chinese Medicine; both are listed as official drugs in the *The Pharmacopeia of the People's Republic of China.*[10] Peony and plum flowers are cultural floral symbols in China.[10] The Qing Dynasty declared peony the national flower in 1903. Mongolian nomads consumed peony roots as food. It was believed that *P. lactiflora* was introduced to European gardens from Siberia in 1558. They were grown in Virginia as early as 1771.[10]

Native Americans administered *P. brownii* to treat a variety of digestive complaints, including nausea, stomachaches, indigestion, constipation, and diarrhea.[14] The root was also employed for colds, coughs, pneumonia, tuberculosis, heart and kidney problems, chest pain, venereal disease, and sore eyes.[14] A wash was used to relieve headaches and sore eyes. The root was used to fatten people and horses. A poultice of crushed roots was applied to cuts, wounds, sores, burns, and boils. The Diegueno consumed sliced, baked roots of *P. californica* to alleviate indigestion.[10,14]

CONSTITUENTS: *P. lactiflora* contains monoterpenoid glycosides (paeoniflorin, albiflorin, lactiflorin, benzoylpaeoniflorin, oxypaeoniflorin, and (Z)-(1S,5R)-β-pinen-10-yl-vivianoside), acetophenones (paeonol), phytosterols (5-sterols: β-sitosterol, β-sitosterol-α-glucoside), volatile oil (with benzoic acid), palmitic acid, *cis*-9,12-octadecadienoic acid, alkanes ($C_{24} - C_{26}$), daucosterol, tannins (gallotannins), methyl gallate, glucogallin, D-catechin, myoinositol, and carbohydrates (starch, sucrose, and water-soluble polysaccharides: paeonans).[11,15,16]

NUTRITIONAL PROPERTIES: None known.

MEDICINAL PROPERTIES: Analgesic, antiatherosclerotic, anticoagulant, anticonvulsant, antihyperglycemic, anti-inflammatory, antimutagenic, antioxidant, antispasmodic, liver decongestant, hepatoprotectant, nervine, sedative (mild), tranquilizer, uterine tonic, diuretic (mild), antifungal, antibacterial, antiviral, and antipyretic.

TEMPERATURE AND FLAVOR: Cool, sour, and bitter.

MEDICINAL USES

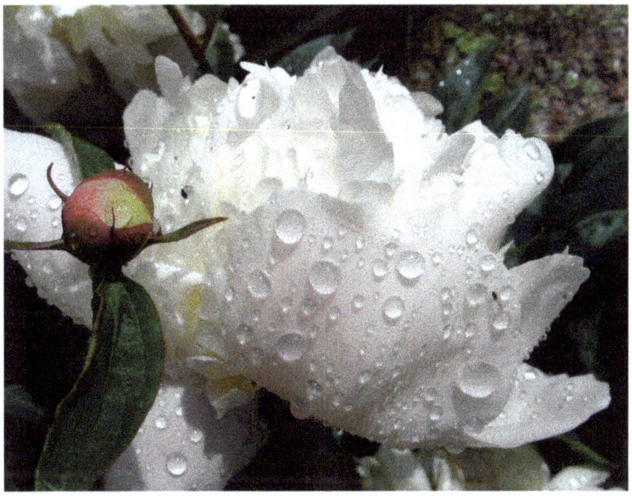

CHINESE WHITE PEONY ROOT (PAEONIA LACTIFLORA)

White peony root is highly beneficial for a variety of female reproductive concerns. It nourishes blood and restores menstruation in women with amenorrhea resulting from blood deficiency.[11,15,16] It is often combined with dong quai *(Angelica sinensis),* shu di huang *(Rehmannia glutinosa),* and chuan xiong *(Ligusticum striatum)* as a blood tonic.[11] White peony root also has uterine tonic actions, as well as antispasmodic and analgesic properties.[15,16,18] White peony (not red) can be used during pregnancy one to two months prior to the due date as a uterine tonic, blood tonic, partus preparator, and parturient. It is a long-term anti-inflammatory, analgesic, and uterine tonic for treating conditions that manifest with heat and pain, such as dysmenorrhea, endometriosis, ovarian cysts, uterine cysts, fibroids, and mittelschmerz.[10,15,16,18,21] White peony root reduces uterine bleeding from cysts or fibroids, and decreases excessive vaginal discharge due to leukorrhea.[10,11,18,21] The cooling attributes help to reduce night sweats and hot flashes.[11,15] White peony root also has benefits for male reproductive concerns, such as prostatic or testicular pain (orchitis, hydroceles, and prostatitis).[18,19,21]

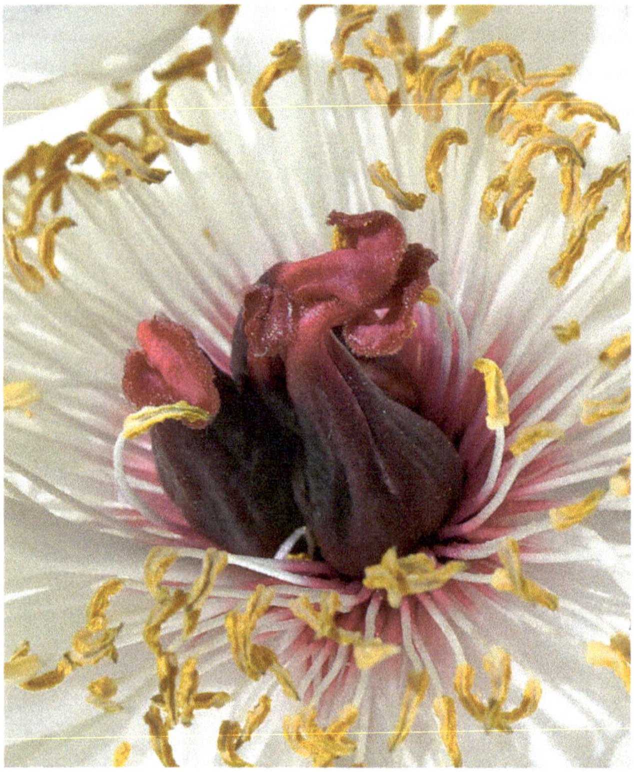

White peony root contains a number of actions beneficial for the gastrointestinal tract. The tea is helpful for decreasing excess gastric secretions, and may prevent gastric ulcers resulting from nervousness.[10] The root's antispasmodic actions are useful for treating cramping in the stomach and intestines, abdominal pain due to bloating, diarrhea, and dysentery.[10] It can be used to manage painful spasms accompanying irritable bowel syndrome, colitis, and Crohn's disease.[11] The antispasmodic actions are also useful for treating systremma and respiratory spasms, although the effects on the respiratory tract are mild.[10,11,20,21]

According to Traditional Chinese Medicine, white peony root "softens and comforts the liver," and is often used to reduce stagnation of liver qi, and curb liver yang.[11,15] The root treats constrained liver qi, which can cause pain and spasms in the chest, flank, abdomen, hands, or feet.[10,11,15] It is often combined with chai hu *(Bupleurum)* for this purpose.[11] White peony root is highly beneficial as a long-term tonic for women with premenstrual syndrome, breast tenderness, menstrual cramping, irregular menses, or night sweats.[10,15] According to Western herbal theory, many of these symptoms result from a combination of liver congestion and excess estrogen. The liver metabolizes estrogen. Excess estrogen strains the liver, compromising its filtration capacity due to the increased load. This results in liver stagnation, and when prolonged, can result in "liver heat." Thus, white peony root is also indicated for headaches, migraines, and dizziness resulting from liver yang rising (liver heat).[10,11,16] The subtle liver cooling actions are beneficial for recovery from hepatitis, jaundice, and skin conditions resulting from liver heat, such as hot, dry eczema.[16]

Peony has very gentle nervine and tranquilizing actions.[10] It is not a potent sedative, and can be consumed throughout the day by individuals prone to anxiety, irritability, and insomnia.[10] It also acts as a mild mood elevator for individuals with depression caused by liver stagnation (melancholia).[18,19] Peony has mild muscle relaxant actions, especially when a headache or muscle tension is present due to excess caffeine or chocolate consumption, physical activity, or stress.[21]

White peony root protects and preserves yin.[11] It alleviates night sweats, hot flashes, and spontaneous sweating due to yin deficiency.[11]

Research indicates that the glycosides in white peony root (especially paeoniflorin), also known as the total glucosides of peony (TGP), are responsible for many of the medicinal properties.[17] *In vitro* and *in vivo* experiments were completed with water- and ethanol-based extracts of *Paeonia lactiflora* root. For instance, the glycosides have antibacterial, antifungal, antiviral, anti-inflammatory and immune modulating properties, as well as analgesic, tranquilizing, sedative, and antispasmodic actions.[10,15,17] The glycosides also enhance phagocytosis of macrophages, reduce platelet aggregation, have antimutagenic and tumor inhibiting actions, elevate cyclic AMP levels, have antifatigue actions, and improve memory.[15,17]

The glycosides have numerous modes of actions for decreasing inflammation and modulating immune function. They decrease prostaglandin E2 (PGE2), leukotriene B4 (LTB4), inflammatory cytokines, and nitric oxide (NO), and suppress the increase of intercellular calcium levels in macrophages.[17] They protect cells from oxidative stress. The glycosides had an inhibitory effect in the delayed-type hypersensitivity in immuno-activated mice, and improved delayed-type hypersensitivity in immunosuppressed mice.[17] TGP showed promising effects in suppressing an overactivated immune response.[17] It had inhibitory effects on lymphocyte proliferation, balanced the differentiation between T-helper cells and T-suppressor cells, and stimulated apoptosis of lymphocytes.[17] The immune modulating effects can be beneficial for autoimmune conditions, such as rheumatoid arthritis, systemic lupus erythematosis, Sjögren syndrome, ankylosing spondylitis, and chronic urticaria.[17]

WESTERN PEONY (PAEONIA BROWNII, P. CALIFORNICA), EUROPEAN PEONY (P. OFFICINALIS)

P. brownii (western peony), *P. californica* (California peony), and *P. officinalis* (European peony) have smooth muscle antispasmodic actions on the uterus and bronchioles.[20,21] Consuming 20 – 60 drops of root extract is effective for treating acute menstrual cramps.[20] Some sources claim that it is a menstrual stimulant helpful for treating slow-starting, crampy menses.[20,21] This is similar to the use of wild varieties of red peony or chi shao *(P. lactiflora)* in Tradition Chinese Medicine, administered as "blood movers" for stagnant or delayed menstruation.[11] Western peony and California peony roots seem more energetic in their actions, with greater potential to stimulate the uterus than white peony. Western peony is beneficial for treating a dry, unproductive cough, although other herbs have been more effective.[21] It also possesses mild smooth muscle and skeletal muscle antispasmodic actions for muscular twitching.[20,21] According to herbalist Michael Moore, the root improves the quality of uterine mucosa and submucosa, increases endothelial muscle tone, and "cools" the uterine lining.[18]

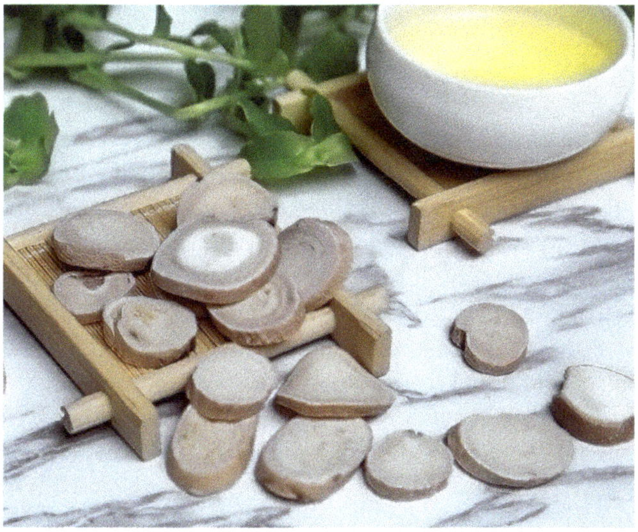

CONTRAINDICATIONS

White peony root should be avoided in individuals with diarrhea resulting from cold due to deficiency.[11] Some sources caution against combining peony root with shi hu *(Dendrobium)*, mang xiao *(Mirabilitum)*, bie jia *(Amyda sinensis)*, xiao ji *(Cephalanoplos segeti)*, and li lu *(Veratrum)*.[11] Due to the potential inhibition of platelet aggregation, it should be avoided two weeks before and after surgery, and in individuals consuming warfarin (Coumadin) or other potent blood thinners.[19]

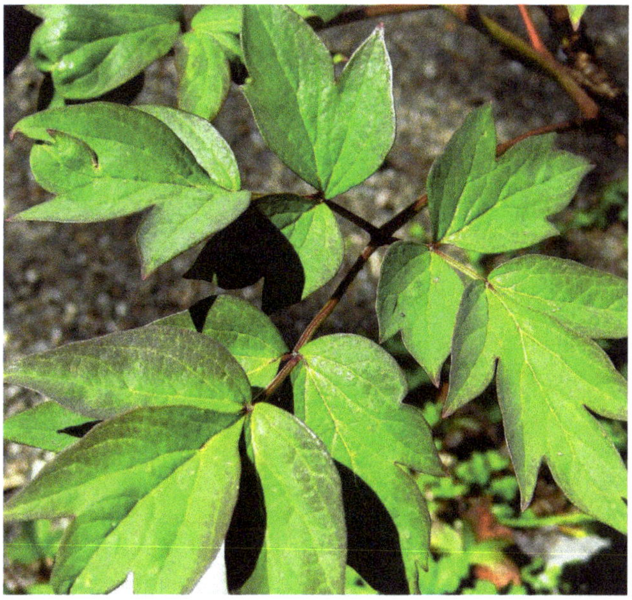

Western peony *(P. brownii)*, California peony *(P. californica)*, European peony *(P. officinalis)*, Chinese red peony *(P. lactiflora)*, and wild peony *(P. officinalis, P. brownii, P. californica*, and *P. veitchii)* should be avoided during pregnancy, based on the potential blood moving and emmenagogue effects.[16,19,20,21] However, the white peony form of *P. lactiflora* is not contraindicated during pregnancy in any Chinese materia medica references.[11]

PREPARATION AND DOSAGE

TINCTURE: Fresh roots [1:2, 70 - 95% alcohol]; dry roots [1:5, 60% alcohol]; consume 10 - 30 drops for tonic use, or 30 - 60 drops as an antispasmodic, up to four times daily.

CAPSULES: Consume 2 - 4 "00" capsules, up to three times daily.

TEA: Prepare a decoction; consume 8 - 12 ounces, three to four times daily.

CULINARY USE: Place 4 - 8 roots in a muslin bag, and cook in soup stock. Remove before serving.

ROOT PREPARATION: To prepare the root after harvesting, place in hot water until the interior is no longer white, or until slightly sticky and fragrant. The root bark is removed after boiling. Dry in the sun for one day, pile in heaps to sweat until root is dry, then slice.

PLANTAIN

DESCRIPTION

BOTANICAL NAMES:
Plantago major, P. lanceolata

COMMON NAMES:
Plantain, broadleaf plantain, narrow leaf plantain, English plantain, common plantain, ripple grass, waybread, slan-lus, snake weed, snake plantain, snakebite, cuckoo's bread, Englishman's foot, white man's foot, ribwort plantain, ribwort, black plantain, long plantain, ripple grass, ribwort, black jack, quinquenervia, jackstraw, lamb's tongue, hen plant, buckhorn
piharatamo (Finnish)
breitwegerich, wegbreit (German)
plantaggine (Italian)
shazenshi (Japanese)
ch'ajônja (Korean)
che qían zi (Mandarin)
lahuriya (Sanskrit)
groblad (Swedish)

FAMILY NAME:
Plantaginaceae

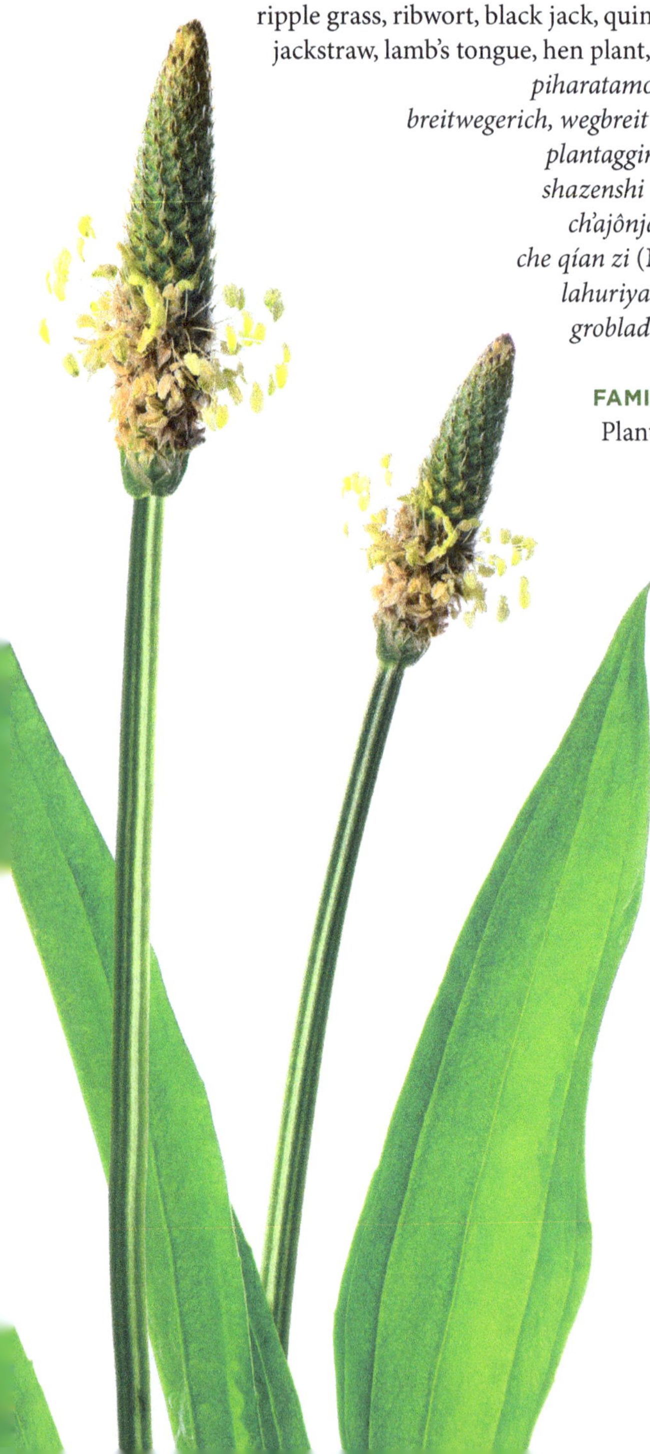

PART USED: The leaves.

BOTANICAL DESCRIPTION AND HABITAT: Plantain is a weedy annual or perennial growing worldwide. It can be found in grassy lawns or meadows, gardens, edges of farms, sidewalk cracks, roadsides, pathways, trails, and

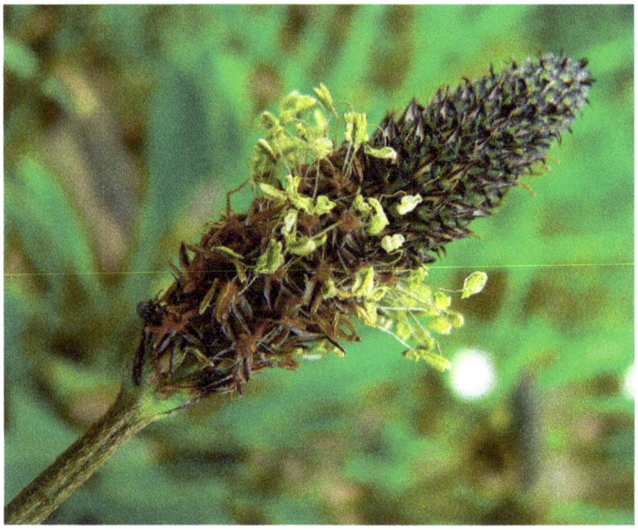

abandoned urban lots. *P. major* has fibrous roots; *P. lanceolata* has a long taproot.[1,2] Both species have basal rosettes of simple, sturdy, fibrous leaves with prominent parallel veins. *P. major* has ovate, mostly glabrous leaves (5 – 18 cm long) with wavy and sometimes finely dentate margins. *P. lanceolata* has narrowly lanceolate, sometimes pubescent leaves (5 – 25 cm long) with flat, finely dentate margins.[2-4] The inflorescence is a dense spike of many tiny flowers on a long peduncle (5 – 60 cm long in *P. major;* 20 – 80 cm long in *P. lanceolata;* both measurements include the peduncle).[3,4] A four-lobed calyx and four-lobed salverform corolla comprise the perianth of the flowers.[5,6] Within the flower are four stamens and a superior ovary that matures into a dry, circumscissile capsule.[5,6]

THE NAME: The common name plantain derives from the Latin *Plantago* — a derivative of the Latin *planta* ("sole of the foot").[5,7] As with other ubiquitous plants with universally esteemed, yet gentle medicinal qualities, plantain has many common names. *Costa canina* refers to the rib-like, parallel mid-veins *(costa* is Latin for "rib"*)*, as do the names ribwort and the medieval name quinquinervia.[8] The name kemps derives from the Anglo-Saxon word for soldier *("cempa")*. This refers to a game in rural England, in which children played with the long, sword-like inflorescences until they broke.[8] Englishman's foot and white man's foot allude to the plant's weedy nature, and how seeds were carried with European colonists who introduced the plant to the American continent.[8] It continues to be called *slan-lus* ("plant of healing") in the Scottish Highlands.[8] It acquired the name snake weed, snakebite, and snake plantain in the U.S. because it was used to treat venomous bites.[8]

The following common names correspond with the Latin binomials: English plantain, narrow leaf plantain, buckhorn, black plantain, long plantain, ribble grass, ribwort, black jack, jackstraw, lamb's tongue, snake plantain, quinquenervia, hen plant, cocks, wendles, kemps, costa canina *(Plantago lanceolata);* and common plantain, broadleaf plantain, ripple grass, waybread, waybroad, snakeweed, cuckoo's bread, Englishman's foot, white man's foot, slan-lus *(Plantago major).*[8]

HISTORICAL USES: The Saxons highly regarded plantain (known as weybroed), deeming it one of the nine most sacred herbs.[8] It was included in an Anglo-Saxon salve to treat irritation from flying ointment.[8] Plantain was used to treat bleeding in the lungs (consumption) and dysentery.[8] Plantain tea or juice mixed with lemon juice was considered an effective diuretic for treating kidney disorders.[8] Up to one quart of the infusion was consumed throughout the day to ease diarrhea and bleeding hemorrhoids.[8] The fresh leaves were consumed as a salad or pot herb.

Plantain poultices were considered effective for treating venomous snakebites and rabid dog bites.[8] Fresh bruised leaves were applied to insect bites, rashes, burns, and abrasions, and to staunch bleeding wounds.[8] A poultice was applied to ease toothache pain.[8] Due to their demulcent quality, plantain seeds were decocted or prepared as syrup to treat coughing.[8] Seed tea was used to stiffen muslin and woven fabrics.[8]

CONSTITUENTS: Plantain contains iridoid glycosides (aucubin = aucubingenin-glucoside and catalpol), tannins, mucilaginous polysaccharides, phenylethanoid glycosides (verbascoside), flavonoids (flavones), phenolic acids (caffeic acid derivatives), plant acids (oleanic, benzoic, fumaric, chlorogenic, and protocatechuic), minerals, saponins, and coumarins.[9,10]

NUTRITIONAL PROPERTIES: Plantain contains high amounts of calcium, protein, crude and dietary fiber, and fat. It contains low to average amounts of ash, chromium, iron, magnesium, manganese, niacin, phosphorus, potassium, selenium, silicon, sodium, and zinc.[11]

MEDICINAL PROPERTIES: Anti-inflammatory, astringent, demulcent, depurative, diuretic (mild), emollient, expectorant (mild), and vulnerary.

TEMPERATURE AND FLAVOR: Cool, astringent, and bitter.

MEDICINAL USES

Plantain is a soothing astringent and subtle demulcent that reduces inflammation in mucous membranes. When it grows near water, it has a higher mucilage content; when it grows in dry, disturbed soil, it has a higher tannin content.[10] Gargling with plantain tea or juice relieves a sore throat or ulcerated mouth. Ingesting the tea or fresh juice aids in treating gastric and duodenal ulcers, and diarrhea.[10] In order to soothe the digestive tract, prepare an infusion containing peppermint *(Mentha piperita)*, chamomile *(Matricaria)*, fennel *(Foeniculum)*, and smaller amounts of meadowsweet *(Filipendula)*, plantain, calendula *(Calendula)*, and a pinch of licorice.

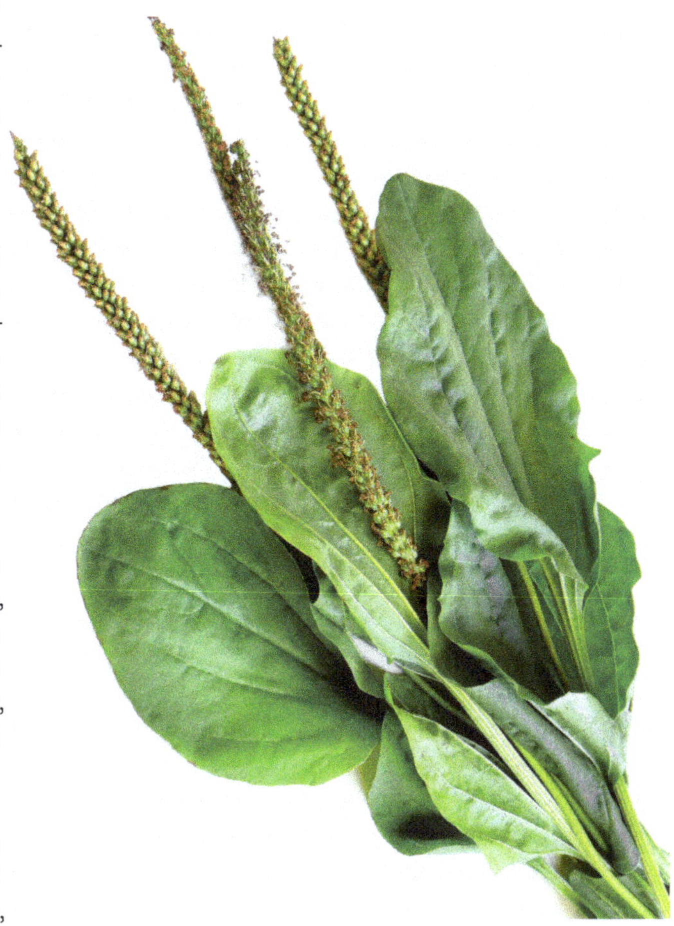

Plantain is a subtle hemostatic that reduces passive bleeding in mucous membranes of the digestive and respiratory tracts. Prepare a hemostatic tea by combining yarrow *(Achillea)*, cinnamon *(Cinnamomum)*, comfrey *(Symphytum)*, plantain, and rose *(Rosa)* or Lady's mantle *(Alchemilla)*.

Rinsing the eyes with well strained, cooled plantain tea reduces inflammation. Combine plantain with chamomile *(Matricaria)* and calendula *(Calendula)* to soothe tired or inflamed eyes. Apply a fresh plant poultice directly to the gums or jaw to relieve a toothache or gum abscess. Add yarrow and/or chamomile to a plantain poultice to ease gum pain.

A poultice prepared from fresh, minced leaves is a very effective drawing agent. Apply the poultice for insect bites (wasp, spider, or mosquito), bee stings, or nettle stings, or to reduce residual inflammation from snakebites.[8-10] The fresh poultice is also effective for drawing splinters, abscesses, boils, zits, and acne, and for easing mastitis pain. Additional anti-infective agents are necessary for treating abscesses and mastitis. Prepare a drawing poultice by blending fresh plantain leaves with ample amounts of clay, enough distilled water to create a thick paste, and several drops of lavender and blue chamomile essential oil. Apply ample amounts to the affected area, wrap with a bandage, and leave in place 15–30 minutes.

A topical vulnerary, astringent, styptic, and emollient, fresh plantain can be applied to soothe cuts, abrasions, ulcers, diaper rash, sunburn, poison oak, poison ivy, dermatitis, eczema, psoriasis, and hemorrhoids.[8-10] Combine fresh plantain and chickweed *(Stellaria)* for the aforementioned conditions. The vulnerary and anti-inflammatory effects are due to the tannins.[9] Plantain has mild antibacterial and moderate antibiofilm effects, although it should not be used as the sole anti-infective agent.[9,12] It contains luteolin and apigenin, known as multiple drug resistant efflux pump inhibitors. They help to prevent bacteria from transporting harmful substances out of their cells. As these bacterial efflux pumps are a critical tool by which bacteria develop antibiotic resistance, inhibiting the efflux pumps with herbs like plantain allows other antimicrobials to be more effective against bacteria.[12] The aucubigenin in plantain contributes to its antimicrobial action, but the plant must be used fresh, as aucubigenin is destroyed by heat.[9] The synergism of plantain's local anti-inflammatory, vulnerary, antiseptic, and immune stimulating qualities contribute to its efficacy in disrupting chronic, pathogenic biofilm infections.[12]

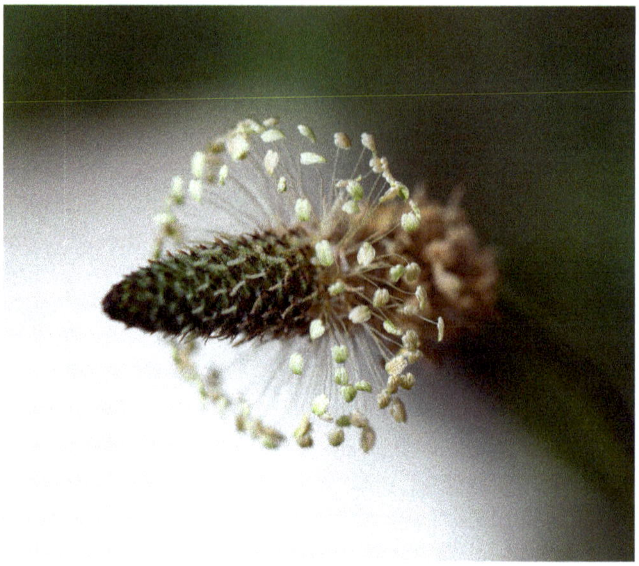

CONTRAINDICATIONS

There are no known contraindications.

PREPARATION AND DOSAGE

TINCTURE: Fresh leaves [1:2–1:3, 70–95% alcohol]; consume 30–90 drops, up to three times daily.

SUCCUS: Consume 1–2 tablespoons of fresh or frozen juice, up to four times daily. Or apply frozen juice topically to soothe inflamed skin conditions.

TEA: Prepare a hot infusion; consume 8–12 ounces, three to four times daily.

TOPICAL USE: Prepare infused oil with recently dried leaves using the alcohol intermediary method, or prepare oil with fresh, wilted leaves using the double boiler method. Apply oil or salve to the affected area. Prepare a fresh leaf poultice or fomentation, and apply to the affected area.

CULINARY USE: Small amounts of young tender leaves may be added to soup or salad in the spring. They become more astringent with age.

PRICKLY ASH

BOTANICAL NAMES:
Zanthoxylum americanum (syn. *Xanthoxylum americanum*), *Z. clava-herculis* (syn. *Z. clavus-herculis, Z. macrophyllum*)

COMMON NAMES:
Prickly ash, northern prickly ash, southern prickly ash, toothache tree, toothache bark, sutterberry, Hercules' club, angelica tree, pepper wood, yellow wood, prickly yellow wood
clavalier d'Amerique, frene epineux (French)
Amerikanische, stachelesche, gebholz, zahnwehholz (German)
tambura (Sanskrit)
Amerikanskt peppartrád (Swedish)

FAMILY NAME:
Rutaceae

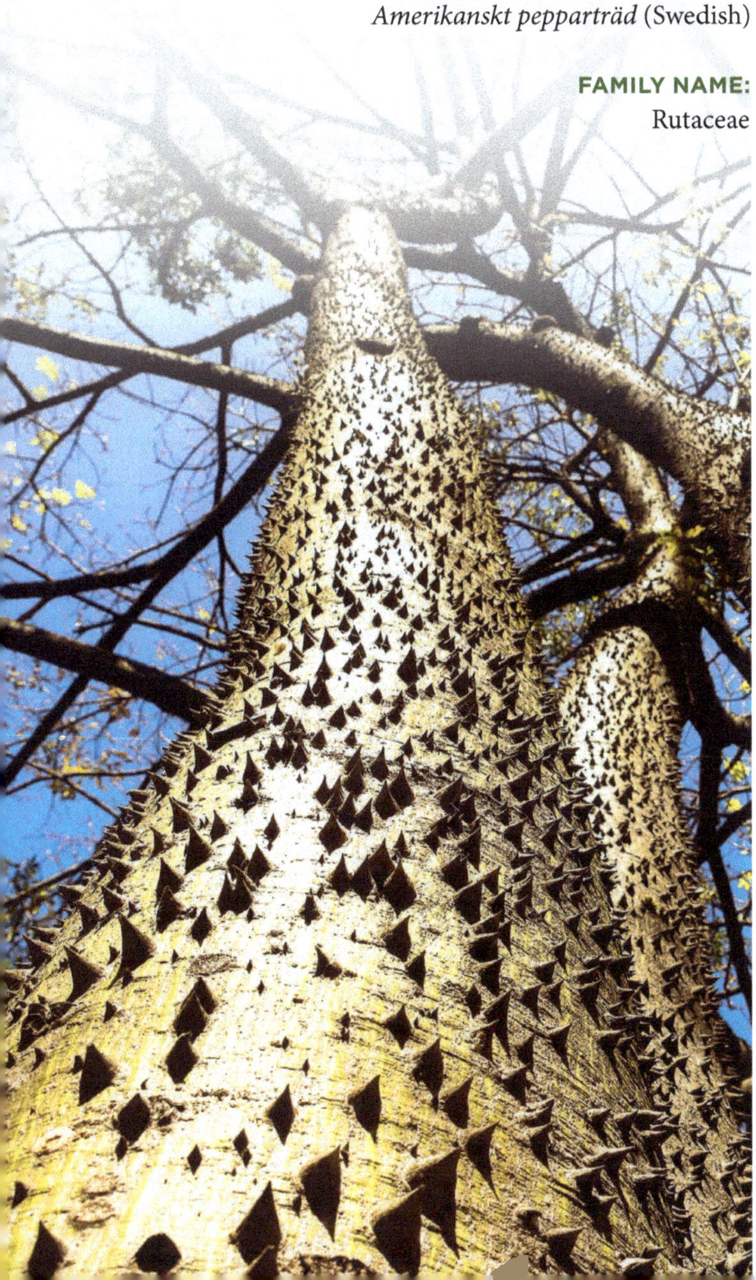

DESCRIPTION

PARTS USED: The bark, berries, and root bark (less common).

BOTANICAL DESCRIPTION AND HABITAT: Northern prickly ash *(Z. americanum)* grows in North America, from Quebec to Mississippi, and west to Oklahoma. It is found in moist valleys, low-lying river areas, bluffs, rocky hillsides, and open forests.[1] Southern prickly ash *(Z. clava-herculis)* grows in the South, from southern Virginia to Florida, and west to Texas.

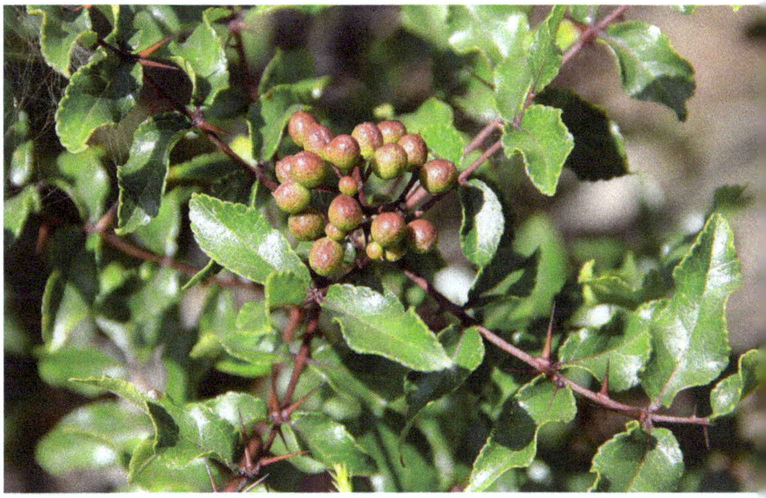

Imbued with a citrusy aroma, northern prickly ash is a thicket-forming, dioecious shrub (3 – 6 m tall).[2] The pale brown stem-bark is smooth; the twigs are pubescent and deep red.[2] Pairs of short, sharp spines (5 – 15 mm long) cover the branch and trunk surfaces.[2] Alternating up the stem, the pinnately compound leaves have 5 – 11 leaflets (2 – 8 cm long by 1 – 4 cm wide) that are elliptic to oblong, with somewhat oblique bases, obtuse apices, and crenate to entire margins.[2] The upper surface is dark green; the underside is paler green.

The small, yellowish-green flowers bloom before the leaves break bud in the spring, and are found in auxiliary cymes on older branches.[1,2] The flowers lack calyces. The male flower has five exserted stamens and a vestigial carpel. The female flower has three to five pistils and minute vestigial staminodes.[2] The female flower produces a deep brown, globose follicle (4 – 5 mm long) with one to two black seeds.[1,2]

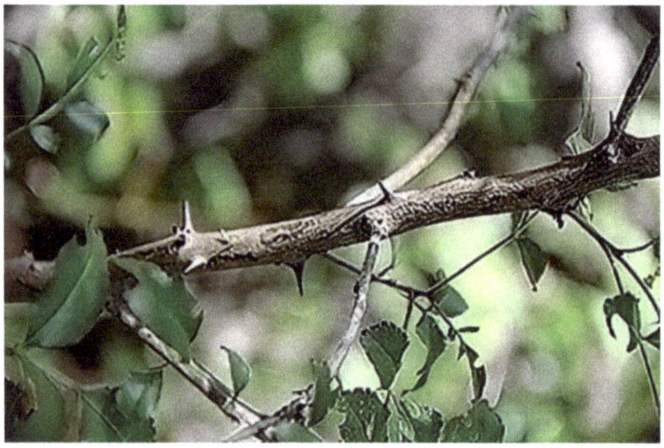

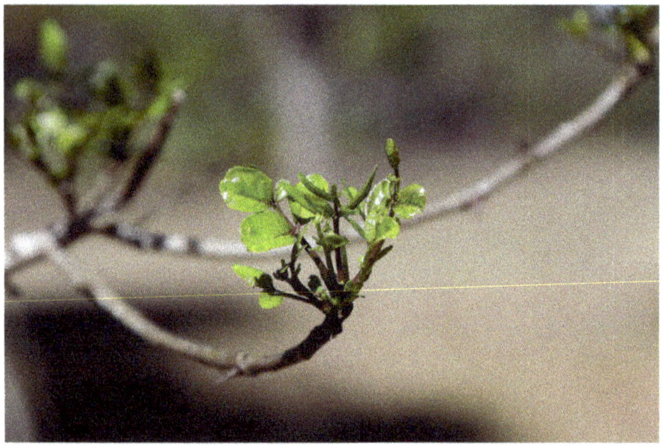

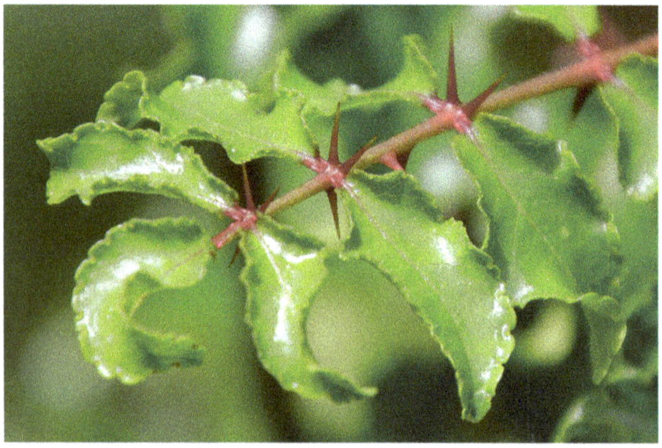

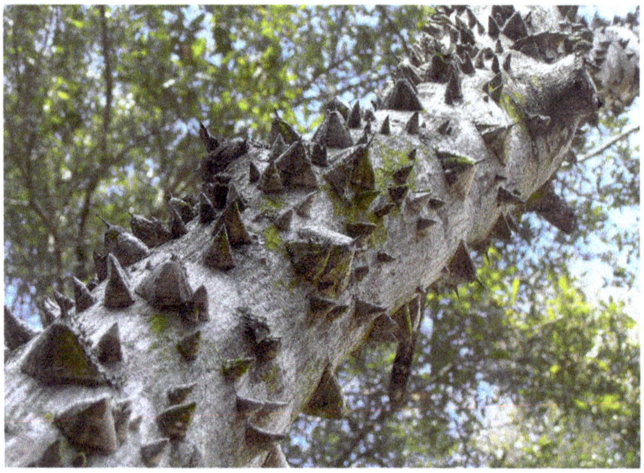

Southern prickly ash *(Z. clava-herculis)* is similar to the northern species described above, except for a few characteristics. Southern prickly ash is less shrubby, taller, and more tree-like, growing up to 10 m tall.[3] The spines on the bark also differ, as they are surrounded by pyramidal, corky warts.[4] The leaves are divided into numerous leaflets (7 – 17) with a narrower ovate shape, and an acute apex that has wavier margins.[3] The flowers grow in larger, showier clusters at axils and the ends of branches.[3]

THE NAME: *Zanthoxylum* derives from two Greek words: *xanthos* ("yellow") and *xylum* ("wood").[5] The epithet *americanum* indicates its origin in North America. The epithet *clava-herculis* translates as "Hercules' club."[5] The common names of *Z. americanum* include northern prickly ash, angelica tree, pepper wood, toothache tree, and yellow wood. The common names of *Z. clava-herculis* include southern prickly ash, sea ash, Hercules' club, prickly yellow wood, and toothache tree. Prickly ash refers to the prickly spines on the bark and stem.

HISTORICAL USES: Prickly ash was administered by Eclectic physicians to treat muscle pain, lower back pain, and chronic rheumatism.[6-9] Because it increases salivary, stomach, intestinal, pancreatic, and hepatic secretions, low doses (5 – 15 drops) were recommended for atonic dyspepsia, belching, flatulence, catarrhal gastritis, and constipation.[6-9] Prickly ash was given to restore digestive tone and secretions, and as an antispasmodic to patients convalescing from dysentery or Asiatic cholera.[6-8] Based on Dr. John King's recommendation, it was often compounded with goldenseal *(Hydrastis)*, and sometimes cayenne *(Capsicum)* as a restorative agent following a debilitating fever, diarrhea, dysentery, or cholera. This remedy was consumed one hour before and after meals.[7-9] Although the berries and bark were used interchangeably, the berries were considered a more potent carminative and antispasmodic. The bark was preferred as a tonic, stimulant, diaphoretic, sialagogue, and alterative.[6,7,10]

Prickly ash was prescribed as a stimulant for the heart, circulation, and sluggish mucous membranes.[7-9,11] Larger doses (20 – 60 drops) were recommended as a nervous system stimulant.[7,8] Prickly ash was widely utilized as an alterative to treat conditions such as scrofula, chronic skin disorders, and "disordered" blood.[7,8] As an alterative, it was typically combined with pink root *(Stillingia)*, yellow dock *(Rumex)*, poke root *(Phytolacca)*, and potassium iodide or acetate to treat torpid conditions.[6,8] Due to the diuretic properties, it was recommended for dropsy.[6,7,9]

A poultice of ground bark was applied to treat toothaches, tongue paralysis, paralytic afflictions, and nervous headaches.[6,7,9,10] Poultices or fomentations also were applied to reduce uterine cramping and neuralgia.[7] Prickly ash was considered a panacea by North American Indians.[12] At least 12 tribes used prickly ash to treat colds, coughs, fevers, and toothaches.[12]

CONSTITUENTS: Northern prickly ash bark contains coumarin (xanthyletin, xanthoxyletin, and alloxanthoxyletin), alkaloids (laurifoline, nitidine, chelerythrine, tembetarine, magnoflorine, and candicine), resins, tannins, and an acrid volatile oil (3 – 4%). The root bark also contains a coumarin (8-(3,3-dimethylallyl)-alloxanthoxyletin), and the leaves contain two furoquinoline alkaloids (γ-fagarine and skimmianine).[10,11,13]

Southern prickly ash bark contains benzophenathridine alkaloids (laurifoline, magnofoline, tembetarine, and candicine). The stem bark contains chelerythrine, nitidine, tembetarine, pungent principles including amides (herculin, neoherculin, and a cinnamamide), pluviatilol γ, γ-dimethylallyl ether, η-acetylanonaine, lignans (asarinin and sesamin), tannins, resins, and an acrid volatile oil (3 – 4%).[10,11,13]

NUTRITIONAL PROPERTIES: Not applicable.

MEDICINAL PROPERTIES: Alterative, antimicrobial, astringent, bitter tonic, carminative, carrier, circulatory stimulant, cholagogue, choleretic, diaphoretic, diuretic, lymphatic, pelvic decongestant, sialagogue, vasodilator, counterirritant, rubefacient, anodyne, and local anesthetic.

TEMPERATURE AND FLAVOR: Hot, bitter, acrid, astringent, and salty.

MEDICINAL USES

Prickly ash is a sialagogue, digestive bitter tonic, choleretic, cholagogue, and carminative.[6,7,9,14] It stimulates upper digestive function, increasing salivary, mucus, and hydrochloric acid secretions.[7,9,14] Prickly ash also stimulates pancreatic, hepatic, and gallbladder secretions.[6,7,9,14] It enhances hepatic function and metabolism.[6,7,9,14] Consume up to one-half hour before meals to improve the digestion of fats, proteins, and carbohydrates.[7,14] Because prickly ash facilitates fat digestion, it decongests the lacteals (lymphatic tissue that absorbs fat in the small intestinal microvilli).[14] It is beneficial for sluggish, torpid, phlegmatic (cool and damp) conditions in the digestive tract.[6,7] Prickly ash aids in treating belching, colic, flatulence, atonic dyspepsia, constipation, chronic diarrhea, and stomach and bowel spasms.[6-8,10]

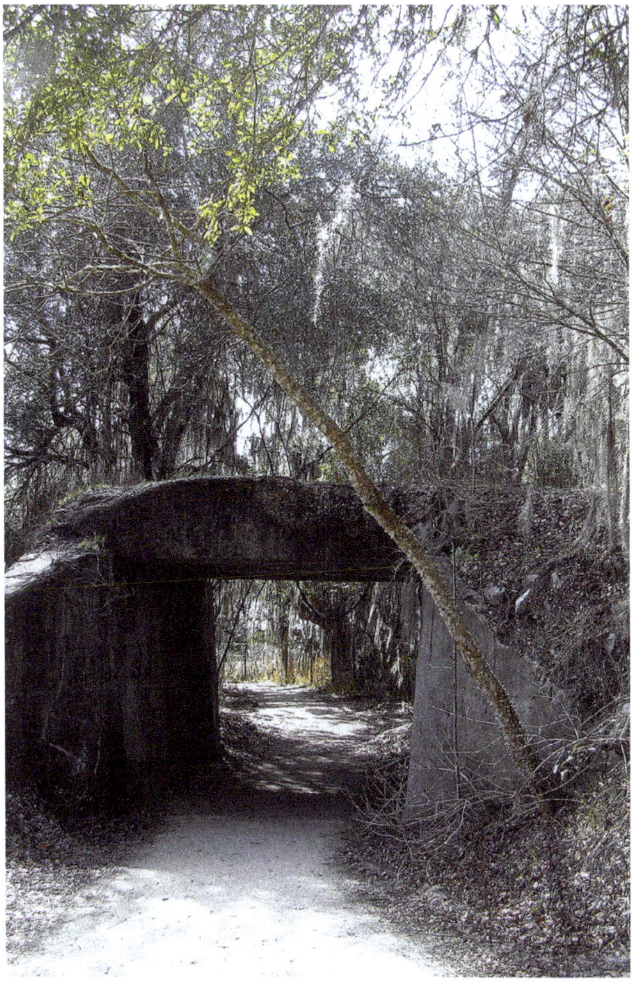

Prickly ash is a vasodilator, circulatory stimulant, energizing stimulant, and carrier.[7-10] It has a tonic effect on the heart, and improves overall microcirculation.[8,10] Internal and topical applications (hand and foot baths) are beneficial for treating Raynaud's phenomenon and intermittent claudication.[13,15] Prickly ash increases cerebral blood flow, oxygenating the brain and supporting individuals with Alzheimer's disease and global dementia (especially in the early stages). It also reduces portal congestion, treating varicose veins, spider veins, and hemorrhoids.[14] Because it reduces blood stasis and congestion, it hastens the healing of bruises and pain due to sluggish circulation.[8]

A hot infusion of prickly ash has warming expectorant and heating diaphoretic actions.[6,9,10,13] It aids in treating a cold or flu accompanied by thick, clear, or cloudy, congested mucus. Gargling with prickly ash tea or extract anesthetizes a sore throat, and aids in treating chronic laryngitis and pharyngitis.[7,8,13]

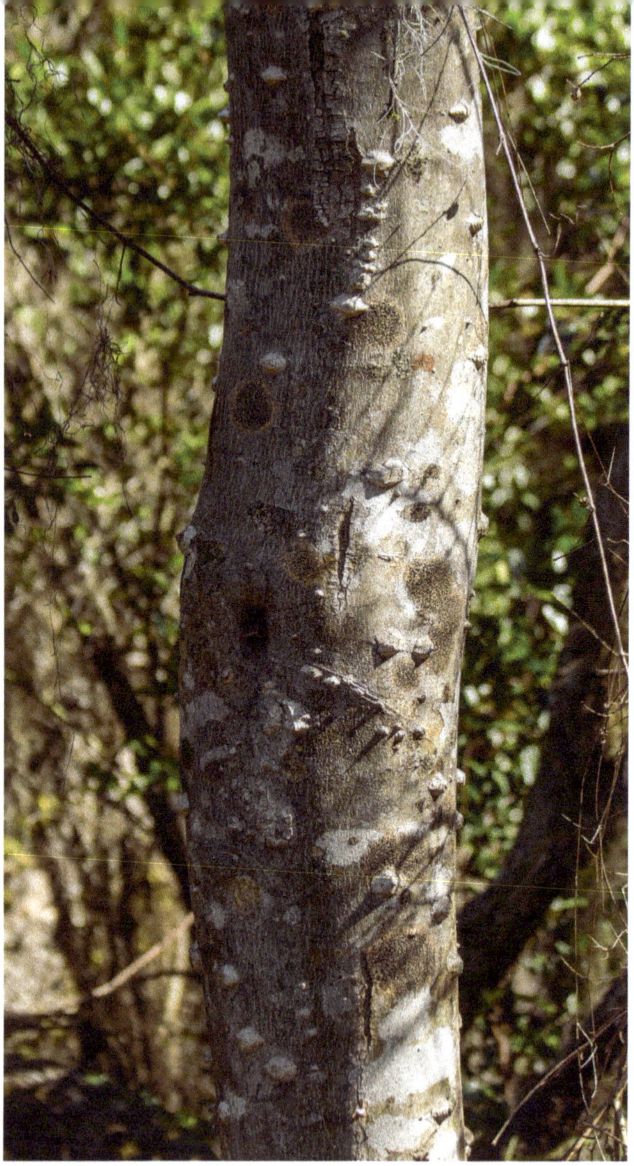

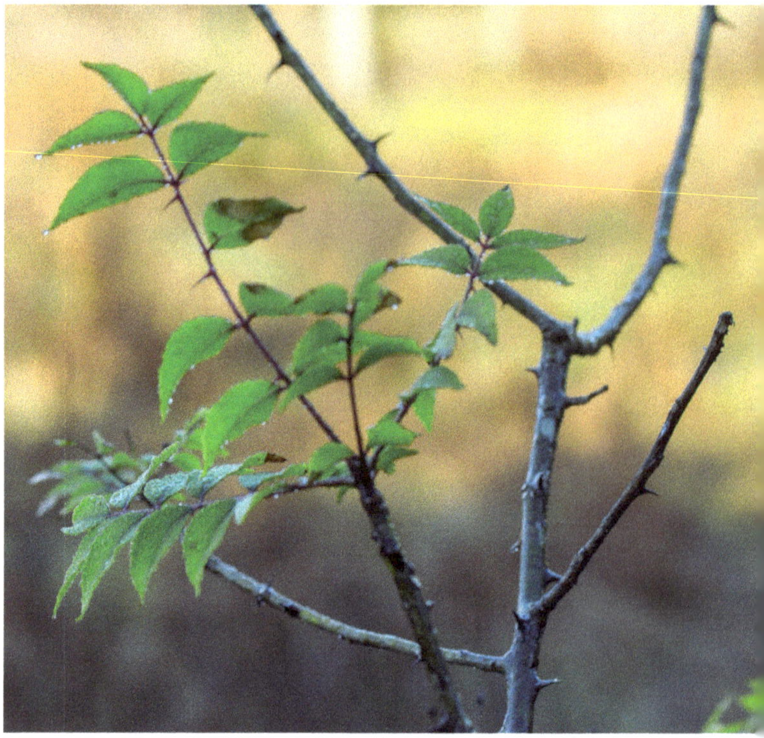

CONTRAINDICATIONS

Avoid internal use of both species during pregnancy. Southern prickly ash is contraindicated during pregnancy and lactation because it contains pungent amides.[13] Avoid use with acute stomach or intestine inflammation. Discontinue use if it causes acid indigestion, hot flashes, or night sweats. There is no known toxicity.

Prickly ash is a counterirritant, rubefacient, and numbing agent that decreases chronic muscle and nerve pain internally and locally.[6,7,13] It aids in treating myalgia, lumbago, tendonitis, and neuralgia.[6,7,9,10,13] Apply prickly ash tea, poultice, liniment, or salve as a counterirritant for sore muscles or joints, carpel tunnel, bruises, varicose veins, spider veins, or chronic rheumatism.[6-11,13,14] Apply powdered bark as a poultice to stimulate the healing of indolent ulcers and slow-healing wounds.[6,10,13] It contains herculin, an alkylamide with a local anesthetizing effect.[15]

Apply powdered bark as a poultice, or diluted extract to anesthetize the gums, reducing a toothache and teething pain.[6,7,9,11,13] Gargling with the diluted extract improves circulation to the gums, treating weak or bleeding gums, as well as gingivitis.

Prickly ash contains several constituents that poison fish, including asarinin, sesamin, neoherculin, pluviatilol γ,γ-dimethylallyl ether, and N-acetylanonanaine.[11]

PREPARATION AND DOSAGE

TINCTURE: Fresh bark or berries [1:2, 80–95% alcohol]; dry bark [1:5, 70% alcohol]; consume 5–30 drops before meals, up to three times daily.

CAPSULES: Consume 1–2 capsules, one to three times daily.

TEA: Prepare a decoction of bark or berries; consume 4–8 ounces, one to three times daily. Prepare a hot infusion of berries, and consume 4–8 ounces, one to three times daily.

TOPICAL USE: Prepare an oil or salve with the alcohol intermediary method. Apply diluted tincture, liniment, poultice, oil, or salve to the affected area.

PROPOLIS

DESCRIPTION

BOTANICAL NAME:
Propolis

COMMON NAMES:
Propolis, bee hive resin, bee glue, hive dross
propolisio (Esperanto)
kittivaha (Finnish)
cire de propolis, propolis d'abeille, résine de propolis (French)
tzori (Hebrew)
méhszurok (Hungarian)
propoli (Italian)
propolim (Latin)
pierzga (Polish)
própolis (Portuguese)
pénicilline Russe (Russian)
propóleos (Spanish)
keo ong (Vietnamese)

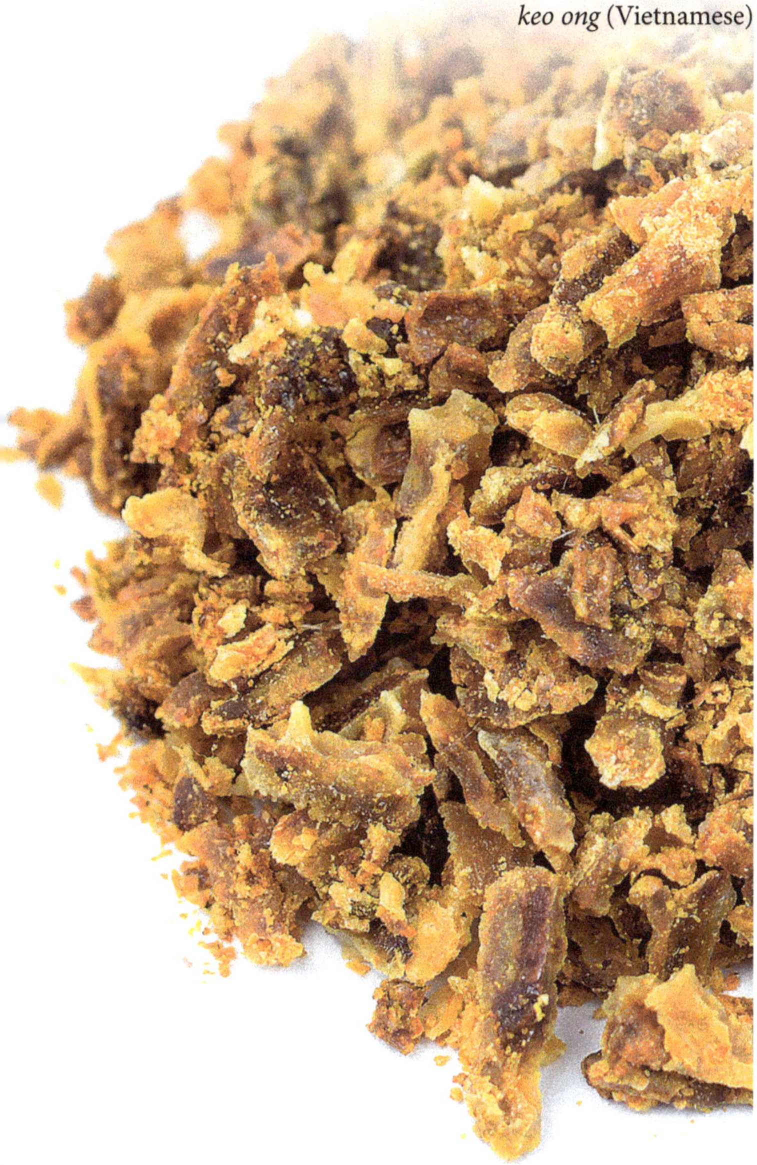

PART USED: Bee hive resin.

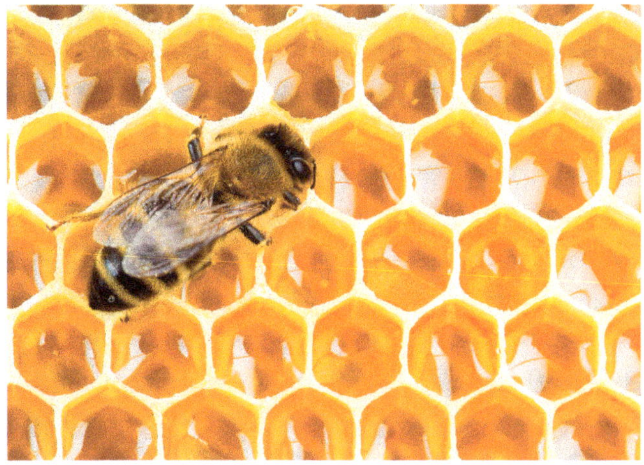

BOTANICAL DESCRIPTION AND HABITAT: Propolis is an orange to reddish-brown resinous material collected by honey bees *(Apis* spp.*)* from the viscid buds of a variety of trees, especially conifers and poplars, as well as ash, cherry, willow, birch, and alders. Bees use it to seal cracks and gaps in their hives, reduce the size of the hive entrance, prevent parasitic, fungal, or bacterial infections, prevent cold air from entering, and strengthen cells. Propolis also is used by guard bees to entomb hive trespassers.

THE NAME: Propolis derives from two Greek words: *pro* ("before or in front of") and *polis* ("a town with walls").[1]

HISTORICAL USES: Propolis was used by ancient Greeks and Romans as a topical application for bruises, ulcers, and sores.[2] The Hebrew word for propolis, *tzori*, is mentioned in the Old Testament for its therapeutic properties.[2] As early as the 12th century, propolis was administered to treat mouth and throat infections, as well as dental cavities.[2] Propolis was an official drug in the pharmacopeias of London until the 17th century.[3]

CONSTITUENTS: Propolis is comprised of 55% resinous compounds and balsams, 30% beeswax, 10% volatile oil, and 5% bee pollen.[2] It contains flavonoids (pinocembrin, pinostrobin, pinobanksin, galangin, kaempferol, quercetin, and pinobanksin-3-acetate), cinnamic acid, cinnamic alcohol, vanillin, benzyl alcohol, benzoic acid, benzyl ester, *p*-coumaric acid, caffeic acid, protein, amino acids, and vitamins (see below).[2,3] *Note:* The chemical composition of propolis varies according to the plant sources from which it is collected by honey bees.

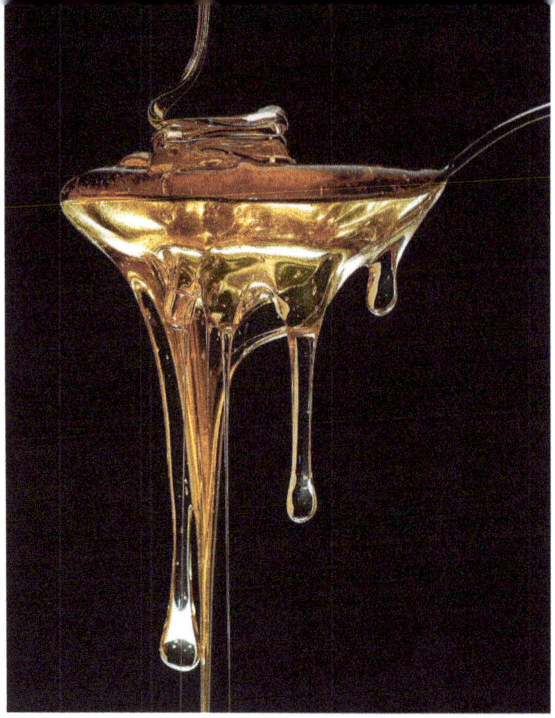

NUTRITIONAL PROPERTIES: Propolis contains small amounts of proteins, amino acids, minerals, and sugars, as well as vitamins A, B_1, B_2, B_6, C, and E.[2] The small quantities of these nutrients have insignificant nutritional value.[2]

MEDICINAL PROPERTIES: Antibacterial, antifungal, anti-inflammatory, antimicrobial, antitussive, antiviral, expectorant, immune stimulant, local anesthetic, lymphatic, counter irritant, and vulnerary.

TEMPERATURE AND FLAVOR: Warm, sweet, pungent, and bitter.

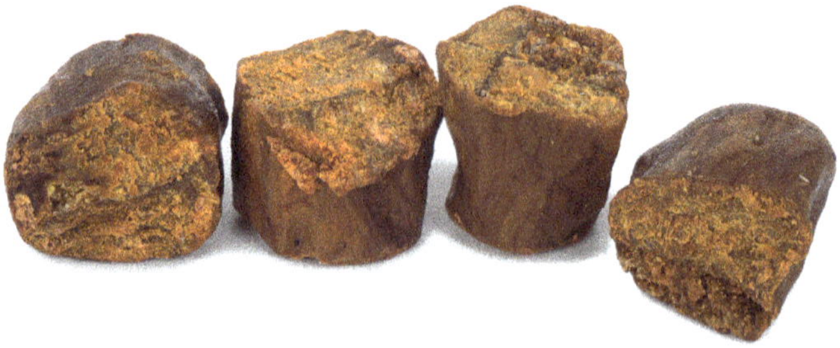

MEDICINAL USES

Propolis extract has potent antiviral, antibacterial, and antifungal properties.[2-4] It also increases phagocytosis, stimulating an immune response.[2,4,5] Propolis reduces lymphatic swelling, and anesthetizes mucous membranes in the throat, reducing pain and irritation.[4,5] It is highly effective for treating a sore, scratchy throat, laryngitis, pharyngitis, strep throat, a cold or flu, herpes, and mononucleosis.[2,4-6] The antiviral effects are attributed to the caffeic acid, luteolin, and quercetin.[2] Pinocembrin, galangin, caffeic acid, and ferulic acid have antibacterial actions.[2] Pinocembrin, pinbanksin, caffeic acid, benzyester, sakuranetin, and pterostilbene are attributed to the antifungal effects.[2] Consume 30 – 90 drops of the extract, gargle with the diluted extract, or apply a throat spray. Combine propolis with echinacea *(Echinacea)*, spilanthes *(Acmella)*, elder berry *(Sambucus)*, red root *(Ceanothus)*, and/or licorice *(Glycyrrhiza)* for the aforementioned conditions.

Propolis is an expectorant and antitussive.[2,4,5] Combined with other aromatic expectorants and antimicrobials, it is an adjunct for treating sinusitis and lower respiratory conditions, such as asthma, bronchitis, and pneumonia.[2,4,5] Propolis inhibits inflammatory prostaglandins that trigger bronchial spasms.[2] Combine propolis with yerba santa *(Eriodictyon)*, yerba mansa *(Anemopsis)*, bayberry *(Morella)*, and/or oshá *(Ligusticum)* to reduce profuse mucus secretions in upper or lower respiratory conditions. For spasmodic conditions of the lungs, such as asthma or a dry cough, combine propolis with thyme *(Thymus)*, anise *(Pimpinella)*, gumweed *(Grindelia)*, and licorice *(Glycyrrhiza)*.

Propolis has antibacterial actions helpful in treating *Helicobacter pylori* infections that cause gastric and duodenal ulcers.[2,6] It also stimulates epithelial regeneration, and hastens the healing of gastric tissues.[2,6] Propolis has antiseptic actions in the gastrointestinal tract, and aids in treating diarrhea resulting from *Giardia* infections, irritable bowel syndrome, and diverticulosis.[2,6] Combine with anti-inflammatory, antispasmodic, and vulnerary herbs such as calendula *(Calendula)*, chamomile *(Matricaria)*, licorice (*Glycyrrhiza*), and meadowsweet *(Filipendula)* to treat ulcers and digestive inflammation. *In vitro* studies also demonstrate that propolis inhibits protozoa growth.[2,3]

Propolis is a topical antimicrobial and anesthetic that alleviates teething and gum pain. It hastens the healing of canker sores and mouth ulcers.[6] Propolis protects mucous

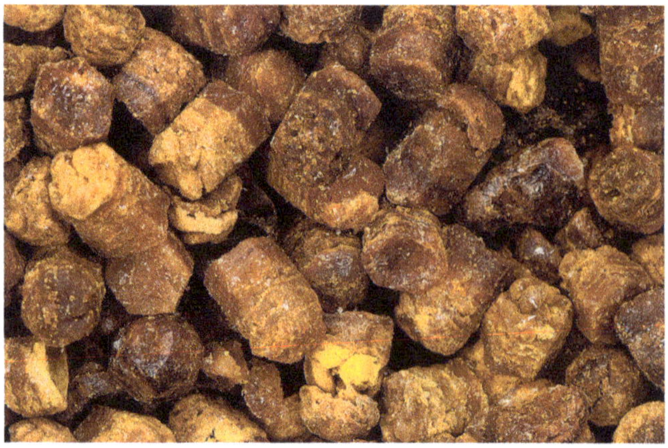

membranes and encourages leucocytosis.[2,6] Gargling with a diluted propolis solution aids in treating gingivitis; it also inhibits plaque formation and bacteria growth that cause dental caries.[2] Combine with calendula *(Calendula)*, yerba mansa *(Anemopsis)*, clove *(Syzygium)*, and/or myrrh *(Commiphora)* as a mouth rinse to treat mouth ulcers, canker sores, and gingivitis, and to reduce plaque. Combine extracts of spilanthes *(Acmella)*, yerba mansa *(Anemopsis)*, myrrh *(Commiphora)*, clove *(Syzygium)*, and/or cow parsnip seeds *(Heracleum)* to alleviate teething pain, a toothache, or gum abscess until dental care is obtained.

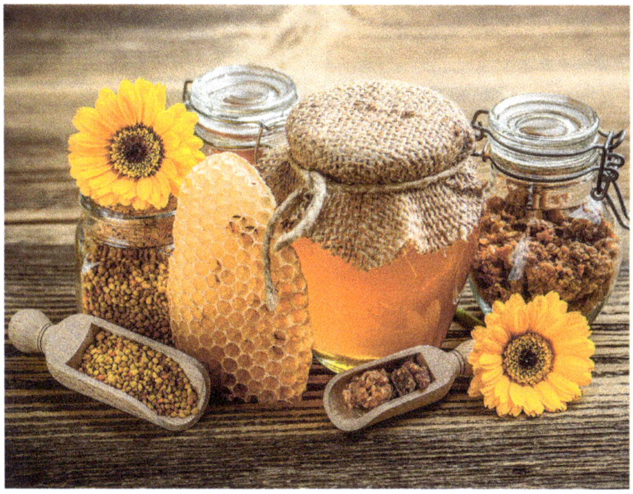

Propolis has topical antibacterial, antifungal, and vulnerary properties.[2-5] Apply diluted tincture, salve, or cream topically to cuts, burns, abrasions, broken skin, abscesses, infected wounds, herpes zoster (shingles), herpes simplex type I, fungal infections (ringworm, athlete's foot, and thrush), and staph infections.[2-5] The antifungal and antibacterial properties are attributed to the flavonoid

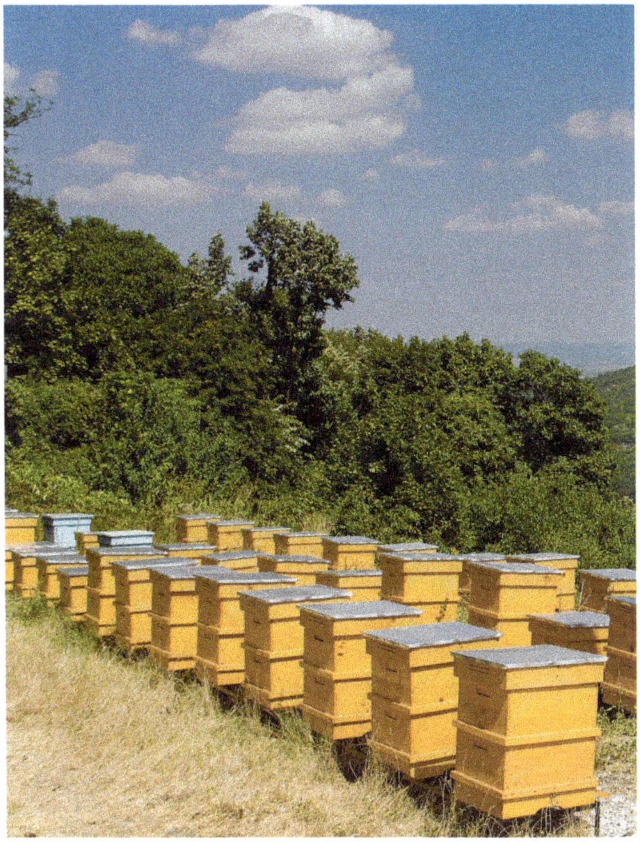

pigments.[2,3] Propolis creates a protective coating, and aids in sealing wounds and stimulating epithelial regeneration. However, after applying propolis medicaments, cover the wound, as particulate matter can adhere to the resin.[2,3] Additionally, propolis has topical counterirritant properties.[4] Apply cream to alleviate sore muscles, sprains, strains, bruises, and arthritic pain.

CONTRAINDICATIONS

Individuals with prior sensitivy to propolis should avoid consuming or applying propolis. Discontinue internal use if it causes a dull lower backache, as it may irritate the kidneys. Because propolis is a resin, individuals with kidney disease, kidney inflammation, or kidney damage should avoid using propolis internally. In rare cases, some individuals develop contact dermatitis; to test, apply a small amount topically to the inner crease of the elbow, and wait 24 – 48 hours.[2] If no skin irritation is present, it should be safe to apply to a larger surface area.

PREPARATION AND DOSAGE

TINCTURE: Resin [1:5, 95% alcohol]; consume 10 - 90 drops, up to four times daily.

HONEY AND SYRUP: Combine propolis tincture with equal parts honey to make syrup; consume ½ - 1 teaspoon, up to four times daily.

TOPICAL USE: Mix 30 - 90 drops of propolis tincture into a two-ounce salve, oil, or cream, and apply to affected area. Or dilute the extract (1:10) with distilled or spring water, and apply as a topical wash.

RASPBERRY LEAF

DESCRIPTION

BOTANICAL NAMES:
Rubus idaeus (syn. *Rubus idaeus* ssp. *idaeus*), *R. leucodermis, R. strigosus* (syn. *Rubus idaeus* ssp. *strigosus*)

COMMON NAMES:
Red raspberry, trefoil, wild raspberry, American red raspberry, whitebark raspberry, blackcap raspberry, black raspberry, blue raspberry

FAMILY NAME:
Rosaceae

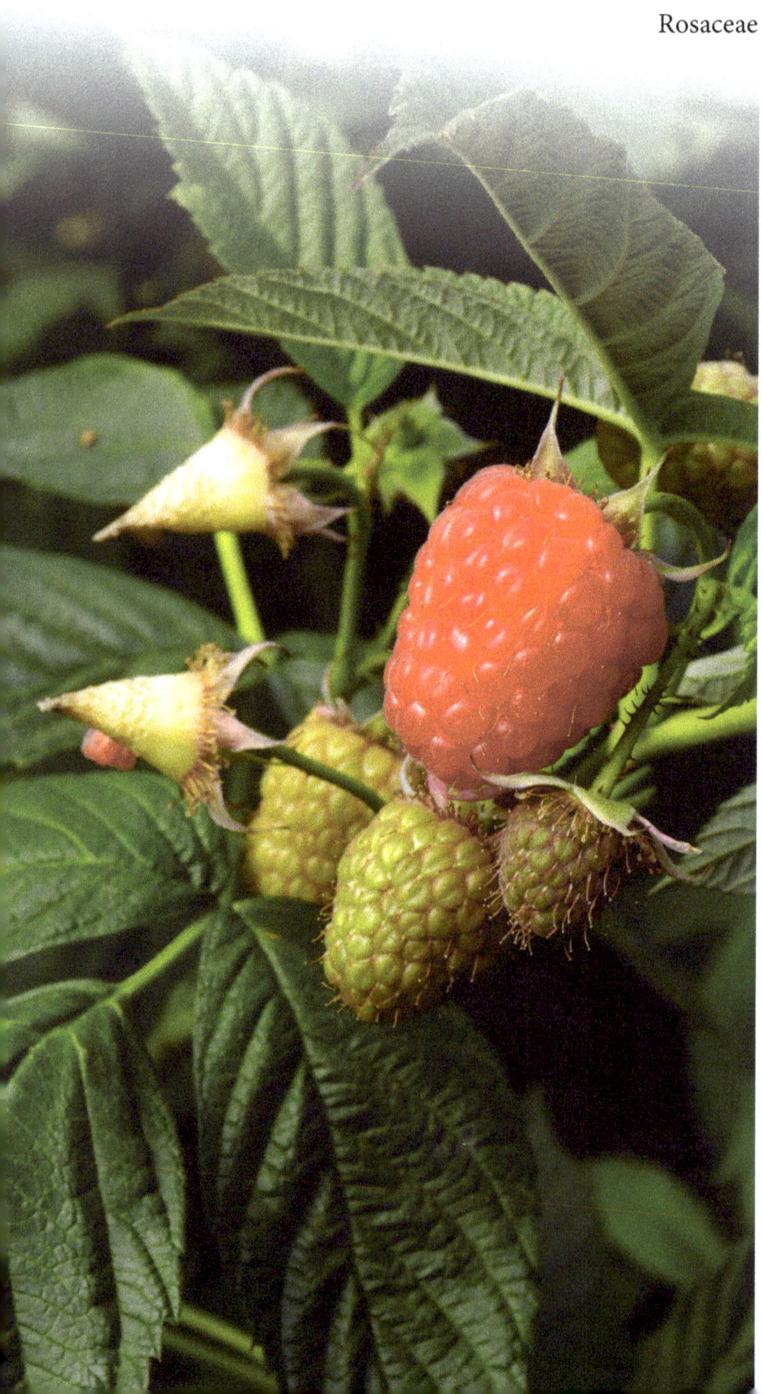

PART USED: The leaves are used for medicinal purposes.

BOTANICAL DESCRIPTION AND HABITAT: *Rubus idaeus* is native to Europe, temperate Asia, and northern Africa.[1] It has been domesticated and is currently cultivated as a crop worldwide. *R. strigosus* is a wild species of raspberry that grows in North America. *R. leucodermis* grows throughout the Mountain West and the western coast of North America.

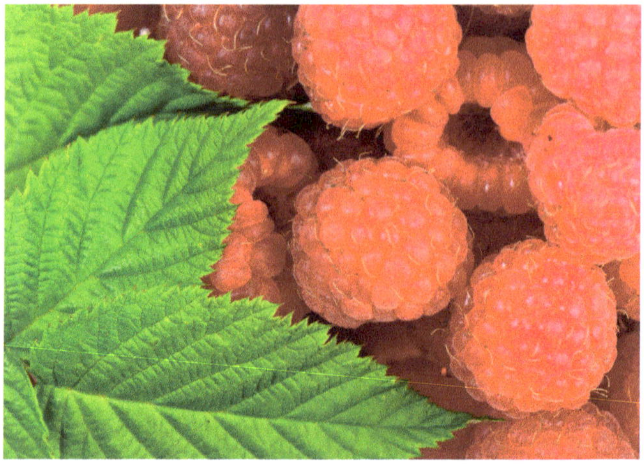

Rubus idaeus is a sparsely prickly, woody shrub (1 – 2 m tall), with biennial canes and perennial rootstock.[1] First-year stems have a dense coating of hair.[1] The stems bear odd-pinnate leaves with pubescent, linear stipules.[1] The elliptic to ovate leaflets (3 – 8 cm by 1.5 – 4.5 cm) are densely hairy on the lower sides, and glabrous or pilose on the upper sides, with doubly serrate margins.[1] The terminal inflorescences consist of flowers (1 – 1.5 cm diameter) on hairy, sparsely prickly pedicels (1 – 2 cm).[1] The flowers have white petals, many stamens, and many pistils with hairy ovaries.[1] The ovaries mature into hairy, red or orange, sweet, fleshy fruit consisting of aggregates of drupes (1 – 1.4 cm diameter).[1]

Rubus strigosus is closely related to *Rubus idaeus.* They have small physical differences, including glandular hairs on the stems of *R. strigosus* that are missing on *R. idaeus.*

Rubus leucodermis has arching biennial canes (1 – 3 meters tall) that root at the tips and bear wide, sturdy prickles.[3,4] When young, the stems are covered with a thick, glaucous

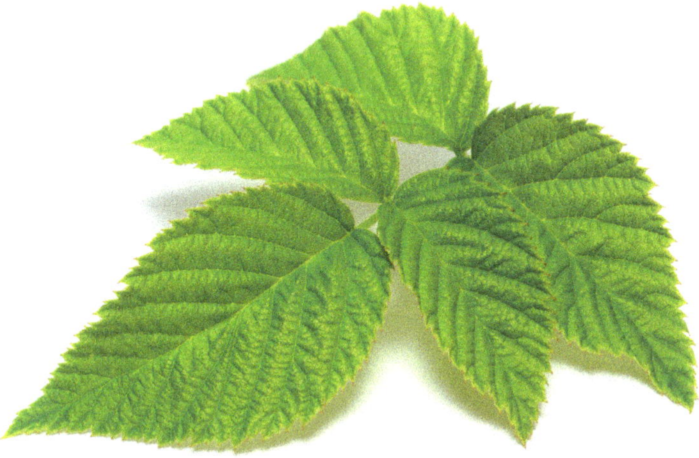 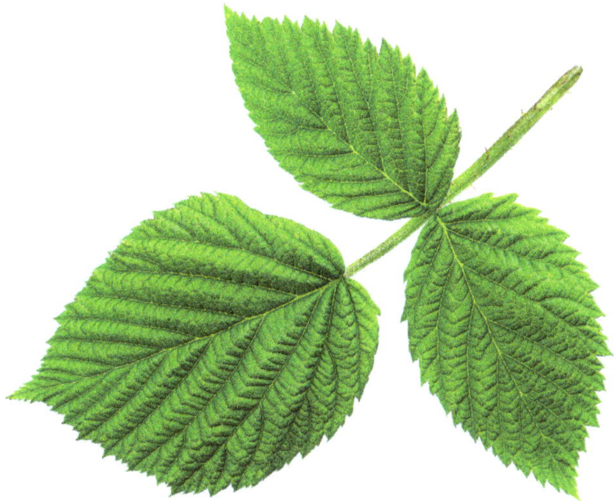

coating. The compound leaves consist of five dentate leaflets with a dense layer of white hairs on the undersides, and thin stipules.[3] In the second year, the stem's bark begins to shred, and the canes produces leaves that are simple or compound with three leaflets.[3,4] The inflorescence is a cyme of 3 – 12 flowers with hairy, prickly sepals, white petals, many separate pistils, and densely hairy ovaries.[3] The fruit is maroon to black.[3]

THE NAME: *Rubus* ("brambles") derives from Latin.[5] *Idaeus* derives from the Latin *Ida,* a mountain in Phrygia where the plant was abundant.[5] The epithet *strigosus* derives from the Latin *striga* ("a row of bristles"). The epithet *leucodermis* is composed of two Latin words: *leuco* ("pale or white") and *dermis* ("skin"), referencing the pale color of the stem.

HISTORICAL USES: The Blackfoot used raspberry leaves to treat diarrhea, sore throats, and lung disorders. The Shoshone applied a poultice of powdered stems on cuts and wounds.[6] Other tribes used raspberry leaves as a pregnancy or postpartum tonic.[5]

CONSTITUENTS: Tannins (gallotannins and ellagitannins), flavonoids (rutin), fragarine, organic acids (citric, succinic, lactic, and malic acids), ferric citrate, volatile oil, fixed oil, resin, and pectin.[7,8]

NUTRITIONAL PROPERTIES: Raspberry leaf contains high amounts of calcium, iron, magnesium, manganese, niacin, selenium, tin, and vitamins A, C, and E. It contains moderate to low amounts of aluminum, ash, chromium, cobalt, crude fiber, dietary fiber, fat, phosphorus, potassium, protein, riboflavin, silicon, sodium, thiamine, and zinc.[7]

MEDICINAL PROPERTIES: Astringent, galactagogue, hemostatic, nutritive, partus preparator, and uterine tonic.

TEMPERATURE AND FLAVOR: Neutral, astringent, sour, sweet, and bitter.

MEDICINAL USES

Raspberry leaf is a traditional women's reproductive tonic and partus preparator.[9,10] The leaves contain fragarine, a uterine tonic (strawberry and blackberry leaves also have fragarine).[9,10] Fragarine relaxes and tones the uterine pelvic muscles.[9,10] Raspberry leaf tea can be consumed daily during pregnancy to prevent a miscarriage, strengthen the uterus, and promote a smooth delivery.[9,10] It helps to tone the uterus following a birth. Raspberry leaf is also beneficial as a structural tonic to improve the integrity of the reproductive organs for women with uterine cysts, dysmenorrhea, or fibroids.[10]

The tea can be beneficial for reducing morning sickness during pregnancy; however, in some individuals the tannins can aggravate the stomach.[5] Combine two parts peppermint leaf with one part raspberry leaf, and prepare as a tea to alleviate morning sickness.

Raspberry leaf has hemostatic properties that can be used during and following a birth to prevent hemorrhage and reduce excessive bleeding.[9] It aids in cleansing afterbirth.[9] Raspberry leaf decreases excessive blood flow following a miscarriage or abortion.[10] It reduces heavy menstrual flow and mid-cycle spotting, as well as menopausal spotting. Prepare a hemostatic compound by combining it with lady's mantle *(Alchemilla),* yarrow *(Achillea),* shepherd's

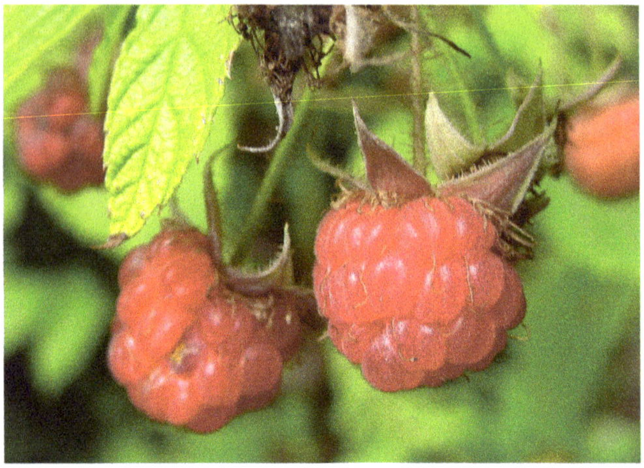

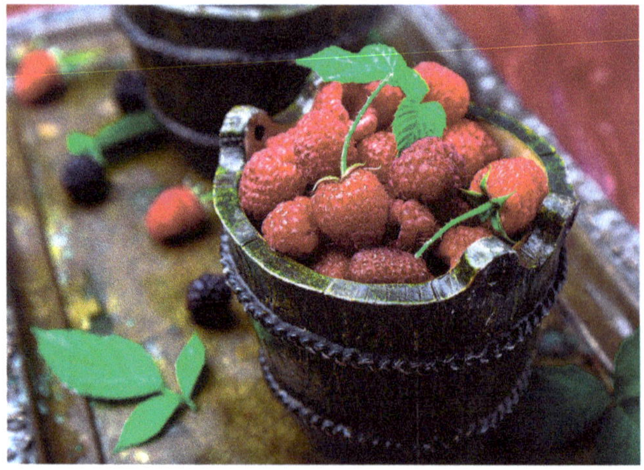

purse *(Capsella)*, nettle leaf *(Urtica)*, and/or cinnamon *(Cinnamomum)*.

Raspberry leaf is a nutritive agent rich in vitamins and minerals.[9,10] It also supports individuals with iron deficiency anemia. The calcium and magnesium content aid in preventing osteoporosis and strengthening bones.[9] Combine raspberry leaf with nettle *(Urtica)*, oat straw *(Avena)*, alfalfa *(Medicago)*, and/or red clover *(Trifolium pratense)* for a deeply nourishing tea blend.

Similar to many plants in the rose family, raspberry leaf decreases inflammation in mucous membranes. It can be used as a sore throat gargle.[8] Consuming the tea reduces excess mucus secretions, and helps to treat diarrhea and dysentery.[8,9] If the cause of diarrhea is microbial, as in dysentery, it is essential to combine raspberry leaf with appropriate antimicrobial herbs. The tea can be used as an enema to astringe tissues and reduce local inflammation. Apply a wash or compress of tea to wounds, ulcers, skin inflammation, or hemmorhoids.[8]

Irrigating the vaginal canal with raspberry leaf reduces excessive vaginal secretions, and decreases localized inflammation. A vaginal irrigation prepared in combination with antifungal herbs also aids in treating non-specific vaginitis and yeast infections. A sitz bath is useful for treating hemorrhoids and anal fissures, and for healing following a birth. The tea also can be used as an eye wash for conjunctivitis, allergies, or eye inflammation. *Note:* For all of the previously listed applications, strain the tea through a coffee filter to remove particulate matter.

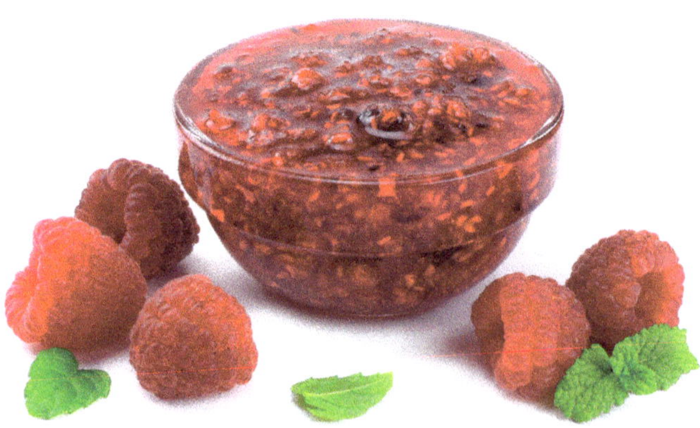

Raspberry leaf has mild bitter tonic properties that gently stimulate digestion.[9] It also has a mild effect on lowering blood glucose levels.[9]

CONTRAINDICATIONS

Raspberry leaf is drying and may exacerbate dry conditions. Avoid using it as a tonic in individuals with dry mucous membranes.

PREPARATION AND DOSAGE

TINCTURE: Fresh leaves [1:2-1:3, 70-95% alcohol]; dry leaves [1:5, 50-60% alcohol]; consume 10-60 drops, up to four times daily.

TEA: Prepare a hot or cold infusion; consume 8-12 ounces, up to four times daily. The tea may taste bitter if the leaves steep longer than five to ten minutes, especially when boiling water is used. The tea is less bitter and astringent when hot, rather than boiling, water is used.

TOPICAL USE: Cool the tea to room temperature, then strain through a coffee filter and use as a vaginal irrigation, enema, eye wash, mouthwash, fomentation, or poultice.

RED CLOVER

DESCRIPTION

BOTANICAL NAME:
Trifolium pratense

COMMON NAMES:
Red clover, purple clover, trefoil, cow clover, meadow clover, pea vine clover, honeysuckle trefoil, king's crown, sweet kitty clover, sleeping Maggie, bee bread
puna-apila (Finnish)
triolet (French)
rose klaver, rotklee (German)
moscino, trifoglio dei prati (Italian)
trepatra (Sanskrit)
trebol rojo (Spanish)
rödklöver (Swedish)

FAMILY NAME:
Fabaceae (Leguminosae)

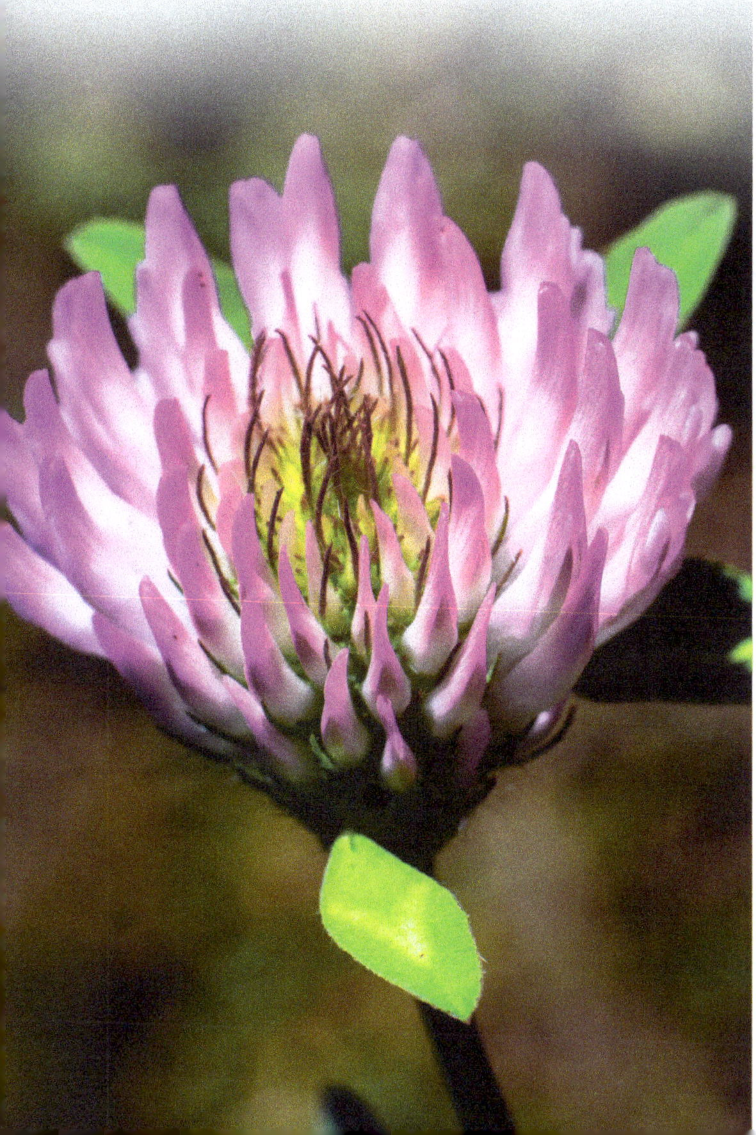

PARTS USED: The blossoms or flowering herb.

BOTANICAL DESCRIPTION AND HABITAT: Red clover is a commonly cultivated perennial; escapees grow wild in meadows with sandy soil and good drainage. It is native to southwest Asia, northern Africa, and Europe.[1]

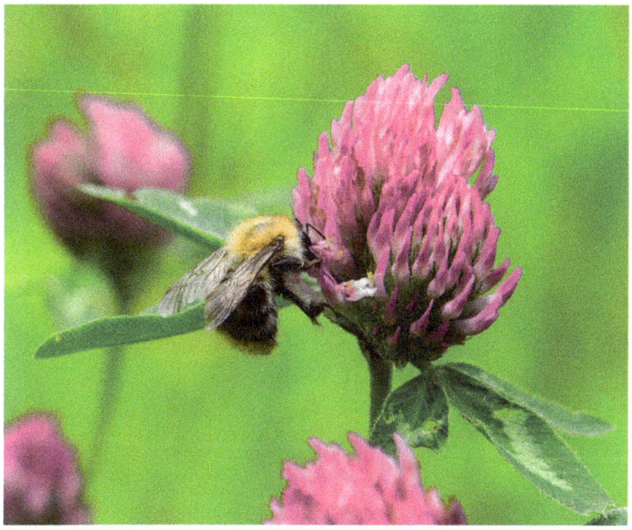

Red clover is an herbaceous, pubescent, short-lived perennial (20 – 70 cm) with trifoliate leaves and petioles that shorten as the leaves climb the stem.[1,2] The obovate to elliptic leaflets (1 – 3 cm long by 1 – 2 cm wide) have bristle-tipped stipules and a distinctive pale chevron pattern on the upper side of the blades.[1,2] Subtended by reduced leaves and lacking a peduncle, the beautiful inflorescence is a dense globose, terminal head (2 – 3 cm wide) of 30 – 70 flowers.[1,2] The tubular calyx has awl-shaped lobes tipped by bristles.[2] The small, purple to white tubular corollas (12 – 14 mm long) resemble a tiny, slender pea flower.[1] Red clover produces an ovoid legume with one or two seeds.[1]

THE NAME: The genus name *Trifolium* derives from two Latin words: *tri* ("three") and *folium* ("leaf"). The epithet *pratense* derives from the Medieval Latin *praetensa* ("to pretend"), or from the Middle Dutch *praten* ("to chatter"). *Trefoil* means "three-leaved plant." Clover derives from the Latin *clava* ("club").

HISTORICAL USES: Red clover is planted as a cover crop to fix nitrogen, rejuvenate the soil, and prevent erosion. The roots contain symbiotic bacteria that can fix nitrogen. Red

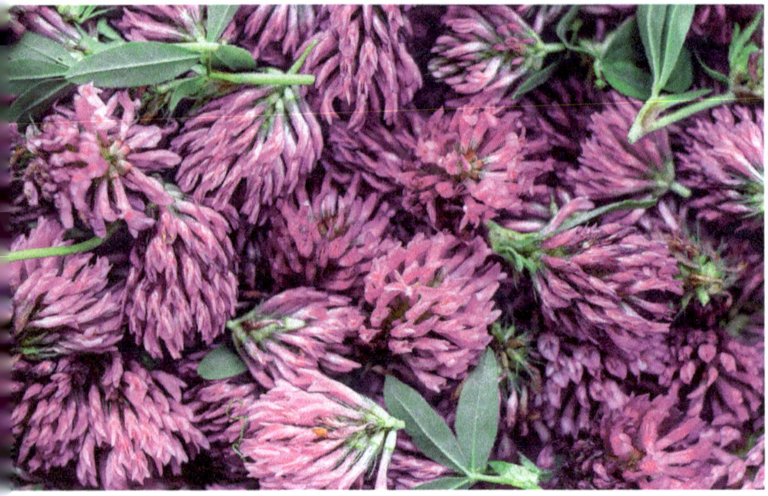

clover is grown on pastureland as fodder for cattle and poultry. Because rural communities believed that clover fattened cattle, the common idiom "to be (or, to live) in clover," referred to living a carefree life in comfort or prosperity. Most clovers have three leaves; finding a four leaf clover was considered good luck. Clovers were symbols of the earth, sea, and heaven for ancient Druid priests, and the Holy Trinity.[3]

In Traditional Chinese Medicine, red clover was used to treat coughs.[3] Russians employed red clover for asthma.[3] Europeans used red clover to ease digestion.[3] Native Americans consumed it as food, and applied it to treat sore eyes and burns.[3] American Eclectic physicians administered red clover as an alterative, blood purifier, expectorant, and antitussive agent.[3] They used the herb to treat cancerous ulcers and whooping cough.[3] Red clover is an important source of nectar for honey bees, their primary pollinators.

CONSTITUENTS: Red clover contains flavonoids (isoflavones: formononetin, biochanin A, daidzein, genistein, pratensein, and trifoside), flavones (pectolinarin), coumarin and coumestrol, saponins (trifolanol), heptacosane, hentriacontane, trifoliin (isoquercitrin), trifolitin, phaselic acid, a galactomannan, mucilaginous polysaccharides, *trans-* and *cis-*clovamides (L-dopa conjugated with *trans-* and *cis-*caffeic acids), allantoic acid, β-sitosterol, campesterol, soyasapogenol, volatile oil (with furfural), glucosides, phenols, eugenol, isoleucine, isorhamnetin, medicagol, α-tocopherol, ononin, pratenol, trifolianol, resin, and methyl salicylate (salicylic acid).[4-6]

NUTRITIONAL PROPERTIES: Red clover contains high amounts of β-carotene, vitamin C, niacin, riboflavin, thiamine, calcium, chromium, magnesium, manganese, phosphorus, potassium, and tin. It contains moderate amounts of protein, pantothenic acid, cobalamin, biotin, choline, inositol, amino acids, α-tocopherol, cobalt, copper, iron, selenium, silicon, sodium, and zinc.[4,6,7]

MEDICINAL PROPERTIES: Alterative, anti-inflammatory, antioxidant, antitumor, antitussive (mild), expectorant, nutritive, lymphatic, and blood thinner.

TEMPERATURE AND FLAVOR: Neutral, sweet, salty, and astringent (mild).

MEDICINAL USES

Red clover is a gentle lymphatic, alterative, depurative, and nutritive agent that can be used long-term to treat chronic conditions.[4,6,8,9] Rich in vitamins and minerals, red clover tea can be consumed daily as a nourishing tonic. Red clover reduces glandular swelling due to acute or chronic debilitating illnesses. It is a subtle adjunct therapy for chronic fatigue syndrome, mononucleosis (Epstein Barr virus), and hepatitis.[6] It enhances detoxification by improving the elimination of metabolic waste products. This aids in treating conditions such as gout and rheumatoid arthritis, and chronic skin conditions such as eczema, psoriasis, and acne.[4,6,8,9] Apply the fomentation or poultice as a topical anti-inflammatory treatment for a burn, rash, dermatitis, or any skin conditions mentioned above.[4,9] Prepare a gentle alterative and lymphatic tea by combining red clover, violet *(Viola)*, cleavers *(Galium)*, nettle *(Urtica)*, alfalfa *(Medicago)*, and a flavoring agent such as mint *(Mentha)*.

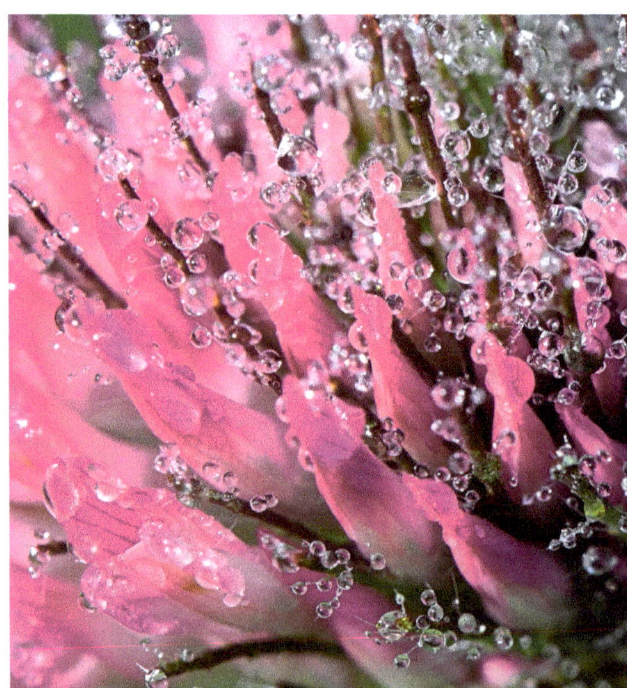

Red clover is a mild expectorant and antitussive agent.[4,6,8] It reduces inflammation in mucous membranes.[9] Consume red clover tea to hasten recovery from respiratory infections including whooping cough, bronchitis, and asthma.[4] To make the tea, combine red cover with mullein *(Verbascum)*, coltsfoot *(Tussilago* or *Petasites)*, tulsi basil *(Ocimum sanctum)*, thyme *(Thymus)*, peppermint *(Mentha piperita)*, and/or eucalyptus *(Eucalyptus)*.

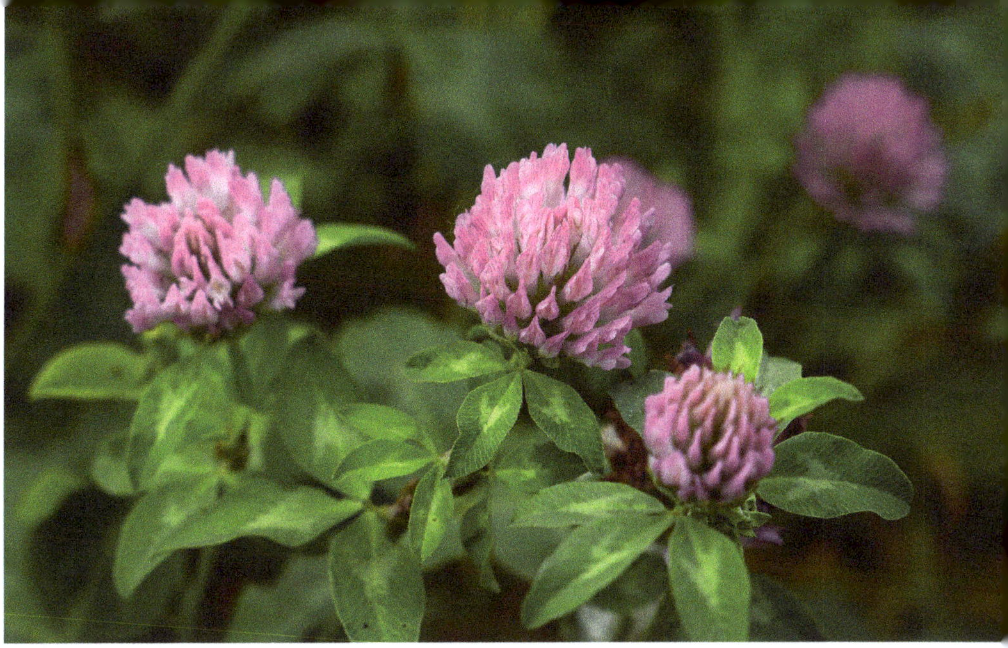

Red clover enhances oxygen and nutrient delivery to the brain. It increases mental alertness, and reduces confusion, memory loss, and senility. A tea that enhances mental clarity includes red clover, ginkgo *(Ginkgo)*, mint *(Mentha)*, lemon verbena *(Aloysia)*, smaller amounts of gotu kola *(Centella)*, rosemary *(Salvia rosmarinus)*, and a pinch of stevia *(Stevia)* as a sweetener.

Red clover has mild blood thinning properties. It reduces blood reactivity, which is helpful in preventing migraine headaches and seasonal allergies. Red clover also increases artery elasticity.[3]

Red clover was incorporated into the Hoxsey formula, an herbal treatment for cancer created by Harry Hoxsey, a holistic practitioner.[3,4] It contains genistein, reported to inhibit the growth and spread of cancer. It is indicated as a preventive and supportive therapy for individuals with estrogen-related breast or uterine cancer.[9] However, the plant actions are subtle. Other than supporting the lymph and providing nutrients to the tissues, the anticancer claims for this plant are overestimated.

CONTRAINDICATIONS

Red clover can be consumed during pregnancy, but due to the potential blood thinning properties, it should be avoided two to four weeks before the due date, or if there are any potential complications. Avoid consuming red clover two weeks prior to, and two weeks following surgery. It is safe for nursing mothers and children.

PREPARATION AND DOSAGE

TINCTURE: Fresh blossoms [1:3-1:4, 60-95% alcohol]; dry blossoms [1:5-1:7, 50% alcohol]; consume 10-60 drops, up to four times daily.

GLYCERITE: Dry blossoms [1:5, 40% glycerin, 30% alcohol, 30% water]; consume 10-60 drops, up to three times daily.

TEA: Prepare a hot or cold infusion; consume 8-12 ounces, three to four times daily.

TOPICAL USE: Apply the fresh plant poultice or fomentation topically.

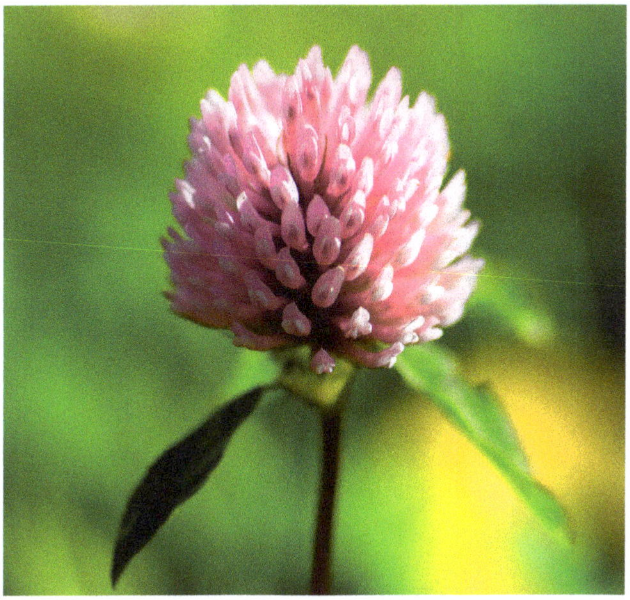

RED ROOT

DESCRIPTION

BOTANICAL NAMES:
Ceanothus americanus, C. cuneatus, C. fendleri, C. greggii, C. herbaceus, C. integerrimus, C. sanguineus, C. thyrsiflorus, C. velutinus, C. spp.

COMMON NAMES:
California lilac, buckbrush, whitethorn, mountain white balm, tobacco brush, sticky laurel, New Jersey tea, Jersey tea, red root, pine mat, deer brush, blue blossom, wild snowball, Walpole tea, mountain sweet
céanothe (French)
säckelblume (German)
ceanoto (Italian)
zeres cayt (Turkish)

FAMILY NAME:
Rhamnaceae

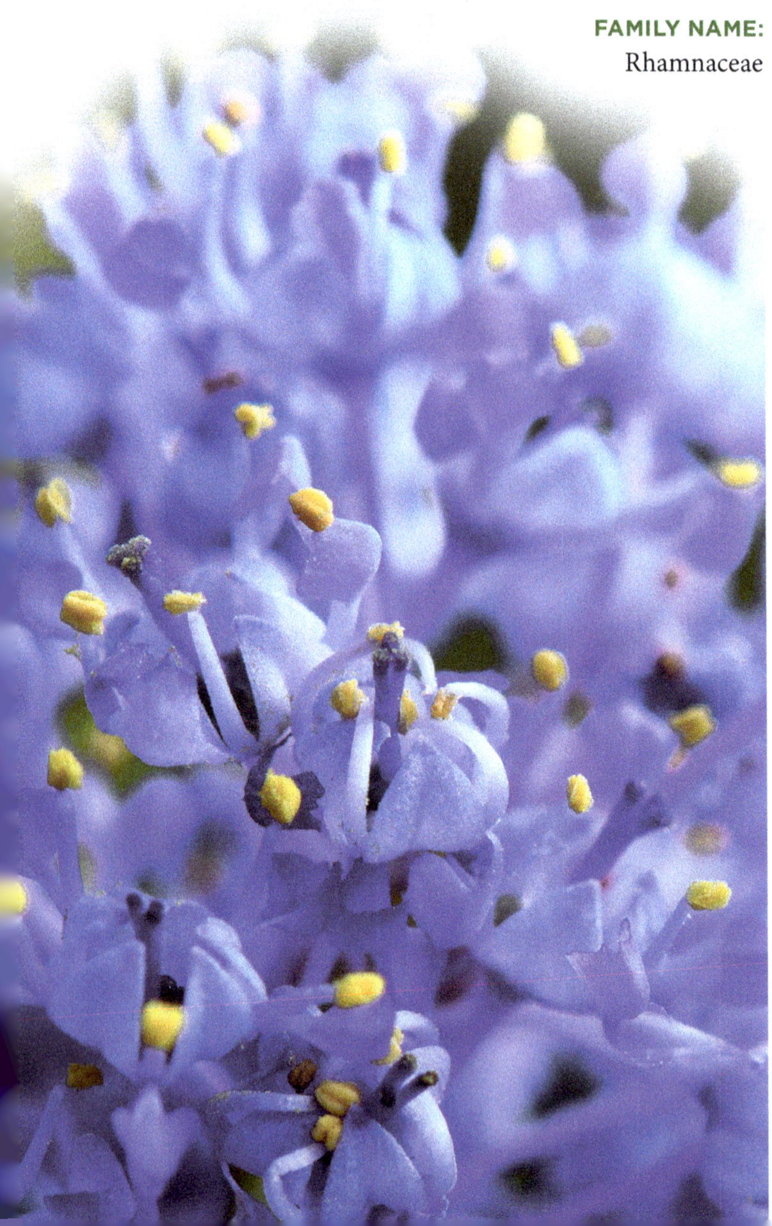

PARTS USED: The root and root bark are the primary portions of the plant used medicinally.

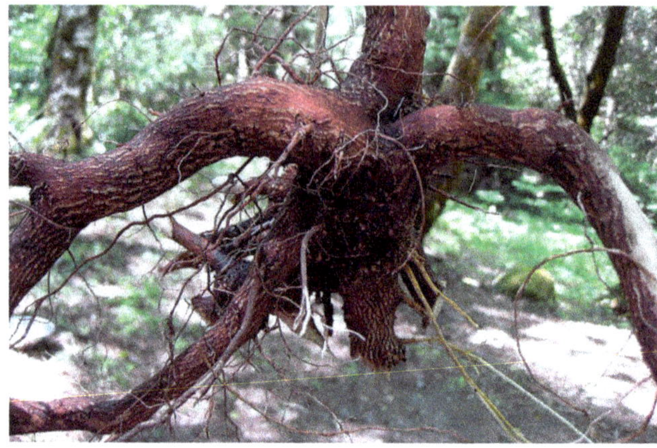

BOTANICAL DESCRIPTION AND HABITAT: Red root grows in sandy soil at various elevations throughout the U.S. Most *Ceanothus* species grow from California to the Rocky Mountains. It often grows on dry, open slopes in wooded clearings, as well as in chaparral and coastal scrub.[1] Red root also can be found in areas that have been clear cut or burned. The seeds can remain dormant up to 200 years; fires cause the seeds to germinate.[2] Red root fixes nitrogen in soil.[2]

Ceanothus is a genus of over 55 species of woody perennials; at least 41 grow in California.[3] Hybridization is common and hybrid forms may not key properly.[3] The habit and vegetative characteristics vary significantly among species; the two subgenera *(Ceanothus* subgenus *Ceanothus* and *Ceanothus* subgenus *Cerastes)* have broad distinctions. *Ceanothus* is either a small tree or shrub, with an erect or mat-forming prostrate habit.[4] Some species have thorns.[3] Depending on the species, the leaves can be alternate or opposite, deciduous or evergreen, with varied margins. Leaves range from dark green to yellow-green to gray-green.[1] Members of the subgenus *Ceanothus* have opposite leaves that tend to have three prominent midribs radiating from the base of the blade, although some species have only one prominent midrib.[3] They have deciduous stipules.[1] Many species have fire-resistant basal burls with dormant buds that can resprout after a fire.[1] Members of the second subgenus, *Cerastes,* bear smaller, thicker alternate leaves with white, splotchy stomatal crypts visible on the underside of the blade; the leaves have only one prominent midrib.[1,3,4] The stipules are persistent and cork-like, and these species lack burls.[1]

The tiny flowers (less than 5 mm across) are relatively consistent from species to species, with small differences.[3] The inflorescences are panicle-like in the *Ceanothus* subgenus, and umbel-like in the *Cerastes* subgenus, bearing many groupings of three-flowered clusters.[3] The base of

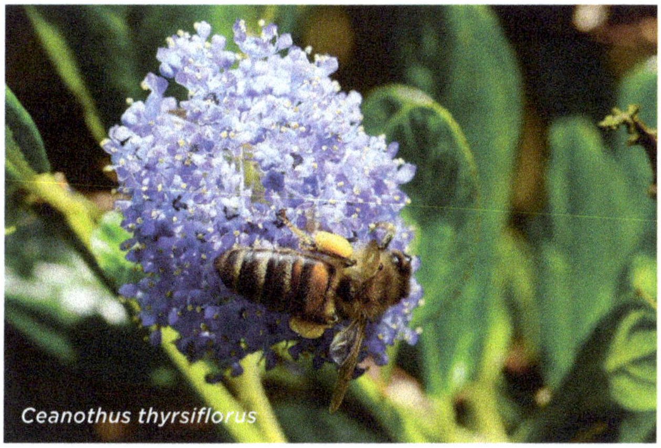

Ceanothus thyrsiflorus

the sepals, petals, and stamens are fused into a hypanthium, with the ovary superior.[1,3] There are five persistent, lanceolate-deltate sepals the same color as the petals, often incurved and larger than the petals.[3] The five spatulate, hooded petals vary in color between, and sometimes within species, from white to deep blue, or lavender.[3] The style generally has three prominent lobes at the tip.[3] The three-lobed ovary becomes a three-valved capsule, with three seeds per fruit.[3]

THE NAME: *Ceanothus* derives from the Greek name for a spiny shrub.[2,5] The epithet *cuneatus* means "web-shaped."[6] The epithet *fendleri* was named in honor of August Fendler (1813 – 1883) who collected plants in North America and Central America.[7] The epithet *greggii* was named after Josiah Gregg (1806 – 1850), frontier trader, author, and plant collector.[8] The epithet *herbaceus* means "not woody."[9] The epithet *integerrimus* means "undivided or with a smooth edge."[10] The epithet *thyrsiflorus* refers to flowers in a thyrse, "a compact cylindrical or ovate panicle with an indeterminate main axis and cymose sub-axes."[11] The epithets *sanguineus* ("bloody red") and *velutinus* ("velvety or with a soft, silky covering") derive from Latin.[2,5]

The common names correspond with the following Latin binomials: New Jersey tea, wild snowball *(Ceanothus americanus);* buckbrush *(C. cuneatus);* mountain white balm *(C. integerrimus);* Jersey tea *(C. herbaceus);* redstem ceanothus, snowbush *(C. sanguineus);* California lilac, blue blossom *(C. thyrsiflorus);* and tobacco brush, sticky laurel, snow brush, cinnamon brush, and mountain balm *(C. velutinus).*

HISTORICAL USES: Native Americans consumed a tea of *C. americanus* and *C. integerrimus* root to treat lung ailments, stomachaches, snakebites, and fever, and as a diuretic.[5,12] It was administered to women during childbirth.[12] A tea prepared from twigs was used to wash newborns.[12] Twig and leaf tea of *C. velutinus* were consumed to treat arthritis, diarrhea, rheumatism, coughs, and gonorrhea, and to aid weight loss.[12] A wash of the tea was applied to treat sores, eczema, broken limbs, arthritis, rheumatism, and pain.[12] Mixing the flowers with water created a soapy lather to wash the skin and hair, treat dandruff, and prevent diaper rash.[5,12] The dried, powdered leaves were mixed with pitch and applied to sores. A tea made from the whole plant was used as a folk treatment for cancer.[12]

New Jersey tea *(C. americanus)* was substituted for black tea during the American Revolutionary War.[13] The leaves were added to smoking mixtures as a tobacco substitute.[5] In Canada, the roots were used to dye wool brownish-red.[13] Red root was administered to treat stomach, liver, and spleen ailments.[12]

Eclectic physicians used red root as an astringent, alterative, lymphatic, and expectorant.[14,15] They prescribed *C. americanus* to improve lymphatic and portal circulation.[14,15] Red root was recommended for patients who had chronic, suboptimal liver function with edematous, sallow skin, and pain in the liver or spleen.[14,15] It was administered for patients with syphilis, scrofula, glandular problems, ovarian and uterine irregularities, bronchitis, asthma, and pneumonia.[13-15] Doctors John King and Harvey Felter administered *C. americanus* as an astringent, antispasmodic, sedative, and expectorant, and to reduce

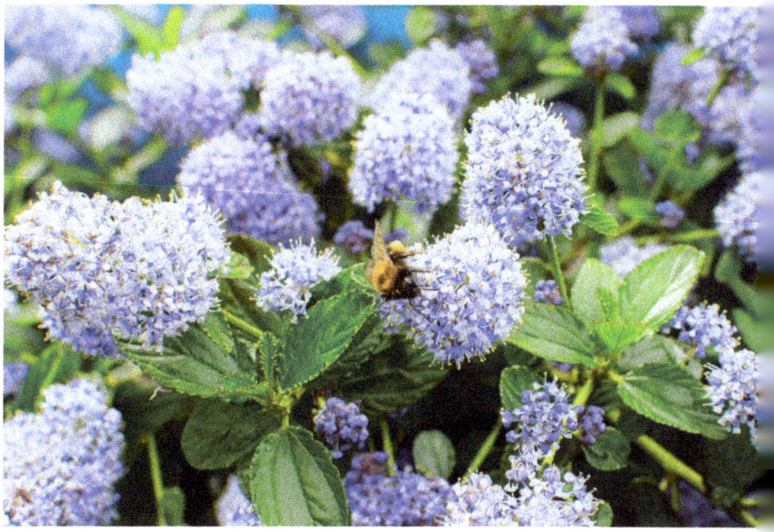

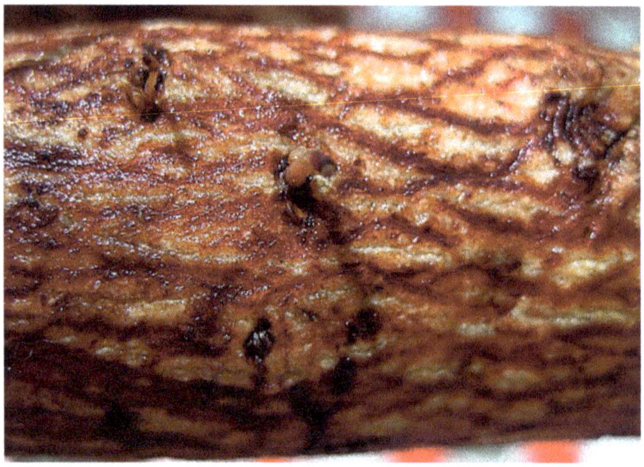

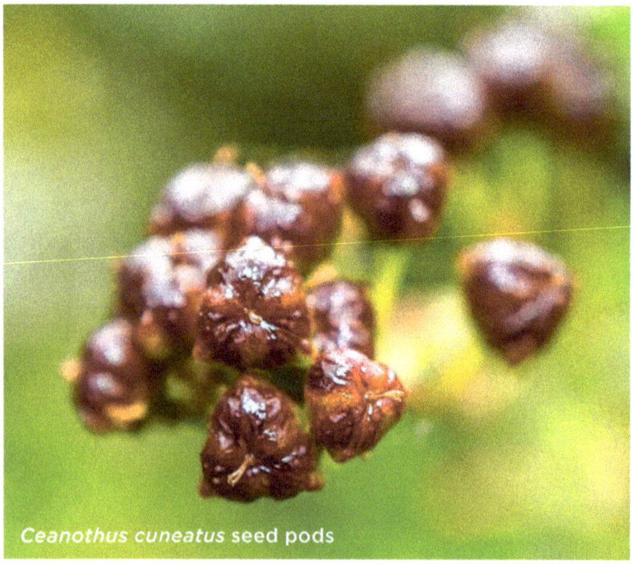

Ceanothus cuneatus seed pods

spleen enlargement, congestion, and pain.[14,16] During the American Civil War, the decoction was consumed by soldiers to treat malarial splenitis.[14,16] Eclectic physician Dr. Henderson, applied an infusion of *C. thyrsiflorus* leaves to treat conjunctivitis. He administered the nearly ripened berries to reduce hoarseness, ease swallowing, and treat a dry, burning sensation in the throat.[15] He also used the berries to treat pharyngitis and tonsillitis, and reduce nasal catarrh. A wash was applied topically to ulcers and sores.[15] Vaginal irrigation was used to treat gonorrhea, gleet, and leukorrhea.[13,15]

CONSTITUENTS: Red root contains tannins, discarine B, 5-β-indolyl-menthyl-8-η-methylvalyl-9-phenyl, 5-iso-butyl-8-η-methyl-iso-leucyl-9-phenyl, 9-benzyl-8-η-n-dimethyl-iso-leucyl-9-phenyl, asparagine, aspartic acid, β-sitosterol, betulinic acid, ceanothenic acid, glutamic acid, organic acids (malonic, gallic, oxalic, succinic, pyrophosphoric, orthophosphoric, and malic), phenolic acids (vanillic and syringic), alkaloids (ceanothines, ceanothamine, integerressine, integerrenine, integerrine, and americine), glutamine, resin, starch, mucilage, and the alkaloid ceanothine.[14,17-19]

The leaves contain tannins, flavonoids (flavonols: quercetin, rutin, and kaempferol; anthocyanins: cyanidin, and delphinidin glycosides), paracoumaric acid, cinnamic acid ethyl ester, nonacosane, 1-hexacosanol, velutin, a soft resin, a bitter substance, a volatile substance, lignin, and ceanothine.[14,17-19]

NUTRITIONAL PROPERTIES: The roots are inedible; the nutritional properties of the leaves are unknown.

MEDICINAL PROPERTIES: Alterative, anti-inflammatory, astringent, hemostatic, lymphatic, and portal decongestant.

TEMPERATURE AND FLAVOR: Cool, astringent, and bitter.

MEDICINAL USES

Red root is a lymphatic alterative that reduces lymph swelling in the throat, armpits, breasts, and groin. It improves fluid drainage from congested tissues, and promotes the movement of lymphatic fluid. Red root strengthens structural cells that form the lymphatic vessels and lymph nodes.[18] It reduces swelling in lymphatic organs (including the spleen and liver) due to infectious illnesses, such as mononucleosis and hepatitis.[14-18] Red root is not an anti-infective agent; however, it can be combined with antimicrobial herbs. It reduces lymphatic swelling accompanying tonsillitis, strep throat, mononucleosis (Epstein Barr virus), pharyngitis, sinusitis, cold, flu, boils, and herpes.[15,17,18,20]

Red root is a long-term lymphatic tonic that reduces fluid stagnation in breast tissue.[18,29] It aids in treating fibrocystic breast disease and benign breast cysts, as well as breast tenderness and swelling prior to menses.[18] When combined with echinacea *(Echinacea)*, cleavers *(Galium)*, and small amounts of wild indigo *(Baptisia)*, red root can be helpful in treating mastitis. Red root can be used as a followup treatment for breast cancer survivors. It is also useful for treating ovarian, uterine, or testicular cysts.[18,20]

Red root is beneficial for reducing acute or chronic inflammatory conditions, such as seasonal allergies, food allergies, migraine headaches, and inflammatory arthritis.[17,18] When excessive dietary fats are consumed in conjunction with other dietary substances that trigger inflammation, fats move rapidly from the digestive tract, into the portal vein, through the liver, and into systemic circulation.

Excess circulating fats (and/or poor quality fats) stimulate mast cells that reside in the capillary beds, triggering a histamine response in tissues.[18] Histamines are pro-inflammatory agents that increase capillary permeability and dilate capillaries, aggravating allergic reactions. Red root tightens capillary beds, and stabilizes mast cells, countering the effects of inflammation. It also improves the quality of blood charge, enhances capillary cells repelling capacity, prevents red blood cells from adhering together, reduces blood viscosity, and improves blood osmolality.[17,18] This improves the fluid transport of non-protein fractions of blood into the interstitium and lymph, and eases blood passage through capillary beds.[17,18] Red root also decreases the capacity for blood fats to trigger inflammation.[18]

Red root decreases congestion of the portal vein that carries blood from the digestive tract and spleen to the liver, where it is filtered.[15,18] Portal vein congestion can result in blood stagnation from the waist down, causing a dull, achy sensation in the venous system and reproductive region. Red root reduces congestion in the reproductive organs, decreasing testicular hydroceles and prostate congestion in men, and cervical or uterine congestion in women.[15,18] It also aids in treating hemorrhoids, varicose veins, and spider veins.[18]

Red root is an astringent hemostatic that decreases capillary fragility and bleeding.[18] It reduces bleeding hemorrhoids, nosebleeds, and bleeding gums, as well as blood in the mucus, urine, or stools.[18,19] It is also beneficial for treating excessive menstrual bleeding, postpartum bleeding, and bleeding cysts, as well as bleeding caused by menopausal hormone imbalances.[17,18] *Warning:* If an individual is hemorrhaging, seek medical attention immediately.

Red root is an astringent, reducing mucous membrane inflammation in the respiratory mucosa, stomach, and intestines.[14,17-19] It can be used as a gargle for treating a sore throat resulting from laryngitis, strep β, or mononucleosis.[18,19] Red root aids in treating watery eyes and a runny nose caused by seasonal allergies.[16,19] It also reduces acute inflammation in the gastrointestinal tract, and is helpful for treating diarrhea.[19] Vaginal irrigation with tea aids in treating leukorrhea, yeast infections, and non-specific vaginitis.[15,19] A sitz bath is useful following a birth and for treating hemorrhoids.[19] Discontinue use if it is too drying to the tissues. Although the leaves have a milder action than the root, they can be used interchangeably as an astringent.[19]

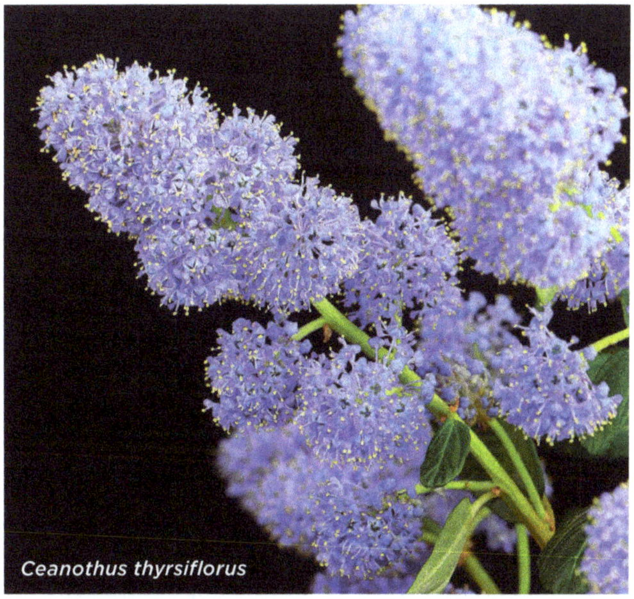

Ceanothus thyrsiflorus

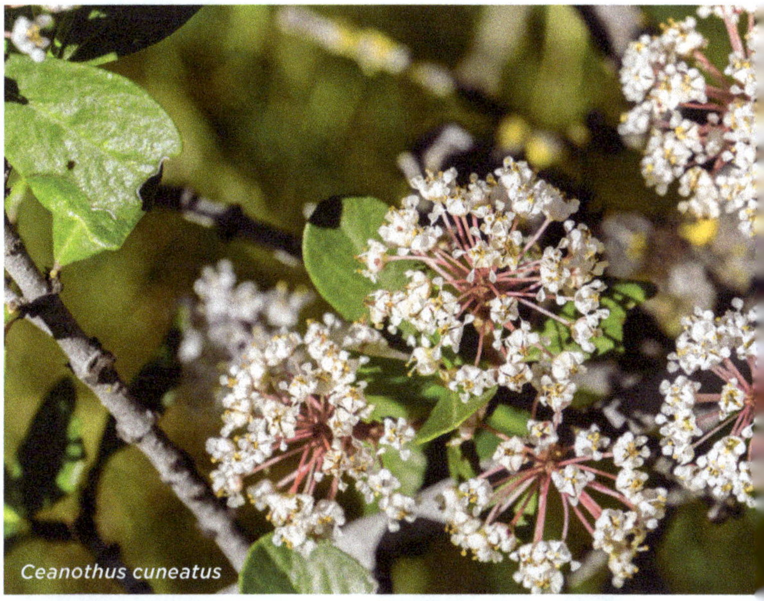

Ceanothus cuneatus

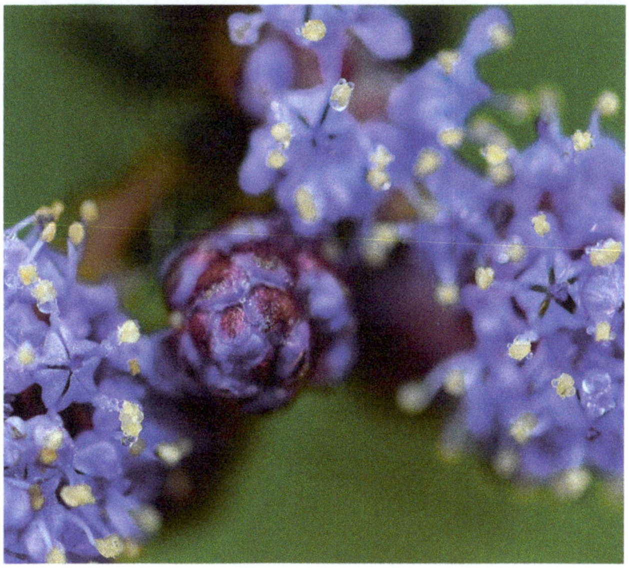

The leaves contain flavonoids with antioxidant actions.[19] They can be used as a non-caffeinated substitute for black tea.[13,20] Macerating fresh flowers in warm water forms suds that can cleanse the hair or skin.[5,12,17]

CONTRAINDICATIONS

Red root should be used in moderation during pregnancy and lactation; however, one source contraindicates internal use during pregnancy or lactation.[18,19] Avoid consuming red root one to two weeks prior to, and following any surgical procedure. Avoid use with blood-clotting disorders.[18] Red root is contraindicated with prescription or over-the-counter drugs that affect blood clotting (warfarin, aspirin, etc.).[18] Exercise caution (or avoid use) in individuals with an overt disease or undergoing chemotherapy.[18] There are no known side effects from the leaves.[19]

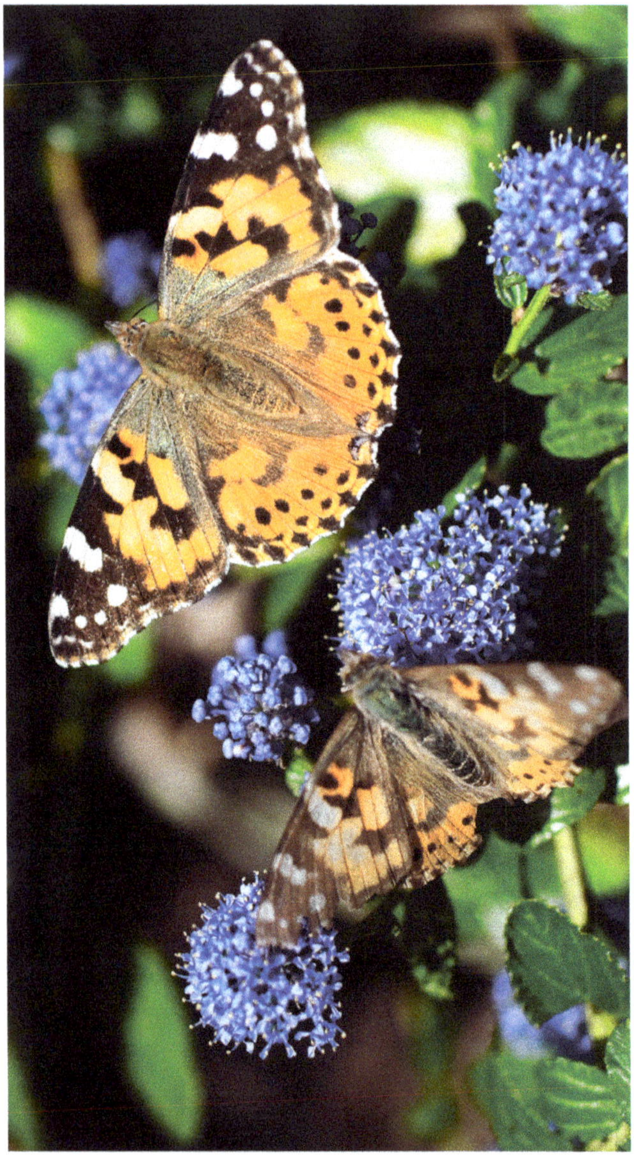

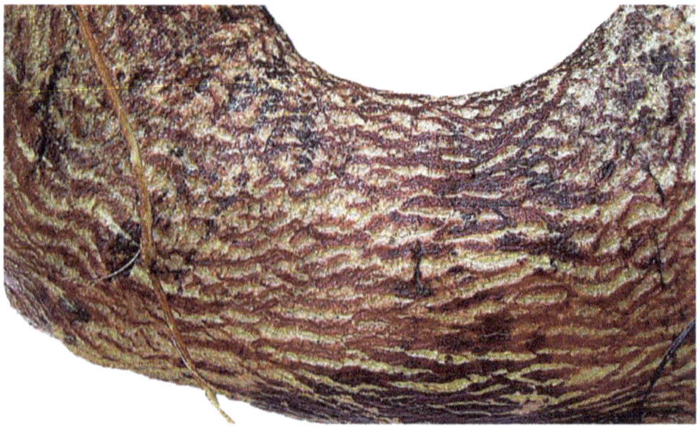

PREPARATION AND DOSAGE

TINCTURE: Fresh roots [1:2–1:3, 70–95% alcohol]; dry roots [1:5, 60% alcohol]; consume 15–90 drops, up to four times daily.

CAPSULES: Consume 2–4 "00" capsules, up to four times daily.

TEA: Prepare a cold infusion or decoction of the roots; consume 8 ounces, up to four times daily. Prepare a hot infusion of the leaves; consume 8 ounces, up to four times daily, or use topically.

HONEY AND SYRUP: Prepare a decoction and add sufficient simple syrup to sweeten. Consume 1 teaspoon to 1 tablespoon, up to four times daily.

TOPICAL USE: Apply a fomentation, poultice, wash, or sitz bath to the affected area.

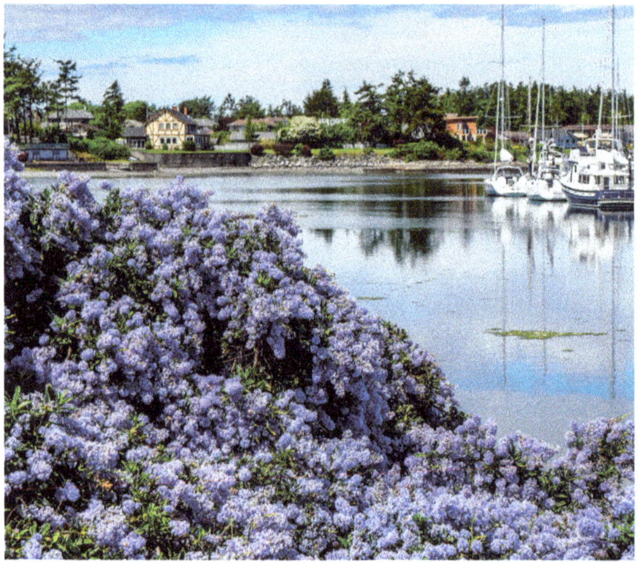

REISHI MUSHROOM

DESCRIPTION

BOTANICAL NAMES:
Ganoderma lucidum (syn. *Polyporus japonicum*), *G. japonicum* (syn. *G. sinense*), *G. capense*, *G. applanatum*, *G. oregonense*, *G. tsugae*

COMMON NAMES:
Reishi, reishi mushroom, ambrosia polypore, mannentake, holy mushroom, miraculous chi, ten-thousand-year mushroom, good omen plant, auspicious herb, plant of immortality, varnished conk, red reishi
ling chi, ling zhi, chi zhi, (red) *ling zhi,* (purple) *ling zhi, zi zhi, zi chih* (Mandarin)[1]

FAMILY NAME:
Ganodermataceae
(formerly Polyporaceae)

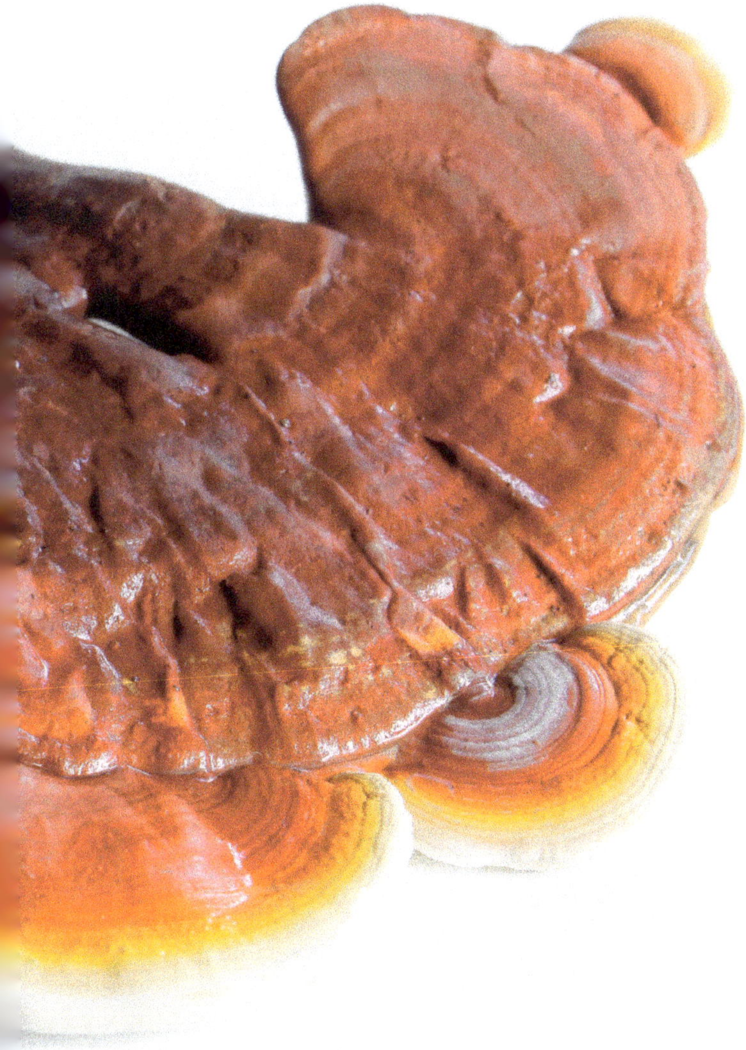

PARTS USED: The fruiting body and mycelium.

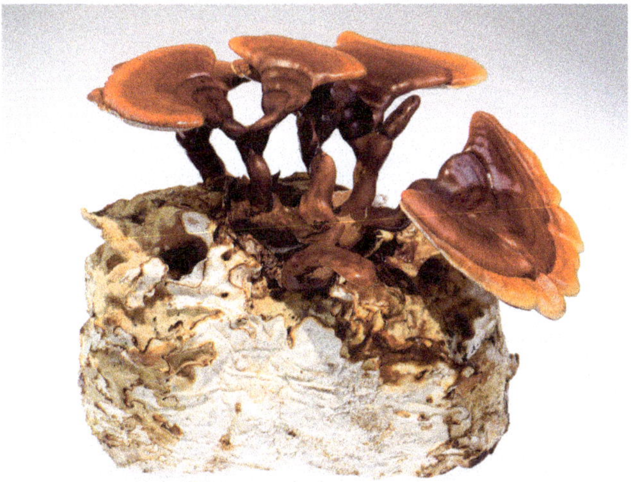

BOTANICAL DESCRIPTION AND HABITAT: Usually found at the base of hardwood trees (rarely on conifers), *Ganoderma lucidum* is an annual polypore mushroom found worldwide in tropical and temperate locales.[2] It commonly grows on maples on the U.S. East Coast, and can be parasitic or saprophytic.[2] The cap (2 – 20+ cm wide and 4 – 8 cm thick) has a soft, corky texture when fresh, and a highly variable shape including circular, fan, and kidney, depending on the climate and location.[2,3] The smooth, shiny upper surface crust, commonly described as "varnished," is sometimes concentrically grooved. It is mostly dark reddish-brown, although when young it can also be yellowish to whitish towards the margin.[2,3] The inner flesh is brown.[2]

Brown spores are released through pores on the underside of the cap, which is whitish when fresh, but turns brown as the mushroom ages or is bruised.[2] The shiny smooth, dark red stipe (3 – 14 cm long, 0.5 – 3 cm thick) is usually offset, although it occasionally grows out of the center underside.[2] Under conditions of high carbon dioxide levels, low light, and high humidity, reishi can grow in an antler form with many branching stipes and no obvious cap. In this form the spores are released through pores at the apex of the stalks.[4]

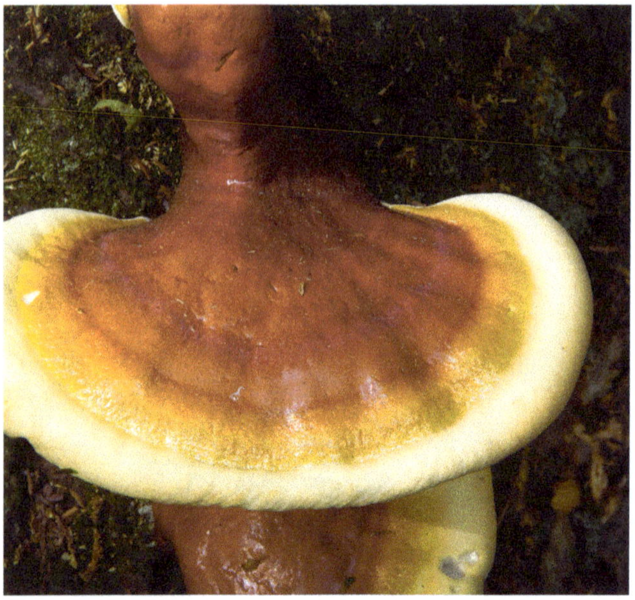

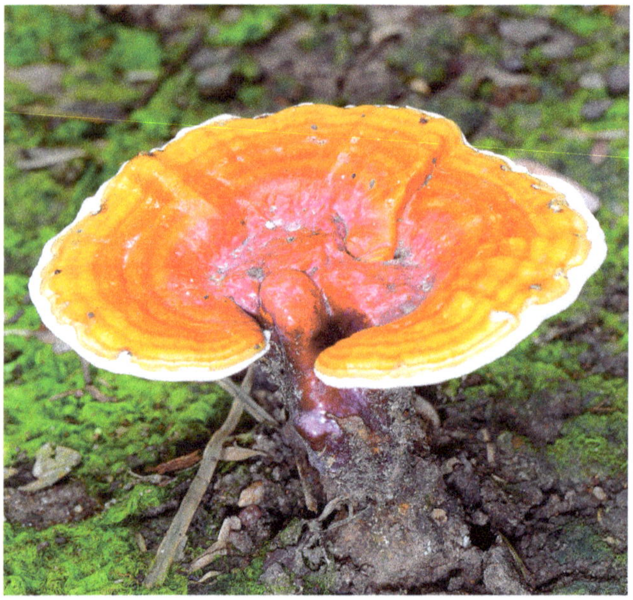

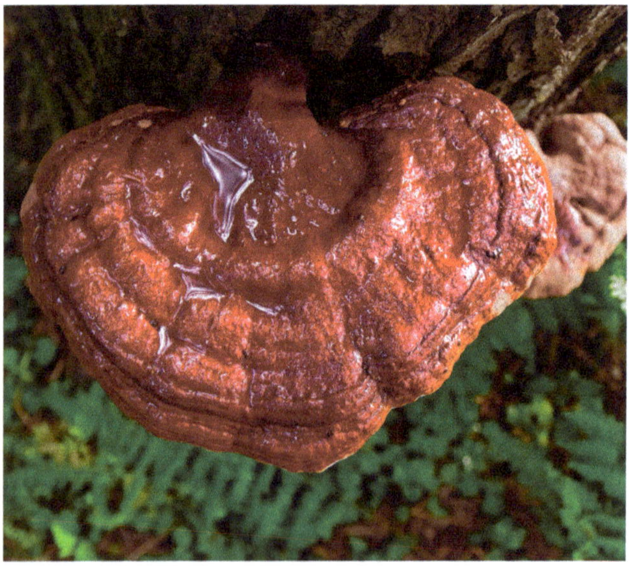

THE NAME: The genus *Ganoderma* means "lustrous skin," and the epithet *lucidum* means "shiny" or "brilliant."[1] The Latin binomial *G. lucidum* refers to the glossy, smooth coating on the top portion of the mushroom. The epithets *sinense* ("Chinese") and *japonicus* ("Japanese") indicate the origin of the mushroom. Reishi is a Japanese name for *G. lucidum.* The Chinese name for *G. lucidum,* ling zhi, is loosely translated as spirit, spiritual, shaman's tree fungus, or spiritual potency.[2] In Japan, reishi is also called mannentake ("ten-thousand-year mushroom"), referring to its use in promoting longevity.[1] *G. lucidum* is known as ling zhi, chi zhi, and red reishi; *G. japonicum* is known as zi zhi, zi chih, purple ling zhi, and black reishi.[5]

HISTORICAL USES: The earliest uses of reishi (ling zhi) were recorded in the *Shen Nong Ben Cao Jing* (200 BCE – 100 CE).[1] From this period on, emperors enlisted the efforts of thousands of laborers to search for reishi mushrooms on the Eastern Sea islands, and in their imperial palaces.[1] In China, reishi was revered as an "elixir of life" and a "fungus of immortality" reserved for emperors and the affluent.[5] The virtues of reishi were later extolled in the *Supplement to Classic of Materia Medica* (502 – 536 CE) and the *Ben Cao Gang Mu* (1590 CE) by Li Shin-Zhen.[6]

Japanese and Chinese herbalists administered reishi to treat insomnia and nervousness.[1] Reishi was prescribed to increase stamina and intellectual capacity, improve memory, and reduce forgetfulness and chronic fatigue.[1,6] It was recommended to improve musculoskeletal afflictions, such as a stiff neck, stiff shoulders, muscle weakness, and rheumatism, and to strengthen tendons and bones.[1,5] Reishi also was administered to treat a cough, asthma, debility, and general weakness.[1,5] By the 1930s, reishi was prescribed to treat bronchitis, liver diseases, kidney inflammation, hypertension, gastric ulcers, and poisoning.[1,5] Reishi was used as a talisman to protect individuals and their homes against evil.[7]

CONSTITUENTS: Red reishi mushroom *(G. lucidum)* contains ergosterol, sterols (β-sitosterol, 24-methylcholestra-7,22-dien-3-β-ol, and others), fungal lysozyme, enzymes (acid protease, laccase, endopolygalacturonase, cellulase, and amylase), water-soluble protein, polypeptides, amino acids, sugars, mannitol, betaine, adenosine, alkanes (tetracosane and hentriacontane), fatty acids (tetracosanoic, stearic, palmitic, nonadecanoic, and behenic acids), triterpenes of the lanostane type (ganoderic acids A-Z), lucidenic acids (A-G, and others), lucidones (A-C), ganolucidic acids (A-E), ganoderal A, ganoderiols (A-I), ganoderol A = ganodermanonol and B = ganodermadiol, ganodermanontriol, ganodermatriol, and polysaccharides (arabinoxyloglucan, heterolglycan, heteroglucan, and ganoderans A and B).[1,5,7] Reishi spores contain choline, betaine, tetracosanoic acid, stearic acid, palmitic acid, ergosta-7,22-dien-3β-ol, nonadecanoic acid, behinic acid, tetracosane, hentriacontane, ergosterol, and β-sitosterol.[7] *G. lucidum* mycelium contains sterols, lactones, alkaloids, polysaccharides, and triterpenenes.[7]

Purple reishi *(G. japonicum)* contains ergosterol, ergosta-7,22-dien-3-β-ol, trehalose, alkaloids (betaine and γ-butyrobetaine), 14 free amino acids, glucosamine, resin, and polysaccharides.[5]

NUTRITIONAL PROPERTIES: Red reishi contains amino acids, riboflavin, calcium, magnesium, sodium, manganese, iron, zinc, copper, germanium, ascorbic acid, and a small amount of protein.[5,7]

MEDICINAL PROPERTIES: Adaptogen, antiallergenic, antibacterial, anti-inflammatory, antioxidant, antitumor, antiviral, calmative, cardiotonic, hepatodetoxifier, hepatoprotectant, immune modulator, immune stimulant, vasodilator, qi tonic, and shen tonic.

TEMPERATURE AND FLAVOR: Warm, bitter, and mildly sweet.

MEDICINAL USES

An adaptogen, reishi enhances immune function and homeostatic mechanisms, and counters the detrimental effects of stress.[1] The adaptogenic actions are attributed to the triterpenes.[7] Reishi is a qi tonic that increases energy and decreases fatigue. It works most effectively when consumed long-term. The studies mentioned in this monograph were completed using *G. lucidum,* unless otherwise noted. *G. japonicum, G. capense, G. applanatum, G. oregonense,* and *G. tsugae* have qualitative and quantitative differences from *G. lucidum.*[7] They have therapeutic actions; however, they should not be considered substitutes for *G. lucidum* until further studies are completed.

Reishi increases resistance to pathogens and chronic disease. It contains immune modulating polysaccharides that stimulate macrophage, monocyte, and helper T cell response. These immune cells aid in destroying bacteria, viruses, and tumor cells.[1,8] The polysaccharides have anti-carcinogenic and desmutagenic properties.[1] They increase cancer-inhibiting compounds, including tumor necrosis factor, interleukins 1, 2, and 6, and Th1 T lymphocytes.[6-8] The polysaccharides also increase DNA synthesis of spleen cells in mixed lymphocyte culture, and RNA and DNA synthesis in the bone marrow of mice.[7] Combining reishi with vitamin C may improve outcomes, demonstrated by Japanese surgeon and researcher, Dr. Fukumi Morishige, who frequently collaborated with Linus Pauling to research vitamin C. Morishige found that combining ten grams of vitamin C per day (a very high dose, as most American medical sources advise a maximum of two grams daily) with polysaccharides increased their bioavailability.[1] β-d-glucan is an antitumor and immune stimulating polysaccharide.[1,7] β-D-glucan binds with specific neutrophil receptors, activating receptor recognition of cancer

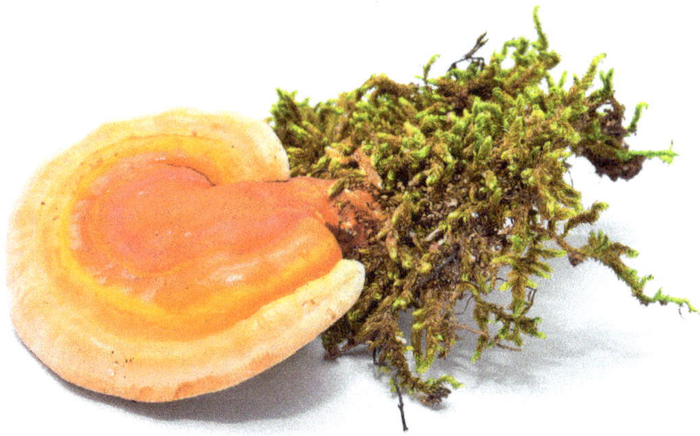

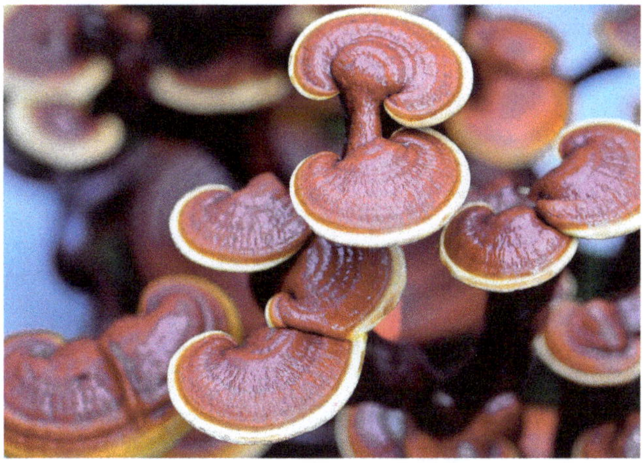

as foreign. Monoclonal antibodies and the complement system encourage activated neutrophils to invade the cancer site, improving the immune system's defenses.[6] Reishi increases total T cell counts, and restores helper T cell to suppresser T cell ratios.[1]

Reishi can be utilized as an adjunct for conventional cancer treatment. It reduces surgical complications, hastens surgical wound healing, restores blood cell counts, and shortens recovery time in cancer patients following surgery.[1] Reishi improves the tolerance and effectiveness of chemotherapy, and helps to treat leucopenia induced by

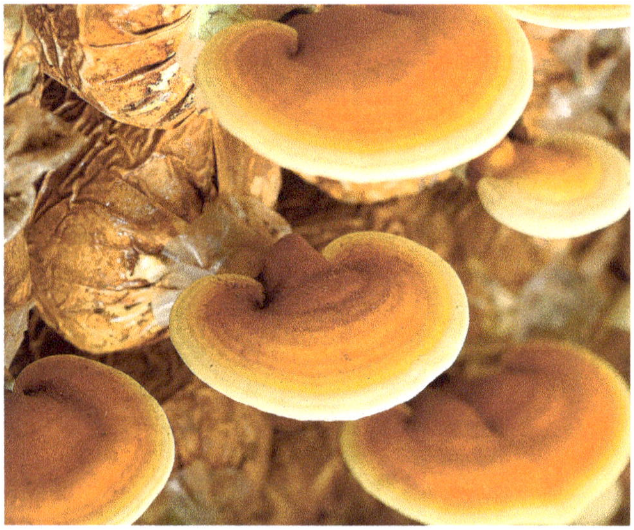

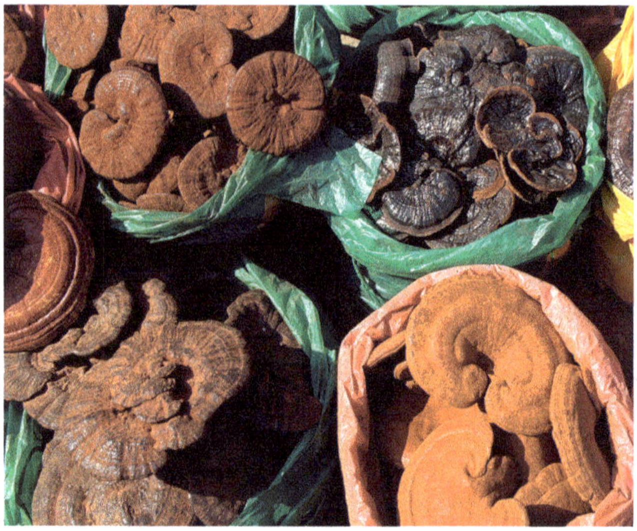

chemotherapy or radiation.[1,6] It reduces the toxicity and side effects of chemotherapy and radiation therapy, such as dizziness, weakness, and insomnia.[1,6] It also decreases the incidence of secondary infections.[1] Combining vitamin C (6 – 12 grams daily) with reishi extract following surgery aids in treating cancer in the lungs, brain, breasts, rectum, liver, pancreas, and kidneys.[1] Patients with myeloblastic leukemia undergoing conventional treatments consumed three grams of reishi extract, three times daily for three months. Their blood cell counts were nearly restored, and remission continued eight months following treatment.[1] Ganoderic acids T-Z demonstrated antitumor activity against hepatoma (liver tumor) cells.[7] Hundreds of studies have been conducted confirming multiple modes of action of *G. lucidum* and its constituents against numerous types of cancer.

Reishi is a superb long-term treatment for reducing the severity of inflammatory conditions such as allergy-induced rhinitis, asthma, and eczema, and for autoimmune conditions.[1,5,7] It has antiallergenic actions inhibiting the release of histamines and passive cutaneous anaphylaxis reaction that aid in treating asthma and contact dermatitis.[1,5] Ganoderic acids A, C, and D, as well as oleic acid and cyclooctasulphur are attributed to the antihistaminic actions.[5,7] Reishi has a stabilizing effect on immunoglobulins. It decreases the allergic response by lowering elevated immunoglobulin E (IgE) levels in individuals with allergies.[1,7] Additionally, reishi restores the beneficial immunoglobulins (IgA, IgG, and IgM) in individuals with lower levels.[1,7] IgG is an antibody that neutralizes toxins and enhances cell digesting activity of the macrophages. IgG deficiency is associated with recurring upper respiratory tract infections, as well as endocrine gland abnormalities. Reishi increases secretory IgA levels, a beneficial immunoglobulin in the respiratory tract. IgA deficiency is associated with severe allergies and recurring respiratory tract infections such as bronchitis.[1] In clinical studies, patients with chronic bronchitis consumed a tablet form of reishi syrup; 60 – 90% of them, especially those with bronchial asthma, experienced marked improvement in two weeks.[7]

Reishi's potent anti-inflammatory actions may be due in part to its free radical scavenging effects.[1] Studies at the Beijing College of Traditional Chinese Medicine demonstrated that large doses of reishi enhance the blood's free radical scavenging action (by 50.4%) against the free radical hydroxyl. Ganoderic acids A, B, C_2, and D exhibit the most potent anti-inflammatory actions.[1]

Reishi has potent antiviral actions that aid in treating subacute and chronic viral conditions. It also hastens recovery from the Epstein Barr virus.[7] Reishi contains substances that significantly decrease HIV activity by inhibiting the ability of the virus to multiply.[1,7] It aids in treating human papilloma virus (HPV) which causes chronic genital inflammation, and is associated with cervical cancer in females, and infertility in males.[1] Reishi also has antibacterial effects on *Bacillus pneumonia, Staphylococcus,* and *Streptococcus.*[7,8]

Reishi is a hepatoprotective agent. Three isolated substances found in the mycelium, ganoderic acids R and S (and the less active ganoderic T), stimulate liver cell function and have potent antihepatotoxic actions.[1] Ganodosterone was also found to stimulate liver function. In China, reishi is administered to treat acute and chronic hepatitis. It is most effective in treating acute hepatitis with less severely impaired liver function.[1] Optimal results were obtained in treatments of acute hepatitis when 20 ml of reishi syrup were consumed twice daily for four to 12 weeks.[1] In Japan, scientists found that extract of reishi mycelium, administered in 50 gram doses three times daily for six months, successfully treated liver failure.[1] At the MARA Institute of Technology in Malaysia, reishi extract (two grams in capsules, three times daily for three months) was administered to patients with hepatitis B. Blood tests revealed that their liver enzyme levels (SGOT and SGPT levels) were restored to normal, and all patients showed seroconversion and production of the antibodies to virus.[1,7]

Reishi has subtle calming effects on the nervous system, reducing anxiety, insomnia, and stress-related symptoms.[7] In Traditional Chinese Medicine, reishi is administered to treat shen disturbance that results in anxiety, insomnia, dream-disturbed sleep, poor memory, and moodiness.[8] Studies in China demonstrated that consuming reishi extract for four months calmed nervous excitability in 90% of patients.[1] Reishi also has muscle relaxant, sedative, anticonvulsive, and analgesic effects attributed to adenosine; however, it is not a narcotic or hypnotic.[1,5] Long-term consumption of reishi extract promotes slow wave sleep.[1] In China, reishi extract is prescribed for neurological afflictions characterized by muscular weakness, such as weakness and lassitude following prolonged illness or anorexia, as well as neurasthenia.[1] Japanese studies demonstrate that extracts of reishi aid in treating Alzheimer's disease and neuroses caused by "environmental stress."[1]

Reishi is a cardiotonic, improving coronary blood flow, and reducing oxygen consumption in the heart muscles.[1,5] It is beneficial for treating hypotension, hypertension, arrhythmia (irregular heartbeat), dyspnea (difficulty breathing), and angina (heart pain), as well as reducing a sensation of fullness in the chest.[1,5,7] Reishi aids in treating hyperlipidemia (elevated concentration of blood fats and cholesterol).[7,8] It reduces low density lipids (LDLs), very low density lipids (VLDLs), total cholesterol, and triglyceride levels.[8] Reishi contains triterpenes, ganoderols A and B, and ganoderic acids B, D, F, H, K, S, and Y that have hypotensive effects.[1,5] The triterpenes also lower cholesterol. Adenosine and triterpenes inhibit platelet aggregation.[1,5,7] In one study, nearly three-fourths of patients experienced restored cholesterol levels after consuming two to three tablets of reishi extract and mandarin peel extract, three times daily for three months. Three tablets contained one gram of reishi extract and two grams of mandarin orange peel extract.[1] Studies in Japan indicate that consuming six reishi extract tablets (240 mg each) per day for six months lowered total cholesterol in patients with essential (congenital) hypertension. The reishi extract tablets reduced mild hypertension, restoring normal blood pressure in systolic and diastolic readings.[1] Reishi also demonstrated antiatherosclerotic actions, preventing the accumulation of fatty deposits (plaque) on arterial walls, aiding in preventing heart attack and stroke.[1] It is a vasodilator, increasing circulation and enhancing oxygen and nutrient delivery to tissues.[5]

Consuming a concentrated reishi extract a minimum of six weeks reduces altitude sickness.[1] Reishi improves tolerance to low oxygen environments.[1] Studies demonstrated that prophylactic consumption of reishi extract tablets (three tablets, twice daily) significantly decreased altitude sickness and associated symptoms such as headaches and vomiting.[1]

In rodent studies, reishi demonstrated hypoglycemic actions in hyperglycemic mice attributed to polysaccharides (especially ganoderans A and B).[1,5,7] These studies found that ganoderan B caused the increase in plasma insulin levels.[1] Further studies are necessary to determine the effects *in vivo*.

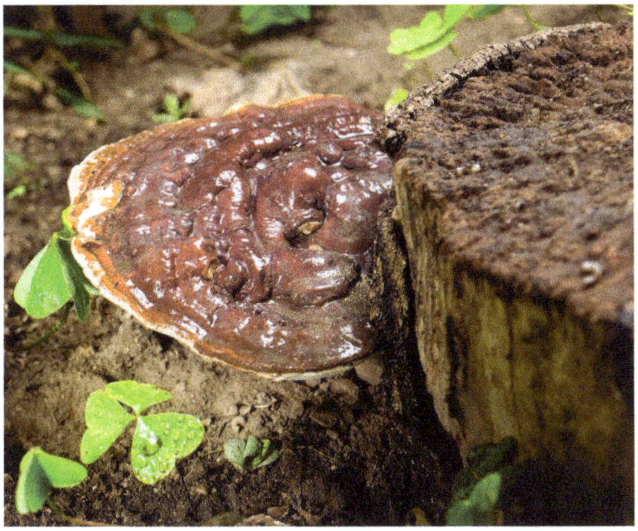

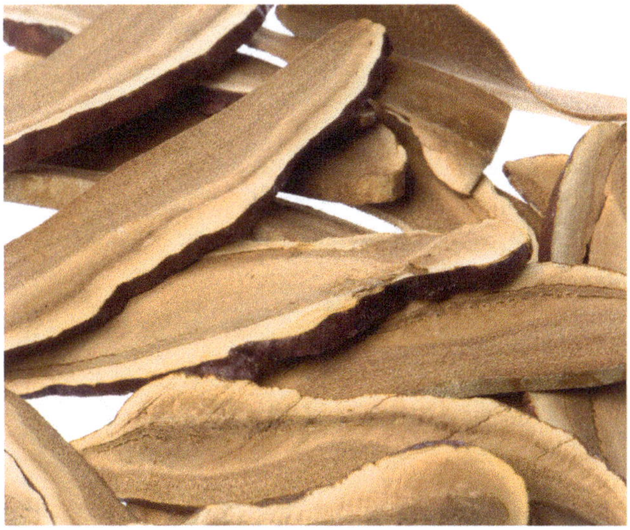

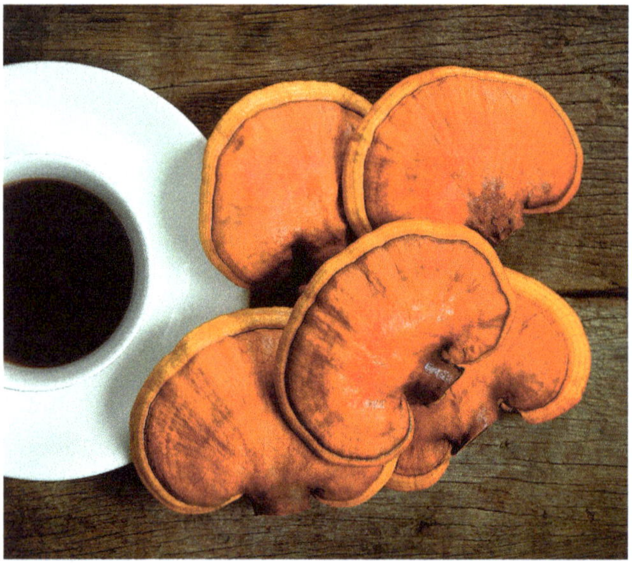

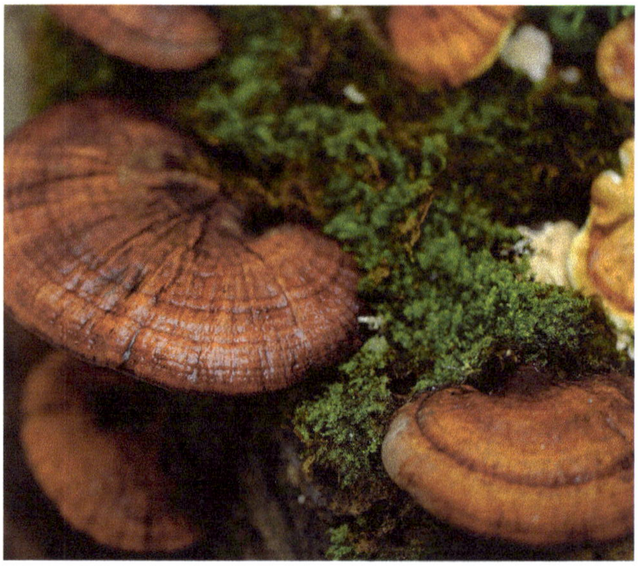

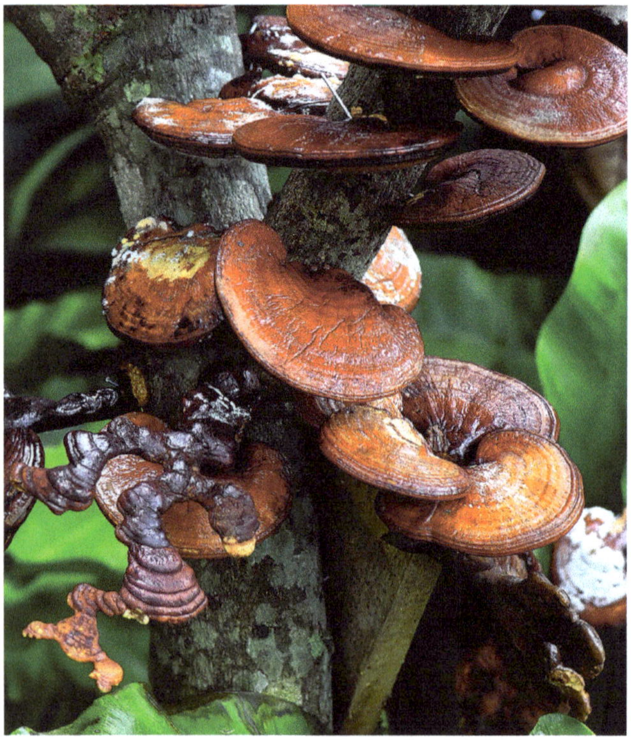

CONTRAINDICATIONS

Side effects are extremely rare; however, symptoms including dry mouth, dry throat, nosebleeds, dizziness, stomach upset, bloody stools, and pruritus have been noted following continuous long-term consumption (3 - 6 months).[5] Some individuals have allergic reactions to the fruiting body and/or spores.[7] Avoid consuming reishi during an acute infectious illness or menstruation.

PREPARATION AND DOSAGE

TINCTURE: Fresh fruiting bodies or mycelia [1:2 - 1:4, 50 - 60% alcohol]; dry fruiting bodies or mycelia [1:5, 20 - 30% alcohol] or [1:5, 50% alcohol, 30% water and 20% glycerin]; consume 20 - 90 drops, up to three times daily.

POWDERED EXTRACT: According to herbalist Donald Yance, "for optimal therapeutic activity [reishi] should be used in a powdered extract [15:1] whereby the water-soluble polysaccharides have been pulled out, followed by an alcohol extraction to extract the triterpenes. It should then be concentrated to yield 10 - 14 percent polysaccharides and 4 percent triterpenes."[6] Consume 1 - 4 grams of powdered extract daily.

CAPSULES: Consume 2 - 6 capsules of the fruiting body or mycelium, one to three times daily. Consume 3 - 9 tablets, up to three times daily. Consuming reishi with up to three grams of vitamin C per day increases its bioavailability.

TEA: Prepare a decoction; consume 8 - 12 ounces, one to three times daily.

HONEY AND SYRUP: Consume 4 - 6 milliliters of reishi syrup daily.

ROSE

DESCRIPTION

BOTANICAL NAMES:
Rosa canina, R. californica, R. centifolia, R. damascena, R. gallica, R. rugosa, R. villosa, R. spp.

COMMON NAMES:
Rose, rose petals, rose buds, rose hips, rosehips, hip berries, queen of flowers
ward (Arabic)
vard, vart (Armenian)
roza (Bulgarian)
roos (Dutch)
gul, gol (Farsi)
ruusu (Finish)
triantafillo (Greek)
vered (Hebrew)
gulab (Hindi)
rózsa (Hungarian)
rós (Icelandic)
mawar (Indonesian)
rosa (Italian)
rozu (Japanese)
roju (Korean)
mei gwai (Mandarin)
gulaf (Nepali)
gul (Persian)
róża (Polish)
rosa (Portguese)
roza (Russian)
śata-patrī (Sanskrit)
rosa (Spanish)
ros (Swedish)
kulaap-on (Thai)
hoa hu'ò'ng (Vietnamese)
royz (Yiddish)

FAMILY NAME:
Rosaceae

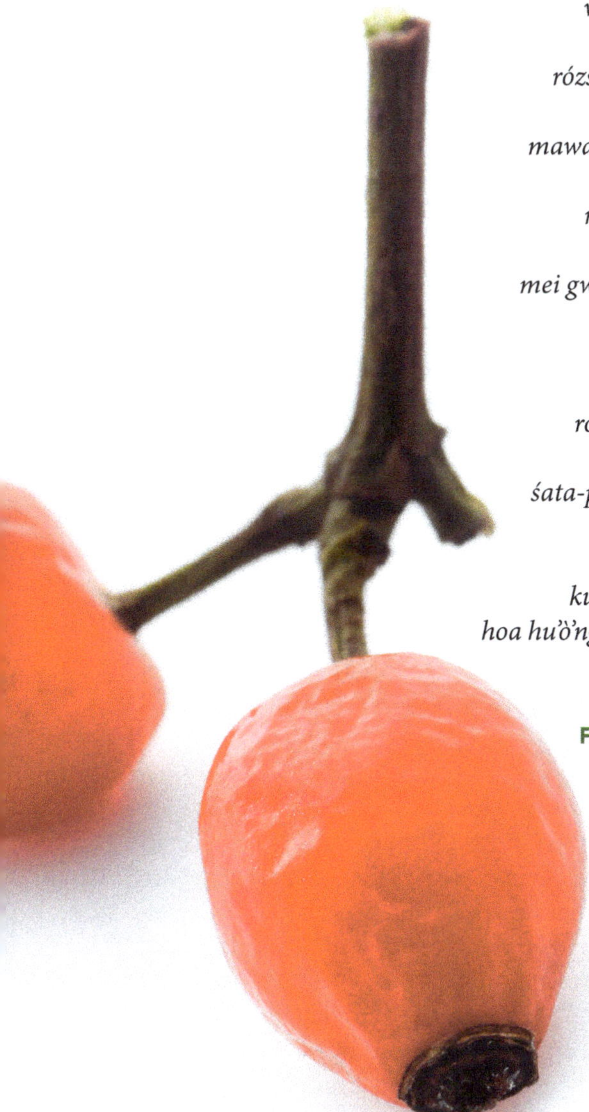

PARTS USED: The buds, petals, leaves, and fruit (rose hips). Rose leaves are a substitute if budding flowers or petals are not available.

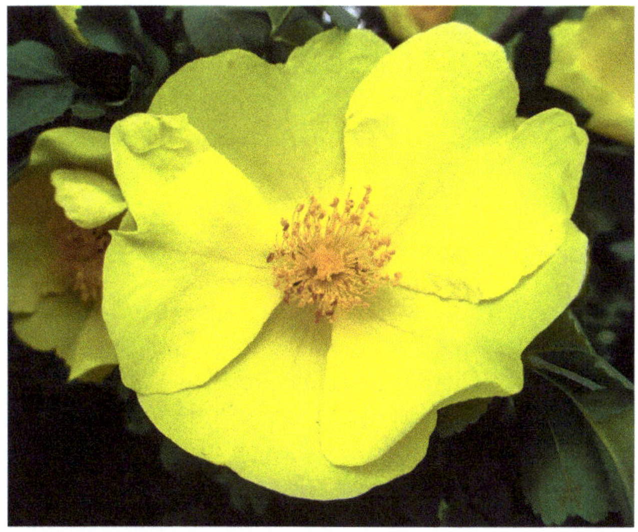

BOTANICAL DESCRIPTION AND HABITAT: Wild rose grows in shady, moist areas such as stream banks and mixed evergreen forests throughout the northern hemisphere. *Rosa* is a large genus of woody shrubs and vines usually bearing sturdy prickles.[1] The odd-pinnate leaves have distinctive stipules fused to the petiole.[2]

Found solitary or in clusters, the flower has an urn-shaped hypanthium and five sepals. Wild roses have a simple elegance, bearing five petals; cultivated varieties may have many more. California natives have pink petals; those from other regions can be white, yellow, pink, or red.[1,3] They have many stamens and separate pistils. Numerous seed-like achenes, the true fruits, are found inside the fleshy red rose hip. The hip is a false fruit, globose to ellipsoid, usually crowned by remnants of the sepals.

THE NAME: *Rosa* derives from the Greek *rodon* ("red").[4] The epithet *canina* originates from the Latin *caninus* ("pertaining to a dog or dogs"), referring to the belief that rose roots could cure rabies.[5] *Gallica* derives from the Latin *gallicus* ("pertaining to gaul or the gauls"). *Rugosa* stems from the Latin *rugosus* ("wrinkled"), referring to the leaves' reticulate venation prominent underneath, with corresponding creases on the upper side. The epithet *villosa* originates from the Latin *villosus* ("shaggy"). Hip, the name

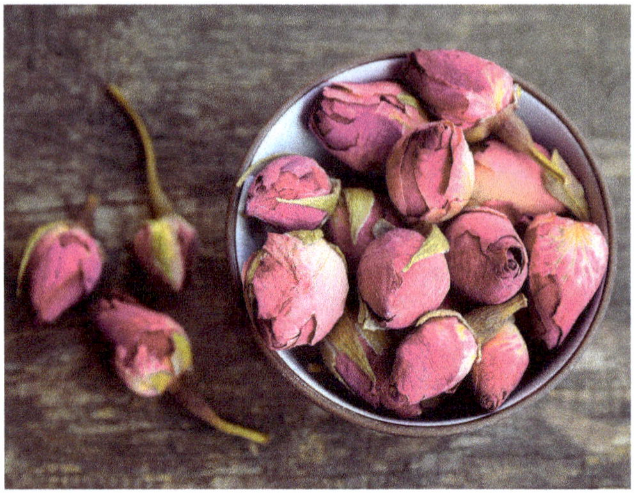

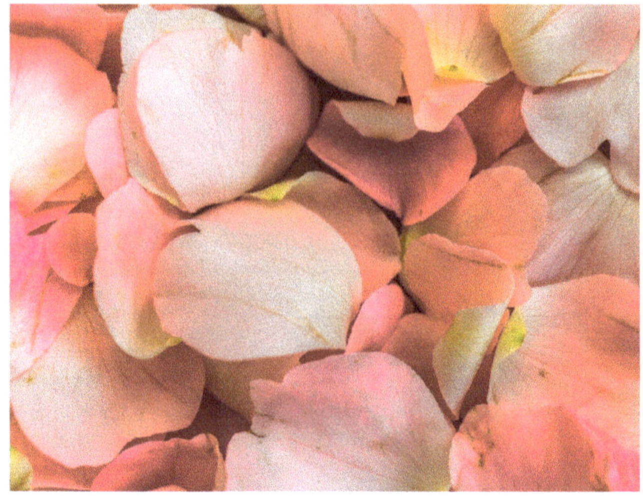

for the fruit, derives from the Anglo-Saxon *hiope* ("flask shaped").[4]

HISTORICAL USES: Ancient Greeks, Romans, and Persians used roses for food and medicine. The ancient Greeks were believed to introduce roses to southern Italy.[5] Romans decorated banquets with roses, floated rose petals in wine, and strewed rose petals on floors.[4] Brides and grooms were adorned with rose crowns. Roses decorated the prows of war vessels, and were cast before victors and their chariots. Romans believed that wearing rose garlands at lavish feasts would prevent drunkenness.[4] Suspending a rose above a dinner table was believed to assure confidentiality.[4] Romans introduced roses to England where they became the national emblem.[5] In one English custom, a rose bush was planted on the grave of a lover who died before marriage.[5]

Prepared rose confection (made by pulverizing one pound of fresh rose petals in three pounds of sugar) was administered to alleviate a cough or pulmonary bleeding.[4] Rose was given to treat pharyngitis and stomatitis.[4] Rose syrup and infusion were used to flavor less pleasant tasting medicines. The lotion was applied for ophthalmia.[4] A fomentation containing roses steeped in distilled vinegar was applied to the head to treat a headache caused by sun overexposure. The French prepared rose liqueur by distilling wine infused with rose petals, then mixing it with sugar.[4] Cold cream, an ointment made with rose water, was applied to reduce inflammation and soothe chapped hands, face, and abrasions.[4] Rose water was used topically to reduce eye inflammation.[4] An ointment or poultice was applied to pimples and sores.

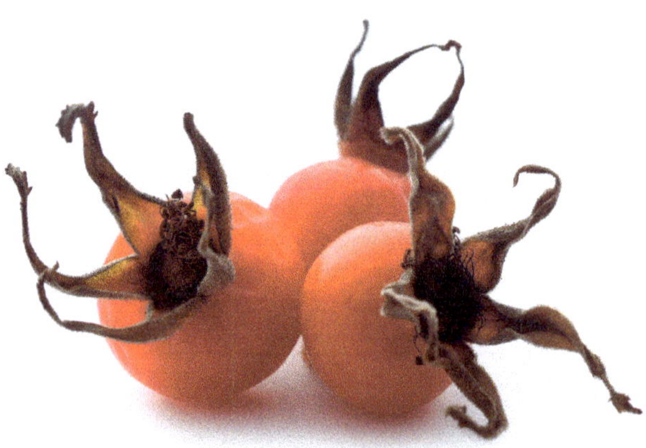

Europeans gathered and consumed wild rose hips during World War II to prevent scurvy.[5] Rose hips were recognized as a rich source of vitamin C.

Culpeper administered rose electuary to treat fevers, jaundice, and joint pain.[4] He prescribed rose syrup to cool an overheated liver, comfort the heart, and treat putrefaction and infection.[4] Rose conserve was given to strengthen the heart and spirit. Rose honey was diluted and gargled, and applied to mouth and throat sores. Culpeper prescribed rose hips as a restorative and expectorant in patients with consumption, and for its binding effects in digestion.[4]

A popular and elegant fragrance, rose perfume was originally prepared by infusing rose petals in lard (pomade). In the 10th century, Avicenna prepared distilled rose water.[4] Rose oil (rose otto) was developed in the late 1500s in Persia.[4]

Native Americans consumed rose hip tea to treat a sore throat, cold, fever, indigestion, kidney problems, and diarrhea, and to cleanse sores.[6] The Blackfoot prepared a root decoction to treat diarrhea, worms, dysentery, and flu.[7] The roots and leaves were ingested as a spring tonic.[7] Rose petal tea was consumed by the Okanagan-Colville in sweat lodges, and applied as a body and hair wash.[6] In the spring, tender leaf shoots were consumed.[8] Leaf poultices were applied to bee stings and abscesses.[8] An eye wash was used to treat sore eyes and cataracts, and improve eyesight.[8] Roots were applied to alleviate headaches and rheumatism.[7] Rose galls were valued for burns; they were charred, powdered, and dusted onto the skin.[7] Dried rose leaves were added to smoking mixtures.[8]

When ripe, rose hips were consumed sparingly by Pacific Northwest coastal tribes, including the Cowichan, Saanich, Ditidaht, Nuu-chah-multh, and Makah.[8] The fruits were steamed, mashed, and fed to infants with diarrhea.[8] The fruit's outer rind was consumed, but not the seeds which are covered in tiny hairs that aggravate the digestive tract.[8]

CONSTITUENTS

ROSE PETALS: Rose petals contain tannins, volatile oil (geraniol, citronellol, nerol, and highly aromatic 2-phenylethanol), flavonoids (anthocyanins and flavonols), quercitrin, quercetin, organic acids (quinic acid), sugar, gum, and fat.[4,9,10] Rose leaves contain squalene, ethane, 1,1-diethoxy, β-D-glucopyranose, 1,6-anhydro, furfural, and 2-furancarboxaldehyde 5-(hydroxymethyl).

ROSE ESSENTIAL OIL: Rose essential oil contains geraniol, citronellol, nerol, β-phenethyl alcohol, geranic acid, and eugenol. It contains smaller amounts of terpene hydrocarbons (α- and β-pinene, and myrcene), esters, C_{14} to C_{23} η-paraffins, nerol oxide, (4R)-*cis*-rose oxide, (4R)-*trans*-rose oxide, 3-(4-methyl-3-pentenyl)-2-buten-4-olide, 3-methyl-4(3-methyl-2-butenyl)-2-buten-4-olide, *cis*- and *trans*-2-(3-methyl-2-butenyl)-3-methyl tetrahydrofuran, β-damascenone, 3-hydroxy-β-damascenone, and β-damascone.[9]

ROSE HIPS: Rose hips are rich in vitamin C (ascorbic acid). They also contain carotenoids (β-carotene, lutein, and lycopene), flavonoids (chiefly flavonols: quercetin, rutin, hesperidin, and kaempferol), pectin, organic acids (malic and citric acid), polyphenols, leucoanthocyanins, catechins, sugars (glucose, fructose, and sucrose), tannins (proanthocyanidins), 2-furancarboxaldehyde 5-(hydroxymethyl), β-D-glucopyranose, 1,6-anhydro, 4H-pyran-4-one, 2,3-dihydro-3,5-dihydroxy-6-methyl, 2,5-furandione, dihydro-3-methylene, furfural, and riboflavin.[9-12]

NUTRITIONAL PROPERTIES: Rose hips contain vitamin C (ascorbic acid), flavonoids (see above), and carotenoids. They also contain high amounts of β-carotene, chromium, niacin, riboflavin, selenium, sodium, thiamine, tin, crude fiber, and dietary fiber. Rose hips contain average amounts of calcium, fat, and phosphorus, and low amounts of cobalt, iron, magnesium, manganese, potassium, silicon, and zinc.[9-11]

MEDICINAL PROPERTIES: Rose petals are antibacterial, anti-inflammatory, astringent, and hemostatic. Rose hips are antioxidant, antiscorbutic, demulcent, nutritive, refrigerant, and mildly antibacterial and diuretic.

TEMPERATURE AND FLAVOR: Rose petals are cool, astringent, pungent, sweet, and sour. Rose hips are cool, sour, sweet, and salty.

MEDICINAL USES

Rose petals, buds, and leaves are astringent; rose hips are demulcent and emollient. Coined by herbalist Michael Moore, the acronym YARFA ("yet another rose family astringent") refers to the medicinal interchangeability of most medicinal plants in the Rosaceae family. Some examples of astringent herbs in this family include: red raspberry leaves *(Rubus idaeus)*, blackberry leaves and root

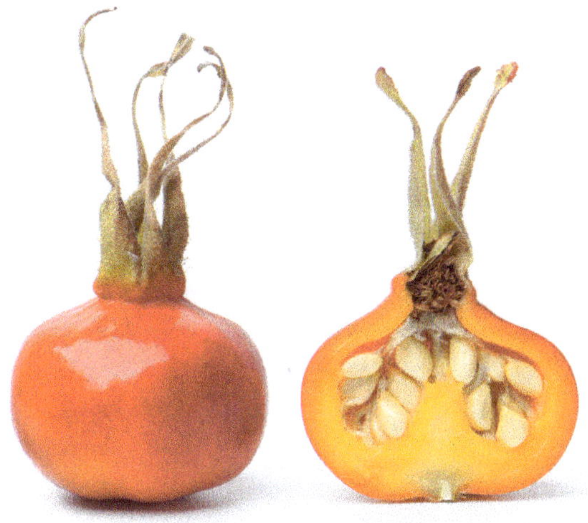

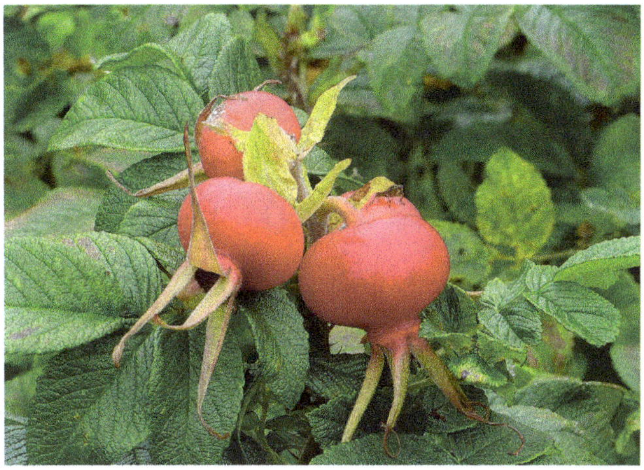

(Rubus villosus), lady's mantle *(Alchemilla)*, quinquefoil *(Potentilla)*, and agrimony *(Agrimonia)*.

ROSE PETALS: Rose petals, buds, and leaves are astringent, reducing inflammation in mucous membranes. A water-based preparation such as tea is a preferable application. Rose petal tea eases heartburn, stomach hyperacidity, ulcers, and enteritis.[13] Consuming a potent tea aids in treating diarrhea due to dysentery, giardia or candida.[13,14] However, additional anti-infective herbs are necessary to treat a microbial infection. Rose petals also decrease excessive secretions in the lungs and sinuses.

A local anti-inflammatory, rose petal tea can be utilized as a gargle, eye wash, vaginal irrigation, enema, fomentation, or poultice. An eye wash reduces inflammation in the eyelids, treating blepharitis, conjunctivitis, and watery eyes.[13,14] Additional anti-infectives are necessary to treat microbial infections. Gargling with tea eases a sore throat and mouth sores.[5] Vaginal irrigation reduces inflammation and leucorrhoea due to non-specific vaginitis, yeast infections, and excess vaginal secretions.[13] An enema reduces colon and rectal inflammation, and internal hemorrhoids. A sitz bath eases irritation in the labia, rectum, fissures, and hemorrhoids, and soothes tissues after childbirth. Topical applications of the fomentation, poultice, or hydrosol reduce itching and alleviate moist, weeping sores caused by acne, eczema, psoriasis, poison oak, and poison ivy.[13] Those applications also aid in treating rosacea, diaper rash, and varicose veins.

Rose is a hemostatic, reducing heavy menstrual, mid-cycle, postpartum, and menopausal bleeding. In Ayurvedic medicine, rose is used to clear *pitta* from the uterus and blood, treating dysmenorrhea, metrorrhagia, endometriosis, and fibroids.[13] It is used during the luteal phase (days 14–28) of the menstrual cycle to ease PMS symptoms, including irritability, emotional hypersensitivity, and heat.[13]

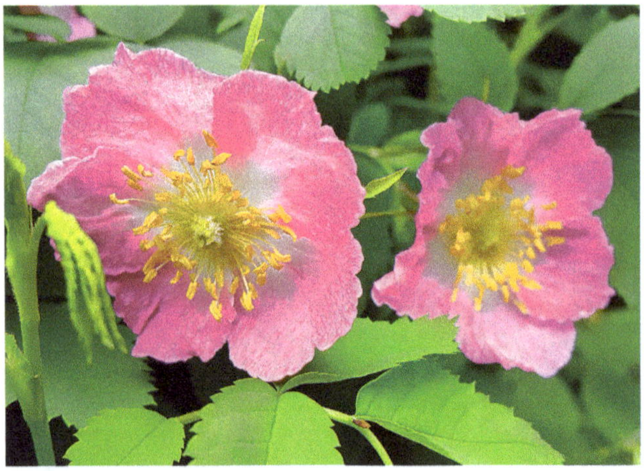

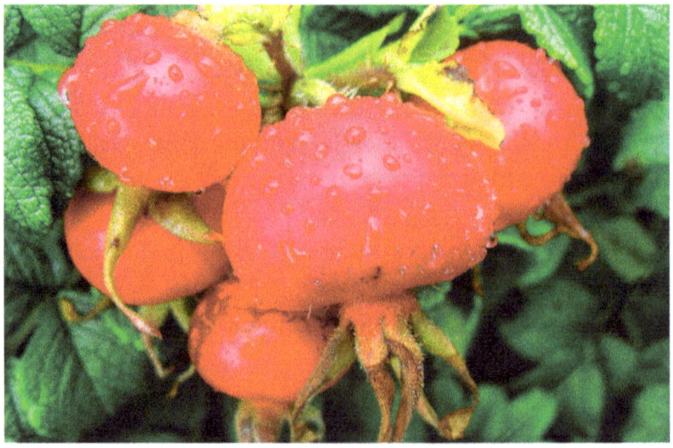

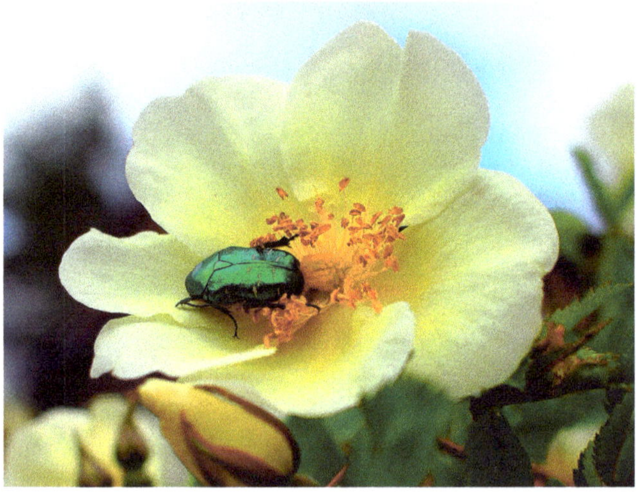

Rose has an affinity for the heart. It lifts the spirits, calms emotions, and soothes nerves.[13] It also eases anxiety and nervous depression.[13] According to Ayurvedic practitioner Sebastian Pole, "It opens the heart chakra *(anāhata)*, thus increasing patience, compassion, and love." Rose can be incorporated into cordials and elixirs as an aphrodisiac and to enhance flavor. Gulkand, rose petal jam, is used as a spread or added to tea.

ROSE ESSENTIAL OIL: Rose oil is obtained from the steam distillation of fresh flowers (rose otto), or petroleum ether extraction (rose absolute).[9,10] Due to the relatively low yield of essential oil, rose otto, rose absolute, and rose concrete are very expensive, but worth their attributes. Rose otto is more precious than absolute or concrete. Approximately 10,000 pounds of roses are distilled to obtain one pound of oil. However, a solvent extraction yields 10 pounds of concrete oil from the same poundage of fresh petals.[4] Thirty roses yield one drop of rose otto; 180 pounds of flowers are required to produce one ounce of rose otto.[4] Rose hydrosol (rose water) is the water portion of the distillate following the removal of rose oil. Its uses are similar to rose oil, but it is gentler and safer.

The following essential oil names correspond with the Latin binomials: Bulgarian rose oil, Bulgarian otto of rose, and Bulgarian attar of rose *(R. damascena* var. *alba);* Moroccan rose oil and Moroccan otto of rose *(R. centifolia);* Turkish rose oil, Turkish otto of rose, and Turkish attar of rose *(R. damascena);* French rose absolute and rose de mai absolute *(R. centifolia).*[9]

Rose oil or hydrosol calms the nervous system and aids in treating nervous exhaustion and anxiety. It is uplifting, easing nervous depression and heartbreak. Rose oil eases premenstrual and menopausal anxiety and irritability. The nervous system stabilizing effects are attributed to the monoterpene alcohol citronellol.[15]

Throughout the ages, rose was a symbol of love, sensuality, and sweetness. An aphrodisiac, rose aids in treating impotence and frigidity. Apply diluted rose oil or hydrosol to conjure its romantic virtues. Prepare an exotic aphrodisiac perfume by combining rose oils with neroli, jasmine, vanilla, tuberose, and/or sandalwood.

Topical applications of diluted rose oil or hydrosol soothe and regenerate the skin.[16] Rose is beneficial for all complexion types; however, the hydrosol is especially beneficial for treating moist skin conditions such as acne and eczema. Rose oil has potent antibacterial actions.[16] Spray rose hydrosol on the eyelids to alleviate eye inflammation; the spray is also helpful in easing hot flashes.[13]

ROSE HIPS: Rose hips provide a rich source of vitamin C, flavonoids, and carotenoids.[7,10] Flavonoids synergize vitamin C. Vitamin C and flavonoids support immune function and counter the adrenal-depleting effects of stress. Vitamin C enhances the integrity of connective tissue and reduces inflammation. Consumption of powdered *R. canina* decreases pain and inflammation from osteoarthritis.[5] Consuming rose hips improves skin elasticity and moisture, reducing age-related skin conditions and crow's feet wrinkles.[17] Rose hips prevent scurvy due to the vitamin C content.

Rose hips are a potent antioxidant. Vitamin C and flavonoids enhance the integrity of the vascular system and improve blood vessel elasticity, supporting heart and cardiovascular function. Rose hips reduce capillary fragility and permeability.[10] Long-term, daily consumption of rose hips aids in treating rosacea, varicose veins, allergies, atherosclerosis, hypertension, and diabetic complications. It also hastens bruise and wound healing. Rose hips are cytotoxic against cervical cancer (HeLa) and breast cancer (T47D) cells.[18] *Rosa rugosa* hips has moderate antibacterial actions.[18]

A decoction of rose hips is mucilaginous, coating and soothing the mucous membranes. A demulcent, the tea is beneficial for treating a sore throat, cold, or flu. The mucilage coats the mucous membranes throughout the digestive tract. The tea soothes digestive tissues after stomach flu, antibiotic use, dysentery, or giardiasis. It also has mild laxative effects. The organic acids (citric and malic) and pectin account for rose hips' subtle laxative and diuretic properties.[5,9]

Rose hips are high in pectin. Pectin is highly ionic and enhances the excretion of heavy metals (lead and mercury).[9] In laboratory animals, pectin demonstrated antihypercholesterolemic activity, and may aid in lowering cholesterol.[9]

Rose hips cool the body in feverish states and hot weather.[10] Consume a tea containing rose hips, hibiscus *(Hibiscus),* lemon grass *(Cymbopogon),* fresh lemon juice *(Citrus limon),* a pinch of sea salt, and a dab of honey for a refreshing, hydrating summer beverage. Rose hips (especially the seeds) have subtle diuretic actions.[9]

CONTRAINDICATIONS

Rose petals can be too astringent and drying for some individuals. Discontinue use if the mucous membranes become too dry, or in dehydrated individuals.

Strain rose hips tea through a paper or fine mesh filter, as the seeds are covered with fine hairs that can irritate the throat. *Note:* After commercial processing of rose hips, the remaining vitamin C content is questionable.

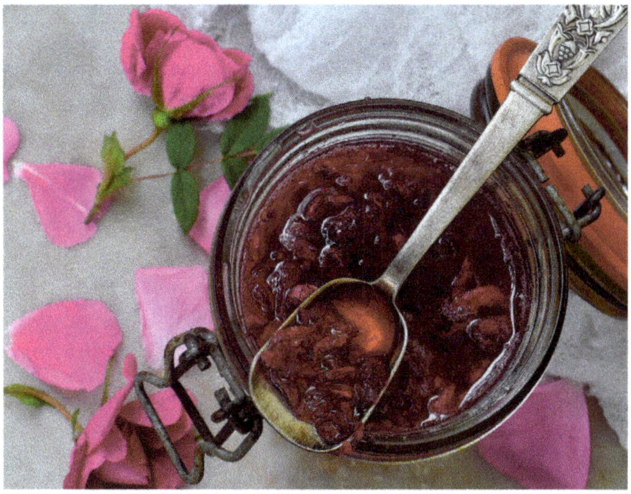

PREPARATION AND DOSAGE

TINCTURE: Fresh petals or hips [1:2-1:3, 60-95% alcohol]; dry petals or hips [1:5, 50-60% alcohol]; consume 10-60 drops, one to three times daily.

GLYCERITE: Fresh petals [1:2, 50% glycerin, 50% alcohol]; dry petals [1:5, 40% glycerin, 30% water, 30% alcohol]; consume 10-30 drops, up to three times daily.

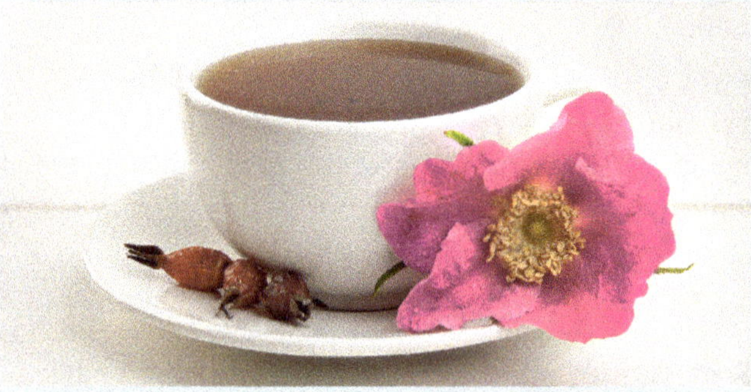

TEA: Prepare a hot infusion of the petals; consume 4-12 ounces, up to four times daily. For the hips, consume 8-12 ounces of the hot or cold infusion, or decoction three to four times daily. To obtain the nutrient content, the hot or cold infusion is ideal; however, the decoction extracts the most mucilage.

HONEY: Infuse fresh or recently dried rose petals in honey two to four weeks; strain the rose petals. Store in a cool, dark place. Add 1 teaspoon to tea, or use topically.

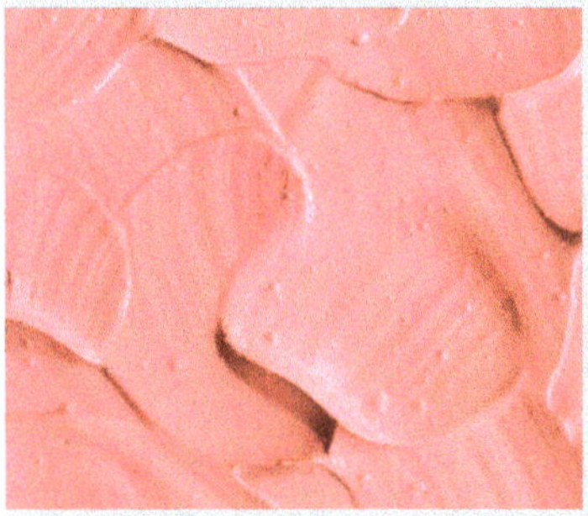

TOPICAL USE: Infuse the wilted or dry petals in oil. Use the oil to make a cream, salve, or lotion. Add dried petals to facial scrubs and body care products. Apply the infusion as a topical wash, eye wash, mouth rinse, gargle, vaginal irrigation, enema, or sitz bath. *Note:* Make sure to cool the tea to room temperature when treating sensitive areas such as the eyes, vagina, or rectum. Strain the tea through a coffee filter so the particulates do not irritate the tissues.

CULINARY USES: The fresh petals are edible and delicious. Prepare rose petal preserves (gulkand) by layering fresh rose petals with fine sugar; the sugar will draw fluid out of the petals, creating a fragrant preserve. Store and age in a closed container at least one month. Add ½-1 teaspoon to hot tea. Herbalist Terry Willard recommends wrapping a stick of butter in fresh rose petals, storing a few days, and spreading on baked goods.

Infuse fresh or dry petals in white wine overnight, strain, and drink. Infuse in brandy, tequila, or vodka; steep two to four weeks, strain and add honey or agave syrup for desired sweetness. The peeled, tender spring shoots are edible.

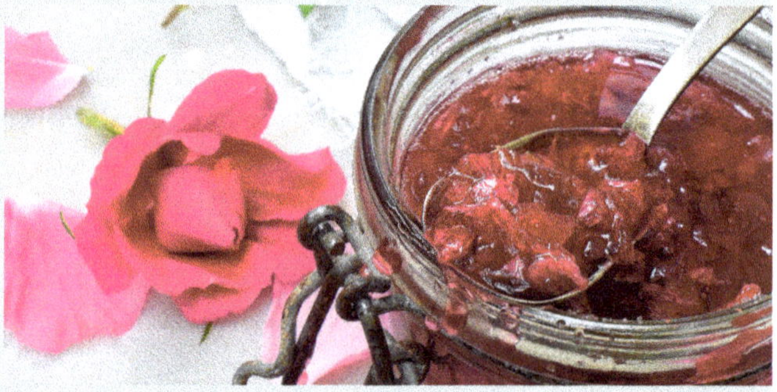

Prepare rose hips jam by placing one cup of cut, sifted, deseeded rose hips in a clean, dry mason jar. Cover with two cups of apple juice (or any non-citrus, unsweetened fruit juice) and steep overnight. Blend and store in a sealed container in the refrigerator one to two months. Consume 1 tablespoon, one to three times daily. Rose hips jam is a very effective way to obtain the nutrients and mucilage.

ROSEMARY

DESCRIPTION

BOTANICAL NAME:
Salvia rosmarinus (syn. *Rosmarinus officinalis*)

COMMON NAMES:
Rosemary, Our Lady's rose, dew of the sea, sea dew, old man, polar plant, compass weed, compass plant
ikleel al-jabal (Arabic)
khngooni (Armenian)
rozmarin (Bulgarian, Romanian, Russian, Yiddish)
maih diht heung (Cantonese)
ruzmarin (Croatian, Serbian)
rozmaryn lékarsky (Czech)
rosmarin (Danish)
rosemarijn (Dutch)
rosmareno (Esperanto)
rosmariin (Estonian)
rosmariini (Finnish)
insensier, romarin, rosmarin (French)
rosmarin (German)
rozmari (Greek)
rosmarin (Hebrew)
rozmaring (Hungarian)
rósmarín (Icelandic)
ramerino, rosmarino (Italian)
rozmarinas (Lithuanian)
mi die xiang (Mandarin)
rosmarin (Norwegian)
rozmaryn (Polish, Ukranian)
alacrim (Portuguese)
rusmari (Sanskrit)
romero, romerillo del llano, rosmario (Spanish)
rosmarin (Swedish)
rosmari (Thai)
biberiye, hasalban (Turkish)
lá hu'o'ng thao (Vietnamese)[1,2]

FAMILY NAME:
Lamiaceae (Labiatae)

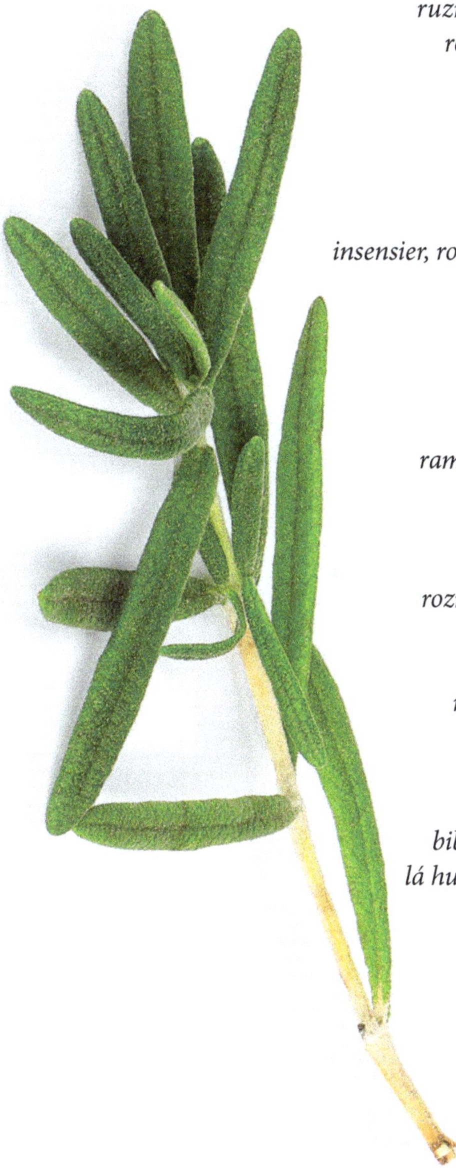

PARTS USED: The leaves and flowering tops.

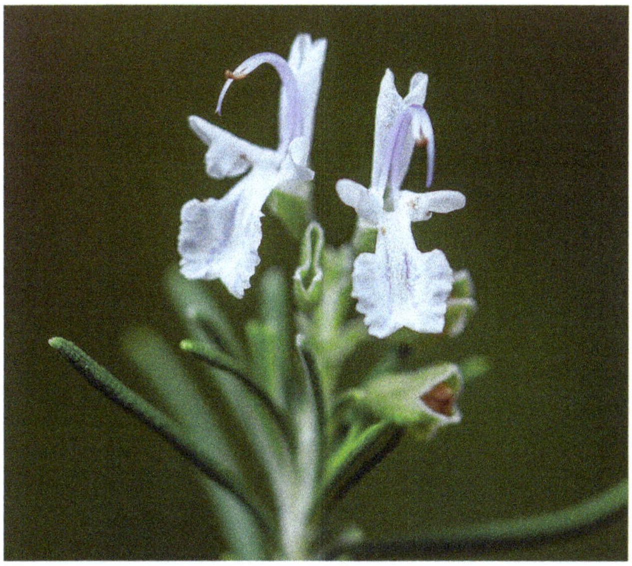

BOTANICAL DESCRIPTION AND HABITAT: A perennial herb native to the Mediterranean, rosemary thrives in temperate climates. It is an extremely drought resistant, erect, evergreen shrub (up to two meters tall). The dark gray bark is irregularly furrowed and flakes off the branches. The potent aromatic, linear leaves (10 – 20 mm long and 1 – 2 mm wide) grow opposite on the stem, in fascicles of four to six leaves. The dark green leaves are glabrous above and densely stellate-tomentose below, with entire, revolute margins. Multiple flowers are borne in numerous small clusters in the center of the fascicle clusters at the ends of branchlets. The small, pale, blue-purple flower has a pubescent calyx consisting of three triangular lobes, a bilabiate corolla with a large, cupped lower lip, a bilobed upper lip, and two wings, as well as two curved, epipetalous, exserted stamens. The single style is exserted, and has an ovary consisting of two fused carpels. Characteristic of the mint family, the fruit has four tiny nutlets.[3-5]

THE NAME: The genus *Salvia* derives from the Greek *salvare* ("to be saved") referring to the plant's healing properties.[2] *Rosmarinus,* derive from two Latin words: *ros* ("dew") and *marinus* ("belonging to the sea"), alluding to the plant's natural habitat on the Mediterranean coast.[1] The epithet *officinalis* denotes the inclusion of the plant in the official pharmacopoeia.

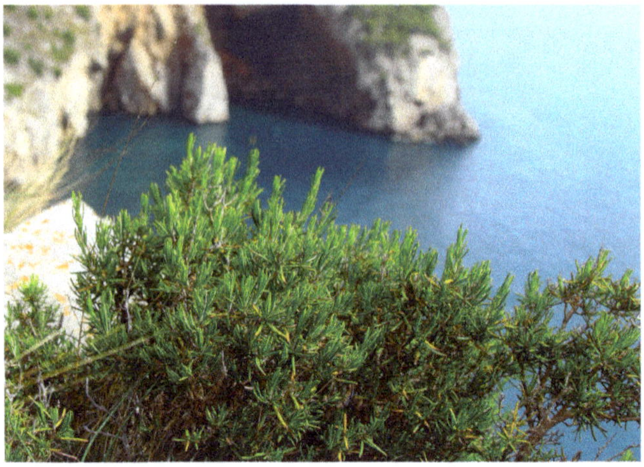

HISTORICAL USES: Rosemary has been utilized since antiquity to enhance memory and concentration; it symbolized remembrance.[2] Ancient Greek scholars wore rosemary around their necks during tests.[6] In Greek mythology, rosemary was affiliated with Minerva, the goddess of knowledge.[6] In *Hamlet,* Shakespeare referenced rosemary when Ophelia handed Hamlet a sprig and proclaimed, "There's rosemary, that's for remembrance: pray, love, remember." In wedding ceremonies, rosemary sprigs were woven into a wreath worn by the bride to symbolize fidelity.[7] Rosemary branches entwined with brightly colored silk ribbons were given as wedding favors to symbolize love and loyalty.[2] It was reputed that when rosemary plants thrived in the garden, the woman was the dominant influence of the house. This elicited the saying, "Where rosemary flourished, the woman ruled."[2]

Fresh rosemary was used to decorate churches and banquet halls during festivals and Christmas.[2] The herb was burned as incense for an affordable alternative to resins such as

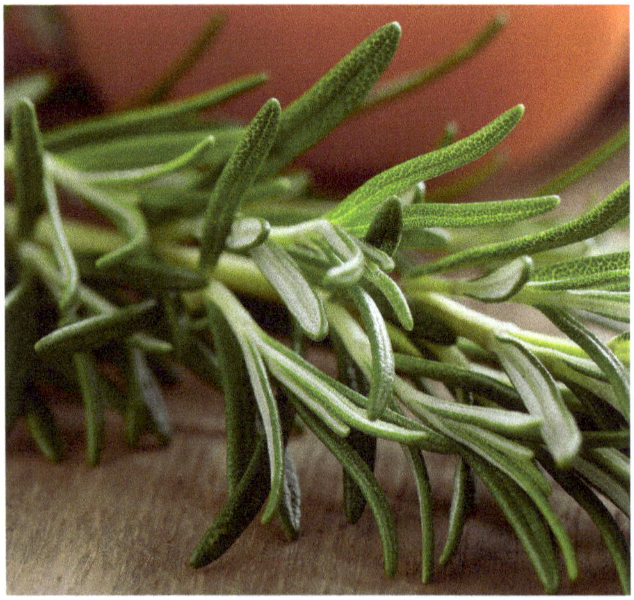

frankincense and myrrh; hence, the French name for rosemary, incensier.[2] It was customary to burn rosemary in sick rooms. In France, hospitals were fumigated with burning rosemary and juniper to purify the air and prevent infections.[2] In Spain, rosemary branches were used to fumigate houses for protection and cleansing. In Spain and Italy, rosemary was hung over doors or planted near entrances to protect against evil influences and witches. Placing rosemary under the bed was believed to protect against nightmares.[2] Sprigs of rosemary were held by mourners at funerals, and cast onto coffins as they were lowered into graves.[2]

Rosemary was consumed to lift the spirits, invigorate and calm the nerves, and treat nervous depression.[6] Hot tea was ingested to alleviate a headache, cold, colic, or dyspepsia, and increase the appetite.[2,6,7] Rosemary wine was ingested as a tonic for a weak heart, to reduce palpitations, and alleviate dropsy.[2] It was also infused in wine and ale to improve the flavor and avoid spoiling.[2] Eclectic physician John Scudder recommended rosemary for uterine obstruction, chlorosis, and nervous conditions associated with the female reproductive system.[8] Rosemary was applied to the scalp to stimulate hair growth, prevent premature balding, and treat dandruff.[2] Fomentations and liniments were applied topically to relieve gout, rheumatism, and arthritic pain.[2,9] Rosemary continues to be included in soaps, creams, lotions, perfumes, and toilet waters.[7-9]

CONSTITUENTS: Rosemary contains a volatile oil with monoterpene hydrocarbons (α- and β-pinenes, camphene, and limonene), cineole = eucalyptol, borneol, camphor, linalool, verbenol, terpineol, 3-octanone, and isobornyl acetate.[7] Rosemary also contains flavonoids (diosmetin, diosmin, genkwanin, genkwanin-4'-methyl ether, 6-methoxygenkwanin, luteolin, 6-methoxyluteolin, 6-methoxyyluteolin-7-glucoside, 6-methoxyluteolin-7-methyl ether, hispidulin, and apigenin), phenolic acids (rosmarinic, labiatic, chlorogenic, neochlorogenic, and caffeic acids), carnosic acid, rosmaricine and isorosmaricine, triterpenic acids (ursolic and oleanolic acids), rosmanol, 7-ethoxyrosmanol, betulinic acid, and carnosol.[7,9]

NUTRITIONAL PROPERTIES: Rosemary contains vitamin C, β-carotene, calcium, magnesium, phosphorus, potassium, iron, and zinc.[10,11]

MEDICINAL PROPERTIES: Antibacterial, antidepressant, antifungal, anti-inflammatory, antioxidant, aromatic stimulant, astringent, antiviral, bitter tonic, carminative, carrier, cholagogue, choleretic, circulatory stimulant, diaphoretic, diuretic, hypocholesterolemic (mild), vasodilator, preservative, and counterirritant.

TEMPERATURE AND FLAVOR: Warm, pungent, astringent, and bitter.

MEDICINAL USES

Rosemary is a warming circulatory stimulant and vasodilator.[8] It increases nutrient and oxygen delivery, and enhances the removal of waste products from tissues.

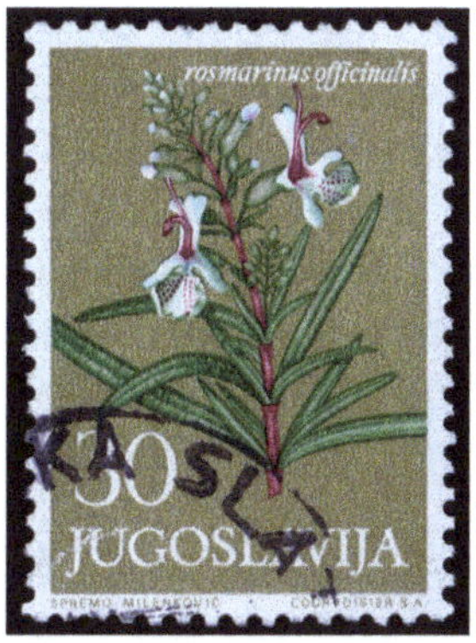

Rosemary aids in treating circulatory weakness, and conditions such as varicose veins, spider veins, Raynaud's phenomenon, and poor circulation. It enhances circulation in young, slender, low energy, pale individuals with underactive skin.[12] Rosemary can be administered to treat individuals with minor hypotension (low blood pressure).[9,12] It has a positive inotropic effect, increasing coronary blood flow.[7,12] It contains flavonoids (including diosmin) that improve the integrity of blood vessels by decreasing capillary permeability and fragility.[7] The volatile oil contains camphor that improves circulation and has a tonic effect on the vascular nerves.[12]

Rosemary increases blood flow to the brain, improving concentration and mental clarity. It aids in treating cerebral anoxia (lack of oxygen to the brain), enhancing memory, and alleviating headaches caused by poor cerebral circulation.[2,6] Rosemary is a potent antioxidant, reducing free radical destruction. It contains more than 12 antioxidant compounds that decrease oxidation in cells and reduce inflammation.[6] Increasing oxygenation supports individuals with conditions such as Alzheimer's disease, global dementia, cerebral arteriosclerosis, attention deficit hyperactivity disorder (ADHD), or seizure disorders.[6,12] The antioxidant actions are attributed to the carnosic acid, labiatic acid, and rosmarinic acid.[6,7] These compounds also inhibit the formation of leukotrienes and prostaglandins, reducing inflammation.[9]

Rosemary is a subtle nervous system stimulant that reduces sluggishness, fatigue, and depression, and improves mood.[6] Compound rosemary with additional non-caffeinated herbal stimulants to ease caffeine withdrawals or reduce caffeine consumption. Combine with tulsi basil *(Ocimum sanctum)*, gotu kola *(Centella asiatica)*, ginkgo *(Ginkgo

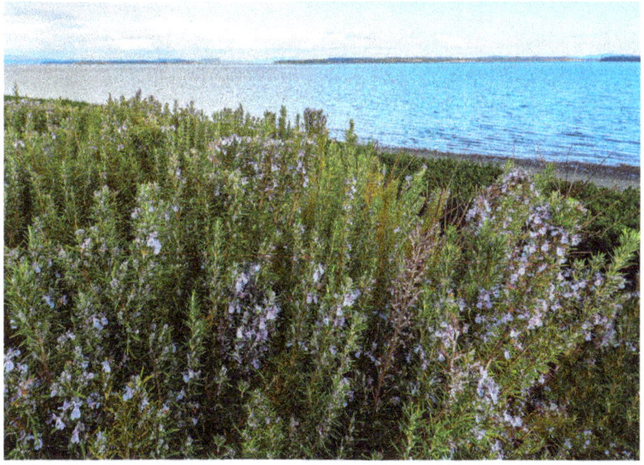

biloba)*, brahmi *(Bacopa* spp.), and/or bay laurel *(Laurus)* to improve circulation, concentration, and clarity, combat fatigue, reduce depression, and elevate mood. When compounded, rosemary is a carrier herb that improves the delivery of herbs to tissues. It is more easily tolerated than other circulation enhancing herbs, such as cayenne *(Capsicum)*, cinnamon *(Cinnamomum)*, and ginger *(Zingiber)* because it is less heating.

Rosemary is an aromatic digestive stimulant, carminative, stomachic, bitter tonic, choleretic, and cholagogue.[9,10] It increases the appetite, aids in treating nonulcer dyspepsia, and enhances digestion — especially in individuals with insufficient bile flow.[9] Rosemary reduces gallbladder and intestinal spasms, an action attributed to the rosemary galenicals and a rosmaricine derivative.[7] The

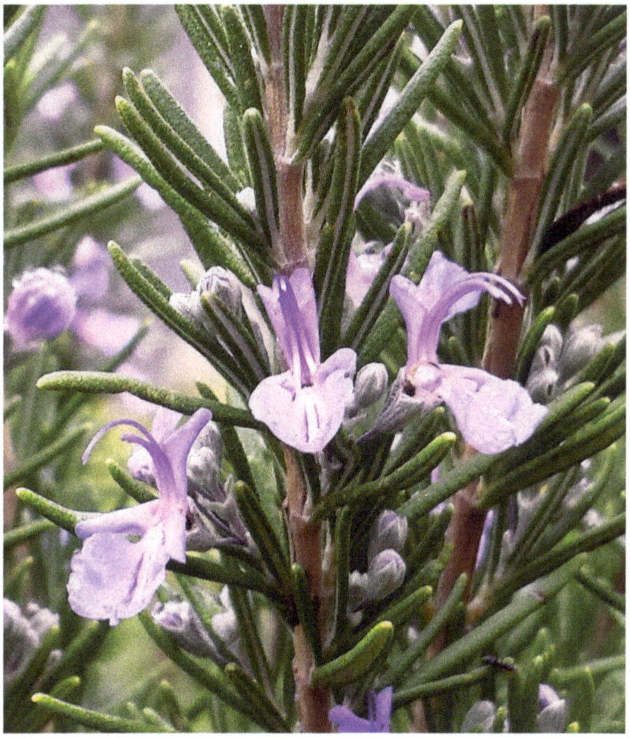

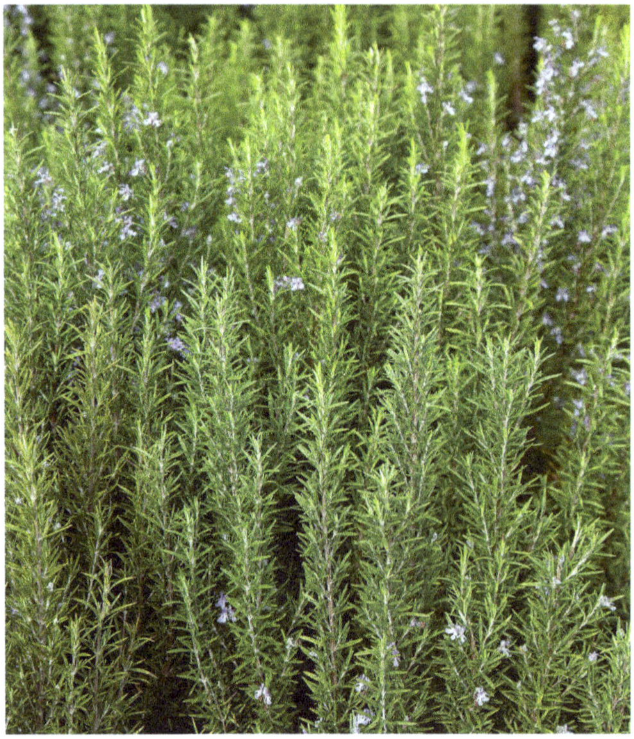

constituents carnosol and triterpene have bitter tonic effects.[9] Rosmarinic acid, caffeic acid derivatives, carnosol, and luteolin have choleretic effects, and lower cholesterol and triglyceride levels.[9] A delicious pungent culinary herb, rosemary enhances flavor and facilitates the digestion of lamb, mutton, goat, veal, red gamey meats, pork, chicken, fish, potatoes, and root vegetables. It is often combined with other Mediterranean herbs to cure and preserve meats. Rosemary mouthwash, tea, or fresh herb freshens the breath, and heals mouth ulcers and canker sores.[10]

The volatile oil of rosemary has potent antimicrobial actions.[7,9,11] Rosmarinic acid and related caffeic acid derivatives are attributed to the antiviral, antibacterial, and antifungal properties.[6,9,11] Borneol also has antifungal and antibacterial actions.[6,9,11] Rosemary inhibits fungal growth and aids in treating *Candida albicans* overgrowth in the digestive and vaginal tracts. Incorporate rosemary tea or extract into formulas as a broad spectrum antimicrobial for treating a cold, flu, sinusitis, sore throat, or digestive infection. Rosemary is an expectorant and astringent, reducing excess mucus. Steaming with rosemary, mint *(Mentha)*, and/or eucalyptus *(Eucalyptus)* decreases respiratory congestion. Combine extracts of usnea *(Usnea)* and thyme *(Thymus vulgaris)* with smaller quantities of orange peel *(Citrus sinensis)*, cinnamon *(Cinnamomum)*, clove *(Syzygium)*, licorice *(Glycyrrhiza)*, and rosemary as an all-purpose warming antimicrobial and diaphoretic compound for respiratory or digestive infections. Consume 30 – 90 drops, four to five times daily.

Rosemary invigorates sluggish, underactive skin. External applications rejuvenate the skin, supporting dry, mature skin and preventing wrinkles. Rinse the hair and scalp with a rosemary infusion, or massage the scalp with a rosemary-infused oil to improve circulation to the scalp, and reduce dandruff, graying, thinning hair, balding, and alopecia.[8] Rosemary adds a glossy sheen to dark hair, stimulates hair growth, and prevents balding.[10] Combine with nettle leaf *(Urtica dioica)* and horsetail *(Equisetum)* for use as a hair and scalp rinse.

Rosemary has counterirritant and rubefacient actions that improve circulation, treating varicose veins, bruises, sprains, strains, muscle pain, muscle spasms, neuralgia, arthritis, and rheumatic pain.[6-8,10] Rosemary foot and hand baths stimulate local circulation, warming cold hands and feet. A topical antimicrobial, rosemary inhibits fungal and bacterial growth, disinfects wounds, and treats athlete's foot, ringworm, skin tinea, and staph.[9] Add rosemary leaves or essential oil to a medicinal oil or salve to prevent rancidity.

Spray a rosemary infusion or diluted essential oil, or spread rosemary leaves in the home or garden to repel ants, other insects, and deer.[10]

ROSEMARY ESSENTIAL OIL
ROSEMARY (CINEOLE TYPE)

Rosemary cineole chemotype is cultivated in North Africa.[13] Rosemary cineole is a mucolytic that aids in treating congestion caused by sinus and lower respiratory infections.[13,14] It also stimulates digestive secretions, enhances the appetite, and energizes.[13] Consume one to

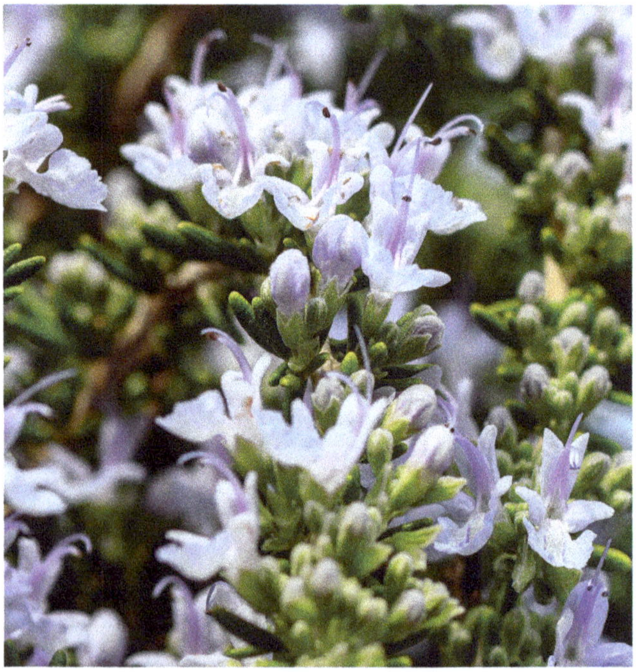

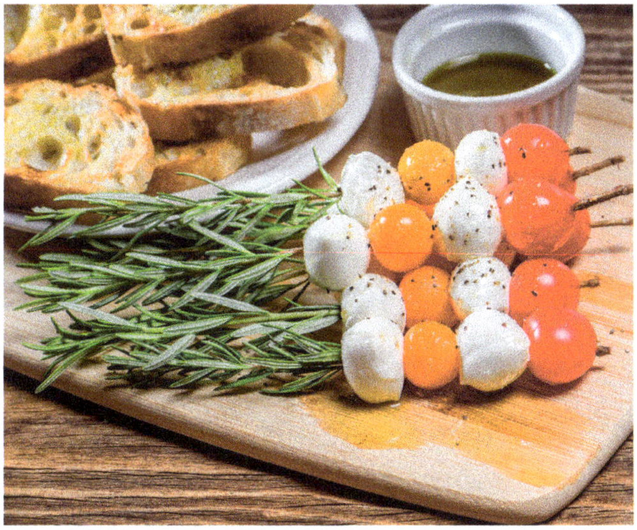

two drops, or add several drops into a diffuser or chest rub ointment. The active principles are cineole and terpene hydrocarbons.[13] *Note:* Avoid internal use during pregnancy. Otherwise, there are no known contraindications.[13]

ROSEMARY (CAMPHOR TYPE)

Rosemary camphor chemotype is cultivated in Croatia and Spain.[13] Consume one drop in a capsule before meals to enhance digestion and stimulate bile flow.[13] Small doses relieve nervous tension; higher doses counteract nervous tension and exhaustion.[13] Topical use of the essential oil has neuromuscular effects, reducing muscle cramping, pain, and tension, and enhancing circulation in the tissues.[13] Rosemary is a vascular decongestant that aids in treating varicose veins, spider veins, and bruises.[14] It also has mucolytic and diuretic actions.[14] Terpene ketone (camphor), terpene oxide (cineole), and terpene hydrocarbons are the active constituents.[13] *Note:* Rosemary camphor type contains ketones; avoid internal use during pregnancy and lactation, in children under 10 years of age, and individuals with seizure disorders.[13]

ROSEMARY (VERBENONE TYPE)

Rosemary verbenone type is cultivated in Corsica.[13] It is a mucolytic that aids in treating upper and lower respiratory conditions, including sinusitis, bronchitis, colds, and flu.[13,14] It energizes the nervous system, and combats adrenal fatigue.[13] Rosemary verbenone stimulates digestion and assimilation.[13] Topical use is indicated for oily skin conditions such as acne, blackheads, and zits.[13] Apply diluted essential oil as a skin regenerative.[13] The essential oil contains ketones (verbenone), cineole, and terpene hydrocarbons.[13] *Note:* Due to the ketone content, avoid internal use during pregnancy and lactation, and in children under 10 years of age.[13]

CONTRAINDICATIONS

Avoid use during pregnancy; however, culinary use is permissible. Rosemary is contraindicated with a blocked bile duct.[9] It can increase blood pressure; therefore, moderate to high doses should be avoided in individuals with high blood pressure. There is no recorded toxicity of the herb in any literature reviewed.[11] Internal use of essential oil (rosemary camphor and verbenone type) is contraindicated during pregnancy and lactation, in children under 10 years of age, and individuals with epilepsy.[13]

PREPARATION AND DOSAGE

TINCTURE: Fresh leaves [1:2-1:3, 70-95% alcohol]; dry leaves [1:5-1:7, 60% alcohol]; consume 15-60 drops, up to three times daily.

ACETUM EXTRACT: Fresh leaves [1:3-1:4, apple cider vinegar]; consume in food preparations such as vinaigrettes or oil, or apply diluted rosemary acetum topically.

CAPSULES: Consume 2-3 capsules, one to three times daily. Add 1-2 drops of essential oil to a charcoal tablet, or a capsule containing a powdered binding agent; and consume 1-2 capsules, one to three times daily.

TEA: Prepare a hot infusion; consume 8-12 ounces, one to three times daily.

HONEY AND SYRUP: Prepare simple syrup by dissolving one part by volume of sugar into one part of a strained rosemary infusion, or infuse rosemary directly into simple syrup.

TOPICAL USE: Apply the tea as a fomentation, poultice, hair rinse, hand or foot bath. Prepare infused oil using the alcohol intermediary method. Dilute essential oil in cream, oil, salve, liniment, soap, or lotion.

CULINARY USE: Freshly chopped or ground rosemary is a seasoning for beef, lamb, veal, venison, rabbit, poultry, soup, gravy, sauces, or root vegetable dishes.

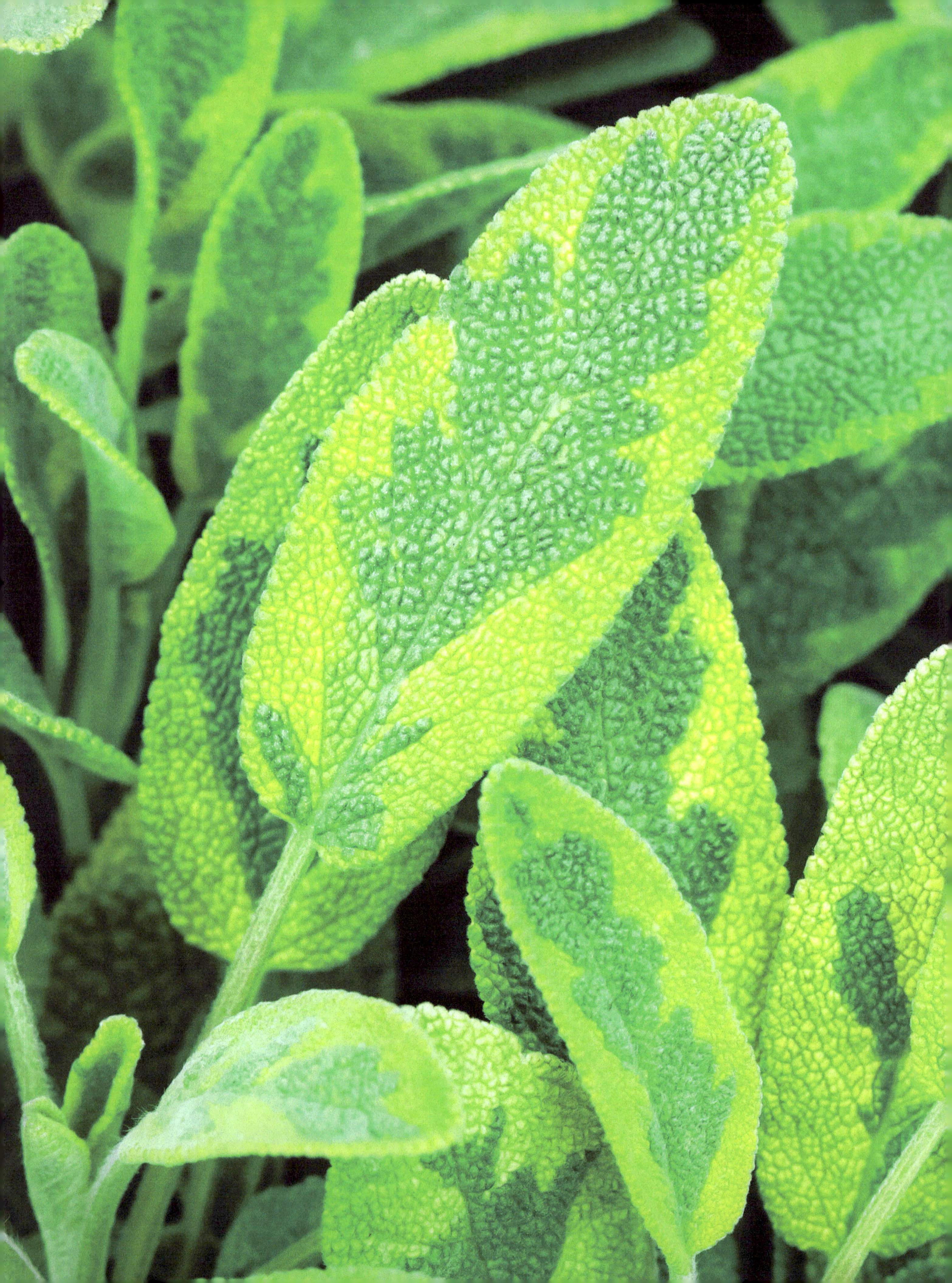

SAGE

DESCRIPTION

BOTANICAL NAME:
Salvia officinalis

COMMON NAMES:
Sage, garden sage, true sage, Dalmatian sage, sawge
marameeah (Arabic)
eghespak, yeghesbag (Armenian)
chaj gradinski (Bulgarian)
lóuh méih chóu (Cantonese)
zilfija (Croatian)
salvej (Czech)
salvie (Danish)
Franse thee (Dutch)
salvio (Esperanto)
salvei (Estonian)
mariam goli (Farsi)
salvia (Finnish)
sauge thé de la Grèce (French)
salbei (German)
alisfakia, foskomilo (Greek)
marva (Hebrew)
zsálya (Hungarian)
salvía (Icelandic)
salvia (Italian)
sarubia, sezi (Japanese)
seiji, selbieo (Korean)
shu wei cao (Mandarin)
salvie (Norwegian)
swalwia lekarska (Polish)
salva-mansa (Portuguese)
salvie (Romanian)
shalfej (Russian)
shati (Sanskrit)
kadulja (Serbian)
salvia (Spanish)
salvia (Swedish)
adacayi (Turkish)
sholvie, shalfey (Yiddish)[1]

FAMILY NAME:
Lamiaceae (Labiatae)

PART USED: The leaves.

BOTANICAL DESCRIPTION AND HABITAT: *Salvia officinalis* is an erect, mounding perennial shrub native to the Mediterranean's northern shores.[2] The white tomentose stem is woody at the base.[3] It has oblong to elliptic

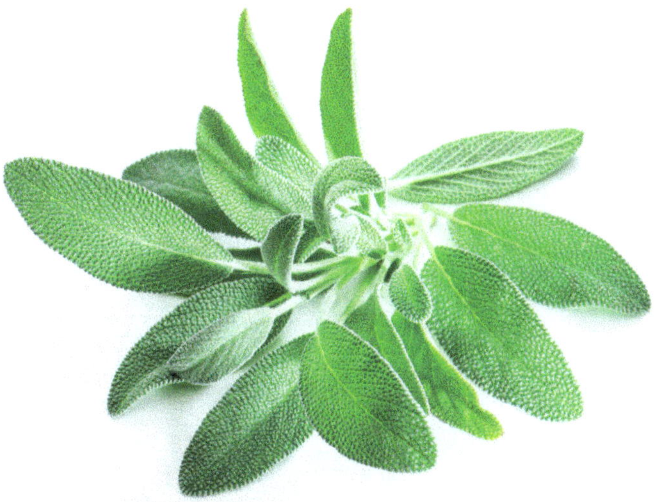

opposite gray-green leaves (1 – 8 cm long by 0.5 – 3.5 cm wide) covered in a dense layer of short white hairs.[3] The leaves have rounded bases, scalloped margins, and acute to mucronate apices.[3]

Terminal racemes (4 – 18 cm long) of verticillasters bear 2 – 18 purple to blue flowers.[3] The flowers have campanulate calyces (1 – 1.5 cm) and bilabiate tubular corollas (2 cm) with spreading, three-lobed lower lips.[3,4] The stamens in the *Salvia* genus are unique; each of the two stamens is forked, with the curved upper fork bearing a fertile anther, and the shorter lower fork bearing a sterile anther. When a bee presses down on the lower fork, a lever action moves the upper fork down as it deposits pollen on the bee's back. The single style is also forked, and sits atop an ovary consisting of two fused carpels.[4] The fruits consist of four dark brown nutlets.[3]

THE NAME: The genus *Salvia* derives from the Greek *salvare* ("to be saved"), referring to the plant's healing properties.[2]

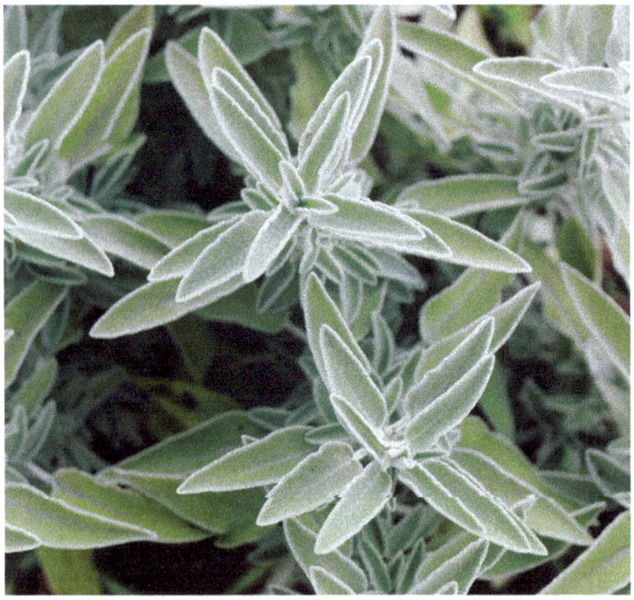

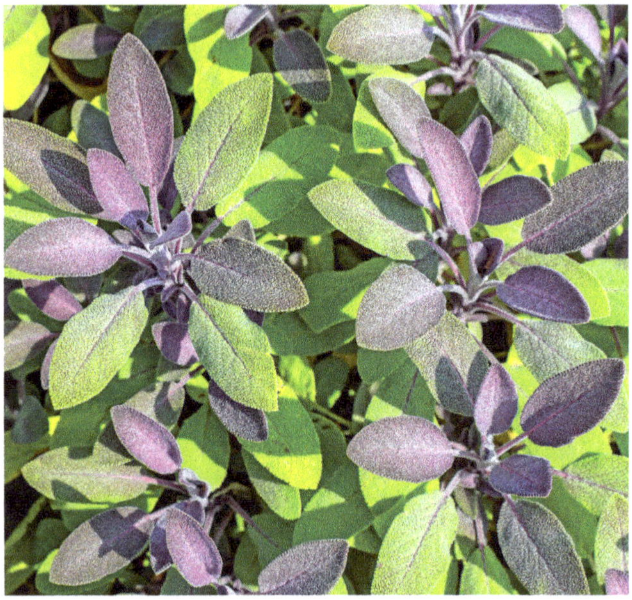

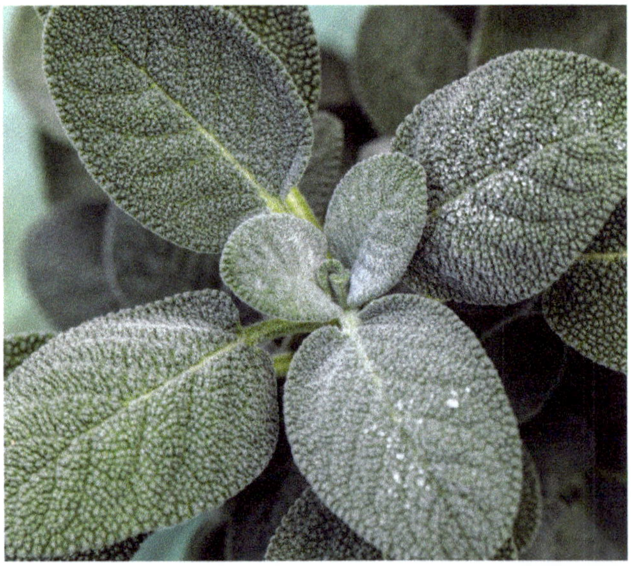

HISTORICAL USES: In early folklore, it was believed that sage would wither or thrive, depending on one's business success.[2] Another popular belief was that sage thrived in homes dominated by women.[2] It was customary to plant sage on graves, as it was used to mitigate grief. Sage was used as an antidote for snakebites.[2] Sage ale was a popular beverage containing sage, betony (*Stachys betonica*), spikenard *(Nardostachys)*, fennel *(Foeniculum)*, and other herbs.[2]

Ancient Greeks administered sage infusions to treat fevers.[2] Italian peasants consumed sage and believed it preserved health.[2] Sage tea was consumed as a stimulant, increasing alertness and heightening the senses.[2] The tea was gargled for sore gums, mouth ulcers, and hoarseness.[2] Fresh leaves were rubbed into gums and teeth to cleanse the breath and strengthen the gums.[2] The leaves were powdered and included in snuff.[2]

Eclectic physicians administered sage as an astringent, diaphoretic, stimulant, antispasmodic, digestive tonic, and anthelmintic.[5,6] Hot sage tea was recommended to improve circulation in cold hands and feet. Sage tea was given as a carminative to treat poor gastric function and flatulence.[5,6] Administered as a hot tea, sage was used to promote sweating; cold sage tea was given to restrain excessive sweating and night sweats.[5,6] An infusion was gargled to treat a sore, ulcerated throat.[6] Sage was one of the few remedies recommended to treat individuals with low specific gravity urine.[6]

CONSTITUENTS: Sage contains volatile oil (α- and β-thujones, 1,8-cineole, borneol, viridifloral, 2-methyl-3-methylene-5-heptene, and sesquiterpenes), bitter principles (picrosalvin and carnosol), salvin, salvin monomethyl ether, carnosic acid, and flavonoids (genkwanin, 6-methoxygenkwanin, luteolin, luteolin-7-methyl ether, 6-methoxyluteolin, 6-methoxyluteolin-7-methyl ether, hispidulin, and salvigenin), Lamiaceae tannins, also known as phenolic acids (rosmarinic, labiatic, caffeic, and chlorogenic acids), and salviatannin.[7,8]

NUTRITIONAL PROPERTIES: Sage contains high amounts of calcium, crude fiber, fat, magnesium, potassium, sodium, thiamine, vitamin A, and zinc. It contains low to average amounts of aluminum, ash, dietary fiber, iron, manganese, niacin, phosphorus, protein, riboflavin, silicon, tin, and vitamin C. It contains trace amounts of chromium.[9]

MEDICINAL PROPERTIES: Antibacterial, antifungal (fungistatic), anti-inflammatory, antioxidant, antiviral (virustatic), aromatic, astringent, carminative, diaphoretic, digestive, perspiration inhibitor (antihidrotic), secretory stimulant, antispasmodic, stomachic, and stimulant.

TEMPERATURE AND FLAVOR: Warm, astringent, pungent, and bitter.

MEDICINAL USES

Sage is an antimicrobial agent with antibacterial, antifungal, and antiviral properties.[7,8,10,11] The antibacterial actions aid in treating sinusitis, pharyngitis, laryngitis, strep throat, tonsillitis, tracheitis, bronchitis, staph infections, and bacterial vaginosis.[7,8,11,12] Sage has antiviral actions against herpes, and virustatic actions that aid in treating a cold and flu.[5,7,8,11] It is an antifungal, inhibiting the growth of *Candida albicans* in the digestive and vaginal tracts, and aids in treating yeast infections.[7,8,10] Sage's astringent properties reduce mucus secretion, and aid in treating upper and lower respiratory infections. The phenolic acids salvin and salvin monomethyl ether have antimicrobial actions that are especially effective against *Staphylococcus aureus*.[7] The antibacterial and antifungal actions are attributed to thujone and 1,8-cineole.[8] The Lamiaceae tannins and thujone contribute to the antiviral and virustatic effects; the tannins have astringent effects.[8]

An astringent, sage reduces inflammation in mucous membranes and skin.[5] Consuming sage tea or extract aids in treating diarrhea.[10] Gargling with the tea or diluted tincture reduces inflammation in the mouth and throat, in addition to treating bleeding gums, gingivitis, and mouth or throat ulcers.[10] Irrigating the vaginal canal with sage tea decreases excessive vaginal secretions (leukorrhea), and soothes irritation caused by non-specific vaginitis and yeast infections.[10] Additional antifungal herbs are necessary for the latter condition. A sage enema, sitz bath, and compress reduce hemorrhoid bleeding and inflammation. *Note:* For all of the aforementioned applications, the tea must be strained through a coffee filter or very fine cloth in order to remove all particulate matter. A fresh batch of tea must be prepared daily to prevent the potential introduction of microbes.

Depending on how sage is administered, it can act as a diaphoretic or antihidrotic (perspiration inhibitor).[5,6] Consume hot sage tea or sage-infused chicken broth as a diaphoretic, and to encourage mucous membrane secretions.[5,6] Hot sage tea or soup stock containing sage, thyme *(Thymus)*, oregano *(Origanum vulgare)*, marjoram *(Origanum majorana)*, and garlic *(Allium)* is highly effective for breaking a fever, treating a cold or flu, and clearing respiratory passages. Consume the cold infusion or room temperature tea as an antihidrotic and astringent.[5,6,12] The latter preparation aids in treating night sweats, hot flashes, and excessive sweating.[8] It also aids in drying excessive secretions of the mucous membranes.

Sage is an aromatic carminative, stomachic, and mild choleretic.[5,8,10,11] It has subtle antispasmodic properties affecting the smooth muscles in the digestive tract.[7] Sage contains bitter components that stimulate digestive secretions and enhance fat digestion.[2] It aids in treating sluggish digestion, nonulcer dyspepsia, gastritis, gas, bloating, and diarrhea.[2,5,6,8,10] One study demonstrated that consuming a sage decoction on an empty stomach lowered blood sugar levels in diabetics.[15]

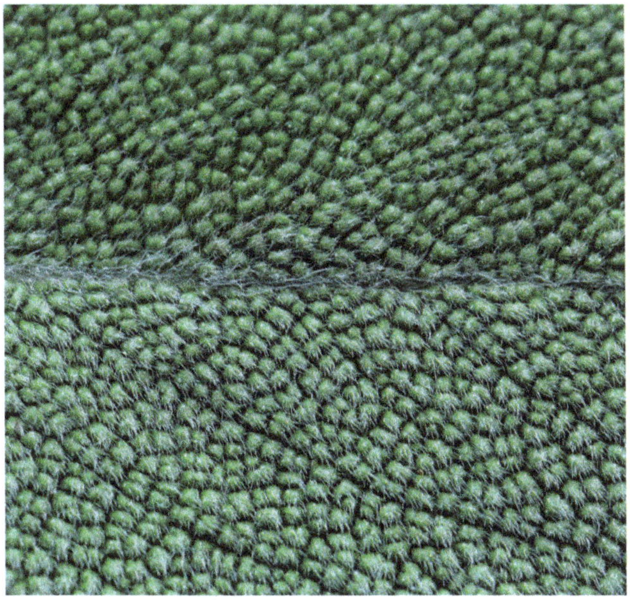

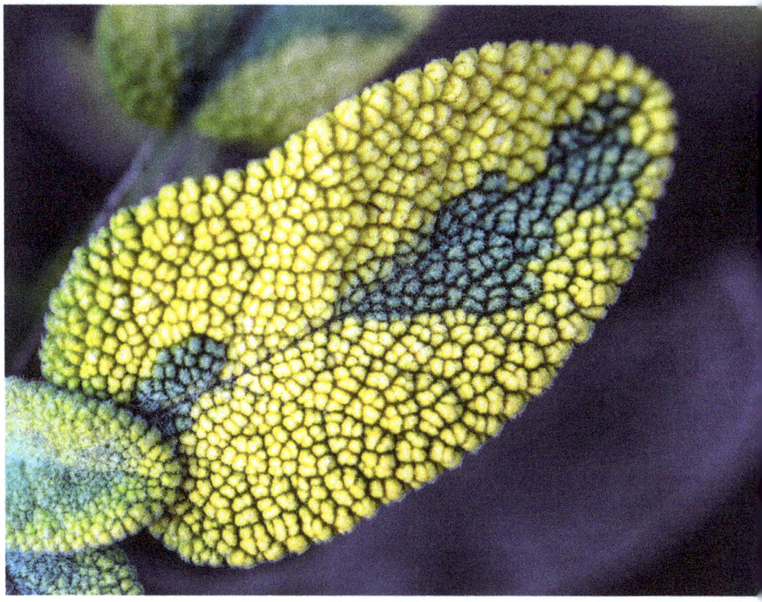

Sage is a delicious pungent culinary herb used to season sausage, ground meat, lamb, beef, pork, poultry, cheese, stuffing, gravy, soup, and sauce. It has potent antioxidant properties that prevent oil rancidity and preserve meat. The antioxidant activity is attributed to the labiatic and carnosic acid.[10]

An antigalactagogue, sage dries up milk flow in order to cease nursing.[9,10] Combine sage with parsley leaf to enhance the antigalactagogue effects.

Sage is a hemostatic, reducing bleeding in mucous membranes. It also reduces excessive menstrual flow, as well as mid-cycle and menopausal spotting.

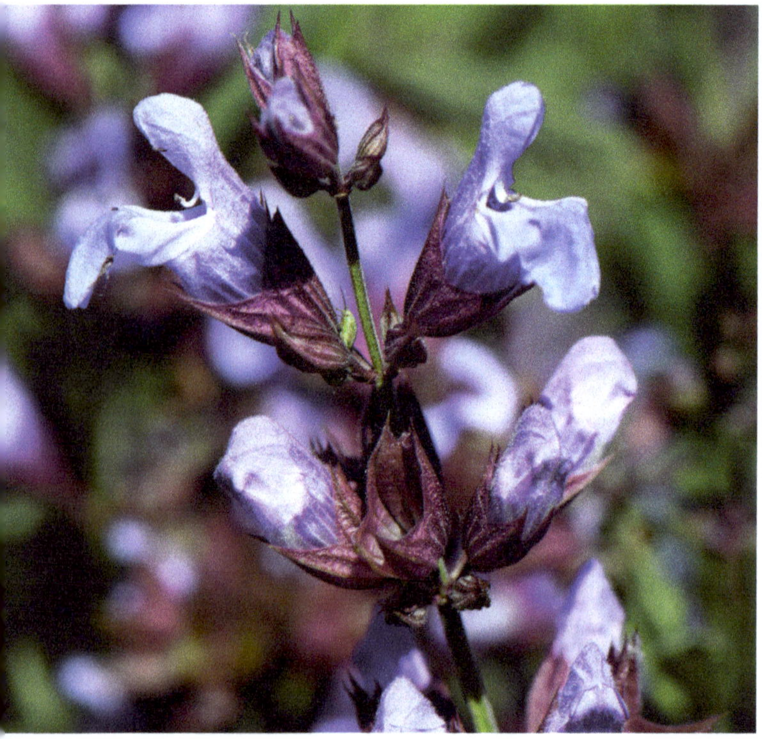

When compounding sage extract, combine it with tannin-containing antimicrobial herbs, rather than alkaloid-containing herbs, because alkaloids precipitate tannins out of solution when combined in alcohol-based compounds.

Sage can be applied topically as an antimicrobial to treat staph infections, ringworm, athlete's foot, cuts, abrasions, and wounds. A bath, wash, fomentation, or compress disinfects and reduces skin inflammation. Washing the face or skin with sage tea or applying a sage toner is highly effective for treating acne, oily skin, or oily hair. Sage hair rinse encourages hair growth, darkens hair, and aids in treating dandruff.[2] Combine sage with nettle (*Urtica*) and horsetail (*Equisetum*) to create a hair tonic.

SAGE ESSENTIAL OIL (SALVIA OFFICINALIS)

Sage essential oil contains α- and β-thujones, 1,8-cineole, borneol, viridifloral, 2-methyl-3-methylene-5-heptene, camphor, and sesquiterpenes.[7,8,10] Depending on where it is cultivated, the chemical composition of the essential oil is highly variable; however, it typically contains high amounts of the ketone thujone.[11]

A broad spectrum antimicrobial agent, sage essential oil is an antibacterial and antifungal.[11,13] It is highly effective against *Staphylococcus aureus* and *Streptococcus* bacteria; it also has an antiviral effect against herpes simplex virus type I.[11,13] Sage essential oil has antispasmodic actions *in vitro*.[7]

Diffusing sage oil is stimulating and invigorating, and improves mental focus.[14] Topically, sage is a skin regenerative.[13] Add several drops to astringent facial toners to treat acne or oily skin.[14] Sage also helps to dissolve cellulite; add several drops to a salve or body cream, and massage into the affected area.[14] Prepare a topical antimicrobial oil or salve by adding one to five drops of sage oil per ounce to treat staph infections, ringworm, athlete's foot, cuts, abrasions, and wounds.[11]

Note: Due to the high ketone content, sage essential oil should not be used during pregnancy or lactation, or in children less than 10 years old.[11] Thujone is a neurotoxic ketone; therefore, sage oil should be avoided by individuals

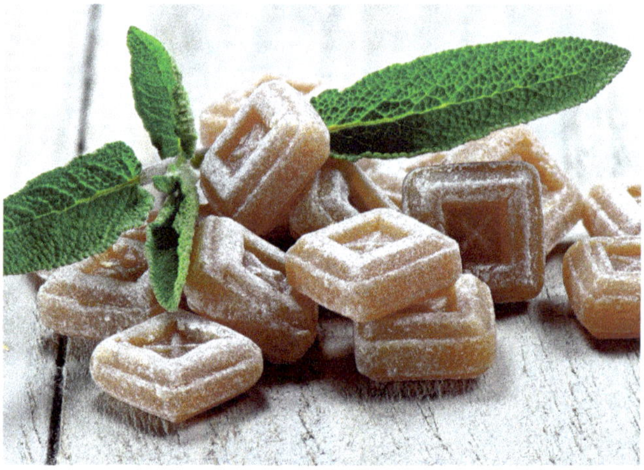

prone to seizures.[14] Thujone also can have acute hepatotoxic properties.[13] Avoid using the essential oil internally more than ten days. Sage oil can be very irritating to the skin; it must be highly diluted for topical applications.[14] Before applying a product containing sage oil, test it on the inner portion of the elbow, and wait 24 – 48 hours. Do not apply if a rash occurs.

CONTRAINDICATIONS

Except for culinary use, avoid sage during pregnancy and lactation.[10] When used in the recommended dosages, there are no reported side effects.[10] Large doses can cause dryness in the mouth and mucous membranes. See the *Note* listed on previous page for essential oil contraindications.

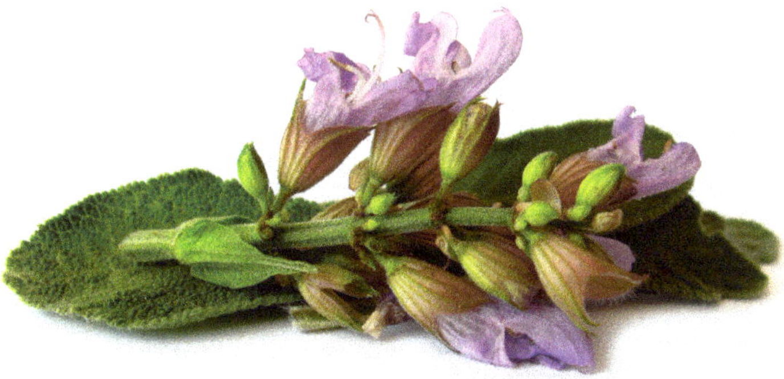

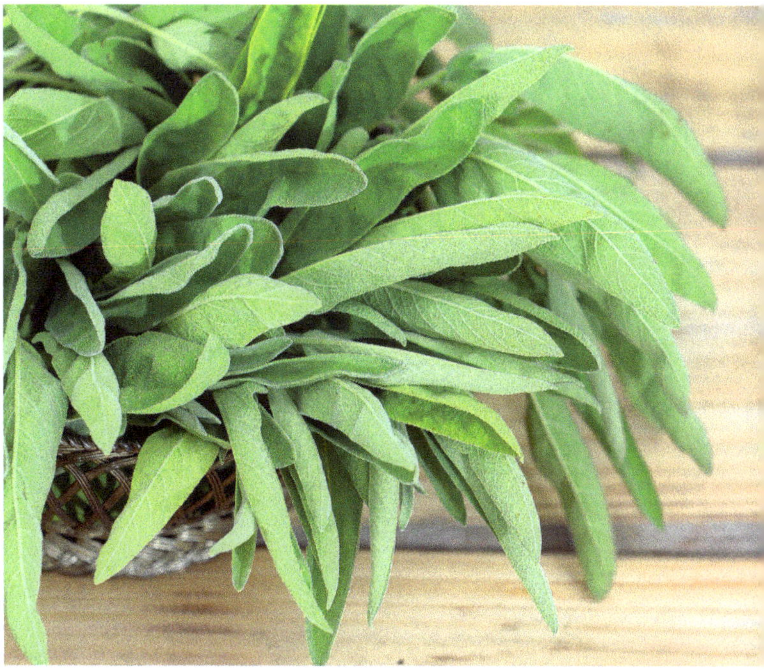

PREPARATION AND DOSAGE

TINCTURE: Fresh leaves [1:2-1:3, 70-95% alcohol]; dry leaves [1:5, 60% alcohol]; consume 15-60 drops, up to three times daily.

ACETUM EXTRACT: Fresh leaves [1:2-1:3, apple cider vinegar]; consume in food preparations such as vinaigrettes or oil, or apply diluted sage acetum topically.

CAPSULES: Consume 2-4 capsules, one to three times daily. Add 1-2 drops of essential oil to a charcoal tablet or capsule containing a powdered binding agent; consume 1-2 capsules, one to three times daily.

TEA: Prepare a hot or cold infusion; consume 8-12 ounces, one to three times daily.

HONEY AND SYRUP: Simple syrup can be prepared in two ways: dissolve one part by volume of sugar into one part of a strained sage infusion, or infuse sage directly into prepared simple syrup. Or, add 1-2 drops of sage essential oil to 1 teaspoon to 1 tablespoon of simple syrup or honey, and mix with a toothpick. Add 1 teaspoon to 1 tablespoon infused honey or syrup to one cup of tea or hot water; consume up to four times daily.

TOPICAL USE: Apply the tea as a fomentation, poultice, wash, or foot bath. Prepare medicinal oil using the alcohol intermediary method. Dilute the essential oil in cream, oil, salve, liniment, soap, or lotion.

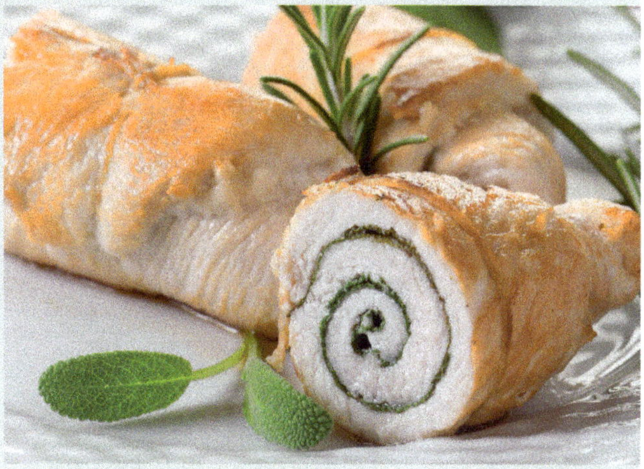

CULINARY USE: Freshly chopped or ground sage is a seasoning for beef, lamb, veal, venison, rabbit, poultry, soup, gravy, sauce, cheese, and stuffing.

SAW PALMETTO

DESCRIPTION

BOTANICAL NAMES:
Serenoa repens (syn. *S. serrulata, Sabal serrulata*)

COMMON NAMES:
Saw palmetto, palmetto, palmetto berry, sabal palm, sabal, American dwarf palm tree, cabbage palm, old man's friend
sahapalmu (Finnish)
palmier de l'Amérique du Nord (French)
zwegpalme, sabalfruchte (German)
sagpalmetto (Swedish)

FAMILY NAME:
Arecaceae (Palmae)

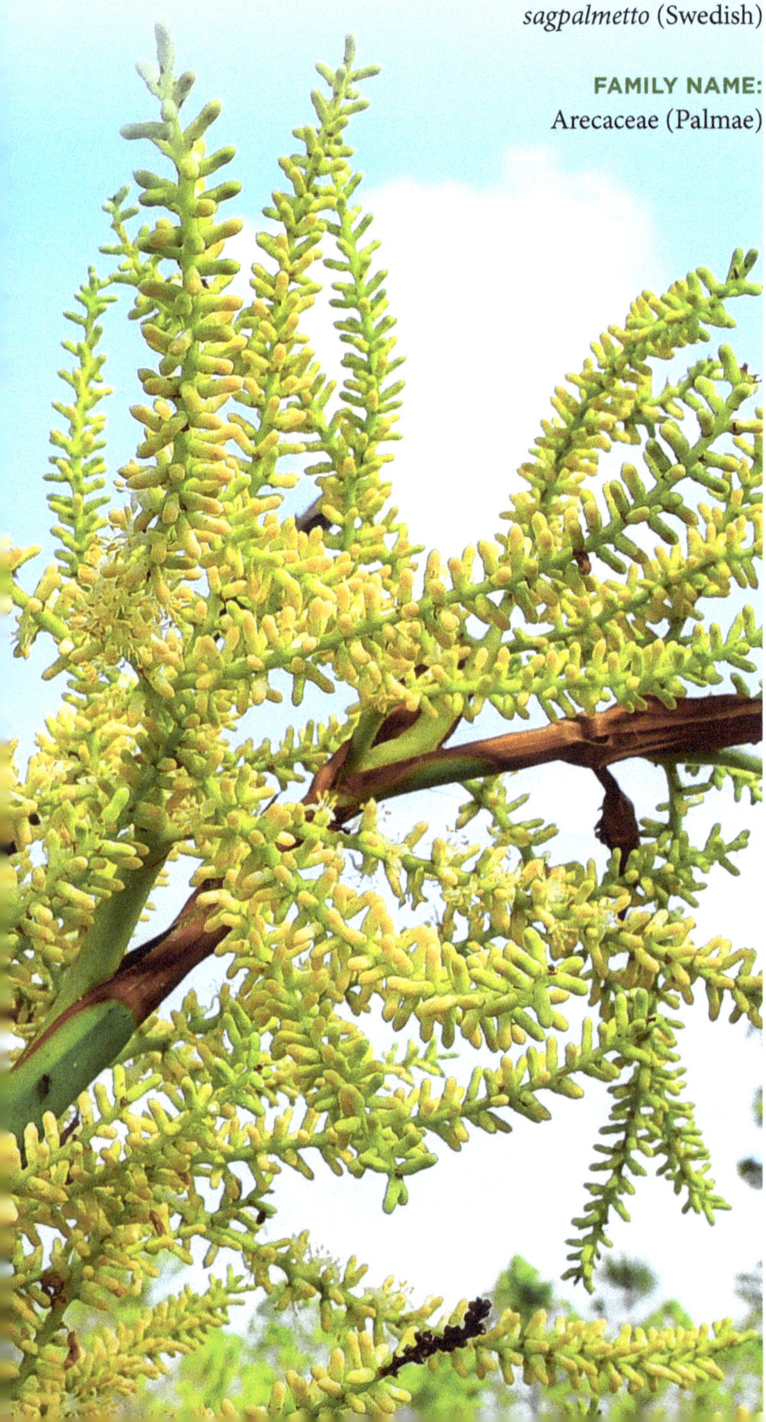

PART USED: The fruits.

BOTANICAL DESCRIPTION AND HABITAT: Saw palmetto is a long-lived, shrubby palm endemic to the southeastern U.S. It grows in sand pine scrub, mesic hammocks, coastal sand dunes, and pinelands, often in large homogenous stands.[1,2]

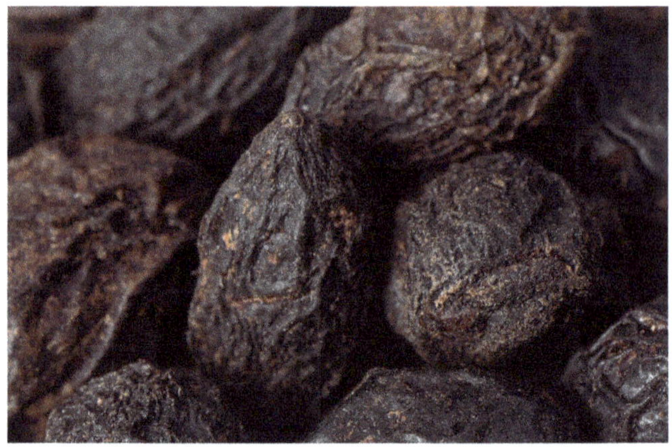

Usually reaching 1 – 3 meters tall, the plants have a sprawling, colonizing habit, and rarely have upright trunks.[2] The stiff, yellow-green, green, or silver-green palmate leaves lack a costa (midrib).[1] The lanceolate leaf segments are fused at their bases, with acute or forked apices, and serrate margins.[1,2] Obtuse hastula are present on both sides of the leaf, and the base of the petiole is particularly armed with teeth.[1]

Long axillary panicles are borne in the leaf crown.[1] Tiny sessile, fragrant, white flowers (4 – 5 mm) bloom in the spring, each consisting of a cup-shaped, three-lobed calyx, three elliptic petals, two whorls of three stamens, with triangular filaments fused to the petals at the base, and three pistils.[1,2] There are also three nectaries that attract bees.[1,2] When ripe, the fruit is a dark reddish-brown to black ellipsoid drupe (2 cm long by 1 cm wide) with brown ellipsoid seeds. It is coveted by black bears, whitetail deer, raccoons, foxes, opossums, and birds.[1,2]

THE NAME: The genus *Serenoa* was named in honor of botanist Sereno Watson (1826 – 1892).[3] The epithet *repens* ("creeping") derives from Latin. The common name saw palmetto ("saw-like palm") refers to the sharp stems that can cut clothing or skin.

HISTORICAL USES: Saw palmetto berries were consumed as food by Native Americans in Florida.[3] They also utilized the herb for urinary problems.[3] Borrowing from indigenous tribal knowledge, early American settlers also supplemented their diet with saw palmetto berries.[3]

Eclectic physician Dr. Goss observed the beneficial effects of animal consumption of the mature berries, noting that these animals grew fat with sleek hair.[4] This attracted the attention of Eclectic physician Dr. J. B. Read, who began utilizing saw palmetto in his practice.[4] In 1879, he published an article in the *American Journal of Pharmacy,* extolling the digestive benefits of saw palmetto, in addition to its ability to increase flesh, strength, and weight, and soothe irritated mucous membranes — especially in the respiratory tract.[3,4] Saw palmetto was later included in the *U.S. Pharmacopoeia* (1906).[3,5] Eclectic physician Finley Ellingwood administered saw palmetto as a nutritive that also increased the appetite and enhanced assimilation. He prescribed saw palmetto for men suffering from an enlarged prostate with dull aching pain, bladder irritability, and conditions related to prostate enlargement, including sexual weakness, epididymitis, orchitis, and orchalgia.[3] He also recommended the herb for women to reduce irritability of the ovaries and treat dysmenorrhea resulting from atonicity, in addition to increasing the size and secreting capacity of small, inactive mammary glands. He mentions its use for treating sterility, and noted that saw palmetto restored ovarian action. Dr. Hale considered the herb among the most effective uterine remedies.[4] As the use and popularity of herbs declined in the U.S., saw palmetto was excluded from the National Formulary. However, it continued to be used in Europe, and studies of standardized extracts were conducted, confirming its therapeutic applications.[3] By 1998, the herb was reintroduced in the U.S. National Formulary.[3]

CONSTITUENTS: Saw palmetto berry has a high lipid content. It is rich in a fixed oil with free fatty acids (including capric, caprylic, caproic, lauric, myristic, isomyristic, palmitic, stearic, and oleic acids); triglycerides, diglycerides, and monoglycerides; phytosterols (β-sitosterol, β-sitosterol 3-O-β-D-glucoside, campesterol, β-sitosterolin = β-sitosterol-glucoside, esterified β-sitosterol, stigmasterol, cycloartenol, lupeol, lupenone, 24-methylene-cycloartenol, hexacosanol, and 1-octacosanol); and fatty alcohols (phytol, farnesol, and geranylgeraniol). Additional components include carotenes, flavonoids, lipase, polysaccharides (S1, S2, S3, and S4, glucose, galactose, mannose, fucose, arabinose, rhamnose, and glucuronic acid), invert sugars, tannins, and mucilaginous compounds (pectin).[3,5-9]

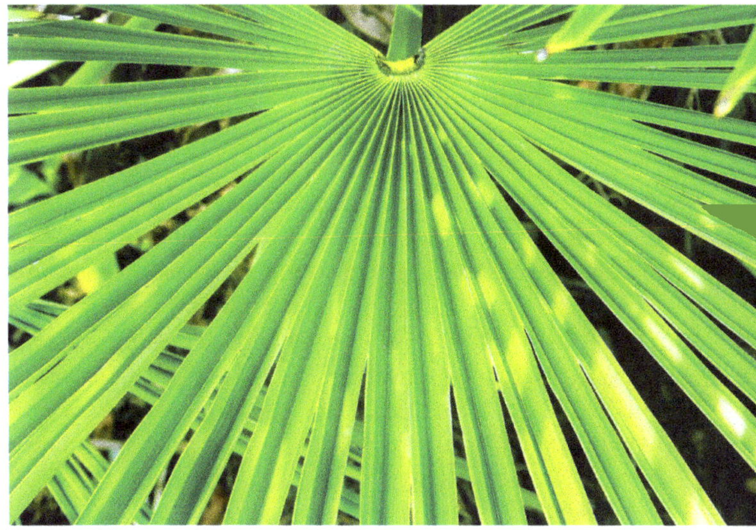

NUTRITIONAL PROPERTIES: Saw palmetto contains high amounts of chromium, fiber, iron, magnesium, manganese, niacin, phosphorus, potassium, riboflavin, selenium, silicon, thiamine, and zinc. It contains low to average amounts of calcium, cobalt, protein, sodium, and vitamins A and C.[9]

MEDICINAL PROPERTIES: Soothing anabolic tonic, antiandrogenic, anti-inflammatory, aperient, aphrodisiac, diuretic, expectorant, galactagogue, nutritive, restorative, urinary antiseptic, and uterine tonic.

TEMPERATURE AND FLAVOR: Warm, bitter, salty, and sweet.

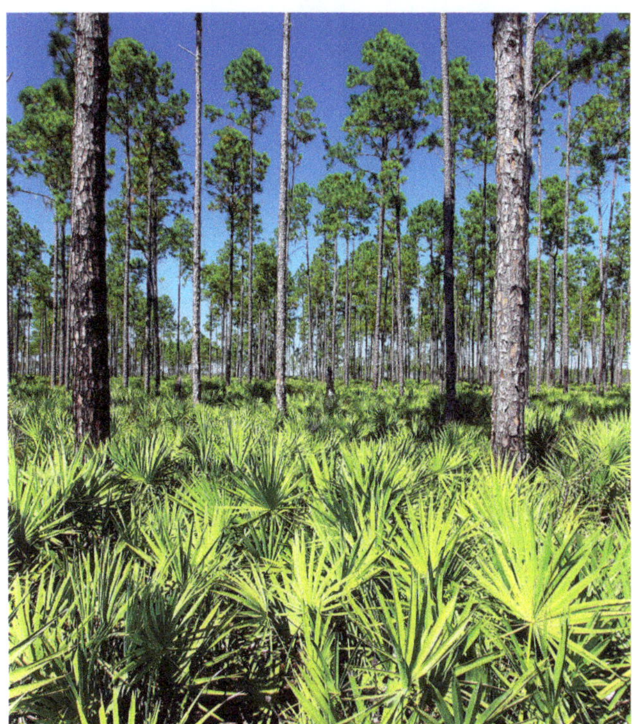

MEDICINAL USES

Saw palmetto aids in treating the early stages of benign prostatic hypertrophy (BPH), characterized by enlargement of the epithelial and fibromuscular structures in the prostate gland.[4,5,7,8,10,11] The accumulation of testosterone in the prostate is considered the primary cause of BPH.[7] Testosterone is converted to 5-α-diyhydrotestosterone (DHT) by the enzyme 5-α-reductase in the prostate.[5,7] DHT causes prostatic cells to multiply excessively, resulting in an enlarged prostate.[5,7] DHT has five times the biological potency of testosterone.[5] The liposterolic extract of saw palmetto limits intraprostatic conversion of testosterone to DHT, and prevents intracellular binding and transport of DHT.[5,7,8,11]

Clinical studies demonstrate that the liposterolic extract of saw palmetto (LESP) reduces the symptoms of BPH in nearly 90% of patients.[5,7] LESP is a standardized extract containing 85 – 95% free fatty acids and sterols. When administered in a dosage of 160 mg twice daily, it increases urinary flow, alleviates or decreases difficulty initiating urinary flow, and reduces the frequency of urination and residual urine, dysuria, and nocturia.[5-8] LESP also exerts

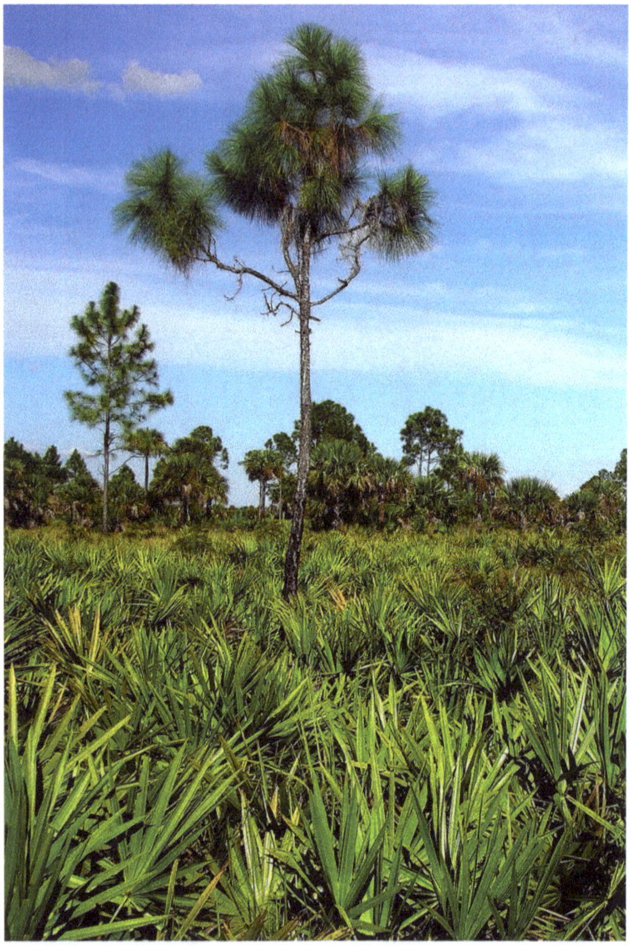

an antiestrogenic effect in prostatic cells.[7] Estrogen inhibits the hydroxylation and elimination of DHT, thus contributing to BPH.[7] Saw palmetto has additional effects on the prostate, reducing inflammation, edema, and spasms by inhibiting the biosynthesis of prostaglandins and leukotrienes.[8] Clinical studies indicate that LESP is more effective, faster acting, and has considerably fewer side effects than the prescription drug finasteride, commonly used to treat BPH.[3,7] However, LESP has no significant influence on prostate volume or serum PSA (prostate specific antigen), the clinical markers used to evaluate BPH (although finasteride does, indicating that LESP has minimal action on 5-α-reductase inhibition).[5] The antispasmodic effects that decrease urethral obstruction caused by increased smooth muscle tone are attributed to the α-adrenoceptor and calcium-blocking actions.[5] In summary, the combined therapeutic properties of LESP, including the androgen inhibitory, antispasmodic, anti-inflammatory, and anti-edemic actions, contribute to the efficacy of saw palmetto for treating BPH.[5]

Saw palmetto strengthens the reproductive organs and bladder, improving the overall tone and function of the genitourinary organs.[10] It is a reproductive tonic that aids in treating uterine hypertrophy and dysmenorrhea resulting from poor tissue and muscle tone.[4,10] It is an adjunct for treating ovarialgia and ovaritis.[10] Saw palmetto reduces congestion in the pelvic region, and can relieve dull, achy sensations associated with congestion in the uterus and ovaries.

Saw palmetto enhances bladder tone, and aids in treating urinary incontinence, and decreasing urinary dribbling and leakage.[10,11] It is a soothing diuretic that reduces inflammation in the mucous membranes lining the urinary tract. In addition to Kegels and other bladder tonics, saw palmetto aids in treating stress incontinence or a cystocele (bladder hernia) resulting from injuries related to childbirth.

Saw palmetto is a valuable adjunct for treating cystitis or urethritis, as well as long-term interstitial cystitis.[3,5,11] It decreases dysuria, is a mild urinary tract antibacterial, and strengthens tissues. These actions are especially helpful for women with difficulty resolving a urinary tract infection, in spite of repeated use of antibiotics.[11]

Saw palmetto is a nourishing anabolic tonic — a substance that encourages tissue building. It contains numerous lipids, vitamins, and minerals that are essential building blocks of healthy cells and tissues.[5,9] Additionally, it enhances digestion and assimilation, improving nutrient metabolism and utilization.[4,10] Saw palmetto aids in replenishing women

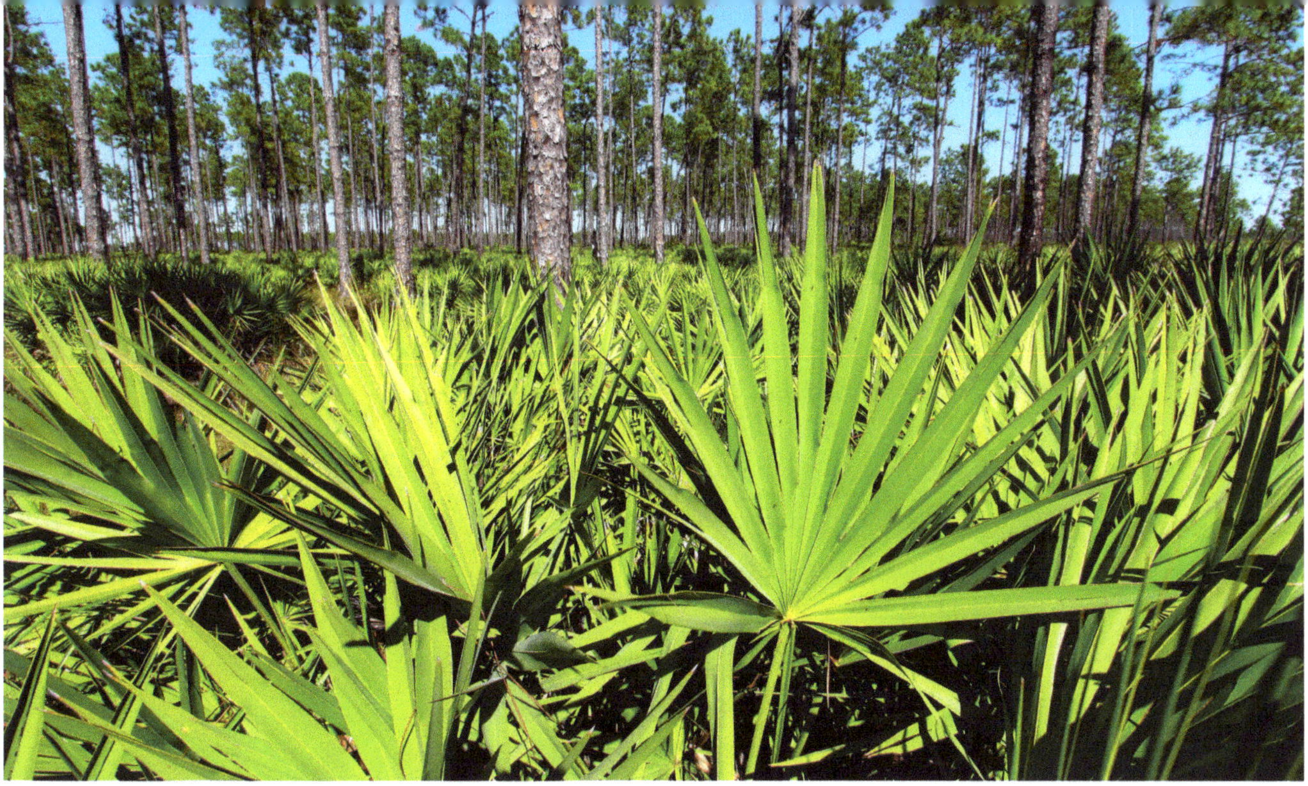

depleted from childbearing and nursing, those who are malnourished, thin-bodied, or catabolic. It is an adjunct treatment for women with a prolapsed uterus or bladder following a birth, and is also a mild galactagogue.

Saw palmetto promotes fertility, and can be incorporated into formulas for women having difficulty conceiving, or who have had miscarriages.[4] It can enhance conception in women who are undernourished or malnourished when combined with making appropriate dietary modifications. Saw palmetto increases fertility most effectively when it is consumed at least six months to one year. *Note:* Many factors influence fertility in women, including progesterone deficiency, hypothyroidism, hyperthyroidism, insulin resistance, stress, severe depletion, and structural abnormalities. In order to obtain optimum results when treating infertility, each of these potential factors must be considered and addressed.

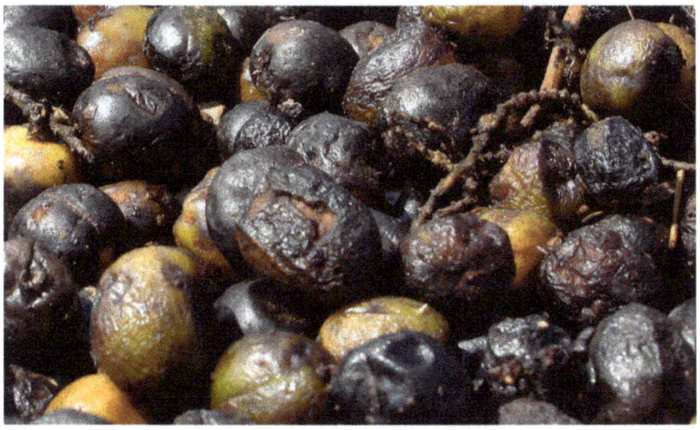

CONTRAINDICATIONS

Saw palmetto is considered safe, and has no toxic effects.[5,7] There are no known contraindications with saw palmetto.[5,7,8] In rare cases, the extracts may cause gastrointestinal problems, including nausea or stomach upset if taken on an empty stomach.[5,8] Before self-prescribing saw palmetto for BPH, consult a physician to rule out prostate cancer.[3]

PREPARATION AND DOSAGE

TINCTURE: Tinctures and fluid extracts are considered inferior because the berries have limited alcohol solubility.[5,7] Fresh berries [1:2-1:3, 95% alcohol]; dry berries [1:5, 80% alcohol]; consume 20-90 drops, up to three times daily.

CAPSULES: Consume 160 mg of standardized liposterolic extracts of saw palmetto (containing 85-95% free fatty acids and sterols) twice daily.[7]

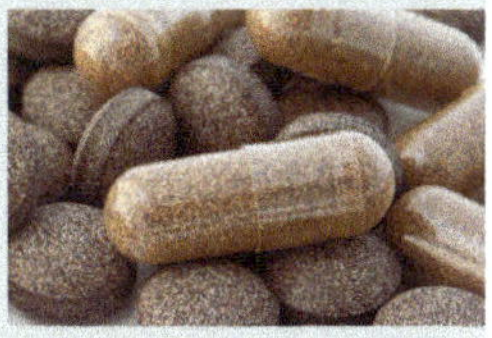

Consume 2-3 "00" capsules containing freeze-dried berry or standardized extract, two to three times daily. Consume 2-10 grams of dried berry powder, up to three times daily.

SCHISANDRA

DESCRIPTION

BOTANICAL NAMES:
Schisandra chinensis, S. sphenanthera, S. glabra (syn. *S. coccinea*), *S.* spp.

COMMON NAMES:
Schisandra, schisandra fruit, fructus schisandrae, five-flavor fruit, five-taste berry, Chinese magnolia vine, magnolia vine, star vine, bay star vine
ng mei ji (Cantonese)
palsamiköynnös (Finnish)
gomishi (Japanese)
omija, omicha, o mi cha (Korean)
wu wei zi, wu wei tza (Mandarin)
limonnik, limonka (Russian)
fjärilsranka (Swedish)

FAMILY NAME:
Schisandraceae (formerly Magnoliaceae)

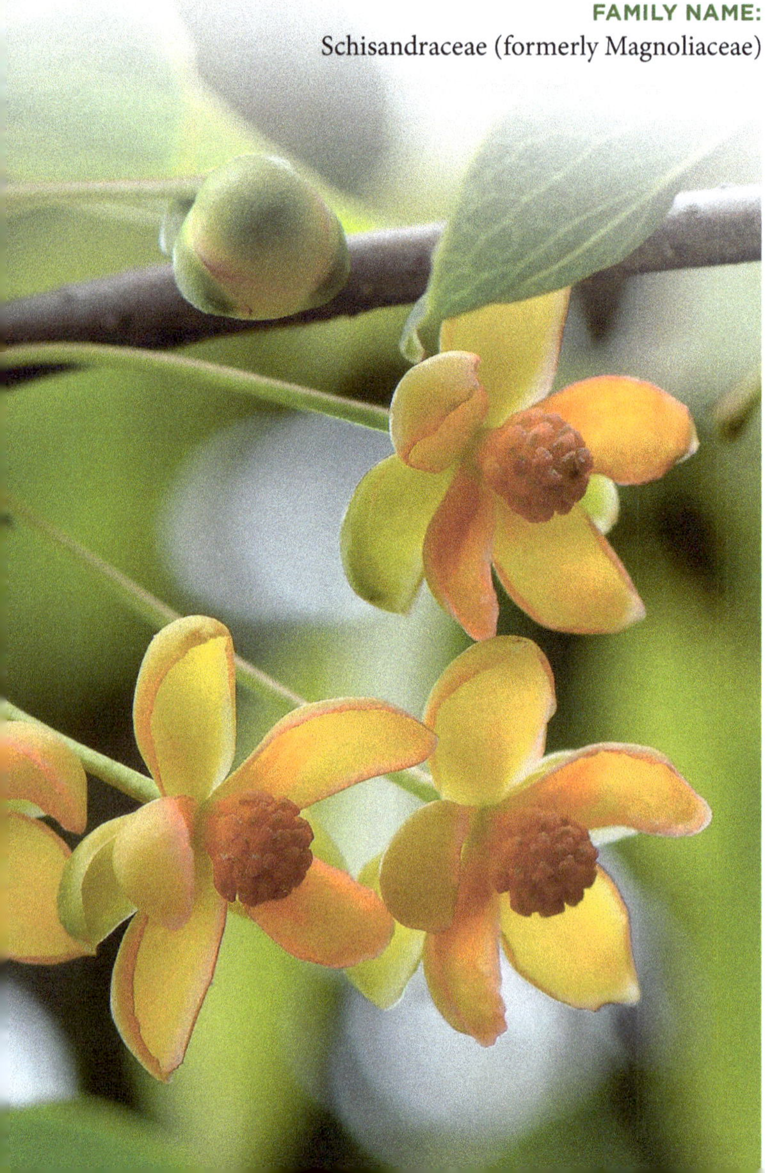

PARTS USED: The fruits and seeds.

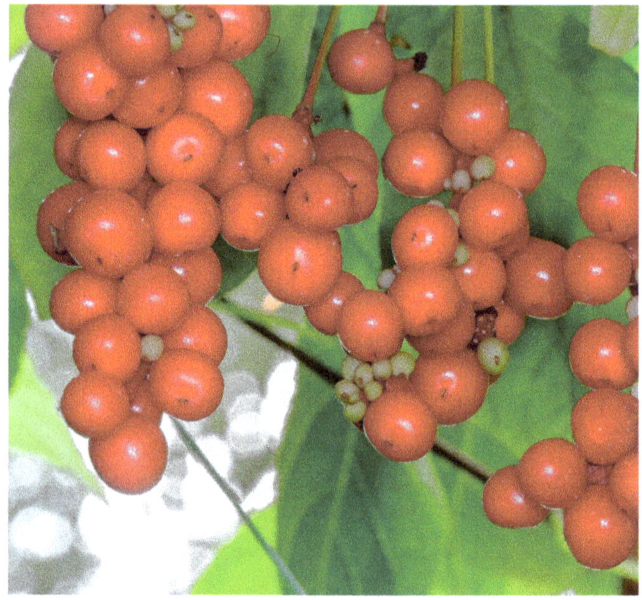

BOTANICAL DESCRIPTION AND HABITAT: *Schisandra chinensis* is a dioecious woody vine native to northern China, northern Japan, Korea, and Russia.[1] Its deciduous leaves have a glabrous petiole (1 – 4 cm long), and a delicate, elliptic blade (3.5 – 8 cm long by 2.5 – 6.5 cm wide) with a short, tapered apex and minutely serrated margin.[1] The solitary flowers are found at the axils of short-lived bracts.[1] Pistillate flowers have longer peduncles than male flowers (up to 2.8 cm in staminate flowers, and up to 3.5 cm in pistillate flowers), while both male and female flowers have five to nine yellow to white tepals (up to 1 cm long).[1] Staminate flowers usually have five stamens, while the pistillate flowers have 14 – 40 separate carpels.[1] These carpels develop into a unique fruit on a long peduncle (2 – 8 cm). The fruit (1.5 – 9.5 cm long) consists of many berry-like units, and appears similar to a cluster of grapes, suggesting origination from multiple flowers. In fact, the entire fruit cluster originates from one flower, making it a single aggregate fruit comparable to an elongated blackberry, rather than a cluster of separate fruits.[2] Each red berry-like unit is called an apocarp; it is referred to as the fruit or berries in this monograph.[2] The dried berries have a deep red to reddish-purple color, with one to two yellow-brown, kidney-shaped seeds.

Schisandra sphenanthera is found in southern and western China.[3] The whole plant is fully glabrous.[3] Compared to *S. chinensis,* it has longer leaf blades (4 – 11 cm long by 2 – 6 cm wide), and longer peduncles (up to 5.4 cm in staminate flowers and 6.4 cm in pistillate flowers). The staminate flowers also bear many more stamens than *S. chinensis,* up to 25, and the pistillate flowers often contain more carpels, from 25 – 45.

Schisandra glabra is a rare species native to North America. It grows in rich soil in the woods, along undisturbed streams, creeks, and ravines throughout the southeastern U.S. It is a vine and can reach over 20 m long.[4] On older stems (up to 4 cm in diameter), the bark is gray-brown and flakes off, while the younger twigs have smooth, light brown bark.[4] The glabrous leaves bear a long petiole (1 – 7 cm long) and cordate blades (2 – 13 cm by 1 – 8 cm) with mostly entire margins.[4] The plant is monecious, with staminate and pistillate flowers growing on top of a thin peduncle (up to 5 cm long). The ovate tepals (3 – 9 mm by 2 – 5 mm) are arranged in two series, with the outer layer pale green in color, and the inner layer red.[4] The unique staminate flowers have a flat disc, in which five anthers are embedded.[4] The pistillate flowers have 6 – 12 reddish, separate carpels that produce small round berries.[4]

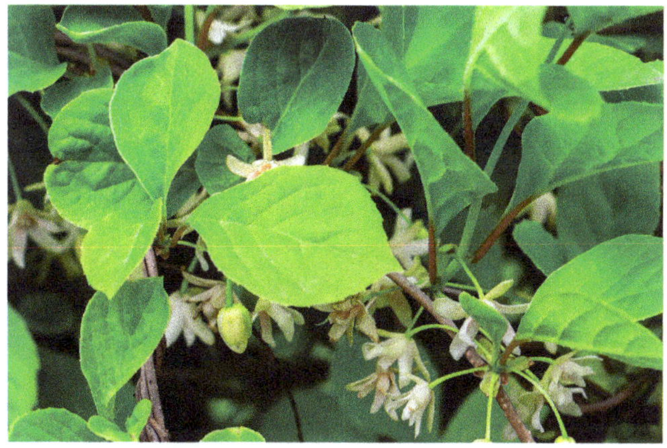

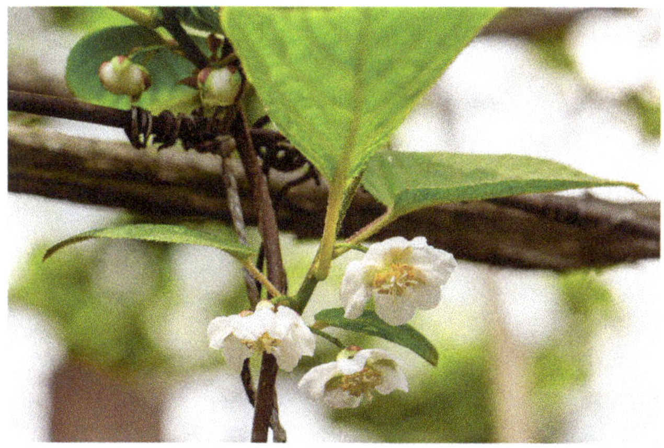

THE NAME: *Schisandra* derives from the Greek words *schizein* ("to cleave") and *andros* ("man"), referring to the cleft or separate anther cells on stamens. Wu wei zi translates as "five-flavor seed."[5] The fruits of *S. chinensis* (northern schisandra) are also referred to as bei wu wei zi; the fruits of *S. sphenanthera* (southern schisandra) are called nan wu wei zi.[5,6] The common names for *Schisandra glabra* include magnolia vine, star vine, and bay star vine.[6]

HISTORICAL USES: Schisandra use began more than 5,000 years ago.[8] It was reserved for the wealthy classes of China, including emperors and royal women because it was rare until recently.[9] Schisandra was used to increase vitality, as a beautifying agent, and a sexual tonic.[9] It was administered to treat nervous conditions, including neurasthenia. Schisandra continues to be used to tonify the lungs, and treat a chronic cough and asthma. It also is used to tonify the kidneys, decreasing excessive urination, night sweats, spontaneous sweating, and impotence.[7] The fruits were stir-fried until black, then powdered and applied as a poultice to ulcerated skin.[7] The vines and roots treated joint pain, rheumatism, and injuries.[6] The leaves were cooked as a vegetable.[8]

CONSTITUENTS: Schisandra contains volatile oil (sesquicarene, citral, β-2-bisabolene, α-ylangene, β-chamigrene, α-chamigrene, and chamigrenal), organic acids (citric, malic, tartaric, ascorbic, and dehydroxysuccinic), monosaccharides, resins, sterols (stigmasterol and β-sitosterol), tannins, pectin, flavonoids, anthocyanins, catechins, and triterpenes, as well as vitamins A, C, and E. It also contains more than 40 lignans including: schizandrin (syn. schizandrol A, wuwiechun A); schizandrin A (syn. deoxyschizandrin, wuwuizisu A); schizandrin B (syn. gammaschizandrin, wuweizisu B); schizandrin C (syn. wuweizisu C); schizandrol B; schisantherin D; pseudo-y-schizandrin; gomisins A-R; wuweizi ester A (syn. gomosin C, schisantherin A, and schizandrer A); wuweizi ester B (syn. gomisin B, schisantherin B, and schizandrer B); wuwiechun B; and others.[5,6,9]

NUTRITIONAL PROPERTIES: Schisandra contains flavonoids, anthocyanins, vitamins A, C, and E, and high amounts of chromium, cobalt, magnesium, and phosphorus. It contains low to average amounts of fiber, iron, manganese, niacin, potassium, protein, riboflavin, selenium, silicon, sodium, thiamine, and zinc.[5,9,10]

MEDICINAL PROPERTIES: Adaptogen, adrenal tonic, immune modulator, jing tonic, kidney qi tonic, kidney yang tonic, kidney yin tonic, lung qi tonic, shen tonic, wei qi tonic, yin tonic, and antiallergenic, antidepressant, antimutagenic, antitussive, calmative, expectorant, euphoric, hepatoregenerative, hepatoprotectant, mild sedative, and vasodilator.

TEMPERATURE AND FLAVOR: Warm, sour, salty, astringent, bitter, sweet, and pungent.

MEDICINAL USES

Schisandra is an extremely effective kidney tonic.[5,12] It increases kidney yin, yang, qi, and jing.[5,9,12] As a kidney yin tonic, schisandra increases sexual fluids. It is a fertility tonic for females with difficulty conceiving. In males, schisandra increases sex drive, seminal fluids, and sexual endurance, and decreases nocturnal emissions and spermatorrhea.[5,9,12,13] Schisandra aids in treating kidney yin deficiency. It inhibits spontaneous sweating, decreases hot flashes and night sweats, reduces incontinence, generates fluids, and aids in treating diabetes insipidus, also known as "thirsting and wasting disorder."[5] As a kidney yang tonic, it increases sexual vitality and libido.[9,13] It aids in treating sexual frigidity and impotence. Schisandra improves circulation to the reproductive organs, increasing genital sensation.[9]

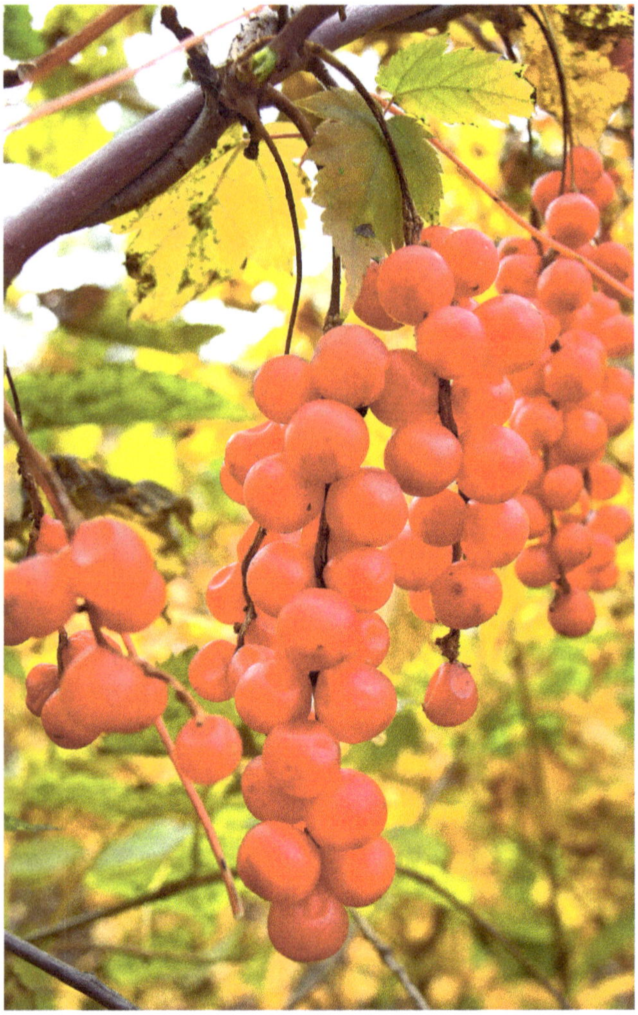

Schisandra is an adrenal tonic and calming adaptogen, enhancing the body's ability to cope with stress.[5,8] It increases endurance, strength, and the non-specific immune response. It also improves work and physical performance.[5,6,8,14] It enhances eyesight, night vision, hearing, mental acuity, reflexes, and tolerance to extreme temperatures.[14] Schisandra can have a calming or stimulating effect on the nervous system.[7] The seed extract stimulates the central nervous system, improving mental and physical capacity, as well as motor coordination and efficiency; however, it does not elicit an excitatory response like caffeine or amphetamines.[14] The seed extract prevents adrenal and thymus gland atrophy in animals experiencing extreme stress.[14]

Schisandra is a lung qi and wei qi tonic.[5,9] The astringent and sour properties improve the lungs' capacity to grasp qi, deepening inhalation.[5] Schisandra aids in treating asthma, wheezing, and a chronic cough resulting from lung qi and kidney deficiency.[5] It increases resistance and prevents respiratory infections in susceptible individuals.[14] It is a convalescing and respiratory recuperative agent following serious infections such as bronchitis, pneumonia, or pleurisy. *Note:* Discontinue use during an acute infection. Consuming schisandra several months prior to allergy season helps to prevent seasonal allergies. The flavonoid-rich berries have antiallergenic actions, as well as immune modulating and anti-inflammatory effects. Schisandra can reduce post-nasal drip and related nighttime snoring. Combine schisandra with huang qi *(Astragalus)*, dang shen *(Codonopsis)*, and smaller amounts of bai zhi *(Atractylodes)* and fang feng *(Saposhnikovia)* to prevent seasonal allergies.

Schisandra is an immune modulator, enhancing non-specific immunity. It increases antibody production in immunized animals, and reduces inflammation by suppressing the arachidonic acid cascade.[14] It protects against the effects of chemotherapy, and inhibits drug resistance in cancer cells.[14]

Schisandra has hepatoprotective, antihepatotoxic, and hepatoregenerative properties.[6,7,13,14] It supports liver function by stimulating the biosynthesis of serum and liver proteins, and encouraging glycogenesis.[6,14] Schisandra increases liver detoxifying enzymes, including glutathione-S-transferase and cytochrome P-450.[14] It is a potent

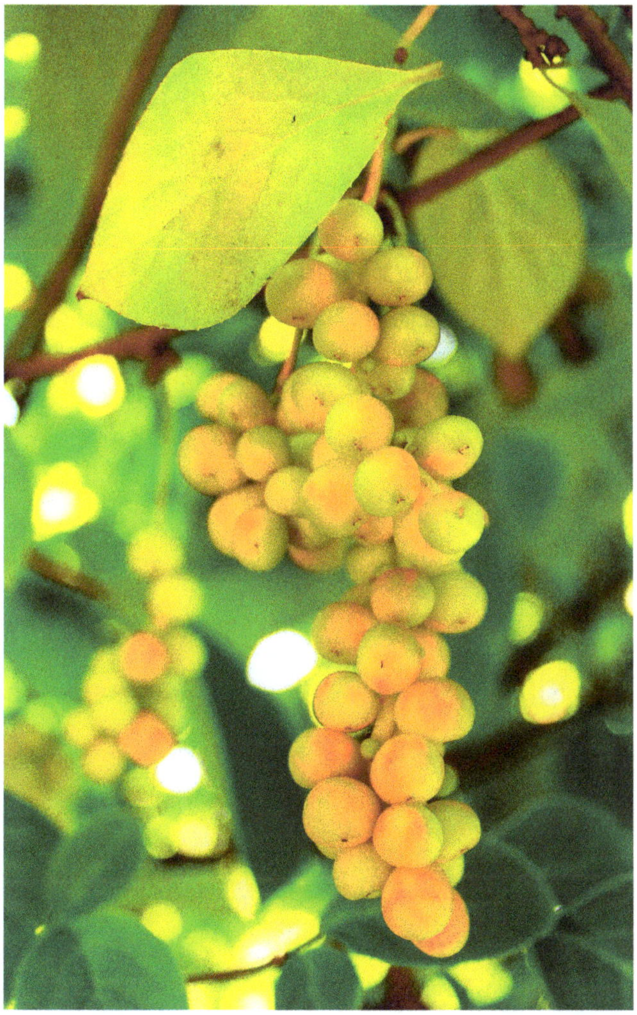

antioxidant that prevents liver damage from a variety of toxic chemical substances.[6,14] Gomisin A, a lignin, inhibits liver lesions caused by hepatotoxins.[6] Schisandra seeds contain additional lignans that inhibit lipid peroxidation induced from carbon tetrachloride and other liver toxins.[6] Studies showed that schisandra reduced the mortality rate in animals poisoned by acetaminophen, digitoxin, and indomethacin.[8] Schisandra accelerates the proliferation of hepatocytes, and the recovery of liver functions after a partial hepatectomy in rats. It also inhibits the development and progression of liver cancer.[14] In one study, a schisandrin-rich extract demonstrated a protective effect against stress-induced liver metastasis of P815 tumor cells in mice.[14]

Schisandra aids in treating viral and chemical hepatitis.[5] It lowers serum alanine amino transferase (ALT) also known as glutamic pyruvic transaminase (SGPT). Elevated liver enzyme levels indicate a fatty liver.[7,14] Schisandra contains more than 14 antihepatotoxic lignans including: wuweizisu C; schisantherin D; gomisin A, C, and N; deoxygomisin A; schizandrin A-C; schizandrol A and B; schizandrer A and B; schisanhenol; and others.[6] The lignin content prevents morphological changes, such as inflammatory filtration and liver cell necrosis. In one study, patients with infectious hepatitis with SGPT levels over 300 IU experienced a 72% success rate in restoring normal liver enzyme counts after consuming powdered schisandra approximately 25 days.[5] Schisandra contains bipheyldimethyldicarboxylate (BDD), an intermediate of schizandrin C synthesis that is more effective than silymarin in treating viral hepatitis.[6] Schisandra's hepatorestorative actions have a positive effect in treating cirrhosis of the liver.[15] Combine schisandra with powdered silymarin, artichoke leaf *(Cynara)*, dandelion *(Taraxacum)*, and reishi mushroom *(Ganoderma)* as a hepatorestorative.

Schisandra enhances the breakdown of estrogen, and aids in treating estrogen-related conditions such as endometriosis and breast cancer.[15] In a double-blind study of perimenopausal and postmenopausal women, the treatment group consumed a supplement containing HMR lignin, indole-3-carbinol, calcium glucarate, milk thistle, schisandra, and stinging nettle. The women receiving the supplement had increased production of estrogen C-2 hydroxylation compared to the control group that received a placebo. Researchers concluded that the supplement may reduce the risk of breast cancer and other estrogen-related cancers.[14]

Schisandra is a shen tonic that calms the heart and quiets the spirit.[5,12] It aids in treating shen disturbance resulting from kidney and heart yin deficiency.[5] Symptoms of shen disturbance include: insomnia, dream disturbed sleep, palpitations, anxiety, and nervous system irritability.[5,12] Schisandra has mild soporific, tranquilizing, and sedative actions.[9] The lignans are attributed to the central nervous system depressant effect.[7] In rodent studies, the constituent schizandrin stimulated cholinergic receptors, having a parasympathomimetic influence.[5] Schisandra also has mood elevating properties that aid in treating depression resulting from nervous system stress, depletion, and exhaustion.[8,14]

Schisandra has vasodilating actions, improving circulation and enhancing oxygen and nutrient delivery to the tissues.[5,6] Adding small quantities of the herb to a tonic formula acts as a carrier. Schisandra has potent antioxidant actions.

Schisandra regulates gastric secretion, increasing pH when the stomach is too acidic, and lowering pH when it is too basic.[5] Alcohol extracts have ulcer preventative actions.[7]

Schisandra also promotes bile secretion and gastric motility.[7,14]

CONTRAINDICATIONS

Avoid use during pregnancy, as it has stimulating effects on the uterus.[5,6] Discontinue consuming schisandra during an acute viral or bacterial infection, such as the early stages of a cold, flu, cough, bronchitis, pneumonia, or skin rash.[5]

Schisandra can cause heartburn or stomach upset due to the tannins.[5,6,9] According to herbalist Ron Teeguarden, digestive upset can be avoided by presoaking the berries several hours, straining and rinsing them, discarding the water, then decocting them for 15 minutes. He recommends adding an equal amount of lycii berries and a few slices of licorice root to the decoction.[9]

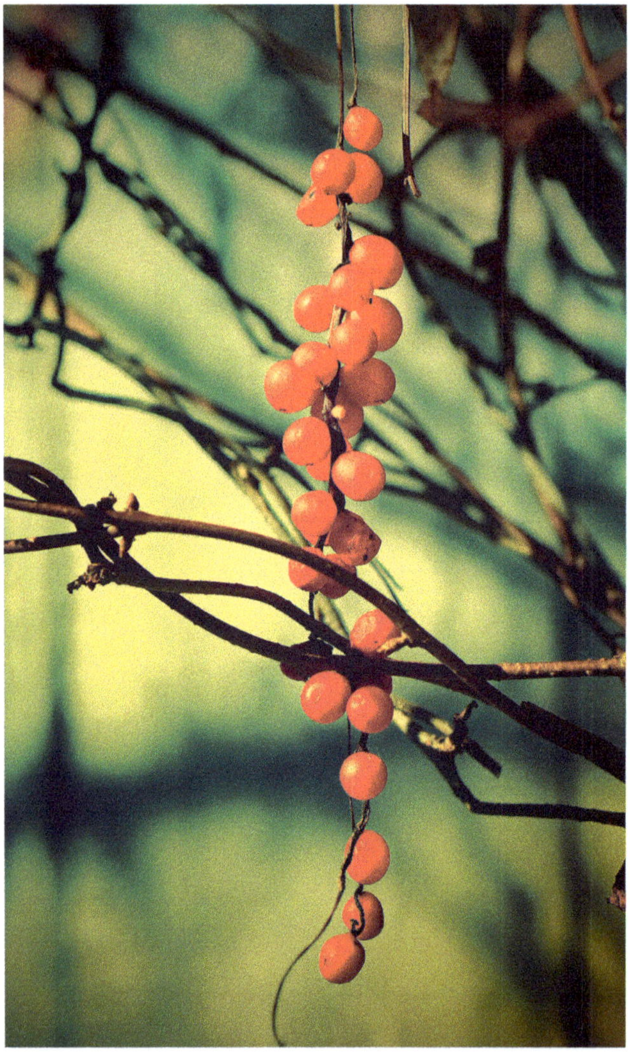

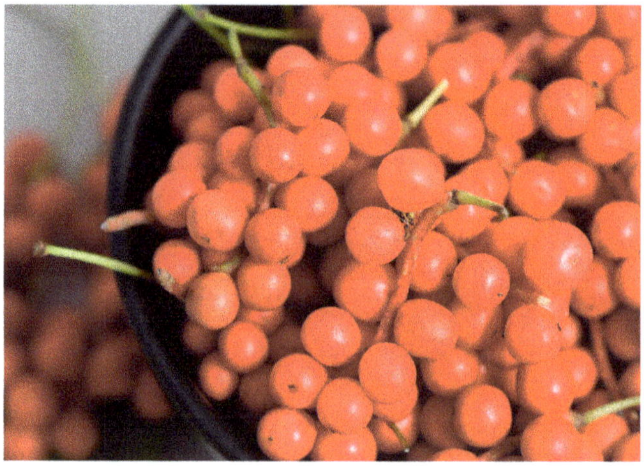

PREPARATION AND DOSAGE

TINCTURE: Fresh berries [1:2, 95% alcohol]; dry berries or seeds [1:5, 60% alcohol]; consume 10-60 drops, up to three times daily.

FLUID EXTRACT: Dry berries or seeds [1:1, 40% alcohol]; consume 10-30 drops, up to three times daily.

GLYCERITE: Dry berries or seeds [1:5, 40% glycerin, 30% alcohol, 30% water]; consume 10-60 drops, up to three times daily.

CAPSULES: Consume 2-4 capsules, two to three times daily.

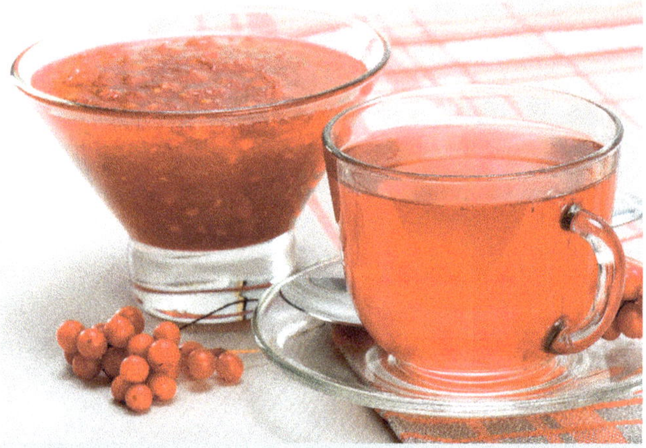

TEA: Prepare a hot or cold infusion, or a decoction; consume 8-12 ounces, up to three times daily.

CULINARY USE: Include a small quantity of schisandra in rose hip jam.

SHEPHERD'S PURSE

DESCRIPTION

BOTANICAL NAME:
Capsella bursa-pastoris

COMMON NAMES:
Shepherd's purse, mother's heart, witch's pouch, rattle pouches, pick pocket, pick purse, poverty weed, shepherd's sprout, shepherd's scrip, shepherd's bag, blind weed, beggar tick, mother's heart, poor man's pharmacy, sanguinary
bourse de pasteur (French)
hirtentasche (German)
clappedepouch (Irish)

FAMILY NAME:
Brassicaceae

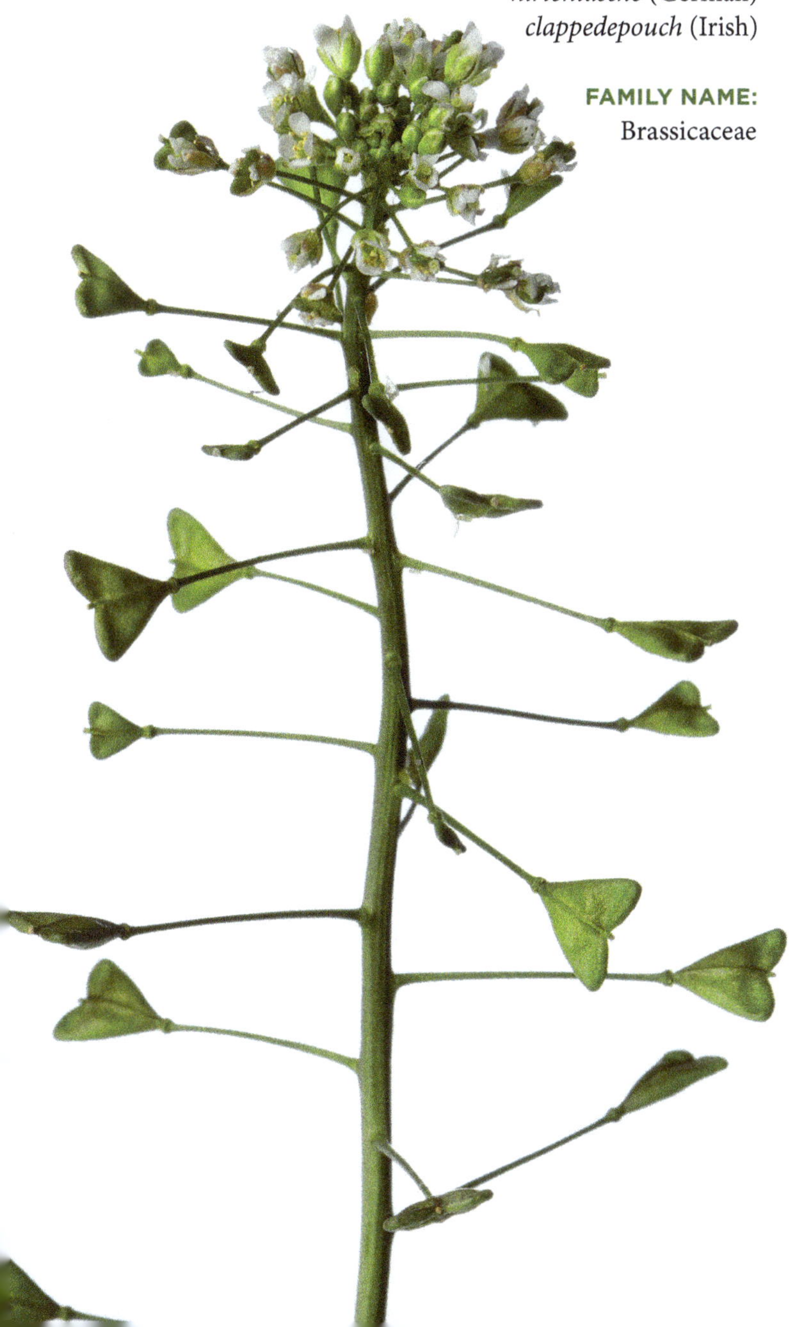

PART USED: The leaves.

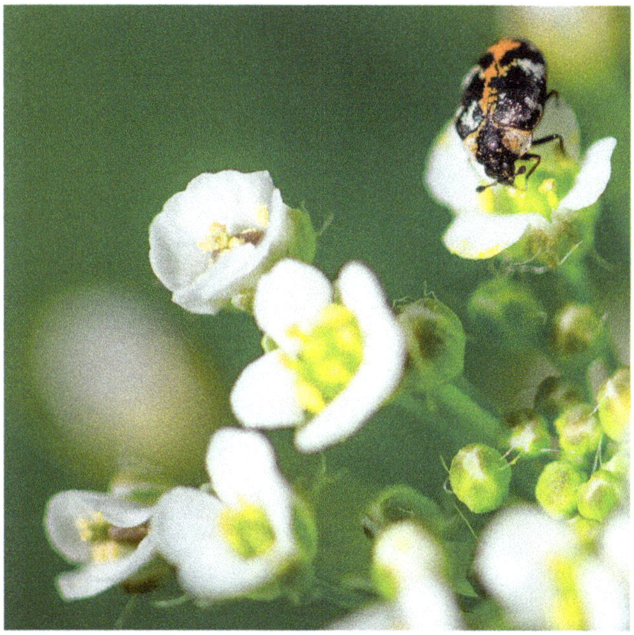

BOTANICAL DESCRIPTION AND HABITAT: Shepherd's purse is an annual or biennial native to Eurasia that has naturalized worldwide, and is known as the world's second most common weed.[1,2] It is often found in farms, fields, pastures and gardens, along roadsides, in waste areas, or on mountain slopes.[2] Covered in stellate hairs, the plant grows 10 – 50 cm tall.[1] The oblancolate basal leaves (3 – 6 cm long) are similar in appearance to other mustard family leaves, and are irregularly lobed.[1] The oblong to linear stem leaves are shorter (1 – 6 cm long).[1] The flower's perianth consists of obovate sepals (about 2 mm long) and white or occasionally pink petals (2 – 4 mm long).[1] Like other members of its family, it has six stamens; two are shorter than the other four. The seedpod (4 – 10 mm by 3 – 7 mm) is a silicle, and is triangular to heart-shaped.[1,2] It is filled with tiny brown seeds, about 1 mm in diameter.[2]

THE NAME: *Capsella* is Latin for "a little box," referring to the fruit.[3] The epithet *bursa-pastoris* was a Latin translation of the common name "shepherd's purse," referring to the purse-shaped fruit. *Bursa* is Latin for a bag, pouch, or purse; *pastoris* refers to the Latin *pastoralis* ("of herdsmen, of shepherds").[4,5]

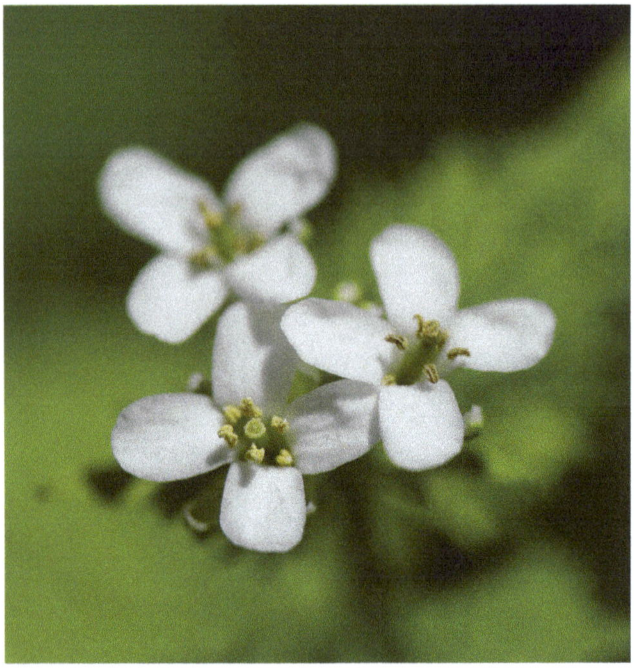

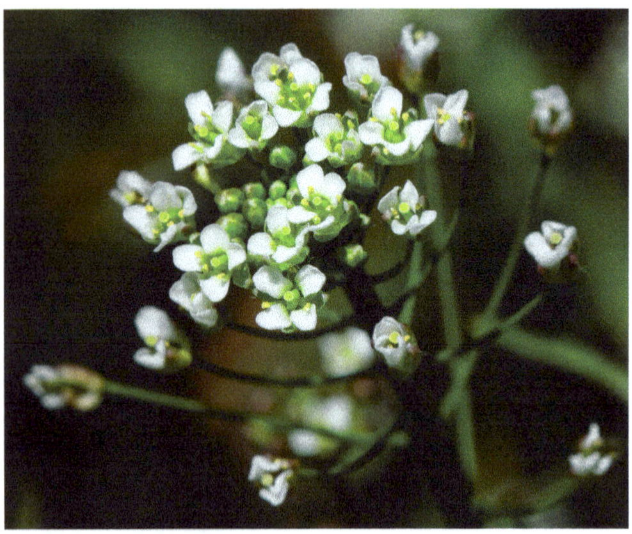

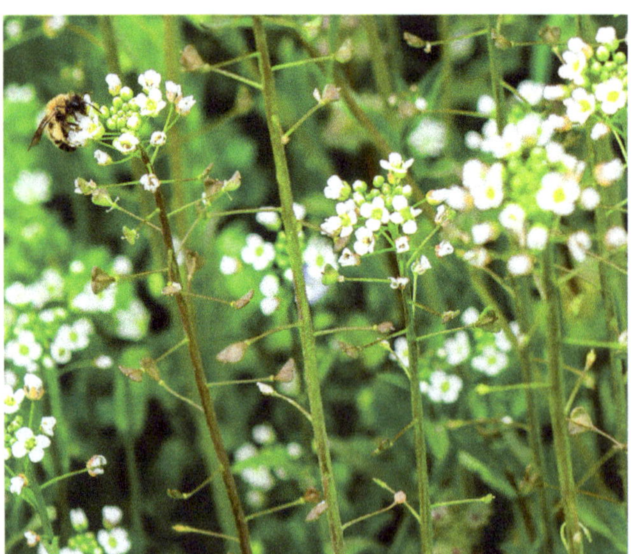

Many of the common names refer to purse and pouch because the seed heads resemble the shape of old fashioned leather purses. The Irish coined the name "clappedepouch," a common name with an intriguing, sorrowful history. In medieval times, lepers were often left to beg for their living. Because people did not want to have contact with them, in some places the lepers would hang a pouch at the end of a long stick, then clap sticks or bells together to draw attention to themselves.[6]

HISTORICAL USES: Shepherd's purse was consumed as a spring green or pot herb.[6] Tea was consumed as an astringent to treat chronic diarrhea and dysentery.[6] Shepherd's purse was administered to reduce hemorrhages from the lungs, stomach, kidneys, or uterus.[6] During World War I, shepherd's purse extract substituted for ergot to reduce bleeding.[6] Wild and domesticated birds feed on its seeds. When poultry eat the fresh plant, their yolks have a more potent flavor and are darker in color.[6]

CONSTITUENTS: Shepherd's purse contains flavonoids (diosmin, luteolin-7-rutinoside, quercetin-3-rutinoside, and scolymoside), choline derivatives (sinapine = sinapic acid choline ester; acetylcholine), minerals (potassium and calcium), tyramine, and phenolic acids (caffeic acid derivatives).[7]

NUTRITIONAL PROPERTIES: Shepherd's purse contains potassium, calcium, and tyramine.

MEDICINAL PROPERTIES: Astringent, diuretic, hemostatic, oxytocin synergist, and counterirritant.

TEMPERATURE AND FLAVOR: Warm, pungent, sweet, astringent, and bitter.

MEDICINAL USES

Shepherd's purse is a hemostatic that can staunch a passive hemorrhage.[6-8] The fresh herbal tea or extract aids in treating postpartum bleeding, menorrhagia (heavy menstruation), and hypermenorrhea (prolonged menstruation) due to uterine or ovarian fibroids, cysts, or mid-cycle bleeding.[7,8] Shepherd's purse also reduces heavy bleeding caused by hormone imbalances during perimenopause, as long as there are no serious complications.[8] Combine extracts of shepherd's purse, red raspberry *(Rubus idaeus)*, lady's mantle *(Alchemilla)*, cinnamon *(Cinnamomum zeylanicum)*, and yarrow *(Achillea)* to reduce uterine bleeding. The hemostatic properties are attributed to

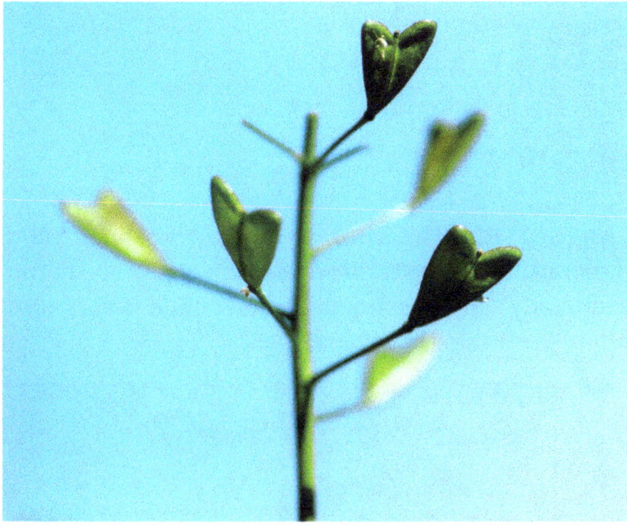

bursinic acid, a vasoconstrictor, and rubinoside that strengthens capillaries.[6]

Shepherd's purse also reduces inflammation and passive bleeding due to gastric or intestinal ulceration from Crohn's disease, ulcerative colitis, irritable bowel syndrome, or hemorrhoids.[7] It aids in treating nosebleeds, bloody sputum, and hematuria (blood in the urine) due to passing kidney stones, interstitial cystitis, and urinary tract bleeding.[6,7] Combine extracts of shepherd's purse, cinnamon *(Cinnamomum zeylanicum)*, yarrow *(Achillea)*, and fleabane *(Erigeron)* as a hemostatic.

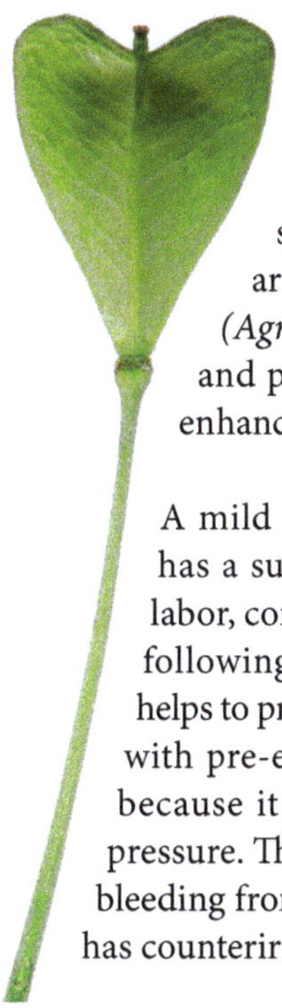

Shepherd's purse has mild diuretic actions.[6,8] It enhances uric acid excretion, and aids in treating conditions caused by excess uric acid, such as kidney stones, gout, and arthritis.[6,8] Combine it with couch grass *(Agropyron)*, dandelion leaf *(Taraxacum)*, and parsley root or seed *(Petroselinum)* to enhance diuresis.

A mild oxytocin synergist, shepherd's purse has a subtle ergot-like effect.[7,8] To stimulate labor, consume 30–60 drops, three times daily following the due date. Shepherd's purse also helps to prevent postpartum hemorrhage. Women with pre-eclampsia should avoid consuming it because it has the potential to increase blood pressure. The fresh plant poultice reduces topical bleeding from cuts and wounds.[7] The poultice also has counterirritant properties that ease joint pain.

CONTRAINDICATIONS

Consult a health professional or go to the hospital immediately for active hemorrhage and/or severe bleeding. Shepherd's purse is only appropriate for treating mild forms of passive hemorrhage.

Shepherd's purse should be avoided during pregnancy unless consumed following the due date. Pregnant women with health complications such as preeclampsia or gestational diabetes should avoid consuming it.

Individuals with hypertension or those medicated for hypertension should avoid consuming shepherd's purse. The vasoconstrictive actions can cause increased blood pressure in individuals with labile hypertension. It also should be avoided by individuals with kidney disease, kidney failure, and those consuming kidney damaging medications.

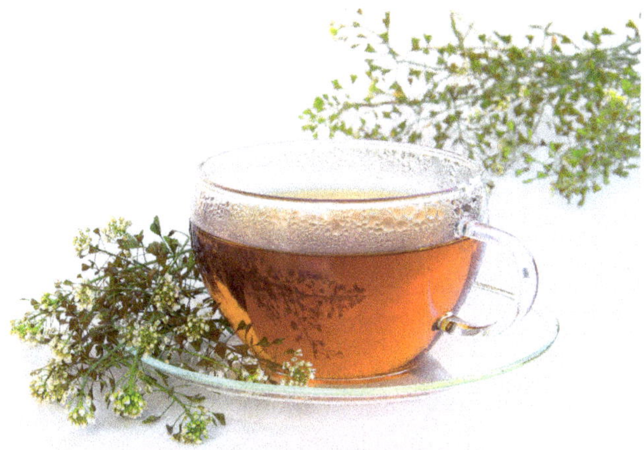

PREPARATION AND DOSAGE

TINCTURE: Fresh leaves [1:2–1:3, 70–95% alcohol]; consume 30–120 drops, up to four times daily.

TEA: Prepare a hot infusion; consume 4–8 ounces, up to four times daily.

TOPICAL USE: Apply a fresh plant poultice to reduce bleeding of cuts, wounds, or abrasions.

CULINARY USE: Use up to 1 teaspoon of chopped, fresh leaves as a pungent, warming green for soups or salads.

SHIITAKE

DESCRIPTION

BOTANICAL NAMES:
Lentinula edodes
(syn. *Lentinus edodes, Tricholomopsis edodes*)

COMMON NAMES:
Shiitake, shiitake mushroom,
golden oak mushroom, black forest mushroom,
oak wood mushroom, forest mushroom, snake butter,
pasania fungus, Chinese mushroom
donku (Japanese)
pasania (Japanese)
shiangu gu, shiang ku, hua gu (Mandarin)[1]

FAMILY NAME:
Marasmiaceae
(formerly Omphalataceae, Tricholomataceae)

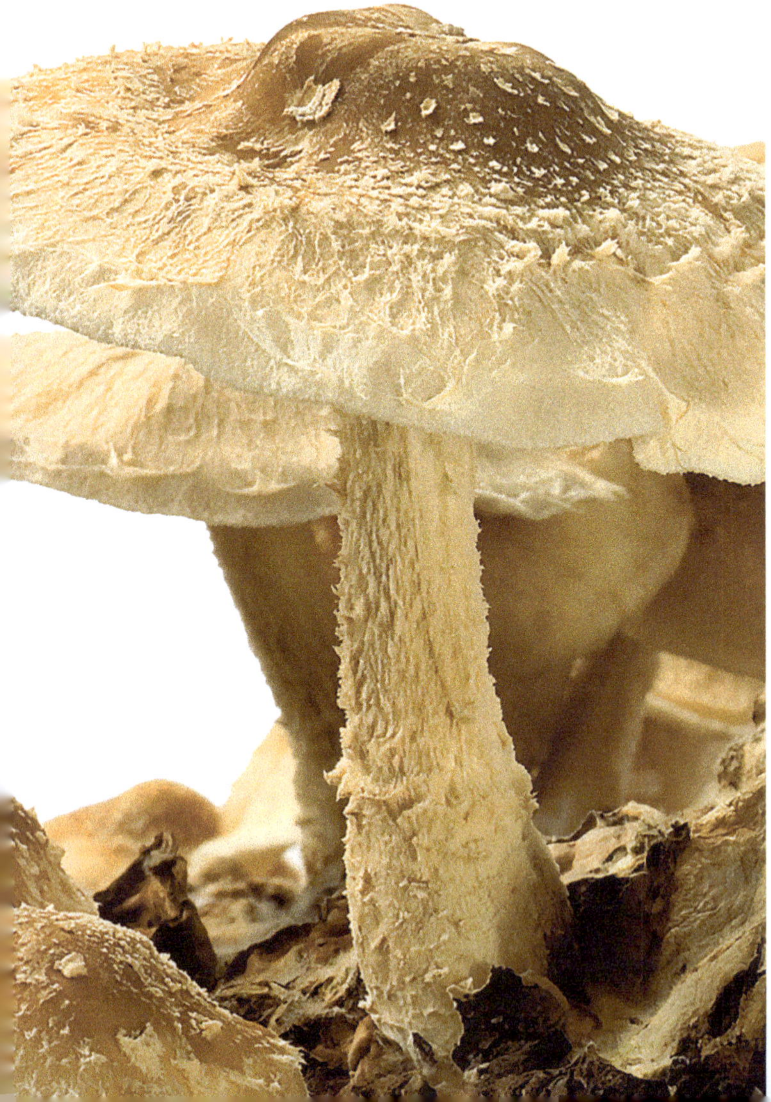

PARTS USED: The mushroom and mycelium. LEM *(Lentinula edodes mycelium extract)* and lentinan are two commonly studied extracts. The mycelium is harvested before the fruiting body develops.

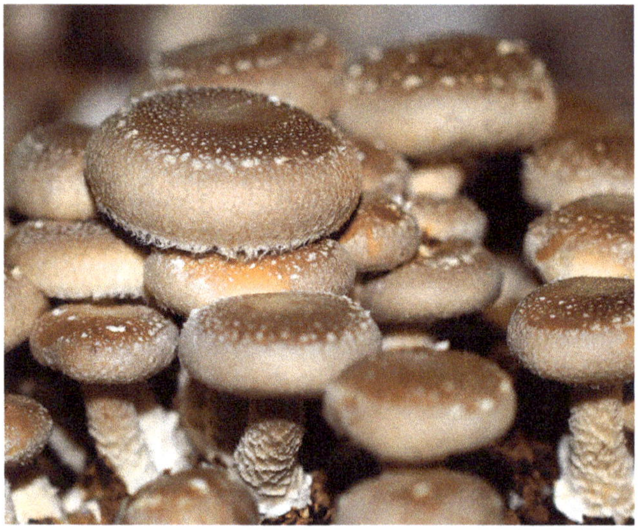

BOTANICAL DESCRIPTION AND HABITAT: Shiitake is native to temperate China, Japan, and Korea.[2,3] *Lentinula edodes* has been cultivated for at least 1,000 years.[2] A wood-decomposing basidiomycete found on dying or fallen hardwood trees, it is cultivated on a variety of species, oaks *(Quercus* spp.*)*, in particular.[2,3] When young, the hemispheric cap (5 – 25 cm diameter) is dark brown or black, with white, smooth, in-rolled margins. Wispy fibrils form a veil stretching across the young gills from the cap to the stipe, leaving white, scaly remnants on the cap. The cap lightens as it ages (or when dried) and flattens; its margins become more ragged as they unroll.[2,3] The fibrous stem occurs centrally or off-center to the cap.[2,3]

THE NAME: The genus *Lentinula* derives from two root words: *lent* ("pliable") and *inus* ("resembling"). The epithet *edodes* means "edible." Shiitake derives from two Japanese words: *shii* ("the trees upon which shiitake grow") and *take* ("mushroom").

HISTORICAL USES: Shiitake has been widely utilized as a food and medicine for thousands of years in China and Japan. It was included in some of the earliest books on botanical medicine. It has been used historically as a symbol of longevity.

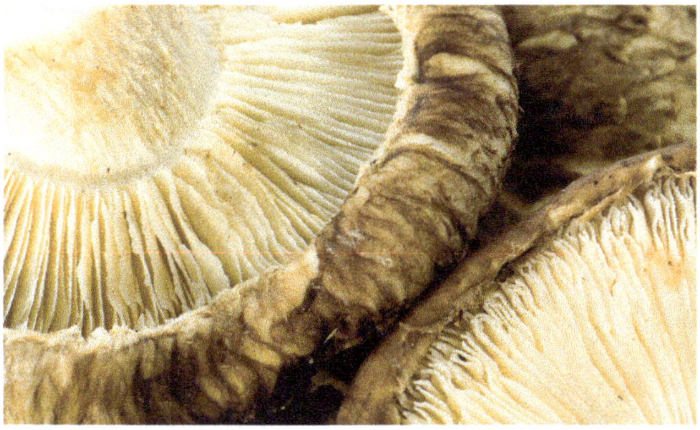

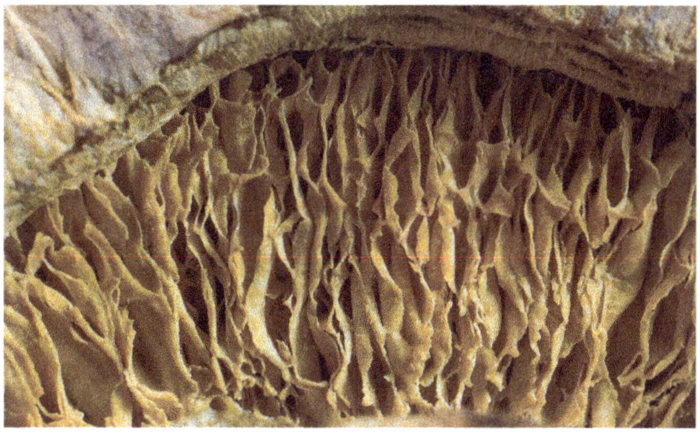

CONSTITUENTS: Shiitake contains high amounts of ergosterol (a provitamin that converts to vitamin D in sunlight), 1-octen-3-ol, ethyl acetate, 2-octenol, and octyl alcohol,1,2,4,5-tetrathiane.[3] It also contains lentinan, a high molecular weight polysaccharide, D-glucan (D-glucose polymer), consisting of a long main chain comprised of β-(1-3) linked D-glucose units, and side chains comprised of β-(1-6) linked D-glucose units.[3,4]

NUTRITIONAL PROPERTIES: Shiitake contains ergosterol, protein, lipids (primarily linoleic acid), carbohydrates, fiber, minerals (potassium, calcium, magnesium, manganese, iron, potassium, zinc, bromine, cadmium, copper, and nickel), and vitamins B_2 and C.[3] It also contains 30 enzymes and more than ten essential amino acids, including lysine, arginine, methionine, and phenylalanine.[3] The mature fruiting bodies contain higher amounts of nutrients than the mycelial cell saps.

MEDICINAL PROPERTIES: Adaptogen, antibacterial, antiparasitic, antitumor, antiviral, hypocholesterolemic, mild hypotensive, and immune modulator.

TEMPERATURE AND FLAVOR: Warm and sweet.

MEDICINAL USES

Shiitake is the source for two well studied preparations, lentinan and *Lentinula edodes* mycelium extract (LEM). LEM is prepared from powdered mycelia extract before the fruiting body emerges.[3] Extracted from the cell wall of fruiting bodies or mycelium, lentinan is a high molecular weight polysaccharide consisting of D-glucan (D-glucose polymer). D-glucan is comprised of a long main chain of β-(1-3) linked D-glucose units, and side chains comprised of β-(1-6) linked D-glucose units.[3,4]

Shiitake is an adaptogen.[4] It increases mental clarity, physical performance, and immune response.[3] Shiitake also has immune restorative and immune modulating actions. Shiitake, LEM, and lentinan aid in treating individuals with compromised immune function. Lentinan and LEM demonstrate potent antitumor activity.[3] Lentinan activates natural killer (NK) cells that inhibit tumor growth.[3] It stimulates helper T cells *in vitro* and *in vivo*.[3] Lentinan stimulates peripheral blood lymphocyte transformation into increased lymphokine-activated killer (LAK) cells, and activates NK cell activity, mediated by interleukin 2 *in vitro* and *in vivo*.[3] It activates the complement cascade, and enhances macrophage activation.[3] Lentinan improves the ratio of activated T cells and killer T cells in the spleen, and inhibits suppressor T cell activity *in vivo*.[3] Oral and injectable doses of lentinan support immune function in immune-compromised individuals, and aid in cancer prevention among high risk individuals.[3] Lentinan increases the effectiveness of chemotherapy and radiation, and counteracts their side effects.[4] It increases cancer survival rates, hastens recovery from chemotherapy and radiation, and prevents secondary infections.[4]

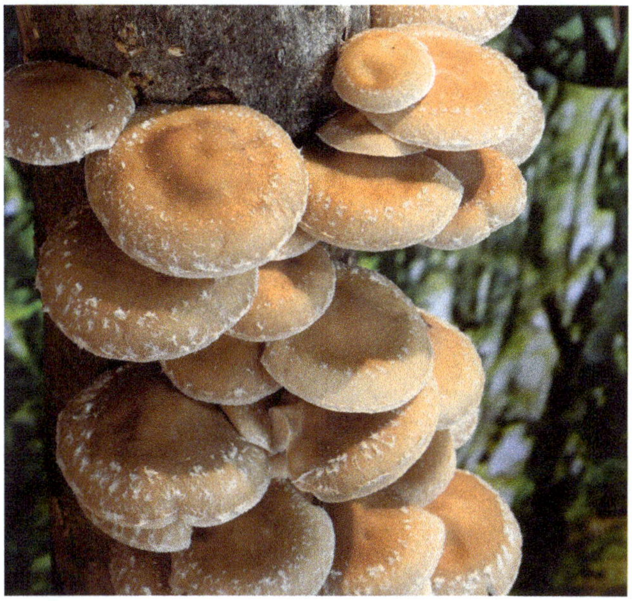

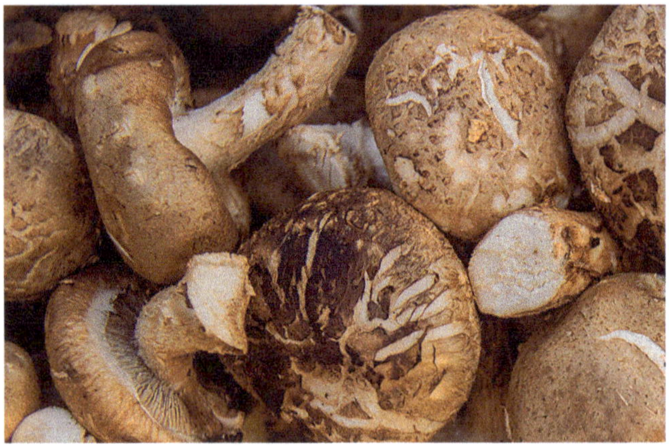

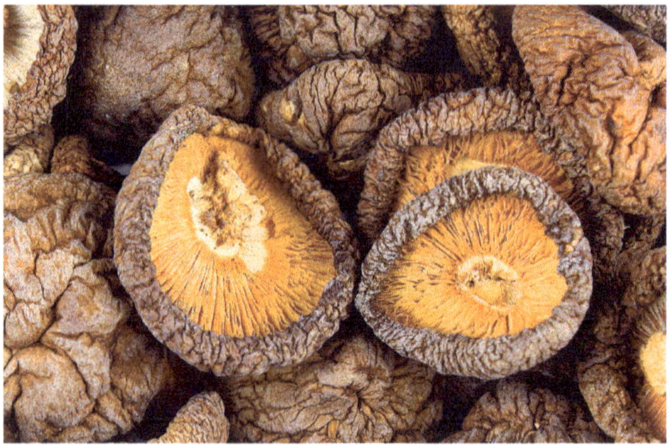

Lentinan enhances humoral and cell-mediated immunity against a variety of cancers, viruses, parasites, and bacteria.[3,4] In rodent studies, lentinan demonstrated antiviral activity against vesicular stomatitis viral encephalitis, adenovirus type 12 virus-induced tumors, and a virulent influenza virus.[3] Lentinan enhances bronchial alveolar macrophage activity, and increases interleukin 6.[3] Combined with LEM, it can be used as a long-term treatment for HIV positive individuals, and those with cancer or viral-induced tumors, chronic fatigue syndrome, herpes, or shingles.[3] LEM inhibits HIV infections in cultured human T cells by potentiating the production of interleukin 1 (lymphocyte-activating factor), encouraging T cell maturation. Lentinan stimulates the mobilization of humoral immunity against antibiotic resistant bacteria.[3] It also strengthens resistance against the parasites *Schistosoma japonicum* and *Schistosoma mansoni.*[3]

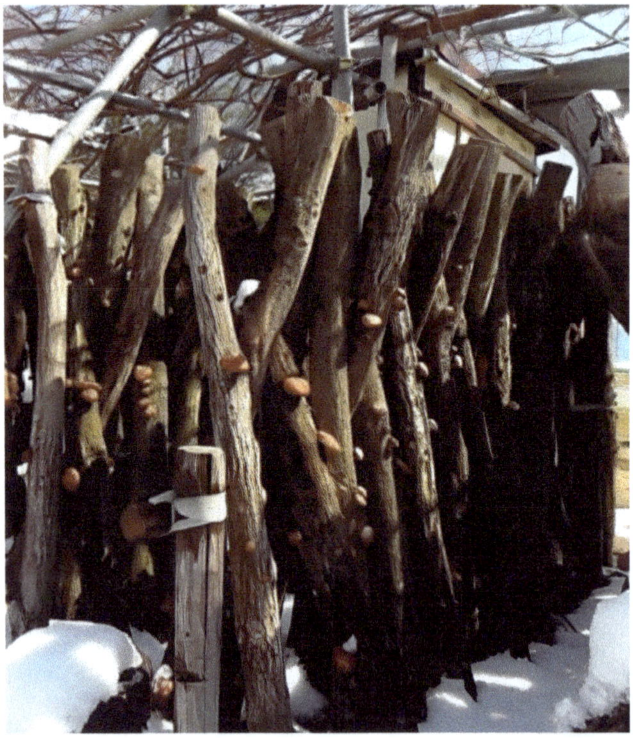

Shiitake can be consumed as a long-term support for individuals with intestinal candida, environmental sensitivity, and chronically reduced immunity.[3]

LEM has hepatoprotective actions.[3] It also enhances liver function, and improves the antibody response to hepatitis B.[3] Lentinan, combined with the polysaccharides from *G. lucidum* and *P. versicolor*, lowered SGPT levels and restored GPT levels *in vivo.*[3] Shiitake also contains adenine and choline that may contribute to the liver-protective effects.

Shiitake has beneficial effects for the cardiovascular system. Eritadenine, a substance contained in shiitake, lowers serum cholesterol and lipids.[3,4] Multiple clinical studies validate the cholesterol-lowering effects. The average dosage was 90 mg of the fresh mushroom or 9 grams of dried shiitake.[3] Shiitake also contains tyronase, which has a blood pressure-lowering effect.[3]

CONTRAINDICATIONS

In some individuals, shiitakes can cause an upset stomach, bloating, or diarrhea. Water-based extracts decrease platelet aggregation.[3] Individuals consuming blood thinners or aspirin should consult a health care practitioner before consuming shiitakes long-term.[3] Avoid consuming shiitakes two weeks prior to, and following surgery or delivery.

In rare cases, individuals may experience minor side effects or allergic reactions, such as shiitake dermatitis. People working indoors cultivating shiitake are prone to immune reactions to spores, called "mushroom worker's lung."[3] LEM can cause diarrhea and skin rashes. Although it is rare, some individuals with cancer receiving lentinan injections have experienced mild side effects including skin eruptions, mild oppression in the chest, mild liver dysfunction, nausea, vomiting, and heat sensations.

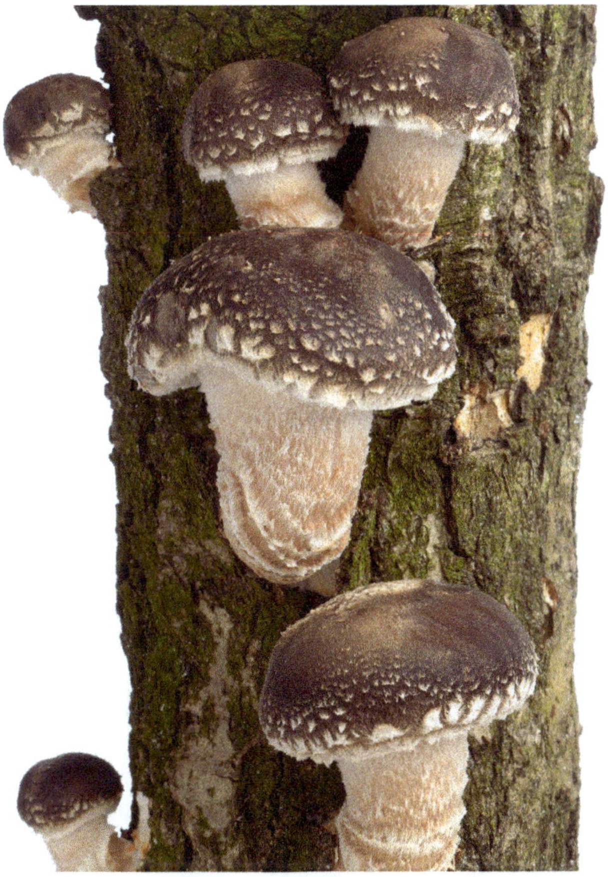

PREPARATION AND DOSAGE

TINCTURE: Fresh fruiting bodies [1:3-1:4+, 70-95% alcohol]; dry fruiting bodies [1:5, 50% alcohol]; consume 30-90 drops, up to three times daily.

CAPSULES: Consume 3-6 "00" capsules, up to three times daily. The dosage of LEM is ½ to 1 gram daily as a prophylactic. When treating individuals with chronic fatigue, hepatitis, HIV, or AIDS, the dose of LEM capsules is 2-6 grams per day consumed in two to three doses daily.

TEA: Decoct the fresh or dried mushrooms in water, bone broth, or chicken broth; consume 8-12 ounces, one to two times daily.

CULINARY USE: Add fresh chopped mushrooms to sautéed onions and garlic, stir fries, meat stews, or miso soup. The dose for the dried fruiting body is 6-16 grams when consumed in soup or other dishes; the dose for the fresh fruiting body is up to 90 grams daily.

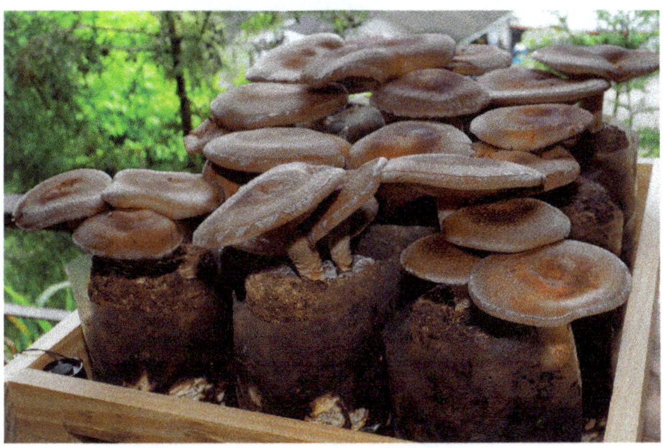

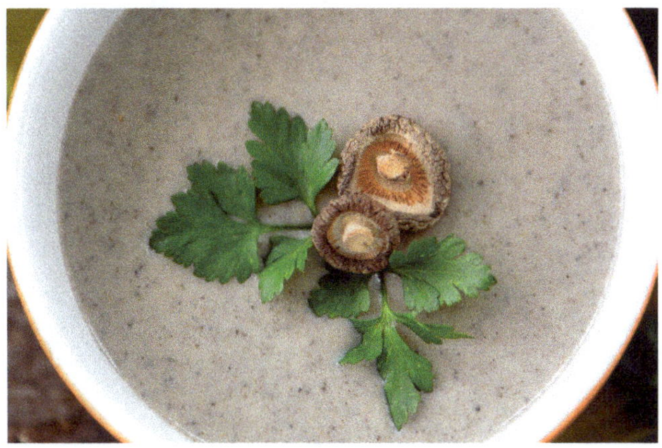

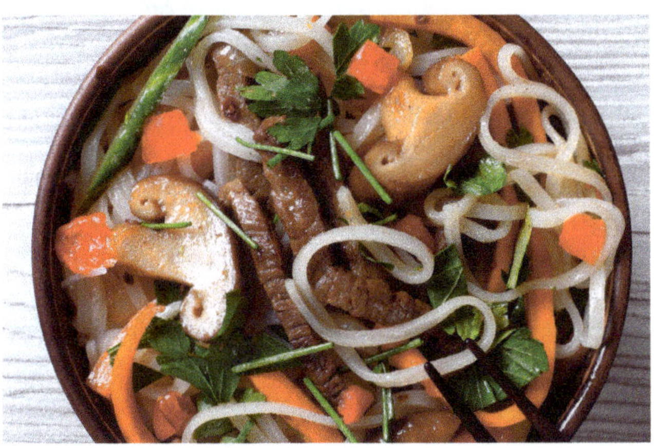

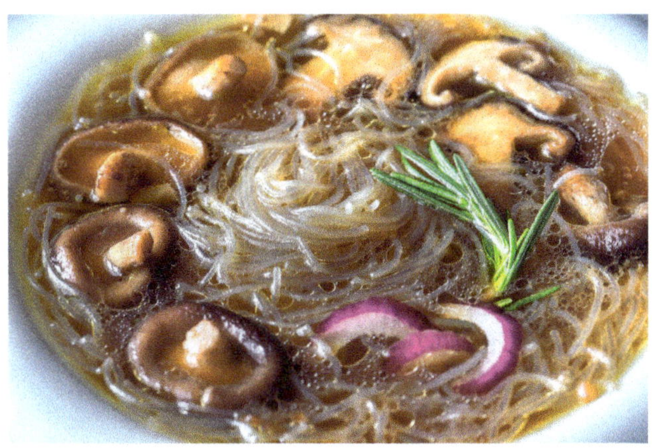

SILK TASSEL

BOTANICAL NAMES:
Garrya elliptica, G. flavescens, G. fremontii, G. wrightii, G. spp.

COMMON NAMES:
Silk tassel, silktassel, quinine bush, bear bush, cuauchichic

FAMILY NAME:
Garryaceae

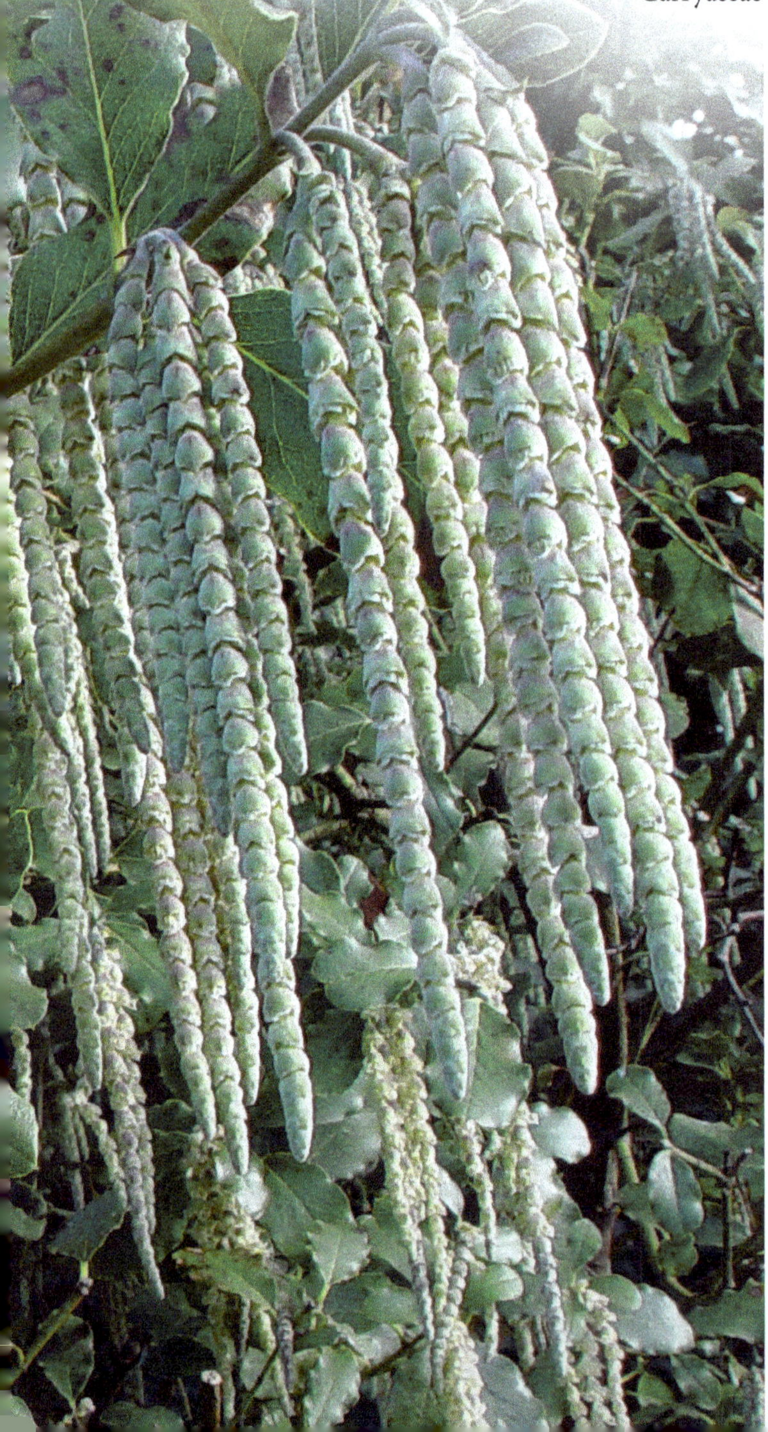

DESCRIPTION

PART USED: The leaves.

BOTANICAL DESCRIPTION AND HABITAT: *Garrya* is the only genus in the *Garryaceae* family, and includes 14 dioecious species that grow in the western U.S., Central America, and the Caribbean.[1] The species range from shrubs to small trees.[1] Silk tassel has simple, opposite, leathery, evergreen leaves, usually ovate to elliptic, and flat

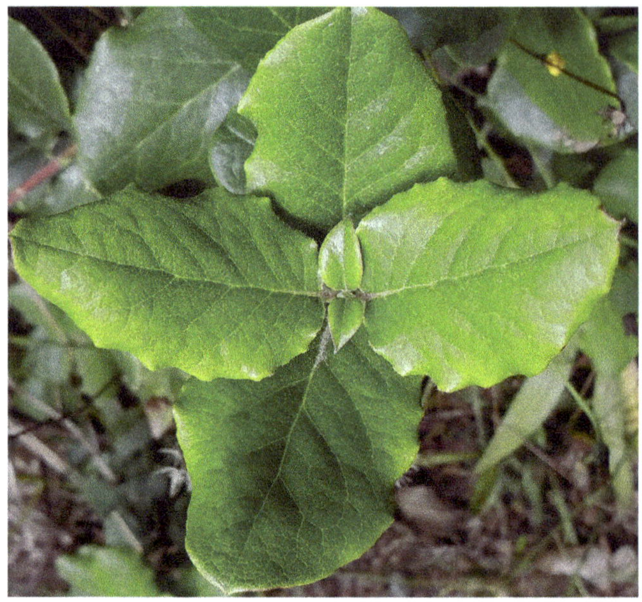

to convex. These margins are entire and vary from flat, to revolute, to wavy.[1] The long, showy catkins are arranged in groups of three or four tiny flowers hidden behind large bracts that are spaced evenly down the floral axis.[1] The male flowers have four stamens. The female flowers lack a perianth, and bear an inferior ovary with one carpel and two styles extending past the fused bracts.[1,2] The fruit is a berry that is initially green and fleshy, but dries and becomes dark blue, black, or whitish gray, and produces two seeds.[1]

Garrya elliptica is a large, tree-like shrub (up to 9 meters tall) usually found on dunes, sea cliffs, and chaparral in coastal Oregon and California. It occasionally grows in the lower elevations of the Sierra foothills.[1] The leaves are usually longer than wide (2 – 10 cm long, 2 – 7 cm wide), and are flat to convex with wavy, sometimes revolute margins.[1] The leaves are dark green and glabrous on the upper surface, with a thick layer of white hairs on the lower surface.[1] The male catkins are 7 – 20 cm long; the female catkins are 5 – 9 cm long, and eventually produce a hairy cluster of dark purple berries.[1-3]

Garrya flavescens, a shrub (up to 3 meters tall), grows in the arid regions of California and the Southwest at elevations from 650 to 2300 meters.[1] The leaves (2 – 8 cm long, 1 – 5 cm wide) range from flat to convex, with flat to wavy margins and a layer of coarse hairs on the undersides.[1] The fruit is generally hairy.[1]

Garrya fremontii is a shrub (up to 3 meters tall) found in foothills, chaparral, and forests (elevations from 300 – 2300 meters) in California, Oregon, Washington, and Nevada.[1] The hairless leaves (2 – 12 cm long and 1 – 7 cm wide) are generally flat, with a shiny upper surface that fades to yellowish-green as it ages.[1,2] The male catkins are 7.5 – 20 cm long, and the female catkins are 4 – 5 cm long, producing mostly hairless clusters of black or purple berries.[1,2]

Garrya wrightii is a one- to three-meter tall shrub found in forests and woodlands in Arizona, New Mexico, Texas, and northern Mexico at elevations of 5000 – 6000 feet.[4] The ovate leaves are flat, with slightly recurved, entire margins; they are yellow-green above, and light green below. The light yellow-green flowers lack petals, and hang in sparse pendent inflorescences.[5] The female flowers develop into mostly hairless fruit that hang individually, or in small, loose clusters.[5]

THE NAME: *Garrya* was named after Nicholas Garry, the first secretary of the Hudson Bay Company.[1] The epithet *flavescens* ("becoming golden yellow") derives from Latin. The epithet *elliptica* means "elliptic," and refers to an oval "about twice as long as wide."[6] The epithet *fremontii* was named for John Charles Fremont (1813 – 1890), an Army officer and presidential candidate who explored the western U.S. and collected plants on hazardous journeys.[7] The epithet *wrightii* was named for Charles Wright (1811 – 1885), an American botanical collector and teacher.[8]

HISTORICAL USES: *Garrya flavescens* was used by the Kawaiisu to treat colds, fevers, stomachaches, constipation, and gonorrhea.[9,10] The Pomo consumed tea of *G. elliptica* to stimulate menses.[9] Decoctions prepared from *G. fremontii* leaves were administered for gallbladder problems, to reduce fever, and as a digestive tonic.[9] Due to the bitter flavor, this herb was also used as a substitute for quinine by early American settlers.[9] Throughout rural New Mexico, silk tassel was known to inhibit diarrhea, and Native Americans administered it to reduce fever.[10] Whole plant extracts contain gutta-percha, a natural rubber.[10]

CONSTITUENTS: Silk tassel contains alkaloids (garryine, garryfoline, veatchine, delphinine, cuauchichicine, and diterpene).[11]

NUTRITIONAL PROPERTIES: It is not safe to consume as food.

MEDICINAL PROPERTIES: Analgesic, anodyne, and smooth muscle antispasmodic.

TEMPERATURE AND FLAVOR: Cool and bitter.

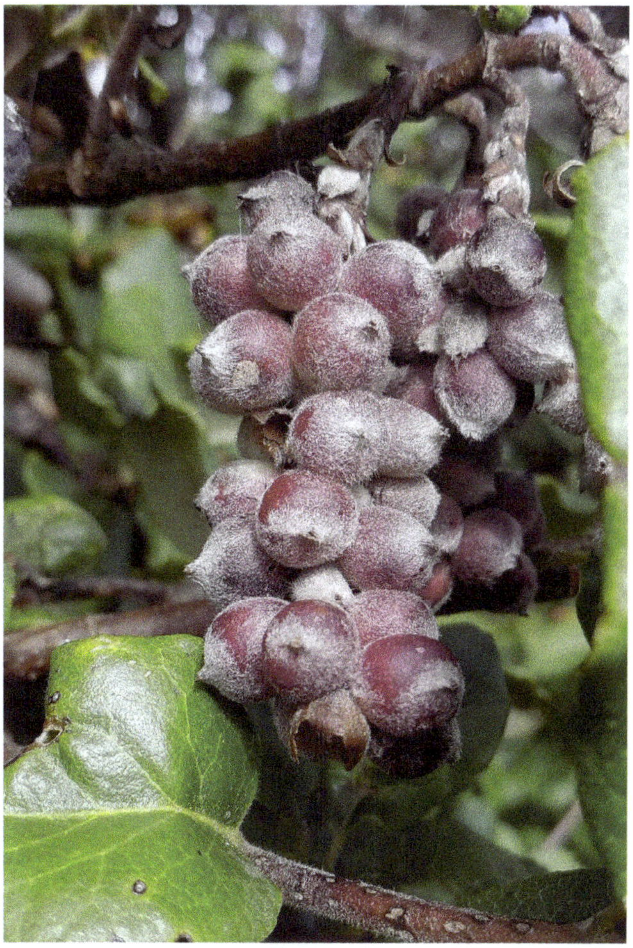

MEDICINAL USES

Silk tassel is a potent smooth muscle antispasmodic. It decreases digestive cramping, and aids in treating gas pains, diarrhea, dysentery, and pain from digestive infections.[11,12] It is a remedy for acute pain resulting from gastritis, irritable bowel syndrome, Crohn's disease, or colitis.[11-13] It also reduces referred pain and spasms from passing kidney stones or gallstones, as well as cholecystitis.[11-13] Silk tassel

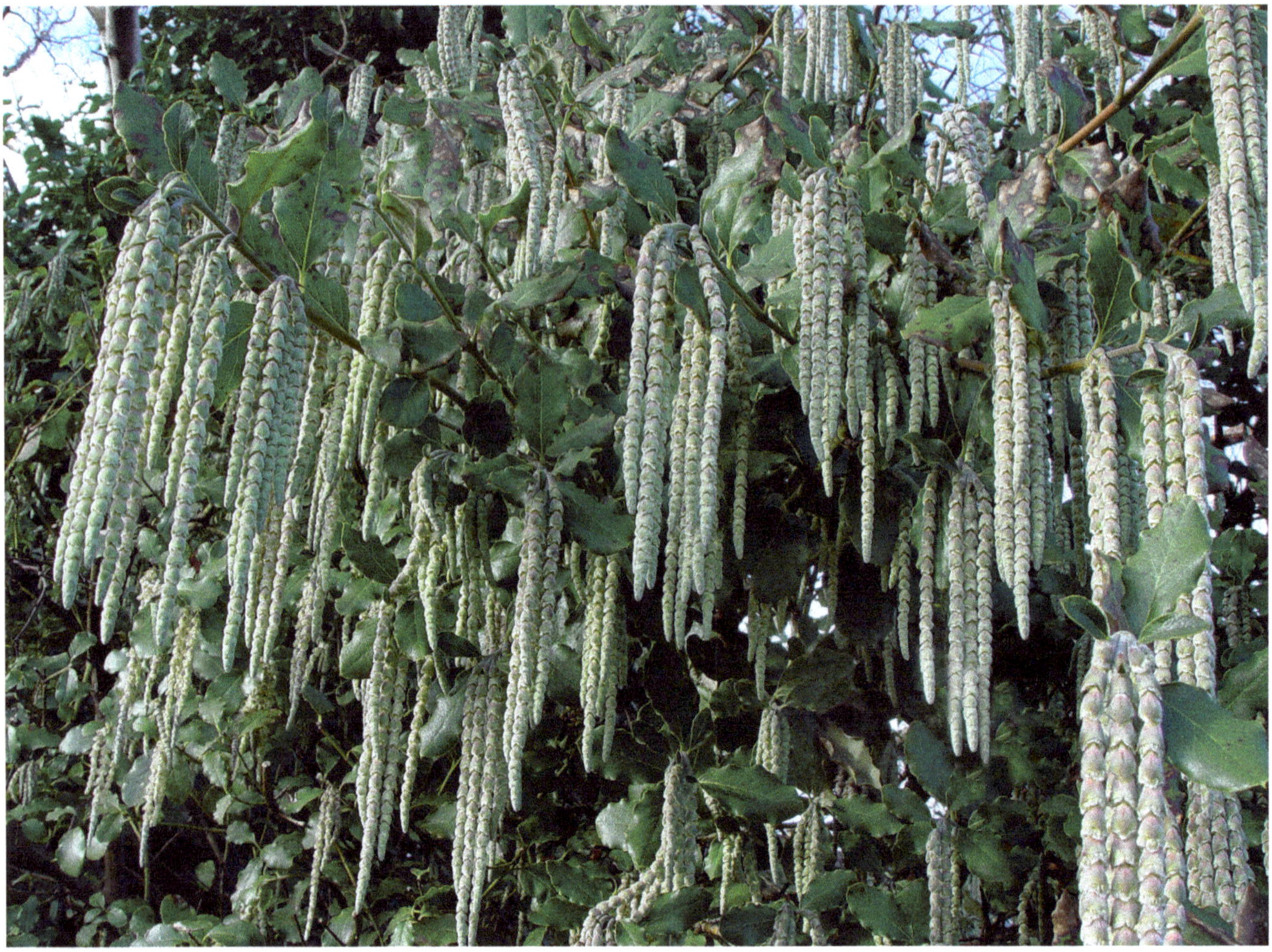

decreases cramping in the uterus and bladder, and relieves menstrual cramps and spasmodic pain from endometriosis, ovarian and uterine cysts, and fibroids. The water-soluble alkaloid garryine facilitates smooth muscle antispasmodic actions.[9]

Silk tassel can have mild sedative actions, as well as analgesic and anodyne effects. Apply a fomentation, poultice, or liniment to reduce pain from recently injured tissues caused by bruises, sprains, strains, cuts, and burns.

CONTRAINDICATIONS

Avoid use during pregnancy or lactation, and with younger children.[11] Use of prescription and over-the-counter anti-inflammatory drugs is contraindicated.[11] An overdose of silk tassel can cause nausea, vomiting, shortness of breath, and a cold, clammy feeling.[11-13] Consumption of silk tassel is contraindicated with biliary obstruction.

PREPARATION AND DOSAGE

TINCTURE: Fresh leaves [1:2-1:3, 70-95% alcohol]; dry leaves [1:5, 50% alcohol]; consume 30-60 drops, up to four times daily.

CAPSULES: Consume 1-3 capsules, up to three times daily.

TEA: Prepare a hot or cold infusion; consume 2-4 ounces, up to four times daily.

TOPICAL USE: Apply a poultice or fomentation of leaves to the affected area.

SKULLCAP

DESCRIPTION

BOTANICAL NAMES:
Scutellaria lateriflora, S. antirrhinoides, S. californica, S. galericulata, S. minor, S. tuberosa, and wild *Scutellaria* spp.

COMMON NAMES:
Skullcap, scullcap, blue skullcap, American skullcap, Virginia skullcap, California skullcap, hooded skullcap, marsh skullcap, greater skullcap, lesser skullcap, nose skullcap, snapdragon skullcap, mad-dog skullcap, mad-dog weed, madweed, hoodwort, helmet flower, quaker bonnet, hooded willow herb, blue pimpernel, side flower
rohtovuohennokka (Finnish)
scutellaire, toque (French)
fieberkraut, helmkraut, schildkraut (German)
escutelaria (Spanish)

FAMILY NAME:
Lamiaceae (Labiatae)

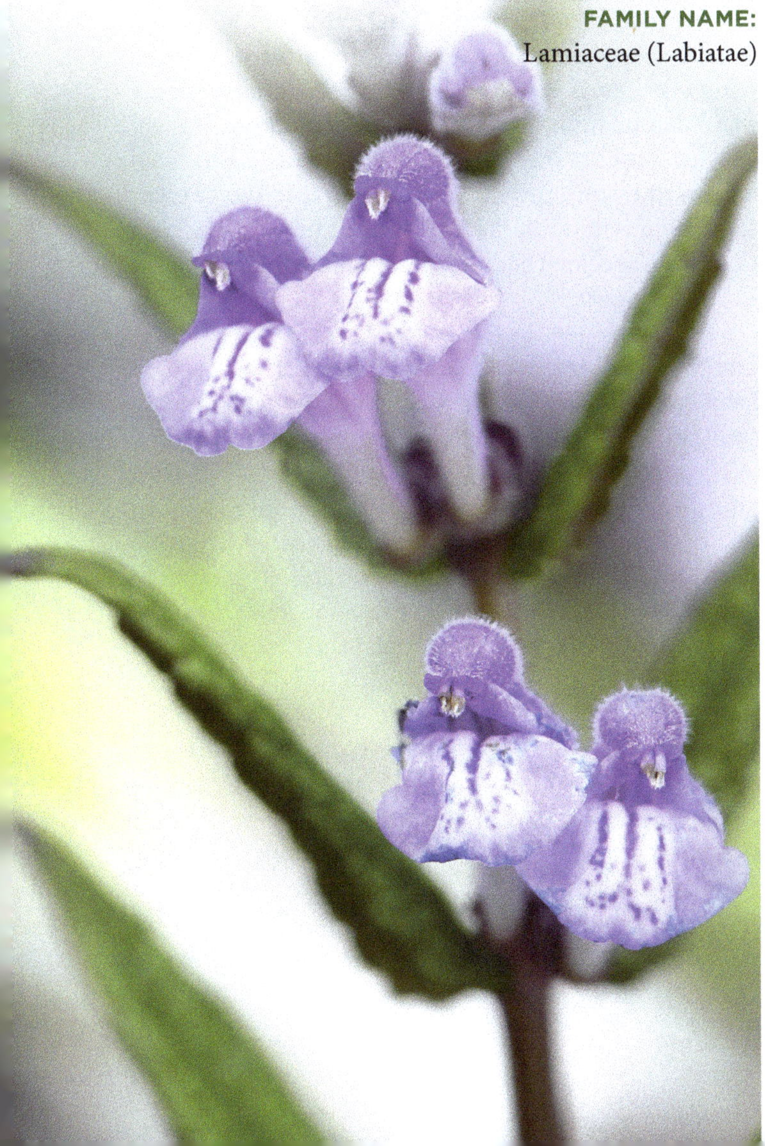

PARTS USED: The foliage, stems, and flowers.

BOTANICAL DESCRIPTION AND HABITAT: Skullcap is an herbaceous perennial that grows in temperate climates worldwide. There are approximately 350 species throughout the world, and 24 species native to the U.S.[1]

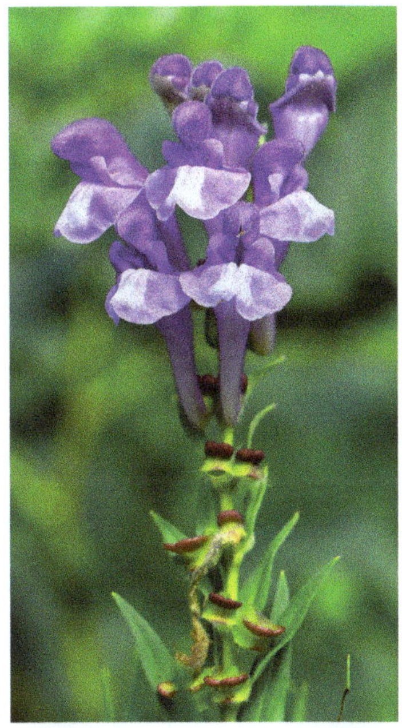

Wild species of skullcap grow along the banks of streams, rivers, and lakes, often in damp woodlands, grassy clearings, and moist mountain meadows. Native *Scutellaria* species found in the wild throughout the U.S. are used interchangeably as medicine.[2] Among the native species in the U.S., *S. lateriflora* is the largest, the least bitter tasting, and the most prolific. *Scutellaria lateriflora* is indigenous to eastern North America. *S. antirrhinoides* grows along drier, rocky slopes of oak or conifer forests, from northern California to Washington.[3] *S. californica* is found in open shrubland and woods in northern California mountains.[4] *Scutellaria galericulata* is circumboreal.[5] Most wild species of skullcap can be transplanted and cultivated easily, although they have a lower yield than *S. lateriflora.*

Scutellaria lateriflora has slender beige rhizomes. This herb (20 – 80 cm tall) has hairy, quadrangular branching stems with opposite, vibrant green, oblong-lanceolate or ovate pointed leaves with serrated margins.[6] The numerous deep violet-blue or pinkish-purple (occasionally white or pink), one-sided flowers are arranged in axillary racemes originating from the leaf axil.[7] The tubular, two-lipped corollas (6 – 8 mm long) of *S. lateriflora* are encircled by fused sepals (1.5 – 3 mm long); the upper lip is hooded with raised appendages.[6] The four stamens and a four-lobed ovary produces four yellow, warty fruits.

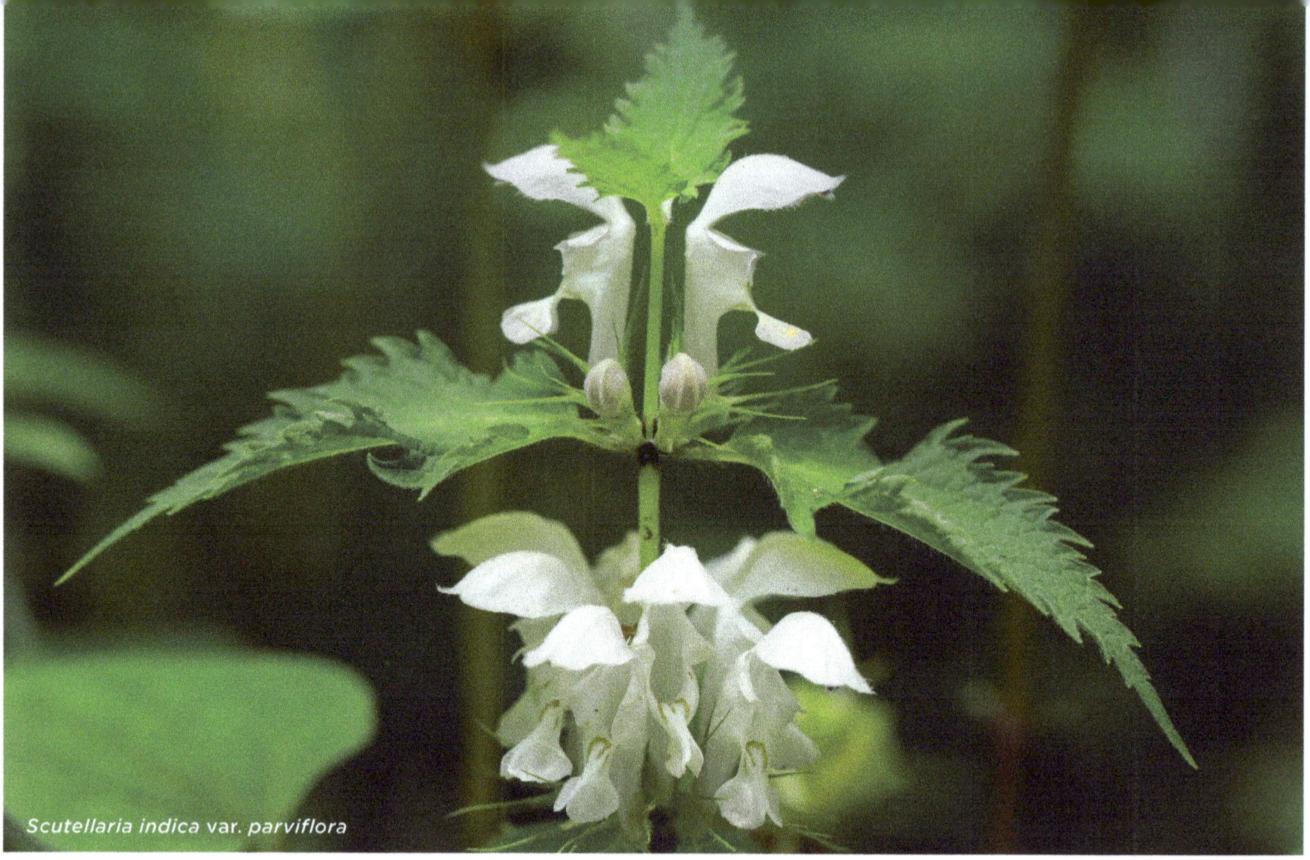

Scutellaria indica var. *parviflora*

Scutellaria antirrhinoides is smaller (10 – 35 cm tall), and its smaller, more delicate ovate to oblong leaves have smooth margins.[3] The violet-blue flower, held singly at the leaf axil, is larger than that of *S. lateriflora,* with the calyx 3 – 4 mm and the corolla 13 – 21 mm.[3] *Scutellaria californica* (15 – 40 cm tall) also has delicate ovate to oblong leaves with smooth margins; the flowers are cream-colored (calyx 3.5 – 5 mm, corolla 16 – 19 mm).[4] *Scutellaria galericulata* differs from *S. lateriflora* in that it has more narrow leaves, and larger, solitary flowers stemming from the leaf axil. The calyx is 3.5 – 4.5 mm long; the violet-blue corolla is 15 – 20 mm long.[5]

THE NAME: The genus name *Scutellaria* derives from the Latin *scutella* ("a small dish"), referring to the tray or cap-like appearance of the appendage on the upper side of the calyx that forms as it seeds. The epithet *antirrhinoides* derives from the Greek *antirrhinum* ("nose-like") because the flowers have a nose-shaped appearance.[8,9] The epithet *californica* indicates the plant's origin in California; *galericulata* ("helmet-shaped") derives from Latin. The epithet *lateriflora* ("flowering on the side") refers to the growth of flowers on the one-sided racemes. The epithet *minor* means "smaller" or "lesser;" *tuberosa* implies that "the rhizomes have tubers," or a "tuberous shape."[8]

The common names mad-dog skullcap, mad-dog weed, and madweed originated because of the plant's reputation for curing hydrophobia (canine rabies).[2] Hoodwort referred to the hooded appearance of the flowers. Native Americans designated the term skullcap because the hooded, two-lobed flowers resembled military helmets worn by early American soldiers.[2] In numerous herbal books, skullcap is erroneously spelled "scullcap." To clarify this common misspelling: a scull refers to a long rowboat, a long oar used at the stem of a boat, or two short-handled oars used by one rower.[10] A skull refers to the bony or cartilaginous framework of a vertebrate head.[11] The name "skullcap" was coined because the flower resembles a helmet, not a boat or oar.

The following common names correspond with these Latin binomials: skullcap, scullcap, blue skullcap, American skullcap, Virginia skullcap, mad-dog skullcap, mad-dog weed, madweed, hoodwort, helmet flower, blue pimpernel, and side flower *(Scutellaria lateriflora);* nose skullcap and snapdragon skullcap *(S. antirrhinoides);* California skullcap (*S. californica*); hooded skullcap, marsh skullcap, greater skullcap, helmet flower, and hoodwort *(S. galericulata);* lesser skullcap *(S. minor);* and Dannie's skullcap *(S. tuberosa).*[12]

HISTORICAL USES: Native American tribes in the eastern U.S. treated menstrual problems and other female conditions with skullcap.[2] It was mixed with pennyroyal *(Hedeoma pulegioides)* as tea for menstrual cramps and pain caused by colds.[13] They also used skullcap as a substitute for quinine to treat fevers.[14] The Cherokee gave skullcap to calm the nerves, aid kidney problems, promote menstruation, and expel the placenta after birth.[2] Poultices were applied topically for breast pain.[13] The Iroquois administered preparations of powdered roots to prevent smallpox and cleanse the throat.[2] The Ojibwa regarded skullcap as a heart medicine.[13] Native American tribes used *Scutellaria tuberosa* as a sedative, nerve tonic, antispasmodic, and digestive aid.[14]

In 1773, physician Lawrence Van Derveer popularized the use of skullcap in the U.S., claiming that it could cure rabies due to its nervine effects.[2] While skullcap did not cure rabies, folk use of the herb for this purpose continued. Subsequently, skullcap was employed as a nervine, tonic, and antispasmodic. It was historically used to treat St. Vitus' dance, neuralgia, insomnia, restlessness, headaches, rickets, spastic coughing, hiccups, hysteria, hypertension, snakebites, and seizures.[2,12,15]

Skullcap was listed in *The United States Pharmacopeia* (1863 – 1916), and in *The National Formulary* (until 1947.)[16] In the early 1900s, Eclectic physicians administered skullcap to treat nervous excitability, restlessness, insomnia, irritability, and mental illness such as schizophrenia.[2] Dr. Finley Ellingwood recommended consuming high doses of skullcap to treat delirium tremens.[17]

CONSTITUENTS: Skullcap contains flavonoids (scutellarein, scutellarin, scutellonin, baicalein, baicalin, and wogonin), tannins (rosmarinic acid and other caffeic acid derivatives), iridoids (catalpol), chrysin-7-glucoronide, volatile oil (caryophyllene, *trans*-β-farnesene, menthone, β-cubenene, α-humulene, germacrene-d, limonene, and apigenin), luteolins, oroxylin-a, wax, β-carotene, 2-methyl-alkanes, 3,9-dimethyl-alkanes, 3-methyl-alkanes, alkanes, η-hentriacontane, η-nonacosane, η-penta-triacontane, η-tritriacontane, lignan, fat, resins, sugar, and cellulose.[12,15,18-20]

NUTRITIONAL PROPERTIES: Skullcap contains high amounts of potassium, zinc, and vitamin C. It contains average amounts of aluminum, ash, carbohydrates, dietary fiber, fat, iron, manganese, niacin, phosphorus, protein, riboflavin, silicon, thiamine, and vitamin A. It contains low amounts of calcium, chromium, crude fiber, magnesium, and sodium.[21]

MEDICINAL PROPERTIES: Antispasmodic, euphoric, mood elevator, nervine, sedative, trophorestorative, bitter tonic, and stomachic.

TEMPERATURE AND FLAVOR: Cool and bitter.

MEDICINAL USES

Skullcap is a gentle nervine and mild sedative. It is a nervous system restorative (trophorestorative), and among the most effective herbs for nervous debilitation. Skullcap calms the central nervous system, and reduces patterns of sympathetic (adrenalin) stress.[22] It is a relaxant that reduces anxiety, agitation, and premenstrual irritability.[22] Skullcap also decreases caffeine or adrenalin induced jitters. While further research is necessary, the flavonoid scutellarein is attributed to skullcap's nervine, sedative, and antispasmodic properties.[2,15,21] Most individuals are capable of consuming skullcap (especially *S. lateriflora*) throughout the day without experiencing sedation. *Scutellaria lateriflora* has mild calming effects; wild skullcap species have more potent sedative effects. To prepare a trophorestorative and nervine tonic, combine skullcap extract with equal parts of wild oats *(Avena)* and St. John's wort *(Hypericum)*, and/or one-half the quantity of lemon balm *(Melissa)*.

Skullcap is a beneficial sedative for treating chronic insomnia. It encourages more restful, deep sleep, but does not cause morning sleepiness. Skullcap improves sleep in individuals withdrawing from prescription antidepressants, analgesics, anxiolytics, or sedatives; however, it can intensify one's dreams. As a sedative, skullcap may require repeated doses prior to bedtime — once in the early evening, and one hour before going to sleep. Individuals with insomnia accompanied by hypervigilance, anxiety disorders, an easily excitable nervous system, or chronic pain may experience more effective results from consuming skullcap throughout

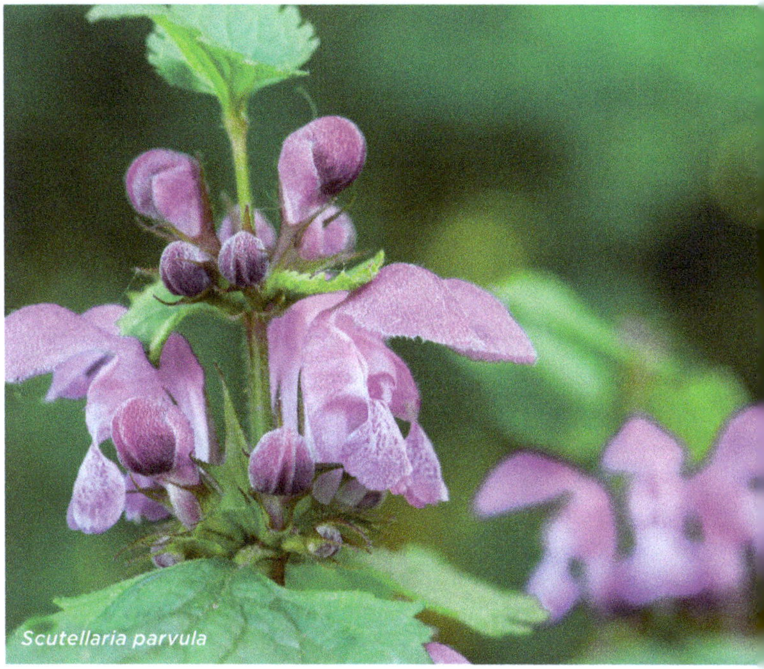
Scutellaria parvula

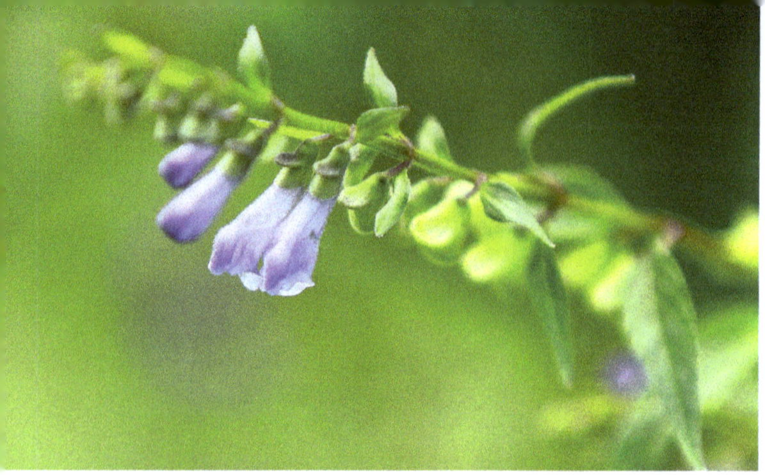

the day as a mild relaxant. More potent nervines can then be consumed in the early evening, and again before bed.

Skullcap has mood elevating and euphoric properties. It aids in treating milder forms of depression, especially when accompanied by anxiety or nervous depletion. Skullcap also supports the nervous system during pharmaceutical or recreational drug withdrawal. It reduces agitation, and has mood enhancing actions for individuals withdrawing from nicotine, marijuana, caffeine, alcohol, morphine, heroin, methadone, barbiturates, antidepressants, or cocaine.[22] Skullcap stimulates mood enhancing endorphins that enhance its euphoric affects.

Skullcap can be used to reduce nerve hypersensitivity and treat nerve related conditions.[22] For instance, it can be beneficial for reducing pain associated with herpes and shingles.[22] It is also helpful to reduce pain from a pinched nerve or misaligned spine, as well as neuralgia or sciatica.[22] This herb reduces nerve spasms and tremors associated with the early stages of multiple sclerosis and Parkinson's disease.

Skullcap has antispasmodic properties that reduce smooth muscle spasms, alleviating intestinal and menstrual cramps.[22] It also eases skeletal muscle spasms and muscle twitching. Skullcap reduces pain associated with trigeminal neuralgia.[22] Consuming skullcap prior to a visit to the dentist or an invasive examination (i.e., a rectoscopy, proctoscopy, or pelvic exam) eases anticipatory tension and aids relaxation.[22] Skullcap also reduces muscular guarding and pain when consumed prior to receiving a deep tissue massage, Rolfing, Heller work, myofacial release, or other structural massage.[22] It can be effective for treating tension headaches. Combine it with pedicularis *(Pedicularis)*, hops *(Humulus)*, and/or Jamaican dogwood *(Piscidia)* to ease muscular tension.

Wild skullcap species have stomachic properties and bitter tonic actions that encourage digestive secretions. They reduce nerve related digestive problems, such as loss of appetite, nonulcer dyspepsia, and irritable bowel syndrome. They also reduce digestive cramping. The bitter properties in the wild species of skullcap can aggravate acid indigestion in some individuals, and may induce hunger in those with hypoglycemic tendencies. This rarely occurs from consuming *S. lateriflora* because it is less bitter.

CONTRAINDICATIONS

Discontinue using skullcap if it causes acid indigestion. There are no reports of contraindications, side effects, or toxicity.[19] However, excessive dosing of the tincture can cause giddiness, stupor, or mental confusion. In the herb industry, skullcap has sometimes been adulterated with germander *(Teucrium)*, an herb with hepatotoxic effects.[19] To avoid this concern, find a reputable source.

PREPARATION AND DOSAGE

TINCTURE: Fresh aerial portions [1:2-1:4, 70-95% alcohol]; recently dried aerial portions [1:5, 60% alcohol]; consume 15-90 drops, up to four times daily. Ideally, when preparing a dry plant tincture, use skullcap harvested in the last six to twelve months.

GLYCERITE: Fresh aerial portions [1:2-1:4, 50% glycerin, 50% alcohol]; consume 10-60 drops, up to three times daily. A smaller ratio can be used, but it is difficult to obtain with sufficient menstruum to cover the plant.

SUCCUS: Prepare a succus and preserve with 20% ethanol; consume ½-1 teaspoon, up to four times daily.

CAPSULES: Consume 2-4 "00" freeze-dried herb capsules, one to three times daily.

TEA: Prepare the infusion with hot water that has not been boiled. Consume 8-12 ounces, one to four times daily.

TOPICAL USE: Apply the poultice, fomentation, paste, tincture, or liniment topically.

CULINARY USE: An adventurous herbalist could incorporate small amounts of fresh *S. lateriflora* leaves in salad, pesto, or paté.

SPILANTHES

DESCRIPTION

BOTANICAL NAMES:
Acmella oleracea
(syn. *Spilanthes acmella, Spilanthes oleracea*)

COMMON NAMES:
Spilanthes, toothache plant, buzz buttons, Brazil cress, Szechuan buttons, sansho buttons, electric buttons, pellitary, para cress
pará cress, jambú, jambú do rio (Brazilian Portuguese)
plamatka (Czech)
parakarse (Danish)
huzarenknoop, paratuinkers, ABC kruid (Dutch)
harilik nööpkakar (Estonian)
parakrassi, spilantes (Finnish)
cresson de Para, spilanthe des potagers (French)
parakresse, prickelknöpfchen, prickelblume (German)
akarkara (Hindi)
abécefű, szenyefű, huszárgomb (Hungarian)
jotang (Indonesian)
spilante (Italian)
kibana-oranda-senniti, oranda-senniti (Japanese)
parakuresu (Korean)
spilantė, indienų kresonas (Lithuanian)
brèdes mafanes, brède mafana (Madagascar)
pokok jotang (Malay)
jin chou kou, liu shen cao (Mandarin)
lato ghans, marati, bhuin timur (Nepali)
agrião do Brasil, agrião do Pará, pimenteira (Portuguese)
jambu (Spanish)
tandvärksplanta, parakrasse (Swedish)
phak khrat hua hewan, phak phet (Thai)
cúc áo, cúc nút áo, núc áo rau (Vietnamese)[1]

FAMILY NAME:
Asteraceae

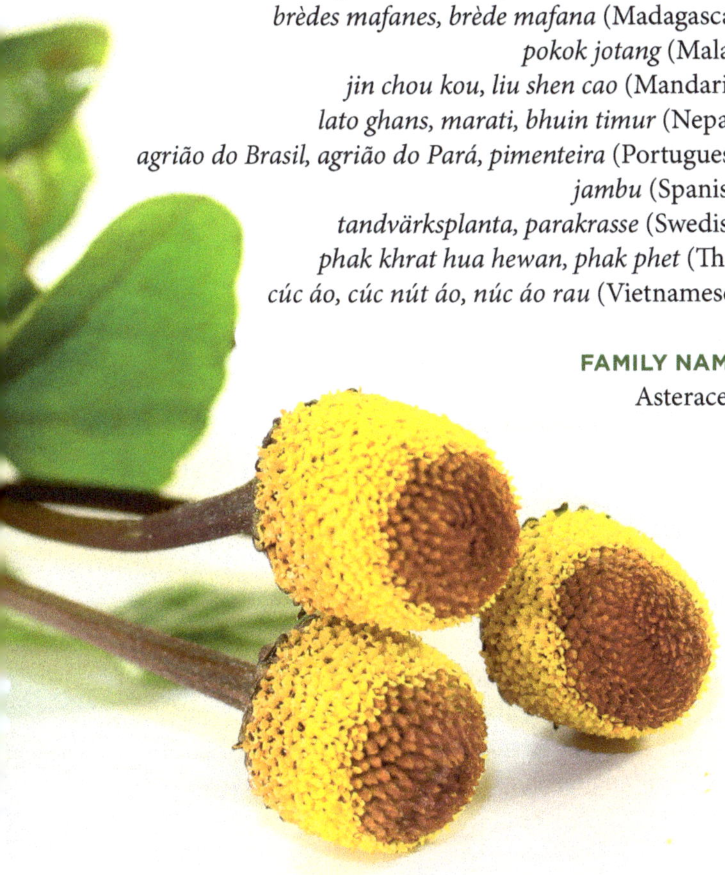

PARTS USED: The flowering heads or whole plant.

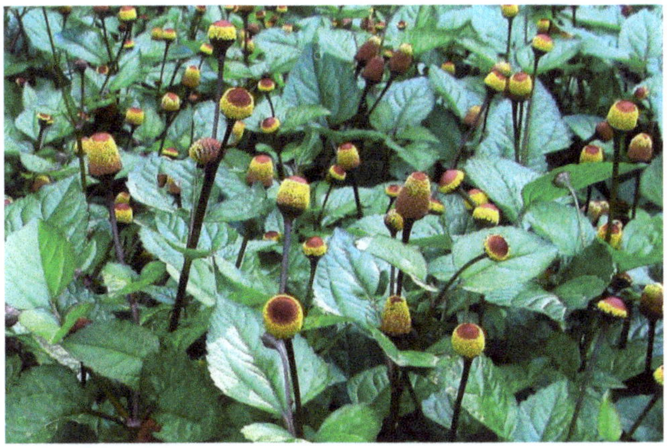

BOTANICAL DESCRIPTION AND HABITAT: Spilanthes is an annual or delicate perennial herb from South America, domesticated from the wild species *Acmella alba,* a native of Peru and Brazil.[2] It has naturalized in East Africa, and has been cultivated worldwide.[2,3]

The smooth, low growing stems (20 – 50 cm long) vary from green to red, and are usually erect, but can also lie flat on the soil.[3,4] The shiny leaves (5 – 10 cm long by 4 – 8 cm wide) are ovate to triangular, with flattened bases, acute tips, and dentate margins.[3] Each leaf has a narrowly winged petiole (2 – 6.4 cm).[3] The beautiful inflorescence, a yellow discoid head (10 – 24 by 11 – 17 mm), grows on a long peduncle (3.5 – 12.5 cm) and flaunts a crimson spot on top.[3] Each head consists of 400 – 600 minute, yellow, five-lobed, tubular florets (3 mm long). The fruit is a tiny hairy achene (2 mm long by 1 mm wide) shouldering two bristles.[3]

THE NAME: The genus and former epithet *Acmella* derives from the Greek *acme* ("point, peak, or sharp"), referring to the plant's pungency. The genus name *Spilanthes* ("stained flower") derives from two Greek words: *spiloma* ("stain") and *anthos* ("flower"), referring to the dark pollen that stains the petals.[1] The epithet *oleracea* derives from the Latin *holus* — a leaf vegetable.[1] The common name pará cress comes from the Brazilian province Pará, and like cress, is eaten as a pungent green or spice.[1] The name toothache plant alludes to the anesthetic properties that ease a toothache.

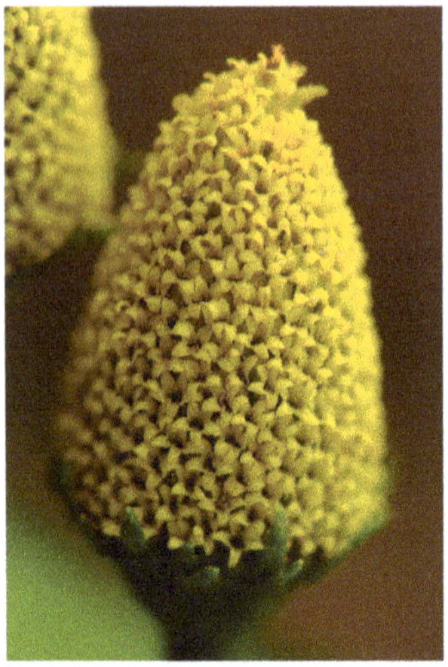

HISTORICAL USES: Spilanthes, also known as paracress, is native to Brazil's tropical regions. It was used as a culinary herb by indigenous people in the provinces Acre, Amazonas, Pará, and Ceará. The salty, pungent fresh leaves were cooked and consumed alone, or included as a flavoring agent in dishes containing manioc, a bland, starchy vegetable.[1] Spilanthes was used to treat a sore throat, dry mouth, or stomachache.[5] In India, spilanthes was administered to treat rheumatism, fever, wounds, gum and dental problems, and stammers in children.[6,7] Poultices were applied to the gums to alleviate toothaches.[5] In Cameroon, it was used to treat a snakebite and rheumatism.[7] Bangladesh tribes administered spilanthes to women in order to alleviate leukorrhea.[7]

CONSTITUENTS: Spilanthes contains pungent principles (isobutylamides: spilanthol = η-isobutylamide; undeca-2E,7Z,9E-trienoic acid; undeca-2E-en-8,10-diynoic acid; 2E-N-(2-methylbutyl)-2-undecene-8,10-diynamide; 2E,7Z-η-isobutyl-2,7-tridecadiene-10,12-diynamide; 7Z-η-isobutyl-7-tridecene-10,12-diynamide; and C9 polyunsaturated alkamides), volatile oil (limonene, β-caryophyllene, Z-β-ocimene, γ-cadinen, thymol, germacrene D, and myrcene), pungent nonvolatile sesquiterpenoids (polygodial and eudesmanolide II), tannins, resin, a biogenic amine (choline), α- and β amyrin, 3-acetylaleuritolic acid, vanillic acid, β-sitostenone, scopoletin, *trans*-ferulic acid, *trans*-isoferulic acid, and phytosterols (β-sitosterol and stigmasterol).[6,7] The pungent flavor and tingly sensation are due to spilanthol, other pungent alkylamides (isobutylamides), and nonvolatile sesquiterpenoids.[1,7]

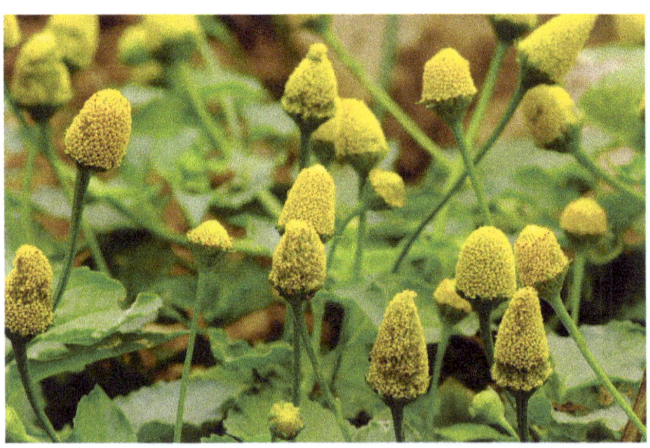

NUTRITIONAL PROPERTIES: Unknown.

MEDICINAL PROPERTIES: Antibacterial, antifungal, anti-inflammatory, antioxidant, antipyretic, antiviral, astringent, lymphatic, bioinsecticidal, potential antispirochetal, mild diuretic, and local anesthetic.

TEMPERATURE AND FLAVOR: Cool, pungent, bitter, salty, and sweet.

MEDICINAL USES

Spilanthes has antimicrobial and immune stimulating properties.[6] Similar to echinacea *(Echinacea)*, it contains isobutylamide bands and caffeic acid derivatives that stimulate immunity, increasing mononuclear leukocytes. Its constituent spilanthol has antibacterial, antifungal, antipyretic, anti-inflammatory, and anesthetic actions.[8] Spilanthes' antibacterial actions complement more potent herbal antibacterial agents that treat sinusitis, strep throat, sore throat, laryngitis, pharyngitis, ear infections, urinary tract infections, and food poisoning.[6] Extracts of spilanthes have antibacterial activity against *Pseudomonas aeruginosa, Streptococcus salivarius, S. viridans, S. mutans, Bacillus megaterium, Neisseria catarrhalis, Bacillus megaterium, B. subtilis, B. cereus, Escherichia coli, Klebsiella pneumoniae, Micrococcus luteus,* and *Pseudomonas aeruginosa.*[6]

An antifungal agent, spilanthes aids in treating intestinal and vaginal yeast infections by reducing *Candida albicans* growth. It also has antifungal activities against *Aspergillus niger, A. parasiticus, Fusarium oxysporum,* and *F. moniliforme.*[7] Topical applications aid in treating skin tineas such as athlete's foot and ringworm. Combine it with usnea *(Usnea)*, echinacea *(Echinacea)*, calendula *(Calendula)*, and/or Oregon grape *(Berberis)* for internal or topical antifungal use.

Spilanthes has antiviral actions that aid in treating a cold, influenza, enteritis, viral gastritis, and mononucleosis (Epstein Barr syndrome). It likely increases interferon, an endogenous antiviral compound. Combine with additional antiviral herbs such as echinacea *(Echinacea)*, elder berry *(Sambucus)*, thyme *(Thymus)*, cinnamon *(Cinnamomum)*, and clove *(Syzygium)* during the first stages of a cold, flu, or viral enteritis.

Spilanthes has antipyretic activity attributed to the flavonoids that inhibit cyclo-oxygenase or lipo-oxygenase.[7] It contains tannins, flavonoids, and phenolic compounds that have antioxidant activities.[7] In animal studies,

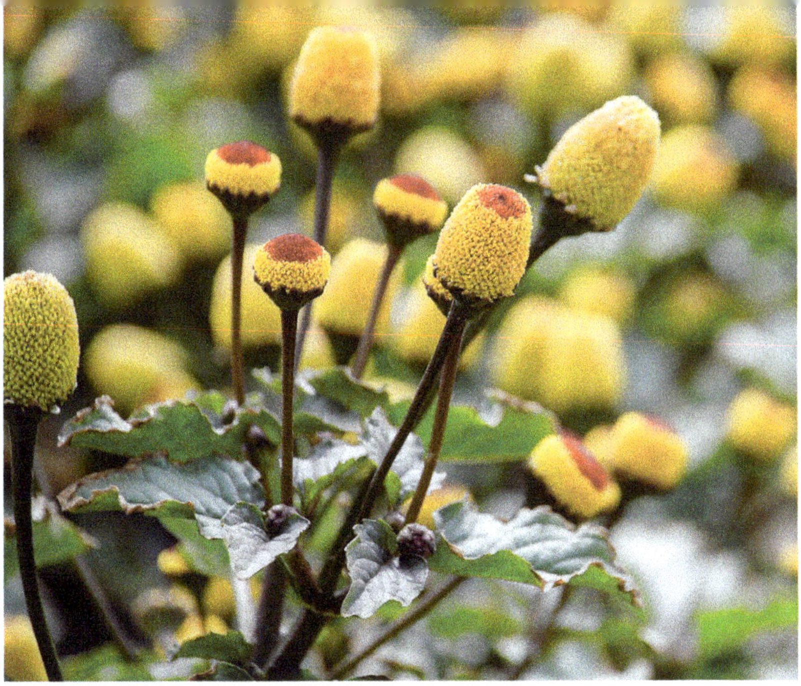

concentration of 7.5 ppm.[7] Multiple constituents demonstrate insecticidal actions, including spilanthol, alkamides, and sesquiterpenoids.[7] Spilanthol was found to have antimalarial and larvicidal action even in low doses.[7] Following a short span of exposure, pupae mortality indicates that spilanthol also disrupts the process of histolysis and histogenesis.[7] Spilanthol extracts are also effective against the larvae of *Culex quinquefasciatus* and *Aedes aegypti*, the neonates of *Helicoverpa zea* (corn earworm moth), *Plutella xylostell*, and *P. americana*.[5,7] In *Plutella americana* adults, spilanthol is more effective as an insecticide than conventional pesticides (carbaryl, lindane, and bioresmethrin).[7]

spilanthes was found to have anti-inflammatory and peripheral analgesic activities due to flavonoids that inhibit prostaglandins.[7]

Spilanthes is a lymphatic that reduces glandular swelling accompanying acute or subacute infections. Consume in the first phase of an infection, and in the clean-up phase of a slowly resolving infection. Combine with echinacea *(Echinacea)*, red root *(Ceanothus)*, yerba mansa *(Anemopsis)*, and calendula *(Calendula)* as an immune stimulating lymphatic compound.

A local anesthetic and sialagogue, spilanthes stimulates salivary secretions. Upon contact, it stimulates mucous membranes and increases blood flow to local tissues. Animal studies demonstrate that spilanthes has potent local anesthetic actions attributed to the alkylamides.[7] A gargle and mouthwash aid in treating gum infections such as gingivitis, abscessed tooth, canker sores, and teething pain.[6] Add two to three droppers of the extract to four ounces of water as a mouth rinse. Apply the fresh plant poultice to a toothache.

Apply spilanthes liniment, poultice, alcohol intermediary oil, or salve as a counterirritant and anesthetic for bruises, sprains, strained muscles, muscular or rheumatic pains, arthritis, and minor wounds.[6] The antimicrobial actions of topical applications help to heal herpes, staph, athlete's foot, and ringworm.

Spilanthes has insecticidal properties that can kill mosquitoes. Extracts of *S. acmella* flowering heads demonstrate potent ovicidal, insecticidal, and pupacidal activity. In one study, 100% of *Anopheles*, *Culex*, and *Aedes aegypti* mosquitoes were killed by a solution containing a spilanthes

CONTRAINDICATIONS

There are no known contraindications or side effects from consuming spilanthes during pregnancy or lactation.

PREPARATION AND DOSAGE

TINCTURE: Fresh flowering herb or flowers [1:2-1:3, 95% alcohol]; dry flowering herb or flowers [1:5, 60% alcohol]; consume 10-60 drops, up to four times daily.

GLYCERITE: Fresh flowering herb or flowers [1:3-1:4, 50% glycerin, 50% alcohol]; consume 10-60 drops, up to four times daily.

CAPSULES: Consume 2-4 capsules, up to four times daily.

SUCCUS: Juice the fresh herb and add 20% alcohol to the total volume. Consume 1 teaspoon, up to four times daily.

TEA: Prepare a hot infusion and consume 8-12 ounces, up to four times daily.

TOPICAL USE: Prepare medicated oil using the alcohol intermediary method. Apply the poultice, fomentation, liniment, diluted tincture, oil, or salve to the affected area. Apply the fresh plant poultice, extract, or glycerin extract to the gums.

ST. JOHN'S WORT

DESCRIPTION

BOTANICAL NAMES:
Hypericum perforatum, H. formosum

COMMON NAMES:
St. John's wort, St. Johnswort, Johnswort, western St. John's wort, St. Joan's wort, Klamath weed, goatweed, goat weed, hardhay, amber
mäkikuisma (Finnish)
chasse-diable, herbe de Saint Jean, herbe aux piqures, millepertuis perfore (French)
echtes Johanniskraut, hexenkraut, wundkraut (German)
iperico, perforata (Italian)
hung-st'ao-lien (Mandarin)
corazoncillo, hierba de San Juan, hiperico (Spanish)
johannesört (Swedish)
yara out (Turkish)

FAMILY NAME:
Clusiaceae
(formerly Hypericaceae)

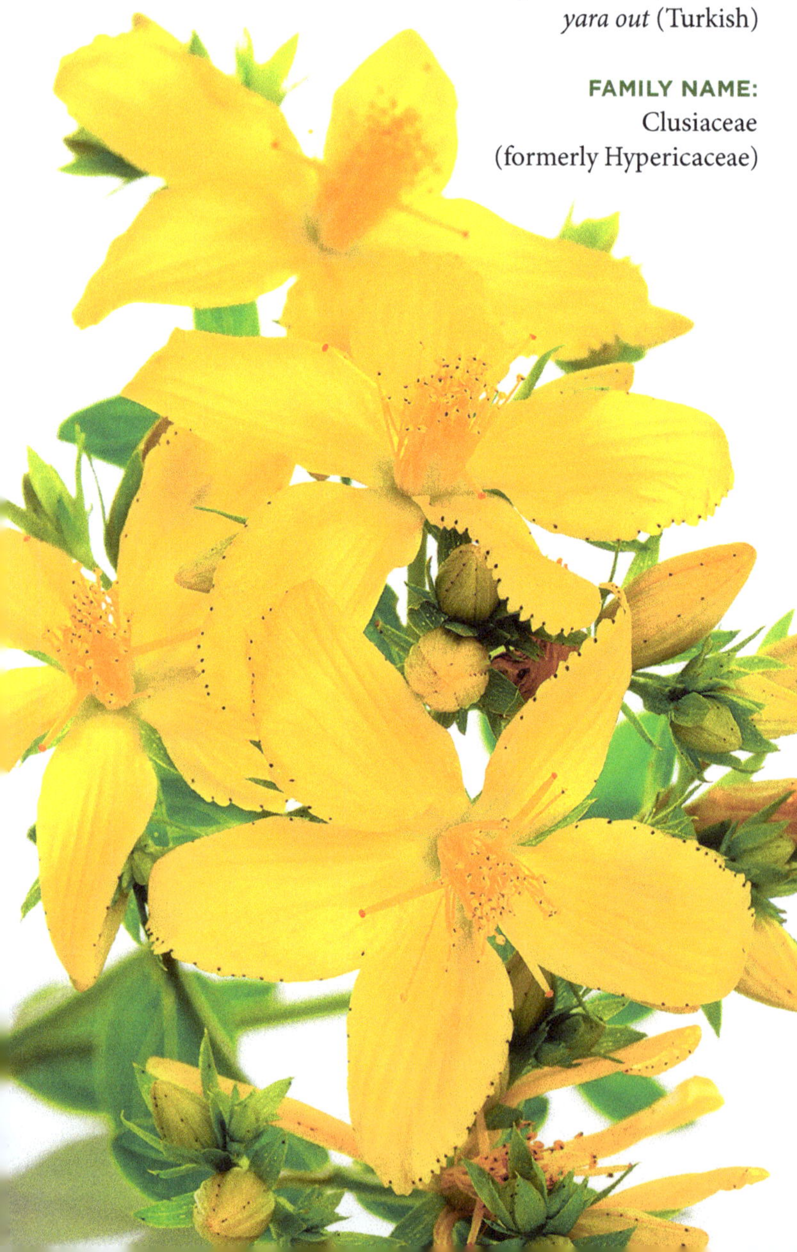

PARTS USED: The flowering tops including buds, flowers, and leaves.

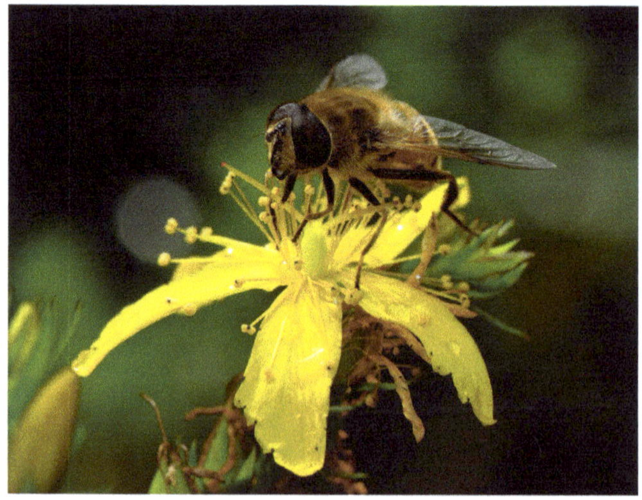

BOTANICAL DESCRIPTION AND HABITAT: St. John's wort is a perennial herb native to Europe and Asia. It has become endemic throughout the U.S. following its introduction by European settlers.[1] It grows in full sun, in disturbed areas including roadsides, pastures, and fields. St. John's wort is self-seeding and easily cultivated. It is considered an invasive weed; seed distribution is not permitted in some states. In an effort to eradicate and control St. John's wort, *Chrysolina quadrigemina* and *C. hyperici,* two leaf-eating beetles, have been introduced.[2]

Hypericum perforatum is a hairless perennial that grows 10 – 80 cm tall. It has numerous upright, cylindrical, hollow stems that are simple to branched, with two raised lines down the stem. The deep green, perforated, entire, oblong to lanceolate leaves (2.5 cm long) are opposite and somewhat clasping at the base. *H. formosum* has narrower ovate to oblong-elliptic leaves. When held up to the light, the leaves show oil glands appearing as tiny pin-like perforations or translucent dots. The vibrant yellow, showy flowers (2.5 cm wide) have five lanceolate to egg-shaped sepals, with five petals, dark dots along the margins, and numerous showy stamens. The flowers appear on the terminal corymbs. When the flowers or leaves are pinched, they stain fingers purple-blue. *Hypericum perforatum* has three-chambered, brownish fruits with rows of pits. *H. formosum* has yellowish fruits that are not veined or pitted.[1,3-5]

THE NAME: The genus name *Hypericum* ("over a picture or icon") derives from Greek, and refers to the traditional use of placing flowers above religious images to ward off evil.[2,3] The epithet *perforatum* refers to tiny holes in the leaves. The common name is associated with St. John the Baptist because the herb bloomed around his birthday, June 24.[1]

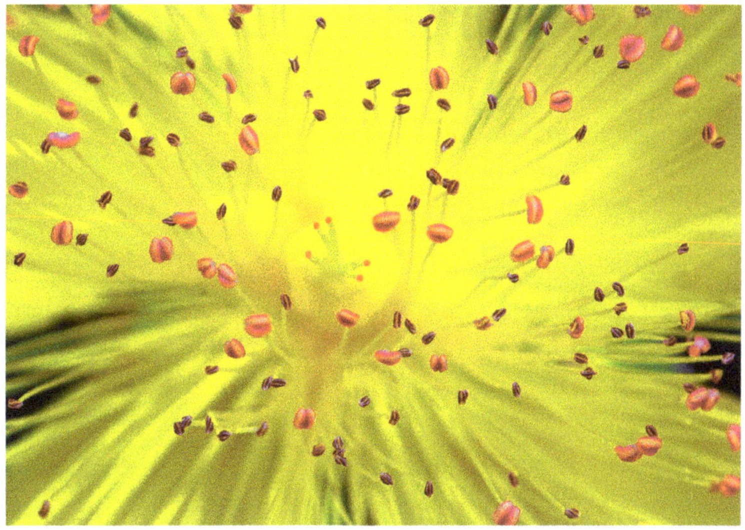

HISTORICAL USES: St. John's wort was treasured by ancient Greeks and Romans as a vulnerary for healing cuts, bruises, sprains, nerve pain, and burns.[1] The Knights of St. John of Jerusalem believed that the perforations in the leaves resembled wounds, so they used the plant to heal the Crusaders' wounds.[1] St. John's wort was a popular folk remedy throughout Europe during the Middle Ages for pulmonary and bladder problems, diarrhea, dysentery, worms, jaundice, and cancer.[1,5] It was administered for nervous exhaustion, nervous depression, insomnia, epilepsy, hysteria, and madness.[1] This herb was given as a remedy for bedwetting.[2,3]

Eclectic physician Harvey Felter recommended consuming St. John's wort to treat shock, concussions, and spinal injuries, as well as irritation, lacerations, and puncture wounds in the extremities.[6] Dr. Finley Ellingwood also recommended using St. John's wort for muscular bruising, deep soreness, and burning pain in the spine.[7] Internal use was recommended to treat piles and diarrhea.[7] Eclectic physicians applied fomentations or ointments of St. John's wort topically as a vulnerary agent for various injuries and acute mastitis.[6]

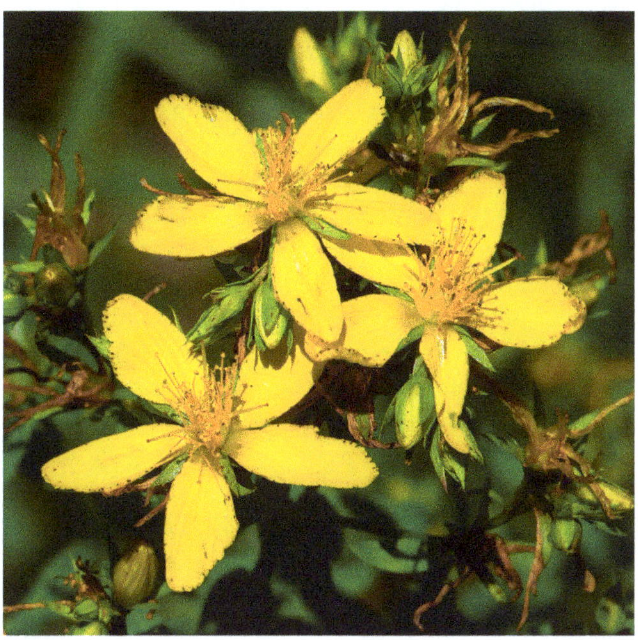

Many folkloric superstitions relate to this herb. St. John's wort was believed to dispel demons and witches, and offer protection from thunderbolts and lightning.[1] Flowers were placed above icons to ward off evil, especially on Midsummer's Day.[1] The tiny leaf perforations were believed to be caused by the devil who attempted to stab the plant to death with a needle.[3] Another name for the plant, *Fuga daemonium,* translates as "devil's flight" because the devil was believed to flee, as he abhorred the plant's scent.[1] When gathered by a childless woman, this herb was believed to aid conception.[1]

Following the introduction of St. John's wort by European settlers, Native American tribes including the Cherokee, Iroquois, and Montagnais used St. John's wort medicinally.[5] The Cherokee used St. John's wort to treat fever, suppressed menstruation, digestive concerns, and bloody diarrhea.[8] A poultice was applied to snake bites and venereal sores.[8] The Montagnais consumed the tea to treat coughs. The Iroquois used the roots to enhance fertility, and the whole plant to reduce fever.[8]

CONSTITUENTS: St. John's wort contains napthodianthrones (hypericin and psedohypericin), flavonols (hyperin = hyperoside, quercetin, isoquercetin, quercitrin, isoquercitrin, rutin, and kaempferol), flavanols ((+)-catechin, leucocyanidin, (-)-epicatechin, and 13-II8-biapigenin), acylphloroglucinols (hyperforin and adhyperforin), volatile oil (including monoterpenes α-pinene, β-pinene, myrcene, and limonene; and the sesquiterpenes caryophyllene and humulene), xanthones (kielcorin, magniferin, and 1,3,6,7-tetrahydroxy-xanthone), tannins (including oligomeric proanthocyanidins = OPCs), nicotinic acid, vitamins A and C, β-sitosterol, choline, pectin, phlobaphene, rhodan, a resin, and others.[1,5,9]

NUTRITIONAL PROPERTIES: St. John's wort contains vitamins A and C.

MEDICINAL PROPERTIES: Antibacterial, antidepressant, anti-inflammatory, anxiolytic, astringent, antiviral, calmative, nervine, (mild) sedative, trophorestorative, and vulnerary.

TEMPERATURE AND FLAVOR: Cool, astringent, bitter, and sweet.

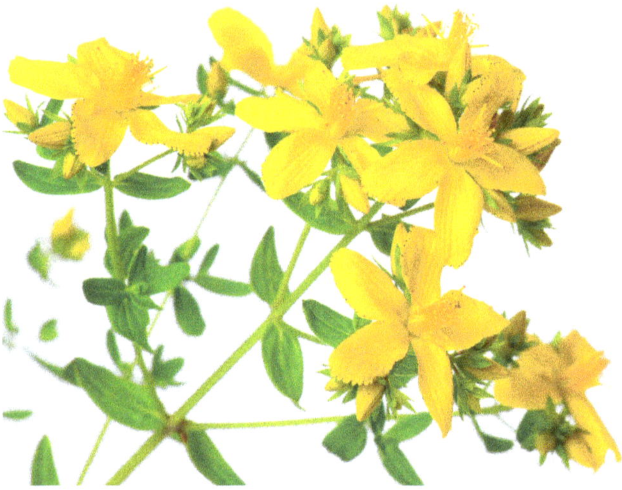

MEDICINAL USES

St. John's wort is a nervine and anxiolytic. It has gentle calmative actions, reducing anxiety, nervousness, and agitation. St. John's wort is a nervous system restorative agent (trophorestorative) for nervous exhaustion. Consuming St. John's wort throughout the day can aid in treating insomnia, although stronger nervines and sedatives may be needed in the evening to encourage sleep. Hypericin is attributed to the tranquilizing actions.[5] St. John's wort also aids in treating hyperactive or anxious children, unless they already take medications such as Ritalin.

St. John's wort acts as an antidepressant and mood elevator to treat mild to moderate forms of depression and seasonal affective disorder (SAD). It reduces premenstrual depression and symptoms of premenstrual syndrome, such as anxiety and irritability. Clinical studies validate the improvement of symptoms associated with depression, including insomnia, hypersomnia, anxiety, dysphoric mood, and anorexia.[2] The antidepressant effects are attributed to the hyperforin, and to a lesser degree, hypericin.[1] While the specific effects are still being studied, it is postulated that hyperforin blocks neurotransmitter reuptake in the brain.[1] Depression is associated with a deficiency of neurotransmitters, or excessively rapid reabsorption of them. Some antidepressant medications inhibit the enzymes causing the reabsorption of neurotransmitters. The inhibition of neurotransmitter reuptake increases the amount of time they are in contact with nerve receptors. St. John's wort has similar actions as SSRI antidepressant drugs that inhibit monoamine oxidase (MAO) A and B. Studies indicate that hypericin, a constituent in St. John's wort, inhibits type A and B monamine oxidase (MAO) in rat brain mitochondria.[2] St. John's wort works most effectively as an antidepressant when it is ingested consistently for three months. Consume 30 – 90 drops of the extract, or 2 – 3 freeze-dried capsules, two to three times daily. For longstanding cases of depression, it may be necessary to consume a higher dose range of the extract (90 drops), two to three times daily.

St. John's wort has potent anti-inflammatory actions. It reduces inflammation in the nerves, muscles, and joints. It sedates nerve fibers, reducing rapid nerve firing. St. John's wort decreases nerve pain caused by herpes, shingles, and neuralgia, including sciatica and trigeminal pain, tendonitis, and carpal tunnel syndrome.[10] Internal and topical applications decrease joint inflammation and aid in treating rheumatism and osteoarthritis. It is one of few herbs that stimulate nerve regeneration; therefore, it aids in treating recent nerve damage (in the past 6 – 12 months). Consuming one teaspoon to one tablespoon of the oil on an empty stomach acts as a vulnerary to the gastrointestinal tract lining, and hastens the healing of gastric and duodenal ulcers.[10,11]

St. John's wort oil has antibacterial and antiviral properties.[1,2] It contains hyperforin, an antibacterial agent against *Staphylococci* and *Streptococci*.[2] The hypericin and pseudohypericin have demonstrated potent antiretroviral activity *in vivo* and *in vitro*.[2] According to Leung and Foster, "It is postulated that the compounds interfere with viral infections and/or spread by direct inactivation of the virus or prevent virus shedding, budding, or assembly at the cell membrane."[2] Clinical trials using oral doses of hypericin with HIV-positive subjects are underway. Leung and Foster note that "hypericin achieves complete inactivation of more than five logs (more than 100,000 HIV particles/ml of blood) of infectious HIV."[2] Hypericin also exhibits antiviral activity against herpes and hepatitis.[1] St. John's wort shows promise as an antibacterial against gram-positive organisms such as *Micrococcus bacillus,* and as an antiviral against *Influenza* A/PR8.[5]

St. John's wort can be applied topically as an astringent anti-inflammatory and antimicrobial agent. It contains numerous flavonoids that stimulate tissue and capillary regeneration, reduce capillary permeability, and prevent scar formation.[10] Even small amounts of hypericin have been found to increase blood flow to constricted tissues.[5] Topical applications of St. John's wort infused oil (or diluted tincture applied as a liniment) reduce local pain and inflammation. It is an effective vulnerary for treating first-aid conditions such as myalgia, neuralgia, joint pain, sprains, strains, bruises, abrasions, broken bones, cuts, thermal burns, sunburns, and surgical wounds. Apply oil or salve to hemorrhoids, fistulas, varicose veins, and rectal or vaginal fissures, as well as tears of the vagina, labia, or perineum resulting from birth.

To prepare St. John's wort oil, macerate fresh flowering tops in oil and steep in sunlight for two to four weeks. It can be strained when it acquires a deep reddish hue, attributed to the hypericin or lipophilic compounds. Hyperiforin is also found in the freshly macerated oil, but is unstable and can degrade in 30 – 90 days, although storage time may be increased with limited exposure to air.[2]

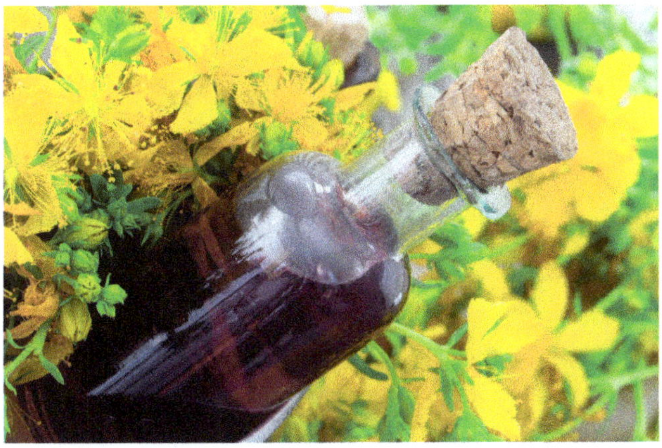

CONTRAINDICATIONS

St. John's wort contains hypericin that is absorbed in the intestines, and concentrates near the skin. The photosensitizing effects were first noticed in cattle, sheep, and other livestock. While moderate doses of hypericin do not cause photodermatitis in humans, fair-skinned individuals should avoid direct exposure to sunlight after ingesting the herb.[2] Avoid internal use during pregnancy until further studies are conducted. Nursing mothers consuming this herb are cautioned to protect infants from direct or prolonged exposure to sunlight, as the photosensitizing effects may pass through the milk.

St. John's wort lowers the bioavailability of pharmaceutical 3A4/P-glycoprotein cosubstrates by stimulating 3A4 enzyme production. Therefore, coadministration is contraindicated with the following medications: Alprozalam,

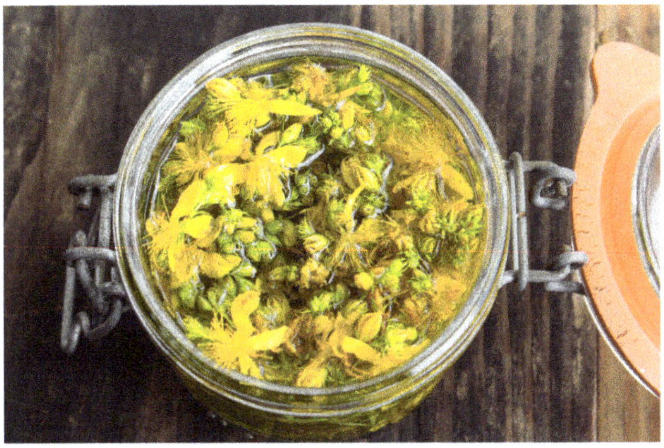

Amitriptyline (a tricyclic antidepressant), Antiretrovirals, and immune suppressive agents such as Cyclosporine or Tacrolimus, Digoxin (a cardiac glycoside), Verapamil (a calcium channel blocker), Etoposide, Fexofenidrine, oral contraceptives, and Variconazole (an antifungal).[12]

PREPARATION AND DOSAGE

TINCTURE: Fresh flowers and leaves [1:2-1:3, 60-95% alcohol]; consume 10-90 drops, up to four times daily.

GLYCERITE: Fresh flowers and leaves [1:2-1:3, 60% glycerin, 40% water] or [1:2-1:3, 50% glycerin and 50% alcohol]; consume 10-90 drops, up to four times daily.

CAPSULES: Consume 2-4 freeze-dried capsules, up to three times daily.

TEA: Prepare a hot infusion; consume 8-12 ounces, up to three times daily.

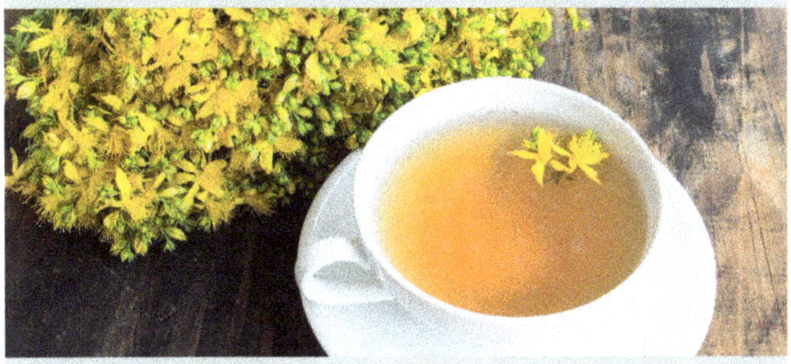

TOPICAL USE: Infuse wilted flowers in oil using the solar infused oil method. Apply the oil topically, or consume 1 teaspoon to 1 tablespoon, up to three times daily on an empty stomach.

STONE ROOT

DESCRIPTION

BOTANICAL NAME:
Collinsonia canadensis

COMMON NAMES:
Stone root, stoneroot, horsebalm, northern horse balm, horseweed, richleaf, richweed, knob root, knobweed, hardback, heal-all, oxbalm, knot root
Baume de Cheval, häst mynta (Swedish)

FAMILY NAME:
Lamiaceae (Labiatae)

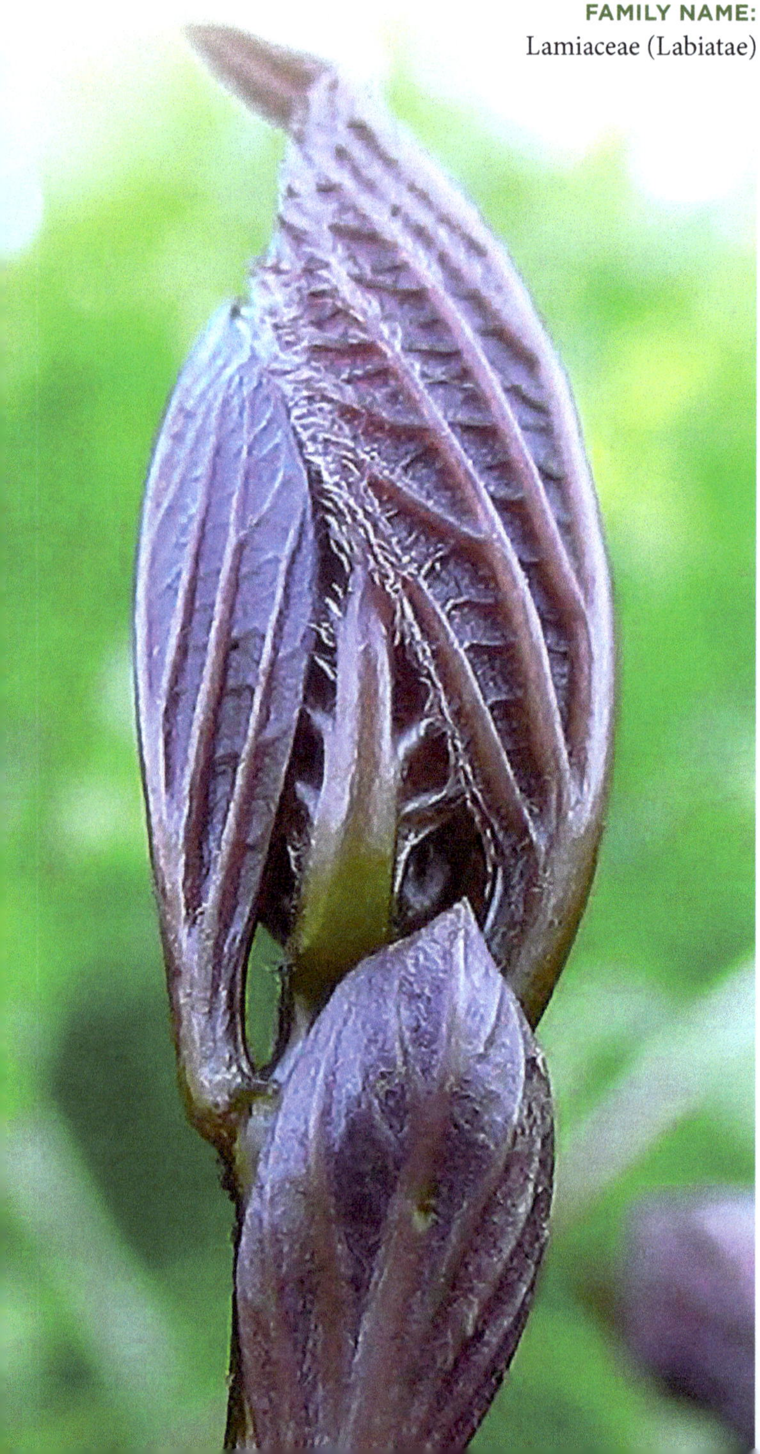

PARTS USED: The whole plant (aerial portions and roots).

BOTANICAL DESCRIPTION AND HABITAT: Stone root grows at lower elevations east of Mississippi in the Appalachian Mountains, along shady hillsides and creek beds. The fresh leaves have a citron-lemon-custard or melon-like scent.

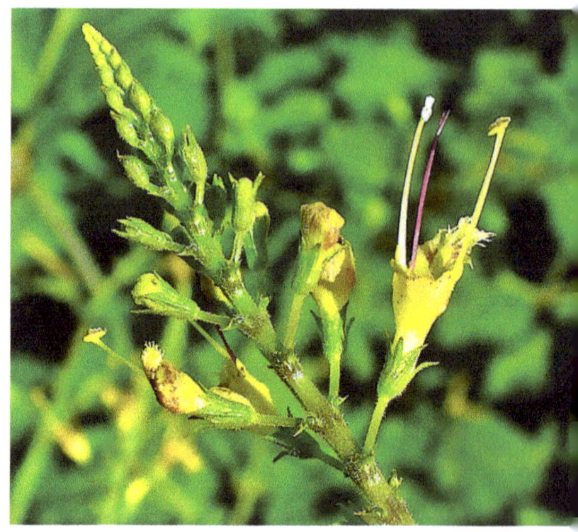

Stone root is an herbaceous perennial with square stems (60 – 120 cm tall). It has thick, hard, knotty roots, with brown bark and white flesh (15 – 20 cm long). The roots resemble river rocks. Stone root's opposite, ovate, sharply dentate leaves are 10 – 20 cm long, with an acuminate apex and a truncate to rounded base. The terminal inflorescence of loose, branching clusters bears many small, lemon-scented, yellow flowers. The bilabiate flowers (8 – 13 mm long) have five fused sepals, five fused petals, two exserted stamens, and an exserted, forked pistil. The flower's upper lip is yellow, with small red stripes. The larger lower lip is cream-colored and strongly fringed; the throat is somewhat hairy. Stone root blooms from mid to late summer.[1,2]

THE NAME: The genus *Collinsonia* was named for Peter Collinson.[3] The epithet *canadensis* means "of or referring to Canada."

HISTORICAL USES: Eclectic physicians recommended using stone root to treat a sore throat, laryngitis, pharyngitis, thracheitis, or hoarseness caused by excessive speaking or singing, ("minister's sore throat").[4-6] Stone root also was used to alleviate venous stasis, and hemorrhoid pain and inflammation.[4-6] Stone root was given to enhance the appetite and digestion.[5,6] Some Eclectics prescribed stone root to treat chorea and mucoenteritis, and to follow up on dysentery symptoms.[5] Physician John Scudder considered stone root an esteemed diuretic, although he was skeptical of its use as a lithotriptic. He suggested that stone root had a soothing influence, reducing irritation from urinary stones.[6] Maude Grieves noted that the fresh root was administered to treat gravel, dropsy, leucorrhoea, and bladder catarrh.[3]

Physician Finley Ellingwood recommended stone root for "enfeebled structure of the heart," and claimed that it directly influenced atonic or dilated veins and arteries. He administered stone root to strengthen the heart, especially if the muscle was debilitated due to fever, rheumatic inflammation, or strain.[5] A poultice or fomentation of the leaves was applied for cuts, abrasions, bruises, and boils.[3]

CONSTITUENTS: Stone root contains volatile oil (α- and β-pinene, limonene, and caryophyllene), tannins (rosmarinic acid and caffeic acid derivatives), triterpenoid saponins, mucilaginous polysaccharides, alkaloids, resins, bitter principles (diterpenoid lactones), and organic acids.[3-5,7]

NUTRITIONAL PROPERTIES: Unknown.

MEDICINAL PROPERTIES: Anti-inflammatory, antilithic, antispasmodic (smooth muscle), aromatic, bitter tonic, portal decongestant, soothing diuretic, and astringent.

TEMPERATURE AND FLAVOR: Cool, sweet, bitter, and mildly astringent.

MEDICINAL USES

Stone root improves digestion and assimilation.[5] The herb acts as a mild digestive bitter tonic, increasing the appetite. It also has mild smooth muscle antispasmodic actions.[4] Stone root is an astringent anti-inflammatory that increases mucous membrane tone in the digestive tract. Long-term use as a bitter tonic improves bowel movements, and aids in treating atonic dyspepsia, gas, loose stools, and chronic digestive inflammation.[4,7] Consume a decoction to extract the mucilage content that coats and soothes the digestive tract, calms the nerve plexus in the gut, and reduces digestive spasms. Long-term consumption of the tea is beneficial for individuals with chronic inflammatory digestive conditions such as irritable bowel syndrome, Crohn's disease, and ulcerative colitis.[7]

Stone root reduces venous stasis and portal congestion.[4,5,8] It aids in treating varicose veins, hemorrhoids, spider veins, fistulas, inner thigh veins, and cervical erosion.[4,5,8] It also reduces hemorrhoidal symptoms in the rectum and anus.[4,5]

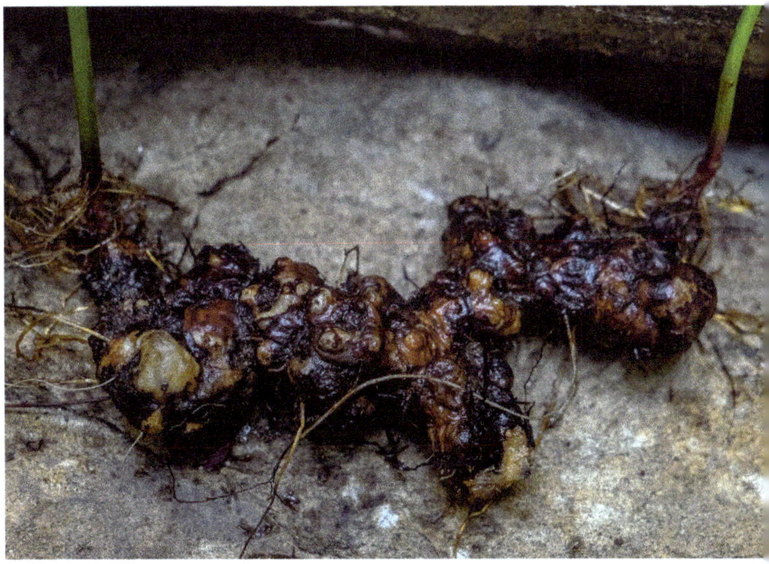

Stone root helps to reduce prostate engorgement resulting from insufficient venous function.[8] Prepare a tannin-based extract by combining stone root, red root *(Ceanothus)*, yellow dock *(Rumex)*, dandelion root *(Taraxacum)*, and/or witch hazel *(Hamamelis)*. Alternatively, prepare an alkaloid-based extract by combining stone root, horse chestnut *(Aesculus hippocastanum)*, ocotillo *(Fouquiera)*, and dandelion root *(Taraxacum)*.[4,5] Consume 60 – 90 drops of either compound, three times daily to ease hemorrhoid flareups, or consume long-term for varicose veins and spider veins.

CONTRAINDICATIONS

Avoid use with obstructive urinary stones or bile stones. An excessive dose, especially of the fresh herb, can cause digestive irritation in some individuals.[7] Most sources consider this herb safe to consume during pregnancy and lactation; however, a few authors caution against it.[4,5,7]

PREPARATION AND DOSAGE

TINCTURE: Fresh whole plant or roots [1:2, 70 - 95% alcohol]; consume 20 - 60 drops, up to three times daily. Dry roots [1:5, 50 - 60% alcohol]; consume 45 - 60 drops, up to three times daily.

CAPSULES: Consume 2 capsules, two to three times daily.

TEA: Prepare tea as a decoction or cold infusion; consume up to 8 ounces, two to four times daily.

THYME

BOTANICAL NAMES:
Thymus vulgaris, T. serpyllum, T. × *citriodorus* (syn. *T. serpyllum* var. *vulgaris*), *T. zygis*

COMMON NAMES:
Thyme, common thyme, garden thyme, lemon thyme, creeping thyme, wild thyme, mother thyme, mother-of-thyme, English thyme, German thyme, French thyme, Spanish thyme
satr, zatr (Arabic)
cotor, dzotor (Armenian)
mashterka gradinska (Bulgarian)
baak leih heung (Cantonese)
timijan (Croatian)
tymián (Czech)
timian (Danish)
tjim (Dutch)
tüümian (Estonian)
timjami (Finnish)
thym (French)
thymian (German)
thymari (Greek)
timin, koranit (Hebrew)
timián (Hungarian)
timjan (Icelandic)
timi (Indonesian)
timo (Italian)
taimu (Japanese)
taim (Korean)
bia li xiang (Mandarin)
timian (Norwegian)
tymianek (Polish)
tomilho (Portuguese)
cimbru (Romanian)
timyan (Russian)
ipar (Sanskrit)
timijan (Serbian)
tomillo (Spanish)
timjan (Swedish)
taymat (Thai)
dag kekigi (Turkish)
chebrets (Ukrainian)
feldkiml (Yiddish)[1,2]

FAMILY NAME:
Lamiaceae (Labiatae)

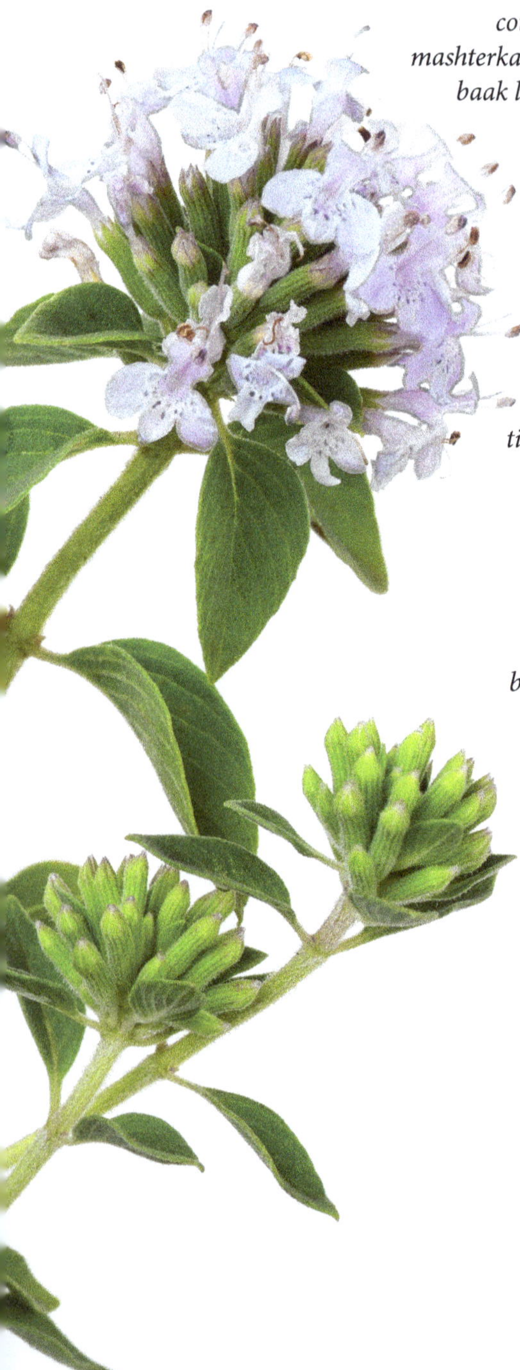

DESCRIPTION

PARTS USED: The leaves and flowering tops.

BOTANICAL DESCRIPTION AND HABITAT: *Thymus* is a large genus of woody perennials native to Africa, Europe, and temperate Asia.[3] *T. vulgaris,* a mounding perennial shrub (15 – 30 cm tall and wide), originated in southern

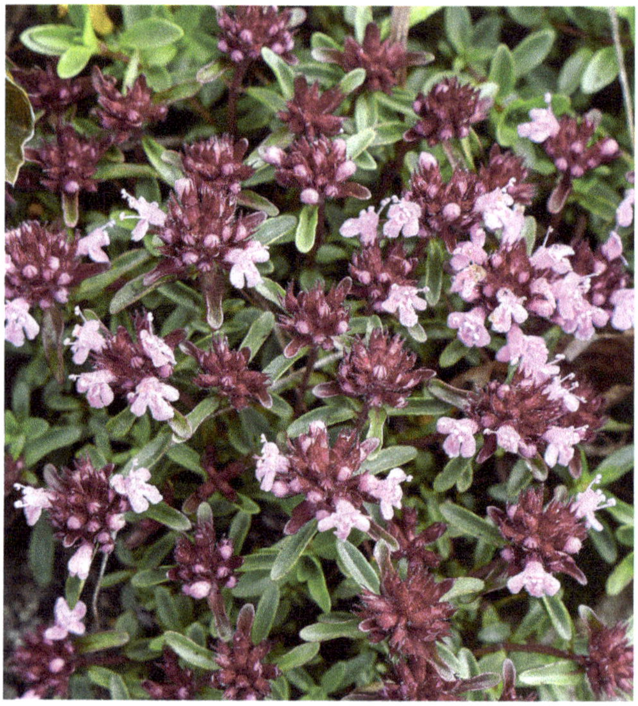

Europe. New stems are herbaceous but become woody as they age.[4] The small, opposite, strongly aromatic, greenish-gray leaves (3 mm long by 1.5 mm wide) are linear to elliptic, with an acute apex and entire, revolute margins.[2,4] In locales with mild winters, the plants keep their leaves year round.[4] Small, terminal spike-like inflorescences produce many tiny bilabiate, tubular flowers with five-toothed calyces, and pale, purplish-white corollas.[2] Four exserted stamens (two short and two long), and a two-lobed style atop a four-lobed ovary comprised of two carpels comprise the inner whorls.[3,5] The fruits are four tiny, smooth nutlets.[3]

THE NAME: The genus *Thymus* and common name thyme have two possible origins. The first derives from Greek, meaning "to fumigate," due to its balsamic odor, or because it was burned as incense.[2] The second derives from the Greek *thumos* ("courage") because in ancient and medieval times, the plant was considered invigorating.[2] The epithet *serpyllum* ("to creep") derives from Greek.[2] The epithet *vulgaris* ("ordinary or common") derives from Latin. The common names, mother thyme and mother-of-thyme, allude to the domestic use of the plant for uterine disorders.[2]

The following common names correspond with the Latin binomials: garden thyme, common thyme, and French thyme *(T. vulgaris)*; creeping thyme, wild thyme, mother thyme, and mother-of-thyme *(T. serpyllum)*; lemon thyme *(T. × citriodorus)*; and Spanish thyme *(T. zygis)*.

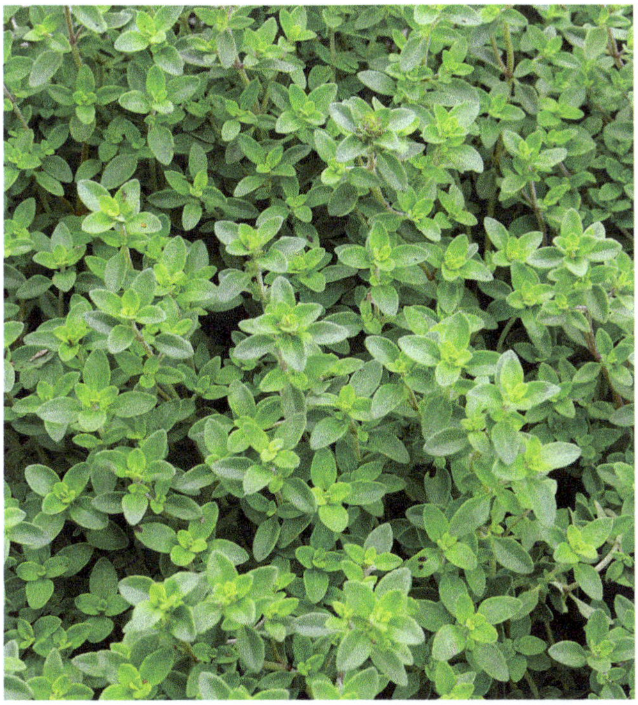

HISTORICAL USES: Thyme was burned in ancient times to fumigate sick rooms.[2] In Greece, it was considered a compliment "to smell of thyme." Ancient Greeks prized the unique flavor of honey from Mount Hymettus near Athens, where wild thyme covered the hillsides.[2] Romans used thyme to flavor cheese and liqueur. They also administered wild thyme to melancholic individuals. Thyme was a symbol of bravery and energy. It was customary for women to embroider scarves with the image of a bee hovering over a sprig of thyme, and present them to their knights.[2] Thyme was a symbol of republicanism in southern France.[2] Fresh thyme prepared as a syrup was administered to treat whooping cough, a sore throat, and catarrh.[2] Thyme tea was consumed to reduce gastric fermentation, and treat colic, flatulence, and intestinal spasms.[2] Hot tea also was consumed to encourage perspiration, and resolve a fever or cold. Ointments containing thyme were applied to relieve sciatica, gout, swelling, and warts.[2] Thyme oil was applied as a counterirritant and rubefacient for rheumatism, and to embalm corpses. Dried thyme flowers were included in sachets in linen drawers to protect the contents from moths and other insects. Thyme was used as a culinary herb to flavor stuffing, sauces, pickles, soups, stews, and olives.[2]

Wild thyme was believed to be among the herbs that formed the Virgin Mary's bed.[2] In Wales, wild thyme was associated with death, and planted on graves. Thyme sprigs were brought to funerals and tossed on graves.[2] Wild thyme was also considered a favored flower of fairies who played on flower tufts.[2] It was used medicinally as an aromatic, carminative, antiseptic, stimulant, antispasmodic, diuretic, and emmenagogue.[2] Wild thyme and rosemary tea were administered to alleviate headaches and nervous afflictions.[2]

Thymol, a thyme derivative, was used internally and externally as an antiseptic.[2] A germicidal, it medicated gauze and wool for surgical dressings. Thymol was added to ointments to treat ringworm, chilblains, parasitic skin infections, burns, eczema, and psoriasis.[2] Combined with one-half lavender essential oil, it was used to repel gnats and mosquitoes. Thymol spirits were inhaled or applied to respiratory passages to treat nasal catarrh, sore throat, laryngitis, bronchial infections, and whooping cough.[2] Thymol was consumed internally to expel parasites. It also was used to preserve meat.[2]

CONSTITUENTS: *Thymus vulgaris* contains volatile oil consisting of phenols (thymol and carvacrol), monoterpene hydrocarbons (*p*-cymene and γ-terpinene), and alcohols (linalool, α-terpineol, and thujan-4-ol). It also contains tannins (rosmarinic, caffeic, labiatic, ursolic, and oleanolic acids), triterpene saponins, bitter principles, and flavonoids.[6,7]

T. serpyllum contains a volatile oil consisting of phenols (carvacrol and thymol), alcohols, and monoterpene hydrocarbons. It also contains tannins (rosmarinic acid and other caffeic acid derivatives), bitter principles, flavonoids, and triterpene saponins.[7]

NUTRITIONAL PROPERTIES: Thyme contains high amounts of aluminum, ash, calcium, chromium, crude fiber, fat, iron, magnesium, manganese, riboflavin, selenium, silicon, sodium, and thiamine. It contains average to low amounts of carbohydrates, dietary fiber, niacin, phosphorus, potassium protein, tin, zinc, and vitamins A.[8]

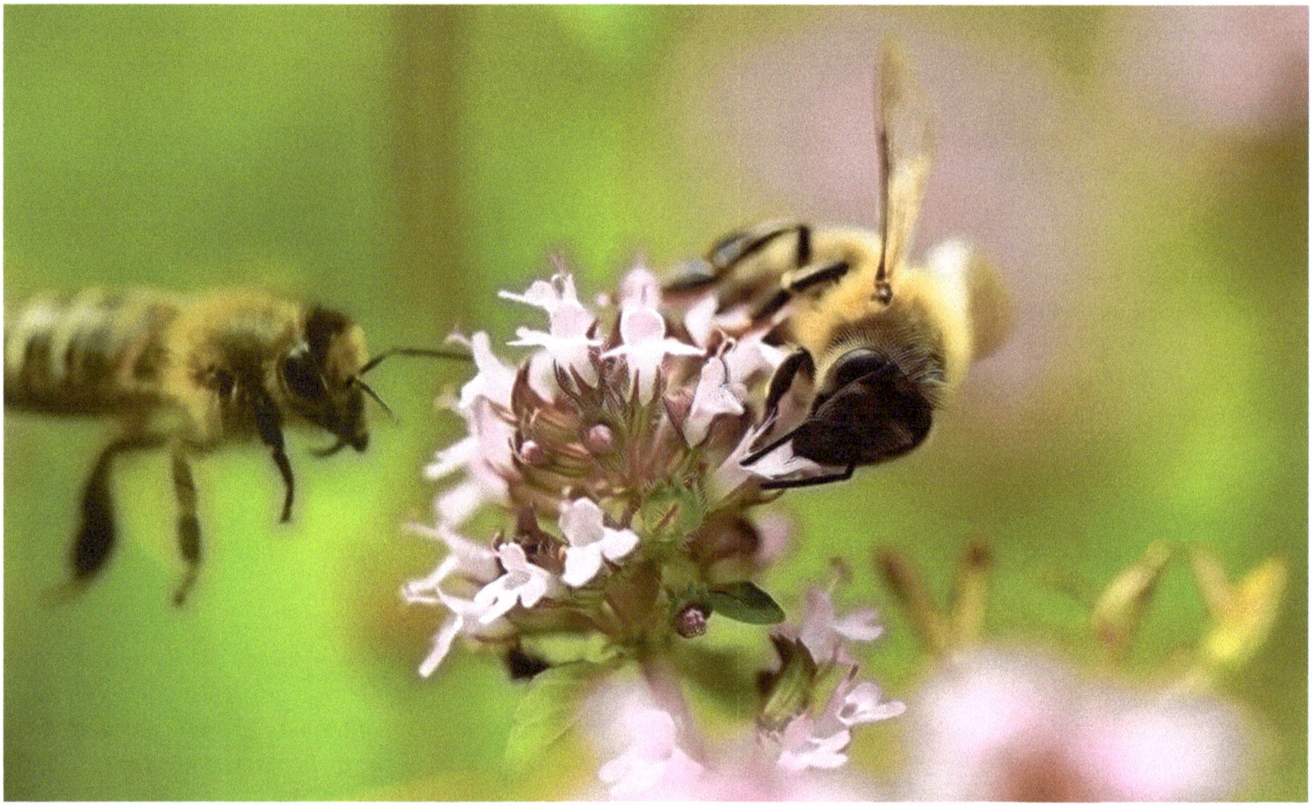

MEDICINAL PROPERTIES: Anthelmintic, antibacterial, antifungal, antioxidant, antiseptic, antispasmodic, antitussive, antiviral, aromatic, bronchodilator, carminative, carrier, circulatory stimulant, counterirritant, expectorant, mild astringent, mild diuretic, rubefacient, and vermifuge.

TEMPERATURE AND FLAVOR: Hot, pungent, sweet, and mildly astringent.

MEDICINAL USES

Thyme is a highly effective antimicrobial agent.[6] Its antiviral actions aid in treating a cold, flu, stomach flu, and mononucleosis.[7] Thyme has antibacterial properties that help to treat sinusitis, laryngitis, strep throat, and staph infections.[7] Due to the antimicrobial, expectorant, and antitussive properties, thyme is excellent for treating lower respiratory conditions, such as whooping cough, pertussis, bronchitis, pleurisy, and pneumonia.[6-8] The antimicrobial properties are attributed to the thymol and carvacrol.[6] The antitussive properties also aid in treating a dry cough, asthma, and emphysema.[8] Steaming with thyme, eucalyptus *(Eucalyptus)*, and/or peppermint *(Mentha piperita)* decreases respiratory congestion. Consume hot thyme tea or thyme-infused chicken broth as a diaphoretic. Combine extracts of thyme, usnea *(Usnea)*, and oregano *(Origanum vulgare)* with smaller quantities of orange peel *(Citrus sinensis)*, cinnamon *(Cinnamomum)*, clove *(Syzygium)*, licorice *(Glycyrrhiza)*, and rosemary *(Salvia rosmarinus)* as a broad spectrum, warming antimicrobial and diaphoretic compound for respiratory or digestive infections. Consume 30 – 90 drops, four to five times daily.

Although thyme is heating, it is an antibacterial agent that treats urinary tract infections, including cystitis and urethritis. It also serves as an adjunct antibacterial agent against bacterial vaginosis and β-strep infections. Thyme is an antifungal that aids in treating *Candida albicans* overgrowth in the digestive and vaginal tracts.[6] It also has anthelmintic properties to treat hookworms and pinworms.[7] Thymol is attributed to the fungicidal, bactericidal, and anthelmintic properties.[6,7]

Thyme is a stomachic and aromatic carminative, reducing gas and bloating.[6,7] It has antispasmodic properties affecting smooth muscles in the trachea and digestive tract.[6] Thyme stimulates digestive secretions, and is a choleretic, supporting healthy digestive function.[7] It aids in treating sluggish digestion, nonulcer dyspepsia, and diarrhea.[7] The stomachic and choleretic actions are attributed to the bitter principles and phenolic acids.[7]

A delicious, pungent culinary herb, thyme enhances the flavor and facilitates the digestion of lamb, mutton, goat, veal, red gamey meats, pork, poultry, fish, egg dishes, gravy, stuffing, vinaigrettes, potatoes, and root vegetables. Due to its potent antioxidant properties, it is often combined with other Mediterranean herbs to cure and preserve meat.[2]

Thyme mouthwash, tea, and fresh herb freshen the breath, and heal mouth ulcers and canker sores.[7] The antimicrobial properties aid in treating gingivitis and halitosis. Thyme essential oil is included in cough drops, toothpaste, mouth rinses such as Listerine, and vapor rubs such as Vicks.[6]

Thyme has counterirritant and rubefacient actions that improve circulation, treating varicose veins, bruises, sprains, strains, muscle pain, muscle spasms, neuralgia, arthritis, and rheumatic pain. A topical antimicrobial, thyme inhibits fungal and bacterial growth, disinfects wounds, and treats athlete's foot, ringworm, skin tinea, and staph.[7] Add thyme leaves or *Thymus* × *citriodorus* essential oil to a medicinal oil or salve to prevent rancidity.

THYME ESSENTIAL OIL
THYMUS VULGARIS, THYME OIL

There are several different chemotypes of thyme *(Thymus vulgaris);* the same species cultivated in different regions produce essential oils with different chemical compositions. The chemotypes include: thymol type, thujanol type, linalool type, geraniol type, and carvacol type.[10] Most of the chemotypes are described in the text that follows. How the oil was distilled also influences how it should be used; red thyme is distilled once and is very harsh; white thyme is distilled twice, and is somewhat less irritating. Generally, *Thymus vulgaris* oil is a potent broad spectrum antimicrobial for infectious illnesses.[11] It is an expectorant, antibacterial, antifungal, antiviral, anthelmintic, and antispasmodic.[7]

THYMUS VULGARIS, RED THYME

Named for its color, red thyme essential oil has been distilled once.[2] It is extremely heating and irritating to the skin and mucous membranes. It is used primarily in cleaning products to disinfect mold, bacteria, and fungi. *Note:* It should not be used internally or topically.

THYMUS VULGARIS, WHITE THYME

White thyme is distilled twice, yielding a clear oil.[2,12] Although it is less irritating than red thyme, it can still irritate the skin and mucous membranes. It is used primarily in cleaning products to disinfect mold, bacteria, and fungi. *Note:* Avoid internal use of white thyme during pregnancy or lactation, and in children under the age of ten.[7] White thyme should only be consumed internally with caution, and is best diluted in vegetable oil in capsules.[10] Discontinue internal use if it is too irritating to the mucous membranes. Avoid topical use, as it is highly irritating to the skin.

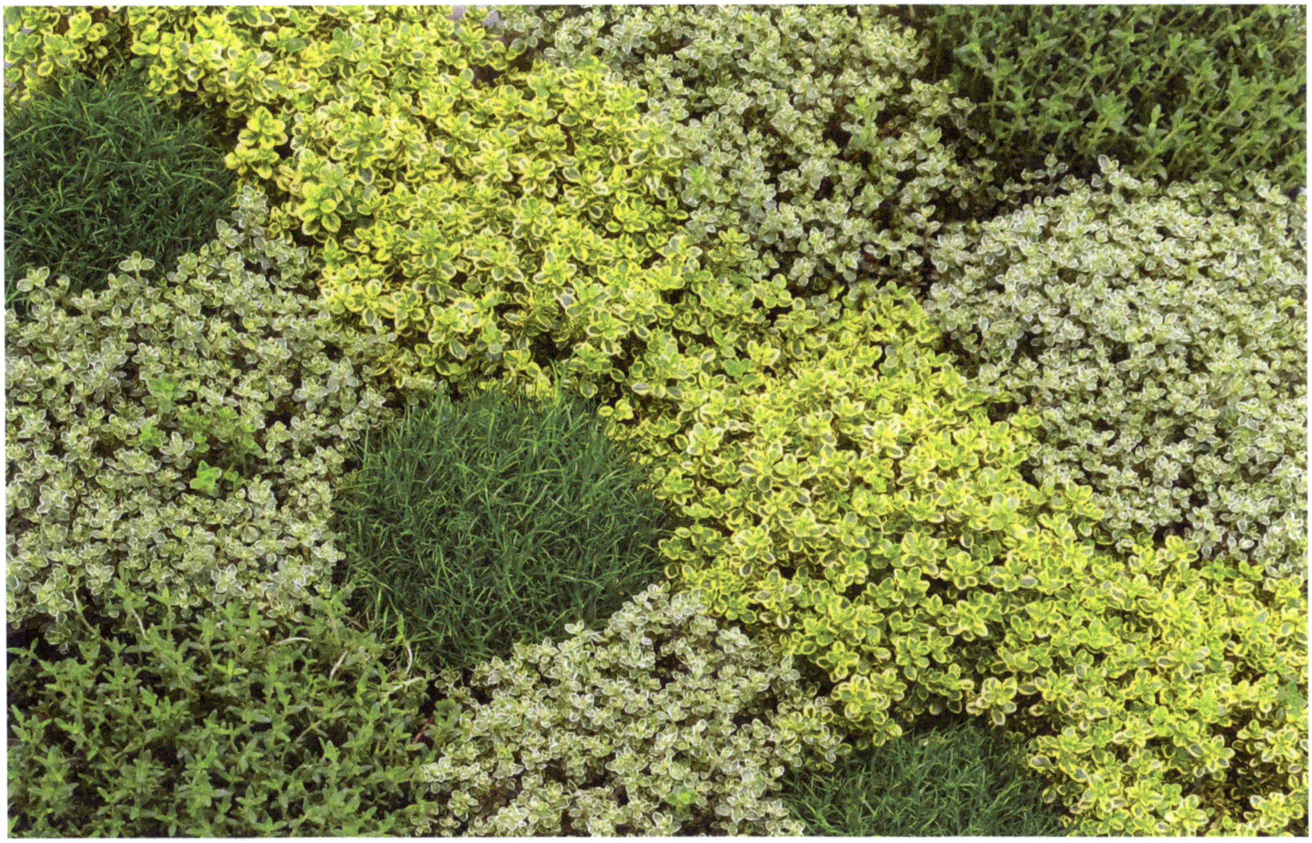

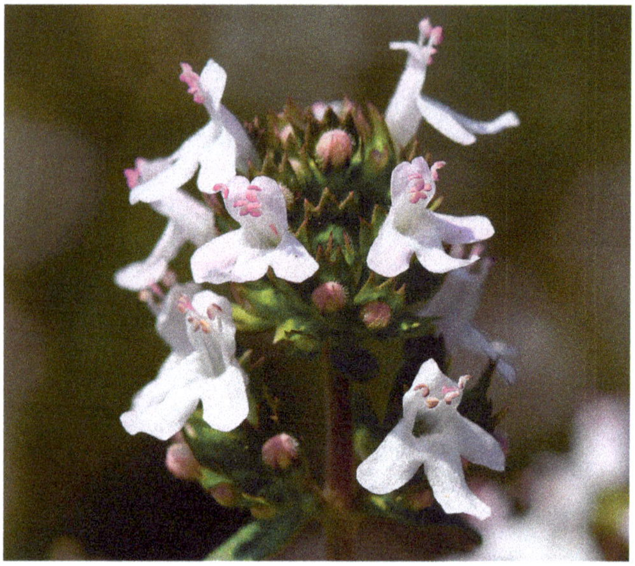

THYMUS VULGARIS, THYMOL TYPE

Thyme thymol type contains a higher quantity of thymol, as well as *p*-cymene and carvacol.[7,11] Sometimes it is distilled from *Thymus zygis.*[11] The constituent thymol has potent fungicidal, bactericidal, and anthelmintic properties; however, it can irritate mucous membranes and skin.[6,10,12] Thyme thymol can be used internally to treat digestive infections, including intestinal candida, hookworms, pinworms *(Oxyuris* spp.*),* food poisoning, and bacterial or viral digestive infections.[7] An antimicrobial and expectorant, it also aids in treating upper and lower respiratory tract infections. Thyme thymol is stimulating and energizing.[10] *Note:* Avoid internal use of thyme thymol type in pregnancy, lactation, and with children under the age of ten.[7] Thyme thymol is best diluted in vegetable oil in capsules.[10] Discontinue internal use if it is too irritating to the mucous membranes. Do not apply topically, as it can be highly irritating to the skin.[7,10]

THYMUS VULGARIS, THUJANOL TYPE

Thyme thujanol contains high amounts of thujanol and terpenes; however, it is lower in phenols.[12] It is a broad spectrum antimicrobial, and is extremely effective against viruses due to its immune stimulating properties. Thyme thujanol type aids in treating upper and lower respiratory infections such as a cold, flu, or bronchitis.[11] Vaginal suppositories containing thyme thujanol aid in treating cervicitis (due to human papilloma virus), bacterial vaginitis, and vaginal candida.[11] Combine one to three drops for every 2 – 3 grams of cocoa butter when making suppositories. Thyme thujanol is a rare essential oil that is effective against chlamydia and condyloma.[11,12] It is also a hepatoregenerative.[11] Topical use is nonirritating and effective against microbial skin infections.[12] *Note:* Avoid internal use of thyme thujanol type during pregnancy and lactation, and with children under the age of ten. In some individuals, topical use irritates the skin.

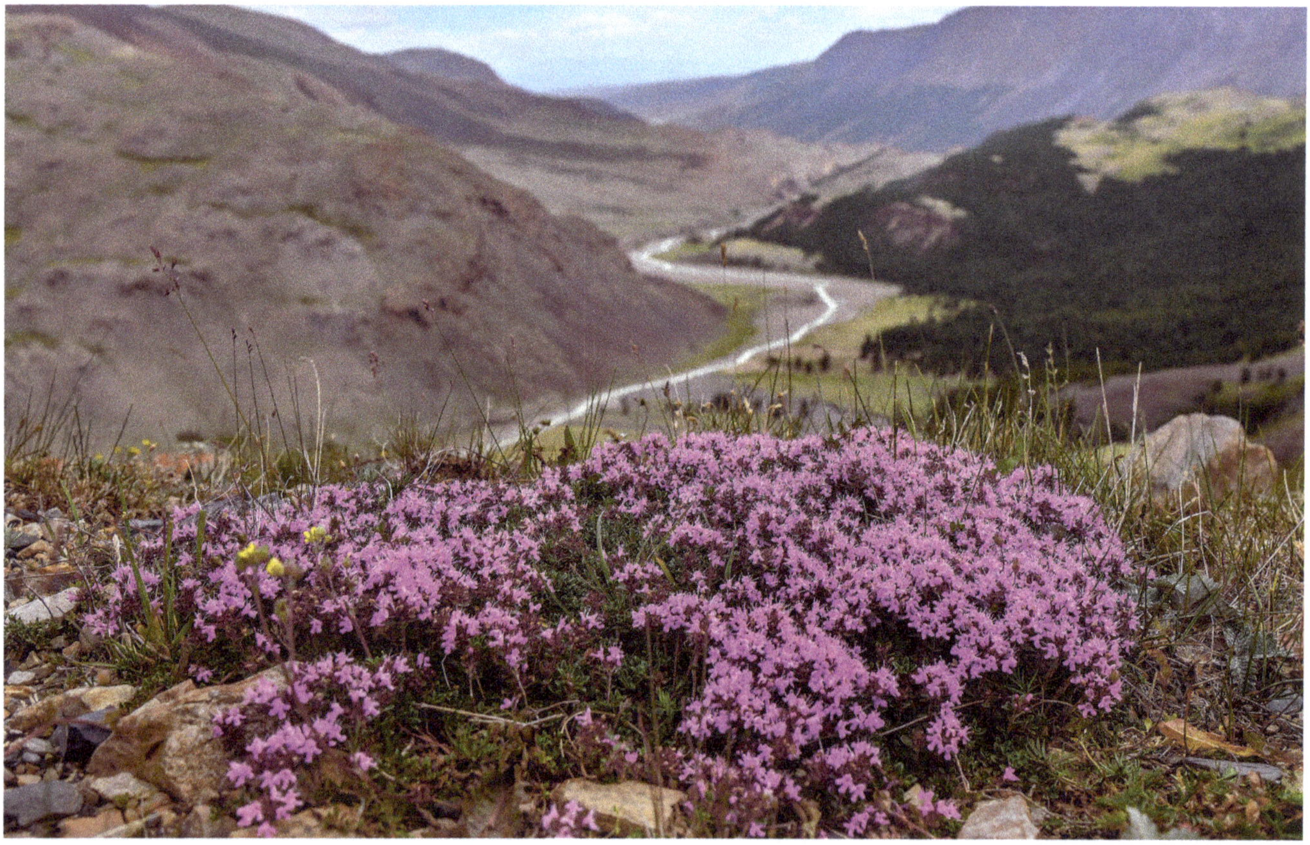

THYMUS VULGARIS, LINALOOL TYPE

Thyme linalool is a gentle, non irritating, highly effective antimicrobial agent.[11] It is high in terpene alcohols (linalool) and esters (linalyl acetate).[11] Internal use aids in treating upper and lower respiratory infections such as a cold, flu, strep throat, or bronchitis, as well as urinary tract infections.[12] Inhaling the essential oil aids in treating sinus and lung congestion. Internal and topical applications (including suppositories for vaginal infections) aid in treating candida, β-strep, bacterial vaginosis, and staph infections.[11] Apply topically to treat acne, wounds, and skin tineas.[10,11] Thyme linalool is also soothing to the nervous system, and helpful for treating nervous exhaustion.[11]

THYMUS VULGARIS, GERANIOL TYPE

Similar to thyme linalool, thyme geraniol is gentle and nonirritating; however, it is rarely available commercially.[10] It is high in terpene alcohols, predominantly geraniol.[11] Thyme geraniol is a broad spectrum antimicrobial against bacteria, viruses, and fungi.[11] Internal use aids in treating upper and lower respiratory infections such as a cold, flu, strep throat, bronchitis, and viral enteritis.[10,11] Internal and topical applications (i.e., a suppository) aid in treating candida, β-strep, bacterial vaginosis, and staph infections.[10,11] Thyme geraniol calms the nervous system and has sedative properties.[11] Apply topically to treat skin tineas and acne, and to disinfect wounds.[10-12]

THYMUS × CITRIODORUS, LEMON THYME

Lemon thyme is a gentle, safe form of thyme essential oil. It contains higher amounts of geraniol and citral than other species or chemotypes. Consume 1 – 2 drops as an aromatic carminative, stomachic, and mild antimicrobial.[7] The geraniol and citral contribute to the antimicrobial actions, as well as the calming effects on the nervous system.[7] Suppositories containing lemon thyme oil aid in treating vaginal infections, including candida, bacterial vaginosis, and β-strep. Add lemon thyme to bug repellants.

Directions for internal use: Take care to note that only some chemotypes of thyme oil (thyme linalool, citriodorus, and geraniol) are safe to consume internally. Place 1 – 2 drops in a charcoal tablet or capsule containing a carrier powder (such as marshmallow) or oil (such as olive oil). Consume 1 – 2 tablets, up to three times daily.

Note: There are no known contraindications for thyme linalool, citriodorus, or geraniol when used in the physiologic dosage (1 – 3 drops).[11]

THYMUS SERPYLLUM, WILD THYME

Wild thyme contains higher amounts of carvacrol and lesser amounts of thymol than *T. vulgaris*.[7] It is milder in action, but can be used interchangeably with *T. vulgaris* thymol type.

CONTRAINDICATIONS

Culinary use of thyme is permissible during pregnancy; however, limit internal use of the extract during pregnancy. See *Note* section for essential oil before using.

PREPARATION AND DOSAGE

TINCTURE: Fresh leaves [1:3 - 1:4, 80 - 95% alcohol]; dry leaves [1:5 - 1:7, 60% alcohol]; consume 15 - 90 drops, three to four times daily.

ACETUM EXTRACT: Fresh leaves [1:3 - 1:4, apple cider vinegar]; consume in food preparations such as vinaigrettes or oil, or apply diluted thyme acetum as a topical preparation.

CAPSULES: Add 1 - 3 drops of essential oil to a charcoal tablet or capsule containing a binding agent; consume 1 - 2 capsules, one to three times daily.

TEA: Consume 8 - 12 ounces of the hot infusion, one to three times daily.

HONEY AND SYRUP: Simple syrup can be prepared by dissolving one part by volume of sugar into one part of a strained thyme infusion, or by infusing thyme directly into prepared simple syrup. Add 1 - 2 drops of thyme essential oil to 1 teaspoon to 1 tablespoon of honey, and mix with a toothpick. Add the honey to one cup of tea or hot water; consume up to four times daily.

TOPICAL USE: Apply the tea as a fomentation, poultice, or foot bath. Prepare infused oil using the alcohol intermediary method. Dilute the essential oil in cream, oil, salve, liniment, soap, or lotion.

CULINARY USE: Freshly chopped or ground thyme is a seasoning for beef, lamb, veal, venison, rabbit, poultry, soup, gravy, sauces, potatoes, or root vegetable dishes.

TULSI BASIL

DESCRIPTION

BOTANICAL NAMES:
Ocimum tenuiflorum (syn. *O. sanctum*), *O. gratissimum*

COMMON NAMES:
Holy basil, tulsi basil, sacred basil, queen of herbs
tulsi, Rama tulsi, Sri tulsi, Krishna tulsi, vana tulsi (Hindi)
tulasī, visnu-priyā, divyā (Sanskrit)
bai gkaprow, kaphrao daeng (Thai)

FAMILY NAME:
Lamiaceae

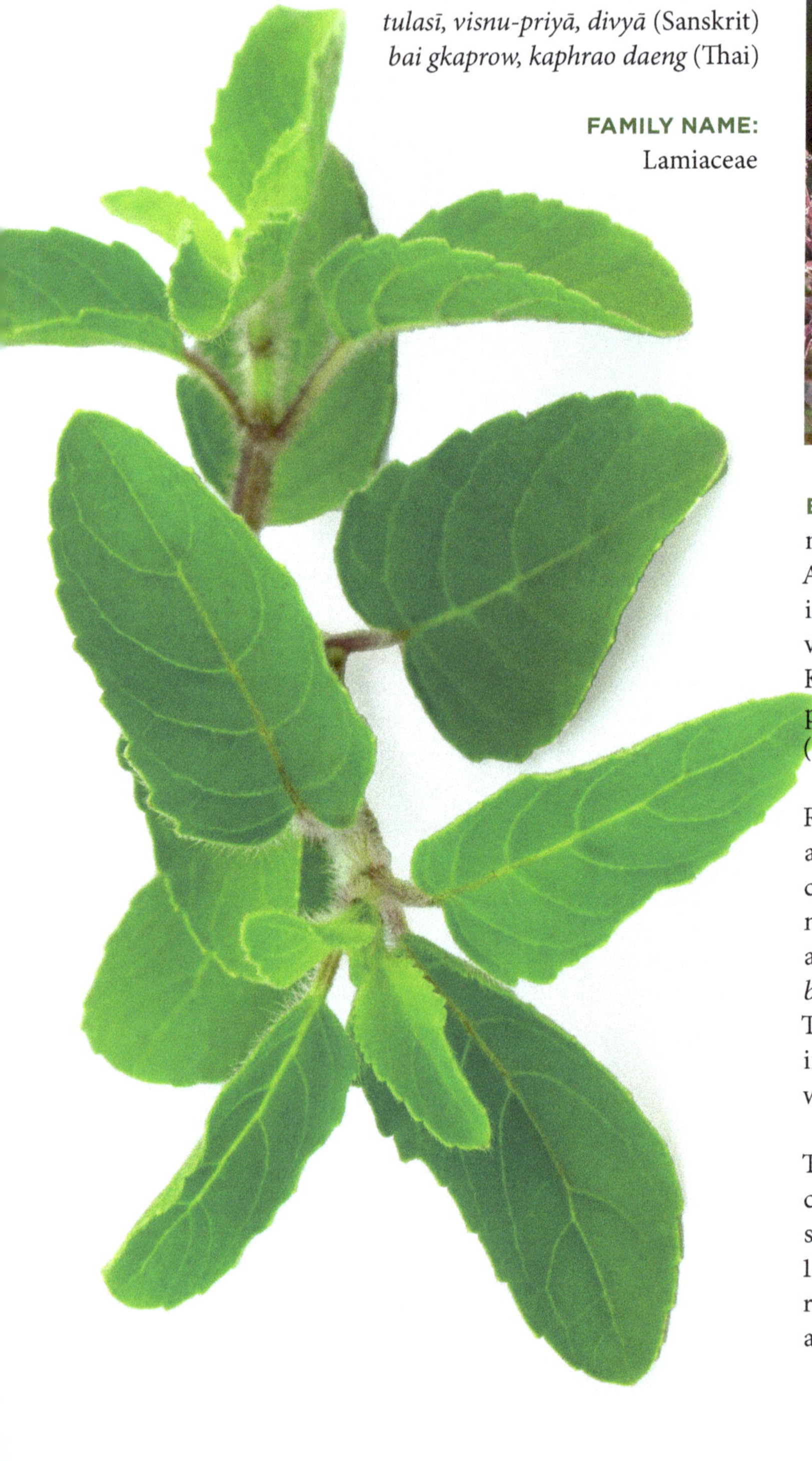

PARTS USED: The leaves, flowers, and small stems.

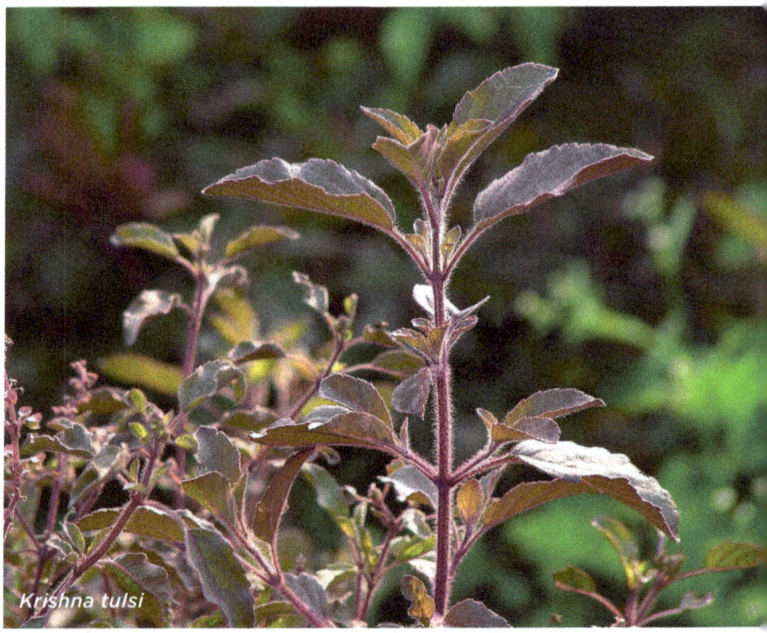

Krishna tulsi

BOTANICAL DESCRIPTION AND HABITAT: Tulsi is native to lower elevations in India and other Southeast Asian countries. The three most well-known types of tulsi include: Rama tulsi or Sri tulsi *(O. tenuiflorum)*, with vibrant green leaves and white flowers; Krishna tulsi or Krishna *(O. tenuiflorum)*, with deep green to purple leaves, purple flowers, and a more pungent aroma; and vana tulsi (*O. gratissimum*) that grows wild in woodlands.

Richly scented of clove and basil, tulsi is cultivated widely, and prefers dry, sandy soil.[1] When found in tropical climates, tulsi is a perennial with a woody base (up to 1 meter tall).[1] However, it is frost sensitive, and in temperate areas of the world, grows as an annual, similar to *Ocimum basilicum* (basil). The plant is mainly covered in fine hairs. The leaf blade (2.5 – 5.5 cm long by 1 – 3 cm wide) varies in shape according to the variety, but is generally oblong, with shallowly serrated margins.[1]

The inflorescences (about 7 cm long) are stacked verticillasters of six small, hairy flowers, with each whorl subtended by sessile, heart-shaped bracts (1.5 mm long by 1.5 mm wide).[1] The bell-shaped, vaguely two-lipped, villous, red-tinged calyces (1.5 mm long) have spine-tipped teeth and strong veins.[1] The white to purplish corollas (about 2 mm long) extend past the calyx; four stamens and a style with a two-cleft stigma extend past the corolla margin.[2] Two carpels bear four brown nutlets at maturity.[2]

THE NAME: The genus name *Ocimum* is the Latin version of the Greek name for basil *(okimon),* derived from the Greek *ozien* ("smell").[3] In Sanskrit, tulsi translates as "the incomparable one."[4] Throughout India, tulsi is known as the "queen of herbs." Basil derives from the Greek *basileus* ("royal or kingly").

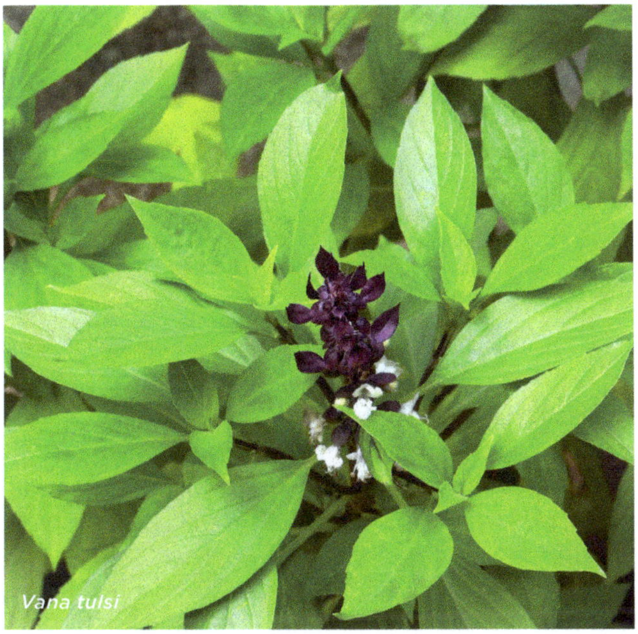
Vana tulsi

HISTORICAL USES: Considered by some to be the most sacred plant in India, tulsi is worshiped in the Hindu tradition as a representation or avatar of the goddess Lakshmi. She is denoted by the common name *haripriya* ("dear to Lord Vishnu"), as well as *tulsi mata* (tulsi mother).[5] The wood, sometimes unfamiliar to tulsi growers in temperate climates, is made into *mala* beads, or prayer beads. One hundred and eight beads are used to create a necklace on which mantras are counted and recited.[5] Tulsi beads are especially renowned by devotees of Vishnu.[6] Tulsi is often planted in Hindu courtyards, and integrated into the daily ritual of praying to Vishnu (the Lord of Preservation) for health, well being, and spiritual purity.[7,8] The spiritual importance of tulsi is perhaps most clearly illustrated in the practice of placing the leaves and water from the Ganges River into the mouth of a dying person, in faith that it will lead the spirit on its journey.[5] Tulsi also was believed to ward off evil spirits, perhaps due to its antimicrobial qualities.[5]

Tulsi was widely utilized as an expectorant; juice from the leaves was combined with honey to treat coughs, colds, and bronchitis.[9] Anthropological records describe the use of tulsi by the Nicobarese, indigenous people of Katchal Island, India. They indicate its use combined with common medicine-plant *(Adenostemma lavenia)* and ngai camphor *(Blumea balsamifera),* pounded in pig blood, and consumed twice daily to address chronic chest pain.[10] The powdered leaves were prepared as snuff to reduce nasal congestion.[8] Tulsi tea was consumed to ease nausea, vomiting, upset stomach, gas, and biliousness.[8] A poultice of fresh roots and leaves was applied to treat insect bites, snakebites, and scorpion stings.[8] Juice from the leaves was also used to treat ringworm infections.[11]

CONSTITUENTS: Tulsi basil contains volatile oil (eugenol, methyl eugenol, estragole, carvacrol, linalool, limatrol, and caryophyllene), sterols (β-sitosterol and stigmasterol), a triterpene (ursolic acid), flavonoids (orientin = 8-C-β-glucopyranosyl-3',4',5,7-tetrahydroxyflav-2-en-3-one; vicenin = 6-C-β-D-xylopyranosyl-8-C-β-D-glucopyranosyl apigenin; and molludistin), phenolic compounds (rosmarinic acid, propanoic acid, apigenin, cirsilenol, cirsimaritin, isothymusin, and isothymonin), ocimumoside A and B, ocimarin, and fatty acids.[4,7,8,12,13]

NUTRITIONAL PROPERTIES: Tulsi contains vitamins A and C, carotenoids, calcium, iron, zinc, and chlorophyll.[4]

MEDICINAL PROPERTIES: Adaptogen, antibacterial, antidepressant, antifungal, anti-inflammatory, antioxidant, antispasmodic, antiulcerogenic, antiviral, aromatic, carminative, diaphoretic, diuretic, expectorant, febrifuge, galactagogue, hypoglycemic, immune modulator, neuroprotective, nervine, and radioprotective.

TEMPERATURE AND FLAVOR: Warm, sweet, pungent, and bitter.

MEDICINAL USES

An expectorant and mucolytic, tulsi has an affinity for the respiratory system. It clears mucus from the upper and lower respiratory tracts.[7] Tulsi basil is an antiallergenic, a mild bronchodilator, and a subtle antitussive that aids in treating allergies, allergic rhinitis, asthma, bronchitis, and labored breathing.[7,8,12] It increases lung capacity and strengthens the vital force *(prāna).*[7] An immune modulator, tulsi regulates antibody production, increasing antibodies when they are low, while reducing an allergy-related increase in antibodies.[8] It enhances immune function and

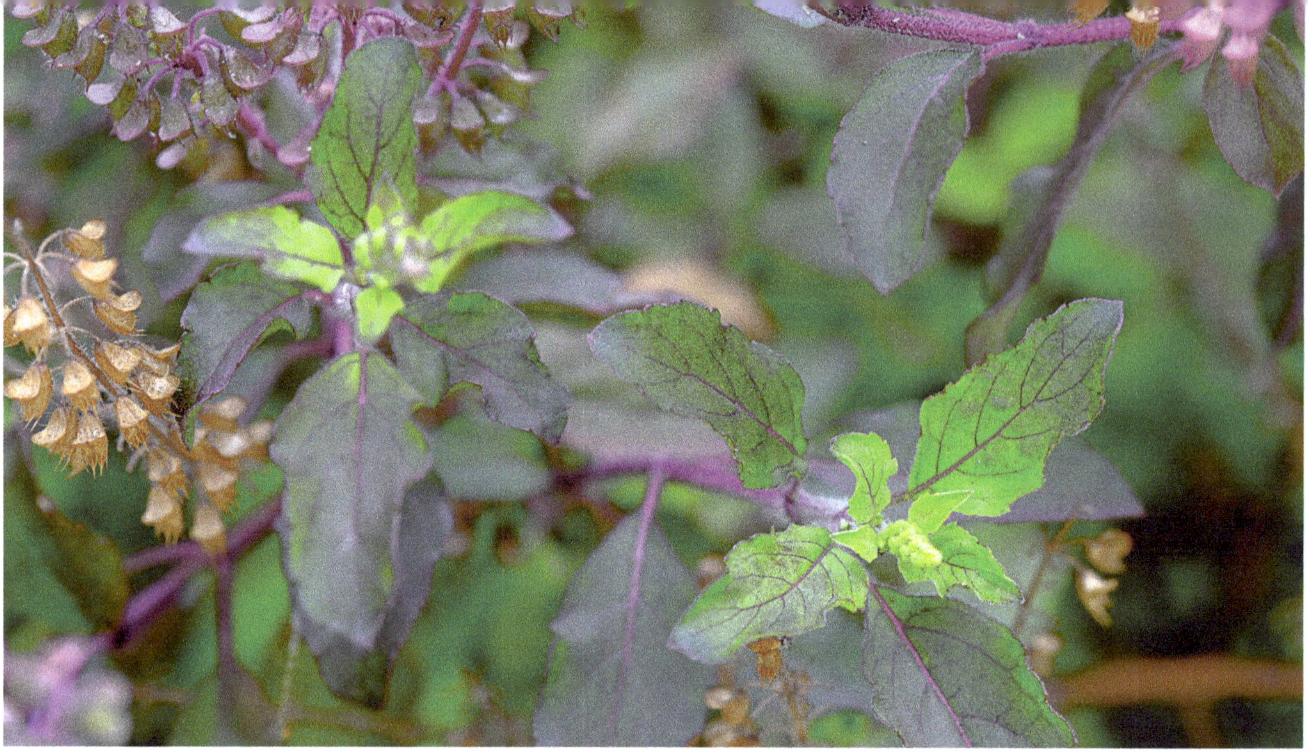

humoral immunity. Consuming hot tulsi tea encourages diaphoresis, alleviating a fever.[7,12] Tulsi also has antibacterial and antiviral properties. The volatile oil has antibacterial activity against *Staphylococcus aureus, Bacillus pumilus,* and *Pseudomonas aeruginosa.* Aqueous extracts inhibited the growth of *Klebsiella, E. coli, Proteus, S. aureus,* and *Candida albicans.*[4] In preliminary studies, tulsi extract inhibited *Neisseria gonorrhoeae,* with activity comparable to penicillin and ciprofloxacin.[4]

An antinauseant and aromatic carminative, tulsi reduces gas and bloating, and enhances digestion.[7] Prepare a delicious digestive tea by combining tulsi with carminatives, such as coriander *(Coriandrum),* orange peel *(Citrus sinensis),* and cardamom *(Elettaria),* and smaller amounts of allspice *(Pimenta),* clove *(Syzygium),* licorice *(Glycyrrhiza),* and vanilla *(Vanilla).* Additionally, tulsi extract has antiulcerogenic activity.[4,8] Consuming 100 mg/kg of the extract was found to reduce pepsin secretion and lipid peroxidation, and to have a protective effect by increasing mucin secretion, protecting mucosal cells, and increasing their lifespan.[4]

Tulsi increases cerebral circulation, improving mental focus, alertness, and clarity. It aids in treating individuals with a poor memory, ADD, and ADHD, and hastens recovery from a head trauma.[8] A nootropic, neuroprotective, and antioxidant, tulsi may delay the onset and prevent the progression of Alzheimer's and dementia.[4] Tulsi is a stimulant and energizer, combating fatigue. Combine tulsi with gotu kola *(Centella)* and smaller amounts of rosemary *(Salvia rosmarinus),* brahmi *(Bacopa),* and ginkgo *(Ginkgo)* to increase mental clarity and memory, and as a stimulant. It is a subtle nervine that eases anxiety and headaches caused by tension or congestion.[7] Tulsi is a mood elevator that aids in treating mild to moderate depression and seasonal affective disorder (SAD). Tulsi's ability to improve neurotransmitter levels associated with mood has been affirmed in rodent studies. The research found that tulsi leaf extract increased dopamine levels, serotonin (5-HT), and 5-HT turnover when the rodents were stressed.[4] Combine tulsi with other mood elevating herbs such as St. John's wort *(Hypericum),* damiana *(Turnera),* aralia berry *(Aralia californica),* and smaller amounts of rosemary *(Salvia rosmarinus)* and lavender *(Lavandula).*

Tulsi is an adaptogen that counters the detrimental effects of stress, and prevents a stress-related increase in cortisol levels.[4,8,13] It improves motor activity and physical performance.[13] The stress alleviating effects are attributed to ocimumoside A and B.[13] Consuming a tulsi infusion consistently over time is effective for reducing the negative effects of stress. Prepare a gentle adaptogen tea by combining tulsi, gotu kola *(Centella),* spearmint *(Mentha spicata),* and a nutritive, such as oatstraw *(Avena).* Tulsi aids in regulating cortisol levels and lowering elevated blood glucose levels.[4,8] It lowers post-prandial blood glucose levels and cholesterol levels, and can be useful for long-term management of metabolic syndrome and diabetes mellitus. In one study, tulsi lowered blood glucose levels up to 17.6% in type 2 diabetics.[8]

Tulsi is an antioxidant and anti-inflammatory. It increases the activity of the antioxidant enzymes superoxide dismutase and superoxide catalase, and prevents lipid peroxidation.[4,8] It protects against radiation-induced hepatic lipid peroxidation.[13] When consumed before and after mercury intoxication, tulsi leaf extract (10 mg/kg of body weight) protected rodents from mercury toxicity, and decreased hepatic lipid peroxidation.[4] Rosmarinic acid, propanoic acid, apigenin, cirsimaritin, eugenol, isothymusin, isothymonin, civsilineol, and civsimavatine are attributed to the antioxidant and anti-inflammatory actions.[4] The cyclooxygenase inhibitory activity of these isolated components was comparable to over-the-counter drugs such as Ibuprofen, Naproxen, and aspirin.[4]

A radioprotective, tulsi contains two water-soluble flavonoids, orientin and vicenin, that help to protect human blood lymphocytes from radiation-induced chromosomal damage.[4] These flavonoids also protect against radiation damage to the liver, and chromosomal damage to cells (in rodent studies.)[8]

Tulsi may have thyroid-modulating effects; however, its influence on the thyroid warrants further scientific and clinical studies. As an adjunct, it has been useful for modifying symptoms in individuals with hypothyroidism and hyperthyroidism. This may be due to tulsi's adaptogenic and cortisol-regulating actions that support the adrenals and reduce symptoms of stress-aggravated autoimmune conditions, such as Hashimoto's and Grave's disease. Currently, it is not known whether it directly influences the thyroid gland. Based on clinical observation, tulsi tea has reduced symptoms of hypothyroidism in numerous patients by lowering elevated cortisol levels, reducing inflammation and allergies, improving mental clarity, and reducing depression. Some patients with Grave's disease have found it calming and energy sustaining, in addition to addressing some of the aforementioned symptoms. In one study, tulsi leaf extract (consumed at a dose of 0.5 g/kg body weight for 15 days) significantly decreased serum T4 concentration in male rats.[4] However, no changes were observed in the serum T3 level.[4] It has been suggested that the method in which the herb is employed could be the determining factor. Tulsi extract could exert a hypothyroidal effect, while the tea may have more thyroid stimulating actions.

Tulsi is a vulnerary agent that supports wound healing.[13] It decreases the formation of keloids and hypertrophic scars.[13] Tulsi contains ursolic acid that inhibits the formation of wrinkles and age spots by improving skin's elasticity and enhancing collagen fiber structures.[13] Ursolic acid also inhibits the action of elastase, an enzyme that attacks structural proteins in the skin.[13]

CONTRAINDICATIONS

Women attempting to conceive should avoid consuming tulsi, as it may have an antifertility effect.[8] Minimize or avoid use during pregnancy until further studies are completed.[8,12] Individuals with hypothyroidism and those medicated with thyroid hormones may want to avoid long-term daily consumption of tulsi extract.

Regular use should be avoided by individuals consuming glutathione-depleting medications such as paracetamol, due to its eugenol content that may further deplete glutathione from the liver.[7]

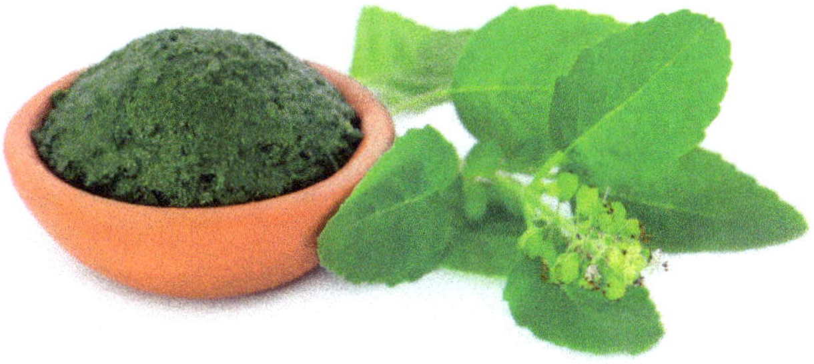

PREPARATION AND DOSAGE

TINCTURE: Fresh herb [1:2-1:3, 70-95% alcohol]; or recently dried herb [1:5, 50% alcohol]; consume 20-60 drops, up to three times daily.

SUCCUS: Consume ½-1 ounce of fresh juice in the morning or before lunch.

CAPSULES: Consume 2-3 freeze-dried capsules, one to three times daily.

TEA: Prepare a hot or cold infusion; consume 8-12 ounces, one to three times daily.

HONEY AND SYRUP: Prepare syrup by combining the tincture or hot infusion with honey to taste. Add fresh leaves to prepare an infused honey. Consume 1 teaspoon to 1 tablespoon, up to four times daily.

TOPICAL USE: Apply a fresh plant poultice to boils and a wash, soak, or fomentation to fungal infections.

CULINARY USE: Add small amounts of fresh tulsi to foods as a carminative.

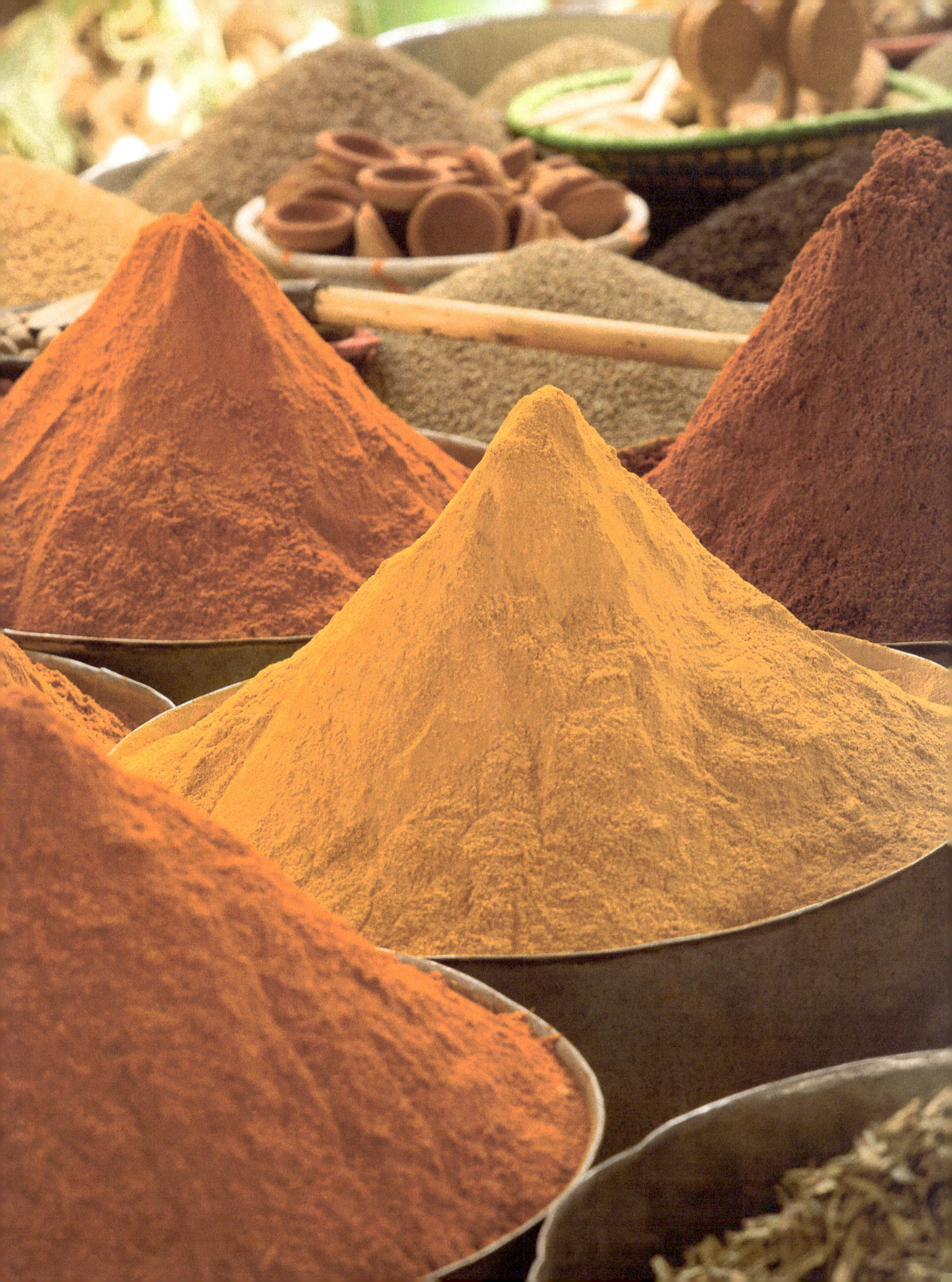

TURMERIC

DESCRIPTION

BOTANICAL NAMES:
Curcuma longa (syn. *C. domestica*)

COMMON NAMES:
Turmeric, curcuma, yellow ginger, Indian saffron
gurkemeje (Danish)
rhizome de curcuma, safran des Indes (French)
kurkumawurzelstock, gelbwurzel (German)
haldi (Hindi)
jiang huang (Mandarin)
haridra, shati (Sanskrit)

FAMILY NAME:
Zingiberaceae

PART USED: The rhizomes.

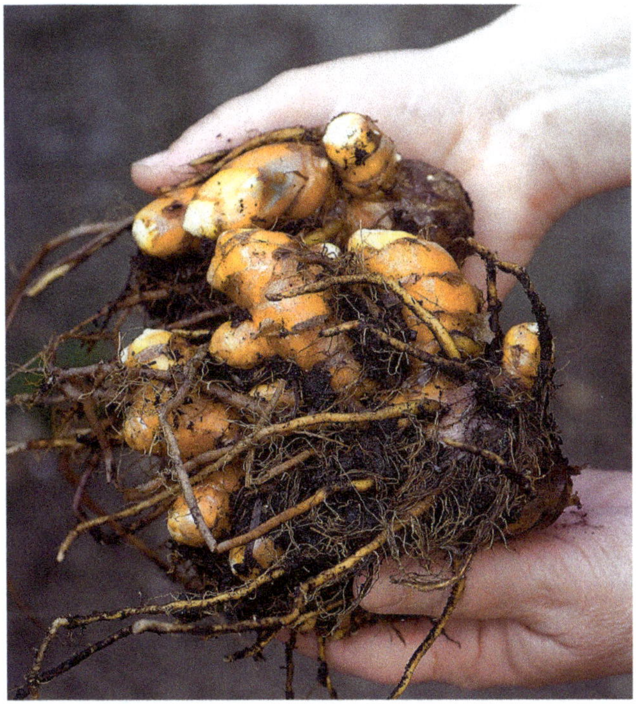

BOTANICAL DESCRIPTION AND HABITAT: A perennial herb, turmeric is indigenous to Southeast Asia. It is propagated from root cuttings or divisions, and thrives in tropical climates, growing in moist, well-drained soil. However, it can be cultivated in greenhouses in temperate climates. India produces 94% of the world's supply of turmeric. It is also cultivated in China, Taiwan, Burma, Indonesia, Jamaica, Haiti, Japan, and Hawaii.[1,2]

Turmeric grows up to 1.5 meters tall. It has vibrant green, glabrous, oblong or lanceolate leaf blades (35 – 45 cm long by 15 – 18 cm wide) on top of long petioles (20 – 45 cm long).[1] The orange-yellow, branching, oblong rhizomes superficially resemble ginger, and are covered with light brown skin with transverse parallel rings. Dense spikes arising from the rhizomes display tubular flowers. Each flower is surrounded by a pale green bract sometimes tinged with purple. The flowers have white calyces (about 1 cm long) and pale yellow, three-lobed corollas (3 cm long).[1] Sterile staminodes grow on either side of the short, wide, centrally located, fertile stamen.[2] The ovary consists of three fused carpels that develop into a three-valved capsule.[2]

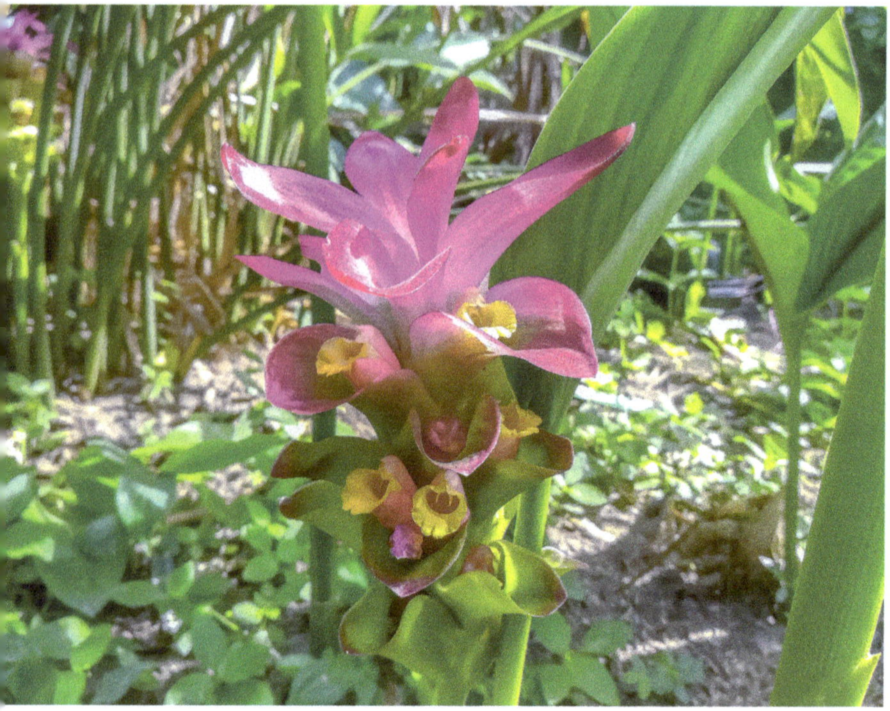

THE NAME: *Curcuma* derives from the Persian *kurkum* ("saffron") because the orange-yellow rhizome hue resembles that of saffron.[3] The epithet *longa* refers to the long, tubular roots. The Chinese name jiang huang means "ginger yellow." Haridra means "yellow." Turmeric derives from the Latin *terra merita,* referring to the yellow mineral pigment.[2]

HISTORICAL USES: In India, turmeric is a venerated herb used as a spice, medicine, and dye; it is also used in Hindu religious ceremonies. Today, it continues to be used to dye priests' holy robes, as well as silk, cotton, and wool.[4,6] Traditionally, turmeric was consumed as a digestive aid, blood purifier, tonic, antispasmodic, and diaphoretic.[4] It was also used to treat morning sickness and liver disorders. Turmeric was applied externally for skin infections, sores, sprains, arthritis, conjunctivitis, eczema, cancer, and hemorrhoids.[4,8] It was considered a preventative and a treatment for intestinal worms and parasites.[9] In Ayurvedic medicine, turmeric is used to eliminate excess kapha.[5] Ayurvedic practitioner Vasant Lad explains that turmeric "gives the energy of the Divine Mother to grant prosperity" and "cleanses the chakras *(nadi-shodhana)*."[6] Historically, turmeric has been incorporated into facial cosmetics to impart a golden glow.[4] It has been cultivated and harvested in India since 3000 BCE.[5] More than 100,000 acres of turmeric were cultivated in 1950.[5] Today, turmeric sales continue to increase. In 2006, 846,700 tons of rhizomes were cultivated.

India introduced turmeric to China by 700 CE. It was mentioned in the *Tang Pen Tsao* (1578) for its medicinal effects on the liver and digestion.[5] In Traditional Chinese Medicine, turmeric was used to treat flatulence, colic, abdominal pain, liver problems, menstrual cramping, afterbirth pain, chest pain, blood in the urine, hemorrhaging, toothaches, bruises, and sores.[3,4] It was also used to invigorate the blood, remove deficiency cold, and dispel wind.[8] Due to its "wind-dispelling actions," turmeric has been used to treat epilepsy and febrile seizures. Topical applications were administered to relieve pain and itching, and eliminate ringworm.[3]

In Polynesia, turmeric was used to treat asthma, skin diseases, and constipation, and was employed in religious rituals.[3] It has been an important traditional medicine in Thailand, where it was used as a carminative, appetite stimulant, antidiarrheal, and astringent.[4] It was also used to treat dizziness, gonorrhea, and peptic ulcers. Turmeric was applied topically to insect bites, ringworm, wounds, bleeding, and inflamed gums.[8]

In the 13th century, Arab traders introduced turmeric to Europe; however, it was not popular in Western cultures until recently. European and Western herbalists recommended turmeric as a mild aromatic stimulant and stomachic for dyspepsia, flatulence, and jaundice. It was believed to have effects similar to ginger. Turmeric was used as a test for alkalies, and to color ointments and pharmaceutical products.

CONSTITUENTS: Turmeric contains volatile oil (turmerone, ar-turmerone, α-atlantone, γ-atlantone, zingiberene, 1,8-cineole, α-phellandrene, D-sabinene, borneol, dehydroturmerone, aneole, and monoterpines), orange-yellow pigment (curcumin, monodesmethoxycurcumin, and didesmethoxycurcumin), *p*-coumaroylferuloylmethane, and di-*p*-coumaroylmethane. It also contains sugars (glucose, fructose, and arabinose), protein, polysaccharides (starch and ukonanes), minerals, and vitamins A and C. Some sources suggest that turmeric contains β-carotene, rather than vitamin A.[3,11]

NUTRITIONAL PROPERTIES: Turmeric rhizome contains high amounts of iron, magnesium, manganese, niacin, potassium, selenium, silicon, and sodium. It also contains moderate to low amounts of calcium, chromium, cobalt, crude fiber, dietary fiber, phosphorus, protein, riboflavin, thiamine, vitamin A (β-carotene), vitamin C, and zinc.[12]

MEDICINAL PROPERTIES: Antiarthritic, antibacterial, anticarcinogenic, antihepatotoxic, anti-inflammatory, antimetastatic, antimutagenic, antioxidant, antispasmodic, antiviral, aromatic, bitter tonic, carminative, cholagogue, choleretic, depurative, hepatoprotectant, hypolipidemic, immune modulator, and vulnerary.

TEMPERATURE AND FLAVOR: Warm, bitter, and pungent.

MEDICINAL USES

Turmeric is a potent anti-inflammatory. The rhizomes contain curcumin that reduces prostaglandins and leukotrienes synthesis.[3] A dual inhibitor of arachidonic acid metabolism, curcumin inhibits the enzymes 5-lipoxygenase and cyclooxygenase (to a lesser degree).[13] In acute tests, curcumin's anti-inflammatory actions were comparable to phenylbutazone, and nearly as potent as cortisone. In chronic tests, it was only one-half as potent as phenylbutazone.[7,13] In one study, 400 mg of curcumin was comparable to 100 mg of phenylbutazone and 400 mg of ibuprofen in treating rheumatoid arthritis.[7] Turmeric does not have NSAID-related side effects such as ulcer formation, intestinal bleeding, and suppression of white blood cells.[13] Essential oil of turmeric (in doses of 0.1 ml/kg) has antihistaminic activities. [13] Long-term consumption of turmeric aids in treating osteoarthritis, rheumatoid arthritis, gout, asthma, tendonitis, allergies, and other inflammatory conditions such as acne, psoriasis, eczema, and urticaria.[3,4,11,13,14] It reduces joint swelling, stiffness, and tenderness, and increases mobility.[4] Ingesting turmeric on an empty stomach between meals is most effective as an anti-inflammatory. Frequent, consistent consumption of the herb (three to four times daily) is recommended to manage pain and inflammation. According to Ayurvedic practitioners, adding small amounts of black pepper (1:10) catalyzes turmeric's anti-inflammatory effects.[14]

Turmeric is a carminative and smooth muscle antispasmodic that alleviates digestive cramping, gas, bloating, and nonulcer dyspepsia.[4,11] The antispasmodic actions are due to prostaglandin and leukotriene inhibition. Consuming turmeric one week prior to menstruation eases cramping and decongests the pelvic region.[11,14,15] Daily turmeric consumption decreases chronic uterine cramping, and aids in pain management due to conditions such as endometriosis or fibroids.[14] Turmeric also decreases allergy related respiratory spasms, and can be used as a long-term treatment for asthma.[4] It combines effectively with ginger *(Zingiber)*, wild yam *(Dioscorea)*, white peony *(Paeonia)*, and smaller amounts of cinnamon *(Cinnamomum)* to prevent or treat uterine cramping. Turmeric also can be combined with gumweed *(Grindelia)*, elecampane *(Inula)*, anise *(Pimpinella)*, aralia *(Aralia)*, senega snakeroot *(Polygala)*, and smaller amounts of licorice *(Glycyrrhiza)* for long-term treatment of asthma and respiratory spasms.

A warming aromatic and mildly bitter tonic, turmeric enhances fat and protein digestion.[4,6,11] It reduces nausea and indigestion due to simultaneously consuming too many different types of food.[5] Turmeric extract increases gastric wall mucus production protecting the stomach cells.[13] Turmeric hastens recovery from digestive infections, such as stomach flu, food poisoning, salmonella, dysentery, and parasitic infections (i.e., *Giardia*).[14] A closely related species, *Curcuma zedoary*, is one of the most effective herbs for killing amoebae such as *Entamoeba histolytica*, a major cause of amoebic dysentery.[5] Prepare a digestive bitter tonic compound by combining turmeric with additional bitter herbs including gentian *(Gentiana)*, artichoke leaf *(Cynara)*, or berberis root *(Berberis)*, and aromatic herbs such as fennel *(Foeniculum)*, cardamom *(Elettaria)*, anise *(Pimpinella)*, and/or citrus peel *(Citrus)*.

Turmeric alcohol extract, curcumin, and its volatile oil have demonstrated weak antibacterial activity against gram-positive bacteria.[3,13] Turmeric improves intestinal microflora and reduces pathogenic bacteria, supporting the digestive tract following recent use of antibiotics.[6,14] It also addresses digestive flora imbalances such as *Candida albicans* overgrowth. The diluted volatile oil (1:500) has potent antifungal activity.[13] Adding small amounts of fresh turmeric rhizome to lacto-fermented foods such as sauerkraut and kimchi supports the growth of beneficial microbes in the digestive tract. Turmeric aids in the long-term treatment of difficult or painful digestion, peptic ulcers, irritable bowel syndrome (IBS), colitis, Crohn's disease, food sensitivities, and celiac disease.[4,8,14] It also alleviates hemorrhoid flareups.

Turmeric contains hepatoprotective compounds with actions similar to those in milk thistle seeds. Curcumin, *p*-coumaroylferuloylmethane, and di-*p*-coumaroylmethane protect hepatocytes against injury caused by carbon tetrachloride and galactosamine exposure.[3] Turmeric enhances hepatic detoxification of heavy metals and environmental toxins.[5] The liver-detoxifying effects are beneficial for individuals with alcohol-induced liver toxicity, and those consuming over-the-counter and prescription drugs that negatively affect liver function.[4,8] Curcumin also enhances liver detoxification from cancer-causing compounds.[7] Turmeric aids in treating liver conditions such as jaundice and hepatitis.

Turmeric is a cholagogue and choleretic.[3,4,11] It regulates bile viscosity and shrinks engorged hepatic ducts. The choleretic and bile regulating actions are attributed to tolmethyl carbinol, a component of the essential oil.[3] Sodium curcuminate also increases bile excretion; however, aqueous extracts of turmeric do not demonstrate this effect.[13] Turmeric and curcumin are highly effective for treating gallbladder disorders such as cholecystitis, cholangitis, and nonobstructive gallstones, as well as for providing support following a cholecystectomy (gallbladder removal).[11] To thin bile and reduce gallbladder inflammation, combine turmeric with dandelion root *(Taraxacum)*, gentian *(Gentiana)*, and/or berberis *(Berberis)*, as well as carminatives such as fennel *(Foeniculum)* or cardamom *(Elettaria)*. To aid the passing of nonobstructive gallstones, combine with dandelion root *(Taraxacum)*, celandine *(Chelidonium)*, fringe-tree *(Chionanthus)*, and fennel *(Foeniculum)*. Potent analgesic herbs such as silk tassel *(Garrya)*, California poppy *(Eschscholzia)*, opium poppy *(Papaver)*, and *Cannabis* also ease the passing of gallstones.

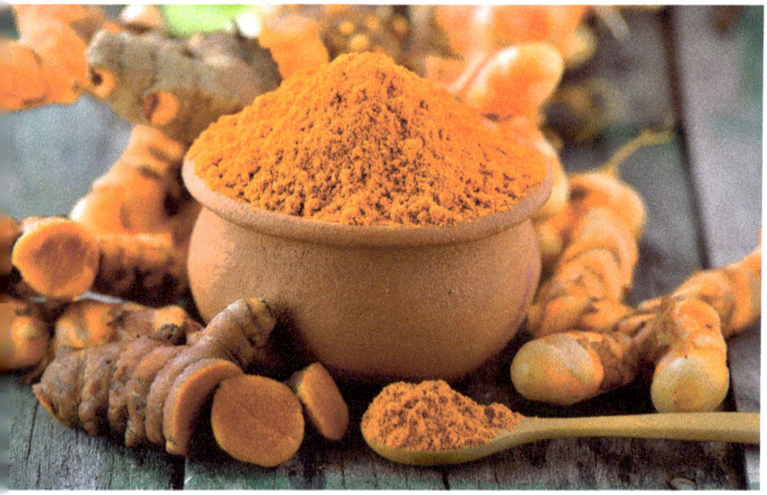

Turmeric aids in preventing and treating hypercholesterolemia and atherosclerosis.[4,7] A hypocholesterolemic, curcumin lowers serum cholesterol levels, including low density lipids (LDLs), very low density lipids (VLDLs), and triglycerides.[3,4,13] It also increases the ratio of high density lipid levels (HDL) to total cholesterol.[13] Curcumin enhances fecal excretion of bile acids and cholesterol in normal and hypercholesterolemic individuals, and counteracts an increase in the body and liver weights induced by cholesterol intake.[13] It also prevents the oxidation of cholesterol that damages blood vessels and leads to the buildup of plaque on the arterial walls. Turmeric extracts and curcumin increase fibrinolytic activity and inhibit platelet aggregation.[13] Curcumin inhibits ADP-, collagen-, and epinephrine-induced platelet aggregation, with effects comparable to aspirin *in vitro* and *ex vivo*.[13] It selectively lowers thromboxane production from platelets, but unlike aspirin, curcumin spares prostacyclin activity in the aorta.[13] Turmeric improves circulation, and is a carrier agent in herbal compounds.

Turmeric has numerous benefits for treating cancer. Curcuminoids impede cancer development in the initiation, promotion, and progression stages.[13] Numerous *in vitro* and *in vivo* studies have confirmed the anticarcinogenic, antimutagenic, and antimetastatic activities.[7,13] Curcumin has inhibitory effects on epidermal growth factor (EGF) receptor sites. Two-thirds of all cancers produce an abundance of EGF receptor sites, causing increased sensitivity to EGF which stimulates cellular proliferation.[7] Curcumin decreases the cellular tendency to proliferate by decreasing the number of EGF receptors.[7] It also inhibits tumor growth by limiting angiogenesis, preventing the formation of new blood vessels that feed the tumor. It prevents excessive production of the enzyme cyclooxygenase 2 (COX-2) that contributes to tumor development.[7] Curcumin inhibits nuclear factor kappa beta (NF-kb), a protein that cancer cells produce to stimulate cancer cell proliferation.[7] It also inhibits cancerous growth-promoting enzymes.[7] Curcumin encourages the destruction of unhealthy cells by increasing the nuclear p53 protein that is essential for apoptosis.[7]

Turmeric exhibits further mechanisms for fighting cancer. A potent antioxidant and anti-inflammatory, curcumin inhibits lipid peroxide formation, and protects cells from oxidative damage to DNA.[7,13] Curcumin enhances the cellular destruction of mutated cancer cells, and increases the body's production of the carcinogen-detoxifying enzyme, glutathione.[13] In a controlled study, a diet containing 1% turmeric fed to rats reduced lipid peroxidation by increasing antioxidant enzyme activity of superoxide dismutase, catalase, and glutathione peroxidase.[13] Mice fed a diet containing 1% turmeric had fewer benzo (alpha) pyrene (BAP)-induced stomach tumors, and fewer spontaneous mammary tumors.[13] Turmeric, turmeric extract, and curcumins decreased the incidence of BAP metabolite binding to calf thymus DNA.[13] Three curcuminoids were found to inhibit BAP-DNA adduct formation in mouse liver microsomes.[13] Curcumin and genistein (from soybeans) prevented the growth of estrogen-positive human breast cells induced by pesticides and/or estradiol.[13] Turmeric decreases the incidence of cell mutation in tobacco smokers, and significantly reduces the levels of cancer causing compounds measured in the urine.[7,8] It inhibits various stages of colon cancer.[7] Curcumin reduced the incidence of colon adenocarcinomas and the growth of invasive and non-invasive tumors, and decreased colon tumor volume in rats.[13] Turmeric exhibits anticancerous activity against Dalton's lymphoma cells in rodents.[3] Via similar mechanisms stated above, curcumin slows the progression of Alzheimer's and multiple sclerosis in rodents.[7]

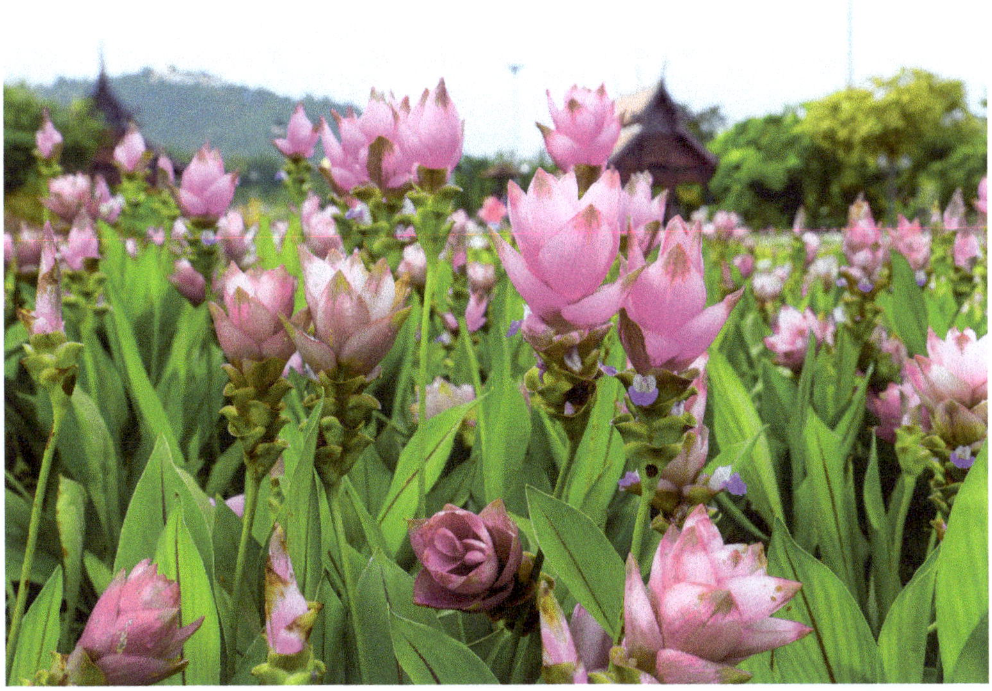

Internal and topical preparations of turmeric aid in treating precancerous and cancerous skin conditions.[4] There are three stages of cancerous growth: initiation, promotion, and progression. In the promotion phase when cancer begins to grow, repeated topical applications of turmeric or curcumin reduced DMBA-induced skin papillomas in mice.[13] A topical preparation for precancerous skin conditions combines three parts turmeric *(Curcuma),* one part each calendula *(Calendula)* and cannabis *(Cannabis).* Prepare this as a salve (using the alcohol intermediary method), extract, or paste (made with powdered herbs and honey). Apply it twice daily to the affected area. *Note:* Turmeric is not a substitute for medical treatment of skin cancer, a condition that should be monitored by a dermatologist or doctor.

Turmeric is highly effective for healing bruises, sprains, strains, contusions, tendonitis, and burns.[6,14] It is a deobstruent that moves stagnant blood, and reduces swelling due to physical trauma. Externally, it stimulates circulation in the tissues, reducing congestion and decreasing inflammation. Topical applications, such as a fresh or dry rhizome poultice, turmeric honey, or salve, effectively reduce pain and swelling. Apply a thick poultice or paste to treat mastitis, benign breast lumps, arthritis, and abscesses.[6,8] A traditional preparation of powdered turmeric combined with slaked lime was applied as a topical anti-inflammatory; the addition of slaked lime likely increases turmeric's water solubility.[13] A similar preparation, sodium curcuminate, demonstrates significantly more potent anti-inflammatory activity than curcumin or hydrocortisone.[13]

Turmeric hastens wound healing and prevents infection.[4,14] Due to the volatile oil and curcumin, it has antibacterial actions, especially against *Staphylococcus aureus.* The volatile oil is antiseptic against strains of gram-positive bacteria and yeast.[13] Turmeric is an antifungal, effective against ringworm and other skin tineas.[4,6] Combine it with neem *(Azadirachta)* to treat fungal infections.[14]

CONTRAINDICATIONS

Avoid turmeric consumption in individuals with obstructive gallstones.[11,13] High doses of turmeric are contraindicated during pregnancy or attempts to conceive, and for individuals with hair loss.[3,11,13] Based on clinical observation, consuming small quantities of turmeric during pregnancy is not known to be problematic. Excessive doses, especially when not combined with carminatives, may cause nausea and/or vomiting.[11] Based on theoretical concerns, avoid high doses of turmeric in patients taking antiplatelet or anticoagulant medications. However, no clinical evidence of interactions has been reported.[13] According to Traditional Chinese Medicine, turmeric is contraindicated for individuals with yin deficiency with heat signs (e.g., hot flashes or night sweats), and for blood deficiency with stagnant qi or congealed blood.[10]

Note: Purchasing organically cultivated turmeric is recommended, as it is less likely to be irradiated.

Warning: Preparations of turmeric impart a vivid yellow hue that can stain skin, fabric, clothing, countertops, and wooden and plastic utensils. Consider wearing nitrile gloves to prevent staining hands when processing turmeric.

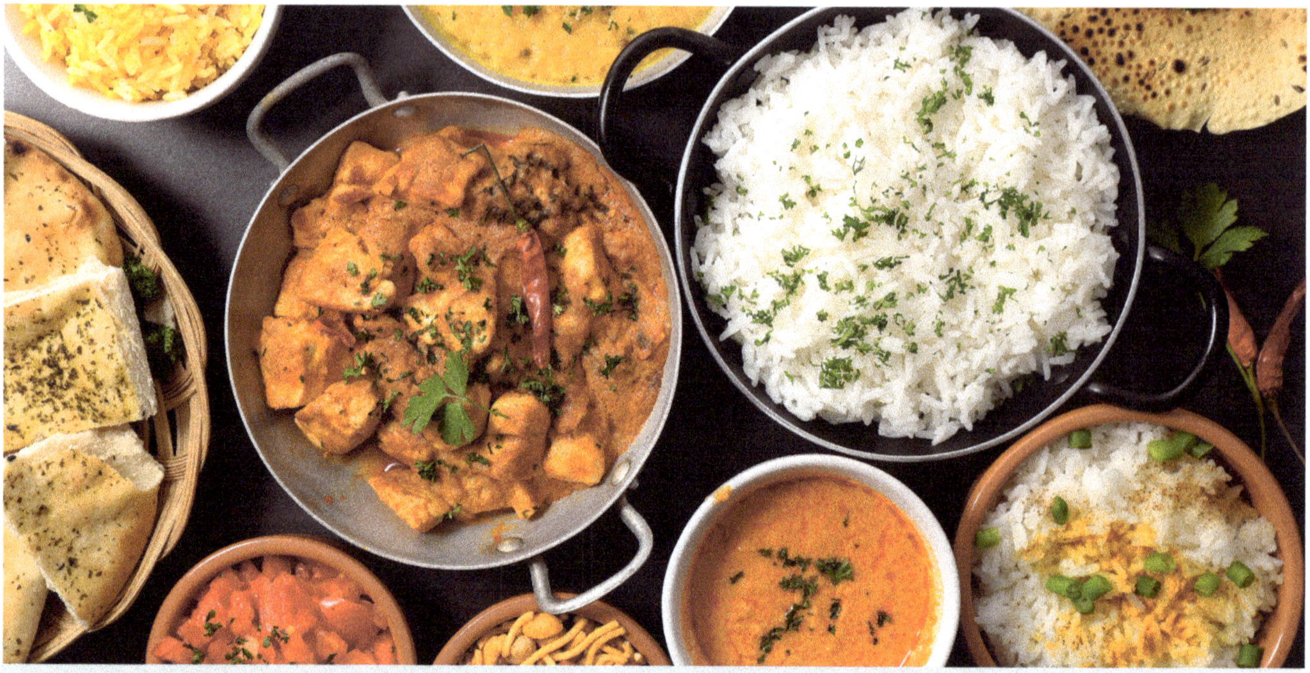

PREPARATION AND DOSAGE

TINCTURE: Fresh rhizomes [1:2, 70 - 95% alcohol]; recently dried rhizomes [1:5, 60% alcohol]; consume 30 - 90 drops, up to four times daily.

FLUID EXTRACT: Dried rhizomes [1:1, 50% alcohol]; consume 15 - 60 drops, up to four times daily.

GLYCERITE: Fresh rhizomes [1:2, 60% glycerin, 40% water] or [1:2, 50% glycerin, 50% alcohol]; consume 15 - 60 drops, up to three times daily.

ACETUM EXTRACT: Fresh rhizomes [1:2, apple cider vinegar]; consume 1 teaspoon, up to four times daily.

CAPSULES: Consume 2 - 6 "00" capsules, up to three times daily, or consume 250 - 500 mg standardized capsules, up to three times daily.

TEA: Prepare a hot or cold infusion, or decoction; consume 8 - 12 ounces, up to three times daily. Alternatively, mix 1 heaping teaspoon vigorously into 6 - 8 ounces of hot water, and consume twice daily.

HONEY AND SYRUP: Prepare turmeric honey by mixing the powdered or fresh root in honey. Only the fresh root requires straining. For a delicious treat, add 1 teaspoon to 1 tablespoon of medicated honey to warm goat, cow, almond, cashew, or coconut milk. The powdered root and honey mixture is ideal as a topical application.

TOPICAL USE: Turmeric can be applied as a fresh or dry plant poultice. Prepare an oil of fresh, wilted rhizomes using the double boiler method, or prepare an oil of dry rhizomes using the alcohol intermediary method.

CULINARY USE: The flavor of the fresh root is reminiscent of ginger, and complements most recipes containing ginger. Fresh turmeric retains more of the aromatic and pungent qualities than the dry root, and is slightly less bitter. Add ½ - 1 teaspoon of turmeric to smoothies, or fresh vegetable or fruit juice. As a preventative or long-term tonic, add up to 1 teaspoon daily of the powder in food. Grate or mince the herb, and add to soups, salad dressing, kraut, kimchi, rice, beans, or protein dishes. *Note:* A little bit goes a long way. It's easy to overdo.

Turmeric is used as a flavoring and coloring agent in the food industry and culinary practice. It is an ingredient in curry blends, relishes, pickles, fats, oils, butter, margarine, cheese, egg products, mustard, baked goods, soups, sauces, Worcestershire sauce, gravies, meat and meat products, microwave popcorn, cakes, icings, gelatins, and desserts.[3] Turmeric's antioxidant properties preserve food and prevent rancidity in oils and fats. It also can be used as an Easter egg dye.

USNEA

BOTANICAL NAMES:
Usnea barbata, U. californica, U. ceratina, U. dasypoga, U. florida, U. hirta, U. longissima (syn. *Dolichousnea longissima*), *U. wirthii, U.* spp.

COMMON NAMES:
Usnea, old man's beard, beard lichen, beard moss, bear's beard, moose moss, Methuselah's beard, tree moss, woman's long hair, witches broom, tree's dandruff
naava (Finnish)
barbe decaucin, usnee barbue (French)
bart-flechte (German)
barba di bosco (Italian)
kayu angin, saruogase (Japanese)
hia feng teng, son luo, sun lo (Mandarin)
grå slägglav (Swedish)

FAMILY NAME:
Parmeliaceae
(formerly Usneaceae)

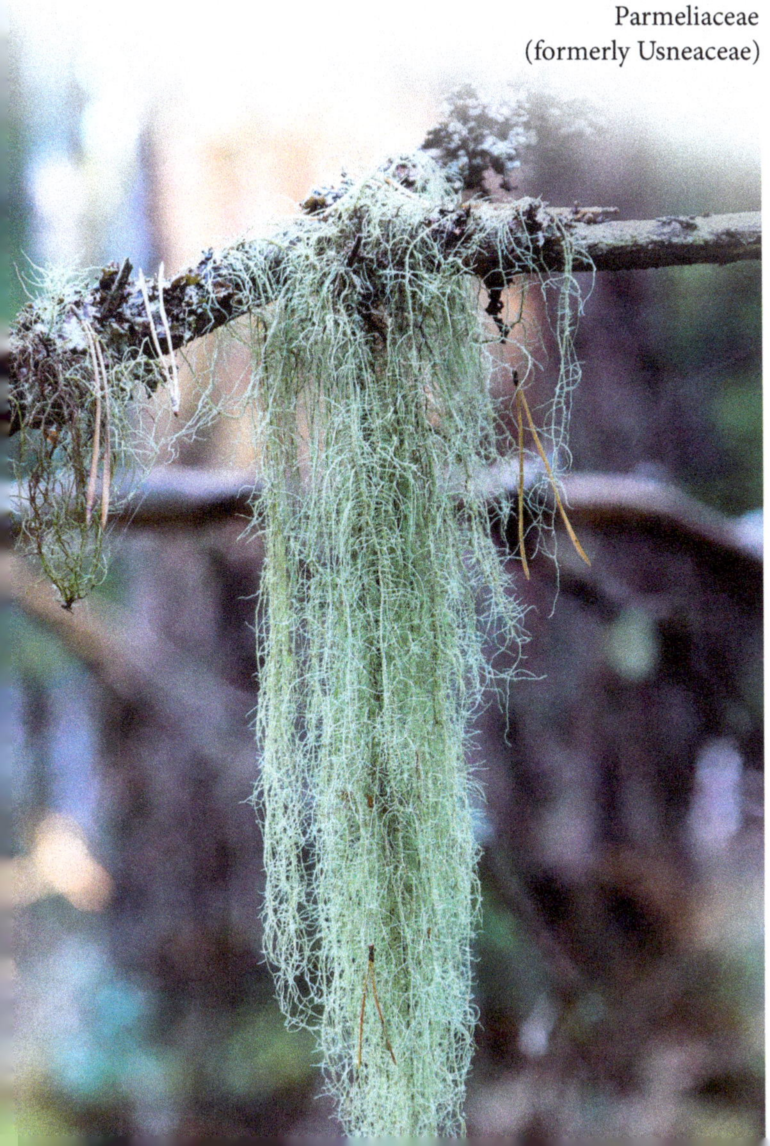

DESCRIPTION

PART USED: The thallus (lichen).

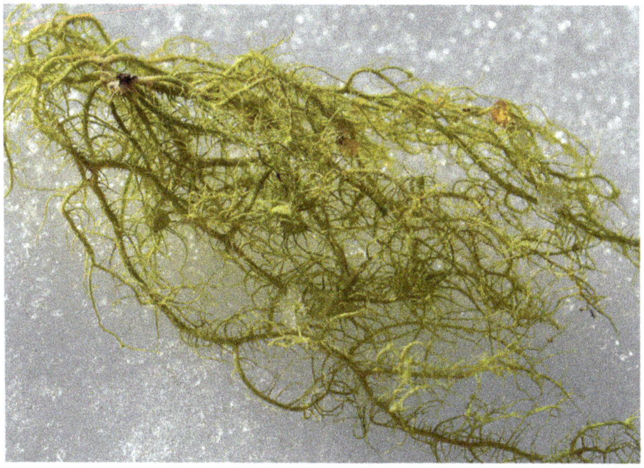

BOTANICAL DESCRIPTION AND HABITAT: Usnea is a slow growing, tufted or pendulous fruticose lichen consisting of branching, round strands with a gray-green to yellow-green outer cortex, and a white, elastic core. The cortex is covered with dense papillae, and/or long hair-like fibrils. Strands do not usually grow longer than 25 cm in most species, but can reach up to 3 meters long or more in *Usnea longissima*, a species threatened by logging of old growth forests and air pollution.[1] Usnea grows attached to the branches of shrubs and trees, including spruces, firs, Douglas firs, birches, cottonwoods, oaks, manzanitas, and pines, especially on the edges or well-lit interiors of open, old-growth forests.[1-4]

Two lichens are commonly mistaken for Usnea: *Alectoria sarmentosa* (witches' hair) and *Evernia prunastri* (ramalina). Both lichens lack the central, threadlike white cord.[4]

THE NAME: *Usnea* derives from the Arabic *usna* ("moss").[4] The epithet *barbata* derives from the Latin *barba* ("beard, barbed"); *florida* ("flowery, in bloom") derives from Latin; and *longissima* means "longest."[4,5]

HISTORICAL USES: *Usnea longissima*, known in Mandarin as sun lo (son luo), has been prescribed as an expectorant, and applied externally as a powder to heal skin ulcers.[3] The alcohol extract continues to be used to treat tubercular lymphadenitis.[3] In Romania, *Usnea barbata* was listed as medicine in the *Farmacia Naturii* and *Flora Medicinal a Romaniei* (1929).[6] Prior to the 1700s, physicians grouped together most lichens, mosses, and liverworts, classifying them all as "lichen," "moss," or "musci" in pharmacopeias. This makes it difficult to determine which genera and species they described.[3] Based on the "Doctrine of Signatures" and usnea's resemblance to hair, it was used as a hair and scalp remedy.[3] Haida Indians used fibers of *U. longissima* to filter impurities from hot pitch prior to using pitch medicinally.[4]

CONSTITUENTS: Usnea contains dibenzofurans (rich in usnic acid), depsidones (lichenic acid including usnaric and barbatic acids), fatty acids (linoleic, oleic, and arachidonic acids), and polysaccharides (D-glucans: lichenin — water insoluble, and isolichenin — water-soluble).[3,7,8]

NUTRITIONAL PROPERTIES: Not applicable.

MEDICINAL PROPERTIES: Antibacterial, antifungal, immune modulator, anti-inflammatory, and antitumor.

TEMPERATURE AND FLAVOR: Cool, bitter, and sweet.

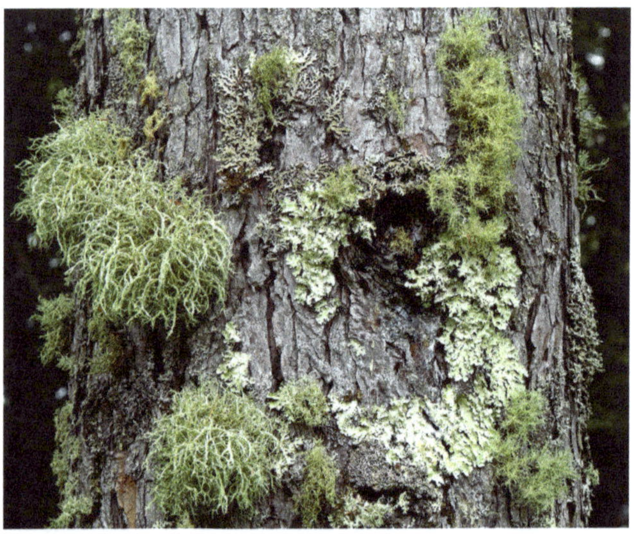

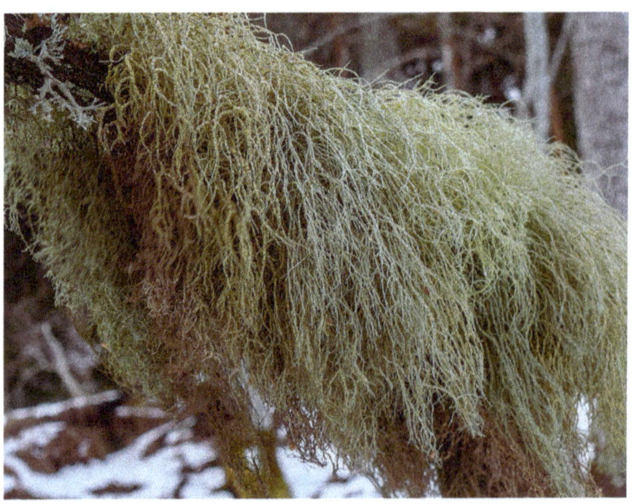

MEDICINAL USES

Usnea has potent antibacterial, antifungal, and immune modulating actions.[5] The antibacterial actions are attributed to usnic acid, the bitter principle contained in the outer gray-green cortex.[3,6-8] According to animal studies, usnic acid is more effective than penicillin against some bacterial strains.[3] In a dilution of 1:20,000, usnic acid inhibited the growth of gram-positive bacterial infections, such as *Streptococcus* (strep throat), *Staphylococcus* (impetigo and staph), and *Pneumococcus*.[3,7,8] It also inhibited the growth of *Mycobacterium tuberculosis* in a dilution of 1:20,000 to 1:50,000, and weakened their growth in a solution of 1:200,000 to 1:2,000,000.[3] Scientists believe that usnic acid disrupts cellular metabolism by preventing the formation of ATP from ADP, or by uncoupling oxidative phosphorylization.[3] Alcohol-based extracts of usnea have antitumor and anti-inflammatory actions.[6] Usnic acid also increases resistance to colds and influenza.[6] The immune stimulating polysaccharides are contained in the white inner core.[3]

Usnea aids in treating sinusitis, strep throat, bronchitis, pleurisy, pneumonia, and lingering lung infections.[3] Combine extracts of usnea, thyme *(Thymus)*, oshá *(Ligusticum)*, aralia *(Aralia)*, lomatium *(Lomatium)*, yerba santa *(Eriodictyon)*, and/or licorice *(Glycyrrhiza)* in order to treat respiratory infections. Usnea is an effective antibacterial agent for urinary tract infections, including cystitis and urethritis.[3] Combine extracts of usnea, uva ursi *(Arctostaphylos)*, yarrow *(Achillea)*, and corn silk *(Zea)* to treat urinary tract infections. Usnea also aids in treating bacterial vaginosis and β-strep infections. To treat all of the aforementioned infections, consume 60 – 90 drops of the extract, three to five times daily, or include it in a compound.

Usnea is an effective antifungal agent that aids in treating intestinal and vaginal candida. Combining usnea with berberis root *(Berberis)* prevents candida overgrowth resulting from the use of conventional antibiotics. Consume 60 – 90 drops three times daily for two to four weeks following antibiotic use. Probiotics are also recommended to support the growth of beneficial bacteria that inhibit candida overgrowth. When treating vaginal candida, internal consumption of usnea extract works most effectively, and is best used in addition to vaginal irrigation (using other herbs). For internal use, combine with additional antifungal herbs, such as echinacea *(Echinacea)*, calendula *(Calendula)*, yerba mansa *(Anemopsis)*, thyme *(Thymus vulgaris)*, and/or oregano *(Origanum vulgare)*. Usnea also can be combined with astringent herbs, such

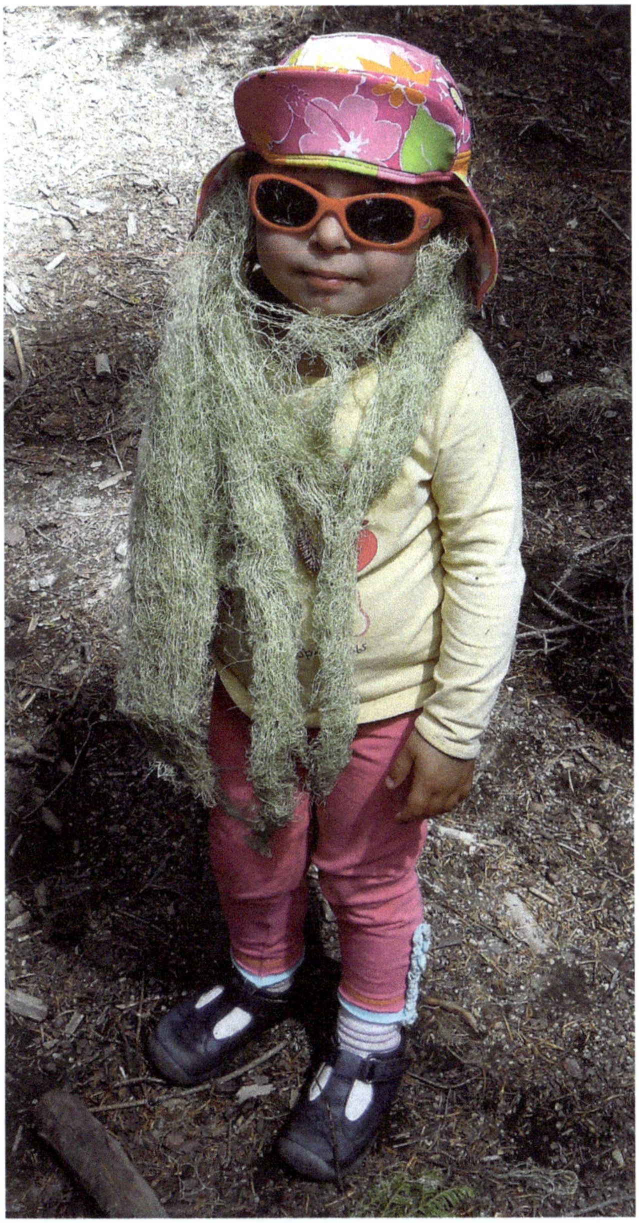

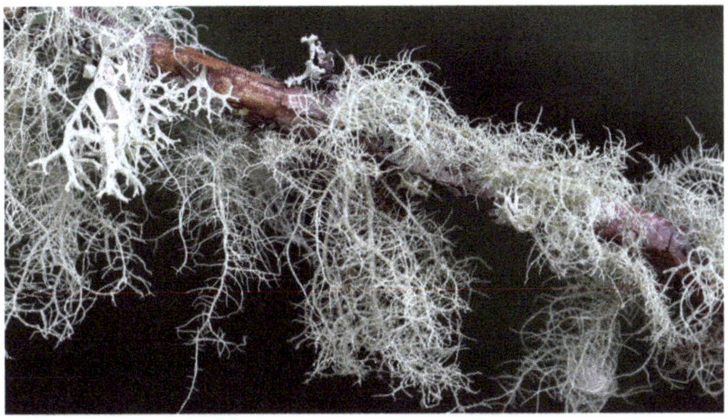

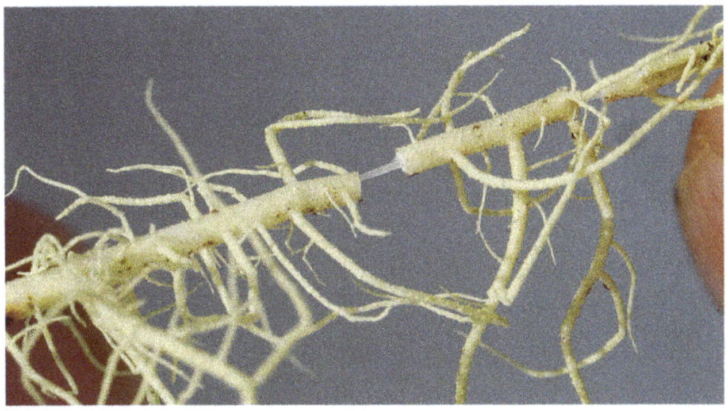

as yerba mansa *(Anemopsis)* or bayberry *(Morella)* to reduce excess vaginal secretion. It can be effective against *Trichomonas,* a parasitic vaginal infection.[3]

Usnea is a topical antifungal agent that aids in treating skin tineas, including athlete's foot, beard rot, cradle cap, jock itch, and ringworm. An internal antifungal protocol may be necessary if diligent external applications are not effective.

CONTRAINDICATIONS

There are no known contraindications.[7] In rare cases, topical applications can cause skin irritations following prolonged sun exposure.[7]

PREPARATION AND DOSAGE

TINCTURE: Fresh, moist lichen [1:3-1:5, 80-95% alcohol]; dry lichen [1:5-1:10, 70% alcohol]; consume 30-120 drops, up to five times daily.

ACETUM EXTRACT: Usnea is partially soluble in vinegar. Prepare dry lichen [1:7-1:10, apple cider vinegar]; consume 30-120 drops, up to five times daily.

CAPSULES: Consume 3-6 capsules, up to four times daily. However, capsules are not as effective as alcohol-based preparations.

TEA: Presoaking usnea in alcohol before adding to water-based preparations increases its water-solubility; the alcohol evaporates as the tea is decocted. To do this, moisten usnea in a small amount of alcohol (just enough to coat it lightly), and store in a glass container with a lid. Steep this preparation a minimum of 12-24 hours. Use this method to prepare a decoction. Consume 8-12 ounces of the decoction, up to four times daily.

TOPICAL USE: Prepare an oil or salve using the alcohol intermediary oil method. Apply to the affected area as needed.

UVA URSI AND MANZANITA

DESCRIPTION

BOTANICAL NAMES:
Arctostaphylos uva-ursi, A. manzanita, A. spp.

COMMON NAMES:
Uva ursi, uva-ursi, bearberry, common bearberry, bear grape, bear's grape, pinemat, hogberry, hog cranberry, rockberry, chipmunks' apples, mealberry, mountain cranberry, sandberry, upland cranberry
kinnikinnick (Algonquian)
sianpuola (Finnish)
arbousier, abre aux fraises, arctostaphyle, loonier (French)
harnkraut, moosebeere, wolfsbeere (German)
uva d'orso (Italian)
manzanita, coralillo, gayuba, pinguica (Spanish)

FAMILY NAME:
Ericaceae

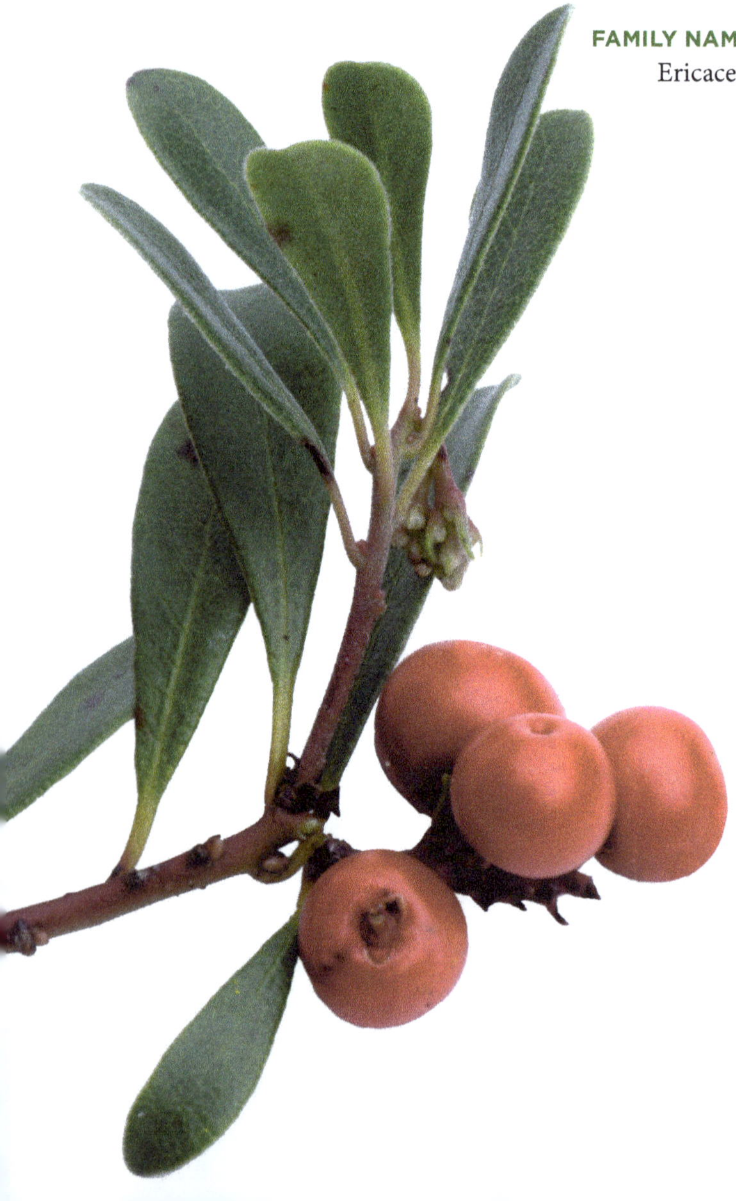

PART USED: The leaves.

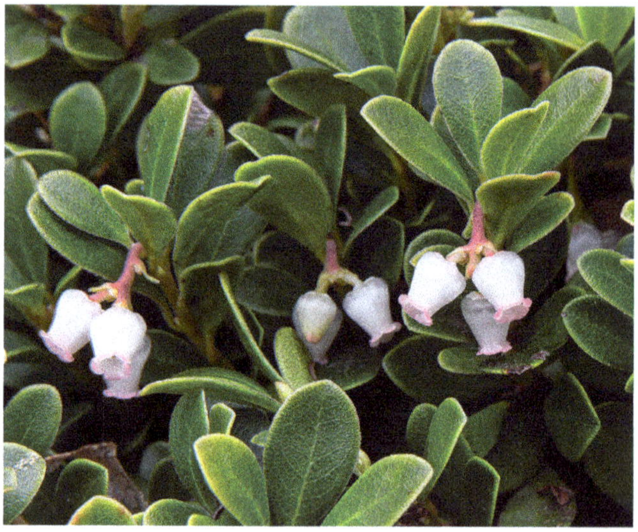

BOTANICAL DESCRIPTION AND HABITAT: *Arctostaphylos* is a large genus of evergreen, prostrate to erect shrubs and small trees; there are more than 60 species, and much hybridization occurs between species.[1] Manzanitas are usually found in dry, fire prone areas; some species have adapted by growing a burl of fire resistant wood at the base.[1]

Members of *Arctostaphylos* have reddish bark, sometimes consisting of many shredding layers. The outer layers can be rough and gray; the inner bark is red, thin, and smooth.[1] The leathery, alternate leaves are glabrous or very finely pubescent, and have entire margins that are curled under or flat.[1] As a whole, the leaves can be very flat or convex. In many species, the leaves are isofacial, with little distinction between the upper and lower sides, although the undersides can vary in color and hairiness.[1] The terminal racemes bear clusters of tiny flowers with five free sepals, a white or pink urceolate corolla with five lobes, ten stamens, and five fused carpels in a superior ovary.[1] The fruit is a bright red, leathery, berry-like drupe.[1]

Arctostaphylos uva-ursi (uva ursi) is a prostrate to decumbent, mat-like shrub (less than 50 cm tall).[1] The oblanceolate leaves are not isofacial; the upper surface is a shiny, dark green convex; the underside is light green and slightly puberulent.[1] The flower has a glabrous ovary.[1] The fruit is also glabrous.[1]

Arctostaphylos manzanita (manzanita) consists of at least six subspecies of shrubs and trees (2 – 8 meters high).[1] One subspecies has a fireproof burl.[1] The twigs range from smooth to tomentose, depending on the subspecies.[1] Erect, widely ovate, isofacial leaves with round or wedge-shaped bases and entire margins grow on short petioles.[1] The surfaces are bright green and shiny, except in one subspecies.[1] The open inflorescence has tomentose branches.[1] The flowers have a glabrous or glandular ovary.[1] The fruit is glabrous or pubescent.[1]

THE NAME: The genus name *Arctostaphylos* derives from two Greek words: *arctos* ("bear") and *staphyles* ("a bunch of grapes").[2,3] The Spanish epithet manzanita ("little apple") refers to the appearance of small, scarlet fruits.[2] The epithet *uva-ursi* derives from two Latin words: *uva* ("cluster") and *ursus* ("bear").[4] The Latin binomial *(A. uva-ursi)* and common name bearberry refer to the bear's consumption of the fruit, or because the tough, flavorless berries were only fit for a bear to eat. Kinnikinnick ("that which is mixed") is Algonquian, originating from Chippewa and Cree dialects.[2,3,5]

HISTORICAL USES: More than 12 Native American tribes used uva ursi medicinally. Many tribes consumed it as a urinary antiseptic, astringent, and diuretic for kidney and urinary ailments.[5] The Haida consumed the tea as a diuretic for urinary tract infections and kidney diseases.[2] A hair wash made from tea was massaged into the scalp to treat dandruff and scalp disorders. A paste made from ground leaves and stems was applied in order to hasten the healing of burns, sores, cuts, boils, and pimples.[5] A tea was consumed, or a poultice was applied to alleviate back pain.[5] The leaves were used to tan animal hides due to the high tannin content.[3]

Uva ursi was included in smoking mixtures and substituted for tobacco, or blended to extend tobacco supply.[2,4] Numerous coastal tribes smoked the herb, including the Salish, Nuu-chah-nulth, Haida, Nuxalk, Tsimshian, and Kwakawaka'wakw.[2] In the Southwest, decoctions of uva ursi and a *piloncillo* (a small, compressed cone of unrefined sugar) were recommended to treat syphilis and gonorrhea; one cup was consumed every morning for ten days.[4] Consuming the tea was believed to reduce body fat. Rheumatic joints were bathed in a decoction of the tea.[4]

Uva ursi berries or leaves were chewed to prevent thirst because the bitter flavor was believed to stimulate saliva flow.[3,5] The edible fruits were consumed when food was scarce, although they caused severe constipation.[2] The fruits were mixed with animal fat and administered to children for diarrhea.[5] The berries were incorporated into preserves, pemmican, stews, and wine.

Eclectic physicians administered the herb to treat urinary tract disorders, including infections, pyelonephritis, incontinence, dysuria, urinary calculi, and prostate problems.[6,7] The herb was thought to impart tone to the urinary tract.[6,7] David Culbreth dispensed uva ursi extract and tea for diarrhea, dysentery, hemorrhoids, profuse menstruation, uterine hemorrhage, bronchitis, and cardiac dropsy.[7] Finley Ellingwood prescribed the herb for gonorrhea.[6]

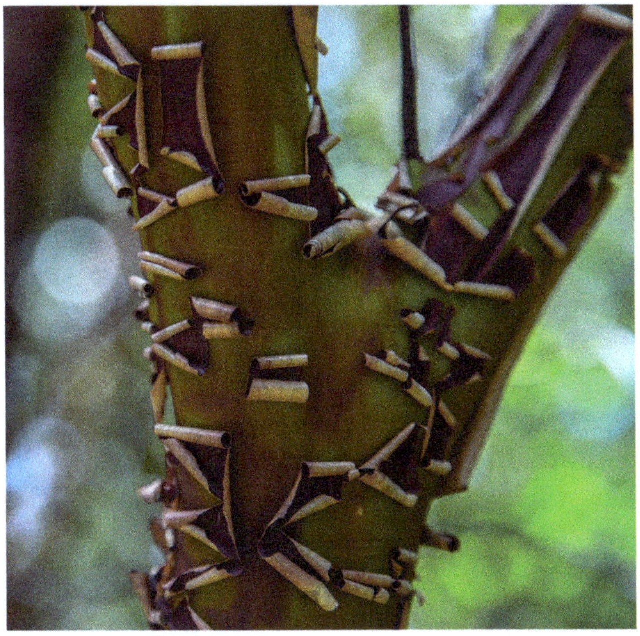

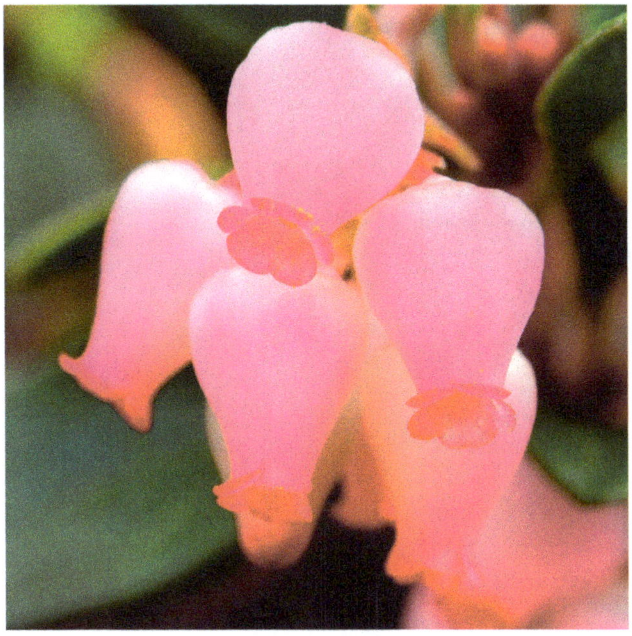

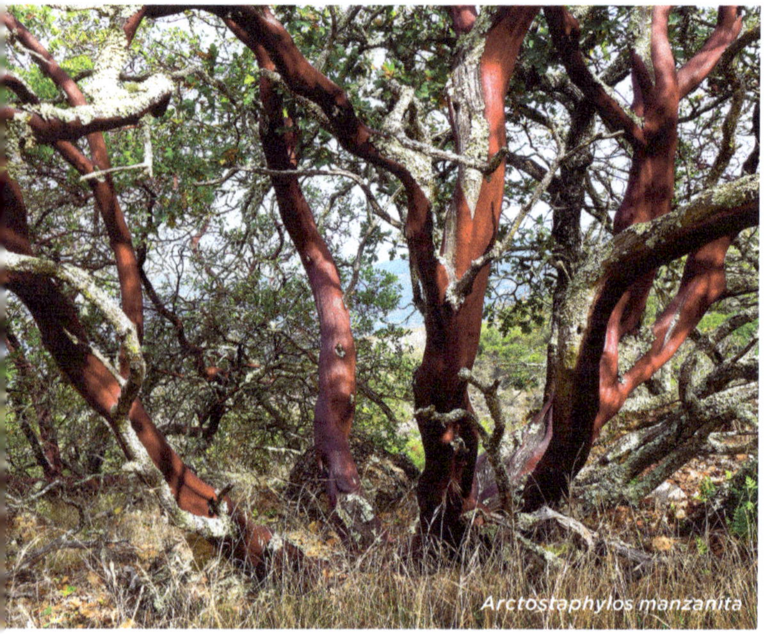

Arctostaphylos manzanita

CONSTITUENTS: Uva ursi contains arbutin (hydroquinone β-glucoside, methylarbutin, and piceoside), flavonoids (quercetin monoglucosides and diglucosides, myricetin, quercitrin, and hypericin, a flavonol), tannins (gallotannin and ellagitannin), triterpenes (ursolic acid), phenolic acids (gallic, ellagic, and quinic acids), an iridoid glycoside (monotropein), uvaol, ursone (a resinous substance), allantoin, ericolin, lupeol, taraxasterol, betulinic acid, and a trace of volatile oil.[8-10,12]

NUTRITIONAL PROPERTIES: Unknown.

MEDICINAL PROPERTIES: Antibacterial, astringent, diuretic, and fungistatic.

TEMPERATURE AND FLAVOR: Cool, astringent, and bitter.

MEDICINAL USES

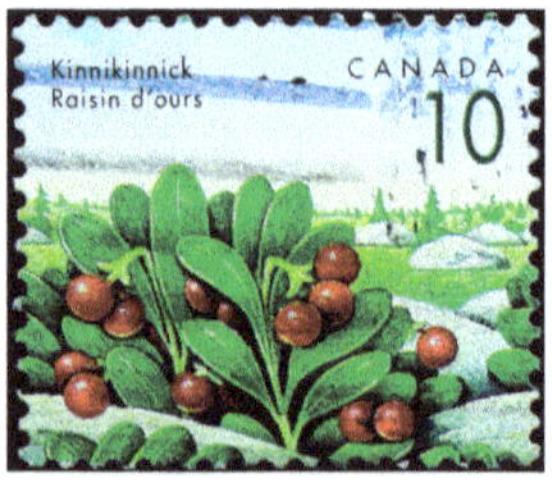

Arctostaphylos uva-ursi, A. manzanita, and *Vaccinium* spp. can be used interchangeably. Unless otherwise noted, all uses listed for uva ursi also apply to *A. manzanita* and *Vaccinium.*

Uva ursi is extremely effective as an antibacterial, diuretic, and anti-inflammatory for urinary tract infections.[3,8,9] It has antibacterial actions against *Staphylococcus* spp., *Pseudomonas* spp., *Proteus* spp., and *Escherichia coli (E. coli)* attributed to the hydroquinone.[10] *E. coli* is the most common bacterial cause of cystitis. Normally, urine is slightly acidic (6 – 6.5 pH), preventing *E. coli* growth in the urinary tract. Urine's acidity results from hydrogen ions, a byproduct of metabolized dietary proteins. Insufficient consumption of dietary proteins and excessive consumption of alkalinizing foods can result in alkaline urine (with a 7+ pH), increasing the propensity for *E. coli* bacterial growth in the lower urinary tract.[8] Uva ursi is a urinary tract antibacterial; it also creates an acidic environment in the urinary tract that discourages the growth of *E. coli.* Uva ursi contains the glycosides arbutin and ericolin that are metabolized in the intestines, and excreted in the urine as hydroquinone and methylhydroquinone. These antibacterial byproducts aid in treating alkaline urinary tract infections. [8,9] Uva ursi contains tannins that astringe mucous membranes and reduce inflammation. It also has diuretic properties that flush the urinary tract.

When treating urinary tract infections, uva ursi can be combined with antibacterial agents such as usnea *(Usnea),* yarrow *(Achillea),* corn silk *(Zea),* and/or yerba mansa *(Anemopsis).* The soothing effects of marshmallow *(Althaea),* parsley root *(Petroselinum),* and licorice *(Glycyrrhiza)* counter the drying actions of uva ursi, yarrow, and yerba mansa in water-based preparations.

Uva ursi has diuretic actions that aid in passing kidney stones and the short-term treatment of benign prostatic hypertrophy.[3,6,7,10] Additional demulcent and analgesic herbs are beneficial for reducing pain and discomfort associated with kidney stones. The hyperin content is attributed to the diuretic actions.[10]

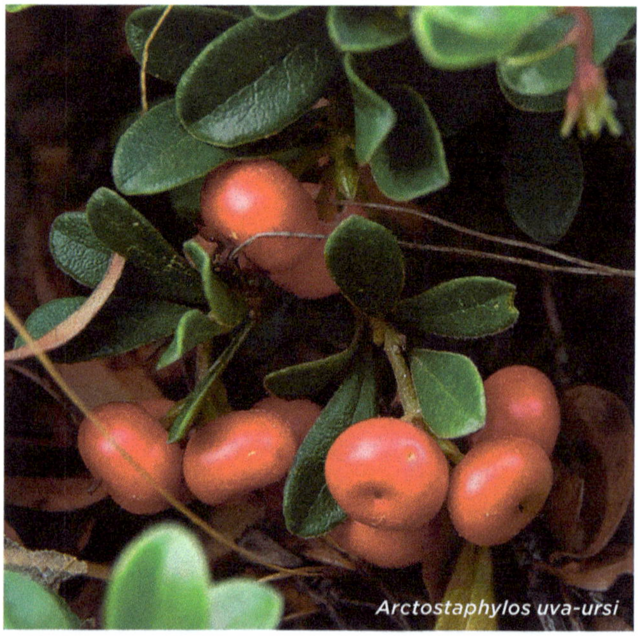

Arctostaphylos uva-ursi

Uva ursi contains astringent tannins that reduce inflammation of the mucous membranes.[7,10] Consuming the tea internally (or as an enema) aids in treating diarrhea.[7] It also has gastrointestinal antibacterial properties that inhibit digestive bacteria causing diarrhea.

Relative to other medicinal members of the Ericaceae family, uva ursi *(Arctostaphylos uva-ursi)* contains the highest content of tannins. Comparatively, manzanita *(Arctostaphylos manzanita)*, huckleberry *(Vaccinium)*, and madrone *(Arbutus menziesii)* contain fewer tannins; Ericaceae family relatives such as shinleaf *(Pyrola)* and pipsissewa *(Chimaphila)* contain the least amount of tannins.[8]

Topical applications made from the decocted herb (a wash, bath, fomentation, or poultice) are superior treatments for poison oak or poison ivy. Prepare a decoction, strain, and cool; then soak or apply frequently to the affected area. This treatment reduces inflammation, itching, pain, and skin blistering, and dries poison oak or poison ivy rashes. It also aids in treating inflamed skin, hives, heat rash, and thrush.[8] Discontinue use if the tissues become dry or cracked. A sitz bath reduces vaginal or rectal inflammation, and relieves itching and swollen hemorrhoids, as well as inflamed vaginal tissues resulting from childbirth, vaginitis, yeast infections, or genital herpes.[3,8] Herbalist Terry Willard recommends soaking one's feet in a decoction the night before hiking in order to prevent blisters.[3]

CONTRAINDICATIONS

Avoid internal preparations using the fresh leaves, as they contain higher amounts of hydroquinone. Consuming concentrates of hydroquinone or one-half ounce of fresh leaves has demonstrated toxicity.[9,12] Symptoms of toxicity include shortness of breath, vomiting, nausea, tinnitus, delirium, collapse, and convulsions.[9,12] Consuming preparations of dry uva ursi is considered safe.

Avoid consuming large quantities during pregnancy, because uva ursi can cause vasoconstriction of the uterine endometrium, potentially decreasing blood supply to the fetus.[3,8] Limit consumption during lactation, as the tannins potentially decrease the flow of breast milk. Due to the hydroquinone content, children under the age of 12 should avoid consuming uva ursi.[5,10]

Excessive or long-term consumption of tannin-containing plants can cause an upset stomach or constipation, or aggravate the kidneys, causing a dull lower backache.[8,10] Because of the high tannin content, do not consume uva ursi more than 14 consecutive days. Gentler alternatives such as shinleaf *(Pyrola)* or pipsissewa *(Chimaphila)* are preferable if kidney irritation or digestive upset occur. These herbs can be consumed for longer periods of time. *Note:* Seek a health care practitioner for the treatment of kidney infections.

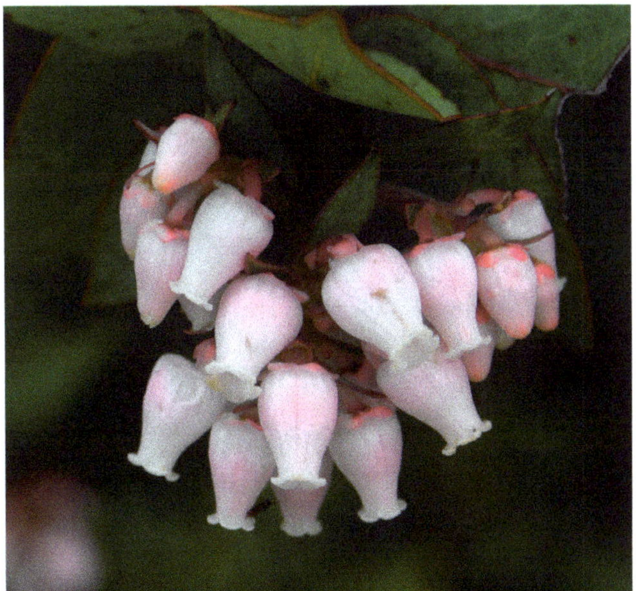

Arctostaphylos manzanita

PREPARATION AND DOSAGE

TINCTURE: Dry leaves [1:5, 60% alcohol]; consume 30-60 drops, up to four times daily.

ACETUM EXTRACT: Prepare a vinegar-based extract, dilute, and apply topically to affected areas.

TEA: Prepare a hot infusion or decoction and consume 8-12 ounces, three to four times daily.

TOPICAL USE: Apply a poultice, fomentation, tea, or acetum extract to the affected areas. To prepare a sitz bath, pour 8-32 ounces of strained tea into warm water; bathe once in the morning and evening. Administer strained, lukewarm tea as a vaginal irrigation or enema. Combine decocted tea with powdered clay, mix thoroughly, and apply to bites, stings, chicken pox, poison oak, or poison ivy.

CULINARY USE: Berries are edible (raw or cooked), but taste rather bland and may cause constipation.

VALERIAN

DESCRIPTION

BOTANICAL NAMES:
Valeriana officinalis, V. acutiloba, V. californica, V. diversiloba, V. dioica, V. edulis, V. occidentalis, V. scandens, V. scouleri, V. septentrionalis, V. sitchensis, V. spp.

COMMON NAMES:
Valerian, Belgian valerian, English valerian, German valerian, common valerian, fragrant valerian, garden valerian, great wild valerian, wild valerian, marsh valerian, sharpleaf valerian, Florida valerian, Sitka valerian, valeriane, all heal, setwall, moon root, all-heal, setewale, Capon's tail, garden heliotrope
baldroin (Danish)
racine de valériane (French)
baldrianwurzel, katzenwurzel, balderbrackenwurzel (German)
amantilla (Italian)

FAMILY NAME:
Valerianaceae

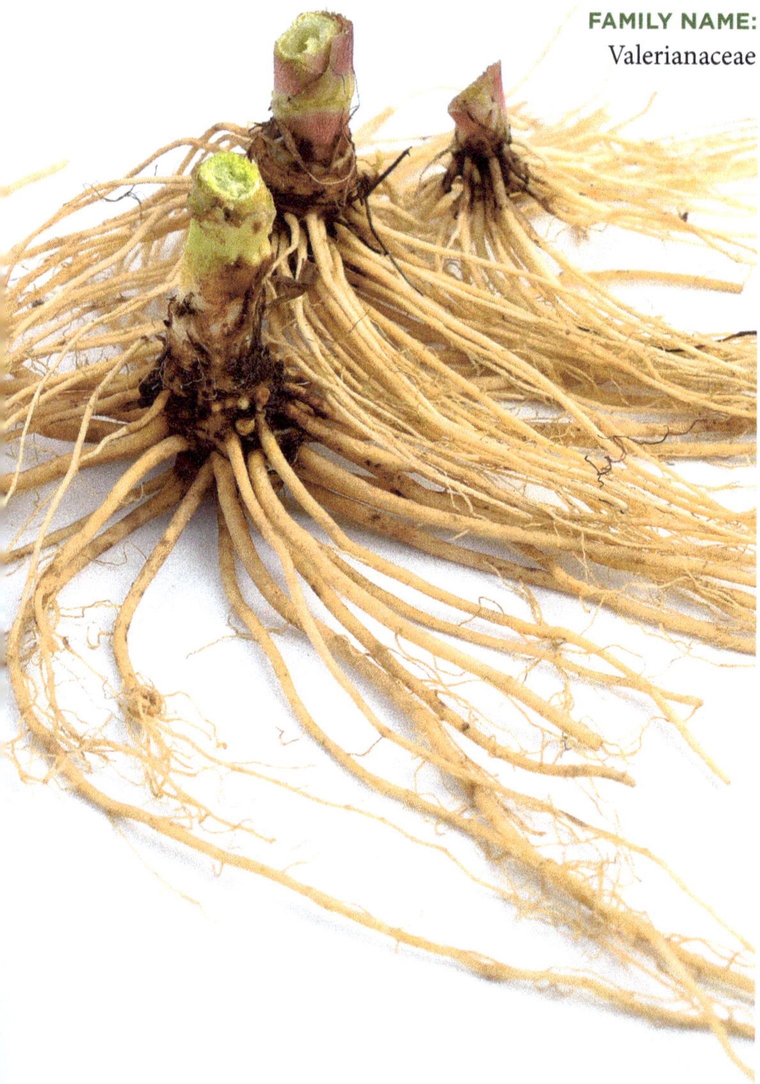

PARTS USED: The roots and rhizomes.

BOTANICAL DESCRIPTION AND HABITAT: The genus *Valeriana* includes approximately 285 species worldwide; 16 species grow in North America.[1] This perennial is native

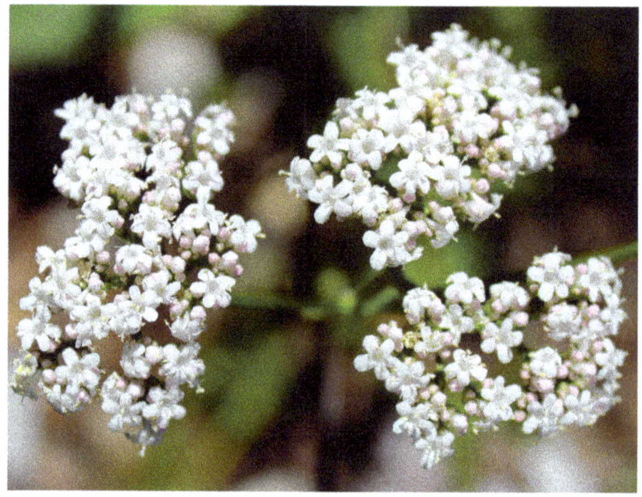

to Eurasia and North America.[1-3] Valerian grows wild in moist mountain meadows and marshes, and along the edges of rivers and ditches. It thrives in moist, rich soil that is heavy in loam.

Valeriana species are herbaceous perennials with distinctively scented rootstock. Basal leaves can be simple, pinnatifid, or pinnate. The opposite stem leaves that often clasp the stem are pinnatifid or pinnate.[4,5] The complex inflorescences are corymb-like, and bear many tiny white to pink flowers.[4,6] The in-rolled, urn-shaped calyx unfurls and becomes feathery in fruit. The tubular to funnel-shaped corolla has five spreading lobes. Three epipetalous stamens and an inferior ovary of three fused carpels are inside the corolla; only one is fertile.[4,6] The ovary yields an achene topped by the plumose calyx (up to 8 mm long).[5,6]

Valeriana officinalis has beige-brown roots (up to 2.5 cm in diameter) with a sweet, pungent, musky, earthy fragrance.[7] The vibrant green, pinnately compound, ovate leaves (5 – 15 cm long by 3 – 8 cm wide) bear 7 – 10 pairs of lanceolate leaflets with a few coarsely-cut teeth. Basal leaves have petioles (up to 8 cm long); stem leaves may be sessile.[7] Valerian has erect, hollow stems with longitudinal grooves (up to 200 cm tall). Pairs of flowering stems are arranged in right angles along the main stems. The stems terminate with large, tight cymose clusters of white flowers with tubular corollas (4 – 6 mm long) that are often tinged with pink, and have a musky, sweet, mildly intoxicating fragrance.[7] The fruit contains one pale brown, four-ribbed, oblong seed (4 – 5 mm long).[7] The stems begin to die back after flowering.

THE NAME: *Valeriana* derives from the Latin *valere* ("to be in health" or "to be healthy"). However, according to some botanists and the *Oxford English Dictionary,* it is named after Valerius, reportedly the first individual to use the herb as medicine.[8] Another source claims that the common name valerian derives from Valeria, a part of Hungary where *V. officinalis* grows.[9] The epithet *officinalis* ("official") derives from Latin, and refers to the plant's pharmaceutical use.[10] The epithet *acutiloba* means "sharp leaved;" *californica* indicates the plant's origin in California; and *diversiloba* means "many shaped lobes," or "diversely lobed." The epithet *dioica* derives from two Greek words: *dis* ("double or twice") and *oikos* ("family or dwelling"). The botanical term *dioica* ("two houses") refers to the plant as dioecious, or having staminate and pistillate flowers on separate plants of a species.[11] The epithet *edulis* derives from the Latin *edere* ("edible" or "to eat, consume, or devour").[12] *Occidentalis* means "of or pertaining to the west;" *septentrionalis* ("of the north") originates from Latin.[13] *Scandens* derives from the Latin *scandere* ("to climb, mount, ascend, get up, or clamber").[14] *V. scouleri* is named after botanist John Scouler who discovered the plant. The Alaskan Tlingit name for *V. sitchensis* plant means "medicine that stinks."[9]

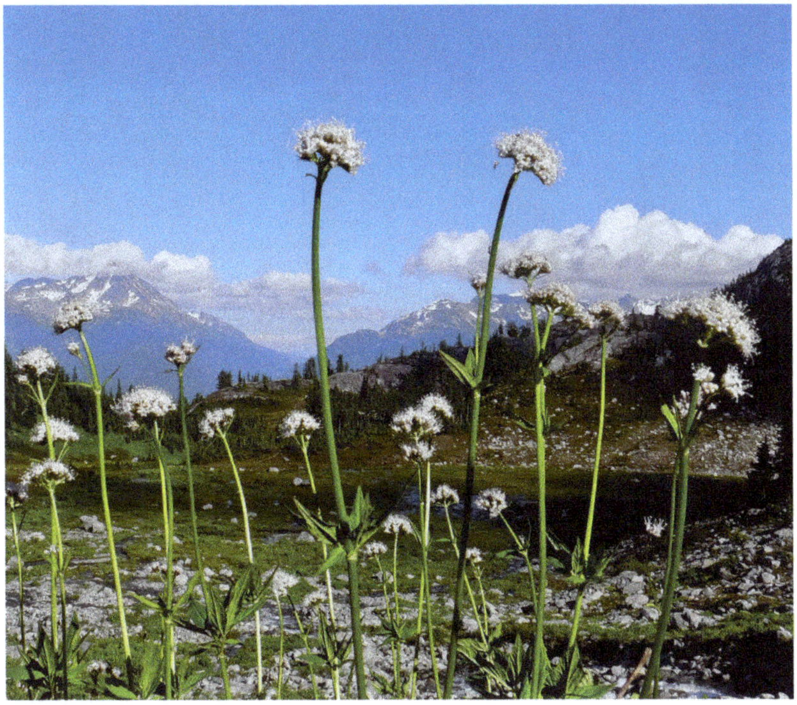

The following common names correspond with these Latin binomials: common valerian, fragrant valerian, garden valerian, all heal, setwall, moon root, all-heal, setewale, Capon's tail, amantilla, racine de valériane, baldrianwurzel, katzenwurzel, balderbrackenwurzel, and baldroin *(Valeriana officinalis);* sharpleaf valerian *(V. acutiloba);* California valerian *(V. californica);* woods valerian and marsh valerian *(V. dioica);* Mexican valerian and tobacco root *(V. edulis);* western valerian *(V. occidentalis);* Florida valerian *(V. scandens);* Scouler's valerian *(V. scouleri);* northern valerian *(V. septentrionalis);* and Sitka valerian *(V. sitchensis).*[15]

During medieval times, valerian synonyms included phu, fu, or amantilla. Capon's tail is another medieval name referring to the impressive spread of the white flowers. The herb was also referred to as "all heal" during that era, because it was revered as a potent medicine for numerous conditions.[8] Additional names included theriacaria, marinella, genicularis, and terdina.[8] Chaucer and earlier writers referred to the herb as setwall or setewale; the derivation is unknown.[8] The common name valerian was not applied until the 11th century.

HISTORICAL USES: Ancient Greeks and Romans administered valerian for digestive problems, nausea, liver complaints, and urinary tract disorders.[16] Galen, a Greek physician, was the first to describe its use for insomnia.[16] He also administered the herb to treat epileptic children and adults. During the Middle Ages, valerian was believed to cure nearly every condition under the sun, for which it earned the common name "all heal."[16] Valerian root was used as a medicine, spice, and perfume. Commoners considered the root a valuable culinary herb to be added to broths and pottages.[17] The roots were placed with clothing to add fragrance. Valerian was also used as an aphrodisiac in Europe.[8,9] During the 14th century, Professor Henslow mentions a recipe translated as follows: "Men who begin to fight and when you wish to stop them, give to the juice of *Amantilla id est Veleriana* and peace will be made immediately."[8]

Throughout the 1700s to 1900s, valerian root gained popularity in Europe as a nervine and sedative.[16] It was administered for insomnia, nervous unrest, neuralgic pains, hysteria, hypochondriasis, St. Vitus' dance, and epilepsy.[8] The juice of fresh valerian root was administered as a narcotic for insomnia.[8,16] In the 17th century, Nicholas Culpeper recommended decocting valerian roots with licorice, anise, and raisins to treat coughs and the plague. He also recommended applying a poultice of ground leaves to the head in order to relieve pain. Gerard prescribed valerian to treat croup, bruising, and injury.[8]

Eclectic physicians employed valerian as a nervine, sedative, and carminative. It was included in the *U.S. Pharmacopoeia* (1820 – 1936), and the *National Formulary* (1888 – 1946).[17,18] Physician Harvey Felter recommended valerian to stimulate gastrointestinal secretions, and as a carminative to relieve flatulence and unpleasant abdominal fullness after a meal. He also prescribed valerian as a calmative agent for hysteria, hypochondria, and nervous headache, and to relieve heart palpitations. He stated that valerian was one of the best medicines for chorea, and recommended consuming equal quantities of valerian and *Macroytes* (black cohosh) in 10 – 15 drop increments, three to four times daily.[19] In the *American Materia Medica, Therapeutics, and Pharmacognosy,* Finley Ellingwood wrote about valerian:

> Its influence upon the nervous system is best obtained when the circulation of those centers is inactive and feeble, especially when there is paleness of the face and the skin is cool. It is directly indicated in hysterical conditions of whatever character with feebleness; with nervous excitement, morbid vigilance, hysterical epilepsy, and in nervous headaches with some pallor. It controls distress and imaginary pain and produces quiet, permitting sleep and rest.[20]

In addition to the aforementioned applications by the Eclectics, English physician David Culbreth also recommended using valerian for nervous coughs, whooping cough, delirium tremens, typhoid state, vertigo, epilepsy, and reflex neuralgia.[21]

Valerian was consumed to calm civilian nerves during World War II air raids.[8] Oil of valerian was a popular remedy for cholera at that time. It was also used in soap perfumery.

More than six species of valerian were used by North American tribes to treat headaches, constipation, colds, cuts, and inflammation.[22] Native American and Canadian tribes considered valerian a cure for distempered horses.[13] They also gathered the spring roots of *Valeriana edulis* and cooked them in fire pits or stews as a nutritious food.[13]

Contemporary Ayurvedic practitioners Dr. Vasant Lad and Dr. David Frawley assert that valerian is one of the best herbs for *vatagenic* nervous disorders. They recommend the root tea to clear nerve channels of *vata* accumulation, and as an antispasmodic. They also recommend valerian to clear *ama* (toxins) from the colon, blood, joints, and nerves.[23] In traditional Ayurvedic medicine, *V. officinalis* and *V. wallichii* were used to treat hysteria, neurosis, and epilepsy.[24]

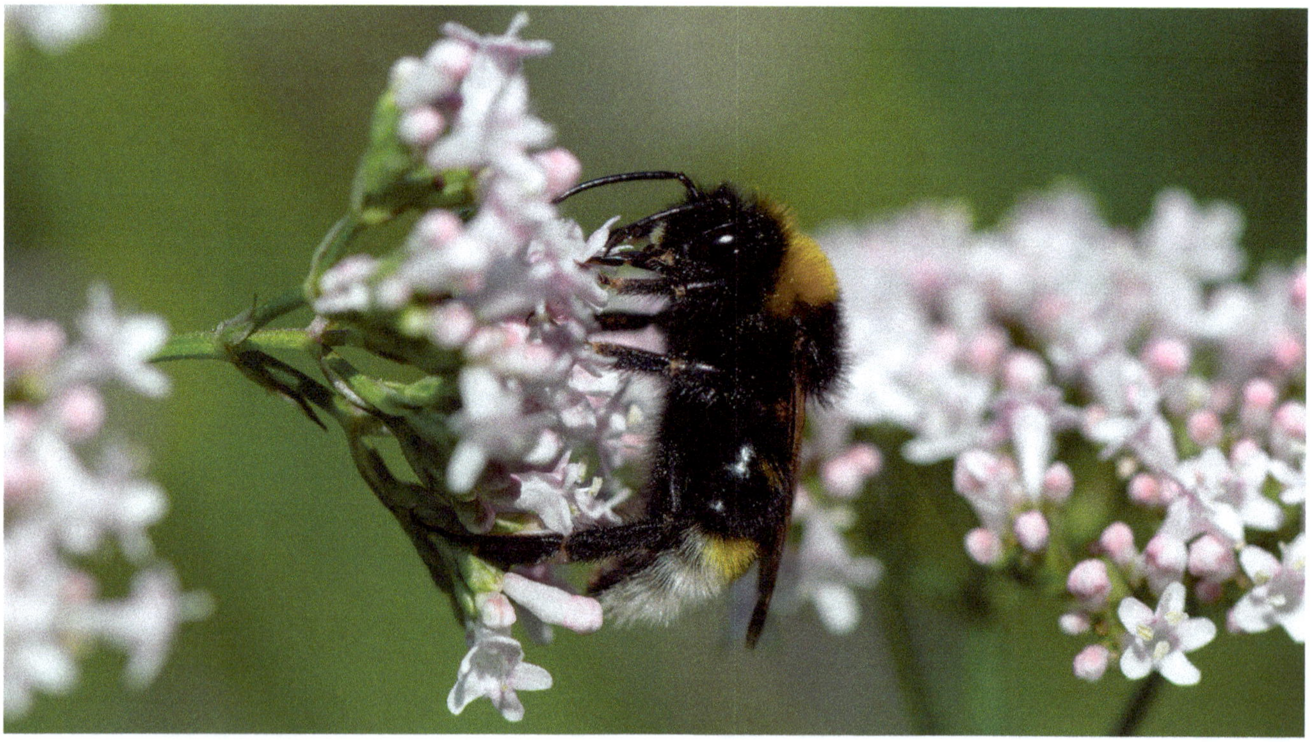

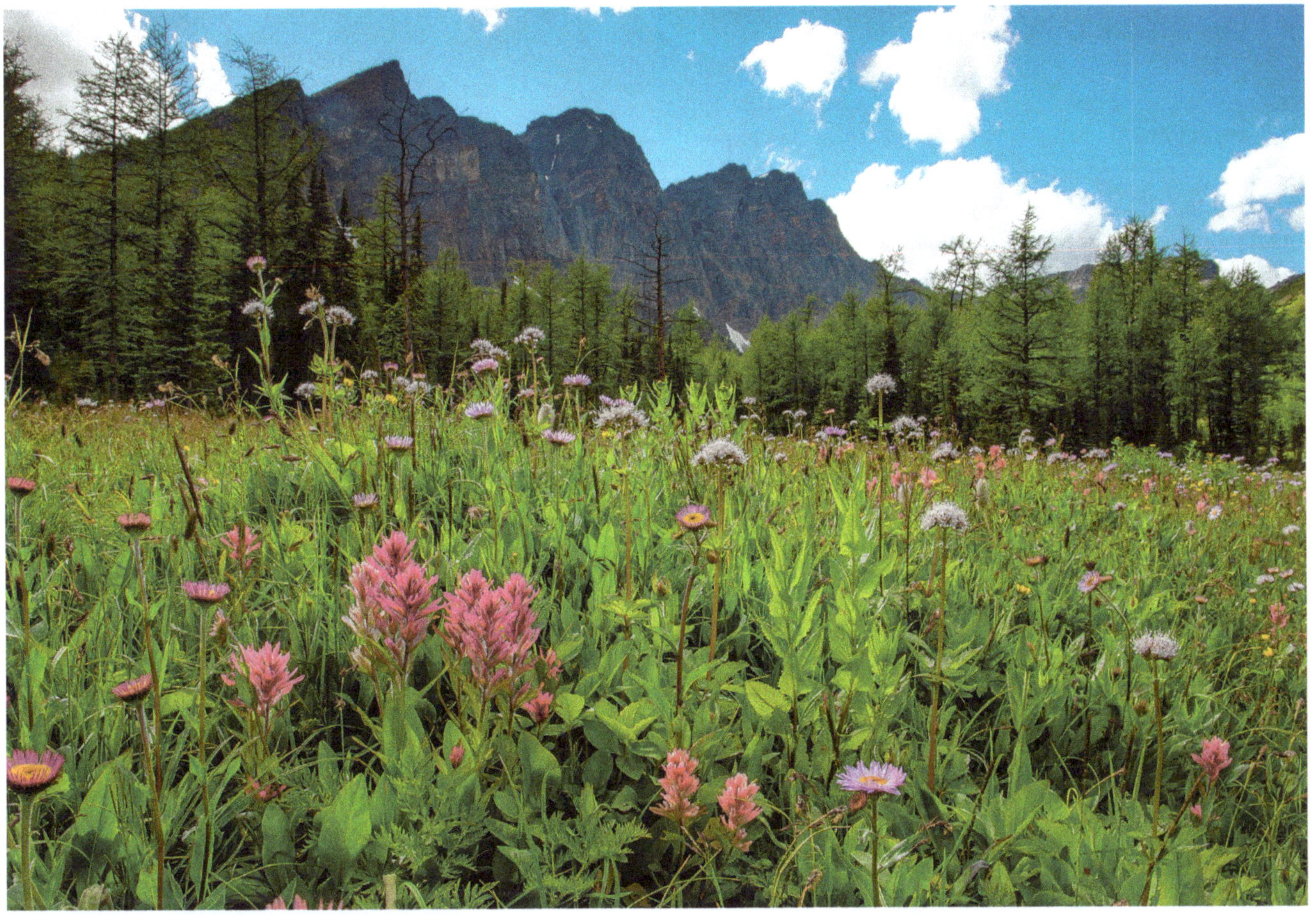

Valerian affects the nervous systems of animals. Like catnip *(Nepeta cataria),* it has an intoxicating effect on cats, likely due to the monoterpene (iridoid) — actinidine; a similar constituent is present in catnip.[25] Valerian was used for bait in rat traps. According to the German myth, the Pied Piper of Hamelin, who was a musician and herbalist, attributed his power over rats to the emission of valerian odor, a common perfume when this myth was created.[8]

CONSTITUENTS: Valerian consists of iridoids known as valepotriates (valtrate, isovaltrate, isovaleroxyhydrin, acevaltrate, valechlorine, 7-epi-deacetylisovaltrate, and others), didrovaltrates (didrovaltrate, homodidrovaltrate, deoxydodidrovaltrate, homodeoxydodidrovaltrate, and isovaleroxyhydroxydidrovaltrate), an iridoid glycoside (valerosidatum), volatile oil (bornyl acetate, borneol, isovalerate, caryophyllene, α- and β-pinene, valerenal, valerenic acid, valerone, valeranone, β-ionone, eugenyl isovalerate, isoeugenyl isovalerate, patchouli alcohol, valerianol, borneol, camphene, β-bisabolene, ledol, terpinolene, and isovaleric acid), alkaloids (actinidine valerianine, valerine, and chatinine), flavonoids (quercetin, rutin, and others), choline, methyl 2-pyrrolyl ketone, chlorogenic acid, caffeic acid, valeric acid, valerodeatrum, β-sitosterol, tannins, gums, and others. The dried root (not alcoholic extracts) contains gamma-aminobutyric acid (GABA).[1-3,22,24-27] The valepotriates are unstable compounds that are thermolabile and decompose in alcoholic solutions, as well as under acid or alkaline conditions.[24,25] The potent odor of dried valerian is due to the release of isovaleric acid and its relatives as the valepotriates decompose.[24,28] These constituents are referred to as baldrinals, and are only present in the dried root or dry root extract.[24,27]

NUTRITIONAL PROPERTIES: Valerian root contains high amounts of aluminum, ash, calcium, chromium, iron, magnesium, selenium, and tin. It contains low to average amounts of cobalt, crude fiber, dietary fiber, fat, manganese, niacin, potassium, protein, riboflavin, silicon, sodium, and thiamine, as well as trace amounts of phosphorus, zinc, and vitamins A and C.[2]

MEDICINAL PROPERTIES: Analgesic, anodyne, antispasmodic, calmative, carminative, hypnotic, nervine, relaxant, sedative, and stomachic.

TEMPERATURE AND FLAVOR: Warm, pungent, sweet, and mildly bitter.

MEDICINAL USES

Valerian sedates the central nervous system, treating anxiety and insomnia, as well as sleeplessness due to pain. It improves sleep quality, reducing sleep latency (the time required to fall asleep) and nighttime awakening.[3] While the mechanism of action and active components are not fully understood, several compounds are attributed to valerian's sedative effects. These include iridoid-based compounds known as valepotriates, valeric acid, and volatile oil.[2,3,29] A recent double-blind study indicated that a combination of valerian (160 mgs) and lemon balm *(Melissa officinalis)* (80 mgs) had sedative effects comparable to a benzodiazepine (triazolam, 0.125 mg). In another study, valerian reduced sleep latency as effectively as barbiturates and benzodiazepines, without the negative side effects.[3] Valerian contains valepotriates and valeric acid that are capable of binding to the same receptors as Valium and other benzodiazepine drugs.[3] Valerian can modify the symptoms of withdrawal from benzodiazepines.[26] One study recommended consuming valerian consistently for two to four weeks to improve sleep patterns.[18]

Fresh and dry valerian roots have sedative actions, although based on clinical observation, the dry roots are more sedating. Dry roots are more likely to cause morning sleepiness; however, lowering the dosage can eliminate this problem. Valerian can intensify dreams in some individuals. As a sedative, valerian can be consumed as a single extract or combined with equal parts of hops *(Humulus)*, California poppy *(Eschscholzia)*, motherwort *(Leonurus)*, and passion flower *(Passiflora)* extracts. When treating insomnia, consume 20 – 90 drops of valerian extract, one to two hours before going to sleep, and again one-half hour before bedtime. Or infuse 16 ounces of hot water with one to two tablespoons of valerian root and one tablespoon of orange peel or two tablespoons of orange flower blossoms. Consume one to two cups several hours before sleeping, and if needed, another cup up to one hour before going to bed. To improve the palatability of the tea, sweeten with a small amount of honey, orange syrup, or neroli syrup.

Valerian root is a potent analgesic and antispasmodic. It reduces smooth muscle or skeletal muscle cramping. Valerian sedates respiratory spasms, relieving a dry cough, whooping cough, croup, bronchitis, or asthma. It is useful for treating menstrual or intestinal cramps caused by flatulence, irritable bowel syndrome, or diarrhea. Valerian also alleviates referred pain from passing gallstones or kidney stones. The antispasmodic actions are attributed to the valerianic acid.[2] Valerian is specifically indicated when pain or cramping improves with the application of heat and warmth. Combine extracts of valerian, California poppy *(Eschscholzia)*, passion flower *(Passiflora)*, and hops *(Humulus)* to treat the aforementioned conditions.

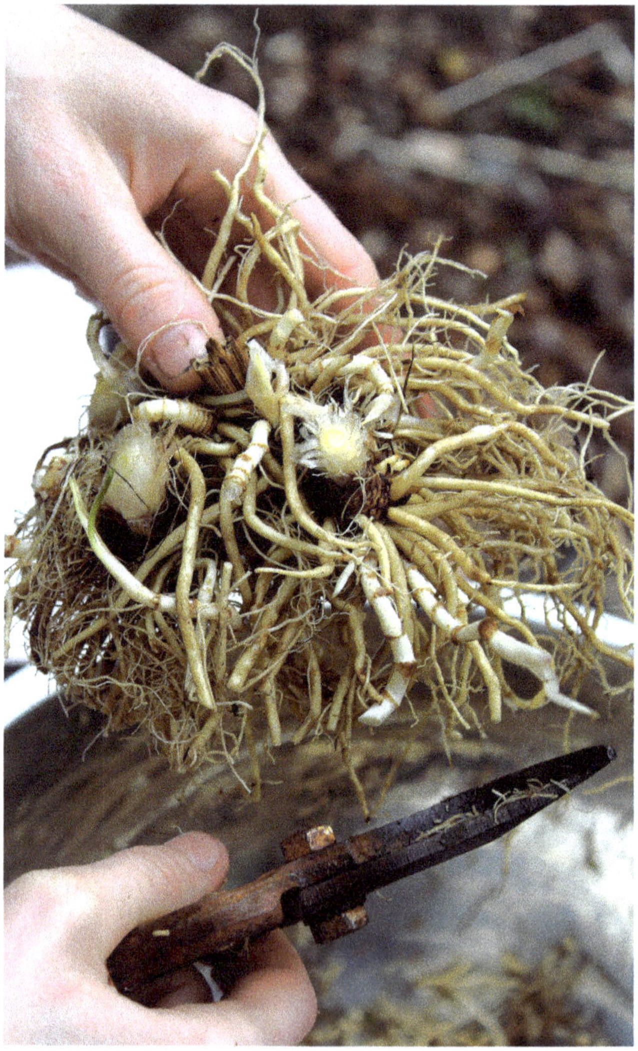

Valerian can be highly effective for reducing skeletal muscle spasms. It sedates rapid nerve firing, and reduces neuralgia caused by an abscessed tooth, sciatica, or an injury. Valerian can be used to reduce muscle spasticity and pain caused by tension headaches, trigeminal neuralgia, or multiple sclerosis. Start with a low to moderate dose (10 – 60 drops) for pain management, and repeat throughout the day; increase the dose as necessary. Consume a combination of extracts of valerian, California poppy *(Eschscholzia)*, passion flower *(Passiflora)*, hops *(Humulus)*, and cannabis *(Cannabis)* for pain relief. Apply valerian oil or root poultice topically to reduce muscle spasms and pain resulting from muscle strains and sprains. For topical relief of pain, valerian can be combined with other topical analgesic or anti-inflammatory herbs, such as hops *(Humulus)*, chamomile *(Matricaria)*, poplar *(Populus)*, cannabis *(Cannabis)*, arnica *(Arnica)*, yarrow *(Achillea)*, or figwort *(Scrophularia)*.

CONTRAINDICATIONS

Valerian may potentiate the effects of CNS depressants including sedative, hypnotic, and antidepressant prescription drugs, as well as alcoholic beverages.[26] Consult a health professional before combining them with valerian. Avoid consuming valerian when operating heavy machinery or vehicles.

Valerian root can exacerbate symptoms of heat, such as heartburn, acid indigestion, gastric or duodenal ulcer, hot flashes, or night sweats. It also can increase stomach and intestinal secretions, and peristalsis.[2,28] In rare cases, valerian can have idiosyncratic actions; for example, it can act as a stimulant, cause heart palpitations, or increase heart rate and circulation.[24] The few individuals who experience any of these reactions should discontinue or avoid use.

Fresh root preparations are best tolerated for long-term use, and are less heating than dry root preparations. Long-term use of the dry root can cause rapid emotional shifts, melancholy, or depression in some individuals.[28] Large doses can cause giddiness, restlessness, agitation, headaches, mental excitation, or hallucinations.[2,13,24]

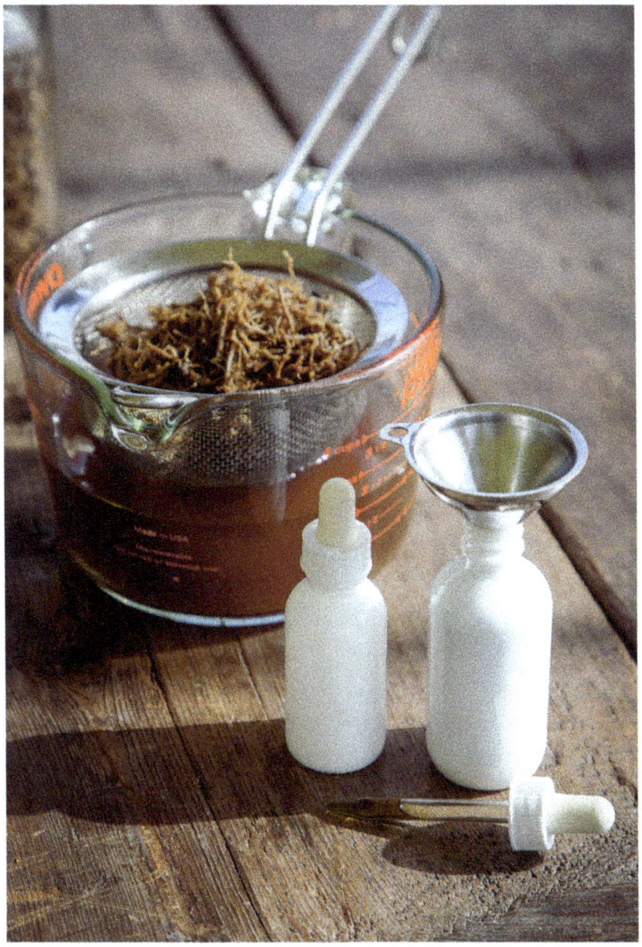

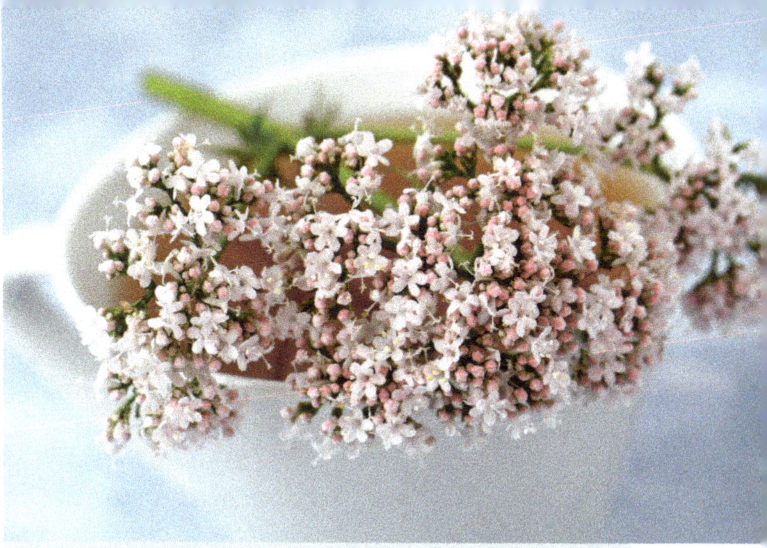

PREPARATION AND DOSAGE

TINCTURE: Fresh roots [1:2, 70-95% alcohol]; dry roots [1:5, 60-70% alcohol]; consume 10-120 drops as necessary, up to four times daily. Many European sources recommend consuming higher doses (½-2 teaspoons or up to 7-8 ml) for effective use.[24,25]

GLYCERITE: Fresh roots [1:2, 50% glycerin and 50% alcohol]; dry roots [1:5, 40% water, 30% glycerin, and 30% alcohol]; consume 10-60 drops, up to four times daily.

CAPSULES: Consume 2-3 "00" capsules, up to four times daily. The powder can be incorporated into capsules, lozenges, cough drops, or pills.

TEA: Consume 4-8 ounces of the hot or cold infusion, or the root decoction, one to two times in the evening. Consume 4-8 ounces of the flower infusion, one to four times daily. Herbalist Terry Willard cautions against boiling the root.[13]

HONEY AND SYRUP: Prepare fresh root honey [1:4, volume of root to honey]; consume 1 teaspoon, up to five times daily. Syrup can be prepared by simmering a root decoction [1:4, volume of root to volume of water] to half the volume. Add honey to desired sweetness; consume 1 teaspoon, up to five times daily. Add 20% alcohol to the total volume of syrup to increase shelf life. Refrigerate either preparation.

TOPICAL USE: Apply the fomentation or poultice topically, or the tincture or glycerite as a liniment. Infuse the fresh wilted root or dry root in oil via the alcohol intermediary or double boiler method. Prepare as a salve and apply.

VITEX

DESCRIPTION

BOTANICAL NAME:
Vitex agnus-castus

COMMON NAMES:
Chaste tree, chaste tree berry, monk's pepper, Abraham's balm, sage tree
kaf marim, ghar bari azraq (Arabic)
viteks (Bulgarian)
sing git muih (Cantonese)
konopljika (Croatian)
drmek obecny (Czech)
kyskhedstrae (Danish)
monnikenpeper, kuisboom (Dutch)
harilik mungapipar (Estonian)
munkinpippuri, siveydenpuu (Finnish)
arbre au poivre, gattilier, poivre des moines, agneau caste (French)
keuschlamm, mönchspfeffer (German)
angos, lygos (Greek)
siah Avraham mazui (Hebrew)
barátcserje (Hungarian)
agnocasto (Italian)
itarianinjin-boku (Japanese)
jing li, sheng ji mei (Mandarin)
niepokalanek, pieprzowy (Polish)
lemmul lui Avram (Romanian)
avraamovo derevo, viteks (Russian)
rakita (Serbian)
kyskheträd, munkpeppa (Swedish)
ayit, hayit (Turkish)
viteks (Yiddish)[1]

FAMILY NAME:
Lamiaceae
(formerly Verbenaceae)[2]

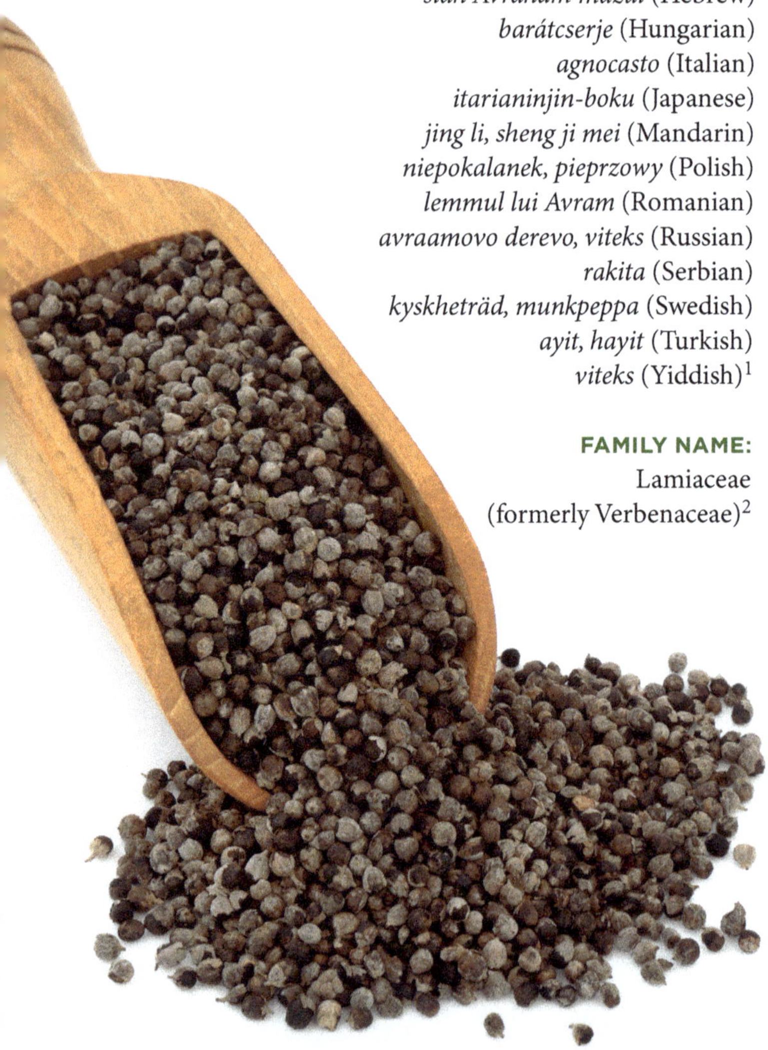

PART USED: The berries.

BOTANICAL DESCRIPTION AND HABITAT: *Vitex agnus-castus* is a deciduous shrub usually growing 1 – 2 meters high, but it can reach up to 4 meters in hot, dry climates.[3]

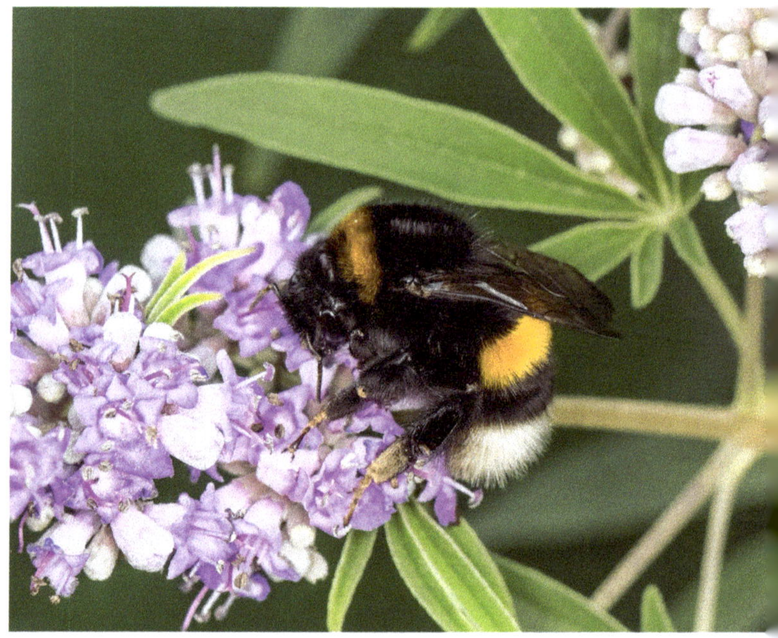

The stems are covered in a fine down; the young shoots are square, and the older shoots are round. The opposite, petiolate leaves are palmately compound; each leaf usually has five to seven lanceolate leaflets with acuminate apices. The two outer leaflets are much smaller than the others. The leaflet undersides are also covered in a fine, whitish layer of hair.

The beautiful terminal inflorescences (10 – 20 cm long) consist of whorls of flowers climbing a central axis, forming a verticillaster adherent to the mint family pattern.[3] The flowers have a campanulate calyx (3 mm long), and a lilac to violet, somewhat bilabiate, five-lobed corolla (7 – 10 mm long).[3,4] Inside, the flowers have two pairs of epipetalous stamens.[4] There are two carpels with two chambers, each producing two seeds.[4] Diverging from the usual mint family pattern, the fruit is a small, round drupe (up to 2.5 mm wide) that remains partially enclosed within the persistent calyx.[4]

THE NAME: The genus *Vitex* derives from the Latin *vitilis* ("made by plaiting"), referring to the use of branches to construct plaited fences.[1] The epithet *agnus* means "lamb;" *castus* means "chaste." The names chaste tree berry and monk's pepper originate from the plant's use as an anaphrodisiac and symbol of chastity.

HISTORICAL USES: As early as the 6th century BCE, vitex was used as a relaxant and analgesic.[5] Hippocrates administered it to staunch bleeding after childbirth, and aid in passing afterbirth.[5] Pliny the Elder administered the herb to encourage normal menstruation and lactation, and as an anaphrodisiac.[5,6] Eventually, it was used to stimulate menstruation and alleviate menstrual cramping.[6] Vitex was also given as a carminative to ease flatulence and constipation.[5,6] A tea was used to treat rheumatism and colds.[7] Vitex fruit was substituted for pepper. The branches were woven into baskets.[7] The leaves were combined with wine or vinegar and water to treat spider bites and snakebites.[6]

In ancient Greece, vitex was considered an anaphrodisiac. In initiation ceremonies, vitex flowers were strewn in front of novice monks.[5] Vitex fruit was used as a libido-lowering condiment in monasteries; hence, the name "monk's pepper."[7] In French convents, a syrup of the fruit was prepared from seeds and distributed to encourage chastity.[6] Persians believed that it cured madness and epilepsy; they continue to use the fruit as a calming agent for "hysteria."[6] Vitex tea was administered as an emmenagogue, diaphoretic, and carminative.[6] It also was used to treat impotence, nervousness, and memory loss.[7] Eclectic physicians prescribed it to treat menstrual disorders, and as a galactagogue.[7]

CONSTITUENTS: Vitex berries contain volatile oil (α- and β-pinene, 1,8-cineole, bornyl acetate, β-caryophyllene, α-terpinyl acetate, and limonene), flavonoids (casticin, penduletin, 6-hydroxykaempferol-3,6,7,4'-tetramethylether, 3,6,7-trimethylether of 6-hydroxykaempferol, 3,6,7-trimethylether of quercetagetin, chrysosplenol-D, isovitexin, luteolin-7-glucoside, orientin, isoorientin, and homoorientin), iridoid glycosides (aucubin, eurostoside, and agnuside), diterpenoids (rotundifuran, vitexilactone, and 6β, 7β-diacetoxy-13-hydroxy-labda-8,14-diene), and triterpenoids (3β-acetoxyolean-12-en-27-oic acid, 2α,3α-dihydroxyolean-5,12-dien-28-oic acid, 2β-3α-diacetoxyolean-5,12-dien-28-oic acid, and 2α,3β-diacetoxy-18-hydroxylean-5,12-dien-28-oic acid).[6,8,9] The flower extracts contain ketosteroids, including progesterone, 17-α-hydroxyprogesterone, testosterone, and epitestosterone.[8] The leaves contain three iridoid glycosides (aucubin, agnuside, and eurotoside), flavonoids (homoorientin and luteolin-7-glucoside), and volatile oil; the leaf extracts contain androstenedione.[6,8]

NUTRITIONAL PROPERTIES: Other than the flavonoids previously mentioned, the nutritional properties of vitex are unknown.

MEDICINAL PROPERTIES: Hormone balancing agent, progesterone agonist, anti-inflammatory, antibacterial, and antifungal.

TEMPERATURE AND FLAVOR: Warm, pungent, and bitter.

MEDICINAL USES

Vitex is an extremely effective hormone-balancing herb. It influences the anterior lobe of the pituitary gland by increasing luteinizing hormone (LH) production, and mildly inhibiting the release of a follicle-stimulating hormone (FSH).[6,8-11] FSH stimulates the maturation of the follicle that increases estrogen production. LH causes the mature follicle to rupture, releasing the ovum (ovulation), and transforming the ruptured follicle into the corpus luteum. Progesterone and smaller amounts of estrogen are secreted from the corpus luteum following the release of the ovum. During this phase of the menstrual cycle, progesterone is the dominant hormone; estrogen is the dominant hormone prior to ovulation. The first day of menses until ovulation is the follicular phase or estrogen phase. From ovulation to the first day of menses is the luteal or progesterone phase. Vitex strengthens the luteal or progesterone phase, and restores estrogen-to-progesterone balance.[10,11] It may also exert its hormone-balancing effects by reducing pituitary gland secretion of prolactin,

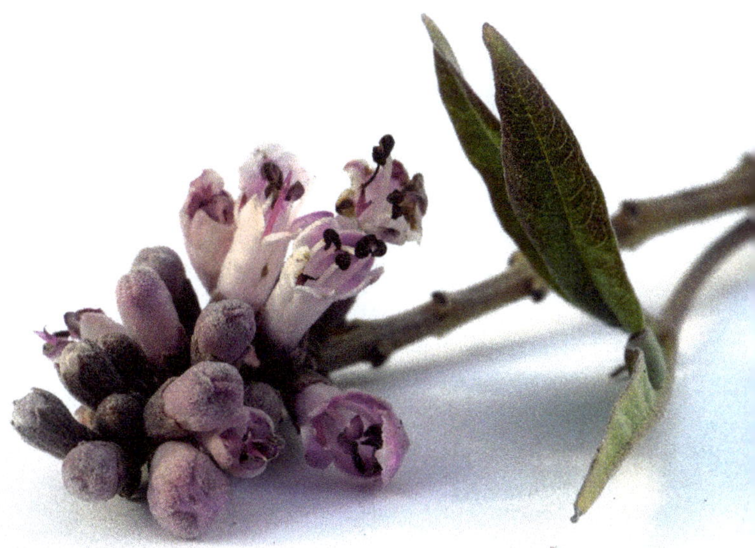

and a dopamine-agonistic effect by binding with dopamine receptors.[9] See below for further information on the effect of vitex on prolactin levels.

Vitex is a progesterone agonist that aids in treating primary and secondary corpus luteum insufficiency and estrogen-dominant conditions.[7,8,10] Women with corpus luteum insufficiency, a relative deficiency of progesterone and excess of estrogen, are likely to experience the following symptoms: premenstrual syndrome, slow-starting, crampy menses, vaginal or uterine inflammation or congestion, cystic hyperplasia, increased inflammation before menses and during ovulation, and long menstrual cycles.[10,12] Women in menopause with corpus luteum insufficiency may experience hot flashes, night sweats, depression, dizziness, or dry vaginal mucosa. The flavonoids and alkaloids are steroidal hormone precursors attributed to the hormone-balancing effects.[5]

Vitex normalizes the menstrual cycle. Treating polymenorrhea (shortened cycle) and oligomenorrhea (infrequent menstruation), it can lengthen short menstrual cycles (21 – 24 days), and organize and consolidate menstrual cycles in women with lengthy (35 days or longer) or irregular menstrual cycles.[5,6,8-14] Vitex aids in regulating menstrual cycles following the discontinuation of birth control pills.[6-8] It also restores hormone balance after an abortion or miscarriage. Taken as a long-term tonic, vitex alleviates symptoms of premenstrual syndrome (PMS) attributed to excess estrogen.[6-10] It reduces premenstrual water retention, breast pain, tenderness, and swelling, and aids in treating fibrocystic breast disease.[6,8-11,15] Consumed as a long-term tonic, vitex aids in treating hormone-related headaches, migraines, dysmenorrhea, joint pain, anxiety, mood swings, bloating, and flareups of acne and eczema.[5,6,10,12,] Clinical studies have confirmed its effectiveness for dysfunctional uterine bleeding, amenorrhea, endometrial hyperplasia, anovulatory cycles, and polymenorrhea.[9,10,13,14] Vitex should be consumed consistently a minimum of three to six months for optimal hormone-balancing effects.

Due to the progesterone agonist actions, vitex may aid in reducing and/or resolving uterine or ovarian cysts and fibroids.[6,9,10] Combine vitex with reproductive tonifying herbs, such as saw palmetto *(Serenoa)*, white peony *(Paeonia lactiflora)*, yellow pond lily *(Nuphar)*, or blue cohosh *(Caulophyllum)* to treat these conditions. Vitex can be helpful for reducing endometrial hyperplasia, and discomfort and bleeding caused by endometriosis.[13]

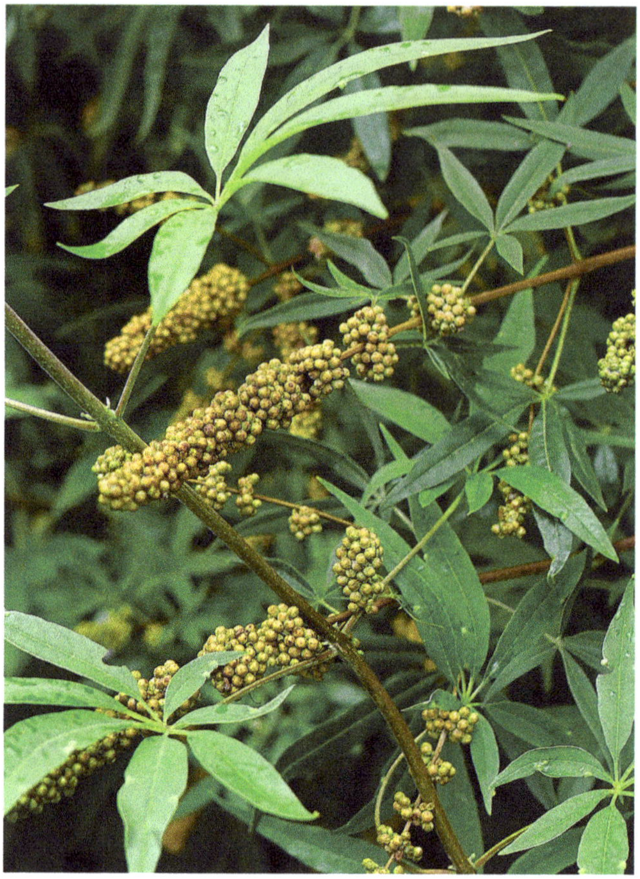

Vitex aids in re-establishing ovulation and treating infertility resulting from corpus luteum insufficiency.[5,9,10,13] Because it increases gestagens, it can be consumed three to six months prior to conception, and while attempting to conceive.[11] Consume with other reproductive tonics, such as wu wei zi *(Schisandra)*, shatavari *(Asparagus root)*, and saw palmetto *(Serenoa)*. Also consume tea blends of reproductive and nourishing tonics such as red raspberry leaf *(Rubus idaeus)*, partridge berry *(Mitchella)*, oat straw *(Avena)*, alfalfa *(Medicago)*, and nettle *(Urtica)*. According to German research, vitex aids in preventing miscarriages in women with low progesterone levels.[6]

Numerous menopausal maladies are eased by vitex, including hot flashes, depression, mood swings, and anxiety.[6,10,16] Its effects are attributed to its influence on the pituitary gland.[16] Use it alone, or in combination with other hormone-balancing herbs, such as black cohosh *(Actaea racemosa)*, dong quai *(Angelica sinensis)*, motherwort *(Leonurus)*, white peony *(Paeonia)*, and/or licorice root *(Glycyrrhiza)*. In animal studies, vitex demonstrated osteoprotective effects, maintaining cortical and trabecular bone.[17] It also was found to have cancer-suppressing effects.[17]

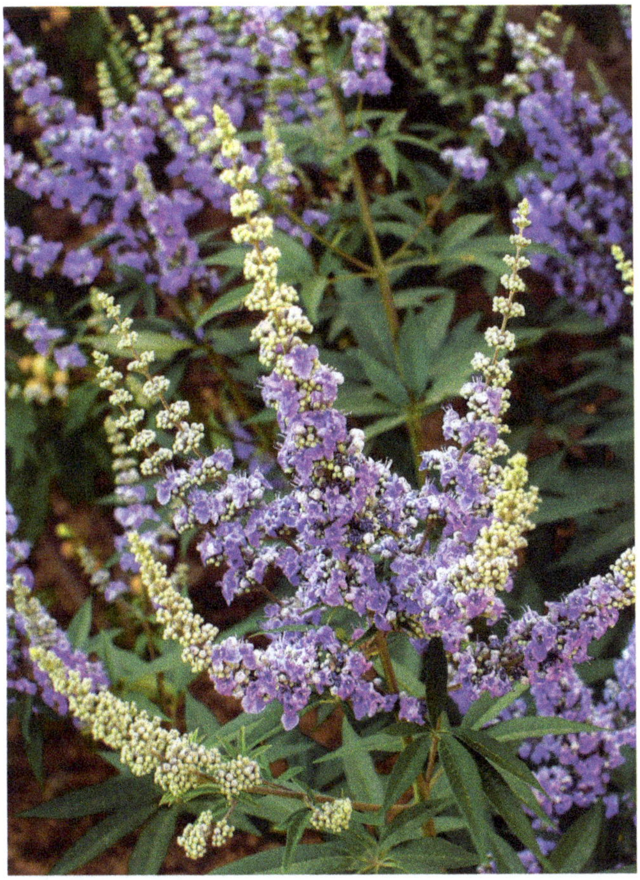

Breastfeeding women with insufficient milk production can benefit from vitex, as it increases prolactin secretion resulting in a galactagogue effect.[5-8,11] Consume the herb several months to obtain the best results.[11] In a controlled study of 817 patients, milk production tripled within 20 days for patients in the vitex group.[10] In another study of 125 patients, it increased milk production in 80% of the subjects.[10] A study using low doses of Agnolyt, a 1:10 homeopathic solution, confirmed vitex's prolactin-stimulating effect.[13] In order to enhance the galactagogue actions, combine with blessed thistle *(Cnicus)*, fennel *(Foeniculum)*, and anise *(Pimpinella)*. Vitex also aids in restoring postpartum hormone balance.

Alternate studies have reported that higher doses of vitex lowered prolactin levels when elevated levels resulted from stress.[13,14] This action was attributed to enhanced binding to dopamine receptors that inhibited prolactin secretion.[13,14] A three-month, double-blind study was conducted to determine the effects of a 20 mg daily dose of vitex in women with luteal phase defects resulting from hyperprolactinaemia (elevated prolactin levels).[14] The study concluded that prolactin levels were reduced, the short luteal phase was normalized, and progesterone production was normalized in the vitex group.[14] In a clinical study of men, low doses resulted in a rise in prolactin; higher doses reduced secretion.[13] This suggests that the influence of vitex on prolactin secretion is dose dependent; however, further clinical studies are necessary to better understand the influence of this herb.

Vitex aids in treating benign prostatic hyperplasia (BPH), impotence, and male infertility.[10] It also reduces acne in teenage men.[6]

Although it is not typically used as an antimicrobial, vitex has antibacterial actions against *Bacillus cereus, B. megaterium, Escherichia coli, Staphylococcus aureus, S. faecalis,* and *Salmonella* spp.[8,10] The iridoids (aucubin and agnuside) and flavonoids are attributed to the antibacterial effects.[7] Vitex has antifungal actions against *Candida albicans, C. tropicalis, C. pseudotropicalis,* and *C. krusei.*[8,10] It also is toxic against the mycelia growth of *Trichophyton mentagrophytes, Epidermophyton floccosum, Microsporum canis, M. gypseum,* and *Penicillium virdicatum.*[10]

CONTRAINDICATIONS

According to German research, vitex is safe to consume during the first trimester of pregnancy to prevent a miscarriage.[6,10] However, other sources recommend avoiding use during pregnancy unless recommended by a health care practitioner.[15] Consult a health care practitioner before consuming this herb during lactation.[15] Vitex is contraindicated with the birth control pill, hormone replacement therapy, and progesterone drugs.[10,13] Avoid consuming with antipsychotic drugs (domamine-2 receptors), as it can counteract them.[15] Vitex can cause a headache, upset stomach, nausea, or diarrhea in some individuals.[14] Although it is rare, it can cause itching and urticaria.[8,10,14]

PREPARATION AND DOSAGE

TINCTURE: Fresh berries [1:2, 70-95% alcohol]; dry berries [1:5, 70% alcohol]; consume 30-120 drops, up to three times daily.

CAPSULES: Consume 2-6 "00" capsules, up to three times daily.

TEA: Prepare a hot infusion or decoction and consume 8-12 ounces, three to four times daily. *Note:* The active constituents of vitex are not entirely water-soluble.

WILD CHERRY BARK

DESCRIPTION

BOTANICAL NAMES:
Prunus virginiana, Prunus serotina, Prunus spp.

COMMON NAMES:
Wild cherry, choke cherry, chokecherry, western chokecherry, bitter-berry, Virginia bird cherry, common chokecherry, black chokecherry, wild black cherry, rum cherry, rum cherry bark, wild rum cherry, mountain black cherry
kiitotuomi, virginiahägg (Finnish)
cerisier (French)
kirsche, spätblühende traubenkirsche (German)
celiegio, pruno (Italian)
cerezo, capulín (Spanish)
glanshägg (Swedish)
kiraz ag (Turkish)

FAMILY NAME:
Rosaceae

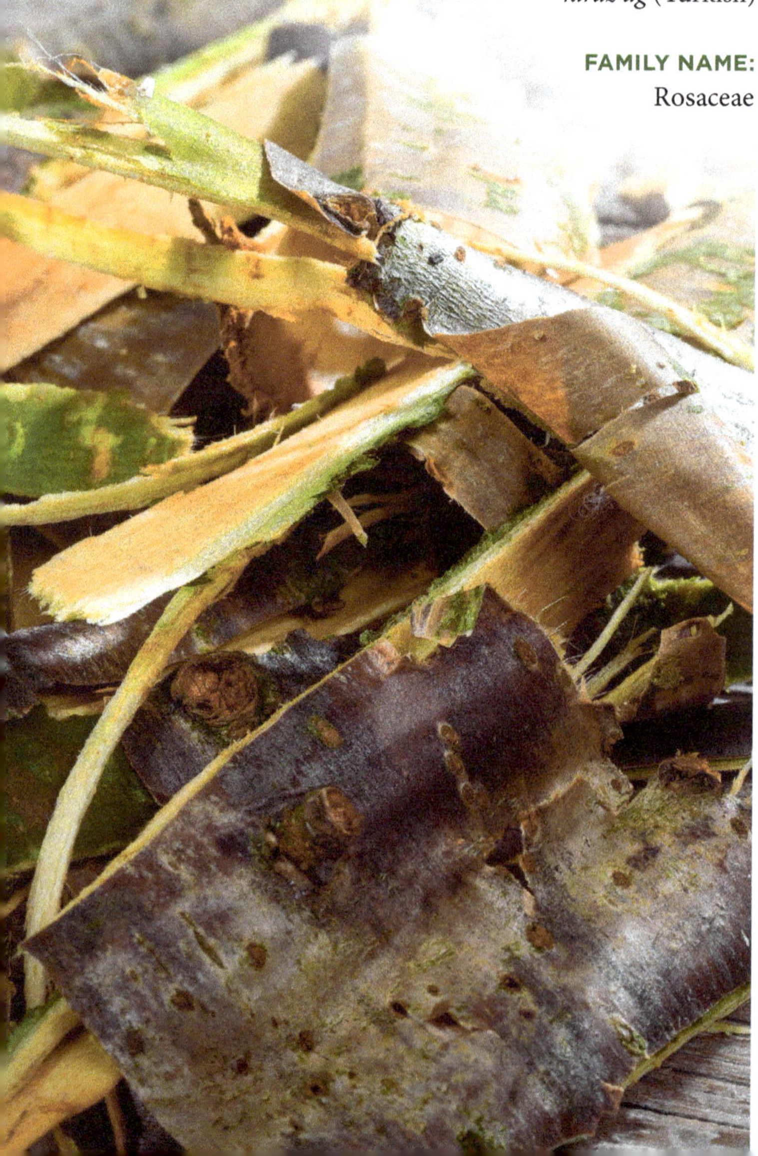

PART USED: The inner bark, harvested (preferably) in the fall or late summer.

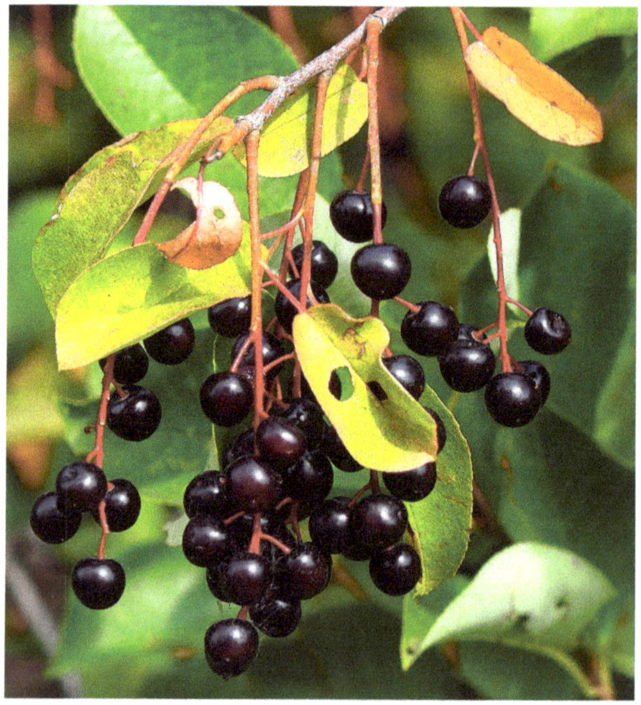

BOTANICAL DESCRIPTION AND HABITAT: There are 200 species of the genus *Prunus.*[1] Wild cherry grows as a deciduous shrub or small tree.[2] *P. serotina* typically grows 50 – 70 feet tall, while *P. virginiana* usually reaches up to 30 feet tall, often forming thickets.[3,4] The simple glabrous, alternate leaves have membranous stipules that fall off early in development.[5] The leaf margins are serrated and can be finely wavy.[2] Other features of the leaf include a shortly acuminate tip, and a pair of tiny nectaries at the junction of the blade and petiole.[2] A raceme inflorescence displays tiny white flowers; each has a campanulate hypanthium with five sepals, five petals, and 20 – 30 stamens.[5] The superior ovary has a single carpel and two ovules. The ovary develops into a reddish-black, glabrous, spheric, fleshy drupe.[2,4]

Prunus virginiana grows throughout the U.S. in dry and rocky soils, ravines, canyons, and wooded slopes.[4] *Prunus serotina* is native to the eastern U.S., growing in moist, fertile soils in forests and along streams.[3]

THE NAME: *Prunus* is New Latin for plum tree, derived from the Greek *proumnē* ("plum tree").[6] The epithet *virginiana* ("of or from Virginia") also derives from New Latin.[5] The epithet *serotina* derives from the Latin *serotinus* ("late"), referring to the *Prunus serotina* habit of fruiting and flowering later than other cherry species.[3]

The following common names correspond with the Latin binomials: wild cherry, wild black cherry, rum cherry, wild rum cherry, and mountain black cherry *(Prunus serotina);* wild cherry, choke cherry, chokecherry, bitter berry, Virginia bird cherry, western chokecherry, black chokecherry, and common chokecherry *(Prunus virginiana).*

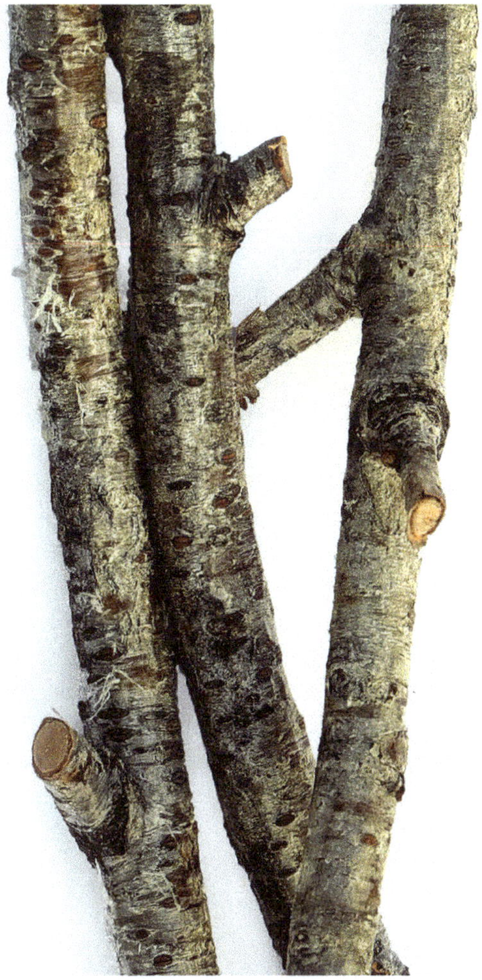

HISTORICAL USES: Native Americans were the first to utilize wild cherry bark medicinally.[8] They prepared tea and syrup to treat laryngitis, coughs, colds, bronchitis, and pneumonia, to lower fever, and ease childbirth. They also consumed the tea as a blood tonic, and to treat digestive conditions such as an upset stomach, lack of appetite, and diarrhea.[8] Preparations of the root were consumed to expel worms, treat burns, and heal ulcers.[8] The people of Peña Blanca harvested the roots in September, simmered them in water, and added a little sugar. This beverage was consumed on an empty stomach to relieve stomach inflammation.[9] A tea prepared from the roots also was used to treat rheumatism; a small glass was consumed, and the rest was used in a bath.[9]

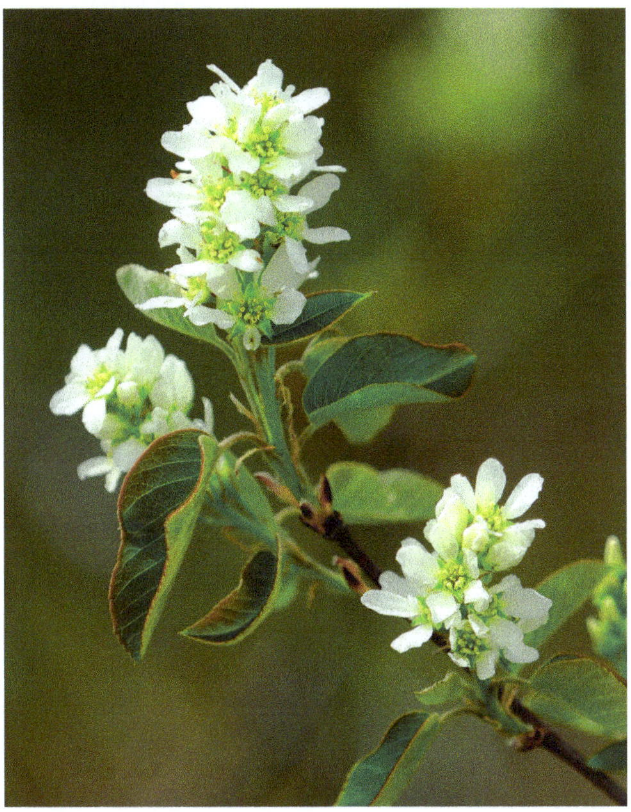

Early colonists learned about wild cherry from Native Americans and adopted similar medicinal uses.[8] They administered preparations of wild cherry bark to treat catarrh, cold, cough, whooping cough, consumption, and lung problems.[10] Wild cherry bark was eventually incorporated into American pharmacopeias. It was added to lozenges (wild cherry cough drops), and cough preparations known as wild cherry bark syrup and white pine compound.[1,8] Eclectic physicians Harvey Felter and Finley Ellingwood administered wild cherry bark for uncomplicated heart palpitations, heart pain, and difficulty breathing.[11,12] Dr. John Scudder and Ellingwood recommended wild cherry bark syrup tonic for dyspepsia, stomach irritability, and general debility following inflammatory diseases.[11,13]

The dark, bittersweet fruits of wild cherry were simmered, then prepared in jelly, jam, marmalade, pie, and pudding.[8] They also were added as a flavoring to spirits and liqueurs, such as rum and a southern liqueur known as cherry bounce.[8] Wild cherry wine was prepared by adding cherry juice to sugar, water, and yeast.[9] A purplish-red dye was obtained from wild cherries.[9]

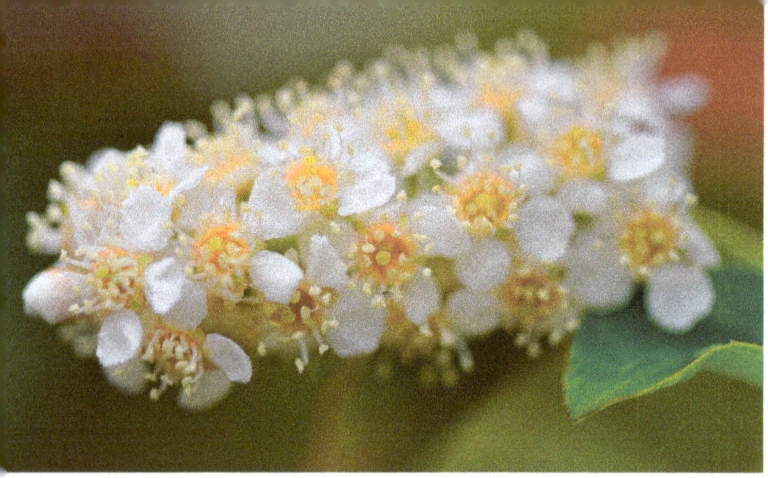

MEDICINAL USES

A water-based preparation of wild cherry bark is a highly effective antitussive that sedates the tracheal nerves, decreasing respiratory spasms.[1,13] Wild cherry bark deepens respiration, reduces cardiopulmonary excitability, and is an expectorant. It aids in treating dry, spastic, percussive coughing resulting from thracheitis, bronchitis, pneumonia, smoker's cough, allergies, or asthma.[1,13] Due to the almond-like flavor, wild cherry bark syrup is administered as a harmonizing flavoring agent in cough syrups. Wild cherry bark also has astringent actions that tone mucous membranes in the respiratory tract, decreasing inflammation. The medicinal actions of wild cherry bark are inert unless it is macerated with room temperature water for 12 – 24 hours. This process allows prunasin to be hydrolyzed by prunase, releasing hydrocyanic acid, benzaldehyde (this gives the characteristic almond scent and flavor), and glucose.[13] Boiling the herb destroys the medicinal properties.[10,14]

Herbalist Ed Smith, co-founder of Herb Pharm, comments about the potential concerns of the cyanogenic acid content, and describes common misconceptions about consuming cherry bark:

> Wild cherry (bark) is a very misunderstood medicinal herb and is most often incorrectly harvested, processed, and administered. Even though it contains a deadly poison (cyanide), it can still be safely used as an effective cough medicine.
>
> Wild cherry bark contains the glycoside amygdalin, which upon hydrolysis by the endogenous enzyme emulsin, decomposes into cyanide, benzaldehyde, and glucose. It's the benzaldehyde that gives the characteristic odor of almond extract.
>
> Many plants contain cyanide, especially those in the rose family, which contain cyanide in the form of amygdalin (e.g., almonds, bitter almonds — especially high in amygdalin — apple seeds, the pits, leaves and bark of peach, plum and apricot). In fact, peach leaves and seeds are Traditional Chinese Medicine cough remedies.
>
> Wild cherry bark is best harvested in the fall, instead of the usual spring harvest as with other barks. The highest quality bark is harvested from the south-facing side of the tree in order to get greener bark that is richer in amygdalin. To judge the quality of wild cherry bark, powder a sample of the bark, mix

CONSTITUENTS: Wild cherry bark contains prunasin (D-mandelonitrile glucoside), prunase (an enzyme), emulsin, eudismic acid (3,4,5-trimethoxybenzoic acid), *p*-coumaric acid, scopoletin, trimetnhoxy-benzoic acid, tannins, sugars, lanthamum, benzaldehyde, β-glycosidase, cyanidin, kaempferol, quercetin, and ursolic acid.[1,13-15] Prunasin is a cyanogenic glucoside hydrolyzed by the enzyme prunase, liberating hydrocyanic acid (HCN, prussic acid), glucose, and benzaldehyde. Bark collected in the fall yields the highest content of HCN (0.15%); bark collected in the spring has a lower yield of HCN (0.05%).[1] Fresh spring leaves contain the highest amount of HCN (0.25%).[1]

NUTRITIONAL PROPERTIES: The bark has no known nutritional properties.

MEDICINAL PROPERTIES: Antitussive, astringent, expectorant, and bitter tonic.

TEMPERATURE AND FLAVOR: Warm, bitter, sweet, and astringent.

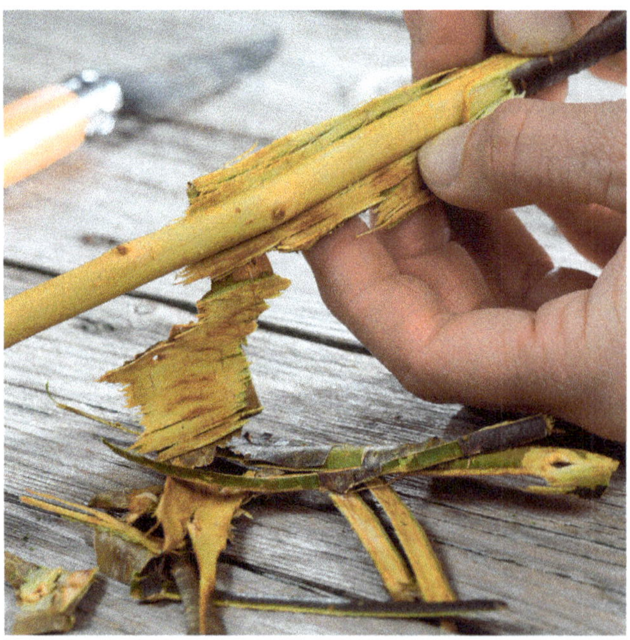

with room temperature water to a slurry, then let set for several hours. Good quality wild cherry bark should give off an obvious, nice-smelling aroma of benzaldehyde; the stronger the aroma, the better quality the bark. However, I find most wild cherry bark on the market has very little, to no aroma of benzaldehyde, and contains way too much adhering wood.

Even the best quality wild cherry bark can easily lose it medicinal properties if prepared incorrectly. Heating the bark denatures its emulsin enzyme needed to hydrolyze amygdalin, thus the bark is rendered therapeutically inert. The same thing happens when alcohol is added to wild cherry bark, but here it's the alcohol that denatures the emulsin. This is why I always ferment my wild cherry bark before making a tincture. The best organoleptic test for quality wild cherry bark tincture is the tell-tale aroma of benzaldehyde (smells like almond extract). By the way, almond extract has the cyanide removed, although the aromatic benzaldehyde remains.

So how poisonous is wild cherry bark? Paracelsus taught us that "The dose makes the poison." Toxic substances can be harmless in small doses, while ordinarily-harmless substances can be deadly if over-consumed. The amount of cyanide in wild cherry bark is relatively small, and smaller still in a dose of wild cherry bark tincture. In all my years of studying herbal medicine, I have never read or heard of a death due to taking wild cherry bark or any medicines made from it.

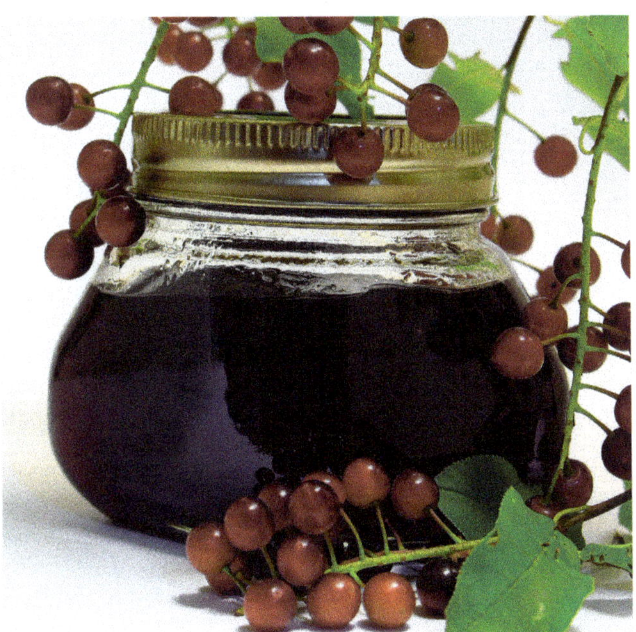

Although numerous herbs have more prominent actions in the digestive tract, wild cherry bark is a bitter tonic that restores the appetite following an infectious illness of the digestive or respiratory system. It also aids in treating general debility of the digestive tract, as well as atonic or nervous dyspepsia.[11,12]

Wild cherry bark can be classified as a minor topical medicine. Applying a poultice of the ground or powdered bark acts as an astringent, reducing bleeding from cuts and wounds. Gargling with the herbal tea treats a sore throat.[13]

CONTRAINDICATIONS

Avoid consumption during pregnancy or lactation.[13] Herbalist Michael Moore considers wild cherry completely safe — even for small children.[15] The maximum daily dose of hydrocyanic acid for adults is 0.002 grams (2 mg), and as a single dose, 0.006 grams (6 mg).[13] Individuals with extremely low blood pressure, or cardiovascular or respiratory depression should avoid consuming the bark.

PREPARATION AND DOSAGE

TINCTURE: Fresh bark [1:3 - 1:4, 60 - 95% alcohol] or [1:3 - 1:4, 60% alcohol, 10% glycerin]; dry bark [1:5, 50% alcohol, 10% glycerin]; consume 30 - 60 drops, up to five times daily. *Note:* Tincturing this herb is less effective medicinally than consuming the cold infusion or syrup.

TEA: Prepare a cold infusion of the bark and consume 4 - 8 ounces, up to three times daily.

HONEY AND SYRUP: Prepare syrup using a water-based percolation (1:10); add an equal volume of simple syrup and 10% alcohol to the total volume; consume 1 teaspoon, up to four times daily. Traditional wild cherry syrup was prepared from a mixture of wild cherry bark extract, glycerin, sucrose, alcohol, and water. This preparation was used as an adjuvant for less palatable drugs.[1]

CULINARY USE: Wild cherry fruits are edible. They can be cooked and added to wine, liqueur, jam, jelly, pie, pudding, or pemmican. They also can be dried for later consumption.

WILD YAM

DESCRIPTION

BOTANICAL NAME:
Dioscorea villosa

COMMON NAMES:
Wild yam, colic root, rheumatism root, devil's bones, yuma
igname (French)
yamswurzel, wilde yam wurzel (German)

FAMILY NAME:
Dioscoreaceae

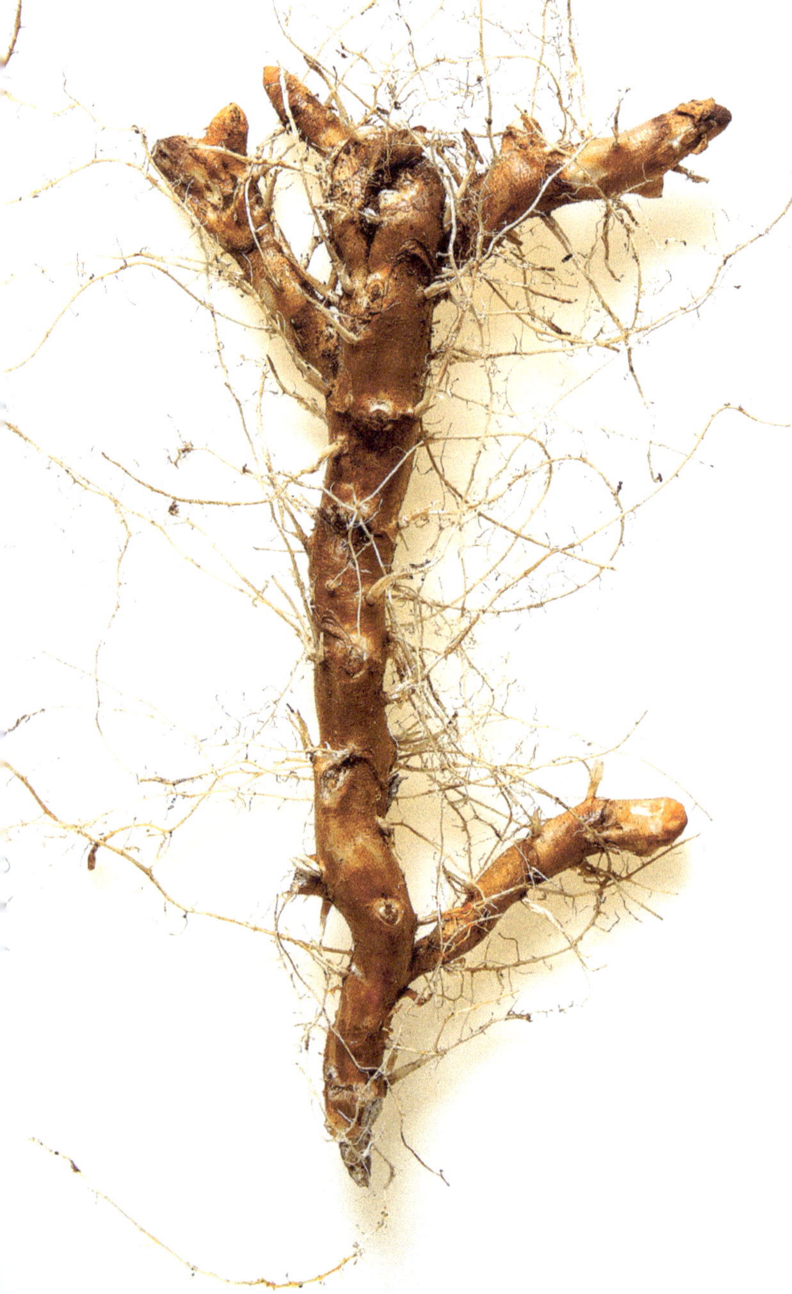

PART USED: The rhizome.

BOTANICAL DESCRIPTION AND HABITAT: More than 800 species of *Dioscorea* grow in tropical and subtropical regions worldwide.[1] *Dioscorea villosa* is a perennial native in the midwestern, northeastern, and southeastern U.S. *Dioscorea villosa* is highly variable across its geographical and ecological range, displaying drastic differences depending on where it grows.[1] Rather than the usual tuber-like roots of the *Dioscorea* genus, *D. villosa* has

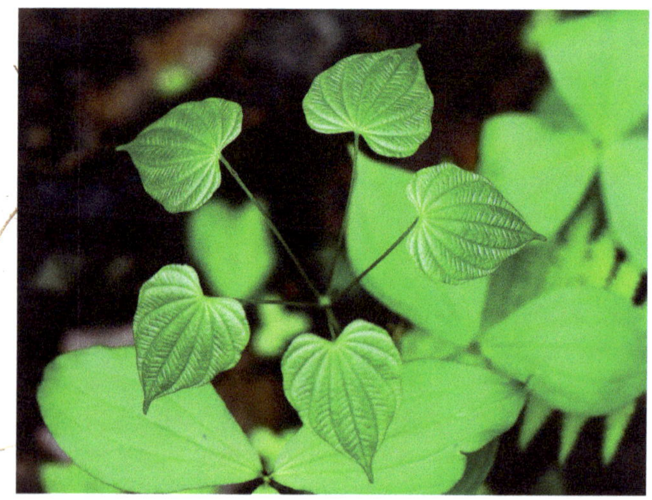

dense, slender, gnarled brown rhizomes. These horizontal creeping rhizomes (0.5 to 1.5 cm in diameter) bear numerous stem scars on the tops, and thin, fibrous rootlets below. This lovely vining herb (up to 7 meters high) has vibrant green, cordate leaves with prominent parallel veins.[1] The leaves vary from pubescent to glabrous or glaucous.[1] Multiple leaves (3 – 13 cm long and wide) with long petioles (3 – 14 cm long) grow in whorls of three to six at the base of the plant, but as the thin, green vine ascends, the leaves are alternate.[1] This dioecious herb has inconspicuous greenish-yellow flowers, with the male flowers growing in drooping, axillary panicles, and the female flowers growing in spicate racemes. The fruit has sharp three-angled sides, with three chambers, each containing two flat, winged seeds.

Note: The medicinal uses of *D. villosa* are not necessarily interchangeable with other species of *Dioscorea*. Also, wild yam should not be confused with the delicious, bright orange sweet potato *(Ipomoea batatas)* known as yam. Sweet potatoes are part of the morning glory family (Convolvulaceae); true yams are in the Dioscoreaceae family.

THE NAME: The genus *Dioscorea* was named in honor of Dioscorides, Roman physician and naturalist.[2] The epithet *villosa* derives from the Latin *villōsus* ("hairy" or "shaggy").[3] The word yam derives from the Portuguese *inhame,* or the Spanish *name,* both of which come from the West African *nyami* ("to eat").[4] Except *D. villosa,* many members of the *Dioscorea* genus are edible, starchy tubers; the name yam refers to their long history as a food source. Colic root was coined because the plant was adopted by European settlers who used the root as a remedy for colic.[2,4] Rheumatism root signifies its traditional use for joint pain.

HISTORICAL USES: Numerous Native American tribes administered the root tea to relieve menstrual cramps and labor pain.[4] Fox Indians employed wild yam as an analgesic and a gynecological aid.[5] Wild yam was used in folk medicine for rheumatism, inflammation, muscle spasms, digestive complaints, asthma, hiccups, and morning sickness.[4,5]

Eclectic physicians recommended using wild yam to treat bilious colic, dysenteric tenesmus, indigestion, painful vomiting, chronic hepatic congestion, ovarian neuralgia, spasmodic dysmenorrhea, and afterbirth pains, and to reduce the pain of cholera infantum.[6-8] The following indications are listed in *King's American Dispensatory*: bilious colic with spasmodic contractions; yellow skin and conjunctiva with nausea and colicky pains; coated tongue; frequent flatulent passages; colic with tenderness upon pressure; and sharp abdominal pain worsened by motion.[8] Priest and Priest recommend the following indications for using wild yam:

> ... autonomic nerve relaxant, especially for gastrointestinal conditions, vegetative neuroses and hyperaesthesiae. Rheumatic syndromes arising from hepatic and intestinal function.[9]

CONSTITUENTS: Wild yam root contains saponins (dioscin, gracillarin, and an aglycone: diosgenin), dioscorin, polysaccharides (rich in starch and mucilage), tannins, and minerals.[6,10]

NUTRITIONAL PROPERTIES: Wild yam root contains low to average amounts of aluminum, ash, calcium, dietary fiber, fat, iron, magnesium, niacin, phosphorus, potassium, protein, riboflavin, selenium, silicon, thiamine, tin, and vitamins A and C. It contains high amounts of carbohydrates, chromium, cobalt, crude fiber, manganese, sodium, and zinc.[11]

MEDICINAL PROPERTIES: Anti-inflammatory, antispasmodic, bitter tonic, cholagogue, expectorant, stomachic, and antirheumatic.

TEMPERATURE AND FLAVOR: Warm, bitter, and mildly sweet.

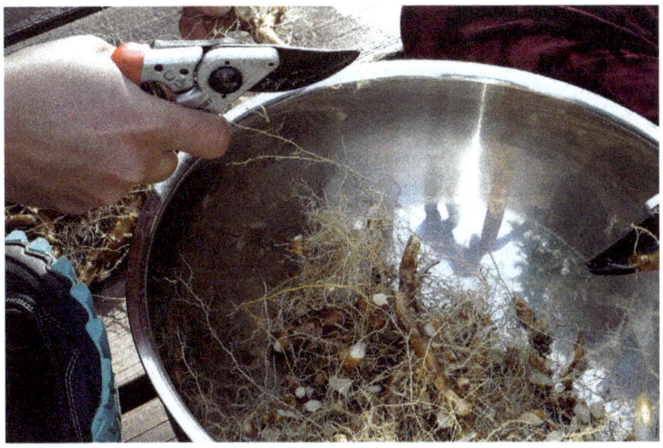

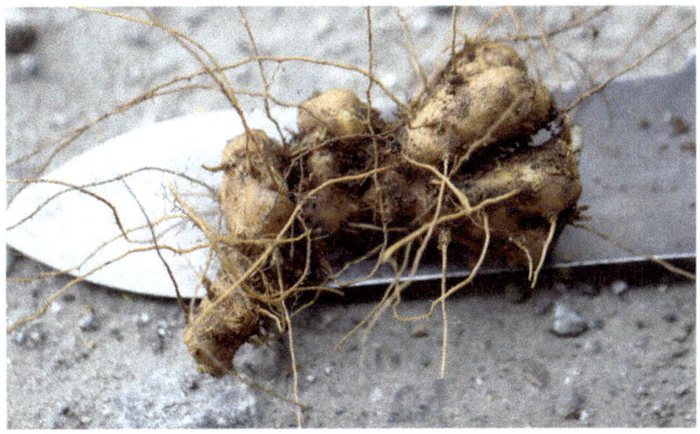

MEDICINAL USES

Wild yam is an impressive non-sedating, smooth muscle antispasmodic.[6-8,12,13] It is used to treat gastrointestinal and reproductive tracts cramps, and can be used short- or long-term.[6-8] Wild yam is one of the few herbs that reduces hiatal hernia pain and spasms, and ceases burping and hiccups.[13] The root reduces spasms of the stomach, intestines, and gallbladder.[6-8,13] It can be used daily to manage pain and spasms from irritable bowel syndrome (IBS), Crohn's disease, diverticulitis, or ulcerative colitis.[6-8,13] Wild yam also reduces griping and colicky pain associated with food poisoning, diarrhea, and dysentery.[6-8] The cholagogue and antispasmodic properties decrease gallbladder spasms, and aid in passing gallstones.[6-8,13]

Wild yam has digestive bitter tonic properties and carminative actions, decreasing gas and bloating. A cholagogue, wild yam stimulates bile excretion from the gallbladder. Consuming the extract or tea 15 – 30 minutes prior to a meal enhances fat and protein digestion. It combines well with extracts of fresh turmeric *(Curcuma longa),* fresh ginger *(Zingiber officinale),* orange peel *(Citrus sinensis),* and fennel *(Foeniculum vulgare)* in digestive bitter tonic formulas. The herb is also beneficial for allaying morning sickness and nausea in pregnant women.[13] It can be used alone or with extracts of fresh ginger *(Zingiber officinale)* and orange peel *(Citrus sinensis).*

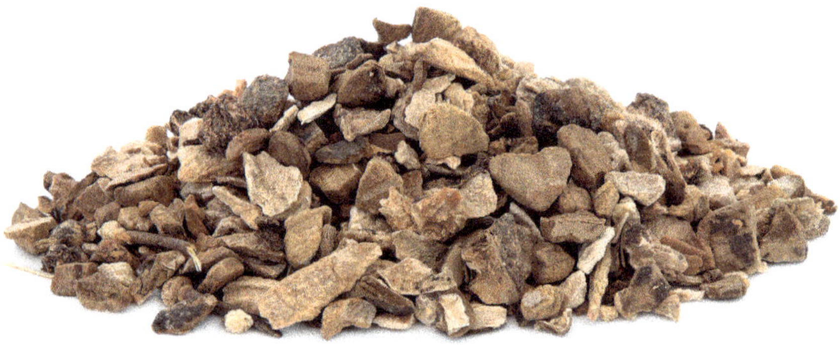

Wild yam addresses a variety of gynecological issues. It is a reliable antispasmodic for treating dysmenorrhea and ovaralgia, as well as ovulatory, labor, and afterbirth pain.[6-8,13] Long-term use helps to manage the pain of endometriosis, as well as uterine and ovarian cysts. Consuming 20 – 60 drops of wild yam extract is effective to alleviate uterine cramping, although up to 100 drops is sometimes needed. While a single extract of this medicine is very useful, it also combines well with tannin-based antispasmodics such as cramp bark *(Viburnum opulus)* or black haw *(Viburnum prunifolium).* Cramp bark compound contains these aforementioned antispasmodic herbs, with the addition of skullcap and several other circulatory stimulants, such as cinnamon, orange peel, and clove. For more information, review the recipe listed in the black haw monograph. When tannin-based analgesics are ineffective for pain management, additional antispasmodic and analgesic herbs such as kava *(Piper methysticum)* or Jamaican dogwood *(Piscidia erythrina),* or alkaloid-based herbs such as California poppy *(Eschscholzia californica),* valerian *(Valeriana officinalis),* or black cohosh *(Actaea racemosa)* are recommended alternatives. *Note:* Tannin and alkaloid-based extracts should not be combined.

Wild yam herb relaxes the uterus, and has been effective for treating a threatened miscarriage.[13] The following formula has been helpful in stopping uterine spasms during pregnancy and uterine bleeding that may occur during a threatened miscarriage. Combine equal parts of wild yam, black haw *(Viburnum prunifolium),* Chinese white peony *(Paeonia alba),* and red raspberry *(Rubus idaeus);* consume 30 – 60 drops of the tincture or eight ounces of the decoction, three to four times daily. Wild yam also can be used alone, or with black haw *(Viburnum prunifolium)* and cramp bark *(Viburnum opulus)* to reduce uterine cramping and bleeding following a miscarriage or abortion.

Wild yam reduces referred pain patterns from passing kidney stones.[13] It can be effective in treating bladder spasms, and as a tonic to reduce pain associated with a spastic or irritable bladder, as well as pain caused by interstitial cystitis. It has mild antispasmodic actions in the respiratory tract, and can alleviate asthma symptoms.[8]

Wild yam has anti-inflammatory properties.[4,13,14] Herbalist Michael Moore recommends using the herb to reduce inflammatory prostaglandins that can cause pain and cramping of smooth muscles.[13] Wild yam reduces acute inflammation associated with rheumatoid arthritis and other inflammatory related pain.[4] Extracts of *D. villosa* administered to rodents inhibited neurogenic and inflammatory pain, as well as leukocyte migration.[14] This study confirmed the anti-inflammatory and antinociceptive effects, while no acute or subacute toxicity was observed.[14] Consuming 30 – 90 drops three to four times daily of the following anti-inflammatory compound has been effective for managing muscle and joint pain: two parts each of wild yam *(Dioscorea villosa)* and Jamaican dogwood *(Piscidia erythrina),* and one part each of turmeric *(Curcuma longa)* and ginger *(Zingiber officinale).*

Although the tea tastes bitter, water-based preparations (decoctions) of wild yam extract the mucilaginous qualities of the root.[8,10] This mucilage soothes tissues and decreases inflammation of the mucous membranes lining the digestive, renal, respiratory, and reproductive tracts. Wild yam has been used with limited success in treating tinnitus (ringing in the ears).

Due to the emollient properties, topical applications are beneficial for decreasing inflammation.[10] Water-based preparations such as a compress, fomentation, or poultice are most effective for decreasing irritated skin conditions such as eczema, psoriasis, or dermatitis.[10] Oil- or water-based preparations decrease inflammation in muscles and joints.[10]

WILD YAM SCAM

In 1940, American biochemist Russell E. Marker published the results of his work on diosgenin, a saponin isolated from wild yam. Beginning with diosgenin, Marker chemically synthesized the hormones progesterone and testosterone. American pharmaceutical companies were uninterested in the project at the time, and Marker moved his laboratory to Mexico, where he began to synthesize progesterone from the Mexican species *(Dioscorea macrostachya, D. barbasco,* and *D. mexicana)* of wild yam. He succeeded in producing 6½ pounds of the hormone, which attracted the attention of a small Mexican pharmaceutical company, Laboratorios Hormona. The owners created a partnership with Marker in 1944, and Syntex was formed to synthesize progesterone for the pharmaceutical industry. Within one year, Marker left the company due to a fight with his partners, and took the secrets of his synthesis process with him. Syntex replaced Marker with Hungarian chemist, George Rosenkranz, who determined the missing steps, and Syntex patented the diosgenin-to-progesterone process. In a few years, they discovered how to synthesize testosterone and the female hormones estrone and estradiol, as well as cortisol. In 1952, they created the active ingredient for what would soon become the birth control pill. Eventually, diosgenin was synthesized in the laboratory, but prior to 1970, wild yam was the sole source of this precursor.[2,4]

Wild yam contains the saponin diosgenin, a precursor for synthetic hormones; however, the root is not a source of steroid hormones such as estrogen, progesterone, and testosterone. These hormones can be chemically synthesized from diosgenin, but diosgenin is not converted to these hormones in the body. Although there is no evidence proving direct hormonal actions of wild yam, and some studies have proven that it has no hormonal effects for hormone-related disorders, wild yam products were marketed as a hormone-balancing agent for menopause related disorders. This marketing ploy was dubbed the "wild yam scam."[2,4]

CONTRAINDICATIONS

Wild yam is a cholagogue and should be avoided in individuals with a blocked bile duct. One study suggests that individuals with compromised renal function and those who take medications altering kidney function should avoid using *D. villosa* longer than one month.[15]

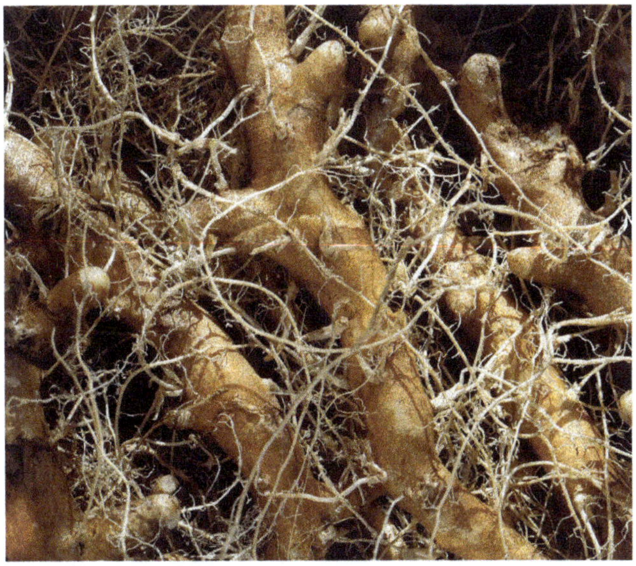

PREPARATION AND DOSAGE

Note: It is important to chop the dense, rock-hard root immediately after harvesting, as it is difficult to process the next day. Use caution when processing the root in non-industrial blenders, as it can break the blades or burn out the motors. This is one of the few herbs that should be purchased in powdered form, as most home appliances cannot adequately powder the chopped root.

TINCTURE: Fresh roots [1:2, 70-95% alcohol]; dry roots [1:5, 60% alcohol]; consume 30-100 drops, up to four times daily.

FLUID EXTRACT: Dry roots [1:1, 50% alcohol]; consume 10-60 drops, up to three times daily.

CAPSULES: Consume 2-4 "00" capsules, up to four times daily.

TEA: Prepare a decoction or cold infusion; consume 4-8 ounces, up to four times daily. The tea tastes very bitter and may be difficult to palate.

TOPICAL USE: Apply the poultice, fomentation, cream, or salve topically. Prepare the oil using the alcohol intermediary oil method.

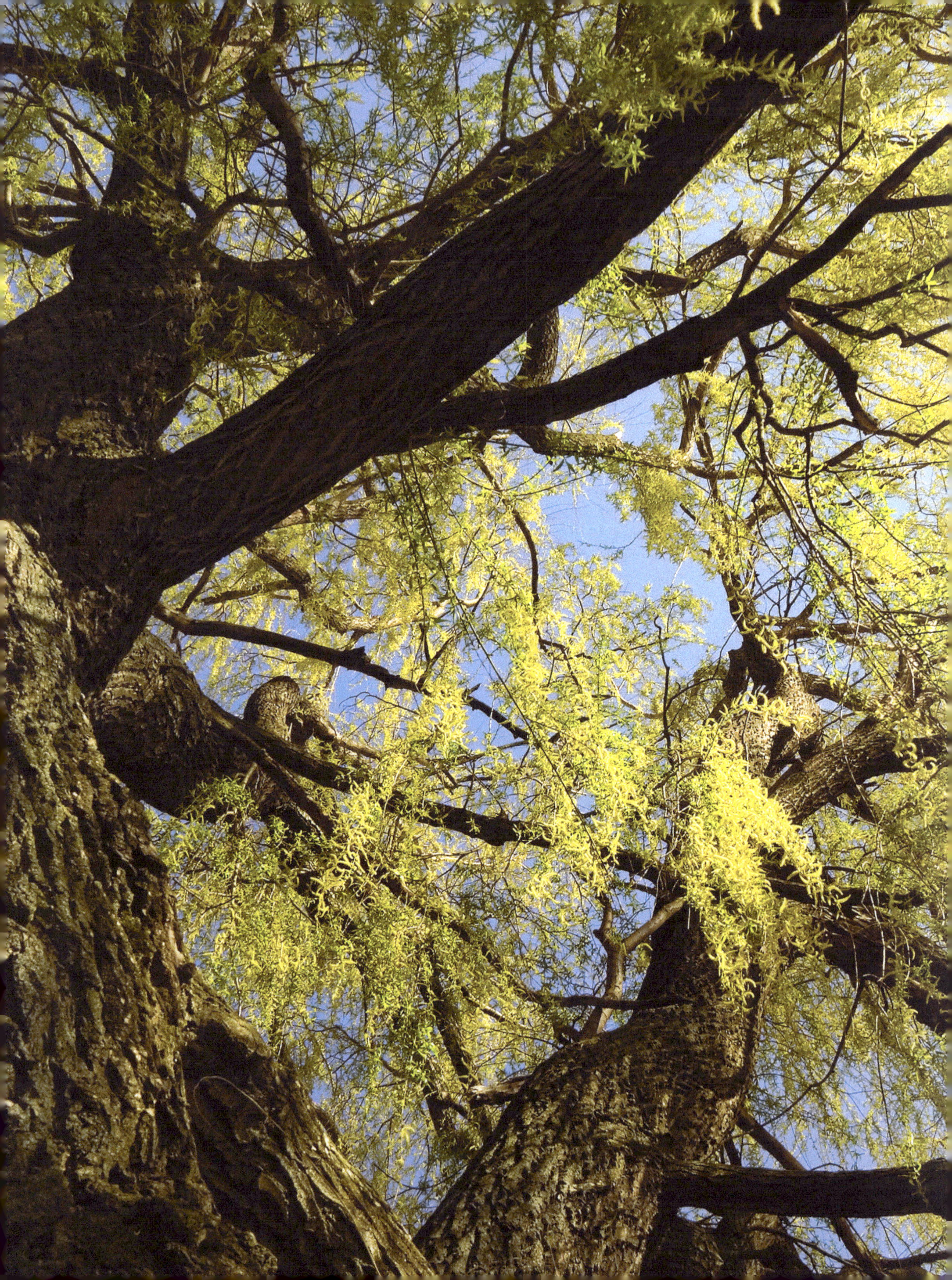

WILLOW BARK

BOTANICAL NAMES:
Salix alba, S. fragilis, S. nigra, S. pentandra, S. purpurea, Salix spp.

COMMON NAMES:
White willow, European willow, black willow, pussy willow, purple willow, purple osier, catkins willow, basket willow, crack willow, brittle willow, withe, withy
hvidpil (Danish)
valkopaju (Finnish)
saule, osier (French)
felbinger, weide, wilgenbaum (German)
salice, salcio (Italian)
kvitpil (Norwegian)
jara, jarita, sauz (Spanish)
vitpil (Swedish)
ak sogut, soynd (Turkish)

FAMILY NAME:
Salicaceae

DESCRIPTION

PART USED: The bark from young branches.

BOTANICAL DESCRIPTION AND HABITAT: Willow is a prolific deciduous, perennial tree or shrub that thrives in damp soil on the banks of rivers, creeks, streams, lakes, swamps, and marshes. It grows wild throughout North

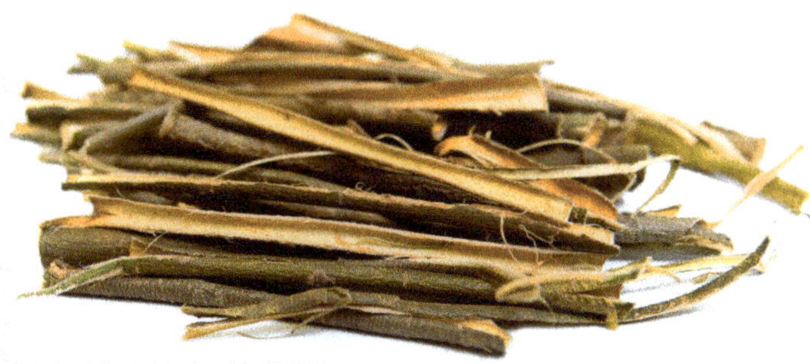

America, Central America, Europe, central Asia, and northern Africa. *Salix alba, S. fragilis, S. purpurea,* and *S. pentandra* are native to Britain, and central and southern Europe. These species have naturalized throughout North America following their introduction in eastern North America by European settlers.[1,2] *S. nigra* is native to the eastern and western U.S.[3]

Salix is a large genus with significant variation between species that often hybridize. Generally, *Salix* species have alternate lanceolate, oblanceolate, or ovate leaves with entire, serrated, or toothed margins; the upper surface is dark green, and the underside is pale.[4] The leaf surface varies from glabrous to tomentose, depending on the species.[4] The bark ranges from yellow to brownish-red in younger trees, and turns brownish-gray in older specimens.[4] The young branches are flexible, and the leaf buds are protected by a single scale.[4] Willow is dioecious, and flowers of both sexes are found in catkins, with a brown, black, or two-toned, sometimes deciduous bract subtending each flower.[4] The flowers lack a traditional perianth that is replaced by a single nectary.[4] Male flowers usually have two stamens; female flowers consist of a single pistil with two stigmas, each with two lobes.[4] Female flowers yield a two-valved fruit.[4]

THE NAME: *Salix* derives from the Celtic *sal lis* ("near water").[1] The epithet *alba* ("white") refers to the fine white hairs on the leaves. The following epithets derive from Latin: *fragilis* ("brittle" or "fragile"), *nigra* ("black"),

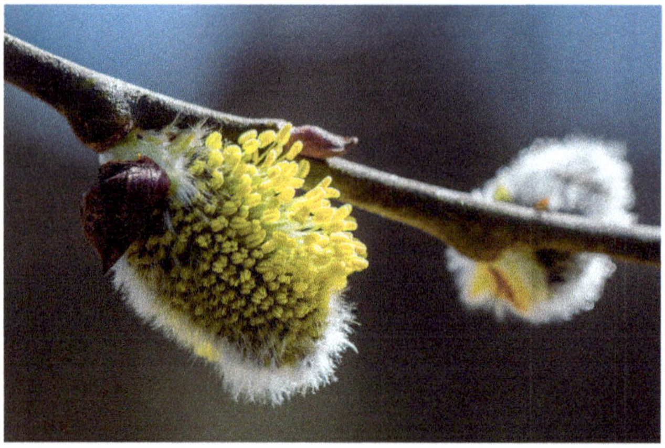

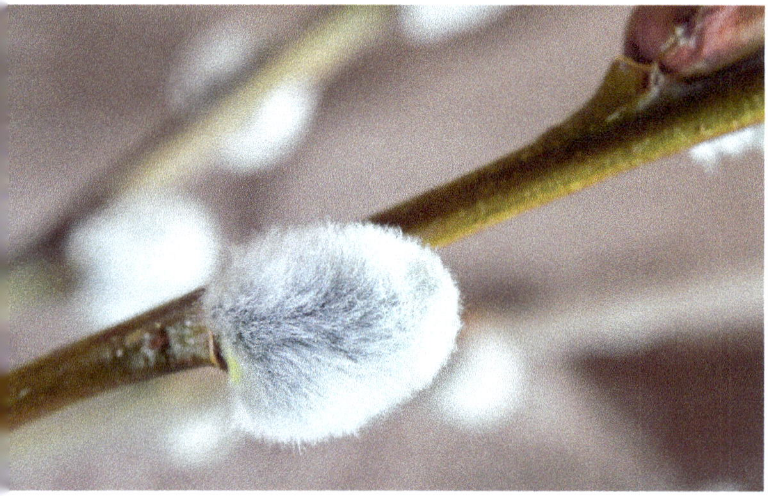

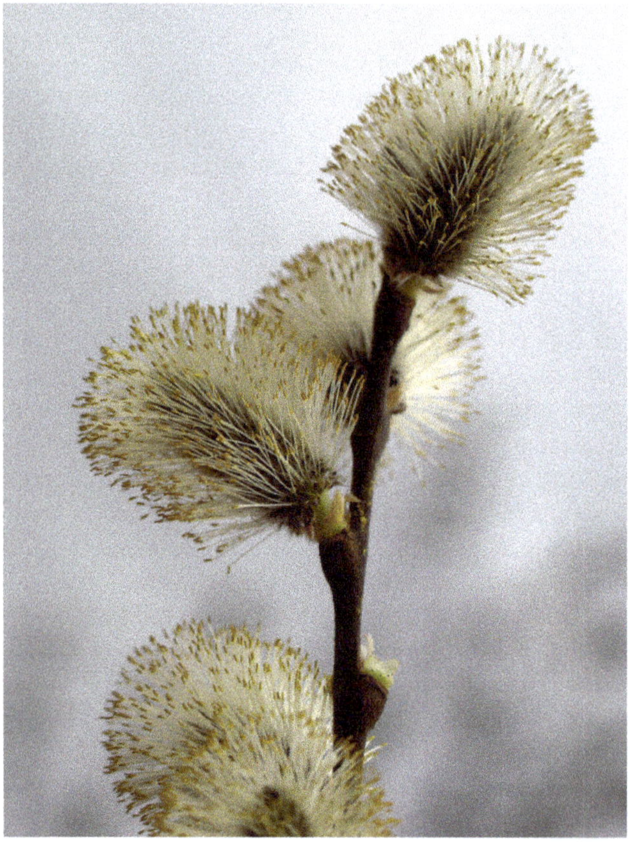

and *purpurea* ("purple"). The epithet *pentandra* refers to the male flowers having five stamens. The common name willow derives from the Old English name for the tree: *welig*.

The following common names correspond with the Latin names: white willow and European willow *(Salix alba);* crack willow and brittle willow *(S. fragilis);* black willow, catkins willow, and pussy willow *(S. nigra);* European willow and bay willow *(S. pentandra);* and purple willow, purple osier, and basket willow *(S. purpurea).* Jara and jarita derive from the old Spanish *xara* ("shaft"), or from the Arabic *xara* ("branch").[5] Willow is commonly known as *jarita* in New Mexican Spanish.[5]

HISTORICAL USES: Willow was used medicinally in early Egypt, Greece, and Assyria.[1] Ancient Greek practitioners, including Dioscorides, Hippocrates, and Galen advised patients to chew on the bark to relieve a fever or inflammation.[1] In medieval Europe, the herb was used to treat headaches, pain, arthritis, gout, colds, heartburn, and fever.[1] Topical preparations were applied to treat burns, sores, cuts, and rashes.[1]

In medieval times, wearing sprigs of willow signified grief and mourning. Rejected or forsaken lovers wore garlands of the leaves and branches.[1] Magic wands made from willow were said to be sorcerers' favorites. Willow baskets carried the offerings and sacrifices of ancient Druid priests.[1] The word "witchcraft" derives from willow, as willow branches were used to bind birch twigs on ash stakes for witches' brooms.[1] Willow branches were kept in homes for protection and to guard against evil; some people believed that evil could be averted by knocking on a willow tree.[1]

Native American tribes including the Cherokee, Blackfoot, and Iroquois administered willow bark to relieve headaches, fever, and muscle and joint pain.[1] In the southwestern U.S., the leaves and small willow branches *(S. exigua)* were chewed to firm gums and treat pyorrhea.[5] Pima, Apache, Mohave, Winnebago, and Dakota consumed a decoction of willow leaves and bark as a febrifuge.[5] A bath of crushed willow bark infused in water was used for dye and to cure the hides of goats, dogs, deer, and cows; tanned hides were used to make shoes.[5] Willow was used to make structures, sweat lodges, baskets, and other woven surfaces.

Eclectic physicians prepared fresh willow catkins (aments), claiming that they were medicinally superior to any other portion of the tree. Finley Ellingwood describes the uses of *Salix nigra* catkins that differ from the current uses of willow bark:

> This agent was brought to the attention of the profession through its influence in controlling sexual hyperesthesia and undue sexual excitement. It is a remedy for satyriasis, erotomania and nymphomania, more particularly from local irritation. It relieves spermatorrhea when dependent upon these or similar causes, and quiets the general nervous system. It is a remedy for ovarian congestion, ovarian neuralgia and hyperesthesia, also for ovarian irritation and hysteria. It will exercise a direct and satisfactory influence in many cases of hysteria, overcoming the extreme excitability and nervousness, headache, and the globus hystericus, and will permit quiet, restful sleep. It will serve an excellent purpose in these cases in combination with general nerve tonics and restoratives, greatly enhancing their influence.[6]

Eclectic physician Harvey Felter describes similar uses for catkins:

> *Salix nigra* is a remedy of great value in a restricted field in therapeutics. While the bark and its preparations have long been recognized as possessing antiseptic and detergent properties, the use of the aments is of more recent date and confined almost wholly to the generative organs. Above all other uses, its greatest value is in that form of sexual erethism, and irritability due chiefly to an irritative condition of the urethra resulting in spermatorrhoea…it proves a decided and valuable anaphrodisiac and tonic. The mental emotions play a lesser part in the disorders requiring *Salix nigra,* but when the genital tract is sensitive, when the bladder becomes more involved, and when sexual excesses and masturbation are the causal factors, it is a remedy of first importance. Secondarily…it will be found to moderate passion and strengthen the reproductive tract when pollutions are the result of sexual intemperance, libidinous thoughts by day, and lascivious dreams by night.[7]

Unfortunately, during that era, the sexist attitudes of some medical practitioners subjugated women by diagnosing them with conditions such as "hysteria" and "neurasthenia."

The constituent salicin, the active ingredient in aspirin, was isolated in Munich in 1828 by Johann Buchner. In 1838, Raffaele Piria prepared the first pure form of salicylic acid from willow bark when he was a student in Paris.[8] German chemist, Hermann Kolbe, synthesized salicylic acid in Marburg and Leipzig in 1860.[8] In the late 1900s, acetylsalicylic acid (aspirin) was synthesized.[1] The use of willow declined following the introduction of aspirin.

CONSTITUENTS: Willow bark contains tannins, catechin tannins, and phenol glycosides (salicin = salicyl alcohol, salicortin, 2'-acetyl-salicortin, and populin), flavonoids (isosalipurposide and isoquercitrin), phenolic acids (caffeic, syringic, and ferulic acids), apigenin, and fragilin. The content of salicin and related compounds of willow bark varies among species and according to harvesting period.[1,9,10]

NUTRITIONAL PROPERTIES: Willow bark contains average to high amounts of ash, calcium, calories, carbohydrates, cobalt, crude fiber, dietary fiber, iron, magnesium, manganese, niacin, phosphorus, riboflavin, selenium, silicon, tin, and zinc. It contains low amounts of aluminum, potassium, protein, sodium, tin, and vitamins C.[11]

MEDICINAL PROPERTIES: Anti-inflammatory, astringent, analgesic, antipyretic, cooling diaphoretic, sudorific, antioxidant, and antiseptic.

TEMPERATURE AND FLAVOR: Cool, astringent, bitter, and mildly sweet.

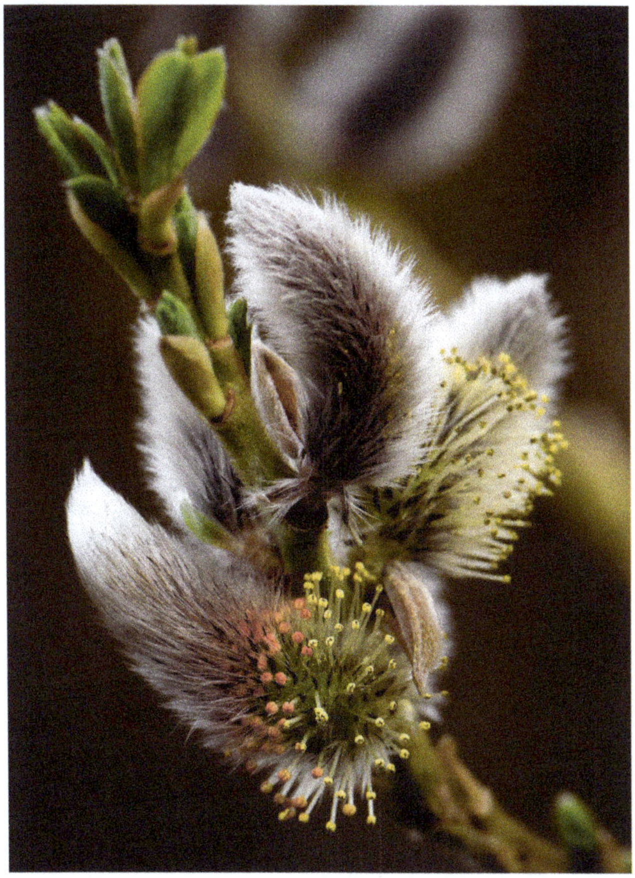

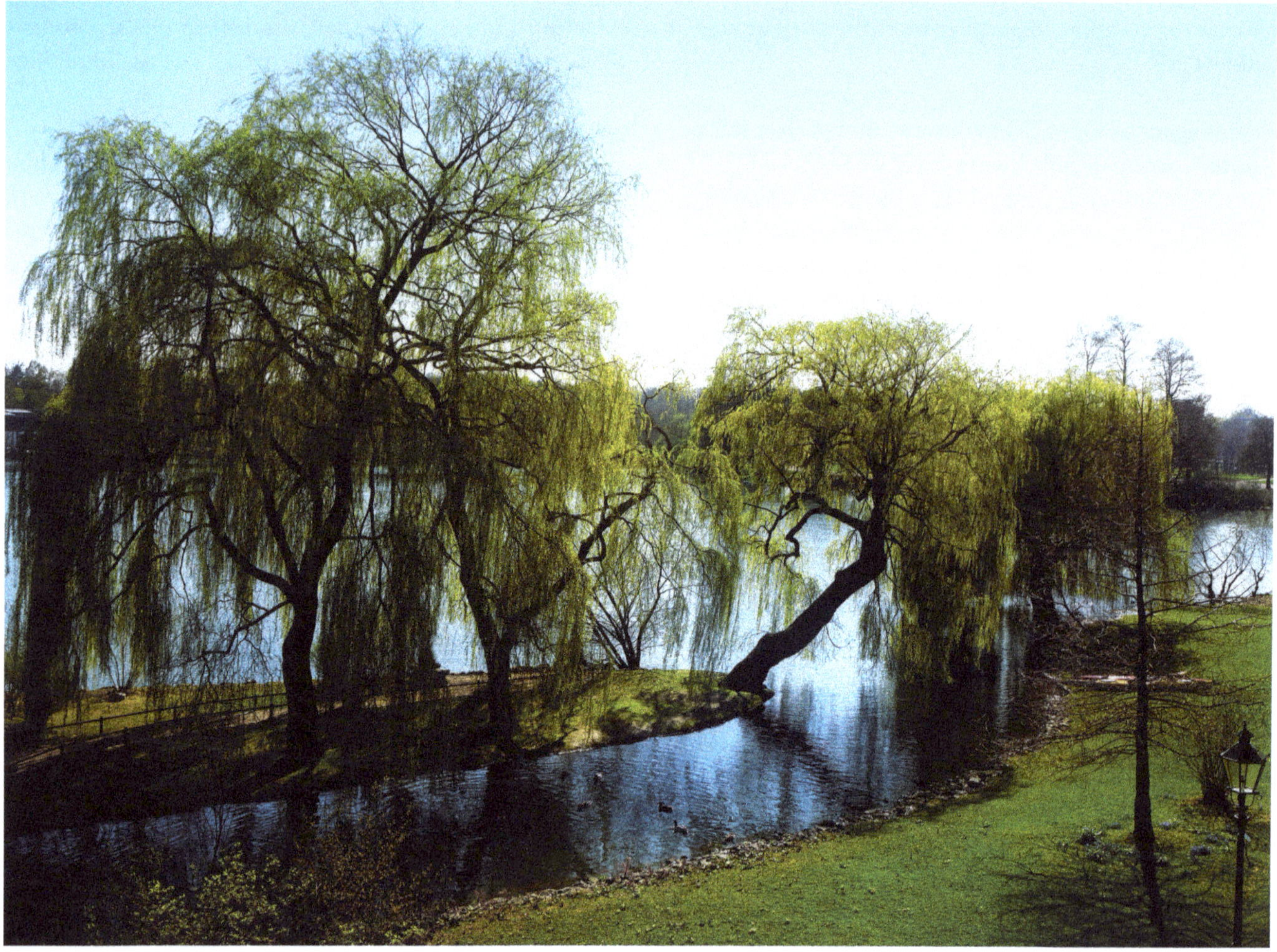

MEDICINAL USES

Willow bark has subtle anti-inflammatory and analgesic actions. The anti-inflammatory actions aid in treating acute and chronic muscle or joint pain, fever, and headache. Willow bark also can be useful for reducing inflammation caused by conditions such as fibromyalgia, arthritis, and rheumatic pain. Willow bark can be combined with meadowsweet *(Filipendula)*, Jamaican dogwood *(Piscidia)*, and St. John's wort *(Hypericum)* as an internal anti-inflammatory compound for pain management. A hot willow bark bath or fomentation has an astringent anti-inflammatory action, and can be applied directly to the affected area.

Willow bark contains the glycoside salicin and related glycosides that liberate salicyl alcohol in the intestinal tract. The salicyl alcohol is then converted in the liver to the active principle salicylic acid, the precursor to acetylsalicylic acid (aspirin).[1,9] Acetylsalicylic acid is the active principle in aspirin. Because salicin lacks the acetyl residue of aspirin that binds to thromboxane synthetase of platelets, willow bark doesn't influence the biosynthesis of platelets (thrombocytes). Therefore, willow bark does not have a blood-thinning effect. The salicin content of willow inhibits prostaglandins and reduces the inflammatory response. However, as a result of the conversion in the liver, the actions are more subtle, but longer lasting than aspirin, and without the side effects.[1]

Willow is a sudorific, antipyretic, and cooling diaphoretic that aids in reducing fever. Consume one cup of hot willow bark tea every hour or two to treat a fever. Alternatively, prepare two quarts of a hot decoction, and strain the tea into a lukewarm bath to reduce a fever and accompanying aches and pains. Make a cooling sudorific tea by combining willow bark with meadowsweet *(Filipendula)*, elder flowers *(Sambucus nigra)*, yarrow *(Achillea)*, chamomile *(Matricaria)*, and/or peppermint *(Mentha piperita)*.

Willow bark is an astringent and mild hemostatic. Consuming the tea reduces inflammation or bleeding in the digestive tract. The tea also aids in treating diarrhea. Gargling with the tea alleviates a sore throat. A sitz bath of willow bark tea soothes inflammation of the labia and rectum. Apply the wash as a topical astringent for poison oak, poison ivy, cuts, abrasions, skin ulcers, bruises, sprains,

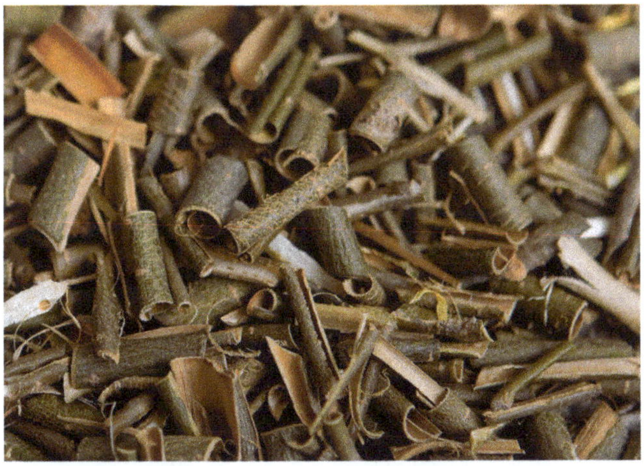

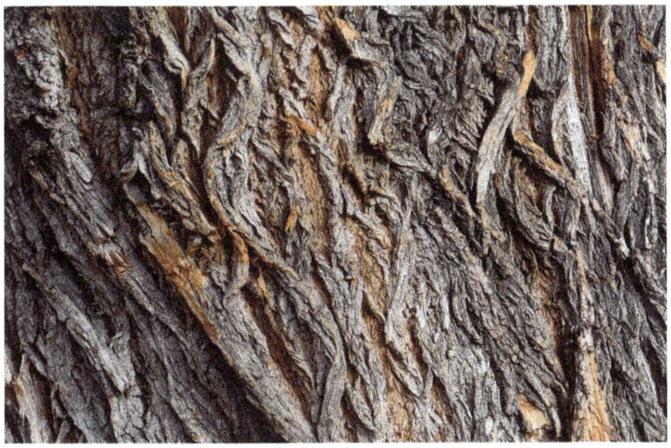

and moist skin conditions such as eczema. A tea or wash also has mild antiseptic properties for infected wounds, lacerations, or ulcerations.

A decoction made from willow bark or a cold infusion of the fresh twig tips enhances rooting when propagating plants. Dip freshly cut stems in cooled tea before planting; continue watering the plants with willow tea daily until they root.

CONTRAINDICATIONS

Although willow bark contains salicin (not salicylic acid), it does not contain the acetyl residue of aspirin that prevents blood clotting. However, to err on the side of caution, avoid consuming willow bark two weeks prior to, and following surgery and delivery. Also consider avoiding internal use of willow bark in individuals consuming anticoagulant medications or involved in immunosuppressant organ transplant therapy. In all cases, avoid internal use of willow bark in individuals with aspirin allergies.[10] The salicylates can cause an allergic reaction in hypersensitive individuals. High doses of willow bark can cause gastrointestinal irritation including nausea, upset stomach, or constipation.

PREPARATION AND DOSAGE

TINCTURE: Fresh bark [1:2-1:3, 70-95% alcohol] or [1:3, 50% alcohol, 40% water, 10% glycerin]; dry bark [1:5, 60% alcohol]; consume 30-90 drops, up to four times daily.

CAPSULES: Willow bark capsules or tablets standardized to the phenol glycosides content are preferable for optimum anti-inflammatory effects. Consume 2-4 "00" capsules, up to three times daily.

TEA: Prepare a decoction or cold infusion; consume 8-12 ounces, up to four times daily.

TOPICAL USE: Apply a hot fomentation, poultice, wash, or bath.

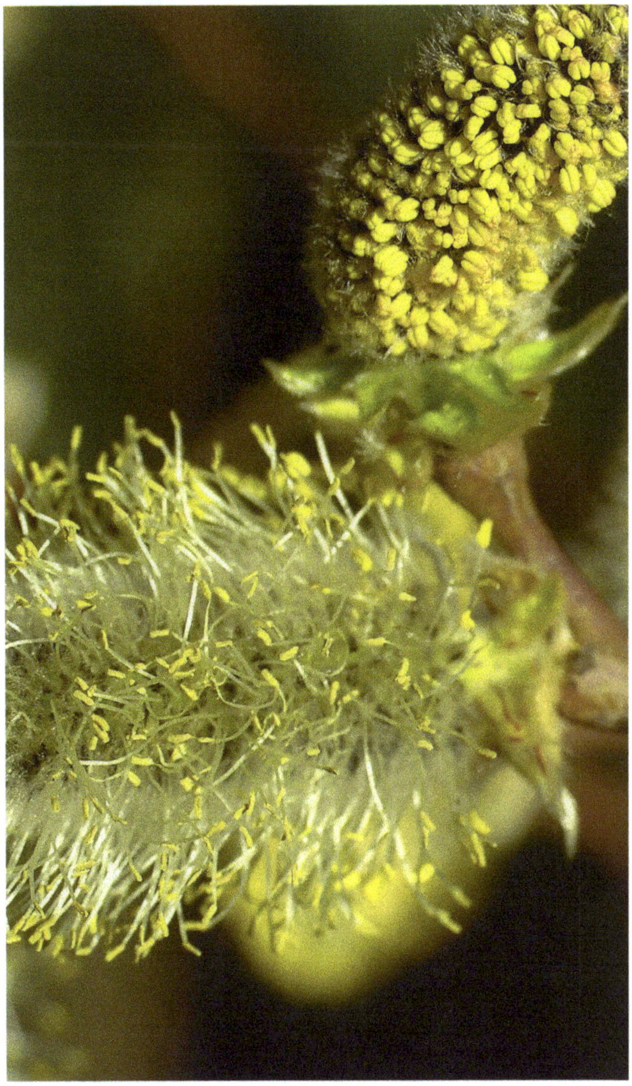

YARROW

DESCRIPTION

BOTANICAL NAME:
Achillea millefolium

COMMON NAMES:
Yarrow, yarroway, milfoil, knight's milfoil, woundwort, soldier's woundwort, carpenter's weed, staunchweed, nosebleed, devil's nettle, devil's plaything, bad man's plaything, old man's pepper, thousand weed, sanguinary
yerw (Dutch)
herba millitaris (Latin)
gearwe (Saxon)
plumajillo (Spanish)
field hop (Swedish)[1]

FAMILY NAME:
Asteraceae (Compositae)

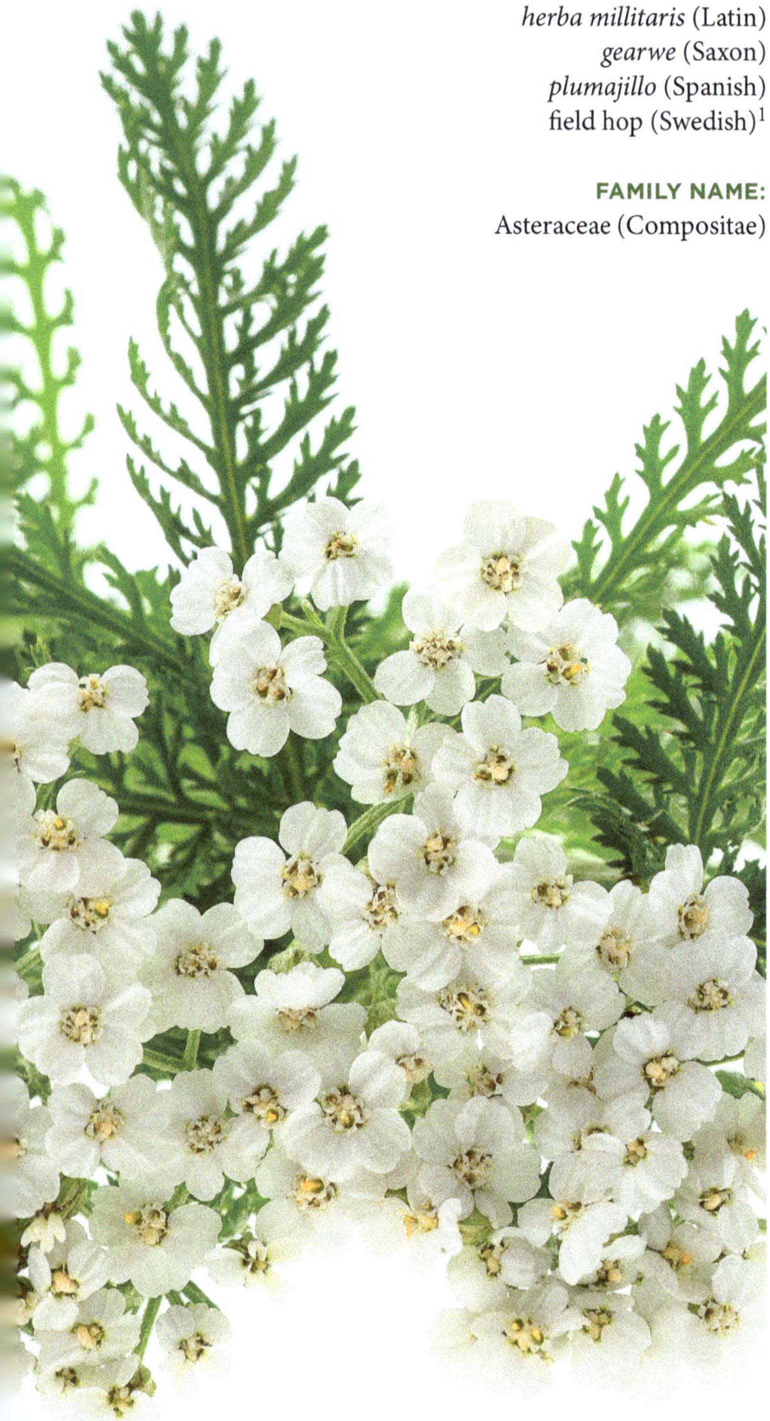

PARTS USED: The flowers and foliage (above ground parts of the plant).

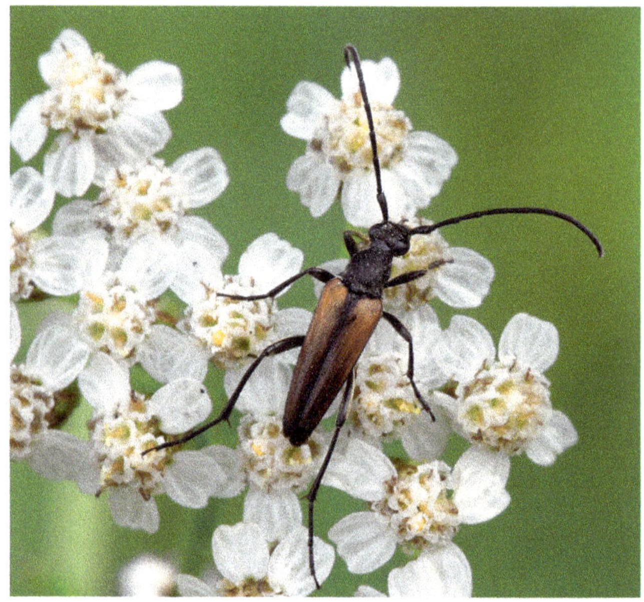

BOTANICAL DESCRIPTION AND HABITAT: Yarrow grows in Europe, and throughout the U.S. West Coast and inland mountains. Yarrow also grows in dry, sandy soil, and in sunny meadows throughout the Midwest and East Coast. It has a circumboreal distribution, and grows up to 3,500 meters in elevation.[2]

Yarrow displays significant variation in size, depending on its local habitat. It usually grows 30 – 75 cm tall, but can be as short as 10 cm when exposed to the harsh environment of salt spray and ocean wind, or in high elevations with short growing seasons, late snow melt, or high winds.[3] The *Jepson Manual* also states that it can grow up to 200 cm tall.[2]

Yarrow is an herbaceous perennial with a distinct aroma. It has alternate, lacey, thrice-pinnately compound leaves with leaf bases that sheath around the stem. When not flowering, yarrow forms a basal rosette; otherwise, it has a caulescent form. The fine downy hairs on the stem and leaves vary in quantity.

The inflorescence is a corymb of many radiate heads; each head bears several series of phyllaries (4 – 9 mm long).[2] There are 3 – 8 ray flowers per head (2.5 to 4 mm long), with ovate to round ligules, each with three lobes.[2] There are 15 – 40 disk flowers per head, each with five-petalled, connate corollas (2 – 3 mm long).[2] Each flower in the head is associated with a chaff, a small, narrow bract attached to the receptacle.[2] It has no pappus, unlike many other Asteraceae flowers.[4] The ligules and corollas range from white to pink, with the white considered most medicinally active.[2] The fruit is a small oblong to ovate achene (about 2 mm long).[2]

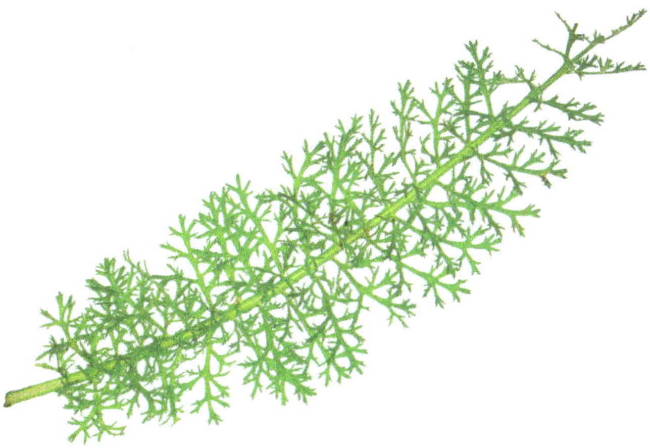

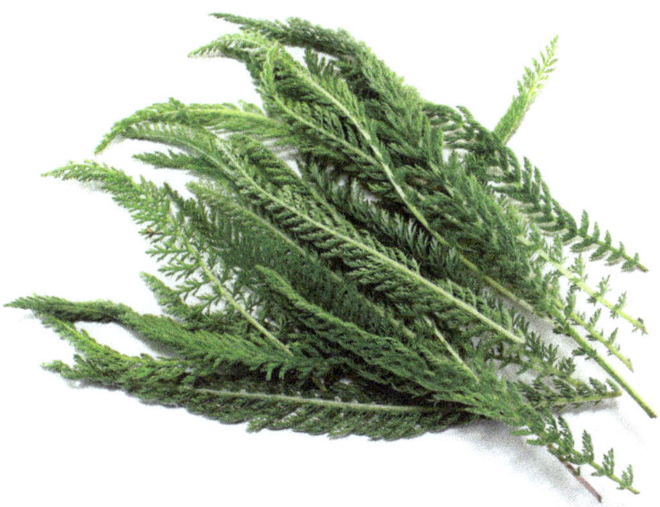

THE NAME: The Latin name *Achillea* derives from Achilles, the famous Greek mythological warrior who used the plant to staunch soldiers' bleeding during the Trojan War.[1,5] The epithet *millefolium* ("many leaves") refers to the finely divided leaves, as do milfoil and thousand weed.[1] The common name yarrow originated from the Anglo-Saxon and Dutch gearwe and yerw.[1,5] Many common names, including woundwort, bloodwort, staunchweed, and carpenter's weed refer to the plant's use for treating bleeding wounds. The names soldier's wound wort and knight's milfoil attest to the plant's use as a vulnerary.[1] Yarrow also was referred to as herba militaris, the military herb, due to its use in staunching soldiers' bleeding wounds.[1] Devil's nettle, devil's plaything, and bad man's plaything refer to the plant's association with divination and the devil.[1] Swedes refer to the plant as field hop because it was an ingredient in beer.[1] The Spanish name, plumajillo ("little feather"), refers to the feather foliage.[6]

HISTORICAL USES: Linnaeus applied fresh, bruised leaves as a vulnerary and styptic.[1] Culpeper recommended yarrow as an antispasmodic, and for ague. In Scotland, an ointment made from the fresh herb was applied to piles.[1] In Norway, fresh leaves were chewed to cure a toothache. The herb was used as snuff and referred to as "old man's pepper." The Swedes called yarrow "field hop" due to its use in brewing beer. Yarrow was an ingredient in salads in the 17th century. Washing the scalp with yarrow tea was believed to prevent baldness.[1]

Yarrow was among the witches' herbs brought to weddings to ensure seven years of love.[6] It was regarded as a love charm, especially when gathered by a lovelorn maiden from the grave of a young man.[6] Yarrow was used for divining.[1]

Yarrow was widely utilized medicinally throughout North America. Native Americans consumed yarrow tea to alleviate fevers, headaches, and stomachaches, and to purify blood.[7] The tea was administered to treat bronchitis, colds, coughs, diarrhea, and measles.[8] Zunis believed that the leaves produced a cooling sensation when applied to the skin. They chewed yarrow blossoms and roots, and anointed their bodies with yarrow prior to ceremonies involving fire dancing.[6]

Yarrow tea was consumed as a childbirth medicine and applied to desensitize breasts following childbirth.[7,8] It was gargled to alleviate a sore throat.[8] A poultice prepared from chopped leaves was applied to bruises, sprains, swellings, wounds, sores, burns, rheumatic joints, and broken bones,

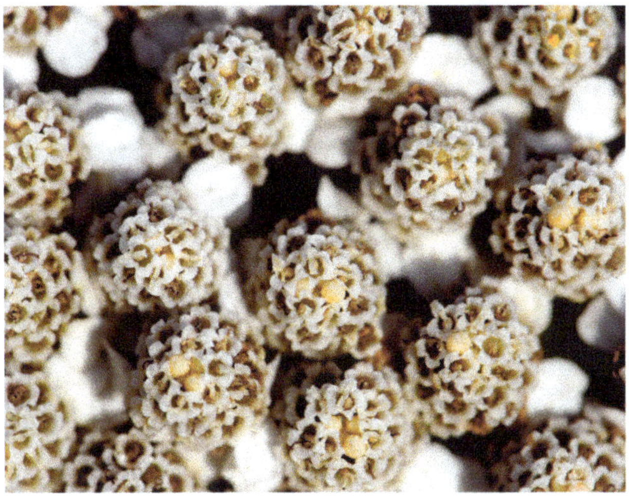

and to stop the bleeding of wounds.[6-8] Root and leaf poultices were applied to reduce toothaches.[7] A wash of the tea was applied to insect stings, snakebites, and sore eyes.[7]

Eclectic physicians prescribed yarrow to allay passive hemorrhaging. They administered the herb for hematuria, sanguineous discharge, and menorrhagia, as well as uterine and intestinal bleeding.[9-11] Yarrow was given as an astringent for bleeding piles, dysentery, profuse mucus secretion, and leukorrhea; it was often combined with *Lycopus virginicus* for this purpose.[10] Yarrow was used as a diaphoretic, and to alleviate tonsillitis or a chronic cough.[9] Additionally, it was administered to treat delayed menses, nervous debility, incontinence, and flatulent colic, to remove obstructions, and as a blood purifier for autotoxemia.[9,10] Yarrow was believed to tone the urinary tract, alleviate irritation, and encourage urine flow when suppressed.[9,12] Dr. Cole, an Eclectic physician, considered yarrow an effective remedy for epididymitis, especially if the patient had a fever of at least 100 degrees.[9]

CONSTITUENTS: Yarrow contains volatile oil (azulene, α- and β-pinene, caryophyllene, borneol, terpineol, cineole, bornyl acetate, camphor, camphene, *p*-cymene, limonene, sabinene, and isoartemisia ketone), lactones (achillin, millefin, and deacetylmatricarine), flavonids (rutin), tannins, resin, coumarins, saponins, sterols (β-sitosterol), alkanes (tricosane, heptadecane, and pentacosane), fatty acids (linoleic, palmatic, and oleic acids), sugars (glucose, sucrose, arabinose, inositol, dulcitol, and mannitol), alkaloids or bases (achilleine, betaine, choline, trigonelline, betonicine, and stachydrine), amino acids (alanine, leucine, lysine, histidine, and glutamic acid), and acids (salicylic acid and succinic acid).[5,13-15]

NUTRITIONAL PROPERTIES: Yarrow contains average to high amounts of ash, calcium, chromium, dietary fiber, magnesium, manganese, phosphorus, protein, potassium, riboflavin, selenium, silicon, thiamine, tin, and vitamin C. It contains low amounts of aluminum, crude fiber, and sodium.[16]

MEDICINAL PROPERTIES: Antibacterial, anti-inflammatory, amphoteric, antipyretic, astringent, bitter tonic, carminative, cholagogue, diaphoretic, diuretic, emmenagogue, expectorant, hemostatic, hypotensive, mild immune stimulant, sudorific, vasodilator, and vulnerary.

TEMPERATURE AND FLAVOR: Cool, bitter, pungent, astringent, salty, and mildly sweet.

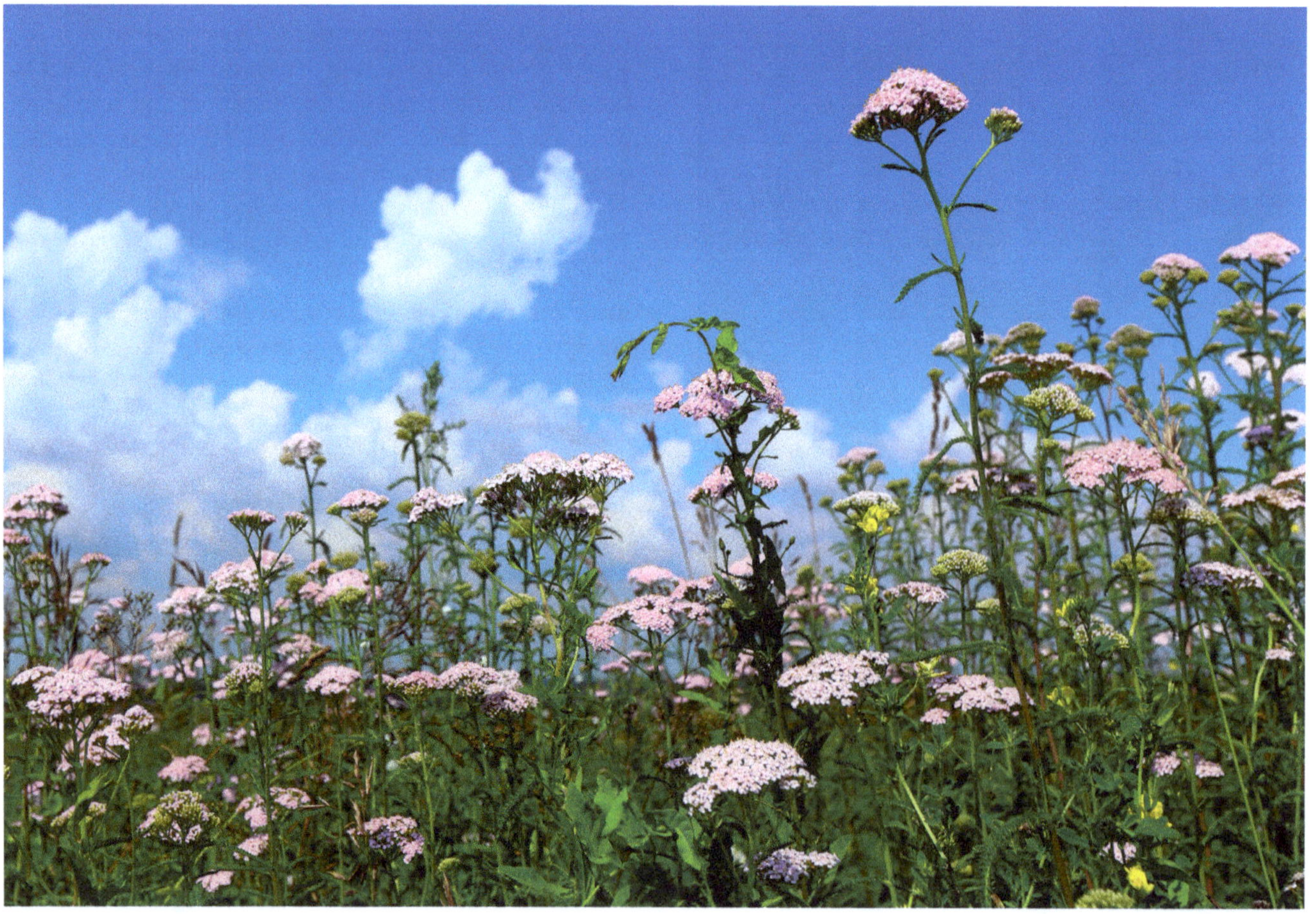

MEDICINAL USES

Yarrow has a wide range of medicinal actions. It is a cooling diaphoretic and sudorific. Consuming the hot tea frequently (or placing the tincture in hot water) works most effectively to break a fever. Yarrow was specifically indicated for sthenic fevers with a hot, dry, burning sensation in the skin and suppressed secretion.[9,15] Yarrow encourages secretions and causes skin to become moist, soft, and supple. Eclectic physician Dr. John Fearn stated:

> [Yarrow] has a stimulating action which will be a revelation to those who have not used it. It causes the sudoriferous glands to literally pour out their secretions. In fevers of the sthenic type, when we desire to arouse the skin, nothing can surpass this remedy. The patient is covered warmly in bed and a hot infusion of yarrow is given in frequent doses... In cases of severe fever, intermittent or bilious fever, it will cause the secretions to be poured out so freely as to discolor the bed clothes.[9]

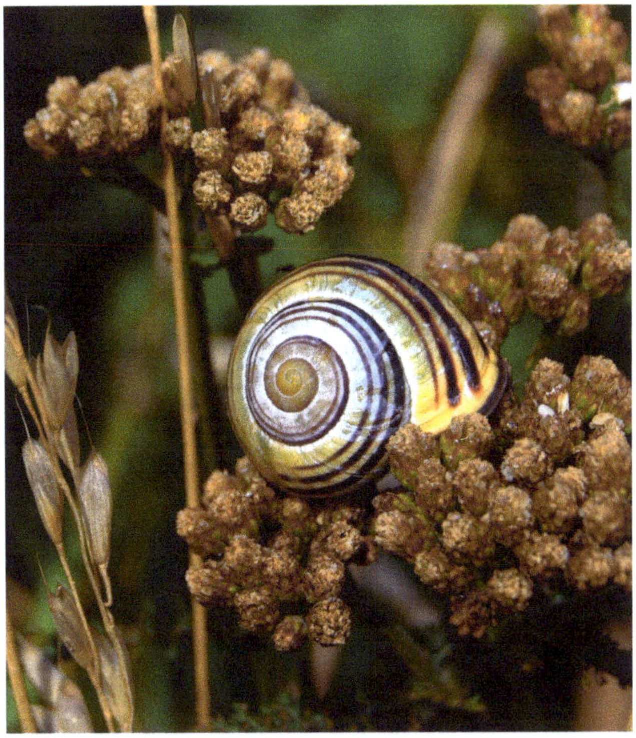

Yarrow contains volatile oils and bitters that stimulate secretions in the respiratory mucosa. It has expectorant actions that reduce lung congestion.[5] Due to its astringent properties, yarrow also reduces excessive mucus secretion. It balances and restores secretions in the upper and lower respiratory mucosa, and aids in treating sinusitis, allergies, hay fever, and colds.[5] Yarrow is a mild antibacterial and white blood cell stimulant.

Yarrow has mild choleretic, cholagogue, and bitter tonic actions that stimulate digestive secretions.[13,18] When consumed prior to a meal, it aids in digesting fats and proteins. The bitter tonic and hepatobiliary actions are attributed to the bitter sesquiterpene lactones, proline-betaines, phenolic acids, and alkaloid content.[13,18]

Yarrow has astringent anti-inflammatory properties that tone mucous membranes. It reduces inflammation in the digestive tract, treating mild forms of diarrhea, and decreasing residual inflammation following stomach flu, food poisoning, gastroenteritis, chronic dysentery, and giardia.[9] Consuming yarrow tea (warm or room temperature) aids in treating flareups of colitis, diverticulitis, irritable bowel syndrome, and hemorrhoids. The tea or tincture reduces bleeding in the digestive tract, ulcers, and hemorrhoids.

Yarrow tea and tincture have many properties for treating urinary tract infections such as cystitis and urethritis.[17] It is a mild antibacterial agent and diuretic, and soothes the urinary tract.[11] It astringes mucous membranes and reduces inflammation, pain, and hematuria (small amounts of blood in the urine). Some patients can treat urinary tract infections solely with yarrow; however, it is important to include several additional antibacterial agents, such as usnea *(Usnea)*, uva ursi *(Artcostaphylos)*, and corn silk *(Zea)*. Additionally, teas containing diuretic and demulcent herbs such as parsley root *(Petroselinum)* and corn silk *(Zea)* soothe the urinary tract.

The tincture, cold infusion, and tepid tea have vasodilating and blood pressure-lowering properties.[5] Also useful for calming the mind, it works for temperamental, anabolic individuals prone to patterns of heat or a flushed face with a full, bounding pulse. It works well when combined with other blood pressure-lowering herbs such as hawthorn *(Crataegus)* and dandelion leaf *(Taraxacum)*. Yarrow contains alkaloids that have hypotensive actions.[13]

Yarrow tea (cold infusion or hot infusion served at room temperature) or tincture is effective as a hemostatic for a passive hemorrhage. Yarrow reduces bleeding in the intestinal and urinary tracts.[9,10] It also reduces excessive bleeding resulting from menstruation, ovarian or uterine cysts, fibroids, or Mettelschmertz.[9,17] Yarrow staunches postpartum bleeding and bleeding resulting from menopausal hormone imbalances. It can be used to reduce nosebleeds, as well as bloody sputum.[9] Mouth rinses containing yarrow reduce bleeding in the gums. Yarrow contains the alkaloid achilleine that reduces clotting time.[5]

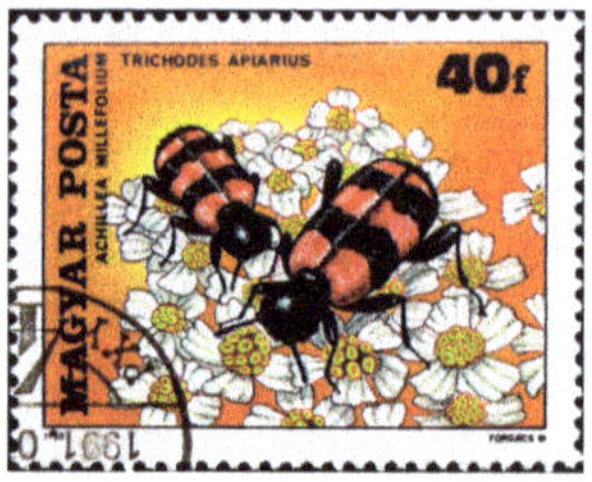

Yarrow can be combined with cinnamon *(Cinnamomum)*, shepherd's purse *(Capsella)*, and Canadian fleabane *(Erigeron)* as a hemostatic. Consuming the herb works best for internal bleeding; topical applications reduce bleeding from cuts and bruises.

Conversely, frequently consuming small quantities of a hot infusion of yarrow tea acts as an emmenagogue that stimulates suppressed or delayed menstruation.[10,17] Yarrow reduces stagnation of blood in the uterus and decreases menstrual blood clotting.[17] It also stimulates the expulsion of suppressed lochia.[10]

Yarrow was administered by the Ancient Greeks for its vulnerary (wound-healing) actions.[9] Topical applications of yarrow aid in treating varicose veins, spider veins, and hemorrhoids.[15,17] Yarrow contains flavonoids that strengthen the vasculature and reduce venous distention.[5] It contains anti-inflammatory tannins.[5] Yarrow aids in treating most first aid skin conditions, such as cuts, bruises, abrasions, sprains, and strains, as well as carpal tunnel and tendonitis flareups.[15,17,19,20] A poultice of yarrow leaf or root reduces a toothache or gum pain.[15,17]

YARROW ESSENTIAL OIL

Yarrow essential oil has cooling anti-inflammatory and analgesic actions. It stimulates cell regeneration and helps to prevent scarring.[19] Yarrow essential oil can be applied neat, diluted in a carrier oil, or added to a salve to treat bruises, sprains, strained muscles, tendonitis, neuralgia, arthritis, carpal tunnel, and varicose veins.[19,20] Topical applications of yarrow essential oil also aid in treating inflammatory skin conditions, including eczema, dermatitis, acne, psoriasis, and poison oak.[20] Applying the diluted essential oil reduces gum inflammation, treating dental abscesses, gingivitis, and canker sores.[19] Yarrow essential oil with a blue hue contains chamazulene, a calming constituent also found in blue chamomile.[19] *Note:* If the essential oil is light yellow or green, it doesn't contain chamazulene.[19]

CONTRAINDICATIONS

Avoid consumption during pregnancy, except during delivery. Avoid long-term use of yarrow in high doses. Yarrow can cause contact dermatitis in individuals who are hypersensitive to Asteraceae family plants; discontinue use if this occurs.[13]

Note: Although yarrow is a hemostatic, individuals with severe bleeding or a hemorrhage should seek immediate medical attention. Yarrow can be effective for treating urinary tract infections; however, if the infection travels into the kidneys causing a high fever or severe back pain, seek immediate medical attention.

Yarrow essential oil contains ketones; therefore, it should not be used by children younger than 10, or by pregnant women.[19]

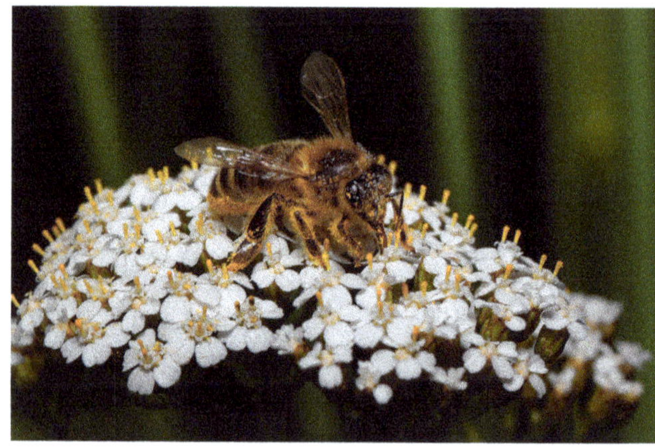

PREPARATION AND DOSAGE

TINCTURE: Fresh flowers and leaves [1:2-1:3, 75-95% alcohol]; dry flowers [1:5-1:6, 60% alcohol]; consume 10-60 drops, up to four times daily.

GLYCERITE: Fresh flowers and leaves [1:3, 50% glycerin, 50% alcohol]; consume 10-60 drops, up to four times daily.

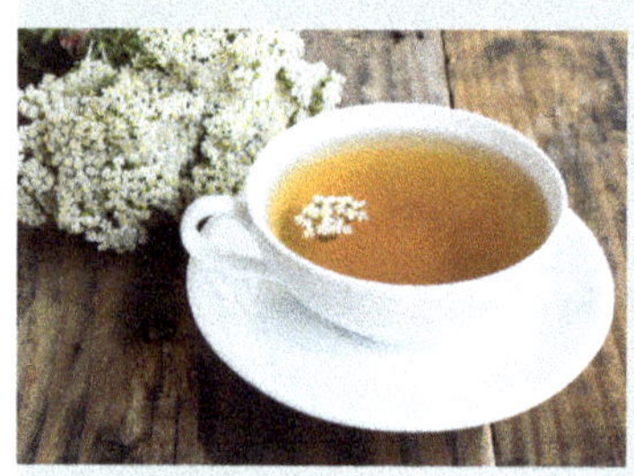

TEA: Prepare a hot or cold infusion; consume 4-8 ounces, up to four times daily. Avoid boiling the herb, or the volatile oil will be destroyed. Keep the lid on the vessel to prevent aromatic oils from evaporating.

TOPICAL USE: Infuse the fresh wilted leaf and flower in oil using the Simpler's method, or use the alcohol intermediary method to infuse the dry leaf and flower in oil. Apply 1-2 drops of the essential oil neat, or dilute in a base oil or salve.

YELLOW DOCK

DESCRIPTION

BOTANICAL NAMES:
Rumex crispus, R. obtusifolius, R. aquatica

COMMON NAMES:
Yellow dock, dock, curly dock, curled dock, sour dock, narrow dock, garden patience, water dock, butter dock, common wayside dock
poimuhierakka (Finnish)
churelle, herbe britannique, oreille de vache, parielle, rhubarbe sauvage (French)
gelber ampfer, grindampfer, krauser ampfer, mengelwurz, wilder mangolt, zitterwurz (German)
erba britannica, romice (Italian)
amlavetasa (Sanskrit)
acedera, lengua de vaca (Spanish)
krusskräppa, krussyra (Swedish)

FAMILY NAME:
Polygonaceae

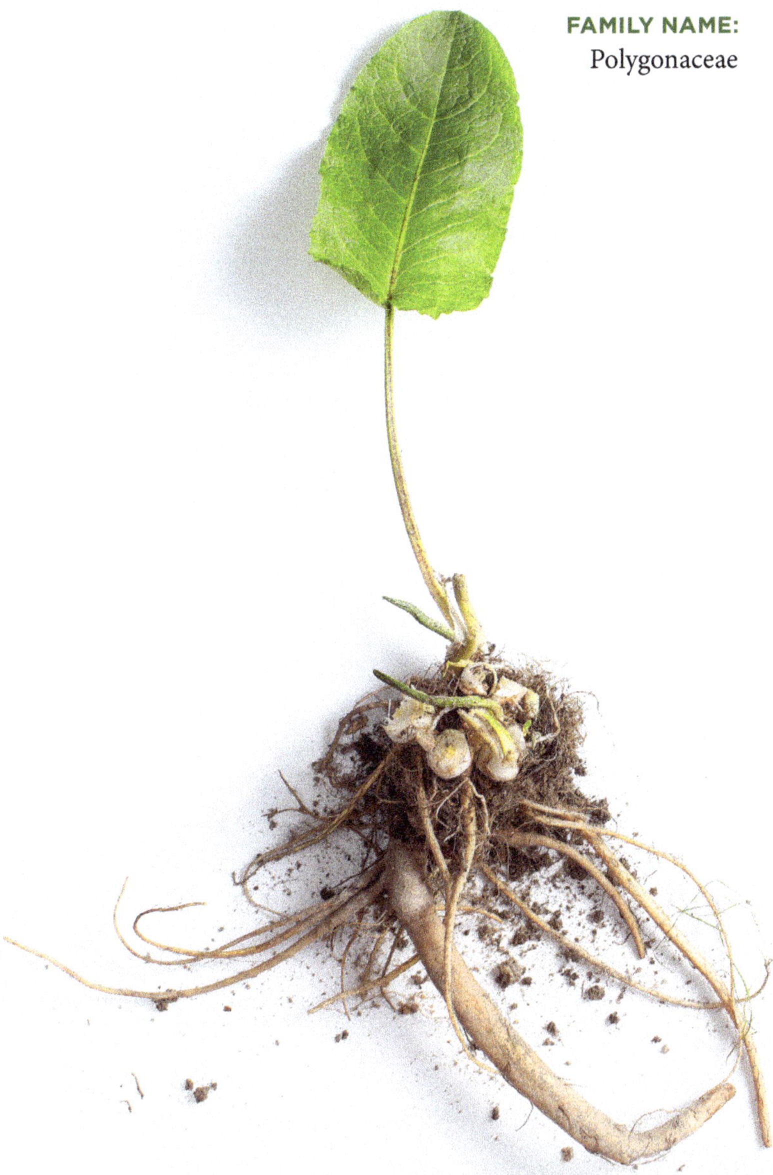

PART USED: The roots.

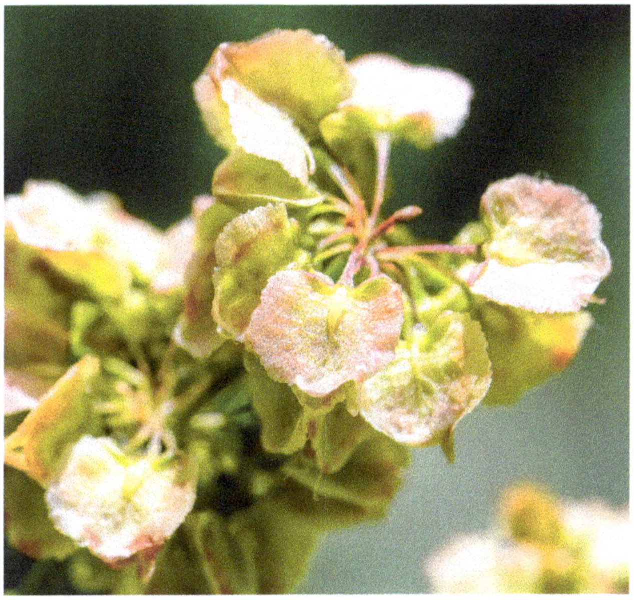

BOTANICAL DESCRIPTION AND HABITAT: Yellow dock is a prolific perennial weed (up to 120 cm tall) that grows in moist soils.[1] It is native to Europe and Africa, and has naturalized throughout the U.S.[2] Yellow dock has a large, slender, fibrous taproot with a brown cork and yellow cortex. The dark green, lanceolate leaves (15 – 30 cm long by 2 – 6 cm wide) have a truncate to cordate base, wavy margins, and acute tips; older leaves are often covered with reddish-brown spots.[3] Leaves growing toward the base of the erect stems have longer petioles, and are larger than the upper leaves. Whorls of drooping, pale green flowers consisting of six tepals (4 – 6 mm long by 3 – 5 mm wide), six stamens, and three plumose styles grow in loose panicles.[3,4] The small, heart-shaped fruit is a three-angled achene (2 – 3 mm long by 2 mm wide) enclosed by three papery wings ranging from red to light green.[4]

THE NAME: The genus *Rumex* ("a lance") derives from Latin, and refers to the leaf shape.[5] The former genus name *Lapathum* was derived from the Greek *lapazien* ("to cleanse").[2,6] The epithet *crispus* ("crisped") derives from Latin, referring to the leaves' crisped edges.[6] The epithet *obtusifolius* derives from two Latin words: *obtusus* ("blunt") and *folius* ("leaf"). The epithet *aquaticus* ("relating to water") derives from Latin, referring to the plant growing in moist places. The common name dock has

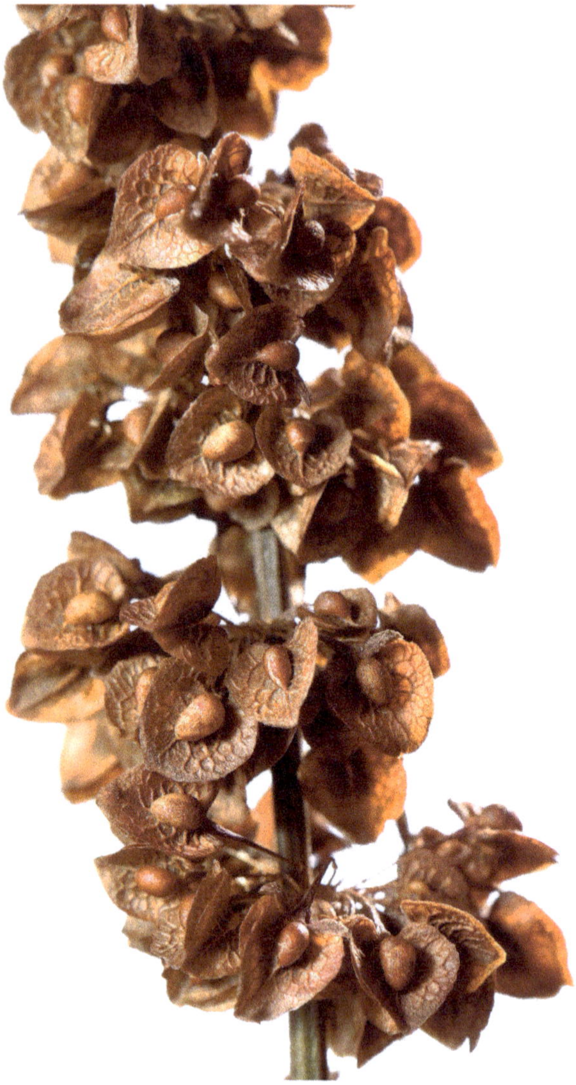

several potential origins. One is from the Middle Dutch or German word *docke* ("ship's berth"), indicating the plant's presence near boating docks where grounded vessels bank in the mud. Another origin refers to the Scandinavian *dokk* ("low ground").[7]

HISTORICAL USES: Yellow dock root has been administered as a blood purifier for liver disorders and skin diseases since the Middle Ages.[2,6,8] Teas and tinctures of the roots were consumed to treat skin conditions including acne, eczema, and boils.[6] Yellow dock was also used as a laxative, a stomach tonic, to relieve a congested liver, and an astringent for bleeding piles.[6] Yellow dock was used to treat chronic enlarged lymph glands, jaundice, gallbladder ailments, diarrhea, constipation, indigestion, dysentery, and anemia.[9]

An ointment was prepared by boiling the root in vinegar until the fibers were soft, then infusing the root pulp in lard.[6] The ointment or poultice was applied topically for scabies, mouth sores, boils, ulcers, burns, itching, athlete's foot, cuts, bruises, and wounds.[9] Native Americans applied poultices of fresh crushed leaves to boils, and pulverized roots to cuts.[8]

Yellow dock was valued by folk herbalists and Eclectic physicians, including Finley Ellingwood, who suggests these uses:

> The alterative properties of this agent are underestimated. It is a renal depurant and general alterative of much value when ulceration of mucous surfaces or diseases of the skin result from impure blood. It acts directly in its restorative influence, purifying the blood, removing morbific material and quickly cures the disease conditions. It is valuable in ulcerative stomatitis, in nursing sore mouth, and in ulceration of the stomach with lack of tone. It has cured exceedingly persistent cases of exhaustive morning diarrhea…it has also been used in the treatment of syphilis and scrofula with good results.[7]

Eclectic physician Harvey Felter describes the conditions in which he administers yellow dock:

> Rumex is decidedly alterative…it should especially be brought into requisition in depraved states of body fluids with tendency to chronic skin disorders, with glandular engorgement, tendency to ulceration, and slow recuperative powers. It is especially valuable in strumous patients with low deposits in the cellular and glandular tissues which break down easily but are slow to repair.[8]

Felter's specific indications for yellow dock are:

> Vitiated blood with chronic skin disorders; low glandular and cellular deposits with tendency to indolent ulcers; feeble recuperative power; chronic sore throat with glandular engorgement and hypersecretion; cough with shortness of breath and prae cordial fullness; dry, irritative laryngo-tracheal cough; stubborn dry summer cough; nervous dyspepsia with epigastric fullness and pain extending into the chest.[11]

Dr. John Scudder recommended yellow dock as an alterative, resolvent, and depurative to strengthen the constitution when treating cutaneous eruptions resulting from scabies, herpes, or syphilis. Additionally, he administered the herb for cancerous tumors or ulcers, scrofula, dental carries, necrosis, morbid conditions of the bones, scurvy, and scorbutic afflictions.[12]

CONSTITUENTS: Yellow dock root contains anthraquinone glycosides (emodin, chrysophanol, oxymethylanthraquinone, and 1,8-dihidroxy-3-methyl-9-anthrone), tannin, 1,8-naphthalenediol (nepodin and its glycoside), brassidinic acid, oxalic acid, rumicin, calcium oxalate, chrysophanein, chrysophanic acid, chrysophanin, erucic acid, lapatinic acid, nepodin, fatty acids, mucilaginous polysaccharides, starch, physcion, rheochrysin, and rumicin.[13-15] The leaves contains avicularin, calcium acetate, calcium maleate, hyperoside, and rumicin.[14]

NUTRITIONAL PROPERTIES: Yellow dock root contains aluminum, ash, calcium, cobalt, crude fiber, dietary fiber, iron, magnesium, manganese, niacin, phosphorus, potassium, protein, riboflavin, selenium, sodium, thiamine, tin, and vitamins A and C.[5] Yellow dock leaves contain ascorbic acid and oxalate crystals, likely potassium oxalate, which should be consumed in limited quantities due to its potential for irritating the kidneys.[5]

MEDICINAL PROPERTIES: Alterative, astringent, bitter tonic, cholagogue, laxative, and nutritive.

TEMPERATURE AND FLAVOR: Cool, bitter, astringent, and sour.

MEDICINAL USES

Yellow dock is a digestive bitter tonic and cholagogue.[13] Consuming the tea or tincture 15–30 minutes prior to a meal aids digestion. Yellow dock primarily stimulates lower digestive secretions, although it has a mild stimulating effect on upper digestive secretions. It enhances the digestion and assimilation of nutrients, including fat, fat-soluble vitamins (A, D, E), proteins, amino acids, B vitamins, and minerals.[14,16] It indirectly helps to prevent osteoporosis by enhancing calcium and magnesium absorption.[16] Vegetarians can consume yellow dock to enhance the assimilation of vitamin B_{12} and other B vitamins.[16] Additionally, yellow dock root contains a considerable quantity of minerals and vitamins A and C, and is therefore considered a nutritive herb.[5] Yellow dock contains moderate quantities of iron and enhances iron absorption; therefore, it is an excellent adjunct for treating iron-deficiency anemia when consumed with iron rich foods or herbs and iron supplements.[16,17] Some herbalists assert that in addition to enhancing iron absorption, yellow dock facilitates the release of iron stores, making it available for hemoglobin production.[16]

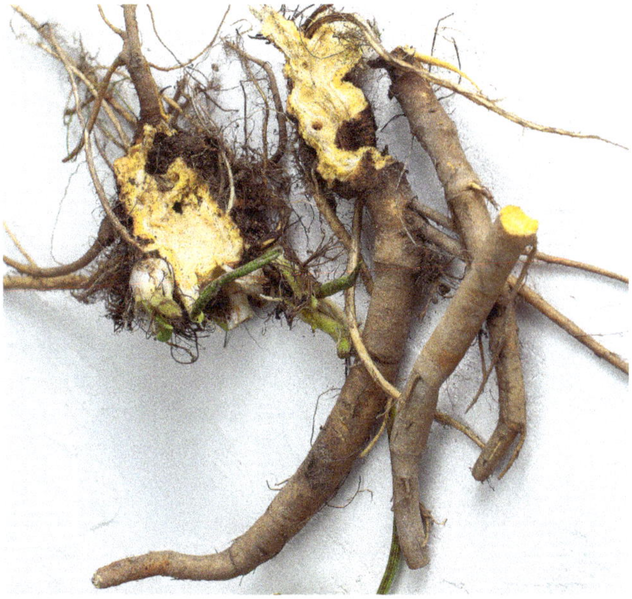

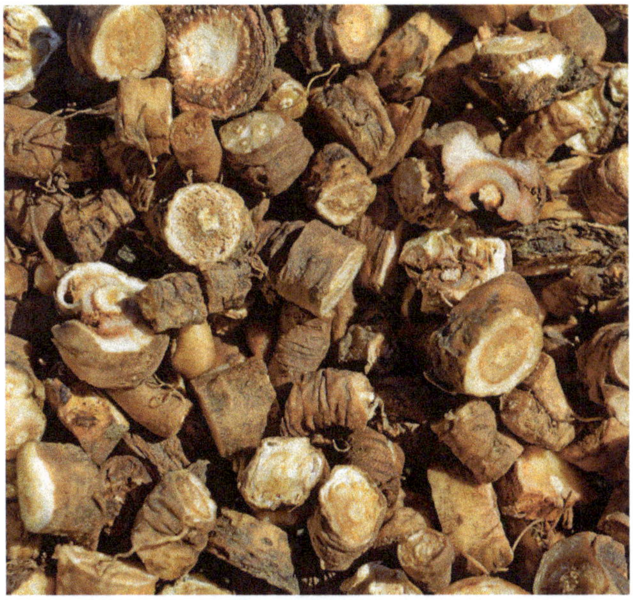

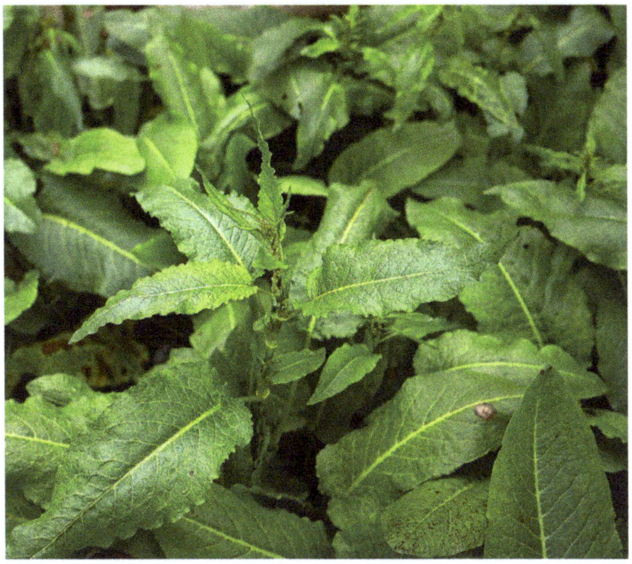

Yellow dock acts as a digestive alterative that normalizes digestive processes. The dosage determines whether the herb has astringent, anti-inflammatory, or laxative actions.[17] Consuming low doses of yellow dock (5 – 15 drops or four ounces of tea) reduces inflammation of the small and large intestines.[17] The astringent actions aid in treating digestive conditions such as irritable bowel syndrome, leaky gut syndrome, food sensitivities, dysbiosis, candida, ulcerative colitis, and diverticulitis.[14,16] Lower

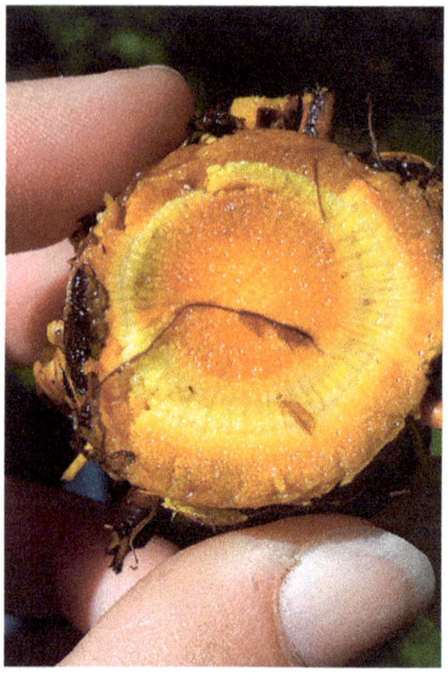

doses reduce loose stools, and improve conditions such as poor digestion and spleen qi deficiency, as well as gas and bloating.[16,17] When treating these conditions, start by consuming five drops and increase the dosage in five-drop increments, up to 15 drops. Do not exceed 15 drops if loose stools are present. Yellow dock also has mild antibacterial effects against *E. coli, Salmonella,* and *Staphylococcus.*[15] The constituent neopodin has demonstrated an antibacterial effect.[13]

A higher dose range of yellow dock (20 – 60 drops or 8 – 10 ounces of tea) has laxative properties.[13-15] Yellow dock is a cholagogue that increases bile flow and softens the stools. It also contains small amounts of anthraquinone glycosides (emodin and chrysophanic acid) that stimulate intestinal motility.[2,13,14]

When treating chronic constipation, it is initially best to use gentle therapies. Make sure the patient is adequately hydrated and consuming healthy amounts of fiber. Identify any food allergies or sensitivities (i.e., dairy or gluten), and eliminate the allergen from the diet. Consume probiotic foods or supplements to establish beneficial bacteria in the digestive tract. The next step is to consume mucilaginous herbs, aperient herbs (bulking agents), and carminative and bitter herbs. If the above measures are unsuccessful in facilitating a bowel movement, consume yellow dock before meals. Increase the dosage in five-drop increments with each meal until the bowel movement is stimulated. Carminative herbs such as fennel or cardamom prevent potential intestinal cramping that can occur from the laxative properties. Yellow dock is recommended before

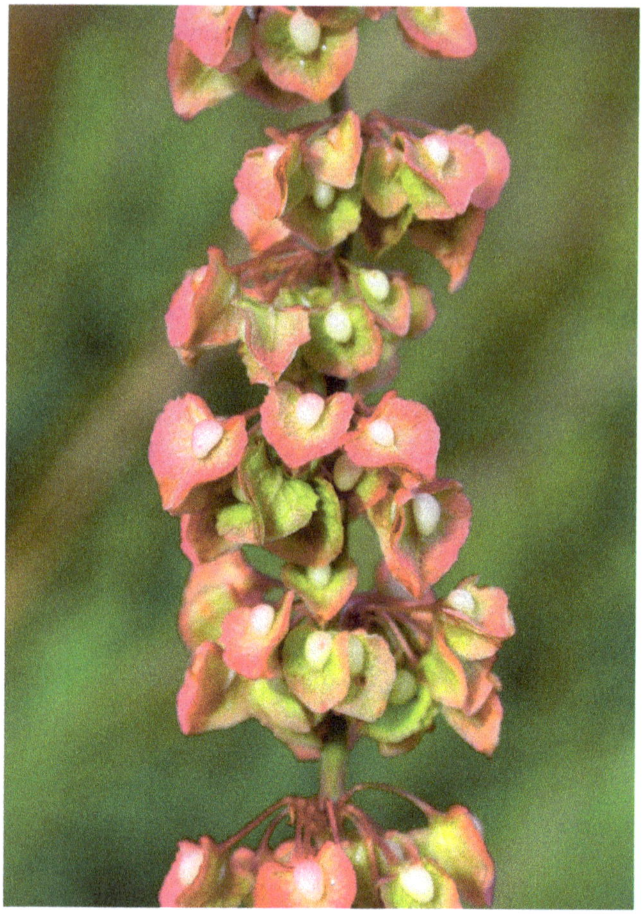

trying more potent purgative herbs, such as turkey rhubarb *(Rheum palmatum),* cascara sagrada *(Rhamnus purshiana),* or senna *(Senna alexandrina).*

Yellow dock acts as a gentle liver cleanser, enhancing detoxification.[6,13,15] It reduces inflammation and improves liver-related skin conditions such as acne, boils, eczema, and psoriasis.[6,13-15] Yellow dock can be used as a long-term tonic by individuals with liver congestion and liver disease.[14] The tea or capsules support the liver when treating jaundice and hepatitis.[6,14] From a Traditional Chinese Medicine perspective, yellow dock decreases damp-heat in the intestines, liver, and gallbladder.

Yellow dock reduces congestion of the portal vein, and can be used as a tonic for individuals with varicose veins, spider veins, and hemorrhoids.[6,14] It also reduces blood stagnation in the pelvic region. Some women have noticed less menstrual cramping after using a yellow dock tonic two to three months. Yellow dock is not an antispasmodic; it simply reduces blood stagnation in the reproductive organs.

Topical applications of the root have astringent and antiseptic actions for treating cuts, wounds, boils, burns, bleeding hemorrhoids, ulcers, and insect and animal

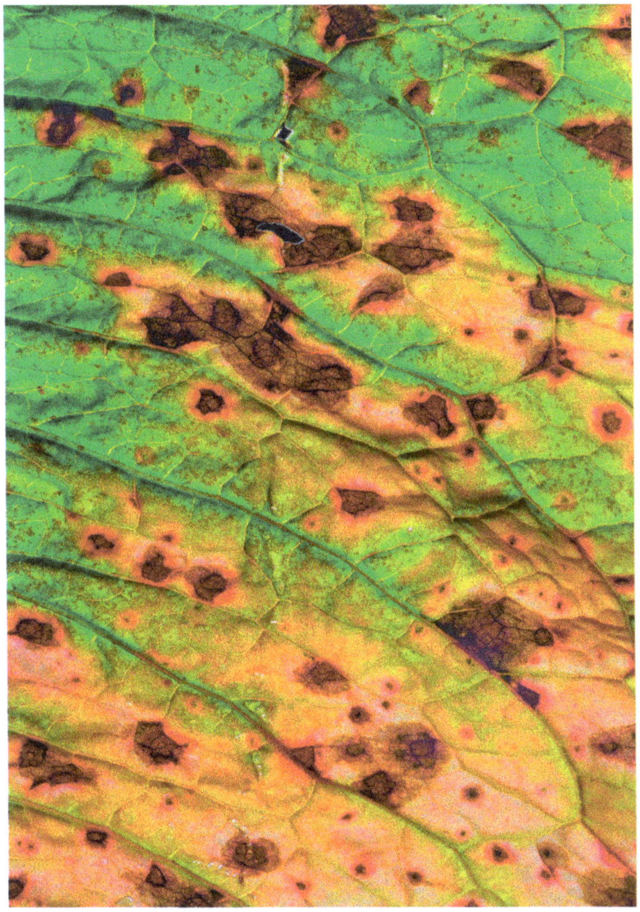

bites.[13-15] Gargle with the tea to reduce inflammation of the oral cavity, including bleeding gums and sore throat.[13]

Yellow dock leaves are a topical astringent and styptic for treating cuts, wounds, boils, burns, and bleeding hemorrhoids.[17] Apply a fresh leaf poultice to reduce the painful burning sensation of nettle stings, bee stings, and insect bites; this gives validity to the herbal adage "nettle in, dock out."[17]

CONTRAINDICATIONS

Pregnant and lactating women should avoid consuming high doses of yellow dock.[14] Avoid consumption when bowel or gallbladder obstruction is present.[13] Large doses can cause loose stools, diarrhea, intestinal cramping, nausea, or polyuria.[15] Individuals with conditions caused or aggravated by oxalate crystals, such as kidney stones, kidney or bladder sensitivity, should avoid using yellow dock consistently. No toxicity has been recorded from the recommended doses of yellow dock.[13]

PREPARATION AND DOSAGE

TINCTURE: Fresh roots [1:2, 70-95% alcohol] or [1:2, 70-90% alcohol and 10% glycerin]; dry roots [1:5, 60% alcohol] or [1:5, 50% alcohol, 40% water, and 10% glycerin]; consume 10-90 drops, up to three times daily.

ACETUM EXTRACT: Fresh roots [1:2-1:3, apple cider vinegar]; consume 1 teaspoon to 1 tablespoon, up to three times daily.

CAPSULES: Consume 2-4 "00" capsules, up to three times daily.

TEA: Prepare a decoction of the root; consume 4-12 ounces, up to three times daily.

HONEY AND SYRUP: Prepare a decoction of yellow dock, and cook to one-half the original volume; then add the desired amount of a sweetening agent such as molasses, honey, or simple syrup. Consume 1 teaspoon to 1 tablespoon, up to three times daily.

TOPICAL USE: Apply the fresh leaf poultice topically to nettle stings, insect stings, bites, or wounds.

CULINARY USE: Young, fresh yellow dock leaf is edible; small amounts can be included in salads or as a pot herb. Some herbalists recommend boiling the leaves once, discarding the water, and then boiling them again to remove the bitterness.

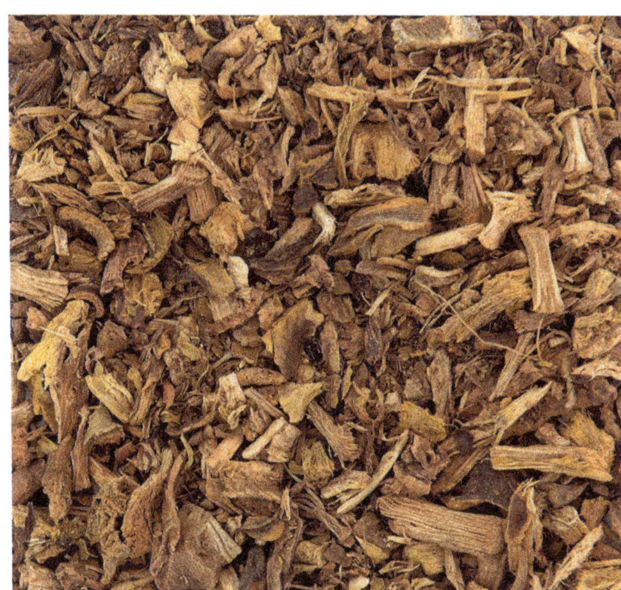

YELLOW POND LILY

BOTANICAL NAMES:
Nuphar lutea, N. polysepala, N. variegatum

COMMON NAMES:
Yellow pond lily, alligator bonnet, bonnet lily, bullhead lily, yellow cowlily, brandy-bottle, alligator-bonnet, Indian pond lily, cow lily, spatterdock

FAMILY NAME:
Nymphaeaceae

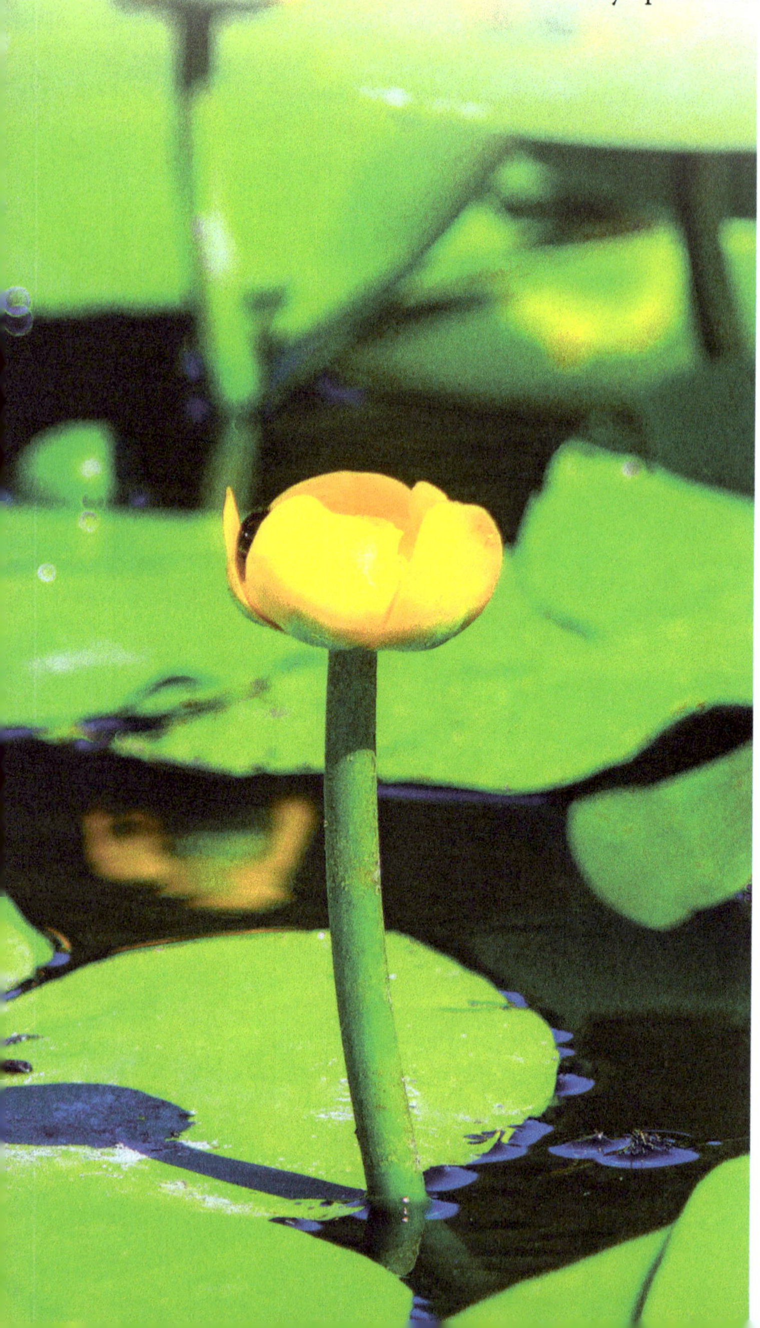

DESCRIPTION

PARTS USED: The rhizomes and seeds.

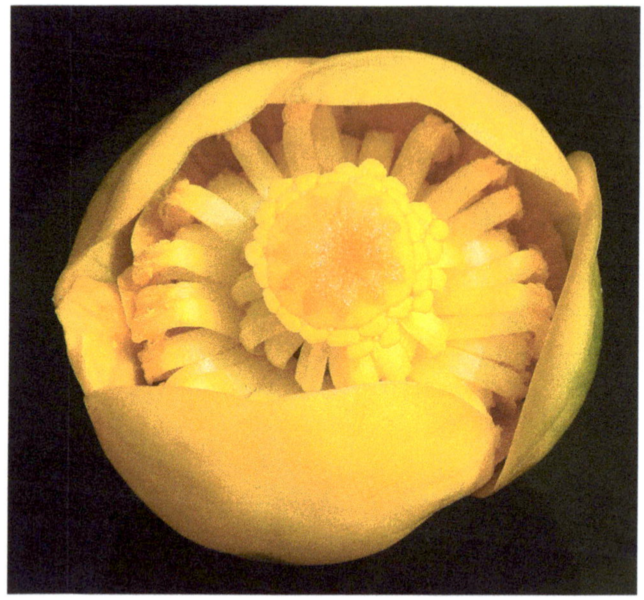

BOTANICAL DESCRIPTION AND HABITAT: Yellow pond lily is a perennial aquatic herb that grows in colonies in ponds, shallow lakes, and marshes. It can be found in still waters at lower and middle elevations throughout the Midwest and Mountain West. The thick, spongy, yellow, tuberous, prehistoric-looking rhizomes have spiraling leaf scars. The branching, prostrate rhizomes attach to the bottom of the lake or pond, deep in the mud. Species of *Nuphar* usually have ovate to round leaves that float on the water surface. The leaves are distinguished by the round basal lobes, and a deep notch where the petiole attaches. The cup-shaped flowers emerge out of the water with 5 – 9 large, reddish-yellow or greenish-yellow, petal-like sepals (10 – 20 thick), spatulate petals, numerous yellow or reddish stamens, and a single, large, knob-like stigma.[1,2] The spongy, berry-like fruit produces fleshy, ovoid seeds.[2]

THE NAME: *Nuphar* is adapted from *new-far,* the Persian name for water lily.[3] The epithet *luteum* means "yellow;" *polysepala* means "many sepals." *Variegatum* ("irregularly colored") derives from Latin. [3] Spatterdock integrates two words: spatter ("strewn about") and dock ("a coarse weed"), referring to the leaves strewn across a pond or lake.[4]

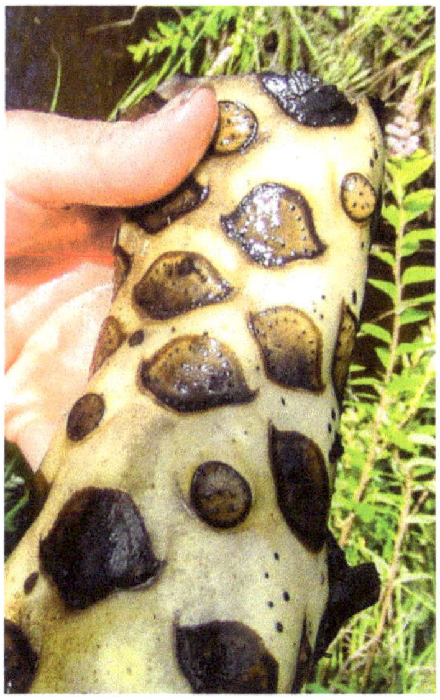

HISTORICAL USES: The seeds were an important source of medicine and food for many tribes in California and Oregon. The seeds were called *wokas* by Klamath Indians, and were dried, stored, or ground into flour. They were also used to thicken soups or gruel.[3-5] The young, tender leaves were incorporated into stews and soups.[4]

Numerous Native American tribes harvested the rhizomes in early spring; the root skins were removed, and the inner root was incorporated into food.[4] However, the rhizomes are difficult to palate; they are astringent and bitter, and sometimes taste like murky pond water. Despite this, in times of famine or out of desperation, young rhizomes may be foraged for food, but the tannins must be leached in warm water repeatedly before consumption.[4]

Yellow pond lily rhizome was used medicinally by many tribes. Sioux prepared rhizome poultices as a styptic for wounds; other tribes prepared leaf poultices for wounds.[3] Montana Indians consumed rhizome tea, and applied poultices to treat venereal diseases. [3] Pond lily was used by Yukon Tagish to treat gallstones.[3] Tsimshian consumed the boiled heart of the rootstock, or drank an infusion made from roasted rootstock for bleeding in the lungs, and as a contraceptive.[5] Haida used the root for a wide range of conditions, including colds, tuberculosis, chest pains, internal pains, heart problems, ulcers, rheumatism, and cancer.[5] Nuxolk treated tuberculosis, rheumatism, heart disease, and gonorrhea with the rhizomes.[5] Kwakwaka'wakw ingested the decoction for edema, sickness in the bones, asthma, and chest pain.[5] Quinault prepared a hot poultice of rhizomes to reduce rheumatic pain.[5] Hesquiat called the herb "west wind" because it was said to bring calmer weather from westerly storms if the leaves were slapped against the water while yelling "West wind! West wind!"[5] The rhizomes were employed as an analgesic, and used in tanning due to the high tannin content.[4] Menominee Indians believed that yellow pond lily belonged to the "Underneath Spirits." They thought it was the source of lake fog, and represented "great medicine."[4]

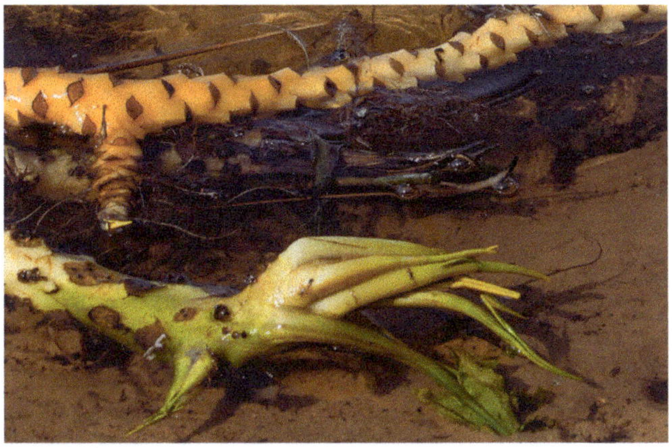

Yellow pond lily leaves protect a variety of wildlife, including fish, turtles, snakes, frogs, crayfish, aquatic insects, and other water creatures.[6] The leaves are consumed by beavers, muskrats, deer, and nutria.[4] The seeds are ingested by Canadian geese, mallards, and wood ducks.[6] Frogs and aquatic insects attach their eggs to pond lily leaves and stems.[4] The leaves provide resting places for frogs, dragonflies, and bees.[6]

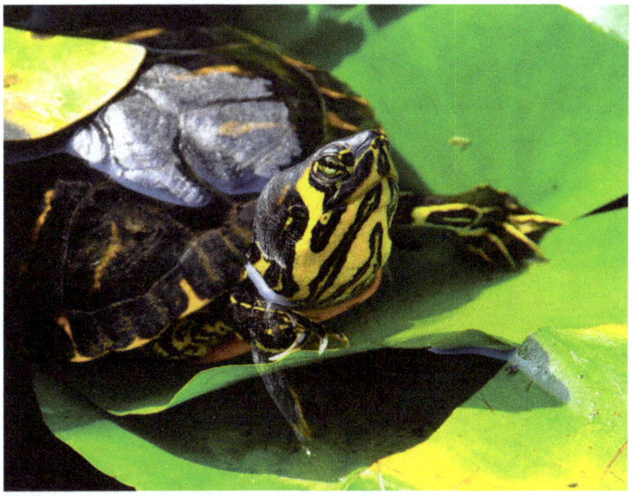

CONSTITUENTS: Yellow pond lily rhizome contains alkaloids (nuphacristine, nupharidine, thiobinupharidine, pseudothiobinupharidine, thiobidesoxy-nupharidine, and allothiobinupharidine), phytosterols, two gallotannins, two ellagitannins, and mucilage.[7]

NUTRITIONAL PROPERTIES: Pond lily seeds and roots are edible, but the nutritional properties have not been documented.

MEDICINAL PROPERTIES: Anti-inflammatory, astringent, bladder tonic, and reproductive tonic.

TEMPERATURE AND FLAVOR: Cold, astringent, bitter, sour, and mildly sweet.

MEDICINAL USES

Yellow pond lily rhizome is a reproductive structural tonic.[8] It enhances uterine tone, and reduces tissue inflammation and swelling.[7,8] Yellow pond lily can be used as a long-term cooling tonic to treat conditions such as endometriosis, ovarian cysts, uterine cysts, fibroids, cervical dysplasia, ovarialgia, and mittelschmerz that present with inflammation and heat.[7,8] It can be used as a postpartum tonic to restore uterine tone and decrease uterine bleeding.

Yellow pond lily reduces inflammation associated with vaginitis and pelvic inflammatory disease; however, additional anti-infectives are necessary to treat an infection.[7] Due to the astringency, using the decoction in a sitz bath or vaginal irrigation aids in treating leukorrhea.[7,8]

Yellow pond lily rhizome improves bladder tone and decreases urinary inflammation.[7] It is beneficial as a long-term tonic to treat interstitial cystitis, but also can be used with other antibacterial agents to treat urinary tract infections. The root reduces testicular and prostate swelling and inflammation.[8] The tonic is useful for treating pain resulting from urination due to benign prostatic hypertrophy and testicular hydroceles. It also decreases residual inflammation following recovery from prostatitis.[7,8]

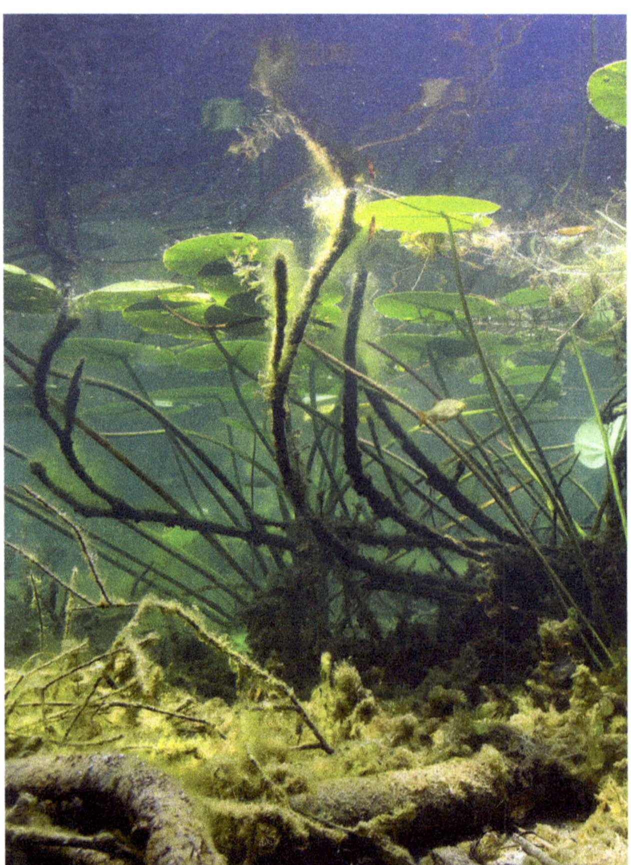

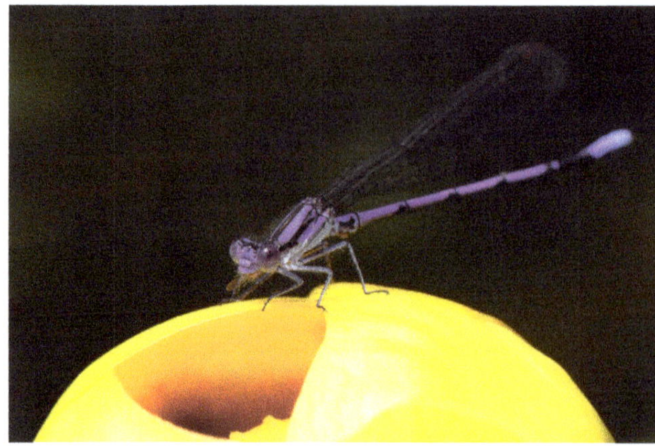

Yellow pond lily rhizomes or seeds can be used as a cooling astringent to decrease digestive tract inflammation.[7,8] The decoction or diluted tincture alleviates acute flareups of digestive conditions, such as esophagitis, gastritis, irritable bowel syndrome, Crohn's, ulcerative colitis, rectal inflammation, and hemorrhoids. Yellow pond lily sitz baths aid in treating hemorrhoids.[7] The rhizome poultice or tea bath is an anti-inflammatory that reduces acute flareups of rheumatoid arthritis or osteoarthritis.[7,8]

CONTRAINDICATIONS

Avoid using rhizome preparations when treating congested tissues with a dull ache.[7,8] Yellow pond lily is specific for hot, inflamed tissues that need cooling and shrinking.[7,8]

PREPARATION AND DOSAGE

TINCTURE: Fresh rhizomes [1:2–1:3, 70–95% alcohol]; consume 10–60 drops, up to three times daily.

CAPSULES: The seeds or rhizomes can be ground and encapsulated into capsules; consume 2–4 "00" capsules, up to two times daily.

TEA: Prepare a rhizome decoction; consume 4–8 ounces, up to four times daily.

TOPICAL USE: Prepare the root decoction and strain through a fine filter. Use the tea as a vaginal irrigation, sitz bath, enema, poultice, or wash.

CULINARY USE: The seeds are edible. Herbalist Janet Schofield recommends making pond lily popcorn by popping ¼ cup of seeds in 2 tablespoons of oil.

YERBA MANSA

DESCRIPTION

BOTANICAL NAME:
Anemopsis californica

COMMON NAMES:
Yerba mansa, yerba del manso, lizard tale, bear root, swamp root, manso, apache beads

FAMILY NAME:
Saururaceae

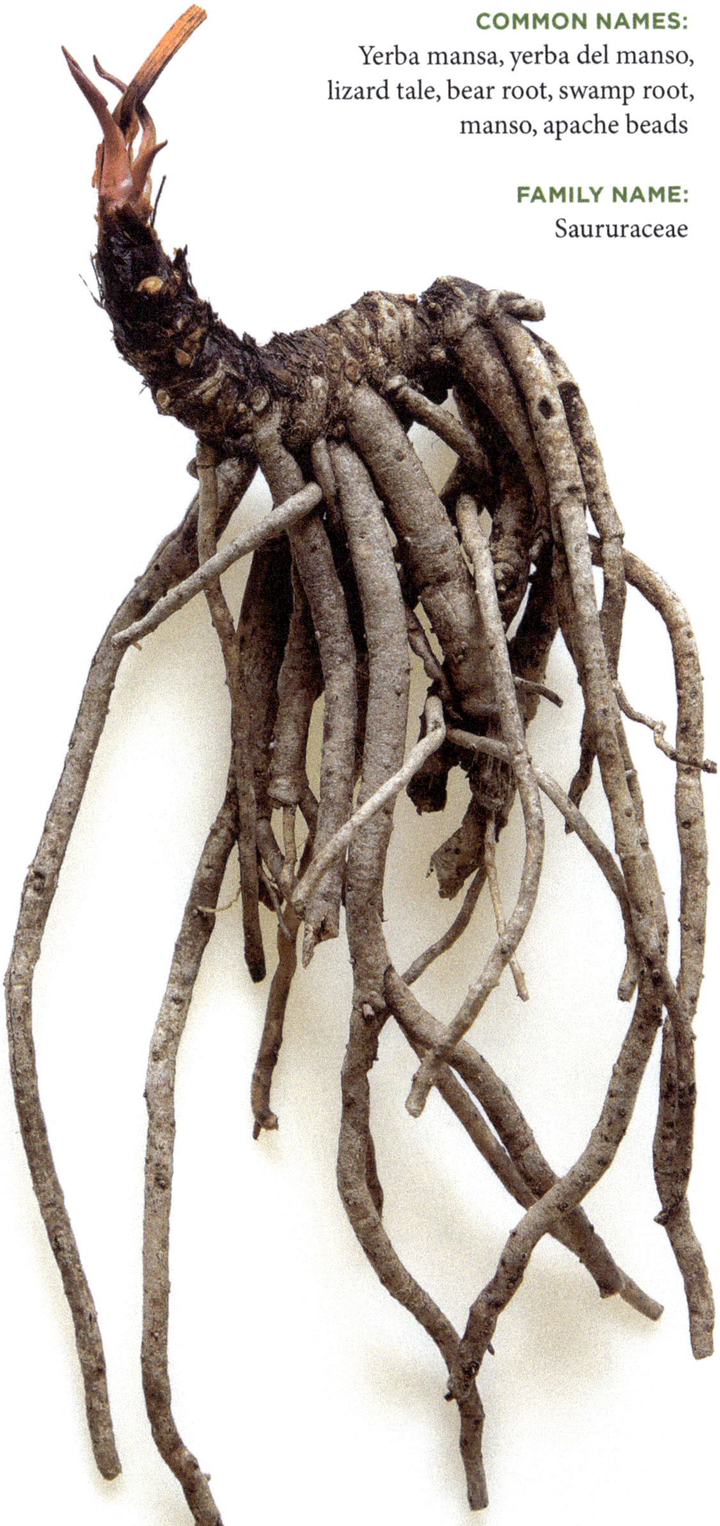

PART USED: The roots.

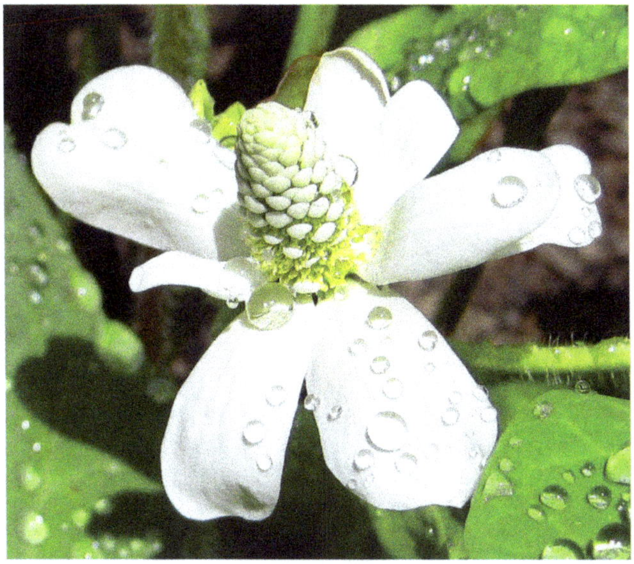

BOTANICAL DESCRIPTION AND HABITAT: The *Anemopsis* genus consists of only one species, *A. californica*, which grows in saline or alkaline seeps and springs in the Sierra Nevada, southern California, Oregon, Kansas, Texas, and northwest Mexico.[1] It is a rhizomatous, perennial ground cover that spreads via stolons.[1,2] The plant can be glabrous or densely pubescent.[2] The simple alternate leaves are elliptic to oblong with a rounded apex. Sometimes the base is cordate; the blades are 3 – 20 cm long, and the petioles are 2 – 40 cm long.[1] The leaves are predominantly basal, although a few may be sessile and cauline; they can assume an unusual dimorphic form in which a second leaf grows at the axil.[2]

What appears to be a large, beautiful, white flower is actually a conical inflorescence (1 – 4 cm long).[2] It is a spike subtended by four to nine white or red-tinged, petal-like involucre bracts (0.3 – 3.5 cm long).[2] Small spatulate, white bracts subtend the individual flowers (3.5 – 6 mm long).[1] Spikes bear 75 – 150 apetalous flowers that contain six to eight stamens, one fused pistil with three carpels, and three distinct styles.[3] The fruit is a fleshy capsule producing many brown seeds.[1]

THE NAME: *Anemopsis* derives from two Greek words: *anemone* (the Greek name and current genus name for a group of plants in the Ranunculaceae family) and *opsis*

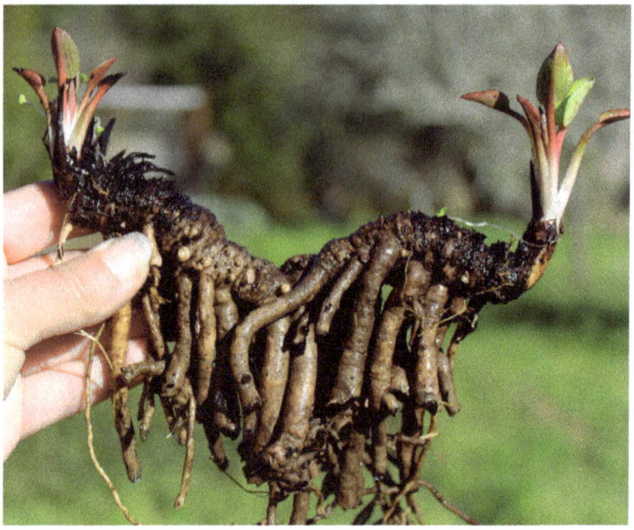

("like"), referring to the flower's anemone-like appearance.[4] The epithet *californica* ("of or from California") indicates the plant's origin.[5] In Spanish, the name of the plant translates as *yerba* ("herb") and *mansa* ("calm, peaceful, tame"). In *Healing Herbs of the Upper Rio Grande — Traditional Medicine of the Southwest,* author Leslie Curtin mentions that yerba mansa was loosely translated as "herb of the tamed Indian." The plant was never traditionally used as a sedative; it was frequently used to treat infections by enslaved Native Californians, who were forced to live in closely confined encampments.[6]

HISTORICAL USES: Yerba mansa was a highly esteemed herb among Native Americans in southern California, Arizona, New Mexico, and Mexico.[7] They administered the root to treat malarial fevers, diarrhea, and dysentery.[7] The roots were chewed and the juice was swallowed for coughs, tuberculosis, and pulmonary infections.[7] Native Americans gargled with the tea to alleviate a sore throat, ulcers, or mouth and throat sores.[6,8] A decoction was consumed as a blood purifier, for digestive disturbances, colic, and dysentery, and to tone mucous membranes.[6] Pima and Maricopa Indians consumed a decoction to treat syphilis.[6] Yerba mansa tea was consumed regularly, and a poultice was applied to treat arthritis and rheumatoid arthritis.[6,7] The root poultice was applied to ulcerated gums, abrasions, burns, sores, and swellings.[6] A wash made from the tea was applied to saddle and collar galls on horses.[7]

Native Americans in southern California shared their uses of yerba mansa with Eclectic physician Dr. William H. George, who introduced the herb to the Eclectics.[7] He described the herb as having astringent, carminative, stimulant tonic, and antiemetic properties.[7] The Eclectics prescribed the herb to treat nasal catarrh, gonorrhea, painful diarrhea, dysentery, a cough, and typhoid.[7,9] Yerba mansa was administered as an aromatic, astringent tonic for mucous membranes in the gastrointestinal, renal, and respiratory tracts.[9] A poultice was applied to severe bruises, skin ulcers, arthritic joints, and syphilitic sores.[9]

CONSTITUENTS: Yerba mansa contains volatile oil (eugenol methyl ether, thymol, piperitone, estragole = methylchavicol, 1,8-cineole, linalool, and related compounds), tannins, *p*-cymene, and lignans (asarinin = sesamin isomer).[10,11]

NUTRITIONAL PROPERTIES: Unknown.

MEDICINAL PROPERTIES: Antibacterial, antifungal, anti-inflammatory, antiseptic, astringent, diuretic, and expectorant.

TEMPERATURE AND FLAVOR: Warm, astringent, pungent, sour, and bitter.

MEDICINAL USES

Yerba mansa has antibacterial and antifungal properties.[9-11] It aids in treating infectious conditions with glandular swelling and/or profuse mucus secretion, such as strep throat, pharyngitis, sinusitis, and bronchitis.[6,9-11] It has subtle lymphatic actions for stagnant, swollen lymphatic tissues or lymph nodes. Gargling with the tea or diluted extract treats a sore throat, swollen glands, strep throat, a cold, or flu.[8]

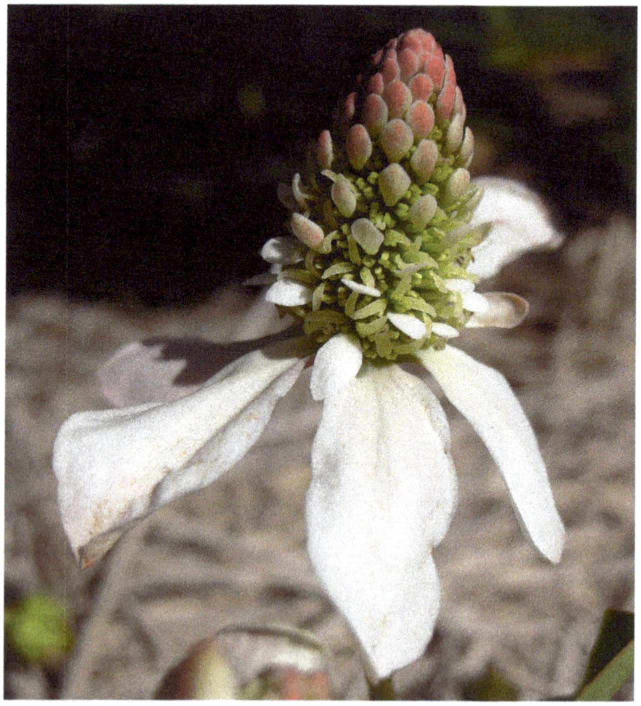

The antibacterial and astringent properties aid in treating bacterial digestive infections, diarrhea, dysentery, and chronic digestive ulcers in the stomach, intestine, and colon.[6,7,9,10] Yerba mansa is also a hemostatic, reducing gastrointestinal bleeding. Topical preparations, such as a sitz bath, poultice, or salve alleviate hemorrhoid pain and bleeding, as well as anal fissures.[6,10] Yerba mansa also has antifungal properties, reducing *Candida albicans* overgrowth in the mouth, digestive tract, and vagina.[8,10] The antibacterial and antifungal actions are attributed to the thymol.[11] The lignans are also attributed to the antimicrobial, anti-inflammatory, and immune modulating effects.[11]

Yerba mansa contains tannins that reduce excessive mucus formation. It is also an expectorant that alleviates seasonal allergies, allergic rhinitis, sinusitis, and lingering hypersecretory lung infections.[8,9] Herbalist Michael Moore recommends preparing a water percolation (1:10), then adding 20% glycerin and 10% alcohol to the finished product as a nasal spray.[10] This treatment has worked very effectively for patients with sinus infections, allergic rhinitis, and nasal polyps.

Yerba mansa has an aromatic astringent, anti-inflammatory effect that is highly beneficial for treating chronically inflamed, swollen, congested mucous membranes.[9,10] It is a resolvent, hastening the removal of waste products from tissues following an infection. Yerba mansa contains volatile oil that increases circulation into the tissues, improving blood flow and enhancing nutrient and oxygen delivery. It also contains tannins that reduce capillary permeability, preventing the leakage of fluids and proteins from the bloodstream into the tissues due to inflammation. The volatile oil has an initial warming effect, but the tannins ultimately have cooling and constricting actions in the tissues that decrease inflammation.

Yerba mansa is a diuretic that enhances the excretion of nitrogenous acids, including uric acid that aids in treating gout.[10] It also has anti-inflammatory effects that treat joint pain, arthritis, and rheumatoid arthritis.[10] In the Southwest, the poultice was widely used to alleviate arthritic pain.[6,10] Yerba mansa has diuretic, astringent, anti-inflammatory, and antibacterial actions that alleviate lingering urinary tract infections such as cystitis or urethritis.[9-11]

Gargling with the tea or diluted tincture, or applying a poultice is beneficial for periodontal diseases. Yerba mansa is highly effective for treating indolent gum sores, gingivitis, bleeding gums, and gum abscesses.[10,11] It also aids in treating gum conditions resulting from methamphetamine addiction. Yerba mansa has anesthetizing qualities that reduce teething pain and toothaches.

Yerba mansa is a very effective first aid herb. Topical applications of the leaf or root tea, fomentation, poultice, or salve is a superior antimicrobial, astringent, styptic, and drawing agent. Yerba mansa hastens the healing of wounds, abscesses, cat scratches, diabetic ulcers, staph infections, skin tinea, cystic acne, moist eczema, poison oak, poison ivy, boils, and diaper rash.[8,10,11] A poultice, oil, or salve reduces hemorrhoidal inflammation and bleeding.[6,8] A drawing agent, the root poultice can be applied alone or mixed with clay for insect bites and stings. Yerba mansa also has counterirritant, anti-inflammatory, and analgesic properties that reduce the pain of bruises, sprains, strains, contusions, arthritis, gout, and muscle and joint discomfort.[6,10] A sitz bath alleviates hemorrhoids and perineum, vaginal, or labial tears following birth.[11] Vaginal irrigation with a well-strained tea aids in treating leukorrhea, candida, and vaginitis.[8]

CONTRAINDICATIONS

There are no known side effects or contraindications when consumed in recommended doses.[11] No toxicity has been reported; however, consuming large quantities can cause the gag reflex, nausea, vomiting, or an upset stomach.[11] Discontinue use if the mucous membranes become too dry. Avoid consuming large amounts while lactating, because the astringent properties potentially reduce the flow of breast milk.

PREPARATION AND DOSAGE

TINCTURE: Fresh roots [1:2-1:3, 70-95% alcohol]; dry roots [1:5, 60% alcohol]; consume 20-60 drops, up to five times daily.

TEA: Prepare a cold infusion or decoction of the roots; consume 4-8 ounces, four times daily. Prepare a hot infusion of the leaves; consume 4-8 ounces, four times daily.

TOPICAL USE: Dry the leaves and prepare medicinal oil using the alcohol intermediary oil method. Apply the powdered leaves or roots as a dust, or to make a poultice. Decoct the roots or infuse the leaves, strain, and apply as a wash, fomentation, or poultice.

YERBA SANTA

DESCRIPTION

BOTANICAL NAMES:
Eriodictyon angustifolium, E. californicum, E. crassifolium, E. spp.

COMMON NAMES:
Yerba santa, mountain balm, bear's weed, bear plant, consumptive weed, tarweed, sacred herb, holy herb, wild balsam, gum bush, mountain balm
santakraut (German)
yerba santa (Spanish)

FAMILY NAME:
Boraginaceae (formerly Hydrophyllaceae)

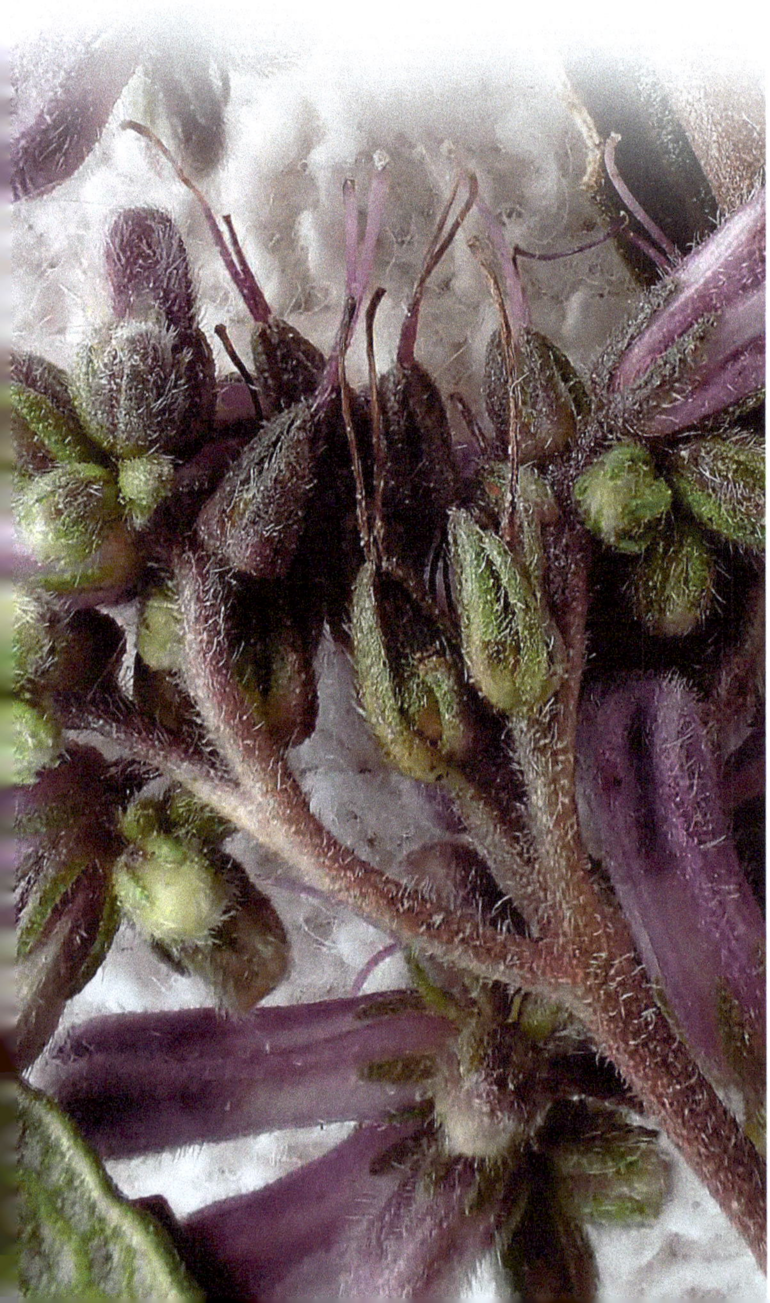

PARTS USED: The leaves and upper portions of the stems and flowers.

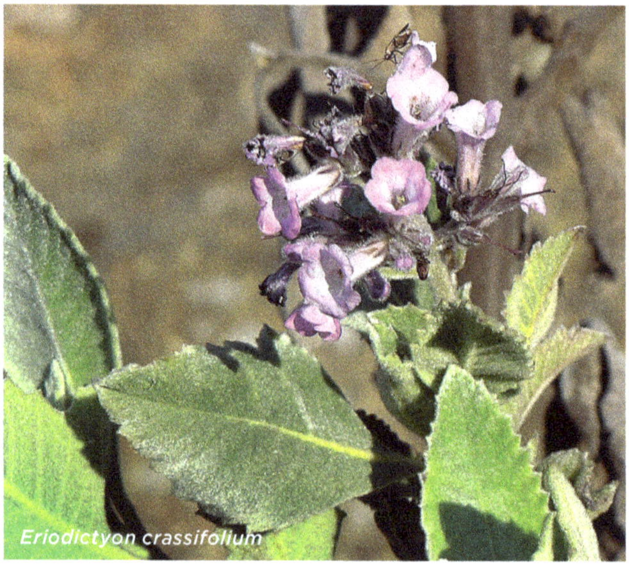

Eriodictyon crassifolium

BOTANICAL DESCRIPTION AND HABITAT: Yerba santa is an evergreen shrub that grows one to three meters tall.[1] It thrives in sunny, well-drained soil, and often grows along slopes or roadsides. *Eriodictyon angustifolium* is native to the southwestern U.S., and grows at elevations of 1500 – 1900 meters.[1] *E. californicum* grows throughout much of California at elevations of 20 – 1800 meters.[2] *E. crassifolium* grows from central to southern California at elevations of 30 – 2500 meters; other species grow in Mexico.[1]

Eriodictyon is a genus of erect evergreen shrubs with shredding bark and simple, leathery, alternate leaves.[1] The leaf upper surface varies species to species, with sticky, hairy, shiny, or glabrous characteristics. The lower surface of the leaf is generally tomentose. The open inflorescences grow at the ends of branches.[1] The hairy flowers have funnel- to bell-shaped corollas with five white to purple lobes.[1] Each flower has two carpels and two styles, and the stamen ovary and filaments are usually hairy.[1] The fruit is a small capsule (1 – 3 mm wide) with four valves that produce dark brown or black, striate seeds.[1]

E. angustifolium is an uncommon species growing to a height of less than two meters.[1] It has sticky stems bearing linear leaves (2 – 10 cm long by 0.2 – 1 cm wide) with entire to roughly toothed revolute margins.[1] The leaves are sessile or short-petioled, with a glabrous and sticky upper surface. The undersides are covered in a fine white down, excluding the prominent network of veins.[1] It has mostly glabrous calyx lobes (1 – 4 mm) and hairy corollas with recurved white petals (3 – 6 mm).[1] The fruit bears 1 – 8 seeds.[1]

E. californicum grows up to 3 meters tall.[2] The elliptic to lanceolate leaves (4 – 15 mm long by less than 5 cm wide) sometimes have fine teeth on revolute margins.[2] The upper surface is dark green and sticky glandular; the lower surface is pale green to whitish, and finely hairy with a prominent network of veins.[3] The sparsely hairy flower has a calyx with lobes 2 – 4 mm long.[4] The corolla ranges from white to purple (8 – 17 mm long).[2] The fruit bears 2 – 20 seeds.[2]

E. crassifolium grows 1 – 3 meters tall with densely hairy stems.[1] The lanceolate-ovate to oblong leaf (3 – 17 cm long, 1 – 6 cm wide) has short petioles and entire to toothed margins.[1,3] The upper surface varies from sparsely hairy to white-tomentose; the underside is tomentose.[1] The hairy calyx lobes are 2 – 6 mm long; the hairy lavender, campanulate corolla is 5 – 16 cm long.[1] The fruit bears 8 – 14 seeds.[1]

THE NAME: The genus *Eriodictyon* derives from two Greek words: *erion* ("wool") and *diktuon* ("a net or seine for fishing"), referring to the appearance of the leaf undersides.[5] The epithet *angustifolium* means "narrow-leaved."[6] The epithet *californicum* means "of or from California." The epithet *crassifolium* derives from two Latin words: *crassus* ("thick") and *folium* ("leaf"), referring to the thick, fleshy leaves.[7] The common name *yerba santa* is comprised of two Spanish words: yerba ("herb") and santa ("saint").

HISTORICAL USES: Yerba santa tea was consumed by more than 12 Native American tribes to treat coughs, colds, asthma, pleurisy, and pneumonia.[8] It also was used to alleviate nausea, indigestion, and a stomachache.[8] The leaves were applied as a poultice for poison oak, insect bites, sores, wounds, and sprains.[8] Yerba santa vapor was inhaled for dizziness.[8]

Eclectic physicians learned how to use yerba santa from Native Americans. The extract or syrup was administered as a stimulating expectorant to treat a moist cough, asthma, pneumonia, and acute and chronic bronchitis.[9,10] Yerba santa was used to strengthen digestion and reduce catarrh in the stomach and bladder.[9] Yerba santa syrup was used to mask the bitter taste of quinine and other herbs.[10]

CONSTITUENTS: Yerba santa contains eriodictyonine (homoeriodictyol), eriodictyol (5, 7, 4', 3' -tetrahydroxyflavanone), 3', 4', 5, 7-tetrahydroxyflavone, chrysoeriodictyol, xanthoeriodictyol, 5, 4'-dihydroxy-6, 7-dimethoxyflavone, 5, 7, 4'-trihydroxy-6, 3'-dimethoxyflavone, 3'-methyl-4'-isobutyryleriodictyol, pinocembrin, sakuranetin, cirsimaritin, chrysoeriol, hispidulin, chrysin, eriodictyonic acid, acetic acid, formic acid, butyric acid, resin (triacontane, pentatriacontane, cerotic acid, chyrsoeriodictyol, xanthoeriodictyol=xanthoeriodol, and eriodonol=eriodonal), naringenin 4'-methyl ether, phytosterols, tannin, gum, sugars, fats, and a trace of volatile oil.[11-14]

NUTRITIONAL PROPERTIES: Yerba santa contains high amounts of chromium, cobalt, crude fiber, fat, iron, magnesium, manganese, niacin, phosphorus, selenium, silicon, and vitamins A and C. It contains low to average amounts of ash, calcium, dietary fiber, potassium protein, sodium, and zinc.[15]

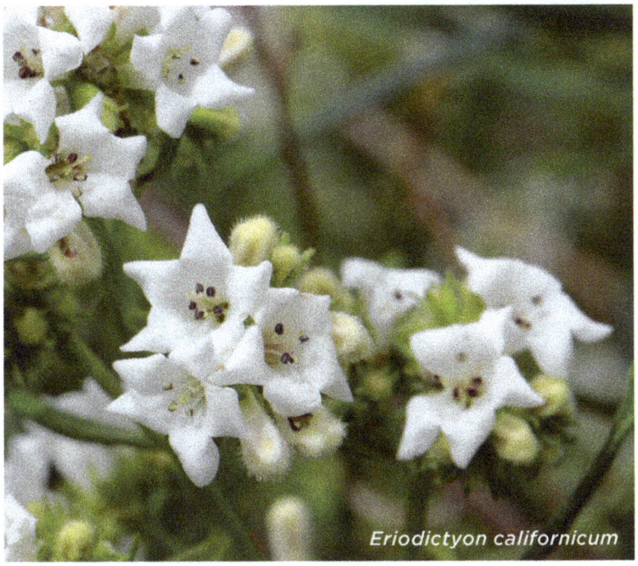
Eriodictyon californicum

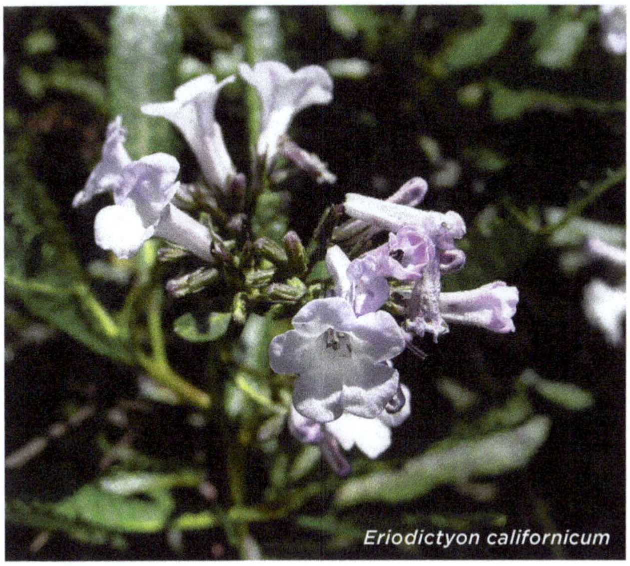
Eriodictyon californicum

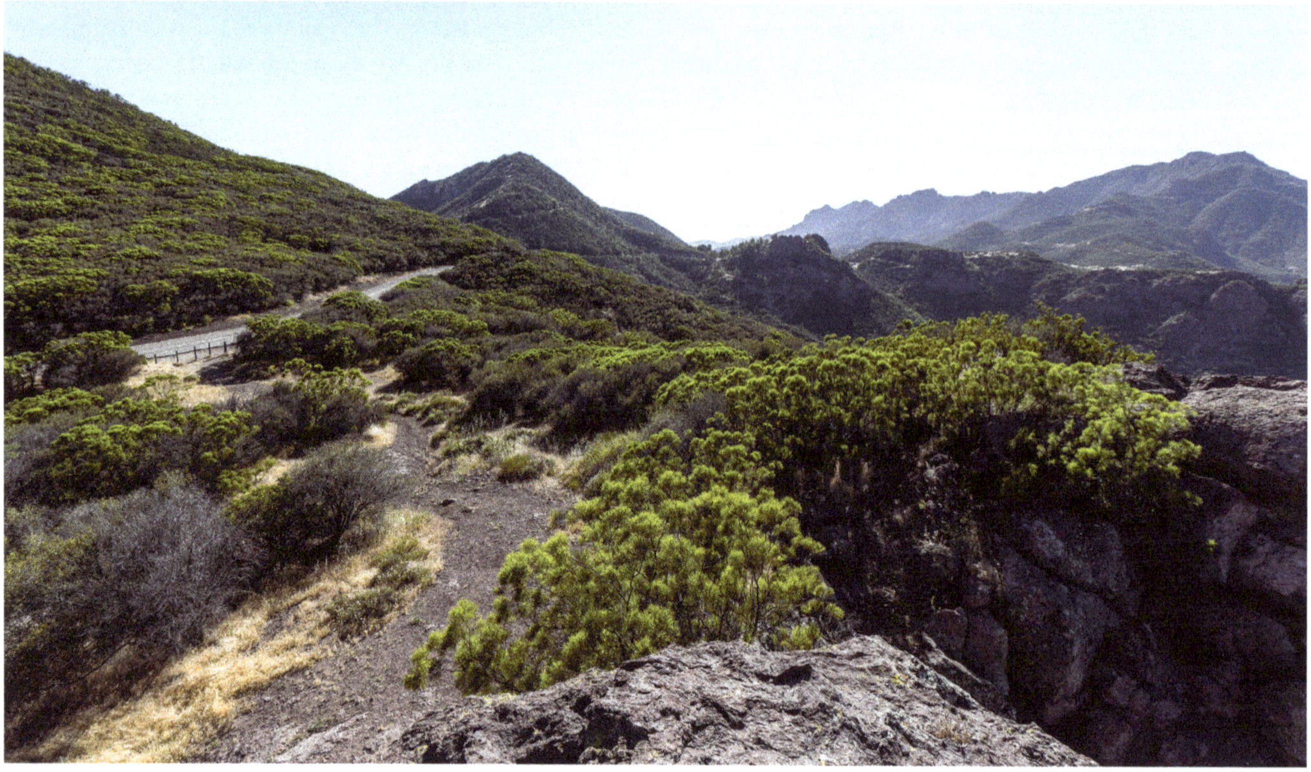

MEDICINAL PROPERTIES: Anti-inflammatory, (mild) antimicrobial, antitussive, astringent, bronchodilator, decongestant, expectorant, harmonizer, and mild diuretic.

TEMPERATURE AND FLAVOR: Warm, sweet, pungent, astringent, and mildly bitter.

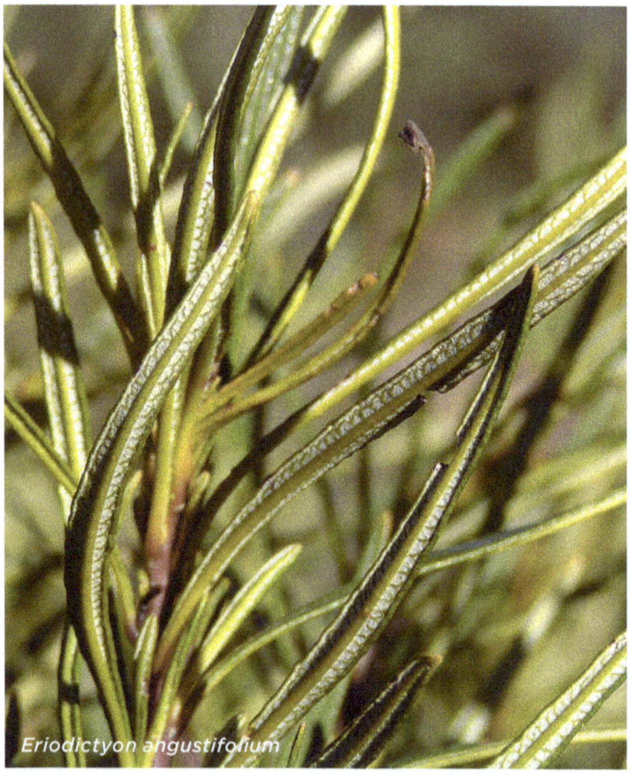

Eriodictyon angustifolium

MEDICINAL USES

Yerba santa is a warming, resinous, expectorant herb with astringent and decongestant properties.[11,12,16] It decreases mucous membrane swelling, and helps to shrink engorged tissues.[9,12] Yerba santa contains flavonoids that stabilize leaky capillaries and reduce inflammation.[12,16] Eriodictyol is attributed to the expectorant properties.[13] Yerba santa is a mild bronchodilator.[11] It is extremely beneficial for reducing secretions in the upper and lower respiratory systems, and aids in treating seasonal allergies, sinusitis, cold, flu, bronchitis, pneumonia, and asthma.[9,11,12,14,16] When treating seasonal allergies or upper respiratory infections, combine yerba santa extracts with bayberry *(Morella)*, ragweed *(Ambrosia)*, and/or goldenrod *(Solidago)*. The following tea recipe is also effective: one part each of yerba santa, yerba mansa *(Anemopsis), and* Mormon tea *(Ephedra nevadensis);* one-half part each of cinnamon *(Cinnamomum)* and bayberry *(Morella);* and one-eighth to one-quarter part licorice *(Glycyrrhiza)*. If the tea is too drying, add two to three parts of marshmallow root *(Althaea)*. For lower respiratory infections and asthma, combine yerba santa with yerba mansa *(Anemopsis)*, aralia *(Aralia californica)*, gumweed *(Grindelia)*, and a small portion of licorice *(Glycyrrhiza)* to harmonize the flavor. Smokers can add small portions of dried, ground leaves to smoking blends for flavor. Smoking the leaves also has antitussive and expectorant properties.[11]

Yerba santa resin is excreted in the urinary tract, serving as an antibacterial agent and anti-inflammatory for slowly resolving urinary tract infections.[9,11,14,16] Combine extracts of yerba mansa *(Anemopsis)*, usnea *(Usnea)*, juniper berries *(Juniperus)*, gumweed *(Grindelia)*, and/or buchu *(Barosma)* to treat recurring urinary tract infections.

Yerba santa extract is a harmonizer and flavoring agent.[10] It increases the palatability of bitter herbs in compounds.[10] Yerba santa blocks a bitter taste without interfering with sweet, salty, or sour tastes.[14]

An alcohol-based spray (tincture diluted in water) can be applied topically to reduce itching and dry out poison oak or poison ivy.[16] Combine the extracts of yerba santa, gumweed *(Grindelia)*, yerba mansa *(Anemopsis)*, and/or uva ursi *(Arctostaphylos)*. Topically, yerba santa acts as an antimicrobial for cuts, abrasions, wounds, and insect bites. It also is a mild counterirritant for sprains, strains, bruises, and rheumatism.[14]

CONTRAINDICATIONS

Although the side effects have not been thoroughly researched, yerba santa is considered safe. High frequent doses can cause dryness in tissues, and the resins can potentially irritate the kidneys. Use moderate doses during pregnancy and lactation.

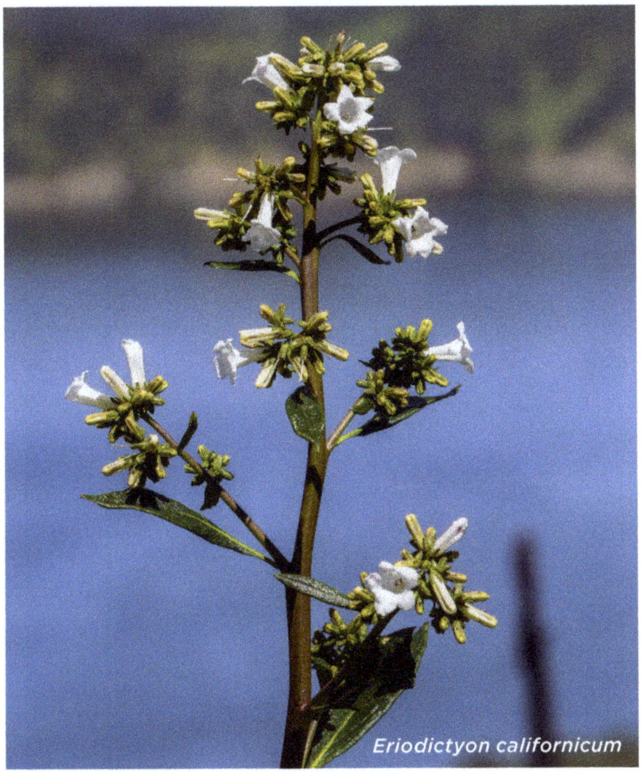

Eriodictyon californicum

PREPARATION AND DOSAGE

TINCTURE: Fresh leaves [1:2-1:3, 95% alcohol]; dry leaves [1:5, 70% alcohol]; consume 15-90 drops, up to four times daily.

GLYCERITE: Fresh leaves [1:3, 50% glycerin, 50% alcohol]; dry leaves [1:5, 40% alcohol, 30% glycerin, and 30% water]; consume 15-60 drops, up to four times daily.

CAPSULES: Consume 2-4 "00" capsules, up to four times daily.

TEA: Prepare a hot infusion or decoction; consume 8-12 ounces, up to four times daily.

HONEY AND SYRUP: Consume 1 teaspoon to 1 tablespoon of yerba santa syrup or honey.

TOPICAL USE: Dry the leaves and prepare using the alcohol intermediary oil method. Apply the oil, salve, or diluted tincture topically.

MEDICINE MAKING

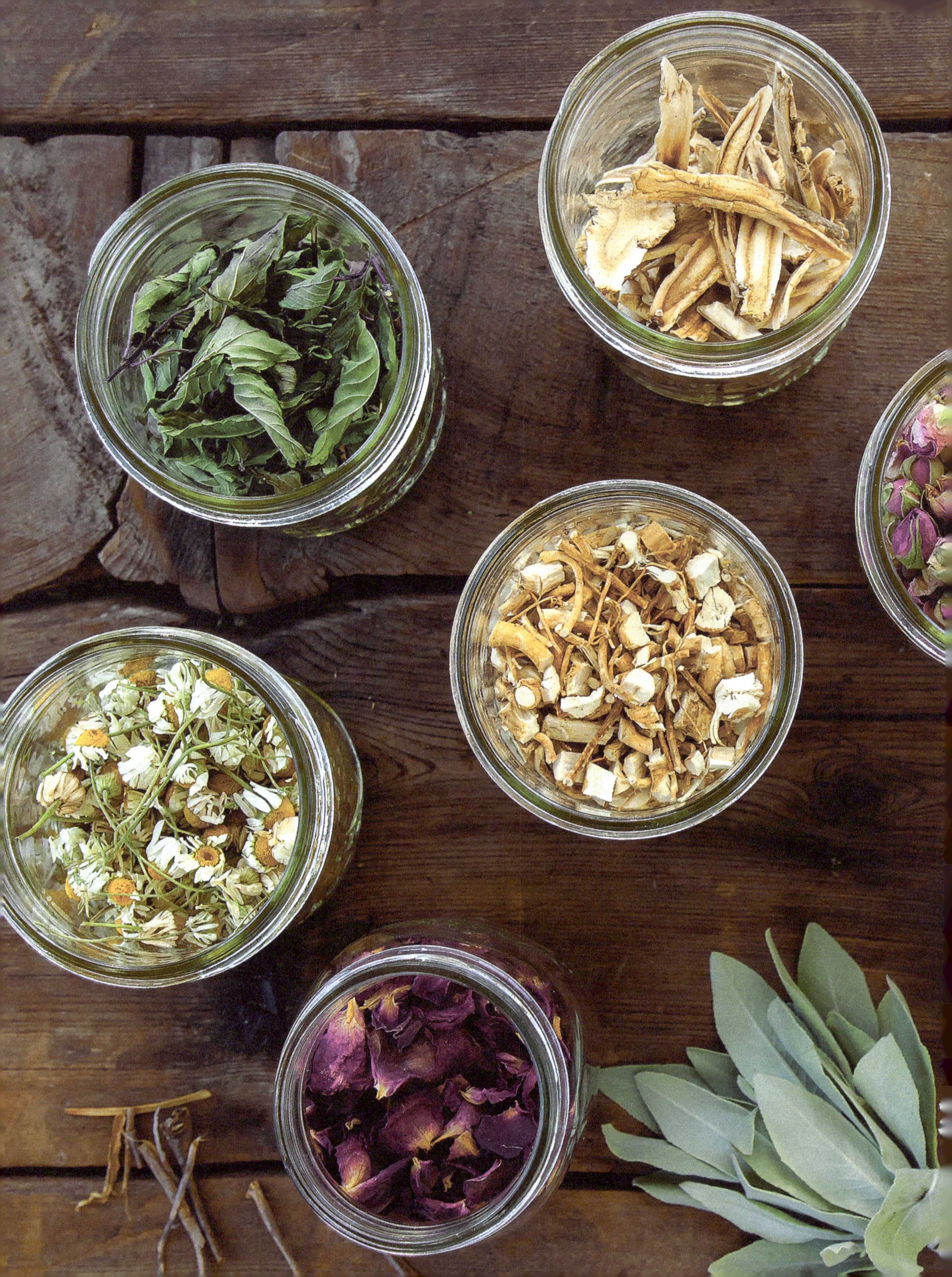

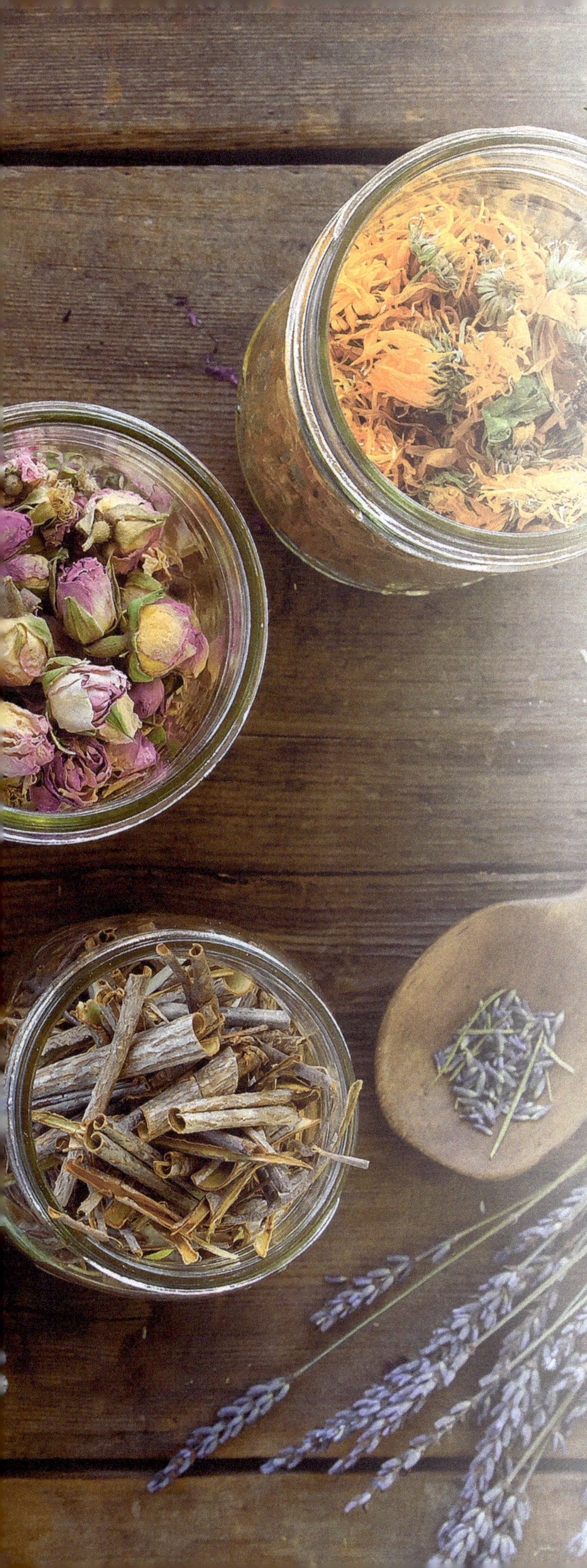

WATER-BASED PREPARATIONS

HERBAL TEA

One of the most ancient and simple healing preparations of medicinal plants, herbal tea is made by combining herbs with water. Depending on the preparation method, herbal teas can be called infusions, tisanes, or decoctions. Teas are ideal for treating a wide variety of acute and chronic conditions. In contrast to the potentially harsh effects of alcohol extracts on the mucous membranes, internal organs, and other tissues, teas are soothing and widely tolerated. Teas are relatively affordable as a long-term therapy, and can be effective vehicles for delivering potent medicine.

Preparing and drinking herbal tea helps individuals to slow down and pay more attention to their bodies and health. This critical component of healing is often missing in modern medicine.

THE VESSEL: Herbal tea should be prepared in a closed vessel, ideally with a tight-fitting lid. The vessel should be made of glass, porcelain, glazed earthenware, or stainless steel. Avoid using aluminum, tinned iron, or other metallic vessels that can leach into the preparation.

DRY HERBAL TEA PROPORTIONS: Depending on the therapeutic goal or the herb's strength, age, or condition, different proportions may be utilized to prepare a tea. In this text, preparations assume the following proportion: for infusions and decoctions, combine one ounce of herb (by weight) to 30 ounces of water (by volume).

Other methods can be employed. The standard pharmacopoeia method is to combine one part herb to 20 parts water, or 50 gm of herb to 1000 ml of water. The Simpler's method combines 6 – 8 tablespoons of herb with each quart of water.

FRESH HERB TEA PROPORTIONS: Fresh herbs have high water content, and tend to be less concentrated than dry herbs. Thus, when preparing tea with fresh herbs, it is best to use larger volumes of plant material than when using dry herbs. For an infusion, pack the vessel one-half to three-quarters full with fresh herbs, then fill it with water. For decoctions that are generally made with denser plant material, only fill the vessel one-quarter to one-third full with fresh herbs.

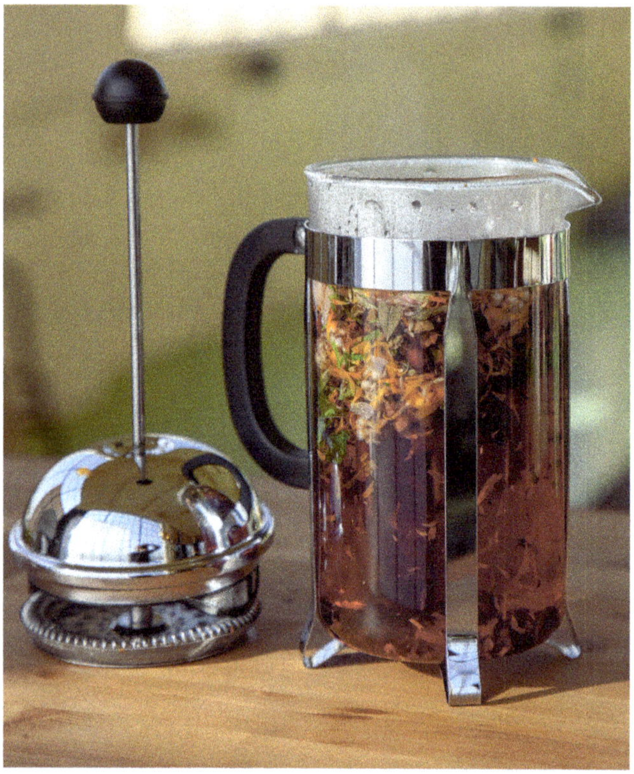

STORAGE: Herbal tea is often made in one-quart batches and is best prepared fresh each day. However, if the tea is refrigerated or stored in a very cool environment, it can last up to 48 hours before it begins to taste flat or starts fermenting.

DOSAGE FOR ACUTE AND CHRONIC CONDITIONS: When treating acute health conditions, it is best to drink small doses of tea frequently — about four to six ounces every one to two hours throughout the day. When treating chronic health conditions, less frequent dosing is acceptable; drink two to three 10-ounce cups (up to one quart) of tea daily. Teas are most quickly absorbed on an empty stomach.

Tea can be prepared as an infusion or a decoction, depending on the type of herb and part of the plant used. Infusions are usually made with the more delicate parts of the plants, including the flowers, leaves, soft stems, and buds. Boiling these parts of the plants will often destroy or injure their medicinal properties. Infusions extract vitamins, minerals, volatile oil, mucilage, and other constituents from the plants.

Dried herbs are best prepared for extraction by water when they are cut and sifted or sliced. Fine powders are more difficult to strain, and should be avoided when making infusions. Although it is not imperative, fresh herbs can be chopped or bruised to release the volatile oil.

HOT INFUSIONS

Hot infusions are made from plants with medicinal components that can be extracted in a relatively short amount of time.

STEEPING TIME: A medicinal infusion should steep at least 30 to 60 minutes; with teas containing minerals or mucilage, the ideal steeping time is even longer. Infusions can steep all day; however, do not steep it so long that the tea begins to spoil. One option is to prepare herbal tea before going to bed, allow it to steep overnight, and re-warm it for consumption the next day. This is recommended for nutritive herbs.

HERBS CONTAINING TANNINS: Tannins can be extracted in two to five minutes. If plants with large quantities of tannins are allowed to steep longer, they can become very astringent, and sometimes bitter or sour. Tannins can upset the stomach; reduce the possibility of this by infusing the herbs for a short amount of time in hot water that is slightly below boiling temperature.

Examples of plants that contain tannins are black and green tea *(Camilla sinensis)*, oak bark *(Quercus)*, and raspberry leaf *(Rubus)*. When combining these plants with other herbs, steep the non-tannin containing herbs at least 30 to 60 minutes, then add the tannin-containing herbs to the infusion up to five minutes before the tea is ready to strain. Alternately, these herbs can be prepared as a single herb tea or cold infusion.

METHODS OF PREPARATION: To prevent a glass or porcelain vessel from cracking, run hot water into the vessel and leave for several minutes before draining.

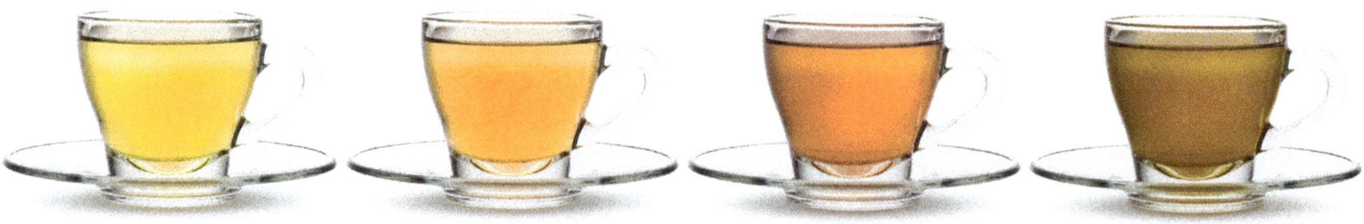

Method One — Place the herbs in a pre-warmed vessel such as a mason jar, and pour hot water over them. Cover and steep at least 30 minutes. Strain the herbs and serve. **Method Two** — Place the herbs in a pot with cold water and cover. Slowly bring the water close to a boil and remove the vessel from heat. Allow to steep at least 30 minutes. Strain the herbs and serve.

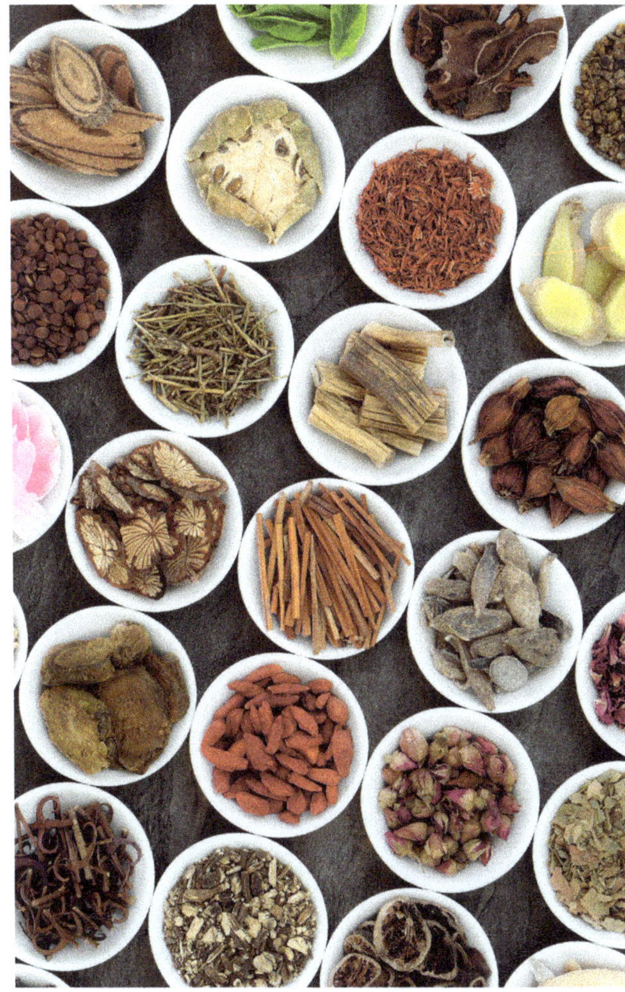

COLD INFUSIONS

Cold infusions are made from plants with medicinal components that need longer infusion times. This method is also useful for herbs containing constituents that are destroyed in the process of heating. To prepare, place the herbs in a muslin tea bag, moisten with a small amount of water and submerge moistened herbs by using the lid to suspend the tea bag. This passive circulation process enhances extraction. Steep overnight and consume the infusion the following day.

SOLAR AND LUNAR INFUSIONS

Solar and lunar infusions are subtle preparations that imbibe the majestic forces of nature. Use the cold infusion method when preparing solar and lunar infusions, as the tea will be more potent.

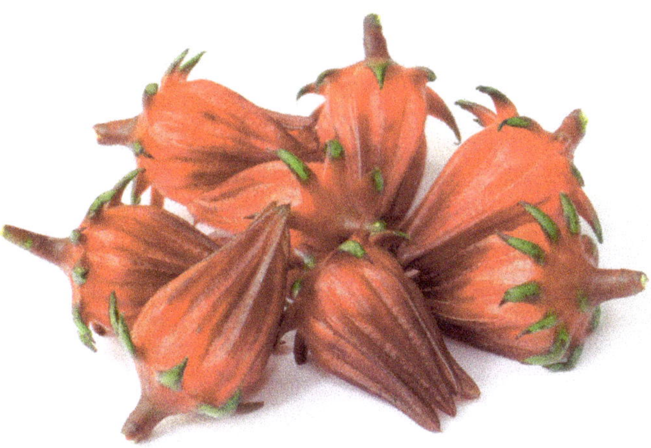

Solar Infusions — Place the herbs and water in a glass jar, cover with a lid and steep in the sun one to four hours. **Lunar Infusions** — Place the herbs and water in a glass jar, cover with a lid and steep in the moonlight overnight.

DECOCTIONS

A decoction effectively extracts dense plant material such as roots, rhizomes, bark, nuts and seeds. Place the herbs in a vessel with room-temperature water, cover with a tight-fitting lid. Bring the water and herbs to a gentle boil and turn the heat down to a low rolling simmer; cook at least 30 to 60 minutes, though the herbs can be decocted for hours. Generally, the longer the tea simmers, the sweeter and more harmonious the result. To ensure the water level does not drop too low, increase the initial water volume by fifty to one hundred percent, especially when simmering the tea for hours. After removing from the heat, strain the tea immediately or allow the herbs to steep in water up to 12 hours before consuming.

The herbs may be brewed twice before discarding the remaining plant material (referred to as the marc), although the tea becomes weaker with consecutive brewings. Optionally, add new herbs to the reused herbs to increase decoction potency.

COMBINING DENSE AND DELICATE PLANT PARTS:

Some recipes call for combining herbs that need different preparation methods. To prepare, separate the herbs into two groups: denser herbs that need decoction, and delicate herbs that need infusion. To proceed, decoct the denser herbs; then remove the tea from the heat source, add the delicate herbs to the pot, and replace the lid. Infuse the herbs at least 30 minutes, then strain and drink.

EXAMPLES OF HOT INFUSION HERBS

Achillea (yarrow)
Acmella (spilanthes)
Agrimonia (agrimony)
Alchemilla (lady's mantle)
Ambrosia (ragweed)
Anaphalis (pearly everlasting)
Antennaria (cat's paw, pussy toes)
Anthemis nobilis (Roman chamomile)
Avena (wild oats, oat straw)
Bidens (tickseed)
Borago (borage)
Calendula (calendula)
Cassia marilandica (American senna)
Centella (gotu kola)
Chamaenerion angustifolium (fireweed)
Cinnamomum (cinnamon)
Clematis (virgin's bower)
Cornus (dogwood)
Cynara (artichoke)
Daucus carota (carrot seed)
Ephedra viridis (Mormon tea)
Ephedra vulgaris (ma huang)
Equisetum (horsetail)
Eucalyptus (eucalyptus)
Filipendula (meadowsweet)
Foeniculum (fennel)
Fragaria (strawberry)
Galega (goat's rue)
Galium aparine (cleavers)
Geum (avens)
Ginkgo biloba (ginkgo)
Gnaphalium (cudweed)
Hibiscus (hibiscus)
Humulus (hops)
Hyssopus (hyssop)
Illicium (star anise)
Juniperus (juniper)
Lactuca (wild lettuce)
Lavandula (lavender)
Ledum (Labrador tea)
Leonurus (motherwort)
Leucanthemum (ox eye daisy)
Malva neglecta (mallow, malva)
Medicago sativa (alfalfa)
Melilotus (sweet clover)
Melissa officinalis (lemon balm)
Mentha arvensis (brook mint)
Mentha piperita (peppermint)
Mentha pulegium (pennyroyal)
Mentha spicata (spearmint)
Mitchella repens (partridge berry)
Monarda (bee balm)
Nepeta (catnip)
Ocimum (basil or holy basil)
Olea europaea (olive leaves)
Origanum majorana (marjoram)
Origanum vulgare (oregano)
Passiflora (passion flower)
Pedicularis (pedicularis)
Petasites (western coltsfoot)
Pimenta (allspice)
Pimpinella (anise)
Pinus (pine)
Potentilla (cinquefoil, silverweed)
Rosa (rose)
Rubus (raspberry or blackberry leaves)
Salvia (sage)
Salvia rosmarinus (rosemary)
Sambucus (elder flower or berry)
Sapindus saponaria (soapberry)
Satureja douglasii (yerba buena)
Schisandra (wu wei zi)
Scrophularia (figwort)
Scutellaria (skullcap)
Sphaeralcea (yerba de la negrita)
Stachys (hedge nettle or wood betony)
Stellaria (chickweed)
Symphytum (comfrey leaves)
Taraxacum (dandelion leaves)
Thelesperma gracile (cota)
Thymus (thyme)
Tilia (linden)
Trifolium pratense (red clover)
Turnera (damiana)
Tussilago (European coltsfoot)
Urtica (nettle)
Vaccinium (blueberry or huckleberry)
Verbascum (mullein)
Verbena (blue vervain)
Viola odorata (violet)
Zea mays (corn silk)

EXAMPLES OF COLD INFUSION HERBS

Agropyron (couch grass)
Ailanthus (tree of heaven)
Althaea officinalis (marshmallow)
Amygdalus persica (peach leaf)
Anthemis (Roman chamomile)
Arctium (burdock)
Argemone (prickly poppy)
Artemisia absinthium (wormwood)
Artemisia californica (sagebrush)
Artemisia douglasiana (mugwort)
Artemisia vulgaris (mugwort)
Asclepias tuberosa (pleurisy root)
Astragalus (huang qi)
Barosma (buchu)
Castela (chaparro amargoso)
Ceanothus (red root)
Chilopsis (desert willow)
Chionanthus (fringetree)
Cnicus benedictus (blessed thistle)
Cornus (dogwood bark)
Curcuma (turmeric)
Dicentra (bleeding heart or turkey corn)
Echinacea (echinacea)
Eleutherococcus (Eleuthero, Siberian ginseng)
Fucus (bladderwrack)
Hamamelis (witch hazel)
Hydrangea (hydrangea)
Hyssopus (hyssop)
Marrubium (horehound)
Matricaria (German chamomile)
Mentha piperita (peppermint)
Oplopanax (devil's club)
Prunus (wild cherry bark)
Rhamnus californica (California buckthorn)
Rhamnus purshiana (cascara sagrada)
Rhus aromatica (sweet sumach)
Smilax (sarsaparilla)
Swertia (American columbo)
Symphytum (comfrey)
Tabebuia (pau d'arco)
Tanacetum parthenium (feverfew)
Ulmus fulva (slippery elm)
Urtica dioica (nettle)
Viburnum opulus (cramp bark)
Viburnum prunifolium (black haw)

EXAMPLES OF DECOCTION HERBS

Althaea officinalis (marshmallow)
Angelica (angelica)
Aralia californica (aralia)
Arctium (burdock)
Arctostaphylos uva-ursi (uva ursi)
Asparagus (asparagus root)
Astragalus (huang qi)
Atractylodes (bai zhu)
Chionanthus (fringe tree)
Cichorium (chicory)
Cinnamomum (cinnamon)
Codonopsis (dang shen)
Collinsonia (stone root)
Coptis chinensis (huang lian)
Corydalis (yan hu suo)
Crataegus (hawthorn berry)
Dioscorea batatas (shan yao)
Echinacea (echinacea)
Elettaria cardamomum (cardamom)
Eleutherococcus (eleuthero)
Eutrochium (gravel root)
Glycyrrhiza (licorice)
Hydrangea (hydrangea)
Inula (elecampane)
Levisticum (lovage)
Ligusticum porteri (oshá)
Ligusticum striatum (chuan xiong)
Ligustrum lucidum (nu zhen zi)
Morella californica (bayberry)
Oplopanax (devil's club)
Paeonia alba (white peony, bai shao)
Panax (ginseng)
Phellodendron (huang bai)
Pimenta (allspice)
Piper methysticum (kava)
Rubus villosus (blackberry root)
Rumex crispus (yellow dock)
Salix (willow bark)
Sassafras (sassafras)
Smilax (sarsaparilla)
Symphytum (comfrey root)
Syzigium (clove)
Urtica dioica (nettle)
Viburnum opulus (cramp bark)
Viburnum prunifolium (black haw)

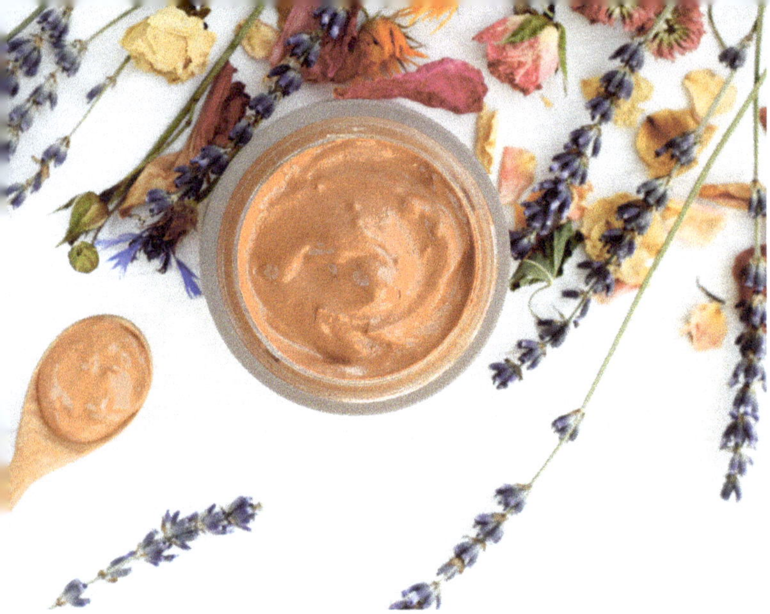

rubefacient herbs such as mustard or toxic plants should not be in contact with the skin longer than 20 minutes. After using an irritating poultice, wash the treated area using chamomile or mugwort tea.

TOPICAL PREPARATIONS

FOMENTATION: A fomentation is a cloth soaked in tea that is applied topically to reduce inflammation, pain, and irritation, or to draw out toxins such as bee venom. To prepare a fomentation, strain the herbal tea. Next, place a natural fabric such as flannel, gauze, cotton wool, or muslin into the liquid until saturated. Wring the cloth out until it no longer drips, and place on the affected area. The fomentation should be applied as hot as can be tolerated. Cover the fomentation with a towel to keep it warm. As it cools or dries, continue to re-soak the cloth and re-apply.

POULTICE: A poultice is usually a heated, moist, herbal mass spread on a cloth and applied to the skin. It can be prepared using at least three different methods: utilizing the marc of an herbal infusion or decoction; pulverizing fresh herbs; or combining powdered herbs with water. After applying to the skin, cover it with a towel to help retain the heat. As it dries or cools, remoisten as needed. Non-irritating poultices can be left in contact with the skin for long periods of time. However, poultices containing

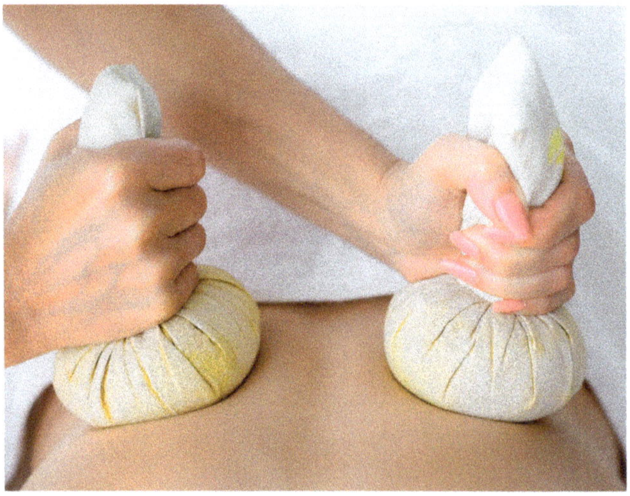

VAGINAL IRRIGATION AND ENEMA: Vaginal irrigation or enema can be effective for reducing local irritation in vaginal or rectal areas. Vaginal irrigation can be particularly beneficial for treating a yeast infection. Prepare a douche or enema by straining herbal tea (infusion or decoction) through a coffee filter to remove any potentially irritating particles. Cool to room temperature and pour the tea into a hot water bottle, then attach a hose and nozzle designated for rectal or vaginal insertion. Control the flow rate with the clamp on the hose, and allow the tea to flush the affected area.

When using vaginal irrigation, allow two to four cups of tea to flow in a slow, steady stream in and out of the vagina. When administering an enema, allow one to two cups of tea to flow into the rectum in a slow, steady stream. In some cases, such as with inflammatory bowel disease, up to one quart can be used. Hold in the contents five to ten minutes, then sit on the toilet and release the contents. If an individual is very dehydrated, there may be little or no liquid released, especially if they have had a high fever.

Caution: Only use lukewarm tea as a vaginal irrigation or enema. Never use hot tea!

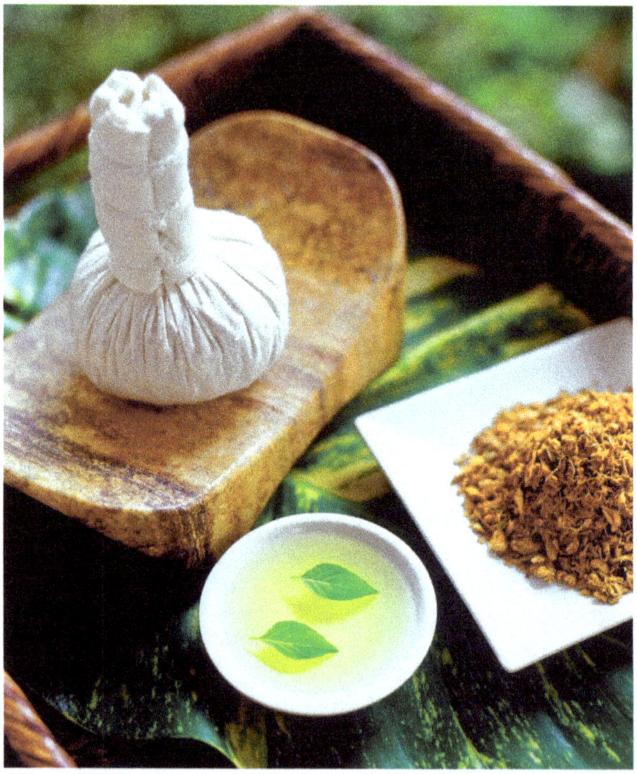

ALCOHOL-BASED EXTRACTS

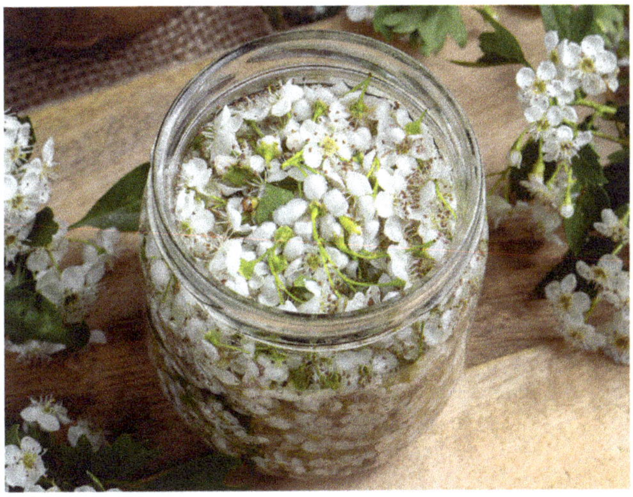

Tinctures (extracts) are best prepared from fresh plant material because the vital energy is still present. Aromatic essential oils in fresh plants are often more potent than in dry plants. However, because some plants may not be available to harvest fresh year-round or may come from distant regions of the world, dry plants can be used as an alternative. Some plants, including cascara sagrada *(Rhamnus)* or iris *(Iris),* should not be prepared as tinctures while fresh — they must be dried first.

FRESH PLANT EXTRACTS

Fresh plant tinctures are usually made with 190 proof or 95% pharmaceutical grade ethyl alcohol (ethanol), ideally organic. The water within the plant material is drawn into the menstruum as it macerates, resulting in a more dilute tincture. Some plants call for a diluted menstruum that can be prepared by combining 95% alcohol with water. When using dilute spirits such as vodka or brandy (generally containing only 40% alcohol), it is not necessary to further dilute the menstruum with water. While labels should indicate the proof and percentage of alcohol, percentage of alcohol is determined by dividing the proof in half; for example, 80 proof spirits contain 40% alcohol.

According to U.S. National Pharmacopoeia Standards, the standard ratio for making a fresh plant tincture is 1:2, or one part by weight of the plant, to two parts by volume of menstruum. This holds true for the standard U.S. system (weight by ounce to fluid ounce) or the metric system (grams to milliliters). It is important to ensure that the plant material is fully submerged in the menstruum. Roots are easily extracted with the 1:2 ratio; however, whole plants or their aerial parts may require higher ratios. Due to their bulk, some fresh plants will require a 1:3 or 1:4 ratio for the menstruum to fully cover the plant material. If necessary, the material can be weighed down with a clean rock or other heavy object that will not leach into the preparation.

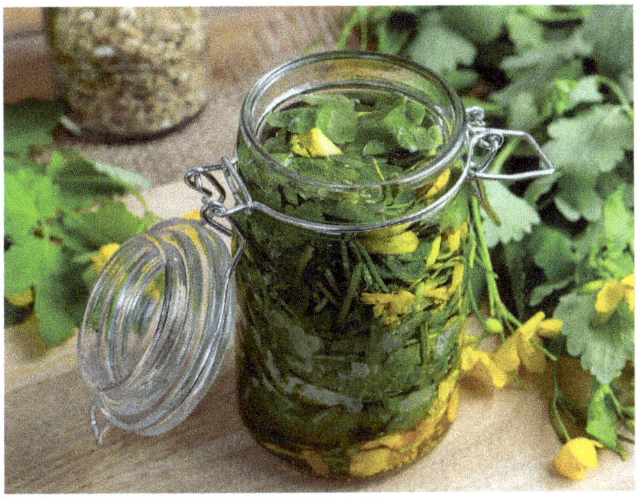

To prepare a fresh plant tincture, begin with fresh, washed plant material chopped into small pieces. While it is not necessary to chop foliage unless it is bulky, it is easier to press the tincture when the leaves are chopped. Place the fresh plant material in a clean, dry glass mason jar and pour alcohol over the herbs. The extraction process is

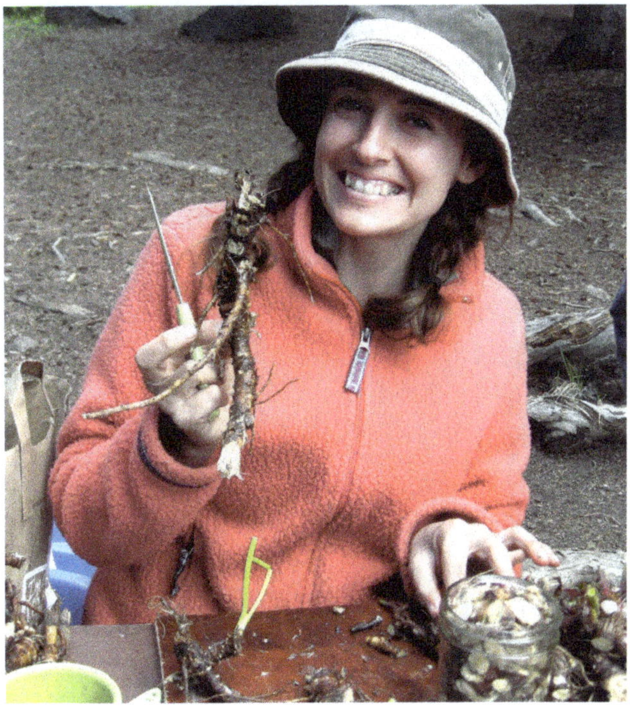

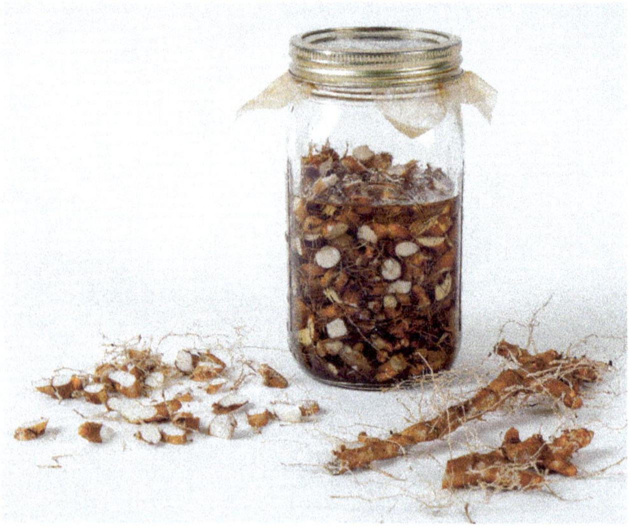

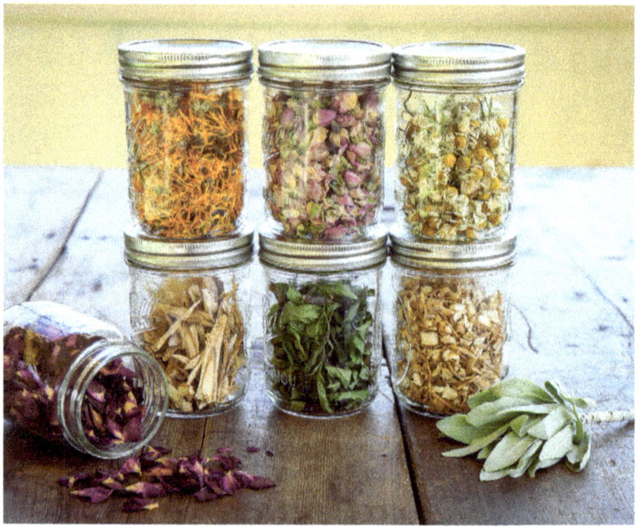

maximized by increasing the surface area of the herbs. Press and pound the herbs in the alcohol with a wooden spoon to make sure all of the air bubbles are released. Avoid pressing so hard as to excessively compact the herbs, which can prevent contact with the alcohol. If the plant matter is not covered by approximately one inch of menstruum over the plant's surface, the ratio needs to be increased to 1:3 – 1:4 for bulkier fresh plants. These ratios are noted in the *Preparations and Dosage* section. Place a piece of wax paper between the jar and the lid, and tightly close the lid. Label the preparation clearly.

Tinctures should be stored in a cool, dark place until they are ready to be pressed. *Note:* Fresh plant tinctures are formed passively as a result of dehydration, so there is no reason to shake the jar while steeping. Fresh plant tinctures should steep two to six weeks in order to extract all of the properties from the plant. When ready, strain and press the tincture, then store it in an amber bottle in a cool, dark place. Always label finished tinctures immediately after they are pressed. Alcohol-based tinctures can last many years.

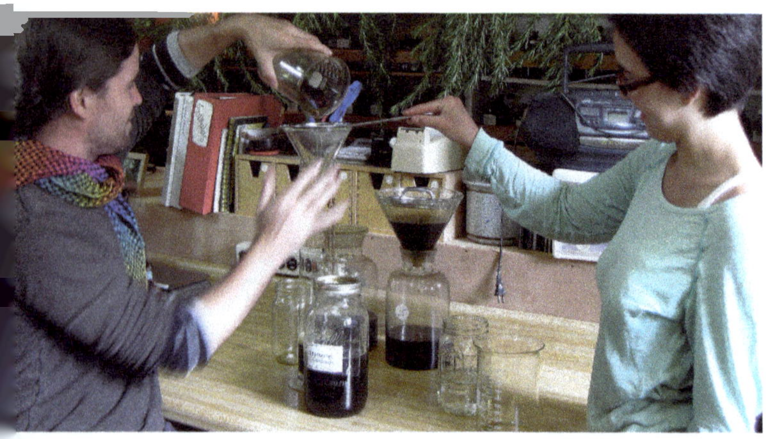

DRY PLANT EXTRACTS

A dry plant extract, also known as a maceration or tincture, is usually prepared with coarsely ground (but not powdered) material. Most dry plant extracts are made with a 1:5 ratio — one part by weight of plant to five parts by volume of menstruum.

Dry plants do not contain water; thus, it is necessary to add a portion of water to the menstruum. When using dilute alcohols such as vodka or brandy, further dilution is generally unnecessary. The most commonly recommended percentage ratio is 60% alcohol to 40% water. However, plants may require different proportions based on their level of solubility in alcohol, and the percentage of water lost from a plant during the drying process. Specific recommendations for the composition of menstruum for each plant are listed in *Preparation and Dosage.*

Plants rich in oleoresins or aromatic resins, such as *Lomatium* (lomatium), require a higher percentage of alcohol, generally 70% and above. However, some highly resinous plants, pure resins, or pitches require 80 – 95% alcohol, including *Commiphora* (myrrh), propolis, and *Cannabis* (marijuana). On the other hand, plants with high levels of mucilage can be extracted with 30 – 50% alcohol.

COMPLETING THE EXTRACT: Mix the alcohol and water to create the menstruum, and pour the menstruum over the herbs. Shake dry plant tinctures once daily. Tinctures are ready after two to six weeks, when they can be strained and bottled. Always label tinctures with the appropriate information.

CALCULATIONS FOR PREPARING THE MENSTRUUM

The volume of alcohol, water, and/or glycerin appropriate to a menstruum can be calculated as follows: First refer to the *Preparation and Dosage* section for the herb you are using. Determine the appropriate herb-to-menstruum ratio, as well as the percentages of alcohol, water, and/or glycerin. Ascertain the weight of herb to be used.

STEP 1—Find the total menstruum volume (TMV) using the herb-to-menstruum ratio:
Herb-to-menstruum ratio 1:Y (1 part herb to Y parts of menstruum)
Multiply quantity of herb (ounce) x Y parts of menstruum = TMV (fluid ounces)

STEP 2—Determine the quantities of alcohol and water:
Multiply TMV x % of alcohol = total quantity of alcohol in menstruum
Multiply TMV x % of water = total quantity of water in menstruum
Multiply TMV x % of glycerin = total quantity of glycerin in menstruum

Alcohol plus water plus glycerin quantities should equal TMV.

AN EXAMPLE: Begin with 3 ounces of dry herb. The tincture calls for an herb-to-menstruum ratio of 1:5, with a menstruum composed of 60% alcohol and 40% water:

STEP 1—Find the total menstruum volume (TMV):
1:5 means 1 part herb to 5 parts menstruum
3 ounces herb x 5 parts menstruum = 15 fluid ounces TMV

STEP 2—Determine the quantities of alcohol and water:
Multiply TMV (15 oz) by % of alcohol (60%)
15 x .60 = 9 ounces alcohol

Multiply TMV (15 ounces) by % of water (40%)
10 x .40 = 6 ounces water

Alcohol plus water total should equal TMV, in this case, 15 ounces
9 ounces alcohol + 6 ounces water = 15 ounces TMV

PRESSING THE EXTRACT: After a tincture has steeped two to six weeks, it is ready to be pressed. Pre-moisten a fine, unbleached muslin cloth with filtered or spring water, then squeeze the excess water out of the cloth. Place a strainer lined with the moistened cloth over a glass measuring cup. Strain the liquid contents of the extract through the cloth, and allow all of the liquid to drain. Then place a fist-size wad of saturated herbal material (marc) into the cloth, and squeeze out any remaining liquid, taking care to keep the marc securely inside so it does not burst out under the pressure. Consider wearing nitrile gloves while pressing the tincture. Continue to press the liquid out of the marc until no more can be extracted. Compost the remaining marc, or bury it if it is a semi-toxic or toxic plant to protect animal life. Next, pour the strained herbal material through a coffee filter to further remove particulate matter. The tincture is ready to be bottled and labeled. Store the tincture in an amber bottle in a cool, dark place.

QUANTITIES AND YIELDS: When learning to prepare tinctures, it is easy to yield too much product, so it is best to start by making smaller quantities. Usually, 4 – 16 ounces of herbal material is sufficient.

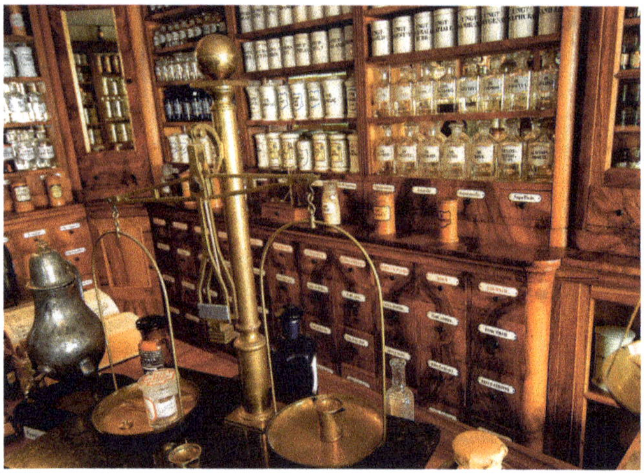

MEASUREMENTS FOR A PINT JAR (16 OUNCES):
Fresh Plant Extracts (1:2) — use 4–5 ounces of fresh plant material and 8–10 ounces of 95% ethanol menstruum. **Dry Plant Extracts (1:5)** — use 2 ounces of dry herb and 10 ounces of menstruum. **Yields** — one pint yields an average of 6–10 ounces of tincture.

MEASUREMENTS FOR A QUART JAR (32 OUNCES):
Fresh Plant Extracts (1:2) — use 8–10 ounces of fresh plant material and 16–20 ounces of menstruum. **Dry Plant Extracts (1:5)** — use 4–5 ounces of dry plant material and 20–25 ounces of menstruum. **Yields** — one quart yields an average of 14–23 ounces of tincture.

LABELING THE EXTRACT

Include the following information on a tincture label:

- The Latin name including the genus and species.
- The common name and part of the plant used for the tincture.
- Information about whether the plant is organic, wildcrafted, biodynamic, or G.M.P. certified.
- The ratio and percentage of ethanol (EtOH), water, and/or glycerin, including type of alcohol and/or glycerin, and whether it is organic.
- The date it was made and/or when it was pressed on the final bottle.
- Optional: note the phase of the moon or occurrence of a solar eclipse.

LABEL EXAMPLE

Glycyrrhiza glabra
Dry, organic licorice root
1:5, 60% organic cane sugar alcohol
9/8/2025 Lunar Eclipse

TINCTURE WORKSHEET

BOTANICAL NAME ____________________

COMMON NAME ____________________

PART USED ____________________ **DATE** ____________________

Weight of dried herb ______ ounces
Recommend herb-to-menstruum ratio ______ : ______ (weight to volume)

1) ______ ounce herb weight × ______ parts menstruum = ______ Total Menstruum Volume (TMV)

2) Menstruum ______ % alcohol ______ % water ______ % glycerin

3) ______ % alcohol × ______ fluid ounce TMV = ______ fluid ounce alcohol in menstruum
______ % water × ______ fluid ounce TMV = ______ fluid ounce water in menstruum
______ % glycerin × ______ fluid ounce TMV = ______ fluid ounce glycerin in menstruum

4) ______ fluid ounce alcohol + ______ fluid ounce water + ______ fluid ounce glycerin = ______ = TMV

PRESSING DATE ____________________ **FINISHED TINCTURE QUANTITY** ____________________ ounces

GLYCERIN EXTRACTS

GLYCERIN AS MENSTRUUM

Glycerin is a sweet-tasting, viscous substance derived from plant or animal sources that can be used as a solvent. For sensitive individuals and children, it can be easier to palate than alcohol extracts. Glycerin is also used as a preservative, a sweetener, a syrup-base, and as a humectant in cosmetic products.

Glycerin is inferior to alcohol as a solvent; however, it extracts polyphenols, flavonoids, chlorophyll and volatile compounds (although it does not extract resinous aromatic oils). Combining glycerin with distilled water as a menstruum increases its extraction capacity to include: mucopolysaccharides, phenols, anthocyanins, proanthocyanidins, ascorbic acid, carotenoids, vitamins (B and K) and minerals (calcium, copper, iron, magnesium, manganese, and zinc). in addition to the aforementioned ingredients.

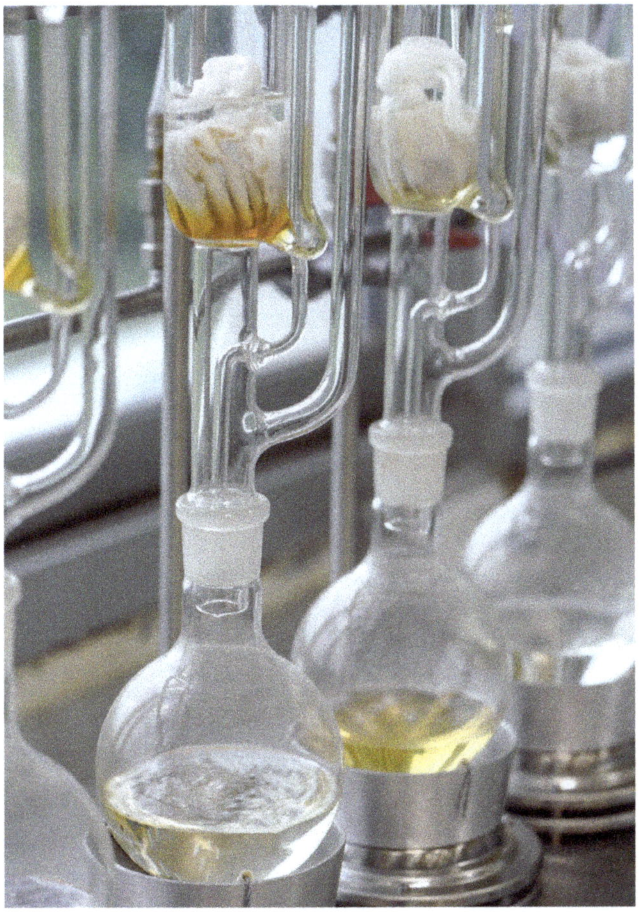

USE WITH HIGH-TANNIN SOLUTIONS: Glycerin prevents tannins from precipitating out of solution. When preparing alcohol-based extracts of plants that contain high amounts of tannins, consider adding 10% glycerin to the total menstruum volume. Otherwise, tannins tend to precipitate out of solution and form solids that settle at the bottom of the liquid.

EXAMPLES OF PLANTS WITH HIGH AMOUNTS OF TANNINS

Anemopsis (yerba mansa root)
Arctostaphylos (uva ursi leaf)
Ceanothus (red root)
Ephedra (ma huang or Mormon tea stem)
Heuchera (alum root)
Juglans (black walnut leaf or hull)
Krameria (rhatany twig or bark)
Morella (bayberry root bark)
Quercus (oak leaf or bark)
Rheum palmatum (Turkey rhubarb root)
Rubus (blackberry or raspberry root or leaf)
Rumex crispus (yellow dock root)
Viburnum opulus (cramp bark)
Viburnum prunifolium (black haw bark)

CONTRAINDICATIONS: Individuals with liver or digestive diseases who must avoid alcohol-based extracts may use glycerin extracts as an alternative. Although glycerin is low glycemic, it is not always well tolerated by individuals with blood sugar disorders, such as hypoglycemia or hyperglycemia (prediabetes or diabetes). Glycerin is metabolized by the liver, and for those with blood sugar disorders or impaired liver function, herbal teas, capsules, or tablets are preferable for long-term use.

PREPARING GLYCERIN EXTRACTS: It is best to use kosher vegetable glycerin rather than animal glycerin to prepare glycerites. Vegetable glycerin is readily available through several prominent herbal companies. Glycerin stores well in a cool, dark place.

Glycerin is very viscous and must be diluted with distilled water and/or alcohol, as it can irritate the throat when used alone. Tap water and unfiltered water should always be avoided since they can encourage microbial growth and shorten shelf life.

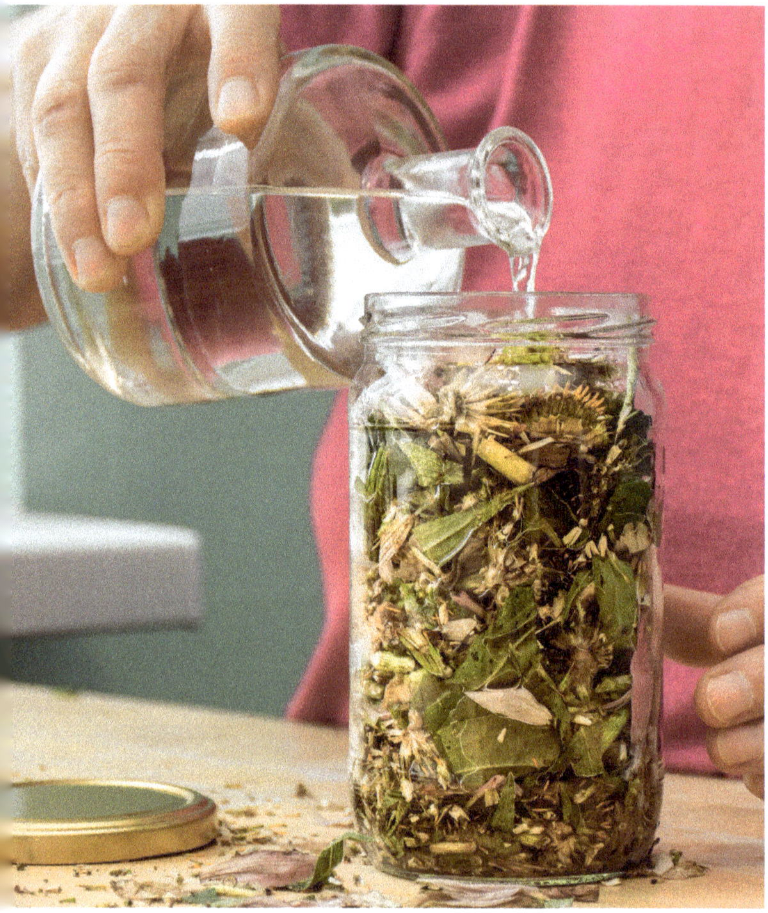

Menstruum ingredients should be measured and blended before pouring over the herbs. It is important to wash and finely chop fresh herbs before covering with the menstruum. Dry herbs should be ground, not powdered. It can be beneficial to grind the herbs and menstruum in a blender or food processor.

After combining the herbs and menstruum, pour them into a clean, dry glass jar. Place a piece of wax paper between the jar and lid. Seal tightly. Label the jar and allow the herbs to steep four weeks. The glycerite can then be strained, pressed, labeled, and stored in a cool, dark place.

PROPORTIONS: The ratio for fresh herb glycerin extract is 1:2 or 1:3 (one part by weight of herb to two or three parts volume of menstruum). Sometimes, a higher ratio is needed to adequately cover the herb. The ratio for dry herb glycerin extract is 1:5; a higher ratio may be necessary to adequately cover the herb with menstruum.

Three options for preparing a menstruum solution for a glycerin extract follow:

USING FRESH OR DRY PLANTS: Prepare a menstruum with 60% glycerin and 40% distilled water. Place glycerin-water-based extracts in a hot water bath for two to four hours to enhance extraction.

Note: The following second and third options should be avoided by individuals who cannot consume alcohol.

USING FRESH PLANTS: Prepare a menstruum with 50% glycerin and 50% alcohol (composed of 95% pure ethanol). The portion of alcohol ensures that most of the medicinal constituents are properly extracted, but may not be ideal for individuals sensitive to alcohol.

USING DRY PLANTS: Prepare a menstruum with 40% glycerin, 30% alcohol (composed of 95% pure ethanol), and 30% distilled water. Dry plants must be rehydrated, so it is important that a percentage of the menstruum contains water. This solution extracts the majority of dry plant constituents.

STORAGE: Glycerites have a shorter shelf life than alcohol extracts, with an average of six months to three years for glycerin-water-based extracts. Fresh plant glycerites contain more water, and therefore, spoil more quickly. Pressed extracts can be refrigerated to extend their shelf life. A glycerite is spoiled if it smells fermented, bubbles, or grows bacteria or mold. Discard the glycerite at the first signs of spoilage.

Glycerites with 40 – 50% alcohol have an extended shelf life because the alcohol inhibits microbial growth and prevents spoilage. The shelf life of a glycerin-alcohol-based extract ranges from one to ten years, depending on the conditions in which they are stored. Glycerites may be stored in the refrigerator or in an amber bottle in a cool, dark place away from direct sunlight.

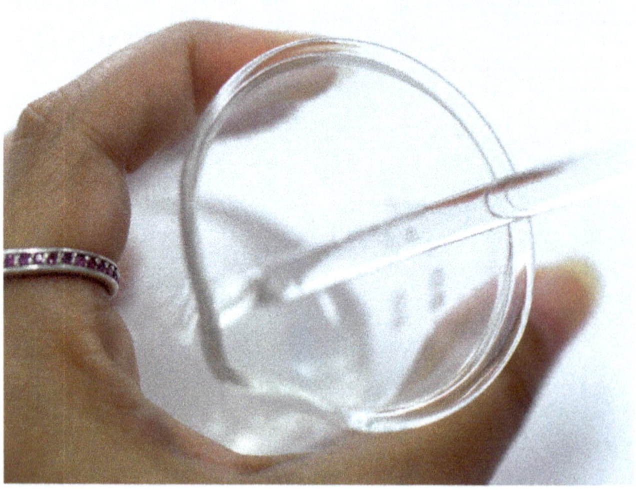

EXAMPLES OF ALCOHOL-FREE FRESH PLANT GLYCERITES

Fresh plants prepared with a menstruum ratio of 1:2 or 1:3, 60% glycerin and 40% distilled water:

Astragalus membranaceus (huang qi roots)
Curcuma (turmeric rhizomes)
Echinacea (echinacea roots or flowers)
Lavandula (lavender flowers)
Matricaria (chamomile flowers)
Melissa (lemon balm leaves)
Piper methysticum (kava roots)
Salvia rosmarinus (rosemary leaves)
Sambucus (elder berries)
Taraxacum (dandelion roots)
Thymus (thyme leaves)
Urtica (nettle leaves)
Zingiber (ginger rhizomes)

EXAMPLES OF ALCOHOL-FREE DRY PLANT GLYCERITES

Dry plants prepared with a menstruum ratio of 1:5, 60% glycerin and 40% distilled water:

Astragalus membranaceus (huang qi roots)
Echinacea (echinacea roots or flowers)
Foeniculum (fennel seeds)
Inula (elecampane roots)
Lavandula (lavender flowers)
Matricaria (chamomile flowers)
Mentha piperita (peppermint leaves)
Mentha spicata (spearmint leaves)
Piper methysticum (kava roots)
Salvia rosmarinus (rosemary leaves)
Sambucus (elder berries)
Trifolium pratense (red clover flowers)
Verbascum (mullein leaves or flowers)

EXAMPLES OF GLYCERIN-ALCOHOL FRESH PLANT EXTRACTS

Fresh plants prepared with a menstruum ratio of 1:2 or 1:3, 50% glycerin and 50% alcohol:

Achillea (yarrow flowers)
Aralia californica (aralia roots or berries)
Avena (milky oat seeds)
Echinacea (echinacea roots or flowers)
Eriodictyon (yerba santa leaves)
Eschscholzia (California poppy roots or whole plant)
Foeniculum (fennel seeds)
Heracleum (cow parsnip seeds)
Humulus (hops strobiles)
Hypericum (St. John's wort flowers)
Inula (elecampane roots)
Matricaria (chamomile flowers)
Melissa (lemon balm leaves)
Mentha piperita (peppermint leaves)
Rosa (rose buds or petals)
Sambucus (elder berries)
Scutellaria (skullcap leaves)
Taraxacum (dandelion roots)
Thymus (thyme leaves)
Urtica (nettle leaves)
Verbascum (mullein leaves or flowers)
Zingiber (ginger rhizomes)

EXAMPLES OF GLYCERIN-ALCOHOL DRY PLANT EXTRACTS

Dry plants prepared with a menstruum ratio of 1:5, 40% glycerin, 30% alcohol, and 30% distilled water:

Astragalus membranaceus (huang qi roots)
Cinnamomum (cinnamon bark)
Echinacea (echinacea roots)
Elettaria (cardamom seeds)
Eriodictyon (yerba santa leaves)
Foeniculum (fennel seeds)
Glycyrrhiza (licorice roots)
Humulus (hops strobiles)
Inula (elecampane roots)
Lavandula (lavender flowers)
Mentha piperita (peppermint leaves)
Pimpinella (anise seeds)
Piper methysticum (kava roots)
Rosa (rose buds or petals)
Sambucus (elder berries)
Schisandra (wu wei zi, five flavor berries)
Syzygium (clove buds)
Trifolium pratense (red clover flowers)
Verbascum (mullein leaves)
Vitex (vitex berries)
Zingiber (ginger rhizomes)

ACETUM EXTRACTS

VINEGAR AS MENSTRUUM

Herbal vinegar (acetum) extracts can be used as an alternative to alcohol extracts, especially to address digestive and liver concerns. These extracts retain the medicinal properties of plants for many years. Vinegar stimulates the digestive process, and is an ideal base for digestive bitters. It reduces the glycemic index of food when consumed before or with a meal. Apple cider vinegar helps to maintain an optimal internal pH balance.

When preparing a vinegar extract, it is best to use raw, organic, apple cider vinegar. Other types of vinegar used for culinary purposes may be substituted, such as rice vinegar, wine vinegar, white or red balsamic vinegar, and sherry vinegar. Do not use distilled white vinegar as a menstruum.

MENSTRUUM ACTIONS: Vinegar extracts are great alternatives for individuals who cannot consume alcohol-based extracts. When used as a menstruum, vinegar effectively extracts the following plant constituents: minerals, vitamins, alkaloids, and some aromatic compounds. It is ideal for extracting alkaloids because the acidic menstruum makes them more bioavailable.

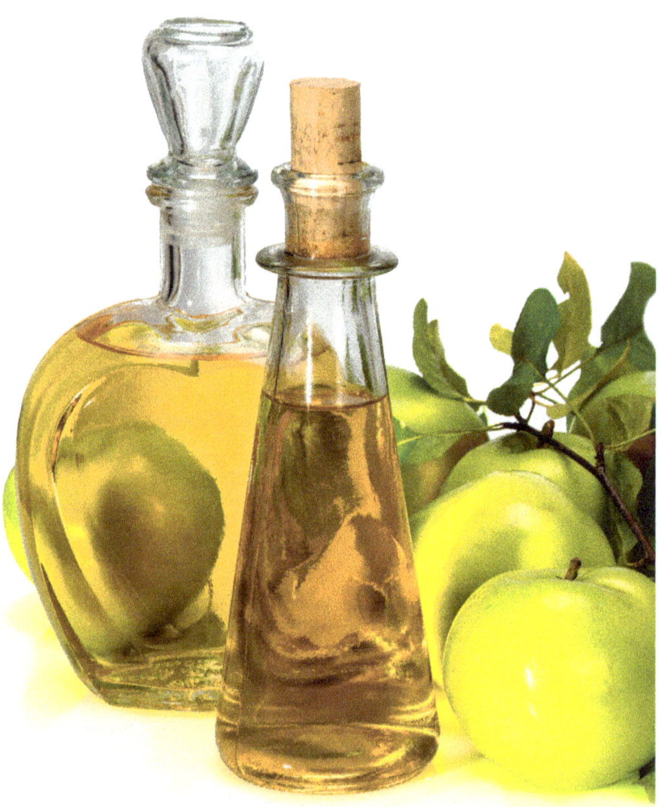

INTERNAL USE

Vinegar extracts are usually prepared using Simpler's method. Pack a clean, dry mason jar with fresh or dry plant material one inch below the shoulder of the jar, then cover the herb with vinegar. Press and stir the herb with a utensil to eliminate all air bubbles. Next, place a piece of wax paper between the jar and lid. Seal tightly. The vinegar menstruum doesn't need to be diluted with water, as it is already a dilute substance. Ideally, the vinegar should contain 5 – 7% acetic acid.

The extract should steep four weeks prior to being strained, pressed, bottled, and labeled. Alternatively, prepare an oxymel by adding 1/6 to ⅓ warmed honey to the total volume of the strained acetum extract to temper the tartness and increase palatability. Store it in a cool, dark place, or in the refrigerator. Vinegar extracts last six months to ten years, depending on the plant and its water content. It is best to use the extract sooner, rather than later.

Vinegar extracts can be incorporated into any recipe requiring vinegar, as long as the herb is palatable and non-toxic. Add vinegar extracts to salad dressings, stir fries, marinades, and sweet and sour recipes. Drizzle on baked or French fried potatoes, or consume ½ to 1 teaspoon up to three times daily.

FIRE CIDER

Fire cider is an herbal compound made with raw, organic, apple cider vinegar that enhances immune function. The herbs traditionally used in this recipe include: fresh *Allium cepa* (onion), *Allium sativum* (garlic), *Capsicum frutescens* (cayenne or other hot peppers), *Cochlearia armoracia* (horseradish), and *Zingiber officinale* (ginger); however, the formula can be modified in various ways. Mediterranean herbs such as *Petroselinum* (parsley), *Origanum* (marjoram, oregano), *Salvia* (sage), *Salvia rosmarinus* (rosemary), *Satureja* (savory), *Thymus* (thyme), and *Laurus nobilis* (bay leaves) can be added to enhance the flavor and nutritional value. Herbs such as *Arctium lappa* (burdock root, gobo), *Curcuma* (turmeric), and *Alpinia* (galangal) also make wonderful additions to fire cider. Add small amounts of seaweed to increase the vitamin and nutrient content. Add honey to enhance flavor.

DOSAGE: Consume one to four droppers (up to one teaspoon), three to five times daily for acute conditions. Consume one to three droppers, one to three times daily for chronic conditions, or as a tonic. Fire cider can substitute for vinegar in most recipes. It tastes great with a variety of foods, such as vinaigrettes, sweet and sour soups, stir-fries, and marinades.

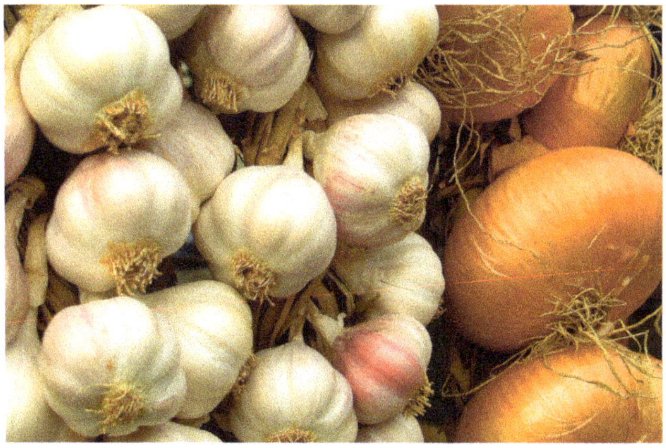

FIRE CIDER RECIPE

A one-quart batch:
2" x 1" x 1" piece of ginger
3" x 1" piece of horseradish
1 small onion
1 head of garlic
2 - 3 small hot peppers
Raw, organic, apple cider vinegar
Any additional herbs of your choosing

Peel onions and garlic. Chop onions, garlic, and peppers, being careful not to touch your eyes. The horseradish and ginger should be grated or finely chopped. Place the ingredients in a sterilized quart mason jar, filling the jar one to two inches below the mouth. Pour the vinegar over the herbs, making sure that there are no air bubbles. Leave at least one-half to one inch between the lid and the vinegar. Add a layer of wax paper between the jar and the lid, and seal the lid. Allow the herbs to steep in a dark place two weeks to one month. Strain, press, and store in an amber bottle.

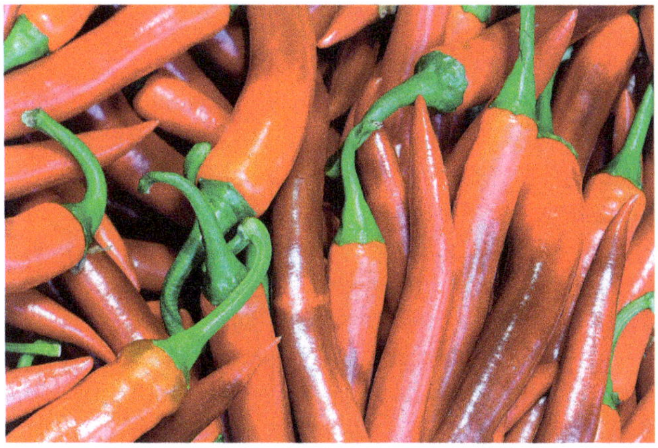

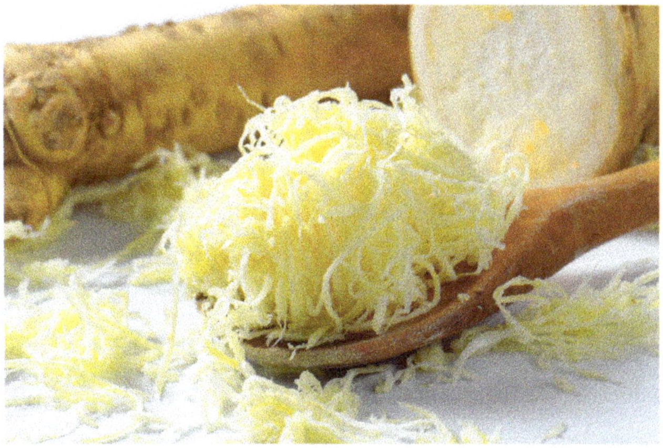

MEDICINAL USES: Fire cider can be consumed in the early stage of a cold or flu, or anytime to boost resistance. It has antibacterial, antifungal, and antiviral propterties. Fire cider enhances immune functions by stimulating neutrophils, T cells, and natural killer cells. In addition, it has diaphoretic and vasodilating properties that aid in treating a fever. Due to the expectorant properties of the herbs, fire cider is an adjunct treatment for sinusitis, bronchitis, and allergies.

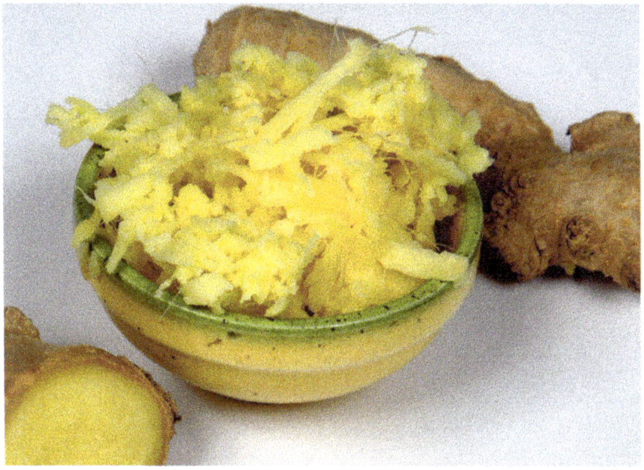

A circulatory stimulant, fire cider increases blood flow to the tissues and enhances their oxygenation. It also aids in removing waste products from tissues.

Many herbs used in fire cider help to lower elevated cholesterol levels and low density lipids (LDLs). They also increase high density lipids (HDLs) that can be beneficial in preventing and treating atherosclerosis. Some of the herbs used in this formula have blood-thinning properties that can be beneficial for people with elevated blood pressure and cholesterol levels.

CONTRAINDICATIONS: The herbs in this formula can affect individuals taking blood-thinning medications or aspirin. Anyone undergoing surgical procedures should stop taking blood-thinning herbs at least two weeks prior to, and two weeks following surgery. This formula should be used with caution by individuals with a sensitive stomach, acid reflux, chronic heartburn, gastric ulcers, irritable bowel syndrome, Crohn's disease, or flatulence.

MEDITERRANEAN VINEGAR

Mediterranean herbs can be used in salad dressings, gargles, or tonics. These herbs stimulate the digestive and immune systems. Examples of Mediterranean herbs that can be used for vinegar extracts include: *Allium cepa* (onion), *Allium sativum* (garlic), *Artemisia dracunculus* (tarragon), *Laurus* (bay leaves), *Origanum* (marjoram, oregano), *Salvia* (sage), *Salvia rosmarinus* (rosemary), *Satureja* (savory), and *Thymus* (thyme). In general, these herbs have the following medicinal properties: antimicrobial, immune stimulant, expectorant, carminative, cholagogue, and circulatory stimulant.

DIGESTIVE BITTERS

To stimulate digestive secretions, consume 2 – 3 droppers, 15 to 30 minutes prior to a meal. Examples of herbs that can be incorporated into a digestive bitters formula include: *Arctium* (burdock), *Berberis* (berberis), *Citrus* (orange peel), *Cnicus* (blessed thistle), *Cynara* (artichoke leaf), *Foeniculum* (fennel), *Gentiana* (gentian), *Menyanthes* (bogbean), *Rumex* (yellow dock), *Salvia rosmarinus* (rosemary), *Taraxacum* (dandelion), *Zanthoxylum* (prickly ash), and *Zingiber* (ginger).

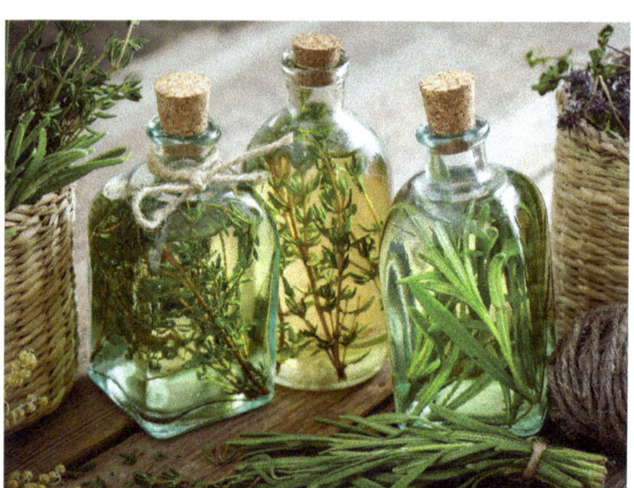

PICKLED HERBS AND SEAWEED

Pickled *Allium* (onions, garlic), *Arctium* (burdock), and *Urtica* (nettle) are delicious. Pickling seaweed decreases the low tide flavor. Chop the fresh herbs and place in a jar. Pour in enough vinegar to coat the herbs. Seal the jar and let pickle for 2 to 4 weeks before consuming.

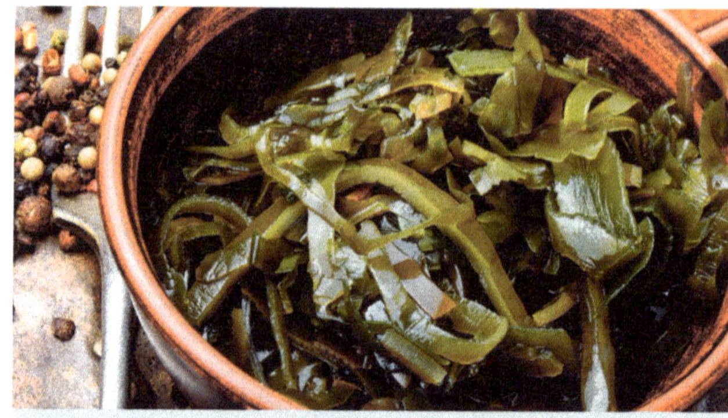

PICKLED SEAWEED RECIPE

PREPARATION DIRECTIONS: Rinse seaweed in filtered or spring water to remove sand and particulate matter. Remove tough stems. Slice kelp into thin ribbons or cut feather boa into 1 - 2 inch length pieces, then soak them in warm water for five minutes until they soften. Strain excess water and place the seaweed in a sterile one quart jar.

Combine water, vinegar, sugar, and spices in a saucepan and bring to a low rolling simmer. Cook until the sugar dissolves, then remove from the heat. Pour the liquid over the seaweed and cover the jar with a lid. Allow the jar to cool to room temperature. Store pickled seaweed in the refrigerator.

8 ounces of kelp *(Laminaria)* or feather boa *(Cystoseira)*
320 ml or 12 fluid ounces filtered or spring water
120 ml or 4 fluid ounces white wine or unseasoned rice vinegar
50 grams cane sugar
1 teaspoon allspice berry
1 teaspoon black pepper
1 teaspoon coriander seed
1 teaspoon mustard seed
1 teaspoon red pepper flakes (optional for spice)
2 bay leaves
1 - 2 cinnamon sticks
6 clove buds
1 - 2 cloves garlic (optional)

TOPICAL PREPARATIONS

Externally, vinegar extracts can be used as a base for liniments. Use on the scalp and hair to stimulate hair growth, reduce dandruff, and add luster. They can also be diluted and used topically as a facial astringent.

VINEGAR LINIMENTS

Liniments are liquid preparations for the skin that are, in most cases, either rubefacient or locally anesthetic. Vinegar extracts make great liniments; prepare as previously described. Traditionally, vinegar-based extracts used as liniments include: *Achillea* (yarrow), *Equisetum* (horsetail), *Hamamelis* (witch hazel), *Lobelia* (lobelia), *Pedicularis* (pedicularis), *Quercus* (oak bark), *Rosa* (roses), *Salvia rosmarinus* (rosemary), *Umbellularia* (California bay leaves), *Valeriana* (valerian), and *Zingiber* (ginger).

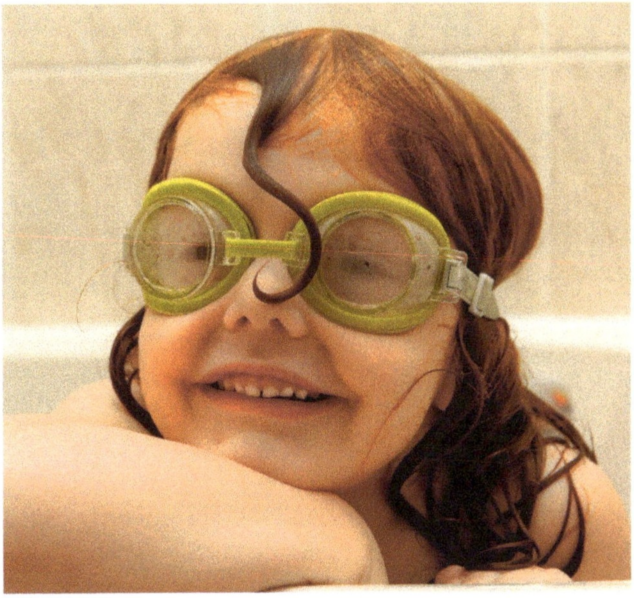

PAIN RELIEF LINIMENT RECIPE

PREPARATION DIRECTIONS: Place herbal ingredients in a clean, dry quart glass jar. Cover with 16 ounces of raw apple cider vinegar. If necessary, add enough vinegar to completely cover the herbs. Steep for four weeks; strain, press, and bottle.

DIRECTIONS FOR USE: Apply the liniment topically for sore muscles, sprains, strains, arthritic joints, neuralgia, and sciatica. *Warning:* Do not apply to broken skin.

1½ ounces valerian root *(Valeriana)*
½ ounce tobacco leaf *(Nicotiana)*
½ ounce lobelia leaf *(Lobelia)*
¼ ounce prickly ash bark *(Zanthoxylum)*
¼ ounce cayenne fruit *(Capsicum)*
16 ounces raw apple cider vinegar

HAIR RINSES

Vinegar extracts classically used as rinses for blond or red hair include: *Achillea* (yarrow flowers), *Calendula* (calendula flowers), and *Matricaria* (chamomile flowers). Vinegar extracts of *Equisetum* (horsetail), *Urtica* (nettle leaves), *Salvia rosmarinus* (rosemary leaves), and *Salvia* (sage leaves) are beneficial for brunettes, and helpful for treating dandruff. Vinegar extract can be used directly on the scalp, or after dilution with water. Apply extract to the hair and scalp, comb it in, and leave it on for 10 minutes before shampooing and conditioning.

HAIR RINSE RECIPE FOR BLONDES OR REDHEADS

½ ounce chamomile flowers *(Matricaria)*
½ ounce calendula flowers *(Calendula)*
½ ounce yarrow flowers *(Achillea)*
½ ounce pink rose petals *(Rosa)*
10 - 12 ounces raw apple cider vinegar

HAIR RINSE RECIPE FOR BRUNETTES

½ ounce nettle leaves *(Urtica)*
½ ounce rosemary leaves *(Salvia rosmarinus)*
½ ounce sage leaves *(Salvia)*
½ ounce horsetail *(Equisetum)*
10 - 12 ounces raw apple cider vinegar

PREPARATION: Place herbal ingredients in a clean, dry pint glass jar. Cover with 10 - 12 ounces of raw apple cider vinegar. (If necessary, add more vinegar to completely cover the herbs.) Steep for four weeks; strain, press, and bottle.

DIRECTIONS FOR USE: Moisten hair and scalp in the shower or bath. Apply hair rinse to hair and scalp using a squirt-bottle. Massage into the scalp and comb into hair. Rinse hair and scalp after 10 minutes. (Optional: shampoo and condition hair after hair treatment.) *Note:* Directions for use and preparation applies to both hair rinses.

HERBAL HONEY AND SYRUP

HONEY

MEDICINAL PROPERTIES: Honey is most medicinal when it is raw and unpasteurized. It has antimicrobial properties and helps to prevent infections.

Used internally, honey also has expectorant actions, and soothes mucous membranes, especially in the upper respiratory system. For internal use, add one teaspoon to one tablespoon of plain or medicinal honey to one cup of boiled water or tea. If you have a sweet tooth, you can consume the undiluted honey.

An effective topical treatment for burns and wounds, honey reduces inflammation, encourages tissue healing, and prevents scarring. It has hydrophilic (water-drawing) properties that prevent blistering, and help to soothe inflamed, irritated tissues. It prevents scarring and promotes smooth healing of tissues. Raw honey also has antimicrobial properties that prevent infection. Undiluted, raw honey is applied directly to the affected area.

HONEY FACIAL: Honey is useful as a rejuvenating facial mask. First tie your hair back and wear a headband to keep hair from sticking to your face. Next, open your pores using an herbal facial steam, then wipe all moisture from your face and apply the honey mask for 15 to 30 minutes, then rinse with warm water. Your skin will have a warm, radiant glow, and sweet honey fragrance.

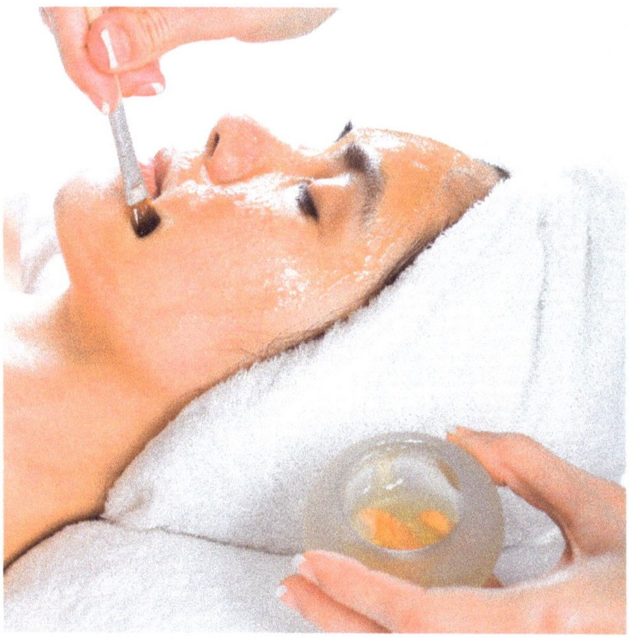

CONTRAINDICATIONS: Honey has a high glycemic index. Regular consumption of honey is not recommended for individuals with type I or type II diabetes, syndrome X, hypoglycemia, or any blood sugar-related disorders.

All kinds of sugar, including pasteurized honey, have immune suppressant qualities. Individuals with severely compromised immunity may want to avoid regular or frequent consumption of honey.

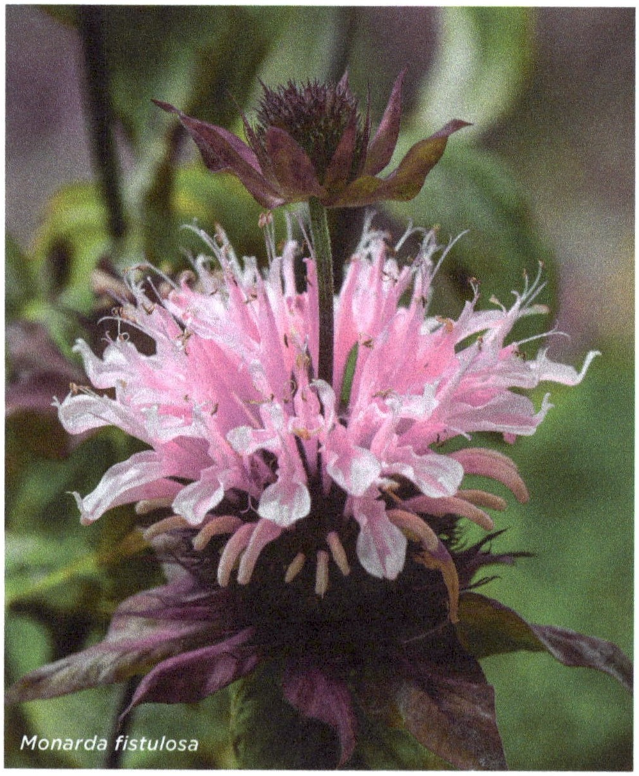

Monarda fistulosa

FRESH HERBAL HONEY

Fresh herbal honey can be made with a plant's aerial parts or roots, each requiring a different method of preparation.

INFUSING FRESH LEAVES OR FLOWERS

Fresh aerial parts should be wilted one to two days on a cardboard tray or in a paper bag before preparation. After they are wilted, the herbs can be coarsely chopped and placed in a clean, dry mason jar, filling the jar one inch below the lid. Next, pour honey over the herbs and stir the mixture, making sure that all air bubbles are released. If the honey is solid or too thick to pour, heat at a low temperature to liquefy; otherwise, heating is unnecessary. The herbs should be fully submerged. Wipe off any honey on the upper lip or outside threads of the jar, and dry. Cover with a piece of wax paper and tighten the lid.

Place the container on a window sill or elsewhere in the sun, as heat speeds the extraction process. Steep the mixture two to six weeks, watching closely to make sure no mold develops. If you notice moisture forming on the inside of the jar, wipe with a paper towel. Consider placing the jar in warm (not boiled) water to liquefy the honey before straining. If the jar is heated too quickly, it will crack. Strain the herbs through a stainless-steel mesh strainer; no cloth is needed for straining. Bottle, label, and store in a cool dark place or in the refrigerator.

FRESH HERB EXAMPLES

Allium (garlic bulbs)
Capsicum (cayenne fruits)
Citrus (orange peels)
Curcuma (turmeric rhizomes)
Echinacea (echinacea flowers)
Jasminum (jasmine flowers)
Lavandula (lavender flowers)
Melissa (lemon balm leaves)
Mentha piperita (peppermint leaves)
Monarda (bee balm flowers)
Origanum (oregano and marjoram leaves)
Rosa (rose petals)
Salvia (sage leaves)
Salvia rosmarinus (rosemary leaves)
Thymus (thyme leaves)
Umbellularia (California bay leaves)
Viola (violet leaves and flowers)
Zingiber (ginger rhizomes)

MEDICINAL USES: Infusing garlic in honey tempers the garlic's heating qualities. It tastes delicious, and can be consumed by the spoonful during the first stage of a cold or flu, or for upper or lower respiratory infections.

Lavender honey and lemon balm honey have a subtle, aromatic flavor. Consume one teaspoon in hot water, or in your favorite nervine tea for a calming effect.

Bee balm flower honey has diaphoretic and expectorant actions. It is also beneficial as an antimicrobial during the first stage of a cold or flu, and has throat-numbing actions. Mediterranean herbal honey containing any combination of thyme, oregano, marjoram, sage, and/or bay leaves is excellent during the first stages of a cold, flu, sore throat, or upper/lower respiratory infection. The honey has a delicious pungent flavor. Add one teaspoon of honey in hot water to your favorite immune and respiratory tea, or consume small amounts by the teaspoonful.

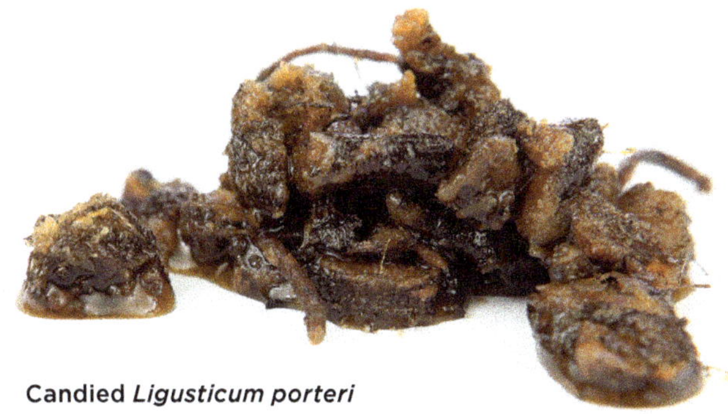

Candied *Ligusticum porteri*

INFUSING FRESH ROOTS

To prepare fresh root honey, clean and chop the roots into quarter-inch to half-inch slices. The ratio is 1:4—one part of fresh root (by volume) to four parts honey (by volume). For example, combine one cup of fresh chopped roots with four cups (one quart) of honey.

Place ingredients in a large stainless-steel, glass, or porcelain pot with a lid. Make sure the pot accommodates at least two to three times the total honey volume, as the honey will expand when heated. Slowly bring the honey to a low rolling simmer, then turn it down to the lowest possible setting. Check the honey and stir frequently to make sure it doesn't boil and bubble over the pan. Place a lid on the pot after the honey bubbles slightly and a consistent cooking temperature is reached. Cook on low three to four hours. Turn the heat off; allow the honey to cool overnight. Another option is to place the herbs in a crockpot, cover, and cook on a low temperature 12 to 24 hours.

The next day, warm the honey until it liquefies. Place a stainless-steel strainer over a glass measuring cup and pour the honey, straining out the roots. Make sure the volume is the same or less than the original volume. If there is more liquid than the original volume, continue to cook the honey until the initial volume is obtained. This occasionally occurs with roots that have high water content. If the extra water is not evaporated off by cooking, the honey can ferment.

Sometimes it is necessary to strain the roots twice to pull out the particulate matter. If the honey becomes too thick to strain, reheat it. After the honey is thoroughly strained,

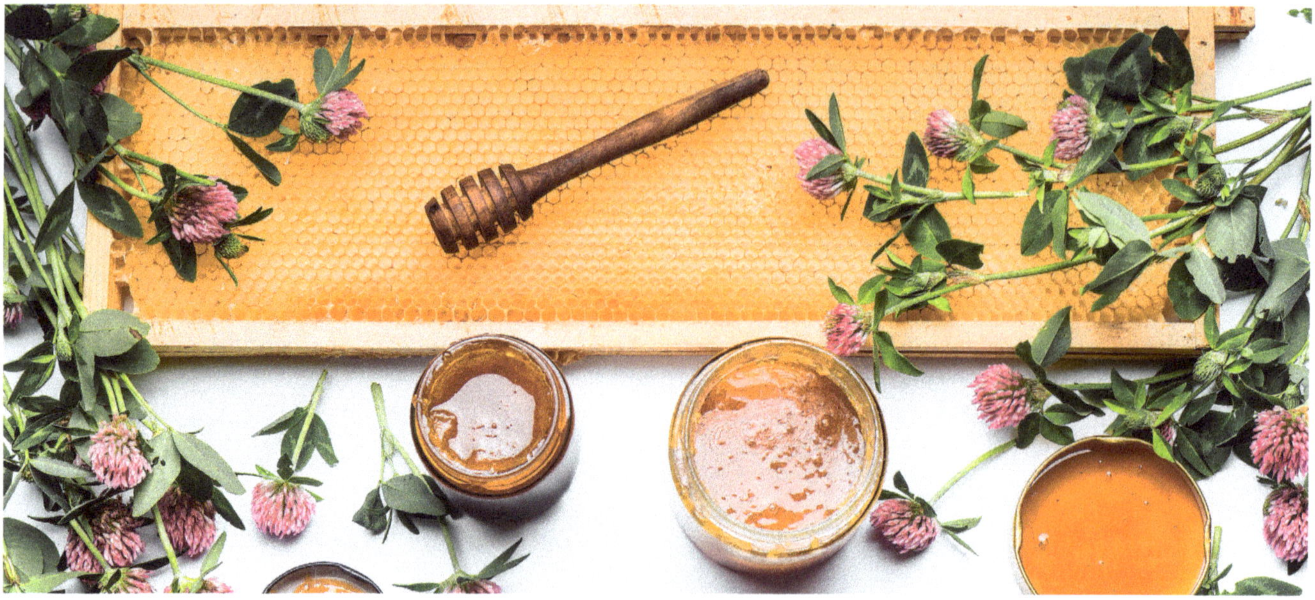

pour into a clean, dry glass mason jar — preferably a wide-mouth jar for easier removal. Cover with a lid and store in a cool, dark cupboard. It is not necessary to refrigerate the honey; it can be stored for many years. Root honeys can last a decade and remain delicious and potent.

MEDICINAL USES: Angelica, balsam root, elecampane, lomatium, and oshá honey are extremely beneficial for treating lower respiratory infections, as they have antimicrobial properties and expectorant actions. Angelica and oshá encourage diaphoresis during the first stage of a cold or flu. Angelica, elecampane, and aralia have expectorant and antitussive actions. They can be used as respiratory tonics to reduce asthmatic spasms and deepen respiration.

FRESH ROOT EXAMPLES

Althaea (marshmallow)
Angelica (angelica)
Aralia (aralia)
Arctium (burdock)
Armoracia syn. *Cochlearia* (horseradish)
Astragalus (huang qi)
Balsamorhiza (balsam root)
Echinacea (echinacea)
Inula (elecampane)
Levisticum (lovage)
Ligusticum (oshá)
Lomatium (lomatium)
Taraxacum (dandelion)
Zingiber (ginger)

IMPORTANT TIPS

TEMPERATURE: Gas stoves are ideal for the honey-making process. Sometimes, electric stoves are too hot on the lowest setting, and can burn honey.

CHECK THE HONEY FREQUENTLY: Do not walk away from the honey while it is heating up. Within minutes, honey can go from just starting to bubble, to completely boiling over, resulting in a sticky mess.

BEES LOVE HONEY: Bees, most humans, and many animals find the smell of honey irresistible. Thus, it is best to close all doors and windows without screens. It does not take much time for nearby bees to locate honey being heated. They will fill your kitchen, and even plunge themselves into the liquid. If you are in bear country, keep windows and doors closed until your honey-making process is complete. This is one reason to avoid making fresh root honey in the field.

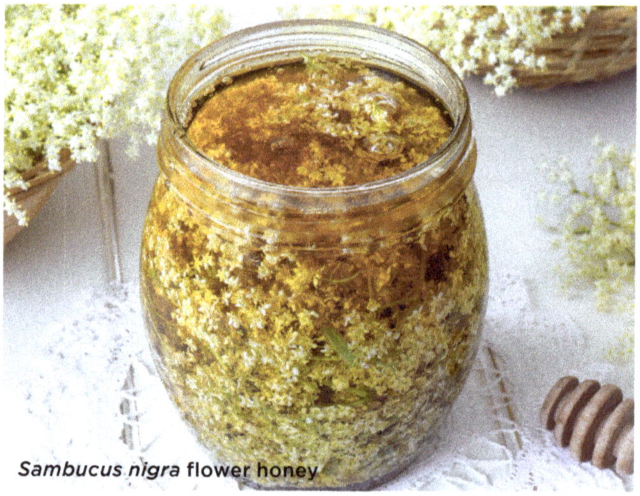

Sambucus nigra flower honey

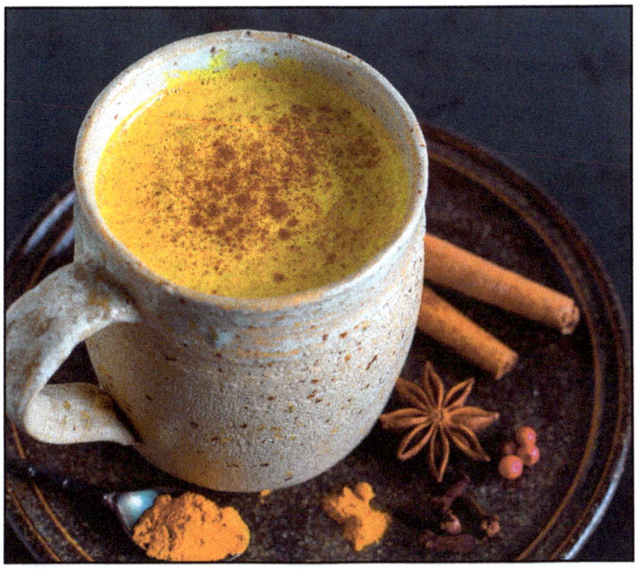

DRY HERBAL HONEY

INFUSING ROOTS, SEEDS, AND BARK

Dried, chopped roots and additionally dry seeds, barks, and berries can be prepared similarly to fresh root honey; however, dry plants are often better suited for preparing syrups. See section on *Herbal Syrups* for further instruction.

INFUSING POWDERED HERBS

Herbal honeys can be easily prepared with powdered herbs. Measure approximately one quarter cup of powdered herbs for every cup of honey and place in a clean, dry glass jar. Gently warm the honey using a double boiler, and pour into the jar with the powdered herbs. Place a lid on the jar and allow the mixture to infuse at least two weeks; the honey is then ready to consume. There is no need to strain out the herbs unless desired. Label the jar and store in a cool, dark place.

SPICED HONEY RECIPE

Place the following in a clean, dry pint glass jar and cover with a lid: 2 cinnamon sticks, 1 teaspoon of clove, ½ of a thinly-sliced orange peel or tangerine peel, and 1 teaspoon of allspice.

Pour honey over the herbs and stir to release all air bubbles. Thoroughly coat the herbs with honey and cover the jar. Steep the honey on a warm window sill four weeks. Warm the honey until it liquefies and strain out the herbal material. Bottle, label, and store in a cool, dark place, or in the refrigerator.

HERBAL SYRUP

Syrups are generally sweetened, water-based preparations that incorporate an herbal infusion or decoction. They are more efficient than honey at extracting water-soluble constituents, including some vitamins, minerals, and mucilage, but they have a shorter shelf life and require refrigeration. Honey is often used as a base for herbal syrups, though other liquid sweeteners such as molasses, simple syrup, agave, and brown rice syrup also can be used as sweetening agents. Syrups also can be prepared by combining any of these liquid sweeteners with an alcohol- or vinegar-based extract.

PREPARING SIMPLE SYRUP: Place one cup each of sugar and distilled water (or use herbal tea for an infused simple syrup) in a pot. Heat the water or tea until it simmers, then turn heat to low. Heat and stir until the sugar dissolves in the water. Place in a clean, dry bottle with a lid. Label, date, and store in the refrigerator up to one month. Discard if the liquid has a fermented or moldy smell.

Simple syrup is a sweetener that can be added to teas or tinctures. Two to ten drops of essential oils also can be added to simple syrup.

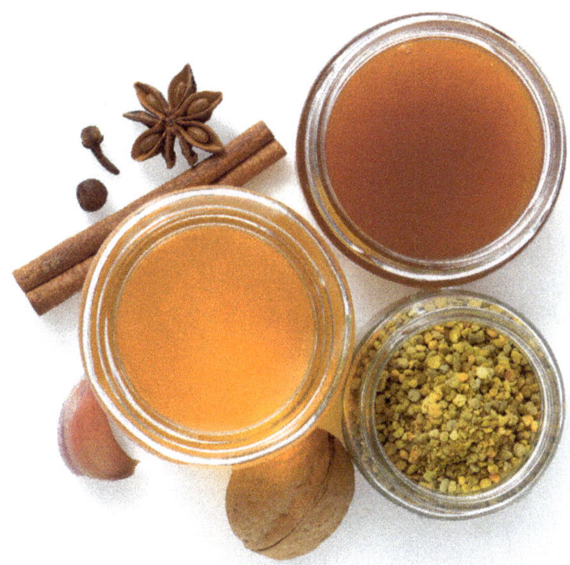

INFUSING WATER-BASED HERBAL SYRUP

Method One — Prepare an infusion from the aerial portions of the plants. **Method Two** — Prepare a decoction using roots and other dense plant materials. The two methods only differ in the first part of the preparation.

USING AERIAL PARTS: Aerial plant material (leaves, flowers, and delicate seeds) high in volatile oil should not be simmered. To make syrup with the aerial portions of the plants, place one ounce by weight of herbs in a vessel and cover with 8 – 16 ounces of distilled, boiled water. Use distilled water to prevent spoilage. Cover and steep the herbs in a covered vessel four to eight hours.

USING DENSER PARTS: For roots and other dense plant materials, place one ounce of herbs by weight in a vessel with a lid and add 16 ounces of distilled water. Bring the water to a boil and immediately turn down to a low rolling simmer until the volume is reduced to one-half the original amount (8 ounces). Combine aerial portions of the herbs with decocted herbs, after the decoction has been removed from the heat, and cover with a tight-fitting lid. Steep the herbs with the lid on for several hours, until the liquid is warm or room temperature.

COMPLETING THE SYRUP: Strain the infusion or decoction through a cloth, and press out remaining liquid from the herbs. Compost or discard the exhausted herbal material (marc).

After the infusion or decoction has been strained and pressed, reheat the liquid, but do not boil. Remove from the heat, then add enough honey or simple syrup to desired sweetness. Usually, one-third to one-half of the final product volume (3 – 4 ounces by volume) is sufficient.

Refrigerate the syrup to prevent spoilage. It will last two to eight weeks. To extend the shelf life of the syrup, add 15 – 20% grain, grape, or cane sugar alcohol (190 proof) of the total syrup volume and mix thoroughly. The syrup should last up to six months or more with this method, and should still be refrigerated.

INFUSING TINCTURE-BASED SYRUP

Another simple method of making syrup is to add plain honey, infused honey, or simple syrup to an alcohol-based extract. Measure the extract volume. Add an equal amount of honey or simple syrup (if using honey, liquefy it by using a double boiler to ensure easy mixing). Stir until completely mixed with the extract. Consume one-half to one teaspoon, three to five times daily.

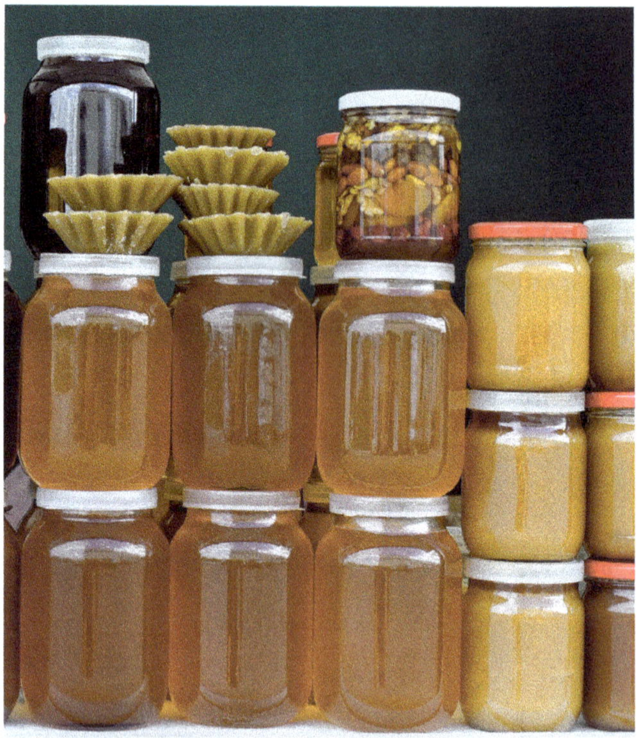

ELDER BERRY SYRUP

½ cup dried elder berries
½ cup echinacea root
3 tablespoons fresh grated ginger rhizome
2 - 3 cinnamon sticks
2 tablespoons cardamom pods (whole)
2 tablespoons orange peel
1 teaspoon clove buds

Combine ingredients in a pot and cover with one quart of distilled or spring water. Bring to a water to a boil, then turn down to a low rolling simmer for 40 to 60 minutes or until the liquid is approximately half the original volume. Remove from the burner and allow the tea to cool down. Strain the herbs through a cheesecloth or muslin, and then press the remaining liquid. Add one quarter to one third the total volume in honey. *Note:* If the honey is solid, heat in a double boiler until it liquefies. Mix the honey and tea with a whisk until the honey is completely dissolved. Pour into containers, label and date them. Store in the refrigerator for up to two months.

MEDICINAL OILS AND SALVES

BASE OILS

Base oil is the liquid medium used to extract medicinal properties from herbs in order to make oils and salves. The base oils least likely to become rancid are cold pressed vegetable, nut, and seed oils. Avoid using hydrogenated oils. When purchasing base oils, it is important to ensure that they are hexane-free. Hexane is a toxic solvent used to extract apricot, castor, and grapeseed oil.

Extra virgin olive oil is ideal for making salves, since it will store well for a long time. Derived from the first pressing of the olives, it is the purest grade. On the other hand, olive oil can be too heavy for facial and massage oils; instead, use cosmetic-grade bases for massage oils, creams, and lotions. Oils with a lighter texture and milder scent include: almond, apricot, grapeseed, jojoba, sunflower, and safflower.

PREVENTING RANCIDITY: Oils degrade and become rancid when they are exposed to oxygen, light, or heat. An antioxidant, vitamin E improves the shelf life of oils and salves. Add one to two drops of vitamin E oil to every ounce of medicinal oil to prevent rancity. It should be added to the oil after it is pressed and ready to be stored, or several drops may be added to each container before the salve is poured.

Rosemary *(Salvia rosmarinus)* or chaparral *(Larrea tridentata)* also can be added to a medicinal oil or salve recipe to prevent rancidity. Chaparral has a rather potent scent, but is a highly-effective antioxidant.

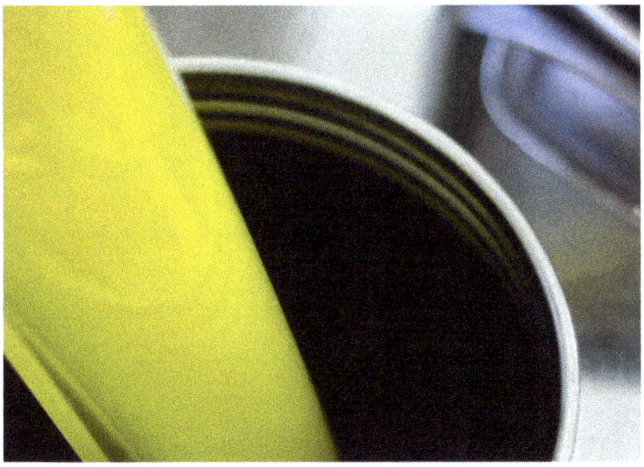

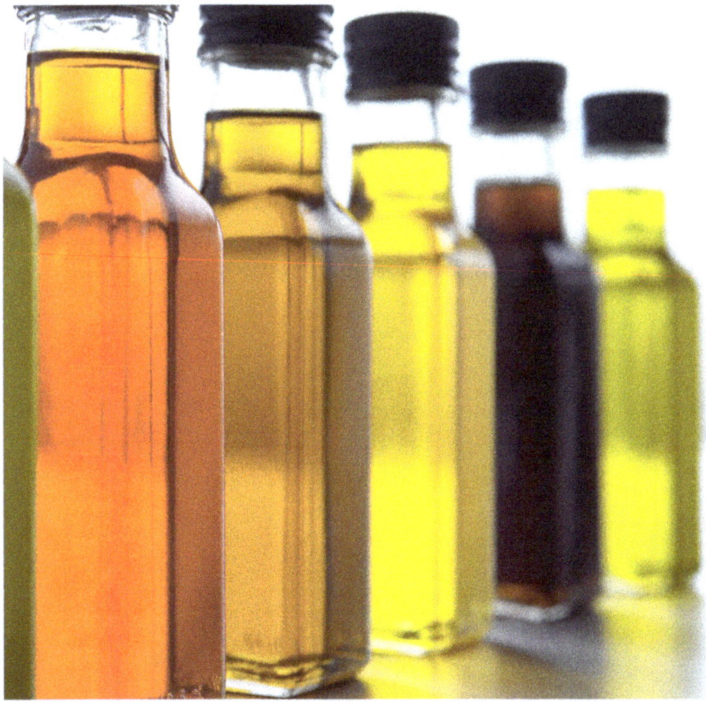

PREPARING MEDICINAL OILS

Several methods can be used to make medicinal oils. The solar infusion method takes the longest amount of time; the double boiler and alcohol intermediary methods are the fastest processes.

SIMPLER'S METHOD—FRESH OR DRY PLANTS

The Simpler's method is a traditional way of determining the amount of herb to use in making herbal oils, and does not require weighing the plant material. It is ideal when working with fresh herbs.

PASSIVE INFUSION—FRESH HERBS: The first step is to wilt the fresh plants one to three days, as they contain water that can cause the oil to mold. Chop the herbs into small pieces and place them in a clean glass jar. Cover the herbs with oil and press with a large spoon making sure there are no air bubbles. Next, pour an additional one to two inches of oil on top to completely submerge the herbs; exposed plant material will oxidize and encourage bacterial growth, resulting in oil spoilage. A round, flat rock can be placed on top of the plant material to ensure it stays under the liquid. Place a piece of wax paper between the jar and lid. The oil should be checked every one to two days to make sure there is no water condensation. If water appears in the oil, soak it up with a paper towel, or suction it out with a turkey baster or glass dropper. Steep the oil two to four weeks, then strain it through unbleached cheesecloth or muslin.

SOLAR INFUSION METHOD—FRESH: The solar infusion method incorporates the vital energy of the sun, and is useful when making fresh plant oils. Fill a clean, dry mason jar with wilted, chopped fresh herbs one inch below the shoulder of the jar. Cover the herbs with oil, press with a wooden spoon to release all air bubbles. Pour one extra inch of oil on top, then place a piece of wax paper between the jar and lid, and cover tightly. It is important to avoid pouring the oil past the shoulder of the jar, as it can expand and make a mess. Place the jar in a warm, sunny spot. It looks lovely in a garden or on a windowsill. Allow the mixture to infuse two to four weeks. The oil will not go rancid in the sun while it steeps. Strain out the herbs and rebottle the oil, then store it in a cool, dark place or refrigerate. After the mixture is strained, it will go rancid quickly if left in the sun.

BLENDER METHOD—FRESH OR DRY: Chop and wilt fresh herbs. Use the Simpler's Method or weigh herbs. If using the latter, add four ounces of vegetable oil for each ounce of herb. Pulse the herbs and oil in a blender. Pour the mixture into a jar and cover with a layer of wax paper and a lid; steep two to four weeks. Strain and press the oil. Pour into an amber bottle, and add vitamin E oil to prevent rancidity. Label and store in a cool, dark place.

EXAMPLES OF FRESH PLANTS IN OIL

Arnica (arnica flowers)
Galium (cleavers leaves)
Hypericum (St. John's wort flowers)
Lavandula (lavender flowers)
Matricaria (chamomile flowers)
Plantago (plantain leaves)
Prunella (self-heal leaves)
Scrophularia (figwort leaves)
Stellaria (chickweed leaves)
Viola (violet leaves)
Zingiber (ginger rhizomes)

DOUBLE BOILER METHOD—FRESH OR DRY: Place the herbs and oil in a double boiler and cover with a tight-fitting lid. Gently bring the water in the bottom pan to a low simmer. Slowly cook the herbs in the oil for 30 minutes to four hours. It is important to check and maintain the water levels in the bottom pan, and check the oil frequently to make sure it is not overheating. If the oil gets too hot, it will be ruined. Strain, press, and bottle the oil after it cools.

CROCKPOT METHOD—FRESH OR DRY: Place herbs and oil in the crockpot and turn it to the lowest heat setting. Cover the pot and steep the mixture one to four hours. The amount of time the oil cooks will depend on the temperature of the lowest setting. Check the oil frequently.

FRESH PLANTS FOR DOUBLE BOILER OR CROCKPOT METHOD

Anaphalis (pearly everlasting aerial parts)
Artemisia (mugwort leaves)
Calendula (calendula flowers)
Curcuma (turmeric rhizomes)
Lavandula (lavender flowers)
Matricaria (chamomile flowers)
Rosa (rose petals)
Salvia rosmarinus (rosemary leaves)
Symphytum (comfrey roots or leaves)
Trifolium (red clover flowers)
Urtica (nettle leaves)

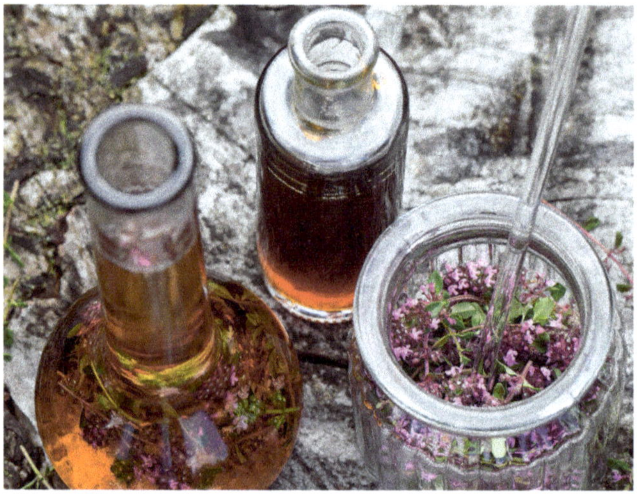

BODY OIL RECIPE

Combine one ounce each of calendula, chamomile, lavender, and roses, and place in a double boiler. Add 40 ounces of base oil (i.e., almond, apricot, or safflower). Use the double boiler or crock pot method. This oil has a 1:10 ratio of herb (by weight) to oil (by volume). This is a luxurious massage or body oil. Experiment with other herbs that delight the senses, relax the body, improve circulation, or reduce pain.

ALCOHOL INTERMEDIARY OIL METHOD (AIOM) —DRIED PLANTS

Some plants are inadequately soluble in oil and require added alcohol to pull out the alcohol soluble constituents. In these cases, the alcohol intermediary method is highly effective for making medicinal oils or salves; it is also a very rapid process. One must not use dilute alcohol like vodka for this process, only 95% ethanol.

PREPARING A MEDICINAL OIL USING ALCOHOL INTERMEDIARY OIL METHOD: Grind up one part of dry herb (by weight) and place it in a measuring cup to determine its total volume. Take ⅓ to ½ of the total volume to determine the maximum amount of pure ethanol to be used for moistening the plant material. Place the herb in a bowl, then slowly mix in a few ounces of alcohol at a time. Pour in enough alcohol to cover all of the herbal material, but do not saturate it (it is not a tincture). The ideal texture is obtained when the soaked herb holds the shape of your hand if it is picked up and compressed, but does not drip with alcohol. Place the herb and alcohol mixture in a glass or plastic container with a tight-fitting lid. Allow it to steep 12 to 24 hours. Place the mixture in a blender, cover it with seven parts (by volume) of vegetable oil, and blend until the blender is warm. Pour the herb-saturated oil through muslin draped over a strainer, strain and press the oil into a measuring cup, then bottle and label.

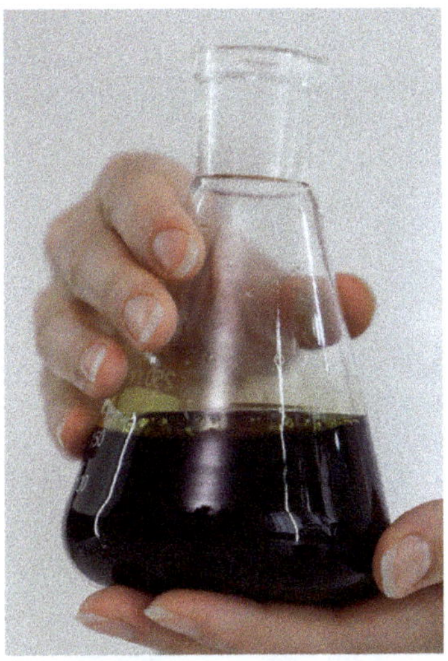

EXAMPLE: Begin with two ounces (by weight) of pre-ground herb (not powdered). The herb occupies a volume of six ounces when placed in a measuring cup. One-half of that volume is three ounces, the maximum volume of alcohol that should be used to moisten the herb. After mixing the herb and alcohol (less alcohol is preferable), place the mixture in a sealed container. After 12 to 24 hours, place the contents in a blender with seven parts by volume (14 ounces) of oil. The medicinal oil has a 1:7 herb-to-oil ratio. Blend, strain, and bottle the oil or make a salve.

EXAMPLES OF DRIED PLANTS USING ALCOHOL INTERMEDIARY OIL METHOD

Achillea (yarrow flowers)
Anemopsis (yerba mansa leaves)
Arnica (arnica leaves)
Balsamorhiza (balsam leaves)
Berberis (berberis leaves)
Boswellia (frankincense)
Calendula (calendula flowers)
Cannabis (cannabis leaves)
Centella (gotu kola leaves)
Commiphora (myrrh)
Curcuma (turmeric rhizome)
Echinacea (echinacea leaves)
Equisetum (horsetail leaves)
Eriodictyon (yerba santa leaves)
Filipendula (meadowsweet leaves)
**Garrya* (silk tassel leaves)
Grindelia (gumweed flowers)
Hydrastis (goldenseal leaves or roots)
Larrea (chaparral leaves)
Leonurus (motherwort leaves and flowers)
**Lobelia* (lobelia aerial parts)
Melissa (lemon balm leaves)
Myroxylon (balsam of Peru resin)
Myroxylon (balsam of Tolu resin)
Piper methysticum (kava roots)
Populus (poplar buds)
Propolis resin (beehive resin)
Salvia (sage leaves)
Salvia rosmarinus (rosemary leaves)
Sanguinaria (bloodroot)
Symphytum (comfrey leaves)
Thuja (western red cedar leaves)
Thymus (thyme leaves)
Umbellularia (California bay leaves)
Usnea (usnea lichen)
Valeriana (valerian roots)
Verbena (blue vervain leaves and flowers)
Zanthoxylum (prickly ash bark)
Zingiber (ginger roots)

*Use these herbs on a surface area no larger than 3 square feet, as extensive use can cause toxicity.

SALVES

BEESWAX: The primary agent used to solidify oils when making salves is beeswax. Cocoa butter, shea butter, and coconut oil also can be used as additional solidifying agents; however, they can create a slightly chunky or grainy texture when they solidify in oil. Beeswax is more reliable for producing a smooth salve, and adds a lovely subtle scent.

The ratio of beeswax to oil depends on the desired consistency of the salve; the higher the ratio of oil to beeswax, the softer the consistency. For a more solid salve, use a 1:5 ratio (weight of beeswax to volume of herbal-infused medicinal oil). For a creamier salve, use a 1:10 ratio of beeswax to oil.

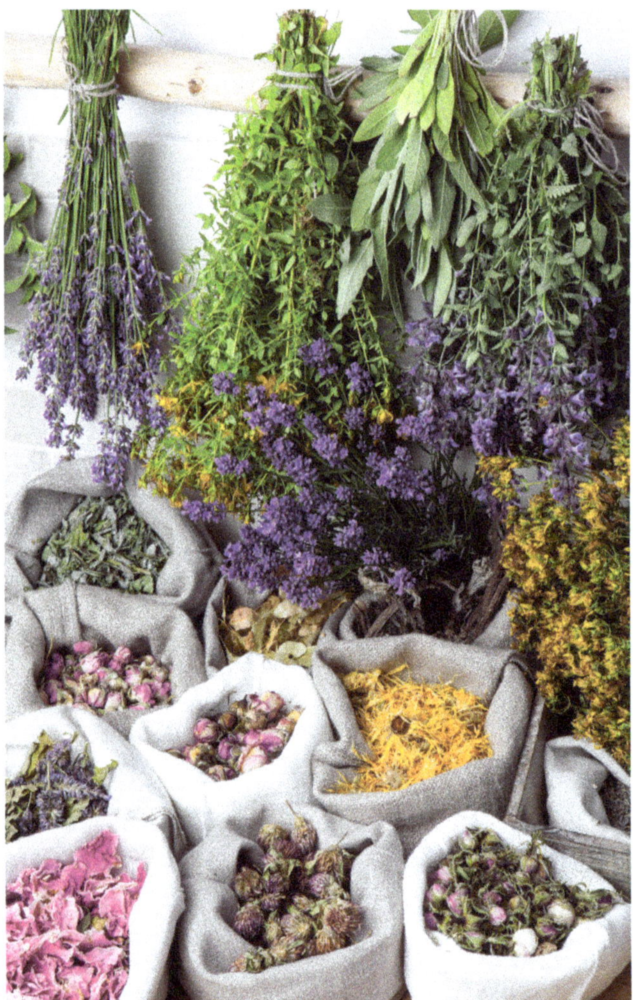

EXAMPLE: If you have 20 ounces of oil and a 1:10 ratio of beeswax to oil is desired, add two ounces of beeswax.

Caution: Beeswax should be avoided by individuals with known allergies to propolis.

PREPARING SALVES: Heat beeswax and strained medicinal oil in a double boiler on low heat. When the beeswax has melted into the oil, pour into salve jars. Add essential oil into the salve before it cools. Depending on the potency and type of essential oil, add 2 to 10 drops per ounce of salve. Wait until the mixture cools before covering.

ESSENTIAL OILS: Highly concentrated, distilled aromatic plant extracts are unrelated to the base oils. They are much more potent than herbal-infused medicinal oils. Some essential oils can irritate, burn, or cause blistering when used directly on the skin. Others can be used directly in low doses, but they should be studied extensively before using them directly and topically in oils and salves. *Note:* Many pounds of a plant are required to produce one ounce of essential oil.

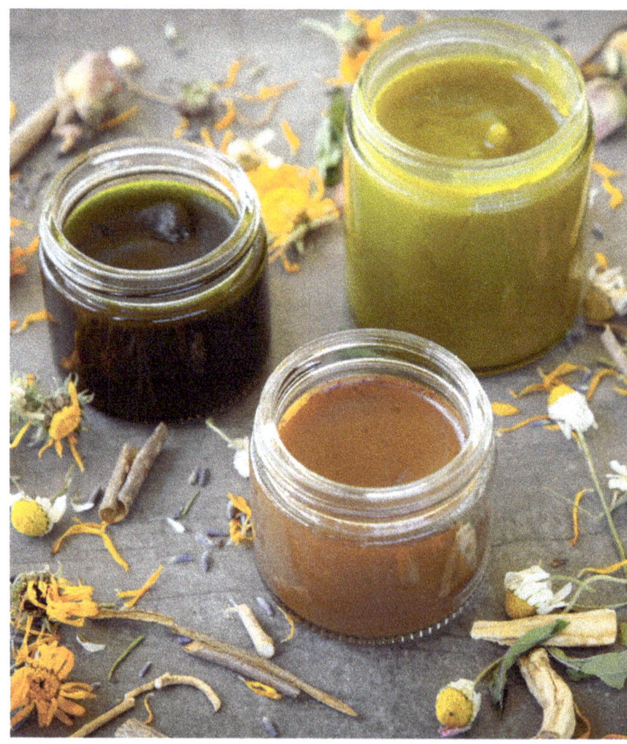

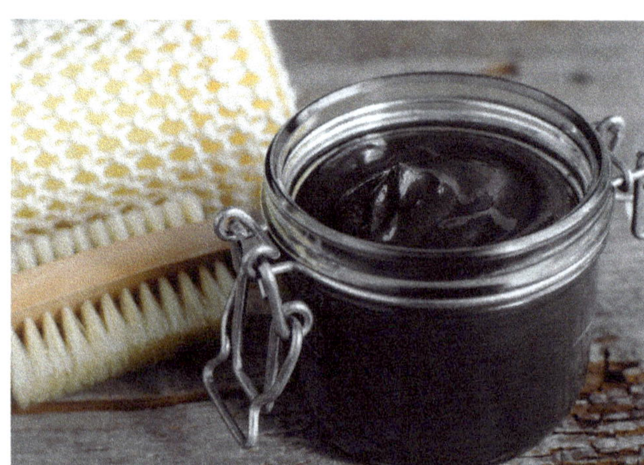

SALVE RECIPES

Prepare the following recipes first as a single or combination oil, then make a salve by adding beeswax. Use the ratios described in the *Preparing Medicinal Oils* section, and vary the weight of herbs to match the quantity of desired salve. Each ounce of herb will produce an average five to seven ounces of oil.

For example, if four herbs are listed as one part each, and you want to make less than ten ounces of salve, only use ¼ ounce of each herb. Single infused oils can also be combined and then utilized to prepare salve.

MUSCLE AND JOINT SUPPORT SALVE: This salve contains equal parts of arnica leaves, calendula flowers, chamomile flowers, comfrey leaves, St. John's wort flowers, and yarrow flowers. Prepare arnica, calendula, and comfrey using the alcohol intermediary oil method. Prepare the St. John's wort as fresh plant oil, and add it to the blend after the other oil is pressed and strained. Prepare chamomile and yarrow oil as fresh plant oil, or with the alcohol intermediary oil method. This salve is very effective for treating sprains, strains, sore muscles and joints, arthritis, and bruises.

ANTIBACTERIAL/ANTIFUNGAL FIRST AID SALVE: Combine equal parts of dried calendula, comfrey, chaparral, and rosemary. Prepare an oil with these herbs using the alcohol intermediary oil method, then make a salve. This salve can be used to treat athlete's foot, ringworm, skin tinea, staph, cuts, abrasions, rashes, and bruises. Other antibacterial herbs can be substituted.

ANTI-INFLAMMATORY OIL OR SALVE: Prepare the oil using the double boiler or crock-pot method. Combine equal parts of dry or fresh calendula, chickweed, comfrey root, figwort, licorice, and marshmallow root. After the oil is infused and strained, add one to two parts of fresh St. John's wort oil. Prepare a salve if desired. This preparation can be helpful for diaper rash, dermatitis, dry eczema, psoriasis, cradle cap, poison oak, or poison ivy (in the dry stage).

MOLES AND BASAL CELL CARCINOMA SALVE: Prepare the oil using the alcohol intermediary oil method. Include two parts dried turmeric, and one part each of dried chaparral, calendula, and cannabis leaf. Apply only to affected area.

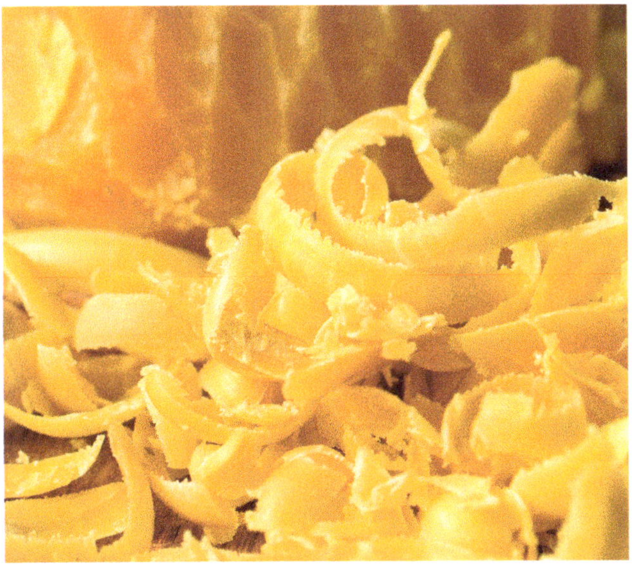

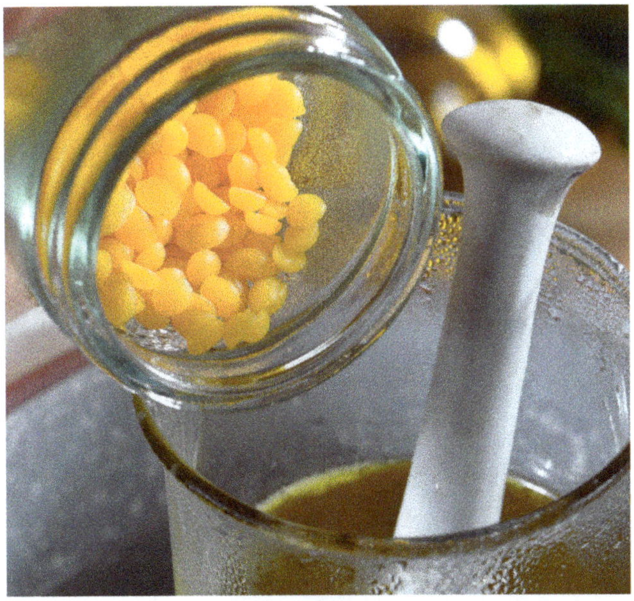

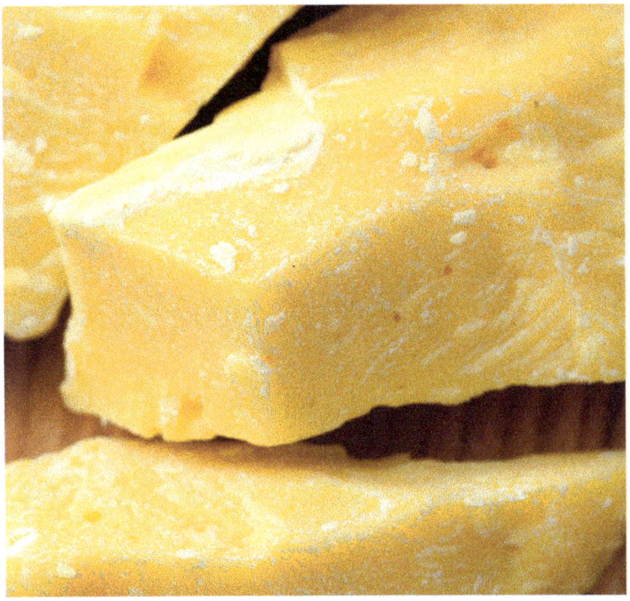

HERBAL THERAPEUTIC FORMULAS

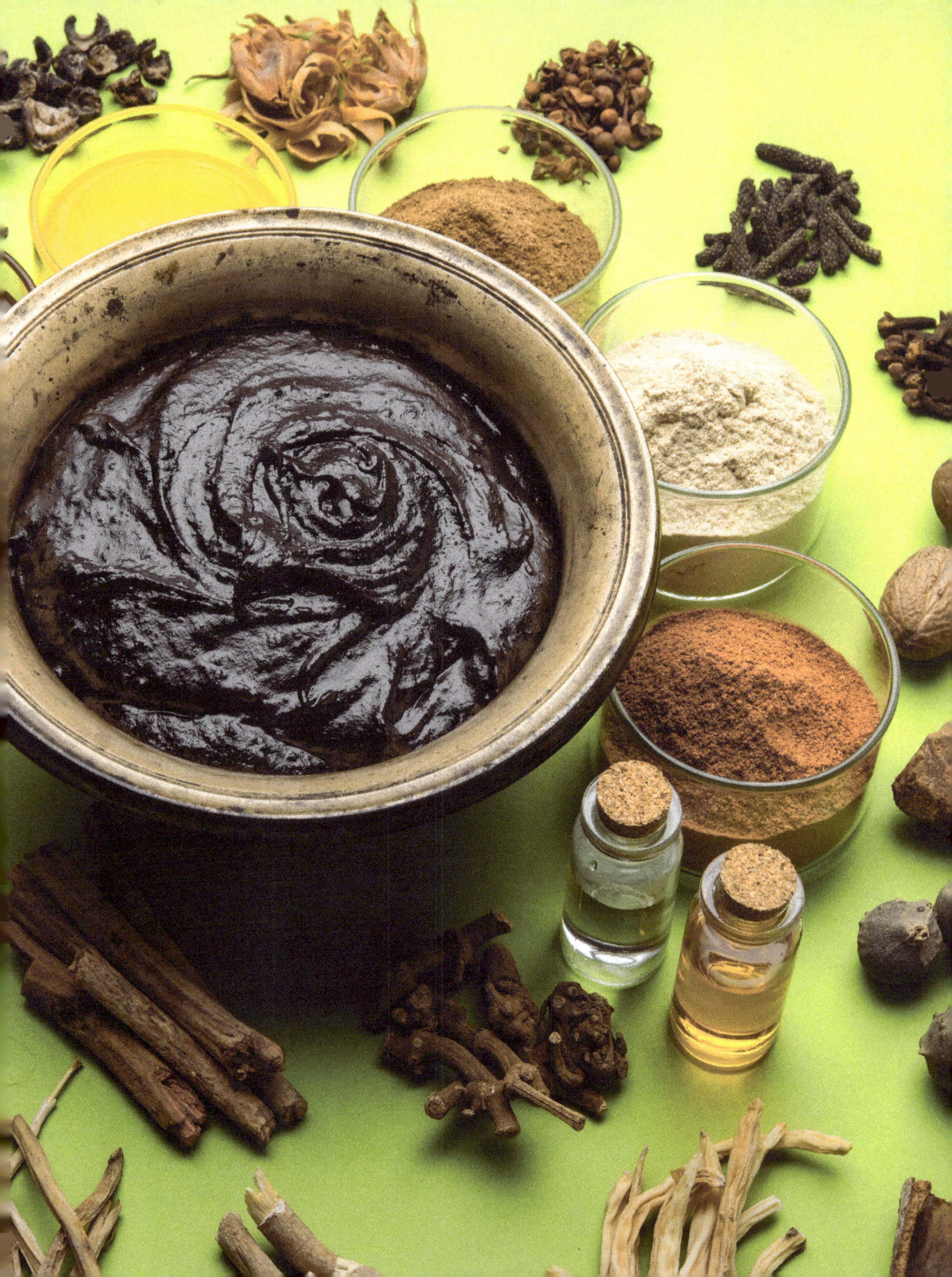

ADRENAL AND IMMUNE SUPPORT

ADAPTOGENIC COMPOUNDS AND TEAS

ADAPTOGEN AND ADRENAL TONIC COMPOUND

DIRECTIONS: Combine the following single extracts. Consume 30-90 drops, up to three times daily.

2 parts tulsi basil *(Ocimum sanctum)*
2 parts reishi *(Ganoderma)*
1½ parts eleuthero *(Eleutherococcus)*, American ginseng *(Panax quinquefolius)*, or uncured Chinese ginseng *(Panax ginseng)*
1½ parts shu di huang *(Rehmannia)*
1 part devil's club *(Oplopanax)*
1 part white peony *(Paeonia lactiflora)*
½ part ashwagandha *(Withania)*
¼-½ part schisandra *(Schisandra)*
¼ part licorice *(Glycyrrhiza)*—omit with high blood pressure and/or edema

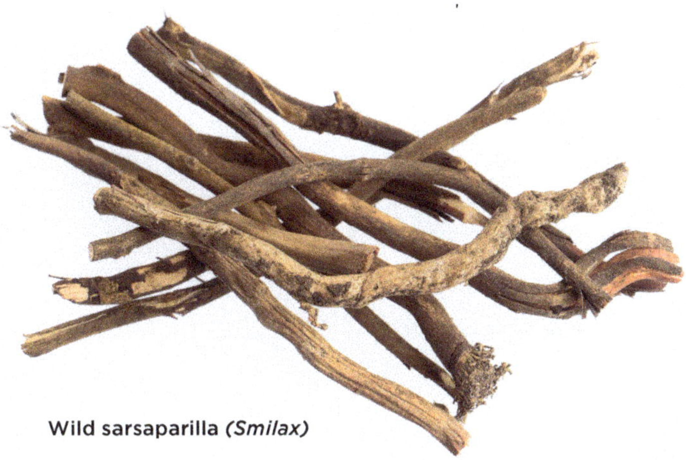

Wild sarsaparilla *(Smilax)*

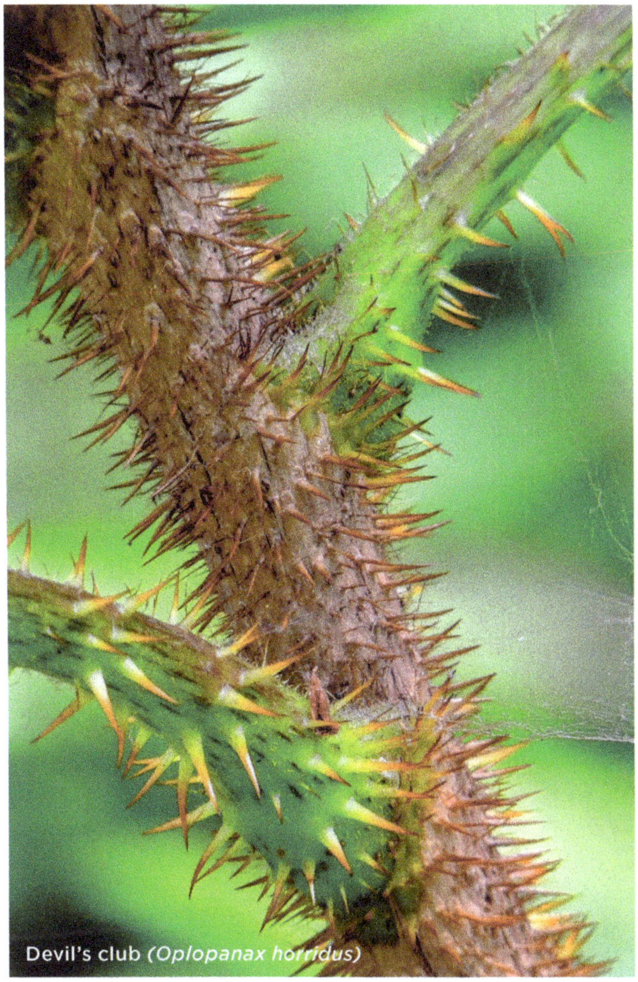

Devil's club *(Oplopanax horridus)*

ADAPTOGEN AND ADRENAL TONIC TEA I

DIRECTIONS: Prepare a decoction or cold infusion containing the herbs below. Consume 8-12 ounces in the morning and early afternoon. *Note:* Some individuals may have difficulty sleeping if they drink this tea after 2 pm.

2 parts shatavari *(Asparagus)*
1 part eleuthero *(Eleutherococcus)*—omit if it overstimulates
1 part devil's club *(Oplopanax)*
1 part wild sarsaparilla *(Smilax)*
1 part carob pods *(Ceratonia)*
½ part muira puama *(Ptychopetalum)*
½ part Indian sarsaparilla *(Hemidesmus)*
½ part ashwagandha *(Withania)*
¼ part licorice *(Glycyrrhiza)*—omit with high blood pressure and/or edema

ADAPTOGEN AND ADRENAL TONIC TEA II

DIRECTIONS: Prepare a decoction containing the following herbs. Consume 8–12 ounces in the morning and early afternoon. *Note:* Some individuals may have difficulty sleeping if they drink this tea after 2 pm.

2 parts shatavari *(Asparagus)*
1 part rehmannia, prepared *(Rehmannia)*
1 part Chinese ginseng *(Panax ginseng)*, American ginseng, woods-grown *(Panax quinquefolius)*, or eleuthero *(Eleutherococcus)* (optional)
1 part Jamaican sarsaparilla *(Smilax)*
½ part Indian sarsaparilla *(Hemidesmus)*
½ part ashwagandha *(Withania)*
½ part anise *(Pimpinella)*
½ part allspice *(Pimenta dioica)*
½ part fennel *(Foeniculum)*
¼ part vanilla *(Vanilla)* (optional)
¼ part licorice *(Glycyrrhiza)*—omit with high blood pressure and/or edema

ADAPTOGEN DELIGHT

DIRECTIONS: Prepare an infusion containing the following herbs. Consume 8–12 ounces in the morning and early afternoon.

2 parts tulsi basil *(Ocimum sanctum)*
1 part oat straw *(Avena)*
½ part gotu kola *(Centella)*
1/16 part stevia *(Stevia)*

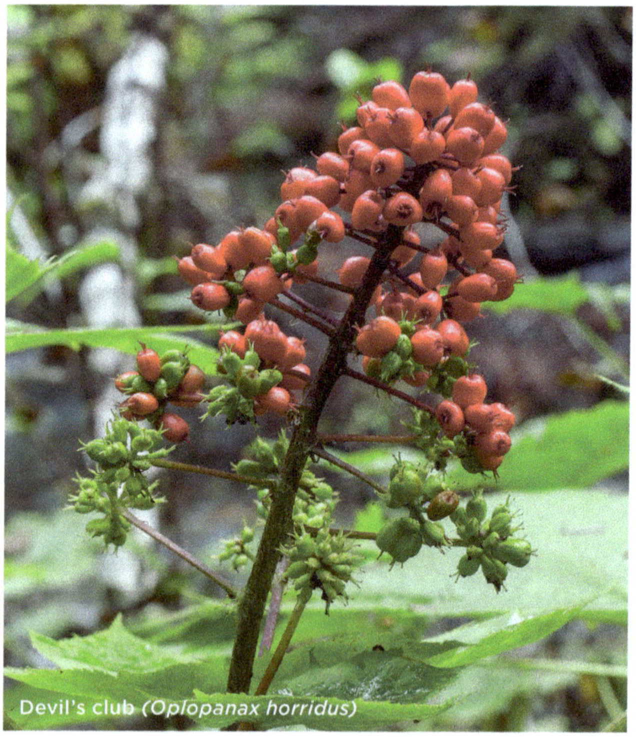

Devil's club *(Oplopanax horridus)*

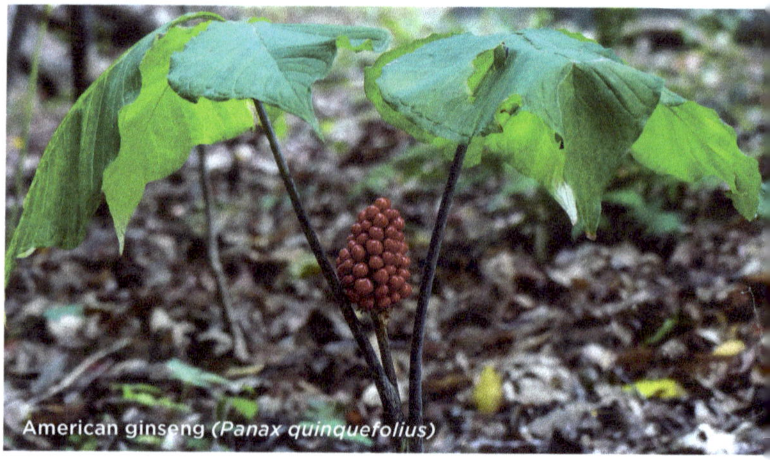

American ginseng *(Panax quinquefolius)*

CALMING ADAPTOGEN COMPOUND

DIRECTIONS: Combine the following single extracts. Consume 30–90 drops, up to three times daily.

2 parts reishi mushroom *(Ganoderma)*
2 parts shu di huang, prepared *(Rehmannia)*
1½ parts American ginseng, woods-grown *(Panax quinquefolius)*
1½ parts devil's club *(Oplopanax)*
1½ parts ashwagandha *(Withania)*
1½ parts white peony root *(Paeonia lactiflora)*
½ part wu wei zi *(Schisandra)*
½ part licorice *(Glycyrrhiza)*—omit with high blood pressure and/or edema

The following information applies to all of the aforementioned *Adaptogen and Adrenal Tonic Teas and Compounds*.

ACTIONS

Adaptogen
Adrenal tonic
Energizing
Qi tonic

APPLICABLE CONDITIONS

Adrenal burnout
Chronic allergies
Chronic fatigue
Chronic stress
Decreased resistance to stress
Endocrine disorders
Hyperinsulinemia
Hypoglycemia
Insulin resistance
Low libido
Lowered resistance

TONIFYING TEAS

DELICIOUS IMMUNE TONIC TEA

DIRECTIONS: Prepare a decoction containing the following herbs. Consume 8–10 ounces, up to three times daily. For short- or long-term use. For acute infections, omit astragalus and codonopsis.

2 parts marshmallow root *(Althaea)*
2 parts astragalus *(Astragalus)*
2 parts codonopsis *(Codonopsis)*
1 part jie geng *(Platycodon)*
1 part fu ling *(Poria)*
1 part cinnamon *(Cinnamomum)*
1 part cardamom *(Elettaria)*
½ part Indian sarsaparilla *(Hemidesmus)*
½ part allspice *(Pimenta dioica)*
½ part licorice *(Glycyrrhiza)*—omit with high blood pressure and/or edema, or substitute 1 part red jujube date *(Ziziphus jujuba)*

ACTIONS

Energizing
Immune modulator
Qi tonic (lung and spleen qi tonic)
Recuperative (after infection has cleared)

APPLICABLE CONDITIONS

Fatigue, weakness
Lowered resistance
Qi deficiency (lung and spleen qi deficiency)

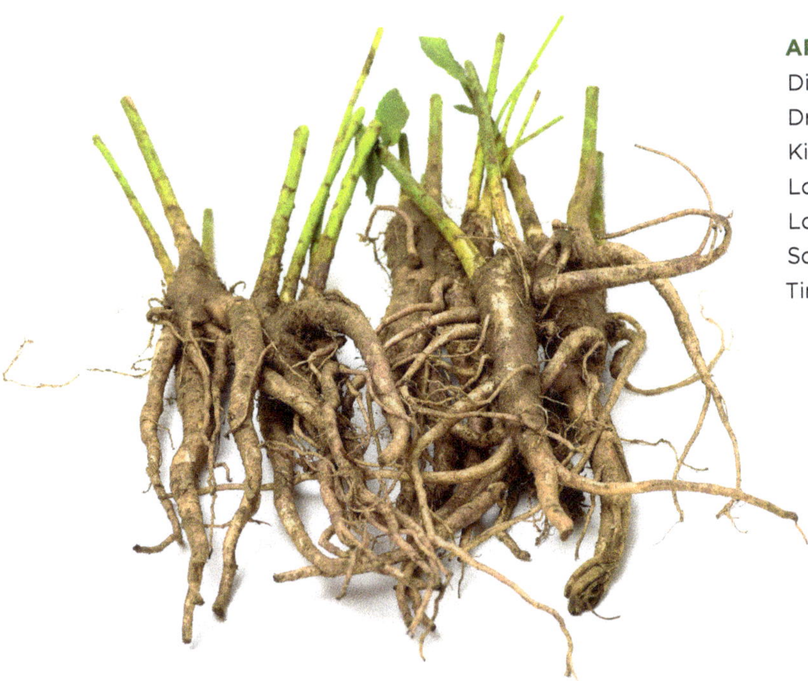

Jie geng *(Platycodon grandiflorum)*

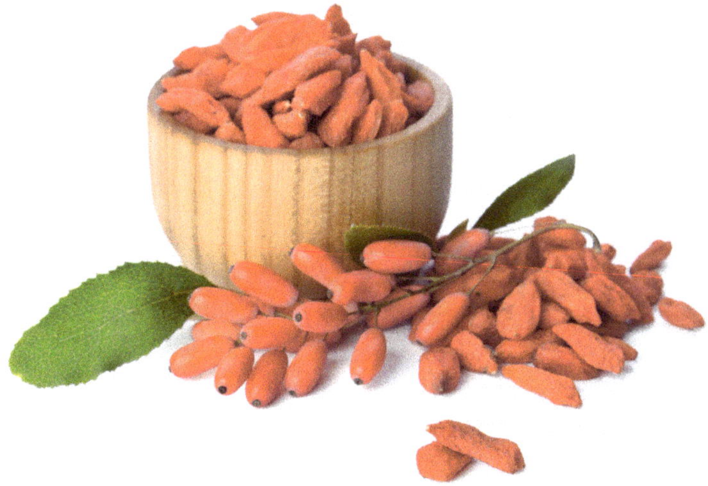

Lycii berry, gogi berry, gou qi zi *(Lyciium barbarum)*

KIDNEY AND LIVER YIN TONIC TEA

DIRECTIONS: Prepare a decoction containing the following herbs. Consume 8–12 ounces in the morning and early afternoon.

1 part shan yao *(Dioscorea batatas)*
1 part fu ling *(Poria)*
1 part sheng di huang *(Rehmannia)*
1 part lycii berry or gogi berry *(Lyciium barbarum)*
½ part mountain peony *(Paeonia suffruticosa)*
½ part ze xie *(Alisma plantago)*
¼ part licorice *(Glycyrrhiza)*

ACTIONS

Yin tonic (kidney and liver yin tonic)

APPLICABLE CONDITIONS

Dizziness
Dry or cracked red tongue
Kidney and liver yin deficiency
Low libido
Lower back weakness
Scant urination
Tinnitus

LUNG QI TONIC TEA

DIRECTIONS: Prepare a decoction containing the following herbs. Consume 8–12 ounces in the morning and early afternoon. *Note:* Some individuals may have difficulty sleeping if they drink this tea after 2 pm.

2 parts astragalus *(Astragalus)*
2 parts codonopsis *(Codonopsis)*
1 part fu ling *(Poria)*
1 part jie geng *(Platycodon)*
1 part asparagus tuber *(Asparagus)*
1 part mai men dong *(Ophiopogon)*
½ part orange peel *(Citrus)*
½ part fresh ginger *(Zingiber)*

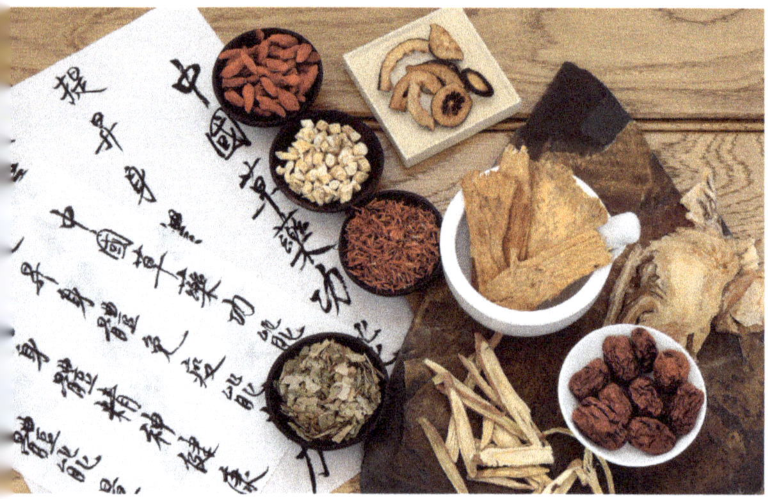

ACTIONS

Deepens respiration
Demulcent
Energizer
Expectorant
Immune modulator
Increases resistance
Lung qi tonic
Lung yin tonic
Regulates respiratory mucus secretion

APPLICABLE CONDITIONS

Allergies (preventative)
Asthma (preventative)
Chronic cough
Chronic obstructive pulmonary disease
Difficulty breathing
Dyspnea
Immune deficiency
Shallow breathing
Shortness of breath
Wheezing

SPLEEN AND LUNG QI TONIC TEA

DIRECTIONS: Prepare a decoction containing the following herbs. Consume 8–12 ounces in the morning and early afternoon. Discontinue use during an acute infection or fever. *Note:* Some individuals may have difficulty sleeping if they drink this tea in the late afternoon.

2 parts astragalus *(Astragalus)*
2 parts codonopsis *(Codonopsis)*
2 parts red jujube dates *(Ziziphus)*
1 part fu ling *(Poria)*
½ part orange peel *(Citrus)*
¼–½ part ginger, fresh *(Zingiber)*
¼ part licorice *(Glycyrrhiza)*—omit with high blood pressure and/or edema

SPLEEN QI TONIC TEA

DIRECTIONS: Prepare a decoction containing the following herbs. Consume 8–12 ounces in the morning and early afternoon. Discontinue use during an acute infection or fever. *Note:* Some individuals may have difficulty sleeping if they drink this tea in the late afternoon.

2 parts astragalus *(Astragalus)*
2 parts shan yao *(Dioscorea batatas)*
2 parts fu ling *(Poria)*
2 parts codonopsis *(Codonopsis)*
1 part jie geng *(Platycodon)*
1 part red jujube dates *(Ziziphus)*
½–1 part bai zhu *(Atractylodes)*
¼–½ part licorice *(Glycyrrhiza)*—omit with high blood pressure and/or edema

Note: The following actions and applicable conditions apply to the two aforementioned teas.

ACTIONS

Energizer
Enhances digestion
Expectorant
Immune modulator
Increases resistance
Qi tonic (lung and spleen qi)
Regulates mucus secretion

APPLICABLE CONDITIONS

Abdominal distension
Chronic fatigue
Lack of appetite
Loose stools and non-infectious diarrhea
Weakness in the extremities

CARDIO-VASCULAR SUPPORT

CIRCULATORY COMPOUNDS

ATHEROSCLEROSIS COMPOUND

DIRECTIONS: Combine the following single extracts. Consume 60 - 90 drops, up to three times daily.

4 parts hawthorn fruit or flower and leaf *(Crataegus)*
3 parts dandelion root *(Taraxacum)*
1 part red root *(Ceanothus)*
1 part dan shen *(Salvia miltiorrhiza)* or ginkgo *(Ginkgo)*
1⁄16 - 1⁄8 part cayenne *(Capsicum)*

ACTIONS

Blood thinner
Circulatory stimulant
Deobstruent
Diuretic
Hypocholesterolemic
Hypotensive
Increases blood vessel elasticity
Vasodilator

APPLICABLE CONDITIONS

Atherosclerosis
Elevated triglycerides, phospholipids, or LDLs
Hypercholesterolemia
Hypertension
Type II diabetic complications

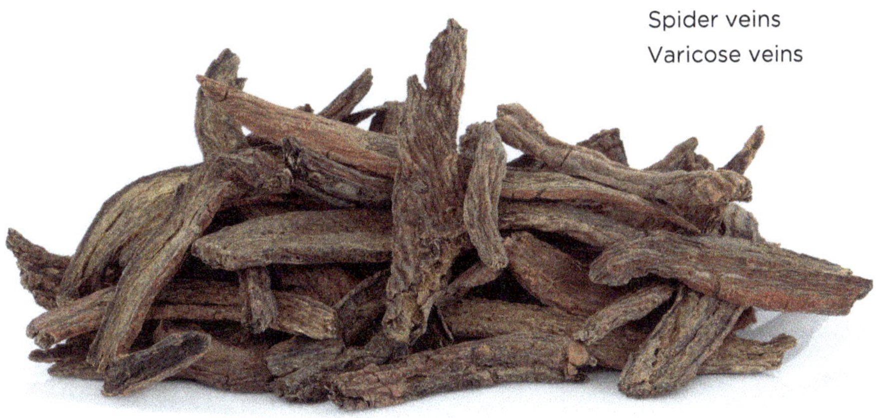

Dan shen *(Salvia miltiorrhiza)*

CIRCULATORY STIMULANT COMPOUND

DIRECTIONS: Combine the following single extracts. Consume 15 - 60 drops, up to three times daily.

2 parts ginkgo *(Ginkgo)*
1 part gotu kola *(Centella)*
1 part ginger *(Zingiber)*
½ - 1 part cinnamon *(Cinnamomum)*
½ part orange peel *(Citrus)*
½ part rosemary *(Salvia rosmarinus)*
1⁄16 - 1⁄8 part cayenne *(Capsicum)*

CIRCULATORY STIMULANT TEA

DIRECTIONS: Prepare an infusion containing the following herbs. Consume 8 - 12 ounces in the morning and early afternoon. *Note:* Some individuals may have difficulty sleeping if they drink this tea in the late afternoon.

2 parts tulsi basil *(Ocimum sanctum)*
2 parts hawthorn flower and leaf *(Crataegus)*
1 part ginkgo *(Ginkgo)*
½ part orange peel *(Citrus)*
¼ - ½ part gotu kola *(Centella)*
¼ part rosemary *(Salvia rosmarinus)*
1⁄16 part stevia *(Stevia)*

Note: The following actions and applicable conditions apply to the two aforementioned formulas.

ACTIONS

Circulatory stimulant
Vasodilator

APPLICABLE CONDITIONS

Enhances circulation
Increases mental clarity
Raynaud's phenomenon
Slow healing bruises
Spider veins
Varicose veins

DIURETIC HYPERTENSION COMPOUND

DIRECTIONS: Combine the following single extracts. Consume 30-90 drops, up to three times daily.

4 parts dandelion leaf or whole plant *(Taraxacum)*
4 parts hawthorn fruit or flower and leaf *(Crataegus)*
1-2 parts yarrow *(Achillea)*
1-2 parts parsley seed or root *(Petroselinum)*
⅞-1 part horsetail *(Equisetum)*
⅛-1⁄16 part cayenne *(Capsicum)*

ACTIONS

Blood thinner (mild)
Circulatory stimulant
Deobstruent
Diuretic
Increases blood vessel elasticity
Hypocholesterolemic
Hypotensive
Vasodilator

APPLICABLE CONDITION

Hypertension (especially sodium-related)

NERVINE HYPERTENSION COMPOUND

DIRECTIONS: Combine the following single extracts. Consume 30-90 drops, up to three times daily.

4 parts hawthorn fruit or flower and leaf *(Crataegus)*
3 parts motherwort *(Leonurus)*
2 parts bugleweed *(Lycopus)*
2 parts dandelion leaf or whole plant *(Taraxacum)*
1 part yarrow *(Achillea)*

ACTIONS

Circulatory stimulant
Deobstruent
Diuretic (mild)
Hypocholesterolemic
Hypotensive
Increases blood vessel elasticity
Nervine
Vasodilator

APPLICABLE CONDITIONS

Cardiac irritability
Hypertension (anxiety- or hyperthyroid-related)
Palpitations

HYPOTENSION RELIEF COMPOUND

DIRECTIONS: Combine the following single extracts. Consume 30-60 drops, up to three times daily. *Note:* Individuals with difficulty sleeping should avoid consuming this compound after 2 pm.

3 parts eleuthero *(Eleutherococcus)*
3 parts shu di huang *(Rehmannia)*
2 parts astragalus *(Astragalus)* or fu ling *(Poria)*
2 parts codonopsis *(Codonopsis)*
1-2 parts anise *(Pimpinella)*
½ part licorice *(Glycyrrhiza)*
½ part rosemary *(Salvia rosmarinus)*

ACTIONS

Adaptogen
Adrenal tonic
Circulatory stimulant
Hypertensive (mild)
Kidney and qi tonic

APPLICABLE CONDITIONS

Dizziness
Fatigue
Hypotension
Labile hypotension
Low blood pressure due to cardiovascular and/or renal deficiency

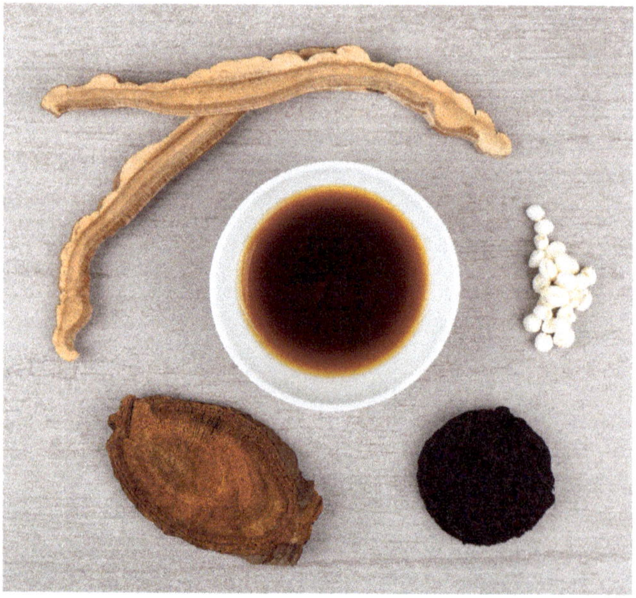

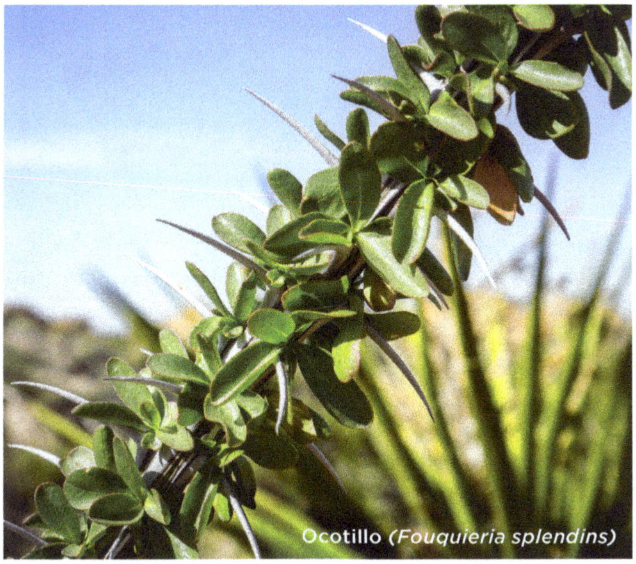

Ocotillo *(Fouquieria splendins)*

VARICOSE VEIN TONIC (ALKALOID-BASED)

2 parts turmeric *(Curcuma)*
2 parts dandelion *(Taraxacum root)*
1 part ocotillo *(Fouquieria)*
½ part horse chestnut *(Aesculus)*
¼ - ½ part prickly ash *(Zanthoxylum)*

VARICOSE VEIN TONIC (TANNIN-BASED)

DIRECTIONS: Combine the following single extracts. Consume 60 - 90 drops, up to three times daily.

4 parts stone root *(Collinsonia)*
2 parts dandelion root *(Taraxacum root)*
1 - 2 parts red root *(Ceanothus)*
1 part yarrow *(Achillea)*
1 part yellow dock *(Rumex)*
½ - 1 part rosemary *(Salvia rosmarinus)*

Note: The following actions and applicable conditions apply to the two aforementioned compounds.

ACTIONS

Anti-inflammatory
Astringent
Hepatic
Laxative (mild)
Pelvic and portal decongestant
Venous tonic

APPLICABLE CONDITIONS

Chronic dull ache in pelvic region
Hemorrhoids
Spider veins
Varicose veins

DIGESTIVE SUPPORT

CARMINATIVE FORMULAS

CALM BELLY COMPOUND

2 parts peppermint *(Mentha piperita)*
1 part fennel *(Foeniculum)*
1 part anise *(Pimpinella)*
1 part chamomile *(Matricaria)*
1 part lemon balm *(Melissa)*

ACTIONS

Anti-inflammatory
Antispasmodic (smooth muscles)
Aromatic
Carminative
Nervine

APPLICABLE CONDITIONS

Anxiety
Colic
Crohn's disease
Digestive cramping
Gas and bloating
Irritable bowel syndrome
Nerve-related digestive disorders
Stomachache
Ulcerative colitis

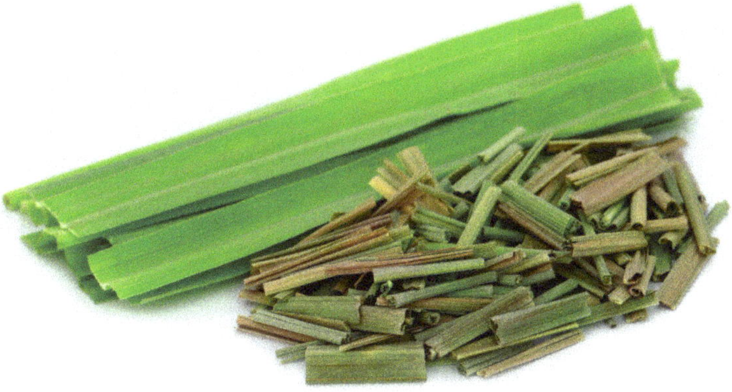

Lemon grass *(Cymbopogon citratus)*

CARMINATIVE TEA

DIRECTIONS: Prepare a decoction containing the following herbs. Consume 8-10 ounces, up to three times daily.

4 parts marshmallow *(Althaea)*
1 part anise *(Pimpinella)*
1 part cardamom *(Elettaria)*
1 part coriander *(Coriandrum)*
1 part fennel *(Foeniculum)*
1 part orange peel *(Citrus sinensis)*
½ part allspice *(Pimenta)*
½ part fresh ginger *(Zingiber)*
¼-½ part licorice root *(Glycyrrhiza)*—omit with high blood pressure and/or edema

ACTIONS

Anti-inflammatory
Antispasmodic (smooth muscles)
Aromatic
Carminative
Diaphoretic (mild)

APPLICABLE CONDITIONS

Digestive cramping
Gas and bloating
Irritable bowel syndrome
Nonulcer dyspepsia
Stomachache

DIGESTIVE DELIGHT TEA

DIRECTIONS: Prepare an infusion containing the following herbs. Consume 8-10 ounces, up to three times daily.

2-3 parts fresh grated ginger *(Zingiber)*
2-3 parts fresh sliced lemon grass *(Cymbopogon)*
1 part allspice *(Pimenta)*
¼-½ part licorice *(Glycyrrhiza)*—omit with high blood pressure and/or edema

ACTIONS

Antibacterial
Anti-inflammatory
Antispasmodic (smooth muscles)
Aromatic
Carminative
Diaphoretic (mild)

APPLICABLE CONDITIONS

Digestive cramping
Gas and bloating
Stomachache

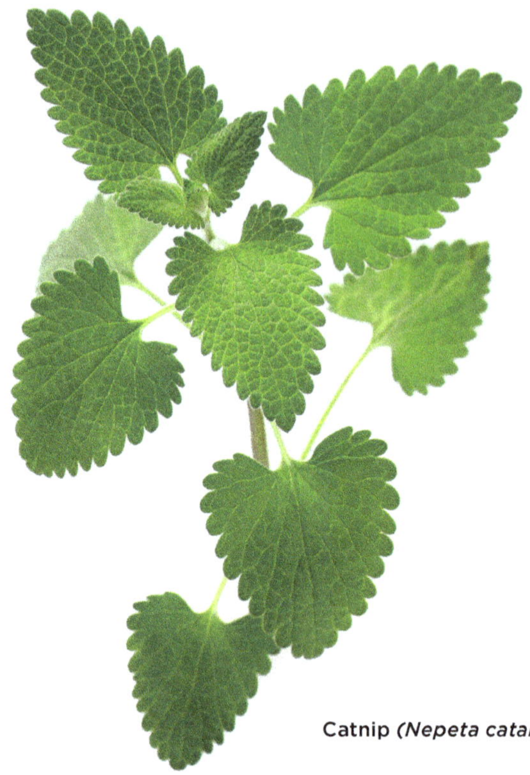

Catnip *(Nepeta cataria)*

DIGESTIVE SOOTHING AND CALMING TEA

DIRECTIONS: Prepare an infusion containing the following herbs. Consume 8-10 ounces, up to three times daily.

2 parts spearmint *(Mentha spicata)*
1 part chamomile *(Matricaria)*
½ part lemon balm *(Melissa)*
½ part catnip *(Nepeta)*
¼ part meadowsweet *(Filipendula)*
¼ part rosemary *(Salvia rosmarinus)*
¼ part lavender *(Lavandula)*
1/16 part stevia *(Stevia)*

ACTIONS

Anti-inflammatory
Antispasmodic (smooth muscles)
Aromatic
Carminative
Nervine

APPLICABLE CONDITIONS

Anxiety
Colic
Crohn's disease
Digestive cramping
Gas and bloating
Irritable bowel syndrome
Nerve-related digestive disorders
Stomachache
Ulcerative colitis

DIGESTIVE FORMULAS

ANTIDIARRHEA COMPOUND

DIRECTIONS: Combine the following extracts. Consume 30 - 90 drops, up to four times daily.

1 part yerba mansa *(Anemopsis)*
1 part blackberry root *(Rubus)*
1 part cinnamon *(Cinnamomum)*
If digestive cramping is present, add 1 part fennel *(Foeniculum)*, or 1 part wild yam *(Dioscorea villosa)*.

ACTIONS

Antibacterial
Astringent
Hemostatic

APPLICABLE CONDITIONS

Diarrhea (additional anti-infective herbs may be necessary)
Hemorrhoids (bleeding)
Intestinal bleeding (passive)
Loose stools

ASTRINGENT TEA

DIRECTIONS: Prepare an infusion containing the following herbs. Consume 8 - 12 ounces, up to three times daily.

2 parts spearmint *(Mentha spicata)*
1 part chamomile *(Matricaria)*
½ part meadowsweet *(Filipendula)*
½ part rose petals *(Rosa)*
⅛ - 1/16 part licorice *(Glycyrrhiza)* — omit with high blood pressure and/or edema or substitute stevia *(Stevia)*
If this tea is too astringent, add 2 parts marshmallow root *(Althaea)*.

ACTIONS

Anti-inflammatory to mucous membranes
Astringent
Carminative
Hemostatic

APPLICABLE CONDITIONS

Diarrhea (additional anti-infective herbs may be needed)
Hemorrhoids (bleeding)
Intestinal bleeding (passive)
Loose stools
Reduces inflammation throughout the digestive tract

COATING AND SOOTHING TEA

DIRECTIONS: Prepare a decoction containing the following herbs. This tea is best consumed for one to three months. For best results, consume one cup of tea on an empty stomach one-half to one hour before meals, or two hours after a meal, three times daily. Due to the pyrrolizidine alkaloids contained in comfrey root, long-term use (more than 2 - 6 weeks) should be avoided by individuals with liver deficiency or disorders. Long-term use of slippery elm bark should also be avoided, as it is threatened in the wild.

2 - 4 parts marshmallow root *(Althaea)*
1 - 2 parts slippery elm bark *(Ulmus)*
1 part anise seed *(Pimpinella)*
1 part fennel seed *(Foeniculum)*
½ part comfrey root *(Symphytum)*
¼ - ½ part licorice root *(Glycyrrhiza)* — omit with high blood pressure and/or edema

ACTIONS

Anti-inflammatory to mucous membranes
Carminative
Demulcent
Laxative

APPLICABLE CONDITIONS

Acid indigestion
Crohn's disease
Gastric or duodenal ulcers
Gastroesophageal reflux disease
Inflammation in the upper or lower digestive tract
Irritable bowel syndrome
Ulcerative colitis

COATING AND SOOTHING TEA (PYRROLIZIDINE ALKALOID FREE)

DIRECTIONS: Prepare a decoction containing the following herbs. Consume 8 - 12 ounces on an empty stomach (20 - 30 minutes before meals), up to three times daily. *Note:* This tea has the same actions and applicable conditions as the previously listed tea.

4 parts marshmallow *(Althaea)*
1 - 2 parts carob pods *(Ceratonia)*
1 part anise seed *(Pimpinella)*
1 part fennel seed *(Foeniculum)*
1 part cardamom *(Elettaria)*
¼ - ½ part licorice root *(Glycyrrhiza)* — omit with high blood pressure and/or edema

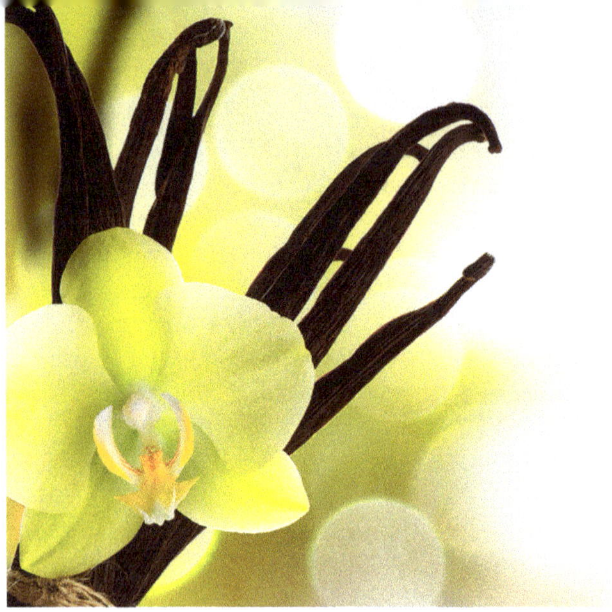

DELICIOUS DIGESTIVE TEA

DIRECTIONS: Prepare a decoction containing the following herbs. Consume 8–12 ounces on an empty stomach.

4 parts marshmallow *(Althaea)*
2 parts carob pods *(Ceratonia)*
1 part anise seed *(Pimpinella)*
1 part fennel seed *(Foeniculum)*
1 part cardamom *(Elettaria)*
1 part roasted dandelion root *(Taraxacum)*
¼ part vanilla *(Vanilla)*
¼ part licorice *(Glycyrrhiza)* — omit with high blood pressure and/or edema

ACTIONS

Anti-inflammatory to mucous membranes
Antispasmodic (smooth muscles)
Aromatic
Carminative
Demulcent
Laxative

APPLICABLE CONDITIONS

Colic
Constipation
Crohn's disease
Digestive cramping
Digestive ulcers
Gas and bloating
Gastritis
Gastroenteritis
Gastroesophageal reflux disease
Inflammation from gluten intolerance
Irritable bowel syndrome
Nonulcer dyspepsia
Stomachache
Ulcerative colitis

DIGESTIVE HEALING TEA I

DIRECTIONS: Prepare an infusion containing the following herbs. Consume 8–12 ounces on an empty stomach, up to three times daily.

2 parts peppermint *(Mentha piperita)* or spearmint *(M. spicata)*
1 part chamomile *(Matricaria)*
½ part meadowsweet *(Filipendula)*
½ part comfrey leaf *(Symphytum)*
¼ part chickweed *(Stellaria)*
¼ part calendula *(Calendula)*
1/16 part licorice *(Glycyrrhiza)* or stevia *(Stevia)*

DIGESTIVE HEALING TEA II

DIRECTIONS: Prepare an infusion containing the following herbs. Consume 8–12 ounces on an empty stomach, up to three times daily.

2 parts peppermint *(Mentha piperita)*, spearmint *(Mentha spicata)*, or tulsi *(Ocimum sanctum)*
1 part chamomile *(Matricaria)*
1 part anise *(Pimpinella)*
1 part fennel *(Foeniculum)*
½ part meadowsweet *(Filipendula)*
½ part alfalfa *(Medicago)*
¼–½ part licorice *(Glycyrrhiza)* — omit with high blood pressure and/or edema

Note: The following actions, applicable conditions, and contraindications apply to the two aforementioned teas.

ACTIONS

Anti-inflammatory to mucous membranes
Carminative
Demulcent
Vulnerary

APPLICABLE CONDITIONS

Constipation
Crohn's disease
Digestive cramping
Digestive ulcers
Gas and bloating
Gastritis
Gastroenteritis
Gastroesophageal reflux disease
Irritable bowel syndrome
Inflammation from gluten intolerance
Nonulcer dyspepsia
Stomachache
Ulcerative colitis

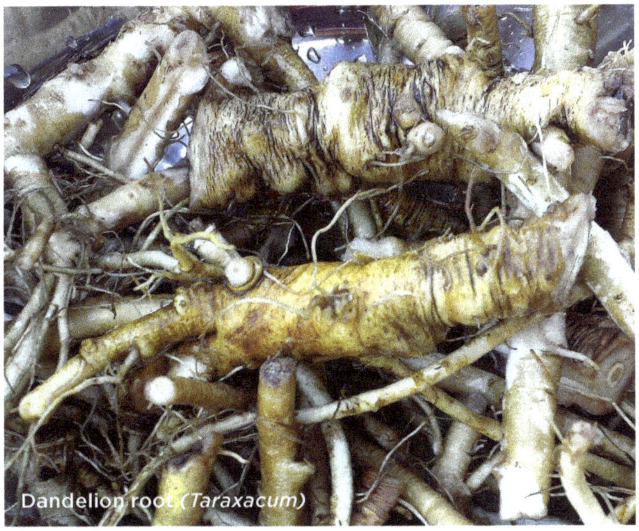

Dandelion root (*Taraxacum*)

LIVER AND GALLBLADDER SUPPORT

BLOOD SUGAR BALANCING FORMULA

DIRECTIONS: Combine the following powdered herbs and encapsulate. Consume 3 - 4 capsules before meals, up to three times daily. Omit *Panax ginseng* if anxiety, insomnia, or nervousness is present.

1 part Asian ginseng *(Panax ginseng)*
1 part gymnema *(Gymnema)*
1 part devil's club *(Oplopanax)*
1 part fenugreek *(Trigonella)*
1 part cinnamon *(Cinnamomum)*
1 part dandelion *(Taraxacum)*
1 part Oregon grape *(Berberis)*

ACTIONS

Cholagogue
Hepatodetoxifier
Hypoglycemic
Reduces sugar craving

APPLICABLE CONDITIONS

Hyperglycemia
Syndrome X
Prediabetes
Type II Diabetes

CHRISTA'S FAVORITE LIVER SUPPORT TEA

DIRECTIONS: Prepare a decoction containing the following herbs. Consume 8 - 10 ounces, up to three times daily.

1 part unroasted dandelion root *(Taraxacum)*
1 part roasted dandelion root *(Taraxacum)*
1 part burdock root *(Arctium)*
1 part Jamaican sarsaparilla *(Smilax)*
1 part Indian sarsaparilla *(Hemidesmus)*
1 part anise *(Pimpinella)*
1 part fennel *(Foeniculum)*
1 part carob pods *(Ceratonia)*
¼ - ½ part licorice *(Glycyrrhiza)* — omit with high blood pressure and/or edema

ACTIONS

Bitter tonic
Carminative
Cholagogue
Choleretic
Demulcent
Hepatic
Hepatodecongestant
Hepatodetoxifier
Laxative

APPLICABLE CONDITIONS

Acne
Cholangitis
Cholecystitis
Cholestasis
Cholethiasis
Cirrhosis
Constipation
Dermatitis
Eczema
Hepatitis
Jaundice
Psoriasis
Steatorrhea

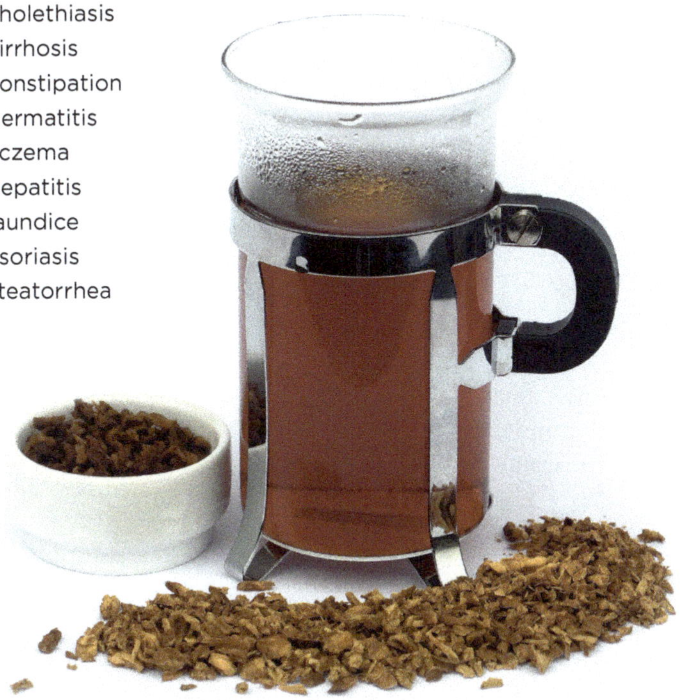

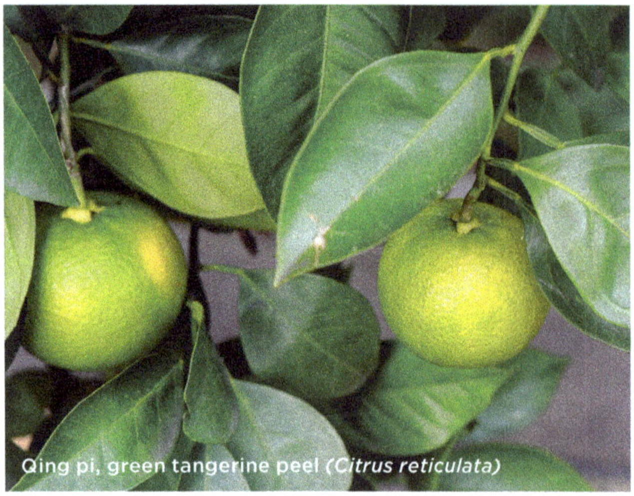

Qing pi, green tangerine peel *(Citrus reticulata)*

COOLING BITTERS COMPOUND

DIRECTIONS: Combine the following single extracts. Consume 30-90 drops, 15 to 30 minutes before meals, up to three times daily.

2 parts Oregon grape *(Berberis)*
2 parts artichoke leaf *(Cynara)*
2 parts dandelion *(Taraxacum)*
1 part orange peel *(Citrus sinensis)* or
green tangerine peel *(Citrus reticulata)*
½-1 part cardamom *(Elettaria)*
½-1 part fennel *(Foeniculum)* or anise *(Pimpinella)*

ACTIONS

Bitter tonic
Carminative
Cholagogue
Choleretic
Depurative
Hepatic
Hepatodecongestant
Hepatodetoxifier
Laxative

APPLICABLE CONDITIONS

Acne
Cholangitis
Cholecystitis
Cholestasis
Cholethiasis
Cirrhosis
Dermatitis
Eczema
Hepatitis
Jaundice
Psoriasis
Steatorrhea

DIGESTIVE BITTER ACETUM COMPOUND

DIRECTIONS: Combine the following single extracts or combine the herbs and prepare using the Simpler's method. Consume 60-90 drops, 15 to 30 minutes before meals, up to three times daily.

2 parts dandelion, fresh *(Taraxacum)*
2 parts burdock root, fresh *(Arctium)*
2 parts orange peel *(Citrus sinensis)*
2 parts artichoke leaf, fresh *(Cynara)*
1 part cardamom *(Elettaria)*
1 part yellow dock root, fresh *(Rumex)*

DIGESTIVE BITTER COMPOUND

DIRECTIONS: Combine the following single extracts. Consume 30-90 drops, 15 to 30 minutes before meals, up to three times daily.

6 parts artichoke *(Cynara)*
4 parts turmeric *(Curcuma)*
3 parts orange peel *(Citrus sinensis)*
3 parts cardamom *(Elettaria)*
2 parts anise *(Pimpinella)*
1 part fennel *(Foeniculum)*
1 part fresh ginger *(Zingiber)*
½-1 part licorice root *(Glycyrrhiza)*—omit with high blood pressure and/or edema

Note: The following actions and applicable conditions apply to the two aforementioned compounds.

ACTIONS

Bitter tonic
Carminative
Increases appetite
Increases digestive secretions

APPLICABLE CONDITIONS

Anorexia
Constipation
Gas and bloating
Hypochlorhydria
Nonulcer dyspepsia
Poor digestion
Post-meal nausea

GALLBLADDER AND LIVER-COOLING COMPOUND

DIRECTIONS: Combine the following single extracts. Consume 30 - 90 drops, up to three times daily.

4 parts milk thistle *(Silybum)*
2 parts dandelion *(Taraxacum)*
1 part gentian *(Gentiana)*
1 part artichoke leaf *(Cynara)*
1 part white peony root *(Paeonia lactiflora)*
1 part cardamom *(Elettaria)* or turmeric *(Curcuma)*
½ - 1 part fennel seed *(Foeniculum)* or anise *(Pimpinella)*
¼ - ½ part licorice root *(Glycyrrhiza)*—omit with high blood pressure and/or edema

ACTIONS

Anti-inflammatory
Bitter tonic
Cholagogue
Choleretic
Hepatic
Hepatodecongestant
Hepatodetoxifier
Laxative

APPLICABLE CONDITIONS

Acne
Cholangitis
Cholecystitis
Cholestasis
Cholethiasis
Cirrhosis
Dermatitis
Eczema
Hepatitis
Jaundice
Liver heat
Psoriasis
Steatorrhea

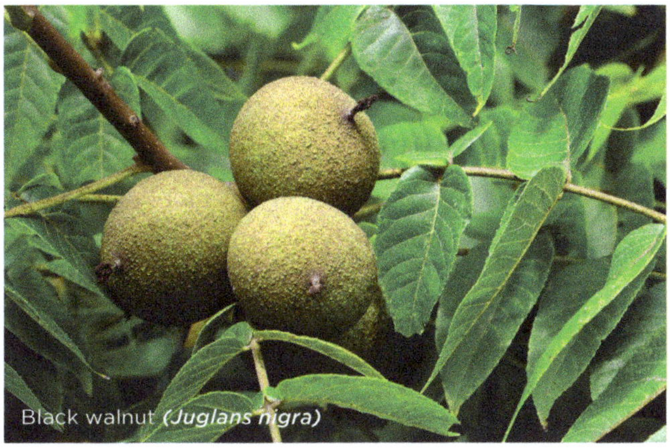
Black walnut *(Juglans nigra)*

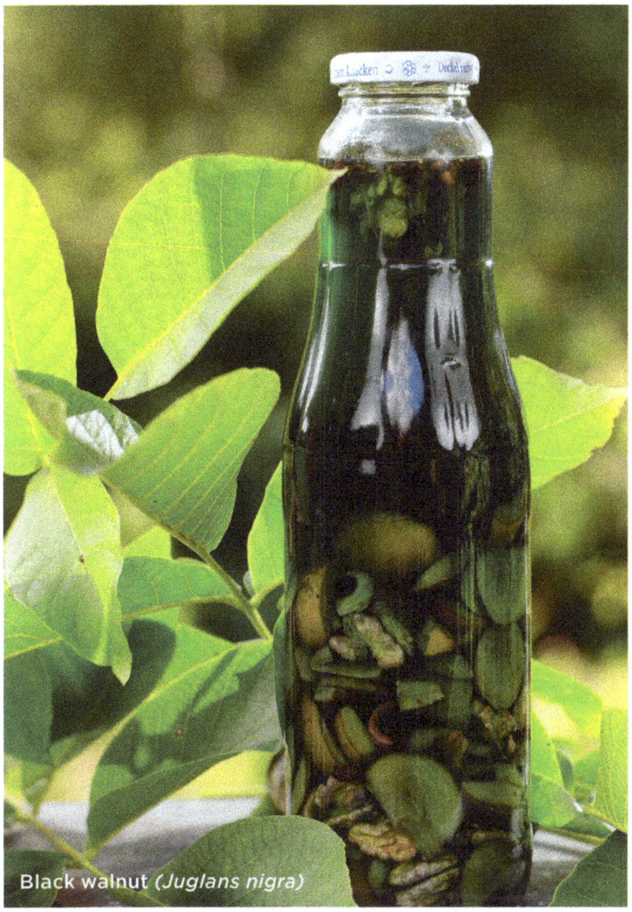
Black walnut *(Juglans nigra)*

HEMORRHOID COMFORT COMPOUND

DIRECTIONS: Combine the following single extracts. Consume 30 - 90 drops, up to three times daily.

2 parts dandelion *(Taraxacum)*
2 parts milk thistle *(Silybum)*
1 - 2 parts yellow dock *(Rumex)*
1 part red root *(Ceanothus)*
1 part black walnut leaf *(Juglans)*
1 part turmeric *(Curcuma)*
1 part fennel *(Foeniculum)*

ACTIONS

Cholagogue
Choleretic
Hepatodetoxifier
Hepatoprotectant
Lymphatic (lower body)
Pelvic/portal decongestant

APPLICABLE CONDITIONS

Hemorrhoids
Liver stagnation
Spider veins
Varicose veins

HEPATODETOXIFYING COMPOUND

DIRECTIONS: Combine the following single extracts. Consume 30–90 drops, 15 to 30 minutes before meals, up to four times daily.

4 parts milk thistle *(Silybum)*
4 parts turmeric *(Curcuma)*
3 parts dandelion root *(Taraxacum)*
3 parts burdock root *(Arctium)*
1–2 parts yellow dock *(Rumex)*
1–2 parts anise *(Pimpinella)* or cardamom *(Elettaria)*
1 part red root *(Ceanothus)*
½ part licorice *(Glycyrrhiza)*—omit with high blood pressure and/or edema

ACTIONS

Bitter tonic
Cholagogue
Choleretic
Hepatic
Hepatodecongestant
Hepatodetoxifier
Hypocholesterolemic
Laxative

APPLICABLE CONDITIONS

Constipation
Hypercholesterolemia
Dermatitis
Eczema
Fatty liver
Hepatitis
Hives
Liver heat
Jaundice
Pelvic congestion
PMS
Psoriasis

LIVER DECONGESTANT COMPOUND

DIRECTIONS: Combine the following single extracts. Consume 30–90 drops, up to three times daily.

2 parts turmeric *(Curcuma)*
1½ parts anise *(Pimpinella)*
1 part fennel *(Foeniculum)*
1 part white peony *(Paeonia)*
1 part devil's club *(Oplopanax)*
1 part orange peel *(Citrus sinensis)* or green tangerine peel *(Citrus reticulata)*
½ part licorice *(Glycyrrhiza)*—omit with high blood pressure and/or edema

ACTIONS

Cholagogue
Choleretic
Hepatic
Hepatodecongestant
Hepatodetoxifier
Laxative

APPLICABLE CONDITIONS

Dermatitis
Eczema
Fatty liver
Hemorrhoids
Hepatitis
Hives
Jaundice
Premenstrual syndrome
Psoriasis
Varicose veins and spider veins

LIVER-HEAT CLEARING COMPOUND

DIRECTIONS: Combine the following single extracts. Consume 10–60 drops, up to three times daily.

4 parts huang bai *(Phellodendron amurense)*
2 parts huang qin *(Scutellaria baicalensis)*
1–1½ parts huang lian *(Coptis chinensis)*
¼–½ part licorice *(Glycyrrhiza)*—omit with high blood pressure and/or edema

ACTIONS

Cholagogue
Choleretic
Depurative
Hepatic
Hepatodecongestant
Hepatodetoxifier

APPLICABLE CONDITIONS

Acne
Boils
Cholangitis
Cholecystitis
Cholethiasis
Cirrhosis
Dermatitis
Eczema
Fatty liver
Hepatitis
Hives
Jaundice

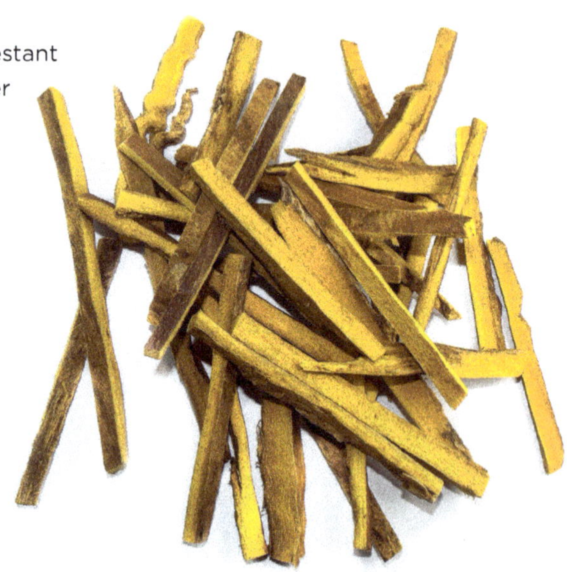

Huang bai *(Phellodendron amurense)*

NERVOUS SYSTEM SUPPORT

ANALGESIC, ANTISPASMODIC, AND ANTI-INFLAMMATORY COMPOUNDS

ANALGESIC, ANTISPASMODIC, AND SEDATIVE COMPOUND I (ALKALOID-BASED)

DIRECTIONS: Combine the following single extracts. When treating insomnia, consume 30 - 90 drops, two hours before going to sleep; if necessary, repeat one-half hour before bedtime. Avoid operating heavy machinery or driving.

1 part valerian *(Valeriana)*
1 part California poppy *(Eschscholzia)*
1 part hops *(Humulus)*
1 part passion flower *(Passiflora)*

ANALGESIC, ANTISPASMODIC, AND SEDATIVE COMPOUND II (ALKALOID-BASED)

DIRECTIONS: Combine the following single extracts. Consume 30 - 90 drops, up to four times daily. Avoid operating heavy machinery or driving.

1 part kava *(Piper methysticum)*
1 part passion flower *(Passiflora)*
1 part California poppy *(Eschscholzia)*

The following actions and applicable conditions apply to the two aforementioned compounds.

ACTIONS

Analgesic
Anodyne
Antispasmodic (smooth and skeletal muscles)
Anxiolytic
Hypnotic
Nervine
Sedative

APPLICABLE CONDITIONS

Anxiety
Insomnia
Pain
Passing gallstones or kidney stones
Skeletal or smooth muscles spasms
Tension headaches

ANTI-INFLAMMATORY COMPOUND (SHORT-TERM)

DIRECTIONS: Combine the following single extracts. Consume 30 - 90 drops, three to four times daily.

2 parts Jamaican dogwood *(Piscidia)*
2 parts St. John's wort *(Hypericum)* — omit when taking SSRI antidepressants
2 parts feverfew *(Tanacetum)*
1 part meadowsweet *(Filipendula)*
1 part willow bark *(Salix)*

ACTIONS

Analgesic
Anodyne
Anti-inflammatory
Nervine

APPLICABLE CONDITIONS

Fibromyalgia flareups
Headaches, acute
Muscle and joint inflammation
Osteoarthritis flareups
Pain
Rheumatoid arthritis flareups

ANTI-INFLAMMATORY COMPOUND (LONG-TERM)

DIRECTIONS: Combine the following single extracts. Consume 30 - 90 drops, two to three times daily.

2 parts turmeric *(Curcuma)*
1 - 2 parts chamomile *(Matricaria)*
1 part St. John's wort *(Hypericum)* — omit when taking SSRI antidepressants
½ - 1 part meadowsweet *(Filipendula)*
¼ - ½ part licorice root *(Glycyrrhiza)* — omit with high blood pressure and/or edema

ACTIONS

Analgesic
Anti-inflammatory

APPLICABLE CONDITIONS

Fibromyalgia
Headaches (chronic)
Muscle and joint inflammation
Myalgia
Osteoarthritis
Rheumatoid arthritis

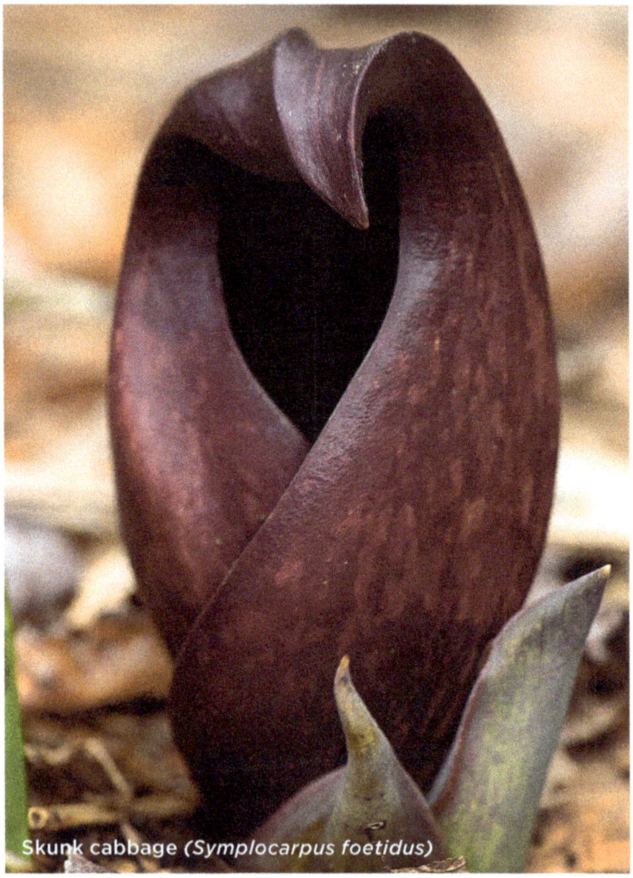

Skunk cabbage *(Symplocarpus foetidus)*

CRAMP BARK COMPOUND

DIRECTIONS: Combine the following single extracts, then add ¼ part of the total compound volume of honey. Consume 30–120 drops, up to four times daily. *Note:* This is a modified version of *Hayden's Viburnum Compound.*

3 parts black haw *(Viburnum prunifolium)*
2 parts cramp bark *(Viburnum opulus)*
2 parts cinnamon *(Cinnamomum)*
1 part wild yam *(Dioscorea villosa)*
1 part skullcap *(Scutellaria)*
1 part orange peel *(Citrus sinensis)*

ACTIONS

Anti-inflammatory
Antispasmodic (smooth muscles)
Astringent
Calmative
Hemostatic
Nervine

APPLICABLE CONDITIONS

Colic
Intestinal cramping
Menorrhagia
Uterine cramping

HEADACHE RELIEF COMPOUND

DIRECTIONS: Combine the following single extracts. Consume 30–90 drops, three to five times daily.

1 part feverfew *(Tanacetum parthenium)*
1 part Jamaican dogwood *(Piscidia)*
1 part pedicularis *(Pedicularis)*

ACTIONS

Analgesic
Anti-inflammatory
Antispasmodic (skeletal muscle)
Nervine

APPLICABLE CONDITIONS

Headaches, migraine
Headaches, muscle tension
Muscle and joint inflammation

SAMUEL THOMSON'S COMPOUND TINCTURE OF LOBELIA AND CAPSICUM

DIRECTIONS: Combine the following single extracts. Consume 2–10 drops, up to three times daily, or apply topically.

1 part skunk cabbage *(Symplocarpus* or *Lysichiton)*
1 part lobelia *(Lobelia)*
1 part cayenne *(Capsicum)*

ACTIONS

Analgesic
Antispasmodic (smooth and skeletal muscle)
Antitussive
Counterirritant
Expectorant
Nervine

APPLICABLE CONDITIONS

Asthma, wheezing
Myalgia
Pain
Skeletal muscle spasms
Smooth muscle spasms
Spastic cough

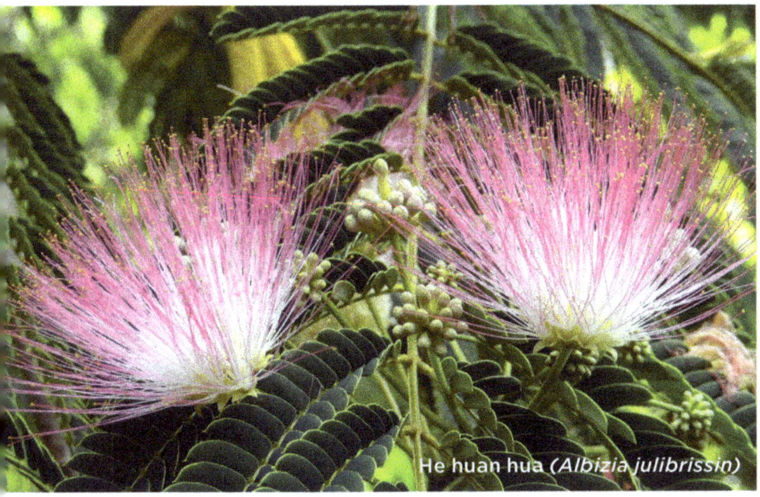

He huan hua *(Albizia julibrissin)*

ANTIDEPRESSANT, ANXIOLYTIC, AND NOOTROPIC COMPOUNDS

ANTIDEPRESSANT COMPOUND

DIRECTIONS: Combine the following single extracts. Consume 30-90 drops, up to three times daily.

4 parts St. John's wort *(Hypericum)*—omit when taking SSRI antidepressants
2 parts fresh milky oats *(Avena)*
1 part aralia berry *(Aralia californica)*
1 part gotu kola *(Centella)*
1 part lemon balm *(Melissa)*
1 part bacopa *(Bacopa)*
¼-½ part lavender *(Lavandula angustifolia)*
¼-½ part rosemary *(Salvia rosmarinus)*

ACTIONS

Antidepressant
Anxiolytic
Circulatory stimulant (mild)
Mood elevator
Nervine, gentle
Trophorestorative

APPLICABLE CONDITIONS

Adrenal burnout
Anxiety
Depression (mild to moderate)
Insomnia
Nervous system burnout

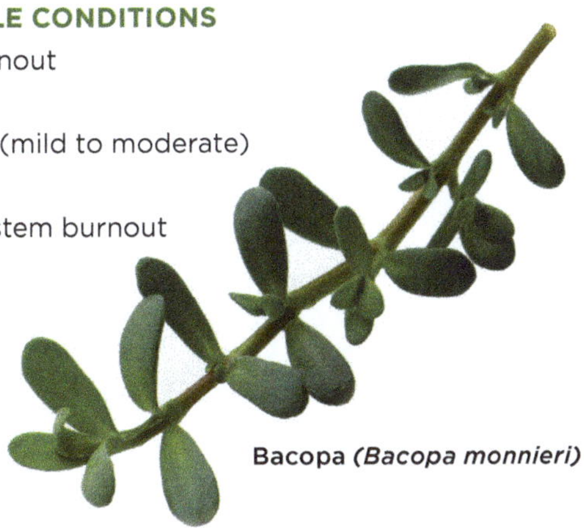

Bacopa *(Bacopa monnieri)*

ANXIOLYTIC COMPOUND (ALKALOID-BASED)

DIRECTIONS: Combine the following single extracts. Consume 30-90 drops, up to three times daily.

2 parts motherwort *(Leonurus)*
2 parts fresh milky oats *(Avena)*
1 part kava *(Piper methysticum)*
1 part passion flower *(Passiflora)*
⅛-¼ part pulsatilla *(Anemone)* (optional)

ACTIONS

Antispasmodic
Anxiolytic
Deepens respiration
Nervine
Sedative

APPLICABLE CONDITIONS

Anxiety
Heart palpitations
Insomnia
Irritability
Panic attacks
Prementrual Syndrome

ANXIOLYTIC COMPOUND (TANNIN-BASED)

DIRECTIONS: Combine the following single extracts. Consume 30-90 drops, up to three times daily.

2 parts motherwort *(Leonurus)*
1-2 parts bugleweed *(Lycopus)*
1 part hawthorn fruit *(Crataegus)*
1 part he huan hua *(Albizia)*
1 part lemon balm *(Melissa)*

ACTIONS

Antispasmodic
Anxiolytic
Cardiotonic
Nervine (heart-specific)
Sedative

APPLICABLE CONDITIONS

Anxiety
Heart palpitations
Insomnia
Panic attacks
Premenstrual syndrome

GENTLE NERVINE TEA

DIRECTIONS: Prepare an infusion containing the following herbs. Consume 8–12 ounces, up to three times daily.

2 parts spearmint *(Mentha spicata)*
1 part chamomile *(Matricaria)*
1 part oat straw *(Avena)*
½ part lemon balm *(Melissa)*
½ part of catnip *(Nepeta)*
1/16–⅛ part lavender *(Lavandula)* (optional)
1/16 part stevia *(Stevia)*

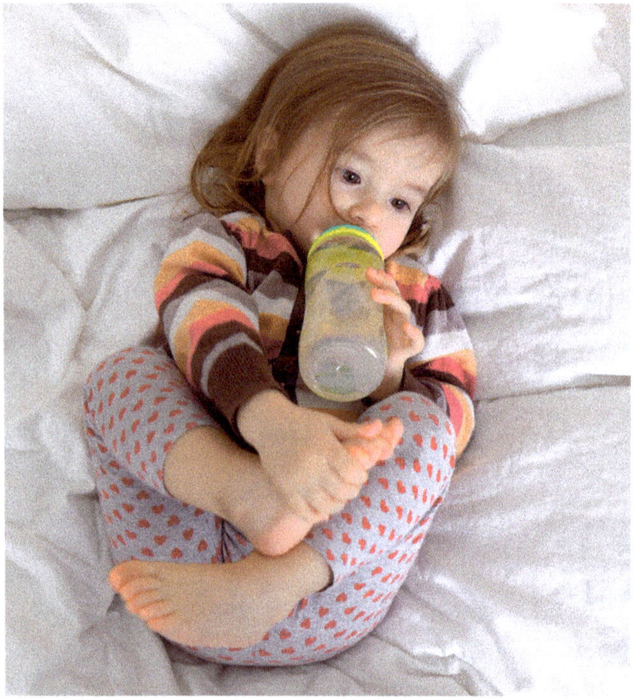

ACTIONS

Antidepressant
Anti-inflammatory
Anxiolytic
Calmative
Carminative
Mood elevator
Nervine, gentle
Sedative, very mild

APPLICABLE CONDITIONS

Anxiety
Depression (mild)
Digestive cramping
Headaches
Insomnia
Irritability
Pain
Premenstrual syndrome

MENTAL CLARI-TEA

DIRECTIONS: Prepare an infusion containing the following herbs. Consume 8–12 ounces, in the morning and early afternoon.

2 parts tulsi basil *(Ocimum sanctum)*
1 part gingko *(Ginkgo)*
½–1 part gotu kola *(Centella)*
½–1 part oat straw *(Avena)*
½ part red clover *(Trifolium)*
¼–½ part rosemary *(Salvia rosmarinus)*
1/16–⅛ part stevia *(Stevia)*

MENTAL CLARITY COMPOUND

DIRECTIONS: Combine the following single extracts. Consume 30–90 drops in the morning and early afternoon. Avoid consuming in the late afternoon or evening, as it can cause difficulty sleeping.

2 parts tulsi basil *(Ocimum sanctum)*
1–2 parts reishi mushroom *(Ganoderma)*
1–2 parts eleuthero *(Eleutherococcus)*
1 part gingko *(Ginkgo)*
½–1 part gotu kola *(Centella)*
½ part bay laurel *(Laurus nobilis)*
½ part bacopa *(Bacopa)*
¼–½ part rosemary *(Salvia rosmarinus)*

Note: The following actions and applicable conditions apply to the two aforementioned formulas.

ACTIONS

Antidepressant
Circulatory stimulant
Energizer
Improves focus
Non-caffeinated stimulant
Vasodilator

APPLICABLE CONDITIONS

Attention deficit hyperactivity disorder
Caffeine or stimulant withdrawal
Cerebral anoxia
Depression (asthenic)
Fatigue
Hypothyroid-related mental fogginess
Lethargy
Poor circulation

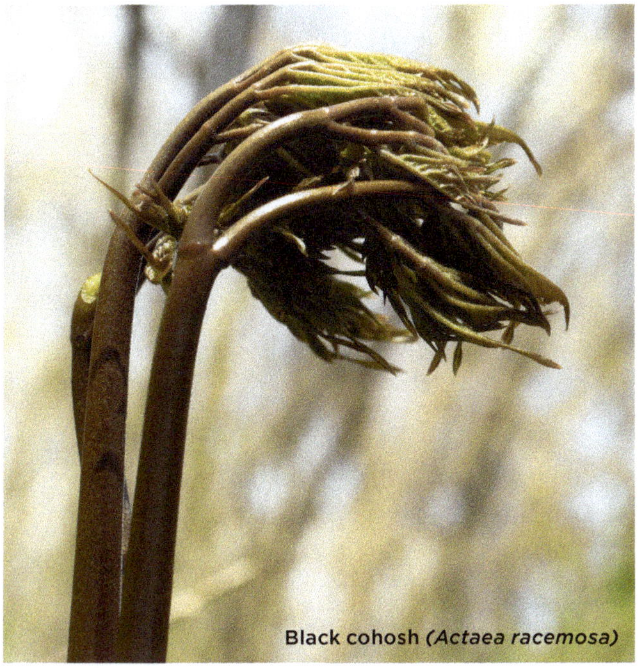

Black cohosh *(Actaea racemosa)*

REPRODUCTIVE SYSTEM SUPPORT, FEMALE

PERIMENOPAUSE SUPPORT

PERIMENOPAUSE COMPOUND (WITH ADRENAL DEPLETION)

DIRECTIONS: Combine the following single extracts. Consume 30-90 drops, three times daily.

4 parts chaste tree berry *(Vitex)*
2-4 parts black cohosh *(Actaea racemosa)*
2 parts white peony *(Paeonia lactiflora)*
1-2 parts American ginseng *(Panax quinquefolius)* or ashwagandha *(Withania)*
1-2 parts rehmannia, prepared *(Rehmannia)*
1 part dong quai *(Angelica sinensis)*—omit with menorrhagia
½-1 part schisandra berry *(Schisandra)*
½ part licorice *(Glycyrrhiza)*—omit with high blood pressure and/or edema

ACTIONS

Adaptogen
Adrenal support
Hepatodetoxifier
Hormone support
Kidney yin tonic
Reproductive tonic

APPLICABLE CONDITIONS

Adrenal burnout
Hormone-related mood swings
Hot flashes and night sweats
Irritability
Low libido
Perimenopause
Vaginal dryness

MOOD ELEVATING, TROPHORESTORATIVE, AND GENTLE NERVINE COMPOUND

DIRECTIONS: Combine the following single extracts. Consume 30-90 drops, up to three times daily.

4 parts St. John's wort *(Hypericum)*—omit when taking SSRI antidepressants
3 parts fresh milky oats *(Avena)*
2 parts skullcap *(Scutellaria)*
1 part lemon balm *(Melissa)*

ACTIONS

Analgesic
Antidepressant
Anxiolytic
Nervine, mild
Trophorestorative

APPLICABLE CONDITIONS

Adrenal burnout
Anxiety
Attention deficit hyperactivity disorder
Depression
Insomnia
Nervous tension
Pain
Premenstrual syndrome

PERIMENOPAUSE COMPOUND (CALMING AND LIVER-DECONGESTING)

DIRECTIONS: Combine the following single extracts. Consume 30 - 90 drops, three times daily.

4 parts chaste tree berry *(Vitex)*
2 parts white peony *(Paeonia lactiflora)*
1 - 2 parts black cohosh *(Actaea racemosa)*
1 - 2 parts dandelion root *(Taraxacum)*
1 - 2 parts motherwort *(Leonurus)* and/or blue vervain *(Verbena)*
½ - 1 part dong quai *(Angelica sinensis)* — omit with menorrhagia
½ part licorice *(Glycyrrhiza)* — omit with high blood pressure and/or edema

ACTIONS

Anti-inflammatory
Anxiolytic
Blood tonic
Hepatodecongestant
Hepatodetoxifier
Hormone support
Hypothalamic and pituitary regulator
Nervine

APPLICABLE CONDITIONS

Anxiety
Depression
Hormone-related mood swings
Hot flashes and night sweats
Irritability
Low libido
Mood swings
Perimenopause
Vaginal dryness

PREGNANCY SUPPORT

PREGNANCY-SAFE HEMOSTATIC TEA

DIRECTIONS: Prepare an infusion containing the following herbs. Consume 8 - 10 ounces, up to three times daily.

1 - 2 parts mint *(Mentha)*
1 part alfalfa *(Medicago)*
1 part nettle leaf *(Urtica)*
1 part raspberry leaf *(Rubus idaeus)*
½ part lady's mantle *(Alchemilla)*
½ part rose petals *(Rosa)*

UTERINE CALMING COMPOUND I (FOR THREATENED MISCARRIAGE)

DIRECTIONS: Combine the following single extracts. Consume 30 - 60 drops of the tincture, three to four times daily. Evaporate the alcohol by placing in 4 ounces of boiled water.

4 parts black haw *(Viburnum prunifolium)*
2 parts wild yam *(Dioscorea villosa)*
1 - 2 parts raspberry leaf *(Rubus idaeus)*
1 part partridge berry *(Mitchella repens)*
1 part cramp bark *(Viburnum opulus)*

ACTIONS

Antispasmodic (smooth muscle)
Hemostatic
Partus preparator
Uterine tonic

APPLICABLE CONDITIONS

Breakthrough bleeding
Threatened miscarriage
Uterine cramping

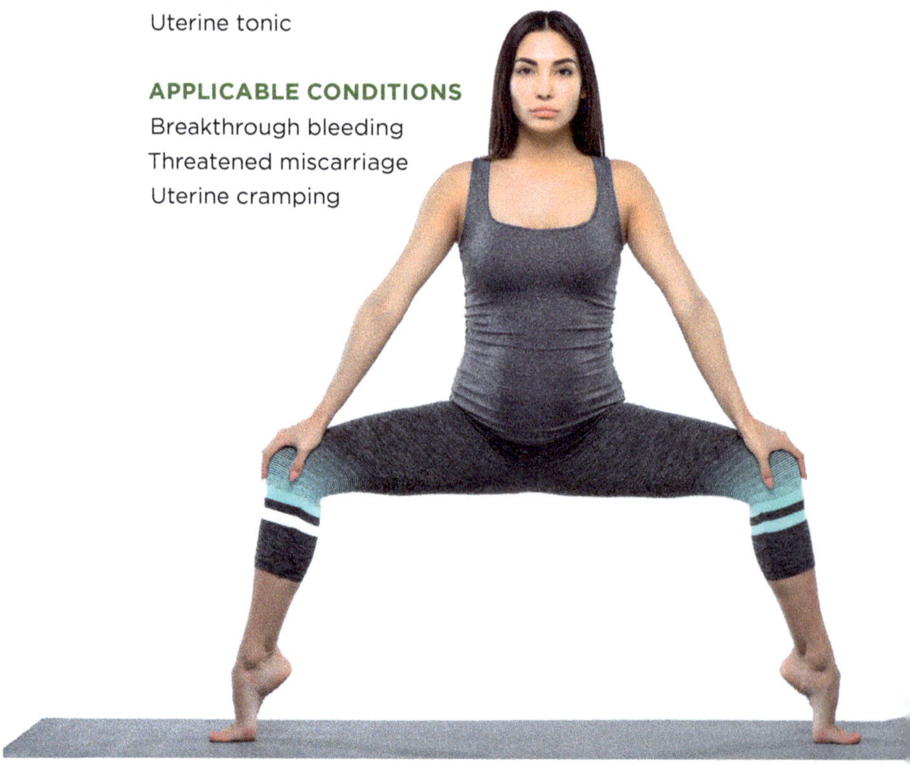

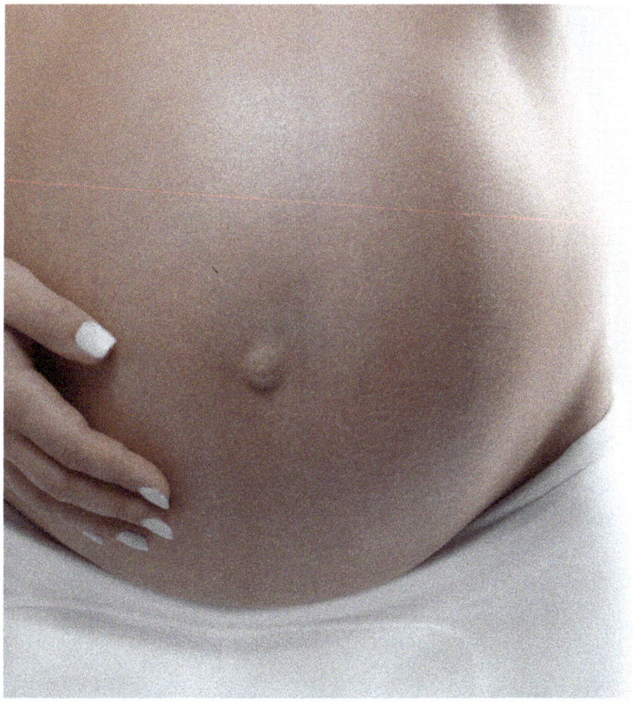

UTERINE CALMING COMPOUND II (FOR THREATENED MISCARRIAGE)

DIRECTIONS: Combine the following single extracts or prepare a decoction. Consume 30 - 60 drops of the tincture, or 8 ounces of the decoction, three to four times daily. Evaporate the alcohol by placing in 4 ounces of boiled water.

2 parts wild yam *(Dioscorea villosa)*
2 parts black haw *(Viburnum prunifolium)*
1 part white peony *(Paeonia lactiflora)*
1 part raspberry leaf *(Rubus idaeus)*

ACTIONS

Antispasmodic (smooth muscle)
Hemostatic
Partus preparator
Uterine tonic

APPLICABLE CONDITIONS

Breakthrough bleeding
Threatened miscarriage
Uterine cramping

UTERINE TONIC PARTUS PREPARATOR COMPOUND

DIRECTIONS: Combine the following single extracts. Consume 30 - 60 drops, two to three times daily. Evaporate the alcohol by placing the extract in 2 - 4 ounces of boiled water for 5 to 15 minutes.

2 parts black haw *(Viburnum prunifolium)*
2 parts white peony *(Paeonia lactiflora)*
1 part raspberry leaf *(Rubus idaeus)*
1 part partridge berry *(Mitchella repens)*

ACTIONS

Partus preparator
Uterine tonic

APPLICABLE CONDITIONS

Pregnancy and uterine tonic
Threatened miscarriage

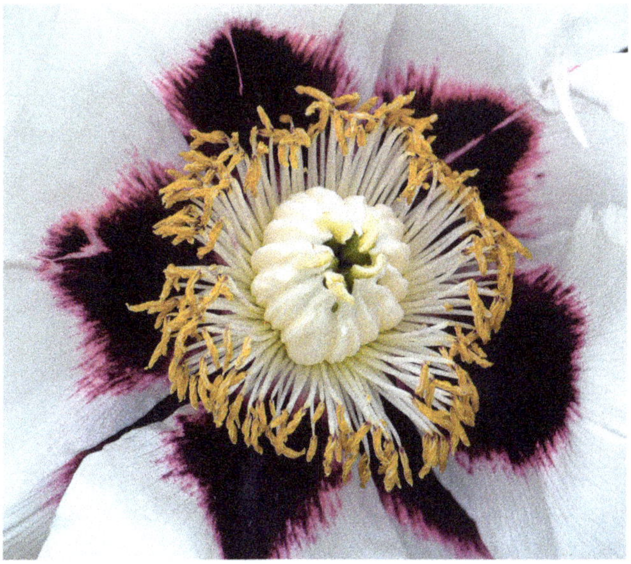

PREMENSTRUAL SYNDROME AND MENSTRUAL SUPPORT

REPRODUCTIVE AND HORMONE DEFICIENCY PHASE I COMPOUND

DIRECTIONS: Combine the following single extracts. Consume 30-90 drops, two to three times daily. Consume during the estrogen/follicular phase (after menstruation ceases, through ovulation).

1 part dong quai *(Angelica sinensis)*—omit with menorrhagia
1 part black cohosh *(Cimicifuga)*
1 part devil's club *(Oplopanax)*
1 part ashwagandha *(Withania)* or eleuthero *(Eleutherococcus)*
1 part Oregon grape *(Berberis)*
½ part fennel *(Foeniculum)*
½ part gotu kola *(Centella)*

REPRODUCTIVE AND HORMONE DEFICIENCY PHASE II COMPOUND

DIRECTIONS: Combine the following single extracts. Consume 30-90 drops, two to three times daily. Consume during the progesterone/luteal phase (post-ovulation, until menstruation begins).

4 parts chaste tree berry *(Vitex)*
1 part devil's club *(Oplopanax)*
1 part Oregon grape root *(Berberis)*
1 part dandelion root *(Taraxacum)*
1 part peony root *(Paeonia lactiflora)*
1-1½ parts motherwort *(Leonurus)*
½ part fennel *(Foeniculum)*
½ part turmeric *(Curcuma)* or ginger *(Zingiber)*—omit with heat present

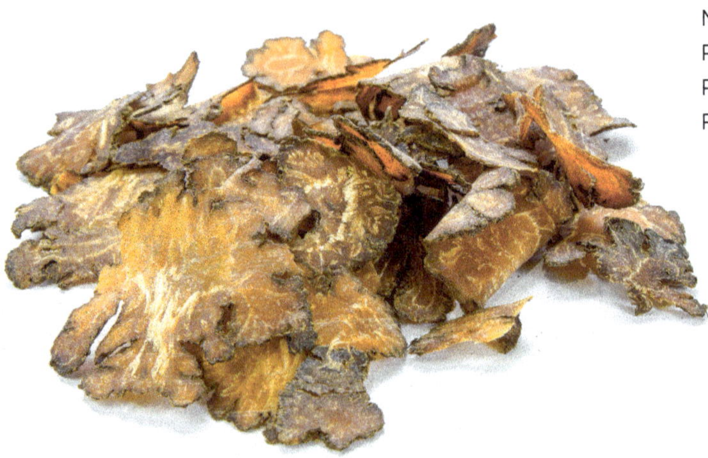

Chuan xiong *(Ligusticum striatum)*

REPRODUCTIVE AND BLOOD TONIFYING TEA

DIRECTIONS: Prepare a decoction containing the following herbs. Consume 8-12 ounces two to three times daily, throughout the month. Avoid use during menstruation.

2 parts shu di huang *(Rehmannia glutinosa)*
2 parts white peony *(Paeonia lactiflora)*
2 parts fu ling *(Poria cocos)*
1 parts donq quai *(Angelica sinensis)*
1 parts huang qi *(Astragalus)*
1 parts dang shen *(Codonopsis)*
1 parts jujube dates *(Zizuphus jujuba)*
½ part chuan xiong *(Ligusticum striatum)*
½ part chai hu *(Bupleurum falcatum)*

Note: The following actions and applicable conditions apply to the three aforementioned formulas.

ACTIONS

Anti-inflammatory
Antispasmodic (smooth muscle)
Anxiolytic
Carminative
Hepatodecongestant
Hepatodetoxifying
Hormone balancing
Nervine
Progesterone agonist

APPLICABLE CONDITIONS

Amenorrhea
Anxiety
Breast tenderness
Estrogen excess
Gas and bloating
Hormone-related liver stagnation
Menstrual cramping (long-term support)
Premenstrual syndrome
Progesterone deficiency
Reduces sugar cravings

ESTROGEN DOMINANCE RELIEF COMPOUND

DIRECTIONS: Combine the following single extracts. Consume 60-90 drops, two to three times daily.

4-6 parts chaste tree berry *(Vitex)*
2 parts dandelion root *(Taraxacum)*
2 parts white peony *(Paeonia lactiflora)*
1-2 parts motherwort *(Leonurus)*
1 part devil's club *(Oplopanax)*
1 part turmeric *(Curcuma)* or artichoke *(Cynara)*

ACTIONS

Anti-inflammatory
Anxiolytic
Endometriosis
Hepatodecongestant
Hormone balancing
Nervine

APPLICABLE CONDITIONS

Anxiety
Breast tenderness
Irritability
Menstrual cramps (long-term support)
Premenstrual syndrome

HORMONE EXCESS COMPOUND

DIRECTIONS: Combine the following extracts. Consume 30-90 drops, two to three times daily, except during menstruation.

2 parts dandelion root *(Taraxacum)*
2 parts white peony *(Paeonia lactiflora)*
1-2 parts bugleweed *(Lycopus)*
1-2 parts devil's club *(Oplopanax)*
1 part red root *(Ceanothus)*
1 part yellow dock *(Rumex)*

ACTIONS

Anti-inflammatory
Anxiolytic
Hemostatic (mild)
Hepatodecongestant
Hepatodetoxifier

APPLICABLE CONDITIONS

Decreases salty, fatty food cravings
Edema
Heavy bleeding
Irritability and anger
Short menstrual cycles (21-27 days or fewer)

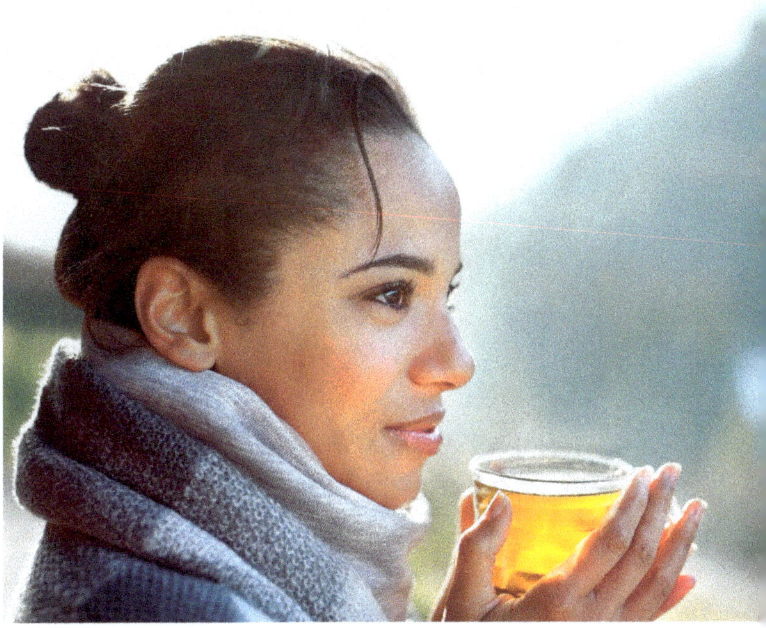

PREMENSTRUAL SYNDROME RELIEF COMPOUND

DIRECTIONS: Combine the following single extracts. Consume 30-90 drops, two to three times daily, as needed for PMS.

4-6 parts kava *(Piper methysticum)*
2-3 parts white peony *(Paeonia lactiflora)*
2-3 parts motherwort *(Leonurus)*
2 parts fresh milky oats *(Avena)*
2 parts damiana *(Turnera)* and/or cannabis *(Cannabis)* (optional)

ACTIONS

Antidepressant
Antispasmodic (smooth muscle)
Anxiolytic
Hepatodecongestant
Nervine
Relaxant
Sedative (mild)

APPLICABLE CONDITIONS

Anxiety
Irritability
Menstrual cramping
Premenstrual depression
Premenstrual syndrome

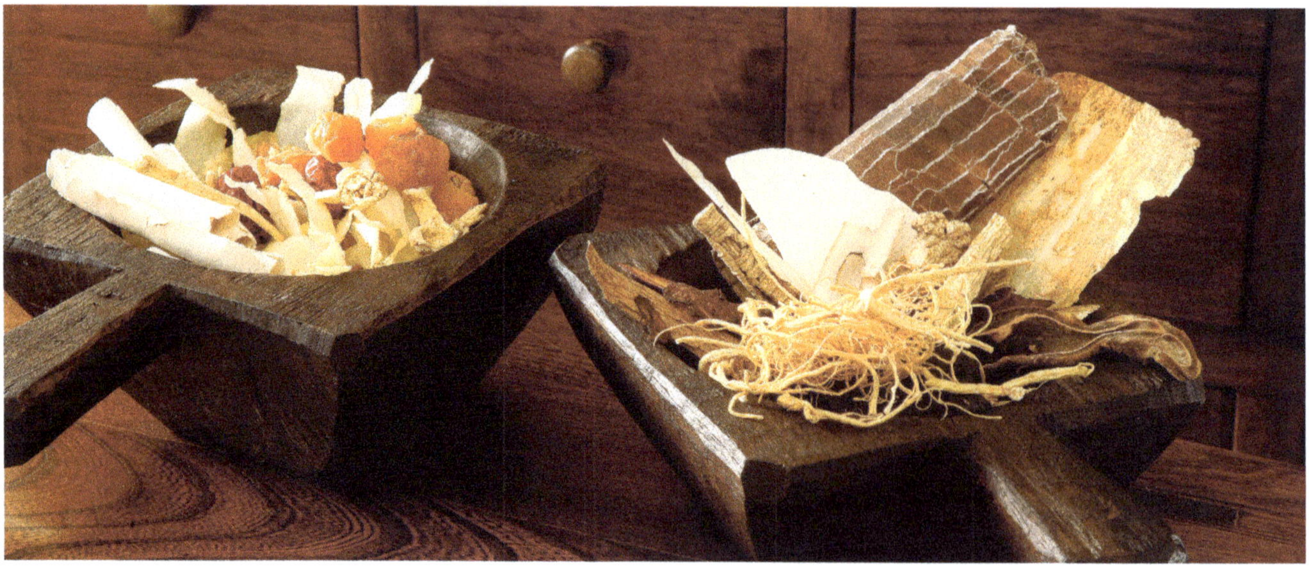

REPRODUCTIVE SYSTEM SUPPORT, MALE

MALE REPRODUCTIVE TONIC TEA

DIRECTIONS: Prepare a decoction or cold infusion containing the following herbs. Consume 8-12 ounces in the morning and early afternoon.

1 part eleuthero *(Eleutherococcus)*
1 part sarsaparilla *(Smilax)*
1 part white peony *(Paeonia)*
1 part nettle root *(Urtica)*
½-1 part allspice *(Pimenta)*
½ part muira puama *(Ptychopetalum)*
½ part ashwagandha *(Withania)*
½ part licorice *(Glycyrrhiza)*—omit with high blood pressure and/or edema
½ part Indian sarsaparilla *(Hemidesmus)*

BENIGN PROSTATIC HYPERTROPHY COMPOUND

DIRECTIONS: Combine the following single extracts. Consume 30-90 drops, up to three times daily.

4 parts nettle root *(Urtica)*
4 parts pygeum *(Prunus africanum)*
2 parts yellow pond lily rhizome *(Nuphar)*
2 parts mullein root *(Verbascum)*
2 parts peony *(Paeonia lactiflora)*
2 parts fu ling *(Poria)*

Additionally, consume 160 mg of standardized liposterolic extracts of saw palmetto (containing 85-95% free fatty acids and sterols) twice daily. Consume 2-3 "00" capsules containing either freeze-dried berry or standardized extract, two to three times daily. Alternatively, consume 2-10 grams of dried berry powder, up to three times daily.

Note: The following actions and applicable conditions apply to the two aforementioned formulas.

ACTIONS

Anti-inflammatory
Antispasmodic (smooth muscles)
Bladder and urinary tract tonic
Decreases residual urine
Decreases urinary frequency
Dribbling
Dysuria
Incontinence
Increases urinary flow and volume
Nocturia
Soothing diuretic

APPLICABLE CONDITIONS

Benign prostatic hypertrophy
Difficulty urinating
Prostate engorgement

RESPIRATORY, IMMUNE, AND LYMPHATIC SUPPORT

ACUTE IMMUNE AND LYMPHATIC TREATMENTS

IMMUNE STIMULANT COMPOUND I

DIRECTIONS: Combine the following single extracts. Consume 30-90 drops, three to four times daily in 2-4 ounces of water.

4 parts echinacea *(Echinacea)*
4 parts elder berry *(Sambucus)*
2 parts propolis *(Propolis)*
1½ parts spilanthes *(Acmella)*
¼-½ part licorice *(Glycyrrhiza)*—omit with high blood pressure and/or edema

ACTIONS

Anesthetize throat
Antibacterial
Antiviral
Astringent
Demulcent
Immune stimulant
Lymphatic

APPLICABLE CONDITIONS

Cold or flu
Mononucleosis recovery
Sore throat or strep throat
Swollen glands or lymph

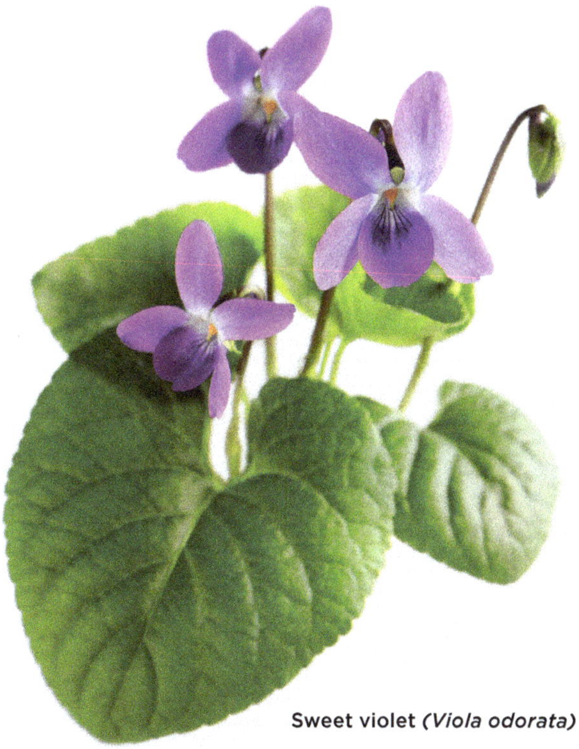

Sweet violet *(Viola odorata)*

IMMUNE STIMULANT COMPOUND II

DIRECTIONS: Combine the following single extracts. Consume 30-90 drops, three to four times daily, in 2-4 ounces of water.

4 parts echinacea *(Echinacea)*
2 parts spilanthes *(Acmella)*
2 parts usnea *(Usnea)*
1 part yerba mansa *(Anemopsis)*
½ part calendula *(Calendula)* or balsam root *(Balsamorhiza)*
½ part thyme *(Thymus)*
⅛-¼ part clove *(Syzygium)*
⅛-¼ part licorice *(Glycyrrhiza)*—omit with high blood pressure and/or edema

ACTIONS

Anesthetize throat
Antibacterial
Antiviral
Astringent
Demulcent
Immune stimulant
Lymphatic

APPLICABLE CONDITIONS

Cold or flu
Mononucleosis recovery
Sore throat or strep throat
Swollen glands or lymph

LYMPHATIC COMPOUND

DIRECTIONS: Combine the following single extracts. Consume 30-90 drops, up to four times daily.

4 parts echinacea *(Echinacea)*
2 parts spilanthes *(Acmella)*
1-2 parts red root *(Ceanothus)*
1-2 parts cleavers *(Galium)*
1 part yerba mansa *(Anemopsis)*
½ part false indigo *(Baptisia)* (optional)

ACTIONS

Anesthetize throat
Antibacterial
Antiviral
Astringent
Demulcent
Immune stimulant
Lymphatic

APPLICABLE CONDITIONS

Cold or flu
Mononucleosis recovery
Sore throat
Resolve lymph swelling or swollen glands

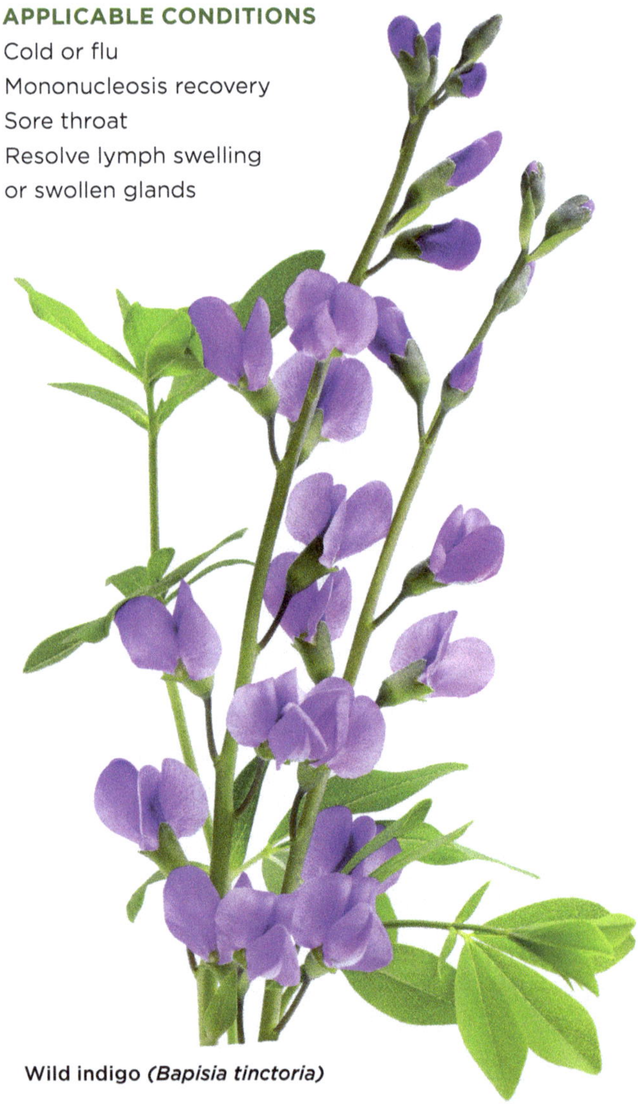

Wild indigo *(Bapisia tinctoria)*

LYMPHATIC ALTERATIVE COMPOUND I

DIRECTIONS: Combine the following single extracts. Consume 30-90 drops, three to four times daily in 2-4 ounces of water.

4 parts echinacea *(Echinacea)*
2 parts elder berry *(Sambucus)*
1-2 parts cleaver *(Galium)*
1 part burdock root, fresh *(Arctium)*
1 part red root *(Ceanothus)*
½-1 part red clover *(Trifolium)*
½-1 part figwort *(Scrophularia)*

LYMPHATIC ALTERATIVE COMPOUND II—HOXEY FORMULA (MODIFIED)

Harry Hoxsey was a holistic practitioner who offered a natural cancer treatment, "The Hoxsey Formula," as an alternative to conventional therapy. The original formula also contained barberry bark *(Berberis vulgaris)*, licorice root *(Glycyrrhiza glabra)*, cascara sagrada bark *(Rhamnus purshiana)*, buckthorn bark *(Rhamnus frangula)*, poke root and berry *(Phytolacca americana)*, potassium iodide, zinc chloride, and antimony trisulfide. Due to the extreme physiologic actions of the cathartic laxatives and caustic properties, these ingredients have been replaced with gentler herbs.

DIRECTIONS: Combine the following single extracts. Consume 30-90 drops, three to four times daily in 2-4 ounces of water.

4 parts red clover *(Trifolium pratense)*
2 cleavers *(Galium aparine)*
2 parts burdock root *(Arctium lappa)*
2 parts dandelion root *(Taraxacum officinale)*
1 part yellow dock *(Rumex crispus)*
1 part queen's root *(Stillingia sylvatica)*

Note: The following actions and applicable conditions apply to the two aforementioned compounds.

ACTIONS

Alterative
Depurative
Detoxifier (gentle)
Lymphatic
Resolvent
Vulnerary

APPLICABLE CONDITIONS

Gentle cleansing
Resolve lymph swelling or swollen glands

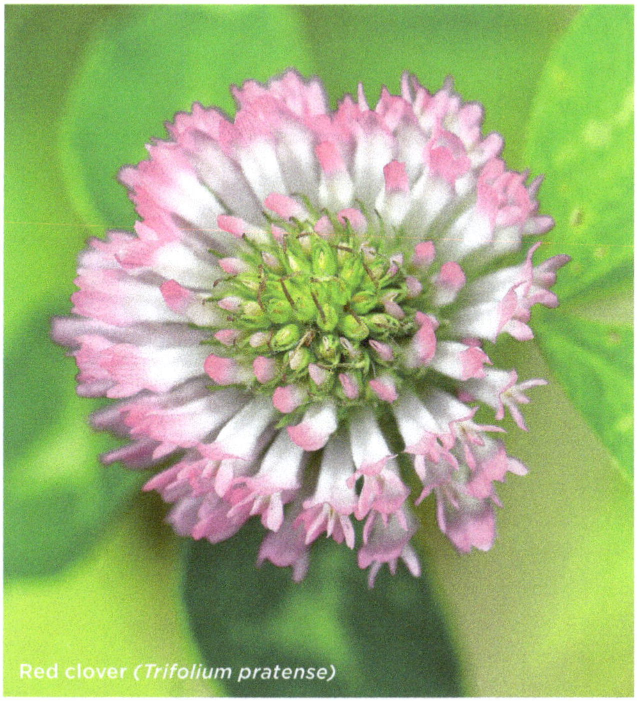
Red clover *(Trifolium pratense)*

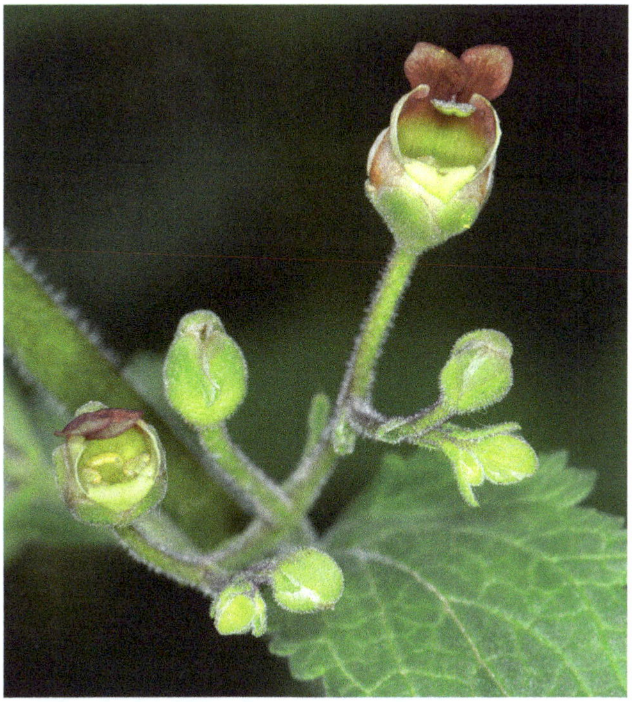

LYMPHATIC ALTERATIVE TEA I

DIRECTIONS: Prepare an infusion containing the following herbs. Consume 8-10 ounces, up to three times daily.

2 parts mint *(Mentha)* or tulsi basil *(Ocimum sanctum)*
2 parts violet leaves *(Viola)*
1 part red clover *(Trifolium)*
½ part cleavers *(Galium)*
½ part chickweed *(Stellaria)*
1⁄16 part stevia *(Stevia)*

ACTIONS

Alterative
Depurative
Detoxifier (gentle)
Lymphatic
Resolvent
Vulnerary

APPLICABLE CONDITIONS

Gentle cleansing
Resolve lymph swelling
Sore throat
Swollen glands

LYMPHATIC ALTERATIVE TEA II

DIRECTIONS: Prepare an infusion containing the following herbs. Consume 8-10 ounces, up to three times daily.

2 parts mint *(Mentha)* or tulsi basil *(Ocimum sanctum)*
½ part red clover *(Trifolium)*
½ part violets *(Viola)*
¼ part alfalfa *(Medicago)*
¼ part calendula *(Calendula)*
¼ part chickweed *(Stellaria)*
¼ part cleavers *(Galium)*
¼ part figwort *(Scrophularia)*
1⁄16 part stevia *(Stevia)*

ACTIONS

Alterative
Depurative
Detoxifier (gentle)
Lymphatic
Resolvent
Vulnerary

APPLICABLE CONDITIONS

Aids recovery from throat infections or mononucleosis
Dermatitis
Eczema
Gentle cleansing
Psoriasis
Resolve lymph swelling

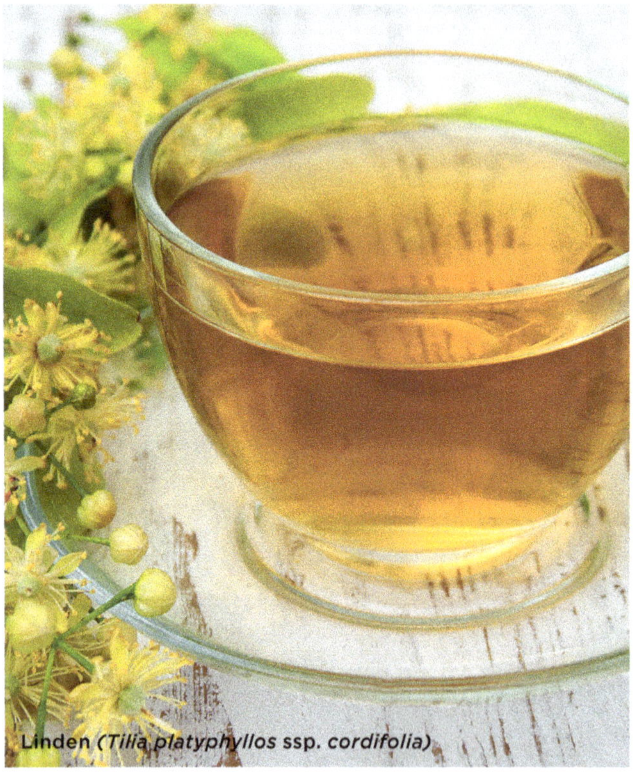

Linden (*Tilia platyphyllos* ssp. *cordifolia*)

SUDORIFIC COLD AND FLU TEA

DIRECTIONS: Prepare a hot infusion containing the following herbs. Consume one cup every hour up to five times daily. Add raw honey to increase palatability.

2 parts peppermint *(Mentha piperita)*
1 part elder flower *(Sambucus)*
½ part yarrow *(Achillea)*
½ part chamomile *(Matricaria)*
½ part linden *(Tilia platyphyllos* ssp. *cordifolia)*
½ part boneset *(Eupatorium perfoliatum)* (optional)
¼ part meadowsweet *(Filipendula)*
¹⁄₁₆ part stevia *(Stevia)*

ACTIONS

Anti-inflammatory
Antibacterial
Antiviral
Diaphoretic
Sudorific
Vasodilating

APPLICABLE CONDITIONS

Cold
Fever
Flu

RESPIRATORY, LOWER

HACK-AWAY COMPOUND

DIRECTIONS: Combine the following single extracts. Consume 30–90 drops, three to four times daily in 2–4 ounces of water. Alternatively, add ¼ of the total tincture volume of honey to make syrup. Consume ½–1 teaspoon, up to four times daily.

4 parts usnea *(Usnea)*
2 parts aralia *(Aralia californica)*
2 parts gumweed *(Grindelia)*
1 part yerba santa *(Eriodictyon)*
1 part anise seed *(Pimpinella)*
½ part elecampane *(Inula)*
½ part oshá *(Ligusticum porteri)* or lovage *(Levisticum)*
½ part biscuit root *(Lomatium)*
½ part licorice *(Glycyrrhiza)*—omit with high blood pressure and/or edema

ACTIONS

Antibacterial
Antitussive
Antiviral
Decongestant
Deepens respiration
Demulcent
Expectorant
Immune stimulant

APPLICABLE CONDITIONS

Bronchitis
Dry cough
Lingering cough
Lower respiratory infection
Pneumonia
Whooping cough

QUITTER'S CRUTCH—SMOKER'S MIX

DIRECTIONS: Remove stems from the herbs, combine herbs in a bowl, store in a jar. Roll the blend in paper or place herbs in a pipe. Smoke as an alternative to tobacco.

1 part yerba santa *(Eriodictyon)*
1 part coltsfoot *(Tussilago)*
1 part raspberry leaf *(Rubus idaeus)*
¼ part mullein leaf *(Verbascum)*
¼ part damiana *(Turnera)*
¼ part spearmint *(Mentha spicata)*
¼ part peppermint *(Mentha piperita)*

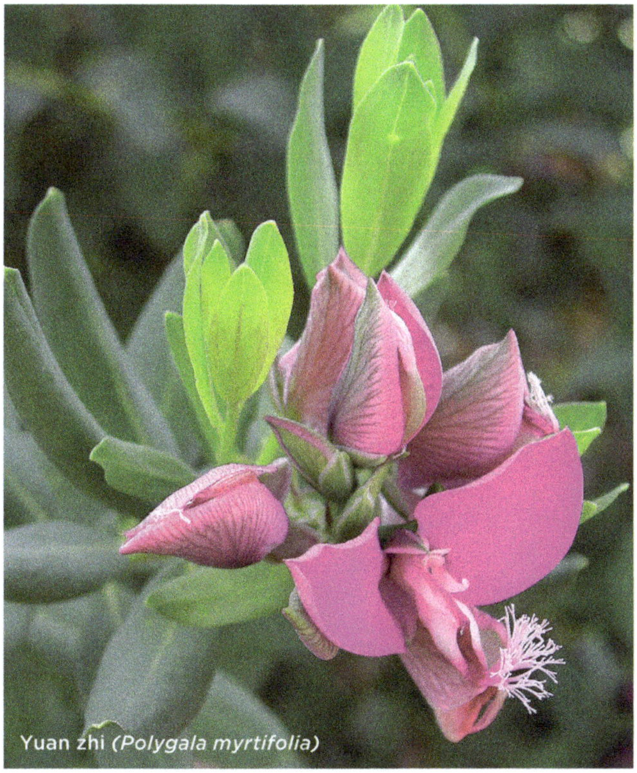

Yuan zhi *(Polygala myrtifolia)*

RESPIRATORY ANTISPASMODIC COMPOUND

DIRECTIONS: Combine the following single extracts. Consume 30-90 drops, three to four times daily in 2-4 ounces of water.

2 parts gumweed *(Grindelia)*
1 part aralia *(Aralia californica)*
1 part elecampane *(Inula)*
1 part anise *(Pimpinella)*
½ part yuan zhi *(Polygala tenuifolia)*
½ part licorice *(Glycyrrhiza)* — omit with hypertension and edema

ACTIONS

Antispasmodic
Antitussive
Bronchodilator
Decongestant
Deepens respiration
Demulcent
Expectorant

APPLICABLE CONDITIONS

Asthma
Chronic obstructive pulmonary disease
Dyspnea
Wheezing

RESPIRATORY RELIEF TEA

DIRECTIONS: Prepare an infusion containing the following herbs. Consume 8-12 ounces, three to four times daily.

2 parts peppermint *(Mentha piperita)*
1 part coltsfoot *(Tussilago farfara* or *Petasites frigidus* var. *palmatus)*
½ part hyssop *(Hyssopus)*
½ part mullein *(Verbascum)*
½ part marjoram *(Origanum majorana)* or thyme *(Thymus)*
½ part eucalyptus *(Eucalyptus)*
¼ part licorice *(Glycyrrhiza)* — omit with hypertension and edema

ACTIONS

Antitussive
Astringent (mild)
Bronchodilator (mild)
Demulcent
Diaphoretic
Expectorant

APPLICABLE CONDITIONS

Cold
Cough
Dyspnea
Wheezing

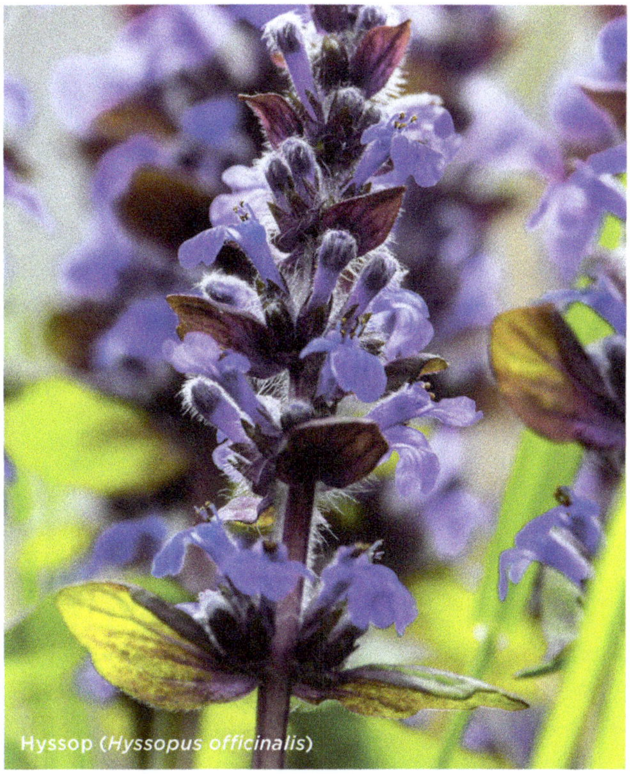

Hyssop *(Hyssopus officinalis)*

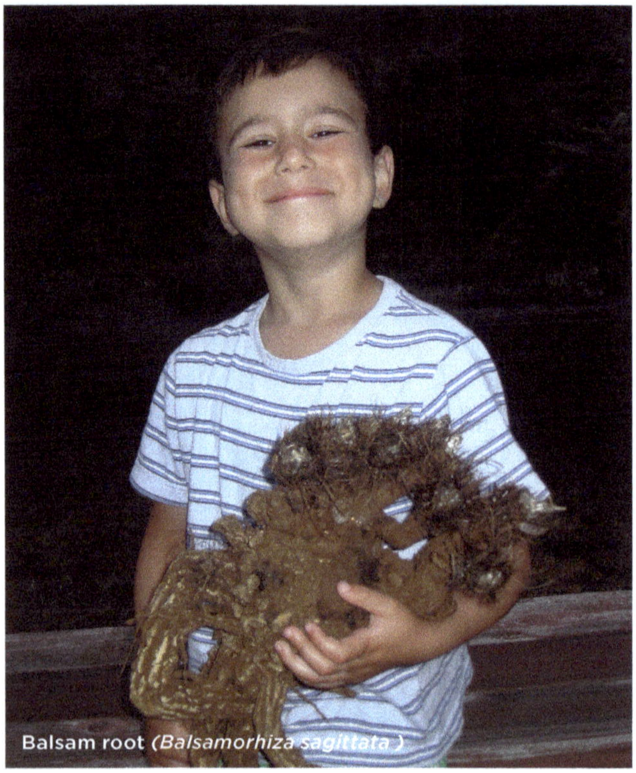

Balsam root *(Balsamorhiza sagittata)*

RESPIRATORY ROOTS BLEND

DIRECTIONS: Prepare a decoction containing the following herbs. Consume 8-12 ounces, three to four times daily.

4 parts marshmallow root *(Althaea)*
2 parts anise seed *(Pimpinella)*
1 part balsam root *(Balsamorhiza)*—if available
½-1 part cinnamon bark *(Cinnamomum)*
¼-½ part oshá root *(Ligusticum)*
¼-½ part licorice *(Glycyrrhiza)*—omit with high blood pressure and/or edema

ACTIONS

Antibacterial
Antitussive
Antiviral
Bronchodilator (mild)
Demulcent
Diaphoretic
Expectorant

APPLICABLE CONDITIONS

Bronchitis
Cold
Cough
Dyspnea
Lower respiratory infection

RESPIRATORY, UPPER

ALLERGY-EASE COMPOUND

DIRECTIONS: Combine the following single extracts. Consume 30-90 drops, three to four times daily in 2-4 ounces of water.

4 parts yerba mansa *(Anemopsis)*
4 parts yerba santa *(Eriodictyon)*
2 parts ambrosia *(Ambrosia)*
2 parts gumweed *(Grindelia)*
1 part bayberry *(Morella)*
1 part goldenrod *(Solidago)*

ACTIONS

IgE response
Antibacterial
Anti-inflammatory
Astringent
Decongestant
Expectorant
Lymphatic

APPLICABLE CONDITIONS

Allergies
Allergic rhinitis
Sinusitis

RESPIRATORY DECONGESTANT TEA

DIRECTIONS: Prepare a decoction containing the following herbs. Consume 8-12 ounces, three to four times daily.

2 parts marshmallow root *(Althaea)*
1 part Mormon tea *(Ephedra)*
½ part yerba santa *(Eriodictyon)*
½ part cinnamon *(Cinnamomum)*
½ part yerba mansa *(Anemopsis)* (optional)
⅛-¼ part licorice *(Glycyrrhiza)*—omit with high blood pressure and/or edema

ACTIONS

Antibacterial
Anti-inflammatory
Astringent
Decongestant
Expectorant

APPLICABLE CONDITIONS

Allergic rhinitis
Asthma
Sinus or lung congestion
Sinusitis

SINUS DECONGESTANT COMPOUND

DIRECTIONS: Combine the following single extracts. Consume 30 - 90 drops, up to four times daily.

4 parts yerba mansa *(Anemopsis)*
4 parts yerba santa *(Eriodictyon)*
2 parts usnea *(Usnea)*
1 part bayberry *(Morella)*
1 part ambrosia *(Ambrosia)*

ACTIONS

Antibacterial
Anti-inflammatory
Astringent
Decongestant
Expectorant
Lymphatic

APPLICABLE CONDITIONS

Allergic rhinitis
Sinus or lung congestion
Sinusitis

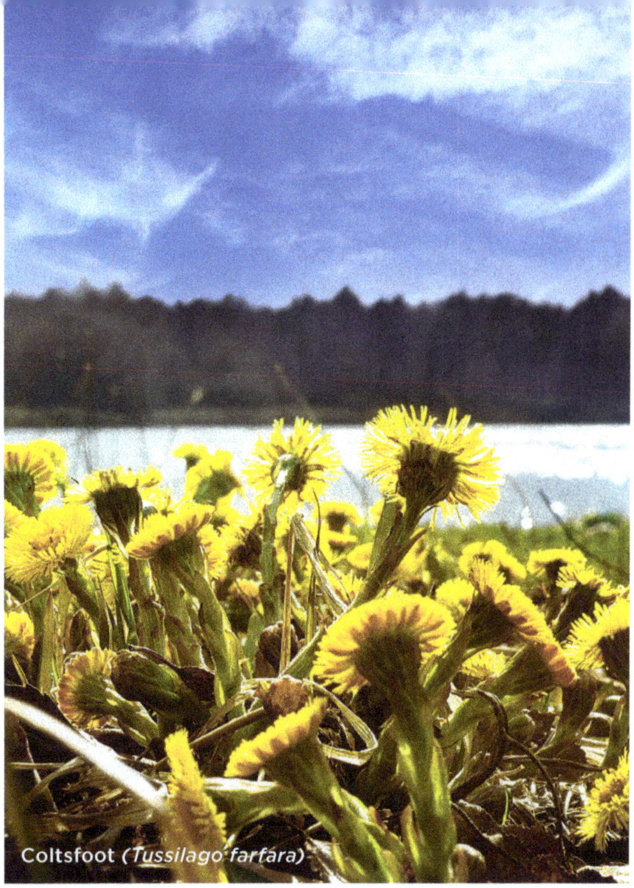

Coltsfoot *(Tussilago farfara)*

SINUS DECONGESTANT TEA

DIRECTIONS: Prepare a decoction containing the following herbs. Consume 8 - 12 ounces, three to four times daily.

3 parts marshmallow root *(Althaea)*
1 part yerba santa *(Eriodictyon)*
1 part cinnamon *(Cinnamomum)*
½ part bayberry *(Morella)*
½ part oshá *(Ligusticum)*
½ part elecampane root *(Inula)*
¼ - ½ part licorice *(Glycyrrhiza)* — omit with high blood pressure and/or edema

ACTIONS

Antibacterial
Antiviral
Astringent
Decongestant
Demulcent
Expectorant
Immune stimulant

APPLICABLE CONDITIONS

Allergic rhinitis
Sinus or lung congestion
Sinusitis

SINUS DECONGESTANT STEAM

DIRECTIONS: Combine the herbs in a bowl, pour boiled water over them. Place a towel over the head to form a steam tent. Steam 15 - 20 minutes, up to four times daily using a fresh batch of herbs each time.

2 parts peppermint *(Mentha piperita)*
2 parts eucalyptus *(Eucalyptus globulus)*
1 part hyssop *(Hyssopus officinalis)* or thyme *(Thymus)*
1 part bee balm *(Monarda fistulosa)*

ACTIONS

Antitussive
Bronchodilator
Expectorant

APPLICABLE CONDITIONS

Cold
Cough
Dyspnea
Wheezing

THROAT COAT AND SOOTHE TEA I

DIRECTIONS: Prepare a decoction containing the following herbs. Consume 8-12 ounces, three to four times daily.

4 parts marshmallow *(Althaea)*
1 part orange peel *(Citrus)*
1 part fenugreek *(Trigonella)*
1 part cinnamon *(Cinnamomum)*
¼-½ part licorice *(Glycyrrhiza)*—omit with high blood pressure and/or edema

THROAT COAT AND SOOTHE TEA II

DIRECTIONS: Prepare a decoction containing the following herbs. Consume 8-10 ounces, up to four times daily.

4 parts marshmallow *(Althaea)*
2 parts echinacea *(Echinacea)*
2 parts slippery elm *(Ulmus)*
1 part anise *(Pimpinella)*
½-1 part cinnamon *(Cinnamomum)*
¼-1⁄16 part licorice *(Glycyrrhiza)*—omit with high blood pressure and/or edema

Note: The following actions and applicable conditions apply to the two aforementioned teas.

ACTIONS

Antibacterial
Antiviral
Astringent (mild)
Demulcent
Expectorant
Immune stimulant
Lymphatic

APPLICABLE CONDITIONS

Dry cough
Laryngitis
Sore throat
Strep throat
Swollen lymph
Whooping cough

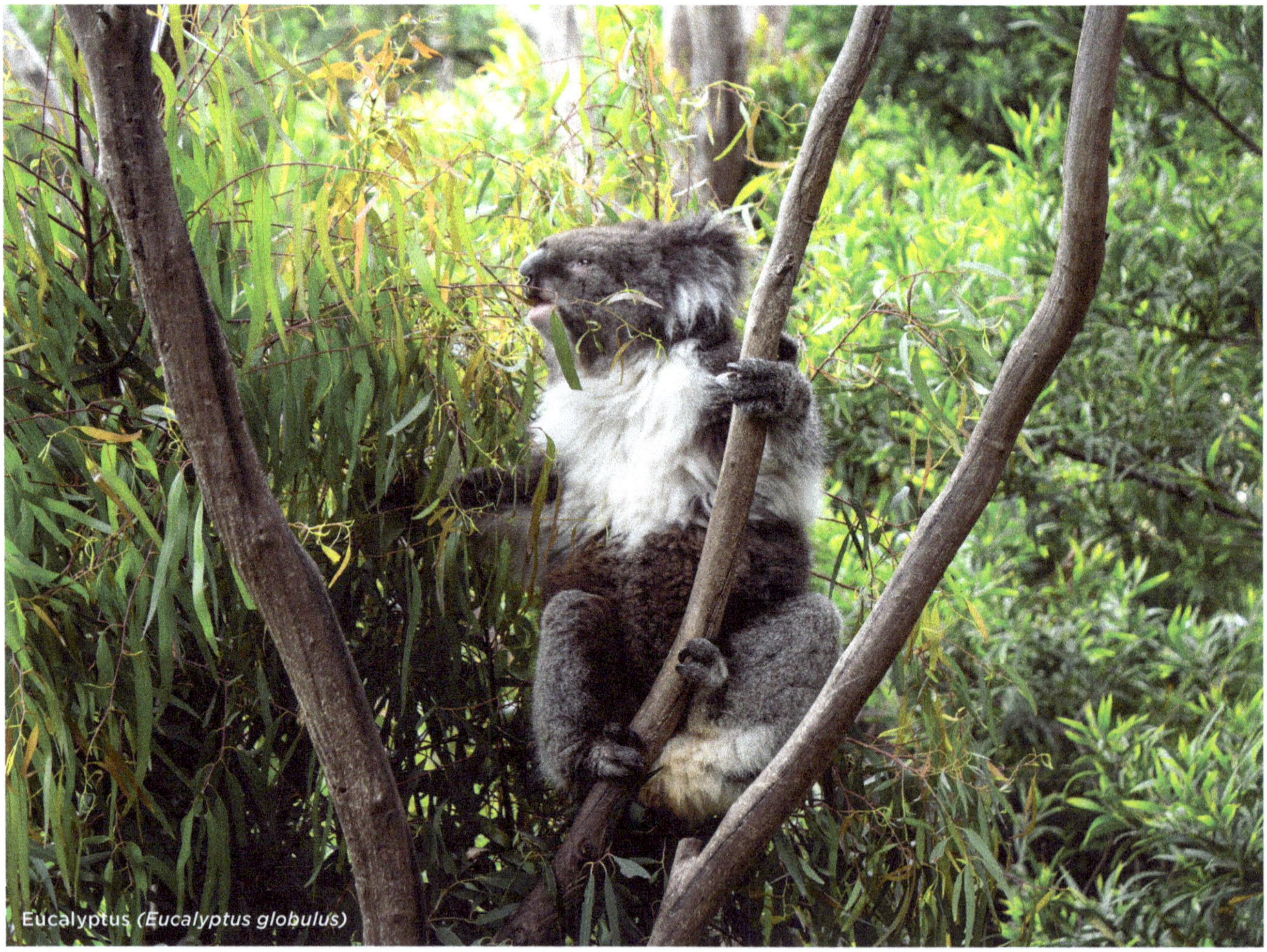

Eucalyptus *(Eucalyptus globulus)*

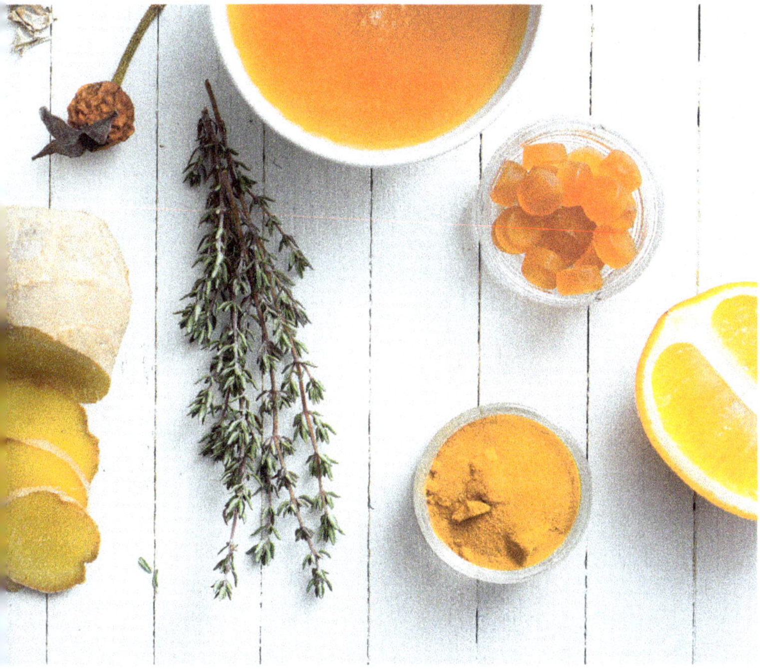

THROAT EASE COMPOUND

DIRECTIONS: Combine the following single extracts. Consume 30 - 90 drops, up to four times daily.

4 parts echinacea *(Echinacea)*
2 parts red root *(Ceanothus)*
2 parts propolis *(Propolis)*
2 parts spilanthes *(Acmella)*
2 parts usnea *(Usnea)*
½ part licorice *(Glycyrrhiza)* — omit with high blood pressure and/or edema
½ part lomatium *(Lomatium)*

ACTIONS

Anesthetizes throat
Antibacterial
Antiviral
Demulcent
Immune stimulant
Lymphatic

APPLICABLE CONDITIONS

Laryngitis
Sore throat
Strep throat
Swollen lymph

THROAT PASTILLES

DIRECTIONS: Weigh powders and stir together until thoroughly mixed. Add one tablespoon of honey and mix into the powders until a piecrust dough-like consistency is obtained. If necessary, add another one-half tablespoon of honey. Roll into ¼ - ⅓ inch size balls. Place one tablespoon of cinnamon or licorice powder on a plate and roll the balls in the powder until they are lightly coated. Place pastilles in a small glass container, in single layers on parchment paper, cap and store in the refrigerator.

12 grams marshmallow powder *(Althaea)*
12 grams echinacea powder *(Echinacea)*
3 grams cinnamon powder *(Cinnamomum)*
¾ gram clove powder *(Syzigium)*
¾ gram ginger powder *(Zingiber)*
½ gram licorice powder *(Glycyrrhiza)* — omit with high blood pressure and/or edema
1 - 1½ tablespoon raw honey
5 - 10 grams licorice or cinnamon powder to coat pastilles

THROAT SPRAY

DIRECTIONS: Combine the following single extracts in a spray-top bottle. Spray 2 - 4 times in the back of the throat, up to five times daily.

4 parts echinacea *(Echinacea)*
3 parts propolis *(Propolis)*
2 parts spilanthes *(Acmella)*
½ part yerba mansa *(Anemopsis)* or bayberry *(Morella)*
½ part clove powder *(Syzigium)* or ½ part licorice *(Glycyrrhiza)* — omit with high blood pressure and/or edema

ACTIONS

Anesthetic
Antibacterial
Antiviral
Astringent
Demulcent
Immune stimulant
Lymphatic

APPLICABLE CONDITIONS

Laryngitis
Sore throat
Strep throat
Swollen lymph

THYROID SUPPORT

HYPERTHYROID SUPPORT COMPOUND

DIRECTIONS: Combine the following single extracts. Consume 30–90 drops, two to three times daily.

3–4 parts bugleweed *(Lycopus)*
1–2 parts motherwort *(Leonurus)*
1–1½ parts lemon balm *(Melissa)*
1–1½ parts blue vervain *(Verbena)*

ACTIONS

Anxiolytic
Cardiotonic
Hypotensive
Hypothyroidal (mild)
Nervine

APPLICABLE CONDITIONS

Anxiety
Hypertension
Hyperthyroid
Insomnia
Irritability
Palpitations
Panic attacks

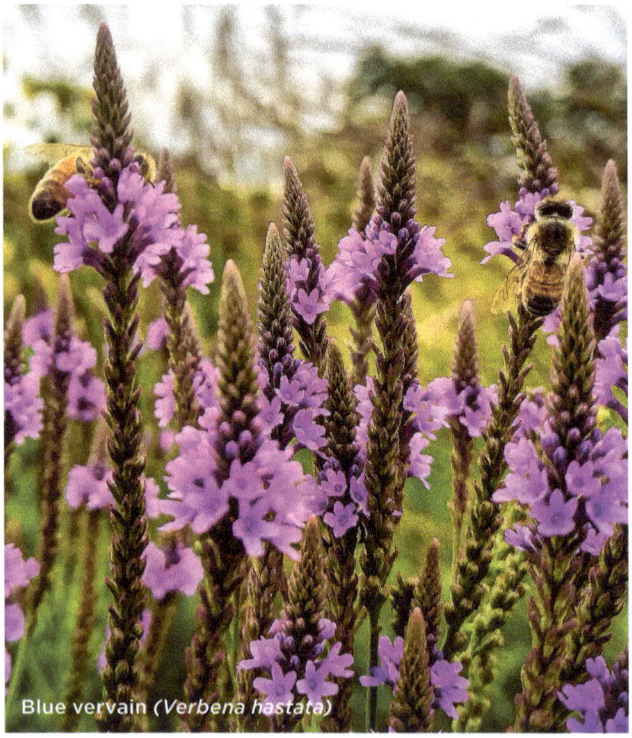

Blue vervain *(Verbena hastata)*

HYPOTHYROID SUPPORT COMPOUND

DIRECTIONS: Combine the following single extracts. Consume 60–90 drops, two to three times daily, in 3–4 ounces of water. *Note:* Some individuals may have difficulty falling asleep when they consume this compound after 2 pm. This is due to the eleuthero, ginseng, and/or gotu kola.

3 parts ashwagandha *(Withania)*
2 parts gotu kola *(Centella)*
2 parts eleuthero *(Eleutherococcus)* or white ginseng *(Panax ginseng)*
2 parts devil's club *(Oplopanax)*
1 part Oregon grape *(Berberis)* or dandelion *(Taraxacum)*
½–1 part ginger, fresh *(Zingiber)*

ACTIONS

Adaptogen
Anti-inflammatory
Blood sugar regulating
Circulatory stimulant
Energizing
Hepatic
Immune modulator
Qi tonic
Thyroid stimulant
Vasodilator

APPLICABLE CONDITIONS

Hypothyroidism, Hashimoto's thyroiditis, and related symptoms:
Adrenal burnout
Connective tissue weakness
Increase libido
Kidney yin and yang deficiency
Reduce fatigue and lethargy
Slow mentation and mental fogginess

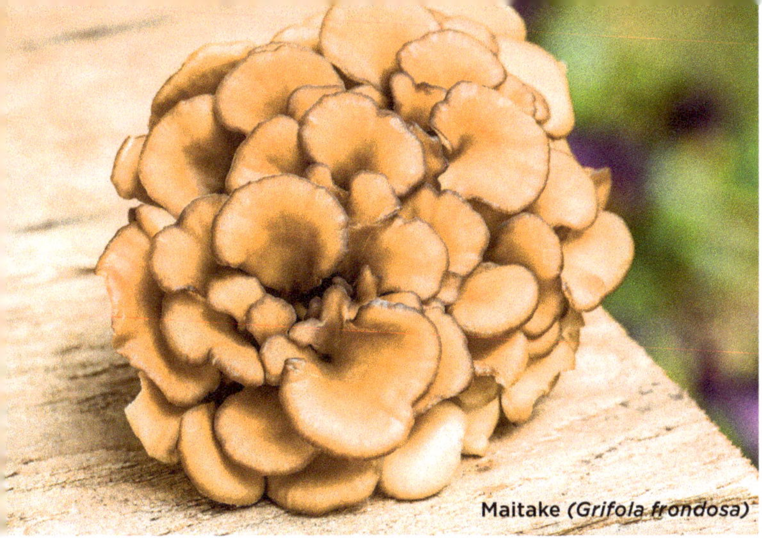

Maitake *(Grifola frondosa)*

URINARY SYSTEM SUPPORT

HASHIMOTO'S THYROIDITIS AND HYPOTHYROIDISM IMMUNE MODULATING COMPOUND

DIRECTIONS: Consume 60 - 90 drops, two to three times daily, in 3 - 4 ounces of water.

4 parts ashwagandha *(Withania)*
4 parts astragalus *(Astragalus)*
4 parts reishi *(Ganoderma)*
2 parts maitake *(Grifola frondosa)*
2 parts eleuthero *(Eleutherococcus)*
2 parts devil's club *(Oplopanax)*
1 - 2 parts gotu kola *(Centella)*
1 part wu wei zi *(Schisandra)*
1 part licorice (*Glycyrrhiza*) — omit with high blood pressure and/or edema

ACTIONS

Adaptogen
Anti-inflammatory
Blood sugar regulating
Circulatory stimulant
Energizing
Hepatodetoxifying
Immune modulator
Kidney yin and yang tonic
Qi tonic
Strengthen connective tissue
Thyroid stimulant
Vasodilator

APPLICABLE CONDITIONS

Hypothyroidism, Hashimoto's thyroiditis, and related symptoms:
Adrenal burnout
Connective tissue weakness
Fatigue and lethargy, or low libido
Kidney yin and yang deficiency
Slow mentation and mental fogginess

CHILDREN'S BLADDER STRENGTHENING COMPOUND

DIRECTIONS: Combine the following single alcohol or glycerin extracts. Consume 30 - 60 drops, two to three times daily.

2 parts mullein root *(Verbascum)*
1 part corn silk *(Zea mays)*

ACTIONS

Bladder tonic
Soothing diuretic

APPLICABLE CONDITIONS

Urinary incontinence
Bedwetting due to physical causes

DIURETIC TEA

DIRECTIONS: Prepare an infusion containing the following herbs. Consume 8 - 10 ounces, up to three times daily.

2 parts spearmint (*Mentha spicata*) or peppermint *(Mentha piperita)*
1 part nettle *(Urtica)*
½ - 1 part parsley seed or root *(Petroselinum)*
½ part cleavers *(Galium)*
½ part chickweed *(Stellaria)*
½ part horsetail *(Equisetum)*

ACTIONS

Diuretic

APPLICABLE CONDITIONS

Edema
Flush kidney stones
Sodium-related hypertension
Water-related weight gain

DIURETIC SOOTHING TEA

DIRECTIONS: Prepare a decoction containing the following herbs. Consume 8–10 ounces, up to three times daily.

3 parts marshmallow root *(Althaea)*
1 part gravel root *(Eutrochium purpureum)*
1 part hydrangea root *(Hydrangea)*
1 part stone root *(Collinsonia)*
1 part parsley root *(Petroselinum)*
1 part dandelion root *(Taraxacum)*
1 part roasted dandelion root *(Taraxacum)*
1 part burdock root *(Arctium)*
1 part carob pod *(Ceratonia)*

ACTIONS

Anti-inflammatory
Antilithic
Demulcent
Diuretic, soothing

APPLICABLE CONDITIONS

Bladder irritation
Concentrated urine
Edema
Flush kidney stones
Post-urinary tract or kidney infections
Reduces kidney stone formation
Sodium-related hypertension
Urinary tract inflammation
Water-related weight gain

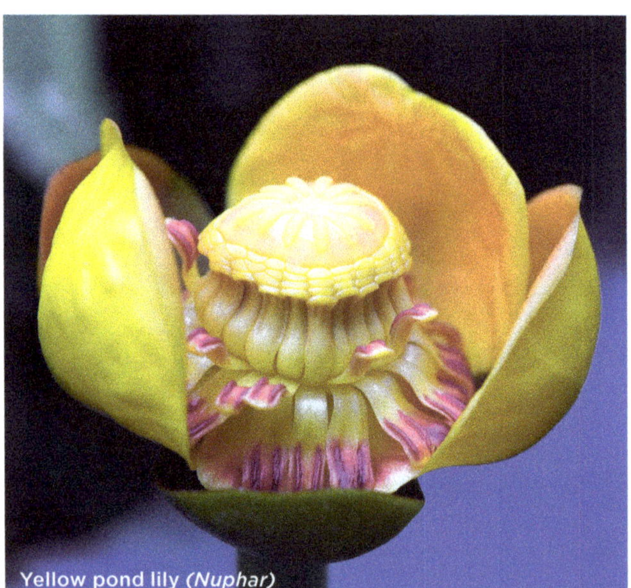

Yellow pond lily *(Nuphar)*

INTERSTITIAL CYSTITIS SUPPORT COMPOUND

DIRECTIONS: Combine the following single extracts. Consume 30–90 drops, two to three times daily with two capsules of saw palmetto, one to three times daily. Best used long-term.

4 parts mullein root *(Verbascum)*
2 parts fresh corn silk *(Zea mays)*
2 parts nettle root *(Utica dioica)*
2 parts yellow pond lily *(Nuphar)*
2 parts peony, white *(Paeonia lactiflora)*

ACTIONS

Anti-inflammatory
Antispasmodic
Bladder tonic
Diuretic, soothing

APPLICABLE CONDITIONS

Bladder weakness
Dribbling
Dysuria (painful urination)
Sense of urgency
Urinary tenismus (painful straining)

KIDNEY AND BLADDER SOOTHING TEA

DIRECTIONS: Prepare a decoction containing the following herbs. Consume 8–10 ounces, up to three times daily.

3 parts marshmallow *(Althaea)*
2 parts mullein root *(Verbascum)*
1 part stone root *(Collinsonia)*
1 part parsley root *(Petroselinum)*
1 part gravel root *(Eutrochium purpureum)*
⅛–½ part licorice (*Glycyrrhiza*)—omit with high blood pressure and/or edema

ACTIONS

Anti-inflammatory
Antilithic
Bladder tonic
Demulcent
Diuretic, soothing

APPLICABLE CONDITIONS

Bladder or kidney inflammation
Flush kidney stones
Reduce kidney stone formation
Urinary tract inflammation

TOPICAL FORMULAS

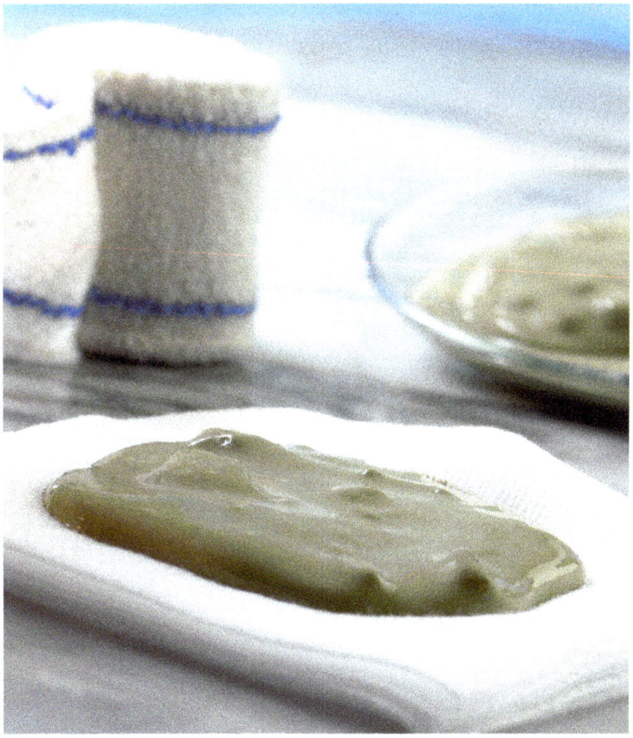

BURN RELIEF OIL

DIRECTIONS: Combine the following infused oils, then add essential oils. Apply to the affected area. The oil works most effectively when applied following a fresh aloe vera leaf or gel application, and after the burn has cooled for several hours.

2 parts St. John's wort *(Hypericum)*
1 part calendula *(Calendula)*
10–15 drops lavender essential oil *(Lavandula angustifolia)*
5–15 drops peppermint essential oil *(Mentha piperita)*
2 drops blue chamomile essential oil *(Matricaria recutita)*

ACTIONS

Anti-inflammatory
Vulnerary

APPLICABLE CONDITIONS

Sunburns
Thermal burns

BURN RELIEF SPRAY

DIRECTIONS: Combine the following hydrosols. If one or more aren't available, use equal parts of what is available.

1 part peppermint hydrosol *(Mentha piperita)*
1 part calendula hydrosol *(Calendula)*
1 part cucumber hydrosol *(Cucurbita)*
1 part rose hydrosol *(Rosa)*

ACTIONS

Anti-inflammatory
Vulnerary

APPLICABLE CONDITIONS

Sunburns
Thermal burns

ECHINACEA CLAY POULTICE

DIRECTIONS: Prepare a drawing poultice by combining ½–1 cup of clay (any type), enough echinacea extract or glycerite to create a thick paste, 5–10 drops of lavender essential oil, and 1–3 drops of blue chamomile essential oil. Apply a sufficient amount of this poultice to cover two to three times the surface area of the insect sting or bite. Apply two to three times daily until the swelling decreases.

ACTIONS

Anti-infective
Anti-inflammatory
Antinecrotic
Drawing

APPLICABLE CONDITIONS

Abscesses
Acne, blackheads, boils, zits
Bee, wasp, and hornet stings
Insect bites (spider, bug, mosquito)

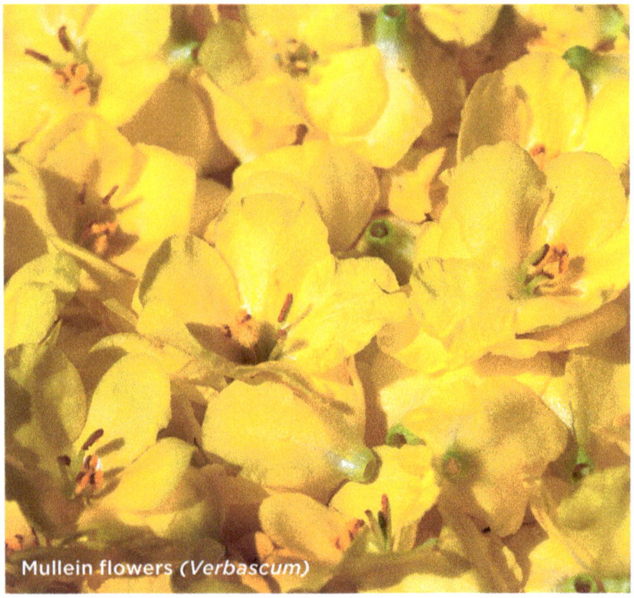

Mullein flowers *(Verbascum)*

EARACHE EASE GLYCERIN- OR OIL-BASED COMPOUND

DIRECTIONS: Combine the following single plant oils or glycerin and alcohol-based extracts. Place 3 - 5 drops of finished oil in the ear canal, three times daily.

1 part mullein flower *(Verbascum)*
1 part echinacea *(Echinacea)*
1 part St. John's wort *(Hypericum)*

EARACHE EASE OIL

DIRECTIONS: Combine the following single plant oils, then infuse the blend with fresh chopped garlic 8 to 12 hours before straining the mixture. Add 1 - 2 drops of blue chamomile essential oil *(Matricaria recutita)* per 1 - 2 ounces of the blend. Place 2 - 4 drops in the affected ear canal, and cover with a warm towel and/or hot water bottle.

1 part mullein flower *(Verbascum)*
1 part St. John's wort *(Hypericum)*

ACTIONS

Analgesic
Antibacterial
Anti-inflammatory

APPLICABLE CONDITIONS

Earache
Early stage of ear infection

PLANTAIN CLAY POULTICE

DIRECTIONS: Gather, clean, and wipe dry fresh plantain leaves. Prepare a drawing poultice by blending one cup of fresh plantain leaves with two cups of clay, enough distilled water to create a thick paste, and several drops of lavender and blue chamomile essential oil. If consistency is too watery, add more clay. Apply ample amounts to the affected area, wrap with a bandage, and leave in place 15 - 30 minutes.

ACTIONS

Anti-infective
Anti-inflammatory
Antinecrotic
Drawing

APPLICABLE CONDITIONS

Abscesses
Acne, blackheads, boils, zits
Bee, wasp, and hornet stings
Blisters
Insect bites (spider, bug, mosquito)
Mastitis pain
Nettle sting
Reduce residual inflammation from snakebites
Splinters

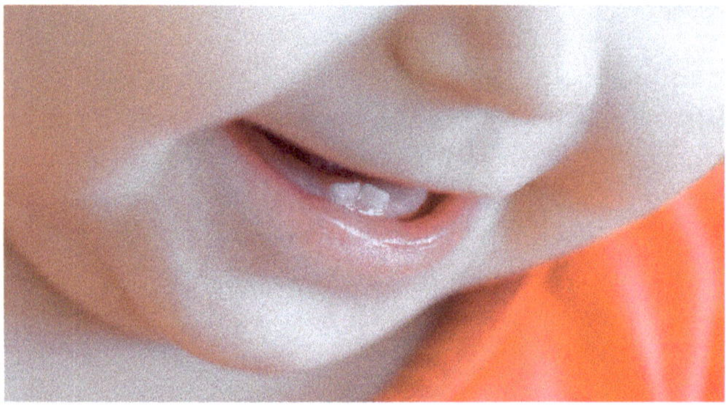

TOPICAL TEETHING COMPOUND

DIRECTIONS: Combine the following single plant alcohol, or glycerin and alcohol-based extracts. Place three - five drops onto the affected area of the gums, three to five times daily.

5 parts spilanthes *(Acmella)*
4 parts St. John's wort *(Hypericum)*
4 parts clove *(Syzygium)*
2 parts yarrow *(Achillea)*
1 part cow parsnip seeds *(Heracleum)*

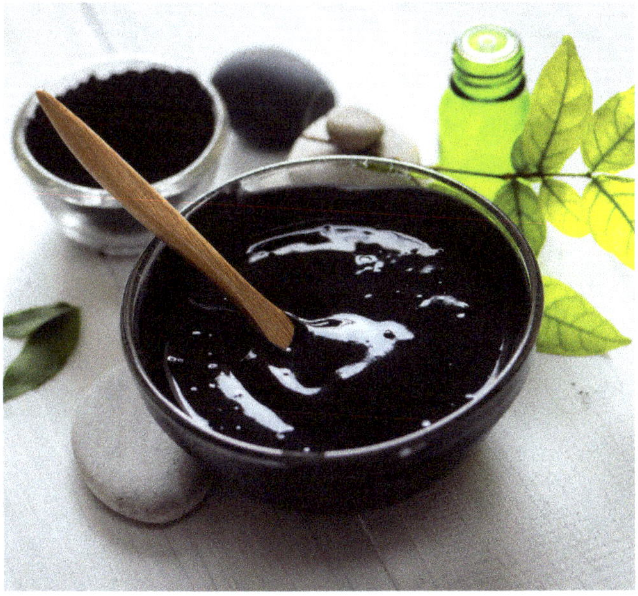

SALVES

BLACK DRAWING SALVE

DIRECTIONS: Measure, combine, and mix activated charcoal and powdered clay in a bowl. Add lavender essential oil to the combined powders and blend with a whisk. Measure oils, shea butter, beeswax, and vitamin E. Combine and heat them in a double boiler until wax and butter dissolve. Whisk charcoal and clay powders into the oil until they are smoothly blended with the oils; then cook on low for 30 minutes in a double boiler. Pour into clean, dry salve jars. This recipe makes 9–10 ounces of salve.

Apply to insect bites, bee stings, splinters, zits, boils, skin tags, and moles.

3 tablespoons castor oil
3 tablespoons herb-infused oil (calendula, chamomile, comfrey, plantain)
2 tablespoons shea butter
2 tablespoons beeswax
1 teaspoon vitamin E oil
3 tablespoons activated charcoal
3 tablespoons bentonite and kaolin clay
20–30 drops lavender essential oil

CAYENNE AND CINNAMON SALVE

DIRECTIONS: Weigh and whisk powders in a bowl. Weigh beeswax shavings or granules and set aside in a bowl. Measure olive and coconut oil, place oils in a double boiler and cook on low until the coconut oil liquifies. Add powdered ingredients, stir, and cook for 30 minutes. Allow the oil to cool before pressing. Pour the oil through a cloth-lined strainer. Wear nitrile gloves to strain remaining oil from the herbs. Place oil in a clean, dry double boiler with beeswax and heat until the beeswax dissolves. Pour into clean, dry salve jars. This recipe makes 9–10 ounces of salve.

Apply topically to bruises, sprains, strains, sore muscles, neuralgia, or myalgia.

8 ounces (1 cup) olive oil, cold pressed, extra-virgin
4 ounces (½ cup) coconut oil
1½ ounces beeswax (granules or shavings)
2 tablespoons cayenne powder *(Capsicum annuum)*
2 tablespoons ginger powder *(Zingiber officinale)*
2 tablespoons cinnamon powder *(Cinnamomum cassia)*
1 tablespoon clove powder *(Syzigium aromaticum)*

Note: See the medicinal oils and salve portion of the *Medicine Making* section for muscle and joint support, first aid, and anti-inflammatory salve recipes.

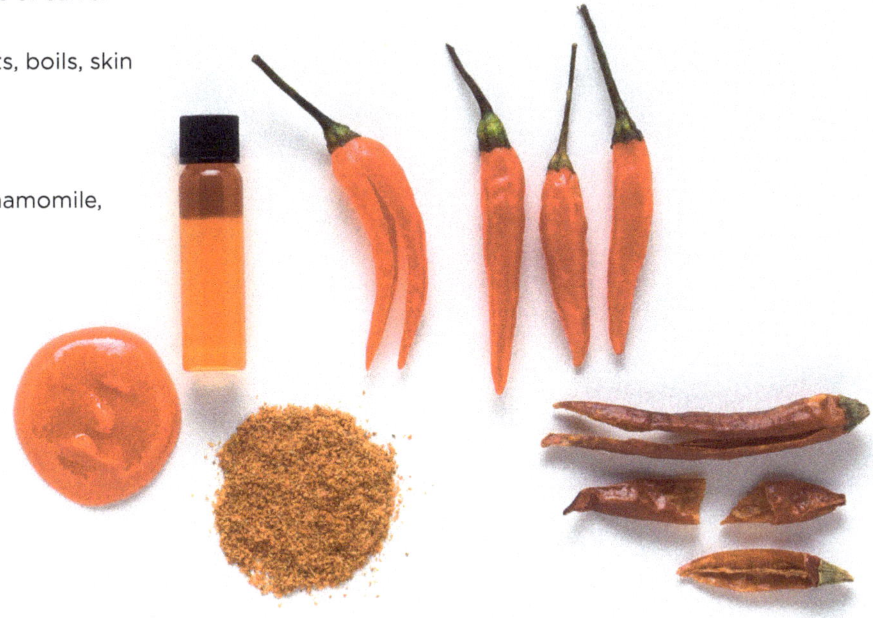

APPENDICES AND INDEXES

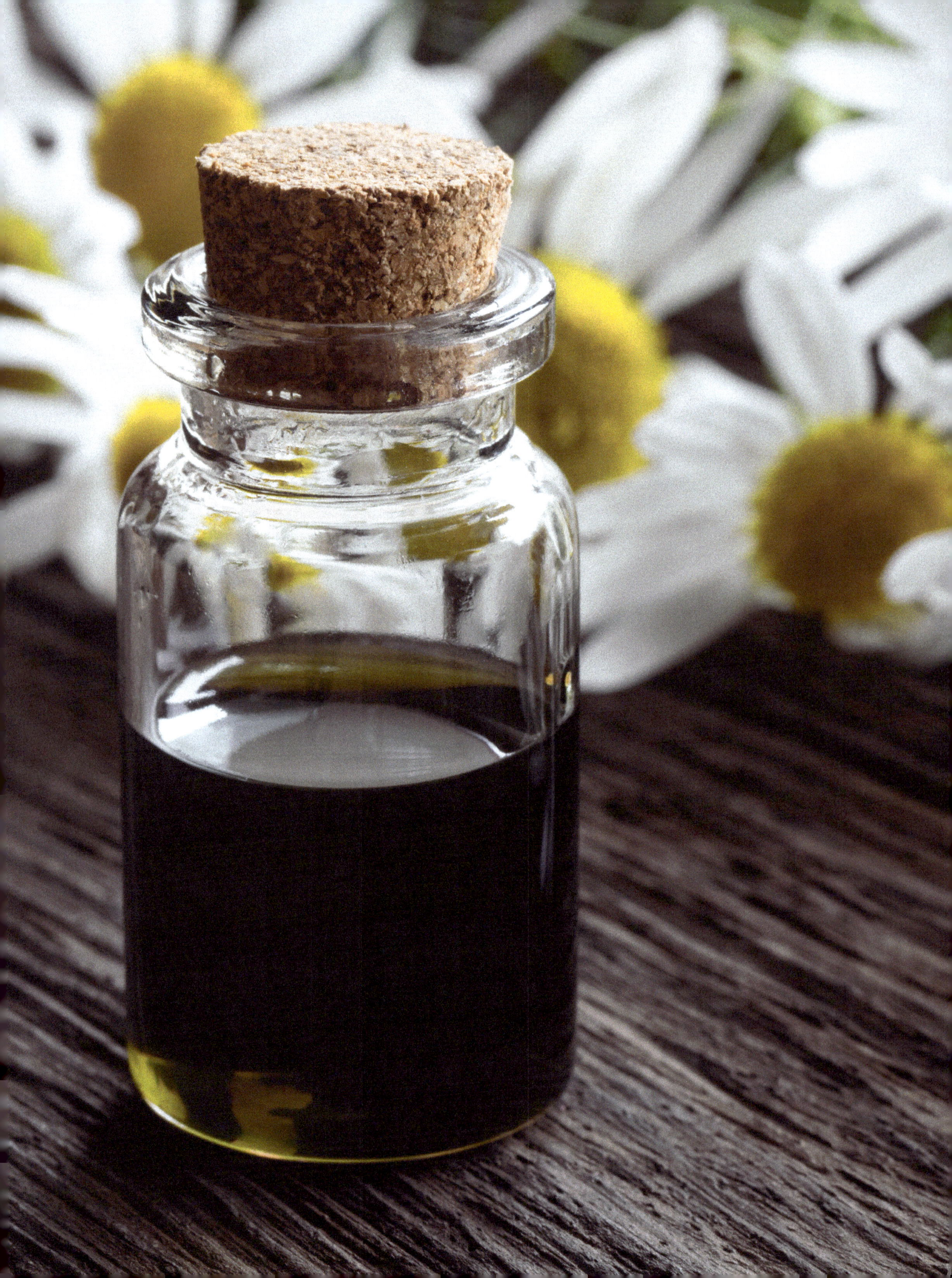

COMPENDIUM OF HERBAL THERAPEUTIC USES AND CONDITIONS

ABSCESSES, INTERNAL

Astragalus
Bayberry
Berberis
Burdock
Calendula
Chickweed
Dandelion
Echinacea
Fenugreek
Gentian
Ginger
Marshmallow
Plantain
Propolis
Red cedar
Red root
Spilanthes
Thyme
Turmeric
Usnea
Wild indigo
Yarrow
Yerba mansa

ABSCESSES, TOPICAL

Berberis
Burdock root (fresh)
Calendula
Chaparral
Chickweed (fresh)
Echinacea
Fenugreek
Ginger
Goldenseal
Lavender EO (topical)
Myrrh
Plantain
Salt
St. John's wort
Turmeric
Wild indigo
Yarrow
Yerba mansa

ACNE, INTERNAL

(see Bitter Tonics; Cholagogues; Choleretics; Hepatics)

Alfalfa
Artichoke leaf
Berberis
Blue flag
Burdock
Calendula
Dandelion
Gentian
Gotu kola
Milk thistle
Nettle
Red clover
Turmeric
Vitex
Yellow dock
Yerba mansa

ACNE, TOPICAL

Aloe
Agrimony
Chamomile, blue EO
Chickweed
Clay
Drawing poultice
Echinacea
Goldenseal
Helichrysum EO
Lavender EO
Plantain
Rose
Rosemary EO
Sage
Thyme geraniol EO
Thyme linalool EO
Turmeric
Witch hazel
Yarrow EO
Yerba mansa

ACRID

Anemone
Aralia
Bayberry (fresh)
Cayenne
Cinnamon
Clove
Cow parsnip
Garlic
Ginger
Horseradish
Lobelia
Orange peel
Oregano
Skunk cabbage

ADAPTOGENS

Aralia
Ashwagandha
Asparagus tuber
Astragalus
Codonopsis
Cordyceps
Eleuthero
Ginseng, American
Ginseng, Asian
Gotu kola
Licorice
Reishi
Rhodiola
Schisandra
Shiitake
Tulsi
Turkey tail

ADRENERGICS

(see Stimulants)

ALLERGIC REACTIONS

(seek immediate medical attention, if severe)

Burdock
Chlorophyll
Coffee
Dandelion root (fresh)
Ephedra
Eyebright
Ginger (fresh)
Licorice
Nettle (freeze-dried)
Turmeric

ALLERGIES, LONG-TERM

Ashwagandha
Astragalus
Blueberry fruit
Bogbean
Burdock root
Chamomile
Codonopsis
Cordyceps

Dandelion root
Devil's club
Dong quai
Echinacea
Feverfew
Flavonoids
Ginger
Ginkgo
Ginseng, Asian
Grindelia
Hawthorn
Licorice
Maitake
Nettle (freeze-dried)
Orange peel
Oregon grape
Red clover
Red root
Reishi
Rose hips
Saposhnikovia
Schisandra
Shiitake
Tulsi
Turkey tail
Turmeric
Vitamin C

ALLERGIES, SHORT-TERM

Acerola berry
Ambrosia (extract)
Bayberry
Burdock root
Dandelion root
Echinacea
Elder flower
Ephedra
Eyebright
Ginger
Ginkgo
Goldenrod
Goldenseal
Grindelia
Licorice
Mormon tea
Nettle (freeze-dried)
Ox eye daisy
Peppermint
Red clover
Red root
Turmeric

Yerba mansa
Yerba santa

ALTERATIVES

Alfalfa
Aralia
Bayberry
Berberis
Bleeding heart
Blue flag
Buckbean
Burdock (mild)
Calendula
Chickweed
Cleavers
Dandelion
Devil's club
Echinacea
Elecampane
Figwort
Gotu kola
Kelp
Nettle
Oregon grape
Prickly ash
Red clover
Red root
Sarsaparilla
Stillingia
Viola
Wild indigo
Yellow dock
Yerba mansa

AMENORRHEA, LONG-TERM

(see Emmenagogues; Thyroid, Hypoactive)

Ashwagandha
Asparagus tuber
Black cohosh
Chuan xiong
Cinnamon
Dong quai
Eleuthero
Ginger
Ginseng, Asian
Kelp
Motherwort
Partridge berry
Peony, white
Rehmannia, prepared
Schisandra
Vitex

AMENORRHEA, SHORT-TERM

Anemone
Angelica
Black cohosh
Blue cohosh
Chamomile
Cotton root
Damiana
Dong quai
Feverfew
Ginger
Motherwort
Mugwort
Pennyroyal
Vervain
Yarrow

ANABOLIC COOLERS

Burdock
Dandelion
Devil's club
Eleuthero
Ginseng, American
Mugwort
Peony, white
Puncture vine

ANABOLIC STIMULANTS

Ashwagandha
Asparagus tuber
Blue cohosh
Devil's club
Dong quai
Eleuthero
Ginseng, American
Ginseng, Asian
Licorice
Peony, white
Saw palmetto
Vitex

ANALGESICS

(see Anesthetics; Neuralgia)

Anemone
Arnica
Ashwagandha
Black cohosh
Bleeding heart
Blue cohosh
California poppy
Cannabis
Cayenne (topical)
Chamomile

Chamomile, blue EO (topical)
Clove
Corydalis
Cow parsnip
Dong quai
Dutchman's breeches
Ginger
Helichrysum EO (topical)
Hops
Jamaican dogwood
Kava
Lobelia
Meadowsweet
Passion flower
Pedicularis
Peony, white
Peppermint EO (topical)
Prickly ash
Silk tassel
Skullcap
St. John's wort
Valerian
Wild yam
Willow
Yarrow EO (topical)
Yerba mansa (topical)

ANAPHRODISIACS

Caffeine
Cannabis (for some)
Coffee
Hops (for some)
Stimulants

ANEMIA

Alfalfa
Ashwagandha
Astragalus
Blackberry fruit
Codonopsis
Cordyceps
Dong quai
Elder berry
Fenugreek
Iron
Kelp
Liver
Molasses
Nettle leaf
Oat straw
Raspberry leaf
Yellow dock

ANESTHETICS, INTERNAL

(see Analgesics; Neuralgia)

Alcohol
Cannabis
Kava
Poppy
St. John's wort

ANESTHETICS, TOPICAL

Cannabis
Cayenne
Clove
Cow parsnip
Echinacea
Ice
Kava
Peppermint EO (topical)
Prickly ash
Propolis
Spilanthes
St. John's wort
Tobacco
Valerian
Yarrow

ANGINA PECTORIS

(seek immediate medical attention)

Black cohosh
Bugleweed
Cayenne
Cereus
Hawthorn
Lobelia
Motherwort

ANODYNES

(see Analgesics; Anesthetics; Neuralgia)

ANTHELMINTICS

Berberis
Black walnut
Chaparro
Chenopodium
Coptis
Elecampane
Epazote
Garlic
Ginger
Oregano
Oregon Grape
Quassia
Sage
Thyme
Wormseed
Wormwood

ANTIBACTERIALS

(see specific conditions)

Andrographis
Aralia (respiratory)
Arnica
Baikal skullcap
Balsam root
Bay laurel
Berberis
Bursera
Calendula
California bay
Cardamom
Chaparral
Cinnamon
Coptis
Echinacea
Elecampane
Eucalyptus
Forsythia
Garlic
Ginger
Goldenseal
Juniper
Kava
Lavender
Licorice
Lomatium
Madrone
Marjoram
Myrrh
Oregano
Oregon grape
Oshá
Phellodendron
Plantain
Propolis
Rosemary
Sage
Spilanthes
Spruce
Thuja
Thyme
Turmeric
Usnea
Uva ursi
Western red cedar
Wild indigo

Yarrow
Yerba mansa
Yerba santa

ANTIDEPRESSANTS, ESSENTIAL OILS

Basil
Bay laurel
Chamomile, Roman
Citrus
Frankincense
Jasmine
Lavender
Lemon grass
Lemon verbena
Neroli
Orange
Palmarosa
Petitgrain
Rose
Rose geranium
Rosemary
Tulsi

ANTIDEPRESSANTS, INTERNAL

Anemone
Aralia berry
Black cohosh
Damiana
Devil's club
Eleuthero
Ginkgo
Gotu kola
Kava
Lavender
Lemon balm
Oats (fresh milky seed)
Orange peel
Passion flower
Peony, white
Reishi
Rhodiola
Rosemary
Schisandra
Skullcap
St. John's wort
Tulsi

ANTIEMETICS

(see Nausea)

ANTIFUNGALS

Balsamroot leaf
Bay laurel
Berberis
Black walnut
Bursera
Calendula
California bay
Cardamom
Chaparral
Coptis
Echinacea
Eucalyptus
Garlic
Ginger
Goldenseal
Hops
Juniper
Kava
Lavender EO (topical)
Lomatium
Madrone
Marjoram EO (topical)
Mugwort
Myrrh
Neem
Olive leaf
Oregano
Oregon grape
Pau d'arco
Rosemary
Sage
Spilanthes
Spruce
Tea tree EO (topical)
Thyme
Turmeric
Usnea
Uva ursi
Western red cedar
Yerba mansa

ANTI-INFLAMMATORIES, MUCOUS MEMBRANES

(see Astringents; Demulcents; Digestive Lining Damage)

ANTI-INFLAMMATORIES, INTERNAL FOR MUSCLES AND JOINTS

(see Analgesics; Anesthetics; Arthritis; Antispasmodics)

Arnica
Ashwagandha
Black cohosh
Black haw
Bogbean
Cannabis
Chamomile
Cramp bark
Echinacea
Feverfew
Figwort
Ginger
Gotu kola
Gymnema
Hawthorn
Hedge nettle
Jamaican dogwood
Meadowsweet
Peony, white
Poplar bud
Red root
Skullcap
St. John's wort
Tulsi
Turmeric
Wild yam
Willow
Wood betony

ANTI-INFLAMMATORIES, TOPICAL

Arnica
Cannabis
Chamomile
Chamomile, blue EO (topical)
Figwort
Ginger
Hedge nettle
Helichrysum EO (topical)
Jamaican dogwood
Lavender EO (topical)
Meadowsweet
Nettle leaf
Peppermint EO (topical)
Poplar bud
St. John's wort
Turmeric

Willow
Wood betony
Yarrow

ANTILITHICS

(see Kidney Stones)

ANTIOXIDANTS

Acerola
Alfalfa
Allspice
Artichoke
Astragalus
Berberis
Bilberry
Blackberry fruit
Blueberry fruit
Cacao
Cannabis
Cayenne
Clove
Cordyceps
Cress
Currant
Dandelion
Dogwood
Echinacea
Elder flower
Eleuthero
Fennel
Garlic
Ginger
Ginkgo
Ginseng, Asian
Gotu kola
Grape
Grindelia
Hawthorn
Honeysuckle
Horseradish
Jujube
Kelp
Lemon
Lemon grass
Licorice
Lycii
Marjoram
Milk thistle
Mustard
Nettle leaf
Oat straw
Olive leaf
Orange peel
Oregano
Peony, white
Radish, black
Red clover
Red root
Rehmannia
Reishi
Rooibos
Rose
Rose hips
Rosemary
Sage
Savory
Schisandra
Sea buckthorn
Spilanthes
Spruce
Strawberry
Thyme
Tomato
Tulsi
Turmeric

ANTIPARASITICS

(see specific parasite, Anthelmintics

Andrographis
Berberis
Black walnut hull
Chaparro amargosa
Clove
Coptis
Forsythia
Garlic
Ginger
Goldenseal
Myrrh
Oregano EO
Quassia
Quinine bark
Spilanthes
Sweet Annie
Thyme EO
Turmeric
Wormseed
Wormwood

ANTIPHLOGISTICS

(see Allergies; Anti-inflammatories)

ANTIPYRETICS

(see Diaphoretics)

ANTITUSSIVES

(see Coughs)

ANTIVIRALS

(see specific virus)

Aloe
Andrographis
Astragalus
Baikal skullcap
Berberis
Boneset
Calendula
Cinnamon
Clove
Coptis
Cordyceps
Cypress
Echinacea
Elder berry
Forsythia
Frankincense
Garlic
Ginger
Isatis
Kalmia
Lavender, spike
Lemon balm
Licorice
Lomatium
Marjoram
Myrrh
Olive leaf
Oregano
Oregon grape
Oshá
Pau d'arco
Peppermint EO (topical)
Phellodendron
Propolis
Red cedar
Reishi
Rosemary
Sage
Shiitake
Spilanthes
St. John's wort
Thuja
Thyme
Tulsi
Turmeric
Usnea
Western red cedar

White sage
Wild indigo

ANTISPASMODICS, SMOOTH MUSCLE

(see Aromatics; Coughs; Uterine Cramping)

Angelica
Black cohosh
Black haw
Blue cohosh
Bugleweed
Calamus
California poppy
Chamomile (mild)
Cramp bark
Damiana
Elecampane (mild)
Hops
Jamaican dogwood
Kava
Lavender (mild)
Lemon balm (mild)
Marjoram (mild)
Motherwort
Passion flower
Silk tassel
Turmeric
Valerian
Wild yam

ANTISPASMODICS, SKELETAL MUSCLE

Black cohosh
Bleeding heart
California poppy
Cannabis
Hops
Jamaican dogwood
Kava
Lobelia
Passion flower
Pedicularis
Poppy
St. John's wort
Skullcap
Turmeric
Valerian

ANXIETY (ANXIOLYTICS)

(see Nervines)

Anemone
Bleeding heart
Bugleweed
Cannabis (CBDs)
Cereus
Chamomile
Lemon balm
Motherwort
Oats (fresh milky seed)
Passion flower
Skullcap
St. John's wort
Vervain

APERIENTS

(see Constipation; Demulcents)

APHRODISIACS

Allspice
Anise
Ashwagandha
Asparagus tuber
Basil
Cardamom
Cinnamon
Clove
Cotton root
Damiana
Ginger
Ginseng, American
Ginseng, Asian
Horny goat weed
Kava
Licorice root
Muira puama
Sarsaparilla
Schisandra
Shatavari
Vanilla
Yohimbe

APPETITE

(see Aromatics; Bitter Tonics; Carminatives; Cholagogues)

AROMATICS

Allspice
Angelica
Anise
Basil
Black pepper
Caraway
Cardamom
Chamomile
Cinnamon
Clove
Coriander
Cumin
Dill
Fennel
Ginger
Hops
Lavender
Lemon balm
Lemon verbena
Marjoram
Orange peel
Oregano
Peppermint
Rosemary
Savory
Spearmint
Thyme
Turmeric

ARTHRITIS, OSTEO

(see Anti-inflammatories)

Arnica
Ashwagandha
Black cohosh
Cannabis
Chamomile
Ginger
Jamaican dogwood
Meadowsweet
Nettle
St. John's wort
Turmeric
Willow

ARTHRITIS, RHEUMATOID

(see Anti-inflammatories; Autoimmunity)

Alfalfa
Arnica
Ashwagandha
Black cohosh (fresh)
Bogbean
Burdock
Cannabis
Chamomile
Chamomile EO (topical)
Dandelion root
Devil's club
Feverfew
Figwort
Ginger
Hawthorn

Jamaican dogwood
Meadowsweet
Nettle
Parsley leaf
Peony, white
Red clover
Turmeric
Wild yam
Willow
Yerba mansa

ASTHMA, GENERAL

Ammi
Angelica
Anise
Aralia californica
Calamus
Cubeb
Ephedra
Ginger
Grindelia
Licorice
Lobelia
Mullein
Orange peel
Platycodon
Polygala
Schisandra
Thyme
Turmeric
Yerba santa

ASTHMA, DRY COUGH

Angelica (short-term)
Anise
Aralia
California poppy
Cherry bark
Coltsfoot, Eastern
Coltsfoot, Western
Grindelia
Licorice
Marshmallow
Mullein flower
Thyme

ASTHMA, MOIST COUGH

Aralia
Bayberry
Cinnamon
Cubeb
Ginger
Grindelia
Mullein leaf
Polygala
Poria
Turmeric
Yerba mansa
Yerba santa

ASTRINGENTS

Agrimony
Allspice
Bayberry
Black tea
Blackberry leaf and root
Calendula
Catnip
Chamomile
Cinnamon
Comfrey leaf
Coptis
Fireweed
Geranium
Goldenseal
Lady's mantle
Madrone
Manzanita
Meadowsweet
Oak
Pearly everlasting
Plantain
Potentilla
Raspberry leaf
Red root
Rose family herbs
Rose petals
Sage
Salal
Schisandra
Shepherd's purse
St. John's wort
Strawberry leaf
Tea, green or black
Uva ursi
Willow
Witch hazel
Yarrow
Yellow dock
Yerba mansa
Yerba santa

ATHLETE'S FOOT

(see Antifungals)

AUTOIMMUNITY

(see specific conditions)

Ashwagandha
Astragalus
Baikal skullcap
Burdock root
Codonopsis
Cordyceps
Dandelion root
Devil's club
Maitake
Reishi
Schisandra
Shiitake
Turkey tail
Turmeric

BACK PAIN

(see Analgesics; Antispasmodics, Skeletal Muscle; Neuralgia)

BAD BREATH

(see Halitosis)

BENIGN PROSTATIC HYPERTROPHY (BPH)

Black cohosh
Blue cohosh
Dong quai
Hydrangea
Kegel exercise
Mullein root
Nettle root
Peony, white
Poria
Pygeum
Saw palmetto
Stone root
Yellow pond lily
Ze xie

BILE

(see Cholagogues; Choleretics)

BITES, INTERNAL

Activated charcoal
Burdock root
Chickweed
Dandelion root
Echinacea
Plantain
Turmeric

BITES, TOPICAL

(see Astringents; Drawing Agents)

Chickweed
Clay poultice
Echinacea
Fireweed
Lavender
Madrone
Manzanita
Plantain
Turmeric
Yellow dock leaf
Yerba mansa

BITTER TONICS

(see Cholagogues; Choleretics; Hepatics)

Angelica
Artichoke leaf
Black walnut
Blessed thistle
Blue flag
Bogbean
Bugleweed
Burdock
Calamus
Cascara sagrada
Celandine
Chaparral
Chicory
Coptis
Dandelion
Elecampane
Feverfew
Fringe tree
Gentian
Goldenseal
Hops
Licorice
Milk thistle
Motherwort
Mugwort
Orange peel
Oregon grape
Prickly ash
Red root
Sweet Annie
Tangerine peel
Turmeric
Vervain
Wild yam
Yellow dock

BLADDER INFECTIONS

(see Urinary Tract Infections)

BLADDER TONICS

Corn silk
Horsetail
Kegel exercise
Peony, moutan
Mullein root
Nettle leaf
Nettle root
Poria
Rehmannia
Saw palmetto
Yellow pond lily
Ze xie

BLEEDING

Cayenne
Cinnamon
Comfrey
Erigeron
Horsetail
Nettle leaf
Plantain
Raspberry leaf
Red root
Red sage
Shepherd's purse
Tienchi ginseng
Yarrow

BLISTERS

(see Astringents; Vulneraries)

Aloe gel
Calendula
Chickweed (fresh)
Comfrey root (fresh)
Plantain (fresh)
St. John's wort
Yerba mansa

BLOATING

(see Aromatics; Bitter Tonics; Carminatives)

BLOOD BUILDERS

(see Anemia)

Alfalfa
Astragalus
Beets
Bone broth
Chlorophyll
Chuan xiong
Codonopsis
Dong quai
Iron
Liver
Molasses
Nettle leaf
Oat straw
Rehmannia, prepared

BLOOD CLEANSING

(see Alteratives)

BLOOD MOVERS

Cayenne
Dong quai
Garlic
Ginger
Mugwort
Peony, red
Red sage
Tienchi ginseng
Turmeric
Yarrow

BLOOD PRESSURE

(see Heart Disease; Hypertension; Hypotension; Vasodilators)

BLOOD THINNERS, REDUCE PLATELET AGGREGATION FACTOR

Cayenne
Feverfew
Garlic
Ginger, fresh
Ginkgo
Mugwort
Red clover
Red sage

BOILS, INTERNAL

Baikal skullcap
Burdock
Coptis
Dandelion
Echinacea
Phellodendron
Red root
Wild indigo
Yerba mansa

BOILS, TOPICAL COMPRESS OR POULTICE

(see Antibacterials)

Berberis
Burdock, fresh poultice
Clay poultice
Coptis
Echinacea
Ginger poultice
Lavender EO (topical)
Neem
Plantain poultice
Thyme linalool EO (topical)
Turmeric compress
Wild indigo
Yerba mansa

BONES, BROKEN

(see Nutritives)

Alfalfa
Bone broth
Comfrey
Gotu kola
Horsetail
Nettle
Oat straw

BPH

(see Benign Prostatic Hypertrophy)

BREASTFEEDING

(see Galactagogues; Mastitis; Weaning)

BRONCHITIS

(see Antivirals; Antibacterials; Coughs; Expectorants)

Angelica
Anise (dry cough)
Aralia californica
Balsam root
California poppy (dry cough)
Cordyceps (recovery phase)
Elecampane
Ephedra (moist cough)
Fenugreek (dry cough)
Garlic (moist cough)
Ginger (moist cough)
Grindelia
Jamaican dogwood (dry cough)
Licorice (dry cough)
Lobelia (dry cough)
Lomatium
Marjoram (dry cough)
Myrrh (moist cough)
Orange peel (moist cough)
Oregano (moist cough)
Oshá (moist cough)
Pleurisy root
Polygala
Reishi (recovery)
Thyme (dry cough)
Tulsi
Usnea
Wild cherry bark (dry cough)
Yerba santa

BRUISES

(see Anemia; Antioxidants)

Arnica
Calendula
Chamomile
Chamomile, blue EO (topical)
Comfrey
Elecampane
Figwort
Ginger
Goldenrod
Gotu kola
Hawthorn
Helichrysum EO (topical)
Hops
Horsetail
Jamaican dogwood
Lavender EO (topical)
Marjoram
Meadowsweeet
Myrrh EO (topical)
Prickly ash
Rosemary
St. John's wort
Turmeric
Willow
Yarrow
Yerba mansa

BURNS

(see Anti-inflammatories; Astringents; Sunburns; Vulneraries)

Aloe gel
Calendula
Chamomile
Chamomile EO (topical)
Chickweed
Comfrey
Figwort
Gotu kola
Hawthorn
Helichrysum EO (topical)
Honey
Lavender EO (topical)
Plantain
Peppermint EO (topical)
Rose (hydrosol, tea)
St. John's wort
Willow
Witch hazel
Yarrow

CAFFEINE WITHDRAWAL

(see Adaptogens; Nervines; Stimulants; Vasodilators)

Allspice
Cardamom
Chai tea
Cinnamon
Eleuthero
Ginger
Ginkgo
Gotu kola
Guarana (short-term)
Kola (short-term)
Licorice
Rhodiola (short-term)
Rosemary
Skullcap
Tulsi

CARDIAC STIMULANTS

Caffeine
Coffee
Ginkgo
Guarana
Inmortal
Kola nut
Pleurisy root
Rhodiola
Stillingia

CARMINATIVES

Allspice
Angelica
Anise
Basil
Black pepper
Caraway
Cardamom
Catnip
Chamomile

Cilantro
Cinnamon
Clove
Coriander
Cumin
Dill
Fennel
Ginger
Hops
Lavender
Lemon balm
Lemon verbena
Licorice
Marjoram
Mint
Orange peel
Oregano
Parsley leaf and seed
Peppermint
Rosemary
Spearmint
Thyme
Turmeric
Wild yam
Yerba buena

CATHARTICS

(see Constipation; Purgatives)

CHOLAGOGUES

(see Bitter Tonics)

Angelica
Artichoke leaf
Baikal skullcap
Beet
Berberis
Blessed thistle
Bogbean
Bupleurum
Bugleweed
Burdock
Calamus (low dose)
Celandine
Coptis (short-term)
Dandelion
Elecampane
Feverfew
Fringe tree
Gentian
Goldenseal (short-term)
Hops
Motherwort
Mugwort
Oregon grape
Phellodendron
Prickly ash
Red root
Turmeric
Vervain
Wild yam
Yellow dock

CHOLERETICS

Aloe (juice)
Angelica
Artichoke leaf
Berberis
Bogbean
Burdock
Calendula (mild)
Celandine
Chelidonium
Coptis
Dandelion
Elecampane
Feverfew
Fringe tree
Gentian
Ginger
Lavender
Licorice
Milk thistle
Mint
Oregano
Peppermint EO
Prickly ash
Rosemary
Sage (mild)
Thyme (mild)
Turmeric
Yarrow (mild)
Yellow dock (mild)

CHOLESTEROL, HIGH

Alfalfa
Artichoke leaf
Burdock
Cayenne
Coptis
Dandelion
Fenugreek
Flax seed
Garlic
Ginger
Ginkgo
Hawthorn
Kelp
Mugwort
Olive leaf
Omega 3 fatty acids
Onion
Turmeric

CIRCULATION PROBLEMS

(see Circulatory Stimulants; Varicose Veins; Vasodilators)

CIRCULATORY STIMULANTS

Angelica
Bayberry
Cardamom
Cayenne
Cinnamon
Clove
Dong quai
Garlic
Ginger
Ginkgo
Gotu kola
Hawthorn
Horseradish
Lovage
Oshá
Peppermint
Prickly ash
Rosemary
Tulsi
Turmeric
Wafer ash
Wild ginger
Yarrow

COLDS

(see Antivirals; Congestion; Coughs; Diaphoretics; Expectorants; and specific symptoms)

Angelica
Aralia
Balsam root
Bayberry
Baikal skullcap
Burdock seed
Cayenne
Clove
Coptis
Echinacea
Elder berry
Elder flower

Fire cider
Forsythia
Garlic
Honeysuckle
Lemon balm (mild)
Lomatium
Mint
Oregano
Oshá
Prickly ash
Propolis
Red root
Sage
Thyme
Tulsi
Wild cherry (dry cough)
Willow (fever)
Yarrow
Yerba mansa
Yerba santa

COLD SORES

(see Herpes)

COLIC

(see Aromatics; Antispasmodics, Smooth Muscle; Carminatives)

CONGESTION, RESPIRATORY

(see Astringents; Expectorants; Sinus Congestion)

Bayberry
Cayenne
Garlic
Golden seal
Horseradish
Marjoram
Oregano
Thyme
Yerba mansa
Yerba santa

CONJUNCTIVITIS

Berberis
Calendula
Chamomile
Coptis
Elder flower
Goldenseal
Licorice
Myrtle hydrosol
Rose
Saline eye wash

CONSTIPATION, DRY

(see Demulcents)

Bladderwrack
Chia seed
Flax seed
Kelp
Marshmallow
Slippery elm

CONSTIPATION, LACK OF BULK

Carob pod
Chia seed
Fiber
Flax seed
Marshmallow
Psyllium

CONSTIPATION, WEAK PERISTALSIS

Alder buckthorn
Aloe juice
Buckthorn
California buckthorn
Cascara sagrada
Senna
Triphala
Turkey rhubarb
Yellow dock

COUGHS, DRY; ANTITUSSIVES

(see Bronchitis; Demulcents; Expectorants)

Angelica
Anise
Aralia
Asparagus tuber
Balsam root
Black cohosh
Butterbur
California poppy
Coltsfoot, Eastern
Coltsfoot, Western
Elecampane
Grindelia
Horehound
Hyssop
Jamaican dogwood
Jimson weed (smoked)
Licorice
Lobelia
Marjoram
Marshmallow
Mullein
Oshá
Passion flower
Platycodon
Pleurisy root
Polygala
Poppy
Slippery elm
Thyme
Turmeric
Valerian
Wild cherry
Yerba santa

COUGHS, MOIST

(see Astringents; Bronchitis; Expectorants)

Ambrosia
Aralia
Elecampane
Eucalyptus
Grindelia
Horehound
Mullein
Polygala
Yerba mansa
Yerba santa

COUNTERIRRITANTS

(see Rubefacients)

Angelica
Cayenne
Cinnamon
Clove
Garlic
Ginger
Horseradish
Mustard
Prickly ash
Rosemary
Turmeric

CUTS

(see Vulneraries)

CYSTITIS

(see Urinary Tract Infections; Interstitial Cystitis)

DANDRUFF

(see Bitter Tonics; Cholagogues; Demulcents; Emollients)

Aloe
Asparagus tuber
Berberis

Burdock
Calendula
Chickweed
Dandelion
Licorice
Marshmallow
Milk thistle
Nettle
Omega 3 fatty acids
Oregon grape
Rosemary
Sage
Yellow dock

DEMULCENTS

Bladderwrack
Chamomile
Chia seed
Chickweed
Cinnamon
Coltsfoot, Eastern
Coltsfoot, Western
Comfrey
Fenugreek
Flax seed
Fucus
Gum tragacanth
Hibiscus
Irish moss
Jujube dates
Kelp
Kudzu
Licorice
Marshmallow
Meadowsweet (mild)
Mullein flower
Pearly everlasting
Psyllium
Rose hips
Shatavari
Slippery elm
Violet

DENTAL INFECTIONS

(seek immediate medical attention)

(see Gum Infections; Toothaches)

DEPRESSION

(see Antidepressants)

DIAPHORETICS, COOLING (SUDORIFICS)

Andrographis
Boneset
Catnip
Chamomile
Elder flower
Eucalyptus
Feverfew
Forsythia
Isatis
Lemon balm
Linden
Meadowsweet
Mugwort
Pennyroyal
Peppermint
Spearmint
Willow
Yarrow

DIAPHORETICS, HEATING (SUDORIFICS)

Angelica
Basil
Cayenne
Cinnamon
Elecampane
Garlic
Ginger
Horseradish
Juniper
Marjoram
Mustard seed
Oregano
Oshá
Rosemary
Sage
Thyme
Tulsi
White sage

DIARRHEA

(see Antibacterials; Antiparasitics; Antivirals; Astringents)

Activated charcoal
Baikal skullcap
Berberis
Blackberry root
Chamomile
Coptis
Curing Pills
Goldenseal
Plantain
Probiotics
Rose family (astringents)
Yarrow
Yerba mansa
Yogurt

DIGESTION

(see Aromatics; Bitter Tonics; Carminatives; Cholagogues; Choleretics; Hepatics)

DIGESTIVE LINING DAMAGE

(see Vulneraries)

Alfalfa
Bone broth
Calendula
Chamomile
Chickweed
Comfrey
Corn silk
Licorice
Marshmallow
Meadowsweet
Plantain
St. John's wort

DIURETICS, GENERAL

Blueberry leaf
Buchu
Burdock seed
Celery seed
Cleavers
Corn silk
Couch grass
Cubeb pepper
Dandelion leaf
Elecampane
Goldenrod
Gravel root
Horsetail
Huckleberry
Hydrangea
Juniper berry
Madrone
Manzanita
Mormon tea
Mullein root
Nettle root and seed
Parsley root and seed
Pearly everlasting
Prince's pine
Pygeum

Raspberry leaf
Shin leaf
Stone root
Uva ursi
Yarrow

DIURETICS, LONG-TERM

Blueberry leaf
Burdock seed
Celery seed
Cleavers
Corn silk
Couch grass
Dandelion leaf
Gravel root
Horsetail
Huckleberry leaf
Hydrangea
Nettle
Parsley root
Parsley seed
Pearly everlasting
Prince's pine
Pygeum
Shinleaf
Stone root
Wild yam

DIURETICS, SHORT-TERM

Buchu
Cubeb pepper
Juniper berry
Madrone
Manzanita
Mormon tea
Uva ursi

DIZZINESS

Chrysanthemum (ju hua)
Electrolytes
Hydration
Licorice
Lycii berry
Peony, white
Poria
Rehmannia
Salt
Shatavari
Six flavor teapills

DRAWING AGENTS, TOPICAL

(see Astringents)

Burdock root, fresh
Calendula
Castor oil packs (hard, lumpy masses)
Chickweed
Clay
Comfrey
Echinacea
Epsom salt baths
Ginger, fresh
Marshmallow
Plantain
Tobacco
Turmeric, fresh
Yellow dock
Yerba mansa

DYSPEPSIA

(see Demulcents; Indigestion)

DYSPNEA

(see Antispasmodics—Smooth Muscle; Antitussives; Expectorants)

EAR INFECTIONS, INTERNAL

Baikal skullcap
Berberis
Coptis
Echinacea
Goldenseal
Oregon grape
Phellodendron
Usnea

EAR INFECTIONS, TOPICAL

Echinacea extract
Echinacea glycerite
Garlic oil
Garlic and onion poultice, sautéed
Mullein flower
St. John's wort

EARS, RINGING

(see Tinnitus)

ECZEMA, EXTERNAL

(see Emollients)

Aloe
Asparagus tuber
Calendula
Chamomile
Chamomile, blue EO (topical)
Comfrey
Chickweed
Elder flower
Licorice
Marshmallow
St. John's wort

ECZEMA, INTERNAL

(see Anti-inflammatories; Bitter Tonics; Cholagogues; Choleretics; Demulcents; Hepatics; Nutritives)

Alfalfa
Aloe
Artichoke leaf
Asparagus tuber
Berberis
Burdock
Calendula
Chickweed
Coptis
Dandelion
Gentian
Gotu kola
Licorice
Marshmallow
Milk thistle
Nettle
Oregon grape
Parsley leaf
Red clover
Turmeric
Vitex
Yellow dock
Yerba mansa

EDEMA

(see Diuretics)

EMMENAGOGUES

(see Amenorrhea)

Aloe juice (not gel)
Anemone
Angelica
Baneberry
Black cohosh
Blue cohosh
Calamus
Corn smut
Cotton root
Cow parsnip
Damiana
Dong quai
Feverfew

Inmortal
Lovage
Motherwort
Mugwort
Oshá
Parsley seed
Pennyroyal
Peony, red
Pleurisy root
Red sage
Rue
Sagebrush
Tansy
Wild carrot
Wild ginger
Yarrow

EMOLLIENTS

(use water-based preparations)

Bladderwrack
Chamomile
Coltsfoot, Eastern
Coltsfoot, Western
Comfrey root
Fenugreek
Flax seed
Fucus
Gum tragacanth
Irish moss
Kelp
Licorice
Marshmallow
Rose hips
Slippery elm
Violet

EXPECTORANTS

(see Bronchitis; Coughs)

Allspice
Angelica
Anise
Aralia
Balsam root
Bay
Bayberry
Calamus
Cardamom
Chickweed
Cinnamon
Coltsfoot
Comfrey leaf
Cordyceps
Damiana
Devil's club
Elder flower
Elder berry
Elecampane
Ephedra
Eucalyptus
Fennel
Fenugreek
Garlic
Ginger
Grindelia
Hyssop
Lavender
Licorice
Lobelia
Lomatium
Marjoram
Mullein
Myrrh
Orange peel
Oregano
Oshá
Parsley seed
Peppermint
Propolis
Red clover (mild)
Rosemary
Saw palmetto
Spilanthes
Thyme
Tulsi
Wild cherry
Yerba mansa
Yerba santa

EYE DISORDERS

(see Conjunctivitis; Retinal Degeneration)

Acerola
Blueberry
Calendula
Cannabis
Chrysanthemum (ju hua)
Gotu kola
Ginkgo
Huckleberry
Lycii
Rose hips
Turmeric

EYE WASHES

(see Conjunctivitis)

Berberis
Black tea
Calendula
Chamomile
Chickweed
Coptis
Elder flower
Goldenseal
Rose family astringents
Saline eye wash

FACE, SWELLING

Aloe
Calendula
Chamomile
Clay
Comfrey
Honey, raw
Marshmallow
Plantain
Rose family astringents
Witch hazel

FACE, ZITS

(see Acne)

FAINTNESS

Peppermint EO

FATIGUE

(see Adaptogens; Nutritives; Qi Tonics; Trophorestoratives)

FEVER

(see Diaphoretics)

FLATULENCE

(see Aromatics; Carminatives; Antispasmodics, Smooth Muscle)

FLAVONOIDS

(see Antioxidants)

Blueberry
Bilberry
Calendula
Ginkgo
Hawthorn
Horsetail
Huckleberry
Prickly pear
Rose hips

FOOD POISONING

(see Antibacterials; Aromatics; Carminatives; Diarrhea; Digestive Lining Damage; Nausea)

FUNGISTATICS/FUNGI

(see Antifungals)

GALACTAGOGUES

Alfalfa
Anise
Asparagus tuber
Blessed thistle
Caraway
Dill
Fennel
Goat's rue
Marshmallow
Motherwort
Nettle leaf
Shatavari
Vervain

GALLSTONES

(see Antispasmodics, Smooth Muscle; Cholagogues)

Artichoke leaf
Berberis
Blue flag
Boldo
Burdock
Celandine
Coptis
Dandelion
Fringe tree
Gentian
Milk thistle
Olive leaf
Oregon grape
Peony, white
Phellodendron
Rosemary
Turmeric
Wahoo
Wild yam
Yellow dock

GANGRENE

Baikal skullcap
Calendula
Coptis
Echinacea
Goldenseal
Phellodendron
Red root
Wild indigo
Yerba mansa

GOUT

(see Anti-inflammatories; Diuretics; Nutritives)

Alfalfa
Angelica (compress)
Blackberry fruit
Bogbean
Burdock
Cannabis
Celery seed
Cherry fruit
Chickweed
Cleavers
Comfrey
Dandelion
Gravel root
Hawthorn
Nettle
Parsley
Red clover
Turmeric
Willow
Yerba mansa

GRAVE'S DISEASE

(see Thyroid, Hyperactive)

GUM DISEASE

(see Toothaches/Gum Absesses)

H. PYLORI

(see Helicobacter pylori)

HALITOSIS

(see Gum Disease)

Anise
Basil
Chlorophyll
Fennel
Mint
Parsley leaf
Peppermint
Probiotics
Spearmint

HASHIMOTO'S DISEASE

(see Thyroid, Hypoactive)

HAY FEVER

(see Allergies)

HEADACHES

(see Analgesics; Anti-inflammatories, Internal for Muscles, Joints, and Headaches; Migraines)

Black cohosh
Feverfew
Ginger
Ginkgo
Jamaican dogwood
Kava
Lavender
Meadowsweet
Pedicularis
Peony, white
Skullcap
Vervain
Willow
Wood betony

HEART DISEASE

(see Antioxidants; Blood Thinners; Flavonoids; Hypertension)

Bugleweed
Cordyceps
Ginkgo
Hawthorn
Motherwort

HEART STIMULANTS

(see Cardiac Stimulants)

HEARTBURN

(see Digestive Lining Damage; Helicobacter pylori; Indigestion)

Calendula
Comfrey
Fennel
Licorice
Marshmallow
Meadowsweet
Slippery elm
St. John's wort

HELICOBACTER PYLORI

(see Heartburn; Indigestion)

Baikal skullcap
Berberis
Coptis
Garlic
Goldenseal

Licorice
Oregano
Oregon grape
Phellodendron
Turmeric

HEMORRHOIDS

Agrimony
Calendula
Chamomile
Plantain
Rose family astringents
Witch hazel
Yarrow

HEMOSTATICS

(see Bleeding)

HEPATICS

(see Bitter Tonics)

Artichoke leaf
Beet
Berberis
Blessed thistle
Blue flag
Bupleurum
Burdock root
Celandine
Dandelion
Dong quai
Fringe tree
Gentian
Licorice
Milk thistle
Oregon grape
Peony, white
Peppermint EO
Schisandra
Turmeric
Yellow dock

HEPATITIS

Artichoke leaf
Baikal skullcap
Berberis
Blessed thistle
Burdock root
Coptis
Dandelion
Dong quai
Gentian
Licorice
Milk thistle
Oregon grape
Peony, white
Phellodendron
Red root
Reishi
Schisandra
Shiitake
Turmeric
Yellow dock

HEPATOPROTECTANTS

Artichoke leaf
Astragalus
Bogbean
Cordyceps
Dong quai
Garlic
Licorice
Milk thistle
Peony, white
Reishi
Schisandra
Turmeric

HEPATOREGENERATIVES

Artichoke leaf
Cordyceps
Milk thistle
Schisandra

HERPES

Aloe
Baikal skullcap
Berberis
Calendula
Coptis
Echinacea
Eleuthero
Garlic
Lemon balm
Licorice
Lomatium
Marjoram EO (topical)
Myrrh
Pau d'arco
Propolis
Reishi
Self heal
Shiitake
Spilanthes
St. John's wort
Thuja
Thymus

HIVES, INTERNAL

(see Rashes; Skin Inflammations)

Baikal skullcap
Berberis
Burdock root
Dandelion root
Licorice
Phellodendron
Turmeric

HOARSENESS

(see Demulcents; Sore Throat)

Anise
Calendula
Chickweed
Clove
Comfrey root
Echinacea
Elder berry
Fenugreek
Hyssop
Licorice
Marshmallow
Propolis
Red root
Sage
Slippery elm
Spilanthes

HOT FLASHES

Baikal skullcap
Black cohosh
Chrysanthemum (ju hua)
Coptis
Ginseng, American
Motherwort
Peppermint
Phellodendron
Sage
Schisandra
Shatavari
Yin tonics

HYPERGLYCEMIA, HYPOGLYCEMIC HERBS

Bitter melon
Blueberry leaves and fruits
Brickellia
Cacalia
Carob
Cinnamon
Cordyceps
Damiana, under investigation

Dandelion
Devil's club
Eleuthero
Fenugreek
Garlic
Ginseng, Asian
Gymnema
Huckleberry leaves and fruits
Reishi
Tulsi basil

HYPERTENSION (HIGH BLOOD PRESSURE)

(see Anxiolytics; Diuretics; Nervines; Vasodilators)

Bugleweed
Burdock seed
Cereus
Dandelion leaf
Dong quai
European mistletoe
Garlic
Gotu kola
Gravel root
Hawthorn
Horsetail
Motherwort
Notoginseng
Olive leaf
Onion
Passion flower
Rauwolfia (use with caution)
Reishi
Yarrow

HYPOTENSIVES, GRAVE'S DISEASE

(see Thyroid, Hyperactive)

HYPOTENSION (LOW BLOOD PRESSURE)

Anise
Eleuthero
Licorice
Rehmannia
Rhodiola
Rosemary

HYPOTHALAMUS AND PITUITARY STIMULANTS

Ashwagandha
Cotton root
Damiana
Ginseng
Eleuthero
Motherwort
Muira puama
Pulsatilla
Vitex

HYPOTHYROID

(see Thyroid, Hypoactive)

IMMUNE MODULATORS

Aloe gel
Angelica
Aralia
Artist conk
Ashwagandha
Asparagus tuber
Astragalus
Atractylodes
Berberis
Bladderwrack
Bogbean
Calendula
California snakeroot
Cannabis
Chinese wild yam
Codonopsis
Cordyceps
Devil's club
Dong quai
Echinacea
Elder berry
Elecampane
Eleuthero
Garlic
Ginger
Ginseng, American
Ginseng, Asian
Gotu kola
He shou wu
Iris
Kalmia
Kelp
Lycii
Maitake
Marshmallow
Nettle
Pau d'arco
Peony, white
Poria
Rehmannia
Reishi
Sarsaparilla, Jamaican
Schisandra
Shiitake
Tulsi basil
Turkey tail
Turmeric
Usnea

IMMUNE STIMULANTS, INNATE IMMUNITY

Andrographis
Angelica
Aralia
Arnica
Balsam root
Bee balm
Berberis
Boneset
Bursera
Calendula
California bay
Clove
Coptis
Cypress
Echinacea
Elder
Elecampane
Eucalyptus
Forsythia
Frankincense
Garlic
Ginger
Horseradish
Juniper
Kalmia
Lomatium
Lovage
Marjoram
Marshmallow
Myrrh
Oregano
Oshá
Pine
Propolis
Rosemary
Spilanthes
Spruce
Stillingia
Thyme
Usnea
Western red cedar
Wild ginger

Wild indigo
Yarrow
Yerba mansa

IMPOTENCE

(see Adaptogens)

Ashwagandha
Asparagus tuber
Cardamom
Cinnamon
Cnidium
Damiana
Eleuthero
Epimedium
Ginseng, Asian
Lycii
Muira puama
Schisandra
Tribulus
Vanilla
Yohimbe (caution)

INCENSE

Angelica
Balsam of Peru
Balsam of Tolu
Benzoin
Cedar
Copal
Douglas fir resin
Fir needles
Frankincense
Juniper
Lavender
Lovage
Mugwort
Myrrh
Oshá
Palo santo
Pine resin
Rose
Rosemary
Sandalwood
Sweetgrass
White sage
Yerba santa

INCONTINENCE

Corn silk
Horsetail
Mullein root
Nettle root
Peony, white
Poria
Rehmannia
Saw palmetto
Schisandra
Six flavor tea pills
Yellow pond lily
Ze xie

INDIGESTION, ACID

(see Demulcents; Helicobacter pylori; Vulneraries)

Alfalfa
Aloe gel
Anise
Asparagus
Calendula
Catnip
Chamomile
Chickweed
Comfrey root
Fennel
Meadowsweet
Wild yam

INDIGESTION, NONULCER DYSPEPSIA

(see Aromatics; Bitter Tonics)

Angelica
Anise
Berberis
Bogbean
Cardamom
Chamomile
Cinnamon
Cow parsnip
Elecampane
Fennel
Fenugreek
Gentian
Ginger
Hibiscus
Licorice
Lime
Marshmallow
Mugwort
Orange peel
Peppermint
Prickly ash
Trikatu
Turmeric
Wild yam

INFECTIONS

(see Anthelmintics; Antibacterials; Antifungals; Antivirals; Antiparasitics; Diaphoretics; and Lymphatics)

INFLAMMATION

(see Anti-inflammatories)

INJURIES

(see Anti-inflammatories; Antispasmodics, Skeletal Muscles; Bones, Broken; Bruises; Sprains; Vulneraries)

Arnica
Calendula
California poppy
Chamomile
Chamomile, blue EO (topical)
Comfrey
Cow parsnip
Echinacea
Figwort
Ginger
Gotu kola
Helichrysum EO (topical)
Horsetail
Lavender
Lobelia
Moxibustion (topical)
Mugwort (topical)
Poplar
Self heal
St. John's wort
Tobacco (topical)
Turmeric
Willow
Yarrow

INSECT BITES

(see Bites)

INSECT REPELLENTS, TOPICAL—DILUTED

Citronella EO (topical)
Eucalyptus EO (topical)
Lavender EO (topical)
Lemon grass EO (topical)
Pennyroyal EO (topical)
Rose geranium EO (topical)

INSOMNIA

(see Nervines; Sedatives; Trophorestoratives)

INTERSTITIAL CYSTITIS

(see Antispasmodics—Smooth Muscles; Bladder Tonics)

Blue cohosh
Cannabis
Corn silk
Cramp bark
Damiana
Gravel root
Horsetail
Hydrangea
Jamaican dogwood
Kava
Mullein root
Nettle
Peony, white
Saw palmetto
Wild yam
Yellow pond lily

INTESTINAL SPASMS

(see Antispasmodics; Aromatics; Carminatives; Diarrhea; Digestive Lining Damage)

IRRITABLE BOWEL SYNDROME

(see Anti-inflammatories, Mucous Membranes; Antispasmodics, Smooth Muscles; Carminatives; Digestive Lining Damage)

ITCHING

(see Poison Ivy and Poison Oak; Hives; Rashes; Skin Inflammations)

Baikal skullcap
Burdock root
Chickweed (fresh, topical)
Coptis
Dandelion root
Gentian
Licorice
Milk thistle
Oats (gruel, topical)
Oregon grape
Phellodendron
Plantain (fresh, topical)
Turmeric

JAUNDICE

(seek immediate medical attention)

Artichoke leaf
Baikal skullcap
Berberis
Chamomile
Chrysanthemum (ju hua)
Coptis
Dandelion
Gentian
Milk thistle
Oregon grape
Peony, white
Phellodendron
Red root
Turmeric
Yellow dock

JOINT INFLAMMATION

(see Anti-inflammatories, Muscle and Joints)

JOINT PAIN AND STIFFNESS

(see Anti-inflammatories)

Angelica (topical)
Black cohosh
Calamus (topical)
Cannabis
Chamomile
Chamomile, blue EO (topical)
Comfrey (topical)
Figwort
Ginger
Jamaican dogwood
Meadowsweet
Poplar
St. John's wort
Stachys
Turmeric
Wild yam
Willow
Wintergreen
Wood betony
Yerba mansa

KIDNEY FAILURE

(seek immediate medical attention)

Cordyceps
Nettle seed

KIDNEY INFLAMMATION

(seek immediate medical attention)

(see Bladder Tonics; Demulcents; Diuretics; Kidney Stones)

KIDNEY STONES, ANTISPASMODICS AND ANALGESICS

(see Diuretics)

Black cohosh
Bleeding heart
California poppy
Cannabis
Cramp bark
Corydalis
Jamaican dogwood
Kava
Poppy
Prickly poppy
Silk tassel
Wild yam

KIDNEY STONES, DIURETICS

Celery seed
Cleavers
Couch grass
Dandelion
Goldenrod
Gravel root
Hydrangea
Madder
Marshmallow
Nettle
Parsley
Stone root
Yarrow

KIDNEY STONES, DEMULCENTS

Asparagus tuber
Chickweed
Comfrey root
Corn silk
Fenugreek
Licorice
Marshmallow
Parsley root
Rose hips
Slippery elm
Stone root
Violet

LACTAGOGUES

(see Galactagogues)

LAXATIVES

(see Constipation)

LEAKY GUT SYNDROME
(see Digestive Lining Damage)

LITHOTRIPTICS
(see Kidney Stones)

LIVER CONGESTION—STAGNATION
(see Bitter Tonics; Cholagogues; Choleretics; Hepatics)

Artichoke leaf
Berberis
Bidens
Burdock
Chai hu
Chamomile
Dandelion
Devil's club
Gentian
Milk thistle
Mugwort
Oregon grape
Peony, white
Yellow dock

LIVER METABOLISM ENHANCERS

Artichoke leaves
Blessed thistle
Blue flag
Bogbean
Calamus
Dandelion
Gentian
Milk thistle
Oregon grape
Prickly ash
Turmeric
Wild yam
Yellow dock

LIVER SWELLING

Berberis
Dandelion
Oregon grape
Red root
Wild indigo

LOW BLOOD PRESSURE
(see Hypotension)

LUNG CONGESTION
(see Expectorants)

LYMPHATICS

Bayberry
Berberis
Burdock (mild)
Calendula
Cleavers
Echinacea
Elder berry
Figwort
Myrrh
Prickly ash
Propolis
Red clover
Red root
Spilanthes
Stillingia
Viola (mild)
Wild indigo
Yerba mansa

MASTITIS, INTERNAL

Baikal skullcap
Berberis
Calendula
Echinacea
Oregon grape
Phellodendron
Red root
Spilanthes
Yerba mansa

MASTITIS, EXTERNAL

Chickweed
Calendula
Echinacea
Hot water
Plantain
Yerba mansa

MEMORY PROBLEMS

Bacopa
Calamus
Eleuthero
Ginkgo
Gotu kola
Lion's mane
Prickly ash
Red clover
Reishi
Rhodiola
Rosemary
Tulsi basil
Turkey tail

MENOPAUSE
(see Hot Flashes)

Aloe gel (internal)
Anemone
Asparagus tuber
Black cohosh
Bugleweed
Chrysanthemum (ju hua)
Dandelion root
Dong quai
Ginseng, American
Ginseng, Asian
Motherwort
Oats (fresh milky seed)
Peony, white
Schisandra
St. John's wort
Vitex

MENORRHAGIA
(see Bleeding; Uterine Bleeding)

MENSTRUAL CRAMPS
(see Uterine Cramping)

MIGRAINES, GENERAL

Anemone
Cannabis
Clematis
Feverfew
Ginger
Guarana
Hedge nettle (mild)
Jamaican dogwood
Kola nut
Lavender (mild)
Pedicularis
Periwinkle
Pulsatilla
Wood betony (mild)

MIGRAINES DUE TO LIVER HEAT

Baikal skullcap
Berberis
Chrysanthemum (ju hua)
Coptis
Feverfew
Gentian
Peony, white
Phellodendron
Turkey rhubarb

MISCARRIAGE, THREATENED

(seek immediate medical attention)

Black haw
Partridge berry
Peony, white
Raspberry leaf

MOOD ELEVATORS

(see Antidepressants)

MORNING SICKNESS

Cardamom
Chamomile
Ginger (fresh)
Mint
Orange peel
Peppermint
Spearmint

MUCILAGE

(see Demulcents)

MUSCLE ACHES

(see Anesthetics; Analgesics; Anti-inflammatories; Antispasmodics; Injuries; Muscle Stiffness)

Arnica
Black cohosh
Cannabis
Ginger
Jamaican dogwood
Lobelia
Meadowsweet
Pedicularis
St. John's wort
Turmeric
Valerian
Willow

MUSCLE SPASMS, SKELETAL MUSCLE

(see Antispasmodics, Skeletal Muscle)

MUSCLE STIFFNESS

Arnica
Black cohosh
Ginger
Jamaican dogwood
Pedicularis
Peony, white
Turmeric
Valerian

NASAL CONGESTION

(see Sinus Congestion)

NAUSEA

(see Morning Sickness)

Anise
Cannabis
Cardamom
Chamomile
Fennel
Ginger
Lemon zest and peel
Lime zest and peel
Mint
Orange peel
Peppermint
Peppermint spirits
Spearmint

NECK PROBLEMS

Black cohosh
California poppy
Cannabis
Jamaican dogwood
Kava
Lobelia
Passion flower
Pedicularis
Peony, white
Valerian

NERVINES, GENTLE

Black haw
Catnip
Chamomile
Lavender
Lemon Balm
Linden
Oats (fresh milky seed)
Wood betony

NERVINES, MODERATE

Black cohosh
Black haw
Bleeding heart
Bugleweed
California poppy
Cannabis
Cereus
Cramp bark
Hops
Kava
Lemon balm
Motherwort
Passion flower
Skullcap
St. John's wort

NERVINES, POTENT

Anemone
Black cohosh
Bleeding heart
California poppy
Corydalis
Dutchman's breeches
Hops
Jamaican dogwood
Kava
Motherwort
Passion flower
Poppy
Valerian
Vervain

NERVINES, HEART SPECIFIC

Anemone
Bugleweed
Cereus
Hawthorn
Motherwort
Passion flower

NERVOUSNESS

(see Anxiety; Nervines; Sedatives; Trophorestoratives)

NEURALGIA

(see Counterirritants)

Aconite (topical)
California poppy
Camphor (topical)
Cannabis
Cayenne
Cow parsnip
Dong quai
Jamaican dogwood
Kava
Lavender EO (topical)
Meadowsweet
Peppermint EO (topical)
Prickly ash
Skullcap
St. John's wort
Wintergreen

NIGHTMARES

Anemone
Bleeding heart
California poppy
Cereus
Chamomile
Lavender
Lemon balm
Passion flower
Rose
Shen tonics
Skullcap
St. John's wort

NIGHT SWEATS

Aloe gel
Asparagus tuber
Baikal skullcap
Black cohosh
Bugleweed
Cereus
Chickweed
Chrysanthemum (ju hua)
Dandelion
Dong quai
Ginseng, American
Marshmallow
Motherwort
Peony, white
Phellodendron
Sage
Vervain
Vitex
Yin tonics

NUMBNESS

(see Counterirritants)

Cow parsnip
Prickly ash

NURSING

(see Galactagogues, Mastitis)

NUTRITIVES

(see Antioxidants, Flavonoids)

Alfalfa
Blueberry
Bilberry
Celery
Chicory
Chlorophyll
Cilantro
Dandelion
Ginger
Horsetail
Nettle
Oat straw
Parsley
Raspberry leaf
Red clover
Rooibos
Rose hips
Sage

PAIN RELIEVERS

(see Analgesics; Anesthetics; Anti-Inflammatories; Antispasmodics; Joint Pain and Stiffness; Muscle Aches; Neuralgia)

PARALYSIS, MINOR

Cow parsnip (topical)
Prickly ash
St. John's wort

PELVIC DECONGESTANTS

Angelica
Black cohosh
Blue cohosh
Damiana
Dandelion
Dong quai
Ginger
Ocotillo
Prickly ash
Red root
Stone root
Turmeric

PERIODONTAL DISEASE

(see Gum Disease)

POISON OAK AND POISON IVY, TOPICAL

(see Rashes; Skin Inflammations)

Calendula
Grindelia
Jewel weed
Manzanita
Oats (gruel)
Plantain
Sassafras
Uva Ursi
Witch hazel

PORTAL DECONGESTANTS

Berberis
Black walnut leaf
Blue flag (low dose)
Buckeye, Ohio
Burdock root
Dandelion
Hop tree
Milk thistle
Ocotillo
Oregon grape
Prickly ash
Red root
Stone root
Wahoo
Yellow dock

POTENTIALLY TOXIC HERBS

(Warning: Avoid internal use during pregnancy, lactation, and with children. Seek immediate medical attention if poisoning occurs. Use in low doses only, under the supervision of a health care practitioner.)

Aconite
Alder
Apocynum
Aristolochia
Asarum
Aspidum
Baneberry
Bittersweet
Blood root
Blue flag
Bryonia
Bryony
Buttercup
Chaparral
Convallaria
Corn smut
Cow parsnip
Culver's root
Datura
Delphinium
Digitalis
Elder bark
False hellebore
Foxglove
Gelsemium
Yellow jasmine
Henbane
Hyocyamus

Indian tobacco
Ipecac
Iris
Jack in the pulpit
Jimson weed
Larkspur
Leptandra
Lily of the valley
Lobelia
Male fern
Mistletoe
Monkshood
Nicotiana
Peyote
Phytolacca
Poke
Pukeweed
Ranunculus
Rue
Snakeroot
Syrian Rue
Tansy
Tobacco
Veratrum
Western skunk cabbage
Wild ginger
Wormwood

POULTICES/COMPRESSES

(see Anti-inflammatories; Arthritis, Topical; Astringents; Bites; Counterirritants; Drawing Agents)

Angelica
Arnica
Calendula
Chamomile
Chickweed
Clay
Cleavers
Figwort
Fireweed
Ginger
Jimson weed
Mallow
Marshmallow
Mugwort
Parsley leaf
Passion flower
Pedicularis
Plantain
Prickly ash
Red clover
Shepherd's purse
Silk tassel
Tobacco
Tulsi
Turmeric
Uva ursi
Valerian
Willow
Yarrow
Yellow pond lily
Yellow dock leaf
Yerba mansa

PREGNANCY

(see Morning Sickness; Miscarriage; Nutritives; Uterine Contractions; Uterine Tonics)

Alfalfa
Black haw
Chickweed
Dandelion
Lady's mantle
Nettle leaf
Oat straw
Partridge berry
Raspberry leaf

PROSTATE

(see Benign Prostatic Hypertrophy)

PSORIASIS

(see Bitter Tonics; Cholagogues; Demulcents; Emollients; Hepatics; Nutritives)

Alfalfa
Aloe gel
Asparagus tuber
Berberis
Blue flag
Bogbean
Burdock root
Calendula
Chickweed
Cleavers (mild)
Dandelion
Gentian
Gotu kola
Licorice
Marshmallow
Milk thistle
Omega 3 fatty acids
Oregon grape
Rosemary (topical)
Sarsaparilla, Jamaican
Turmeric
Yellow dock

PURGATIVES

Cascara sagrada
Ipecac
Poke root (toxic)
Senna
Turkey rhubarb
Yellow dock (high doses)

PYRROLIZIDINE ALKALOID-CONTAINING HERBS

Boneset
Borage
Coltsfoot, Eastern/Western
Comfrey
Liferoot plant
Senecio

RASHES, TOPICAL

Aloe gel
Calendula
Chamomile
Chickweed
Corn silk
Fenugreek
Kelp
Licorice
Mallow
Marshmallow
Plantain
St. John's wort

RECUPERATIVES

(see Alteratives; Nutritives)

Alfalfa
Aloe gel
Aralia (respiratory)
Bayberry
Burdock
Calendula
Chickweed
Dandelion
Echinacea
Elecampane (respiratory)
Horsetail
Kelp
Nettle
Prickly ash
Red clover
Red root

Schisandra
Yellow dock
Yerba mansa

REFRIGERANTS

Chickweed
Chrysanthemum (ju hua)
Hibiscus
Lemon juice
Lemon grass
Marshmallow
Mint

REPRODUCTIVE STRUCTURAL TONICS

Black cohosh
Blue cohosh
Dong quai
Partridge berry
Peony, white
Pygeum
Raspberry leaf
Saw palmetto
Stone root
Yellow pond lily

RESOLVENTS

(see Alteratives; Lymphatics; Recuperatives)

RESPIRATORY CONGESTION

(see Bronchitis; Colds; Congestion, Respiratory; Coughs; Expectorants; Sinus Congestion)

RETINAL DEGENERATION

(see Antioxidants)

Bilberry
Blueberry
Ginkgo
Gotu kola
Hawthorn
Lycii

RHEUMATISM

(see Arthritis)

RUBEFACIENTS

(see Counterirritants)

Cayenne
Cow parsnip seeds
Garlic
Ginger
Horseradish
Mustard seed
Onion
Oregano
Prickly ash
Thyme

SCIATICA

Aconite (topical)
Bleeding heart
California poppy
Cannabis
Chamomile, blue EO (topical)
Corydalis
Dutchman's breeches
Jamaican dogwood
Kava
Lobelia
Passion flower
Poppy
Skullcap
St. John's wort
Valerian

SCURVY

(see Vitamin C)

SEASICKNESS

(see Nausea)

SEDATIVES

(see Nervines)

Anemone
Ashwagandha (long-term)
Black cohosh
Black haw (mild)
Bleeding heart
Bugleweed
California poppy
Cannabis
Cramp bark (mild)
Dutchman's breeches
Hops
Jamaican dogwood
Kava
Lemon balm
Lobelia
Motherwort (mild)
Nutmeg
Passion flower
Peony, white (mild)
Poppy
Schisandra (long-term)
Skullcap
Valerian
Vervain

SIALAGOGUES

Angelica (mild)
Calamus (mild)
Echinacea
Kava
Lobelia
Prickly ash
Rudbeckia
Spilanthes

SINUS CONGESTION

Ambrosia
Baikal skullcap
Balsam root
Bay laurel EO
Bay, California
Bayberry
Berberis
Black radish
Calamus (local)
Cayenne
Ephedra
Eucalyptus
Eyebright
Garlic
Goldenrod
Goldenseal
Horseradish
Hyssop
Lomatium
Marjoram EO
Mustard
Myrrh
Myrtle
Nettle
Onion
Oshá
Peppermint
Phellodendron
Saline flush (Neti pot)
Stillingia
Yarrow
Yerba mansa
Yerba santa

SKIN, DRY

(see Demulcents; Emolleints; Choleretics; Cholagogues)

Aloe gel
Anise
Bladderwrack
Calendula
Chickweed
Comfrey root
Fenugreek
Kelp
Licorice
Marshmallow
Oatmeal (gruel)
Omega 3 Fatty Acids
Oregon grape
Rehmannia
Shatavari
Shiitake

SKIN INFLAMMATIONS, INTERNAL

(see Hives; Rashes)

Baikal skullcap
Berberis
Burdock root
Calendula
Chamomile
Chickweed
Chrysanthemum (ju hua)
Coptis
Dandelion root
Echinacea
Gentian
Honeysuckle flower
Licorice
Marshmallow
Nettle
Okra
Oregon grape
Peony, white
Phellodendron
Red clover
Verbena

SKIN INFLAMMATIONS, EXTERNAL

(see Emollients; Hives; Rashes; Poison Oak and Poison Ivy; Vulneraries)

Agrimony
Aloe gel
Avens
Bladderwrack
Borage
Calendula
Chamomile
Chamomile, blue EO (topical)
Chickweed
Cleavers
Coltsfoot, Eastern
Coltsfoot, Western
Comfrey root
Cucumber
Elder flower
Fenugreek
Figwort
Kelp
Licorice
Mallow
Oats (gruel)
Plantain
Rose
Yarrow

SKIN, FLUSHED

(see Anti-inflammatories)

Aloe
Baikal skullcap
Berberis
Bladderwrack
Calendula
Chamomile
Chickweed
Chrysanthemum (ju hua)
Coptis
Cucumber
Dandelion root
Gentian
Honeysuckle flower
Kelp
Oregon grape
Peony, white
Phellodendron
Sea buckthorn

SKIN, OILY

(see Astringents; Bitter Tonics; Cholagogues; Choleretics)

Baikal skullcap
Beet root
Berberis
Burdock
Dandelion
Gentian
Mugwort
Nettle
Oregon grape
Peony, white
Phellodendron
Vitex

SLEEP PROBLEMS

(see Nervines; Sedatives; Trophorestoratives)

SMOKING, HERBS FOR

California poppy
Cannabis
Coltsfoot
Damiana
Jimson weed (asthma)
Mint
Mugwort
Mullein leaf
Lavender
Lobelia
Pearly everlasting leaf
Pedicularis
Raspberry leaf
Rose
Skullcap
Tobacco
Uva ursi
Yerba santa

SMUDGING

(see Incense)

SORE THROATS

Anise
Aralia root
Arnica (obstinate)
Balsam root
Bayberry
Berberis
Calendula
Cinnamon
Cleavers
Echinacea
Honey
Hyssop
Licorice
Lomatium
Marshmallow
Myrrh
Oregano
Oshá
Plantain

Propolis
Red root
Sage (gargle)
Spilanthes
Usnea
Wild indigo
Willow (gargle)
Yerba mansa

SPASMOLYTICS

(see Antispasmodics)

SPRAINS, EXTERNAL

(see Anti-inflammatories; Injuries)

Arnica
Calendula
Chamomile, blue EO (topical)
Comfrey
Epsom salt
Figwort
Ginger
Helichrysum EO (topical)
Horsetail
Jimson weed
Moxibustion
Mugwort
Poplar
St. John's wort
Tobacco
Turmeric
Willow

SPRAINS, INTERNAL

Arnica
Comfrey
Echinacea
Gotu kola
Horsetail
Meadowsweet
Poplar
St. John's wort
Willow
Turmeric

STIMULANTS

Cacao
Caffeine
Coca leaf
Cocaine
Coffee
Eleuthero
Ephedra
Ginseng, Asian
Gotu kola
Guarana
Kola nut
Maté
Muira puama
Rhodiola
Rosemary
Tea, black or green
Yohimbe

STINGS

(see Bites)

STOMACH, BURNING AND INFLAMMATION

(see Demulcents; Digestive Lining Damage; Indigestion; Helicobacter pylori; Ulcers; Vulneraries)

Aloe gel
Chamomile
Chickweed
Fenugreek
Licorice and DGL
Marshmallow
Slippery elm

STRESS

(see Adaptogens; Anxiolytics; Nervines; Sedatives; Trophorestoratives)

SUDORIFICS

(see Diaphoretics)

SUNBURN

(see Astringents; Emollients)

Aloe
Calendula
Chickweed
Lavender hydrosol
Marshmallow
Rose hydrosol
Self heal
St. John's wort
Witch hazel

THROAT, DRY

(see Demulcents; Sore Throats)

THROAT, SORE

(see Sore Throats)

THYROID, HYPOACTIVE

(see Autoimmunity)

Ashwagandha
Astragalus
Devil's club
Eleuthero
Ginseng, Asian
Gotu kola
Reishi
Schisandra

THYROID, HYPERACTIVE

(see Adaptogens; Autoimmunity; Trophorestoratives)

Bugleweed
Lemon balm
Motherwort
Vervain

TINNITUS

Bupleurum
Chrysanthemum (ju hua)
Ginkgo
Lycii berry
Peony, white
Poria
Rehmannia
Six flavor tea pills

TOOTHACHES/GUM ABSCESSES

(seek immediate medical attention)

Bayberry
Calendula
Clove
Cow parsnip seed (topical)
Echinacea
Goldenseal
Kava
Myrrh
Peppermint
Plantain (poultice)
Prickly ash (topical)
Spilanthes
Valerian
Yarrow (poultice)
Yerba mansa

TROPHORESTORATIVES

Ashwagandha
Oats (fresh milky seed)
Skullcap
St. John's wort

ULCERS, DIGESTIVE

(see Digestive Lining Damage; Helicobacter pylori; Indigestion)

Cabbage juice
Irish moss
Licorice
Marshmallow
Meadowsweet
Mugwort
Rose family astringents
Shatavari
Slippery elm
St. John's wort

URINARY TRACT INFECTIONS, GENERAL

Baikal skullcap
Berberis
Burdock root
Chickweed
Cleavers
Corn silk
Dandelion
Echinacea
Goldenrod
Grindelia
Horsetail
Kava
Madrone
Manzanita
Marshmallow
Oregon grape
Parsley root and seed
Phellodendron
Pipsissewa
Pyrola
Usnea
Uva ursi
Yarrow

URINARY TRACT INFECTIONS, ANTIBACTERIALS

Baikal skullcap
Berberis
Buchu
Coptis
Corn silk
Cubeb
Echinacea
Grindelia
Huckleberry leaf
Juniper
Kava
Madrone
Manzanita
Oregon grape
Phellodendron
Prince's pine
Shin leaf
Usnea
Uva ursi
Yarrow
Yerba mansa
Yerba santa

UTERINE BLEEDING

Avens
Bugleweed
Cinnamon
Erigeron
Nettle leaf
Raspberry leaf
Red root
Rose
Shepherd's purse
Strawberry leaf
Yarrow

UTERINE CRAMPING

Angelica
Black cohosh
Black haw
Bleeding heart
Blue cohosh
Bugleweed
Bupleurum
California poppy
Chamomile
Clary sage
Cotton root
Cow parsnip
Cramp bark
Damiana
Dong quai
Ginger
Hops
Jamaican dogwood
Kava
Lemon balm
Lobelia
Motherwort
Passion flower
Pedicularis
Pennyroyal
Peony, white
Silk tassel
Skullcap
Turmeric
Valerian
Valerian
Verbena
Wild yam

UTERINE TONICS

Black cohosh
Black haw
Blue cohosh
Dong quai
Lady's mantle
Partridge berry
Peony, white
Raspberry leaf
Rose
Saw palmetto
Strawberry leaf
Yellow pond lily

UTERINE-CONTRACTING STIMULANTS

Black cohosh
Blue cohosh
Cotton root
Damiana

VAGINAL YEAST INFECTIONS

(see Antifungals)

Baikal skullcap
Berberis
Calendula
Coptis
Garlic
Oregano
Pau d'arco
Phellodendron
Thyme
Usnea
Yerba mansa

VARICOSE VEINS, INTERNAL

(see Portal Decongestants)

Blue flag
Buckeye, Ohio
Burdock
Calendula
Dandelion root
Flavonoids
Ginger
Ginkgo
Gotu kola

Hawthorn
Ocotillo
Prickly ash
Red root
Rose hips
Rosemary
Stone root
Vitamin C
Wahoo
Witch hazel
Yarrow
Yellow dock

VARICOSE VEINS, TOPICAL

Arnica
Calendula
Ginger
Prickly ash
Rosemary
St. John's wort
Witch hazel
Yarrow

VASODILATORS

Angelica
Arnica
Bayberry
Cayenne
Cinnamon
Clematis
Garlic
Ginger
Ginkgo
Hawthorn
Horseradish
Prickly ash
Rosemary
Wild ginger
Yarrow

VERMICIDES AND VERMIFUGES

(see Anthelmintics; Antiparasitics)

VERTIGO

(see Dizziness)

VITAMIN C DEFICIENCY

Acerola
Aloe
Artichoke leaf
Ashwagandha
Berberis fruit
Black haw fruit
Blackberries
Burdock
Cayenne
Chickweed
Cleavers
Cramp bark berries
Cress
Currant, black
Elder berries
Hawthorn berries
Jujube
Lemon
Lime
Orange
Paprika
Rose hips

VOMITING

(see Nausea)

VULNERARIES

(see Wounds)

Aloe
Calendula
Chickweed
Comfrey
Marshmallow
Plantain
St. John's wort

WARTS, TOPICAL

(see Antivirals)

Bloodroot
Calendula
Celandine (sap)
Garlic (fresh)
Milkweed (sap)
Thuja EO

WATER RETENTION

(see Diuretics)

WEANING, BREASTFEEDING

Parsley leaf
Sage

WHOOPING COUGH

(see Antivirals; Bronchitis; Cough; Demulcents; Expectorants)

WOUNDS, TOPICAL

(see Burns, Bruises, Strains)

Berberis
Calendula
Comfrey
Echinacea
Goldenrod
Gotu kola
Lavender
Myrrh
Plantain
Propolis
Rose family astringents
St. John's wort
Turmeric
Yarrow
Yerba mansa

WHEEZING

(see Asthma)

Anise
Aralia
Elecampane
Ephedra
Grindelia
Licorice
Lobelia
Marjoram
Passion flower
Polygala
Thyme

YIN TONICS

Aloe
Asparagus Tuber
Bladderwrack
Chamomile
Chia seed
Chickweed
Chrysanthemum (ju hua)
Comfrey root
Fenugreek
Flax seed
Irish moss
Jujube dates
Kelp
Licorice
Lycii berry
Marshmallow
Mullein flower
Peony, white
Poria
Rehmannia
Rose hips
Shatavari
Shiitake
Slippery elm
Violet

HERBAL THERAPEUTIC GLOSSARY

ACRID
A term used to describe a plant with a pungent, sharp, or harsh taste. Acrid plants irritate the mucous membranes; circulation increases to the tissues when applied. Acrid plants can be used to treat respiratory congestion or sluggish circulation.

ACUTE
A type of disease or disorder featuring a sudden onset with severe symptoms, and generally a short or self-limited duration, such as a cold. See the opposite term, chronic.

ADAPTOGEN
An adaptogen reduces the body's negative responses to stress. Adaptogens maintain and/or enhance the adrenal stress response, decrease hypothalamic and pituitary overreactions to perceived stress, and increase non-specific resistance. A remedy that improves adaptability.

ADJUVANT
An ingredient that facilitates and/or enhances the effectiveness of a compound formula, principal ingredient, or medical treatment.

ADRENERGIC
An activity or structure that responds to epinephrine (adrenaline).

AGONIST
A substance that binds with cellular receptors activating a biological response.

ALKALOID
A nitrogen-containing constituent found in some plants, usually with potent pharmacological actions. Alkaloid-containing plants should not be combined with plants high in tannins. Examples of alkaloids are caffeine, nicotine, and cocaine.

ALTERATIVE
A plant that gradually alters metabolic function, enhancing nutrient delivery to the tissues and waste removal. Alterative herbs improve the elimination of waste products from tissues. An alterative can aid in treating chronic conditions, such as autoimmune diseases, immune deficiency, allergies, inflammatory skin conditions, arthritis, lymphatic swelling, or stagnation.

AMPHOTERIC
An herb, substance, or activity that normalizes tissue or organ function.

ANALGESIC
A substance that relieves pain without a loss of consciousness.

ANESTHETIC
A substance that decreases nerve sensitivity to pain, producing a numbing effect.

ANABOLISM
The metabolic building of simple compounds into more complex substances needed by the body.

ANODYNE
A pain-relieving substance.

ANTHELMINTIC
A remedy that eliminates parasites from the gut. Many anthelmintic herbs have strong purgative effects and very bitter flavors.

ANTIBACTERIAL
An agent that inhibits bacterial growth, also termed a "bacteriostatic."

ANTIBILIOUS
An agent that is useful against biliousness or minor health disturbances related to liver dysfunction.

ANTICARCINOGENIC
An agent with a positive influence against cancer.

ANTICATARRHAL
A substance that eliminates or counteracts mucus formation.

ANTICHOLINERGIC
An agent that impedes the impulses or actions of the nerve fibers of the parasympathetic ganglia, competing with, and blocking the release of acetylcholine at the muscarinic receptor sites. Cholinergic functions affected include those that induce spasms and cramps in the intestinal tract and allied ducts. Examples are atropine and datura.

ANTIDEPRESSANT
An agent that alleviates or prevents depression.

ANTIEMETIC
A substance that can prevent or alleviate vomiting.

ANTIFUNGAL
An agent that inhibits fungal growth, also termed a "fungistatic."

ANTIHISTAMINE
A substance that opposes the action of, and/or inhibits the release of histamines, used for symptomatic relief of allergies and inflammation.

ANTI-INFLAMMATORY
An agent that counteracts inflammation.

ANTILITHIC
An agent that aids in the dissolution of calculi such as kidney stones, joint and muscle deposits, and in some cases, gallstones.

ANTIMICROBIAL
An agent that inhibits or destroys microorganisms.

ANTIOXIDANT
An agent that inhibits oxidation, and slows the formation of lipid peroxides and other free radical oxygen forms. This prevents the rancidity of oils or blocks cellular damage resulting from peroxides.

ANTIPHLOGISTIC
An agent that decreases or prevents inflammation, usually an anti-inflammatory or antihistamine.

ANTIPYRETIC
A fever-reducing agent.

ANTISEPTIC
A substance that can be applied topically to the skin to prevent the growth of microorganisms. Most volatile oils are considered antiseptics. Many plants with high levels of tannins, resins, alkaloids, and acrid properties also can prevent microbial growth.

ANTISPASMODIC
A substance that can prevent or relieve muscle spasms and reduce muscle tension. Antispasmodics can be consumed internally, or applied externally for pain relief, relaxing smooth muscles and/or skeletal muscles.

ANTITUSSIVE
A substance that acts as an antispasmodic in the respiratory tract, inhibiting a cough.

ANTIVIRAL
An agent that inhibits viral growth.

ANXIOLYTIC
A substance that reduces anxiety.

APERIENT
A mild laxative that encourages healthy bowel movements. Aperients include agar-agar, psyllium seed, marshmallow, seaweed gums, and dietary fiber.

APHRODISIAC
A substance that stimulates sexual function and performance, and/or increases blood flow to erogenous zones. An **anaphrodisiac** has the opposite function.

AQUARETIC
Diuretic agents that excrete water from the body, often associated with potassium excretion, but not other electrolytes. They may exert their effects through increased blood flow to the kidneys. Most herbal diuretics are in this class.

AQUEOUS
Pertaining to water; an aqueous solution is one in which water is the solvent.

AROMATICS
Fragrant or spicy-tasting herbs that stimulate the gastrointestinal mucous membranes. Aromatics are often used to cover strong, bitter, and unpleasant tasting herbs.

ASTRINGENT
A substance that constricts tissues, reducing inflammation of the mucous membranes and aiding in waste product removal. Most astringents are high in tannins. Astringents are commonly used as gargles, mouthwashes, sitz baths, and vaginal irrigation. Overuse can be excessively drying to the tissues. Plants with high amounts of tannins should not be combined with plants that contain high quantities of alkaloids.

BACTERIOSTATIC
An agent that inhibits bacterial growth.

BITTER TONIC
Plants with a prominent bitter taste due to the presence of a variety of chemical constituents, including volatile oils, alkaloids, sesquiterpene lactones, and monoterpene iridoids, also termed "bitter principles." Bitter tonics stimulate digestive secretions, enhancing digestive processes, and aiding elimination.

CALMATIVE
An agent with a mild sedative effect.

CARMINATIVE
A substance that eases flatulence and colic in the gut. Many volatile oils have carminative actions. Carminatives prevent intestinal pains that can occur while using cathartics and cholagogues. Examples of carminatives are anise, fennel, cardamom, and ginger.

CATABOLISM
The metabolic breakdown of substances into simpler substances, including the digestion of food and the oxidation of nutrient molecules for energy.

CATALYST
A circulatory stimulant herb that enhances the delivery of herbs in a compound formula to the tissues where they are needed. For example, adding a small quantity of cayenne *(Capsicum)* to a formula increases circulation of antimicrobial and immune-stimulating herbs to the respiratory mucosa. Adding ginger *(Zingiber)* or prickly ash *(Zanthoxylum)* increases circulation of bitter tonics and cholagogue to the digestive system; rosemary *(Salvia rosmarinus)* improves blood flow to the brain and increases the effectiveness of nootropic herbs. This class of herbs are also referred to as "carriers" or "directors."

CATHARTIC
A purgative that causes evacuation of the bowels, and encourages the elimination of waste from the liver, gallbladder, and alimentary canal by excreting waste.

CATARRH
Excessive mucus secretion; this term is frequently used in reference to the respiratory mucosa, but can also refer to mucus in the bowels or bladder.

CHOLAGOGUE
A substance that stimulates bile flow from the gallbladder. A cholagogue has a laxative effect, and is often used to cleanse the liver and gallbladder.

CHOLERETIC
A substance that stimulates bile production in the liver.

CHOLINERGIC
An activity or structure that responds to acetylcholine and pertains to functions controlled by the parasympathetic nervous system.

CHRONIC
A long-lasting disease or imbalance. Chronic conditions may exhibit little overall change, and are characterized by periods of remission, interspersed with acute episodes.

CIRCULATORY STIMULANT
A substance that enhances blood circulation through the tissues, increasing oxygen and nutrient delivery, and speeding waste product removal. Most circulatory stimulants have vasodilating actions. The prominent constituents in plants that stimulate circulation include volatile oils, alkaloids, and mustard oil glycosides.

COMMINUTION
The grinding of herbal material to convenient size, powdered or in large pieces. The mortar and pestle were traditionally used, but modern machinery is often used today.

CONCOCTION
A preparation made from a mixture of ingredients.

COUNTERIRRITANT
A substance that stimulates blood flow when applied locally.

DECOCTION
A preparation made by boiling plant parts (usually root or bark) in water at least 30 minutes.

DEFICIENCY
A condition of weakness or hypofunction of the whole body, an organ, or the endocrine system. According to Traditional Chinese Medicine, a deficiency can be caused by a lack of qi, blood, fluids, yin, yang, or essence.

DEMULCENT
A soothing substance containing mucilage that reduces mucous membrane inflammation. Demulcents have a protective and cooling action on the mucous membranes, that has a pronounced effect on the respiratory, gastrointestinal, and urinary systems. Many demulcents are considered yin tonics.

DEPRESSANT
A sedative.

DEPURATIVE
(see diuretic depurative)

DIAPHORETIC
A substance that increases perspiration by dilating the peripheral blood vessels. Diaphoretics work by directly stimulating the nerves affecting the sweat glands, or by introducing volatile oil into the bloodstream that performs both actions.

DIURETIC
A substance causing an increase in urine output.

DIURETIC DEPURATIVE
A substance that increases urine output, and aids in the excretion of water, as well as metabolite and waste product removal.

ELECTUARY
A medicinal paste comprised of powders and liquid sweeteners.

ELIMINATIVE
A substance that encourages one or more eliminatory functions or organs to increase the removal of metabolites and toxic material from the body. Bodily toxicity is the accumulation of cellular waste products and ingested toxins that result from inadequate eliminatory function, poor tissue circulation, poor liver or kidney function, poor digestion, or excessive ingestion of chemicals, additives, adulterants, drugs, and other toxins.

ELIXIR
A flavored liquid preparation of herbs or other medicines, often heavily sweetened.

EMETIC
A substance that induces vomiting. Emetics should only be used with caution and only by individuals with robust constitutions. Emetics are sometimes used when a toxic substance is accidentally ingested.

EMMENAGOGUE
A substance that stimulates menstruation.

EMOLLIENT
A substance used on the skin to create a soothing, softening effect.

EXCESS

In western herbology, a person with an excess condition or body type will demonstrate a constitutional tendency for the hyperfunction of an organ, metabolism, or endocrine system. Excess conditions can also result from the frequent use of alcohol, caffeine, fatty or refined foods, sugar, stimulants, and certain drugs, as well as from a lack of exercise or stagnation. In Traditional Chinese Medicine, excess is a condition resulting from the accumulation of too much of something, including yin, yang, heat, cold, or fluids.

EXPECTORANT

A substance that stimulates the expulsion of mucus from the respiratory mucosa.

FLAVONOIDS

A group of brightly pigmented compounds found in many plants. They account for the yellow, orange, red, and purple pigments of fruits, berries, and vegetables. Flavonoids improve the integrity of blood vessels.

FEBRIFUGE

An agent that reduces or eliminates fever.

FOMENTATION

A hot, moist cloth saturated in strained tea and applied to painful, inflamed, or swollen tissue.

FUNGISTATIC

An agent that inhibits fungal growth.

GALACTAGOGUE

A substance that increases the flow of breast milk; synonymous with the term "lactagogue."

HAEMOSTATIC OR HEMOSTATIC

A substance that stops or slows bleeding internally and/or externally.

HARMONIZER

A pleasant tasting herb that enhances the palatability of bitter, cathartic, purgative, or acrid herbs in compound formulas. Examples include: anise seed *(Pimpinella)*, carob pod *(Ceratonia)*, cinnamon *(Cinnamomum)*, fennel *(Foeniculum)*, jujube date *(Zizuphus jujuba)*, licorice root *(Glycyrrhiza)*, longan fruit *(Dimocarpus)*, mulberry *(Morus alba)*, stevia *(Stevia robusta)*, and/or vanilla bean *(Vanilla planifolia)*.

HEPATIC

A term used for a remedy that enhances liver function. Many hepatic herbs stimulate the liver through metabolic, regulatory, and detoxifying functions.

HEPATOPROTECTIVE

An agent that protects liver tissue from damage.

HEPATOREGENERATIVE

An agent that regenerates liver cells.

HYPERTENSIVE

An agent that increases blood pressure.

HYPNOTIC

A sleep-inducing agent.

HYPOTENSIVE

An agent that lowers blood pressure.

IATROGENIC

An illness, disease, or imbalance created by medical treatment.

IMMUNE STIMULANT

An immune-stimulating agent used to prevent and treat infections.

INFUSION

A preparation made by steeping plant parts (usually leaves or flowers) in hot water a minimum of 30 minutes.

LACTAGOGUE

A substance that promotes lactation or increases the flow of breast milk.

LAXATIVE

A substance that promotes bowel movements.

LINIMENT

A liquid or semi-liquid preparation for the skin; either rubefacient or locally anesthetic in most cases, although it can include soothing preparations.

LITHOTRIPTIC

An agent that affects the dissolution of kidney stones (calculus).

LYMPHATIC

A substance that enhances fluid drainage from the tissues and decreases lymphatic swelling. It has potential immune-enhancing function.

MENSTRUUM

A solvent used to extract plant properties.

MUCILAGE

A substance with a slimy texture that can act as a simple soothing demulcent.

MUCOLYTIC

A substance that reduces mucus production.

NARCOTIC

A powerful anodyne and/or hypnotic.

NERVINE

An agent with a calming effect on the nervous system.

NOOTROPIC
A substance that enhances cognitive function, memory, and concentration. Examples include: bacopa *(Bacopa)*, ginkgo *(Ginkgo)*, gotu kola *(Centella)*, lion's mane *(Hericium)*, and reishi mushroom *(Ganoderma)*.

NUTRITIVE
A substance that supplies the body with the elements necessary for metabolism. Most nutritive herbs are high in minerals, vitamins, or both.

PARASYMPATHETIC NERVOUS SYSTEM
The craniosacral division of the autonomic nervous system; generally reverses the flight-or-fight response and encourages digestion and relaxation.

PARASYMPATHOMIMETIC
An agent that stimulates the parasympathetic nervous system. See also cholinergic.

PHOTODERMATITIS
A skin eruption resulting from exposure to sunlight after ingesting or contacting a phototoxic substance.

PHOTOSENSITIZATION
Sensitivity to sunlight after ingesting or contacting a plant or plant substance.

PILL
A coated or uncoated ball of herbs and other medicinal agents with binding agents, designed to hold together for dispensing, dissolving easily in the stomach. Pills are a useful means of applying herbs with an unpleasant taste, but inappropriate when relying on the bitter tonic effect.

POULTICE
A pack of herbs applied to the skin, often over a wound or other damaged tissue. A poultice can be made by mixing hot water with chopped or ground herbs in a muslin bag, and is often used to draw pus and other debris from a wound.

PROPHYLACTIC
A substance or action taken to prevent disease.

PURGATIVE
A substance with a drastic laxative action; most purgatives should only be used by individuals with a robust constitution. Purgatives should never be used during pregnancy.

RECUPERATIVE
An herb that works most effectively in the clean-up, or post-infectious stage of an illness to encourage the complete healing of tissues and prevent scar tissue.

REFRIGERANT
A substance that gives a sensation of coolness or relieves feverishness.

RESTORATIVE
An herb that restores health or strength.

RUBEFACIENT
A topical agent that increases circulation in local tissues. Rubefacients are similar to counterirritants; however, they can potentially be more irritating to the skin, and can cause blistering if in excessive contact with the skin. An example of a rubefacient is mustard seed powder.

RESOLVENT
An agent that eliminates or reduces inflammation. Herbs such as bayberry and yerba mansa with aromatic astringent properties are often effective resolvents.

SEDATIVE
A substance that calms or tranquilizes by reducing functional activity. Sedatives can be used to reduce nervous tension, pain, neuromuscular spasms, and insomnia.

SIALAGOGUE
A substance that excites salivary secretions.

SOPORIFIC
A sleep-inducing substance.

SPASMOLYTIC
A substance that decreases or eliminates spasms or cramping.

STIMULANT
A substance that increases functional activity of a specific organ or general organism.

STOMACHIC
A substance that tones or stimulates the action of the stomach.

SUDORIFIC
A remedy that induces profuse sweating by stimulating the sudoriferous glands when ingested as a hot tea.

SUPPOSITORY
A small cone made by suspending medicine in a soft base readily dissolved at body temperature in order to apply medicines via the rectum or vagina.

SYMPATHOMIMETIC
An agent that stimulates the sympathetic nervous system. See adrenergic.

SYMPATHETIC NERVOUS SYSTEM
The thoracolumbar division of the autonomic nervous system; stimulates a flight-or-fight response.

SYRUP
A solution of water and sugar often used to preserve and act as a vehicle for herbal extracts. Syrups are particularly suited to children, and for disguising unpleasant flavors.

TABLET

A compressed preparation of medicaments with binding agents and other substances designed to aid in digesting and assimilating the contents.

TANNINS

A class of phenolic plant constituents usually found in inactive plant tissues, such as old and drying leaves, outer cork, heartwood, and galls. Tannins precipitate proteins in solution, which tends to curdle the solution; their effect on the body is to astringe the tissues. Tannins are a common constituent of many rose family plants. Plants containing high amounts of tannins should not be combined with plants high in alkaloids.

TCM

The abbreviation for Traditional Chinese Medicine.

TINCTURE

A preparation made by steeping plant material in a menstruum of alcohol and, oftentimes, water. The average steeping time for a tincture is two to four weeks. Tinctures have a longer shelf life than teas, and the alcohol is more effective than water for extracting resins, alkaloids, and volatile oils. A tincture is a more concentrated extract than an aqueous preparation.

TONICS

A remedy that repletes the body; tonics are nourishing, restorative, and supportive. They are often used long term, although most of them should be avoided during an acute illness or when menstruating.

TROPHORESTORATIVE

A nourishing, revitalizing herb or food that restores normal functioning in hypo- or hyperfunctioning tissues, organs, and glands.

VASOCONSTRICTOR

A substance causing blood vessels to constrict.

VASODILATOR

A substance causing blood vessels to dilate.

VERMICIDE

A substance that kills intestinal worms.

VERMIFUGE

A substance causing the expulsion of intestinal worms.

VULNERARY

A substance that promotes wound healing.

BOTANY GLOSSARY

ACHENE
A single-seeded dry fruit that does not break open at maturity.

ACTINOMORPHIC
A radially symmetrical flower.

ACUMINATE
Having a long, tapered tip.

ACUTE
Having a short, tapered tip.

ADNATE
One floral part fused to a different floral part (i.e., the stamens are fused to the petals).

ADVENTITIOUS ROOTS
Secondary roots growing from any part of the plant except the main root system.

AGGREGATE FRUIT
A cluster of fruitlets formed from a single flower with many separate carpels; e.g., blackberry *(Rubus* spp.*)*, raspberry *(Rubus idaeus)*, and wu wei zi *(Schisandra chinensis)*.

ALTERNATE LEAVES
One leaf per node.

ANDROECIUM
The male parts of a flower; the stamens.

ANNUAL
A plant with a life cycle completed within one year, from germination, through flowering and seed production, to death.

ANTHER
The pollen-producing portion of the stamen, found at the tip.

APETALOUS
Lacking petals.

APEX (LEAF APEX)
The tip of the leaf.

APOCARPOUS
A flower with two or more separate carpels.

ASCOMYCETE
A member of Ascomycota, a division of the fungus kingdom.

ASEPALOUS
Lacking sepals.

ASYMMETRIC FLOWER
A flower in which the parts within one or more whorls show no symmetry.

AWNED
An abrupt, hard, bristle-like point.

AXILLARY
Arising from the leaf axil.

AXILLARY BUD
A bud borne in an axil between the twig and a subtending leaf.

AXIS, FLORAL
The stem on which flowers attach in an inflorescence.

BASIDIOMYCETE
A member of Basidiomycota, a division of the fungus kingdom.

BASAL ROSETTE
Leaves arising only from the base of the plant, with reduced internodes along the short stem.

BIENNIAL
A plant with a life cycle completed within two years.

BILABIATE FLOWER
A flower with the perianth arranged into two lip-shaped structures.

BILATERAL SYMMETRY
A flower with one line of symmetry; zygomorphic.

BIRADIAL SYMMETRY
A flower with two lines of symmetry.

BLADE (LAMINA)
The expanded portion of a leaf, petal, or other structure, generally flat, but sometimes cylindrical.

BRACT
A leaf-like or scale-like structure associated with a flower, inflorescence, or cone.

BRACTEOLE (BRACTLET)
A small bract associated with an individual flower within an inflorescence.

BUD
An immature shoot, protected by tough scale leaves from which the stem and leaves or flowers may develop.

BULB
A short, underground bud composed of reduced fleshy leaves or leaf bases attached to, and surrounding the stem.

CALYX
All of the sepals of one flower.

CAMPANULATE/BELL SHAPED
Pertaining to a fused calyx, corolla, or perianth that is shaped like a bell: it widens abruptly at the base, then widens more gradually towards the tips of the petals.

CAPSULE
A dry, multi-chambered fruit arising from multiple fused carpels that breaks open at maturity to release seeds.

CARPEL
The female reproductive unit of a flower. There may be one or more per pistil.

CARPELLATE/PISTILLATE
A flower with fertile carpels but sterile or missing stamens.

CARYOPSIS
A dry, one-seeded fruit typical of the grass family, that does not split open at maturity, in which the fruit wall is fused to the seed coat; e.g., oats *(Avena)*, corn *(Zea)*.

CAULINE
Growing on an aerial stem.

CAULESCENT
Having aerial stems.

CIRCUMBOREAL
Occurring throughout the far northern regions of North America and Eurasia.

COMPLETE FLOWER
A flower with all four series of whorls (sepals, petals, stamens, carpels).

CONNATE
Where a flower part is fused to another part within the same whorl.

CORDATE
Heart-shaped.

CORM
A short, thick, unbranched, underground stem, often surrounded by dry (not fleshy) leaves or leaf bases; e.g., *Crocosmia*.

COROLLA
All of the petals of one flower.

CORONA
A ring of often showy structures arising from the perianth, found between the petals and the stamens.

CORTEX
The outer layer or "skin" of lichen; the outer layer of a plant stem or root.

CORYMB
A raceme-like inflorescence in which the floral branches reach approximately the same height, lending a flat-topped appearance.

COSTA
The specialized midrib of the leaves of an Araceae (Palm) family plant.

CRENATE
Scalloped.

CUPULE
Fused involucral bracts subtending a flower or fruit, as in an acorn cup.

CYME
An inflorescence in which the central or uppermost flower opens before the flowers on the edge or bottom of the stalk.

DECIDUOUS
Plants with leaves that fall off naturally at the end of a growing period.

DECUMBENT
Mainly lying flat on the ground.

DECURRENT
When the leaf base or mushroom gill extends downward along the stem or stipe.

DELTOID
Somewhat triangular.

DENTATE
Having teeth projecting at right angles perpendicular (outward) to the leaf margin.

DETERMINATE GROWTH
Plant growth that stops after a genetically predetermined structure has fully formed.

DIOECIOUS
Plants with unisexual flowers in which female and male flowers grow on separate plants.

DISCOID HEAD
A characteristic of Asteraceae family members; a flower head consisting solely of disc florets and lacking ray florets. See radiate head, ligulate head.

DOUBLE SERRATE
Having serrations that are also serrated.

DRUPE
A fleshy fruit with a single large, stony seed.

ELLIPTIC/AL
Shaped like a flattened circle.

ENTIRE MARGINS

Not indented; having smooth edges.

EPHEMERAL

A plant that completes its life cycle very rapidly. In favorable environments, an ephemeral species may germinate, bloom, set seed, and die several times in one year. Many weeds are ephemerals.

EPICALYX

A set of sepal-like bracts; e.g., strawberry *(Fragaria)*.

EPIPETALOUS STAMENS

Stamens with bases fused to the petals.

EVERGREEN

Plants that always have living leaves. Evergreen species have leaves that remain green more than one season and do not fall all at once.

EXSERTED

When one floral part projects beyond the surrounding parts; usually describes when the stamens or pistils extend beyond the length of the corolla.

FIBRILS

Tiny fibers.

FIBROUS

A root system comprised of many thinner roots similar in length and thickness. No clearly dominant root is present; e.g., grasses, annuals, monocots.

FILAMENT

The stalk of the stamen.

FOLLICLE

A fruit arising from a single carpel that breaks open at maturity, usually along a suture, to release its seeds. It also can form as an aggregate fruit, consisting of a cluster of follicles arising from multiple separate carpels of a single flower; e.g., aconite *(Aconitum)*, columbine *(Aquilegia)*.

FRUTICOSE

Of lichen, having a shrubby or bushy growth structure.

FUNNEL SHAPED

A calyx or corolla narrower at the base, and wider at the petal tips.

FUSED

When a flower part is attached to, or merged with, another flower part.

GLABRESCENT

Becomes hairless over time or at maturity.

GLABROUS

Hairless.

GLAND

A secretory structure often found on the plant surface.

GLANDULAR HAIR

A gland-tipped hair that often secretes essential oils or resinous substances.

GLAUCOUS

Having a whitish, waxy coating.

GLOBOSE

Spherical.

GYNOECIUM

The female parts of a flower.

GYNOPHORE

A specialized reproductive structure consisting of a stem that supports the gynoecium above the point of attachment to the other whorls.

HASTULA

The single or pair of specialized triangular structures where the petiole meets the base of the leaf blade specific to the Palm family.

HEAD

An inflorescence in which hundreds to thousands of tiny flowers are grouped to form a single, flower-like structure, often comprising two kinds of florets (ray florets and disk florets); capitulum; pseudoanthium.

HERBACEOUS

Not woody.

HYPANTHIUM

A flower structure in which the base of the calyx, corolla, and stamens are fused into the shape of a cup or tube.

IMBRICATE

Overlapping; usually referring to bracts, sepals, or petals.

IMPERFECT FLOWER (UNISEXUAL)

Having either fertile stamens or pistils.

INCOMPLETE

A flower with one or more series of whorls missing.

INDETERMINATE GROWTH

Plant growth that does not have a genetically predetermined termination point.

INFERIOR OVARY

The base of the ovary is below where the base of the other floral parts attach to the flower. Compare to superior ovary.

INFLORESCENCE

A cluster of two or more flowers.

INVOLUCRE

A set of bracts at the base of an inflorescence separate from each other, or fused to form a cup.

IRREGULAR FLOWER
A flower that is not radially symmetrical.

ISOFACIAL
Identical upper and lower sides of a leaf.

LACTIFEROUS
Producing milky latex.

LANCEOLATE
Lance-shaped; much longer than wide, and tapered at either end (especially towards the apex).

LEAF AXIL
The upper angle between a leaf and the stem on which it grows, just above where the leaf attaches to the stem.

LEAFLET
One leaf-like unit of a compound leaf.

LENTICEL
Pores on the surface of tree or shrub bark that enable the exchange of gases between the inner plant tissues and the atmosphere.

LIGULE
The strap-like, fused corolla found in some flower forms in the Asteraceae family.

LIGULATE HEAD
Found in members of Asteraceae, a flower head solely consisting of ligulate or ray florets, and lacking discoid florets. See radiate head, discoid head.

LINEAR
Elongated and very narrow, with nearly parallel sides.

LOBED
Deeply indented.

LOCULE
A compartment of an ovary; one or more locules may be present.

MARGIN
In plants, the edge of a structure, such as a leaf blade or flower petal; in mushrooms, the edge of the cap.

MIDRIB
The rib-like strip of vascular tissue running through the middle of the leaf blade.

MONOECIOUS
Plants with unisexual flowers in which male and female flowers grow on the same plant.

MYCELIUM
The interwoven, branching, thread-like structures that comprise the "vegetative" or non-reproductive mass of a fungus. Mycelium is usually submerged in the soil or host substrate. Mycelium specializes to form fungal fruiting bodies.

NECTAR
A sweet fluid secreted in many flowers to attract pollinators.

NECTARIES
Specialized structures that produce nectar; they may comprise a modified portion of a petal, sepal, stamen, carpel, or receptacle.

OBLANCEOLATE
Upside-down lance shaped; the leaf blades are widest above the middle.

OBLONG
Longer than wide, with nearly parallel sides and rounded corners.

OBOVATE
Upside-down egg-shaped; ovate, but the narrower end is at the base, towards the attachment to the petiole.

OBTUSE
Having a blunt tip or base with an angle wider than 90 degrees.

OLEORESIN
A resin suspended in a fatty oil or essential oil base; naturally occurring oleoresins are also called balsams.

OLEO-GUM RESIN
Similar to an oleoresin, but also contains a water-soluble gum component.

ONE- (ONCE-) PINNATE
A compound leaf with one series of leaflets.

OPPOSITE LEAVES
Two leaves per node directly across from each other on the stem.

OVARY
The basal portion of the pistil that produces ovules, and matures into fruit.

OVATE
Egg-shaped, with a wider end at the base.

OVULE
The structure containing the female germ cell that when fertilized becomes the seed.

PALMATE
Radiating from a common point; generally describes leaf veins, lobes, or leaflets.

PALMATELY COMPOUND
Leaflets radiating from a common point on the leaf.

PANICLE
A compound raceme in which the central axis branches out, and each branch is arranged as a raceme.

PAPILLAE
Tiny protrusions on the surface of a plant or lichen.

PAPPUS
In members of Asteraceae, a specialized structure at the apex of an achene that derives from the sepals of individual flowers. It may take the form of tufts of hair or bristle-like protrusions.

PARASITIC
An organism (plant, fungus, animal, etc.) depending partially or wholly on another living organism for basic survival needs, including nutrients and/or water. Parasites do not usually kill their hosts, but the relationship is detrimental for the host. Fully parasitic plants usually have no green parts, as they don't need to photosynthesize in order to obtain sugars.

PARALLEL VEINS
Leaf veins that run parallel to the margins.

PEDICEL
The stem of an individual flower in an inflorescence.

PEDUNCLE
The stem of a single flower not found in an inflorescence, or the stem of an entire inflorescence.

PELTATE
With the stem (of a leaf, scale, or other flat structure) attached toward the middle of the leaf, not at the margin.

PERENNIAL
A plant that lives at least three years.

PERFECT FLOWER (BISEXUAL)
Flowers with fertile stamens and pistils.

PERIANTH
The calyx and corolla as a collective unit.

PERSISTENT
Floral parts that don't fall off after the fruit matures.

PETAL
An individual member of the corolla, fused or not, often colored. They are sometimes indistinguishable from the sepals; in those cases, the petals and sepals are called tepals.

PETIOLATE
Having a petiole.

PETIOLE
The stalk of the leaf connects the blade to the stem.

PHYLLARIES
The sepal-like bracts forming the involucre that surrounds and protects the flower heads in some members of Asteraceae.

PINNATE VENATION
Venation consisting of a central mid-vein, with many secondary veins emerging on both sides to form a feathered pattern.

PINNATELY COMPOUND
Featherlike; more than three leaflets arranged in two rows along a common rachis.

PISTIL
The female flower structure, typically consisting of an ovary, style, and stigma. There may be one or more per flower. It consists of one or more carpels.

PISTILLATE FLOWER
A flower with fertile pistils having sterile, rudimentary, or missing stamens.

PLACENTA
Where ovules are attached in the ovary.

PLUMOSE
Featherlike.

POLLEN
A powder released by the anther that contains the male gamete which fertilizes the ovule to create a seed; the collective mass of pollen grains produced in the anthers.

POLYGAMOUS
A species in which the plants have both perfect and imperfect flowers.

POLYPORE MUSHROOMS
An evolutionarily unrelated group of mushrooms that release spores through downward-facing tubes. Some of the most common, medicinally significant polypores form durable, shelf-like fruiting bodies called conks; e.g., reishi *(Ganoderma),* turkey tail *(Trametes);* others grow in a flattened, crust-like form, or a more traditional mushroom shape.

PROSTRATE
Lying flat on the ground.

PUBESCENT
Covered in hairs.

RACEME
An unbranched cluster of flowers with pedicels on a single axis that have indeterminate growth, in which the lower flowers open up before the top ones.

RACHIS
The central axis of a compound leaf.

RADIAL SYMMETRY
A flower with three or more lines of symmetry; a flower with roughly identical parts; actinomorphic.

RADIATE HEAD
Of members of Asteraceae, a flower head consisting of ray florets and disc florets. See discoid head, ligulate head.

RAY
A primary branch in a compound umbel.

RECEPTACLE
The structure on the pedicel to which flower parts attach.

REGULAR FLOWER
A radially symmetrical flower.

RESIN
A highly viscous, strongly scented substance secreted by plants rich in phenolic compounds and terpenes.

REVOLUTE
Rolled under.

RHIZOME
An underground, horizontal stem usually persisting from season to season. Distinguished from a root by the presence of leaves, leaf scars, scales, and buds.

ROTATE
Wheel- or saucer-shaped.

SAGITTATE
An arrowhead-shaped leaf or leaf base, triangular, with basal lobes extending below the attachment of the blade to the petiole.

SALVERFORM
Having a slender tube and tips that abruptly flare out with a flat face.

SCAPE
A leafless flowering stalk.

SCAPOS
Having a scape.

SCHIZOCARP
A dry, multisegmented fruit arising from a flower with multiple carpels, in which the segments break apart at maturity; e.g., members of the carrot family *(Apiaceae)* and marshmallow *(Althaea)*.

SEPAL
An individual member of the calyx, fused or not, generally green. They are sometimes indistinguishable from the petals, and in those cases, both the petals and the sepals are called tepals.

SEPTUM
An interior wall in the ovary or fruit that divides the locules.

SERRATE
Having a sawtoothed margin with teeth pointing forward toward the tip.

SESSILE
Lacking a stalk (petiole, peduncle, or pedicel).

SIMPLE LEAF
A leaf composed of a single part, undivided, unbranched.

SINUATE
A sinuous, wavy margin.

SOLITARY
A single flower per peduncle; a flower not grouped in a cluster.

SPADIX
A spike-like inflorescence with a thick, fleshy axis, sometimes bearing innumerable minute flowers.

SPATHE
A relatively large, and sometimes brightly colored bract partially or completely surrounding a spadix; e.g., skunk cabbage *(Lysichiton)*.

SPATULATE
Spoon-shaped.

SPIKE
An unbranched cluster of sessile flowers on a single axis.

STAMEN
The male organ of the flower composed of a filament (stalk) and anther (pollen sacs).

STAMINATE FLOWER
A flower with fertile stamens, but sterile or missing carpels.

STIGMA
The apical part of the pistil receptive to pollen.

STIPE
A stem; often refers to a mushroom or seaweed.

STIPULATE
Having stipules.

STIPULE
The appendage at the base of a petiole, generally paired, variable in form, but often leaf-like or scale-like, sometimes a tendril or spine.

STOLON
A runner or horizontal stem at, or below the ground surface that produces a new plant at its tip; e.g., strawberry *(Fragaria)*.

STROMA
In fungi, a mass of mycelium containing spore-bearing structures.

STYLE
The elongated stalk of the pistil between the ovary and the stigma.

SUPERIOR OVARY
An ovary attached to the receptacle above the point of attachment of the other floral parts.

SYNCARPOUS
A flower with two or more fused carpels in a single pistil.

TAP ROOT
A root system with one main, tapered root that generally grows straight down into the soil, and has smaller lateral branches.

TENDRIL
A twining stem, leaf, or petiole, either terminal or arising from the axil of a leaf, used by climbing plants for support.

TEPAL
A member of the perianth in which the petals are indistinguishable from the petal-like sepals.

TERMINAL
Situated at the apex of a stalk or branch.

TERNATE
In groups of three; a ternately compound leaf branches in patterns of three branches, each bearing three leaflets.

THREE- (THRICE-) PINNATE
Pinnately compound leaves in which the leaflets themselves are bipinnate.

TOMENTOSE
Thickly covered with matted hairs.

TRIFOLIATE (TRIFOLIOLATE)
One leaf composed of three leaflets.

TRUNCATE
Having a blunt base or apex as if cut straight across; e.g., quaking aspen *(Populus tremuloides).*

TUBER
An enlarged, thick, fleshy underground stem for storage of food and/or water; e.g., potato *(Solanum tuberosum).*

TWO- (TWICE-) PINNATE
One leaf composed of one degree leaflets divided into secondary leaflets.

UMBEL
An umbrella-shaped inflorescence; an inflorescence in which three or more pedicels radiate from a common point. Compound umbels are formed when the umbel structural pattern is repeated. Each ray of the umbel then bears its own umbel of flowers.

UNICARPELLATE
Having a single carpel.

URCEOLATE/URN SHAPED
A fused calyx or corolla shaped like an urn: narrowing toward the tip.

VERTICILLASTER
An inflorescence in which the flowers appear to be arranged in a whorl, but actually are pairs of opposite axillary cymes. Many members of the mint family have this form of inflorescence.

WHORL, FLORAL
One of the various rings of floral parts (the sepals, petals, stamens, and pistils).

WHORLED LEAVES
Three or more leaves per node.

ZYGOMORPHIC
Bilateral symmetry.

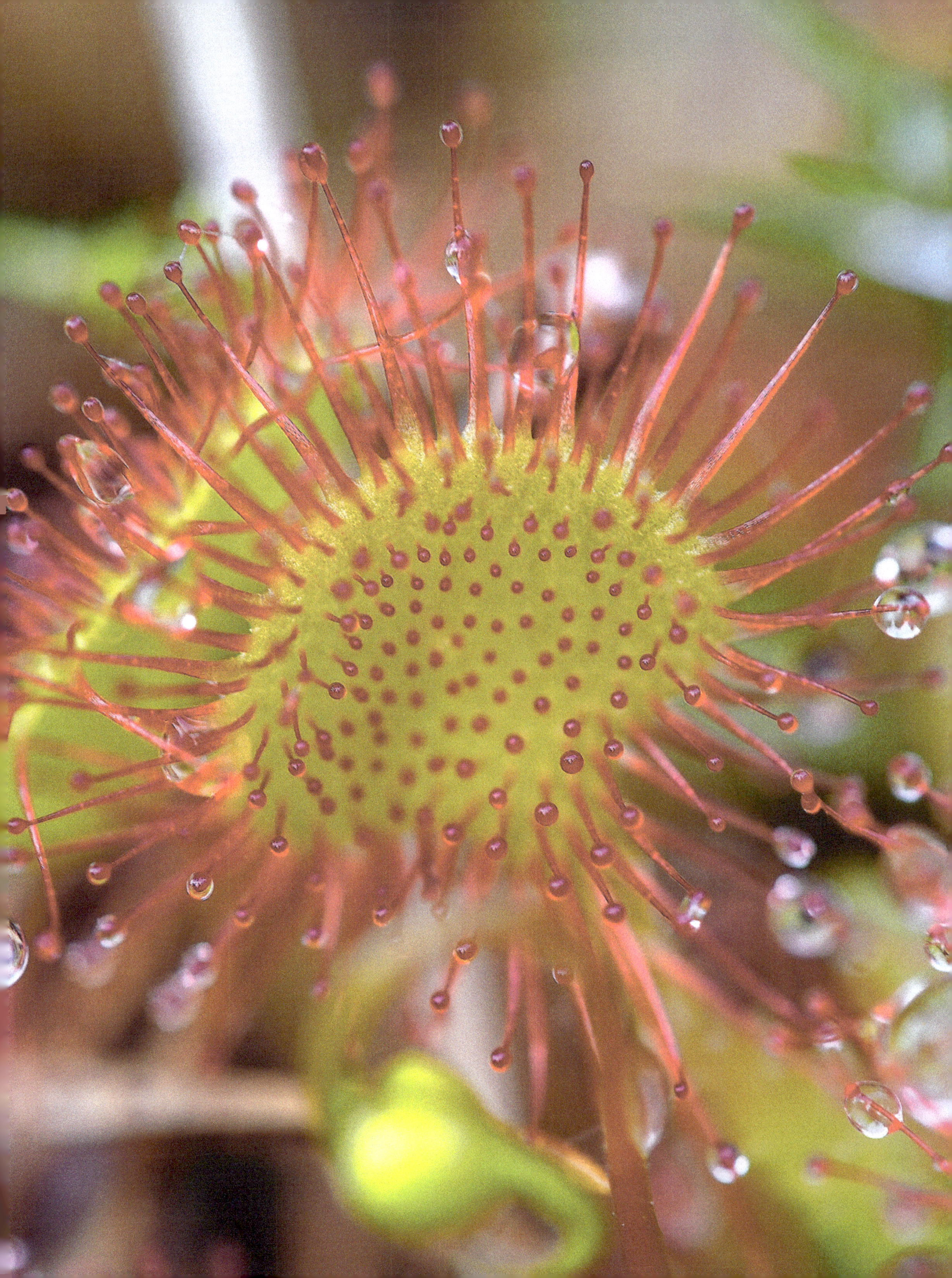

PLANTS BY FAMILY OR GROUP

ALGAE (BY CLASS OR PHYLUM)

CHLOROPHYTA (GREEN ALGAE)

Ulva lactuca (Sea lettuce, green laver)

CYANOBACTERIA (BLUE GREEN ALGAE)

Arthrospira platensis, A. maxima syn. *Spirulina* spp. (Spirulina)
Chlorella spp. (Chlorella)
Nostoc spp. (Star jelly)

PHAEOPHYCEAE (BROWN ALGAE)

Alaria esculent (Murlin)
Ascophyllum nodosum (Knotted wrack)
Eisenia bicyclis (Arame)
Fucus spp. (Bladderwrack)
Hizikia fusiformis (Hijiki)
Laminaria digitata (Kelp)
Laminaria saccharina (Kelp, sugar wrack)
Laminaria spp. (Kombu, oarweed)
Macrocystis pyrifera (Kelp)
Undaria pinnatifida (Wakame)

RHODOPHYTA (RED ALGAE)

Chondrus crispus (Irish moss)
Gelidium spp. (Agar-agar)
Gracilaria spp. (Gracilaria)
Palmaria palmata (Dulse)
Porphyra spp. (Nori, laver)

FUNGI (BY PHYLUM)

ASCOMYCOTA (SAC FUNGI)

Aspergillus flavus (Bread mold)
Aspergillus oryzae (Miso mold)
Candida albicans (Thrush yeast)
Claviceps purpurea (Ergot fungus)
Morchella esculenta (Morel)
Penicillium camemberti (Camembert cheese yeast)
Penicillium chrysogenum (Antibiotic penicillin)
Penicillium notatum (Antibiotic penicillin)
Saccharomyces carlsbergensis (Beer yeast)
Saccharomyces cerevisiae (Baker's yeast)
Saccharomyces ellipsoideus (Wine yeast)
Saccharomyces theobromae (Cacao yeast)
Tuber spp. (Truffle)

BASIDIOMYCOTA (HIGHER FUNGI)

Amanita muscaria (Fly agaric)
Boletus spp. (Bolete mushroom)
Cantharellus cibarius (Chanterelle mushroom)
Flammulina velutipes (Enoki mushroom, velvet shank)
Ganoderma spp. (Reishi mushroom)
Lentinula edodes (Shiitake)
Lycoperdon marginatum (Gi i sa wa)
Lycoperdon spp. (Puffball)
Pleurotus spp. (Oyster mushroom)
Psilocybe cubensis, P. cyanescens, P. azurescens (Teonanacatl, divine mushroom)
Trametes versicolor (Turkey tail mushroom)
Ustilago maydis (Corn smut)

LICHENS

Cetraria islandica (Iceland moss)
Evernia prunastri (Oak moss)
Usnea spp. (Usnea, old man's beard)

BRYOPHYTES

Sphagnum spp. (Sphagnum, peat moss)

FERNS & FERN ALLIES

Adiantum spp. (Maiden hair fern)
Cyathea spp. (Tree fern)
Dryopteris filix-mas (Male fern)
Equisetum spp. (Horsetail, scouring rush)
Lycopodium alpinum (Club moss)
Lycopodium clavatum (Club moss)
Pteridium aquilinum (Bracken fern, brake fern)

GYMNOSPERMS (NAKED SEEDED PLANTS)

CUPRESSACEAE (JUNIPER OR CEDAR FAMILY)

Calocedrus decurrens (Incense cedar)
Juniperus communis (Common juniper)
Sequoia sempervirens (Redwood)
Taxodium distichum (Bald cypress)
Thuja occidentalis (Northern white cedar)

Thuja plicata (Western red cedar)
Tsuga canadensis (Eastern hemlock)
Tsuga heterophylla (Western hemlock)

EPHEDRACEAE (EPHEDRA FAMILY)

Ephedra sinica (Ephedra, ma huang, somalata)
Ephedra nevadensis (Mormon tea)
Ephedra viridris (Western ephedra)

GINKGOACEAE (GINKGO OR MAINDENHAIR TREE FAMILY)

Ginkgo biloba (Ginkgo, maidenhair tree)

PINACEAE (PINE FAMILY)

Abies alba (European silver fir)
Abies balsamea (Balsam fir)
Abies concolor (White fir)
Abies grandis (Giant fir, grand fir)
Abies procera (Noble fir)
Cedrus atlantica (Atlantic cedar)
Cedrus deodara (Deodar cedar, devadaru)
Cedrus libani (Cedar of Lebanon)
Larix deciduas (European larch)
Larix laricina (Eastern larch, tamarack)
Picea abies (Norway spruce)
Picea glauca (White spruce)
Picea sitchensis (Sitka spruce)
Pinus edulis, P. monophylla (Piñon pine)
Pinus ponderosa (Ponderosa pine)
Pinus strobus (White pine)
Pinus sylvestris (Scotch pine, Scots pine)
Pinus spp. (Pine)
Pseudotsuga menziesii (Douglas fir)

TAXACEAE (YEW FAMILY)

Taxus baccata (English yew)
Taxus brevifolia (Pacific yew)
Taxus cuspidate (Japanese yew)
Torreya nucifera (Japanese torreya)

ANGIOSPERMS (FLOWERING PLANTS)

ACANTHACEAE (ACANTHUS FAMILY)

Adhatoda vasica syn. *Justica adhatoda* (Vasa, malabar nut)
Andrographis paniculata (Kalamegha, andrographis)

ADOXACEAE (MOSCHATEL FAMILY)

Sambucus spp. (Elder berry)
Viburnum opulus (Cramp bark)
Viburnum prunifolium (Black haw)

AGAVACEAE (CENTURY PLANT FAMILY)

Agave atrovirens (Maguey, pulque)
Agave cantala (Cantala, manila maguey)
Agave tequilana (Mezcal)
Agave (Maguey)
Camassia spp. (Camas)
Chlorogalum pomeridianum (Soaproot)
Dracaena draco (Dragon tree)
Polianthes tuberosa (Tuberose, azucena)
Yucca baccata (Banana yucca)
Yucca brevifolia (Joshua tree)
Yucca mohavensis (Mohave yucca)
Yucca treculeana (Trecul yucca)
Yucca whipplei (Chaparral yucca)
Yucca spp. (Palma istle)

ALISMATACEAE (ARROWHEAD FAMILY)

Alisma orientalis, A. plantago (Water plantain, ze xie)
Sagittaria latifolia (Arrowhead, wapato)
Sagittaria sagittifolia (Arrowhead)

AMARYLLIDACEAE (AMARYLLIS FAMILY)

Allium ampeloprasum (Elephant garlic, leek)
Allium ascalonicum (Shallot)
Allium cepa (Onion)
Allium sativum (Garlic)
Allium schoenoprasum (Chives)

ANACARDIACEAE (CASHEW FAMILY)

Mangifera indica (Mango)
Pistacia vera (Pistachio, green almond)
Rhus coriaria (Sumac)
Rhus integrifolia (Lemonade berry)
Toxicodendron diversilobum (Western poison oak)
Toxicodendron radicans (Poison ivy)

ANNONACEAE (CUSTARD APPLE FAMILY)

Cananga odorata (Ylang ylang)

APIACEAE/UMBELLIFERAE (UMBEL OR CARROT FAMILY)

Anethum graveolens (Dill)
Angelica archangelica (Angelica)
Angelica dahurica (Dahurian angelica)
Angelica sinensis (Dong quai)
Anthriscus cerefolium (Chervil)
Apium graveolens (Celery, celeriac, ajmoda)
Centella asiatica syn. *Hydrocotyle asiatica* (Gotu kola, brahmi, mandukaparni)
Carum carvi (Caraway)
Coriandrum sativum (Coriander, cilantro)
Cuminum cyminum (Cumin)

Daucus carota (Carrot)
Ferula asafoetida (Asafetida, devil's dung, hing)
Ferula galbaniflua (Galbanum)
Foeniculum vulgare (Fennel, finochio)
Heracleum maximum, syn. *H. lanatum* (Cow parsnip)
Levisticum officinale (Lovage)
Ligusticum porteri (Oshá)
Lomatium dissectum syn. *Leptotaenia dissecta* (Lomatium, biscuit root)
Opopanax chironium (Opopanax)
Osmorhiza occidentalis (Sweet root, western sweet cicely)
Pastinaca sativa (Parsnip)
Petroselinum crispum (Parsley)
Pimpinella anisum (Anise)
Saposhnikovia divaricata (Siler, fang feng)
Semecarpus anacardium (Bhallataka, bhilawa, marking nut)
Sium sisarum (Skirret)
Trachyspermum copticum (Ajowan, ajwain, yavani)

APOCYNACEAE (DOGBANE FAMILY)

Apocynum cannabinum (Indian hemp)
Gymnema sylvestre (Gurmar)
Hemidesmus indicus (Indian sarsaparilla)
Holarrhena pubescens (Kutaja)
Rauvolfia serpentina (Indian snakeroot, sarpagandha)
Tabernanthe iboga (Iboga)
Vinca major (Periwinkle)

AQUIFOLIACEAE (HOLLY FAMILY)

Ilex paraguariensis (Yerba mate)
Ilex guayusa (Guayusa)

ARACEAE (AROID OR PHILODENDRON FAMILY)

Acorus calamus (Calamus root, sweet flag, vacha)
Colocasia antiquorum (Taro)
Lysichiton americanus (Skunk cabbage)
Philodendron spp. (Philodendron)
Symplocarpus foetidus (skunk cabbage)

ARALIACEAE (GINSENG FAMILY)

Aralia californica (Aralia, elk clover, spikenard)
Aralia nudicaulis (Wild sarsaparilla)
Aralia racemosa (American spikenard)
Eleutherococcus senticosus (Siberian ginseng, eleuthero)
Oplopanax horridus (Devil's club)
Panax ginseng (Ginseng, sang)
Panax quinquefolius (American ginseng)
Panax notoginseng (Nodoginseng, tienchi ginseng)

ARECACEAE / PALMAE (PALM FAMILY)

Areca catechu (Betel nut, areca nut)
Cocos nucifera (Coconut)
Sabal palmetto (Cabbage palm)
Serenoa repens (Saw palmetto)

ARISTOLOCHIACEAE (BIRTHWORT FAMILY)

Aristolochia spp. (Birthwort)
Asarum caudatum (Wild ginger)

ASCLEPIADACEAE (MILKWEED FAMILY)

Asclepias spp. (Milkweed)
Asclepias tuberosa (Pleurisy root, butterfly weed)
Tylophora indica, T. asthmatica (Antrapachaka, Indian ipecac)

ASPARAGACEAE (ASPARAGUS FAMILY)

Asparagus adscendens (Safed musali)
Asparagus cochinchinensis (Tian men dong)
Asparagus officinalis (Asparagus)
Asparagus racemosus (Shatavari)

ASPHODELACEAE (ALOE FAMILY)

Aloe vera (Aloe, kumari)

ASTERACEAE/COMPOSITAE (ASTER, DAISY OR SUNFLOWER FAMILY)

Achillea millefolium (Yarrow)
Acmella oleracea (Spilanthes)
Ambrosia spp. (Ragweed)
Anaphalis margaritacea (Pearly everlasting)
Anthemis nobilis (Roman chamomile)
Arctium lappa (Burdock, gobo)
Arnica spp. (Arnica)
Artemisia absinthium (Wormwood)
Artemisia californica (California sagebrush)
Artemesia douglasiana (Douglas' mugwort)
Artemisia dracunculus (Tarragon)
Artemisia vulgaris (Common mugwort, damanaka)
Balsamorhiza sagittata (Balsam root)
Bupleurum chinense (Chai hu, thorowax)
Calea zacatechichi (Dream herb, bitter grass)
Calendula officinalis (Calendula, pot marigold)
Carthamus tinctorius (Safflower)
Chrysanthemum indicum, C. x *morifolium* (Chrysanthemum, ju hua, sevanti)
Cnicus benedictus (Blessed thistle)
Echinacea angustifolium, E. purpurea, E. pallida (Echinacea, purple cone flower, Kansas snake root)
Eclipta alba (Bhringaraja, bringraj)
Eriogonum spp. (Buckwheat bush)
Eupatorium perfoliatum (Boneset)

Grindelia spp. (Grindelia, gumweed)
Inula helenium (Elecampane)
Inula racemosa (Indian elecampane, pushkarmoola)
Lactuca spp. (Wild lettuce)
Leucanthemum vulgare (Ox eye daisy)
Matricaria recutita syn. *M. chamomilla, Chamomilla recutita* (German chamomile)
Petasites palmatus (Western coltsfoot)
Saussurea lappa (Kushtha, costus root)
Silybum marianum (Milk thistle)
Tanacetum parthenium (Feverfew)
Taraxacum officinale (Dandelion)
Tussilago farfara (Eastern coltsfoot)

BERBERIDACEAE (BARBERRY FAMILY)

Berberis aquifolium, syn. *Mahonia aquifolium* (Oregon grape)
Berberis aristata, B. chitria (Daruharidra, Indian barberry)
Berberis vulgaris (Barberry)
Caulophyllum thalictroides (Blue cohosh)
Podophyllum emodi (Indian or Himalayan mayapple)
Podophyllum peltatum (American mandrake or mayapple)
Vancouveria hexandra (Inside-out flower, duckfoot)

BETULACEAE (BIRCH FAMILY)

Alnus glutinosa (Black alder)
Alnus rubra syn. *A. oregana* (Red alder)
Betula lenta (Cherry birch)
Betula papyrifera (Paper birch)
Betula pendula (European birch)
Corylus americana (American hazelnut)
Corylus avellana (European hazelnut)
Corylus chinensis (Chinese filbert)
Corylus cornuta (Beaked hazelnut)

BIGNONIACEAE (BIGNONIA FAMILY)

Chilopsis linearis (Desert willow)
Tabebuia avellanedae (Pau d'arco)

BORAGINACEAE (BORAGE FAMILY)

Alkanna tinctoria (Alkanna, alkanet)
Borago officinalis (Borage)
Eriodictyon californicum (Yerba santa)
Pulmonaria officinalis (Lungwort)
Symphytum officinale (Comfrey)

BRASSICACEAE/CRUCIFERAE (MUSTARD FAMILY)

Armoracia lapathifolia (Horseradish)
Barbarea verna (Spring cress)
Brassica chinensis (Chinese cabbage)
Brassica juncea (Brown mustard, mustard greens)
Brassica napus (Rape, rutabaga, swede)
Brassica nigra (Black mustard)
Brassica oleracea (Broccoli, cauliflower)
Brassica oleracea (Cabbage)
Brassica oleracea (Kohlrabi)
Brassica oleracea (Kale, collard greens)
Brassica rapa (Turnip, pak choi)
Camelina sativa (False flax)
Capsella bursa-pastoris (Shepherd's purse)
Eruca sativa (Arugula)
Eutrema wasabi (Wasabi, Japanese horseradish)
Isatis tinctoria (Woad)
Lepidium meyenii (Maca)
Lepidium sativum (Garden cress)
Nasturtium officinale (Water cress)
Raphanus sativus (Radish)
Sinapis alba (White mustard)

BROMELIACEAE (BROMELIAD OR PINEAPPLE FAMILY)

Ananas comosus (Pineapple)
Tillandsia usneoides (Spanish moss)

BURSERACEAE (BURSERA FAMILY)

Boswellia carteri, B. serrata (Frankincense, olibanum)
Bursera microphylla (Elephant tree)
Canarium luzonicum (Elemi)
Commiphora gileadensis (Balm of Gilead)
Commiphora myrrha, C. molmol (Myrrh)
Commiphora mukul (Gugul, Indian bedellium, Indian myrrh)

CACTACEAE (CACTUS FAMILY)

Carnegia gigantea (Saguaro)
Echinopsis pachanoi syn. *Trichocereus pachanoi* (San Pedro cactus)
Lophophora williamsii (Peyote, peyotl cactus)
Opuntia ficus-indica (Prickly pear)
Peniocereus greggii syn. *Cereus greggii* (Night blooming cereus, queen of the night)
Stenocereus stellatus (Pityayo)

CAMPANULACEAE (BLUEBELL FAMILY)

Codonopsis pilosula (Dang shen)
Lobelia cardinalis (Cardinal lobelia)
Lobelia inflata (Indian tobacco)
Lobelia syphilitica (Lobelia)
Lobelia tuba (Tupa)
Platycodon grandiflorus (Balloon flower, Chinese bell flower)

CANNABACEAE (MARIJUANA FAMILY)

Cannabis sativa, C. indica (Hemp, marijuana)
Humulus lupulus (Hops)

CAPPARACEAE (CAPER FAMILY)

Capparis spinosa (Caper bush)

CAPRIFOLIACEAE (HONEYSUCKLE FAMILY)

Lonicera spp. (Honeysuckle)

CARICACEAE (PAPAYA FAMILY)

Carica papaya (Papaya, pawpaw, mamao)

CARYOPHYLLACEAE (CARNATION FAMILY)

Dianthus spp. (Carnation)
Saponaria officinalis (Soapwort)
Stellaria media (Chickweed)

CHENOPODIACEAE (GOOSEFOOT FAMILY)

Beta vulgaris var. *cicia* (Chard, Swiss chard)
Beta vulgaris var. *vulgaris* (Beet, sugar beet, mangei)
Chenopodium ambrosioides (Epazote, Mexican tea)
Chenopodium anthelminticum (Wormseed)
Chenopodium quinoa (Quinoa)
Spinacia oleracea (Spinach)

CISTACEAE (ROCKROSE FAMILY)

Cistus ladaniferus (Rockrose, labdanum)

COLCHICACEAE (COLCHICUM FAMILY)

Colchicum autumnale (Autumn crocus)

COMBRETACEAE (TERMINALIA FAMILY)

Terminalia arjuna (Arjuna, kakubha, arjuna myrobalan)
Terminalia bellirica (Bibhitaki)
Terminalia catappa (Indian almond)
Terminalia chebula (Haritaki)
Terminalia spp. (Myrobalan, terminalia)
Terminalia superba (Afara)

CONVOLVULACEAE (MORNING GLORY FAMILY)

Evolvulus alsinoides (Shankhapushpi)
Ipomoea violacea (Morning glory, tlitliltzin)
Operculina turpethum (Trivrit)

CORNACEAE (DOGWOOD FAMILY)

Camptotheca acuminata (Happy tree, tree of life)
Cornus spp. (Dogwood)
Cornus canadensis (Bunchberry)
Cornus sericea syn. *C. stolonifera* (Red osier)
Nyssa sylvatica (Sour gum, black gum)

CUCURBITACEAE (SQUASH OR GOURD FAMILY)

Momordica charantia (Bitter melon, karella)

CYPERACEAE (SEDGE FAMILY)

Cyperus esculentus (Tiger nut, chufa)
Cyperus papyrus (Papyrus)
Cyperus rotundus (Musta, mustaka, nut grass)
Eleocharis dulcis (Water chestnut)

DIOSCOREACEAE (YAM FAMILY)

Dioscorea alata (Greater Asiatic yam, white yam)
Dioscorea batatas (Chinese yam, Chinese potato, shan yao)
Dioscorea esculenta (Chinese yam, potato yam)
Dioscorea villosa (Wild yam)

DIPSACACEAE (TEASEL FAMILY)

Dipsacus sylvestris (Fuller's teasel)

EBANACEAE (EBONY FAMILY)

Diospyros digyna (Black persimmon, black sapote, chocolate pudding fruit)
Diospyros kaki (Japanese persimmon, kaki)
Diospyros virginiana (American persimmon)
Fraxinus quadrangulata (Blue ash)

ELEGANACEAE (OLEASTER FAMILY)

Elaeagnus angustifolia (Russian olive)
Elaeagnus pungens (Silver berry)
Shepherdia argentea (Buffalo berry)

ERICACEAE (HEATH FAMILY)

Arbutus menziesii (Madrone, madrono)
Arbutus unedo (Strawberry tree)
Arctostaphylos uva ursi (Bearberry)
Arctostaphylos spp. (Manzanita)
Chimaphila menziesii (Little prince's pine)
Gaultheria procumbens (Wintergreen)
Gaultheria shallon (Salal)
Gaylussacia baccata (Huckleberry)
Kalmia latifolia (Mountain laurel)
Ledum glandulosum (Labrador tea)
Vaccinium macrocarpon (Cranberry)
Vaccinium myrtillus (Bilberry)
Vaccinium ovatum (Black huckleberry)
Vaccinium parviflorum (Red huckleberry)
Vaccinium spp. (Blueberry, cowberry, huckleberry)

ERYTHROXYLACEAE (COCA FAMILY)

Erythroxylum coca (Coca)
Erythroxylum novogranatense (Coca)

EUPHORBIACEAE (SPURGE OR EUPHORB FAMILY)

Jatropha spp. (Physic nut, spurge nut, Barbados nut)
Ricinus communis (Castor oil)

FABACEAE/LEGUMINOSAE (LEGUME, BEAN, OR PEA FAMILY)

Acacia catechu (Catechu, black cutch)
Acacia senegal (Gum Arabic)
Albizia lebbeck (Pit shirisha)
Albizia saman (Rain tree)
Aspalathus linearis (Rooibos)
Astragalus gummifer (Gum tragacanth)
Astragalus membranaceus (Astragalus root, huang qi)
Baptisia tinctoria (Wild indigo)
Bauhinia variegata (Kanchanara, mountain ebony)
Butea monosperma (Palasha, flame of the forest)
Cassia angustifolia (Indian senna)
Cassia fistula (Purging cassia, aragvadha)
Cassia occidentalis (Coffee weed)
Ceratonia siliqua (Carob, St. John's bread)
Cicer arietinum (Chickpea, garbanzo bean)
Copaifera officinalis (Copaiba balsam)
Copaifera spp. (Copal)
Cyamopsis tetragonolobus (Guar gum)
Dipteryx odorata (Tonka bean)
Glycine max (Soybean)
Glycyrrhiza glabra (Licorice)
Glycyrrhiza uralensis (Gan cao)
Hymenaea spp. (Madagascar copal, Brazilian copal)
Indigofera tinctoria (Indigo)
Lens culinaris (Lentil)
Medicago sativa (Alfalfa)
Melilotus spp. (Sweet clover)
Mimosa tenuiflora (Jurema)
Myroxylon balsamum (Balsam of Tolu)
Myroxylon pereirae (Balsam of Peru)
Mucuna pruriens (Kapikacchu, velvet bean, cowhage)
Phaseolus aureus (Mung bean)
Phaseolus limensis (Lima bean)
Phaseolus vulgaris (Black bean, chili b., cranberry b., green b., haricot b., kidney b., navy b., pea b. pink b., pinto b., red b., snap b., string b., was b., white b.)
Piscidia erythrina (Jamaican dogwood, fish poison tree)
Pisum sativum (English pea, garden pea)
Prioria copaifera (Copaiba balsam)
Prosopis glandulosa (Mesquite, algarroba)
Psoralea corylifolia (Bakuchi)
Pterocarpus santalinus (Barwood, rosewood, red sandalwood)
Pueraria lobata (Kudzu)
Pueraria tuberosa (Vidarikanda)
Saraca indica (Ashoka)
Sophora secundiflora (Mescal bean, red bean)
Tamarindus indica (Tamarind)
Trifolium pratense (Red clover)
Trifolium spp. (Clovers)
Trigonella foenum-graecum (Trigonella)
Vicia faba (Broad bean, fava bean, horse bean, Windsor bean)
Vigna angularis (Adzuki bean)

FAGACEAE (OAK OR BEECH FAMILY)

Castanea crenata (Japanese chestnut)
Castanea dentate (American chestnut)
Castanea mollissima (Chinese chestnut)
Castanea pumila (Chinquapin)
Castanea sativa (European chestnut)
Fagus crenata (Japanese beech)
Fagus grandifolia (American beech)
Fagus sylvatica (European beech, beechnut)
Lithocarpus densiflorus (Tan oak)
Quercus suber (Cork oak)
Quercus spp. (Oak)

FOUQUIERIACEAE (OCOTILLO FAMILY)

Foquieria splendens (Ocotillo)

GARRYACEAE (SILK TASSEL FAMILY)

Garrya elliptica (Coast silk tassel)
Garrya flavescens (Silk tassel, quinine bush)

GENTIANACEAE (GENTIAN FAMILY)

Gentiana lutea (Yellow gentian)
Swertia chirata (Chiretta)

GERANIACEAE (GERANIUM FAMILY)

Geranium spp. (Cranesbill)
Pelargonium odoratissimum (Rose geranium)

GRAMINAE (GRASS FAMILY)—SEE POACEAE

GROSSULARIACEAE (GOOSEBERRY FAMILY)

Ribes nigrum (Black currant)
Ribes rubrum (Red currant)
Ribes spp. (Gooseberry, currant)

HAMAMELIDACEAE (WITCH HAZEL FAMILY)

Hamamelis virginiana (Witch hazel)
Liquidambar orientalis (Styrax)
Liquidambar styraciflua (Sweet gum)
Loropetalum chinense (Razzleberry)

HIPPOCASTANACEAE (BUCKEYE FAMILY)

Aesculus arguta (Western buckeye)
Aesculus californica (California buckeye, horse chestnut)
Aesculus flava (Yellow buckeye)
Aesculus hippocastanum (Horse chestnut)
Aesculus pavia (Red buckeye)

HYDRANGEACEAE (HYDRANGEA FAMILY)

Hydrangea arborescens (Seven barks)
Hydrangea quercifolia (Oakleaf hydrangea)
Hydrangea macrophylla (Bigleaf hydrangea)
Hydrangea paniculata (Panicled hydrangea)

HYPERICACEAE (ST. JOHN'S WORT FAMILY)

Hypericum perforatum (St. John's wort, St. Johnswort)

ILLICIACEAE (STAR-ANISE FAMILY)

Illicium floridanum (Florida anise, purple anise)
Illicium parviflorum (Yellow star anise)
Illicium verum (Star anise, Chinese star anise)

IRIDACEAE (IRIS FAMILY)

Crocus sativus (Saffron)
Iris florentina (Orris root)
Iris versicolor (Blue flag)

JUGLANDACEAE (WALNUT FAMILY)

Carya illinoensis (Pecan)
Carya spp. (Hickory, pignut, mockernut)
Juglans ailanthifolia (Japanese walnut)
Juglans cinerea (Butternut)
Juglans nigra (Black walnut)
Juglans regia (English walnut)

JUNCACEAE (RUSH FAMILY)

Juncus bufonius (Toad rush)
Juncus effuses (Rush)

LAMIACEAE/LABIATAE (MINT FAMILY)

Coleus blumei, C. forskohlii syn. *Plectranthus barbatus* (Coleus)
Collinsonia canadensis (Stone root, horsebalm)
Hedeoma pulegioides (American pennyroyal, mock pennyroyal)
Hyptis suaveolens (Fat chia, wild spikenard)
Hyssopus officinalis (Hyssop)
Lavandula angustifolia syn. *L. officinalis, L. vera* (English lavender)
Lavandula stoechas (French lavender)
Leonurus cardiaca (Motherwort)
Lycopus europaeus, L. virginicus (Bugleweed)
Marrubium vulgare (Horehound)
Melissa officinalis (Lemon balm)
Mentha arvensis (Wild mint)
Mentha piperita (Peppermint)
Mentha pulegium (Pennyroyal)
Mentha spicata (Spearmint)
Monarda didyma, M. fistulosa, M. spp. (Oswego tea, horsemint, bee balm, bergamot)
Nepeta cataria (Catnip)
Ocimum basilicum (Basil)
Ocimum tenuiflorum (Holy basil, tulsi basil)
Origanum majorana (Marjoram)
Origanum vulgare (Oregano)
Perilla frutescens (Perilla)
Pogostemon cablin (Patchouli)
Prunella vulgaris (Self-heal, xia ku cao)
Salvia columbariae (Chia, chan)
Salvia divinorum (Heirba de la pastora, heirba de la virgen)
Salvia officinalis (Sage)
Salvia rosmarinus (Rosemary)
Salvia sclarea (Clary sage)
Salvia hortensis (Savory)
Scutellaria lateriflora (Skullcap)
Scutellaria baicalensis (Baikal skullcap)
Stachys palustris (Marsh woodwort)
Stachys officinalis (Betony)
Thymus vulgaris (Thyme)
Trigonella foenum-graecum (Fenugreek, methika)
Vitex agnus-castus (Vitex, chaste tree)
Vitex negundo (Nirgundi)

LAURACEAE (LAUREL FAMILY)

Aniba rosaeodora (Rosewood)
Cinnamomum camphora (Camphor, ravintsara)
Cinnamomum cassia (Cassia)
Cinnamomum verum syn. *C. zeylanicum* (Cinnamon)
Laurus nobilis (Bay laurel)
Persea americana (Aguacate, avocado, alligator pear)
Sassafras albidum (Sassafras)
Umbellularia californica (California laurel, pepperwood)

LINACEAE (FLAX FAMILY)

Linum catharticum (Purging flax)
Linum usitatissimum (Flax)

LOGANIACEAE (LOGANIA FAMILY)

Gelsemium elegans (Allspice jessamine)
Gelsemium sempervirens (Yellow jessamine, yellow jasmine)
Strychnos nux-vomica (Nux vomica)

MAGNOLIACEAE (MAGNOLIA FAMILY)

Liriodendron tulipifera (Tulip tree)
Magnolia officinalis (Houpu magnolia, magnolia bark)
Magnolia virginiana (Sweet bay)

MALPIGHIACEAE (MALPIGHIA FAMILY)

Banisteriopsis caapi (Yage, vine of the soul, ayahuasca)

MALVACEAE (COTTON OR MALLOW FAMILY)

Abelmoschus esculentus (Okra, gumbo)
Althaea officinalis (Marshmallow)
Gossypium arboretum (Tree cotton)
Gossypium spp. (Cotton root)
Hibiscus sabdariffa (Roselle, sorrel, hibiscus)
Malva spp. (Mallow)
Sida cordifolia (Bala, Indian country mallow)

MELIACEAE (MAHOGANY FAMILY)

Azadirachta indica (Neem)

MENISPERMACEAE (MOONSEED FAMILY)

Tinospora cordifolia (Guduchi)

MENYANTHACEAE (BOG BEAN FAMILY)

Menyanthes trifoliata (Buckbean, bogbean)

MORACEAE (FIG OR MULBERRY FAMILY)

Ficus carica (Fig)
Ficus hispida (Kakadumbara)
Morus spp. (Mulberry)

MYRICACEAE (MYRICA FAMILY)

Morella californica (California bayberry)
Morella cerifera (Wax myrtle)
Morella pensylvanica (Bayberry)

MYRISTICACEAE (NUTMEG FAMILY)

Myristica fragrans (Mace, Nutmeg)
Virola spp. (Epena, Otoba butter)

MYRSINACEAE (MYRSINE FAMILY)

Embelia ribes (Vidanga)

MYRTACEAE (MYRTLE OR EUCALYPTUS FAMILY)

Eucalyptus globulus, E. spp. (Eucalyptus, blue gum)
Melaleuca alternifolia (Tea tree)
Melaleuca leucadendra (Cajeput)
Melaleuca quinquenervia (Niaouli)
Myrtus communis (Common myrtle)
Pimenta dioica (Allspice, bay)
Pimenta racemosa (Bay leaf, bay rum)
Syzygium aromaticum syn. *Caryophyllus aromaticus, Eugenia caryophyllata, E. aromaticum* (Clove)
Syzygium cumini syn. *Eugenia jambolanum* (Jambul)

NELUMBONACEAE (INDIAN LOTUS FAMILY)

Nelumbo nucifera (Sacred lotus, Indian lotus, padma, kamala)
Nelumbo pentapetala (Water chinquapin)

NYCTAGINACEAE (FOUR O'CLOCK FAMILY)

Boerhaavia diffusia (Punarnava, Indian hogweed)
Mirabilis jalapa (Marvel of Peru)
Mirabilis multiflora (Four o'clock)

NYMPHACEAE (WATER LILY FAMILY)

Nymphaea spp. (Water lily)
Nuphar lutea, N. polysepala (Yellow pond lily)

OLEACEAE (OLIVE FAMILY)

Chionanthus virginicus (Fringe tree)
Fraxinus americana (American ash)
Fraxinus excelsior (European ash)
Fraxinus pensylvanica (Red ash)
Jasminum officinale, J. grandiflorum (Jasmine)
Ligustrum lucidum (Privet, nu zhen zi)
Olea europaea (Olive tree)
Ptychopetalum olacoides (Muira puama)
Syringa vulgaris (Lilac)

ONAGRACEAE (EVENING PRIMROSE FAMILY)

Chamaenerion angustifolium (Fireweed)
Oenothera biennis (Evening primrose)

ORCHIDACEAE (ORCHID FAMILY)

Vanilla planifolia (Vanilla)

OROBANCHACEAE (BROOMRAPE FAMILY)

Pedicularis densiflora (Indian warrior)
Pedicularis groenlandica (Elephant's head)
Pedicularis spp. (Lousewort, betony, pedicularis)

OXALIDACEAE (OXALIS OR SORREL FAMILY)

Oxalis oregana (Redwood sorrel)

PAPAVERACEAE (POPPY FAMILY)

Argemone mexicana (Mexican poppy, prickly poppy)
Chelidonium majus (Greater celandine)
Corydalis ambigua (Yán hú suǒ)
Dicentra formosa (Bleeding heart)
Eschscholzia californica (California poppy)
Papaver somniferum (Opium poppy, poppy)
Sanguinaria canadensis (Bloodroot)

PASSIFLORACEAE (PASSION FLOWER FAMILY)

Passiflora incarnata (Passion flower)
Turnera diffusa (Damiana)

PEDALIACEAE (SESAME FAMILY)

Harpagophytum procumbens (Devil's claw)
Sesamum indicum (Sesame)

PHYLLANTHACEAE (PHYLLANTHUS FAMILY)

Phyllanthus amarus (Bhumiamalaki)
Phyllanthus emblica syn. *Emblica officinalis* (Amla, amalaki, dhatri, Indian gooseberry)

PHYTOLACCACEAE (POKE WEED OR POKE BERRY FAMILY)

Phytolacca americana (Poke, poke weed, poke berry)

PIPERACEAE (PIPER OR PEPPER FAMILY)

Piper betle (Betel pepper)
Piper cubeba (Cubeb pepper)
Piper longum (Long pepper, pippali)
Piper methysticum (Kava, kava kava, grog, yongona)
Piper nigrum (Black pepper, white pepper)

PLANTAGINACEAE (PLANTAGO FAMILY)

Bacopa monnieri (Brahmi)
Digitalis purpurea (Foxglove) *toxic
Picrorhiza kurroa (Kutki)
Plantago afra, P. ovata (Psyllium)
Plantago lanceolatum, P. major, P. minor (Plantain)
Rehmannia glutinosa (Chinese foxwort, di huáng)

PLUMBAGINACEAE (LEADWORT FAMILY)

Plumbago zeylanicum (Chitrak, white leadwort, chita)

POACEAE/GRAMINEAE (GRASS FAMILY)

Andropogon virginicus (Broomsedge)
Avena spp. (Wild oats)
Bambusa spp. (Bamboo, vamsa lochana)
Coix lacryma-jobi (Job's tears, adlay)
Cymbopogon citratus (Lemon grass)
Cymbopogon martinii (Palmarosa)
Cymbopogon nardus (Citronella)
Dendrocalamus spp. (Bamboo)
Guadua angustifolia (Bamboo)
Hierochloe odorata (Sweet grass)
Hordeum vulgare (Barley)
Oryza glaberrima (African rice, red rice)
Oryza sativa (Rice)
Panicum miliaceum (Proso millet)
Pennisetum glaucum (Pearl millet)
Phyllostachys spp. (Bamboo)
Saccharum officinarum (Sugar cane)
Secale cereale (Rye)
Setaria spp. (Foxtail millet)
Sorghum bicolor (Sorghum, milo, Sudan grass, broom corn)
x *Triticosecale* spp. (Triticale, wheat x rye)
Triticum durum (Durum wheat, macaroni wheat)
Vetiveria zizanioides (Vetiver, khus khus)
Zea mays (Corn, maize, teosinte)
Zizania palustris (Wild rice)

POLYGALACEAE (POLYGALA FAMILY)

Polygala senega (Senga snakeroot)
Polygala tenuifolia (Yuan zhi, Chinese polygala)

POLYGONACEAE (SMARTWEED OR KNOTWEED FAMILY)

Polygonum multiflorum (He shou wu, fo ti)
Rheum officinale (Indian rhubarb, Turkish rhubarb)
Rheum palmatum (Chinese rhubarb)
Rheum rhabarbarum (Rhubarb)
Rumex crispus (Yellow dock, dock)
Rumex hymenosepalus (Canaigre, tanner's dock)

PORTULACEAE (PURSLANE FAMILY)

Portulaca oleracea (Purslane)

PUNICACEAE (POMEGRANATE FAMILY)

Punica granatum (Pomegranate)

RANUNCULACEAE (BUTTERCUP OR CROWFOOT FAMILY)

Actaea rubra, A. arguta (Baneberry)
Aconitum columbianum, A. napellus (Monkshood, wolfbane)
Caulophyllum thalictroides (Blue cohosh)
Clematis wrightii (Desert clematis, virgin's bower, barbo de chivo)
Coptis chinensis (Coptis, goldthread)

Hydrastis canadensis (Goldenseal)
Nigella sativa (Nigella, black cumin, Krishna jiraka)
Paeonia lactafloria (White peony, bai shao)
Paeonia rubra (Red peony, chai shao)

RHAMNACEAE (BUCKTHORN FAMILY)

Ceanothus americanus, C. spp. (Red root, New Jersey tea)
Rhamnus cathartica, R. purshiana (Cascara sagrada)
Zizuphus jujuba (Jujube date, Chinese date)
Zizuphus spinosa (Zizuphus seed)

ROSACEAE (ROSE FAMILY)

Alchemilla vulgaris (Lady's mantle)
Agrimonia striata (Agrimony)
Crataegus oxyacantha, C. spp. (Hawthorn)
Cydonia oblonga (Quince)
Eriobotrya japonica (Loquat)
Filipendula ulmaria (Meadowsweet)
Fragaria spp. (Strawberry)
Malus sylvestris (Apple)
Potentilla spp. (Potentilla, cinquefoil, silvergrass)
Prunus africana (Pygeum tree, African pygeum, red stinkwood)
Prunus avium (Wild cherry)
Prunus armeniaca (Apricot)
Prunus domestica (Plum, prune)
Prunus dulcis (Almond, bitter almond)
Prunus emarginata (Bitter cherry, Mad River plant)
Prunus persica (Peach, nectarine)
Prunus serotina (Black cherry)
Pyrus communis (Pear)
Rosa spp. (Rose)
Rosa x *damascena* (Damascus rose)
Rubus chamaemorus (Cloudberry)
Rubus idaeus (Red raspberry)
Rubus occidentalis (Black raspberry)
Rubus parviflorus (Thimbleberry)
Rubus spectabilis (Salmonberry)
Rubus spp. (Boysenberry, loganberry, veitchberry, youngberry)
Rubus ursinus (California blackberry)

RUBIACEAE (MADDER OR COFFEE FAMILY)

Cinchona spp. (Quinine)
Coffea arabica (Arabian coffee)
Gardenia jasminoides (Gardenia)
Galium aparine (Cleavers, bedstraw)
Mitchella repens (Partridge berry, squaw vine)
Morinda citrifolia (Indian mulberry, noni)
Pausinystalia yohimbe (Yohimbe)
Psychotria ipecacuanha (Ipecac)
Psychotria viridis (Chacruna, amiruku panga)
Rubia cordifolia (Manjishtha, Indian madder)
Rubia tinctorum (Madder)
Uncaria spp. (Cat's claw, una de gato)

RUTACEAE (CITRUS FAMILY)

Aegle marmelos (Bilva, bael fruit, Bengal quince, wood apple tree, bel)
Angostura febrifuga (Angostura)
Barosma betulina (Buchu)
Citrus aurantifolia (Lime)
Citrus aurantium (Sour orange, bitter orange, Seville orange)
Citrus bergamia (Bergamot orange)
Citrus hystrix (Kaffir lime)
Citrus limon (Lemon)
Citrus medica (Citron)
Citrus x *nobilis* (Tangerine, sweet orange)
Citrus x *paradise* (Grapefruit)
Citrus reticulata (Clementine, Mandarin orange, tangerine)
Citrus x *tangelo* (Tangelo)
Fortunella spp. (Kumquat)
Galipea officinalis (Angostura)
Phellodendron spp. (Cork tree)
Pilocarpus jaborandi (Jaborandi)
Ruta graveolens (Rue)
Zanthoxylum americanum (Prickly ash)
Zanthoxylum piperitum (Sichuan pepper)

SALICACEAE (WILLOW FAMILY)

Populus alba (White poplar)
Populus balsamifera (Balsam poplar)
Populus grandidentata (Largetooth aspen)
Populus tremula (European aspen)
Populus tremuloides (Quaking aspen)
Salix alba (White willow)
Salix spp. (Willow)

SANTALACEAE (SANDALWOOD FAMILY)

Santalum album (Indian sandalwood)
Santalum spicatum (Australian sandalwood)

SAPINDACEAE (SOAP BERRY FAMILY)

Dimocarpus longan (Longan, lungan)
Litchi chinensis (Litchi nut, lychee nut)
Paullinia cupana, P. spp. (Guarana)
Sapindus saponaria (Soapberry)

SAURURACEAE (LIZARD'S TAIL FAMILY)

Anemopsis californica (Yerba mansa)

SAXIFRAGACEAE (STONE BREAKER FAMILY)

Bergenia ligulata syn. *Saxifraga ligulata* (Pashana bheda)
Heuchera glabra, H. micrantha (Alum root)

SCHISANDRACEAE (MAGNOLIA VINE FAMILY)

Schisandra chinensis (Schisandra, wu wei zi, five flavor berry, magnolia vine)

SCROPHULARIACEAE (SNAPDRAGON FAMILY)

Scrophularia californica (Figwort, California bee plant, carpenters's square)
Scrophularia nodosa (Figwort, woodland figwort)
Verbascum bombyciferum (Giant silver mullein)
Verbascum thapsus (Mullein)

SIMAROUBACEAE (QUASSIA FAMILY)

Castela emoryi, C. texana (Chaparro amargosa, crucifixon thorn)
Quassia amara (Surinam quassia, quassia)
Quassia indica (Quassia)

SIMMONDSIACEAE (JOJOBA FAMILY)

Simmondsia chinensis (Jojoba)

SMILAXACEAE (SMILAX FAMILY)

Smilax spp. (Sarsaparilla)

SOLANACEAE (NIGHTSHADE, POTATO, OR TOMATO FAMILY)

Atropa belladonna (Belladonna)* toxic
Capsicum annuum (Anaheim pepper, banana p., bell p., bird p., chili p., green p., jalapeno p., paprika p., pepperoni p., pimiento p., poblano p., Serrano p.)
Capsicum baccatum (Cayenne pepper, aji pepper)
Capsicum chinense (Aji pepper, habanero p., rocotillo p.)
Capsicum frutescens (Bird pepper, chili p., cayenne p., Tobasco p.)
Datura innoxia (Sacred datura, toloache, toloatzin)
Datura stramonium, D. metel (Dhattura, jimson weed, thorn apple, wyscoccan)
Hyoscyamus niger (Black henbane)
Lycium barbarum, L. chinense (Matrimony vine, wolfberry, goji berry, lycii berry)
Lycopersicon pimpinellifolium (Cherry tomato, wild currant tomato)
Mandragora officinarum (Mandrake, hexenkraut)
Nicotiana rustica (Indian tobacco)
Nicotiana tabacum (Tobacco)
Physalis peruviana (Cape gooseberry)
Solanum melongena (Eggplant, aubergine)
Solanum nigrum (Black nightshade, wonderberry)
Solanum tuberosum (Potato, Irish potato, white potato)
Withania somnifera (Ashwagandha)

STERCULIACEAE (KOLA OR CACAO FAMILY)

Cola acuminata, C. nitida (Kola nut, cola nut)
Theobroma cacao (Cacao)

STYRACACEAE (STYRAX FAMILY)

Styrax spp. (Benzoin)

SYMPLOCACEAE (SWEETLEAF FAMILY)

Symplocos racemosa (Lodhra)

THEACEAE (CAMELLIA OR TEA FAMILY)

Camellia sinensis (Tea)

TILIACEAE (BASSWOOD FAMILY)

Tilia americana (Basswood, linden tree)
Tilia cordifolia syn. *T. platyphyllos* ssp. *cordifolia* (European linden tree, lime tree)

TROPAEOLACEAE (NASTURTIUM FAMILY)

Tropaeolum majus (Nasturtium)

TYPHACEAE (CATTAIL FAMILY)

Typha spp. (Cattail)

ULMACEAE (ELM FAMILY)

Ulmus americana (American elm)
Ulmus fulva, U. rubra (Slippery elm)
Ulmus pumila (Siberian elm)

UMBELLIFERAE (UMBEL OR CARROT FAMILY)—SEE APIACEAE

URTICACEAE (NETTLE FAMILY)

Urtica dioica, U. spp. (Nettle)
Urtica urens (Nettle, dog nettle)

VALERIANACEAE (SPIKENARD FAMILY)

Nardostachys grandiflora syn. *Nardostachys jatamansi, Valeriana jatamansi* (Spikenard, jatamansi)
Valeriana officinalis (Valerian, moonroot)
Valeriana wallichi (Indian valerian, tagarah)

VERBENACEAE (VERVAIN OR VERBENA FAMILY)

Aloysia citriodora syn. *A. triphylla* (Lemon verbena)
Verbena hastata (Verbena, vervain)
Verbena officinalis (Blue vervain, verbena, vervain)

VIOLACEAE (VIOLET FAMILY)

Viola odorata (Sweet violet)
Viola spp. (Violet)

VISCACEAE (MISTLETOE FAMILY)

Phoradendron flavescens (Mistletoe)
Viscum album (Mistletoe)

VITACEAE (GRAPE FAMILY)

Vitis labrusca (Wild grape, Concord grape)
Vitis vinifera (European grape, wine grape, table grape, raisin)

ZINGIBERACEAE (GINGER FAMILY)

Alpinia galanga (Galangal)
Curcuma longa (Turmeric)
Elettaria cardamomum (Cardamom)
Kaempferia galanga (Kampferia galangal)
Zingiber officinale (Ginger)

ZYGOPHYLLACEAE (CALTROP FAMILY)

Guaiacum officinale, G. sanctum (Lignum vitae)
Larrea tridentata, L. spp. (Creosote)
Peganum harmala (Syrian rue, harmel)
Tribulus terrestris (Gokshura, puncture vine)

REFERENCES

- Hickman JC (ed.) *The Jepson Manual—Higher Plants of California.* Berkeley and Los Angeles, CA: University of California Press; 1993.
- Hill A. *Economic Botany.* New York, NY: McGraw-Hill; 1952.
- Pendell D. *Pharmako/Dynamis: Stimulating Plants, Potions and Herbcraft.* San Francisco, CA: Mercury House; 2005.
- Pendell D. *Pharmako/Gnosis: Plant Teachers and the Poison Path.* San Francisco, CA: Mercury House; 2005.
- Pendell D. *Pharmako/Poeia—Plant Powers, Poisons, and Herbcraft.* San Francisco, CA: Mercury House; 1995.
- Pole S. *Ayurvedic Medicine: The Principles of Traditional Practice.* Philadelphia, PA: Churchill Livingstone Elsevier; 2006.
- Smith Jr, JP. *Plants and Civilization.* Humboldt State University, Arcata, CA.
- The Plant List Version 1.1. website. http://www.theplantlist.org. Published 2013.

INDEX OF ALTERNATIVE NAMES (COMMON TO LATIN)

Acanthopanax	*Eleutherococcus*
Acerola	*Malpighia*
Aconite	*Aconitum*
Actaea	*Cimicifuga*
African bird pepper	*Capsicum*
Agathosma	*Barosma*
Agrimony	*Agrimonia*
Alder	*Alnus*
Alder, black	*Prinos*
Alder, buckthorn	*Frangula/Rhamnus*
Alfalfa	*Medicago*
Alisma	*Plantago alisma*
Alkanet	*Alkanna tinctoria*
Allspice	*Pimenta*
Almond	*Prunus amygdalus*
Alum root	*Heuchera*
American aloe	*Agave*
American sarsaparilla	*Aralia nudicaulis*
Amole	*Yucca*
Amur cork tree	*Phellodendron*
Anemone	*Anemone* spp.
Anise seed	*Pimpinella anisum*
Anise, star	*Illicium*
Anisum	*Pimpinella anisum*
Antelope horns	*Asclepias asperula*
Apricot	*Prunus armeniaca*
Arabic gum	*Acacia senegal*
Arbor vitae	*Thuja*
Arbutus, trailing	*Epigaea*
Archangel	*Angelica*
Armoracia	*Cochlearia*
Arrow leaf	*Balsamorhiza*
Artichoke	*Cynara*
Asafetida	*Ferula asafetida*
Ash	*Fraxinus*
Ash, mountain	*Sorbus*
Ash, prickly	*Zanthoxylum*
Ash, wafer	*Ptelea*
Asparagus	*Asparagus officinalis*
Ashwagandha	*Withania somnifera*
Aspen	*Populus tremuloides*
Avens	*Geum*
Avocado	*Persea americana*
Baby's breath	*Gypsophila*
Bai zhu	*Atractylodes*
Baikal skullcap	*Scutellaria baicalensis*
Bai shao	*Paeonia lactiflora*
Balloon bell flower	*Platycodon*
Balm of Gilead	*Populus candicans*
Balmony	*Chelone*
Balsam root	*Balsamorhiza*
Balsam tree	*Myroxylon*
Baneberry	*Actaea*
Barberry	*Berberis/Mahonia*
Barbo de chivo	*Clematis*
Barestem desert parsley	*Lomatium*
Basil	*Ocimum basilicum*
Basswood	*Tilia americana*
Bastard ginseng	*Codonopsis*
Bayberry	*Morella*
Bay laurel	*Laurus nobilis*
Bay leaf	*Laurus nobilis*
Bearberry	*Arctostaphylos*
Bear's foot	*Alchemilla*
Bearsfoot	*Polymnia*
Bear medicine	*Ligusticum porteri*
Bear's weed	*Eriodictyon*
Bedstraw	*Galium*
Bee balm	*Monarda*
Bee plant	*Scrophularia*
Beech	*Fagus*
Beet	*Beta vulgaris*
Belladonna	*Atropa*
Bergamot	*Citrus bergamia*
Bergamot	*Monarda*
Bethroot	*Trillium*
Betony	*Pedicularis*
Betony, wood	*Stachys*
Bilberry	*Vaccinium*
Birch	*Betula*
Birthroot	*Trillium*
Birthwort	*Aristolochia*
Biscuit root	*Lomatium*
Bishop's weed	*Ammi visnaga*
Bistort	*Polygonum bistorta*
Bitter milkwort	*Polygala*
Bittersweet	*Solanum dulcamara*
Blackberry	*Rubus villosus, R.* spp.
Black cohosh	*Actaea/Cimicifuga*
Black current	*Ribes nigrum*
Black elder	*Sambucus nigrum*
Black haw	*Viburnum prunifolium*
Black mustard	*Brassica nigrum*
Black pepper	*Piper nigrum*
Black root	*Leptandra*
Black walnut	*Juglans major*

Common name	Botanical name
Bladderwrack	*Fucus vesiculous*
Blazing star	*Liatris*
Bleeding heart	*Dicentra formosa*
Blessed thistle	*Cnicus benedictus*
Bloodroot	*Sanguinaria*
Blueberry	*Vaccinium*
Blue cohosh	*Caulophyllum*
Blue flag	*Iris*
Blue gentian	*Gentiana*
Blue ginseng	*Caulophyllum*
Blue gum tree	*Eucalyptus*
Blue vervain	*Verbena*
Blue violet	*Viola*
Bogbean	*Menyanthes*
Boneknit	*Symphytum*
Boneset	*Eupatorium perfoliatum*
Bonnet bell flower	*Codonopsis*
Borage	*Borago*
Bouncing bet	*Saponaria*
Brahmi	*Bacopa*
Brahmi	*Centella*
Bricklebush	*Brickellia*
Brookmint	*Mentha arvensis*
Broomrape	*Orobanche*
Broom tops	*Scoparius*
Bruisewort	*Symphytum*
Bryony	*Bryonia*
Buchu	*Barosma*
Buck brush	*Ceanothus*
Buckbean	*Menyanthes*
Buckeye	*Aesculus*
Buckthorn	*Frangula*
Buckthorn	*Rhamnus*
Buckwheat bush	*Eriogonum*
Bugleweed	*Lycopus*
Bunchberry	*Cornus*
Burdock	*Arctium*
Burnet	*Sanguisorba*
Burning bush	*Euonymus*
Bursage	*Ambrosia*
Buttercup	*Ranunculus*
High bush cranberry	*Viburnum opulus*
Butcher's broom	*Ruscus aculeatus*
Butter and eggs	*Linaria*
Butterbur	*Petasites*
Butterfly weed	*Asclepias tuberosa*
Butternut	*Juglans cinerea*
Buttonbush	*Cephalanthus*
Cachana	*Liatris*
Cacao	*Theobroma*
Cactus	*Cereus*
Calamus	*Acorus calamus*
California buckeye	*Aesculus californica*
California laurel	*Umbellularia*
California lilac	*Ceanothus*
California poppy	*Eschscholzia*
California slippery elm	*Fremontia*
California snakeroot	*Aristolochia californica*
California wax myrtle	*Morella californica*
Camphor tree	*Cinnamomum camphora*
Camphor weed	*Pluchea, Heterotheca*
Canada balsam	*Abies*
Canada fleabane	*Erigeron*
Canadian hemp	*Apocynum*
Canada snakeroot	*Asarum*
Canaigre	*Rumex hymenosepalus*
Candlewood	*Fouquieria*
Canela	*Cinnamomum*
Cannabis	*Cannabis sativa*
Canutillo	*Ephedra viridis*
Capers	*Capparis*
Caraway	*Carum*
Cardamom	*Elettaria*
Cardinal lobelia	*Lobelia cardinalis*
Cardo santo	*Argemone*
Carnation	*Dianthus*
Carpenter's square	*Scrophularia*
Carrot	*Daucus carota*
Caryophyllus	*Syzygium*
Cascara sagrada	*Rhamnus purshiana*
Cassia angustifolia	*Senna*
Cassia	*Cinnamomum cassia*
Castor bean	*Ricinus communis*
Cat's paw	*Antennaria*
Cataria	*Nepeta cataria*
Cat's claw	*Acacia greggii*
Catmint	*Nepeta × faassenii*
Catnip	*Nepeta cataria*
Cayenne	*Capsicum*
Cebadilla	*Swertia*
Cedar	*Cedrus*
Celandine	*Cheladonium*
Celery	*Apium*
Cenizio	*Leucophyllum*
Centaury	*Centaurium*
Centaury	*Agave*
Chai hu	*Bupleurum*
Chamomile, German	*Matricaria*
Chamomile, Roman	*Anthemis*
Chaparral	*Larrea*
Chaparro amargosa	*Castela*
Chaste tree berry	*Vitex*
Cheese plant	*Malva*

Chen pi, mature	*Citrus sinensis*
Cherry, wild	*Prunus virginiana*
Chervil	*Anthriscus*
Chestnut	*Castanea*
Chestnut, horse	*Aesculus*
Chickweed	*Stellaria media*
Chicory	*Cichorium*
Chilcuan	*Heliopsis*
Child root	*Pseudostellaria*
Chimaja	*Cymopterus*
Chinese foxglove	*Rehmannia*
Chinese goldthread	*Coptis*
Chinese matrimony vine	*Lycium*
Chinese senega	*Polygala tenuifolia*
Chinese wolfberry	*Lycium*
Chinese yam	*Dioscorea batatas*
Chive	*Allium schoenoprasum*
Chrysanthemum tanace.	*Tanacetum parthenium*
Chuan xiong	*Ligusticum striatum*
Chuchupate	*Ligusticum porteri*
Cilantro	*Coriandrum*
Cinnamon	*Cinnamomum*
Cinquefoil	*Potentilla*
Cistus	*Helianthemum*
Ci wu jia	*Eleutherococcus*
Clary sage	*Salvia sclarea*
Cleavers	*Galium*
Clover, red	*Trifolium pratense*
Clover, sweet	*Melilotus*
Clove	*Syzygium*
Cocoa	*Theobroma cacao*
Cochlearia	*Armoracia*
Cocklebur	*Xanthium*
Coconut	*Cocos nucifera*
Coffee	*Coffea arabica*
Cohosh, black	*Actaea/Cimicifuga*
Cohosh, blue	*Caulophyllum*
Colic root	*Dioscorea villosa*
Coltsfoot, eastern	*Tussilago*
Coltsfoot, western	*Petasites*
Columbine	*Aquilegia*
Columbo	*Swertia*
Comfrey	*Symphytum*
Common ivy	*Hedera helix*
Concha	*Marrubium*
Coneflower	*Echinacea*
Conopholis	*Orobanche*
Consumptive's weed	*Eriodictyon*
Conyza	*Erigeron*
Copaiba	*Copaifera*
Coriander	*Coriandrum*
Corona de Cristo	*Castela*
Cornsilk	*Zea mays*
Corn smut	*Ustilago*
Corydalis canadense	*Dicentra canadense*
Costmary	*Chrysanthemum balsamita*
Cota	*Thelesperma*
Cotton root	*Gossypium*
Cough grass	*Agropyron*
Cough root	*Ligusticum*
Cowboy tea	*Ephedra viridis*
Cow parsnip	*Heracleum*
Cowslip	*Primula*
Cramp bark	*Viburnum*
Cranberry	*Vaccinium oxycoccos*
Cranesbill	*Geranium*
Crawley	*Corallorhiza*
Creosote bush	*Larrea*
Crucifixion thorn	*Castela*
Cuauchichic	*Garrya*
Cubeb	*Piper cubeba*
Cudweed	*Gnaphalium*
Culver's root	*Leptandra*
Cumin	*Cuminum cyminum*
Currant	*Ribes*
Cypress	*Cupressus*
Da qing ye	*Isatis*
Da zao	*Ziziphus jujuba*
Damiana	*Turnera*
Dan shen	*Salvia miltiorrhiza*
Dandelion	*Taraxacum*
Dang shen	*Codonopsis*
Deer brush	*Ceanothus*
Desert anemone	*Anemone tuberosa*
Desert clematis	*Clematis*
Desert cotton	*Gossypium*
Desert lavender	*Hyptis*
Desert tea	*Ephedra viridis*
Desert willow	*Chilopsis*
Devil leaf	*Urtica*
Devil's bush	*Eleutherococcus*
Devil's claw	*Harpagophytum*
Devil's club	*Oplopanax*
Devil's dung	*Asafetida*
Devil's shrub	*Eleutherococcus*
Devil's walking stick	*Aralia hispida*
Dew of the sea	*Rosmarinus*
Dill	*Anethum*
Ditchweed	*Cannabis*
Dock	*Rumex*
Dodder	*Cuscuta*
Dogbane	*Apocynum*
Dog grass	*Agropyron*
Dogwood	*Cornus*

Dogwood, Jamaican	*Piscidia*
Don quai	*Angelica sinensis*
Dong quai	*Angelica sinensis*
Douglas fir	*Pseudotsuga*
Dropwort	*Filipendula*
Dugaldia	*Helenium*
Dusty miller	*Cineraria*
Echinopanax	*Oplopanax*
Ela	*Elettaria*
Elder	*Sambucus*
Elder, dwarf	*Aralia hispida*
Elecampane	*Inula*
Elephant's head	*Pedicularis*
Elephant tree	*Bursera*
Eleuthero	*Eleutherococcus*
Elk clover	*Aralia californica*
English ivy	*Hedera helix*
Epazote	*Chenopodium*
Escoba de la vibora	*Gutierrezia*
Eugenia	*Syzygium*
European mistletoe	*Viscum album*
Evening primrose	*Oenothera biennis*
Everlasting	*Euphrasia*
Everlasting	*Helichrysum*
Everlasting, pearly	*Anaphalis*
Eyebright	*Euphrasia*
Fang feng	*Saposhnikovia divaricata*
False aloe	*Agave*
False Solomon's seal	*Smilacina*
False unicorn root	*Chamaelirium*
Fennel	*Foeniculum*
Fenugreek	*Trigonella*
Fern, maidenhair	*Adiantum*
Fern, male	*Aspidium*
Ferula asafetida	*Asafetida*
Feverfew	*Tanacetum*
Fever wort	*Eupatorium perfoliatum*
Figwort	*Scrophularia*
Fireweed	*Chamaenerion*
Five flavor berry	*Schisandra*
Flag, blue	*Iris*
Flag, sweet	*Acorus*
Fleabane	*Erigeron*
Fleece flower	*Polygonum multiflorum*
Foxglove	*Digitalis*
Fu ling	*Poria cocos*
Fo ti	*Polygonum multiflorum*
Frankincense	*Boswellia*
Fringe tree	*Chionanthus*
Fumitory	*Fumaria*
Fu tze	*Aconitum carmichaelii*
Galangal	*Alpinia*
Gan cao	*Glycyrrhiza*
Gan jiang	*Zingiber*
Garlic	*Allium sativum*
Gay feather	*Liatris*
Gentian	*Gentiana*
Gentian, green	*Swertia*
Giant arbor vitae	*Thuja plicata*
Giant willow herb	*Chamaenerion*
Ginger	*Zingiber*
Ginger, wild	*Asarum*
Ginseng	*Panax*
Ginseng, Siberian	*Eleutherococcus*
Goat's head	*Tribulus*
Goat's rue	*Galega*
Gobernadora	*Larrea*
Gobo	*Arctium japonicum*
Goldenrod	*Solidago*
Goldenseal	*Hydrastis*
Goldthread	*Coptis*
Golden poppy	*Eschscholzia*
Golden smoke	*Corydalis*
Goosegrass	*Galium*
Gotu kola	*Centella*
Gou qi zi	*Lycium*
Grape	*Vitus vinifera*
Gravel root	*Eupatorium*
Guarana	*Paullinia*
Guelder rose	*Viburnum opulus*
Guggul	*Commiphora mukul*
Gum arabic	*Acacia senegal*
Gumweed	*Grindelia*
Gurmar	*Gymnema*
Gypsywort	*Lycopus*
Hair moss	*Usnea*
Hamula	*Brickellia*
Hare's ear root	*Bupleurum*
Hawthorn	*Crataegus*
He shou wu	*Polygonum multiflorum*
Heal all	*Prunella*
Heartsease	*Viola*
Hedge nettle	*Gratiola*
Hedge nettle	*Stachys*
Hediondilla	*Larrea*
Helianthemum	*Cistus*
Hellebore	*Veratrum*
Helleborine	*Epipactis*
Hemlock spruce	*Tsuga canadensis*
Hemp	*Cannabis*
Henbane	*Hyoscyamus*
Henna	*Lawsonia*
Hercules club	*Aralia spinosa*
High cranberry	*Viburnum*

Holacantha	*Castela*
Hollyhock	*Althaea*
Holy thistle	*Cnicus*
Honeysuckle	*Lonicera*
Hong zao	*Ziziphus jujuba*
Hop tree	*Ptelea*
Hops	*Humulus*
Horehound	*Marrubium*
Horehound, water	*Lycopus*
Horse balm	*Collinsonia*
Horse chestnut	*Aesculus*
Horse nettle	*Solanum*
Horsemint	*Monarda*
Horseradish	*Armoracia*
Horsetail	*Equisetum*
Hound's tongue	*Cynoglossum*
Hu lu ba	*Trigonella*
Huang bai	*Phellodendron*
Huang lian	*Coptis*
Huang qi	*Astragalus*
Huang qin	*Scutellaria baicalensis*
Huckleberry	*Vaccinium*
Hydrangea	*Hydrangea arborescens*
Hydrocotyle	*Centella*
Hyssop	*Hyssopus*
Iceland moss	*Cetraria*
Incensier	*Rosmarinus*
Incienso	*Brickellia*
Indian consumption plt.	*Lomatium*
Indian corn	*Zea mays*
Indian root	*Aristolochia*
Indian spinach	*Urtica*
Indian turnip	*Arisaema*
Indian warrior	*Pedicularis*
Indigo	*Isatis*
Indigo, wild	*Baptisia*
Inmortal	*Asclepias*
Ipe roxo	*Tabebuia*
Irish moss	*Chondrus crispus*
Ivy, common	*Hedera*
Ivy, ground	*Glechoma*
Jabin	*Piscidia*
Jaborandi	*Pilocarpus*
Jack in the pulpit	*Arisaema*
Jamaican dogwood	*Piscidia*
Jasmine	*Jasminum officinale*
Jasmine, yellow	*Gelsemium*
Jasmine, white	*Jasminium*
Jatamansi	*Nardostachys*
Jersey tea	*Ceanothus*
Jewel weed	*Impatiens*
Jie geng	*Platycodon*
Jimson weed	*Datura*
Jin yin hua	*Lonicera japonica*
Jojoba	*Simmondsia*
Jujube dates	*Ziziphus jujuba*
Juniper	*Juniperus*
Kava	*Piper methysticum*
Kava kava	*Piper methysticum*
Kelp	*Fucus*
Khella	*Ammi visnaga*
Kinnikinnick	*Arctostaphylos*
Klamath weed	*Hypericum*
Knotgrass	*Polygonum*
Kola	*Cola*
Labrador tea	*Ledum*
Lady's mantle	*Alchemilla*
Lamb's quarters	*Chenopodium*
Lapacho	*Tabebuia*
Lappa	*Arctium*
Larkspur	*Delphinium*
Laurel, California	*Umbellularia*
Lavender	*Lavandula*
Leafcup	*Polymnia*
Lechuguilla	*Agave*
Leek	*Allium porrum*
Lemon	*Citrus limon*
Lemon balm	*Melissa*
Lemon grass	*Cymbopogon*
Lemon thyme	*Thymus* x *citriodorus*
Lemon verbena	*Aloysia*
Leopard's bane	*Arnica*
Leptotaenia	*Lomatium*
Lettuce, wild	*Lactuca*
Lian qiao	*Forsythia*
Licorice	*Glycyrrhiza*
Licorice fern	*Polypodium*
Life root	*Senecio*
Lilac	*Syringa*
Lily of the valley	*Convallaria*
Lily, tiger	*Lilium tigrinum*
Lime, kaffir	Citrus hystrix
Lime	*Citrus aurantiifolia*
Lime, Persian	*Citrus × latifolia*
Linden	*Tilia cordata*
Ling zhi	*Ganoderma*
Lion's foot	*Alchemilla*
Liriosma	*Ptychopetalum*
Liverwort	*Hepatica*
Lizard tail	*Anemopsis*
Lobaria	*Sticta*
Loosestrife	*Lythrum*
Lotebush	*Condalia*

Lovage	*Ligusticum*
Lovage	*Levisticum*
Love parsley	*Ligusticum porteri*
Lousewort	*Pedicularis*
Lungwort moss	*Sticta*
Lungwort	*Pulmonaria*
Ma huang	*Ephedra*
Macrotis	*Actaea/Cimicifuga*
Madder	*Rubia cordifolium*
Madrone	*Arbutus*
Maguey	*Agave*
Mahonia	*Berberis*
Mai dong	*Ophiopogon*
Mai men dong	*Ophiopogon*
Maidenhair fern	*Adiantum*
Maidenhair tree	*Ginkgo*
Man t'ien hsing	*Centella*
Mandrake, American	*Podophyllum*
Manzanilla	*Matricaria*
Manzanita	*Arctostaphylos*
Maravilla	*Mirabilis*
Marigold, European	*Calendula*
Marijuana	*Cannabis*
Marjoram	*Origanum majorana*
Marsh fleabane	*Pluchea*
Marshmallow	*Althaea*
Mastranzo	*Marrubium*
Mate	*Ilex paraguariensis*
Matico	*Piper angustifolia*
Maturin	*Cacalia*
Maturique	*Cacalia*
May apple	*Podophyllum*
May pop	*Passiflora*
Meadow anemone	*Anemone*
Meadowsweet	*Filipendula*
Mescal buttons	*Lophophora*
Mesquite	*Prosopis*
Methi	*Trigonella*
Milkweed	*Asclepias*
Milfoil	*Achillea*
Milk thistle	*Silybum*
Mimbre	*Chilopsis*
Mint, water	*Mentha aquatica*
Mistletoe	*Viscum*
Monk's pepper	*Vitex*
Monkshood	*Aconite*
Moon root	*Valeriana*
Mormon tea	*Ephedra*
Moss, Iceland	*Cetraria*
Motherwort	*Leonurus*
Mountain balm	*Eriodictyon*
Mountain everlasting	*Antennaria*

Mountain holly	*Berberis*
Mountain laurel	*Kalmia*
Mountain mahogany	*Cercocarpus*
Mugwort	*Artemisia* spp.
Muira puama	*Ptychopetalum*
Mullein	*Verbascum*
Musk root	*Sumbul*
Mustard	*Sinapis*
Myroxylon pereirae	*Balsam of Peru*
Myroxylon toluifera	*Balsam of Tolu*
Myrrh	*Commiphora*
Nasturtium	*Tropaeolum*
Navajo tea	*Thelesperma*
Nettle	*Urtica*
New Jersey tea	*Ephedra*
Night-blooming cereus	*Cereus*
Notoginseng	*Panax notoginseng*
Nutmeg	*Myristica*
Oak	*Quercus*
Oats	*Avena*
Ocotillo	*Fouquieria*
Odontotrichum	*Cacalia*
Odostemon	*Berberis*
Ohio buckeye	*Aesculus*
Old man's beard	*Clematis*
Old man's beard	*Usnea*
Olive	*Olea*
Orange sneezeweed	*Helenium*
Oregano	*Origanum vulgare*
Oregon grape	*Berberis/Mahonia*
Oregon myrtle	*Umbellularia*
Oregon wintergreen	*Gaultheria*
Orris root	*Iris florentina*
Ox eye daisy	*Leucanthemum*
Parrot's beak	*Pedicularis*
Parsley	*Petroselinum*
Partridge berry	*Mitchella*
Pasque flower	*Anemone*
Passion flower	*Passiflora*
Pau d'arco	*Tabebuia*
Pausinystalia	*Corynanthe*
Peach tree	*Prunus persica*
Peniocereus	*Cereus*
Pennyroyal, American	*Hedeoma*
Pennyroyal, European	*Mentha pulegium*
Peony	*Paeonia*
Pepper, black	*Piper nigrum*
Pepper, cayenne	*Capsicum*
Peppermint	*Mentha piperita*
Pepperwood	*Umbellularia*
Periwinkle	*Vinca major*
Peruvian balsam	*Myroxylon balsamum*

Peruvian bark	*Cinchona*
Peyote	*Lophophora*
Phellodendron	*Phellodendron amurense*
Pickpocket	*Capsella*
Picrasma	*Picraena*
Pigweed	*Amaranthus*
Pine	*Pinus*
Pineapple weed	*Matricaria*
Pinkroot	*Spigelia*
Piper cubeba	*Cubeba*
Pipsissewa	*Chimaphila*
Plantain	*Plantago*
Pleurisy root	*Asclepias tuberosa*
Plumajillo	*Achillea*
Poke root, berries	*Phytolacca*
Poleo	*Mentha arvensis*
Poleo Chino	*Hedeoma*
Pomegranate	*Granatum*
Pond lily, white	*Nymphaea*
Pond lily, yellow	*Nuphar*
Ponil	*Cercocarpus*
Poor man's saffron	*Calendula*
Poplar buds	*Populus*
Potency wood	*Ptychopetalum*
Prairie dock	*Parthenium*
Prickly ash	*Zanthoxylum*
Prickly pear	*Opuntia*
Prickly poppy	*Argemone*
Primrose	*Primula*
Primrose, evening	*Oenothera*
Prince ginseng	*Ophiopogon*
Prince's root	*Pseudostellaria*
Privet	*Ligustrum*
Prodigiosa	*Brickellia*
Prunus africanum	*Pygeum africanum*
Pseudoginseng	*Panax notoginseng*
Psyllium	*Plantago ovata*
Pulsatilla	*Anemone*
Punica	*Granatum*
Purple sage	*Leucophyllum*
Pussy toes	*Antennaria*
Pyrethrum	*Chrysanthemum*
Qing pi, green	*Citrus viride*
Quassia	*Picraena*
Quebracho	*Aspidosperma*
Queen of the meadow	*Eutrochium purpureum*
Queen of the meadow	*Filipendula*
Queen's root	*Stillingia*
Quinine bark	*Cinchona*
Quinine bush	*Garrya*
Ragweed	*Ambrosia*
Ragwort	*Senecio*
Raiz del Indio	*Aristolochia watsonii*
Raspberry	*Rubus idaeus*
Rattlesnake master	*Eryngium*
Red osier	*Cornus*
Red root	*Ceanothus*
Red sage	*Salvia miltiorrhiza*
Reishi mushroom	*Ganoderma*
Ren shen	*Panax ginseng*
Resin weed	*Grindelia*
Rhamnus frangula	*Frangula*
Rhatany	*Krameria*
Rheumatism root	*Dioscorea villosa*
Rheumatism root	*Jeffersonia*
Rhodiola	*Rhodiola rosea*
Rhubarb	*Rheum*
Rock rose	*Cistus*
Roman chamomile	*Anthemis*
Rose	*Rosa*
Rosemary	*Salvia Rosmarinus*
Rue	*Ruta graveolens*
Rue, goats	*Galega*
Rue, meadow	*Thalictrum*
Rue, Syrian	*Peganum harmala*
Sabal	*Serenoa*
Safflowers	*Carthamus*
Saffron	*Crocus*
Saffron, American	*Carthamus*
Sage	*Salvia*
Sagebrush	*Artemisia tridentata*
Salvia root	*Salvia miltiorrhiza*
San qi	*Notoginseng*
Sandalwood	*Santalum*
Sangre de drago	*Jatropha*
Sanicle	*Sanicula*
Sarsaparilla, Indian	*Hemidesmus*
Sarsaparilla, true	*Smilax*
Sassafras	*Sassafras albidum*
Saw palmetto	*Serenoa*
Scarlet globe mallow	*Sphaeralcea*
Scarlet pimpernel	*Anagallis*
Schisandra	*Schisandra chinensis*
Scotch broom	*Cytisus scoparius*
Scouring rush	*Equisetum*
Selenicereus	*Cereus*
Self-heal	*Prunella*
Senecio cineraria	*Cineraria*
Senega snakeroot	*Polygala*
Senna	*Cassia, Senna*
Serpentaria	*Aristolochia*
Sha ren	*Amomum villosum*
Shan yao	*Dioscorea batatas*
Shavegrass	*Equisetum*

Shen san qi	*Panax notoginseng*
Sheng di huang	*Rehmannia* (unprocessed root)
Shepherd's purse	*Capsella*
Shinleaf	*Pyrola*
Shiu chiu	*Panax* (cured red)
Shu di huang	*Rehmannia* (prepared root)
Siberian ginseng	*Eleutherococcus*
Siler root	*Saposhnikovia divaricata*
Silk tassel	*Garrya*
Skullcap	*Scutellaria*
Skunk cabbage, eastern	*Symplocarpus*
Skunk cabbage, western	*Lysichiton*
Slippery elm	*Ulmus*
Snakeroot, Missouri	*Echinacea*
Snakeroot, Kansas	*Echinacea*
Snakeroot, Senega	*Polygala*
Snakeroot, Virginia	*Aristolochia serpentaria*
Snowball tree	*Viburnum*
Soapberry	*Sapindus*
Soapwort	*Saponaria*
Solomon's seal	*Polygonatum*
Sourwood	*Oxydendron*
Spearmint	*Mentha spicata*
Spikenard	*Aralia*
Squaw vine	*Mitchella*
Squaw weed	*Senecio*
St. John's wort	*Hypericum*
Stone root	*Collinsonia*
Stramonium	*Datura*
Strawberry	*Fragaria*
Sumach, fragrant	*Rhus aromatica*
Sumach, smooth	*Rhus glabra*
Sumach, sweet	*Rhus aromatica*
Sundew	*Drosera*
Suterberry	*Zanthoxylum*
Swamproot	*Anemopsis*
Sweet Annie	*Artemisia annua*
Sweet cicely	*Osmorhiza*
Sweet clover	*Melilotus*
Sweet flag	*Acorus calamus*
Sweet root	*Osmorhiza*
Sweet sagewort	*Artemisia annua*
Sweet wormwood	*Artemisia annua*
Sweetgum	*Liquidambar*
Syrian rue	*Peganum harmala*
Szechuan lovage	*Ligusticum striatum*
Tag alder	*Alnus*
Taheebo	*Tabebuia*
Tai zi shen	*Pseudostellaria*
Tang kwei	*Angelica sinensis*
Tang shen	*Codonopsis*
Tansy	*Tanacetum*
Tar weed	*Eriodictyon*
Tarragon	*Artemisia dracunculus*
Te de coral	*Bidens*
Teasel	*Dipsacus*
Thlaspi	*Capsella*
Thorn apple	*Datura*
Thorowax root	*Bupleurum*
Thyme	*Thymus vulgaris*
Tian dong	*Asparagus*
Tian men dong	*Asparagus*
Tian qi	*Panax notoginseng*
Tickseed	*Bidens*
Toadflax	*Linaria*
Tobacco	*Nicotiana*
Tobacco brush	*Ceanothus*
Tobacco, Indian	*Lobelia inflata*
Toluifera	*Myroxylon toluifera*
Toothache plant	*Spilanthes*
Toothache tree	*Zanthoxylum*
Tooth of the lion	*Taraxacum*
Torote	*Bursera*
Tree of heaven	*Ailanthus*
Trefoil	*Rubus idaeus*
Triticum	*Agropyron*
Trumpet flower	*Tecoma*
Tsuga	*Abies*
Turkey corn	*Dicentra*
Turkey mullein	*Eremocarpus*
Turkey rhubarb	*Rheum*
Turkey tail mushroom	*Trametes*
Turmeric	*Curcuma*
Turtlehead	*Chelone*
Uña de gato	*Uncaria*
Unicorn root	*Aletris/Chamaelirium*
Uva ursi	*Arctostaphylos*
Vanilla leaf	*Achlys*
Verbena	*Verbena*
Verbena, lemon	*Aloysia*
Veronicastrum	*Leptandra*
Vervain	*Verbena*
Virgin's bower	*Clematis*
Wafer ash	*Ptelea*
Wahoo	*Euonymus*
Water horehound	*Lycopus*
Water mint	*Mentha aquatica*
Water plantain	*Plantago alisma*
Wax myrtle	*Morella*
Western coltsfoot	*Petasites*
Western greenbrier	*Smilax*
White man's foot	*Plantago*
White pond lily	*Nymphaea*
White sage	*Salvia apiana*

White willow	*Salix alba*
Whorehouse tea	*Ephedra viridis*
Widow maker	*Eucalyptus*
Wild cherry	*Prunus virginiana*
Wild ginger	*Asarum*
Wild indigo	*Baptisia*
Wild lettuce	*Lactuca*
Wild oats	*Avena*
Wild spinach	*Urtica*
Wild yam	*Dioscorea*
Willow	*Salix*
Wind flower	*Anemone*
Wintergreen	*Gaultheria*
Witch hazel	*Hamamelis*
Witch's hair	*Usnea*
Witches pouch	*Capsella*
Woad	*Isatis*
Wolf berry	*Lycium*
Wood betony	*Stachys betonica*
Wormseed	*Chenopodium*
Wormwood	*Artemisia absinthium*
Woundwort	*Stachys*
Wu wei zi	*Schisandra*
Xi yang shen	*Panax quinquefolius*
Yan hu suo	*Corydalis*
Yarrow	*Achillea*
Yellow dock	*Rumex crispus*
Yellow jasmine	*Gelsemium*
Yellow pond lily	*Nuphar*
Yellow root	*Coptis*
Yellow vetch	*Astragalus*
Yerba buena	*Satureja*
Yerba de la negrita	*Sphaeralcea*
Yerba de sangre	*Berberis*
Yerba del buey	*Grindelia*
Yerba del lobo	*Helenium*
Yerba del sapo	*Ambrosia*
Yerba mansa	*Anemopsis*
Yerba mate	*Ilex*
Yerba reuma	*Frankenia*
Yerba santa	*Eriodictyon*
Yohimbe	*Corynanthe*
Yuan zhi	*Polygala tenuifolia*
Ze xie	*Plantago alisma*
Zhi shi (immature)	*Citrus × aurantium*

REFERENCE OF ALKALOID- AND TANNIN-CONTAINING HERBS

FORMULA COMBINATIONS: When formulating tincture compounds, it is important to avoid combining tannin- and alkaloid-containing herbs, as tannins precipitate proteins out of solution, reducing the efficacy of a compound. Compounding tannin- and alkaloid-based alcohol extracts into a base of simple syrup or glycerin reduces precipitation; however, tannins won't remain in solution long-term.

ALKALOID-CONTAINING HERBS

Aconitum (aconite)
Anemone (pulsatilla)
Argemone (prickly poppy)
Berberis (barberry)
Berberis (Oregon grape)
Clematis (virgin's bower)
Coptis (gold thread, huang lian)
Corydalis (Dutchman's breeches)
Cytisus scoparius (broom tops)
Datura (jimson weed)
Dicentra (bleeding heart)
Eschscholzia (California poppy)
Fouquieria (ocotillo)
Garrya (silk tassel)
Hydrastis (goldenseal)
Hyocyamus (henbane)
Jeffersonia (twin leaf)
Lactuca (wild lettuce)
Lobelia (puke weed)
Lophophora (peyote)
Lycium (lycii berry)
Nicotiana (tobacco)
Nuphar (yellow pond lily)
Papaver (poppy)
Passiflora (passion flower)
Peganum (Syrian rue)
Petasites (western coltsfoot)
Pilocarpus (jaborandi)
Ptelea (wafer ash, hop tree)
Sanguinaria (blood root)
Senecio (life root)
Solanum carolinense (horsenettle)
Solanum dulcamara (bittersweet)
Tribulus (puncture vine)
Tussilago (eastern coltsfoot)
Ustilago (corn smut)
Vinca (periwinkle)
Zanthoxylum (prickly ash)

TANNIN-CONTAINING HERBS

Abies (spruce)
Agrimonia (agrimony)
Alchemilla (lady's mantle)
Alnus (alder)
Anemopsis (yerba mansa)
Arbutus (madrone)
Arctostaphylos (manzanita, uva ursi)
Betula (birch)
Camillia sinensis (tea)
Ceanothus (red root)
Chamaenarion (fireweed)
Cinnamomum (cinnamon)
Cola nitida (kola nut)
Commiphora (myrrh)
Crataegus (hawthorn)
Ephedra (ma huang, Mormon tea)
Filipendula (meadowsweet)
Fraxinus (ash)
Geranium (cranesbill)
Ginkgo (maidenhair tree)
Granatum (pomegranate)
Guaiacum (lignum vitae)
Hamamelis (witch hazel)
Heuchera (alum root)
Hypericum (St. John's wort)
Jatropha (sangre de drago)
Juglans (walnut, butternut)
Kramaria (rhatany)
Lavandula (lavender)
Ligustrum (privet)
Lycopus (bugleweed)
Melissa (lemon balm)
Morella (bayberry)
Nepeta (catnip)
Orobanche (broomrape)
Paullinia (guarana)
Polygonum (bistort)
Potentilla (cinquefoil)
Prunus (wild cherry bark)
Quercus (oak)
Rheum (rhubarb)
Rhus (sumac)
Rosa (rose)
Rubus (blackberry, raspberry)
Rumex crispus (yellow dock)
Rumex hymenosepalus (canaigre)
Salvia (sage)
Salvia miltiorrhiza (dan shen)
Scutellaria (skullcap)
Trillium (wake robin)
Vaccinium (blueberry, huckleberry, bilberry)
Viburnum opulus (cramp bark)
Viburnum prunifolium (black haw)
Xanthium (cocklebur)

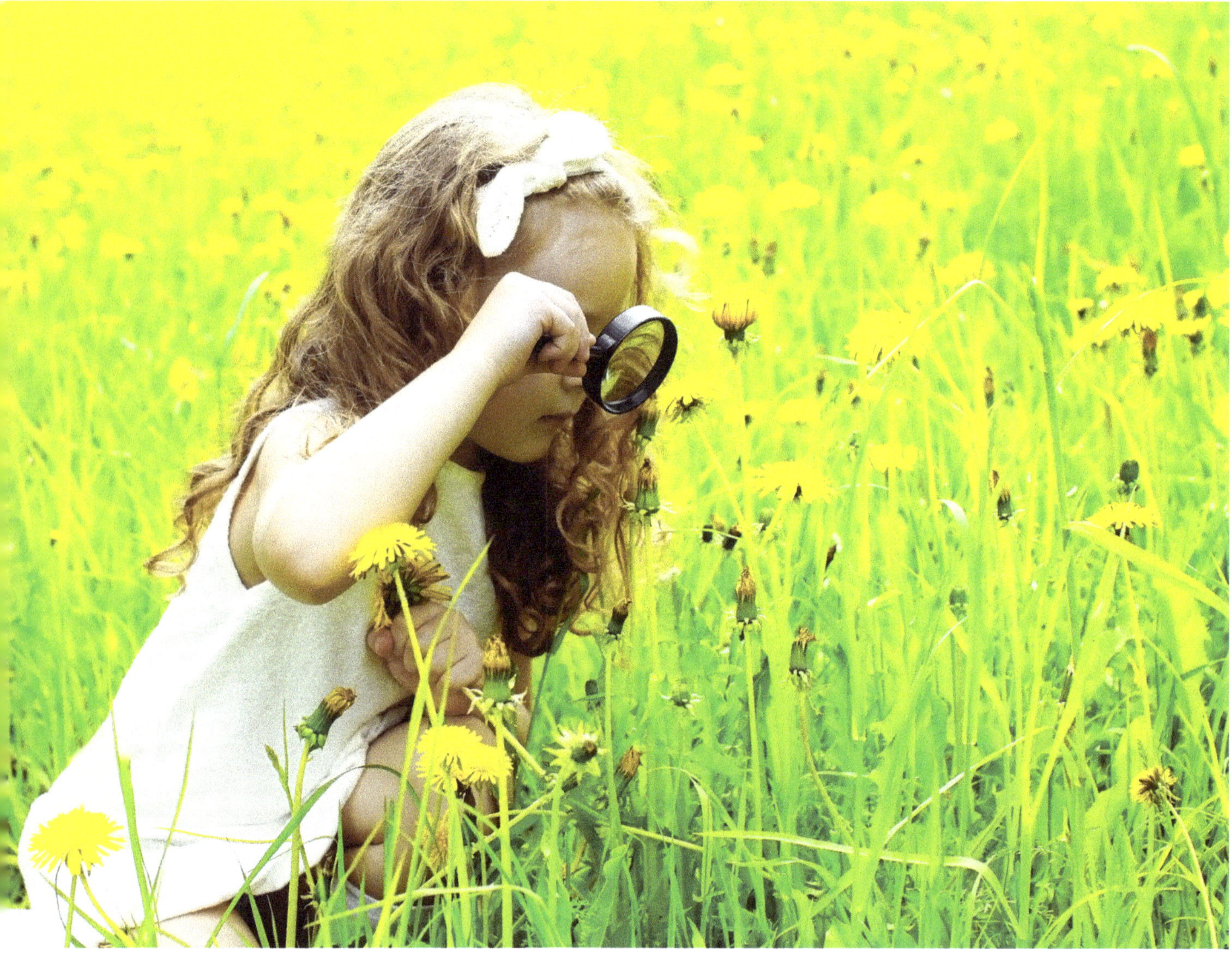

ENDNOTES

ALFALFA

1. Wojciechowski MF, Isely D. Medicago sativa. Flora Project. Jepson eFlora website. http://ucjeps.berkeley.edu/cgi-bin/get_IJMpl?tid=32943. Published 2014. Accessed February 18, 2015.
2. Medicago sativa. Flora of China. eFloras website. Missouri Botanical Garden, St. Louis, MO & Harvard University Herbaria, Cambridge, MA. http://efloras.org/florataxon.aspx?flora_id=2&taxonid=200012215. Published 2008. Accessed February 18, 2015.
3. Grieve M. *A Modern Herbal.* Great Britain: Jonathan Cape Ltd.; 1931: 501-502.
4. Foster S, Johnson R. *Desk Reference to Nature's Medicine.* Washington, D.C.: National Geographic Society; 2006: 12-13.
5. Leung AY, Foster S. *Encyclopedia of Common Natural Ingredients Used in Food, Drugs, and Cosmetics.* 2nd ed. Hoboken, NJ: A John Wiley & Sons, Inc.; 2003: 13-16.
6. Moore M. *Medicinal Plants of the Mountain West.* Santa Fe, NM: Museum of New Mexico Press; 2003: 23-24.
7. Pedersen M. *Nutritional Herbology: A Reference Guide to Herbs.* Warsaw, IN: Wendell W. Whitman Company; 1998: 34.
8. Willard T. *Edible and Medicinal Plants of the Rocky Mountains and Neighboring Territories.* Calgary, AB: Wild Rose College of Natural Healing; 1992: 129.
9. Ellingwood F. *American Materia Medica, Therapeutics, and Pharmacognosy.* Rev. ed. Albuquerque, NM: Southwest School for Botanical Medicine; 1994: 71.
10. Soule D. *The Roots of Healing, A Woman's Book of Herbs.* New York, NY: Carol Publishing Group; 1995: 45-46.

ALOE

1. McNeal DW. Aloe. Jepson Flora Project. Jepson eFlora website. http://ucjeps.berkeley.edu/cgi-bin/get_IJM.pl?tid=82544. Published August 26, 2008. Accessed March 6, 2015.
2. Aloe. Flora of China. eFloras website. Missouri Botanical Garden, St. Louis, MO & Harvard University Herbaria, Cambridge, MA. http://efloras.org/florataxon.aspx?flora_id=2&taxon_id=101163. Published 2008. Accessed March 6, 2015.
3. Aloe Flora of North America. eFloras website. Missouri Botanical Garden, St. Louis, MO & Harvard University Herbaria, Cambridge, MA. http://efloras.org/florataxon.aspx?flora_id=1&taxon_id=101163. Published 2008. Accessed March 6, 2015.
4. Leung AY, Foster S. *Encyclopedia of Common Natural Ingredients Used in Food, Drugs, and Cosmetics.* 2nd ed. Hoboken, NJ: A John Wiley & Sons, Inc.; 2003: 25-29.
5. Tyler V. *The Honest Herbal.* Binghamton, NY: The Hawthorn Press, Inc.; 1993: 25-28.
6. Agaru. Spoken Sanskrit Dictionary website. Version 4.2 http://spokensanskrit.de/index.php?tinput=aguru&script=&direction=SE&link=yes. Accessed March 27, 2015.
7. Ahalim. The Bible Hub website. http://biblehub.com/hebrew/174.htm. Accessed March 27, 2015.
8. Aloe. Online Etymology Dictionary website. http://www.etymonline.com/index.php?term=aloe&allowed_in_frame=0. Accessed March 27, 2015.
9. Ferox. The Latin Dictionary website. http://latindictionary.wikdot.com/adjective:ferox. Accessed March 27, 2015.
10. Pole S. *Ayurvedic Medicine: The Principles of Traditional Practice.* Philadelphia, PA: Churchill Livingstone Elsevier; 2006: 124-125.
11. Foster S, Johnson R. *Desk Reference to Nature's Medicine.* Washington, D.C.: National Geographic Society; 2006: 14-15.
12. Murray M. *The Healing Power of Herbs.* Rocklin, CA: Prima Publishing; 1992, 1995: 29-42.
13. Ellingwood F. *American Materia Medica, Therapeutics, and Pharmacognosy.* Rev. ed. Albuquerque, NM: Southwest School for Botanical Medicine; 1994: 14-15.
14. King J, Felter H, Lloyd J. *King's American Dispensatory* (Volume 1, 19th Edition, Third Revision). Cincinnati, OH: The Ohio Valley Company; 1905: 148-152.
15. Scudder J. *The American Eclectic Materia Medica and Therapeutics* (Twelfth Edition). Cincinnati, OH: The Scudder Brothers Company Publishers; 1898: 170-171.
16. Felter HW. *The Eclectic Materia Medica, Pharmacology and Therapeutics.* Cincinnati, OH: Published by John K. Scudder; 1922: 11.
17. Skenderi G. *Herbal Vade Mecum.* Rutherford, NJ: Herbacy Press; 2003: 10-11.
18. Pedersen M. *Nutritional Herbology: A Reference Guide to Herbs.* Warsaw, IN: Wendell W. Whitman Company; 1998: 36-37.
19. Mills S, Bone K. *Principles and Practice of Phytotherapy.* London, UK: Harcourt Publishers Limited; 2000: 133, 149.
20. Willard T. *The Wild Rose Scientific Herbal.* Calgary, AB: Wild Rose College of Natural Healing; 1998: 11-15.
21. Moore M. Lecture presented at Southwest School for Botanical Medicine residency program. Albuquerque, NM; 1994.
22. Foster S. *An Illustrated Guide to 101 Medicinal Herbs.* Loveland, CO: Interweave Press, Inc.; 1998: 18-19.
23. Weiss, RF. *Herbal Medicine.* Avon, UK: The Bath Press; 1996: 109-110.

AMBROSIA

1. Ambrosia. Flora of North America. eFloras website. Missouri Botanical Garden, St. Louis, MO & Harvard University Herbaria, Cambridge, MA. http://efloras.org/florataxon.aspx?flora_id=1&taxon_id=101325. Accessed May 8, 2015.
2. Keil DJ. Ambrosia. Jepson Flora Project. Jepson eFlora website. http://ucjeps.berkeley.edu/cgi-bin/get_IJM.pl?tid=812. Accessed May 8, 2015.
3. Ambrosia. Flora of China. eFloras website. Missouri Botanical Garden, St. Louis, MO & Harvard University Herbaria, Cambridge, MA. http://efloras.org/florataxon.aspx?flora_id=2&taxon_id=101325. Accessed May 8, 2015.
4. Charters, M. California Plant Names: Latin and Greek Meanings and Derivations website. http://www.calflora.net/botanicalnames/pageAB-AM.html. Accessed November 19, 2015.
5. Charters, M. California Plant Names: Latin and Greek Meanings and Derivations website. http://www.calflora.net/botanicalnames/pageCA-CH.html. Accessed November 19, 2015.
6. Charters M. California Plant Names: Latin and Greek Meanings and Derivations website. http://www.calflora.net/botanicalnames/pageCI-CY.html. Accessed November 19, 2015.
7. Charters M. California Plant Names: Latin and Greek Meanings and Derivations website. http://www.calflora.net/botanicalnames/pagePI-PY.html. Accessed November 19, 2015.
8. Curtin, LSM. revised by Michael Moore. *Healing Herbs of the Upper Rio Grande.* Santa Fe, New Mexico: Western Edge Press; revised edition 1997: 195-196.
9. Foster, SH. Christopher. *Western Medicinal Plants and Herbs.* New York, New York: Peterson Field Guides, Houghton Mifflin Company; 2002: 248.
10. King, J, Felter, H, Lloyd, J. *King's American Dispensatory* (Volume 1, 19th Edition, Third Revision). Cincinnati, OH: The Ohio Valley Company; 1905: 168.
11. Cane C. *Herbal Medicine of the American Southwest.* Lincoln Town Press; 2006; 39-41.
12. Moore M. Lecture notes from Southwest School for Botanical Medicine residency program. Albuquerque, NM: 1994.
13. Seller A. Lecture notes from Pacific School of Herbal Medicine. Oakland, CA: 1995.
14. Wang P, Liang W, Kong C, Jiang Y. Allelopathic potential of volatile allelochemicals of Ambrosia trifida. *Allelopathic Journal.* 2004 Nov: 15(1): 131-136. http://www.researchgate.net/publication/259823647_Allelopathic_potentials_of_volatile_allelochemicals_of_Ambrosia_trifida_L_on_other_plants. Accessed November 19, 2005.
15. Moore M. *Medicinal Plants of the Pacific Northwest.* Santa Fe, NM: Red Crane Books; 1993: 291.

ANEMONE

1. Anemone pulsatilla L., Sp. Pl.:559 (1753). Medicinal Plant Names Service. Kew Royal Botanic Gardens website. http://mpns.kew.org/mpns-portalplantDetail?plantId=638599&query=anemone&filter=&fuzzy=false&nameType=other&dbs=wcsCmp. Accessed February 10, 2017.
2. Simono S. Anemone. Jepson Flora Project. Jepson eFlora website. http://ucjeps.berkeley.edu/eflora/eflora_display.php?tid=10123. Accessed December 30, 2016.
3. Dutton BE, Keener, CS, Ford, BA. Anemone. Flora of North America. eFloras website. Missouri Botanical Garden, St. Louis, MO & Harvard University Herbaria, Cambridge, MA. http://efloras.org/florataxon.aspx?flora_id=1&taxon_id=101733. Accessed December 30, 2016.
4. Pojar J, MacKinnon A. *Plants of the Pacific Northwest Coast.* Vancouver, BC: Lone Pine Publishing; 1994: 172-173.
5. Grieve, M. *A Modern Herbal.* Great Britain: Jonathan Cape Ltd.; 1931: 32-34.
6. Foster S, Johnson R. *Desk Reference to Nature's Medicine.* Washington, D.C.: National Geographic Society; 2006: 294-295.
7. Ellingwood F. *American Materia Medica, Therapeutics, and Pharmacognosy.* Rev. ed. Albuquerque, NM: Southwest School for Botanical Medicine; 1994: 87-88.
8. William, Salmon. *1710 Botanologia, or The English Herbal.* London: Dawks, Rhodes, and Taylor. Republished online by Henriette Kress, 1999. http://www.henriettes-herb.com/eclectic/salmon/anemones-wild.html. Accessed March 31, 2017.
9. Foster, S, Hobbs, C. *Western Medicinal Plants and Herbs.* New York, NY: Peterson Field Guides, Houghton Mifflin Company; 2002: 78-79.
10. King J, Felter H, Lloyd, *J. King's American Dispensatory,* 1898. http://www.henriettes-herb.com/eclectic/kings/anemone-nemo.html. Republished online by Henriette Kress, 1999. Accessed April 7, 2017.
11. Skenderi G. *Herbal Vade Mecum.* Rutherford, NJ: Herbacy Press; 2003: 308.
12. Moore M. *Medicinal Plants of the Pacific Northwest.* Santa Fe, NM: Red Crane Books; 1993: 257-263.
13. Scudder JM. *Specific Medication and Specific Medicines.* Cinncinatti, OH: Wilstach, Baldwin & Co.,1870. Republished online by Henriette Kress, 1999. Available at http://www.henriettes-herb.com/eclectic/spec-med/pulsatilla.html. Accessed April 7, 2017.
14. Seller A. Lecture notes from Pacific School of Herbal Medicine. Oakland, CA; 1995.
15. Felter HW. *The Eclectic Materia Medica, Pharmacology and Therapeutics.* Cincinnati, OH: Published by John K. Scudder; 1922: 95-97.

ANGELICA

1. Constance L, Wetherwax M. Angelica. Jepson Flora Project. Jepson eFlora website. http://ucjeps.berkeley.edu/cgi-bin/get_IJM.pl?tid=10358. Accessed December 3, 2015.
2. Angelica archangelica (angelica). Kew Royal Botanic Gardens Website. http://www.kew.org/science-conservation/plants-fungi/angelica-archangelica-angelica. Accessed December 3, 2015.
3. Grieve M. *A Modern Herbal.* Great Britain: Jonathan Cape Ltd.; 1931: 35-40.
4. Foster, S, Johnson, R. *Desk Reference to Nature's Medicine.* Washington, D.C.: National Geographic Society; 2006: 18-19.
5. Pojar, J, MacKinnon, A. *Plants of the Pacific Northwest Coast.* Vancouver, BC: Lone Pine Publishing; 1994: 218.
6. Foster S, Hobbs C. *Western Medicinal Plants and Herbs.* New York, NY: Peterson Field Guides, Houghton Mifflin Company; 2002: 65-67.
7. Murray M. *The Healing Power of Herbs.* Rocklin, CA: Prima Publishing; 1992: 43-49.
8. Leung AY, Foster S. *Encyclopedia of Common Natural Ingredients Used in Food, Drugs, and Cosmetics.* 2nd ed. Hoboken, NJ: A John Wiley & Sons, Inc.; 2003: 32-34.
9. Willard T. *The Wild Rose Scientific Herbal.* Calgary, AB: Wild Rose College of Natural Healing; 1998: 16-18.
10. Lust J. *The Herb Book.* New York, NY: Bantam Books; 1974: 97-99.
11. Moore M. *Medicinal Plants of the Mountain West.* Santa Fe, NM: Museum of New Mexico Press; 2003: 30-34.
12. Foster S. *Herbal Renaissance.* Layton, UT: Peregrine Smith Books; 1993: 36-38.
13. Moore M. *Medicinal Plants of the Pacific Northwest.* Santa Fe, NM: Red Crane Books; 1993: 41-45.
14. Moore M. Lecture presented at Southwest School for Botanical Medicine residency program. Albuquerque, NM; 1994.
15. Skenderi G. *Herbal Vade Mecum.* Rutherford, NJ: Herbacy Press; 2003: 13-14.
16. Weiss RF. *Herbal Medicine.* Avon, UK: The Bath Press; 1996: 46.

ANISE

1. *Growing Herbs: Bulletin #54.* University of Arizona Cooperative Extension, Yavapai County. http://extension.arizona.edu/sites/extension.arizona.edu/files/resources/growingherbs_0.pdf. Accessed April, 15, 2015.
2. Pimpinella anisum. Flora of China. eFloras website. Missouri Botanical Garden, St. Louis, MO & Harvard University Herbaria, Cambridge, MA. http://efloras.org/florataxon.aspx?flora_id=2&taxon_id=200015767. Accessed April 2, 2015.
3. Apiaceae. Flora of China. eFloras website. Missouri Botanical Garden, St. Louis, MO & Harvard University Herbaria, Cambridge, MA. http://efloras.org/florataxon.aspx?flora_id=2&taxon_id=10052. Accessed April 2, 2015.
4. Grieve M. *A Modern Herbal.* Great Britain: Jonathan Cape Ltd.; 1931: 41-42.
5. Anise (Pimpinella anisum L.). Katzer, Gernot Spice Page. http://gernot-katzers-spice-pages.com/engl/Pimp_ani.html. Accessed April 2, 2015.
6. Willard T. *The Wild Rose Scientific Herbal.* Calgary, AB: Wild Rose College of Natural Healing; 1998: 19.
7. Lust J. *The Herb Book.* New York, NY: Bantam Books; 1974: 99-100.
8. Foster S. *Herbal Renaissance.* Layton, UT: Peregrine Smith Books; 1993: 38.
9. Leung AY, Foster S. *Encyclopedia of Common Natural Ingredients Used in Food, Drugs, and Cosmetics.* 2nd ed. Hoboken, NJ: A John Wiley & Sons, Inc.; 2003: 36-38.
10. Skenderi G. *Herbal Vade Mecum.* Rutherford, NJ: Herbacy Press; 2003: 15.
11. Tierra M. *The Way of Herbs.* New York, NY: Pocket Books; 1990: 107.
12. Moore M. Lecture presented at Southwest School for Botanical Medicine residency program. Albuquerque, NM; 1994.
13. Schnaubelt K. *Advanced Aromatherapy — The Science of Essential Oil Therapy.* Rochester, VT: Healing Arts Press; 1995: 59.
14. Keville K, Green M. *Aromatherapy — A Complete Guide to the Healing Art.* Freedom, CA: The Crossing Press; 1995: 46.

ARALIA

1. Foster S, Johnson R. *Desk Reference to Nature's Medicine.* Washington, D.C.: National Geographic Society; 2006: 336-337.
2. Hickman JC. (ed.). *The Jepson Manual: Higher Plants of California.* Berkeley, CA: University of California Press; 1996: 169.
3. Willard T. *Edible and Medicinal Plants of the Rocky Mountains and Neighboring Territories.* Calgary, AB: Wild Rose College of Natural Healing; 1992: 148-150.
4. Foster S, Hobbs C. *Western Medicinal Plants and Herbs.* New York, NY: Peterson Field Guides, Houghton Mifflin Company; 2002: 69-70.
5. Ellingwood F. *American Materia Medica, Therapeutics, and Pharmacognosy.* Rev. ed. Albuquerque, NM: Southwest School for Botanical Medicine; 1994: 12.
6. Felter HW. *The Eclectic Materia Medica, Pharmacology and Therapeutics.* Cincinnati, OH: Published by John K. Scudder, 1922: 14.
7. Felter HW, Lloyd JU. *King's American Dispensatory.* Vol. 1, 19th ed, 3rd Revision. Cincinnati, OH: The Ohio Valley Company; 1923: 261-264.
8. Scudder J. *The American Eclectic Materia Medica and Therapeutics* (Twelfth Edition). Cincinnati, OH: The Scudder Brothers Company Publishers; 1898: 214; 251; 354; 484; 485.

9. Moore M. *Medicinal Plants of the Pacific Northwest.* Santa Fe, NM: Red Crane Books; 1993: 116-120.
10. Skenderi G. *Herbal Vade Mecum.* Rutherford, NJ: Herbacy Press; 2003: 355-356.
11. Moore M. Lecture presented at Southwest School for Botanical Medicine residency program. Albuquerque, NM; 1994.
12. Seller A. Lecture notes from Pacific School of Herbal Medicine. Oakland, CA; 1995.

ARNICA

1. Wolf SJ, Barkley TM. Arnica. Jepson eFlora website. http://ucjeps.berkeley.edu/cgi-bin/get_IJM.pl?tid=322. Published August 26, 2008. Accessed January 16, 2015.
2. Wolf SJ. Arnica. Flora of North America. eFloras website. Missouri Botanical Garden, St. Louis, MO & Harvard University Herbaria, Cambridge, MA. http://efloras.org/florataxon.aspx?flora_id=1&taxon_id=102636. Published 2008. Accessed January 16, 2015.
3. Foster S, Johnson R. *Desk Reference to Nature's Medicine.* Washington, D.C.: National Geographic Society; 2006: 20-21.
4. Charters ML. Wrightii. California Plant Names: Latin and Greek Meanings and Derivations website. http://www.calflora.net/botanicalnames/pageMI-MY.html. Updated 2014. Accessed January 19, 2015.
5. Online Etymology Dictionary. http://www.etymonline.com/index.php?term=Montana. Accessed January 19, 2015.
6. Ellingwood F. *American Materia Medica, Therapeutics, and Pharmacognosy.* Rev. ed. Albuquerque, NM: Southwest School for Botanical Medicine; 1994: 13-14.
7. Felter HW. *The Eclectic Materia Medica, Pharmacology and Therapeutics.* Cincinnati, OH: Published by John K. Scudder; 1922: 15-16.
8. Foster S, Hobbs C. *Western Medicinal Plants and Herbs.* New York, NY: Peterson Field Guides, Houghton Mifflin Company; 2002: 136-137.
9. Leung AY, Foster S. *Encyclopedia of Common Natural Ingredients Used in Food, Drugs, and Cosmetics.* 2nd ed. Hoboken, NJ: A John Wiley & Sons, Inc.; 2003: 40-42.
10. Willard T. *The Wild Rose Scientific Herbal.* Calgary, AB: Wild Rose College of Natural Healing; 1998: 21-23.
11. Moore M. *Medicinal Plants of the Mountain West.* Santa Fe, NM: Museum of New Mexico Press; 2003: 35-37.
12. Skenderi G. *Herbal Vade Mecum.* Rutherford, NJ: Herbacy Press; 2003: 18.

ARTICHOKE LEAF

1. Mills S, Bone K. *Principles and Practice of Phytotherapy.* London, UK: Harcourt Publishers Limited; 2000: 433-38.
2. Keil DJ, Turner CE. Cynara. Jepson Flora Project. Jepson eFlora website. http://ucjeps.berkeley.edu/cgi-bin/get_IJM.pl?tid=91740. Accessed April 10, 2015.
3. Cynara cardunculus. Flora of North America. eFloras website. Missouri Botanical Garden, St. Louis, MO & Harvard University Herbaria, Cambridge, MA. http://efloras.org/florataxon.aspx?flora_id=1&taxon_id=200023811. Accessed April 10, 2015.
4. Cynara cardunculus *Linnaus* subsp. cardunculus. Flora of North America. eFloras website. Missouri Botanical Garden, St. Louis, MO & Harvard University Herbaria, Cambridge, MA. http://efloras.org/florataxon.aspx?flora_id=1&taxon_id=250068239. Accessed April 10, 2015.
5. Eade S. *The History of Globe Artichoke.* http://gardenofeaden.blogspot.com/2009/06/history-of-globe-artichoke.html. Published online June 9, 2009. Accessed November 30, 2013.
6. Sonnante G, Pignone D, Hammer K. *The Domestication of Artichoke and Cardoon: From Roman Times to the Genomic Age.* http://www.ncbi.nlm.nih.gov/pmc/articles/PMC2759203/Ann Bot. 2007 October; 100(5): 1095-1100. Published online 2007 July 4. doi: 10.1093/aob/mcm127. Accessed November 24, 2013.
7. Murray M. *The Encyclopedia of Healing Foods.* New York, NY: Atria Books; 2005: 154-59.
8. King J, Felter HW, Lloyd, JU. *King's American Dispensatory.* Vol. 1, 19th ed, 3rd Revision. Cincinnati, OH: The Ohio Valley Company; 1923: 641.
9. Leung AY, Foster S. *Encyclopedia of Common Natural Ingredients Used in Food, Drugs, and Cosmetics.* 2nd ed. Hoboken, NJ: A John Wiley & Sons, Inc.; 2003: 42-44.
10. Hobbs C. *Foundations of Health—Healing with Herbs and Foods.* Capitola, CA: Botanica Press; 1992: 214-16.
11. Skenderi G. *Herbal Vade Mecum.* Rutherford, NJ: Herbacy Press; 2003:19-20.
12. Weiss RF. *Herbal Medicine.* Avon, UK: The Bath Press; 1996: 88-89.

ASHWAGANDHA

1. Withania somnifera. Flora of China. eFloras website. Missouri Botanical Garden, St. Louis, MO & Harvard University Herbaria, Cambridge, MA. http://efloras.org/florataxon.aspx?flora_id=2&taxon_id=200020616. Accessed December 2, 2014.
2. Withania somnifera. Flora of Pakistan. eFloras website. Missouri Botanical Garden, St. Louis, MO & Harvard University Herbaria, Cambridge, MA. http://efloras.org/florataxon.aspx?flora_id=5&taxon_id=200020616. Accessed December 2, 2014.
3. Withania. Flora of Pakistan. eFloras website. Missouri Botanical Garden, St. Louis, MO & Harvard University Herbaria, Cambridge, MA. http://efloras.org/florataxon.aspx?flora_id=5&taxon_id=134946. Accessed December 2, 2014.
4. Withania. Flora of China. eFloras website. Missouri Botanical Garden, St. Louis, MO & Harvard University Herbaria, Cambridge, MA. http://efloras.org/florataxon.aspx?flora_id=2&taxon_id=134946. Accessed December 2, 2014.
5. Pole S. *Ayurvedic Medicine: The Principles of Traditional Practice.* Philadelphia, PA: Churchill Livingstone Elsevier; 2006: 133-134.
6. Lad, V, Frawley D. *The Yoga of Herbs.* Twin Lakes, WI: Lotus Press; 1992: Frawley and Lad: 160-161.
7. Skenderi G. *Herbal Vade Mecum.* Rutherford, NJ: Herbacy Press; 2003: 23-24.

ASPARAGUS

1. Asparagus. The Flora of China. eFloras website. Missouri Botanical Garden, St. Louis, MO & Harvard University Herbaria, Cambridge, MA. http://efloras.org/florataxon.aspx?flora_id=2&taxon_id=102837. Published 2008. Accessed December 12, 2014.
2. Asparagus. The Flora of North America. eFloras website. Missouri Botanical Garden, St. Louis, MO & Harvard University Herbaria, Cambridge, MA. http://efloras.org/florataxon.aspx?flora_id=1&taxon_id=102837. Published 2008. Accessed December 12, 2014.
3. Asparagus. The Flora of Pakistan. eFloras website. Missouri Botanical Garden, St. Louis, MO & Harvard University Herbaria, Cambridge, MA. http://efloras.org/florataxon.aspx?flora_id=5&taxon_id=102837. Published 2008. Accessed December 12, 2014.
4. Asparagus cochinchinensis. The Flora of China. eFloras website. Missouri Botanical Garden, St. Louis, MO & Harvard University Herbaria, Cambridge, MA. http://efloras.org/florataxon.aspx?flora_id=2&taxon_id=200027560. Published 2008. Accessed December 12, 2014.
5. Asparagus racemosus. The Flora of China. eFloras website. Missouri Botanical Garden, St. Louis, MO & Harvard University Herbaria, Cambridge, MA. http://efloras.org/florataxon.aspx?flora_id=2&taxon_id=240001105. Published 2008. Accessed December 12, 2014.
6. Asparagus racemosus. The Flora of Pakistan. eFloras website. Missouri Botanical Garden, St. Louis, MO & Harvard University Herbaria, Cambridge, MA. http://efloras.org/florataxon.aspx?flora_id=5&taxon_id=240001105. Published 2008. Accessed December 12, 2014.
7. Caldecott T. Shatavari. Todd Caldecott website. http://toddcaldecott.com/herbs/shatavari/. Updated 2014. Accessed December 12, 2014.
8. Charters M. California Plant Names: Latin and Greek Meanings and Derivations website. http://www.calflora.net/botanicalnames/pageAN-AZ.html. Accessed October 28, 2015.
9. Charters M. California Plant Names: Latin and Greek Meanings and Derivations website. http://www.calflora.net/botanicalnames/pageR.html. Accessed October 28, 2015.
10. Charters M. California Plant Names: Latin and Greek Meanings and Derivations website. http://www.calflora.net/botanicalnames/pageLH-LY.html. Accessed October 28, 2015.

11. Backyard Gardener website. http://www.backyardgardener.com/gardendictionary/cochinchinensis.html. Accessed October 28, 2015.
12. Pole S. *Ayurvedic Medicine: The Principles of Traditional Practice.* Philadelphia, PA: Churchill Livingstone Elsevier; 2006: 271-272.
13. Bensky D, Gamble A. *The Chinese Herbal Medicine Materia Medica.* Rev. ed. Seattle, WA: Eastland Press; 1993: 359-360.
14. Teeguarden R. *Chinese Tonic Herbs.* Tokyo, Japan: Japan Publications, Inc.; 1995: 113-114.
15. Leung AY, Foster S. *Encyclopedia of Common Natural Ingredients Used in Food, Drugs, and Cosmetics.* 2nd ed. Hoboken, NJ: A John Wiley & Sons, Inc.; 2003: 47-49.
16. Winston D, Maimes S. *Adaptogens—Herbs for Strength, Stamina, and Stress Relief.* Rochester, VT: Healing Arts Press; 2007: 198-201.
17. Grieve M. *A Modern Herbal.* Great Britain: Jonathan Cape Ltd.; 1931: 71-72.
18. Yance D. *Adaptogens in Medical Herbalism.* Rochester, VT: Healing Arts Press; 2013: 586-588.
19. Skenderi G. *Herbal Vade Mecum.* Rutherford, NJ: Herbacy Press; 2003: 24.
20. Pedersen M. *Nutritional Herbology: A Reference Guide to Herbs.* Warsaw, IN: Wendell W. Whitman Company; 1998: 40-41.
21. Lad V, Frawley D. *The Yoga of Herbs.* Twin Lakes, WI: Lotus Press; 1992: 183-184.
22. Mills S, Bone K. *Principles and Practice of Phytotherapy.* London, UK: Harcourt Publishers Limited; 2000: 156.

ASTRAGALUS

1. Foster S. Astragalus/Astragalus membranaceus/Huang-qi. Steven Foster Group Inc. website. http://www.stevenfoster.com/education/monograph/astragalus.html. Published 2011. Accessed February 3, 2015.
2. Thayer S. *Nature's Garden: A Guide to Identifying, Harvesting, and Preparing Edible Wild Plants.* Birchwood, WI: Forager's Harvest Press; 2010: 48.
3. Astragalus mongholicus. Flora of China. eFloras website. Missouri Botanical Garden, St. Louis, MO & Harvard University Herbaria, Cambridge, MA. http://efloras.org/florataxon.aspx?flora_id=2&taxon_id=200011902. Accessed February 3, 2015.
4. Schafer P. *The Chinese Medicinal Herb Farm.* White River Junction, VT: Chelsea Green Publishing Company; 2011: 116.
5. Foster S, Yue C. *Herbal Emissaries, Bringing Chinese Herbs to the West.* Rochester, VT: Healing Arts Press; 1992: 27-33.
6. Leung AY, Foster S. *Encyclopedia of Common Natural Ingredients Used in Food, Drugs, and Cosmetics. 2nd ed.* Hoboken, NJ: A John Wiley & Sons, Inc.; 2003: 50-53.
7. Bensky D, Gamble A. *The Chinese Herbal Medicine Materia Medica.* Rev. ed. Seattle, WA: Eastland Press; 1993: 318-320.
8. Skenderi G. *Herbal Vade Mecum.* Rutherford, NJ: Herbacy Press; 2003: 24-25.
9. Pedersen M. *Nutritional Herbology: A Reference Guide to Herbs.* Warsaw, IN: Wendell W. Whitman Company; 1998: 41-42.
10. Yance D. *Adaptogens in Medical Herbalism.* Rochester, VT: Healing Arts Press; 2013: 368-373.
11. Foster S, Johnson R. *Desk Reference to Nature's Medicine.* Washington, D.C.: National Geographic Society; 2006: 28-29.

BAYBERRY

1. Bornstein A. Morella californica. Jepson Flora Project. Jepson eFlora website. http://ucjeps.berkeley.edu/cgi-bin/get_IJM.pl?tid=80350. Accessed February 3, 2015.
2. Myrica californica. Flora of North America. eFloras website. Missouri Botanical Garden, St. Louis, MO & Harvard University Herbaria, Cambridge, MA. http://efloras.org/florataxon.aspx?flora_id=1&taxon_id=233500789. Published 2008. Accessed February 3, 2015.
3. Myrica cerifera. Flora of North America. eFloras website. Missouri Botanical Garden, St. Louis, MO & Harvard University Herbaria, Cambridge, MA. http://efloras.org/florataxon.aspx?flora_id=1&taxon_id=233500790. Published 2008. Accessed February 3, 2015.
4. Myrica pensylvanica. Flora of North America. eFloras website. Missouri Botanical Garden, St. Louis, MO & Harvard University Herbaria, Cambridge, MA. http://efloras.org/florataxon.aspx?flora_id=1&taxon_id=233500794. Published 2008. Accessed February 17, 2015.
5. Charters M. California Plant Names: Latin and Greek Meanings and Derivations. http://www.calflora.net/botanicalnames/pageMI-MY.html. Accessed October 26, 2015.
6. Charters M. California Plant Names: Latin and Greek Meanings and Derivations. http://www.calflora.net/botanicalnames/pageCA-CH.html. Accessed October 26, 2015.
7. Ellingwood F. *American Materia Medica, Therapeutics, and Pharmacognosy.* Rev. ed. Albuquerque, NM: Southwest School for Botanical Medicine; 1994: 76.
8. Felter HW. *The Eclectic Materia Medica, Pharmacology and Therapeutics.* Cincinnati, OH: Published by John K. Scudder, 1922: 80-81.
9. Grieve M. *A Modern Herbal.* Great Britain: Jonathan Cape Ltd.; 1931: 87-88.
10. Leung AY, Foster S. *Encyclopedia of Common Natural Ingredients Used in Food, Drugs, and Cosmetics.* 2nd ed. Hoboken, NJ: A John Wiley & Sons, Inc.; 2003: 73.
11. Skenderi G. *Herbal Vade Mecum.* Rutherford, NJ: Herbacy Press, 2003: 35-36.
12. Pedersen M. *Nutritional Herbology: A Reference Guide to Herbs.* Warsaw, IN: Wendell W. Whitman Company; 1998: 44-45.
13. Moore M. *Medicinal Plants of the Pacific Northwest.* Santa Fe, NM: Red Crane Books; 1993: 100-104.
14. Moore M. Lecture presented at Southwest School for Botanical Medicine residency program. Albuquerque, NM; 1994.

BERBERIS

1. Leung AY, Foster S. *Encyclopedia of Common Natural Ingredients Used in Food, Drugs, and Cosmetics.* 2nd ed. Hoboken, NJ: A John Wiley & Sons, Inc.; 2003: 66-68.
2. Pojar J, MacKinnon A. *Plants of the Pacific Northwest Coast.* Vancouver, BC: Lone Pine Publishing; 1994: 95.
3. Hickman JC. (ed.) *The Jepson Manual: Higher Plants of California.* Berkeley, CA: University of California Press; 1996: 362-363.
4. Grieve M. *A Modern Herbal.* Great Britain: Jonathan Cape Ltd.; 1931: 82-84.
5. Berberis vulgaris. Flora of North America. eFloras website. Missouri Botanical Garden, St. Louis, MO & Harvard University Herbaria, Cambridge, MA. http://efloras.org/florataxon.aspx?flora_id=1&taxon_id=233500244. Published 2008. Accessed January 6, 2015.
6. Berberis vulgaris. Fire Effects Information Database. USDA Forest Service website. http://www.fs.fed.us/database/feis/plants/shrub/bervul/all.html. Accessed January 6, 2015.
7. Berberis. Flora of North America. eFloras website. Missouri Botanical Garden, St. Louis, MO & Harvard University Herbaria, Cambridge, MA. http://efloras.org/florataxon.aspx?flora_id=1&taxon_id=103816. Published 2008. Accessed January 6, 2015.
8. Berberis. Merriam-Webster Dictionary website. www.merriam-webster.com/dictionary/berberis. Updated 2015. Accessed January 5, 2015.
9. Willard T. *Edible and Medicinal Plants of the Rocky Mountains and Neighboring Territories.* Calgary, AB: Wild Rose College of Natural Healing; 1992: 98-99.
10. Mahonia. Fine Dictionary website. Updated 2015. http://www.finedictionary.com/Mahonia.html. Accessed January 5, 2015.
11. Tall Oregon Grape *(Mahonia aquifolium).* European Trees. http://www.european-trees.com/tall-oregon-grape.html. Updated 2015. Accessed January 5, 2015.
12. Cary R. Shining Netvien Barberry, *(Berberis aquifolium* var. *dictyota).* Yosemite National Park. http://www.yosemitehikes.com/wildflowers/dwarf-barberry/dwarf-barberry.htm. Published 2006. Accessed January 5, 2015.
13. Arayne MS, Sultana N, Bahadur SS. The Berberis Story—Berberis vulgaris in Therapeutics. Abstract. Pak. J. Pharm. Sci., 2007; 20(1):83-92.
14. Foster S, Hobbs C. *Western Medicinal Plants and Herbs.* New York, NY: Peterson Field Guides, Houghton Mifflin Company; 2002: 283-285.

15. Balls E. *Early Uses of California Plants.* Berkeley, CA: University of California Press; 1962: 41-42.
16. Curtin LSM, Moore M. *Healing Herbs of the Upper Rio Grande.* Rev. ed. Santa Fe, NM: Western Edge Press; 1997: 128.
17. Ellingwood F. *American Materia Medica, Therapeutics, and Pharmacognosy.* Rev. ed. Albuquerque, NM: Southwest School for Botanical Medicine; 1994: 18-19.
18. Felter HW, Lloyd JU. *King's American Dispensatory.* Vol. 1, 19th ed, 3rd Revision. Cincinnati, OH: The Ohio Valley Company; 1923: 346-349.
19. Felter HW. *The Eclectic Materia Medica, Pharmacology and Therapeutics.* Cincinnati, OH: Published by John K. Scudder; 1922: 21.
20. Skenderi G. *Herbal Vade Mecum.* Rutherford, NJ: Herbacy Press; 2003: 32-33.
21. Moore M. *Medicinal Plants of the Mountain West.* Santa Fe, NM: Museum of New Mexico Press; 2003: 46-47.
22. Murray M. *The Healing Power of Herbs.* Rocklin, CA: Prima Publishing; 1992, 1995: 162-172.
23. Moore M. *Medicinal Plants of the Pacific Northwest.* Santa Fe, NM: Red Crane Books; 1993: 190-194.
24. Guyten A, Hall J. *Textbook of Medical Physiology.* Philadelphia, PA: W.B. Saunders Co.; 1996: 793-843.
25. Moore M. Lecture presented at Southwest School for Botanical Medicine residency program. Albuquerque, NM; 1994.
26. Hoffman D. *Medical Herbalism — The Science and Practice of Herbal Medicine.* Rochester, VT: Healing Arts Press; 2003: 533-534.
27. Bensky D, Gamble A. *The Chinese Herbal Medicine Materia Medica.* Rev. ed. Seattle, WA: Eastland Press; 1993: 77-83.
28. Weiss RF. *Herbal Medicine.* Avon, UK: The Bath Press; 1996: 341.

BLACK COHOSH

1. Actaea racemosa. Missouri Botanical Garden Plant Finder. http://www.missouribotanicalgarden.org/PlantFinder/PlantFinderDetails.aspx?kempercode=j790. Accessed January 6, 2015.
2. Cimicifuga racemosa. Flora of North America. eFloras website. Missouri Botanical Garden, St. Louis, MO & Harvard University Herbaria, Cambridge, MA. http://efloras.org/florataxon.aspx?flora_id=1&taxon_id=233500379. Published 2008. Accessed January 6, 2015.
3. King J, Felter H, Lloyd J. *King's American Dispensatory* (Volume 1, 19th Edition, Third Revision). Cincinnati, OH: The Ohio Valley Company; 1905: 528-533.
4. Willard T. *The Wild Rose Scientific Herbal.* Calgary, AB: Wild Rose College of Natural Healing; 1998: 32-35.
5. Tyler V. *The Honest Herbal.* Binghamton, NY: The Hawthorn Press, Inc.; 1993: 45-46.
6. Foster S, Johnson R. *Desk Reference to Nature's Medicine.* Washington, D.C.: National Geographic Society; 2006: 54-55.
7. Pedersen M. *Nutritional Herbology: A Reference Guide to Herbs.* Warsaw, IN: Wendell W. Whitman Company; 1998: 47-49.
8. Curtin LSM, Moore, M. *Healing Herbs of the Upper Rio Grande.* Rev. ed. Santa Fe, NM: Western Edge Press; 1997: 190.
9. Pojar J, MacKinnon A. *Plants of the Pacific Northwest Coast.* Vancouver, BC: Lone Pine Publishing; 1994: 179.
10. Ellingwood F. *American Materia Medica, Therapeutics, and Pharmacognosy.* Rev. ed. Albuquerque, NM: Southwest School for Botanical Medicine; 1994: 32-34.
11. Scudder J. *The American Eclectic Materia Medica and Therapeutics* (Twelfth Edition). Cincinnati, OH: The Scudder Brothers Company Publishers; 1898: 607-608.
12. Mills S, Bone K. *Principles and Practice of Phytotherapy.* London, UK: Harcourt Publishers Limited; 2000: 303-309.
13. Leung AY, Foster S. *Encyclopedia of Common Natural Ingredients Used in Food, Drugs, and Cosmetics.* 2nd ed. Hoboken, NJ: A John Wiley & Sons, Inc.; 2003: 88-89.
14. Blumenthal M. *The ABC Clinical Guide to Herbs.* Austin, TX: The American Botanical Council; 2003: 15-22.
15. Moore M. *Medicinal Plants of the Pacific Northwest.* Santa Fe, NM: Red Crane Books; 1993: 59-60; 74-79.
16. Skenderi G. *Herbal Vade Mecum.* Rutherford, NJ: Herbacy Press; 2003: 51.
17. Moore M. Lecture presented at Southwest School for Botanical Medicine residency program. Albuquerque, NM; 1994.
18. Weiss RF. *Herbal Medicine.* Avon, UK: The Bath Press; 1996: 318-319.
19. Moore M. *Medicinal Plants of the Mountain West.* Santa Fe, NM: Museum of New Mexico Press; 2003: 44-45.
20. Foster S. *Herbal Renaissance.* Layton, UT: Peregrine Smith Books; 1993: 47-48.

BLACK HAW

1. Missouri Botanical Garden Plant Finder website. http://www.missouribotanicalgarden.org/PlantFinder/PlantFinderDetails.aspx?taxonid=278961&isprofile=1&basic=Viburnum%20prunifolium. Accessed July 7, 2015.
2. Rosatti TJ, Bell CD. Viburnum. Jepson Flora Project. Jepson eFlora website. http://ucjeps.berkeley.edu/cgi-bin/get_IJM.pl?key=10324. Accessed July 7, 2015.
3. Online Etymology Dictionary website. http://www.etymonline.com/index.php. Accessed July 7, 2015.
4. Foster S, Johnson R. *Desk Reference to Nature's Medicine.* Washington, D.C.: National Geographic Society; 2006: 56-57.
5. Ellingwood F. *American Materia Medica, Therapeutics, and Pharmacognosy.* Cincinnati, OH; 1919: 104-105.
6. Felter HW. *The Eclectic Materia Medica, Pharmacology and Therapeutics.* Cincinnati, OH: John K. Scudder; 1922: 117-118.
7. Scudder J. Specific Medications and Specific Medicines. Henriette's Home Page website. http://www.henriettes-herb.com/eclectic/spec-med/viburnum-prun.html. Accessed July 9, 2015.
8. Lydia Pinkham. Wikipedia website. http://en.wikipedia.org/wiki/Lydia_Pinkham. Last modified October 31, 2013. Accessed July 8, 2015.
9. Leung AY, Foster S. *Encyclopedia of Common Natural Ingredients Used in Food, Drugs, and Cosmetics.* 2nd ed. Hoboken, NJ: A John Wiley & Sons, Inc.; 2003: 89-90.
10. Skenderi G. *Herbal Vade Mecum.* Rutherford, NJ: Herbacy Press; 2003: 52.
11. Mills S, Bone K. *Principles and Practice of Phytotherapy.* London: Harcourt Publishers Limited; 2000: 51.
12. Gladstar R. *Herbal Healing for Women.* New York, NY: Simon and Shuster; 1993: 232-233.

BLACKBERRY

1. Alice LA. Rubus armeniacus. Jepson Flora Project. Jepson eFlora website. http://ucjeps.berkeley.edu/eflora/eflora_display.php?tid=87465. Accessed December 10, 2015.
2. Grieve M. *A Modern Herbal.* Great Britain: Jonathan Cape Ltd.; 1931: 108-110.
3. Lust J. *The Herb Book.* New York, NY: Bantam Books; 1974: 123-124.
4. Hoffmann D. *Medical Herbalism — The Science and Practice of Herbal Medicine.* Rochester, Vermont: Healing Arts Press; 2003: 558.
5. Scudder J. *The American Eclectic Materia Medica and Therapeutics* (Twelfth Edition). Cincinnati, OH: The Scudder Brothers Company Publishers; 1898: 548.
6. Felter HW. *The Eclectic Materia Medica, Pharmacology and Therapeutics.* Cincinnati, OH: Published by John K. Scudder; 1922: 100.
7. Ellingwood F. *American Materia Medica, Therapeutics, and Pharmacognosy. Rev. ed.* Albuquerque, NM: Southwest School for Botanical Medicine; 1994: 90.
8. Pojar J, MacKinnon A. *Plants of the Pacific Northwest Coast.* Vancouver, BC: Lone Pine Publishing; 1994: 78.
9. Lyons K, Cooney-Lazaneo M. *Plants of the Coast Redwood Region.* Boulder Creek, CA: Looking Press; 1988: 91.
10. Skenderi G. *Herbal Vade Mecum.* Rutherford, NJ: Herbacy Press, 2003: 52-53.
11. Leung AY, Foster S. *Encyclopedia of Common Natural Ingredients Used in Food, Drugs, and Cosmetics.* 2nd ed. Hoboken, NJ: A John Wiley & Sons, Inc.; 2003: 195.
12. Moore M. Lecture presented at Southwest School for Botanical Medicine residency program. Albuquerque, NM; 1994.
13. Tierra M. *The Way of Herbs.* New York, NY: Pocket Books; 1990: 116-117.

14. Moore M. *Medicinal Plants of the Mountain West.* Santa Fe, NM: Museum of New Mexico Press; 2003: 213-215.
15. Blackberries, raw. SELF Nutrition Data website. http://nutrition data.self.com/facts/fruits-and-fruit-juices/1848/2?print=true. Accessed January 30, 2014.

BLUE COHOSH

1. Caulophyllum. Flora of North America. eFloras website. Missouri Botanical Garden, St. Louis, MO & Harvard University Herbaria, Cambridge, MA. http://efloras.org/florataxon.aspx?flora_id=1&taxon_id=105942. Accessed May 6, 2015.
2. Caulophyllum thalictroides. Flora of North America. eFloras website. Missouri Botanical Garden, St. Louis, MO & Harvard University Herbaria, Cambridge, MA. http://efloras.org/flora taxon.aspx?flora_id=1&taxon_id=233500331. Accessed May 6, 2015.
3. Hilty J. Blue Cohosh. Illinois Wildflowers website. http://www.illinoiswildflowers.info/woodland/plants/blue_cohosh.html. Accessed May 6, 2015.
4. Willard T. *The Wild Rose Scientific Herbal.* Calgary, AB: Wild Rose College of Natural Healing; 1998: 41-42.
5. Felter HW, Lloyd, JU. *King's American Dispensatory.* Vol. 1, 19th ed, 3rd Revision. Cincinnati, Ohio: The Ohio Valley Company; 1923: 468-472.
6. Foster S. *Herbal Renaissance.* Layton, UT: Peregrine Smith Books; 1993: 48-50.
7. Foster S, Johnson R. *Desk Reference to Nature's Medicine.* Washington, D.C.: National Geographic Society; 2006: 60-61.
8. Leung AY, Foster S. *Encyclopedia of Common Natural Ingredients Used in Food, Drugs, and Cosmetics.* 2nd ed. Hoboken, NJ: A John Wiley & Sons, Inc.; 2003: 93.
9. Colby B. *A Guide to Health.* Retrieved from http://chestofbooks.com/health/natural-cure/A-Guide-To-Health/The-Mother-s-Cordial.html. Accessed May 6, 2015.
10. Felter HW. *The Eclectic Materia Medica, Pharmacology and Therapeutics.* Cincinnati, OH: Published by John K. Scudder; 1922: 32.
11. Ellingwood F. *American Materia Medica, Therapeutics, and Pharmacognosy. Rev. ed.* Albuquerque, NM: Southwest School for Botanical Medicine; 1994: 28.
12. Mabey R. *The New Age Herbalist.* New York, NY: Gaia books; 1988: 29.
13. Pedersen M. *Nutritional Herbology: A Reference Guide to Herbs.* Warsaw, IN: Wendell W. Whitman Company; 1998: 53-54.
14. Skenderi G. *Herbal Vade Mecum.* Rutherford, NJ: Herbacy Press; 2003: 54-55.
15. Gladstar, Rosemary. *Herbal Healing for Women.* New York, New York: Simon and Shuster; 1993: 234-235.
16. Moore M. Lecture presented at Southwest School for Botanical Medicine residency program. Albuquerque, NM; 1994.
17. Bergner P. (2001). Caulophyllum: Cardiotoxic effects of blue cohosh on a fetus. *Medical Herbalism,* 12(1), 12-14. Retrieved from http://medherb.com/Materia_Medica/Caulophyllum_Cardiotoxic_effects_of_Blue_Cohosh_on_a_fetus.htm.

BOGBEAN

1. Menyanthes trifoliata. Flora of China. eFloras Web Site. Missouri Botanical Garden, St. Louis, MO & Harvard University Herbaria, Cambridge, MA. http://efloras.org/florataxon.aspx?flora_id=2&taxon_id=200018194. Published 2008. Accessed October 22, 2015.
2. Menyanthes. Flora of China. eFloras Web Site. Missouri Botanical Garden, St. Louis, MO & Harvard University Herbaria, Cambridge, MA. http://efloras.org/florataxon.aspx?flora_id=2&taxon_id=120253. Published 2008. Accessed October 22, 2015.
3. Willard T. *Edible and Medicinal Plants of the Rocky Mountains and Neighboring Territories.* Calgary, AB: Wild Rose College of Natural Healing; 1992: 174.
4. Grieve M. *A Modern Herbal.* Great Britain: Jonathan Cape Ltd.; 1931: 117-18.
5. Plant of the Week: Menyanthes trifoliate. Davis Landscape Architecture Blog. http://davisla.wordpresscom/?s=Plant+of+the Week%3A+Menyanthes+trifoliata++&submit=Search. Accessed October 12, 2013.
6. Pojar J, MacKinnon A. *Plants of the Pacific Northwest Coast.* Vancouver, BC: Lone Pine Publishing; 1994: 339.
7. Foster S, Hobbs C. *Western Medicinal Plants and Herbs.* New York, NY: Peterson Field Guides, Houghton Mifflin Company; 2002: 21.
8. Moore M. *Medicinal Plants of the Pacific Northwest.* Santa Fe, NM: Red Crane Books; 1993: 91-92.
9. Skenderi G. *Herbal Vade Mecum.* Rutherford, NJ: Herbacy Press; 2003: 56.
10. Moore M. Lecture from Southwest School for Botanical Medicine residency program. Albuquerque, NM: 1994.
11. Weiss RF. *Herbal Medicine.* Avon, Great Britain: The Bath Press, 1996: 42-43.

BONESET

1. Eupatorium perfoliatum. Flora of North America. eFloras website. Missouri Botanical Garden, St. Louis, MO & Harvard University Herbaria, Cambridge, MA. http://efloras.org/flora taxon.aspx?flora_id=1&taxon_id=242416531. Published 2008. Accessed January 6, 2015.
2. Eupatorium perfoliatum. Missouri Botanical Garden Plant Finder website. http://www.missouribotanicalgarden.org/Plant Finder/PlantFinderDetails.aspx?kempercode=c730. Accessed January 6, 2015.
3. Tyler V. *The Honest Herbal.* Binghamton, NY: The Hawthorn Press, Inc.; 1993: 49-50.
4. Grieve M. *A Modern Herbal.* Great Britain: Jonathan Cape Ltd.; 1931: 118-119.
5. Willard T. *The Wild Rose Scientific Herbal.* Calgary, AB: Wild Rose College of Natural Healing; 1998: 48-50.
6. Ellingwood F. *American Materia Medica, Therapeutics, and Pharmacognosy. Rev. ed.* Albuquerque, NM: Southwest School for Botanical Medicine; 1994: 50.
7. Felter HW. *The Eclectic Materia Medica, Pharmacology and Therapeutics.* Cincinnati, OH: Published by John K. Scudder; 1922: 48-49.
8. Leung AY, Foster S. *Encyclopedia of Common Natural Ingredients Used in Food, Drugs, and Cosmetics.* 2nd ed. Hoboken, NJ: A John Wiley & Sons, Inc.; 2003: 96-98.
9. Skenderi G. *Herbal Vade Mecum.* Rutherford, NJ: Herbacy Press; 2003: 57-58.
10. Derksen A, Kuhn J, Hafezi W, et al. Antiviral activity of hydro alcoholic extract from Eupatorium perfoliatum L. against the attachment of influenza A virus. *J Ethnopharmacol.* 2016 Jul 21;188:144-52. doi:10.1016/j.jep.2016.05.016. Accessed December 30, 2016.
11. Hensel A, Mass M, Sendker J, et al. Eupatorium perfoliatum L.: phytochemistry, traditional use and current applications. *J Ethnopharmacol.* 2011 Dec 8;138(3):641-51. doi: 10.1016/j.jep.2011.10.002. Epub 2011. Oct. https://www.ncbi.nlm.nih.gov/pubmed/22004891. Accessed December 30, 2016.
12. Bergner P. Materia Medica Intensive lecture. Detroit, OR: Breitenbush Herbal Conference; 2013.

BUGLEWEED

1. Lycopus virginicus: Virginia Water Horehound. Michigan Natural Features Inventory website. http://mnfi.anr.msu.edu/abstracts/botany/Lycopus_virginicus.pdf. Accessed December 2, 2014.
2. Hilty J. Virginia Bugleweed. Illinois Wildflowers website. http://www.illinoiswildflowers.info/wetland/plants/va_bugle weed.htm. Accessed December 2, 2014.
3. Miller JM, Wilken DH. Lycopus americanus. Jepson Flora Project. Jepson eFlora website. http://ucjeps.berkeley.edu/cgi-bin/get_IJM.pl?tid=32313. Accessed November 19, 2015.
4. Hilty J. American Bugleweed. Illinois Wildflowers website. http://www.illinoiswildflowers.info/wetland/plants/am_bugleweed.htm. Accessed November 19, 2015.
5. Gypsywort. LuontoPortii/NatureGate website. http://www.luontoportti.com/suomi/en/kukkakasvit/gipsywort. Accessed December 2, 2014.
6. Lycopus. Charters M. California Plant Names: Latin and Greek Meanings and Derivations website. http://www.calflora.net/botanicalnames/pageLH-LY.html. Accessed November 16, 2015.

7. Virginicus. Charters M. California Plant Names: Latin and Greek Meanings and Derivations website. http://www.calflora.net/botanicalnames/pageV.html. Accessed November 16, 2015.
8. Europaeus. Charters M. California Plant Names: Latin and Greek Meanings and Derivations website. http://www.calflora.net/botanicalnames/pageE.html. Accessed November 16, 2015.
9. Felter HW. *The Eclectic Materia Medica, Pharmacology and Therapeutics.* Cincinnati, OH: Published by John K. Scudder, 1922: 75.
10. Ellingwood F. *American Materia Medica, Therapeutics, and Pharmacognosy.* Rev. ed. Albuquerque, NM: Southwest School for Botanical Medicine; 1994: 72-73.
11. Felter, HW, Lloyd JU. Lycopus. King's American Dispensatory, 1898. http://www.henriettes-herb.com/eclectic/kings/lycopus.html. Accessed November 16, 2015.
12. Skenderi G. *Herbal Vade Mecum.* Rutherford, NJ: Herbacy Press; 2003: 61-62.
13. Moore M. *Medicinal Plants of the Mountain West.* Santa Fe, NM: Museum of New Mexico Press; 2003: 63-64.
14. Foster S, Hobbs C. *Western Medicinal Plants and Herbs.* New York, NY: Peterson Field Guides, Houghton Mifflin Company; 2002: 53.
15. Hoffman D. *Medical Herbalism — The Science and Practice of Herbal Medicine.* Rochester, VT: Healing Arts Press; 2003: 563-564.
16. Bugleweed. Drugs.com website. http://www.drugs.com/npp/bugleweed.html. Accessed November 15, 2015.
17. Mills S, Bone K. *Principles and Practice of Phytotherapy.* London, UK: Harcourt Publishers Limited; 2000: 246.
18. Vonhoff C, Baumgartner A, Hegger M, Korte B, Biller A, Winterhoff H. Extract of Lycopus europaeus L. reduces cardiac signs of hyperthyroidism in rats. *Life Sci.* 2006;78(10): 1063-70. Available from PubMed. http://www.ncbi.nlm.nih.gov/pubmed/16150466. Accessed November 15, 2015.
19. Beer AM, Wiebelitz KR, Schmidt-gayk H. Lycopus europaeus (Gypsywort): effects on the thyroidal parameters and symptoms associated with thyroid function. *Phytomedicine.* 2008;15(1-2):16-22. Available from PubMed. http://www.ncbi.nlm.nih.gov/pubmed/18083505. Accessed November 16, 2015.
20. Fialová S, Slobodníková L, Veizerová L, GranČai D. Lycopus europaeus: phenolic fingerprint, antioxidant activity and antimicrobial effect on clinical Staphylococcus aureus strains. *Nat Prod Res.* 2015;29(24):2271-4. Available from PubMed. http://www.ncbi.nlm.nih.gov/pubmed/25674680. Accessed November 16, 2015.

BURDOCK

1. Leung AY, Foster S. *Encyclopedia of Common Natural Ingredients Used in Food, Drugs, and Cosmetics.* 2nd ed. Hoboken, NJ: A John Wiley & Sons, Inc.; 2003: 107-108.
2. Arctium lappa. Flora of North America. eFloras website. Missouri Botanical Garden, St. Louis, MO & Harvard University Herbaria, Cambridge, MA. http://efloras.org/florataxon.aspx?flora_id=1&taxon_id=200023153. Accessed December 10, 2015.
3. Arctium lappa. Flora of China. eFloras website. Missouri Botanical Garden, St. Louis, MO & Harvard University Herbaria, Cambridge, MA. http://efloras.org/florataxon.aspx?flora_id=2&taxon_id=200023153. Accessed December 10, 2015.
4. Grieve M. *A Modern Herbal.* Great Britain: Jonathan Cape Ltd.; 1931: 143-145.
5. Bensky D, Gamble A. *The Chinese Herbal Medicine Materia Medica.* Rev. ed. Seattle, WA: Eastland Press; 1993: 41-42.
6. Ellingwood F. *American Materia Medica, Therapeutics, and Pharmacognosy.* Rev. ed. Albuquerque, NM: Southwest School for Botanical Medicine; 1994: 12.
7. Willard T. *The Wild Rose Scientific Herbal.* Calgary, AB: Wild Rose College of Natural Healing; 1998: 56-58.
8. Foster S, Hobbs C. *Western Medicinal Plants and Herbs.* New York, NY: Peterson Field Guides, Houghton Mifflin Company; 2002: 181-182.
9. Skenderi G. *Herbal Vade Mecum.* Rutherford, NJ: Herbacy Press; 2003: 63.
10. Moore M. Lecture presented at Southwest School for Botanical Medicine residency program. Albuquerque, NM; 1994.
11. Pedersen M. *Nutritional Herbology: A Reference Guide to Herbs.* Warsaw, IN: Wendell W. Whitman Company; 1998: 57-59.
12. Moore M. *Medicinal Plants of the Mountain West.* Santa Fe, NM: Museum of New Mexico Press; 2003; 64-67.

CALAMUS

1. Acorus calamus. Flora of China. eFloras website. Missouri Botanical Garden, St. Louis, MO & Harvard University Herbaria, Cambridge, MA. http://efloras.org/florataxon.aspx?flora_id2&taxon_id=200027130. Accessed December 3, 2015.
2. Acoraceae. Flora of China. eFloras website. Missouri Botanical Garden, St. Louis, MO & Harvard University Herbaria, Cambridge, MA. http://efloras.org/florataxon.aspx?flora_id=2&taxon_id=20008. Accessed December 3, 2015.
3. Grieve M. *A Modern Herbal.* Great Britain: Jonathan Cape Ltd.; 1931: 726-29.
4. Lad V, Frawley D. *The Yoga of Herbs.* Twin Lakes, WI: Lotus Press; 1992: 107-08.
5. Tierra M. *The Way of Herbs.* New York, NY: Pocket Books; 1990: 131-32.
6. Weiss RF. *Herbal Medicine.* Avon, UK: The Bath Press; 1996: 44-46.
7. Foster S. *Herbal Renaissance.* Layton, UT: Peregrine Smith Books; 1993: 54-56.
8. Leung AY, Foster S. *Encyclopedia of Common Natural Ingredients Used in Food, Drugs, and Cosmetics.* 2nd ed. Hoboken, NJ: A John Wiley & Sons, Inc.; 2003: 111-113.
9. Skenderi G. *Herbal Vade Mecum.* Rutherford, NJ: Herbacy Press; 2003: 69-70.
10. Teeguarden R. *Chinese Tonic Herbs.* Tokyo, Japan: Japan Publications, Inc.; 1995: 132.
11. Tierra M. *The Way of Chinese Herbs.* New York, NY: Pocket Books, 1998: 303.
12. Foster S, Johnson R. *Desk Reference to Nature's Medicine.* Washington, D.C.: National Geographic Society; 2006: 72-73.
13. Foster S, Hobbs C. *Western Medicinal Plants and Herbs.* New York, NY: Peterson Field Guides, Houghton Mifflin Company; 2002: 380.
14. Willard T. *Edible and Medicinal Plants of the Rocky Mountains and Neighboring Territories.* Calgary, AB: Wild Rose College of Natural Healing; 1992: 150.
15. Felter HW. *The Eclectic Materia Medica, Pharmacology and Therapeutics.* Cincinnati, OH: Published by John K. Scudder; 1922: 25.
16. Tyler V. *The Honest Herbal.* Binghamton, NY: The Hawthorn Press, Inc.; 1993: 73-74.

CALENDULA

1. Grieve M. *A Modern Herbal.* Great Britain: Jonathan Cape Ltd.; 1931: 517-518.
2. Calendula officinalis. Flora of China. eFloras website. Missouri Botanical Garden, St. Louis, MO & Harvard University Herbaria, Cambridge, MA. http://efloras.org/florataxon.aspx?flora_id=2&taxon_id=220002139. Accessed March 11, 2015.
3. Keil DJ. Calendula officinalis. Jepson Flora Project. Jepson eFlora website. http://ucjeps.berkeley.edu/cgi-bin/get_IJM.pl?tid=1863. Accessed March 11, 2015.
4. Foster S, Johnson R. *Desk Reference to Nature's Medicine.* Washington, D.C.: National Geographic Society; 2006: 74-75.
5. Leung AY, Foster S. *Encyclopedia of Common Natural Ingredients Used in Food, Drugs, and Cosmetics.* 2nd ed. Hoboken, NJ: A John Wiley & Sons, Inc.; 2003: 113-114.
6. Mabey R. *The New Age Herbalist.* New York, NY: Gaia books; 1988: 46.
7. Skenderi G. *Herbal Vade Mecum.* Rutherford, NJ: Herbacy Press; 2003: 70.
8. Moore M. Lecture presented at Southwest School for Botanical Medicine residency program. Albuquerque, NM; 1994.
9. Dall'Acqua S, Catanzaro D, Cocetta V, et al. Protective effects of esters ψ taraxasterol-3-O-myristate and arnidiol-3-O-myristate isolated from Calendula officinalis on epithelial intestinal barrier. *Fitoterapia.* 2016; 109(3):230-5. doi: 10.1016/j.fitote.2016.01.007. Accessed December 9, 2016.

10. Dinda M, Mazumbdar S, Das S, et al. The water fraction of Calendula officinalis hydroethanol extract stimulates in vitro and in vivo proliferation of dermal fibroblasts in wound healing. *Phytother Res.* 2016; 30 (10): 1696-1707. doi: 10.1002/ptr.5678. Accessed December 9, 2016.

CALIFORNIA POPPY

1. Hannan GL, Clark C. Eschscholzia californica. Jepson Flora Project. Jepson eFlora website. http://ucjeps.berkeley.edu/cgi-bin/get_IJM.pl?tid=25206. Published 2014. Accessed November 5, 2015.
2. Eschscholzia californica. Lady Bird Johnson Wild Flower Center, University of Texas, Austin. www.wildflower.org/plants/result.php?id_plant=ESCA2. Accessed March, 6, 2014.
3. Pojar J, MacKinnon A. *Plants of the Pacific Northwest Coast.* Vancouver, BC: Lone Pine Publishing; 1994: 314.
4. Yosemite Wildflowers: Tufted Poppy (Eschscholzia caespitosa). http://www.yosemitehikes.com/wildflowers/tufted-poppy/tufted-poppy.htm. Accessed March, 6, 2014.
5. Glyptosperma. California Plant Names: Latin and Greek Meanings and Derivations. *A Dictionary of Botanical and Biographical Etymology.* http://www.calflora.net/botanicalnames/pageG.html. Accessed March, 6, 2014.
6. Lobbii. California Plant Names: Latin and Greek Meanings and Derivations. *A Dictionary of Botanical and Biographical Etymology.* http://www.calflora.net/botanicalnames/pageLH-LY.html. Accessed March, 6, 2014.
7. Foster S, Hobbs C. *Western Medicinal Plants and Herbs.* New York, NY: Peterson Field Guides. Houghton Mifflin Company; 2002: 152.
8. Lyons K, Cooney-Lazaneo M. *Plants of the Coast Redwood Region.* Boulder Creek, CA: Looking Press; 1988: 153.
9. Moore M. *Medicinal Plants of the Mountain West.* Santa Fe, NM: Museum of New Mexico Press; 2003: 73-74.
10. Skenderi G. *Herbal Vade Mecum.* Rutherford, NJ: Herbacy Press; 2003: 304.
11. Weiss RF. *Herbal Medicine.* Avon, UK: The Bath Press; 1996: 289.
12. Eschscholzia californica—A Scientific Review on Usage, Dosage, and Side Effects. www.examine.com/supplements/Eschscholzia+californica. Accessed March, 6, 2014.
13. Brinker F. *Herb Contraindications and Drug Interactions.* Sandy, OR: Eclectic Institute, Inc.; 1997: 31-32.

CANNABIS

1. Cannabis sativa. Flora of Pakistan. eFloras website. Missouri Botanical Garden, St. Louis, MO & Harvard University Herbaria, Cambridge, MA. http://efloras.org/florataxon.aspx?flora_id=5&taxon_id=200006342. Accessed March 12, 2015.
2. Cannabis sativa. Flora of North America. eFloras website. Missouri Botanical Garden, St. Louis, MO & Harvard University Herbaria, Cambridge, MA. http://efloras.org/florataxon.aspx?-flora_id=1&taxon_id=200006342. Accessed March 12, 2015.
3. Cannabis sativa. Flora of China. eFloras website. Missouri Botanical Garden, St. Louis, MO & Harvard University Herbaria, Cambridge, MA. http://efloras.org/florataxon.aspx?flora_id=2&taxon_id=200006342. Accessed March 12, 2015.
4. Cannabis. Flora of China. eFloras website. Missouri Botanical Garden, St. Louis, MO & Harvard University Herbaria, Cambridge, MA. http://efloras.org/florataxon.aspx?flora_id=2&taxon_id=105522. Accessed March 12, 2015.
5. Cannabis. Flora of North America. eFloras website. Missouri Botanical Garden, St. Louis, MO & Harvard University Herbaria, Cambridge, MA. http://efloras.org/florataxon.aspx?flora_id=1&taxon_id=105522. Accessed March 12, 2015.
6. Harper D. Etymonline website. http://www.etymonline.com/index.php?allowed_in_frame=0&search=cannabis.
7. Culbreth D. *A Manual of Materia Medica and Pharmacology.* 1917. Bisbee, AZ: Southwest School of Botanical Medicine; 1927: 24-25.
8. Grotenhermen F, Russo E. *Cannabis and Cannabinoids. Pharmacology, Toxicology, and Therapeutic Potential.* Birmingham, NY: The Haworth Press, Inc.; 2002.
9. Ellingwood F. *American Materia Medica, Therapeutics, and Pharmacognosy.* Rev. ed. Albuquerque, NM: Southwest School for Botanical Medicine; 1994: 23-24.
10. Felter HW. *The Eclectic Materia Medica, Pharmacology and Therapeutics.* Cincinnati, OH: Published by John K. Scudder; 1922: 27-29.
11. Skenderi G. *Herbal Vade Mecum.* Rutherford, NJ: Herbacy Press; 2003: 241.
12. Grotenhermen F. Cannabinoids and the endocannabinoid system. *Cannabinoids.* 2006;1(2):10-14. https://www.cannabisinternational.org/info/Cannabinoids-Review.pdf. Accessed April 7, 2017.
13. Spelman K. The Endocannabinoid System: A Basis in Reality (slideshow). Accessible at www.707humboldtcannabiscollege.com/PDFs/Spellman_Endocanabinoid_Basis_in_Reality.pdf. Accessed April 7, 2017.
14. Onaivi ES. Commentary: Functional neuronal CB2 cannabinoid receptors in the CNS. *Curr Neuropharmacol.* 2011 Mar; 9(1): 205-208. doi: 10.2174/157015911795017416. Accessed April 21, 2017.
15. Spelman K. Keeping it together: The other compounds in *Cannabis and the benefits of whole-herb use. Integrative Medicine (Encinitas).* 2015 Jun; 14(3): 18-22. https://www.ncbi.nlm.nih.gov/pmc/articles/PMC4566471. Accessed April 7, 2017.
16. Sulak D, Saneto R, Goldstein B. The current status of artisanal cannabis for the treatment of epilepsy in the United States. *Epilepy Behav.* 2017 Feb 18. Epub. doi: 10.1016/j.yebeh.2016.12.032. Accessed April 7, 2017.
17. Hill MN. Regional alterations in the endocannabinoid system in an animal model of depression: effects of concurrent anti-depressant treatment. *Neurochem.* 2008 Sep; 106(6):2322-36. doi: 10.1111/j.1471-4159.2008.05567.x. Accessed April 7, 2017.
18. Lynskey MT, Glowinsky AL, Torordov AA, et al. Major depressive disorder, suicidal ideation, and suicide attempt in twins discordant for cannabis dependence and early-onset cannabis use. *Arch Gen Psychiatry.* 2004 Oct;61(10):1026-32. https://www.ncbi.nlm.nih.gov/pubmed/15466676. Accessed April 8, 2017.
19. Moore M. Lecture presented at Southwest School for Botanical Medicine residency program. Albuquerque, NM; 1994.
20. Papanastassiou AM, Fields HL, Meng ID. Local application of the cannabinoid receptor agonist, WIN 55,212-2, to spinal trigeminal nucleus caudalis differentially affects nociceptive and non-nociceptive neurons. *Pain.* 2004 Feb;107(3):267-75. https://www.ncbi.nlm.nih.gov/pubmed/14736589. Accessed April 7, 2017.
21. Costa B, Giagnoni G, Franke C, et al. Vanilloid TRPV1 receptor mediates the antihyperalgesic effect of the nonpsychoactive cannabinoid, cannabidiol, in a rat model of acute inflammation. *Br J Pharmacol.* 2004 Sep; 143(2): 247–250. Published online 2001 Aug 16. doi: 10.1038/sj.bjp.0705920. Accessed April 21, 2017.
22. Agarwal N, Pacher P, Tegeder I, et al. Cannabinoids mediate analgesia largely via peripheral type 1 cannabinoid receptors in nociceptors. *Nat Neurosci.* 2007 Jul; 10(7): 870–879. Published online 2007 Jun 10. doi: 10.1038/nn1916. Accessed April 21, 2017.
23. Quartilho A, Mata HP, Ibrahim MM, et al. Inhibition of inflammatory hyperalgesia by activation of peripheral CB2 cannabinoid receptors. *Anesthesiology.* 2003 Oct; 99(4):955-60. https://www.ncbi.nlm.nih.gov/pubmed/14508331. Accessed April 21, 2017.
24. Corey-Bloom J, Wolfson T, Gamst A, Jin S, Marcotte TD, et al. Smoked cannabis for spasticity in multiple sclerosis: a randomized, placebo-controlled trial. *CMAJ.* 2012 Jul 10; 184(10): 1143–1150. doi: 10.1503/cmaj.110837. Accessed April 7, 2017.
25. Courtney W. The Impact of THC on Dietary Intake of Cannab inoid Acids: Cannabis as a Unique Functional Food. *Treating Yourself.* 2010; 24. Accessible at https://www.cannabisinternational.org/info/treatingyourself.pdf. Accessed April 21, 2017.
26. Pazos MR, Mohammed N, Lafuente H, et al. Mechanisms of cannabidiol neuroprotection in hypoxic-ischemic newborn pigs: role of 5HT(1A) and CB2 receptors. *Neuropharmacology.* 2013 Aug;71:282-91. doi: 10.1016/j.neuropharm.2013.03.027. Accessed April 21, 2017.
27. Ruhaak LR, Felth J, Karlsson PC, et al. Evaluation of the Cyclooxygenase Inhibiting Effects of Six Major Cannabinoids Isolated from Cannabis sativa. *Biol. Pharm. Bull.* 2011. 34(5) 774—778. https://www.jstage.jst.go.jp/article/bpb/34/5/34_5_774/_pdf. Accessed April 7, 2017.

28. Yu M, Ives D, Ramesha CS. Synthesis of Prostaglandin E2 Ethanolamide from Anandamide by Cyclooxygenase-2. *The Journal of Biological Chemistry.* 1997; 272, 21181-21186. doi: 10.1074/jbc.272.34.21181. Accessed April 7, 2017.
29. Appendino G, Gibbons S, Giana A, et al. Antibacterial cannabinoids from Cannabis sativa: A structure–activity study. *J. Nat. Prod.,* 2008, *71* (8), pp 1427–1430. doi: 10.1021/np8002673. Accessed April 28, 2017.
30. Cabral GA, Rogers TJ, Lichtman AH. Turning Over a New Leaf: Cannabinoid and Endocannabinoid Modulation of Immune Function. *J Neuroimmune Pharmacol.* 2015; 10(2): 193–203. doi: 10.1007/s11481-015-9615-z. Accessed April 28, 2017.
31. Lukhele ST, Motadi LR. Cannabidiol rather than Cannabis sativa extracts inhibit cell growth and induce apoptosis in cervical cancer cells. *BMC Complement Altern Med.* 2016; 16(1): 335. doi: 10.1186/s12906-016-1280-0. Accessed April 28, 2017.
32. Solinas M, Massi P, Cantelmo AR, et al. Cannabidiol inhibits angiogenesis by multiple mechanisms. *Br J Pharmacol.* 2012 Nov; 167(6): 1218–1231.doi: 10.1111/j.1476-5381.2012.02050.x. Accessed April 28, 2017.
33. Leelawat S, Leelawat K, Narong S, Matangkasombut O. The dual effects of delta(9)-tetrahydrocannabinol on cholangiocarcinoma cells: anti-invasion activity at low concentration and apoptosis induction at high concentration. *Cancer Invest.* 2010 May;28(4):357-63. doi: 10.3109/07357900903405934. Accessed April 28, 2017.
34. Ramer R, Bublitz K, Freimuth N, et al. Cannabidiol inhibits lung cancer cell invasion and metastasis via intercellular adhesion molecule-1. *FASEB J.* 2012 Apr;26(4):1535-48. doi: 10.1096/fj.11-198184. Accessed April 28, 2017.
35. Guzman M, Duarte MJ, Blazquez C, Ravina J, et al. A pilot clinical study of Δ9-tetrahydrocannabinol in patients with recurrent glioblastoma multiforme. *Br J Cancer.* 2006 Jul 17; 95(2): 197–203. doi: 10.1038/sj.bjc.6603236. Accessed April 28, 2017.
36. Blazquez C, Carracedo A, Barrado L, Real PJ, et al. Cannabinoid receptors as novel targets for the treatment of melanoma. *FASEB J.* 2006 Dec;20(14):2633-5. https://www.ncbi.nlm.nih.gov/pubmed/17065222. Accessed April 28, 2017.
37. Naguib M, Xu JJ, Diaz P, et al. Prevention of paclitaxel-induced neuropathy through activation of the central cannabinoid type 2 receptor system. *Anesth Analg.* 2012 May; 114(5): 1104–1120. doi: 10.1213/ANE.0b013e31824b0191. Accessed April 28, 2017.
38. Khasabova IA, Khasabov S, Paz J, et al. Cannabinoid type-1 receptor reduces pain and neurotoxicity produced by chemotherapy. *J Neurosci.* 2012 May 16; 32(20): 7091–7101. doi: 10.1523/JNEUROSCI.0403-12.2012. Accessed April 28, 2017.
39. Pole S. *Ayurvedic Medicine: The Principles of Traditional Practice.* Degenhardt L, Hall W, Lynskey M. Exploring the association between cannabis use and depression. *Addiction.* 2003 Nov;98(11):1493-504. https://www.ncbi.nlm.nih.gov/pubmed/14616175. Accessed April 7, 2017.
40. Kramer JL. Medical marijuana for cancer. *CA: A Cancer Journal for Clinicians*. 2015;65(2): 109–122. 10.3322/caac.21260. Accessed April 28, 2017.
41. Yazulla S. Endocannabinoids in the retina: From marijuana to neuroprotection. *Prog Retin Eye Res.* 2008 Sep; 27(5): 501–526. Published online 2008 Aug 3. doi: 10.1016/j.preteyeres.2008.07.002. Accessed April 21, 2017.
42. Crandall J, Matragoon S, Khalifa YM, et al. Neuroprotective and intraocular pressure-lowering effects of (-)Delta9-tetra hydrocannabinol in a rat model of glaucoma. *Ophthalmic Res.* 2007;39(2):69-75. Epub 2007 Feb 2. https://www.ncbi.nlm.nih.gov/pubmed/17284931. Accessed April 21, 2017.
43. Novack GD. Cannabinoids for treatment of glaucoma. *Curr Opin Ophtalmol.* 2016; 27(2): 146-150. doi: 10.1097/ICU.000000 0000000242. Accessed April 7, 2017.
44. Tomida I, Azuara-Blanco A, House H, et al. Effect of Sublingual Application of Cannabinoids on Intraocular Pressure: A Pilot Study. *J Glaucoma* 2006 15(5):349-353. http://www.cannabis-med.org/studies/ww_en_db_study_show.php?s_id=201. Accessed April 21, 2017.
45. Tomida I, Pertwee RG, Azuara-Blanco A. Cannabinoids and glaucoma. *Br J Ophthalmol.* 2004 May; 88(5): 708–713. doi: 10.1136/bjo.2003.032250. Accessed April 21, 2017.

CARDAMOM

1. Katzer G. The Spice Pages. http://gernot-katzers-spice-pages.com/engl/Elet_car.html. January 20, 2015.
2. Leung AY, Foster S. *Encyclopedia of Common Natural Ingredients Used in Food, Drugs, and Cosmetics.* 2nd ed. Hoboken, NJ: A John Wiley & Sons, Inc.; 2003: 121-122.
3. Anandaraj M, Sudharshan MR. Cardamom, Gingner, and Turmeric. In: Verheye WH, ed. *Soils, plant growth, and crop production.* EOLSS-UNESCO. http://www.eolss.net/Sample-Chapters/C10/E1-05A-49-00.pdf. Accessed January 27, 2015.
4. Sasidharan N. Elettaria cardamomum. India Biodiversity Portal website. http://indiabiodiversity.org/species/show/229602. Accessed January 27, 2015.
5. Harper D. Cardamom. Online Etymology Dictionary website. http://www.etymonline.com/index.php?term=cardamom&allowed_in_frame=0. Accessed January 07, 2015.
6. Grieve M. *A Modern Herbal.* Great Britain: Jonathan Cape Ltd.; 1931: 159-160.
7. Keville K, Green M. *Aromatherapy—A Complete Guide to the Healing Art.* Freedom, CA: The Crossing Press; 1995: 49.
8. Cardamom Seeds History and Uses, Green Tea Recipe. Herbs—Treat and Taste website (http://herbs-treatandtaste.blogspot.com/2010/06/cardamom-seeds-there-are-basically-two.html). Updated June 10, 2010. Accessed January 21, 2015.
9. Felter HW. *The Eclectic Materia Medica, Pharmacology and Therapeutics.* Cincinnati, OH: Published by John K. Scudder; 1922: 30.
10. *British Herbal Pharmacopoeia.* Originally published by the British Herbal Medicine Association. Bisbee, AZ: Southwest School of Botanical Medicine; 2008): 81-82.
11. Pole S. *Ayurvedic Medicine: The Principles of Traditional Practice.* Philadelphia, PA: Churchill Livingstone Elsevier; 2006: 151-152.
12. Skenderi G. *Herbal Vade Mecum.* Rutherford, NJ: Herbacy Press; 2003: 76-77.
13. Bensky D, Gamble A. *The Chinese Herbal Medicine Materia Medica.* Rev. ed. Seattle, WA: Eastland Press; 1993: 220.

CAROB

1. Leung AY, Foster S. *Encyclopedia of Common Natural Ingredients Used in Food, Drugs, and Cosmetics.* 2nd ed. Hoboken, NJ: A John Wiley & Sons, Inc.; 2003: 123-134.
2. Ceratonia siliqua. Flora of Pakistan. eFloras website. Missouri Botanical Garden, St. Louis, MO & Harvard University Herbaria, Cambridge, MA. http://efloras.org/florataxon.aspx?flora_id=5&taxon_id=200012036. Published 2008. Accessed January 6, 2017.
3. Ceratonia. Flora of China. eFloras website. Missouri Botanical Garden, St. Louis, MO & Harvard University Herbaria, Cambridge, MA. http://efloras.org/florataxon.aspx?flora_id=2&taxon_id=106187. Published 2008. Accessed January 6, 2017.
4. Algaroba. Merriam-Webster Dictionary website. https://www.merriam-webster.com/dictionary/algaroba. Accessed January 6, 2017.
5. Carob. Merriam-Webster Dictionary website. https://www.merriam-webster.com/dictionary/carob. Accessed January 6, 2017.
6. Harper D. Locust Tree. Online Etymology Dictionary website http://www.etymonline.com/index.php?search=locust+tree. Accessed January 6, 2017.
7. Coit JE. Carob or St. John's bread. *Economic Botany.* 1951:5(1): 82-96. http://0-www.jstor.org.catalog.multcolib.org/stable/4252012. Accessed January 13, 2017.
8. Carat. Merriam-Webster Dictionary website. https://www.merriam-webster.com/dictionary/carat. Accessed January 6, 2017.
9. Harper D. Karat. Online Etymology Dictionary website. http://etymonline.com/index.php?allowed_in_frame=0&search=karat. Accessed January 6, 2017.
10. Silique. Merriam-Webster Dictionary website. https://www.merriam-webster.com/dictionary/silique. Accessed January 6, 2017.
11. Thompson C. The Assyrian kisal as the origin of the carat-weight. *Iraq.* 1938:5: 23-30. http://www.jstor.org/stable/4241619. Accessed January 13, 2017.

12. Ceratonia. Legumes of the World. Kew Royal Botanic Gardens website. http://www.kew.org/science-conservation/research-data/resources/legumes-of-the-world/genus/ceratonia. Accessed January 13, 2017.
13. Roth CA. Prodigal son eats carob pods. God as a Gardener website. https://godasagardener.com/2013/09/02/prodigal-son-eating-carob-pods. Published September 2, 2013. Accessed January 13, 2017.
14. Skenderi G. *Herbal Vade Mecum.* Rutherford, NJ: Herbacy Press, 2003: 78-79.

CAYENNE

1. Katzer G. The Spice Pages website. http://gernot-katzers-spice-pages.com/engl/Caps_fru.html. Accessed November 30, 2015.
2. Leung AY, Foster S. *Encyclopedia of Common Natural Ingredients Used in Food, Drugs, and Cosmetics.* 2nd ed. Hoboken, NJ: A John Wiley & Sons, Inc.; 2003: 115-118.
3. Foster S. *Herbal Renaissance.* Layton, UT: Peregrine Smith Books; 1993: 62-64.
4. Capsicum. Flora of China. eFloras website. Missouri Botanical Garden, St. Louis, MO & Harvard University Herbaria, Cambridge, MA. www.efloras.org/florataxon.aspx?flora_id=2&taxon_id=105577. Accessed October 29, 2014.
5. Capsicum. Flora of Pakistan. eFloras website. Missouri Botanical Garden, St. Louis, MO & Harvard University Herbaria, Cambridge, MA. http://www.efloras.org/florataxon.aspx?flora_id=5&taxon_id=105577. Accessed December 3, 2015.
6. Capsicum annuum. Flora of Pakistan. eFloras website. Missouri Botanical Garden, St. Louis, MO & Harvard University Herbaria, Cambridge, MA. http://www.efloras.org/florataxon.aspx?flora_id=5&taxon_id=200020513. Accessed December 3, 2015.
7. Capsicum frutescens. Flora of Pakistan. eFloras website. Missouri Botanical Garden, St. Louis, MO & Harvard University Herbaria, Cambridge, MA. http://www.efloras.org/florataxon.aspx?flora_id=5&taxon_id=230000933. Accessed December 3, 2015.
8. Grieve M. *A Modern Herbal.* Great Britain: Jonathan Cape Ltd.; 1931: 175-176.
9. Curtin LSM, Moore, M. *Healing Herbs of the Upper Rio Grande.* Rev. ed. Santa Fe, NM: Western Edge Press; 1997: 48-51.
10. Foster S, Johnson R. *Desk Reference to Nature's Medicine.* Washington, D.C.: National Geographic Society; 2006: 92-93.
11. Ellingwood F. *American Materia Medica, Therapeutics, and Pharmacognosy.* Rev. ed. Albuquerque, NM: Southwest School for Botanical Medicine; 1994: 24-25.
12. Felter HW. *The Eclectic Materia Medica, Pharmacology and Therapeutics.* Cincinnati, OH: Published by John K. Scudder; 1922: 29-30.
13. Skenderi G. *Herbal Vade Mecum.* Rutherford, NJ: Herbacy Press; 2003: 74.
14. Willard T. *The Wild Rose Scientific Herbal.* Calgary, AB: Wild Rose College of Natural Healing; 1998: 68-73.
15. Pedersen M. *Nutritional Herbology: A Reference Guide to Herbs.* Warsaw, IN: Wendell W. Whitman Company; 1998: 61-62.
16. Murray M. *The Encyclopedia of Healing Foods.* New York, NY: Atria Books; 2005: 70-76.
17. Moore M. Lecture presented at Southwest School for Botanical Medicine residency program. Albuquerque, NM; 1994.
18. Just How Hot Are My Chiles? Uncle Steve's Hot Sauce website. http://ushotstuff.com/Heat.Scale.htm. Accessed December 1, 2015.

CHAMOMILE

1. Foster S, Johnson R. *Desk Reference to Nature's Medicine.* Washington, D.C.: National Geographic Society; 2006: 94-95.
2. *British Herbal Pharmacopoeia.* British Herbal Medicine Association. Republished. Bisbee, AZ: Southwest School of Botanical Medicine; 2008: 139.
3. Williams D. *The Chemistry of Essential Oils.* Weymouth, England: Micelle Press; 1997: 92-93.
4. Grieve M. *A Modern Herbal.* Great Britain: Jonathan Cape Ltd.; 1931: 185-188.
5. Keville K, Green M. *Aromatherapy—A Complete Guide to the Healing Art.* Freedom, CA: The Crossing Press; 1995: 50-51.
6. Foster S. *An Illustrated Guide to 101 Medicinal Herbs.* Loveland, CO: Interweave Press, Inc.; 1998: 54-55.
7. Ellingwood F. *American Materia Medica, Therapeutics, and Pharmacognosy.* Rev. ed. Albuquerque, NM: Southwest School for Botanical Medicine; 1994: 73-74.
8. Felter HW. *The Eclectic Materia Medica, Pharmacology and Therapeutics.* Cincinnati, OH: Published by John K. Scudder, 1922: 12; 78-79.
9. Willard T. *The Wild Rose Scientific Herbal.* Calgary, AB: Wild Rose College of Natural Healing; 1998: 74-76.
10. Lad V, Frawley D. *The Yoga of Herbs.* Twin Lakes, WI: Lotus Press; 1992: 111.
11. Leung AY, Foster S. *Encyclopedia of Common Natural Ingredients Used in Food, Drugs, and Cosmetics.* 2nd ed. Hoboken, NJ: A John Wiley & Sons, Inc.; 2003: 145-148.
12. Skenderi G. *Herbal Vade Mecum.* Rutherford, NJ: Herbacy Press; 2003: 91-92.
13. Pedersen M. *Nutritional Herbology: A Reference Guide to Herbs.* Warsaw, IN: Wendell W. Whitman Company; 1998: 67-69.
14. Schnaubelt K. *Advanced Aromatherapy - The Science of Essential Oil Therapy.* Rochester, VT: Healing Arts Press; 1995: 63-64.
15. Schnaubelt K. *Medical Aromatherapy - Healing with Essential Oils.* Berkeley, CA: Frog, Ltd.; 1999: 163-166; 204, 209.
16. Blumenthal M. *The ABC Clinical Guide to Herbs.* Austin, TX: The American Botanical Council; 2003: 53-60.

CHICKWEED

1. Grieve M. *A Modern Herbal.* Great Britain: Jonathan Cape Ltd.; 1931: 195-196.
2. Hartman RL, Rabeler RK. Jepson Flora Project. Jepson eFlora website. http://ucjeps.berkeley.edu/cgi-bin/get_IJM.pl?tid=45497. Accessed March 27, 2015.
3. Stellaria media. Flora of North America. eFloras website. Missouri Botanical Garden, St. Louis, MO & Harvard University Herbaria, Cambridge, MA. http://efloras.org/florataxon.aspx?flora_id=1&taxon_id=200007072. Accessed March 27, 2015.
4. Charters ML. Wrightii. California Plant Names: Latin and Greek Meanings and Derivations website. http://www.calflora.net/botanicalnames. Accessed March 27, 2015.
5. Leung AY, Foster S. *Encyclopedia of Common Natural Ingredients Used in Food, Drugs, and Cosmetics.* 2nd ed. Hoboken, NJ: A John Wiley & Sons, Inc.; 2003: 159-160.
6. Skenderi G. *Herbal Vade Mecum.* Rutherford, NJ: Herbacy Press; 2003: 97-98.
7. Pedersen M. *Nutritional Herbology: A Reference Guide to Herbs.* Warsaw, IN: Wendell W. Whitman Company; 1998: 72-73.
8. Willard T. *The Wild Rose Scientific Herbal.* Calgary, AB: Wild Rose College of Natural Healing; 1998: 79-81.

CINNAMON

1. Foster S, Johnson R. *Desk Reference to Nature's Medicine.* Washington, D.C.: National Geographic Society; 2006: 108-109.
2. Cinnamomum verum. Agroforestry Database 4.0 website. http://www.worldagroforestry.org/treedb/AFTPDFS/Cinnamomum_verum.pdf. Accessed November 12, 2014.
3. Cinnamomum verum. Flora of China website. http://www.efloras.org/florataxon.aspx?flora_id=2&taxon_id=200008735. Accessed November 12, 2014.
4. Gray J. *A Guide to the Study of Pharmacognosy: Or the Essentials of Materia Medica of the Vegetable and Animal Kingdoms.* Buffalo, NY: Peter Paul Book Company and Printers; 1894: 53-54.
5. Verum. California Plant Names: Latin and Greek Meanings and Derivations. http://www.calflora.net/botanicalnames/pageV.html. Accessed January 12, 2015.
6. Aromaticum. California Plant Names: Latin and Greek Meanings and Derivations. http://www.calflora.net/botanicalnames/pageAN-AZ.html. Accessed January 12, 2015.
7. Leung AY, Foster S. *Encyclopedia of Common Natural Ingredients Used in Food, Drugs, and Cosmetics.* 2nd ed. Hoboken, NJ: A John Wiley & Sons, Inc.; 2003: 167-170.
8. Ellingwood F. *American Materia Medica, Therapeutics, and Pharmacognosy.* Rev. ed. Albuquerque, NM: Southwest School for Botanical Medicine; 1994: 34.

9. Felter HW. *The Eclectic Materia Medica, Pharmacology and Therapeutics.* Cincinnati, OH: Published by John K. Scudder, 1922: 35-36.

CLEAVERS

1. Grieve M. *A Modern Herbal.* Great Britain: Jonathan Cape Ltd.; 1931: 206.
2. Hickman JC (ed.). *The Jepson Manual: Higher Plants of California.* Berkeley, CA: University of California Press; 1996: 978-986.
3. Munz PA. *A Flora of Southern California.* Berkeley, CA: University of California Press; 1974: 765.
4. Pojar J, MacKinnon A. *Plants of the Pacific Northwest Coast.* Vancouver, BC: Lone Pine Publishing; 1994: 330.
5. Willard T. *Edible and Medicinal Plants of the Rocky Mountains and Neighboring Territories.* Calgary, AB: Wild Rose College of Natural Healing; 1992: 189.
6. Foster S. *Herbal Renaissance.* Layton, UT: Peregrine Smith Books; 1993: 199-200.
7. Skenderi G. *Herbal Vade Mecum.* Rutherford, NJ: Herbacy Press; 2003: 38.
8. Moore M. Lecture presented at Southwest School for Botanical Medicine residency program. Albuquerque, NM; 1994.
9. Ellingwood F. *American Materia Medica, Therapeutics, and Pharmacognosy.* Rev. ed. Albuquerque, NM: Southwest School for Botanical Medicine; 1994: 53.
10. Mills S, Bone K. *Principles and Practice of Phytotherapy.* London, UK: Harcourt Publishers Limited; 2000: 148.

CLOVE

1. Leung AY, Foster S. *Encyclopedia of Common Natural Ingredients Used in Food, Drugs, and Cosmetics.* 2nd ed. Hoboken, NJ: A John Wiley & Sons, Inc.; 2003: 174-177.
2. Eugenia aromatica. FAO Ecocrop website. http://ecocrop.fao.org/ecocrop/srv/en/cropView?id=2462. Accessed October 21, 2014.
3. Syzygium aromaticum. World Agroforestry Center. http://www.worldagroforestry.org/treedb/AFTPDFS/Syzygium_aromaticum.pdf. Accessed October 21, 2014.
4. Taxonomy: Syzygium aromaticum. Natural History Museum, London website. http://www.nhm.ac.uk/nature-online/species-of-the-day/collections/collecting/syzygium-aromaticum/taxonomy/index.html. Accessed October 21, 2014.
5. Gray J. *A Guide to the Study of Pharmacognosy: Or the Essentials of Materia Medica of the Vegetable and Animal Kingdoms.* Buffalo, NY: Peter Paul Book Company and Printers; 1894: 91-92.
6. Gladen C. Cloves. University of Minnesota. https://www.lib.umn.edu/bell/tradeproducts/cloves. Accessed January 12, 2015.
7. Felter HW. *The Eclectic Materia Medica, Pharmacology and Therapeutics.* Cincinnati, OH: Published by John K. Scudder; 1922: 31.
8. Grieve M. *A Modern Herbal.* Great Britain: Jonathan Cape Ltd.; 1931: 208.
9. Skenderi G. *Herbal Vade Mecum.* Rutherford, NJ: Herbacy Press; 2003: 102-103.
10. Schnaubelt K. *Advanced Aromatherapy—The Science of Essential Oil Therapy.* Rochester, VT: Healing Arts Press; 1995: 65.

CODONOPSIS

1. Codonopsis. Flora of Pakistan. eFloras website. Missouri Botanical Garden, St. Louis, MO & Harvard University Herbaria, Cambridge, MA. http://efloras.org/florataxon.aspx?flora_id=5&taxon_id=107542. Accessed March 10, 2015.
2. Codonopsis. Flora of China. eFloras website. Missouri Botanical Garden, St. Louis, MO & Harvard University Herbaria, Cambridge, MA. http://efloras.org/florataxon.aspx?flora_id=2&taxon_id=107542. Accessed March 10, 2015.
3. Schafer P. *The Chinese Medicinal Herb Farm.* White River Junction, VT: Chelsea Green Publishing Company; 2011: 144.
4. Foster S, Yue C. *Herbal Emissaries, Bringing Chinese Herbs to the West.* Rochester, VT: Healing Arts Press; 1992: 58-64.
5. Charters M. California Plant Names: Latin and Greek Meanings and Derivations—A Dictionary of Botanical and Biographical Etymology website. http://www.calflora.net/botanicalnames/pagePI-PY.html. Updated 2014. Accessed January 19, 2016.
6. Bensky D, Gamble A. *The Chinese Herbal Medicine Materia Medica.* Rev. ed. Seattle, WA: Eastland Press; 1993: 317-318; 327.
7. Leung AY, Foster S. *Encyclopedia of Common Natural Ingredients Used in Food, Drugs, and Cosmetics.* 2nd ed. Hoboken, NJ: A John Wiley & Sons, Inc.; 2003: 185-187.
8. Winston D, Maimes S. *Adaptogens—Herbs for Strength, Stamina, and Stress Relief.* Rochester, VT: Healing Arts Press; 2007: 154-157.
9. Skenderi G. *Herbal Vade Mecum.* Rutherford, NJ: Herbacy Press; 2003: 105-106.
10. Teeguarden R. *Chinese Tonic Herbs.* Tokyo, Japan: Japan Publications, Inc.; 1995: 103-105.

COMFREY

1. Symphytum officinale. Flora of China. eFloras website. Missouri Botanical Garden, St. Louis, MO & Harvard University Herbaria, Cambridge, MA. http://efloras.org/florataxon.aspx?flora_id=2&taxon_id=200019185. Accessed March 11, 2015.
2. Grieve M. *A Modern Herbal.* Great Britain: Jonathan Cape Ltd.; 1931: 215-218.
3. Symphytum Flora of China. eFloras website. Missouri Botanical Garden, St. Louis, MO & Harvard University Herbaria, Cambridge, MA. http://efloras.org/florataxon.aspx?flora_id=2&taxon_id=132030. Accessed March 11, 2015.
4. Kelly RB. Symphytum officinale. Jepson Flora Project. Jepson eFlora website. http://ucjeps.berkeley.edu/cgi-bin/get_IJM.pl?tid=45945. Published 2013. Accessed March 11, 2015.
5. Leung AY, Foster S. *Encyclopedia of Common Natural Ingredients Used in Food, Drugs, and Cosmetics.* 2nd ed. Hoboken, NJ: A John Wiley & Sons, Inc.; 2003: 191.
6. Pedersen M. *Nutritional Herbology: A Reference Guide to Herbs.* Warsaw, IN: Wendell W. Whitman Company; 1998: 73.
7. Foster S. *Herbal Renaissance.* Layton, UT: Peregrine Smith Books; 1993: 76-77.
8. Tyler V. *The Honest Herbal.* Binghamton, NY: The Hawthorn Press, Inc.; 1993: 98-100.
9. Mills S, Bone K. *Principles and Practice of Phytotherapy.* London, UK: Harcourt Publishers Limited; 2000: 180;209;163;165.
10. Weiss RF. *Herbal Medicine.* Avon, UK: The Bath Press; 1996: 334-335.
11. Skenderi G. *Herbal Vade Mecum.* Rutherford, NJ: Herbacy Press, 2003: 109.

COPTIS

1. Coptis. Flora of China. eFloras website. Missouri Botanical Garden, St. Louis, MO & Harvard University Herbaria, Cambridge, MA. http://efloras.org/florataxon.aspx?flora_id=2&taxon_id=107946. Accessed March 10, 2015.
2. Coptis. Flora of North America. eFloras website. Missouri Botanical Garden, St. Louis, MO & Harvard University Herbaria, Cambridge, MA. http://efloras.org/florataxon.aspx?flora_id=1&taxon_id= 107946. Accessed March 10, 2015.
3. Bensky D, Gamble A. *The Chinese Herbal Medicine Materia Medica.* Rev. ed. Seattle, WA: Eastland Press; 1993: 77-80.
4. Charters M. Coptis. California Plant Names: Latin and Greek Meanings and Derivations. A Dictionary of Botanical and Biographical Etymology. http://calflora.net/botanicalnames/pageCI-CY.html. Accessed December 9, 2016.
5. Charters M. Deltoidea. California Plant Names: Latin and Greek Meanings and Derivations. A Dictionary of Botanical and Biographical Etymology. http://calflora.net/botanicalnames/pageD.html. Accessed December 9, 2016.
6. Feng Y, Siu K, Wang N, et al. Bear bile: dilemma of traditional medicinal use and animal protection. *Journal of Ethnobiology and Ethnomedicine.* 2009:5(2). doi: 10.1186/1746-4269-5-2. Accessed December 9, 2016.
7. Huang JI, Shengji P, Chunlin L. An ethnobotanical study of medicinal plants used by the Lisu people in Nujiang, Northwest Yunnan, China. *Economic Botany.* 2004:5: 253-S264. www.jstor.org/stable/4256922. Accessed December 9, 2016.

8. Grieve M. *A Modern Herbal.* Great Britain: Jonathan Cape Ltd.; 1931: 361.
9. Whitmore PM, Cass GR. The ozone fading of traditional Japanese colorants. *Studies in Conservation.* 1988:33(1):29-40. www.jstor.org/stable/1506238. Accessed December 9, 2016.
10. Felter HW. *The Eclectic Materia Medica, Pharmacology and Therapeutics.* Cincinnati, OH: Published by John K. Scudder; 1922: 39-40.
11. Ganjhu RK, Mudgal PP, Maity H, Dowarha D, Devadiga S, et al. Herbal plants and plant preparations as a remedial approach for viral diseases. *Virus Disease.* 2015 Dec; 26(4): 225–236. Published online September 3, 2105. doi: 10.1007/s13337-015-0276-6. Accessed February 16, 2017.
12. Chin LW, Cheng YW, Lin SS, Lai YY, Lin LY, Chou MY, et al. Anti-herpes simplex virus effects of berberine from Coptidis rhizoma, a major component of a Chinese herbal medicine, Ching-Wei-San. *Arch Virol.* 2010 Dec;155(12):1933-41. doi: 10.1007/s00705-010-0779-9. Epub 2010 Aug 5. Accessed February 16 2017.
13. Skenderi G. *Herbal Vade Mecum.* Rutherford, NJ: Herbacy Press, 2003: 111-112; 32-33.

CORDYCEPS

1. Hobbs C. *Medicinal Mushrooms: An Exploration of Tradition, Healing, and Culture.* Summertown, TN: Botanica Press; 1996: 81.
2. Boesi A, Cardi F. Cordyceps sinensis medicinal fungus: Traditional use among Tibetan people, harvesting techniques, and modern uses. *HerbalGram.* 2009;83:52-61. American Botanical Council website. http://cms.herbalgram.org/herbal gram/issue83/article3433.html?Issue=83&ts=1426022898& signature= 60445f37a4d58ecdbec0822f2c36a57f. Accessed March 10, 2015.
3. Lui H, Hu H, Chu C, Li Q, Li P. Morphological and microscopic identification studies of Cordyceps and its counterfeits. *Acta Pharmaceutica Sinica B.* 2011;1(3): 189-195. Elsevier website. http://www.sciencedirect.com/science/article/pii/S2211383511 000669. Accessed March 10, 2015.
4. Bensky D, Gamble A. *The Chinese Herbal Medicine Materia Medica.* Rev. ed. Seattle, WA: Eastland Press; 1993: 338-339.
5. Stamets P, Yao D. *MycoMedicinals—An Informational Treatise on Mushrooms.* Olympia, WA: MycoMedia Productions; 2002: 57-62.
6. Halpern G. *Cordyceps, China's Healing Mushroom.* Garden City Park, NY: Avery Publishing Group; 1999: 1-100.
7. Winston D, Maimes S. *Adaptogens—Herbs for Strength, Stamina, and Stress Relief.* Rochester, VT: Healing Arts Press; 2007: 150-154.
8. Yance D. *Adaptogens in Medical Herbalism.* Rochester, VT: Healing Arts Press; 2013: 397-401.

CORN SILK

1. Curtin LSM, Moore, M. *Healing Herbs of the Upper Rio Grande.* Rev. ed. Santa Fe, NM: Western Edge Press; 1997: 100-103.
2. Zea mays. Missouri Botanical Garden Plant Finder. http://www.missouribotanicalgarden.org/PlantFinder/PlantFinderDetails.aspx?kempercode=b138. Accessed October 14, 2014.
3. Corn. Food for Thought: The Science, Culture, and Politics of Food. website. http://academics.hamilton.edu/foodforthought/Our_Research_files/corn.pdf Accessed October 14, 2014.
4. Grieve M. *A Modern Herbal.* Great Britain: Jonathan Cape Ltd.; 1931: 225.
5. Leung AY, Foster S. *Encyclopedia of Common Natural Ingredients Used in Food, Drugs, and Cosmetics.* 2nd ed. Hoboken, NJ: A John Wiley & Sons, Inc.; 2003: 195.
6. Skenderi G. *Herbal Vade Mecum.* Rutherford, NJ: Herbacy Press; 2003: 112.
7. Tierra M. *The Way of Herbs.* New York, NY: Pocket Books; 1990: 150.
8. Moore M. Lecture presented at Southwest School for Botanical Medicine residency program. Albuquerque, NM; 1994.

COUCH GRASS

1. Grieve M. *A Modern Herbal.* Great Britain: Jonathan Cape Ltd.; 1931: 370-371.
2. Couch grass (Agropyron repens). Plant Profiler. Sigma-Aldrich. http://www.sigmaaldrich.com/life-science/nutrition-research/learning-center/plant-profiler/agropyron-repens.html. Published 2010. Accessed September 26, 2013.
3. Pojar J, MacKinnon A. *Plants of the Pacific Northwest Coast.* Vancouver, BC: Lone Pine Publishing; 1994: 362.
4. Hickman JC (ed.). *The Jepson Manual: Higher Plants of California.* Berkeley, CA: University of California Press; 1996: 1256-1257.
5. Foster S, Hobbs C. *Western Medicinal Plants and Herbs.* New York, NY: Peterson Field Guides, Houghton Mifflin Company; 2002: 383.
6. Moore M. Lecture from Southwest School for Botanical Medicine residency program. Albuquerque, NM; 1994.

COW PARSNIP

1. Cary R. Cow Parsnip (Heracleum lanatum). Yosemite Hikes website. http://www.yosemitehikes.com/wildflowers/cow-parsnip/cow-parsnip.html. Accessed January 8, 2014.
2. Hickman JC. (ed.) *The Jepson Manual: Higher Plants of California.* Berkeley, CA: University of California Press; 1996: 148.
3. Charters ML. Wrightii. California Plant Names: Latin and Greek Meanings and Derivations website. http://www.calflora.net/botanicalnames/pageLA-LE.html). Accessed January 8, 2015.
4. Pojar J, MacKinnon A. *Plants of the Pacific Northwest Coast.* Vancouver, BC: Lone Pine Publishing; 1994: 213.
5. Moore M. *Medicinal Plants of the Pacific Northwest.* Santa Fe, NM: Red Crane Books; 1993: 99-101.
6. Skenderi G. *Herbal Vade Mecum.* Rutherford, NJ: Herbacy Press, 2003: 115-116.

CRAMP BARK

1. Viburnum opulus. Flora of China. eFloras website. Missouri Botanical Garden, St. Louis, MO & Harvard University Herbaria, Cambridge, MA.http://efloras.org/florataxon.aspx?flora_id=2& taxon_id=200022493. Accessed April 24, 2015.
2. Vibunum opulus. Flora of Pakistan. eFloras website. Missouri Botanical Garden, St. Louis, MO & Harvard University Herbaria, Cambridge, MA. http://efloras.org/florataxon.aspx?flora_id=5& taxon_id=200022493. Accessed April 24, 2015.
3. Online Etymology Dictionary website. http://www.etymonline.com/index.php. Accessed November 3, 2013.
4. Willard T. *Edible and Medicinal Plants of the Rocky Mountains and Neighboring Territories.* Calgary, AB: Wild Rose College of Natural Healing; 1992: 194-195.
5. Grieve M. *A Modern Herbal.* Great Britain: Jonathan Cape Ltd.; 1931: 381-382.
6. Foster S, Johnson R. *Desk Reference to Nature's Medicine.* Washington, D.C.: National Geographic Society; 2006: 56-57.
7. Felter HW. *The Eclectic Materia Medica, Pharmacology and Therapeutics.* Cincinnati, OH: Published by John K. Scudder, 1922: 117.
8. Ellingwood F. *American Materia Medica, Therapeutics, and Pharmacognosy.* Rev. ed. Albuquerque, NM: Southwest School for Botanical Medicine; 1994: 104.
9. Pojar J, MacKinnon A. *Plants of the Pacific Northwest Coast.* Vancouver, BC: Lone Pine Publishing; 1994: 68.
10. Willard T. *The Wild Rose Scientific Herbal.* Calgary, AB: Wild Rose College of Natural Healing; 1998: 99.
11. Skenderi G. *Herbal Vade Mecum.* Rutherford, NJ: Herbacy Press; 2003: 117.
12. Maikhuri RK, Dhyani D, Tyagi Y, Singh D, Negi VS, Rawat LS. Determination of nutritional and energy value of Viburnum mullaha Buch.-Ham. Ex D. Don (Indian cranberry). *Ecol Food Nutr.* 2012;51(3):218-26. http://www.ncbi.nlm.nih.gov/pubmed/22632061. Updated May 25th, 2012. Accessed November 20, 2013.
13. Moore M. Lecture presented at Southwest School for Botanical Medicine residency program. Albuquerque, NM; 1994.

DAMIANA

1. Felter HW, Lloyd JU. Damiana. *King's American Dispensatory.* 18th ed, 3rd Rev. Cincinnati: Ohio Valley Co. 1898. Available from Henriette's Herbal website. http://www.henriettes-herb.com/eclectic/kings/ turnera.html. Published 1999. Accessed April 24, 2015.
2. Grieve M. *A Modern Herbal.* Great Britain: Jonathan Cape Ltd.; 1931: 249.

3. Taylor L. *The Healing Power of Rainforest Herbs—A Guide to Understanding and Using Herbal Medicinals.* Garden City Park, NY: Square One Publishers; 2005: 259-262.
4. Moore M. *Los Remedios—Traditional Herbal Remedies of the Southwest.* Santa Fe, NM: Red Crane Books; 1990: 40.
5. Tyler V. *The Honest Herbal.* Binghamton, NY: The Hawthorn Press, Inc.; 1993: 107-108.
6. Ellingwood F. *American Materia Medica, Therapeutics, and Pharmacognosy.* Rev. ed. Albuquerque, NM: Southwest School for Botanical Medicine; 1994: 160-161.
7. Willard T. *The Wild Rose Scientific Herbal.* Calgary, AB: Wild Rose College of Natural Healing; 1998: 104-105.
8. Skenderi G. *Herbal Vade Mecum.* Rutherford, NJ: Herbacy Press, 2003: 127-128.
9. Mabey R. *The New Age Herbalist.* New York, NY: Gaia books; 1988: 116-117.
10. Leung AY, Foster S. *Encyclopedia of Common Natural Ingredients Used in Food, Drugs, and Cosmetics.* 2nd ed. Hoboken, NJ: A John Wiley & Sons, Inc.; 2003: 204-205.
11. Pedersen M. *Nutritional Herbology: A Reference Guide to Herbs.* Warsaw, IN: Wendell W. Whitman Company; 1998: 76-77.
12. Louisiana State Act 159. Wikipedia website. http://en.wikipedia.org/wiki/Louisiana_State_Act_159. Accessed December 4, 2013.
13. Mills S. *The Essential Book of Herbal Medicine.* London, UK: Penguin Books; 1991: 516-518.

DANDELION

1. Taraxacum officinale. Flora of North America. eFloras website. Missouri Botanical Garden, St. Louis, MO & Harvard University Herbaria, Cambridge, MA. Published 2008. Accessed December 10, 2015.
2. Grieve M. *A Modern Herbal.* Great Britain: Jonathan Cape Ltd.; 1931: 249-255.
3. Dandelion (Taraxacum officinale). deviantART website. http://flower-lovers.deviantart.com/journal/Dandelion-Taraxacum-officinale-214198164. Accessed July 13, 2014.
4. Murray M. *The Healing Power of Herbs.* 2nd ed. Rocklin, CA: Prima Publishing; 1995: 86-91.
5. List of Medicinal Herbs. MMS Gardens—Hortus Medicus website. http://www.piam.com/mms_garden/officinalis.html. Accessed July 13, 2014.
6. Willard T. *The Wild Rose Scientific Herbal.* Calgary, AB: Wild Rose College of Natural Healing; 1998: 106-109.
7. Foster S, Johnson R. *Desk Reference to Nature's Medicine.* Washington, D.C.: National Geographic Society; 2006: 230-231.
8. Scudder J. *The American Eclectic Materia Medica and Therapeutics (Twelfth Edition).* Cincinnati, OH: The Scudder Brothers Company Publishers; 1898: 252-253.
9. Ellingwood F. *American Materia Medica, Therapeutics, and Pharmacognosy.* Rev. ed. Albuquerque, NM: Southwest School for Botanical Medicine; 1994: 97.
10. Felter HW. *The Eclectic Materia Medica, Pharmacology and Therapeutics.* Cincinnati, OH: Published by John K. Scudder; 1922: 110-111.
11. *British Herbal Pharmacopoeia.* Originally published by the British Herbal Medicine Association Scientific Committee. Bisbee, AZ: Southwest School of Botanical Medicine; 2008: 206-208.
12. Culbreth D. *A Manual of Materia Medica and Pharmacology.* Bisbee, AZ: Southwest School of Botanical Medicine; 2008: 296-297.
13. Moore M. *Medicinal Plants of the Mountain West.* Santa Fe, NM: Museum of New Mexico Press; 2003: 103-105.
14. Leung AY, Foster S. *Encyclopedia of Common Natural Ingredients Used in Food, Drugs, and Cosmetics.* 2nd ed. Hoboken, NJ: A John Wiley & Sons, Inc.; 2003: 205-207.
15. Pedersen M. *Nutritional Herbology: A Reference Guide to Herbs.* Warsaw, IN: Wendell W. Whitman Company; 1998: 78-79.
16. Skenderi G. *Herbal Vade Mecum.* Rutherford, NJ: Herbacy Press; 2003: 210.
17. Tyler V. *The Honest Herbal.* Binghamton, NY: The Hawthorn Press, Inc.; 1993: 109-110.
18. Moore M. Lecture presented at Southwest School for Botanical Medicine residency program. Albuquerque, NM; 1994.

DONG QUAI

1. Angelica sinensis. Flora of China. eFloras website. Missouri Botanical Garden, St. Louis, MO & Harvard University Herbaria, Cambridge, MA. http://efloras.org/florataxon.aspx?flora_id=2&taxon_id=200015389. Published 2008. Accessed January 6, 2015.
2. Angelica. Flora of China. eFloras website. Missouri Botanical Garden, St. Louis, MO & Harvard University Herbaria, Cambridge, MA. http://efloras.org/florataxon.aspx?flora_id=2&taxon_id=101754. Published 2008. Accessed January 6, 2015.
3. Foster S, Yue C. *Herbal Emissaries, Bringing Chinese Herbs to the West.* Rochester, VT: Healing Arts Press; 1992: 65-73.
4. Mills S, Bone K. *Principles and Practice of Phytotherapy.* London, UK: Harcourt Publishers Limited; 2000: 350-353.
5. Murray M. *The Healing Power of Herbs.* Rocklin, CA: Prima Publishing; 1992, 1995: 43-49.
6. Bensky D, Gamble A. *The Chinese Herbal Medicine Materia Medica.* Rev. ed. Seattle, WA: Eastland Press; 1993: 327; 329-330.
7. Skenderi G. *Herbal Vade Mecum.* Rutherford, NJ: Herbacy Press; 2003: 136-137.
8. Pedersen M. *Nutritional Herbology: A Reference Guide to Herbs.* Warsaw, IN: Wendell W. Whitman Company; 1998: 81-82.
9. Foster S, Johnson R. *Desk Reference to Nature's Medicine.* Washington, D.C.: National Geographic Society; 2006: 136-137.
10. Tricky R. *Women, Hormones and the Menstrual Cycle.* St. Leonards, Australia: Allen and Unwin; 1998: 322-325.
11. Teeguarden R. *Chinese Tonic Herbs.* Tokyo, Japan: Japan Publications, Inc.; 1995: 85-88.
12. Moore M. Lecture presented at Southwest School for Botanical Medicine residency program. Albuquerque, NM; 1994.
13. Circosta C, Pasquale RD, Palumbo DR, Samperi S, Occhiuto F. Estrogenic activity of the standardized extract of Angelica sinensis. Phytother Res. 2006 Aug;20(8):665-9. http://www.ncbi.nlm.nih.gov/pubmed/16691630. Accessed February 4, 2016.

ECHINACEA

1. Echinacea angustifolia. Flora of North America. eFloras website. Missouri Botanical Garden, St. Louis, MO & Harvard University Herbaria, Cambridge, MA. http://www.efloras.org/florataxon.aspx?flora_id=1&taxon_id=242416463. Accessed October 21, 2014.
2. Echinacea purpurea. Flora of North America. eFloras website. Missouri Botanical Garden, St. Louis, MO & Harvard University Herbaria, Cambridge, MA. http://www.efloras.org/florataxon.aspx?flora_id=1&taxon_id=220004561. Accessed October 21, 2014.
3. Willard T. *Edible and Medicinal Plants of the Rocky Mountains and Neighboring Territories.* Calgary, AB: Wild Rose College of Natural Healing; 1992: 211-212.
4. Foster S, Hobbs C. *Western Medicinal Plants and Herbs.* New York, NY: Peterson Field Guides, Houghton Mifflin Company; 2002: 217.
5. Ellingwood F. *American Materia Medica, Therapeutics, and Pharmacognosy.* Rev. ed. Albuquerque, NM: Southwest School for Botanical Medicine; 1994: 42-46.
6. Foster S, Johnson R. *Desk Reference to Nature's Medicine.* Washington, D.C.: National Geographic Society; 2006: 138-139.
7. Felter HW. *The Eclectic Materia Medica, Pharmacology and Therapeutics.* Cincinnati, OH: Published by John K. Scudder; 1922: 43-46.
8. Leung AY, Foster S. *Encyclopedia of Common Natural Ingredients Used in Food, Drugs, and Cosmetics.* 2nd ed. Hoboken, NJ: A John Wiley & Sons, Inc.; 2003: 216-220.
9. Skenderi G. *Herbal Vade Mecum.* Rutherford, NJ: Herbacy Press; 2003: 139-140.
10. Weiss RF. *Herbal Medicine.* Avon, UK: The Bath Press; 1996: 229-230.
11. Moore M. Lecture presented at Southwest School for Botanical Medicine residency program. Albuquerque, NM; 1994.
12. Moore M. *Medicinal Plants of the Desert and Canyon West.* Santa Fe, NM: Museum of New Mexico Press: 45-49.
13. Mills S, Bone K. *Principles and Practice of Phytotherapy.* London, UK: Harcourt Publishers Limited; 2000: 354-362.

ELDER

1. Bell CD. Sambucus. Jepson Flora Project. Jepson eFlora website. http://ucjeps.berkeley.edu/cgi-bin/get_IJM.pl?key=10321. Published 2013. Accessed January 20, 2015.
2. Sambucus nigra. Integrated Taxonomic Information System On-line database. http://www.itis.gov/servlet/SingleRpt/SingleRpt?search_topic=TSN&search_value=35324. Accessed January 20, 2015
3. Sambucus nigra. Flora of Pakistan. eFloras website. Missouri Botanical Garden, St. Louis, MO & Harvard University Herbaria, Cambridge, MA. http://efloras.org/florataxon.aspx?flora_id=5&taxon_id=200022402. Published 2008. Accessed January 20, 2015.
4. Bell CD. Sambucus nigra subsp. caerula. Jepson Flora Project. Jepson eFlora website. http://ucjeps.berkeley.edu/cgi-bin/get_IJM.pl?tid=80587. Published 2013. Accessed January 20, 2015.
5. Charlebois D. Elderberry as a Medicinal Plant. *Issues in New Crops and New Uses Journal.* New Crop Resource Online Program: Purdue University. https://www.hort.purdue.edu/newcrop/ncnu07/pdfs/charlebois284-292.pdf. Published 2007. Accessed January 20, 2015.
6. Brown SH. Taylor K. Sambucus nigra L. subsp. Canadensis. University of Florida: IFAS Lee County Extension website. http://lee.ifas.ufl.edu/Hort/GardenPubsAZ/Elderberry_Sambucus_plant.pdf. Accessed January 20, 2015.
7. Sambucus nigra ssp. canadensis. Ladybird Johnson Wildflower Center Native Plant Database. http://www.wildflower.org/plants/result.php?id_plant=SANIC4. Accessed January 20, 2015.
8. Bell CD. Sambucus racemosa var. melanocarpa. Jepson Flora Project. Jepson eFlora website. http://ucjeps.berkeley.edu/cgi-bin/get_IJM.pl?tid=80590. Published 2013. Accessed January 20, 2015.
9. Grieve M. *A Modern Herbal.* Great Britain: Jonathan Cape Ltd.; 1931: 265-276.
10. Curtin LSM, Moore, M. *Healing Herbs of the Upper Rio Grande.* Rev. ed. Santa Fe, NM: Western Edge Press; 1997: 71-73.
11. Common Elderberry, Sambucus nigra L. ssp. canadensis (L.) R. Bolli. United States Department of Agriculture—Natural Resources Conservation Service. National Plant Data Center & the Biota of North America Program. http://www.plants.usda.gov/plantguide/pdf/cs_sanic4.pdf. Accessed August 24, 2015.
12. Felter HW. *The Eclectic Materia Medica, Pharmacology and Therapeutics.* Cincinnati, OH: Published by John K. Scudder, 1922: 101.
13. Ellingwood F. *American Materia Medica, Therapeutics, and Pharmacognosy.* Rev. ed. Albuquerque, NM: Southwest School for Botanical Medicine; 1994: 91.
14. Leung AY, Foster S. *Encyclopedia of Common Natural Ingredients Used in Food, Drugs, and Cosmetics.* 2nd ed. Hoboken, NJ: A John Wiley & Sons, Inc.; 2003: 220-222.
15. Skenderi G. *Herbal Vade Mecum.* Rutherford, NJ: Herbacy Press; 2003: 141-142.
16. Loizzo MR, Pugliese A, Bonesi M, Tenuta MC, Menichini F, Xiao J, Tundis R. Edible Flowers: A Rich Source of Phytochemicals with Antioxidant and Hypoglycemic Properties. *J Agric Food Chem.* 2015 Aug 19. Available from PubMed. http://www.ncbi.nlm.nih.gov/pubmed/26270801. Accessed August 25, 2015.
17. Foster S, Johnson R. *Desk Reference to Nature's Medicine.* Washington, D.C.: National Geographic Society; 2006: 150-151.
18. Barak V, Halperin T, Kalickman I. The effect of Sambucol, a black-elderberry-based, natural product, on the production of human cytokines: I. Inflammatory cytokines. *Eur Cytokine Netw.* 2001 Apr-Jun;12(2):290-6. Available from PubMed. http://www.ncbi.nlm.nih.gov/pubmed/11399518. Accessed August 24, 2015.
19. Zakay-Rones Z, Thom E, Wollan T, Wadstein J. Randomized study of the efficacy and safety of oral elderberry extract in the treatment of influenza A and B virus infections. 2004 Mar-Apr;32(2):132-40. J Int Med Res. 2004 Mar-Apr;32(2): 132-40. Available from PubMed. http://www.ncbi.nlm.nih.gov/pubmed/15080016. Accessed August 24, 2015.
20. Ho GT, Ahmed A, Zou YF, Aslaksen T, Wangensteen H, Barsett H. Structure-activity relationship of immunomodulating pectins from elderberries. *Carbohydr Polym.* 2015 Jul 10;125: 314-22. http://www.ncbi.nlm.nih.gov/pubmed/25857988. Available from PubMed. doi: 10.1016/j.carbpol.2015.02.057.
21. Anti-Toxoplasma activities of methanolic extract of Sambucus nigra (Caprifoliaceae) fruits and leaves. *Rev Biol Trop.* 2015 Mar;63(1): 7-12. Available from PubMed. http://www.ncbi.nlm.nih.gov/pubmed/26299111. Published March, 2015. Accessed August 25, 2015.
22. Willard T. *Edible and Medicinal Plants of the Rocky Mountains and Neighboring Territories.* Calgary, AB: Wild Rose College of Natural Healing; 1992: 191-192.

ELECAMPANE

1. Grieve M. *A Modern Herbal.* Great Britain: Jonathan Cape Ltd.; 1931: 278-283.
2. Knoke D. Inula helenium. WTU Herbarium Image Collection: Burk Museum of Natural History and Culture website. http://biology.burke.washington.edu/herbarium/imagecollection.php Genus=Inula&Species=helenium. Accessed September 23, 2014.
3. Kowalchik C, Hylton WH. *Rodale's Illustrated Encyclopedia of Herbs.* Emmaus, Pennsylvannia: Rodale Press; 1998: 182.
4. Foster S, Johnson R. *Desk Reference to Nature's Medicine.* Washington, D.C.: National Geographic Society; 2006: 140-141.
5. Felter HW. *The Eclectic Materia Medica, Pharmacology and Therapeutics.* Cincinnati, OH: Published by John K. Scudder; 1922: 64.
6. Ellingwood F. *American Materia Medica, Therapeutics, and Pharmacognosy.* Rev. ed. Albuquerque, NM: Southwest School for Botanical Medicine; 1994: 64-65.
7. Leung AY, Foster S. *Encyclopedia of Common Natural Ingredients Used in Food, Drugs, and Cosmetics.* 2nd ed. Hoboken, NJ: A John Wiley & Sons, Inc.; 2003: 222-224.
8. Skenderi G. *Herbal Vade Mecum.* Rutherford, NJ: Herbacy Press; 2003: 142-143.
9. Pedersen M. *Nutritional Herbology: A Reference Guide to Herbs.* Warsaw, IN: Wendell W. Whitman Company; 1998: 85-86.
10. Pole S. *Ayurvedic Medicine: The Principles of Traditional Practice.* Philadelphia, PA: Churchill Livingstone Elsevier; 2006: 248-249.

ELEUTHERO

1. Mills S, Bone K. *Principles and Practice of Phytotherapy.* London, UK: Harcourt Publishers Limited; 2000: 534-541.
2. Eleutherococcus senticosus. Flora of China. eFloras website. Missouri Botanical Garden, St. Louis, MO & Harvard University Herbaria, Cambridge, MA. http://efloras.org/florataxon.aspx?flora_id=2&taxon_id=220004653. Published 2008. Accessed December 2, 2014.
3. McKenna DJ, Jones K, Hughes K, Tyler VM. *Botanical Medicines: The Desk Reference for Major Herbal Supplements, Second Edition.* New York, NY: Routledge, 2011: 255.
4. Murray M. *The Healing Power of Herbs.* Rocklin, CA: Prima Publishing; 1992, 1995: 314-320.
5. Blumenthal M. *The ABC Clinical Guide to Herbs.* Austin, TX: The American Botanical Council; 2003: 99-106.
6. Foster S, Johnson R. *Desk Reference to Nature's Medicine.* Washington, D.C.: National Geographic Society; 2006: 225-227.
7. Winston D, Maimes S. *Adaptogens—Herbs for Strength, Stamina, and Stress Relief.* Rochester, VT: Healing Arts Press; 2007: 33-37; 157-161.
8. Yance D. *Adaptogens in Medical Herbalism.* Rochester, VT: Healing Arts Press; 2013: 410-418.
9. Leung AY, Foster S. *Encyclopedia of Common Natural Ingredients Used in Food, Drugs, and Cosmetics.* 2nd ed. Hoboken, NJ: A John Wiley & Sons, Inc.; 2003: 225-227.
10. Pedersen M. *Nutritional Herbology: A Reference Guide to Herbs.* Warsaw, IN: Wendell W. Whitman Company; 1998: 158-159.
11. Moore M. Lecture presented at Southwest School for Botanical Medicine residency program. Albuquerque, NM; 1994.
12. Willard T. *The Wild Rose Scientific Herbal.* Calgary, AB: Wild Rose College of Natural Healing; 1998: 316-317.
13. Seller A. Lecture notes from Pacific School of Herbal Medicine. Oakland, CA; 1995.
14. Skenderi G. *Herbal Vade Mecum.* Rutherford, NJ: Herbacy Press; 2003: 173.

EPHEDRA

1. Ephedraceae. Flora of North America. eFloras website. Missouri Botanical Garden, St. Louis, MO & Harvard University Herbaria, Cambridge, MA. http://efloras.org/florataxon.aspx?flora_id=1&taxon_id=10313. Published 2008. Accessed January 6, 2017.
2. Fu L, Yu Y, Riedl H. Ephedraceae. Flora of China. eFloras website. Missouri Botanical Garden, St. Louis, MO & Harvard University Herbaria, Cambridge, MA. http://efloras.org/florataxon.aspx?-flora_id=1&taxon_id=10313. Published 2008. Accessed January 6, 2017.
3. Ephedra nevadensis. Flora of North America. eFloras website. Missouri Botanical Garden, St. Louis, MO & Harvard University Herbaria, Cambridge, MA. http://efloras.org/florataxon.aspx?-flora_id=1&taxon_id=233500607. Published 2008. Accessed January 6, 2017.
4. Ephedra. Flora of North America. eFloras website. Missouri Botanical Garden, St. Louis, MO & Harvard University Herbaria, Cambridge, MA. http://efloras.org/florataxon.aspx?flora_id=1&taxon_id=111784. Published 2008. Accessed January 6, 2017.
5. Ephedra viridis. Flora of North America. eFloras website. Missouri Botanical Garden, St. Louis, MO & Harvard University Herbaria, Cambridge, MA. http://efloras.org/florataxon.aspx flora_id=1&taxon_id=233500611. Published 2008. Accessed January 6, 2017.
6. Ephedra sinica. Flora of China. eFloras website. Missouri Botanical Garden, St. Louis, MO & Harvard University Herbaria, Cambridge, MA. http://efloras.org/florataxon.aspx?flora_id=2&taxon_id=200005521. Published 2008. Accessed January 6, 2017.
7. Charters M. California Plant Names: Latin and Greek Meanings and Derivations website. http://calflora.net/botanicalnames/pageE.html. Accessed January 6, 2017.
8. Harper D. Viridian. Online Etymology Dictionary website. http://etymonline.com/index.php?term=viridian&allowed_in_frame=0. Accessed January 6, 2017.
9. Remington JP, Wood HC. The Dispensatory of the United States of America, 20th ed. 1918. Published online by the Southwest School for Botanical Medicine. http://swsbm.com/Dispensatory/USD-1918-complete.pdf Accessed January 6, 2017.
10. Curtin LSM, Moore, M. *Healing Herbs of the Upper Rio Grande.* Rev. ed. Santa Fe, NM: Western Edge Press; 1997: 35-36.
11. Bensky D, Gamble A. *The Chinese Herbal Medicine Materia Medica.* Rev. ed. Seattle, WA: Eastland Press; 1993: 28-29.
12. Murray M. *The Healing Power of Herbs.* Rocklin, CA: Prima Publishing; 1992, 1995: 108-115.
13. Skenderi G. *Herbal Vade Mecum.* Rutherford, NJ: Herbacy Press; 2003: 144-145.
14. Leung AY, Foster S. *Encyclopedia of Common Natural Ingredients Used in Food, Drugs, and Cosmetics.* 2nd ed. Hoboken, NJ: A John Wiley & Sons, Inc.; 2003: 227-229.
15. Moore M. *Medicinal Plants of the Mountain West.* Santa Fe, NM: Museum of New Mexico Press; 2003: 166-168.
16. Skenderi G. *Herbal Vade Mecum.* Rutherford, NJ: Herbacy Press; 2003: 144-145.
17. Kane C. *Herbal Medicine of the American Southwest.* Lincoln Town Press; 2006: 136-137.

FENNEL

1. Constance J, Wetherwax M. Foeniculus vulgare. Jepson Flora Project. Jepson eFlora website. http://ucjeps.berkeley.edu/cgi-bin/get_IJM.pl?tid=25972. Accessed April 2, 2015.
2. Foeniculum vulgare. Flora of China. eFloras website. Missouri Botanical Garden, St. Louis, MO & Harvard University Herbaria, Cambridge, MA. http://efloras.org/florataxon.aspx?flora_id=2&taxon_id=200015555. Accessed April 2, 2015.
3. Foeniculum. Flora of China. eFloras website. Missouri Botanical Garden, St. Louis, MO & Harvard University Herbaria, Cambridge, MA. http://efloras.org/florataxon.aspx?flora_id=2&taxon_id=112896. Accessed April 2, 2015.
4. Fennel. Online Etymology Dictionary website. http://www.etymonline.com/index.php?term=fennel&allowed_in_frame=0. Accessed July 1, 2013.
5. Grieve M. *A Modern Herbal.* Great Britain: Jonathan Cape Ltd.; 1931: 293-297.
6. Lad, V, Frawley D. *The Yoga of Herbs.* Twin Lakes, WI: Lotus Press; 1992: 117.
7. Leung AY, Foster S. *Encyclopedia of Common Natural Ingredients Used in Food, Drugs, and Cosmetics.* 2nd ed. Hoboken, NJ: A John Wiley & Sons, Inc.; 2003: 242.
8. Foster S, Johnson R. *Desk Reference to Nature's Medicine.* Washington, D.C.: National Geographic Society; 2006: 166-167.
9. Pedersen M. *Nutritional Herbology: A Reference Guide to Herbs.* Warsaw, IN: Wendell W. Whitman Company; 1998: 90.
10. Skenderi G. *Herbal Vade Mecum.* Rutherford, NJ: Herbacy Press; 2003: 151.
11. Willard T. *Edible and Medicinal Plants of the Rocky Mountains and Neighboring Territories.* Calgary, AB: Wild Rose College of Natural Healing; 1992: 118-121.
12. Foster S. *Herbal Renaissance.* Layton, UT: Peregrine Smith Books; 1993: 92-93.
13. Moore M. Lecture presented at Southwest School for Botanical Medicine residency program. Albuquerque, NM; 1994.
14. Mills S, Bone K. *Principles and Practice of Phytotherapy.* London, UK: Harcourt Publishers Limited; 2000: 378-384.
15. Weiss RF. *Herbal Medicine.* Avon, UK: The Bath Press; 1996: 68-69.
16. Keville K, Green M. *Aromatherapy—A Complete Guide to the Healing Art.* Freedom, CA: The Crossing Press; 1995: 54.

FENUGREEK

1. Katzer G. Spice Pages website. http://gernot-katzers-spice-pages.com/engl/Trig_foe.html. Accessed November 12, 2015.
2. Trigonella foenum-graecum. Flora of China. eFloras website. Missouri Botanical Garden, St. Louis, MO & Harvard University Herbaria, Cambridge, MA. http://efloras.org/florataxon.aspx?flora_id=2&taxon_id=200012345. Published 2008. Accessed February 4, 2015.
3. Trigonella foenum-graecum. Flora of Pakistan. eFloras website. Missouri Botanical Garden, St. Louis, MO & Harvard University Herbaria, Cambridge, MA. http://efloras.org/florataxon.aspx?flora_id=5&taxon_id=200012345. Published 2008. Accessed February 4, 2015.
4. Grieve M. *A Modern Herbal.* Great Britain: Jonathan Cape Ltd.; 1931: 299.
5. Leung AY, Foster S. *Encyclopedia of Common Natural Ingredients Used in Food, Drugs, and Cosmetics.* 2nd ed. Hoboken, NJ: A John Wiley & Sons, Inc.; 2003: 243-245.
6. Foster S. *An Illustrated Guide to 101 Medicinal Herbs.* Loveland, CO: Interweave Press, Inc.; 1998: 84-85, 101.
7. Willard T. *The Wild Rose Scientific Herbal.* Calgary, AB: Wild Rose College of Natural Healing; 1998: 122-125.
8. Tyler V. *The Honest Herbal.* Binghamton, NY: The Hawthorn Press, Inc.; 1993: 131-132.
9. Bensky D, Gamble A. *The Chinese Herbal Medicine Materia Medica.* Rev. ed. Seattle, WA: Eastland Press; 1993: 343.
10. Pedersen M. *Nutritional Herbology: A Reference Guide to Herbs.* Warsaw, IN: Wendell W. Whitman Company; 1998: 91-92.
11. Pole S. *Ayurvedic Medicine: The Principles of Traditional Practice.* Philadelphia, PA: Churchill Livingstone Elsevier; 2006: 177-178.
12. Murray M. *The Healing Power of Herbs.* Rocklin, CA: Prima Publishing; 1992, 1995: 359-360.
13. Skenderi G. *Herbal Vade Mecum.* Rutherford, NJ: Herbacy Press; 2003: 152.

FEVERFEW

1. Tanacetum parthenium. Flora of North America website. http://efloras.org/florataxon.aspx?flora_id=1&taxon_id=242101204. Accessed November 26, 2014.
2. Tanacetum parthenium. Flora of Pakistan website. http://efloras.org/florataxon.aspx?flora_id=5&taxon_id=242101204. Accessed November 26, 2014.
3. Foster S, Johnson R. *Desk Reference to Nature's Medicine.* Washington, D.C.: National Geographic Society; 2006: 168-169.
4. Foster S. *Herbal Renaissance.* Layton, UT: Peregrine Smith books; 1993: 93-95.
5. Mills S, Bone K. *Principles and Practice of Phytotherapy*. London, UK: Harcourt Publishers Limited; 2000: 385-393.
6. Grieve M. *A Modern Herbal.* Great Britain: Jonathan Cape Ltd.; 1931: 309-310.

7. Leung AY, Foster S. *Encyclopedia of Common Natural Ingredients Used in Food, Drugs, and Cosmetics.* 2nd ed. Hoboken, NJ: A John Wiley & Sons, Inc.; 2003: 246-247.
8. Blumenthal M. *The ABC Clinical Guide to Herbs.* Austin, TX: The American Botanical Council; 2003: 137-142.
9. Skenderi G. *Herbal Vade Mecum.* Rutherford, NJ: Herbacy Press, 2003: 153.
10. Pedersen M. *Nutritional Herbology: A Reference Guide to Herbs.* Warsaw, IN: Wendell W. Whitman Company; 1998: 93-94.
11. Murray M. *The Healing Power of Herbs.* Rocklin, CA: Prima Publishing; 1992, 1995: 116-120.
12. Moore M. Lecture presented at Southwest School for Botanical Medicine residency program. Albuquerque, NM; 1994.

GARLIC

1. Katzer G. Spice Pages website. http://gernot-katzers-spice-pages.com/engl/Alli_sat.html. Accessed December 8, 2015.
2. Allium sativum. Flora of China. eFloras website. Missouri Botanical Garden, St. Louis, MO & Harvard University Herbaria, Cambridge, MA. http://efloras.org/florataxon.aspx?flora_id=2&taxon_id=200027526. Published 2008. Accessed December 5, 2014.
3. Kamenetsky R, Shafir IL, Baizerman M, Khassanov F, Kik C, Rabinowitch HD. Garlic *(Allium sativum L.)* and its wild relatives from central Asia: Evaluation for Fertility Potential. *ISHS Acta Horticulturae.* 2004; 637: 83-91. http://www.actahort.org/books/637/637_9.htm. Accessed December 5, 2014.
4. Foster S., Yue C. *Herbal Emissaries, Bringing Chinese Herbs to the West.* Rochester, VT: Healing Arts Press; 1992: 86-92.
5. Foster S. *Herbal Renaissance.* Layton, UT: Peregrine Smith Books; 1993: 96-99.
6. Murray M. *The Healing Power of Herbs.* Rocklin, CA: Prima Publishing; 1992, 1995: 121-131.
7. Foster S., Johnson R. *Desk Reference to Nature's Medicine.* Washington, D.C.: National Geographic Society; 2006: 176-177.
8. Leung AY, Foster S. *Encyclopedia of Common Natural Ingredients Used in Food, Drugs, and Cosmetics.* 2nd ed. Hoboken, NJ: A John Wiley & Sons, Inc.; 2003: 260-264.
9. Blumenthal M. *The ABC Clinical Guide to Herbs.* Austin, TX: The American Botanical Council; 2003: 155-170.
10. Pedersen M. *Nutritional Herbology: A Reference Guide to Herbs.* Warsaw, IN: Wendell W. Whitman Company; 1998: 94-96.
11. Skenderi G. *Herbal Vade Mecum.* Rutherford, NJ: Herbacy Press; 2003: 165-166.
12. Pole S. *Ayurvedic Medicine: The Principles of Traditional Practice.* Philadelphia, PA: Churchill Livingstone Elsevier; 2006: 179-180.
13. Lad V., Frawley D. *The Yoga of Herbs.* Twin Lakes, WI: Lotus Press; 1992: 119-120.

GENTIAN

1. Willard T. *Edible and Medicinal Plants of the Rocky Mountains and Neighboring Territories.* Calgary, AB: Wild Rose College of Natural Healing; 1992: 135-37.
2. Foster S, Johnson R. *Desk Reference to Nature's Medicine.* Washington, D.C.: National Geographic Society; 2006: 178-79.
3. Skenderi G. *Herbal Vade Mecum.* Rutherford, NJ: Herbacy Press; 2003: 167-68.
4. Leung AY, Foster S. *Encyclopedia of Common Natural Ingredients Used in Food, Drugs, and Cosmetics.* 2nd ed. Hoboken, NJ: A John Wiley & Sons, Inc.; 2003: 267-68.
5. Grieve M. *A Modern Herbal.* Great Britain: Jonathan Cape Ltd.; 1931: 347-49.
6. Foster S, Hobbs C. *Western Medicinal Plants and Herbs.* New York, NY: Peterson Field Guides, Houghton Mifflin Company; 2002: 193-94.
7. Lust J. *The Herb Book.* New York, NY: Bantam Books; 1974: 423.
8. Ellingwood F. *American Materia Medica, Therapeutics, and Pharmacognosy.* Rev. ed. Albuquerque, NM: Southwest School for Botanical Medicine; 1994: 57.
9. Foster S. *An Illustrated Guide to 101 Medicinal Herbs.* Loveland, CO: Interweave Press, Inc.; 1998: 96-97.
10. Moore M. *Medicinal Plants of the Pacific Northwest.* Santa Fe, NM: Red Crane Books; 1993: 122-25.
11. Hoffman D. *Medical Herbalism — The Science and Practice of Herbal Medicine.* Rochester, VT: Healing Arts Press; 2003: 553.
12. Pedersen M. *Nutritional Herbology: A Reference Guide to Herbs.* Warsaw, IN: Wendell W. Whitman Company; 1998: 97-98.
13. Weiss RF. *Herbal Medicine.* Avon, UK: The Bath Press; 1996: 40-42.
14. Mills S, Bone K. *Principles and Practice of Phytotherapy.* London, UK: Harcourt Publishers Limited; 2000: 38-40.
15. Guyten A, Hall J. *Textbook of Medical Physiology.* Philadelphia, PA: W.B. Saunders Co.; 1996: 824-829.
16. Willard T. *The Wild Rose Scientific Herbal.* Calgary, AB: Wild Rose College of Natural Healing; 1998: 175.
17. Tierra M. *The Way of Chinese Herbs.* New York, NY: Pocket Books, 1998: 177.
18. Bensky D, Gamble A. *The Chinese Herbal Medicine Materia Medica.* Rev. ed. Seattle, WA: Eastland Press; 1993: 81-82.

GINGER

1. Katzer G. The Spice Pages website. http://gernot-katzers-spice-pages.com/engl/Zing_off.html. Accessed December 4, 2015.
2. Bensky D, Gamble A. *The Chinese Herbal Medicine Materia Medica.* Rev. ed. Seattle, WA: Eastland Press; 1993: 36; 300-301.
3. Zingiber officinale. The Flora of China. eFloras website. Missouri Botanical Garden, St. Louis, MO & Harvard University Herbaria, Cambridge, MA. http://efloras.org/florataxon.aspx?flora_id=2&taxon_id=200028468. Published 2008. Accessed December 5, 2014.
4. Ravindran PN, Nirmal Babu K, eds. *Ginger: The Genus Zingiber*. Boca Raton, Florida: CRC Press. 2005. Available from Google Books. https://books.google.com/books?id=w5Echt6km94C&printsec=frontcover#v=onepage&q&f=false. Accessed December 8, 2014.
5. Felter HW, Lloyd JU. Zingiber (U. S. P.)—Ginger. *King's American Dispensatory.* Cincinnatti: Ohio Valley Co. 1898. Available from Henriette's Herbal website. www.henriettes-herb.com/eclectic/kings/zingiber.html. Published 1999. Accessed December 8, 2014.
6. Foster S, Johnson R. *Desk Reference to Nature's Medicine*. Washington, D.C.: National Geographic Society; 2006: 180-181.
7. Mills S, Bone K. *Principles and Practice of Phytotherapy*. London, UK: Harcourt Publishers Limited; 2000: 394-403.
8. Foster S, Yue C. *Herbal Emissaries, Bringing Chinese Herbs to the West.* Rochester, VT: Healing Arts Press; 1992: 92-102.
9. Pole S. *Ayurvedic Medicine: The Principles of Traditional Practice*. Philadelphia, PA: Churchill Livingstone Elsevier; 2006: 183-184.
10. Felter HW. *The Eclectic Materia Medica, Pharmacology and Therapeutics.* Cincinnati, OH: Published by John K. Scudder; 1922: 120.
11. Ellingwood F. *American Materia Medica, Therapeutics, and Pharmacognosy*. Rev. ed. Albuquerque, NM: Southwest School for Botanical Medicine; 1994: 108.
12. Scudder J. *The American Eclectic Materia Medica and Therapeutics (Twelfth Edition).* Cincinnati, OH: The Scudder Brothers Company Publishers; 1898: 215; 354-355; 659.
13. Leung AY, Foster S. *Encyclopedia of Common Natural Ingredients Used in Food, Drugs, and Cosmetics*. 2nd ed. Hoboken, NJ: A John Wiley & Sons, Inc.; 2003: 271-274.
14. Blumenthal M. *The ABC Clinical Guide to Herbs*. Austin, TX: The American Botanical Council; 2003: 173-183.
15. Murray M. *The Healing Power of Herbs*. Rocklin, CA: Prima Publishing; 1992, 1995: 132-142.
16. Pedersen M. *Nutritional Herbology: A Reference Guide to Herbs*. Warsaw, IN: Wendell W. Whitman Company; 1998: 98-101.
17. Willard T. *The Wild Rose Scientific Herbal*. Calgary, AB: Wild Rose College of Natural Healing; 1998: 138-141.
18. Skenderi G. *Herbal Vade Mecum.* Rutherford, NJ: Herbacy Press; 2003: 169.

GINKGO

1. Ginkgo biloba: The Flora of Pakistan. eFloras website. Missouri Botanical Garden, St. Louis, MO & Harvard University Herbaria, Cambridge, MA. http://efloras.org/florataxon.aspx?flora_id=5&taxon_id=200005235. Published 2008. Accessed December 10, 2014.

2. Ginkgo biloba: The Flora of China. eFloras website. Missouri Botanical Garden, St. Louis, MO & Harvard University Herbaria, Cambridge, MA. http://efloras.org/florataxon.aspx?flora_id=2&taxon_id=200005235. Published 2008. Accessed December 10, 2014.
3. Ginkgo biloba: The Flora of North America. eFloras website. Missouri Botanical Garden, St. Louis, MO & Harvard University Herbaria, Cambridge, MA. http://efloras.org/florataxon.aspx?flora_id=1&taxon_id=200005235. Published 2008. Accessed December 10, 2014.
4. Sun C, Dilcher DL, Wang H, Sun G, Ge Y. A study of Ginkgo leaves from the middle Jurassic of Inner Mongolia, China. *International Journal of Plant Science.* 2008. 169(8):1128-1139. http://0-www.jstor.org.catalog.multcolib.org/stable/pdf/10.1086/590474.pdf. Accessed December 18, 2016.
5. Perry L. Ginkgo Trees. University of Vermont Extension, Dept. of Plant and Soil Science. http://pss.uvm.edu/ppp/articles/ginkgo.html. Accessed November 18, 2016.
6. Fernando DD, Quinn CR, Brenner ED, Owens JN. Male gametophyte development and evolution in extant gymnosperms. *International Journal of Plant Developmental Biology.*2010; 4 (1): 47-63. Global Science Books. http://www.esf.edu/efb/faculty/documents/fernandoetal.2010.pdf. Accessed December 10, 2014.
7. Del Tredici P. Ginkgos and people—A thousand years of interaction. *Arnoldia*. 1991. 51(2):2-15. http://www.jstor.org/stable/42954399. Accessed February 17, 2017.
8. Ginkgo. National Center for Complementary and Integrative Health website. https://nccih.nih.gov/health/ginkgo/ataglance.htm. Updated 2016. Accessed February 17, 2017.
9. Murray M. *The Healing Power of Herbs*. Rocklin, CA: Prima Publishing; 1992, 1995: 143-161.
10. Blumenthal M. *The ABC Clinical Guide to Herbs*. Austin, TX: The American Botanical Council; 2003: 187-200.
11. Leung AY, Foster S. *Encyclopedia of Common Natural Ingredients Used in Food, Drugs, and Cosmetics*. 2nd ed. Hoboken, NJ: A John Wiley & Sons, Inc.; 2003: 274-277.
12. Pedersen M. *Nutritional Herbology: A Reference Guide to Herbs*. Warsaw, IN: Wendell W. Whitman Company; 1998: 101-102.
13. Park JW, Kwon HJ, Chung WS, Kim CY, Seong GJ. Short-term effects of Ginkgo biloba extract on peripapillary retinal blood flow in normal tension glaucoma. *Korean J Ophthalmol*. 2011 Oct;25(5):323-8. Epub 2011 Sep 20. doi: 10.3341/kjo.2011.25.5.323. Accessed April 28, 2017.
14. Xu L, Hu Z, Shen J, McQuillan PM. Effects of Ginkgo biloba extract on cerebral oxygen and glucose metabolism in elderly patients with pre-existing cerebral ischemia. *Complement Ther Med*. 2015 Apr;23(2):220-5. doi: 10.1016/j.ctim.2014.12.009. Accessed April 28, 2017.
15. Droy-Lefaix MT. Effect of the antioxidant action of Ginkgo biloba extract (EGB 761) on aging and oxidative stress. *Age*. 1997; 20: 141-149. https://www.ncbi.nlm.nih.gov/pmc/articles/PMC3455891/pdf/11357_1997_Article_13.pdf. Accessed May 12, 2017.
16. Chen JW, Chen YH, Lin FY, Chen YL, Lin SJ. Ginkgo biloba extract inhibits tumor necrosis factor-α–induced reactive oxygen species generation, transcription factor activation, and cell adhesion molecule expression in human aortic endothelial cells. *Arteriosclerosis, Thrombosis, and Vascular Biology*. 2003;23:1559-1566. https://doi.org/10.1161/01.ATV.0000089012.73180.63. Accessed May 12, 2017.
17. Paganelli RA, Benetoli A, Milani H. Sustained neuroprotection and facilitation of behavioral recovery by the Ginkgo biloba extract, EGb 761, after transient forebrain ischemia in rats. *Behav Brain Res*. 2006 Nov 1;174(1):70-7. Epub 2006 August 24. https://www.ncbi.nlm.nih.gov/pubmed/16934342. Accessed April 28, 2017.
18. Mills S, Bone K. *Principles and Practice of Phytotherapy*. London, UK: Harcourt Publishers Limited; 2000: 404-417.
19. Cybulska-Heinrich AK, Mozaffarieh M, Flammer J. Ginkgo biloba: an adjuvant therapy for progressive normal and high tension glaucoma. *Mol Vis*. 2012;18:390-402. Epub 2012 Feb 9. https://www.ncbi.nlm.nih.gov/pubmed/22355250. Accessed May 17, 2017.
20. Fies P, Dienel A. [Ginkgo extract in impaired vision—treatment with special extract EGb 761 of impaired vision due to dry senile macular degeneration]. *Wien Med Wochenschr*. 2002;152(15-16):423-6. https://www.ncbi.nlm.nih.gov/pubmed/12244891. Accessed May 17, 2017.
21. Moore M. Lecture presented at Southwest School for Botanical Medicine residency program. Albuquerque, NM; 1994.
22. Yoshitake T, Yoshitake S, Kehr J. The Ginkgo biloba extract EGb 761® and its main constituent flavonoids and ginkgolides increase extracellular dopamine levels in the rat prefrontal cortex. *British Journal of Pharmacology*. 2010 Feb; 159(3): 659-668. https://www.ncbi.nlm.nih.gov/pubmed/20105177. Accessed May 12, 2017.

GINSENG, ASIAN

1. Leung AY, Foster S. *Encyclopedia of Common Natural Ingredients Used in Food, Drugs, and Cosmetics*. 2nd ed. Hoboken, NJ: A John Wiley & Sons, Inc.; 2003: 277-281.
2. Panax ginseng: The Flora of China. eFloras website. Missouri Botanical Garden, St. Louis, MO & Harvard University Herbaria, Cambridge, MA. http://efloras.org/florataxon.aspx?flora_id=2&taxon_id=200015246. Published 2008. Accessed December 15, 2014.
3. Choi K. Botanical characteristics, pharmacological effects and medicinal components of Korean Panax ginseng CA Meyer. *Acta Pharmacol Sin*. 2008; 29(9): 1109–1118. Nature Publish Group website. http://www.nature.com/aps/journal/v29/n9/pdf/aps2008134a.pdf. Accessed December 15, 2014.
4. Panax: The Flora of China. eFloras website. Missouri Botanical Garden, St. Louis, MO & Harvard University Herbaria, Cambridge, MA. http://efloras.org/florataxon.aspx?flora_id=2&taxon_id=123736. Published 2008. Accessed December 15, 2014.
5. Foster S, Johnson R. *Desk Reference to Nature's Medicine*. Washington, D.C.: National Geographic Society; 2006: 24-25.
6. Ginseng. Dictionary.com website. http://www.dictionary.com/browse/ginseng?s=t. Accessed February 10, 2017.
7. Hu SY. The genus *Panax* (Ginseng) in Chinese Medicine. Economic Botany. 1976; 30(1): 11-28. http://www.jstor.org/stable/4253681. Accessed February 10, 2017.
8. Grieve M. A Modern Herbal. Great Britain: Jonathan Cape Ltd.; 1931: 354-357.
9. Pedersen M. *Nutritional Herbology: A Reference Guide to Herbs*. Warsaw, IN: Wendell W. Whitman Company; 1998: 128-129.
10. Skenderi G. *Herbal Vade Mecum*. Rutherford, NJ: Herbacy Press, 2003: 172-173.
11. Yance D. *Adaptogens in Medical Herbalism*. Rochester, VT: Healing Arts Press; 2013: 438-444.
12. Bensky D, Gamble A. *The Chinese Herbal Medicine Materia Medica*. Rev. ed. Seattle, WA: Eastland Press; 1993: 314-316.
13. Blumenthal M. *The ABC Clinical Guide to Herbs*. Austin, TX: The American Botanical Council; 2003: 213-226.
14. Mills S, Bone K. *Principles and Practice of Phytotherapy*. London, UK: Harcourt Publishers Limited; 2000: 418-432.

GOLDENROD

1. Grieve M. *A Modern Herbal.* Great Britain: Jonathan Cape Ltd.; 1931: 361-362.
2. Hickman JC (ed.). *The Jepson Manual: Higher Plants of California*. Berkeley, CA: University of California Press; 1996: 343.
3. Foster S, Hobbs C. *Western Medicinal Plants and Herbs*. New York, NY: Peterson Field Guides, Houghton Mifflin Company; 2002: 130.
4. Pojar J, MacKinnon A. *Plants of the Pacific Northwest Coast.* Vancouver, BC: Lone Pine Publishing; 1994: 289.
5. Ellingwood F. *American Materia Medica, Therapeutics, and Pharmacognosy*. Cincinnati, OH; 1922: 95-96.
6. Willard T. *Edible and Medicinal Plants of the Rocky Mountains and Neighboring Territories.* Calgary, AB: Wild Rose College of Natural Healing; 1992: 219-222.
7. Skenderi G. *Herbal Vade Mecum.* Rutherford, NJ: Herbacy Press; 2003: 175.

GOTU KOLA

1. Centella. The Flora of China. eFloras website. Missouri Botanical Garden, St. Louis, MO & Harvard University Herbaria, Cambridge, MA. http://efloras.org/florataxon.aspx?flora_id=2&taxon_id=106022. Published 2008. Accessed December 10, 2014.
2. Centella asiatica. The Flora of China. eFloras website. Missouri Botanical Garden, St. Louis, MO & Harvard University Herbaria, Cambridge, MA. http://efloras.org/florataxon.aspx?flora_id=2&taxon_id=200015478. Published 2008. Accessed December 10, 2014.
3. Centella asiatica. The Flora of Pakistan. eFloras website. Missouri Botanical Garden, St. Louis, MO & Harvard University Herbaria, Cambridge, MA. Centella: http://efloras.org/florataxon.aspx?flora_id=5&taxon_id=200015478. Published 2008. Accessed December 10, 2014.
4. Centella. The Flora of Pakistan. eFloras website. Missouri Botanical Garden, St. Louis, MO & Harvard University Herbaria, Cambridge, MA. Centella: http://efloras.org/florataxon.aspx?flora_id=5&taxon_id=106022. Published 2008. Accessed December 10, 2014.
5. Quattrocchi U. *CRC World Dictionary of Medicinal and Poisonous Plants: Common Names, Scientific Names, Eponyms, Synonyms, and Etymology.* Boca Raton, FL: CRC Press; 2012: 881.
6. Pole S. *Ayurvedic Medicine: The Principles of Traditional Practice*. Philadelphia, PA: Churchill Livingstone Elsevier; 2006: 187-188.
7. Lad V, Frawley D. *The Yoga of Herbs.* Twin Lakes, WI: Lotus Press; 1992: 170-172.
8. Yance D. *Adaptogens in Medical Herbalism*. Rochester, VT: Healing Arts Press; 2013: 212-213; 452-457.
9. Murray M. *The Healing Power of Herbs*. Rocklin, CA: Prima Publishing; 1992, 1995: 173-183.
10. Leung AY, Foster S. *Encyclopedia of Common Natural Ingredients Used in Food, Drugs, and Cosmetics.* 2nd ed. Hoboken, NJ: A John Wiley & Sons, Inc.; 2003: 284-286.
11. Pedersen M. *Nutritional Herbology: A Reference Guide to Herbs*. Warsaw, IN: Wendell W. Whitman Company; 1998: 104-105.
12. Skenderi G. *Herbal Vade Mecum.* Rutherford, NJ: Herbacy Press; 2003: 176-177.

GRAVEL ROOT

1. Grieve M. *A Modern Herbal.* Great Britain: Jonathan Cape Ltd.; 1931: 374.
2. Eupatoriadelphus purpureum. Flora of New Zealand Series: Manaaki Whenua- Landcare Research Databases. http://floraseries.landcareresearch.co.nz/pages/Taxon.aspx?id=_b1f39061-c545-456b-a09e-9bad2761f82b&fileName=Flora%204.xml. Accessed October 17, 2014.
3. Eutrochium purpureum. Flora of North America. http://www.efloras.org/florataxon.aspx?flora_id=1&taxon_id=250066769. Accessed October 17, 2014.
4. Ellingwood F. *American Materia Medica, Therapeutics, and Pharmacognosy*. Rev. ed. Albuquerque, NM: Southwest School for Botanical Medicine; 1994: 51.
5. Felter HW. *The Eclectic Materia Medica, Pharmacology and Therapeutics.* Cincinnati, Ohio: Published by John K. Scudder; 1922: 49.
6. Skenderi G. *Herbal Vade Mecum.* Rutherford, NJ: Herbacy Press; 2003: 210-211.

GRINDELIA

1. Grieve M. *A Modern Herbal.* Great Britain: Jonathan Cape Ltd.; 1931: 376-377.
2. Curtin LSM, Moore, M. *Healing Herbs of the Upper Rio Grande.* Rev. ed. Santa Fe, NM: Western Edge Press; 1997: 179-180.
3. Committee on Herbal Medicinal Products. Assessment report on *Grindelia robusta* Nutt., *Grindelia squarrosa* (Pursh) Dunal, *Grindelia humilis* Hook. et Arn., *Grindelia camporum* Greene, herba. European Medicines Agency Web Site. http://www.ema.europa.eu/docs/en_GB/document_library/Herbal_-_HMPC_assessment_report/2013/03/WC500139835.pdf. Published November 20, 2012. Accessed August 28, 2015.
4. Grindelia. Flora of China. eFloras website. Missouri Botanical Garden, St. Louis, MO & Harvard University Herbaria, Cambridge, MA. http://efloras.org/florataxon.aspx?flora_id=2&taxon_id=114086. Published 2008. Accessed December 16, 2014.
5. Moore AJ. Grindelia. Jepson Flora Project. Jepson eFlora website. http://ucjeps.berkeley.edu/cgi-bin/get_IJM.pl?tid=3113. Published August 26, 2008. Accessed December 16, 2014.
6. Grindelia. Flora of North America. eFloras website. Missouri Botanical Garden, St. Louis, MO & Harvard University Herbaria, Cambridge, MA. http://efloras.org/florataxon.aspx?flora_id=1&taxon_id=114086. Published 2008. Accessed December 16, 2014.
7. Charters M. Camporum. California Plant Names: Latin and Greek Meanings and Derivations website. http://www.calflora.net/botanicalnames/pageCA-CH.html. Accessed August 31st, 2015.
8. Charters M. Hi-Hy. California Plant Names: Latin and Greek Meanings and Derivations website. http://www.calflora.net/botanicalnames/pageHI-HY.html. Accessed August 31, 2015.
9. Charters M. Integrifolia. California Plant Names: Latin and Greek Meanings and Derivations website. http://www.calflora.net/botanicalnames/pageI.html. Accessed August 31, 2015.
10. Charters M. Rigida. California Plant Names: Latin and Greek Meanings and Derivations website. http://www.calflora.net/botanicalnames/pageR.html. Accessed August 31, 2015.
11. Robust. Squarosa. Dictionary website. http://dictionary.reference.com/browse/robust. Accessed August 31, 2015.
12. Felter HW. *The Eclectic Materia Medica, Pharmacology and Therapeutics.* Cincinnati, OH: Published by John K. Scudder, 1922: 57-58.
13. Ellingwood F. *American Materia Medica, Therapeutics, and Pharmacognosy*. Rev. ed. Albuquerque, NM: Southwest School for Botanical Medicine; 1994: 59-60.
14. Foster S, Hobbs C. *Western Medicinal Plants and Herbs*. New York, NY: Peterson Field Guides, Houghton Mifflin Company; 2002: 132-133.
15. Willard T. *Edible and Medicinal Plants of the Rocky Mountains and Neighboring Territories.* Calgary, AB: Wild Rose College of Natural Healing; 1992: 215.
16. Moore M. *Medicinal Plants of the Mountain West*. Santa Fe, NM: Museum of New Mexico Press; 2003: 125-126.
17. Skenderi G. *Herbal Vade Mecum.* Rutherford, NJ: Herbacy Press; 2003: 178-179.
18. McLaughlin S. Grindelia. Purdue University Web Site. https://hort.purdue.edu/newcrop/CropFactSheets/grindelia.html. Accessed August 28, 2015.

GYMNEMA

1. Gurmar. Flowers of India website. http://www.flowersofindia.net/catalog/slides/Gurmar.html. Published May 15, 2015. Accessed January 13, 2017.
2. Gymnema. Flora of China. eFloras website. Missouri Botanical Garden, St. Louis, MO & Harvard University Herbaria, Cambridge, MA. http://www.efloras.org/florataxon.aspx?flora_id=2&taxon_id=114243. Published 2008. Accessed January 13, 2017.
3. Gymnema sylvestre. Flora of China. eFloras website. Missouri Botanical Garden, St. Louis, MO & Harvard University Herbaria, Cambridge, MA. http://www.efloras.org/florataxon.aspx?flora_id=2&taxon_id=200018618. Published 2008. Accessed January 13, 2017.
4. Mesler M. Plant Taxonomy. Class Lecture. Arcata, CA: Humboldt State University; 2009.
5. Naked. Merriam-Webster Dictionary website. https://www.merriam-webster.com/dictionary/naked. Accessed January 13, 2017.
6. Nemato. The American Heritage Dictionary website. https://ahdictionary.com/word/search.html?id=N5061400. Accessed January 13, 2017.
7. Sylvan. Merriam-Webster Dictionary website. https://www.merriam-webster.com/dictionary/sylvan. Accessed January 13, 2017.
8. Halpern M. *Textbook of Clinical Ayurvedic Medicine: Part 1.* 6th ed. Nevada City, CA: California College of Ayurveda; 2007: 38-40.
9. Sripathi SK, Sankari U. Ethnobotanical documentation of a few medicinal plants in the Agasthiayamalai Region of Tirunelveli Distric, India. *Ethnobotanical Leaflets.* 2010;14:173-181. http://opensiuc.lib.siu.edu/cgi/viewcontent.cgi?article=1693&context=ebl. Accessed January 20, 2017.

10. Muthu C, Ayyanar M, Raja N, Ignacimuthu S. Medicinal plants used by traditional healers in District of Tamil Nadu, India. *Journal of Ethnobiology and Ethnomedicine.* 2006; 2(43). https://ethnobiomed.biomedcentral.com/articles/10.1186/1746-4269-2-43. Accessed January 20, 2017.
11. Jain SK. Medicinal plant lore of the Tribals of Bastar. *Economic Botany*. 1965; 19 (3): 236-250. http://0-www.jstor.org.catalog.multcolib.org/stable/pdf/4252605.pdf. Accessed January 20, 2017.
12. Bally PRO. Native medicinal and poisonous plants of East Africa. *Bulletin of Miscellaneous Information (Royal Botanic Gardens, Kew).* 1937; 1937(1):10-26. http://0-www.jstor.org.catalog.multcolib.org/stable/pdf/4107637.pdf. Accessed January 20, 2017.
13. The Royal Society. *The British Medical Journal*. 1890; 1 (1538): 1437. http://0-www.jstor.org.catalog.multcolib.org/stable/pdf/20239525.pdf. Accessed January 20, 2017.
14. Tiwari P, Mishra BN, Sangwan NS. Phytochemical and pharma cological properties of Gymnema sylvestre: an important medicinal plant. *Biomed Res. Int.* 2014; 2014 (830285). doi: 10.1155/2014/830285. Accessed January 20, 2017.
15. Skenderi G. *Herbal Vade Mecum.* Rutherford, NJ: Herbacy Press; 2003: 183.
16. Pole S. *Ayurvedic Medicine: The Principles of Traditional Practice*. Philadelphia, PA: Churchill Livingstone Elsevier; 2006: 193-195.
17. Murray M. *The Healing Power of Herbs*. Rocklin, CA: Prima Publishing; 1992, 1995: 358-359.

HAWTHORN

1. Eve M. *A Modern Herbal.* Great Britain: Jonathan Cape Ltd.; 1931: 385-386.
2. Crataegus. Flora of North America. eFloras website. Missouri Botanical Garden, St. Louis, MO & Harvard University Herbaria, Cambridge, MA. http://efloras.org/florataxon.aspx?flora_id=1&taxon_id=108272. Published 2008. Accessed October 29, 2015.
3. Hickman JC. (ed.) . *The Jepson Manual: Higher Plants of California*. Berkeley, CA: University of California Press; 1996: 950.
4. Mitchell L. *Norfolk (Slow Travel): Local. Characterful Guides to Britain's Special Places.* Chalfont St Peter, Eng: Bradt Travel Guides: 2014.
5. Crataegus. Flora of China. eFloras website. Missouri Botanical Garden, St. Louis, MO & Harvard University Herbaria, Cambridge, MA. http://efloras.org/florataxon.aspx?flora_id=2&taxon_id=108272. Published 2008. Accessed November 14, 2014.
6. Crataegus monogyna. Burke Museum of Natural History and Culture: University of Washington website. http://biology.burke.washington.edu/herbarium/imagecollection.php?Genus=Crataegus&Species=monogyna. Accessed November 14, 2014.
7. Crataegus monogyna var. monogyna. Flora of North America. eFloras website. Missouri Botanical Garden, St. Louis, MO & Harvard University Herbaria, Cambridge, MA. Published 2008. http://efloras.org/florataxon.aspx?flora_id=1&taxon_id=250100576. Accessed October 29, 2014.
8. Crataegus laevigata. Flora of North America. eFloras website. Missouri Botanical Garden, St. Louis, MO & Harvard University Herbaria, Cambridge, MA. http://efloras.org/florataxon.aspx?flora_id=1&taxon_id=250100118. Published 2008. Accessed October 29, 2014.
9. Crataegus laevigata: English Hawthorn. University of Floria IFAS Extension: EDIS website. http://edis.ifas.ufl.edu/st210. Accessed November 14, 2014.
10. Charters M. California Plant Names: Latin and Greek Meanings and Derivations. http://www.calflora.net/botanicalnames/pageLA-LE.html. Accessed October 15, 2015.
11. Harper D. Quickset. Online Etymology Dictionary website. http://etymonline.com/index.php?term=quickset&allowed_in_frame=0. Updated 2015. Accessed October 29, 2015.
12. Harper D. Quick. Online Etymology Dictionary website. http://etymonline.com/index.php?term=quick&allowed_in_frame=0. Accessed Updated 2015. October 29, 2015.
13. Foster S, Johnson R. *Desk Reference to Nature's Medicine*. Washington, D.C.: National Geographic Society; 2006: 204-205.
14. Leung AY, Foster S. *Encyclopedia of Common Natural Ingredients Used in Food, Drugs, and Cosmetics*. 2nd ed. Hoboken, NJ: A John Wiley & Sons, Inc.; 2003: 295-297.
15. Ellingwood F. *American Materia Medica, Therapeutics, and Pharmacognosy*. Rev. ed. Albuquerque, NM: Southwest School for Botanical Medicine; 1994: 39-40.
16. Willard T. *The Wild Rose Scientific Herbal*. Calgary, AB: Wild Rose College of Natural Healing; 1998: 164-166.
17. Pojar J, MacKinnon A. *Plants of the Pacific Northwest Coast.* Vancouver, BC: Lone Pine Publishing; 1994: 73.
18. Blumenthal M. *The ABC Clinical Guide to Herbs*. Austin, TX: The American Botanical Council; 2003: 237-245.
19. Murray M. *The Healing Power of Herbs*. Rocklin, CA: Prima Publishing; 1992, 1995: 203-209.
20. Skenderi G. *Herbal Vade Mecum.* Rutherford, NJ: Herbacy Press, 2003: 184-185.
21. Moore M. *Medicinal Plants of the Mountain West*. Santa Fe, NM: Museum of New Mexico Press; 2003: 126-129.
22. Pedersen M. *Nutritional Herbology: A Reference Guide to Herbs*. Warsaw, IN: Wendell W. Whitman Company; 1998: 107-108.
23. Felter HW. *The Eclectic Materia Medica, Pharmacology and Therapeutics.* Cincinnati, OH: Published by John K. Scudder, 1922: 40.
24. Mills S, Bone K. Principles and Practice of Phytotherapy. London, UK: Harcourt Publishers Limited; 2000: 439-447.
25. Weiss RF. *Herbal Medicine*. Avon, UK: The Bath Press; 1996: 162-169.
26. Stargrove M, Treasure J, McKee D. *Herb, Nutrient, and Drug Interactions — Clinical Implications and Therapeutic Strategies*. St. Loius, MS: Mosby Elsevier; 2008: 99-103.
27. Duke J. Crataegus rapidophylla. Dr. Duke's Phytochemical and Ethnobotanical Databases website. https://phytochem.nal.usda.gov/phytochem/plants/show/2174. Accessed October 29, 2015.

HOPS

1. Brinker F. *Herb Contraindications and Drug Interactions.* Sandy, OR: Eclectic Institute, Inc.; 1997: 54.
2. Curtin LSM, Moore M. *Healing Herbs of the Upper Rio Grande.* Rev. ed. Santa Fe, NM: Western Edge Press; 1997: 199.
3. Humulus lupulus L. Information System on the Flora of Rosandra Valley (Trieste Karst, NE Italy) website. http://dryades.units.it/rosandra_en/index.php?procedure=taxon_page&id=294&num=3192. Accessed March 18, 2014.
4. Leung AY, Foster S. *Encyclopedia of Common Natural Ingredients Used in Food, Drugs, and Cosmetics*. 2nd ed. Hoboken, NJ: A John Wiley & Sons, Inc.; 2003: 300-302.
5. Humulus lupulus. Flora of North America. eFloras website. Missouri Botanical Garden, St. Louis, MO & Harvard University Herbaria, Cambridge, MA. http://efloras.org/florataxon.aspx?flora_id=1&taxon_id=200006377. Published 2008. Accessed November 5, 2015.
6. Humulus lupulus. Flora of Pakistan. eFloras website. Missouri Botanical Garden, St. Louis, MO & Harvard University Herbaria, Cambridge, MA. http://efloras.org/florataxon.aspx?flora_id=5&taxon_id=200006377. Published 2008. Accessed November 5, 2015.
7. Whittemore AT, McClintock E. Humulus lupulus. Jepson Flora Project. Jepson eFlora website. http://ucjeps.berkeley.edu/cgi-bin/get_IJM.pl?tid=28532. Published 2014. Accessed November 5, 2015.
8. Humulus. Flora of Pakistan. eFloras website. Missouri Botanical Garden, St. Louis, MO & Harvard University Herbaria, Cambridge, MA. http://efloras.org/florataxon.aspx?flora_id=5&taxon_id=115880. Published 2008. Accessed November 5, 2015.
9. Grieve M. *A Modern Herbal.* Great Britain: Jonathan Cape Ltd.; 1931: 411-415.
10. Foster S, Johnson R. *Desk Reference to Nature's Medicine.* Washington, D.C.: National Geographic Society; 2006: 212-13.
11. Willard T. *The Wild Rose Scientific Herbal*. Calgary, AB: Wild Rose College of Natural Healing; 1998: 167-69.
12. Scudder JM. *The American Eclectic Materia Medica and Therapeutics.* Cincinnati, OH: The Scudder Brothers Company Publishers; 1923: 336.
13. Ellingwood F. *American Materia Medica, Therapeutics, and Pharmacognosy*. Rev. ed. Albuquerque, NM: Southwest School for Botanical Medicine; 1994: 61.

14. Felter HW. *The Eclectic Materia Medica, Pharmacology and Therapeutics.* Cincinnati, OH: Published by John K. Scudder; 1922: 61.
15. Tyler V. *The Honest Herbal.* Binghamton, NY: The Hawthorn Press, Inc.; 1993: 175-76.
16. Foster S. *Herbal Renaissance.* Layton, UT: Peregrine Smith Books; 1993: 106-108.
17. Skenderi G. *Herbal Vade Mecum.* Rutherford, NJ: Herbacy Press; 2003: 196-197.
18. Mills S. *The Essential Book of Herbal Medicine.* London, UK: Penguin Books; 1991: 458-460.
19. Weiss RF. *Herbal Medicine.* Avon, UK: The Bath Press; 1996: 285-286.
20. Pedersen M. *Nutritional Herbology: A Reference Guide to Herbs.* Warsaw, IN: Wendell W. Whitman Company; 1998: 109-110.
21. Gladstar R. *Herbal Healing for Women.* New York, NY: Simon and Shuster; 1993: 243-245.

HORSETAIL

1. Preston RE, Hauke RL. Equisetum. Jepson Flora Project. Jepson eFlora website. http://ucjeps.berkeley.edu/cgi-bin/get_IJM.pl?tid=9816. Accessed February 4, 2015.
2. Equisetum arvense. Flora of North America. eFloras website. Missouri Botanical Garden, St. Louis, MO & Harvard University Herbaria, Cambridge, MA. http://www.efloras.org/florataxon.aspx?flora_id=1&taxon_id=233500616. Accessed February 4, 2015.
3. Equisetum fluviatile. Flora of North America. eFloras website. Missouri Botanical Garden, St. Louis, MO & Harvard University Herbaria, Cambridge, MA. http://www.efloras.org/florataxon.aspx?flora_id=1&taxon_id=233500617. Accessed February 4, 2015.
4. Equisetum hyemale subsp. affine. Flora of North America. eFloras website. Missouri Botanical Garden, St. Louis, MO & Harvard University Herbaria, Cambridge, MA. http://efloras.org/florataxon.aspx?flora_id=1&taxon_id=233500619. Accessed February 4, 2015.
5. Preston RE, Hauke RL. Equisetum hyemale subsp. afine. Jepson Flora Project. Jepson eFlora website. http://ucjeps.berkeley.edu/cgi-bin/get_IJM.pl?tid=50315. Accessed February 4, 2015.
6. Preston RE, Hauke RL. Equisetum laevigatum. Jepson Flora Project. Jepson eFlora website. http://ucjeps.berkeley.edu/cgi-bin/get_IJM.pl?tid=24427. Accessed February 4, 2015.
7. Equisetum palustre. Flora of China. eFloras website. Missouri Botanical Garden, St. Louis, MO & Harvard University Herbaria, Cambridge, MA. http://www.efloras.org/florataxon.aspx?flora_id=2&taxon_id=233500621. Accessed February 4, 2015.
8. Preston RE, Hauke RL. Equisetum palustre. Jepson Flora Project. Jepson eFlora website. http://ucjeps.berkeley.edu/cgi-bin/get_IJM.pl?tid=24434. Accessed February 4, 2015.
9. Equisetum telmateia. Flora of North America. eFloras website. Missouri Botanical Garden, St. Louis, MO & Harvard University Herbaria, Cambridge, MA. http://efloras.org/florataxon.aspx?flora_id=1&taxon_id=233500628. Accessed February 4, 2015.
10. Preston RE, Hauke RL. Equisetum telmateia. Jepson Flora Project. Jepson eFlora website. http://ucjeps.berkeley.edu/cgi-bin/get_IJM.pl?tid=50317. Accessed February 4, 2015.
11. Equisetum variegatum. Flora of North America. eFloras website. Missouri Botanical Garden, St. Louis, MO & Harvard University Herbaria, Cambridge, MA. http://efloras.org/florataxon.aspx?flora_id=1&taxon_id=233500629. Accessed February 18, 2015.
12. Equisetum variegatum. Flora of China. eFloras website. Missouri Botanical Garden, St. Louis, MO & Harvard University Herbaria, Cambridge, MA.http://efloras.org/florataxon.aspx?flora_id=2&taxon_id=233500629. Accessed February 18, 2015.
13. Pojar J, MacKinnon A. *Plants of the Pacific Northwest Coast.* Vancouver, BC: Lone Pine Publishing; 1994: 430-431.
14. Willard T. *Edible and Medicinal Plants of the Rocky Mountains and Neighboring Territories.* Calgary, AB: Wild Rose College of Natural Healing; 1992: 30-31.
15. Leung AY, Foster S. *Encyclopedia of Common Natural Ingredients Used in Food, Drugs, and Cosmetics.* 2nd ed. Hoboken, NJ: A John Wiley & Sons, Inc.; 2003: 306-308.
16. Moore M. Moore M. *Medicinal Plants of the Mountain West.* Santa Fe, NM: Museum of New Mexico Press; 2003: 135-137.
17. Pedersen M. *Nutritional Herbology: A Reference Guide to Herbs.* Warsaw, IN: Wendell W. Whitman Company; 1998: 112-113.
18. Lad V, Frawley D. *The Yoga of Herbs.* Twin Lakes, WI: Lotus Press; 1992: 125.
19. Skenderi G. *Herbal Vade Mecum.* Rutherford, NJ: Herbacy Press; 2003: 201.

HYDRANGEA

1. Hydrangea arborescens. Missouri Botanical Garden Plant Finder. http://www.missouribotanicalgarden.org/PlantFinder/PlantFinderDetails.aspx?kempercode=k520. Accessed October 17, 2014.
2. Smooth Hydrangea. The Herb Hunters Guide. http://www.hort.purdue.edu/newcrop/herbhunters/hydrangea.html. Accessed October 17, 2014
3. Hydrangea arborescens. Missouri Plants. http://www.missouriplants.com/Whiteopp/Hydrangea_arborescens_page.html. Accessed October 17, 2014.
4. Grieve M. *A Modern Herbal.* Great Britain: Jonathan Cape Ltd., 1931: 424-425.
5. Leung AY, Foster S. *Encyclopedia of Common Natural Ingredients Used in Food, Drugs, and Cosmetics.* 2nd ed. Hoboken, NJ: A John Wiley & Sons, Inc., 2003: 309.
6. Ellingwood F. *American Materia Medica, Therapeutics, and Pharmacognosy.* Evanston, IL: Ellingwood's Therapeutist, 1919: 62.
7. Felter HW. *The Eclectic Materia Medica, Pharmacology and Therapeutics.* Cincinnati, OH: John K. Scudder, 1922: 46.
8. Pedersen M. *Nutritional Herbology: A Reference Guide to Herbs.* Warsaw, IN: Wendell W. Whitman Company, 1998: 114.
9. Skenderi G. *Herbal Vade Mecum.* Rutherford, NJ: Herbacy Press, 2003: 201-202.

JAMAICAN DOGWOOD

1. Piscidia piscipula. Atlas of Florida Vascular Plants, Institute for Systematic Botany website. http://www.florida.plantatlas.usf.edu/Plant.aspx?id=3732. Accessed February 5, 2014.
2. Grieve M. *A Modern Herbal.* Great Britain: Jonathan Cape Ltd.; 1931: 261-262.
3. Auxence E. A Pharmacognostic Study of Piscidia Erythrina. Economic Botany. JSTOR database. http://www.jstor.org/discover/10.2307/4287780?uid=3739920&uid=2&uid=4&uid=3739256&sid=21103471423023. Accessed February 6, 2014.
4. Jamaica-dogwood, Florida fishpoison tree. Natives for Your Neighborhood, The Institute for Regional Conservation website. http://www.regionalconservation.org/beta/nfyn/plantdetail.asp?tx=Piscpisc. Accessed February 6, 2014.
5. Nellis D. *Seashore plants of South Florida and the Caribbean: A Guide to Identification and Propagation of Xeriscape Plants.* Sarasota, FL: Pineapple Press Inc.; 1994: 160.
6. Ellingwood F. *American Materia Medica, Therapeutics, and Pharmacognosy.* Rev. ed. Albuquerque, NM: Southwest School for Botanical Medicine; 1994: 82-83.
7. Leung AY, Foster S. *Encyclopedia of Common Natural Ingredients Used in Food, Drugs, and Cosmetics.* 2nd ed. Hoboken, NJ: A John Wiley & Sons, Inc.; 2003: 214-215.
8. Hoffman D. *Medical Herbalism — The Science and Practice of Herbal Medicine.* Rochester, VT: Healing Arts Press; 2003: 573.
9. Skenderi G. *Herbal Vade Mecum.* Rutherford, NJ: Herbacy Press; 2003: 135-136.
10. Mabey R. *The New Age Herbalist.* New York, NY: Gaia books; 1988: 29.
11. Brinker F. *Herb Contraindications and Drug Interactions.* Sandy, OR: Eclectic Institute, Inc.; 1997: 56.

KAVA

1. Cox PA, O'Rourke L. Kava (Piper methysticum, Piperaceae). *Economic Botany.* 1987; 41(3):452-454. http://www.jstor.org/stable/4254999. Accessed November 26, 2014.
2. Orwa C, Mutua A, Kind R, Jamnadass R, Anthony S. Piper methysticum. *Agroforestree Database: a tree reference and selection guide version 4.0.* http://www.worldagroforestry.org/treedb/AFTPDFS/Piper_methysticum.pdf. Published 2009. Accessed November 29, 2014.

3. Lebot V, Lèvesque J. The origin and distribution of kava (Piper methysticum forst. F. Piperaceae): A phytochemical approach. *Allertonia*. 1989; 5(2): 223-281. http://www.jstor.org/stable/23187398. Accessed November 26, 2014.
4. Foster S, Johnson R. *Desk Reference to Nature's Medicine*. Washington, D.C.: National Geographic Society; 2006: 222-223.
5. Murray M. *The Healing Power of Herbs*. Rocklin, CA: Prima Publishing; 1992, 1995: 210-219.
6. Willard T. *The Wild Rose Scientific Herbal*. Calgary, AB: Wild Rose College of Natural Healing; 1998: 190-192.
7. Mills S, Bone K. *Principles and Practice of Phytotherapy*. London, UK: Harcourt Publishers Limited; 2000: 456-464.
8. Leung AY, Foster S. *Encyclopedia of Common Natural Ingredients Used in Food, Drugs, and Cosmetics*. 2nd ed. Hoboken, NJ: A John Wiley & Sons, Inc.; 2003: 330-331.
9. Ellingwood F. *American Materia Medica, Therapeutics, and Pharmacognosy*. Rev. ed. Albuquerque, NM: Southwest School for Botanical Medicine; 1994: 81-82.
10. Felter HW. *The Eclectic Materia Medica, Pharmacology and Therapeutics.* Cincinnati, OH: Published by John K. Scudder; 1922: 89-90.
11. Blumenthal M. *The ABC Clinical Guide to Herbs*. Austin, TX: The American Botanical Council; 2003: 261-269.
12. Skenderi G. *Herbal Vade Mecum.* Rutherford, NJ: Herbacy Press; 213-214.
13. Pendell D. *Pharmako/poeia—Plant Powers, Poisons, and Herbcraft*. San Francisco, CA: Mercury House; 1995: 146-153.

KELP AND BLADDERWRACK

1. Guiry MD. Kelps: Laminaria and Saccharina. The Seaweed Site: Information on Marine Algae. http://www.seaweed.ie/algae/laminaria.php. Accessed March 11, 2015.
2. McConnaughey E. *Sea Vegetables*. Happy Camp, CA: Naturegraph Publishers; 1985: 121-131.
3. Grieve M. *A Modern Herbal.* Great Britain: Jonathan Cape Ltd.; 1931: 111-114.
4. Guiry MD. Fucus vesiculosus. The Seaweed Site: Information on Marine Algae. http://www.seaweed.ie/descriptions/Fucus_vesiculosus.php. Accessed February 18, 2015.
5. Laminaria. Dictionary.com. http://dictionary.reference.com/browse/laminaria Accessed January 20, 2016.
6. Foster S, Johnson R. *Desk Reference to Nature's Medicine*. Washington, D.C.: National Geographic Society; 2006: 224-225.
7. Pedersen M. *Nutritional Herbology: A Reference Guide to Herbs*. Warsaw, IN: Wendell W. Whitman Company; 1998: 116-117.
8. Murray M. *The Encyclopedia of Healing Foods.* New York, NY: Atria Books; 2005: 662-665.
9. Scudder J. *The American Eclectic Materia Medica and Therapeutics (Twelfth Edition).* Cincinnati, OH: The Scudder Brothers Company Publishers; 1898: 653.
10. Ellingwood F. *American Materia Medica, Therapeutics, and Pharmacognosy*. Rev. ed. Albuquerque, NM: Southwest School for Botanical Medicine; 1994: 53.
11. Felter HW. *The Eclectic Materia Medica, Pharmacology and Therapeutics.* Cincinnati, OH: Published by John K. Scudder, 1922: 51.
12. King J, Felter H, Lloyd J. *King's American Dispensatory* (Volume 1, 19th Edition, Third Revision). Cincinnati, OH: The Ohio Valley Company; 1905: 902-903.
13. Leung AY, Foster S. *Encyclopedia of Common Natural Ingredients Used in Food, Drugs, and Cosmetics*. 2nd ed. Hoboken, NJ: A John Wiley & Sons, Inc.; 2003: 16-19.
14. Willard T. *The Wild Rose Scientific Herbal*. Calgary, AB: Wild Rose College of Natural Healing; 1998: 193-195.
15. Seller A. Lecture notes from Pacific School of Herbal Medicine. Oakland, CA; 1995.
16. Drum R. *Medicinal Uses of Seaweeds*. http://www.ryandrum.com/seaweeds.htm. Accessed January 19, 2016.
17. Murray M, Pizzorno J. *The Encyclopedia of Natural Medicine.* Roclin, CA: Prima Publishing; 1998: 456-457; 562.
18. Pitchford P. *Healing with Whole Foods—Oriental Traditions and Modern.* Berkeley, CA: North Atlantic Books; 1993: 548-550.

LADY'S MANTLE

1. Grieve M. *A Modern Herbal.* Great Britain: Jonathan Cape Ltd.; 1931: 462-463.
2. Hawke RG. An Evaluation Study of Alchemilla. The Chicago Botanical Garden website. https://www.chicagobotanic.org/downloads/planteval_notes/no24_alchemilla.pdf. Accessed April 17, 2015.
3. Alchemilla. Flora of China. Missouri Botanical Garden, St. Louis, MO & Harvard University Herbaria, Cambridge, MA website. http://efloras.org/florataxon.aspx?flora_id=2&taxon_id=100964. Accessed April 17, 2015.
4. Online Etymology Dictionary website. http://www.etymonline.com/index.php. Accessed October 3, 2013.
5. Gladstar R. *Herbal Healing for Women.* New York, NY: Simon and Shuster; 1993: 245.
6. Soule D. *The Roots of Healing, A Woman's Book of Herbs.* New York, NY: Carol Publishing Group; 1995: 116-118.
7. Foster S. *Herbal Renaissance.* Layton, UT: Peregrine Smith Books; 1993: 112-113.
8. Skenderi G. *Herbal Vade Mecum.* Rutherford, NJ: Herbacy Press, 2003: 219-220.

LAVENDER

1. Grieve M. *A Modern Herbal.* Great Britain: Jonathan Cape Ltd.; 1931: 467-473.
2. Lavandula angustifolia. School of Horticulture Plant Database: Kwantlen Polytechnic University web site. https://plantdatabase.kwantlen.ca/plant/plantDetail/623. Accessed Sept. 19, 2014.
3. Upson T, Andrews S, Harriott G. *Lavender: The Genus Lavandula.* Ed. Maria Lis-Balchin. New York, NY:Taylor and Francis Inc: 11-42.
4. Lavandula. Cambridge University Botanic Garden website. http://www.botanic.cam.ac.uk/Botanic/Plant.aspx?p=27&ix=63&pid=0&prcid=0&ppid=0. Accessed Sept. 19, 2014.
5. Lavandula x intermedia 'Grosso'. Missouri Botanical Garden Plant Finder. http://www.missouribotanicalgarden.org/PlantFinder/PlantFinderDetails.aspx?kempercode=a393. Accessed Sept. 19, 2014.
6. Sfikas G. *Wildflowers of Crete*. Athens, Greece: Efstathiadis Group; 1998: 204-205.
7. Gledhill D. *The Names of Plants*. Cambridge, UK: The Cambridge University Press; 2002: 286. https://www.academia.edu/10319073/the_names_of_plants_third_edition. Accessed March 25, 2016.
8. Scudder J. *The American Eclectic Materia Medica and Therapeutics (Twelfth Edition).* Cincinnati, OH: The Scudder Brothers Company Publishers; 1898: 362.
9. Felter HW. *The Eclectic Materia Medica, Pharmacology and Therapeutics.* Cincinnati, OH: Published by John K. Scudder; 1922: 68.
10. Leung AY, Foster S. *Encyclopedia of Common Natural Ingredients Used in Food, Drugs, and Cosmetics*. 2nd ed. Hoboken, NJ: A John Wiley & Sons, Inc.; 2003: 339-342.
11. Skenderi G. *Herbal Vade Mecum.* Rutherford, NJ: Herbacy Press, 2003: 221-222.
12. Schnaubelt K. *Advanced Aromatherapy—The Science of Essential Oil Therapy.* Rochester, VT: Healing Arts Press; 1995: 40-41, 75-76; 89.
13. Keville K, Green M. *Aromatherapy—A Complete Guide to the Healing Art.* Freedom, CA: The Crossing Press; 1995: 59.
14. Tisserand RB, Balacs T. *Essential Oil Safety—A Guide for Health Care Professionals.* London, England: Churchill Livingstone (An imprint of Harcourt Publishers Limited); 1999: 144-145.

LEMON BALM

1. Miller JM, Wilken DH. Melissa officinalis. Jepson Flora Project. Jepson eFlora website. http://ucjeps.berkeley.edu/eflora/eflora_display.php?tid=33161. Published 2014. Accessed December 17, 2015.
2. Grieve M. *A Modern Herbal.* Great Britain: Jonathan Cape Ltd.; 1931: 76-77.
3. Foster S, Johnson R. *Desk Reference to Nature's Medicine*. Washington, D.C.: National Geographic Society; 2006: 226-227.

4. Meyers M. *Lemon Balm: An Herb Society of America Guide.* The Herb Society of America. http://www.herbsociety.org/herbs/profiles-and-guides.html. Published 2007. Accessed February 9, 2014.
5. Foster S. *101 Medicinal Herbs.* Loveland, CO: Interweave Press; 1998: 128-129.
6. Foster S, Hobbs C. *Western Medicinal Plants and Herbs.* New York, NY: Peterson Field Guides, Houghton Mifflin Company; 2002: 55-56.
7. Skenderi G. *Herbal Vade Mecum.* Rutherford, NJ: Herbacy Press; 2003: 31.
8. Mabey R. *The New Age Herbalist.* New York, NY: Gaia books; 1988: 68.
9. Hoffman D. *Medical Herbalism — The Science and Practice of Herbal Medicine.* Rochester, Vermont: Healing Arts Press; 2003: 567.
10. Leung AY, Foster S. *Encyclopedia of Common Natural Ingredients Used in Food, Drugs, and Cosmetics.* 2nd ed. Hoboken, NJ: A John Wiley & Sons, Inc.; 2003: 57-59.
11. Weiss RF. *Herbal Medicine.* Avon, UK: The Bath Press; 1996: 31-32.
12. Foster S. *Herbal Renaissance.* Layton, UT: Peregrine Smith Books; 1993: 116-117.

LICORICE

1. Glycyrrhiza glabra. Flora of China. eFloras website. http://www.efloras.org/florataxon.aspx?flora_id=600&taxon_id=242323657. Accessed October 22, 2014.
2. Glycyrrhiza glabra var. glabra. Flora of Pakistan. eFloras website. http://www.efloras.org/florataxon.aspx?flora_id=5&taxon_id=250064889. Accessed October 22, 2014.
3. Hickman JC. (ed.) Glycyrrhiza uralensis. Flora of Pakistan. eFloras website. Missouri Botanical Garden, St. Louis, MO & Harvard University Herbaria, Cambridge, MA. http://efloras.org/florataxon.aspx?flora_id=5&taxon_id=200012145. Accessed June 17, 2016.
4. Glycyrrhiza uralensis. Flora of China. eFloras website. Missouri Botanical Garden, St. Louis, MO & Harvard University Herbaria, Cambridge, MA. http://efloras.org/florataxon.aspx?flora_id=2&taxon_id=200012145. Accessed June 17, 2016.
5. Foster S, Johnson R. *Desk Reference to Nature's Medicine.* Washington, D.C.: National Geographic Society; 2006: 230-231.
6. Bensky D, Gamble A. *The Chinese Herbal Medicine Materia Medica.* Rev. ed. Seattle, WA: Eastland Press; 1993: 323-325.
7. Felter HW. *The Eclectic Materia Medica, Pharmacology and Therapeutics.* Cincinnati, OH: Published by John K. Scudder; 1922: 56.
8. Ellingwood F. *American Materia Medica, Therapeutics, and Pharmacognosy.* Rev. ed. Albuquerque, NM: Southwest School for Botanical Medicine; 1994: 58.
9. Murray M. *The Healing Power of Herbs.* Rocklin, CA: Prima Publishing; 1992, 1995: 228-239.
10. Leung AY, Foster S. *Encyclopedia of Common Natural Ingredients Used in Food, Drugs, and Cosmetics.* 2nd ed. Hoboken, NJ: A John Wiley & Sons, Inc.; 2003: 346-350.
11. Skenderi G. *Herbal Vade Mecum.* Rutherford, NJ: Herbacy Press, 2003: 225.
12. Pedersen M. *Nutritional Herbology: A Reference Guide to Herbs.* Warsaw, IN: Wendell W. Whitman Company; 1998: 118-120.
13. Weiss RF. *Herbal Medicine.* Avon, UK: The Bath Press; 1996: 59-61.
14. Mills S, Bone K. *Principles and Practice of Phytotherapy.* London, UK: Harcourt Publishers Limited; 2000: 465-478.
15. Yance D. *Adaptogens in Medical Herbalism.* Rochester, VT: Healing Arts Press; 2013: 497-502.
16. Tricky R. *Women, Hormones and the Menstrual Cycle.* St. Leonards, Australia: Allen and Unwin; 1998: 220; 312-313.
17. Hudson T. *Women's Encyclopedia of Natural Medicine.* New York, NY: McGraw Hill; 2008: 195-196.

LOBELIA

1. Lobelia. Flora of North America. eFloras website. Missouri Botanical Garden, St. Louis, MO & Harvard University Herbaria, Cambridge, MA. http://www.efloras.org/florataxon.aspx?flora_id=2&taxon_id=118775. Published 2008. Accessed December 16, 2016.
2. Ayers T. Lobelia. Jepson Flora Project. Jepson eFlora website. http://ucjeps.berkeley.edu/eflora/eflora_display.php?tid=60969. Accessed December 16, 2016.
3. Lobelia inflata. Native Plant Database. Lady Bird Johnson Wild Flower Center, University of Texas, Austin. https://www.wildflower.org/plants/result.php?id_plant=LOIN. Accessed December 16, 2016.
4. Tenaglia D. Lobelia inflata. Missouriplants.com website. http://www.missouriplants.com/Whitealt/Lobelia_inflata_page.html. Accessed December 16, 2016.
5. Tenaglia D. Lobelia cardinalis. Missouriplants.com website. http://www.missouriplants.com/Redalt/Lobelia_cardinalis_page.html. Accessed December 16, 2016.
6. Lobelia cardinalis. Native Plant Database. Lady Bird Johnson Wild Flower Center, University of Texas, Austin. https://www.wildflower.org/plants/result.php?id_plant=LOCA2. Accessed December 16, 2016.
7. Lobelia cardinalis. Missouri Botanical Garden: Plant Finder website. http://www.missouribotanicalgarden.org/PlantFinder/PlantFinderDetails.aspx?kempercode=d940. Accessed December 16, 2016.
8. Lobelia siphilitica. Missouri Botanical Garden: Plant Finder website. http://www.missouribotanicalgarden.org/PlantFinder/PlantFinderDetails.aspx?kempercode=i460. Accessed December 16, 2016.
9. Lobelia siphilitica. Missouriplants.com website. http://www.missouriplants.com/Bluealt/Lobelia_siphilitica_page.html. Accessed December 16, 2016.
10. Lobelia. Merriam-Webster website. https://www.merriam-webster.com/dictionary/lobelia. Accessed April 14, 2017.
11. Wood M. *Vitalism: The History of Herbalism, Homeopathy, and Flower Essences.* Berkeley, CA: North Atlantic Books, 2005: 81-106.
12. Griggs B. *Green Pharmacy: The History and Evolution of Western Herbal Medicine.* Rochester, VT: Healing Arts Press, 1997: 155-165.
13. Colby B. *A Guide to Health.* 3rd ed. Milford, NH. John Burns, 1846. Rev. ed. Albuquerque, NM: Southwest School for Botanical Medicine; 1994. http://www.swsbm.com/ManualsOther/Colby-5.pdf. Accessed December 23, 2016.
14. Ellingwood F. *American Materia Medica, Therapeutics, and Pharmacognosy.* Rev. ed. Albuquerque, NM: Southwest School for Botanical Medicine; 1994: 68-72.
15. Felter HW. *The Eclectic Materia Medica, Pharmacology and Therapeutics.* Cincinnati, OH: Published by John K. Scudder; 1922: 70-74.
16. Felter HW, Lloyd JU. *King's American Dispensatory.* 3rd ed. Cincinnati, OH: Ohio Valley Co.; 1898. Republished online by Henriette Kress; 1999. http://www.henriettes-herb.com/eclectic/kings/lobelia.html. Accessed March 17, 2017.
17. Leung AY, Foster S. *Encyclopedia of Common Natural Ingredients Used in Food, Drugs, and Cosmetics.* 2nd ed. Hoboken, NJ: A John Wiley & Sons, Inc.; 2003: 354-355.
18. Skenderi G. *Herbal Vade Mecum.* Rutherford, NJ: Herbacy Press; 2003: 229.

LOMATIUM

1. Hickman JC. (ed.) *The Jepson Manual: Higher Plants of California.* Berkeley, CA: University of California Press; 1996: 150-153.
2. Tilley D, St. John L, Ogle D, Shaw N, Cane J. Plant guide for fern-leaf biscuitroot (Lomatium dissectum). USDA-Natural Resources Conservation Service, Idaho Plant Materials Center. Aberdeen, ID. Published 2001. http://plants.usda.gov/plantguide/pdf/pg_lodi.pdf. Accessed February 5, 2016.
3. Pojar J, MacKinnon A. *Plants of the Pacific Northwest Coast.* Vancouver, BC: Lone Pine Publishing; 1994: 222.

4. Willard T. *Edible and Medicinal Plants of the Rocky Mountains and Neighboring Territories.* Calgary, AB: Wild Rose College of Natural Healing; 1992: 154-155.
5. The History of Lomatium. Harmony Herbs website. http://lomatium.com/history.htm. Accessed February 2, 2016.
6. Foster S, Hobbs C. *Western Medicinal Plants and Herbs*. New York, NY: Peterson Field Guides, Houghton Mifflin Company; 2002: 122-123.
7. Moore M. *Medicinal Plants of the Pacific Northwest.* Santa Fe, NM: Red Crane Books; 1993: 167-168.
8. Chou SC, Everngam MC, Sturtz G, Beck JJ. Antibacterial activity of components from Lomatium californicum. *Phytother Res.* 2006;20(2):153-6. http://www.ncbi.nlm.nih.gov/pubmed/16444670. Accessed January 30, 2016.
9. Vanwagenen BC, Huddleston J, Cardellina JH. Native American food and medicinal plants, 8. Water-soluble constituents of Lomatium. *J Nat Prod.* 1988;51(1):136-41. http://www.ncbi.nlm.nih.gov/pubmed/3373223. Accessed February 2, 2016.
10. Lee TT, Kashiwada Y, Huang L, Snider J, Cosentino M, Lee KH. Suksdorfin: an anti-HIV principle from Lomatium suskdorfii, its structure-activity correlation with related coumarins, and synergistic effects with anti-AIDS nucleosides. *Bioorg Med Chem.* 1994;2(10):1051-6. http://www.ncbi.nlm.nih.gov/pubmed/7773621. Accessed February 2, 2016.
11. McCutcheon AR, Roberts TE, Gibbons E, Ellis SM, Babiuk LA, Hancock RE, Towers GH. Antiviral screening of British Columbian medicinal plants. *J Ethnopharmacol.* 1995;1:49(2): 101-10. http://www.ncbi.nlm.nih.gov/pubmed/8847882. Accessed January 30, 2016.

MARJORAM

1. Katzer G. Spice Pages website. http://gernot-katzers-spice-pages.com/engl/Majo_hor.html. Accessed November 11, 2015.
2. Foster S. *Herbal Renaissance.* Layton, UT: Peregrine Smith Books; 1993: 142-143.
3. Origanum majorana. The Flora of Pakistan. eFloras website. Missouri Botanical Garden, St. Louis, MO & Harvard University Herbaria, Cambridge, MA. http://efloras.org/florataxon.aspx?flora_id=5&taxon_id=242423554. Published 2008. Accessed November 12, 2015.
4. Grieve M. *A Modern Herbal.* Great Britain: Jonathan Cape Ltd.; 1931: 519-521.
5. Charters M. California Plant Names: Latin and Greek Meanings and Derivations—A Dictionary of Botanical and Biographical Etymology website. http://www.calflora.net/botanicalnames/pageMA-ME.html. Accessed November 12, 2015.
6. Foster S. *Herbal Renaissance.* Layton, UT: Peregrine Smith Books; 1993: 142-143.
7. Leung AY, Foster S. *Encyclopedia of Common Natural Ingredients Used in Food, Drugs, and Cosmetics.* 2nd ed. Hoboken, NJ: A John Wiley & Sons, Inc.; 2003: 364-366; 398-400.
8. Skenderi G. *Herbal Vade Mecum.* Rutherford, NJ: Herbacy Press; 2003: 242; 276-277.
9. Schnaubelt K. *Advanced Aromatherapy—The Science of Essential Oil Therapy.* Rochester, VT: Healing Arts Press; 1995: 78-79.
10. Schnaubelt K. *Medical Aromatherapy—Healing with Essential Oils.* Berkeley, CA: Frog, Ltd.; 1999: 195.
11. Keville K, Green M. *Aromatherapy—A Complete Guide to the Healing Art.* Freedom, CA: The Crossing Press; 1995: 61.

MARSHMALLOW

1. Althaea officinalis. Flora of Pakistan. eFloras website. Missouri Botanical Garden, St. Louis, MO & Harvard University Herbaria, Cambridge, MA. http://efloras.org/florataxon.aspx?flora_id=5&taxon_id=200013686. Accessed December 10, 2015.
2. Alcea rosea. Flora of China. eFloras website. Missouri Botanical Garden, St. Louis, MO & Harvard University Herbaria, Cambridge, MA. http://efloras.org/florataxon.aspx?flora_id=2&taxon_id=242302049. Accessed December 10, 2015.
3. Hill SR. Malva. Jepson Flora Project. Jepson eFlora website. http://ucjeps.berkeley.edu/eflora/eflora_display.php?tid=9580. Accessed December 10, 2015.
4. Malva. Flora of China. eFloras website. Missouri Botanical Garden, St. Louis, MO & Harvard University Herbaria, Cambridge, MA. http://efloras.org/florataxon.aspx?flora_id=2&taxon_id=119571. Accessed December 10, 2015.
5. List of Medicinal Herbs. MMS Gardens—Hortus Medicus website. http://www.piam.com/mms_garden/officinalis.html. Accessed March 6, 2014.
6. Leung AY, Foster S. *Encyclopedia of Common Natural Ingredients Used in Food, Drugs, and Cosmetics.* 2nd ed. Hoboken, NJ: A John Wiley & Sons, Inc.; 2003: 29-30; 244-245.
7. Grieve M. *A Modern Herbal.* Great Britain: Jonathan Cape Ltd.; 1931: 507-509.
8. Foster S, Johnson R. *Desk Reference to Nature's Medicine.* Washington, D.C.: National Geographic Society; 2006: 244-245.
9. Lad V, Frawley D. *The Yoga of Herbs.* Twin Lakes, WI: Lotus Press; 1992: 128-129.
10. Ellingwood F. *American Materia Medica, Therapeutics, and Pharmacognosy*. Abr. ed. Albuquerque, NM: Southwest School for Botanical Medicine; 1994: 7.
11. Felter HW. *The Eclectic Materia Medica, Pharmacology and Therapeutics.* Cincinnati, OH: Published by John K. Scudder; 1922: 12.
12. Foster S. *Herbal Renaissance.* Layton, UT: Peregrine Smith Books; 1993: 143-145.
13. Weiss RF. *Herbal Medicine*. Avon, UK: The Bath Press; 1996: 195-196.
14. Moore M. *Medicinal Plants of the Mountain West.* Santa Fe, NM: Museum of New Mexico Press; 2003: 155-157.
15. Curtin LSM, Moore, M. *Healing Herbs of the Upper Rio Grande.* Rev. ed. Santa Fe, NM: Western Edge Press; 1997: 104-105.
16. Willard T. *Edible and Medicinal Plants of the Rocky Mountains and Neighboring Territories.* Calgary, AB: Wild Rose College of Natural Healing; 1992: 139.
17. Felter HW, Lloyd, JU. *King's American Dispensatory*. (Volume 1, 19th Edition, Third Revision). Cincinnati, OH: The Ohio Valley Company; 1923: 157-159.
18. Skenderi G. *Herbal Vade Mecum.* Rutherford, NJ: Herbacy Press; 2003: 242-243.
19. Lust J. *The Herb Book*. New York, NY: Bantam Books; 1974: 93-94.
20. Hoffman D. *Medical Herbalism—The Science and Practice of Herbal Medicine.* Rochester, VT: Healing Arts Press; 2003: 526-527.
21. Kane C. *Herbal Medicine of the American Southwest.* Tuscon, AZ: Lincoln Town Press; 2006: 125-126.
22. Mabey R. *The New Age Herbalist.* New York, NY: Gaia books; 1988: 86.

MEADOWSWEET

1. Grieve M. *A Modern Herbal.* Great Britain: Jonathan Cape Ltd.; 1931: 524-525.
2. Filipendula ulmaria. Flora of China. efloras website. Missouri Botanical Garden, St. Louis, MO & Harvard University Herbaria, Cambridge, MA. http://www.efloras.org/florataxon.aspx?flora_id=2&taxon_id=200010852. Accessed April 17, 2015.
3. Filipendula. Flora of China. efloras website. Missouri Botanical Garden, St. Louis, MO & Harvard University Herbaria, Cambridge, MA. http://efloras.org/florataxon.aspx?flora_id=2&taxon_id=112789. Accessed April 17, 2015.
4. Willard T. *The Wild Rose Scientific Herbal.* Calgary, AB: Wild Rose College of Natural Healing: 1998: 124.
5. Willard T. *Edible and Medicinal Plants of the Rocky Mountains and Neighboring Territories.* Calgary, AB: Wild Rose College of Natural Healing; 1992: 231.
6. Mills S, Bone K. *Principles and Practice of Phytotherapy*. London, UK: Harcourt Publishers Limited; 2000: 480-481.
7. Skenderi G. *Herbal Vade Mecum.* Rutherford, NJ: Herbacy Press; 2003: 245.
8. Mabey R. *The New Age Herbalist.* New York, NY: Gaia books; 1988: 103-104.

MILK THISTLE

1. Silybum marianum. Flora of North America. efloras website. website. http://efloras.org/florataxon.aspx?flora_id=1&taxon_id=200024549. Accessed November 5, 2014.
2. Hickman JC. (ed.) *The Jepson Manual: Higher Plants of California.* Berkeley, CA: University of California Press; 1996: 342.
3. Silybum. Flora of North America. efloras website. http://efloras.org/florataxon.aspx?flora_id=1&taxon_id=130368. Accessed November 5, 2014.
4. Silybum. California Plant Names: Latin and Greek Meanings and Derivations—A Dictionary of Botanical and Biographical Etymology website. http://www.calflora.net/botanicalnames/pagesSI-SY.html. Accessed July 5, 2016.
5. Marianum. California Plant Names: Latin and Greek Meanings and Derivations—A Dictionary of Botanical and Biographical Etymology website. http://www.calflora.net/botanicalnames/pagesMA-ME.html. Accessed July 5, 2016.
6. Foster S, Johnson R. *Desk Reference to Nature's Medicine.* Washington, D.C.: National Geographic Society; 2006: 250-251.
7. Willard T. *The Wild Rose Scientific Herbal.* Calgary, AB: Wild Rose College of Natural Healing; 1998: 233-235.
8. Murray M. *The Healing Power of Herbs.* Rocklin, CA: Prima Publishing; 1992, 1995: 243-252.
9. Leung AY, Foster S. *Encyclopedia of Common Natural Ingredients Used in Food, Drugs, and Cosmetics.* 2nd ed. Hoboken, NJ: A John Wiley & Sons, Inc.; 2003: 366-368.
10. Ellingwood F. *American Materia Medica, Therapeutics, and Pharmacognosy.* Rev. ed. Albuquerque, NM: Southwest School for Botanical Medicine; 1994: 26.
11. Blumenthal M. *The ABC Clinical Guide to Herbs.* Austin, TX: The American Botanical Council; 2003: 287-296.
12. Skenderi G. *Herbal Vade Mecum.* Rutherford, NJ: Herbacy Press, 2003: 248-249.
13. Pedersen M. *Nutritional Herbology: A Reference Guide to Herbs.* Warsaw, IN: Wendell W. Whitman Company; 1998: 123-124.
14. Mills S, Bone K. *Principles and Practice of Phytotherapy.* London, UK: Harcourt Publishers Limited; 2000: 553-562.
15. Desplaces A, Choppin J, Vogel G, Trost W. The effects of silymarin on experimental phalloidine poisoning. *Arzneimittelforschung.* 1975 Jan;25(1):89-96. PubMed website. http://www.ncbi.nlm.nih.gov/pubmed/125090. Published January 25, 1975. Accessed July 18, 2016.
16. Vogel G, Tuchweber B, Trost W, Mengs U. Protection by silibinin against Amanita phalloides intoxication in beagles. *Toxicology and Applied Pharmacology.* 1984 May;73(3):355-62. PubMed website. http://www.ncbi.nlm.nih.gov/pubmed/6719456. Accessed July 18, 2016.

MINT (PEPPERMINT, SPEARMINT, AND BROOK MINT)

1. Hickman JC. (ed.) *The Jepson Manual: Higher Plants of California.* Berkeley, CA: University of California Press; 1996: 716.
2. Grieve M. *A Modern Herbal.* Great Britain: Jonathan Cape Ltd.; 1931: 533-543.
3. Willard T. *The Wild Rose Scientific Herbal.* Calgary, AB: Wild Rose College of Natural Healing; 1998: 263-265.
4. Tyler V. *The Honest Herbal.* Binghamton, NY: The Hawthorn Press, Inc.; 1993: 245-247.
5. Pedersen M. *Nutritional Herbology: A Reference Guide to Herbs.* Warsaw, IN: Wendell W. Whitman Company; 1998: 137-138.
6. Ellingwood F. *American Materia Medica, Therapeutics, and Pharmacognosy.* Rev. ed. Albuquerque, NM: Southwest School for Botanical Medicine; 1994; Original work published 1919: 75.
7. Foster S, Hobbs C. *Western Medicinal Plants and Herbs.* New York, NY: Peterson Field Guides, Houghton Mifflin Company; 2002: 203-204.
8. Pojar J, MacKinnon A. *Plants of the Pacific Northwest Coast.* Vancouver, BC: Lone Pine Publishing; 1994: 244.
9. Willard T. *Edible and Medicinal Plants of the Rocky Mountains and Neighboring Territories.* Calgary, AB: Wild Rose College of Natural Healing; 1992: 177-178.
10. Leung AY, Foster S. *Encyclopedia of Common Natural Ingredients Used in Food, Drugs, and Cosmetics.* 2nd ed. Hoboken, NJ: A John Wiley & Sons, Inc.; 2003: 368-371.
11. Moore M. *Medicinal Plants of the Mountain West.* Santa Fe, NM: Museum of New Mexico Press; 2003: 203-204.
12. Skenderi G. *Herbal Vade Mecum.* Rutherford, NJ: Herbacy Press, 2003: 291-292; 354.
13. Spearmint Essential Oil Information. Esoteric oils website. http://www.essentialoils.co.za/essential-oils/spearmint.htm. Accessed September 30, 2014.
14. Spearmint, Fresh (Mint). Self Nutrition Data. http://nutritiondata.self.com/facts/spices-and-herbs/226/2. Accessed September 30, 2014.
15. Tisserand R. *Essential Oil Safety—A Guide for Health Care Professionals.* London, England: Churchill Livingstone; 1999: 93, 160-161.
16. Weiss RF. *Herbal Medicine.* Avon, UK: The Bath Press; 1996: 28-31.
17. Keville K, Green M. *Aromatherapy—A Complete Guide to the Healing Art.* Freedom, CA: The Crossing Press; 1995: 64-65.
18. Schnaubelt K. *Advanced Aromatherapy—The Science of Essential Oil Therapy.* Rochester, VT: Healing Arts Press; 1995: 85.
19. Moore M. *Medicinal Plants of the Pacific Northwest.* Santa Fe, NM: Red Crane Books; 1993: 200-203.

MOTHERWORT

1. Rogers M. *Herbalpedia.* http://www.herbnet.com. Accessed February 18, 2014.
2. Foster S. *Herbal Renaissance.* Layton, UT: Peregrine Smith Books; 1993: 151-152.
3. Leonurus cardiaca. Flora of Pakistan. eFloras website. Missouri Botanical Garden, St. Louis, MO & Harvard University Herbaria, Cambridge, MA. http://efloras.org/florataxon.aspx?flora_id=5&taxon_id=220007427. Published 2008. Accessed December 10, 2015.
4. Grieve M. *A Modern Herbal.* Great Britain: Jonathan Cape Ltd.; 1931: 555-556.
5. Cardiacs. Dictionary.com website. http://dictionary.reference.com/browse/cardiacs. Accessed February 18, 2014.
6. Ellingwood F. *American Materia Medica, Therapeutics, and Pharmacognosy.* Rev. ed. Albuquerque, NM: Southwest School for Botanical Medicine; 1994: 67.
7. Felter HW. *The Eclectic Materia Medica, Pharmacology and Therapeutics.* Cincinnati, OH: Published by John K. Scudder; 1922: 68.
8. Scudder JM. *The American Eclectic Materia Medica and Therapeutics.* Cincinnati, OH: The Scudder Brothers Company; 1923: 611.
9. Moore M. *Medicinal Plants of the Mountain West.* Santa Fe, NM: Museum of New Mexico Press; 2003: 168-169.
10. Skenderi G. *Herbal Vade Mecum.* Rutherford, NJ: Herbacy Press; 2003: 254.
11. Hoffman D. *Medical Herbalism—The Science and Practice of Herbal Medicine.* Rochester, Vermont: Healing Arts Press; 2003: 562.
12. Gladstar R. *Herbal Healing for Women.* New York, NY: Simon and Shuster; 1993: 248-249.
13. Brinker F. *Herb Contraindications and Drug Interactions.* Sandy, OR: Eclectic Institute, Inc.; 1997: 67.
14. Mills S. *The Dictionary of Modern Herbalism; A Comprehensive Guide to Practical Herbal Therapy.* Rochester, VT: Healing Arts Press; 1988: 153.
15. Moore M. Lecture presented at Southwest School for Botanical Medicine residency program. Albuquerque, NM; 1994.

MULLEIN

1. Grieve M. *A Modern Herbal.* Great Britain: Jonathan Cape Ltd.; 1931: 562-566.
2. Preston RE, Wetherwax. M. Verbascum. Jepson Flora Project. Jepson eFlora website. http://ucjeps.berkeley.edu/cgi-bin/get_IJM.pl?tid=11412. Published Aug 26, 2008. Accessed December 16, 2014.
3. Verbascum. Flora of China. eFloras website. Missouri Botanical Garden, St. Louis, MO & Harvard University Herbaria, Cambridge, MA. http://efloras.org/florataxon.aspx?flora_id=2&taxon_id=134474. Published 2008. Accessed December 16, 2014.

4. Preston RE, Wetherwax M. Verbascum thapsus. Jepson Flora Project. Jepson eFlora website. http://ucjeps.berkeley.edu/cgi-bin/get_IJM.pl?tid=47846. Published Aug 26, 2008. Accessed December 16, 2014.
5. Verbascum thapsus. Flora of China. eFloras website. Missouri Botanical Garden, St. Louis, MO & Harvard University Herbaria, Cambridge, MA. http://efloras.org/florataxon.aspx?flora_id=2&taxon_id=200021301. Published 2008. Accessed December 16, 2014.
6. Preston RE, Wetherwax M. Verbascum bombyciferum. Jepson Flora Project. Jepson eFlora website. http://ucjeps.berkeley.edu/cgi-bin/get_IJM.pl?tid=91790. Published Aug 26, 2008. Accessed December 16, 2014.
7. Felter HW. *The Eclectic Materia Medica, Pharmacology and Therapeutics.* Cincinnati, OH: Published by John K. Scudder; 1922: 117.
8. Ellingwood F. *American Materia Medica, Therapeutics, and Pharmacognosy*. Rev. ed. Albuquerque, NM: Southwest School for Botanical Medicine; 1994: 103-104.
9. Foster S, Johnson R. *Desk Reference to Nature's Medicine*. Washington, D.C.: National Geographic Society; 2006: 254-255.
10. Skenderi G. *Herbal Vade Mecum.* Rutherford, NJ: Herbacy Press; 2003: 259-260.
11. Moore M. *Medicinal Plants of the Mountain West*. Santa Fe, NM: Museum of New Mexico Press; 2003: 170-172.
12. Pedersen M. *Nutritional Herbology: A Reference Guide to Herbs*. Warsaw, IN: Wendell W. Whitman Company; 1998: 124-125.
13. Moore M. Lecture presented at Southwest School for Botanical Medicine residency program. Albuquerque, NM; 1994.

MYRRH

1. Wild H. Flora Zambesiaca. eFlora Project. Kew Royal Botanical Gardens, Kent, England. http://apps.kew.org/efloras/namedetail.do?flora=fz&taxon=1355&nameid=3301. Accessed February 17, 2015.
2. Foster S, Johnson R. *Desk Reference to Nature's Medicine*. Washington, D.C.: National Geographic Society; 2006: 265-266.
3. Tyler V. *The Honest Herbal*. Binghamton, NY: The Hawthorn Press, Inc.; 1993: 221-222.
4. Commiphora. Flora of Pakistan. eFloras website. Missouri Botanical Garden, St. Louis, MO & Harvard University Herbaria, Cambridge, MA. http://efloras.org/florataxon.aspx?flora_id=5&taxon_id=107780. Accessed February 17, 2015.
5. Commiphora myrrha. Agroforestry Database 4.0 Web Site. http://www.worldagroforestry.org/treedb/AFTPDFS/Commiphora_myrrha.pdf. Accessed February 17, 2015.
6. Ellingwood F. *American Materia Medica, Therapeutics, and Pharmacognosy*. Rev. ed. Albuquerque, NM: Southwest School for Botanical Medicine; 1994: 36-37.
7. Felter HW. *The Eclectic Materia Medica, Pharmacology and Therapeutics.* Cincinnati, OH: Published by John K. Scudder; 1922: 81.
8. Leung AY, Foster S. *Encyclopedia of Common Natural Ingredients Used in Food, Drugs, and Cosmetics*. 2nd ed. Hoboken, NJ: A John Wiley & Sons, Inc.; 2003: 382-383.
9. Skenderi G. *Herbal Vade Mecum.* Rutherford, NJ: Herbacy Press; 2003: 263.
10. Schnaubelt K. *Advanced Aromatherapy — The Science of Essential Oil Therapy.* Rochester, VT: Healing Arts Press; 1995: 81.
11. Myrrh. Drugs.com. http://www.drugs.com/npp/myrrh.html. Updated January 15, 2015. Accessed February 13, 2015.
12. Moore M. Lecture presented at Southwest School for Botanical Medicine residency program. Albuquerque, NM; 1994.

NETTLE

1. Preston RE, Woodland DW. Hickman JC, ed. *The Jepson Manual: Higher Plants of California.* Berkeley, CA: University of California Press; 1996: 1082-1083.
2. Preston RE, Woodland DW. Urtica dioica L. subsp. dioica. Jepson Flora Project. Jepson eFlora website. http://ucjeps.berkeley.edu/eflora/eflora_display.php?tid=47575. Published August 26, 2008. Accessed December 6, 2014.
3. Preston RE, Woodland DW. Urtica dioica L. subsp. gracilis. Jepson Flora Project. Jepson eFlora website. http://ucjeps.berkeley.edu/eflora/eflora_display.php?tid=53302. Published Aug 26, 2008. Accessed December 6, 2014.
4. Preston RE, Woodland DW. Urtica dioica L. subsp. holosericea. Jepson Flora Project. Jepson eFlora website. http://ucjeps.berkeley.edu/eflora/eflora_display.php?tid=53303. Published Aug 26, 2008. Accessed December 6, 2014.
5. Urtica urens. Flora of China. eFloras website. Missouri Botanical Garden, St. Louis, MO & Harvard University Herbaria, Cambridge, MA. http://efloras.org/florataxon.aspx?flora_id=2&taxon_id=233501339. Accessed February 19, 2016.
6. Willard T. *Edible and Medicinal Plants of the Rocky Mountains and Neighboring Territories.* Calgary, AB: Wild Rose College of Natural Healing; 1992: 71-74.
7. Grieve M. *A Modern Herbal.* Great Britain: Jonathan Cape Ltd.; 1931: 574-580.
8. Pojar J, MacKinnon A. *Plants of the Pacific Northwest Coast.* Vancouver, BC: Lone Pine Publishing; 1994: 309.
9. Mills S, Bone K. *Principles and Practice of Phytotherapy*. London, UK: Harcourt Publishers Limited; 2000: 490-498.
10. Leung AY, Foster S. *Encyclopedia of Common Natural Ingredients Used in Food, Drugs, and Cosmetics*. 2nd ed. Hoboken, NJ: A John Wiley & Sons, Inc.; 2003: 384-385.
11. Moore M. *Medicinal Plants of the Mountain West*. Santa Fe, NM: Museum of New Mexico Press; 2003: 173-176.
12. Skenderi G. *Herbal Vade Mecum.* Rutherford, NJ: Herbacy Press; 2003: 265-266.
13. Treasure J. Urtica semen reduces serum creatinine levels. *The Journal of the American Herbalists Guild.* 2003; 4(2):22-25. Accessible from http://www.pkdiet.com/pdf/Kcit/nettlecreatinine.pdf. Accessed January 17, 2017.
14. Pedersen M. *Nutritional Herbology: A Reference Guide to Herbs*. Warsaw, IN: Wendell W. Whitman Company; 1998: 125.
15. Gladstar R. *Herbal Healing for Women.* New York, NY: Simon and Shuster; 1993: 250-252.
16. Winston D. Herb of the Season, Stinging Nettle (*Urtica dioica*). Herbalist and Alchemist website. http://www.herbalist-alchemist.com/press/nwsl/may.html. Published 2004. Accessed January 17, 2017.

OATS

1. Wiersema JH, Leon B. *World Economic Plants: A Standard Reference, Second Edition.* Boca Raton, FL: CRC Press; 2016: 86-87, 1057.
2. Baum BR, Smith JP, Wilden DH. Avena. UCJEPS: Jepson Interchange website. http://ucjeps.berkeley.edu/cgi-bin/get_IJM.pl?tid=10991. Published Aug 26, 2008. Accessed January 2, 2015.
3. Avena. Flora of China. eFloras website. Missouri Botanical Garden, St. Louis, MO & Harvard University Herbaria, Cambridge, MA. http://efloras.org/florataxon.aspx?flora_id=2&taxon_id=103247. Published 2008. Accessed January 2, 2015.
4. Baum BR, Smith JP, Wilden DH. Avena sativa. UCJEPS: Jepson Interchange website. http://ucjeps.berkeley.edu/cgi-bin/get_IJM.pl?tid=15323. Published Aug 26, 2008. Accessed December 30, 2014.
5. Avena sativa. Flora of China. eFloras website. Missouri Botanical Garden, St. Louis, MO & Harvard University Herbaria, Cambridge, MA. http://efloras.org/florataxon.aspx?flora_id=2&taxon_id=200024905. Published 2008. Accessed December 30, 2014.
6. Baum BR, Smith JP, Wilden DH. Avena fatua. UCJEPS: Jepson Interchange website. http://ucjeps.berkeley.edu/cgi-bin/get_IJM.pl?tid=15321. Published Aug 26, 2008. Accessed December 30, 2014.
7. Avena fatua. Flora of China. eFloras website. Missouri Botanical Garden, St. Louis, MO & Harvard University Herbaria, Cambridge, MA. http://efloras.org/florataxon.aspx?flora_id=2&taxon_id=200024900. Published 2008. Accessed December 30, 2014.
8. Gibson L, Benson G. Origin, history, and uses of oat (*Avena sativa*), and wheat (*Tritcum astivum*). Iowa State University, Department of Agronomy website. www.agron.ioastate.edu/Courses/agron212/readings/oat_wheat_history.htm. January 2002. Accessed May 1, 2013.

9. Ellingwood F. *American Materia Medica, Therapeutics, and Pharmacognosy*. Rev. ed. Albuquerque, NM: Southwest School for Botanical Medicine; 1994: 16-17.
10. Felter HW. *The Eclectic Materia Medica, Pharmacology and Therapeutics.* Cincinnati, OH: Published by John K. Scudder; 1922: 19.
11. Skenderi G. *Herbal Vade Mecum.* Rutherford, NJ: Herbacy Press; 2003: 272.
12. Pedersen M. *Nutritional Herbology: A Reference Guide to Herbs*. Warsaw, IN: Wendell W. Whitman Company; 1998: 127.
13. Winston D. *Adaptogens: Herbs for Strength, Stamina, and Stress Relief.* Rochester, VT: Healing Arts Press; 2007: 209-210.
14. Moore M. Lecture notes from Southwest School for Botanical Medicine residency program. Albuquerque, NM: 1994.
15. Moore M. *Medicinal Plants of the Desert and Canyon West*. Santa Fe, NM: Museum of New Mexico Press; 2003: 129-131.

ORANGE

1. Citrus. Flora of Pakistan. eFloras website. Missouri Botanical Garden, St. Louis, MO & Harvard University Herbaria, Cambridge, MA. http://efloras.org/florataxon.aspx?flora_id=5&taxon_id=107164. Accessed April 3, 2015.
2. Citrus. Flora of China. eFloras website. Missouri Botanical Garden, St. Louis, MO & Harvard University Herbaria, Cambridge, MA. http://efloras.org/florataxon.aspx?flora_id=2&taxon_id=107164. Accessed April 3, 2015.
3. Khan IA. *Citrus Genetics, Breeding, and Biotechnology.* Cambridge, MA: CAB International; 2007: 49-50.
4. Citrus sinensis. Flora of Pakistan. eFloras website. Missouri Botanical Garden, St. Louis, MO & Harvard University Herbaria, Cambridge, MA. http://efloras.org/florataxon.aspx?flora_id=5&taxon_id=200012428. Accessed April 3, 2015.
5. Citrus aurantium. Flora of Pakistan. eFloras website. Missouri Botanical Garden, St. Louis, MO & Harvard University Herbaria, Cambridge, MA. http://efloras.org/florataxon.aspx?flora_id=5&taxon_id=200012435. Accessed April 3, 2015.
6. Citrus reticulata. Flora of China. eFloras website. Missouri Botanical Garden, St. Louis, MO & Harvard University Herbaria, Cambridge, MA. http://efloras.org/florataxon.aspx?flora_id=2&taxon_id=200012434. Accessed April 3, 2015.
7. Citrus reticulata. Flora of Pakistan. eFloras website. Missouri Botanical Garden, St. Louis, MO & Harvard University Herbaria, Cambridge, MA. http://efloras.org/florataxon.aspx?flora_id=5&taxon_id=200012434. Accessed April 3, 2015.
8. Reticulatis. Online Etymology Dictionary website. www.etymonline.com/index.php?allowed_in_frame=0&search=reticularis&searchmode=none. Accessed December 4, 2015.
9. Grieve M. *A Modern Herbal.* Great Britain: Jonathan Cape Ltd.; 1931: 601-02.
10. Foster S, Johnson R. *Desk Reference to Nature's Medicine*. Washington, D.C.: National Geographic Society; 2006: 264-65.
11. Murray M. *The Encyclopedia of Healing Foods.* New York, NY: Atria Books; 2005: 297-99.
12. Keville K, Green M. *Aromatherapy—A Complete Guide to the Healing Art.* Freedom, CA: The Crossing Press; 1995: 63.
13. Leung AY, Foster S. *Encyclopedia of Common Natural Ingredients Used in Food, Drugs, and Cosmetics*. 2nd ed. Hoboken, NJ: A John Wiley & Sons, Inc.; 2003: 393-97.
14. Weiss RF. *Herbal Medicine.* Avon, UK: The Bath Press; 1996: 289.
15. Tisserand RB. *The Art of Aromatherapy—The Healing and Beautifying Properties of the Essential Oils of Flowers and Herbs.* Rochester, VT: Healing Arts Press; 1977: 261-62.
16. Skenderi G. *Herbal Vade Mecum.* Rutherford, NJ: Herbacy Press; 2003: 275-76.
17. Bensky D, Gamble A. *The Chinese Herbal Medicine Materia Medica.* Rev. ed. Seattle, WA: Eastland Press; 1993: 232-35.
18. Schnaubelt K. *Advanced Aromatherapy—The Science of Essential Oil Therapy.* Rochester, VT: Healing Arts Press; 1995: 61.
19. Hoffman D. *Medical Herbalism—The Science and Practice of Herbal Medicine.* Rochester, VT: Healing Arts Press; 2003: 63.
20. Mabey R. *The New Age Herbalist.* New York, NY: Gaia books; 1988: 110.

OREGANO

1. Katzer G. Spice Pages website. http://gernot-katzers-spice-pages.com/engl/Orig_vul.html. Accessed November 12, 2015.
2. Grieve M. *A Modern Herbal.* Great Britain: Jonathan Cape Ltd.; 1931: 520-521.
3. Origanum vulgare. Flora of China. eFloras website. Missouri Botanical Garden, St. Louis, MO & Harvard University Herbaria, Cambridge, MA. http://www.efloras.org/florataxon.aspx?flora_id=&taxon_id=200019922. Published 2008. Accessed March 6, 2015.
4. Tucker AO. Origanum. Jepson Flora Project. Jepson eFlora website. Updated 2014. Accessed March 6, 2015.
5. Foster S. *Herbal Renaissance.* Layton, UT: Peregrine Smith Books; 1993: 155-157.
6. Vulgare. MyEtymology website. http://www.myetymology.com/latin/vulgare.html. Accessed November 12, 2015.
7. Hirtus. MyEtymology website. http://www.myetymology.com/latin/hirtus.html. Accessed November 12, 2015.
8. Leung AY, Foster S. *Encyclopedia of Common Natural Ingredients Used in Food, Drugs, and Cosmetics*. 2nd ed. Hoboken, NJ: A John Wiley & Sons, Inc.; 2003: 398-400.
9. Skenderi G. *Herbal Vade Mecum.* Rutherford, NJ: Herbacy Press; 2003: 276-277.
10. Schnaubelt K. *Advanced Aromatherapy—The Science of Essential Oil Therapy.* Rochester, VT: Healing Arts Press; 1995: 83.
11. Schnaubelt K. *Medical Aromatherapy—Healing with Essential Oils.* Berkeley, CA: Frog, Ltd.; 1999: 202-203.
12. Keville K, Green M. *Aromatherapy—A Complete Guide to the Healing Art.* Freedom, CA: The Crossing Press; 1995: 61.

OSHÁ

1. Ligusticum. Flora of China. eFloras website. Missouri Botanical Garden, St. Louis, MO & Harvard University Herbaria, Cambridge, MA. http://efloras.org/florataxon.aspx?flora_id=2&taxon_id=118546. Published 2008. Accessed December 16, 2014.
2. Ligusticum. Flora of Pakistan. eFloras website. Missouri Botanical Garden, St. Louis, MO & Harvard University Herbaria, Cambridge, MA. http://efloras.org/florataxon.aspx?flora_id=5&taxon_id=118546. Published 2008. Accessed December 16, 2014.
3. Hickman JC. (ed.) *The Jepson Manual: Higher Plants of California*. Berkeley, CA: University of California Press; 1996: 150.
4. Pojar J, MacKinnon A. *Plants of the Pacific Northwest Coast.* Vancouver, BC: Lone Pine Publishing; 1994: 219.
5. Tilford G. *Edible and Medicinal Plants of the West.* Missoula, MT: Mountain Press Publishing Company; 1997: 204-205.
6. Curtin LSM, Moore, M. *Healing Herbs of the Upper Rio Grande.* Rev. ed. Santa Fe, NM: Western Edge Press; 1997: 121-124.
7. Foster S, Hobbs C. *Western Medicinal Plants and Herbs*. New York, NY: Peterson Field Guides, Houghton Mifflin Company; 2002: 63-64.
8. Willard T. *Edible and Medicinal Plants of the Rocky Mountains and Neighboring Territories.* Calgary, AB: Wild Rose College of Natural Healing; 1992: 154.
9. Moore M. *Medicinal Plants of the Mountain West*. Santa Fe, NM: Museum of New Mexico Press; 2003: 183-186.
10. Skenderi G. *Herbal Vade Mecum.* Rutherford, NJ: Herbacy Press; 2003: 278.

PARSLEY

1. Grieve M. *A Modern Herbal.* Great Britain: Jonathan Cape Ltd.; 1931: 611-614.
2. Hickman JC (ed.). *The Jepson Manual: Higher Plants of California*. Berkeley, CA: University of California Press; 1996: 162.
3. Parsley. Online Etymology Dictionary website. http://www.etymonline.com/index.php?term=parsley&allowed_in_frame=0. Accessed June, 29, 2013.
4. Leung AY, Foster S. *Encyclopedia of Common Natural Ingredients Used in Food, Drugs, and Cosmetics*. 2nd ed. Hoboken, NJ: A John Wiley & Sons, Inc.; 2003: 406-407.
5. Skenderi G. *Herbal Vade Mecum.* Rutherford, NJ: Herbacy Press; 2003: 280-281.
6. Tyler V. *The Honest Herbal.* Binghamton, NY: The Hawthorn Press, Inc.; 1993: 235-236.

7. Pedersen M. *Nutritional Herbology: A Reference Guide to Herbs*. Warsaw, IN: Wendell W. Whitman Company; 1998: 131.
8. Foster S. *Herbal Renaissance.* Layton, UT: Peregrine Smith Books; 1993: 157-159.
9. Foster S, Johnson R. *Desk Reference to Nature's Medicine*. Washington, D.C.: National Geographic Society; 2006: 268-269.
10. Weiss, RF. *Herbal Medicine*. Avon, UK: The Bath Press; 1996: 236-237.
11. Fashori NN, Al-Sheddi ES, Al-Oquail MM, Musarrat J, Al-Khedhairy AA, Siddiqui MA. Anticancer activity of Petroselinum sativum seed extracts on MCF-7 human breast cancer cells. *Asian Pac J Cancer Prev.* 2013; 14 (10):5719-23. http://journal.waocp.org/?sid=Entrez:PubMed&id=pmid:24289568&key=2013.14.10.5719. Published December 18, 2004: 996-999. Accessed July 12, 2016.
12. Allam AA, Moadaa SN, Abo-Eleneen R, Ajarem J. Protective effect of parsley juice (Petroselinum crispum, Apiaceae) against cadmium deleterious changes in the developed albino mice newborns (Mus musculus) brain. *Oxid Med Cell Longevity.* 2016;2016:2646840. http://www.ncbi.nlm.nih.gov/pubmed/26966507. ePublished February 7, 2016. Accessed July 12, 2016.
13. Bolkent S, Yanardag R, Ozsoy-Sacan O, Karabulut-Bulan. Effects of parsley (Petroselinum crispum) on the liver of diabetic rates: a morphological and biochemical study. *Oxid Med Cell Longevity*. 2016;2016:2646840. doi: 10.1155/2016/2646840. ePublished February 7, 2016. Accessed July 12, 2016.
14. Nair VY, Balakrishanan N, Antony Santiago JV. Petroselinum extract attenuates hepatic steatosis in rats fed with fructose enriched diet. *Bratisl Lek Listy.* 2015;116(9):547-53. http://www.ncbi.nlm.nih.gov/pubmed/26435020. Accessed July 12, 2016.
15. Abou Khalil NS, Abou-Elhamd AS, Wasfy SI, El Mileegy IM, Hamed MY, Ageely HM. Antidiabetic and antioxidant impacts of desert date (*Balanites aegyptiaca*) and parsley (*Petroselinum sativum*) aqueous extracts: lessons from experimental rats. *J Diabetes Res.* 2016;2016:8408326. doi: 10.1155/2016/8408326. ePublished February 25, 2016. Accessed July 12, 2016.

PARTRIDGE BERRY

1. Grieve M. *A Modern Herbal.* Great Britain: Jonathan Cape Ltd.; 1931: 766.
2. Stritch L. Plant of the Week: Partridge Berry (Mitchella repens L.) website. http://www.fs.fed.us/wildflowers/plant-of-the-week/mitchella_repens.shtml. Accessed April 17, 2015.
3. Anzelone M. Pretty Partridgeberry: A native groundcover with lots of star potential. Brooklyn Botanic Garden website. http://www.bbg.org/gardening/article/pretty_partridgeberry. Published September 1, 2006. Accessed April 17, 2015.
4. Partridgeberry. Virginia Tech Dendrology Factsheets. Virginia Polytechnic Institute and State University website. http://dendro.cnre.vt.edu/dendrology/syllabus/factsheet.cfm?ID=147. Accessed April 17, 2015.
5. Deane G. Partridgeberry: Split personality. Eat the Weeds website. http://www.eattheweeds.com/partridgeberry-split-personality. Accessed November 2, 2013.
6. Stritch R. Partridge berry (Mitchella repens L.). United States Department of Agriculture website. http://dictionary.reference.com/browse/partridge berry. Accessed November 2, 2013.
7. Strauch B. Herb to know: Partridge berry. Mother Earth News website. http://www.motherearthliving.com/plant-profile/an-herb-to-know-50.aspx. Published August/September 2001. Accessed November 2, 2013.
8. Ellingwood F. *American Materia Medica, Therapeutics, and Pharmacognosy*. Rev. ed. Albuquerque, NM: Southwest School for Botanical Medicine, 1994.
9. Gladstar R. *Herbal Healing for Women.* New York, NY: Simon and Shuster, 1993: 255.
10. Skenderi G. *Herbal Vade Mecum.* Rutherford, NJ: Herbacy Press; 2003: 281-282.

PASSION FLOWER

1. Passiflora incarnata. Flora of Pakistan. eFloras website. Missouri Botanical Garden, St. Louis, MO & Harvard University Herbaria, Cambridge, MA. http://efloras.org/florataxon.aspx?flora_id=5&taxon_id=220009998. Accessed January 28, 2015.
2. Scheper J. Passiflora incarnata. Floridata website. http://www.floridata.com/ref/p/passiflo.cfm. Published December 1, 1996. Updated August 23, 2003. Accessed January 28, 2015.
3. Passiflora incarnata. The Plant List Version 1.1. website. http://www.theplantlist.org/tpl1.1/record/tro-24200150. Published 2013. Accessed January 28, 2015.
4. Dhawan K, Kumar R, Kumar S, Sharma A. Correct identification of Passiflora incarnata Linn., a promising herbal anxiolytic and sedative. *J Med Food.* 2001 Autumn;4(3):137-144. http://www.ncbi.nlm.nih.gov/pubmed/12639407. Accessed January 28, 2015.
5. Charters M. *Passiflora.* http://www.calflora.net/botanicalnames/pagePA-PH.html. Accessed September 28, 2015.
6. Charters M. *Incarnata*. http://www.calflora.net/botanicalnames/pageI.html. Accessed September 28, 2015.
7. Foster S, Johnson R. *Desk Reference to Nature's Medicine*. Washington, D.C.: National Geographic Society; 2006: 280-281.
8. Foster S. *Herbal Renaissance.* Layton, UT: Peregrine Smith Books; 1993: 159-161.
9. Willard T. *The Wild Rose Scientific Herbal*. Calgary, AB: Wild Rose College of Natural Healing; 1998: 257-258.
10. Ellingwood F. *American Materia Medica, Therapeutics, and Pharmacognosy*. Rev. ed. Albuquerque, NM: Southwest School for Botanical Medicine; 1994: 77-78.
11. Felter HW. *The Eclectic Materia Medica, Pharmacology and Therapeutics.* Cincinnati, OH: Published by John K. Scudder; 1922: 86-89.
12. Leung AY, Foster S. *Encyclopedia of Common Natural Ingredients Used in Food, Drugs, and Cosmetics*. 2nd ed. Hoboken, NJ: A John Wiley & Sons, Inc.; 2003: 408-411.
13. Skenderi G. *Herbal Vade Mecum.* Rutherford, NJ: Herbacy Press; 2003: 282-283.
14. Pedersen M. *Nutritional Herbology: A Reference Guide to Herbs*. Warsaw, IN: Wendell W. Whitman Company; 1998: 134-135.
15. Moore M. Lecture presented at Southwest School for Botanical Medicine residency program. Albuquerque, NM; 1994.
16. Moore M. *Medicinal Plants of the Desert and Canyon West*. Santa Fe, NM: Museum of New Mexico Press: 83-85.
17. Pendell D. *Pharmako/poeia—Plant Powers, Poisons, and Herbcraft*. San Francisco, CA: Mercury House; 1995: 146-153.

PEDICULARIS

1. Holmgren NH, Mill RR. Pedicularis. Flora of China. eFloras website. Missouri Botanical Garden, St. Louis, MO & Harvard University Herbaria, Cambridge, MA. http://efloras.org/florataxon.aspx?flora_id=2&taxon_id=124237. Published 2008. Accessed January 14, 2015.
2. Giblin D. Pedicularis bracteosa. Burke Museum of Natural History and Culture: University of Washington website. http://biology.burke.washington.edu/herbarium/imagecollection.php?Genus=Pedicularis&Species=bracteosa. Accessed January 14, 2015.
3. Turner M. Pedicularis bracteosa. Wildflowers of the Pacific Northwest website. http://www.pnwflowers.com/flower/pedicularis-bracteosa. Accessed January 14, 2015.
4. Vorobik LA. Pedicularis densiflora. Jepson Flora Project. Jepson eFlora website. http://ucjeps.berkeley.edu/cgi-bin/get_IJM.pl?tid=36567. Published August 26, 2008. Accessed January 14, 2015.
5. Vorobik LA. Pedicularis groenlandica. Jepson Flora Project. Jepson eFlora website. http://ucjeps.berkeley.edu/cgi-bin/get_IJM.pl?tid=36574. Published August 26, 2008. Accessed January 14, 2015.
6. Oekonom D. Pedicularis oederi. Flora of China. eFloras website. Missouri Botanical Garden, St. Louis, MO & Harvard University Herbaria, Cambridge, MA. http://www.efloras.org/florataxon.aspx?flora_id=2&taxon_id=200021051. Published 2008. Accessed January 14, 2015.

7. Vorobik LA. Pedicularis racemosa. Jepson Flora Project. Jepson eFlora website. http://ucjeps.berkeley.edu/cgi-bin/get_IJM.pl?tid=36606. Published August 26, 2008. Accessed January 14, 2015.
8. Schneider A. Pedicularis groenlandica. Wildflowers, Ferns, and Trees of Colorado, New Mexico, Arizona, & Utah website. http://www.swcoloradowildflowers.com/Pink%20Enlarged%20Photo%20Pages/pedicularis%20groenlandica.htm. Updated August 15, 2014. Accessed August 20, 2014.
9. Pojar J, MacKinnon A. *Plants of the Pacific Northwest Coast.* Vancouver, BC: Lone Pine Publishing; 1994: 252-257.
10. Foster S, Hobbs C. *Western Medicinal Plants and Herbs.* New York, NY: Peterson Field Guides, Houghton Mifflin Company; 2002: 175-176.
11. Willard T. *Edible and Medicinal Plants of the Rocky Mountains and Neighboring Territories.* Calgary, AB: Wild Rose College of Natural Healing; 1992: 184.
12. Lyons K, Cooney-Lazaneo M. *Plants of the Coast Redwood Region*. Boulder Creek, CA: Looking Glass Press; 1988: 49.
13. Moore M. *Medicinal Plants of the Mountain West*. Santa Fe, NM: Museum of New Mexico Press; 2003: 50-52.
14. Skenderi G. *Herbal Vade Mecum.* Rutherford, NJ: Herbacy Press; 2003: 231-232.
15. Moore M. Lecture presented at Southwest School for Botanical Medicine residency program. Albuquerque, NM; 1994.
16. Seller A. Lecture notes from Pacific School of Herbal Medicine. Oakland, CA; 1995.
17. Moore M. *Medicinal Plants of the Pacific Northwest.* Santa Fe, NM: Red Crane Books; 1993: 63-68.

PENNYROYAL

1. Grieve M. *A Modern Herbal.* Great Britain: Jonathan Cape Ltd.; 1931: 624-627.
2. Tucker AO. Mentha pulegium. Jepson Flora Project. Jepson eFlora website. http://ucjeps.berkeley.edu/cgi-bin/get_IJM.pl?tid=33206. Accessed April 24, 2015.
3. Hilty J. American Pennyroyal. Illinois Wildflowers website. http://www.illinoiswildflowers.info/woodland/plants/am_pennyroyal.htm. Accessed April 24, 2015.
4. Lust J. *The Herb Book*. New York, NY: Bantam Books; 1974: 304.
5. Mentha pulegium. Wikipedia website. http://en.wikipedia.org/wiki/Mentha_pulegium. Updated October 1, 2013. Accessed October 31, 2013.
6. Foster S. *Herbal Renaissance.* Layton, UT: Peregrine Smith Books; 1993: 161-163.
7. Foster S, Hobbs C. *Western Medicinal Plants and Herbs*. New York, NY: Peterson Field Guides, Houghton Mifflin Company; 2002: 202.
8. Skenderi G. *Herbal Vade Mecum.* Rutherford, NJ: Herbacy Press; 2003: 286-287.
9. Willard T. *The Wild Rose Scientific Herbal*. Calgary, AB: Wild Rose College of Natural Healing; 1998: 261-262.
10. Moore M. *Medicinal Plants of the Pacific Northwest.* Santa Fe, NM: Red Crane Books; 1993: 128-130.
11. Moore M. Lecture presented at Southwest School for Botanical Medicine residency program. Albuquerque, NM; 1994.

PEONY

1. Paeoniaceae. Flora of North America. eFloras website. Missouri Botanical Garden, St. Louis, MO & Harvard University Herbaria, Cambridge, MA. http://efloras.org/florataxon.aspx?flora_id=1&taxon_id=123659. Published 2008. Accessed October 29, 2015.
2. Tahbaz F. Paeonia californica. Jepson Flora Project. Jepson eFlora website. http://ucjeps.berkeley.edu/cgi-bin/get_IJM.pl?tid=35855. Accessed October 29, 2015.
3. Paeonia lactiflora. Flora of China. eFloras website. Missouri Botanical Garden, St. Louis, MO & Harvard University Herbaria, Cambridge, MA. http://efloras.org/florataxon.aspx?flora_id=2&taxon_id=200008034. Published 2008. Accessed October 29, 2015.
4. Paeonia officinalis (common peony). Go Botany website. New England Wild Flower Society. https://gobotany.newenglandwild.org/species/paeonia/officinalis/. Updated 2015. Accessed October 29, 2015.
5. Paeonia officinalis. Missouri Botanical Garden: Plant Finder website. http://www.missouribotanicalgarden.org/PlantFinder/PlantFinderDetails.aspx?taxonid=286230&isprofile=0&. Accessed October 29, 2015.
6. Tahbaz F. Paeonia brownii. Jepson Flora Project. Jepson eFlora website. http://ucjeps.berkeley.edu/cgi-bin/get_IJM.pl?tid=35854. Accessed October 29, 2015.
7. Paeonia brownii. Flora of North America. eFloras website. Missouri Botanical Garden, St. Louis, MO & Harvard University Herbaria, Cambridge, MA. http://efloras.org/florataxon.aspx?flora_id=1&taxon_id=250065801. Published 2008. Accessed October 29, 2015.
8. Paeonia californica. Flora of North America. eFloras website. Missouri Botanical Garden, St. Louis, MO & Harvard University Herbaria, Cambridge, MA. http://efloras.org/florataxon.aspx?flora_id=1&taxon_id=250065802. Published 2008. Accessed October 29, 2015.
9. Coit JE. *The Peony.* Cornell University, Agricultural Experiment Station of The College of Agriculture. Department of Horticulture. Ithica, NY; A Cornell University Publication. Published 1908. Accessed September 22, 2017.
10. Foster S, Yue C. *Herbal Emissaries, Bringing Chinese Herbs to the West.* Rochester, VT: Healing Arts Press; 1992: 200-207.
11. Bensky D, Gamble A. *The Chinese Herbal Medicine Materia Medica.* Rev. ed. Seattle, WA: Eastland Press; 1993: 331-332.
12. Grieve M. *A Modern Herbal.* Great Britain: Jonathan Cape Ltd.; 1931: 606-607.
13. Lust J. *The Herb Book*. New York, NY: Bantam Books; 1974: 305.
14. Foster S, Hobbs C. *Western Medicinal Plants and Herbs*. New York, NY: Peterson Field Guides, Houghton Mifflin Company; 2002: 179.
15. Leung AY, Foster S. *Encyclopedia of Common Natural Ingredients Used in Food, Drugs, and Cosmetics.* 2nd ed. Hoboken, NJ: A John Wiley & Sons, Inc.; 2003: 544-546.
16. Skenderi G. *Herbal Vade Mecum.* Rutherford, NJ: Herbacy Press; 2003: 288.
17. He DY, Dai SM. Anti-inflammatory and immunomodulatory effects of Paeonia lactiflora Pall., a traditional Chinese herbal medicine. *Front Pharmacol.* 2011;2:10. PMID: 21687505. http://www.ncbi.nlm.nih.gov/pubmed/21687505. Published February 25, 2011. Accessed August 28, 2013.
18. Moore M. Lecture presented at Southwest School for Botanical Medicine residency program. Albuquerque, NM; 1994.
19. Moore M. *Medicinal Plants of the Mountain West*. Santa Fe, NM: Museum of New Mexico Press; 2003: 194.
20. Cane C. *Herbal Medicine of the American Southwest.* Lincoln Town Press; 2006: 204.
21. Moore M. *Medicinal Plants of the Pacific Northwest.* Santa Fe, NM: Red Crane Books; 1993: 260-263.

PLANTAIN

1. Plantago major. Flora of China. eFloras website. Missouri Botanical Garden, St. Louis, MO & Harvard University Herbaria, Cambridge, MA. http://efloras.org/florataxon.aspx?flora_id=2&taxon_id=200022050. Published 2008. Accessed March 27, 2015.
2. Plantago lanceolata. Flora of China. eFloras website. Missouri Botanical Garden, St. Louis, MO & Harvard University Herbaria, Cambridge, MA. http://efloras.org/florataxon.aspx?flora_id=2&taxon_id=200022048. Published 2008. Accessed March 27, 2015.
3. Rosati TJ. Plantago major. Jepson Flora Project. Jepson eFlora website. http://ucjeps.berkeley.edu/eflora/eflora_display.php?tid=38570. Published 2014. Accessed March 27, 2015.
4. Rosati TJ. Plantago lanceolata. Jepson Flora Project. Jepson eFlora website. http://ucjeps.berkeley.edu/eflora/eflora_display.php?tid=38567. Published 2014. Accessed March 27, 2015.
5. Rosati TJ. Plantago. Jepson Flora Project. Jepson eFlora website. Published 2014. Accessed March 27, 2015.
6. Plantago. Flora of China. eFloras website. Missouri Botanical Garden, St. Louis, MO & Harvard University Herbaria, Cambridge, MA. http://efloras.org/florataxon.aspx?flora_id=2&taxon_id=125735. Published 2008. Accessed March 27, 2015.
7. Plantain. Dictionary.com website. http://dictionary.reference.com/browse/plantain. Accessed March 27, 2015.

8. Grieve M. *A Modern Herbal.* Great Britain: Jonathan Cape Ltd.; 1931: 640-644.
9. Skenderi G. *Herbal Vade Mecum.* Rutherford, NJ: Herbacy Press; 2003: 300.
10. Kane C. *Herbal Medicine of the American Southwest.* Lincoln Town Press; 2006: 150-151.
11. Pedersen M. *Nutritional Herbology: A Reference Guide to Herbs.* Warsaw, IN: Wendell W. Whitman Company; 1998: 139-140.
12. Bergner P. Botanicals, Biofilms, and Chronic Infections lecture presented at Breitenbush Herbal Conference. Detroit, OR; 2016.

PRICKLY ASH

1. Zanthoxylum americanum. Missouri Botanical Garden: Plant Finder Web Site. http://www.missouribotanicalgarden.org/PlantFinder/PlantFinderDetails.aspx?kempercode=m900. Accessed November 26, 2014.
2. Zanthoxylum americanum. Oklahoma Biological Survey website. http://www.biosurvey.ou.edu/shrub/zant-ame.htm. Accessed November 26, 2014.
3. Zanthoxylum clava-herculis. Oklahoma Biological Survey website. http://www.biosurvey.ou.edu/shrub/zacl.htm. Accessed November 26, 2014.
4. Comprehensive Report Species—Zanthoxylum clava-herculis. NatureServe Explorer: An Online Encyclopedia of Life website. http://explorernatureserve.org/. Accessed November 26, 2014.
5. Kress H. *King's American Dispensatory* (1898). http://www.henriettes-herb.com/eclectic/kings/xanthoxylum.html. Accessed October 29, 2015.
6. Scudder J. *The American Eclectic Materia Medica and Therapeutics (Twelfth Edition).* Cincinnati, OH: The Scudder Brothers Company Publishers; 1898: 353-354.
7. Felter HW. *The Eclectic Materia Medica, Pharmacology and Therapeutics.* Cincinnati, OH: Published by John K. Scudder; 1922: 119.
8. Ellingwood F. *American Materia Medica, Therapeutics, and Pharmacognosy*. Rev. ed. Albuquerque, NM: Southwest School for Botanical Medicine; 1994: 106.
9. Culbreth D. *A Manual of Materia Medica and Pharmacology*. 1917. Bisbee, AZ: Southwest School of Botanical Medicine; 1927: 135.
10. Grieve M. *A Modern Herbal.* Great Britain: Jonathan Cape Ltd.; 1931: 70-71.
11. Leung AY, Foster S. *Encyclopedia of Common Natural Ingredients Used in Food, Drugs, and Cosmetics*. 2nd ed. Hoboken, NJ: A John Wiley & Sons, Inc.; 2003: 46-47.
12. Willard T. *The Wild Rose Scientific Herbal.* Calgary, AB: Wild Rose College of Natural Healing; 1998: 275-276.
13. Skenderi G. *Herbal Vade Mecum.* Rutherford, NJ: Herbacy Press; 2003: 406-407.
14. Moore M. Lecture presented at Southwest School for Botanical Medicine residency program. Albuquerque, NM; 1994.
15. Foster S. *An Illustrated Guide to 101 Medicinal Herbs*. Loveland, CO: Interweave Press, Inc.; 1998: 160-161.

PROPOLIS

1. Greek Etymology of Propolis. My Etymology website. http://www.myetymology.com/greek/propolis.html. Published 2008. Accessed November 2, 2015.
2. Propolis Research. The Honey Bear website. http://thehoneybear.co.za/propolis-research.htm. Accessed November 2, 2015.
3. Tyler V. *The Honest Herbal*. Binghamton, NY: The Hawthorn Press, Inc.; 1993: 255-256.
4. Moore M. Lecture presented at Southwest School for Botanical Medicine residency program. Albuquerque, NM; 1994.
5. Seller A. Lecture notes from Pacific School of Herbal Medicine. Oakland, CA; 1995.
6. Mills S, Bone K. *Principles and Practice of Phytotherapy*. London, UK: Harcourt Publishers Limited; 2000: 174; 176-180; 215.

RASPBERRY LEAF

1. Rubus idaeus. Natural Resources Conservation Service. United States Department of Agriculture website. http://www.ars-grin.gov/cgi-bin/npgs/html/taxon.pl?32348. Accessed February 20, 2015.
2. Rubus idaeus. Flora of China. eFloras website. Missouri Botanical Garden, St. Louis, MO & Harvard University Herbaria, Cambridge, MA. http://efloras.org/florataxon.aspx?flora_id=2&taxon_id=200011446. Accessed February 20, 2015.
3. Alice LA. Rubus leucodermis. Jepson Flora Project. Jepson eFlora website. http://ucjeps.berkeley.edu/cgi-bin/get_IJM.pl?tid=42027. Accessed February 20, 2015.
4. Rubus idaeus. Fire effects Information Database. USDA Forest Service website. http://www.fs.fed.us/database/feis/plants/shrub/rubida/all.html. Accessed February 20, 2015.
5. Willard T. *Edible and Medicinal Plants of the Rocky Mountains and Neighboring Territories.* Calgary, AB: Wild Rose College of Natural Healing; 1991: 119-122.
6. Foster S, Hobbs C. *Western Medicinal Plants and Herbs*. New York, NY: Peterson Field Guides, Houghton Mifflin Company; 2002: 300.
7. Pedersen M. *Nutritional Herbology: A Reference Guide to Herbs*. Warsaw, IN: Wendell W. Whitman Company; 1998: 145.
8. Skenderi G. *Herbal Vade Mecum.* Rutherford, NJ: Herbacy Press; 2003: 315.
9. Gladstar R. *Herbal Healing for Women.* New York, NY: Simon and Shuster; 1993: 253-254.
10. Soule D. *The Roots of Healing, A Woman's Book of Herbs.* New York, NY: Carol Publishing Group; 1995: 62-63.

RED CLOVER

1. Trifolium pratense. Flora of China. eFloras website. Missouri Botanical Garden, St. Louis, MO & Harvard University Herbaria, Cambridge, MA. http://efloras.org/florataxon.aspx?flora_id=2&taxon_id=200012343. Accessed February 20, 2015.
2. Vincent MA, Isely D. Trifolium pratense. Jepson Flora Project. Jepson eFlora website. http://ucjeps.berkeley.edu/cgi-bin/get_IJM.pl?tid=47160. Published 2013. Accessed February 20, 2015.
3. Foster S, Johnson R. *Desk Reference to Nature's Medicine*. Washington, D.C.: National Geographic Society; 2006: 304-305.
4. Leung AY, Foster S. *Encyclopedia of Common Natural Ingredients Used in Food, Drugs, and Cosmetics*. 2nd ed. Hoboken, NJ: A John Wiley & Sons, Inc.; 2003: 177-178.
5. Willard T. *Edible and Medicinal Plants of the Rocky Mountains and Neighboring Territories.* Calgary, AB: Wild Rose College of Natural Healing; 1992: 280.
6. Moore M. *Medicinal Plants of the Mountain West*. Santa Fe, NM: Museum of New Mexico Press; 2003: 215-218.
7. Pedersen M. *Nutritional Herbology: A Reference Guide to Herbs*. Warsaw, IN: Wendell W. Whitman Company; 1998: 34.
8. Mills S, Bone K. *Principles and Practice of Phytotherapy*. London, UK: Harcourt Publishers Limited; 2000: 148.
9. Skenderi G. *Herbal Vade Mecum.* Rutherford, NJ: Herbacy Press; 2003: 316-317.

RED ROOT

1. Bornstein C. Ceanothus: California's True Blues. San Marcos Growers website. http://www.smgrowers.com/info/ceanothus.asp. Published 2010. Accessed February 3, 2015.
2. Pojar J, MacKinnon A. *Plants of the Pacific Northwest Coast.* Vancouver, BC: Lone Pine Publishing; 1994: 91.
3. Hickman JC (ed.) *The Jepson Manual: Higher Plants of California*. Berkeley, CA: University of California Press; 1996: 932.
4. Mesler M. Plant Taxonomy. Class Lecture. Arcata, CA: Humboldt State University; 2009.
5. Willard T. *Edible and Medicinal Plants of the Rocky Mountains and Neighboring Territories.* Calgary, AB: Wild Rose College of Natural Healing; 1992: 136.
6. Charters M. California Plant Names: Latin and Greek Meanings and Derivations website. http://www.calflora.net/botanicalnames/pageCI-CY.html. Accessed November 4, 2015.
7. Charters M. California Plant Names: Latin and Greek Meanings and Derivations website. http://www.calflora.net/botanicalnames/pageF.html. Accessed November 4, 2015.

8. Charters M. California Plant Names: Latin and Greek Meanings and Derivations website. http://www.calflora.net/botanical names/pageG.html. Accessed November 4, 2015.
9. Charters M. California Plant Names: Latin and Greek Meanings and Derivations website. http://www.calflora.net/botanical names/pageH.html. Accessed November 4, 2015.
10. Charters M. California Plant Names: Latin and Greek Meanings and Derivations website. http://www.calflora.net/botanical names/pageI.html. Accessed November 4, 2015.
11. Charters M. California Plant Names: Latin and Greek Meanings and Derivations website. http://www.calflora.net/botanical names/pageT.html. Accessed November 4, 2015.
12. Foster S, Hobbs C. *Western Medicinal Plants and Herbs*. New York, NY: Peterson Field Guides, Houghton Mifflin Company; 2002: 280-282.
13. Grieve M. *A Modern Herbal*. Great Britain: Jonathan Cape Ltd.; 1931: 673.
14. Felter HW, Lloyd JU. *King's American Dispensatory*. (Volume 1, 19th Edition, Third Revision).. Cincinnati, OH: The Ohio Valley Company; 1923: 472-473.
15. Ellingwood F. *American Materia Medica, Therapeutics, and Pharmacognosy*. Rev. ed. Albuquerque, NM: Southwest School for Botanical Medicine; 1994: 28-29.
16. Felter HW. *The Eclectic Materia Medica, Pharmacology and Therapeutics*. Cincinnati, OH: Published by John K. Scudder, 1922: 32-33.
17. Moore M. *Medicinal Plants of the Mountain West*. Santa Fe, NM: Museum of New Mexico Press; 2003: 220-222.
18. Moore M. *Medicinal Plants of the Pacific Northwest*. Santa Fe, NM: Red Crane Books; 1993: 212-219.
19. Skenderi G. *Herbal Vade Mecum*. Rutherford, NJ: Herbacy Press, 2003: 267-268.
20. Moore M. Lecture presented at Southwest School for Botanical Medicine residency program. Albuquerque, NM; 1994.

REISHI MUSHROOM

1. Jones K. *Reishi—Ancient Herb for Modern Times*. Seattle, WA: Sylvan Press; 1996: 1-38.
2. Aurora D. *Mushrooms Demystified*. Berkeley, CA: Ten Speed Press, 1986: 577-578.
3. Volk T, Engelbrecht K. Ganoderma lucidum, Reishi or Ling Zhi, a fungus used in oriental medicine. Tom Volk Fungi—Department of Biology, University of Wisconsin-La Crosse website. http://botit.botany.wisc.edu/toms_fungi/mar2005.html. Accessed January 28, 2015.
4. Reishi—(Ganoderma lucidum) Sawdust Spawn. Field and Forest Products website. http://www.fieldforest.net/Reishi-Ganoderma-lucidum-Sawdust-Spawn/productinfo/SGL. Accessed January 28, 2015.
5. Leung AY, Foster S. *Encyclopedia of Common Natural Ingredients Used in Food, Drugs, and Cosmetics*. 2nd ed. Hoboken, NJ: A John Wiley & Sons, Inc.; 2003: 255-260.
6. Yance D. *Adaptogens in Medical Herbalism*. Rochester, VT: Healing Arts Press; 2013: 538-543.
7. Hobbs C. *Medicinal Mushrooms*. Santa Cruz, CA: Botanica Press; 1995: 96-107.
8. Winston D, Maimes S. *Adaptogens—Herbs for Strength, Stamina, and Stress Relief*. Rochester, VT: Healing Arts Press; 2007: 35-37; 184-187.
9. Willard T. *The Wild Rose Scientific Herbal*. Calgary, AB: Wild Rose College of Natural Healing; 1998: 286-289.

ROSE

1. Rosa. Flora of China. eFloras website. Missouri Botanical Garden, St. Louis, MO & Harvard University Herbaria, Cambridge, MA. http://efloras.org/florataxon.aspx?flora_id=2&taxon_id=128746. Accessed February 2, 2015.
2. Mesler M. Lecture presented at Humboldt State University's Plant Taxonomy Course. Arcata, CA; 2009.
3. Ertter B. Rosa. Jepson Flora Project. Jepson eFlora website. http://ucjeps.berkeley.edu/cgi-bin/get_IJM.pl?tid=41631. Published 2014. Accessed February 2, 2015.
4. Grieve M. *A Modern Herbal*. Great Britain: Jonathan Cape Ltd.; 1931: 683-694.
5. Foster S, Johnson R. *Desk Reference to Nature's Medicine*. Washington, D.C.: National Geographic Society; 2006: 134-135.
6. Foster S, Hobbs C. *Western Medicinal Plants and Herbs*. New York, NY: Peterson Field Guides, Houghton Mifflin Company; 2002: 298-299.
7. Willard T. *Edible and Medicinal Plants of the Rocky Mountains and Neighboring Territories*. Calgary, Alberta: Wild Rose College of Natural Healing; 1992: 117-118.
8. Pojar J, MacKinnon A. *Plants of the Pacific Northwest Coast*. Vancouver, British Columbia, Canada: Lone Pine Publishing; 1994: 74.
9. Leung AY, Foster S. *Encyclopedia of Common Natural Ingredients Used in Food, Drugs, and Cosmetics, Second Edition*. Hoboken, NJ: A John Wiley & Sons Inc., Publication; 2003: 443.
10. Skenderi G. *Herbal Vade Mecum*. Rutherford, NJ: Herbacy Press; 2003: 321-322.
11. Pedersen M. *Nutritional Herbology, A Reference Guide to Herbs*. Warsaw, IN: Wendell W. Whitman Company; 1998: 147-148.
12. Moustafa M, Alrumman S. First report about pharmaceutical properties and phytochemicals analysis of Rosa abyssinica R. Br. Ex Lindl. (Rosaceae). *Pakistan Journal Of Pharmaceutical Sciences*. 2015;28(6):2009–17. http://www.ncbi.nlm.nih.gov/pubmed/26639478. Accessed July 18, 2016.
13. Pole S. *Ayurvedic Medicine: The Principles of Traditional Practice*. Philadelphia, PA: Churchill Livingstone Elsevier; 2006: 252-253.
14. Moore M. *Medicinal Plants of the Mountain West*. Santa Fe, NM: Museum of New Mexico Press; 2003: 222-225.
15. Schnaubelt K. *Medical Aromatherapy—Healing with Essential Oils*. Berkeley, CA: Frog, Ltd.; 1999: 191.
16. Keville K, Green M. *Aromatherapy—A Complete Guide to the Healing Art*. Freedom, CA: The Crossing Press; 1995: 65.
17. Phetcharat L, Wongsuphasawat K, Winther K. The effectiveness of a standardized rose hip powder, containing seeds and shells of Rosa canina, on cell longevity, skin wrinkles, moisture, and elasticity. *Clinical Interventions In Aging*. 2015;10:1849–56. http://www.ncbi.nlm.nih.gov/pubmed/26604725. Accessed July 18, 2016.
18. Olech M, Nowak R, Pecio L, Malm A, Rzymowska J, Oleszek W. Multidirectional characterization of chemical composition and health-promoting potential of Rosa rugosa hips. *Nat Prod Res*. 2016 May 6:1-5. PubMed website. http://www.ncbi.nlm.nih.gov/pubmed/27153984. Published May 6, 2016. Accessed July 18, 2016.

ROSEMARY

1. Salvia rosmarinus (syn. Rosmarinus officinalis). Gernot Katzer's Spice Pages website. http://gernot-katzers-spice-pages.com/engl/Rosm_off.html. Accessed October 10, 2015.
2. Grieve M. *A Modern Herbal*. Great Britain: Jonathan Cape Ltd.; 1931: 681-683.
3. Salvia rosmarinus (syn. Rosmarinus officinalis). Wildflowers and Other Plants of California Web Site. http://www.calflora.net/bloomingplants/rosemary.html. Accessed November 21, 2014.
4. Salvia rosmarinus (syn. Rosmarinus officinalis). Flora of Pakistan. eFloras website. Missouri Botanical Garden, St. Louis, MO & Harvard University Herbaria, Cambridge, MA. http://efloras.org/florataxon.aspx?floraid=5&taxon_id=200020165. Published 2008. Accessed November 21, 2014.
5. Salvia rosmarinus (syn. Rosmarinus officinalis). Flora of China. eFloras website. Missouri Botanical Garden, St. Louis, MO & Harvard University Herbaria, Cambridge, MA. http://efloras.org/florataxon.aspx?floraid=2&taxon_id=200020165. Published 2008. Accessed November 21, 2014.
6. Foster S, Johnson R. *Desk Reference to Nature's Medicine*. Washington, D.C.: National Geographic Society; 2006: 316-317.
7. Leung AY, Foster S. *Encyclopedia of Common Natural Ingredients Used in Food, Drugs, and Cosmetics*. 2nd ed. Hoboken, NJ: A John Wiley & Sons, Inc.; 2003: 446-448.
8. Scudder J. *The American Eclectic Materia Medica and Therapeutics (Twelfth Edition)*. Cincinnati, OH: The Scudder Brothers Company Publishers; 1898: 613-614.
9. Skenderi G. *Herbal Vade Mecum*. Rutherford, NJ: Herbacy Press; 2003: 322-323.
10. Foster S. *Herbal Renaissance*. Layton, UT: Peregrine Smith Books; 1993: 167-169.

11. Willard T. *The Wild Rose Scientific Herbal*. Calgary, AB: Wild Rose College of Natural Healing; 1998: 296-297.
12. Weiss RF. *Herbal Medicine*. Avon, UK: The Bath Press; 1996: 185-186.
13. Schnaubelt K. *Advanced Aromatherapy—The Science of Essential Oil Therapy.* Rochester, VT: Healing Arts Press; 1995: 87-88.
14. Keville K, Green M. *Aromatherapy—A Complete Guide to the Healing Art.* Freedom, CA: The Crossing Press; 1995: 65-66.

SAGE

1. Katzer G. Spice Pages website. http://gernot-katzers-spice-pages.com/engl/Salv_off.html. Accessed November 12, 2015.
2. Grieve M. *A Modern Herbal.* Great Britain: Jonathan Cape Ltd.; 1931: 700-707.
3. Salvia officinalis. Flora of China. eFloras website. Missouri Botanical Garden, St. Louis, MO & Harvard University Herbaria, Cambridge, MA. http://efloras.org/florataxon.aspx?flora_id=2& taxon-id= 200020236. Accessed March 12, 2015.
4. Salvia. Flora of China. eFloras website. Missouri Botanical Garden, St. Louis, MO & Harvard University Herbaria, Cambridge, MA. http://efloras.org/florataxon.aspx?flora_id=2&taxon_id= 129087. Accessed March 12, 2015.
5. Scudder J. *The American Eclectic Materia Medica and Therapeutics (Twelfth Edition).* Cincinnati, OH: The Scudder Brothers Company Publishers; 1898: 217; 368.
6. Felter HW. *The Eclectic Materia Medica, Pharmacology and Therapeutics.* Cincinnati, OH: Published by John K. Scudder; 1922: 101.
7. Leung AY, Foster S. *Encyclopedia of Common Natural Ingredients Used in Food, Drugs, and Cosmetics*. 2nd ed. Hoboken, NJ: A John Wiley & Sons, Inc.; 2003: 457-460.
8. Skenderi G. *Herbal Vade Mecum.* Rutherford, NJ: Herbacy Press; 2003: 327-330.
9. Pedersen M. *Nutritional Herbology: A Reference Guide to Herbs.* Warsaw, IN: Wendell W. Whitman Company; 1998: 149-150.
10. Foster S. *Herbal Renaissance.* Layton, UT: Peregrine Smith Books; 1993: 170-172.
11. Schnaubelt K. *Advanced Aromatherapy—The Science of Essential Oil Therapy.* Rochester, VT: Healing Arts Press; 1995: 89.
12. Weiss RF. *Herbal Medicine*. Avon, UK: The Bath Press; 1996: 228.
13. Schnaubelt K. *Medical Aromatherapy—Healing with Essential Oils.* Berkeley, CA: Frog, Ltd.; 1999: 174; 198.
14. Keville K, Green M. *Aromatherapy—A Complete Guide to the Healing Art.* Freedom, CA: The Crossing Press; 1995: 66-67.
15. Tyler V. *The Honest Herbal*. Binghamton, NY: The Hawthorn Press, Inc.; 1993: 271-274.

SAW PALMETTO

1. Serenoa. Flora of North America. eFloras website. Missouri Botanical Garden, St. Louis, MO & Harvard University Herbaria, Cambridge, MA. http://efloras.org/florataxon.aspx?flora_id=1&taxon_id=130134. Published 2008. Accessed February 4, 2015.
2. Serenoa repens. Flora of North America. eFloras website. Missouri Botanical Garden, St. Louis, MO & Harvard University Herbaria, Cambridge, MA. http://efloras.org/florataxon.aspx?flora_id=1&taxon_id=222000361. Published 2008. Accessed February 4, 2015.
3. Foster S, Johnson R. *Desk Reference to Nature's Medicine*. Washington, D.C.: National Geographic Society; 2006: 322-323.
4. Ellingwood F. *American Materia Medica, Therapeutics, and Pharmacognosy*. Rev. ed. Albuquerque, NM: Southwest School for Botanical Medicine; 1994: 93-94.
5. Mills S, Bone K. *Principles and Practice of Phytotherapy*. London, UK: Harcourt Publishers Limited; 2000: 523-533.
6. Leung AY, Foster S. *Encyclopedia of Common Natural Ingredients Used in Food, Drugs, and Cosmetics*. 2nd ed. Hoboken, NJ: A John Wiley & Sons, Inc.; 2003: 467-468.
7. Murray M. *The Healing Power of Herbs*. Rocklin, CA: Prima Publishing; 1992, 1995: 306-313.
8. Skenderi G. *Herbal Vade Mecum.* Rutherford, NJ: Herbacy Press; 2003: 337-338.
9. Pedersen M. *Nutritional Herbology: A Reference Guide to Herbs.* Warsaw, IN: Wendell W. Whitman Company; 1998: 153.
10. Felter HW. *The Eclectic Materia Medica, Pharmacology and Therapeutics.* Cincinnati, OH: Published by John K. Scudder, 1922: 105.
11. Moore M. Lecture presented at Southwest School for Botanical Medicine residency program. Albuquerque, NM; 1994.

SCHISANDRA

1. Schisandra chinensis. Flora of China. eFloras website. Missouri Botanical Garden, St. Louis, MO & Harvard University Herbaria, Cambridge, MA. http://efloras.org/florataxon.aspx?flora_id=2& taxon_id=200008486. Accessed March 12, 2015.
2. Schisandra. Flora of China. eFloras website. Missouri Botanical Garden, St. Louis, MO & Harvard University Herbaria, Cambridge, MA. Accessed March 12, 2015.
3. Schisandra sphenanthera. Flora of China. eFloras website. Missouri Botanical Garden, St. Louis, MO & Harvard University Herbaria, Cambridge, MA. http://efloras.org/florataxon.aspx? flora_id=2&taxon_id=200008489. Accessed October 15, 2015.
4. Schisandra glabra. Flora of North America. eFloras website. Missouri Botanical Garden, St. Louis, MO & Harvard University Herbaria, Cambridge, MA. http://efloras.org/florataxon.aspx? flora_id=1&taxon_id=233501218. Accessed October 15, 2015.
5. Bensky D, Gamble A. *The Chinese Herbal Medicine Materia Medica*. Rev. ed. Seattle, WA: Eastland Press; 1993: 376-378.
6. Leung AY, Foster S. *Encyclopedia of Common Natural Ingredients Used in Food, Drugs, and Cosmetics*. 2nd ed. Hoboken, NJ: A John Wiley & Sons, Inc.; 2003: 469-472.
7. Foster S, Yue C. *Herbal Emissaries, Bringing Chinese Herbs to the West.* Rochester, VT: Healing Arts Press; 1992: 146-152.
8. Foster S, Johnson R. *Desk Reference to Nature's Medicine*. Washington, D.C.: National Geographic Society; 2006: 324-325.
9. Teeguarden R. *Chinese Tonic Herbs.* Tokyo, Japan: Japan Publications, Inc.; 1995: 94-96.
10. Pedersen M. *Nutritional Herbology: A Reference Guide to Herbs*. Warsaw, IN: Wendell W. Whitman Company; 1998: 154-155.
11. Tierra M. *The Way of Chinese Herbs*. New York, NY: Pocket Books; 1998: 269-270.
12. Skenderi G. *Herbal Vade Mecum.* Rutherford, NJ: Herbacy Press; 2003: 339-340.
13. Yance D. *Adaptogens in Medical Herbalism*. Rochester, VT: Healing Arts Press; 2013: 579-586.
14. Mills S, Bone K. *Principles and Practice of Phytotherapy*. London, UK: Harcourt Publishers Limited; 2000: 192-195; 244.
15. Winston D, Maimes S. *Adaptogens—Herbs for Strength, Stamina, and Stress Relief.* Rochester, VT: Healing Arts Press; 2007: 195-198.

SHEPHERD'S PURSE

1. Al-Shebaz IA. Capsella bursa-pastoris. Jepson Flora Project. Jepson eFlora website. http://ucjeps.berkeley.edu/cgi-bin/get_IJM.pl?tid=17109. Accessed April 2, 2015.
2. Capsella bursa-pastoris. Flora of North America. eFloras website. Missouri Botanical Garden, St. Louis, MO & Harvard University Herbaria, Cambridge, MA. http://efloras.org/flora taxon.aspx?flora_id=1&taxon_id=200009292. Accessed April 2, 2015.
3. Charters M. Capsella. Plant Names: Latin and Greek Meanings and Derivations website. http://www.calflora.net/botanical-names/pageCA-CH.html. Accessed April 2, 2015.
4. Bursa. Dictionary.com website. http://dictionary.reference.com/browse/bursa?s=ts. Accessed April 2, 2015.
5. Pastoral. Online Etymology website. http://etymonline.com/index.php?allowed_in_frame=0&search=pastoral&searchmode=none. Accessed April 2, 2015.
6. Grieve M. *A Modern Herbal.* Great Britain: Jonathan Cape Ltd.; 1931: 738-739.
7. Skenderi G. *Herbal Vade Mecum.* Rutherford, NJ: Herbacy Press, 2003: 344-345.
8. Moore M. Lecture from Southwest School for Botanical Medicine residency program. Albuquerque, NM: 1994.

SHIITAKE

1. Stamets P, Yao D. *MycoMedicinals—An Informational Treatise on Mushrooms*. Olympia, WA: MycoMedia Productions; 2002: 51-54.
2. Stamets P. *Mycelium Running: How Mushrooms Can Help Save the World.* Berkeley, CA: Ten Speed Press: 2005; 261-262.
3. Hobbs C. *Medicinal Mushrooms: An Exploration of Tradition, Healing, and Culture*. Summertown, TN: Botanica Press; 1996: 125-138.
4. Skenderi G. *Herbal Vade Mecum.* Rutherford, NJ: Herbacy Press; 2003: 42-43.

SILK TASSEL

1. Hickman JC (ed.) *The Jepson Manual: Higher Plants of California*. Berkeley, CA: University of California Press; 1996: 664-666.
2. Stuart JD, Sawyer JO. *Trees and Shrubs of California*. Berkeley, CA: University of California Press; 2001: 243-245.
3. Turner M, Kuhlman E. *Trees and Shrubs of the Pacific Northwest.* Portland, OR: Timber Press; 2014: 321.
4. Uchytil RJ. Garrya wrightii. Fire Effects Information System website. USDA Forest Service, Rocky Mountain Research Station, Fire Sciences Laboratory. http://www.fs.fed.us/database/feis/plants/shrub/garwri/all.html. Published 1990. Accessed September 23, 2014.
5. Kleinman R. Garrya wrightii—Vascular Plants of the Gila Wilderness. Western New Mexico University Department of Natural Sciences website. http://wnmu.edu/academic/nspages/gilaflora/garrya_wrightii.html. Accessed September 23, 2014.
6. Charters ML. Elliptica. California Plant Names: Latin and Greek Meanings and Derivations website. http://www.calflora.net/botanicalnames/pageE.html. Updated 2014. Accessed January 9, 2015.
7. Charters ML. Fremontii. California Plant Names: Latin and Greek Meanings and Derivations website. http://www.calflora.net/botanicalnames/pageF.html. Updated 2014. Accessed January 9, 2015.
8. Charters ML. Wrightii. California Plant Names: Latin and Greek Meanings and Derivations website. http://www.calflora.net/botanicalnames/pageW.html. Updated 2014. Accessed January 9, 2015.
9. Foster S, Hobbs C. *Western Medicinal Plants and Herbs*. New York, NY: Peterson Field Guides, Houghton Mifflin Company; 2002: 266-267.
10. Shepperd, W. Garrya Dougl. ex Lindl. Silktassel. In: Bonner FT, Karrfalt RP, aeds. *The Woody Plant Seed Manual: Agricultural Handbook No. 727*. Washington, D.C.: U.S. Department of Agriculture, Forest Service.; 1948. http://www.fs.fed.us/rm/pubs_other/wo_AgricHandbook727/wo_AgricHandbook727_547_549.pdf. Accessed January 12, 2015.
11. Moore M. *Medicinal Plants of the Pacific Northwest.* Santa Fe, NM: Red Crane Books; 1993: 227-230.
12. Moore M. Lecture presented at Southwest School for Botanical Medicine residency program. Albuquerque, NM; 1994.
13. Seller A. Lecture notes from Pacific School of Herbal Medicine. Oakland, CA; 1995.

SKULLCAP

1. A Worldwide Phylogenetic Analysis of *Scutellaria*. Conference abstract detail. Botany 2013; American Bryological and Lichenological Society (ABLS). http://2013.botanyconference.org/engine/search/index.php?func=detail&aid=332. Accessed March 1, 2014.
2. Foster S, Johnson R. *Desk Reference to Nature's Medicine*. Washington, D.C.: National Geographic Society; 2006: 330-331.
3. Olmstead RG. Scutellaria antirrhinoides. Jepson Flora Project. Jepson eFlora website. http://ucjeps.berkeley.edu/cgi-bin/get_IJM.pl?tid=43877. Published 2014. Accessed November 5, 2015.
4. Olmstead RG. Scutellaria californica. Jepson Flora Project. Jepson eFlora website. http://ucjeps.berkeley.edu/cgi-bin/get_IJM.pl?tid=43883. Published 2014. Accessed November 5, 2015.
5. Olmstead RG. Scutellaria galericulata. Jepson Flora Project. Jepson eFlora website. http://ucjeps.berkeley.edu/cgi-bin/get_IJM.pl?tid=43891. Published 2014. Accessed November 5, 2015.
6. Scutellaria lateriflora. Burke Museum of Natural History and Culture: University of Washington website. http://biology.burke.washington.edu/herbarium/imagecollection.php?Genus=Scutellaria&Species=lateriflora. Accessed November 5, 2015.
7. Olmstead RG. Scutellaria latiflora. Jepson Flora Project. Jepson eFlora website. http://ucjeps.berkeley.edu/cgi-bin/get_IJM.pl?tid=43900. Published 2014. Accessed November 5, 2015.
8. California Plant Names: Latin and Greek Meanings and Derivations; A Dictionary of Botanical and Biographical Etymology website. http://www.calflora.net/botanicalnames/index.html. Accessed March 1, 2014.
9. Anti. Dictionary.com website. http://dictionary.reference.com/browse/anti?s=ts. Accessed March 1, 2014.
10. Scull. Merriam-Webster Dictionary website. http://www.merriam-webster.com/dictionary/scull. Accessed March 1, 2014.
11. Skull. Merriam-Webster Dictionary website. http://www.merriam-webster.com/dictionary/skull. Accessed March 1, 2014.
12. Grieve M. *A Modern Herbal.* Great Britain: Jonathan Cape Ltd.; 1931: 724-725.
13. Willard T. *Edible and Medicinal Plants of the Rocky Mountains and Neighboring Territories.* Calgary, AB: Wild Rose College of Natural Healing; 1992: 181-182.
14. Foster S, Hobbs C. *Western Medicinal Plants and Herbs*. New York, NY: Peterson Field Guides, Houghton Mifflin Company; 2002: 55.
15. Willard T. *The Wild Rose Scientific Herbal*. Calgary, AB: Wild Rose College of Natural Healing; 1998: 310-312.
16. Tyler V. *The Honest Herbal*. Binghamton, NY: The Hawthorn Press, Inc.; 1993: 291-293.
17. Ellingwood F. *American Materia Medica, Therapeutics, and Pharmacognosy*. Rev. ed. Albuquerque, NM: Southwest School for Botanical Medicine; 1994: 92.
18. Moore M. *Medicinal Plants of the Mountain West.* Santa Fe, NM: Museum of New Mexico Press; 2003: 234-236.
19. Skenderi G. *Herbal Vade Mecum.* Rutherford, NJ: Herbacy Press; 2003: 346.
20. Hoffman D. *Medical Herbalism—The Science and Practice of Herbal Medicine.* Rochester, VT: Healing Arts Press; 2003: 582.
21. Pedersen M. *Nutritional Herbology: A Reference Guide to Herbs*. Warsaw, IN: Wendell W. Whitman Company; 1998: 155-156.
22. Moore M. Lecture presented at Southwest School for Botanical Medicine residency program. Albuquerque, NM; 1994.

SPILANTHES

1. Katzer G. Spice Pages website. http://gernot-katzers-spice-pages.com/engl/Spil_acm.html. Accessed November 24, 2015.
2. Bosch CH. Acmella oleracea (L.) R.K. Jansen. Record from PROTA4U. Plant Resources of Tropical Africa Database website. http://database.prota.org/dbtw-wpd/exec/dbtwpub.dll?ac=qbe_query&bu=http%3a%2f%2fdatabase.prota.org%2fsearchhtm&tn=protab~1&qb0=and&qf0=species+code&qi0=acmella+oleracea&rf=webdisplay. Published 2004. Accessed February 3, 2015.
3. Acmella oleracea. Flora of China. eFloras website. Missouri Botanical Garden, St. Louis, MO & Harvard University Herbaria, Cambridge, MA. http://efloras.org/florataxon.aspx?flora_id=2&taxon_id=242412042. Accessed February 3, 2015.
4. Oudhia P. Akarkara (Spilanthes acmella Murr.). New Crop Resource Online Program: Purdue University website. https://www.hort.purdue.edu/newcrop/CropFactSheets/akarkara.html. Published 2004. Accessed February 3, 2015.
5. The Plant Encyclopedia. The Global Guide to Cultivated Plants. http://www.theplantencyclopedia.org/wiki/Acmella_oleracea. Accessed November 27, 2015.
6. Borate P, Disale S. Studies on antibacterial activity of Acmella oleracea (L.) Murr. *International Journal of Pharmaceutical Science and Health Care.* 2013;5(3). http://www.academia.edu/8443889/Studies_on_Antibacterial_Activity_of_Acmella_oleracea_L._Murr. Accessed November 27, 2015.
7. Dubey S, Maity S, Singh M, Saraf S, and Saha S. Phytochemistry, pharmacology and toxicology of Spilanthes acmella: A review. *Advances in Pharmacological Sciences*. 2013. http://www.hindawi.com/journals/aps/2013/423750/. Accessed November 27, 2015.

8. Skenderi G. *Herbal Vade Mecum.* Rutherford, NJ: Herbacy Press; 2003: 356.

ST. JOHN'S WORT

1. Foster S, Johnson R. *Desk Reference to Nature's Medicine.* Washington, D.C.: National Geographic Society; 2006: 338-339.
2. Leung AY, Foster S. *Encyclopedia of Common Natural Ingredients Used in Food, Drugs, and Cosmetics.* 2nd ed. Hoboken, NJ: A John Wiley & Sons, Inc.; 2003: 310-312.
3. Grieve M. *A Modern Herbal.* Great Britain: Jonathan Cape Ltd.; 1931: 707-708.
4. *British Herbal Pharmacopoeia.* Originally published by the British Herbal Medicine Association. Republished Bisbee, AZ: Southwest School of Botanical Medicine; 2008: 115-116.
5. Willard T. *The Wild Rose Scientific Herbal.* Calgary, AB: Wild Rose College of Natural Healing; 1998: 325-327.
6. Felter HW. *The Eclectic Materia Medica, Pharmacology and Therapeutics.* Cincinnati, OH: Published by John K. Scudder, 1922: 64.
7. Ellingwood F. *American Materia Medica, Therapeutics, and Pharmacognosy*. Rev. ed. Albuquerque, NM: Southwest School for Botanical Medicine; 1994: 64.
8. Foster S, Hobbs C. *Western Medicinal Plants and Herbs*. New York, NY: Peterson Field Guides, Houghton Mifflin Company; 2002: 108-109.
9. Skenderi G. *Herbal Vade Mecum.* Rutherford, NJ: Herbacy Press; 2003: 359-360.
10. Moore M. Lecture presented at Southwest School for Botanical Medicine residency program. Albuquerque, NM: 1994.
11. Weiss RF. *Herbal Medicine*. Avon, UK: The Bath Press; 1996: 295-297.
12. Stargrove M, Treasure J, McKee D. *Herb, Nutrient, and Drug Interactions—Clinical Implications and Therapeutic Strategies*. St. Loius, MS: Mosby Elsevier; 2008: 140-159.

STONE ROOT

1. Niering WA. Olmstead. *The Audubon Society Field Guide to North American Wildflowers: Eastern*. New York: Alfred A. Knopf, 1979; 570.
2. Lochman CN. *The American Journal of Pharmacy, Vol. 57. Ed. John M. Maisch.1885.* Henriette's Herbal Homepage website. https://www.henriettes-herb.com/eclectic/kings/collinsonia.html. Accessed October 24, 2014.
3. Grieve M. *A Modern Herbal.* Great Britain: Jonathan Cape Ltd.; 1931: 774-775.
4. Felter HW. *The Eclectic Materia Medica, Pharmacology and Therapeutics.* Cincinnati, OH: Published by John K. Scudder, 1922: 37-38.
5. Ellingwood F. *American Materia Medica, Therapeutics, and Pharmacognosy*. Rev. ed. Albuquerque, NM: Southwest School for Botanical Medicine; 1994: 35-36.
6. Scudder J. *The American Eclectic Materia Medica and Therapeutics (Twelfth Edition).* Cincinnati, OH: The Scudder Brothers Company Publishers; 1898: 248-250.
7. Skenderi G. *Herbal Vade Mecum.* Rutherford, NJ: Herbacy Press, 2003: 362-363.
8. Moore M. Lecture presented at Southwest School for Botanical Medicine residency program. Albuquerque, NM; 1994.

THYME

1. Katzer G. The Spice Pages website. http://gernot-katzers-spice-pages.com/engl/Thym_vul.html. Accessed November 9, 2015.
2. Grieve M. *A Modern Herbal.* Great Britain: Jonathan Cape Ltd.; 1931: 808-815.
3. Thymus. Flora of China. eFloras website. Missouri Botanical Garden, St. Louis, MO & Harvard University Herbaria, Cambridge, MA. http://efloras.org/florataxon.aspx?flora_id=2&taxon_id=132935. Published 2008. Accessed March 6, 2015.
4. Thymus vulgaris. Missouri Botanical Garden: Plant Finder website. http://www.missouribotanicalgarden.org/PlantFinder/PlantFinderDetails.aspx?kempercode=f970. Accessed March 6, 2015.
5. Thymus. Flora of Pakistan. eFloras website. Missouri Botanical Garden, St. Louis, MO & Harvard University Herbaria, Cambridge, MA. http://efloras.org/florataxon.aspx?flora_id=5&taxon_id=132935. Published 2008. Accessed March 6, 2015.
6. Leung AY, Foster S. *Encyclopedia of Common Natural Ingredients Used in Food, Drugs, and Cosmetics.* 2nd ed. Hoboken, NJ: A John Wiley & Sons, Inc.; 2003: 492-495.
7. Skenderi G. *Herbal Vade Mecum.* Rutherford, NJ: Herbacy Press; 2003: 372-374.
8. Pedersen M. *Nutritional Herbology: A Reference Guide to Herbs.* Warsaw, IN: Wendell W. Whitman Company; 1998: 163-164.
9. Weiss RF. *Herbal Medicine.* Avon, UK: The Bath Press; 1996: 208-209.
10. Schnaubelt K. *Medical Aromatherapy—Healing with Essential Oils.* Berkeley, CA: Frog, Ltd.; 1999: 146; 193-194; 202; 237.
11. Schnaubelt K. *Advanced Aromatherapy—The Science of Essential Oil Therapy.* Rochester, VT: Healing Arts Press; 1995: 92-93.
12. Keville K, Green M. *Aromatherapy—A Complete Guide to the Healing Art.* Freedom, CA: The Crossing Press; 1995: 68-69.

TULSI BASIL

1. Ocimum sanctum. Flora of China. eFloras website. Missouri Botanical Garden, St. Louis, MO & Harvard University Herbaria, Cambridge, MA. http://efloras.org/florataxon.aspx?flora_id=2&taxon_id=200019919. Accessed November 18, 2016.
2. Ocimum. Flora of China. eFloras website. Missouri Botanical Garden, St. Louis, MO & Harvard University Herbaria, Cambridge, MA. http://efloras.org/florataxon.aspx?flora_id=2&taxon_id=122604. Accessed November 18, 2016.
3. Katzer G. Spice Pages website. http://gernot-katzers-spice-pages.com/engl/Ocim_bas.html. Accessed November 25, 2016.
4. Pattanayak P, Behera P, Das D, Panda SK. Ocimum sanctum Linn. A reservoir plant for therapeutic applications: An overview. *Pharmacogn Rev*. 2010;4(7): 95-105. *Accessed November 25, 2016.*
5. Upahyaya KD. Indian botanical folklore. *Asian Folklore Studies*. 1964:23(2): 15-34.
6. Francis P Jr. Plants as human adornment in India. *Economic Botany*. 1984:38(2): 194-209.
7. Pole S. *Ayurvedic Medicine: The Principles of Traditional Practice*. Philadelphia, PA: Churchill Livingstone Elsevier; 2006: 280-281.
8. Winston D, Maimes S. *Adaptogens—Herbs for Strength, Stamina, and Stress Relief.* Rochester, VT: Healing Arts Press; 2007: 167-171.
9. Boissya CL, Majumder R, Majumder AK. Some medicinal plants from Darrang District of Assam, India. *Anthropos*. 1981:76(1/2): 220-222.
10. Dagar HS, Dagar JC. Plant folk medicines among the Nicobarese of Katchal Island, India. *Economic Botany*. 1991:45(1): 114-119.
11. Badruzzaman Siddiqui M, Mashkoor Alam M, Husain W. Traditional treatment of skin diseases in Uttar Pradesh, India. *Economic Botany*. 1989:43(4): 480-486.
12. Skenderi G. *Herbal Vade Mecum.* Rutherford, NJ: Herbacy Press; 2003: 194.
13. Yance D. *Adaptogens in Medical Herbalism*. Rochester, VT: Healing Arts Press; 2013: 479-485.

TURMERIC

1. Curcuma longa. Flora of China. eFloras website. Missouri Botanical Garden, St. Louis, MO & Harvard University Herbaria, Cambridge, MA. http://efloras.org/florataxon.aspx?flora_id=2&taxon_id=200028370. Accessed April 23, 2015.
2. Curcuma. Flora of China. eFloras website. Missouri Botanical Garden, St. Louis, MO & Harvard University Herbaria, Cambridge, MA. http://efloras.org/florataxon.aspx?flora_id=2&taxon_id=108706. Accessed April 23, 2015.
3. Leung AY, Foster S. *Encyclopedia of Common Natural Ingredients Used in Food, Drugs, and Cosmetics*. 2nd ed. Hoboken, NJ: A John Wiley & Sons, Inc.; 2003: 499-501.
4. Foster S, Johnson R. *Desk Reference to Nature's Medicine*. Washington, D.C.: National Geographic Society; 2006: 360-361.
5. Hobbs C. *Foundations of Health—Healing with Herbs and Foods.* Capitola, CA: Botanica Press; 1992: 286-89.
6. Lad V, Frawley D. *The Yoga of Herbs.* Twin Lakes, WI: Lotus Press; 1992: 149-150.
7. Murray M. *The Encyclopedia of Healing Foods.* New York, NY: Atria Books; 2005: 521-524.

8. Murray M. *The Healing Power of Herbs*. Rocklin, CA: Prima Publishing; 1992, 1995: 327-335.
9. Foster S. *101 Medicinal Herbs*. Loveland, CO: Interweave Press; 1998: 200-201.
10. Tierra M. *The Way of Chinese Herbs*. New York, NY: Pocket Books, 1998: 229-30.
11. Bensky D, Gamble A. *The Chinese Herbal Medicine Materia Medica*. Rev. ed. Seattle, WA: Eastland Press; 1993: 272-73.
12. Skenderi G. *Herbal Vade Mecum*. Rutherford, NJ: Herbacy Press; 2003: 380-81.
13. Pedersen M. *Nutritional Herbology: A Reference Guide to Herbs*. Warsaw, IN: Wendell W. Whitman Company; 1998: 164-65.
14. Mills S, Bone K. *Principles and Practice of Phytotherapy*. London, UK: Harcourt Publishers Limited; 2000: 569-580.
15. Pole S. *Ayurvedic Medicine: The Principles of Traditional Practice*. Philadelphia, PA: Churchill Livingstone Elsevier; 2006: 282-283.
16. Moore M. Lecture presented at Southwest School for Botanical Medicine residency program. Albuquerque, NM; 1994.

USNEA

1. Ponzetti J, Wittmann E. Species Fact Sheet. Bureau of Land Management: Oregon website. http://www.blm.gov/or/plans/surveyandmanage/files/sfs-li-usnea-longissima-2006.pdf. Accessed January 28, 2015.
2. Public Description of Usnea Dill. ex Adans. Mushroom Observer website. http://mushroomobserver.org/name/show_name_description/755. Accessed January 28, 2015.
3. Hobbs C. *Usnea: The Herbal Antibiotic and Other Medicinal Lichens*. Capitola, CA: Botanica Press, 1990: 8-17.
4. Pojar J, MacKinnon A. *Plants of the Pacific Northwest Coast*. Vancouver, BC: Lone Pine Publishing; 1994: 503.
5. Charters M. Barbata. California Plant Names: Latin and Greek Meanings and Derivations Web Site. http://www.calflora.net/botanicalnames/pageBA-BI.html. Accessed August 31, 2015.
6. Rom J. Contributions to the complex study of some lichens-Usnea genus. Pharmacological studies on Usnea barbata and Usnea hirta species. *Rom J Physiol*. 1993 Jan-Jun;30(1-2):101-7. http://www.ncbi.nlm.nih.gov/pubmed/7982010. Accessed August 12, 2015.
7. Skenderi G. *Herbal Vade Mecum*. Rutherford, NJ: Herbacy Press, 2003: 382-383.
8. Weiss RF. *Herbal Medicine*. Avon, UK: The Bath Press; 1996: 49; 199.

UVA URSI AND MANZANITA

1. Hickman JC (ed.) *The Jepson Manual: Higher Plants of California*. Berkeley, CA: University of California Press; 1996: 545-554.
2. Pojar J, MacKinnon A. *Plants of the Pacific Northwest Coast*. Vancouver, BC: Lone Pine Publishing; 1994: 67.
3. Willard T. *Edible and Medicinal Plants of the Rocky Mountains and Neighboring Territories*. Calgary, AB: Wild Rose College of Natural Healing; 1992: 165-165.
4. Curtin LSM, Moore, M. *Healing Herbs of the Upper Rio Grande*. Rev. ed. Santa Fe, NM: Western Edge Press; 1997: 56-57.
5. Foster S, Hobbs C. *Western Medicinal Plants and Herbs*. New York, NY: Peterson Field Guides, Houghton Mifflin Company; 2002: 276.
6. Ellingwood F. *American Materia Medica, Therapeutics, and Pharmacognosy*. Rev. ed. Albuquerque, NM: Southwest School for Botanical Medicine; 1994: 12-13.
7. Culbreth D. *A Manual of Materia Medica and Pharmacology*. 1917. Republished Bisbee, AZ: Southwest School of Botanical Medicine; 2008: 14.
8. Moore M. *Medicinal Plants of the Mountain West*. Santa Fe, NM: Museum of New Mexico Press; 2003: 250-251.
9. Leung AY, Foster S. *Encyclopedia of Common Natural Ingredients Used in Food, Drugs, and Cosmetics*. 2nd ed. Hoboken, NJ: A John Wiley & Sons, Inc.; 2003: 505-506.
10. Skenderi G. *Herbal Vade Mecum*. Rutherford, NJ: Herbacy Press; 2003: 383.
11. Foster S, Johnson R. *Desk Reference to Nature's Medicine*. Washington, D.C.: National Geographic Society; 2006: 32-33.
12. Murray M. *The Healing Power of Herbs*. Rocklin, CA: Prima Publishing; 1992, 1995: 336-338.

VALERIAN

1. Leung AY, Foster S. *Encyclopedia of Common Natural Ingredients Used in Food, Drugs, and Cosmetics*. 2nd ed. Hoboken, NJ: A John Wiley & Sons, Inc.; 2003: 507-510.
2. Pedersen M. *Nutritional Herbology: A Reference Guide to Herbs*. Warsaw, IN: Wendell W. Whitman Company; 1998: 167-168.
3. Murray M. *The Healing Power of Herbs*. Rev. 2nd ed. Rocklin, CA: Prima Health; 1995: 339-342.
4. Moore AJ, Dempster LT. Valeriana. Jepson Flora Project. Jepson eFlora website. http://ucjeps.berkeley.edu/eflora/eflora_display.php?tid=10572. Published 2014. Accessed December 17, 2015.
5. Valeriana Flora of China. eFloras website. Missouri Botanical Garden, St. Louis, MO & Harvard University Herbaria, Cambridge, MA. http://efloras.org/florataxon.aspx?flora_id=2&taxon_id=134313. Published 2008. Accessed December 17, 2015.
6. Valeriana. Flora of Pakistan. eFloras website. Missouri Botanical Garden, St. Louis, MO & Harvard University Herbaria, Cambridge, MA. http://efloras.org/florataxon.aspx?flora_id=5&taxon_id=134313. Published 2008. Accessed December 17, 2015.
7. Valeriana officinalis. Flora of China. eFloras website. Missouri Botanical Garden, St. Louis, MO & Harvard University Herbaria, Cambridge, MA. http://efloras.org/florataxon.aspx?flora_id=2&taxon_id=200022560. Published 2008. Accessed December 17, 2015.
8. Grieve M. *A Modern Herbal*. Great Britain: Jonathan Cape Ltd.; 1931: 824-829.
9. Pojar J, MacKinnon A. *Plants of the Pacific Northwest Coast*. Vancouver, BC: Lone Pine Publishing; 1994: 333.
10. Santos G. Officinalis. Massachusetts Medical Society Gardens website. http://www.piam.com/mms_garden/officinalis.html. Accessed February 26, 2014
11. Smith J. *Vascular Plant Families*. Eureka, CA: Mad River Press; 1977: 294.
12. Diversiloba. My Etymology website. http://www.myetymology.com/search.php?query=Diversiloba&search=Search. Accessed February 25, 2014.
13. Willard T. *Edible and Medicinal Plants of the Rocky Mountains and Neighboring Territories*. Calgary, AB: Wild Rose College of Natural Healing; 1992: 195-196.
14. William Whitaker Words. University of Notre Dame Archives website. http://www.archives.nd.edu/words.html. Accessed February 25, 2014.
15. Valerian Scientific Names. USDA, Natural Resources Conservation Service. https://plants.usda.gov. Accessed February 25, 2014.
16. Foster S, Johnson R. *Desk Reference to Nature's Medicine*. Washington, D.C.: National Geographic Society; 2006: 362-363.
17. Foster S. *Herbal Renaissance*. Layton, UT: Peregrine Smith Books; 1993: 192-194.
18. Foster S. *101 Medicinal Herbs*. Loveland, CO: Interweave Press; 1998: 202-203.
19. Felter HW. *The Eclectic Materia Medica, Pharmacology and Therapeutics*. Cincinnati, OH: Published by John K. Scudder, 1922: 113.
20. Ellingwood F. *American Materia Medica, Therapeutics, and Pharmacognosy*. Rev. ed. Albuquerque, NM: Southwest School for Botanical Medicine; 1994: 101.
21. Culbreth D. *A Manual of Materia Medica and Pharmacology*. Rev. ed. Albuquerque, NM: Southwest School for Botanical Medicine; 1994: 311.
22. Willard T. *The Wild Rose Scientific Herbal*. Calgary, AB: Wild Rose College of Natural Healing; 1998: 336-338.
23. Lad V, Frawley D. *The Yoga of Herbs*. Twin Lakes, WI: Lotus Press; 1992: 150-151.
24. Mills S, Bone K. *Principles and Practice of Phytotherapy*. London, UK: Harcourt Publishers Limited; 2000: 581-589.
25. Weiss RF. *Herbal Medicine*. Avon, UK: The Bath Press; 1996: 281-285.
26. Skenderi G. *Herbal Vade Mecum*. Rutherford, NJ: Herbacy Press; 2003: 384-385.
27. Hoffman D. *Medical Herbalism — The Science and Practice of Herbal Medicine*. Rochester, Vermont: Healing Arts Press; 2003: 592.

28. Moore M. *Medicinal Plants of the Mountain West.* Santa Fe, NM: Museum of New Mexico Press; 2003: 251-253.
29. Tyler V. *The Honest Herbal*. Binghamton, NY: The Hawthorn Press, Inc.; 1993: 315-317.

VITEX

1. Katzer G. Spice Pages website. http://gernot-katzers-spice-pages.com/engl/Vite_agn.html. Accessed November 11, 2015.
2. Vitex agnus-castus. The Plant List Version 1.1. website. http://www.theplantlist.org/tpl1.1/record/kew-213297. Published 2013. Accessed January 7, 2015.
3. Vitex agnus-castus var. agnus-castus. Flora of Pakistan. eFloras website. Missouri Botanical Garden, St. Louis, MO & Harvard University Herbaria, Cambridge, MA. http://efloras.org/flora taxon.aspx?flora_id=5&taxon_id=250064506. Published 2008. Accessed January 6, 2015.
4. Vitex. Flora of Pakistan. eFloras website. Missouri Botanical Garden, St. Louis, MO & Harvard University Herbaria, Cambridge, MA. http://efloras.org/florataxon.aspx?flora_id=5&taxon_id=134644. Published 2008. Accessed January 6, 2015.
5. Foster S, Johnson R. *Desk Reference to Nature's Medicine*. Washington, D.C.: National Geographic Society; 2006: 98-99.
6. Hobbs C. *Vitex—The Women's Herb*. Capitola, CA: Botanica Press; 1993: 1-34.
7. Foster S. *Herbal Renaissance.* Layton, UT: Peregrine Smith Books; 1993: 67-69.
8. Leung AY, Foster S. *Encyclopedia of Common Natural Ingredients Used in Food, Drugs, and Cosmetics*. 2nd ed. Hoboken, NJ: A John Wiley & Sons, Inc.; 2003: 151-152.
9. Blumenthal M. *The ABC Clinical Guide to Herbs*. Austin, TX: The American Botanical Council; 2003: 61-72.
10. Mills S, Bone K. *Principles and Practice of Phytotherapy*. London, UK: Harcourt Publishers Limited; 2000: 328-334.
11. Weiss RF. *Herbal Medicine*. Avon, UK: The Bath Press; 1996: 317-319.
12. Moore M. Lecture presented at Southwest School for Botanical Medicine residency program. Albuquerque, NM; 1994.
13. Tricky R. *Women, Hormones and the Menstrual Cycle*. St. Leonards, Australia: Allen and Unwin; 1998: 198-199; 202; 217; 253; 345-348.
14. Hudson T. *Women's Encyclopedia of Natural Medicine*. New York, NY: McGraw Hill; 2008: 8-9; 21; 199; 310.
15. Skenderi G. *Herbal Vade Mecum.* Rutherford, NJ: Herbacy Press; 2003: 94-95.
16. Murray M. *The Healing Power of Herbs*. Rocklin, CA: Prima Publishing; 1992, 1995: 375-376.
17. Yance D. *Adaptogens in Medical Herbalism*. Rochester, VT: Healing Arts Press; 2013: 239-240.

WILD CHERRY BARK

1. Leung AY, Foster S. *Encyclopedia of Common Natural Ingredients Used in Food, Drugs, and Cosmetics.* 2nd ed. Hoboken, NJ: A John Wiley & Sons, Inc.; 2003: 155-156.
2. Rohrer JR. Prunus virginiana. Jepson Flora Project. Jepson eFlora website. http://ucjeps.berkeley.edu/cgi-bin/get_IJM.pl?tid=64546. Accessed March 26, 2015.
3. Prunus serotina. Missouri Botanical Garden: Plant Finder website. http://www.missouribotanicalgarden.org/PlantFinder/Plant FinderDetails.aspx?kempercode=a914. Accessed March 26, 2015.
4. Prunus virginiana. Missouri Botanical Garden: Plant Finder website. http://www.missouribotanicalgarden.org/PlantFinder/PlantFinderDetails.aspx?kempercode=c131. Accessed March 26, 2015.
5. Prunus. Flora of China. eFloras website. Missouri Botanical Garden, St. Louis, MO & Harvard University Herbaria, Cambridge, MA. http://www.efloras.org/florataxon.aspx?flora_id=2&taxon_id=126865. Accessed March 26, 2015.
6. *Prunus.* Merriam-Webster Dictionary website. http://www.merriam-webster.com/dictionary/prunus. Accessed March 26, 2015.
7. Charters M. California Plant Names: Latin and Greek Meanings and Derivations website. http://www.calflora.net/botanical names/pageV.html. Accessed March 27, 2015.
8. Foster S, Johnson R. *Desk Reference to Nature's Medicine.* Washington, D.C.: National Geographic Society; 2006: 52-52.
9. Curtin LSM, Moore, M. *Healing Herbs of the Upper Rio Grande.* Rev. ed. Santa Fe, NM: Western Edge Press; 1997: 37.
10. Felter HW. *The Eclectic Materia Medica, Pharmacology and Therapeutics.* Cincinnati, OH: Published by John K. Scudder, 1922: 94.
11. Ellingwood F. *American Materia Medica, Therapeutics, and Pharmacognosy*. Rev. ed. Albuquerque, NM: Southwest School for Botanical Medicine; 1994: 56.
12. Scudder J. *The American Eclectic Materia Medica and Therapeutics (Twelfth Edition).* Cincinnati, OH: The Scudder Brothers Company Publishers; 1898: 442.
13. Skenderi G. *Herbal Vade Mecum.* Rutherford, NJ: Herbacy Press; 2003: 50-51.
14. Grieve M. *A Modern Herbal.* Great Britain: Jonathan Cape Ltd.; 1931: 191.
15. Moore M. *Medicinal Plants of the Mountain West*. Santa Fe, NM: Museum of New Mexico Press; 2003: 82-84.

WILD YAM

1. Dioscorea villosa. Flora of North America. eFloras website. Missouri Botanical Garden, St. Louis, MO & Harvard University Herbaria, Cambridge, MA. http://efloras.org/florataxon.aspx?flora_id=1&taxon_id=242101571. Published 2008. Accessed October 22, 2015.
2. Foster S. *101 Medicinal Herbs*. Loveland, CO: Interweave Press; 1998: 208-209.
3. Charters M. California Plant Names: Latin and Greek Meanings and Derivations website. A Dictionary of Botanical and Biographical Etymology. http://www.calflora.net/botanical names/pageV.html. Accessed November 15, 2015.
4. Foster S, Johnson R. *Desk Reference to Nature's Medicine*. Washington, D.C.: National Geographic Society; 2006: 368-69.
5. Willard T. *The Wild Rose Scientific Herbal.* Calgary, AB: Wild Rose College of Natural Healing; 1998: 343-44.
6. Ellingwood F. *American Materia Medica, Therapeutics, and Pharmacognosy*. Rev. ed. Albuquerque, NM: Southwest School for Botanical Medicine; 1994: 42.
7. Felter HW. *The Eclectic Materia Medica, Pharmacology and Therapeutics.* Cincinnati, OH: Published by John K. Scudder, 1922: 42.
8. King J, Felter HW, Lloyd, JU. *King's American Dispensatory*. (Volume 1, 19th Edition, Third Revision). Cincinnati, OH: The Ohio Valley Company; 1923: 658-661.
9. Hoffman D. *Medical Herbalism—The Science and Practice of Herbal Medicine.* Rochester, VT: Healing Arts Press; 2003: 543.
10. Skenderi G. *Herbal Vade Mecum.* Rutherford, NJ: Herbacy Press, 2003: 210.
11. Pedersen M. *Nutritional Herbology: A Reference Guide to Herbs*. Warsaw, IN: Wendell W. Whitman Company; 1998: 172-73.
12. Grieve M. *A Modern Herbal.* Great Britain: Jonathan Cape Ltd.; 1931: 863.
13. Moore M. Lecture presented at Southwest School for Botanical Medicine residency program. Albuquerque, NM; 1994.
14. Lima CM, Lima AK, Melo MG, Serafini MR, Oliveira DL, de Almeida EB, et al. Bioassay-guided evaluation of Dioscorea villosa—an acute and subchronic toxicity, antinociceptive and anti-inflammatory approach. *BMC Complement Altern Med*. 2013 Jul 28;13: 195. Available from PubMed. http://www.ncbi.nlm.nih.gov/pubmed/23889998. Accessed November 13, 2013.
15. Wojcikowski K, Wohlmuth H, Johnson DW, Gobe G. Dioscorea villosa (wild yam) induces chronic kidney injury via pro-fibrotic pathways. *Food Chem Toxicol*. 2008 Sep;46(9): 3122-31. Available from PubMed. http://www.ncbi.nlm.nih.gov/pubmed/18662738. Accessed November 13, 2013.

WILLOW BARK

1. Foster S, Johnson R. *Desk Reference to Nature's Medicine*. Washington, D.C.: National Geographic Society; 2006: 366-367.
2. *British Herbal Pharmacopoeia*. Originally published by the British Herbal Medicine Association. Rev. ed. Albuquerque, NM: Southwest School for Botanical Medicine; 1994: 184-185.
3. Lust J. *The Herb Book*. New York, NY: Bantam Books; 1974: 402-403.

4. Argus GW. Salix. Jepson Flora Project. Jepson eFlora website. http://ucjeps.berkeley.edu/eflora/eflora_display.php?tid=9887. Published 2014. Accessed December 17, 2015.
5. Curtin LSM, Moore, M. *Healing Herbs of the Upper Rio Grande.* Rev. ed. Santa Fe, NM: Western Edge Press; 1997: 88-89.
6. Ellingwood F. *American Materia Medica, Therapeutics, and Pharmacognosy*. Rev. ed. Albuquerque, NM: Southwest School for Botanical Medicine; 1994: 90-91.
7. Felter HW. *The Eclectic Materia Medica, Pharmacology and Therapeutics.* Cincinnati, OH: Published by John K. Scudder; 1922: 101.
8. Weiss RF. *Herbal Medicine*. Avon, UK: The Bath Press; 1996: 303.
9. Skenderi G. *Herbal Vade Mecum.* Rutherford, NJ: Herbacy Press; 2003: 391-392.
10. Moore M. *Medicinal Plants of the Mountain West*. Santa Fe, NM: Museum of New Mexico Press; 2003: 257-259.
11. Pedersen M. *Nutritional Herbology: A Reference Guide to Herbs*. Warsaw, IN: Wendell W. Whitman Company; 1998: 170-171.

YARROW

1. Grieve M. *A Modern Herbal.* Great Britain: Jonathan Cape Ltd.; 1931: 863-865.
2. Hickman JC (ed.). *The Jepson Manual—Higher Plants of California.* Berkeley and Los Angeles, CA: University of California Press; 1993: 189.
3. Horn E. *Coastal Wildflowers of the Pacific Northwest*. Missoula, MT: Mountain Press Publishing Company; 1994; 102.
4. Mesler M. Plant Taxonomy Course presented at Humboldt State University. Arcata, CA; Spring, 2009.
5. Foster S, Johnson R. *Desk Reference to Nature's Medicine*. Washington, D.C.: National Geographic Society; 2006: 376-377.
6. Curtin LSM, Moore, M. *Healing Herbs of the Upper Rio Grande.* Rev. ed. Santa Fe, NM: Western Edge Press; 1997: 141.
7. Foster S, Hobbs C. *Western Medicinal Plants and Herbs*. New York, NY: Peterson Field Guides, Houghton Mifflin Company; 2002: 86-87.
8. Pojar J, MacKinnon A. *Plants of the Pacific Northwest Coast.* Vancouver, BC: Lone Pine Publishing; 1994: 279.
9. Ellingwood F. *American Materia Medica, Therapeutics, and Pharmacognosy*. Rev. ed. Albuquerque, NM: Southwest School for Botanical Medicine; 1994: 1.
10. Scudder J. *The American Eclectic Materia Medica and Therapeutics (Twelfth Edition).* Cincinnati, OH: The Scudder Brothers Company Publishers; 1898: 556; 612-613.
11. Felter HW. *The Eclectic Materia Medica, Pharmacology and Therapeutics.* Cincinnati, OH: Published by John K. Scudder; 1922: 5.
12. King, J, Felter H, Lloyd J. *King's American Dispensatory* (Volume 1, 19th Edition, Third Revision). Cincinnati, OH: The Ohio Valley Company; 1905: 19-20.
13. Leung AY, Foster S. *Encyclopedia of Common Natural Ingredients Used in Food, Drugs, and Cosmetics.* 2nd ed. Hoboken, NJ: A John Wiley & Sons, Inc.; 2003: 518-519.
14. Willard T. *The Wild Rose Scientific Herbal.* Calgary, AB: Wild Rose College of Natural Healing; 1998: 351-353.
15. Moore M. *Medicinal Plants of the Mountain West*. Santa Fe, NM: Museum of New Mexico Press; 2003: 269-70.
16. Pedersen M. *Nutritional Herbology: A Reference Guide to Herbs*. Warsaw, IN: Wendell W. Whitman Company; 1998: 174-175.
17. Moore M. *Medicinal Plants of the Pacific Northwest.* Santa Fe, NM: Red Crane Books; 1993: 272-275.
18. Skenderi G. *Herbal Vade Mecum.* Rutherford, NJ: Herbacy Press; 2003: 389-399.
19. Schnaubelt K. *Advanced Aromatherapy—The Science of Essential Oil Therapy.* Rochester, VT: Healing Arts Press; 1995: 94.
20. Keville K, Green M. *Aromatherapy—A Complete Guide to the Healing Art.* Freedom, CA: The Crossing Press; 1995: 70.

YELLOW DOCK

1. Rumex crispus. Flora of China. eFloras website. Missouri Botanical Garden, St. Louis, MO & Harvard University Herbaria, Cambridge, MA. http://efloras.org/florataxon.aspx?flora_id=2&taxon_id=200006746. Published 2008. Accessed December 10, 2015.
2. Foster S, Johnson R. *Desk Reference to Nature's Medicine*. Washington, D.C.: National Geographic Society; 2006: 378-379.
3. Rumex crispus. Flora of North America. eFloras website. Missouri Botanical Garden, St. Louis, MO & Harvard University Herbaria, Cambridge, MA. http://efloras.org/florataxon.aspx?flora_id=1&taxon_id=200006746. Published 2008. Accessed December 10, 2015.
4. Rumex. Flora of North America. eFloras website. Missouri Botanical Garden, St. Louis, MO & Harvard University Herbaria, Cambridge, MA. http://efloras.org/florataxon.aspx?flora_id=1&taxon_id=128864. Published 2008. Accessed December 10, 2015.
5. Pedersen M. *Nutritional Herbology: A Reference Guide to Herbs*. Warsaw, IN: Wendell W. Whitman Company; 1998: 176-177.
6. Grieve M. *A Modern Herbal.* Great Britain: Jonathan Cape Ltd.; 1931: 258-260.
7. Harper D. Dock. Online Etymology Dictionary website. http://www.etymonline.com/index.php?term=dock. Accessed February 12, 2014.
8. Lust J. *The Herb Book*. New York, NY: Bantam Books; 1974: 411-412.
9. Foster S, Hobbs C. *Western Medicinal Plants and Herbs*. New York, NY: Peterson Field Guides, Houghton Mifflin Company; 2002: 237.
10. Ellingwood F. *American Materia Medica, Therapeutics, and Pharmacognosy*. Rev. ed. Albuquerque, NM: Southwest School for Botanical Medicine; 1994: 90.
11. Felter HW. *The Eclectic Materia Medica, Pharmacology and Therapeutics.* Cincinnati, OH: Published by John K. Scudder; 1922: 100.
12. Scudder J. *The American Eclectic Materia Medica and Therapeutics.* Cincinnati, OH: The Scudder Brothers Company Publishers; 1898: 482.
13. Skenderi G. *Herbal Vade Mecum.* Rutherford, NJ: Herbacy Press; 2003: 133.
14. Moore M. *Medicinal Plants of the Mountain West*. Santa Fe, NM: Museum of New Mexico Press; 2003: 270-271.
15. Willard T. *Edible and Medicinal Plants of the Rocky Mountains and Neighboring Territories.* Calgary, AB: Wild Rose College of Natural Healing; 1992: 354-355.
16. Moore M. Lecture presented at Southwest School for Botanical Medicine residency program. Albuquerque, NM; 1994.
17. Seller A. Lecture notes from Pacific School of Herbal Medicine. Oakland, CA; 1995.

YELLOW POND LILY

1. Wiersema JH. Nuphar. Jepson Flora Project. Jepson eFlora website. http://ucjeps.berkeley.edu/cgi-bin/get_IJM.pl?tid=34748. Accessed April 23, 2015.
2. Nuphar. Flora of North America. eFloras website. Missouri Botanical Garden, St. Louis, MO & Harvard University Herbaria, Cambridge, MA. http://efloras.org/florataxon.aspx?flora_id=1&taxon_id=122507. Accessed April 23, 2015.
3. Willard T. *Edible and Medicinal Plants of the Rocky Mountains and Neighboring Territories.* Calgary, AB: Wild Rose College of Natural Healing; 1992: 87.
4. Deane G. Yellow Pond Lilly: Raising a Wokas. Eat the Weeds website. http://www.eattheweeds.com/yellow-pond-lilly-raising-a-wokas/. Accessed November 2, 2013.
5. Pojar J, MacKinnon A. *Plants of the Pacific Northwest Coast.* Vancouver, BC: Lone Pine Publishing; 1994: 349.
6. Yellow Pond Lily (*Nuphar luteum*). Study of Northern Virginia Ecology website. http://www.fcps.edu/islandcreekes/ecology/yellow_pond_lily.htm. Accessed August 26, 2013.
7. Moore M. *Medicinal Plants of the Pacific Northwest.* Santa Fe, NM: Red Crane Books; 1993: 275-278.
8. Moore M. Lecture presented at Southwest School for Botanical Medicine residency program. Albuquerque, NM; 1994.

YERBA MANSA

1. Thieret JW, McClintock E. Anemopsis californica. Jepson Flora Project. Jepson eFlora website. http://ucjeps.berkeley.edu/cgi-bin/get_IJM.pl?tid=13392. Published Aug 26, 2008. Accessed December 16, 2014.
2. Anemopsis californica. Flora of North America. eFloras website. Missouri Botanical Garden, St. Louis, MO & Harvard University Herbaria, Cambridge, MA. http://efloras.org/florataxon.aspx?flora_id=1&taxon_id=220000730. Published 2008. Accessed December 16, 2014.
3. Anemopsis. Flora of North America. eFloras website. Missouri Botanical Garden, St. Louis, MO & Harvard University Herbaria, Cambridge, MA. http://efloras.org/florataxon.aspx?flora_id=1&taxon_id=101739. Published 2008. Accessed December 16, 2014.
4. Charters M. California Plant Names: Latin and Greek Meanings and Derivations. http://www.calflora.net/botanicalnames/page AN-AZ.html. Accessed November 16, 2015.
5. Charters M. California Plant Names: Latin and Greek Meanings and Derivations. http://www.calflora.net/botanicalnames/page-CA-CH.html. Accessed November 18, 2015.
6. Curtin LSM, Moore, M. *Healing Herbs of the Upper Rio Grande.* Rev. ed. Santa Fe, NM: Western Edge Press; 1997: 186-188.
7. King J, Felter H, Lloyd, J. *King's American Dispensatory* (Volume 1, 19th Edition, Third Revision). Cincinnati, OH: The Ohio Valley Company; 1905: 202-203.
8. Moore M. *Los Remedios — Traditional Herbal Remedies of the Southwest*. Santa Fe, NM: Red Crane Books; 1990: 83.
9. Ellingwood F. *American Materia Medica, Therapeutics, and Pharmacognosy*. Rev. ed. Albuquerque, NM: Southwest School for Botanical Medicine; 1994: 8.
10. Moore M. *Medicinal Plants of the Desert and Canyon West*. Santa Fe, NM: Museum of New Mexico Press: 132-134.
11. Skenderi G. *Herbal Vade Mecum.* Rutherford, NJ: Herbacy Press; 2003: 401.

YERBA SANTA

1. Hickman JC (ed.) *The Jepson Manual: Higher Plants of California*. Berkeley, CA: University of California Press; 1996: 684.
2. Hannan GL. Eriodictyon californicum. Jepson Flora Project. Jepson eFlora website. http://ucjeps.berkeley.edu/cgi-bin/get_IJM.pl?tid=24668. Accessed November 19, 2015.
3. Stuart JD, Sawyer JO. *Trees and Shrubs of California*. Berkeley, CA: University of California Press; 2001: 231-232.
4. Turner M, Kuhlman E. *Trees and Shrubs of the Pacific Northwest.* Portland, OR: Timber Press; 2014: 146.
5. Page E. Charters M. California Plant Names: Latin and Greek Meanings and Derivations website. http://www.calflora.net/botanical names/pageE.html. Accessed November 13, 2015.
6. Page AN-AZ. Charters M. California Plant Names: Latin and Greek Meanings and Derivations website. http://www.calflora.net/botanical names/pageAN-AZ.html. Accessed November 13, 2015.
7. Page CI-CY. Charters M. California Plant Names: Latin and Greek Meanings and Derivations website. http://www.calflora.net/botanicalnames/pageCI-CY.html. Accessed November 13, 2015.
8. Foster S, Hobbs C. *Western Medicinal Plants and Herbs*. New York, NY: Peterson Field Guides, Houghton Mifflin Company; 2002: 278-279.
9. Felter HW. *The Eclectic Materia Medica, Pharmacology and Therapeutics.* Cincinnati, OH: Published by John K. Scudder; 1922: 46.
10. Ellingwood F. *American Materia Medica, Therapeutics, and Pharmacognosy*. Rev. ed. Albuquerque, NM: Southwest School for Botanical Medicine; 1994: 48.
11. Moore M. *Medicinal Plants of the Mountain West*. Santa Fe, NM: Museum of New Mexico Press; 2003: 276-280.
12. Moore M. *Medicinal Plants of the Pacific Northwest.* Santa Fe, NM: Red Crane Books; 1993: 285-288.
13. Leung AY, Foster S. *Encyclopedia of Common Natural Ingredients Used in Food, Drugs, and Cosmetics*. 2nd ed. Hoboken, NJ: A John Wiley & Sons, Inc.; 2003: 520-521.
14. Skenderi G. *Herbal Vade Mecum.* Rutherford, NJ: Herbacy Press; 2003: 402.
15. Pedersen M. *Nutritional Herbology: A Reference Guide to Herbs*. Warsaw, IN: Wendell W. Whitman Company; 1998: 178.
16. Moore M. Lecture presented at Southwest School for Botanical Medicine residency program. Albuquerque, NM; 1994.

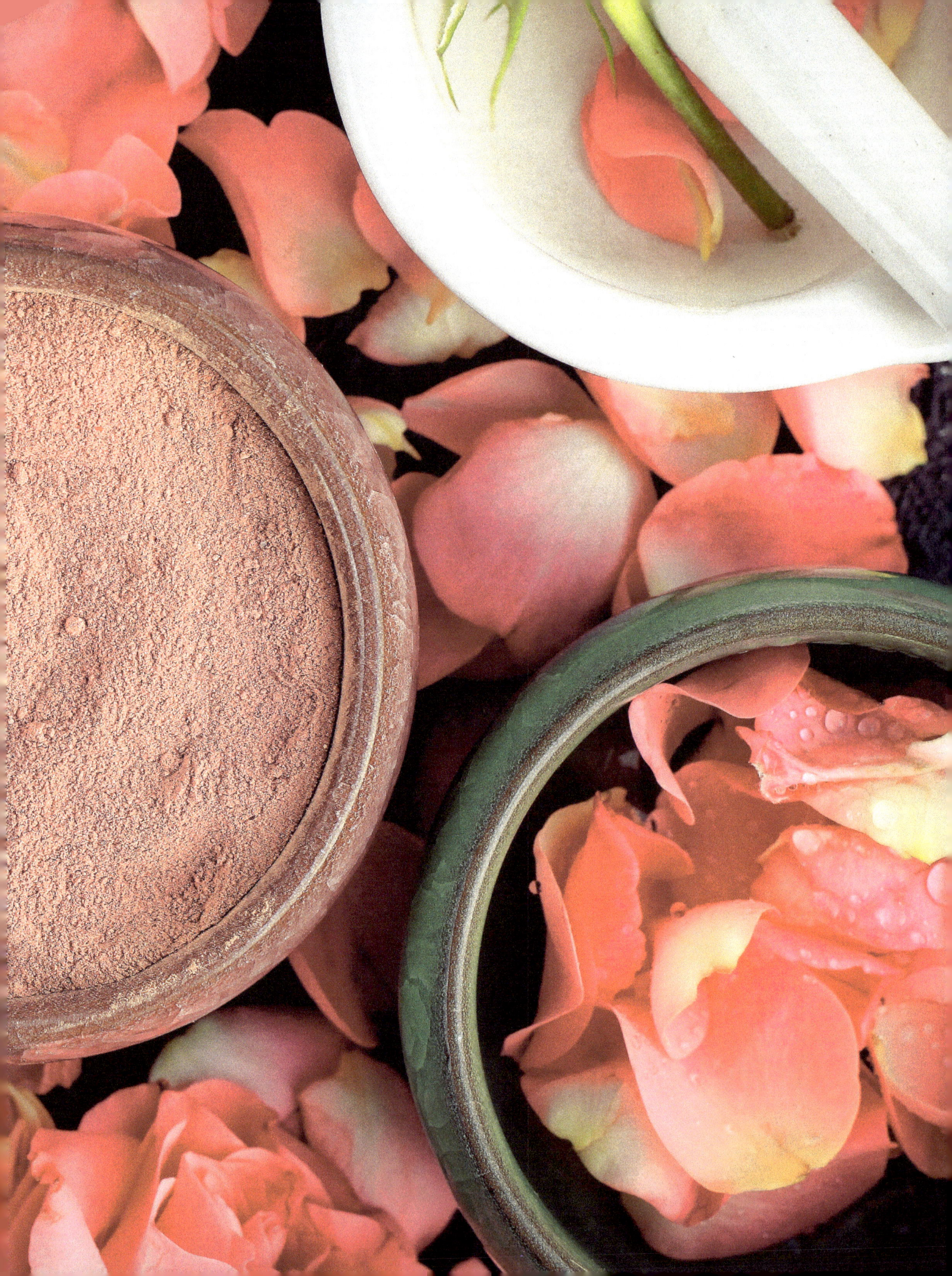

INDEX

Abortion (aids recovery) 65, 71, 388, 400, 419, 516, 524
Abrasions 7, 29, 57, 100, 128, 132, 135, 136, 139, 149, 155, 162, 248, 293, 298, 304, 327, 330, 349, 380, 382, 409, 410, 417, 436, 450, 463, 481, 483, 530, 536, 546, 551, 581
Abscess 32, 48, 51, 56, 88, 89, 100, 132, 142, 148, 154, 155, 156, 166, 176, 178, 186, 189, 217, 229, 235, 279, 284, 327, 339, 340, 352, 410, 417, 437, 477, 499, 512, 536, 547, 620, 621, 622, 627, 652
Acetum extracts (vinegar extracts) 37, 58, 72, 79, 90, 95, 123, 128, 139, 179, 214, 225, 230, 274, 300, 304, 315, 322, 340, 344, 360, 372, 376, 386, 445, 451, 489, 500, 503, 507, 541, **568-571,** 569, 599, 600
Achillea millefolium (see yarrow)
Acid indigestion 3, 21, 43, 131, 149, 217, 326, 593
Acne 27, 36, 55-57, 89, 90, 100, 111, 132, 155, 172, 178, 229, 251, 288, 290, 299, 358, 410, 422, 438, 445, 450, 489, 497, 516, 517, 536, 538, 540, 547, 595-598, 621, 622, 627
Acorus calamus (see calamus)
Actaea racemosa (see black cohosh)
Adaptogens 28, 30, 39, 42, 46, 145, 157, 182, 200-202, 242, 244, 307, 310, 363, 431, 458, 465, 491-493, 585, 586, 590, 603, 618, 619, 627
Adrenals (also see adaptogens) 47, 157, 201, 308, 310, 363, 493
Adrenergic 85, 307, 343, 363, 655
Aesculus hippocastanum (see horse chestnut)
Agropyron repens (see couch grass)
Albizia *(Albizia julibrissin*, he huan hua*)* 601, 674
Alchemilla vulgaris (see lady's mantle)
Alcohol-based extracts (also see tinctures) 561-564
Alcohol intermediary oil method 579
Aldosterone-like 307, 308, 311
Alfalfa *(Medicago sativa)* **1-3,** 89, 212, 358, 383, 420, 422, 516, 558, 594, 604, 611, 627-629, 631, 632, 634-636, 638, 639, 641, 644, 648, 649, 674, 68
Alkaloids 2, 39, 42, 45, 53, 55-57, 60, 70, 74-76, 78, 82, 90, 102, 103, 106, 121, 145, 148, 150, 151, 153, 161, 187, 196, 207-209, 216, 228, 229, 256, 259, 273, 274, 276, 279, 282, 302, 314, 318, 342, 387, 388, 391, 392, 395-397, 413, 426, 431, 450, 469, 470, 483, 511, 516, 524, 534, 535, 543, 565, 568, 593, 598, 600, 649, 655-657, 660
Allergic reaction 11, 24, 135, 208, 213, 239, 257, 340, 427, 434, 466, 531, 627
Allergic rhinitis 39, 51, 208, 356, 432, 491, 547, 614, 615
Allergies 10, 11, 28, 29, 39, 40, 51, 67, 71, 72, 79, 109, 111, 128, 129, 167, 178, 188, 193, 208, 225, 239, 240, 248, 257, 259, 273, 304, 308, 330, 339, 340, 349, 356, 358, 369, 380, 384, 417, 420, 423, 426, 427, 432, 439, 458, 491, 493, 497, 520, 531, 535, 540, 547, 550, 569, 580, 586, 588, 614, 627, 628, 655, 656
Allium sativum (see garlic)
Allspice *(Pimenta dioica)* 135, 492, 570, 585-587, 592, 608, 631-633, 635, 640, 676, 681
Aloe *(Aloe vera, A. ferox)* **4-8,** 306, 339, 351, 621, 627, 631, 634-637, 639, 640, 642-644, 646, 648, 649, 651, 652, 654, 671
Alteratives 2, 14, 27, 28, 50, 55, 57, 61, 81, 89, 138, 176, 182, 186, 187, 192, 197, 250, 287, 288, 310, 355, 356, 412, 413, 422, 425, 426, 538-540, 610, 611, 628, 649, 655
Althaea officinalis (see marshmallow)
Altitude sickness 238, 379, 433
Alzheimer's disease 107, 239, 250, 413, 433, 443, 492, 499
Ambrosia *(Ambrosia* spp.*)* **9-11,** 51, 248, 550, 558, 614, 615, 628, 637, 650, 671, 682, 687, 689
Amenorrhea (absent menstruation) 13, 15, 39, 43, 60, 61, 126, 134, 172, 173, 181, 182, 203, 232, 234, 244, 247, 269, 288, 332, 342, 351, 362, 387, 400, 405, 516, 606, 628, 639
Amur cork tree (see phellodendron)
Anabolic 39, 201, 453, 454, 535, 628
Anabolism 655
Analgesics 32, 39, 56, 61, 63, 75, 81, 102, 103, 106-108, 121-123, 125, 128, 166, 181, 183, 196, 219, 239, 250, 254, 268, 276, 277, 279, 280, 282-285, 293, 314, 315, 338, 357, 390-392, 399, 405, 406, 433, 469, 470, 473, 477, 498, 506, 512, 515, 523, 524, 530, 536, 547, 599, 600, 603, 622, 655
Anaphrodisiacs 284, 515, 529, 656
Anemia 2, 71, 105, 146, 157, 158, 181, 194, 217, 228, 290, 357, 358, 383, 420, 538, 539, 629, 634
Anemone *(Anemone pulsatilla, A.* spp.*)* 12-15, 391, 392, 627, 628, 630, 632, 639, 646, 648, 651, 681, 683, 686, 687, 689
Anemopsis californica (see yerba mansa)
Anesthetics 105, 135, 141-143, 166, 188, 282, 284, 285, 337-339, 413, 416, 475-477, 571, 617, 629, 655, 658
Angelica *(Angelica archangelica)* **16-21,** 197, 212, 280, 302, 344, 379, 559, 574, 628, 632-641, 643-645, 648-650, 653, 654, 670, 681
Angelica sinensis (see dong quai)
Angina (Angina pectoris) 20, 47, 60, 183, 262-264, 314, 433, 629
Anise *(Pimpinella anisum)* 20, **22-25,** 28-30, 55, 114, 117, 118, 131, 150, 197, 208, 212, 214, 217, 257, 303, 309, 326, 336, 379, 416, 423, 497, 510, 517, 559, 567, 586, 590-598, 612-614, 616, 632, 633, 635, 637, 640-644, 647, 651, 654, 656, 658, 671, 681
Anthelmintics 42, 75, 197, 198, 222-224, 233, 267, 287, 374, 375, 448, 486-488, 629, 631, 655
Antiandrogenics 311, 453
Antibacterials 6, 20, 28, 32, 57, 86, 89, 109, 115, 122, 128, 131, 141, 142, 153, 155, 158, 164, 173, 183, 188, 197, 211-213, 224, 235, 264, 267, 269, 285, 303, 309, 318, 321, 327, 338, 339, 351, 357, 358, 369, 375, 410, 416, 417, 432, 437, 439, 444, 449, 450, 486, 492, 497, 499, 502, 506, 535, 540, 546, 547, 551, 569, 581, 592, 593, 609, 610, 612, 614-617, 629, 646, 647, 655
Antibilious 62, 178, 431, 655

Anticarcinogenics 42, 62, 178, 288, 307, 431, 497, 498, 655
Anticatarrhals 13, 176, 248, 351, 356, 655
Anticholinergics 655
Antidepressants 28, 61, 103, 106–108, 128, 172, 173, 202, 209, 238, 240, 251, 270, 282, 284, 285, 298, 302, 370, 371, 391, 392, 442, 458, 473, 474, 480, 481, 491, 513, 601–603, 607, 655
Antiemetics (also see morning sickness or nausea) 120, 142, 232, 233, 546, 655
Antifungals 6, 20, 32, 57, 89, 115, 141, 154, 155, 178, 188, 197, 224, 225, 235, 269, 285, 303, 309, 321, 351, 375, 416, 417, 420, 444, 448, 449, 476, 486, 497, 502, 503, 517, 546, 547, 581, 655
Antihistamines 655
Anti-inflammatories 10, 29, 32, 33, 39, 51, 56, 63, 67, 76, 81, 84, 88, 99, 100, 109, 111, 127, 128, 139, 142, 154, 162, 166, 178, 183, 189, 201, 202, 208, 212, 213, 220, 229, 234, 257, 260, 279, 288, 293, 298, 299, 304, 307, 329, 330, 339, 340, 348, 349, 356, 375, 406, 410, 422, 432, 458, 470, 477, 480, 483, 493, 497, 499, 502, 506, 524, 530, 531, 535, 536, 544, 547, 551, 581, 591–594, 597, 599, 600, 602, 604, 606–608, 612, 614, 615, 617, 618–622, 655
Antilithics 164, 254, 277, 620, 656
Antimicrobials 10, 28, 29, 32, 55, 57, 70, 79, 98, 99, 114, 115, 128, 138, 141, 153, 166, 176, 188, 212, 213, 230, 257, 260, 269, 270, 276, 285, 297, 299, 304, 309, 318, 319, 321, 326, 330, 339, 347, 349, 351, 371, 375, 376, 379, 410, 413, 416, 444, 449, 450, 476, 477, 480, 486–489, 491, 517, 547, 550, 572, 656, 657
Antimutagenics 224, 405, 458, 497, 498
Antinauseants 20, 76, 110, 114, 134, 141, 212, 232, 233, 338, 339, 368, 492
Antioxidants 37, 39, 72, 86, 121, 141, 159, 178, 189, 193, 202, 212, 223, 234, 238, 239, 257, 265, 321, 333, 362, 375, 384, 397, 428, 443, 450, 459, 476, 486, 487, 492, 493, 497, 498, 500, 529, 577, 631, 656
Antiparasitics 57, 141, 224, 232, 352, 375, 376, 465, 631
Antiphlogistics 656
Antipyretics 42, 81, 219, 220, 230, 383, 405, 476, 529, 530, 534, 656
Antiseptics 51, 54, 55, 135, 172, 193, 232, 282, 297, 299, 317, 321, 337, 338, 351, 352, 369, 383, 410, 416, 453, 485, 486, 499, 505, 529, 531, 541, 546, 653, 656
Antispasmodics 19, 20, 24, 56, 60, 63, 66, 67, 75, 94, 103, 108, 114, 120, 127, 128, 142, 166, 167, 169, 181, 183, 212, 248, 268, 269, 181, 183, 212, 248, 268, 269, 279, 280, 283, 285, 296, 298, 303, 313, 321, 337, 338, 342, 344, 375, 392, 396, 400, 405–407, 412, 449, 450, 454, 470, 473, 474, 483, 486, 497, 512, 523, 524, 590, 591, 594, 599–608, 613, 620, 656
Antispasmodic, skeletal muscles 632
Antispasmodic, smooth muscles 632
Antitussives 24, 28, 84, 95, 131, 172, 173, 197, 212, 213, 223, 235, 309, 326, 339, 349, 422, 423, 491, 520, 550, 574, 600, 612–615, 656
Antiulcer (also see ulcers) 6, 135, 145, 224, 307, 340, 491, 492
Antivirals 6, 47, 78, 79, 81, 141, 153, 154, 159, 187, 188, 193, 194, 201, 207, 223, 229, 232, 234, 289, 299, 302, 303, 307, 309, 317, 318, 321, 339, 351, 374, 375, 379, 405, 406, 416, 431, 432, 442, 444, 448–450, 465, 476, 480, 486, 487, 491, 492, 497, 569, 609, 612, 614–617, 631, 656
Anxiolytics 14, 85, 103, 107, 108, 126, 128, 282–285, 297, 302, 314, 342, 343, 371, 391, 599–604, 606, 607, 618, 656
Aperients 111, 131, 176, 307, 383, 453, 540, 656
Aphrodisiacs 24, 39, 134, 172, 173, 244, 283, 284, 370, 438, 439, 509, 532, 656
Apium graveolens (see celery seed)
Appetite 2, 36, 44, 46, 47, 55, 60, 69, 78, 81, 93–95, 110, 114, 120, 127, 146, 177, 207, 211, 212, 219, 227–229, 233, 243, 269, 298, 352, 367, 368, 370, 380, 388, 442, 443, 445, 453, 474, 482, 483, 496, 519, 588, 596
Appetite loss (see nonulcer dyspepsia)
Aquaretics 656
Aqueous 110, 135, 179, 188, 264, 303, 370, 492, 498, 656, 660
Aralia, California spikenard *(Aralia californica)* 20, **26–30,** 93, 197, 202, 208, 257, 309, 318, 379, 492, 497, 502, 550, 559, 567, 574, 602, 612, 613, 627–630, 633, 635–637, 640, 643, 649, 651, 654, 671, 681, 683–685, 688
Arbutus menziesii, madrone (see uva ursi)
Arctium lappa (see burdock)
Arctostaphylos spp. (see uva ursi)
Arnica *(Arnica montana)* **31–33,** 100, 149, 512, 578, 579, 581, 628–630, 632, 635, 643, 644, 647, 649, 651, 652, 654, 671, 685
Aromatics 24, 25, 141, 214, 229, 397, 632, 656
Arrhythmia, cardiac (irregular heartbeat) 264, 433
Arthritis (also see osteoarthritis and rheumatism) 33, 36, 39, 63, 78, 90, 93, 95, 105, 109, 111, 122, 127, 128, 132, 138, 142, 149, 169, 178, 179, 189, 200, 220, 225, 232, 234, 235, 248, 265, 279, 288, 315, 330, 337, 355, 357, 358, 372, 375, 380, 383, 406, 422, 425, 426, 439, 444, 463, 477, 480, 487, 496, 497, 499, 524, 528, 530, 536, 544, 546, 547, 581, 599, 630, 632, 649, 655
Artichoke *(Cynara scolymus)* **34–37,** 114, 212, 369, 459, 497, 558, 570, 596, 597, 607, 627, 631, 634, 636, 639, 641, 642, 645, 646, 654, 681
Ashwagandha *(Withania somnifera)* **38–40,** 61, 62, 182, 201, 203, 244, 251, 585, 586, 603, 606, 608, 618, 619, 627–630, 632, 633, 643, 644, 650, 652, 654, 681
Asian ginseng (see ginseng)
Asparagus *(Asparagus cochinchinensis, A. racemosus)* **41–44,** 182, 217, 244, 270, 516, 559, 585, 586, 588, 627, 628, 632, 637, 639, 641, 643–646, 648, 649, 671, 681, 688
Asthma 13, 15, 20, 23, 24, 27–29, 63, 65, 67, 72, 75, 95, 108, 115, 122, 129, 157–159, 161, 174, 196, 197, 205, 207, 208, 212, 220, 222, 232, 234, 237, 239, 243, 245, 256, 257, 273, 279, 282, 308, 309, 312, 314, 315, 317, 337, 346, 349, 358, 369, 383, 384, 390, 392, 405, 416, 422, 423, 425, 430, 432, 457, 458, 486, 491, 496, 497, 512, 520, 523, 524, 543, 549, 550, 574, 588, 600, 613, 614, 633, 651, 654, 671

Astragalus *(Astragalus membranaceous)* **45–48,** 145, 146, 181, 188, 202, 244, 369, 458, 559, 567, 574, 587, 588, 590, 606, 619, 627, 629, 631, 633, 634, 642, 643, 652, 674, 685, 689
Astringents 10, 25, 39, 50, 51, 55, 57, 58, 61, 65–67, 69–72, 78, 81, 85, 86, 89, 94, 98, 117, 126, 127, 134, 135, 141, 142, 149, 153, 161, 169, 170, 172, 187, 193, 197, 206–209, 216, 217, 238, 248, 254, 256, 259, 262, 263, 268, 273, 279, 291–293, 297, 298, 302–304, 311, 314, 329, 338, 347, 348, 351, 352, 356, 357, 359, 368, 369, 383, 387, 388, 397, 409, 410, 413, 419, 420, 422, 425–427, 437–439, 442–444, 448–450, 458, 562, 476, 480, 483, 486, 496, 502, 505–507, 520, 521, 529, 530, 534, 535, 538–541, 543, 544, 546, 547, 550, 556, 571, 591, 593, 600, 609, 610, 613–617, 633, 656, 659
Atherosclerosis 3, 37, 72, 121, 216, 223, 234, 239, 248, 251, 265, 274, 333, 369, 384, 439, 498, 570, 589
Athlete's foot (see antifungals)
Atractylodes, bai zhu *(Atractylodes macrocephala)* 146, 181, 588, 681
Avena fatua, wild oats (see oats)
Avena sativa, cultivated oats (see oats)
Bacopa *(Bacopa monnieri)* 250, 443, 492, 601, 646, 659, 677, 682
Bacterial vaginosis *(Gardnerella vaginalis)* 98, 188, 299, 319, 375, 377, 486, 489, 502
Bai zhu (see atractylodes)
Baikal skullcap (see skullcap, baikal)
Baldness 533
Balsam root *(Balsamorhiza sagittata)* 28, 257, 574, 609, 614, 629, 635–637, 640, 643, 650, 651, 671, 681
Baptisia tinctoria (see wild indigo)
Bay laurel *(Laurus nobilis)* 139, 443, 602, 629, 630, 650, 681
Bayberry *(Morella californica, M. cerifera,* syn. *Myrica* spp.*)* **49–52,** 208, 248, 313, 318, 352, 416, 503, 550, 565, 614, 615, 617, 627, 628, 633, 636, 637, 640, 646, 649–652, 654, 659, 681
Bee balm *(Monarda fistulosa)* 558, 573, 615, 643, 675, 681, 685
Benign prostatic hypertrophy (BPH) 138, 162, 173, 209, 276, 285, 347, 348, 356, 359, 383, 454, 506, 517, 544, 608, 633
Berberis *(Berberis aquifolium, B.* spp.*)* **53–58,** 188, 212, 334, 369, 375, 476, 497, 498, 502, 570, 579, 595, 596, 606, 610, 618, 627–631, 635, 636–646, 648–651, 653, 654, 672, 681, 686
Bile excretion (see cholagogues)
Bile production (see choleretics)
Biscuit root (see *Lomatium*)
Bitters (bitter tonics) 23, 134, 141, 228, 229, 268, 535, 570, 596, 656
Black cohosh *(Actaea racemosa)* **59–63,** 66, 75, 103, 182, 201, 276, 279, 310, 344, 391, 510, 516, 524, 603, 604, 606, 628–630, 632, 633, 637, 639, 641, 642, 645–648, 650, 653, 681
Black haw *(Viburnum prunifolium)* **64–67,** 169, 170, 280, 388, 524, 559, 565, 600, 604, 605, 630, 632, 647, 649, 650, 653, 654, 670, 681
Black walnut *(Juglans nigra)* 70, 285, 565, 597, 675, 681, 682
Blackberry *(Rubus villosus, R.* spp.*)* **68–72,** 419, 437, 559, 565, 593, 629, 631, 633, 638, 641, 661, 678, 681
Bladder infection (see urinary tract infection)
Bladder problems (also see incontinence and interstitial cystitis) 161, 237, 262, 405, 469, 479
Bladderwrack *(Fucus vesiculosus)* (also see kelp) 286–290, 637, 638, 640, 643, 651, 654, 669, 682
Bleeding (see hemostatics)
Blepharitis (eyelid inflammation) 57, 99, 128, 155, 213, 293, 384, 438
Blisters 193, 202, 256, 262, 507, 622, 634
Bloating (see aromatics and carminatives) 19, 20, 24, 36, 37, 55, 79, 93, 94, 113, 114, 122, 126, 142, 146, 174, 177, 183, 197, 212, 213, 217, 229, 233, 269, 298, 309, 339, 344, 368–370, 378, 384, 400, 406, 449, 466, 486, 492, 497, 516, 524, 540, 591, 592, 594, 596, 606
Blood cells, red (erythrocytes) 3, 7, 181, 427
Blood cells, white (leukocytes) 20, 318, 326, 351, 497
Blood root *(Sanguinaria canadensis)* 314, 579, 648, 675, 677, 681
Blood sugar 48, 55, 75, 76, 111, 202, 203, 259, 260, 298, 358, 449, 565, 595, 618, 619
Blood sugar elevating (see hyperglycemic)
Blood sugar lowering (see hypoglycemic)
Blood sugar stabilizing 48, 55, 135, 202, 203, 259, 260, 298, 358, 595, 618
Blood thinners (anticoagulants) 181, 234, 238, 330, 405, 422, 590, 634
Blood thinners 63, 123, 235, 240, 407, 466, 499, 531
Blue cohosh *(Caulophyllum thalictroides)* **73–76,** 516, 628, 632, 633, 639, 645, 648, 650, 653, 682
Blue vervain, verbena *(Verbena* spp.*)* 580, 604, 618, 679, 682
Bogbean *(Menyanthes trifoliata)* 55, **77–79,** 570, 627, 630, 632, 634, 636, 641–644, 646, 649, 682
Boils 2, 14, 27, 40, 48, 51, 54, 56, 57, 60, 69, 88, 89, 100, 128, 132, 138, 148, 154, 155, 166, 178, 181, 186, 189, 217, 229, 235, 256, 262, 280, 299, 313, 315, 327, 390, 405, 410, 426, 483, 493, 505, 538, 540, 541, 547, 598, 621–623, 634, 635
Bone marrow 47, 145, 159, 181, 431
Bones, broken 148, 149, 251, 273, 318, 358, 481, 635
Boneset *(Eupatorium perfoliatum)* **80–82,** 147, 148, 253, 339, 611, 631, 638, 643, 649, 671, 682
Borage *(Borago officinale)* 649, 651, 672, 682
Brahmi (see bacopa)
Breast cancer 139, 288, 383, 426, 439, 459
Breast lumps (also see fibrocystic breast disease) 90, 139, 499
Breast pain (mastalgia, syn. mastodynia) 61, 86, 473, 516
Breastfeeding (see also galactagogue) 162,
181, 517, 654
Breath, bad; breath freshener (halitosis) 18, 23–25, 93, 114, 141, 142, 154, 214, 225, 338, 384, 444, 448, 487, 641

Bronchitis 17, 18, 20, 23, 24, 28, 29, 57, 60, 75, 95, 103, 131, 146, 149, 158, 192, 196, 197, 207, 212, 216, 217, 223, 235, 243, 256, 273, 280, 309, 314, 317, 318, 321, 326, 337, 351, 358, 369, 375, 376, 379, 416, 423, 425, 430, 432, 445, 449, 458, 486, 488, 489, 491, 502, 505, 512, 519, 520, 533, 546, 549, 550, 569, 612, 614, 635, 637, 640

Bronchitis, chronic 24, 158, 196, 197, 237, 243, 369, 432, 549

Bronchodilators 158, 208, 613-615

Bruises 10, 20, 32, 33, 86, 88, 100, 128, 148, 149, 166, 167, 193, 198, 248, 251, 265, 267, 269, 274, 280, 287, 293, 298, 304, 315, 318, 322, 330, 347, 349, 352, 369, 375, 378, 380, 390, 399, 413-415, 417, 444, 445, 470, 477, 479, 481, 483, 487, 496, 499, 530, 533, 536, 538, 546, 547, 551, 581, 589, 623, 635, 644

Bugleweed *(Lycopus* spp.*)* **83-86,** 264, 304, 343, 363, 590, 601, 607, 618, 629, 632, 634, 636, 641, 643, 646-648, 650, 652, 653, 675, 682

Bupleurum, chai hu *(Bupleurum falcatum)* 606, 636, 642, 652, 653, 671, 682, 684, 688

Burdock *(Arctium lappa)* **87-90,** 183, 308, 319, 334, 383, 559, 568, 570, 574, 595, 596, 598, 610, 620, 627, 628, 632-636, 638, 639, 641-643, 645, 646, 648, 649, 651, 653, 654, 671, 682

Burns (sunburns, thermal burns) 7, 8, 27, 29, 69, 84, 98, 100, 128, 132, 139, 155, 186, 189, 193, 247, 251, 256, 257, 276, 280, 298, 300, 318, 327, 339, 355, 372, 405, 409, 410, 417, 422, 437, 470, 479, 481, 485, 499, 505, 519, 528, 533, 538, 541, 546, 572, 621, 635, 652

Caffeine withdrawal 443, 635

Calamus *(Acorus calamus)* 27, **91-95,** 632-634, 636, 639, 640, 645, 646, 650, 671, 682, 688

Calculi, urinary (see kidney stones)

Calendula (*Calendula officinalis)* **97-100,** 131, 139, 149, 188, 189, 213, 257, 273, 352, 375, 409, 416, 417, 476, 477, 499, 502, 558, 571, 578, 579, 581, 594, 609, 611, 621, 623, 627-631, 633-644, 646, 648, 649, 651-654, 671, 686, 687

California poppy *(Eschscholzia californica)* 56, 75, **101-103,** 108, 254, 268, 277, 315, 392, 498, 512, 524, 567, 599, 628, 632, 633, 635, 637, 644, 645, 647, 648, 650, 651, 653, 677, 682

Calmatives 126, 282, 383, 390, 391, 431, 458, 480, 510, 511, 600, 602, 656

Cancer treatment adjunct (also see chemotherapy) 110, 159, 431, 610

Candida, intestinal and vaginal *(Candida albicans)* 7, 51, 57, 79, 89, 98, 128, 135, 154, 178, 188, 224, 257, 260, 285, 289, 299, 309, 319, 321, 351, 375, 376, 438, 444, 449, 466, 476, 486, 488, 492, 497, 502, 517, 540, 547, 669

Canker sores 155, 309, 352, 416, 417, 444, 477, 487, 536

Cannabis *(Cannabis sativa)* 43, 75, **104-112,** 173, 254, 277, 363, 391, 498, 499, 512, 562, 579, 581, 607, 628-632, 640, 641, 643, 645-647, 650, 651, 671, 682, 683, 685, 686

Capsicum (see cayenne)

Carbuncles (see boils)

Cardamom *(Elettaria cardamomum)* 7, 24, 25, **113-115,** 118, 135, 149, 150, 197, 212, 214, 228, 344, 369, 492, 497, 498, 540, 567, 576, 587, 592, 594, 596-598, 629, 630, 632, 635, 636, 640, 644, 647, 656, 680, 682, 684, 688

Cardiac stimulants 314, 635

Cardioprotectives 251, 263

Cardiotonics 159, 234, 239, 262-264, 343, 601, 618

Cardiovascular disease 121

Carmelite water 18, 302

Carminatives 7, 19, 20, 24, 55, 57, 93, 94, 113, 114, 121, 122, 125-127, 134, 135, 141, 142, 154, 166, 172, 174, 212, 216, 217, 219, 223, 224, 228, 229, 232, 233, 268, 269, 296-298, 303, 321, 337-339, 369, 344, 351, 352, 367-372, 374, 375, 383, 384, 399, 400, 412, 413, 442, 443, 449, 485, 486, 489, 491-493, 496-499, 510, 511, 515, 524, 534, 540, 546, 570, 591-596, 602, 606, 635, 656

Carob pods *(Ceratonia siliqua)* **116-118,** 309, 585, 594, 595, 620, 637, 642, 658, 674

Carpal tunnel 279, 283, 480, 536

Caryophyllus (see clove)

Catabolic 455

Catabolism 656

Cataracts 437

Catarrh 13, 18, 27, 93, 153, 172, 176, 196, 248, 256, 282, 351, 356, 412, 426, 483, 485, 519, 546, 549, 655, 657

Cathartics 5, 7, 20, 24, 27, 81, 132, 194, 212, 233, 327, 657

Catnip *(Nepeta cataria)* 127, 131, 212, 337, 400, 511, 592, 602, 633, 635, 638, 644, 647, 682

Caulophyllum thalictroides (see blue cohosh)

Cayenne *(Capsicum* spp.*)* **119-123,** 313, 314, 412, 443, 568, 571, 573, 589, 590, 600, 623, 627-629, 631, 634, 636-638, 647, 650, 654, 657, 679, 682, 686

Ceanothus spp. (see red root)

Cedar *(Thuja* spp.*)* 579, 629, 631, 642, 654, 669, 670, 681, 684

Celandine *(Cheladonium majus)* 212, 498, 636, 642, 654, 682

Celery seed *(Apium graveolens)* 16, 380, 638, 639, 641, 645, 648, 681

Centella asiatica (see gotu kola)

Central nervous system 14, 103, 106, 108, 110, 126, 128, 145, 207, 208, 251, 268, 283, 297, 315, 458, 459, 473, 512

Ceratonia siliqua (see carob pods)

Cerebral insufficiency 239

Cereus, night blooming *(Cereus gregii)* 343, 629, 632, 643, 647, 648, 672, 682, 686, 687

Cervical dysplasia (also see human papilloma virus) 159, 330, 488, 544

Chai hu (see bupleurum)

Chamomile *(Matricaria recutita, Anthemis nobilis)* 81, 99, 100, 109, **124-129,** 131, 149, 166, 189, 193, 212, 213, 218, 279, 298, 302, 309, 329, 330, 344, 349, 409, 410, 416, 512, 530, 560, 567, 571, 578, 581, 591-594, 599, 602, 612, 620, 621-623, 627-630, 632, 633, 635, 637-640, 642, 644-654, 671, 672, 687

Chaparral *(Larrea tridentata)* 352, 403, 424, 468, 577, 579, 627, 629, 630, 634, 648, 682
Chaparro amargosa *(Castela emoryi)* 57, 559, 629, 631, 679, 682
Chaste tree berry (see vitex)
Cheladonium majus (see celandine)
Chemotherapy (enhances recovery, mitigates side effects; also see antinauseant) 39, 47, 110, 127, 132, 159, 202, 217, 243, 327, 432, 465
Chest pains 84, 283, 306, 405, 491, 496, 543
Chickweed *(Stellaria media)* 99, 100, **130-132,** 138, 139, 357, 410, 578, 593, 610, 618, 627, 628, 633-635, 638-642, 644-654, 682
Chicory *(Cichorium intybus)* 89, 148, 559, 634, 648, 683
Chlorophyll 2, 225, 384, 627, 634, 641, 648
Cholagogues (excretes bile) 19, 20, 24, 36, 37, 55, 56, 78, 79, 81, 89, 94, 114, 141, 153, 154, 172, 174, 176, 177, 181, 182, 197, 211, 212, 219, 229, 232-234, 259, 297, 298, 309, 313, 332, 334, 338, 339, 344, 368, 369, 383, 384, 413, 442, 443, 497, 498, 523-525, 534, 535, 539, 540, 570, 595-598, 636, 656, 657
Cholangitis (bile duct inflammation) 595-598
Cholecystitis (gallbladder inflammation) 55, 56, 154, 197, 229, 469, 498, 595-598
Choleretics (produces bile) 5, 7, 19, 36, 37, 55, 56, 78, 81, 89, 98, 153, 154, 177, 197, 219, 229, 232, 234, 297, 298, 307, 309, 332, 334, 338, 339, 374-376, 413, 442-444, 449, 486, 497, 498, 535, 595-598, 636, 657
Cholestasis (bile stagnation) 37, 50, 56, 177, 229, 334, 596, 597
Cholethiasis (gallstones, nonobstructive) 37, 56, 154, 229, 596-598
Cholinergics 121, 459, 655, 657, 659
Chronic bronchitis (see bronchitis, chronic)
Chronic fatigue syndrome 146, 158, 201, 279, 330, 422, 466, 586, 588
Chrysanthemum (ju hua) *(Chrysanthemum morifolium)* 639, 640, 645, 646, 648, 650, 651, 652, 654
Chuan xiong *(Ligusticum striatum,* syn. *L. wallichii)* 181, 182, 405, 559, 606, 628, 634, 683
Cimicifuga racemosa (see black cohosh)
Cinnamon *(Cinnamomum zeylanicum)* 24, 66, 70, 86, 114, **133-136,** 149, 170, 208, 238, 260, 357, 375, 388, 410, 420, 425, 443, 446, 462, 463, 476, 486, 497, 536, 550, 567, 570, 575, 576, 587, 589, 593, 600, 614-617, 623, 627-629, 631-638, 640, 642, 644, 651, 653, 654, 658, 683
Circulatory problems 234, 265
Circulatory stimulants 19, 20, 32, 51, 94, 115, 121, 122, 134, 135, 141, 142, 172, 173, 181, 183, 223, 232, 234, 238, 250, 251, 263, 368, 380, 413, 442, 443, 486, 524, 569, 570, 589, 590, 601, 602, 618, 619, 636, 657
Cirrhosis 56, 229, 333, 459, 595-598
Citrus x *sinensis, C.* spp. (see orange)
Cleansing 2, 5, 42, 89, 419, 610, 611, 658
Cleavers *(Galium aparine)* 89, **137-139,** 248, 330, 355, 357, 422, 426, 578, 610, 611, 619, 628, 638, 639, 641, 645, 646, 649, 651, 653, 654, 683
Clove *(Syzigium aromaticum)* 66, 114, **140-143,** 166, 296, 302, 524, 559, 570, 576, 627, 632, 636, 637, 683
Codonopsis *(Codonopsis pilosula)* 47, **144-146,** 188, 202, 244, 369, 458, 559, 587-590, 606, 627, 629, 633, 634, 643, 672, 681-683, 688
Coffee *(Coffea arabica)* 176, 627, 629, 635, 652, 678, 683
Coffee substitutes 42, 89, 90, 114, 148, 216
Cognitive function (see nootropics)
Cold sores (see herpes)
Colds 14, 17, 18, 20, 27, 46, 60, 88, 125, 131, 134, 141, 145, 159, 186, 200, 219, 250, 282, 299, 302, 314, 317, 337, 339, 367, 368, 405, 413, 445, 469, 472, 491, 502, 510, 515, 519, 528, 533, 535, 543, 549, 636
Colic 18, 23, 24, 36, 74, 93, 114, 125-127, 129, 172, 196, 211, 212, 219, 225, 232, 298, 303, 320, 321, 337, 339, 371, 372, 375, 382, 413, 442, 485, 496, 522, 523, 534, 546, 591, 592, 594, 600, 656, 683
Colitis (also see ulcerative colitis) 6, 43, 67, 71, 79, 94, 99, 103, 108, 117, 127, 131, 149, 212, 217, 269, 274, 289, 298, 309, 326, 329, 339, 357, 406, 463, 469, 483, 497, 523, 535, 540, 544, 591-594
Collagen 100, 189, 251, 263, 265, 333, 493
Collinsonia canadensis (see stone root)
Coltsfoot, eastern *(Tussilago farfara);* Coltsfoot, western *(Petasites palmatus)* 131, 309, 339, 349, 423, 612, 613, 640, 649, 651, 688
Comfrey *(Symphytum officinale)* 82, 100, 109, **147-151,** 410, 558, 578, 579, 581, 593, 594, 633-635, 636-642, 644, 645, 649, 651, 652, 654, 683
Commiphora myrrha (see myrrh)
Common colds (see colds)
Conjunctivitis (pink eye) 55, 57, 60, 71, 98, 99, 128, 129, 154, 155, 213, 293, 384, 420, 426, 438, 496, 637, 640
Connective tissue 7, 48, 71, 99, 149, 162, 189, 251, 263, 265, 273, 358, 369, 439, 618, 619
Constipation 5, 8, 10, 36, 43, 44, 55, 56, 78, 79, 93, 94, 111, 117, 120, 125, 131, 132, 149, 172, 174, 176, 177, 183, 194, 212, 217, 228, 229, 259, 282, 289, 314, 326, 327, 369, 405, 412, 413, 469, 496, 505, 507, 510, 515, 531, 538, 540, 594-596, 598, 637
Contraceptives 42, 311, 481, 543
Coptis, goldthread *(Coptis chinensis)* 57, 99, **152-155,** 559, 598, 629, 630, 631, 633-643, 645, 646, 651, 653, 677, 683, 684, 685, 689
Cordyceps *(Cordyceps sinensis)* **156-159,** 202, 627, 629, 631, 633, 635, 640-643
Corn silk *(Zea mays)* **160-162,** 164, 188, 212, 273, 276, 348, 358, 502, 506, 535, 619, 620, 634, 638, 639, 644, 645, 649, 653
Coronary heart disease (also see heart disease) 183
Cortisol 158, 307, 308, 492, 493, 525
Cotton root *(Gossypium)* 29, 65, 173, 628, 632, 639, 643, 653, 683
Couch grass *(Agropyron repens)* 138, **163-164,** 212, 248, 463, 638, 639, 645
Cough drops 311, 327, 338, 487, 513, 519
Cough, whooping (see whooping cough)

Coughs 17, 18, 27, 60, 88, 93, 115, 131, 145, 161, 181, 193, 196, 237, 306, 325, 326, 337, 342, 346, 367, 395, 399, 405, 413, 422, 425, 479, 491, 510, 519, 533, 546, 549, 637, 640

Counterirritants 10, 32, 33, 60, 95, 121-123, 135, 141, 142, 166, 167, 198, 225, 232, 233, 235, 248, 297, 299, 314, 321, 338, 355, 358, 375, 380, 413, 414, 417, 443, 444, 462, 463, 477, 485-487, 547, 551, 600, 637, 647, 657, 659

Cow parsnip *(Heracleum lanatum)* 142, **165-167,** 339, 417, 567, 622, 627, 629, 639, 644, 647, 648, 650, 652, 653, 671, 683

Cramp bark *(Viburnum opulus)* 66, 67, **168-170,** 280, 524, 630, 632, 645, 647, 650, 653

Cramps (see antispasmodics)

Crataegus laevigata (see hawthorn)

Crohn's disease 43, 67, 71, 94, 108, 111, 127, 131, 146, 149, 212, 217, 269, 289, 298, 326, 329, 339, 406, 463, 469, 483, 492, 523, 570, 591-594

Curcuma longa (see turmeric)

Cuts 7, 17, 27, 29, 32, 57, 86, 100, 128, 135, 136, 139, 148, 149, 155, 162, 248, 274, 293, 298, 304, 317, 318, 330, 352, 378, 380, 395, 405, 410, 417, 419, 450, 463, 470, 479, 481, 483, 505, 510, 521, 528, 530, 536, 538, 541, 551, 581

Cymbopogon citratus (see lemon grass)

Cynara scolymus (see artichoke)

Cystitis 75, 105, 108, 131, 161, 170, 173, 188, 248, 254, 256, 273, 276, 282, 285, 325, 327, 330, 347, 348, 358, 376, 383, 388, 454, 463, 486, 502, 506, 524, 535, 544, 547, 620, 645

Damiana *(Turnera diffusa)* 24, 29, 108, **171-174,** 251, 349, 492, 607, 612, 628, 630, 632, 639, 643-645, 648, 651, 653, 677, 683

Dandelion *(Taraxacum officinale)* 66, 89, 90, 118, 138, 148, **175-179,** 182, 183, 212, 248, 268, 273, 308, 319, 334, 335, 357, 383, 459, 463, 483, 498, 535, 538, 567, 570, 574, 589-591, 594-598, 604, 606, 607, 610, 618, 620, 627, 628, 631-634, 636, 638, 639, 641-643, 645, 646, 648, 649, 651, 653, 672, 683

Dandelion leaf *(Taraxacum officinale)* 89, 90, 177-179, 212, 248, 357, 463, 535, 590, 638, 639, 643

Dandelion root *(Taraxacum officinale)* 89, 118, 176-178, 182, 183, 308, 319, 383, 483, 498, 589, 591, 594, 595, 598, 604, 606, 607, 610, 620, 627, 628, 632, 633, 642, 645, 646, 651, 653

Dandruff 7, 10, 55, 56, 89, 93, 132, 290, 327, 358, 385, 425, 442, 444, 450, 505, 571, 637, 638

Dementia (global dementia) 239, 250, 413, 444, 492

Demulcents 5, 6, 28, 42-44, 89, 94, 98, 99, 106, 111, 117, 118, 126-128, 131, 134, 135, 149, 161, 162, 164, 193, 216, 217, 250, 277, 288, 289, 306, 307, 309, 325, 326, 329, 349, 379, 387, 388, 409, 437, 439, 506, 535, 588, 593-595, 609, 610, 612-617, 620, 638, 645, 657, 659

Dental 18, 32, 141, 142, 260, 279, 284, 337, 339, 352, 415, 417, 476, 536, 538

Depressants (CNS or neural) 93, 268, 280, 298, 392, 459, 657

Depression (see antidepressant)

Depuratives 36, 90, 131, 138, 186, 538, 596, 598, 610, 611, 657

Dermatitis, alleviates 7, 89, 90, 100, 128, 139, 162, 178, 189, 217, 229, 298, 308, 384, 410, 422, 432, 524, 536, 581, 595-598, 611

Dermatitis, contact/allergic 24, 25, 29, 33, 37, 76, 82, 90, 123, 129, 166, 167, 179, 189, 198, 220, 225, 235, 240, 251, 254, 268, 270, 299, 304, 340, 344, 354, 358, 359, 372, 385, 401, 417, 466, 536

Dermatitis, photo 166, 167, 481, 659

Detoxification 36, 56, 178, 203, 334, 422, 497

Diabetes 118, 244, 259, 260, 262, 352, 384, 458, 492, 595

Diabetes, gestational 76, 463

Diaphoretics 10, 14, 17-20, 27, 28, 32, 60, 65, 75, 81, 82, 89, 98, 114, 121, 122, 125-127, 135, 141, 191-193, 197, 207, 220, 223, 232, 234, 247, 302, 303, 313, 314, 317, 318, 321, 329, 330, 337-339, 342, 374, 375, 379, 384, 399, 400, 412, 413, 442, 444, 448, 449, 486, 491, 496, 515, 529, 530, 534, 535, 569, 573, 592, 612-614, 638, 657

Diarrhea 8, 18, 44, 47, 50, 51, 55, 57, 65-67, 69, 70, 72, 79, 82, 84, 94, 114, 117, 118, 120, 123, 125, 127, 131, 134, 135, 142, 146, 148, 149, 153-155, 170, 183, 194, 198, 207, 208, 212, 217, 223, 227, 229, 230, 232, 233, 240, 243, 248, 267, 293, 306, 309, 321, 325, 326, 329, 337, 339, 351, 352, 355, 357, 367, 369, 375, 387, 405-407, 409, 412, 413, 416, 419, 420, 425, 427, 436, 437, 438, 449, 462, 466, 469, 479, 486, 496, 505, 507, 512, 517, 519, 523, 530, 533, 535, 538, 541, 546, 588, 593, 638

Digestion 3, 13, 19, 25, 36, 37, 55, 56, 58, 89, 94, 95, 122, 146, 154, 174, 181, 196, 197, 211, 214, 217, 229, 232, 233, 309, 321, 337, 340, 351, 368, 370, 375, 388, 413, 443-445, 454, 474, 483, 486, 497, 539, 540, 549, 588, 593, 596, 656, 659

Digestive bitters (see bitters, bitter tonics)

Dioscorea batatas (see shan yao)

Dioscorea villosa (see wild yam)

Diuretics 2, 13, 20, 24, 27, 28, 36, 37, 39, 44, 46, 60, 85, 89, 90, 131, 138, 161, 162, 164, 173, 176, 178, 179, 192, 193, 198, 207, 212, 248, 250, 254, 262, 267, 273, 274, 276, 311, 313, 314, 327, 330, 347, 348, 357, 359, 383, 388, 395, 405, 409, 412, 439, 445, 454, 463, 505, 506, 535, 547, 589, 590, 608, 619, 620, 656, 657

Diverticulitis, diverticulosis 309, 416, 523, 535, 540

Dizziness, alleviates 43, 146, 158, 181, 242, 283, 308, 406, 432, 496, 516, 549, 587, 590, 639

Dizziness, high doses can exacerbate 15, 58, 63, 170, 240, 251, 264, 265, 280, 315, 434

Dong quai *(Angelica sinensis)* 43, 47, 61, 62, 75, **180-183,** 201, 244, 405, 516, 602, 603, 605, 628, 629, 633, 634, 636, 639, 642, 643, 646-648, 653, 669, 683

Douche (also see vaginal irrigation) 560, 656

Dropsy 27, 36, 42, 69, 78, 125, 192, 196, 254, 262, 267, 301, 374, 382, 387, 412, 442, 483, 505

Drowsiness 105, 397

Duodenal ulcers (see ulcers)

Dysentery 43, 50, 54, 65, 69, 70, 93, 120, 131, 135, 148, 153, 154, 208, 222, 224, 232, 233, 250, 325, 326, 337, 355, 399, 406, 409, 412, 420, 436, 438, 439, 462, 469, 479, 482, 497, 505, 523, 534, 535, 538, 546, 547

Dysmenorrhea (painful menstruation) 39, 43, 60, 61, 66, 74, 75, 125, 126, 172, 181, 183, 217, 232, 247, 254, 279, 332, 342, 362, 387, 400, 405, 419, 438, 453, 545, 516, 523, 524
Dyspepsia (see nonulcer dyspepsia)
Dyspnea (shortness of breath) 47, 84, 145, 264, 314, 433, 588, 613-615
Dysuria (painful urination) 105, 108, 138, 282, 348, 454, 505, 608, 620
E. coli (also see *Escherichia coli*) 89, 213, 260, 289, 492, 506, 540
Earaches and ear infections *(Otitis media)* 2, 13, 127, 128, 224, 267, 337, 390, 622
Ears, ringing (see tinnitus)
Echinacea *(Echinacea purpurea)* 81, 89, 99, 100, 139, 142, 145, **185-189,** 309, 318, 349, 352, 379, 416, 426, 476, 477, 502, 559, 567, 573, 574, 576, 579, 609, 610, 616, 617, 621, 622, 627-631, 633-636, 639, 641-644, 646, 649-654, 671, 681, 683, 688
Eczema 2, 7, 33, 36, 44, 55-57, 79, 89, 90, 100, 111, 128, 132, 138, 139, 153, 155, 162, 172, 178, 186, 189, 192, 193, 217, 229, 251, 256, 290, 298, 308, 314, 325, 327, 347, 358, 384, 406, 410, 422, 425, 432, 438, 439, 485, 496, 497, 516, 524, 531, 536, 538, 540, 547, 581, 595-598, 611, 639
Edema 10, 24, 44, 89, 98, 138, 139, 162, 164, 172, 178, 192, 193, 198, 207, 212, 214, 238, 248, 251, 254, 264, 273, 274, 277, 308, 311, 357, 359, 383, 385, 425, 454, 543, 585-588, 592-599, 603, 604, 607-609, 612-617, 619, 620
Elder berry *(Sambucus nigra)* 30, 81, **190-194,** 318, 379, 416, 476, 576, 609, 610, 629, 631, 636, 640, 642, 643, 646
Elder flower *(Sambucus nigra)* 81, 127, 192-194, 330, 339, 400, 530, 558, 612, 628, 631, 636, 637, 639, 640, 651
Elecampane *(Inula helenium)* 20, 29, 131, **195-198,** 209, 257, 497, 567, 612, 613, 615, 628, 629, 632, 635-638, 640, 643, 644, 649, 654, 684
Electuaries 436, 657
Elephant's head (see *Pedicularis*)
Elettaria cardamomum (see cardamom)
Eleuthero *(Eleutherococcus senticosis)* 182, **199-203,** 251, 310, 559, 585, 586, 590, 602, 606, 608, 618, 619, 627, 628, 590, 602, 606, 608, 618, 619, 627, 628, 630, 631, 635, 642-644, 646, 652, 671, 681, 683, 684, 688
Eliminatives 657
Elixirs 249, 302, 367, 430, 657
Emesis 84, 315
Emetics 63, 81, 95, 120, 142, 223, 312-314, 346, 655, 657
Emmenagogues 5, 15, 19, 61, 74-76, 90, 95, 100, 172, 173, 181, 219, 220, 342, 343, 351, 379, 383, 399-401, 407, 485, 515, 534, 536, 628, 655, 657
Emollients 6, 28, 98, 99, 106, 131, 149, 161, 162, 194, 216, 217, 289, 290, 308, 319, 326, 349, 362, 409, 410, 437, 525, 640, 657
Emphysema 28, 29, 158, 197, 256, 257, 286
Endometriosis 21, 60, 66, 75, 108, 169, 254, 293, 387, 405, 438, 459, 470, 497, 516, 524, 544, 607
Endurance 46, 93, 145, 157, 200, 201, 243, 548
Enteritis, gastroenteritis (also see diarrhea) 50, 69, 71, 108, 117, 142, 293, 438, 476, 482, 489, 535, 594
Enuresis (nighttime bed wetting) 158, 273, 282, 348, 358
Ephedra *(Ephedra sinica, E.* spp.*)* **205-209,** 550, 558, 565, 614, 627, 628, 633, 635, 640, 650, 652, 654, 670, 682, 683, 686, 689
Equisetum arvense (see horsetail)
Erectile dysfunction (also see aphrodisiac, impotence, and libido) 244
Erection (also see aphrodisiac and libido) 239
Eriodictyon spp. (see yerba santa)
Erythrocytes (see blood cells, red)
Escherichia coli (also see *E. coli*) 135, 188, 224, 235, 264, 330, 351, 376, 476, 506, 517
Eschscholzia californica (see California poppy)
Eucalyptus *(Eucalyptus globulus)* 423, 444, 486, 558, 613, 615, 616, 630, 638, 640, 643, 644, 650, 676, 682, 689
Eupatorium perfoliatum (see boneset)
Eupatorium purpureum (see gravel root)
Expectorants 20, 24, 27, 28, 30, 95, 135, 149, 158, 173, 193, 196, 197, 212, 213, 223, 232, 235, 256, 257, 299, 313, 314, 318, 321, 339, 346, 349, 351, 369, 375, 379, 383, 395, 400, 409, 413, 416, 423, 436, 444, 491, 535, 547, 549, 550, 569, 572-574, 588, 600, 612-616, 658
Eye, disorders 640
Eyesight (also see vision) 437, 458
Eye washes 55, 58, 71, 72, 99, 154, 169, 194, 214, 293, 330, 420, 437, 438, 440, 640
Face, swelling 640
Fainting 58, 228, 296, 339, 342
Faintness 640
Fatigue (also see chronic fatigue syndrome) 3, 39, 46, 47, 95, 145, 146, 157, 158, 188, 200, 201, 203, 242-245, 264, 279, 282, 285, 288, 289, 309, 330, 339, 358, 406, 422, 430, 431, 443, 445, 466, 467, 492, 586, 588, 590, 602, 618, 619, 664
Fatty liver (see liver, fatty)
Febrifuges 81, 93, 219, 220, 232, 292, 491, 528, 658
Fennel *(Foeniculum vulgare)* 7, 23-25, 54, 55, 57, 89, 110, 114, 117, 118, 149, 154, 197, **210-214,** 217, 277, 303, 306, 309, 329, 344, 369, 383, 409, 448, 497, 498, 517, 524, 540, 558, 567, 570, 586, 591-598, 606, 631, 632, 636, 640, 641, 644, 647, 656, 658, 671, 684
Fenugreek *(Trigonella foenum-graecum)* 24, 66, 212, **215-217,** 260, 593, 595, 616, 627, 629, 635, 636, 638, 640, 642-645, 649, 651, 652, 654, 675, 684
Feverfew *(Tanacetum parthenium)* **218-220,** 240, 279, 330, 599, 600, 628, 630, 632, 634, 636, 638, 639, 646, 684
Fevers (also see diaphoretic and sudorific) 20, 31, 43, 50, 74, 80, 81, 127, 190, 193, 207, 208, 223, 234, 303, 325, 330, 339, 379, 485, 528, 530, 534, 536, 612
Fibrocystic breast disease 288, 426, 516
Fibroids, uterine 21, 62, 66, 75, 135, 169, 293, 387, 405, 419, 438, 462, 470, 497, 516, 535, 544
Figwort *(Scrophularia* spp.*)* 89, 109, 139, 512, 558, 578, 581, 610, 611, 628, 630, 632, 635, 645, 646, 651, 652, 679, 684

Filipendula ulmaria (see meadowsweet)
Fire cider 122, 568, 569, 637
Flatulence 36, 114, 115, 120, 122, 125-127, 135, 166, 177, 197, 222, 225, 232, 267, 289, 296, 298, 303, 321, 375, 412, 413, 448, 485, 496, 510, 512, 515, 570, 656
Flavonoids 23, 32, 36, 46, 55, 66, 70, 71, 72, 74, 78, 81, 84, 88, 98, 100, 106, 121, 126-128, 131, 138, 161, 164, 169, 172, 179, 193, 194, 207, 211, 216, 219, 240, 247, 248, 251, 254, 256, 257, 263-266, 274, 276, 279, 292, 297, 302, 306, 329, 339, 347, 356, 362, 368, 369, 374, 382, 383, 391, 392, 399, 409, 415, 419, 422, 426, 428, 437, 439, 442, 443, 448, 462, 473, 476, 477, 480, 491, 493, 506, 511, 515-517, 529, 536, 550, 628, 640, 653, 658
Flax seed *(Linum usitatissimum)* 636-640
Fluid retention (see diuretics)
Foeniculum (see fennel)
Fomentations 21, 67, 125, 148, 162, 209, 228, 235, 274, 300, 311, 330, 342, 344, 374, 380, 422, 423, 436, 470, 483, 493, 513, 530, 560, 658
Fouquieria splendens (see ocotillo)
Fu ling (see poria)
Fucus vesiculosus (see bladderwrack)
Fungal infections 98, 225, 352, 417, 493, 499
Fungistatics (also see antifungal) 7, 188, 257, 268, 448, 506, 655, 658
Furanocoumarins 166, 319, 380, 385
Furuncles (see boils)
Galactagogues (lactagogues) 2, 3, 24, 42, 86, 211, 212, 216, 217, 269, 356, 358, 419, 453, 455, 491, 515, 517, 641, 658
Galactagogues, anti- (weaning) 86, 383, 384, 450
Galium aparine (see cleavers)
Gallbladder 19, 23, 36, 37, 54-56, 58, 63, 154, 177-179, 211, 212, 227-230, 260, 332, 334, 339, 340, 413, 443, 469, 498, 523, 524, 538, 540, 541, 597, 657
Gallstones, nonobstructive (also see cholelithiasis) 56, 229, 513, 600
Gamma-aminobutyric acid (GABA) 46, 251, 259, 283, 511
Ganoderma lucidum (see reishi)
Gardnerella (see bacterial vaginosis)
Garlic *(Allium sativum)* 37, 57, **221-225,** 232, 327, 349, 384, 449, 467, 568-570, 573, 622, 627, 629-631, 634-643, 650, 653, 654, 670, 684
Garrya spp. (see silk tassel)
Gastric ulcers (see ulcers)
Gastritis 8, 43, 55, 71, 92, 94, 99, 117, 131, 176, 217, 232, 289, 293, 326, 329, 352, 412, 449, 469, 476, 544, 594
Gastroesophageal reflux disease (GERD) (also see acid indigestion) 117, 149, 593, 594
Genitals 128, 228, 282, 432, 458, 507, 529
Gentian *(Gentiana lutea)* 55, 66, 93, 114, 212, **226-230,** 369, 497, 498, 570, 597, 627, 634, 636, 639, 641, 642, 644-646, 649, 651, 674, 682, 684
Gentiana lutea (see gentian)
Giardia *(Giardia lamblia)* 57, 70, 154, 212, 375, 376, 416, 438, 439, 497, 535
Ginger *(Zingiber officinale)* 110, 114, 135, 154, 155, 169, 212, **231-235,** 238, 250, 318, 369, 443, 496, 497, 524, 567, 569, 573, 576, 578, 579, 588, 589, 592, 596, 606, 617, 623, 627-641, 643-650, 652-654, 657, 680, 684
Gingivitis (gum disease) 51, 99, 142, 352, 375, 414, 417, 449, 477, 487, 536, 547
Ginkgo *(Ginkgo biloba)* 108, 202, 236-240, 423, 443, 492, 558, 589, 628, 630, 631, **634-636,** 640, 641, 646, 650, 652, 654, 657, 659, 670, 686
Ginseng, Asian; white ginseng *(Panax ginseng)* 46, 145, 146, 181, 200, 201, 203, **241-245,** 251, 260, 310, 369, 559, 574, 585-586, 595, 604, 618, 627, 628, 632, 643, 644, 646, 648, 652, 671, 684, 687
Ginseng, California (see *Aralia*)
Ginseng, Indian (see ashwagandha)
Ginseng, noto; tienchi *(Panax notoginseng)* 643, 671, 686, 687, 688
Ginseng, poor man's (see codonopsis)
Ginseng, Siberian (see eleuthero)
Glaucoma 110, 209, 238, 239
Globe artichoke (see artichoke)
Glutathione 39, 333, 493, 498
Glycerin extracts 565-567
Glycyrrhiza glabra (see licorice)
Goiter 84-86, 287, 355
Goldenrod *(Solidago* spp.*)* 51, **246-248,** 550, 614, 628, 635, 639, 645, 650, 653, 654, 684
Goldenseal *(Hydrastis canadensis)* 55, 57, 99, 100, 128, 213, 384, 412, 579, 627-631, 633, 634, 636-641, 650, 652, 684
Goldthread (see coptis)
Gonorrhea 206, 282, 543
Gossypium (see cotton root)
Gotu kola *(Centella asiatica)* 95, 108, 203, 238-240, **249-252,** 273, 303, 423, 443, 492, 558, 579, 586, 589, 602, 606, 618, 619, 627, 628, 630, 631, 635, 636, 639, 640, 643, 644, 646, 649, 650, 652-654, 659, 670, 684
Gout 2, 13, 17, 18, 27, 36, 68, 69, 78, 88, 90, 105, 126, 132, 138, 148, 149, 164, 178, 179, 227, 254, 265, 282, 330, 355, 358, 383, 399, 405, 422, 442, 463, 485, 497, 528, 547, 641
Gravel root *(Eutrochium purpureum)* 164, **253-254,** 277, 348, 383, 559, 620, 638, 639, 641, 643, 645, 684
Grave's disease (see hyperthyroidism) 85, 86, 493, 641
Grifola frondosa (see maitake)
Grindelia *(Grindelia robusta)* 20, 28, 29, 164, 197, 208, **255-257,** 309, 318, 379, 416, 497, 551, 579, 612-614, 628, 631, 633, 635, 637, 640, 648, 653, 654, 671, 684, 687, 689
Guarana *(Paullinia cupana)* 209, 635, 646, 652, 678, 684
Gum abscesses 51, 186, 279, 284, 547, 652
Gum disease/inflammation (also see gingivitis) 351, 641, 648
Gum infections (see gum abscesses)
Gumweed (see *Grindelia*)
Gymnema, gurmar *(Gymnema sylvestre)* 258-260, 595, 630, 643, 671, 684
Hair loss 217
Halitosis (see breath, bad; breath freshener)

Hallucinations 111, 513
Hashimoto's thyroiditis 290, 343, 493, 618, 619
Hawthorn *(Crataegus laevigata)* 29, 86, 100, 239, **261-265,** 273, 363, 535, 559, 589, 590, 601, 628-632, 635, 636, 640, 641, 643, 647, 650, 654, 684
Hay fever (also see allergies) 158, 188, 194, 207, 256, 317, 535
He huan hua (see *Albizia julibrissin*)
Headaches (also see migraines) 13-15, 17, 18, 56, 60, 61, 63, 78, 93, 105, 108, 114, 122, 125-127, 172, 182, 186, 203, 207, 209, 219, 220, 222, 228, 230, 240, 247, 279, 282, 283, 293, 296, 297, 302, 315, 321, 325, 330, 337, 339, 342, 362, 363, 390, 392, 396, 399, 401, 405, 406, 413, 423, 426, 433, 437, 443, 473, 474, 485, 492, 510, 512, 513, 516, 528, 533, 599, 600, 602, 641
Hearing, improves 202, 224, 234, 258
Heart attack 223, 308, 433
Heart disease 47, 86, 158, 159, 183, 238, 262, 264, 543, 641
Heart disease, avoid with 58, 203, 209
Heartbeat 14, 86, 260, 264, 343
Heartburn (also see indigestion) 235, 339, 460, 641
Hedeoma pulegoides (see pennyroyal)
Helicobacter pylori (H. pyloria) 224, 416, 641
Hemorrhages 65, 84, 134, 245, 357, 388, 419, 463, 536
Hemorrhoids 5, 10, 52, 71, 149, 420, 547, 591, 593, 598, 642
Hemostatics 2, 3, 20, 66, 67, 71, 85, 86, 134-136, 149, 170, 232, 273, 274, 292, 293, 351, 352, 355-357, 388, 395, 410, 419, 426, 427, 437, 438, 450, 462, 463, 530, 534, 536, 547, 593, 600, 604, 605, 607, 658
Hepatics 36, 37, 55, 60, 85, 121, 125, 159, 176-179, 182, 216, 224, 234, 239, 244, 251, 265, 288, 298, 308, 310, 334, 352, 384, 412, 413, 493, 497, 498, 523, 591, 595-598, 618, 627, 242, 646, 658
Hepatitis 36, 56, 111, 154, 159, 176, 177, 182, 229, 230, 250, 285, 309, 310, 333, 406, 422, 426, 432, 433, 459, 466, 467, 480, 497, 540, 595-598, 642
Hepatodetoxifiers (see liver detoxifier) Hepatoprotectives 37, 48, 203, 260, 309, 334, 384, 432, 466, 497, 658
Hepatoregeneratives 159, 333, 458, 658
Heracleum lanatum (see cow parsnip)
Herbal honey and syrup 572-576
Herpes 6, 98, 109, 141, 154, 186, 201, 202, 223, 289, 303, 309, 321, 339, 344, 417, 450, 474, 480, 642
Herpes simplex (cold sores, genital herpes) 6, 109, 141, 154, 201, 202, 223, 289, 303, 309, 321, 339, 417, 450
Herpes zoster (also see shingles) 98, 309, 417
Hibiscus *(Hibiscus sabdariffa)* 439, 558, 638, 644, 650
High blood pressure (see hypertension)
High density lipids (HDLs) 3, 121, 159, 216, 569
High triglycerides, lowers 223, 260, 333, 498, 589
HIV (human immunodeficiency virus) 6, 37, 158, 178, 201, 245, 289, 308, 309, 318, 432, 466, 467, 480
Hives 319, 598
Hoarseness 81, 483, 642
Honey, herb-infused (see herbal honey)
Hops *(Humulus lupulus)* 17, 50, 103, 126, **266-270,** 302, 392, 474, 512, 567, 599, 629, 630, 632, 634-636, 647, 650, 653, 685
Hormone balancing agents 181, 201, 244, 515-517, 606, 607
Horse chestnut *(Aesculus hippocastanum)* 483, 591, 675, 685
Horseradish *(Armoracia spp.)* 568, 569, 574, 627, 631, 636-638, 643, 650, 654, 672, 685
Horsetail *(Equisetum arvense)* 138, 161, 206, **271-274,** 276, 287, 348, 358, 385, 444, 450, 558, 571, 579, 590, 619, 634, 635, 639, 640, 644, 645, 648, 649, 652, 669, 685
Hot flashes (alleviates) 6, 43, 62, 131, 182, 183, 283, 327, 343, 406, 439, 449, 458, 516, 603, 604, 642, 646
Hot flashes (exacerbates) 21, 48, 123, 135, 146, 235, 245, 380, 414, 499, 513
Huang bai (see phellodendron)
Huang lian (see coptis)
Huang qin (see skullcap, baikal)
Human immunodeficiency virus (see HIV)
Human papilloma virus (HPV; cervical dysplasia) 98, 159, 330, 432, 488, 544
Humulus lupulus (see hops)
Hydrangea *(Hydrangea arborscens)* 164, 254, **275-277,** 559, 620, 633, 638, 639, 645, 675, 685
Hydrastis canadensis (see goldenseal)
Hyperglycemia, treatment 174, 244, 260, 595, 618, 642
Hyperglycemia, use caution with 565, 572
Hyperglycemic effects (elevates blood sugar) 75, 76, 174, 251, 572, 586
Hypericum perforatum (see St. John's wort)
Hypertension, alleviates (high blood pressure) 86, 121, 251, 264, 589, 590, 643
Hypertensives, exacerbates hypertension (elevates blood pressure) 260, 463, 588, 593, 594, 597, 598, 603, 604, 608, 609, 612-620
Hyperthyroidism 14, 67, 85, 110, 245, 251, 303, 304, 343, 391, 445, 493
Hypnotics 40, 103, 157, 268, 280, 599, 658
Hypoglycemia 174, 586
Hypoglycemia, use caution with 174, 251, 272, 572
Hypoglycemic effects 2, 3, 61, 118, 135, 157, 174, 202, 216, 223, 224, 242, 244, 259, 260, 352, 433, 449, 474, 491, 586, 595, 618, 642
Hypotension, treatment (low blood pressure) 63, 265, 308, 433, 443, 590, 643
Hypotensives (blood pressure lowering agents) 15, 47, 57, 63, 85, 93, 146, 202, 203, 223, 264, 289, 311, 357, 392, 433, 535, 589, 590, 618, 658
Hypothalamic-pituitary-adrenal axis (HPA axis) 39, 157, 310, 201
Hypothyroid 39, 67, 86, 158, 202, 203, 244, 251, 288, 302, 303, 304, 343, 344, 455, 493, 602, 618, 619
Hyssop *(Hyssopus officinalis)* 28, 309, 558, 559, 613, 615, 637, 640, 642, 650, 651, 675, 685
Iatrogenic 658

Immune modulators (immunomodulators) 5, 39, 42, 46, 78, 98, 145, 157, 181, 187, 188, 194, 200, 223, 229, 242, 243, 250, 288, 431, 458, 465, 491, 497, 502, 587, 588, 618, 619, 643
Immune stimulants (immunostimulants) 20, 30, 98, 188, 352, 379, 609, 610, 613, 616, 617, 658
Impotence 15, 43, 157, 158, 173, 217, 240, 242, 244, 267, 362, 439, 457, 458, 515, 517, 644
Incontinence 162, 347, 348, 454, 608, 619, 644
Indian warrior (see *Pedicularis*)
Indigestion 13, 58, 340, 474, 497, 593
Infertility 111, 181, 289, 432, 516
Inflammation (see anti-inflammatory)
Influenza 154, 193, 208, 223, 317, 466, 480
Infusions (cold, hot, and solar) 555–559
Injury 7, 31, 32, 47, 107, 283, 307, 396, 497, 510, 512
Insect bites 100, 132, 189, 256, 257, 259, 315, 324, 382, 385, 409, 410, 491, 496, 541, 547, 549, 551, 621–623, 633, 634
Insomnia 14, 18, 39, 44, 61, 63, 84, 85, 103, 105, 107, 126, 128, 154, 174, 208, 209, 240, 243, 245, 251, 264, 267, 268, 279, 280, 284, 297, 302, 314, 315, 325, 343, 363, 370, 371, 390, 392, 406, 430, 432, 433, 459, 473, 479, 480, 509, 512, 595, 599, 601–603, 618, 659
Interstitial cystitis 75, 108, 161, 170, 173, 254, 273, 276, 285, 347, 348, 358, 454, 463, 524, 544, 548, 620, 645
Intestinal infections 98, 149, 376
Intestinal microbes (see individual microbes) 19, 24
Intestinal motility 75, 233, 540
Intestinal spasms (also see antispasmodic, aromatic, and carminative) 166, 212
Inula helenium (see elecampane)
Insulin 118, 159, 202, 203, 216, 224, 244, 245, 259, 260, 384, 433, 455, 586
Irish moss *(Chondrus crispus)* 638, 640, 652, 654, 669, 685
Irritable bowel syndrome (IBS) 67, 71, 79, 94, 103, 108, 117, 127, 131, 146, 149, 212, 217, 233, 269, 289, 298, 308, 326, 329, 339, 406, 416, 463, 469, 474, 483, 497, 512, 523, 535, 540, 544, 570, 591–594, 645
Itching 7, 18, 27, 54, 126, 139, 155, 196, 228, 251, 282, 285, 298, 315, 358, 438, 474, 496, 507, 517, 538, 551, 565
Jamaican dogwood *(Piscidia piscipula)* 66, 103, 107, 108, **278–280,** 281, 302, 315, 330, 391, 474, 524, 530, 599, 600, 629, 630, 632, 633, 635, 637, 641, 645–647, 650, 653, 685
Jaundice 5, 36, 50, 54–56, 105, 111, 125, 126, 154, 176, 177, 227–229, 250, 259, 267, 332, 382, 405, 406, 436, 479, 496, 497, 538, 540, 595–598, 645
Jie jeng (see *Platycodon grandiflorum*)
Joint inflammation 480, 599, 600, 645
Joint pain 2, 20, 63, 93, 95, 109, 149, 169, 232, 235, 259, 330, 436, 457, 463, 481, 516, 523, 524, 528, 530, 547, 645
Ju hua (see chrysanthemum)
Juglans nigra (see black walnut)
Jujube dates *(Zizuphus jujuba)* 145, 587, 588, 606, 631, 638, 654, 658, 678, 685
Juniper *(Juniperus communis)* 164, 317, 442, 551, 558, 629, 630, 638, 639, 643, 644, 653, 669, 685
Kava *(Piper methysticum)* 103, 108, **281–285,** 343, 344, 391, 525, 567, 579, 599, 601, 607, 629, 630, 632, 641, 645, 647, 650, 652, 653, 677, 685
Kelp *(Laminaria digitata)* (also see bladderwrack) **286–290,** 570, 628, 629, 631, 636–638, 640, 643, 649, 651, 654, 685
Kidney failure 157, 158, 359, 463, 645
Kidney inflammation (also see nephritis) 325, 620, 645
Kidney stones (urinary calculi, gravel) 2, 44, 90, 103, 108, 125, 131, 138, 150, 162, 164, 179, 192, 247, 248, 254, 275–277, 285, 325, 327, 330, 355, 372, 383, 385, 463, 469, 506, 512, 524, 541, 599, 619, 620, 645, 656
Kidney trophorestoratives 356, 359
Kidneys 14, 44, 125, 157, 273, 274, 276, 277, 358, 383, 385, 536
Klebsiella pneumoniae 6, 224, 330, 476
Labor 20, 29, 30, 31, 60, 63, 71, 74–76, 126, 170, 173, 174, 217, 254, 280, 313, 325, 343, 344, 384, 387, 388, 463, 491, 523, 524
Lactagogues (see galactagogues)
Lady's mantle *(Alchemilla vulgaris)* 3, **291–293,** 410, 419, 438, 462, 593, 604, 633, 649, 653, 685
Laryngitis 6, 20, 24, 28, 71, 95, 122, 131, 142, 149, 217, 256, 289, 306, 309, 314, 321, 326, 339, 349, 351, 375, 376, 379, 413, 416, 427, 449, 476, 482, 485, 486, 519, 616, 617
Laurus nobilis (see bay laurel)
Lavandin *(Lavandula* x *intermedia)* 269, 297, 299
Lavender, English *(Lavandula angustifolia)* 126, 127, 149, 189, 240, 251, 268, **295–300,** 302, 339, 367, 400, 410, 485, 492, 558, 567, 573, 578, 592, 602, 621–623, 627, 629–632, 634–636, 640, 641, 644, 646–648, 651, 652, 654, 675, 685
Lavender, spike *(Lavandula latifolia)* **295–299,** 631
Laxatives 2, 5–7, 24, 36, 37, 42, 44, 55, 56, 70, 71, 78, 79, 81, 89, 111, 114, 117, 122, 132, 172, 174, 176, 177, 181, 183, 192–194, 212, 216, 217, 229, 233, 306, 307, 324, 326, 327, 332, 334, 344, 369, 370, 384, 439, 538–540, 591, 593–598, 610, 656–659
Lemon balm *(Melissa officinalis)* 29, 85, 107, 108, 126, 202, 240, 251, 264, 298, **301–304,** 343, 344, 363, 473, 512, 558, 567, 573, 579, 591, 592, 601–603, 618, 630–632, 636–638, 642, 647, 648, 650, 652–653, 675, 685
Lemon grass *(Cymbopogon citratus)* 3, 298, 305, 591, 592, 630, 631, 644, 650, 677, 685
Lemon verbena *(Aloysia citriodora)* 423, 630, 632, 636, 679, 685
Leonurus cardiaca (see motherwort)
Lethargy 13, 47, 58, 146, 172, 181, 213, 243, 288, 602, 618, 619
Leukemia 202, 232
Leukocytes (also see blood cells, white) 186, 326
Leukorrhea (excessive vaginal discharge) 10, 51, 60, 69, 71, 237, 254, 287, 293, 351, 405, 426, 427, 449, 476, 534, 544, 547

Libido 35, 39, 43, 157, 158, 173, 182, 201, 217, 243, 244, 458, 515, 587, 603, 604, 618, 619

Licorice root *(Glycyrrhiza glabra)* 20, 24, 25, 28–30, 55, 57, 58, 61, 62, 66, 81, 100, 117, 118, 127, 131, 149, 150, 154, 182, 183, 188, 197, 202, 207, 208, 213, 244, 257, **305–311,** 318, 326, 329, 330, 334, 348, 359, 375, 379, 416, 444, 460, 486, 492, 497, 502, 506, 516, 550, 564, 567, 585–588, 590–599, 603, 604, 608–610, 612–617, 619, 620, 627–629, 631–645, 649, 651–654, 658, 685

Ligusticum porteri (see oshá)

Ligusticum striatum (see chuan xiong)

Linden *(Tilia platypyllos* ssp. *cordifolia)* 612, 638, 647, 679, 685

Liniments 33, 60, 95, 100, 103, 112, 115, 123, 129, 141, 198, 257, 270, 280, 314, 315, 322, 338, 340, 349, 352, 376, 397, 414, 442, 445, 451, 470 474, 477, 481, 489, 513, 571, 658

Lipids, high density (HDLs) 3, 121, 159, 216, 569

Lipids, low density (LDLs) 3, 121, 159, 216, 223, 265, 433, 498, 569

Lithotriptics (also see antilithic) 254, 277, 650, 658

Liver, cirrhosis 56, 229, 333, 459, 595–598

Liver, compromised (herbs to avoid) 30, 36, 76, 82, 150, 151, 285, 340, 376, 400, 401, 593

Liver congestion/stagnation 36, 176, 212, 230, 406, 540, 597, 606, 646

Liver detoxifier (hepatodetoxifier)(also see hepatic) 37, 42, 48, 50, 55–57, 79, 89, 90, 111, 131, 154, 159, 176–178, 182, 201, 203, 212, 224, 227–230, 234, 256, 265, 289, 309, 310, 332–334, 339, 369, 384, 387, 406, 425, 430, 432, 433, 458, 459, 466, 496–498, 509, 538, 540, 565, 568, 587, 595, 597, 598, 606, 629, 633, 646, 655, 657, 658

Liver, fatty 37, 384, 385, 459, 598

Liver heat 230, 406, 597, 598, 646

Liver swelling 57, 646

Lobelia *(Lobelia inflata)* 120, 256, **312–315,** 571, 579, 600, 627, 629, 632, 633, 635, 637, 640, 644, 647, 649, 650, 651, 653, 654, 672, 682, 688

Lomatium *(Lomatium dissectum)* 28, 30, 257, **316–319,** 379, 502, 562, 574, 612, 617, 629–631, 635, 637, 640, 642, 643, 650, 651, 671, 681, 685

Low blood pressure (also see hypotension) 308, 590

Low density lipids (LDLs) 3, 121, 159, 216, 223, 265, 433, 498, 569

Lozenges 196, 325, 327, 513, 519

Lung congestion (also see expectorant) 193, 208, 248, 299, 489, 535, 614, 615

Lung disorders (also see asthma, bronchitis, coughs, pneumonia) 237, 419

Lycii berry *(Lycium barbarum)* 100, 145, 460, 587, 631, 639, 640, 643, 644, 652, 654, 679

Lycopus virginicus (see bugleweed)

Lymphatics 51, 89, 98, 138, 139, 193, 201, 369, 371, 413, 416, 422, 425, 426, 477, 546, 597, 609–611, 614–617, 623, 655, 658

Lymphedema 98

Lymphoma 159, 499

Lysichiton americanus (see skunk cabbage, western)

Ma huang (see ephedra)

Macular degeneration 238, 239

Madder *(Rubia tinctorium)* 254, 645, 678, 686

Madrone (see uva ursi)

Mahonia (see *Berberis*)

Maidenhair tree (see ginkgo)

Maitake *(Grifola frondosa)* 619, 628, 633, 643

Manzanita (see uva ursi)

Marigold (see calendula)

Marjoram *(Origanum majorana)* **320–322,** 374, 449, 573, 613, 629–632, 635–638, 640, 642, 643, 650, 654, 686

Marshmallow *(Althaea officinalis, Malva* spp.*)* 24, 58, 100, 115, 117, 118, 127, 129, 142, 143, 149, 208, 277, 300, 309, **323–327,** 329, 340, 348, 353, 379, 489, 506, 550, 559, 574, 581, 587, 592–594, 614–617, 620, 627, 633, 637, 638–654, 656, 666, 676, 686

Mastalgia or mastodynia (see breast pain)

Mastitis 60, 132, 176, 410, 426, 499, 622, 646

Matricaria recutita (see chamomile)

Meadowsweet *(Filipendula ulmaria)* 99, 127, 149, 279, 293, 309, **328–330,** 409, 416, 530, 558, 579, 592–594, 599, 612, 629, 630, 632, 633, 638, 641, 644, 645, 647, 652, 653, 678, 686

Medicago sativa (see alfalfa)

Medicinal oils (see oils, herb-infused)

Melissa officinalis (see lemon balm)

Memory enhancing (see nootropics)

Memory problems 646

Menopause (perimenopause) 21, 62, 244, 298, 343, 462, 516, 525, 603, 604

Menorrhagia (heavy menstrual bleeding) 21, 43, 60, 75, 146, 170, 181, 287, 462, 534, 600, 603, 604, 606

Menstrual cramping (also see dysmenorrhea) 19, 65, 103, 400, 470, 472, 523, 607

Menstrual disorders 15, 181, 515

Menstruum 474, **561–568,** 658

Mentha arvensis, brookmint (see mint)

Mentha piperita, peppermint (see mint)

Mentha pulegium (see pennyroyal)

Mentha spicata, spearmint (see mint)

Menyanthes trifoliata (see bogbean)

Milk secretion (see galactagogues; antigalactagogues)

Milk thistle *(Silybum marianum)* 37, **331–334,** 459, 497, 597, 598, 627, 631, 634, 636, 638, 639, 641, 642, 645, 646, 648, 649, 672, 686

Miscarriage 43, 65, 67, 71, 100, 135, 170, 385, 387, 388, 419, 455, 516, 517, 524, 604, 605, 647, 649

Mint *(Mentha* spp.*)* 2, 3, 33, 81, 99, 110, 127, 193, 212, 298, 301, 303, 304, 309, 329, 330, **335–340,** 349, 357, 358, 398–400, 409, 419, 422, 423, 444, 492, 530, 558, 559, 567, 573, 591–594, 602, 604, 611–613, 616, 619, 621, 628–632, 635–638, 640–642, 644, 647, 650, 651, 652, 654, 682, 685, 686, 687, 688

Mint family *(Lamiaceae)* 83, 295, 301, 304, 320, 321, 340, 341, 343, 373, 374, 398, 399, 441, 514, 667, **675**

Mitchella repens (see partridge berry)

Monarda fistulosa (see bee balm)

Mononucleosis (Epstein barr virus) 57, 98, 139, 142, 145, 188, 193, 351, 375, 376, 416, 422, 426, 427, 476, 486, 609-611
Mormon tea (see ephedra)
Morning sickness 71, 114, 233, 338, 419, 496, 523, 524, 647
Motherwort *(Leonurus cardiaca)* 62, 66, 85, 86, 182, 264, 303, 310, **341-344,** 363, 391, 512, 516, 579, 590, 601, 604, 607, 618, 628, 629, 632, 634, 636, 640, 641, 643, 646-648, 651-653, 686
Motion sickness 233, 338
Mouth sores 69, 318, 351, 438, 538
Mucilage 89, 94, 116, 121, 131, 134, 148, 149, 164, 197, 216, 217, 289, 324-327, 329, 332, 347, 349, 382, 387, 409, 426, 439, 440, 483, 523, 524, 544, 556, 562, 565, 575, 658
Mucolytics 114, 158, 299, 356, 444, 445, 491, 658
Mucus 10, 20, 28, 43, 44, 51, 71, 81, 114, 196, 197, 199, 208, 237, 248, 273, 342, 416, 420, 449, 491, 497, 534, 535, 546, 547, 588, 655, 657, 658, 727
Mugwort *(Artemisia vulgaris)* 559, 560, 578, 628, 630, 634, 636, 638, 640, 644, 646, 649, 651-653, 671, 686
Muira puama *(Ptychopetalum olacoides)* 201, 585, 586, 608, 632, 643, 644, 652, 676, 685, 686
Mulberry *(Morus alba)* 658, 676
Mullein *(Verbascum thapsus)* 131, 162, 170, 273, 276, 309, 339, **345-349,** 358, 423, 558, 567, 608, 612, 613, 619, 620, 622, 633, 634, 637-640, 644, 645, 651, 654, 679, 686
Mullein flower (also see mullein) 346, 347, 349, 622, 633, 638, 639, 654
Mullein leaf (also see mullein) 309, 339, 346, 347, 349, 612, 633, 651
Mullein root (also see mullein) 161, 170, 273, 276, 347, 348, 358, 608, 619, 620, 633, 634, 638, 644, 645
Muscle aches 81, 647
Muscle pain (see myalgia)
Muscle spasms (skeletal muscle) 44, 65, 103, 109, 279, 283, 315, 321, 392, 396, 444, 474, 487, 512, 523, 600, 656
Muscle spasms (smooth muscle) 7, 128, 181, 321, 474, 512, 600
Muscle stiffness 60, 647
Muscle weakness 76, 430
Mustard seed *(Sinapis alba)* 181, 461, 570, 631, 637, 638, 650, 657, 659, 672, 686
Myalgia (muscle pain) 33, 39, 63, 103, 109, 122, 178, 225, 279, 280, 283, 315, 330, 414, 481, 530, 599, 600, 623
Myrica spp. (see bayberry)
Myrrh *(Commiphora myrrha)* 99, 120, 186, 188, 313, **350-353,** 417, 442, 562, 579, 627, 629-631, 635, 640, 642, 644, 646, 650-652, 654, 672, 686
Nasal congestion (also see sinus congestion) 10, 72, 207, 369, 491
Nasal polyps 95, 547
Nausea 15, 20, 21, 23, 24, 33, 36, 37, 51, 56, 58, 63, 71, 76, 78, 82, 94, 95, 110, 113, 114, 121, 123, 134, 135, 141, 142, 155, 166, 170, 189, 194, 198, 209, 212-214, 219, 225, 229, 230, 232, 233, 240, 280, 285, 296, 312-315, 337-339, 368-370, 400, 401, 405, 455, 466, 470, 491, 492, 497, 499, 507, 509, 517, 523, 524, 531, 541, 547, 549, 596, 647
Nepeta cataria (see catnip)
Nephritis (kidney inflammation) 138, 157, 247, 254, 276, 278, 355, 359, 505
Nerve problems (see neuralgia)
Nervines 14, 39, 60, 61, 63, 67, 75, 85, 102, 103, 106-108, 126, 128, 169, 172, 173, 250, 263, 264, 267, 268, 283, 284, 297, 302, 314, 315, 342, 343, 363, 390, 391, 396, 405, 406, 473, 474, 480, 491, 492, 509-511, 573, 590-592, 599-604, 606, 607, 618, 632, 647, 658
Nervous exhaustion (also see neurasthenia) 14, 39, 282, 363, 439
Nervousness (see nervines)
Nettle *(Urtica dioica)* 2, 3, 19, 89, 132, 138, 170, 273, 274, 276, 314, 330, 348, **354-360,** 383, 385, 410, 420, 422, 444, 450, 459, 516, 532, 533, 541, 558, 559, 567, 570, 571, 578, 604, 608, 619, 620, 622, 627-635, 638, 639, 641, 643-646, 648-651, 653, 679, 686
Neuralgia (nerve pain) 18, 60, 63, 103, 104, 108, 109, 122, 125, 128, 167, 192, 196, 225, 232, 247, 262, 264, 267, 269, 279, 280, 283, 297, 298, 314, 315, 344, 358, 392, 413, 414, 444, 473, 474, 480, 481, 487, 510, 512, 523, 529, 536, 571, 623, 647
Neurasthenia (nervous exhaustion) 157, 173, 362, 433, 457, 529
Nicotiana, tobacco *(Nicotiana tabacum)* 60, 649, 679, 688
Nicotine withdrawal 315
Nicotinic receptors 75, 95, 315
Night blooming cereus (see *Cereus*)
Night sweats 6, 21, 44, 48, 61, 62, 123, 131, 135, 146, 183, 235, 245, 327, 343, 380, 405, 406, 414, 448, 449, 457, 458, 499, 513, 517, 603, 648
Nightmares 14, 127, 405, 442, 648
Nipples, sore 98, 100, 387
Nonulcer dyspepsia 19, 81, 94, 114, 127, 135, 154, 177, 197, 212, 229, 233, 321, 375, 443, 450, 474, 486, 497, 592, 594, 596, 644
Nootropics 243, 601, 657, 659
Nosebleed (also see hemostatics) 86
Nuphar luteum (see yellow pond lily)
Nursing (also see breastfeeding) 23, 86, 102, 203, 211, 225, 244, 299, 348, 358, 385, 423, 450, 455, 481, 538
Nutritives 23, 30, 71, 72, 75, 89, 90, 131, 132, 138, 273, 288, 326, 356, 357, 360, 363, 419, 420, 422, 437, 453, 492, 539, 556, 648, 659
Oats, milky and oat straw *(Avena spp.)* 85, 107, 108, 126, 173, 182, 202, 240, 251, 264, 298, 302, 343, **361-364,** 391, 473, 492, 558, 601, 603, 607, 630, 632, 645, 646-648, 651, 652, 662, 677, 686, 689
Ocotillo (Fouquieria splendens) 483, 591, 648, 654, 674, 686

Oils, herb-infused (medicinal oils; also see salves) **577–581**
Old man's beard (see usnea)
Oligomenorrhea (irregular menstruation) 13, 15, 60, 74, 181, 342
Olive leaf *(Olea europaea)* 558, 630, 631, 636, 641, 643, 676, 686
Oplopanax horridus (see devil's club)
Oral health (also see gingivitis and gum abscesses) 188
Orange peel *(Citrus x sinensis)* 24, 66, 100, 108, 110, 114, 298, 303, **365–372,** 375, 433, 444, 486, 492, 512, 524, 575, 576, 588, 589, 592, 596, 598, 600, 616, 627, 628, 630–636, 640, 644, 647
Oregano *(Origanum vulgare)* 285, 320, **373–376,** 449, 486, 502, 586, 570, 573, 627, 629–632, 635–638, 640, 642, 643, 650, 651, 653, 686
Oregon grape (*see Berberis*)
Origanum majorana (see marjoram)
Origanum vulgare (see oregano)
Oshá *(Ligusticum porteri)* 28, 197, 318, **377–380,** 416, 502, 574, 612, 614, 615, 629, 631, 635–638, 640, 643, 644, 650, 651
Osteoarthritis 33, 39, 63, 109, 234, 235, 279, 357, 440, 480, 497, 544, 599
Otitis media (see earache, ear infection)
Ovarian cysts 66, 75, 135, 169, 387, 405, 516, 524, 544
Paeonia alba (see peony)
Pain relievers (see analgesic, anti-inflammatory, antispasmodic)
Painful menstruation (see dysmenorrhea)
Painful urination (see dysuria)
Palpitations (heart palpitations) 86, 240, 264, 337, 342, 343, 590, 601, 618
Panax ginseng (see ginseng, Asian)
Panax quinquefolius (see ginseng, American)
Panic attacks 14, 85, 343, 391, 601, 618
Paralysis 14, 167, 200, 256, 278, 285, 401, 413, 648
Parasites 57, 222, 232, 233, 466, 486, 496, 655, 665
Parasympathetic nervous system 659
Parasympathomimetics 459, 659
Parsley leaf *(Petroselinum* spp.*)* 86, **381–385,** 450, 633, 636, 639, 641, 649, 654
Parsley root *(Petroselinum* spp.*)* 89, 90, 164, 212, 248, 273, 277, 357, **381–385,** 463, 506, 535, 620, 638, 639, 645, 653
Parsley seed *(Petroselinum* spp.*)* 330, **381–385,** 590, 619, 639, 640
Partridge berry *(Mitchella repens)* 67, 75, 170, **386–388,** 516, 605, 628, 647, 649, 650, 653, 686
Parturients 29, 60, 61, 66, 383, 387, 405
Partus preparators 60, 74, 170, 387, 604, 605
Passiflora incarnata (see passion flower)
Passion flower *(Passiflora incarnata)* 103, 107, 126, 268, 284, 302, 343, **389–392,** 512, 558, 599, 601, 629, 630, 632, 637, 643, 647–650, 653, 654, 677, 686
Pastilles 617
Paullinia cupana (see guarana)
Pedicularis *(Pedicularis* spp.*)* 103, 107, 279, **393–397,** 474, 558, 571, 600, 629, 632, 641, 646, 647, 649, 651, 653, 676, 681, 684–686
Pennyroyal *(Mentha pulegium, Hedeoma pulegioides)* **398–401,** 472, 628, 638, 640, 644, 653, 686
Peony, white *(Paeonia lactiflora)* 61, 62, 67, 75, 244, 310, 388, **403–407,** 497, 516, 524, 559, 585–587, 597, 598, 605–608, 620, 628–631, 633, 634, 639–648, 650–654, 678, 686
Peppermint *(Mentha piperita)*(also see mint) 3, 81, 110, 127, 193, 212, 298, 303, 309, 330, 335–340, 357, 358, 400, 409, 419, 423, 486, 530, 567, 573, 591, 594, 612, 613, 615, 619, 621, 628–632, 635, 636, 638, 640–642, 644, 647, 650, 652, 687
Peptic ulcer (see ulcers)
Perimenopause (see menopause)
Periodontal disease (see toothache) 51, 265, 547
Peristalsis 5, 141
Perspiration 46, 85, 120, 325, 337, 374, 449, 485, 657
Petasites frigidus, P. palmatus (see coltsfoot, eastern)
Petroselinum italicum, P. spp. (see parsley)
Phellodendron, huang bai, amur cork tree *(Phellodendron amurense)* 154, 559, 598, 629, 631, 634, 636, 639, 641, 642, 645, 646, 648, 650, 651, 653, 678, 681, 685, 687
Photodermatitis 167, 481, 659
Photosensitivity 21, 166, 385, 659
Piles (see hemorrhoids)
Pimenta dioica (see allspice)
Pimpinella anisum (see anise)
Pinworms *(Oxyuris* spp.*)* 224, 375, 376, 486, 488
Piper methysticum (see kava)
Piscidia erythrina (see Jamaican dogwood)
Plague 17, 18, 54, 296, 382, 510
Plantain *(Plantago* spp.*)* 356, **408–410,** 578, 622, 623, 627, 629, 633–635, 638–640, 642, 645, 646, 648, 649, 651, 652, 654, 677, 687, 688
Platycodon, jie jing *(Platycodon grandiflorum)* 587, 633, 637, 672, 681, 685
Pleurisy 18, 28, 66, 197, 223, 250, 273, 314, 358, 458, 486, 502, 549, 559, 635, 637, 640, 671, 687
Pleurisy root *(Asclepias tuberosa)* 28, 66, 559, 635, 637, 640, 671, 687
Pneumonia 6, 17, 28, 44, 75, 84, 103, 153, 157, 158, 186, 197, 212, 223, 224, 264, 273, 314, 317, 318, 330, 337, 355, 358, 376, 378, 379, 405, 416, 425, 432, 458, 460, 476, 486, 502, 519, 520, 549, 550, 612
Poison ivy, poison oak 7, 90, 100, 128, 132, 139, 193, 256, 257, 285, 290, 298, 308, 315, 327, 362, 410, 438, 507, 530, 536, 547, 549, 551, 581, 648, 651
Poison oak-like rash, can cause 30, 237
Poisoning, food/alcohol 18, 20, 57, 95, 110, 154, 212, 224, 233, 306, 338, 430, 476, 488, 497, 523, 535, 648
Poisoning, herbicide 72
Poisoning, mushroom/plant 90, 222, 230, 250, 274, 334, 355
Poisoning, pyrrolizidine alkaloid 151
Polygala *(Polygala* spp.*)* 633, 635, 637, 654, 677, 681, 683, 687, 688, 689

Polyps 95, 547
Poplar buds *(Populus* spp.*)* 512, 579, 667, 679, 678, 681, 687
Poria, fu ling *(Poria cocos)* 276, 606, 633, 634, 639, 644, 652, 654, 685
Poultices 2, 10, 14, 17, 21, 27, 32, 33, 40, 51, 63, 67, 78, 79, 86, 88, 89, 95, 98, 100, 102, 126, 132, 145, 148, 155, 162, 167, 179, 186, 189, 211, 217, 219, 225, 232, 235, 247, 267, 270, 272, 274, 279, 280, 283, 290, 292, 293, 300, 304, 311, 315, 318, 320, 322, 324, 325, 330, 337, 346, 349, 356, 374, 382, 385, 390, 395, 397, 399, 405, 409, 410, 413, 414, 419, 422, 423, 436, 457, 463, 470, 477, 479, 483, 491, 493, 499, 505, 510, 512, 513, 521, 524, 533, 536, 538, 541, 543, 544, 546, 547, 549, **560, 621, 622,** 627, 634, 635, 659
Pregnancy (see parturient, partus preparator)
Pregnancy, avoid use during 15, 79, 111, 220, 254, 277, 280, 315, 319, 470, 493
Premenstrual syndrome (PMS) 13, 14, 61, 111, 173, 179, 298, 343, 364, 406, 480, 516, 598, 602, 603, 606, 607
Prickly ash *(Zanthoxylum* spp.*)* **411–414,** 571, 579, 589, 591, 628, 629, 634–637, 646–650, 652, 654, 657, 687
Prophylactics (preventatives) 46, 145, 202, 220, 265, 433, 467, 659
Propolis hive resin *(Propolis)* 81, 310, 318, 379, **415–417,** 579, 609, 617, 627, 629, 631, 637, 640, 642, 643, 646, 652, 654
Prostate swelling (also see benign prostatic hypertrophy) 285, 348, 544
Prostatitis 162, 254, 405, 544
Prunus virginiana (see wild cherry bark)
Prunella vulgaris (see self-heal)
Psoriasis 79, 88, 111, 333, 334, 595–598, 611, 649
Psyllium *(Plantago ovata)* 637, 638, 656, 687
Ptychopetalum olacoides (see muira puama)
Pulsatilla (see anemone)
Purgatives 7, 18, 63, 78, 81, 95, 120, 125, 132, 194, 211, 212, 233, 314, 327, 340, 649, 655–659
Pygeum *(Prunus africana)* 348, 359, 608, 633, 638, 639, 650, 687
Pyrrolizidine alkaloids (PAs) 82, 148–151, 187, 593, 649
Queen's root (see stillingia)
Radiation 6, 7, 44, 47, 100, 110, 127, 132, 149, 159, 189, 200, 202, 217, 243, 288, 289, 327, 432, 465, 493
Rashes 13, 88, 128, 132, 139, 162, 166, 217, 290, 308, 317, 327, 355, 409, 466, 507, 528, 581, 649
Raspberry leaf *(Rubus ideaus)* 2, 3, 67, 68, 71, 149, 170, 274, 349, 357, 358, 388, **418–420,** 437, 462, 516, 524, 556, 558, 565, 604, 605, 612, 629, 633, 634, 639, 647–651, 653, 661, 678, 687
Raynaud's phenomenon 20, 122, 135, 183, 223, 234, 238, 413, 443, 589
Recuperatives 3, 6, 28, 29, 78, 79, 162, 198, 243, 273, 289, 328, 356, 358, 380, 458, 538, 587
Red clover *(Trifolium pratense)* 2, 89, 239, 420, **421–423,** 558, 567, 578, 602, 610, 611, 627, 628, 631, 633, 634, 639, 640, 641, 646, 648, 649, 651, 674
Red root *(Ceanothus* spp.*)* 89, 139, 145, 189, 309, 379, 416, **424–428,** 477, 483, 559, 565, 589, 591, 597, 598, 607, 610, 617, 627, 628, 630, 631, 633, 634, 636, 637, 641, 642, 645, 646, 648, 650, 652–654, 678, 687
Red sage *(Salvia miltiorrhiza,* dan shen*)* 183, 589, 634, 640, 683, 687
Refrigerants 70, 71, 131, 303, 659
Rehmannia glutinosa (shu di huang) 43, 47, 146, 181, 182, 243, 244, 405, 585–587, 590, 603, 606, 628, 631, 634, 639, 643, 644, 651, 652, 654, 677, 683, 688
Reishi 30, 183, 188, 202, 244, 250, **429–434,** 459, 585, 586, 602, 619, 627, 628, 630, 631, 633, 635, 642, 643, 646, 652, 659, 665, 669, 687
Resolvents 51, 88, 188, 538, 547, 610, 611, 659
Respiratory congestion 13, 51, 317, 375, 444, 486
Respiratory depression 315, 521
Restoratives (also see trophorestoratives) 2, 39, 46, 131, 146, 172, 173, 181, 242, 262, 282, 298, 336, 363, 412, 436, 453, 465, 529, 538, 659, 660
Retina 110, 239, 244, 640, 650
Retinopathy 239
Rheumatism 13, 20, 27, 36, 38, 42, 54, 60, 69, 74, 78, 88, 122, 126, 131, 176, 192, 219, 247, 267, 287, 318, 337, 383, 412, 414, 425, 430, 437, 442, 457, 476, 480, 485, 515, 519, 522, 523, 543, 551, 687
Rhinitis (see allergic rhinitis)
Rhodiola *(Rhodiola rosea)* 627, 630, 635, 643, 646, 652, 687
Ringworm (see antifungals)
Rooibos *(Aspalathus contaminates)* 631, 648, 674
Rosa spp. (see rose)
Rose *(Rosa* spp.*)* 70, 89, 100, 150, 261, 293, 337, 339, 357, 410, 420, **435–440,** 460, 520, 567, 571, 573, 578, 593, 604, 621, 627, 628, 630, 631, 633, 635, 637, 638, 640, 642, 644, 645, 648, 651–654, 660, 678
Rose hips *(Rosa* spp.*)* 89, 100, 435–440, 628, 638, 640, 645, 654
Rose petals *(Rosa* spp.*)* 435–440, 571, 573, 578, 593, 604, 633
Rose root (see *Rhodiola rosea*)
Rosemary *(Salvia rosmarinus* syn. *Rosmarinus officinale)* 107, 108, 238–240, 250, 251, 296, 303, 358, 367, 375, 385, 388, 423, **441–445,** 485, 486, 429, 558, 567, 568, 570, 571, 573, 577–579, 581, 589–592, 601, 602, 627, 629–632, 635–638, 640, 641, 643, 644, 646, 649, 652, 654, 675, 688
Rosmarinus (see rosemary)
Roundworm *(Ascaris lumbridoides)* 224
Rubefacients 122, 166, 196, 232, 257, 375, 444, 485, 487, 560, 571, 659
Rubus (see blackberry or raspberry)
Rumex crispus (see yellow dock)
Sabal (see saw palmetto)
Sage *(Salvia officinale)* 86, 267, 384, **447–451,** 558, 559, 568, 570, 571, 573, 579, 627, 629–634, 636–638, 640, 642, 644, 648, 652, 654, 675, 687, 689
Salicin 67, 329, 529–531
Salicylates 141, 329, 330, 422, 531

Salix (see willow)
Salmonella 32, 57, 128, 153, 224, 235, 517
Salve 10, 18, 23, 30, 33, 51, 58, 86, 100, 103, 109, 127–129, 139, 149, 151, 155, 189, 193, 248, 251, 269, 270, 274, 283, 285, 297, 298, 300, 304, 321, 322, 340, 352, 353, 375, 376, 378, 380, 387, 400, 401, 410, 414, 417, 440, 444, 445, 450, 451, 477, 481, 487, 489, 499, 503, 513, 525, 536, 547, 551, **577–581, 623**
Salvia officinalis (see sage)
Sambucus nigra (see elder)
Sandalwood *(Santalum album)* 370, 439, 644, 678, 687
Sarsaparilla, Indian *(Hemidesmus indicus)* 585–587, 595, 608, 687
Sarsaparilla, true *(Smilax* spp.*)* 27, 559, 585–587, 595, 608, 628, 632, 679, 687, 688
Saw palmetto *(Serenoa repens)* 61, 162, 273, 276, 348, 358, 359, **452–455,** 516, 608, 628, 633, 634, 640, 644, 645, 650, 653, 687
Scars, scarring 139, 251, 298, 536, 572
Schisandra *(Schisandra chinense)* 29, 30, 100, 182, 188, 201, 202, 243, 244, **456–460,** 516, 558, 567, 585, 586, 603, 619, 627, 628, 630–633, 642–644, 646, 650, 652, 661, 679, 684, 687, 689
Schisandra (see schisandra)
Sciatica 103, 126, 192, 196, 225, 280, 283, 358, 392, 396, 474, 480, 485, 512, 571, 650
Scrophularia spp. (see figwort)
Scurvy 78, 88, 262, 367, 436, 439, 538, 654
Scutellaria spp. (see skullcap)
Scutellaria baicalensis (see skullcap, baikal)
Seasickness (also sea nausea) 233
Seasonal affective disorder (SAD) 29, 251, 480, 492
Sedatives 14, 40, 57, 60, 61, 66, 84, 85, 93, 102, 103, 106, 107, 126, 127, 157, 169, 264, 267, 268, 270, 276, 279, 280, 283–285, 297, 298, 302, 313–315, 342, 343, 367, 371, 391, 392, 396, 405, 406, 425, 433, 458, 459, 470, 473, 480, 489, 509–513, 599, 601, 602, 607, 650, 656, 658, 659
Self-heal *(Prunella vulgaris)* 578, 675, 684, 687
Serenoa repens (see saw palmetto)
Seven barks (see *Hydrangea*)
Shan yao *(Dioscorea batatas)* 145, 559, 587, 588, 673, 688
Shatavari (see asparagus)
Shepherd's purse *(Capsella bursa-pastoris)* 86, 135, 170, 274, 357, 388, **461–463,** 536, 633, 634, 649, 653, 672, 688
Shigella 57, 89, 153, 264, 330
Shiitake *(Lentinula edodes)* **464–467,** 627, 628, 631, 633, 642, 651, 654
Shingles (herpes zoster) 27, 29, 98, 122, 128, 309, 344, 352, 417, 466, 474, 480
Sialagogues 24, 30, 94, 95, 188, 232, 233, 283, 384, 314, 351, 412, 413, 477, 650, 659
Siberian ginseng (see eleuthero)
Silk tassel *(Garrya* spp.*)* 56, 75, 254, 277, 280, 344, **468–470,** 498, 579, 629, 632, 645, 649, 653, 674, 688
Silybum marianum (see milk thistle)
Sinapis alba (see mustard seed)
Sinus congestion 95, 122, 223, 248, 339, 650
Sinus infection (see sinusitis)
Sinusitis (sinus infection) 51, 57, 208, 223, 351, 375, 379, 416, 426, 444, 445, 449, 476, 486, 502, 535, 546, 547, 550, 569, 614, 615
Skin cancer 581
Skin disorders (also see acne, dermatitis, eczema, and psoriasis) 16, 285, 412, 538
Skin, dry 651
Skin inflammation 71, 208, 330, 420, 450, 645, 651
Skin irritation 90, 167, 214, 227, 376, 417, 503
Skin, flushed 651
Skin, oily 651
Skullcap *(Scutellaria lateriflora)* 66, 107, 108, 126, 173, 302, 363, **471–474,** 524, 567, 600, 603, 629–632, 635, 641, 647, 648, 650–653, 688
Skullcap, baikal *(Scutellaria baicalensis)* 629, 631, 634, 636, 638, 639, 641, 642, 645, 646, 648, 650, 651, 653, 675, 681
Skunk cabbage, eastern *(Symplocarpus foetidus);* skunk cabbage, western *(Lysichiton americanus)* 120, 314, 600, 627, 649, 666, 671, 688
Sleep problems (see insomnia, nightmares)
Slippery elm *(Ulmus fulva)* 89, 115, 129, 143, 326, 340, 353, 593, 616, 637, 638, 640–642, 645, 652–654, 688
Snakebites 14, 60, 186, 228, 378, 409, 622
Solidago spp. (see goldenrod)
Soporifics (also see insomnia, nervines, and sedatives) 126, 127, 268, 283, 459, 659
Sore throat (also see mononucleosis and/or strep throat) 248, 256, 309, 339, 409, 420, 427, 438, 609–611, 616, 617
Sores 10, 17, 27, 29, 32, 42, 51, 54, 56, 69, 88, 98, 102, 131, 132, 155, 186, 189, 196, 202, 222, 247, 257, 292, 303, 304, 306, 308, 309, 317, 318, 327, 337, 351, 352, 378, 395, 405, 415–417, 425, 426, 436, 438, 444, 477, 479, 487, 496, 505, 528, 533, 536, 538, 546, 547, 549
Spasmolytics 40, 213, 220, 298, 299, 321, 339, 347, 376, 659
Spearmint *(Mentha spicata,* also see mint*)* 212, 298, 303, 335–340, 358, 492, 558, 567, 592–594, 602, 612, 619, 632, 636, 638, 641, 647, 675
Spider veins (see varicose veins)
Spikenard (see aralia)
Spilanthes *(Acmella oleracaea,* syn. *Spilanthes)* 98, 142, 166, 188, 285, 309, 352, 375, 379, 416, 417, **475–477,** 609, 610, 617, 622, 627, 629–631, 640, 642, 643, 646, 650, 652, 688
Sprains 10, 20, 32, 33, 98, 100, 125, 128, 142, 148, 149, 166, 167, 189, 193, 198, 248, 251, 269, 276, 279, 280, 287, 298, 304, 315, 318, 322, 330, 375, 385, 417, 444, 470, 477, 479, 481, 487, 496, 499, 512, 530, 533, 536, 547, 549, 551, 571, 581, 623, 644, 652
St. John's wort *(Hypericum perforatum)* 29, 99, 100, 108, 109, 126, 149, 166, 173, 202, 211, 240, 251, 279, 298, 302, 330, 349, 363, 473, **478–481,** 492, 530, 567, 578, 581, 599, 601, 603, 621, 622, 627, 629–635, 638, 639, 641, 642, 644–650, 652–654, 675
Stellaria media (see chickweed)

Stevia *(Stevia rebaudiana)* 423, 586, 592-594, 602, 611, 612, 658
Stillingia *(Stillingia sylvatica*, queen's root, pink root*)* 610, 628, 635, 643, 646, 650, 687
Stimulants 20, 27, 30, 55, 93, 95, 98, 113, 114, 120, 122, 141, 142, 172-174, 176, 183, 188, 223, 228, 229, 234, 238, 290, 314, 339, 351, 370, 379, 407, 412, 443, 492, 496, 546, 589, 590, 601, 602, 609, 610, 612, 615-619, 657, 658, 659
Stomach inflammation (see gastritis)
Stomachics 2, 19, 24, 81, 93, 114, 122, 125, 127, 135, 142, 166, 176, 197, 211, 212, 216, 232, 233, 259, 267, 268, 288, 297, 302, 303, 321, 329, 337, 338, 342, 351, 352, 368, 371, 375, 378, 383, 384, 399, 400, 443, 449, 473, 474, 486, 489, 496, 511, 523, 659
Stone root *(Collinsonia canadensis)* 254, 275-277, **482-483,** 559, 591, 620, 633, 639, 645, 648, 650, 654, 675, 688
Strep throat 51, 57, 71, 141, 142, 188, 223, 309, 318, 321, 326, 351, 375, 376, 379, 416, 426, 449, 476, 486, 489, 502, 546, 609, 616, 617
Sudorifics 27, 81, 106, 121, 122, 126, 127, 193, 279, 302, 330, 339, 529, 530, 534, 535, 612, 659
Sunburn 6, 7, 90, 100, 128, 298, 339, 410, 481, 621, 635, 652
Suppositories 154, 299, 488, 489, 659
Sweating (also see diaphoretic and sudorific) 29, 47, 80, 95, 135, 145, 208, 209, 243, 288, 384, 400, 406, 448, 449, 457, 458, 659
Sweating, excessive 448, 449
Swelling 7, 17, 27, 32, 40, 46, 48, 51, 56, 57, 67, 78, 86, 90, 100, 138, 139, 148, 176-178, 183, 188, 189, 193, 217, 219, 220, 228, 235, 260, 262, 285, 288, 308, 315, 332, 337, 348, 374, 379, 385, 395, 416, 422, 426, 477, 485, 497, 499, 516, 533, 544, 546, 550, 610, 611, 621, 640, 646, 655, 658
Swollen glands (also see lymphatics) 51, 78, 98, 169, 325, 546, 609-611
Sympathomimetics 659
Sympathetic nervous system 122, 172, 201, 207, 659
Symphytum officinale (see comfrey)
Symplocarpus foetidus (see skunk cabbage, eastern)
Syphilis 27, 55, 206, 207, 250, 282, 313, 425, 505, 538, 546
Syrups (also see herbal honey and syrup) 3, 18, 21, 25, 30, 40, 48, 52, 66, 67, 72, 75, 89, 90, 93, 95, 108, 111, 112, 115, 116, 118, 123, 129, 136, 146, 174, 179, 189, 191, 192, 194, 198, 214, 216, 225, 232, 235, 270, 297, 300, 304, 306, 311, 319, 321, 322, 326, 327, 330, 340, 342, 344, 353, 367, 370, 372, 376, 380, 409, 417, 428, 432, 434, 436, 440, 445, 451, 485, 489, 493, 500, 512, 513, 515, 519-521, 541, 549, 551, 565, **575-576,** 612, 659
Tanacetum parthenium (see feverfew)
Tannins 51, 67, 71, 89, 94, 134, 135, 141, 170, 207, 208, 229, 256, 263, 292, 293, 297, 302-304, 321, 329, 330, 338, 374, 387, 405, 419, 437, 449, 450, 473, 479, 483, 485, 506, 507, 543, 547, 556, 565, 656, 660
Tapeworms 81
Taraxacum officinale (see dandelion)
Tea preparation (decoctions and infusions) 555-559
Tendonitis 63, 127, 128, 149, 235, 279, 315, 358, 414, 480, 497, 499, 536
Throat, sore 248, 256, 309, 339, 409, 420, 427, 438, 538, 609-611, 616, 617
Thuja occidentalis, T. plicata (see cedar)
Thyme *(Thymus vulgaris)* 28, 98, 257, 285, 321, 375, 416, 423, 444, 449, 476, **484-489,** 502, 567, 573, 579, 609, 613, 615, 627, 629-633, 635-640, 643, 650, 653, 654, 685, 688
Thymus vulgaris (see thyme)
Thyroid, hyper- (see Grave's disease, hyperthyroidism)
Thyroid, hypo- (see Hashimoto's thyroiditis, hypothyroid)
Tilia platypyllos ssp. *cordifolia* (see linden)
Tinctures 3, 8, 11, 15, 19-21, 25, 30, 32, 33, 37, 40, 45, 48, 51, 52, 57, 58, 63, 67, 70-72, 76, 79, 81, 82, 86, 90, 95, 99, 100, 103, 112, 115, 120, 121, 123, 129, 132, 135, 136, 139, 141-143, 146, 151, 153, 155, 159, 161, 162, 164, 166, 167, 170, 172, 176, 179, 183, 189, 194, 203, 208, 209, 212, 214, 217, 220, 225, 228, 230, 235, 238, 240, 245, 248, 252, 254, 257, 260, 265, 268-270, 273, 274, 277, 280, 284, 285, 292, 293, 300, 304, 311, 315, 319, 331, 334, 339, 340, 344, 349, 352, 353, 355, 360, 361, 363, 364, 372, 376, 379, 380, 385, 387, 388, 392, 397, 401, 407, 410, 414, 417, 420, 423, 428, 434, 440, 445, 449, 451, 455, 460, 463, 467, 470, 474, 477, 481, 483, 489, 493, 500, 503, 507, 513, 517, 521, 524, 525, 531, 535, 536, 538, 539, 541, 544, 547, 551, **561-564,** 575, 576, 600, 612, 660
Tinea spp. (athlete's foot, ringworm, etc.) (also see anti-fungals) 224, 269, 285, 352, 375, 444, 477, 487, 489, 499, 503, 547, 581
Tinnitus (ringing in ears) 43, 239, 507, 524, 587, 652
Tonics 660
Tonics, bitter (see bitters, bitter tonics) 114, 227, 229, 634, 657
Tonics, bladder 170, 634
Tonics, blood (blood tonics) 46, 47, 70, 145, 181, 244, 267, 356, 405, 519, 604
Tonics, kidney yang (kidney yang tonics) 157, 158, 217, 458
Tonics, kidney yin (kidney yin tonics) 44, 157, 458, 603, 618, 619
Tonics, lung (lung qi, respiratory tonics) 29, 574
Tonics, reproductive 6, 39, 42, 60, 61, 71, 181, 388, 419, 454, 516, 543, 603, 608
Tonics, spleen qi (spleen qi tonics) 146, 244
Tonics, yin (yin tonics) 2, 70, 131, 157, 158, 327, 458, 587, 588, 603, 642, 648, 654
Toothaches 13, 32, 74, 93, 120, 128, 142, 186, 235, 247, 279, 280, 324, 337, 346, 399, 413, 476, 496, 534, 547, 652
Tracheitis 20, 24, 131, 309, 326, 349, 449, 482, 520
Tremetes versicolor (see turkey tail)
Tremors 209, 315, 342, 362, 363, 474
Trich, Trichomonas *(Trichomonas vaginalis)* 57, 153, 188, 235, 309, 503
Trifolium pratense (see red clover)

Trigonella foenum-graecum (see fenugreek)
Trophorestoratives 39, 172, 173, 356, 359, 363, 473, 480, 601, 603, 652, 660
Tuberculosis (TB) 14, 17, 32, 54, 60, 102, 128, 157, 222, 224, 237, 267, 282, 314, 317, 318, 390, 405, 502, 543, 546
Tulsi basil *(Ocimum sanctum)* 239, 240, 250, 443, **490-493,** 585, 586, 643, 646
Tumors 18, 25, 88, 93, 105, 110, 120, 150, 159, 176, 213, 222, 287, 337, 466, 498, 538
Turkey rhubarb *(Rheum palmatum)* 7, 89, 540, 565, 637, 646, 649, 688
Turkey tail *(Tremetes versicolor)* 627, 628, 633, 643, 646, 665, 669, 688
Turmeric *(Curcuma longa)* 114, 182, 183, 260, 279, 308, 330, 334, 369, **495-500,** 524, 567, 573, 578, 579, 591, 596-599, 606, 607, 627, 628-637, 639-649, 652-654, 688
Turnera (see damiana)
Tussilago farfara (see coltsfoot, eastern)
Ulcerative colitis 6, 79, 99, 127, 131, 149, 212, 217, 274, 289, 309, 326, 339, 357, 463, 483, 523, 540, 544, 591-594
Ulcers (duodenal, gastric) 6, 7, 10, 27, 33, 43, 51, 76, 79, 99, 115, 117, 123, 127, 131, 134, 142, 145, 146, 148, 149, 179, 181, 186, 217, 225, 230, 233, 235, 274, 289, 308, 311, 325, 326, 329, 406, 409, 416, 430, 438, 480, 496, 497, 535, 547, 570, 593, 594, 652, 653
Urethritis and cystitis (also see urinary tract infection) 108, 131, 150, 161, 173, 188, 248, 254, 256, 276, 282, 285, 327, 330, 348, 376, 454, 486, 502, 535, 547
Urinary calculi (see kidney stones)
Urinary incontinence (see incontinence)
Urinary tract infection 44, 74, 114, 138, 161, 164, 173, 176, 188, 212, 213, 228, 254, 257, 273, 276, 285, 358, 376, 383, 384, 476, 486, 489, 502, 505, 506, 535, 536, 544, 547, 551, 653
Urtica (see nettle)
Usnea *(Usnea spp.)* 98, 100, 131, 161, 164, 188, 212, 257, 285, 318, 327, 352, 375, 379, 444, 476, 486, **501-503,** 506, 535, 551, 579, 609, 612, 615, 617, 627, 629, 630, 631, 635, 639, 643, 652, 653, 669, 684, 686, 689
Uterine bleeding 21, 54, 67, 71, 86, 135, 170, 174, 232, 343, 344, 388, 401, 405, 462, 516, 524, 544, 653
Uterine contractions 60, 74, 75, 173, 181, 217, 280, 343, 396, 653
Uterine cramping 66, 108, 269, 283, 413, 497, 524, 600, 605, 632, 653
Uterine cysts 135, 405, 419, 470, 535, 544
Uva ursi *(Arctostaphylos spp.)* 131, 161, 180, 212, 327, 502, **504-507,** 535, 551, 559, 565, 559, 565, 629, 630, 633, 639, 648, 649, 651, 653, 673, 688
Vaginal discharge (see leukorrhea)
Vaginal discharge, foul (see *Trichomonas vaginalis*)
Vaginal infections, protozoan parasite (see trich, *Trichomonas vaginalis*)
Vaginal infections, yeast (see candida, *Candida albicans*)
Vaginal infections (see bacterial vaginosis, *Gardnerella vaginalis*)
Vaginal irrigation (also see douche) 10, 27, 51, 52, 57, 58, 72, 99, 128, 151, 154, 293, 325, 329, 330, 420, 426, 427, 438, 440, 502, 507, 544, 547, 5600
Vaginitis 51, 71, 149, 293, 319, 325, 420, 427, 438, 449, 488, 507, 544, 547
Vaginosis, bacterial *(Gardnerella vaginalis)* 98, 188, 299, 319, 375, 377, 486, 489, 502
Valerian *(Valeriana officinale)* 63, 103, 109, 127, 254, 268, 277, 315, 344, 367, 392, **508-513,** 524, 571, 579, 599, 629, 632, 637, 647, 649, 650, 652, 653
Valeriana (see valerian)
Vanilla *(Vanilla planifolia)* 24, 115, 118, 492, 586, 594, 632, 644, 658, 676
Varicose veins, spider veins (venous insufficiency) 51, 72, 79, 98, 100, 149, 223, 238, 248, 251, 274, 332, 334, 369, 413, 414, 427, 438, 439, 443-445, 481, 483, 487, 536, 540, 589, 591, 597, 598, 653, 654
Vasoconstrictors 264, 661
Vasodilators 15, 20, 46, 61, 121, 122, 145, 182, 183, 223, 234, 238, 242, 250, 263, 302, 339, 413, 431, 433, 443, 458, 534, 589, 590, 602, 618, 619, 654, 660
Venous insufficiency (see varicose veins)
Verbascum thapsus (see mullein)
Verbena hastata (see blue vervain)
Verbena officinalis (see blue vervain)
Vermicides 660
Vermifuges 660
Vertigo 13, 62, 146, 181, 245, 251, 262, 277, 510
Viburnum opulus (see cramp bark)
Viburnum prunifolium (see black haw)
Vinegar extracts (see acetum extracts)
Violet *(Viola odorata, V. spp.)* 99, 139, 422, 573, 578, 609, 611, 638, 640, 645, 654, 680, 682
Vision 42, 211
Vitex *(Vitex agnus-castus,* chaste tree berry*)* 61, 62, 182, 201, 244, 310, **514-517,** 567, 627, 628, 639, 643, 646, 648, 649, 651, 675, 682, 686
Vomiting, quells (also see antinauseant) 20, 114, 118, 121, 126, 134, 135, 154, 233, 337, 367, 369, 370, 491, 523, 655
Vulneraries 5, 7, 27, 32, 51, 98, 99, 126, 128, 131, 138, 139, 148, 149, 187, 189, 247, 248, 250, 251, 256, 273, 274, 292, 298, 299, 326, 352, 409, 410, 416, 417, 479-481, 493, 497, 533, 534, 536, 594, 611, 621, 660
Water retention (also see diuretics) 89, 273, 308, 357, 383, 516
Weakness 13, 31, 47, 146, 158, 181, 274, 362, 433, 587, 588, 618-620, 657
Whooping cough 17, 20, 131, 326, 612, 616
Wild cherry bark *(Prunus virginiana)* **518-521,** 635
Wild indigo *(Baptisia tinctoria)* 189, 274, 426, 627-629, 632, 634, 635, 641, 644, 646, 652, 685, 689
Wild oats (see oats)
Wild yam *(Dioscorea villosa)* 66, 67, 169, 170, 212, 280, 497, **522-525,** 600, 604, 605, 629, 630, 632-634, 636, 639, 641, 643-646, 653, 673, 689
Wild yam, Chinese (see shan yao)
Willow bark *(Salix spp.)* 330, **527-531,** 559, 599
Withania somnifera (see ashwagandha)

Worms, intestinal (also see hookworms, pinworms, or tapeworms) 81, 164, 196, 198, 219, 222, 224, 227, 342, 375, 376, 436, 479, 486, 488, 496, 629, 631, 660
Wounds (also see vulnerary) 5, 7, 8, 10, 18, 27, 48, 51, 52, 54, 57, 60, 78, 98–100, 132, 145, 148, 151, 181, 186, 189, 196, 198, 208, 247, 248, 251, 256, 257, 265, 269, 272, 274, 276, 292, 296, 299, 302-304, 317, 318, 324, 327, 349, 351, 352, 369, 375, 389, 390, 405, 409, 414, 417, 419, 420, 444, 450, 463, 476, 477, 479, 481, 487, 489, 496, 521, 531, 533, 534, 538, 541, 543, 547, 549, 551, 572, 654
Yarrow *(Achillea millefolium)* 81, 86, 127, 135, 149, 161, 188, 193, 212, 330, 339, 357, 388, 400, 410, 419, 462, 463, 502, 506, 512, 530, **532–536,** 567, 571, 579, 581, 590, 591, 612, 622, 627-631, 633-640, 642-645, 649-654, 689
Yeast infections (see candida, *Candida albicans*)
Yellow dock *(Rumex crispus)* 2, 89, 356, 412, 483, **537–541,** 559, 565, 570, 596-598, 607, 610, 627-629, 633, 634, 636-639, 641, 642, 645, 646, 648-650, 654, 677, 689
Yellow pond lily *(Nuphar luteum)* 75, 276, 348, 358, 516, **542–544,** 608, 620, 633, 634, 644, 645, 649, 650, 653, 689
Yellow root (see coptis)
Yerba mansa *(Anemopsis californica)* 51, 70, 98–100, 139, 188, 189, 208, 248, 257, 318, 352, 416, 417, 477, 502, 503, 506, **545-547,** 550, 551, 565, 579, 593, 609, 610, 614, 615, 617, 627-630, 633-635, 637-641, 644-646, 649, 650, 652-654, 659, 678, 689
Yerba santa *(Eriodictyon* spp.*)* 30, 51, 164, 208, 248, 257, 318, 416, 502, **548-551,** 567, 579, 612, 614, 615, 628, 630, 633, 635, 637, 640, 644, 650, 651, 653, 689
Zanthoxylum americanus (see prickly ash)
Zea mays (see corn silk)
Zingiber officinale (see ginger)

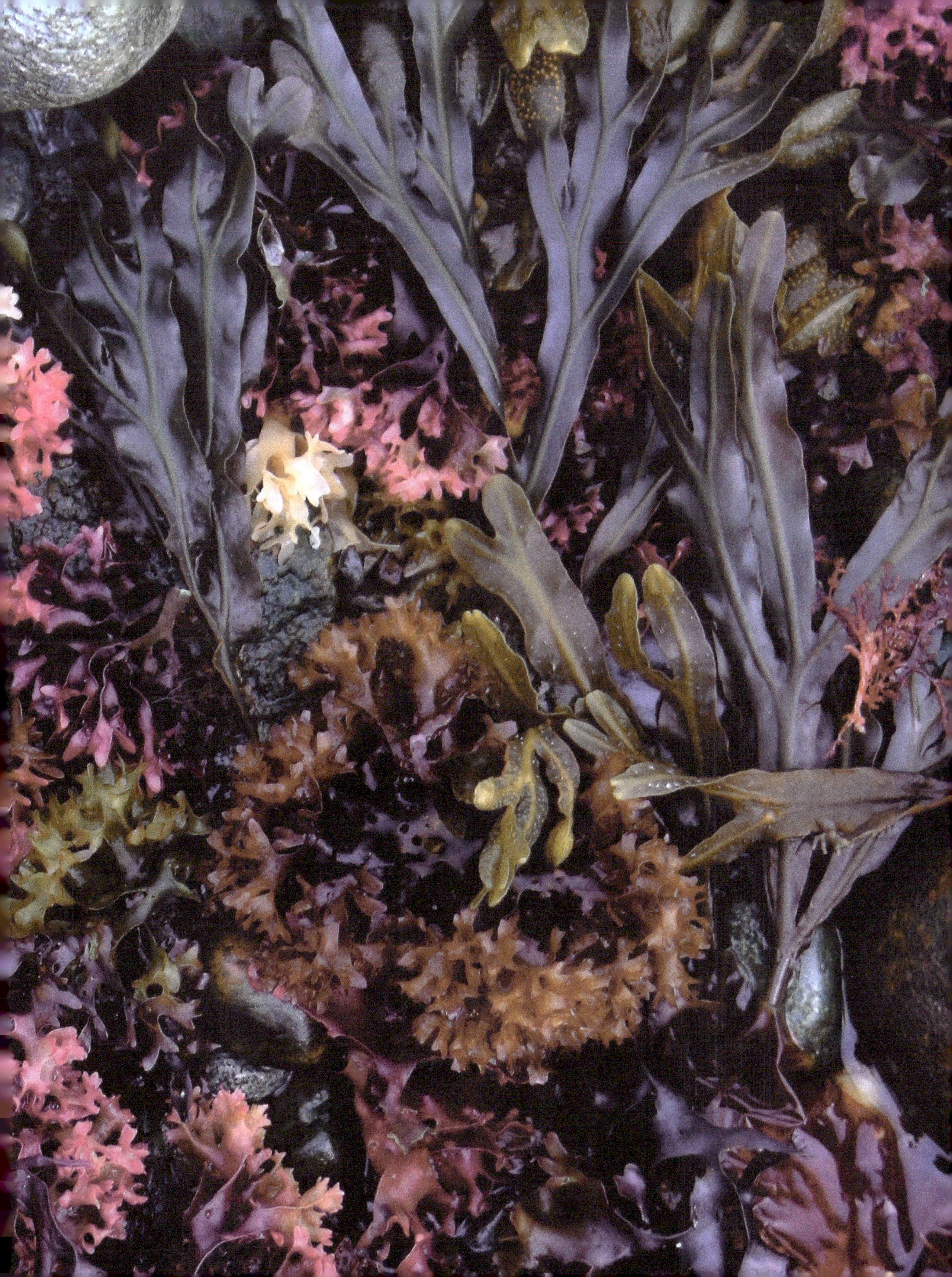

PHOTOGRAPHY CREDITS

7SONG

Page 2, *Medicago sativa* flower (left)
Page 10, *Ambrosia trifida* (left)
Page 10, *Ambrosia artemisiifolia* (right)
Page 52, *Morella cerifera fruits* (left)
Page 64, *Viburnum prunifolium* (both)
Page 66, *Viburnum prunifolium* unripe fruits
Page 73, *Caulophyllum giganteum* (both)
Page 85, *Lycopus americanus* patch (left, middle)
Page 154, *Coptis trifolia* whole plant (left)
Page 155, *Coptis trifolia* rhizomes (top, middle)
Page 180, *Angelica sinensis* seeds (right)
Page 208, *Ephedra fasciculata* (right)
Page 276, *Hydrangea arborescens* (left)
Page 277, *Hydrangea arborescens* (left)
Page 278, *Piscidia erythrina* (left)
Page 279, *Piscidia erythrina* (both)
Page 280, *Piscidia erythrina* (both)
Page 319, *Lomatium dissectum* roots (left)
Page 377, *Ligusticum porteri* roots (right)
Page 378, *Ligusticum porteri* flowers (both)
Page 379, *Ligusticum porteri* roots (top and bottom)
Page 387, *Mitchella repens* leaves (left)
Page 412, *Zanthoxylum clava-herculis* (2nd and 4th left)
Page 413, *Zanthoxylum clava-herculis* (right)
Page 522, *Dioscorea villosa* leaves (right)
Page 523, *Dioscorea villosa* rhizome (lower right)
Page 543, *Nuphar lutea* (upper left)
Page 549, *Eriodictyon angustifolium* flowers (left)
Page 549, *Eriodictyon californicum* flowers (right)
Page 550, *Eriodictyon angustifolium* (lower left)

MAYSUN BLACK

Page 27, *Aralia californica root* (right)
Page 28, *Aralia californica root* (left)
Page 103, *Eschscholzia californica* root (right)
Page 379, *Ligusticum porteri* roots (middle)
Page 503, *Usnea* spp. (lower right)
Page 519, *Prunus virginiana* bark (right)

CANDICE BRUNLINGER

Page 329, *Filipendula ulmaria* leaf (left)

DAVID BUNTING

Page 46, *Astragalus membranaceus* (both)
Page 243, *Panax ginseng* roots (right)
Page 244, *Panax ginseng* cultivators (left)
Page 244, *Panax ginseng* processing (right)
Page 245, *Panax ginseng* berries (left)
Page 455, *Serenoa repens* berries (lower left)

ROSALEE DE LA FORÉT

Page 124, *Matricaria recutita* flower (right)
Page 316, *Lomatium dissectum* (left)
Page 318, *Lomatium dissectum* flower buds (left)
Page 325, *Althaea officinalis* (right)
Page 474, *Scutellaria lateriflora* (left)

AMY KUMLER

Page 26, *Aralia californica* root (left)
Page 29, *Aralia californica* root crown (right)
Page 50, *Morella californica* root (left)
Page 346, *Verbascum bomyciferum* root (top)
Page 513, *Valeriana officinalis* acetum (left)
Page 522, *Dioscorea villosa* rhizome (left)
Page 525, *Dioscorea villosa* (right)
Page 544, *Anemopsis californica* rhizome (left)
Page 554/555, Herb-filled jars
Page 556, Tea in French press
Page 562, *Dioscorea villosa* tincture (top left)
Page 562, Herb-filled jars (top right)
Page 580, Christa's salves (upper right)

RICHARD MANDELBAUM

Page 53, *Berberis thumbergii* rootbark (right)
Page 55, *Berberis thumbergii* (left)
Page 99, *Calendula officinalis* flower (lower right)
Page 363, *Avena fatua* - fresh, milky oat (left)

DARLYNE MURAWSKI/
NATIONAL GEOGRAPHIC COLLECTION

Page 11, *Ambrosia trifida* pollen (lower left)

NEW HAMPSHIRE BOTANICAL GARDENS

Page 81, *Eupatorium perfoliatum* (left)
Page 152, *Coptis trifolia* flower (right)
Page 153, *Coptis trifolia* leaf (left)
Page 153, *Coptis trifolia* flower (right)

SELENA ROWAN

Page 126, *Matricaria recutita* flower (left)
Page 503, *Usnea* and child (left)

COREYPINE SHANE

Page 65, *Viburnum prunifolium* flowers (right)
Page 74, *Caulophyllum* flowers (right)
Page 86, *Lycopus americanus* foliage (middle)
Page 275, *Hydrangea arborescens* (both)
Page 414, *Zanthoxylum clava-herculis* (both)
Page 483, *Collinsonia canadensis* (right)

CHRISTA SINADINOS

Page 27, *Aralia californica* berry (left)
Page 32, *Arnica chamissonis* flower (right)
Page 34, *Cynara scolymus* leaf (right)
Page 49, *Morella californica* leaves (right)
Page 58, *Berberis aquifolium* leaves (left)
Page 76, *Caulophyllum* flowers (left)
Page 98, *Calendula officinalis* flower (right)
Page 99, *Calendula officinalis* flower (top and middle, right)
Page 125, *Matricaria recutita* flowers (right)
Page 128, *Matricaria recutita* flower (left)
Page 139, *Galium aparine* (left)
Page 150, *Symphytum officinale* flower (left)
Page 155, *Coptis trifolia* seed pods (lower left)
Page 210, *Foeniculum vulgare* (right)
Page 218, *Tanacetum parthenium* flowers (right)
Page 248, *Solidago* spp. Goldenrod (left)
Page 255, *Grindelia* buds (right)
Page 257, *Grindelia* buds (left)
Page 265, *Crataegus* berry (right)
Page 276, *Hydrangea arborescens* leaves (right)
Page 317, *Lomatium dissectum* roots (both)
Page 332, *Silybum marianum* (lower left)
Page 342, *Leonurus cardiaca* flowers (left)
Page 343, *Leonurus cardiaca* (right)
Page 344, *Leonurus cardiaca* (both)
Page 346, *Verbascum bombyciferum* root (lower left)
Page 424, *Ceanothus* spp. (right)
Page 426, *Ceanothus* spp. (both)
Page 428, *Ceanothus* spp. (right)
Page 443, *Rosmarinus officinale* (left)
Page 468, *Garrya elliptica* (right)
Page 469, *Garrya elliptica* (right)
Page 508, *Valeriana officinalis* flower (right)
Page 512, *Valeriana officinalis* roots (right)
Page 523, *Dioscorea villosa* (upper right)
Page 544, *Anemopsis californica* flower (right)
Page 546, *Anemopsis californica* (both)
Page 561, Siri Beringer processing oshá
Page 562, Students processing tinctures
Page 595, *Taraxacum officinale* roots (left)
Page 614, Jayden Kaufman with balsam root

RICHARD SPJUT

Page 548, *Eriodictyon trichocalyx* flowers (left)
Page 548, *Eriodictyon crassifolium* flowers (right)

MARIE VAN DER SCHIJFF

Page 38, *Withania somnifera* flower

I'm deeply appreciative to my friends, colleagues, and fellow plant lovers who generously shared their photos: 7Song, Candice Brunlinger, David Bunting, Rosalee de la Forét, Amy Kumler, Richard Mandelbaum, Selena Rowan, CoreyPine Shane, Richard Spjut, and Marie van der Schijff.

Other photos were sourced from online photography providers.

No photographs may be copied or preprinted without the express permission of the photographer.

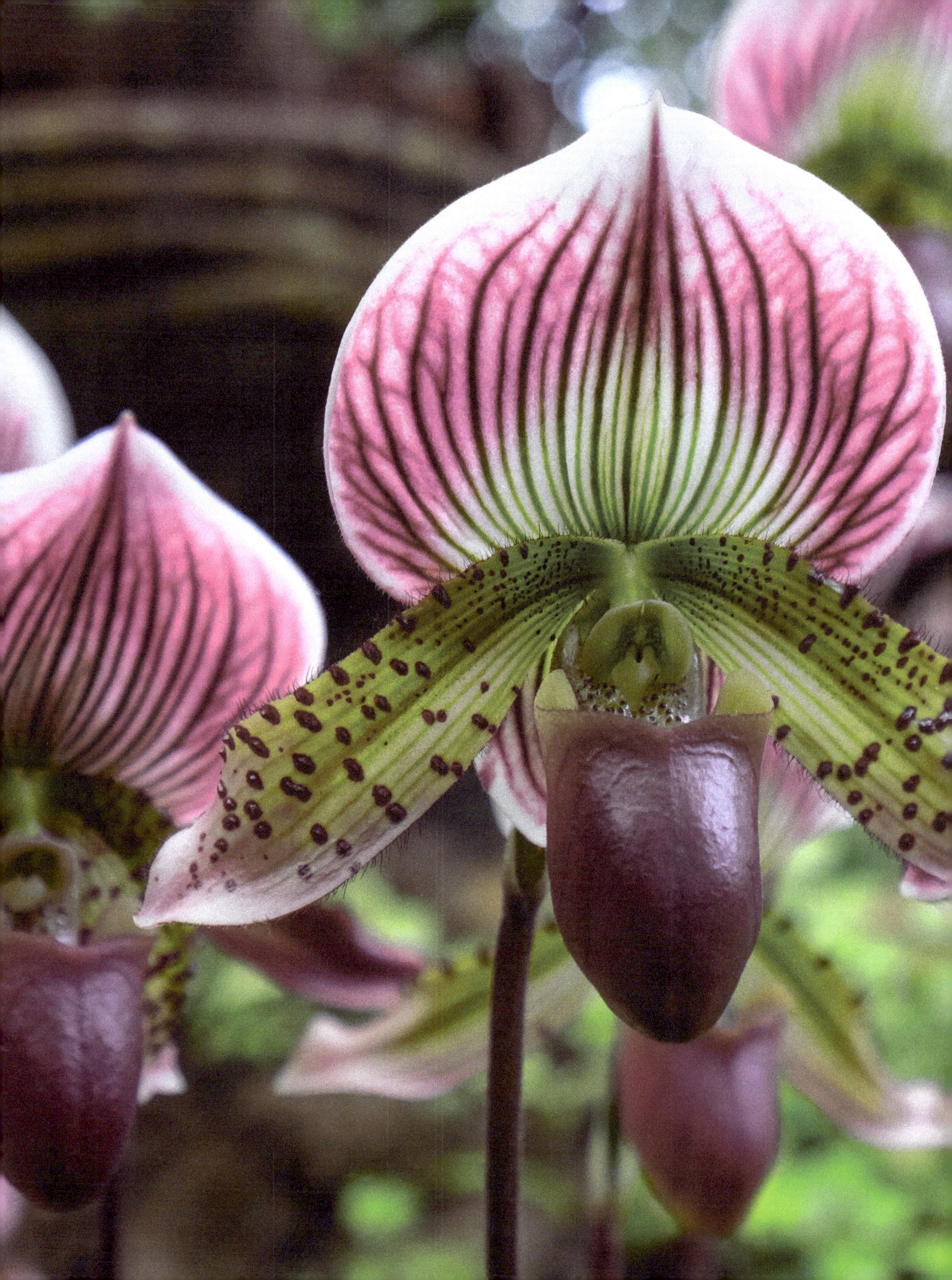

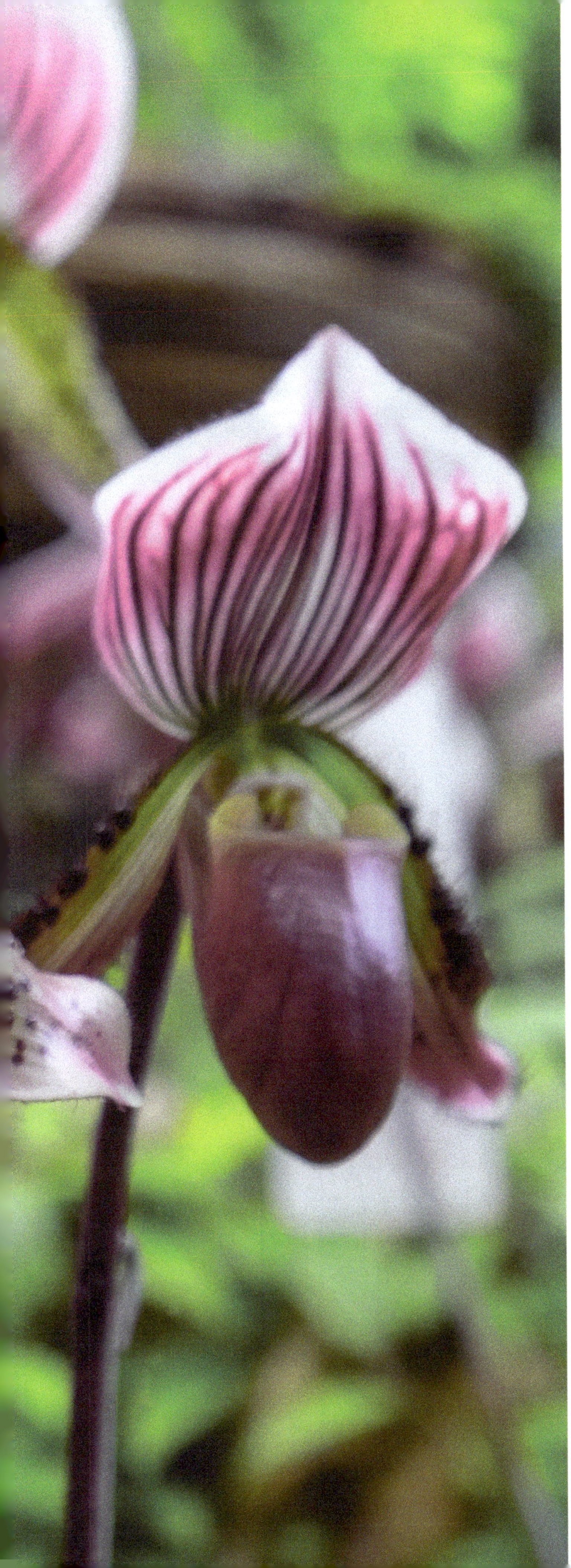

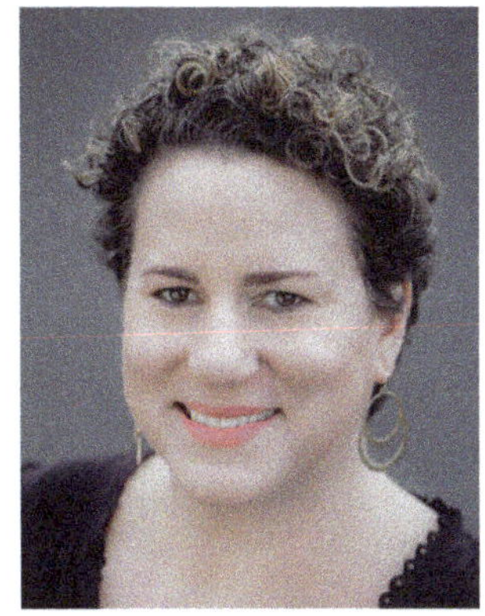

CHRISTA SINADINOS

has more than 30 years of expertise as a clinician, teacher, researcher, and medicine maker. She is the founder and director of the Northwest School for Botanical Studies in California. She has trained hundreds of students who have become the new generation of herbalists. Christa lectures at herbal conferences and schools throughout the United States and maintains an extensive herbal pharmacy and demonstration garden with more than 200 species of medicinal herbs. Her favorite place to write is on her back porch surrounded by plants, and shaded by lilacs and butterfly bushes. She delights in tending her garden, hiking in the lush forests and along the Pacific Coast beaches. Christa lives with her husband, Howie Kaufman, a talented musician, and their entrepreneurial son, Jayden.

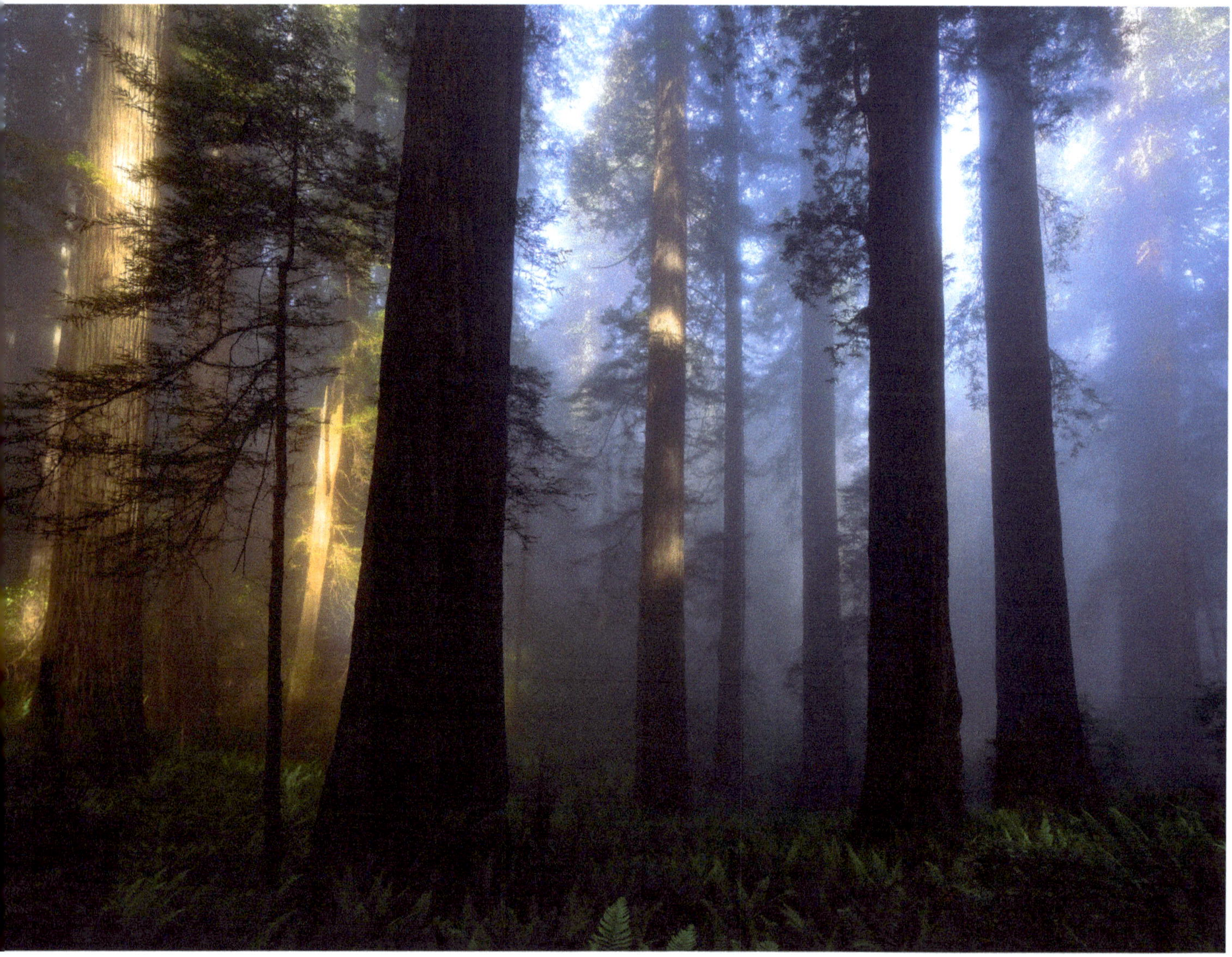

THANK YOU FOR SUPPORTING A SELF-PUBLISHED AUTHOR!

I cannot express how much your support means to me. As an independently-published author, I have dedicated over a decade of time, energy, creativity, and personal resources into every step of this book — from writing and editing, to design, photography, marketing, and distribution. It has been both a rigorous undertaking and a joyful labor of love, made even more meaningful by readers like you.

I chose the self-publishing path to ensure this book remained true to my vision — rich with detailed monographs, therapeutic insights, and abundant photographs — that would otherwise have been greatly reduced in a traditional publishing model.

When you buy directly from an independent author, you help sustain their work, offset the real costs of publication, and keep independent scholarship alive. Every purchase, review, share, and recommendation helps this book reach more readers and ensures diverse voices continue to be heard.

I am also grateful for the partnership of herbal shops and independent bookstores who stock my book. Please support your local businesses!

To purchase additional copies, scan the QR code below or visit christasinadinos.com. For bulk orders, wholesale pricing, or international orders, please send an inquiry through the website contact page.

COLOPHON

Book design by Barbara Lande. Cover photograph by Amy Kumler.
The fonts are Adobe Minion Pro designed by Robert Slimbach
and Gotham designed by Tobias Frere-Jones.

www.ingramcontent.com/pod-product-compliance
Lightning Source LLC
LaVergne TN
LVHW070905210926
848482LV00017B/992

* 9 7 9 8 9 8 9 8 1 8 8 3 9 *